Textbook of
PEDIATRICS

A Textbook for Undergraduate and
A Primer for Postgraduate Students

Textbook of
PEDIATRICS

*A Textbook for Undergraduate and
A Primer for Postgraduate Students*

Editor

Piyush Gupta MD FIAP FNNF FAMS

Professor of Pediatrics
University College of Medical Sciences
University of Delhi, New Delhi, India

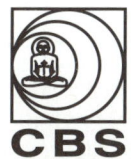

CBS

CBS Publishers & Distributors Pvt Ltd

New Delhi • Bengaluru • Chennai • Kochi • Kolkata • Mumbai
Bhubaneswar • Hyderabad • Jharkhand • Nagpur • Patna • Pune • Uttarakhand

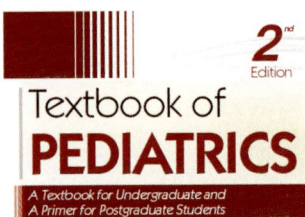

ISBN: 978-93-87964-11-2

Copyright © Piyush Gupta

Second Edition	**2019**
First Edition	2013
Reprint	2016

Published by Satish Kumar Jain and produced by Varun Jain for

CBS Publishers & Distributors Pvt Ltd
4819/XI Prahlad Street, 24 Ansari Road, Daryaganj, New Delhi 110 002
Ph: 23289259, 23266861, 23266867 Fax: 011-23243014 Website: www.cbspd.com
e-mail: delhi@cbspd.com; cbspubs@airtelmail.in

Corporate Office: 204 FIE, Industrial Area, Patparganj, Delhi 110 092
Ph: 4934 4934   Fax: 4934 4935   e-mail: publishing@cbspd.com; publicity@cbspd.com

Branches

- **Bengaluru:** Seema House 2975, 17th Cross, K.R. Road,
  Banasankari 2nd Stage, Bengaluru 560 070, Karnataka
  Ph: +91-80-26771678/79   Fax: +91-80-26771680   e-mail: bangalore@cbspd.com
- **Chennai:** 7, Subbaraya Street, Shenoy Nagar, Chennai 600 030, Tamil Nadu
  Ph: +91-44-26260666, 26208620   Fax: +91-44-42032115   e-mail: chennai@cbspd.com
- **Kochi:** 42/1325, 1326, Power House Road, Opp KSEB Power House, Ernakulam 682 018, Kochi, Kerala
  Ph: +91-484-4059061-65   Fax: +91-484-4059065   e-mail: kochi@cbspd.com
- **Kolkata:** No. 6/B, Ground Floor, Rameswar Shaw Road, Kolkata-700014 (West Bengal), India
  Ph: +91-33-2289-1126, 2289-1127, 2289-1128   e-mail: kolkata@cbspd.com
- **Mumbai:** 83-C, Dr E Moses Road, Worli, Mumbai-400018, Maharashtra
  Ph: +91-22-24902340/41   Fax: +91-22-24902342   e-mail: mumbai@cbspd.com

Representatives

• **Bhubaneswar**	0-9911037372	• **Hyderabad**	0-9885175004	• **Jharkhand**	0-9811541605	• **Nagpur**	0-9021734563
• **Patna**	0-9334159340	• **Pune**	0-9623451994	• **Uttarakhand**	0-9716462459		

Printed at Nutech Print Services, Faridabad, India

to

my students…
who remain
my best teachers

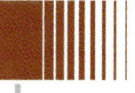

Contributors

Aashima Dabas MD
Assistant Professor
Department of Pediatrics
Maulana Azad Medical College and
Associated Lok Nayak Hospital
New Delhi, India
E-mail: dr.aashimagupta@gmail.com

Abhijeet Saha MD, FISPN, FIPNA, FACEE, FISPD
Professor
Department of Pediatrics
Lady Hardinge Medical College and
Associated Kalawati Saran Children Hospital
New Delhi, India
E-mail: drabhijeetsaha@yahoo.com

Abhishek Jain MD
Resident
Department of Pediatrics
University College of Medical Sciences
New Delhi, India
E-mail: mail2ajain27@gmail.com

Anju Gupta MD
Professor
Department of Pediatrics
Post Graduate Institute of Medical Education and
Research (PGIMER)
Chandigarh, India
E-mail: anjupgi@gmail.com

Anurag Bajpai MD, FRACP, SCE
Pediatric and Adolescent Endocrinologist
Regency Center for Diabetes, Endocrinology, and
Research
Kanpur, UP, India
E-mail: dr_anuragbajpai@yahoo.com

Ashok Kumar MD, FNNF, FIAP, FAMS
Professor
Department of Pediatrics
Institute of Medical Sciences
Banaras Hindu University
Varanasi, India
E-mail: ashokkumar_bhu@hotmail.com

Atul A Kulkarni MD
Assistant Professor
Ashwini Rural Medical College
Solapur, Maharashtra, India
E-mail: dratulkulkarni@rediffmail.com

Devendra Mishra MD, FIAP
Professor
Department of Pediatrics
Maulana Azad Medical College and
Associated Lok Nayak Hospital
New Delhi, India
E-mail: drdmishra@gmail.com

Dheeraj Shah MD, FIAP, MNAMS
Professor
Department of Pediatrics
University College of Medical Sciences
Delhi, India
E-mail: shahdheeraj@hotmail.com

Jaya Shankar Kaushik MD, DNB, MNAMS, DM
Associate Professor
Department of Pediatrics
Pt BD Sharma Postgraduate Institute of Medical Sciences
Rohtak, Haryana, India
E-mail: jayashankarkaushik@gmail.com

Kanika Kapoor MD, FIPNA
Assistant Professor
Department of Pediatrics
Vardhman Mahavir Medical College and
Associated Safdarjung Hospital
New Delhi, India
E-mail: kanikataurus@rediffmail.com

Kausalya Raghuraman MD
Department of Microbiology
Pt BD Sharma Postgraduate Institute of Medical Sciences
Rohtak, Haryana, India
E-mail: kausi_01@yahoo.co.in

Kirti Sudha Mishra MD DNB, FIPNA, FISPN
Associate Professor
Department of Pediatrics
Chacha Nehru Bal Chikitsalaya
Delhi, India
E-mail: kirtisen@gmail.com

Lokesh Guglani MD
Assistant Professor
Pediatric Pulmonary Division
Children's Hospital of Michigan
Wayne State University School of Medicine
Detroit MI, USA
E-mail: lokesh.guglani@gmail.com

Mukta Mantan MD DNB
Professor
Department of Pediatrics
Maulana Azad Medical College and
Associated Lok Nayak Hospital
New Delhi, India
E-mail: muktamantan@hotmail.com

Munesh Tomar MD, FNB
Director
Department of Pediatric Cardiology
Sir Sathya Sai Sanjeevani International Center for Child
Cardiac Care and Research
Palwal, Haryana, India
E-mail: drmuneshtomar@gmail.com

Nidhi Bedi MD
Assistant Professor
Department of Pediatrics
Hamdard Institute of Medical Sciences and Research
New Delhi, India
E-mail: *drnidhibedi@gmail.com*

Niranjan Shendurnikar MD, FIAP
Consultant Pediatrician
KG Patel Children's Hospital
Vadodara, Gujarat, India
E-mail: *drniranjan@rediffmail.com*

OP Mishra MD, FIAP, FAMS
Professor and In-charge
Division of Pediatric Nephrology
Department of Pediatrics
Institute of Medical Sciences
Banaras Hindu University
Varanasi, UP, India
E-mail: *opmpedia@yahoo.co.uk*

Pareshkumar A Thakkar MD, DNB, DCH
Associate Professor
Department of Pediatrics
Medical College Baroda
Maharaja Sayajirao University of Baroda
Vadodara, Gujarat, India
E-mail: *drpareshthakkar123@gmail.com*

Payal Gupta DNB
Senior Resident
Department of Ophthalmology
All India Institute of Medical Sciences
Bhopal, MP, India
E-mail: *drpayal.pg@gmail.com*

Piyush Gupta MD, FIAP, FNNF, FAMS
Professor
Department of Pediatrics
University College of Medical Sciences
University of Delhi, New Delhi, India
E-mail: *prof.piyush.gupta@gmail.com*

Pooja Dewan MD, MNAMS, FIAP
Professor
Department of Pediatrics
University College of Medical Sciences
New Delhi, India
E-mail: *poojadewan@hotmail.com*

PSN Menon MD, MNAMS, FIAP, FIMSA
Consultant and Head
Department of Pediatrics
Jaber Al-Ahmed Armed Forces Hospital
Kuwait
E-mail: *psnmenon@yahoo.com.in*

R Ganesh MBBS, DNB, MRCPCH, PhD
Consultant Pediatrician
Kanchi Kamakoti Childs Trust Hospital
Nungambakkam,Chennai, India
E-mail: *ganeped79@rediffmail.com*

Rachana Dubey MD, DNB, MNAMS, DM
Consultant Pediatric Neurology
Medanta Super-speciality Hospital
Indore, MP, India
E-mail: *rachnadube@gmail.com*

Ranjiti Prasad MD, MAMS, FIAP
Professor
Department of Pediatrics
Institute of Medical Sciences
Banaras Hindu University
Varanasi, India
E-mail: *rajnitip@gamil.com*

Rashmi Sarkar MD
Professor
Department of Dermatology
Maulana Azad Medical College and
Associated Lok Nayak Hospital
New Delhi, India
E-mail: *rashmisarkar@gmail.com*

Richa Jain MD, DM
Assistant Professor
Pediatric Hematology and Oncology
Advanced Pediatrics Center
Postgraduate Institute of Medical Education and Research
Chandigarh, India
E-mail: *docrichajain@gmail.com*

Ruchi Rai MD
Professor of Neonatology
Super Specialty Pediatrics Hospital and Postgraduate
Teaching Institute
Noida, UP, India
E-mail: *ruchiraiald@gmail.com*

Sakshi Sachdeva MD, FNB, DM Fellow
Pediatric Cardiologist
Department of Cardiology
All India Institute of Medical Sciences
New Delhi, India
E-mail: *sakshisachdeva21@gmail.com*

Savitri Srivastava MD, DM, FAMS, FACC, FACA, FICC
Director
Pediatrics and Congenital Heart Disease
Fortis Escorts Heart Institute
Okhla, New Delhi, India
E-mail: *savitri_sh@yahoo.com*

Sheffali Gulati MD, FIAP, FIMSA, FAMS
Professor and Chief
Child Neurology Division
Faculty In-charge, Center of Excellence and
Advanced Research for Childhood Neurodevelopmental
Disorders
Department of Pediatrics
All India Institute of Medical Sciences
New Delhi, India
E-mail: *sheffaligulati@gmail.com*

Shubha R Phadke MD, DM
Professor and Head
Department of Medical Genetics
Sanjay Gandhi Postgraduate Institute of Medical Sciences
Lucknow, UP, India
E-mail: shubharaophadke@gmail.com

Soumya Jagadeesan MD
Assistant Professor
Department of Dermatology
Amrita Institute of Medical Sciences
Cochin, Kerala, India
E-mail: soumyavivek@gmail.com

Soumya Tiwari MD
Associate Professor
Department of Pediatrics
Lady Hardinge Medical College and
Associated Kalawati Saran Children Hospital
New Delhi, India
E-mail: soumyaakshay@gmail.com

Srikanta Basu MD, MAMS, FIAP
Professor
Department of Pediatrics
Lady Hardinge Medical College and
Associated Kalawati Saran Children Hospital
New Delhi, India
E-mail: srikantabasu@gmail.com

Sriparna Basu MD, DCH, FRCPI, FRCPCH
Professor and Head
Department of Neonatology
All India Institute of Medical Sciences
Rishikesh, Uttarakhand, India
E-mail: drsriparnabasu@rediffmail.com

Sriram Krishnamurthy MD, FIPNA
Additional Professor
Department of Pediatrics
Jawaharlal Institute of Postgraduate Medical Education
and Research
Puducherry, India
E-mail: drsriramkris@gmail.com

Utpal Kant Singh MD, FIAP, FRCP, FRCPCH
Professor
Department of Pediatrics
Nalanda Medical College
Patna, Bihar, India
E-mail: utpalkant.singh@gmail.com

Vanny Arora MD
Senior Resident
Department of Pediatrics
University College of Medical Sciences and
Guru Teg Bahadur Hospital
New Delhi, India
E-mail: drvannyarora@gmail.com

Varinder Singh MD, FRCPCH
Director-Professor
Department of Pediatrics
Lady Hardinge Medical College and
Associated Kalawati Saran Children Hospital
New Delhi, India
E-mail: 4vsingh@gmail.com

Vishal Sondhi MD
Assistant Professor
Department of Pediatrics
Armed Forces Medical College
Pune, Maharashtra, India
E-mail: vishalsondhi@gmail.com

Preface to the Second Edition

At the outset, I would like to thank the readers for their steady support to the first edition of this book. The expansion and changing approach to the teaching of the subject at both undergraduate and postgraduate levels necessitated a new orientation for the book. We are happy to present the second edition with fresh flavors, prompted by the wholehearted response from the students, faculty, and practitioners of pediatrics in the country.

This edition represents a thoroughly revised, substantially expanded version. As you would notice, the complete layout is in four colors, with color-coding to highlight treatment of individual conditions. This will aid the practitioners. Another unique feature of this textbook, much appreciated by the critics, are the case studies intended to help reader visualize the presentation in the true clinical context. We have more than doubled their number in this edition; almost every disorder is now explained with a representative case study.

Every chapter has been thoroughly revised and updated. Separate chapters are now included to deal with childhood malignancies and collagen vascular and immune disorders, both penned by experts in respective fields. Another chapter has been added on drug doses; presented thematically and alphabetically to facilitate easy retrieval. Other important additions include focus on severe acute malnutrition, rickettsial diseases, leptospirosis, RMNCH +A strategy, Indian Council of Medical Research (ICMR) food composition charts 2017, recent data pertaining to child health from the Rapid Survey on Children (RSOC), National Family Health Survey-4 (NFHS-4), Sample Registration System (SRS) 2017; and annexures on Indian Academy of Pediatrics (IAP) growth charts for children and adolescents (5–18 years), and International charts for birth size and postnatal growth.

The second edition is intended to serve a dual purpose. Besides being a complete textbook for the undergraduates, it serves the basic building block as a primer for those pursuing postgraduation in pediatrics and allied subjects. Every important topic is followed by a summary of take home messages in a Revision Point Box. The entire book thus, can be revised in a matter of hours.

I thank all the contributing authors; they remain the backbone of this venture. Many new authors have joined in this edition; all stalwarts in their respective fields. I am indebted to them for their hard work, and timely contributions.

I sincerely hope that this revised second edition too will receive the same patronage from readers as the first edition. We welcome any criticism on and suggestions for further improvement of this textbook.

Comments, critical review, and suggestions are welcome at prof.piyush.gupta@gmail.com.

Piyush Gupta
prof.piyush.gupta@gmail.com.

Preface to the First Edition

Oh right … *another* book for undergraduates in pediatrics … ! *But why?* is surely going to be the first reaction. Keeping in view a vital promise that went into the creation of this book, I will get right down to the point without wasting more ink. Well, simply because the existing textbooks are losing their focus on the undergraduate student. The present books are getting bulkier and being converted to tomes, loading further the already overburdened student. Focus is shifting to a fragmented system-based approach branching into excruciating details, with general pediatrics (that is what makes pediatrics different!) taking a backseat. Moreover, the available texts are purely theoretical in nature, in today's world where the word *applied* is in the forefront.

With this book, finally the undergraduate student has something for him/her only. The focus remains on the core pediatric topics; the text is to-the-point, concise and yet complete; and the theory is supplemented by a sprinkling of *Case Studies* highlighting the clinical scenarios and common presentations of common illnesses in children. The language is simple, the paragraphs short, and the jargon simplified for comprehensive readability. The text provides sufficient information, completely independent of the tables, which are interspersed in the text to give an overview of the statistical perspectives. I feel that a void has been filled up for a complete book on pediatrics for the undergraduate medical students.

Though this is a multiauthor book, the reader will never feel that the chapters are written by more than 30 different teachers of pediatrics. The style of editing facilitates understanding. All the chapters have been kept on an even keel and only the material that is absolutely necessary has been included in the text. All these features make this book an invaluable asset in preparing for the professional examinations as well as the MCQ-based competitive examinations. At the same time this treatise has the potential to serve as the basic foundation text for those pursuing specialization in pediatrics.

I remain grateful to all the authors for their contributions. They remain the backbone of this venture.

I thank Mr Satish K Jain, Managing Director, CBS Publishers & Distributors (CBSP&D), for his overall support and belief in this book. A near error-free output was fashioned entirely by the efforts of Mr YN Arjuna, Senior Director—Publishing, CBSP&D.

I welcome comments concerning omissions and errors; healthy reviews regarding content and critical thoughts; and suggestions for further editions.

Enjoy reading!!

Janruary 2013

Piyush Gupta
prof.piyush.gupta@gmail.com.

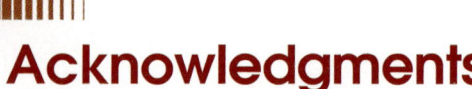

Acknowledgments

Permissions
World Health Organization, *Indian Pediatrics*

Secretarial Assistance
Anju Kumari

Publisher team at CBS
SK Jain (Managing Director), YN Arjuna (Senior Vice President–Publishing, Editorial and Publicity), Ritu Chawla (AGM, Publishing), Jyoti Kaur (Typesetting), Neeraj (Graphics), Kshirod (Proofreading), Abhinandan (Coordination)

Family
Anjali (wife); Payal (daughter); and Aayush (son); for taking pride in whatever I do. Love you all!

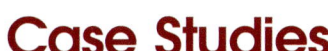

Case Studies

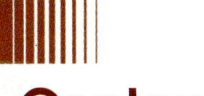

Contents

10. Respiratory Disorders   390

11. Cardiovascular Disorders   429

12. Disorders of Kidneys and Urinary Tract   498

13. Neurological Disorders   544

Growth and Development

1.1 DEFINITIONS

GROWTH

Growth is defined as increase in body size in terms of weight, height, and other measurable domains. It is also defined as measurable change in physical size of body and its parts. It is used to designate all the quantitative changes brought about in structure and function of human anatomy and physiology. Growth reflects an increase in body dimensions and a resultant change in mass of body tissue like fat, muscle, and bone. Examples of growth include change in weight, height, bone density, and dental structure.

During the growth of a child, there is increase in both cell numbers (hyperplasia) and cell size (hypertrophy). The growth is not a steady process; the rate of growth varies with periods of rapid growth and slow growth. For instance, infancy and adolescence are characterized by periods of rapid growth.

DEVELOPMENT

Development is defined as a progressive series of orderly coherent changes that occur as a result of maturity and experience. It may also be defined as behavioral changes in skills and functional abilities. Development refers to gaining of skills in all aspects of child's life like physical development, social and emotional development, intellectual development, communication, and speech development. Hence the development is not easily measurable. The terms maturation and learning are often used along with development.

- *Maturation* refers to process of become fully developed in terms of physiological and behavioral aspects towards attainment of his or her best physical, emotional, intellectual, and social potential.
- *Learning* refers to assimilation of information once the child is mature for particular learning experience resulting in behavioral change.

The terms **growth** and **development** are conceptually different, and denote two altogether different aspects of the change; ie, growth is quantitative while development is qualitative. However, both are interdependent. For instance, to learn to open a door, the child must be able to reach the door knob (physical growth) and also must have a sufficient learning as to how to open the door knob (development).

Revision Point

Growth and Development

Growth: *Quantitative increase* in structure of body (eg, weight gain, height gain)

Development: *Qualitative changes* in body function leading to acquisition of skills in all aspects of child's life like physical development, social and emotional development, intellectual development, communication, and speech development

1.2 PRINCIPLES OF GROWTH

1. Growth and development are *orderly and predictable*. Every child goes through the same process. The growth is considered *sequential* with one stage leading to next stage.
2. Growth progresses in a *cephalocaudal* and *proximodistal* manner. The process starts from the head to toe. Axial functions develop before functions of extremities. *For example:* Arm growth occurs before the finger growth.
3. Growth is considered *cyclic* in the sense that the *rate of growth is not constant*. From birth to 2 years, there is period of rapid growth. This is followed by a period of slow growth till puberty (10–12 years). This phase is followed by a phase of rapid growth again till 15–16 years of age. Periods of rapid growth are called *critical periods* and are most vulnerable to an external insult.
4. *Rate of growth is not similar for all children.* Growth shows wide individual variation and is unique for every child. All children do not grow at same pace. Some children at the age of 1 year weigh 11 kg and a few might weigh 9 kg. Similarly, children reach puberty at different ages. Each child has an individual rate of growth although there might be a lot of variation with a few maturing early and others late.
5. *Different tissues of body grow at different rates. Somatic growth* follows a sigmoid curve with periods of rapid growth during infancy and puberty. The postnatal *brain growth* primarily occurs in the first year of life so that at 1 year infant has 90% adult brain size. In contrast to brain growth, *lymphoid growth* starts after 5 years of age. It peaks during 6–9 years of age and declines steadily, thereafter. *Gonadal development* with both increase in the size and function of reproductive organs starts after the onset of puberty (10–14 years) (Fig. 1.1).

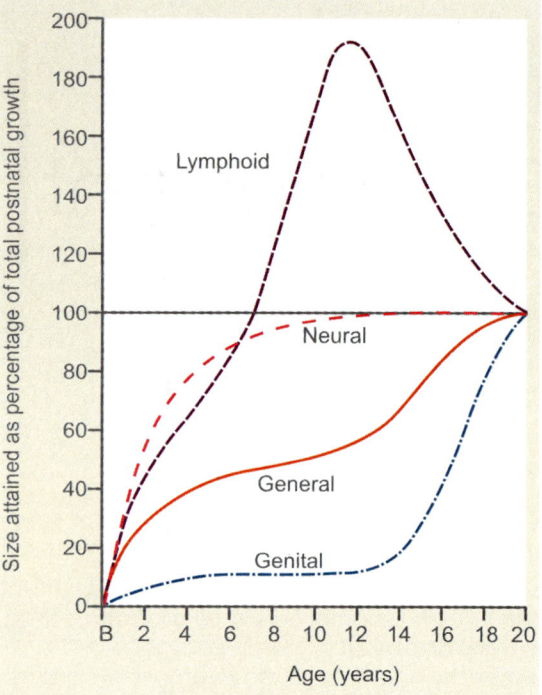

Fig. 1.1 Scammon's curves of systemic growth. Figure depicts the differential growth of body, brain, lymphoid organs, and genital organs, as the child passes through different phases of growth

6. Growth is measurable both in terms of *distance* and *velocity*. The term *linear or distance growth* refers to overall growth at one point of time. Linear growth of a child can be compared to reference standards and it can be interpreted whether the growth at the time of examination is within the normal range or not. But linear growth does not predict the growth pattern in the recent past.

Growth velocity or *rate of growth* is used to determine the growth pattern in recent past and it refers to increment of growth in a unit of time. Growth velocity can predict the ultimate growth potential and helps in early assessment of factors leading to growth retardation.

Why Study Growth and Development?

It is important to study growth and development because of the following reasons:

1. *To know what is expected* of a child at a given age, in terms of physical and mental ability, especially in high-risk babies.
2. *To identify children who may not look apparently sick* but are having a disease process that is affecting growth. For example, a child with celiac disease may remain asymptomatic except for faltering of linear growth. This initial clue for diagnosis can prevent the long-term physical and emotional consequences of the disease (both for the child and the family). Growth charting also helps to monitor the effect of treatment/intervention modalities on the pattern of growth.
3. *Early identification of handicaps.* Developmental assessment helps in early diagnosis of global developmental delay, intellectual disability, cerebral palsy, hearing and visual handicaps, neurological and metabolic disorders, disorders of muscle tone, and physical handicaps.
4. *To assess the general health and nutrition status of the community.* Prevalence of wasting, underweight, and stunting in under-five children serve as indirect indicators of health and nutritional status of the entire community, and may provide a launching pad for advocacy, and planning the most appropriate intervention.
5. *Evaluation of social action.* Effectiveness of medical or social actions for promoting health of the community can be evaluated by comparing the growth data before and after the intervention, such as mid-day meal or preschool children feeding programs.
6. *To assess suitability of a baby for adoption.* Parents may approach pediatrician before adopting a child to assess whether the child has a normal growth and to exclude developmental disabilities.

1.3 PHASES OF GROWTH

It is amazing to realize the transformation of a fertilized egg to develop into an embryo and then into fetus and finally a complete human being. These phases of the growth can be classified into embryonic growth, fetal growth, somatic growth in infancy, preschool years, middle childhood, and adolescent (**Box 1.1**). A few authors have classified the phases of growth into two broad categories: *Prenatal growth* (before the birth) and *postnatal growth* (after birth).

- *The prenatal period is characterized by three phases:* Fertilized ovum or zygote (first 2 weeks), embryo (2–8 weeks), and fetus (9 weeks to birth).
- *Postnatal growth also has three phases:* Infancy, childhood, and adolescence.

Age of viability refers to earliest age at which a fetus could survive, if they were born at that time, generally accepted as 24 weeks, or fetal weight of more than 400 grams.

Conceptus is reserved for growing embryo or fetus and placental structure, throughout the pregnancy.

Puberty refers to that period of life when the ability to reproduce sexually begins. It is characterized by maturation of the genital organs, development of the secondary sex characteristics, and the onset of menstruation (menarche) in girls.

A. PRENATAL GROWTH

1. Embryonic Period (0–8 weeks)

Egg is fertilized by sperm to form a fertilized egg which gets transformed into a blastocyst and gets implanted in

Box 1.1 Phases of Growth	
Embryo	0–8 weeks
Fetus	9 weeks–birth
Early neonatal period	0–7 days
Late neonatal period	7–28 days
Infancy	Birth–1 year
Toddler	1–3 years
Preschool	3–6 years
Middle childhood	6–11 years
Adolescent	11–19 years

uterus with establishment of uteroplacental blood flow by 2 weeks of gestation. By 3 weeks of gestation, all the three germ layers are formed—endoderm, ectoderm, and mesoderm along with formation of primitive neural tube and blood vessels. By the end of embryonic period, rudiments of all major organs are formed. Times of intense development and rapid cell divisions are called *critical period* with development of each organ and tissue being most vulnerable to adverse influences during these periods. For example, critical period for neural tube development is 17–30 days; folate deficiency during this period could predispose to a neural tube defect.

2. Fetal Growth (9 Weeks to Birth)

During the fetal period starting from 9th week, there is consistent increase in cell number and cell size and differentiation of cells into tissues, organs, and systems. There is a rapid increase in fetal weight, length, and head circumference in the last half of gestation. Intrauterine fetal growth can be assessed by ultrasonography in terms of fetal weight, femur length, and biparietal diameter.

In human fetus in the early half of pregnancy, only 10–12% of body weight gain occurs. Early pregnancy is characterized by tissue differentiation, organ formation, and further development of fetal structures. However, there is a steady increase in weight at the rate of 15 g/day from 24–37 weeks of gestation. The weight gain declines in the last 2–3 weeks to 6 g/day. When the pregnancy proceeds beyond 42 weeks of gestation, the weight starts to decline. Similar reduction occurs in growth velocity for length, chest circumference, and head circumference after 37 weeks of gestation. The intrauterine growth curve for fetal body weight is S shaped or sigmoid in shape (*See Annexures for fetal growth curves*).

Fetal length (crown heel length) reaches to half of term length by 20 weeks of gestation. Rate of growth in fetal length reaches a peak of 1 cm/4 weeks by 20 weeks of gestation, and then it decreases. The growth curves for head and chest circumference resemble the fetal weight growth curve, but after 35 weeks of gestation, chest circumference appears to grow more rapidly reducing the difference between chest and head circumference. The normative curves for intrauterine growth have been constructed and any deviation or reduction in expected fetal growth pattern can result in intrauterine growth retardation (IUGR). These normative curves vary with ethnicity, socioeconomic status, parity, and multiple pregnancies. Hence a caution needs to be exercised before labeling a fetus to be having IUGR.

3. Fetal Proportions

The embryo has gross anatomical features of human form. There is differential growth of body segments including the head, trunk, and lower extremity. At 2 months of gestation, the fetus has enormous head in proportion to body. By mid-gestation, growth of trunk and extremities occurs but still head looks proportionally larger. This differential growth continues in the postnatal period (Fig. 1.2).

4. Fetal Differentiation

Early weeks of pregnancy are characterized by differentiation and development of neurons and glial cells with neuronal migration. Major part of 'brain growth spurt' is characterized by rapid multiplication of glial cells in early

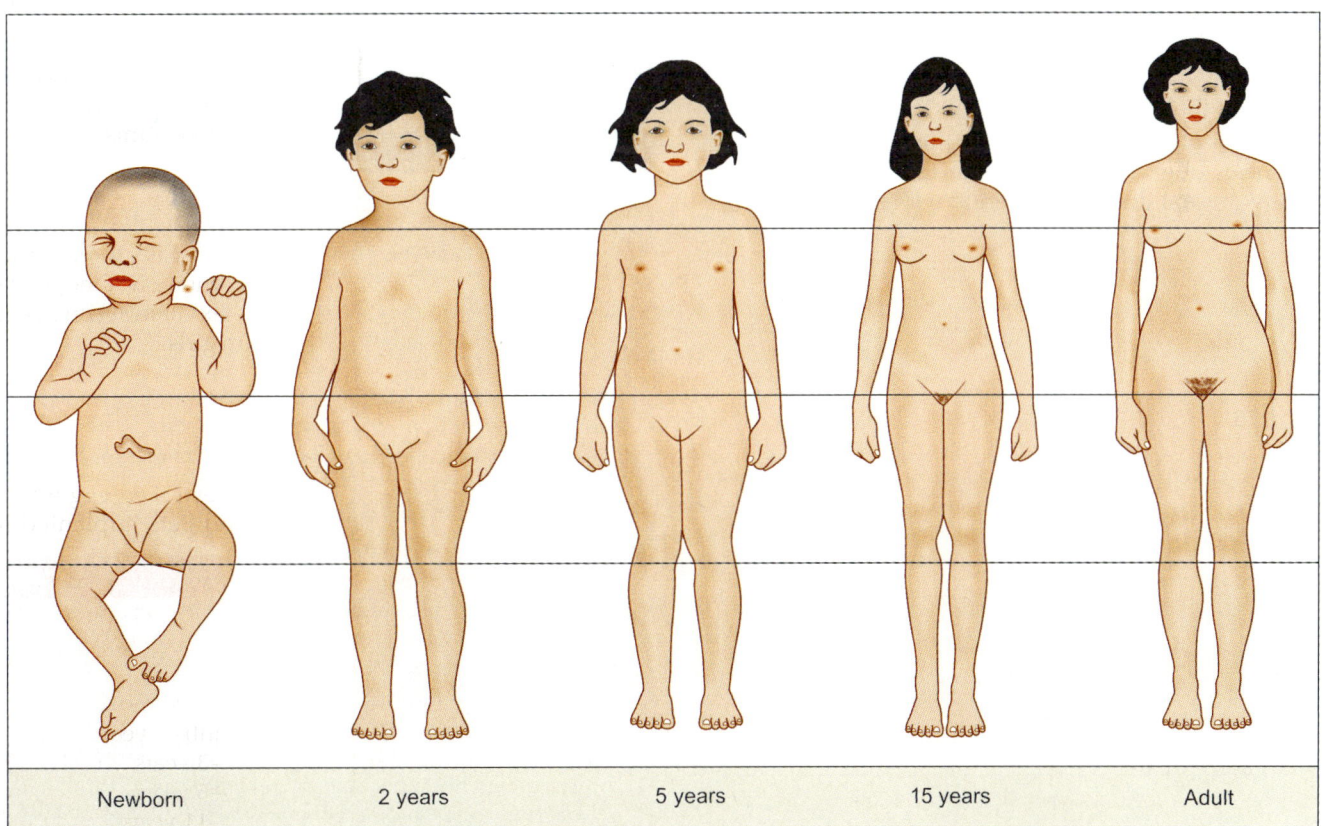

| Newborn | 2 years | 5 years | 15 years | Adult |

Fig. 1.2 Body proportions as the child grows through different phases of growth

stages, followed by myelination of nerve fibers, extending from mid-gestation to 18 months of age. Normal pattern of fetal growth is determined by genetic potential, maternal nutrition, ability of placenta to transfer the nutrients, intrauterine hormones, and growth factors.

5. Fetal Growth Factors

Fetal growth in contrast to postnatal growth is not governed by growth hormones although the growth hormone levels in fetus are high. Hormones like insulin, insulin-like growth factor (IGF), and thyroid hormones have an important role in late gestation for tissue differentiation and growth. Their growth promoting effect is primarily attributed to their anabolic effect on fetal metabolism. Glucocorticoids play an important role near term gestation for initiation and control of maturational events that occur in organs like lung, liver, and gut.

B. POSTNATAL GROWTH

Normal growth pattern in children is shown in Fig. 1.3.

Infancy (birth to 1 year) Infancy comprises of first year of life with maximum rate of growth. Physical, cognitive, and emotional development occurs in the first year of life. There is a rapid growth in most of the body systems and development of neuromuscular system.

Childhood (2–11 years) It consists of two broad groups: *Preschool (2–5 years)* and *schoolgoing* age group (6–11 years). This period is marked by steady progress in growth and maturation with a rapid progress in motor development. The phase of rapid growth in infancy is followed by slower growth rate after one year of age. Child attains to twice his birth length at the end of 2 years. Toddlers have relatively short leg, long torso, and exaggerated lumbar lordosis resulting in a protuberant abdomen. Growth at this stage depends on growth hormone and thyroid hormone. The deficiencies of growth hormone or thyroid hormone will typically present during this period with short stature.

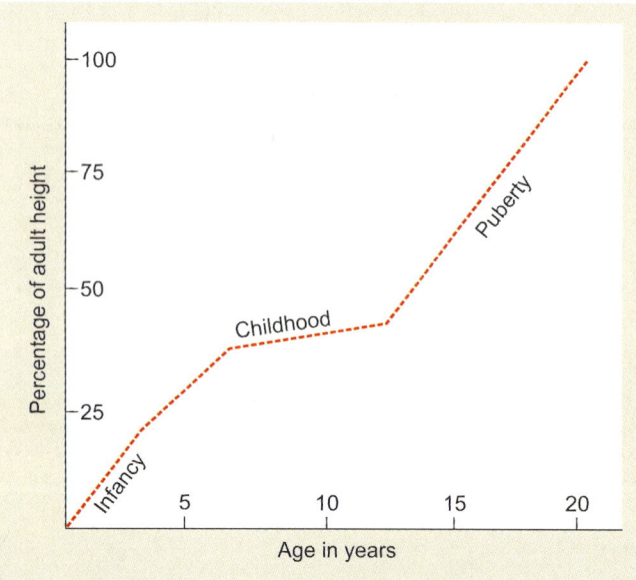

Fig. 1.3 Normal growth pattern in children

Adolescence The period of adolescence extends from age of 11 to 19 years. It is marked by hormonal influences leading to attainment of sexual maturity and adolescent growth spurt. This growth spurt differs by gender, with girls attaining it around 2 years prior to boys. Average age of adolescent growth spurt is 12–15 years in boys. This period is marked by alteration in relative proportion of muscle, fat, and bone resulting in change in body size and shape.

There is marked evolution of reproductive organs during adolescence. Sexual maturity is characterized by development of primary followed by secondary sexual characteristics. By the end of adolescence, boys acquire broader shoulder with deepening of voice; whereas girls acquire a broader pelvis and fat accumulation in buttock and breast region. During puberty, the child achieves almost 40% of peak bone mass. The average gain in height during adolescent period in boys is around 20–35 cm and in girls is around 15–25 cm.

1.4 FACTORS AFFECTING GROWTH AND DEVELOPMENT

Growth at birth is dependent on intrauterine factors that include various maternal, fetal, and placental factors. The transition from intrauterine influence to genetic effect occurs by the age of two years. Postnatal growth is controlled by various genetic, environmental, and endocrine factors. These are broadly classified as *intrinsic factors* (genetic, and endocrinal factors) and *extrinsic factors* (nutritional, sociocultural, psychological, and environmental factors).

Box 1.2 summarizes the factors affecting growth and development.

A. FACTORS AFFECTING FETAL GROWTH

Maternal malnutrition Undernutrition of the mother is identified with intrauterine growth retardation and

---

Box 1.2 Factors Affecting Growth

A. Factors predicting fetal growth

1. *Demographic factors*: Ethnicity/race, infant sex, parity, maternal age, socioeconomic status, history of prior low birth weight
2. *Nutritional factors*: Pre-pregnancy maternal weight, maternal gestational weight gain, maternal height, maternal caloric intake
3. *Substance abuse*: Maternal alcohol/tobacco consumption
4. Maternal infections (toxoplasmosis, rubella, syphilis)
5. Maternal medications (thalidomide, ethanol, antiepileptic medications)
6. Maternal illness (pre-eclampsia, anemia, malnutrition)

B. Factors affecting postnatal growth

1. *Genetic factors*: Race, heredity, sex, genetic disorders
2. *Hormonal factors*: Growth hormone, thyroid and gonadal hormones
3. *Nutritional factors*: Malnutrition
4. *Sociocultural factors*: Socioeconomic status, cultural beliefs, family size and structure
5. *Environmental factors*: Secular trends, geographic factors, physical environment, access to health care
6. *Health factors*: Chronic ailments
7. Psychological factors

consequently small size of the fetus. Fetal nutrition involves three stages: Intake of food by the pregnant woman, placental transfer to fetus, and utilization and metabolism of nutrients by the fetus. The fetal nutrition is affected when any of the maternal, placental, or fetal factors are affected. Adequacy of maternal nutrition is predicted by gestational weight gain and her past nutritional intake (reflected by her weight, height, and body mass index).

Substance abuse Maternal smoking, alcohol, and tobacco consumption leads to direct neurotoxic effect as well as resultant decreased placental blood flow which can adversely affect the fetal growth.

Teratogens Maternal infection (toxoplasmosis, rubella, syphilis), maternal medications (antiepileptic drugs, thalidomide, ethanol) and maternal radiation exposure are teratogens which can adversely affect the fetal growth especially in early gestation which is the period of maximum growth and differentiation.

Maternal illness and obstetric disorders (pre-eclampsia, anemia, malnutrition, heart disease) These could adversely affect the fetal growth leading to intrauterine growth retardation.

B. FACTORS AFFECTING POSTNATAL GROWTH

1. Genetic Factors

Race Genetic influences are responsible for marked variation in body size and structure among different races across the globe. Americans and Europeans are taller while Japanese and Chinese are shorter.

Heredity Genetic makeup of an individual is primarily determined by what has been inherited from previous generation. Final height of a child is influenced by paternal and maternal height. Daughters often reach menarche at a similar age as their mother.

Sex On an average, girls are lighter and shorter than boys. Boys tend to be ahead of girls in terms of weight and height till puberty. Girls achieve puberty earlier than boys hence in 12–14 years age group girls may become taller than boys. Shoulders are wider in boys while hips are broader in girls.

Genetic disorders Defect in chromosomes, single gene, a group of gene or a defect in product of a gene can result in short stature (Turner syndrome) or failure to thrive (inborn errors of metabolism).

2. Hormonal Factors

Prenatal growth is primarily influenced by insulin and insulin-like growth factors; while growth hormone and thyroxine are the most important hormones responsible for postnatal growth.
- *Growth hormone* It is secreted by anterior pituitary, and induces production of insulin-like growth factor-1 (IGF-1) in the liver and skeletal tissue. IGF-1 acts as the final mediator of growth. Thyroxine and cortisol may also influence the IGF plasma levels. The GH–IGF axis is also influenced by nutritional, systemic, and endocrine disorders.

- *Thyroid hormones* These are crucial for epiphyseal development and growth.
- *Gonadal hormones* They play an important role in inducing pubertal growth spurt. Gonadal steroids are responsible for pubertal growth, calcium accretion, and skeletal growth. Estrogens are responsible for epiphyseal closure in both boys and girls.

3. Nutritional Factors

Nutrition is the most important environmental factor influencing growth. Any imbalance in diet might result in either undernutrition or obesity.

Undernutrition Appropriate macronutrient (calorie, protein, fat, etc) and micronutrient (vitamins, minerals) intake is essential for adequate growth of children. Indian Council of Medical Research (ICMR) has outlined recommended dietary allowance (RDA) of all nutrients for sustenance and maintenance of growth. Undernourished children lag behind in attainment of age appropriate weight, height, head circumference, and intellectual scoring.

Obesity Introduction of fast foods, lack of physical activity, excessive and inappropriate dietary choices among children, and food fads could lead to inappropriately high body weight.

4. Sociocultural Factors

Socioeconomic status Children belonging to high socio-economic status tend to be taller and heavier than their counterparts from lower socioeconomic status. In contrast to infancy and toddlers, adolescents belonging to families of higher socioeconomic status are predisposed to developing obesity.

Cultural beliefs Culture influences every aspect of child rearing, nutrition, hygiene, health, and development. The culture is in turn influenced by ethnicity, religion, lifestyle, social class, and geographic location.

Family size and structure Number of children in a family and birth order might have impact on nutritional distribution of family food especially among those from poorer strata of society. Disturbances in family including separated or divorced parents, family quarrels/conflicts, unemployment, and moving homes might deprive the emotional component to child's growth and development.

5. Environmental Factors

Secular Trends

India is following a secular trend of growth and puberty with subsequent generations having better height and early puberty, due to increasing industrialization and changing lifestyle.

Geographic Factors

Growth patterns differ between countries and climates. Iodine deficiency disorder, a widespread nutritional deficiency prevalent in people from mountainous Himalayan regions, may predispose to growth retardation.

Physical Environmental Factors

Air pollutants like carbon monoxide, sulfur dioxide, and chlorofluorocarbons (CFCs) might influence the respiratory system and hence indirectly influence the growth and well-being. Similarly, sanitation, sewage treatment, waste disposal, and provision of safe water have impact on health.

Access to Healthcare

Ease of access to health care along with appropriate health care seeking behavior of parents would influence the growth in a positive direction.

6. Health Factors

Chronic ailments like congenital malformations and chronic infections; progressive renal, cardiac, gastrointestinal, and neurological illness; or malignancy could adversely affect the growth of child either directly or indirectly by interfering with the child's nutritional intake and metabolism.

7. Psychological Factors

Health and growth can be affected by the way the individuals feel about themselves (self-esteem and self-image). Stress may lead to decline of growth hormone levels leading to psychosocial dwarfism.

Crespi B. The evolutionary biology of child health. *Proc Biol Sci.* 2011;278:1441–9.

Jain V, Singhal A. Catch up growth in low birth weight infants: striking a healthy balance. *Rev Endocr Metab Disord.* 2012;13:1417–9.

1.5 ASSESSMENT OF PHYSICAL GROWTH: ANTHROPOMETRY

Anthropometry (Greek *anthropos*—man and *metron*—measure) refers to the measurement of the human. Measurements that can be made on the body are almost limitless but weight and stature (height/length) are the most widely taken growth measurements. Commonly measured parameters are discussed below.

1. Weight

Before the advent of digital electronic scales, two types of weighing scales were commonly used: Beam balance scales (with moving weights) and the spring balance scales. Of these, beam balancing scales were more accurate.

The basket/pan type scale for infants can be used to weigh children up to 10.0 kg. Infants can be placed on the tray, which is supported on a reading frame calibrated for measuring a minimum of 10 g increment. The platform scale is for older children who can climb and stand up on the scale.

- Weigh the child in bare minimum of clothes and without shoes. Infants should be weighed naked (without diapers) and older children can be weighed with a vest and brief.
- Ensure that the scale is resting on firm, stable and even surface, or uncarpeted floor.
- Check the zero of the scale before weighing. Calibrate the weight scale at the beginning and at the end of each measurement.
- *Infants* Place the infant in a manner so as to distribute the weight evenly about the center of the pan. If a diaper is worn, its weight should be subtracted from the observed weight; because the reference data for infants is based on nude weight.
- *Children* Ask them to stand in the center of the platform, with body weight evenly distributed on both feet. Ensure that the child is not holding onto anything.
- A child on follow-up should preferably be weighed on the same scale.
- Read the weight by standing in front of the scale and not from the side.

2. Stature

Stature is ascertained by measuring the length (in children less than 2 years old) or height (in older children).

Harpenden infantometer It is used to measure the length of a newborn and infant. The tool consists of a horizontal wooden board limited by two vertical planks perpendicular to the two ends (Fig. 1.4). At one end, plank is fixed to the wooden board (headpiece); the other end has a movable vertical plank to adjust to the infant's length (foot piece). There is a calibrated reading strip in the middle of the board on which the length of the baby can be read directly. The infantometer is designed to measure lengths between 0 and 100 cm, with a precision of 1 mm.

Stadiometer It is used for measuring standing height. The child stands on a wooden plank with his back against a wooden board that is calibrated in cm/inches. A flat board (wooden, metallic or cardboard) is placed at head end of the child to level off the height. Alternatively, the height can also be measured against a flat wall.

Length

- Place the child supine on the infant measuring board.
- Ask the assistant to hold the child's head in the Frankfort plane, while you steady the legs. The head is positioned in the Frankfort plane when the crown touches the headpiece and a vertical line from the ear canal to the lower border of the eye socket is perpendicular to the horizontal board (ie, positioned vertically). Apply gentle traction to bring the head into contact with the fixed headpiece.

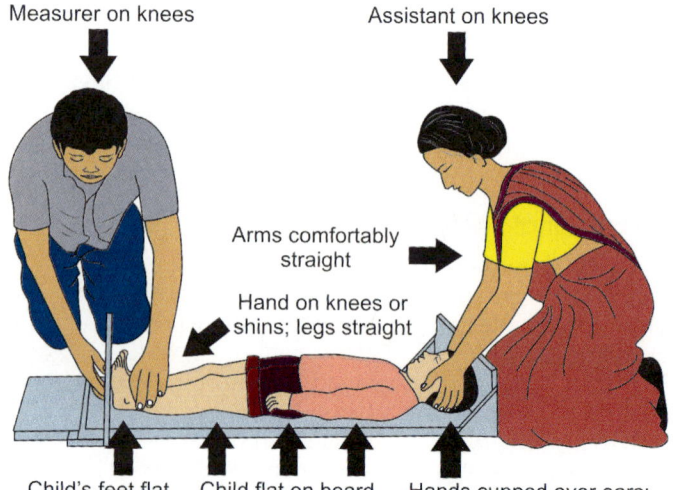

Fig. 1.4 Taking length on an infantometer

- Position the child's shoulders and hips at right angles to the long axis of the body. Apply gentle pressure on the knees to straighten the legs and prevent the knees from flexing.
- Bring the movable footboard to rest firmly against the child's feet with the soles flat on the board and the toes pointing directly upwards.
- Record the measurement to the nearest 0.1 cm from the counter on the measuring board.

Height

- Remove the hair ornaments, undo the buns and braids, and take off the footwear.
- Ask the child to stand on the stadiometer with feet slightly apart at a 60° angle and confirm that the weight is evenly distributed on both feet. The arms hang freely by the sides of the trunk with palms facing the thighs.
- Ensure that the back of the head, shoulder blades, buttocks, calves and heels are touching the vertical board/wall. This can be done by trying to insert a plastic rule at places where these points touch the wall. Inability to insert the rule implies good contact.
- Ask the child to look straight. Position the child's head so that a horizontal line drawn from the external auditory meatus to the lower edge of the eye socket runs parallel to the baseboard (*ie*, the Frankfort plane positioned horizontally) (Fig. 1.5).
- The headpiece is moved down to rest firmly on top of the child's head, compressing the hair; keeping it perpendicular to the wall.
- Record the reading to the last completed 0.1 cm.

3. Body Circumferences

Circumferences are measured to nearest 0.1 cm with a tape made up of a soft and non-shrinkable material.

Head Circumference

The head circumference is recorded between birth to 6 years of age (the period of brain growth) as the maximum circumference of the head with measuring tape overlying the occiput at back and supraorbital ridges in front.

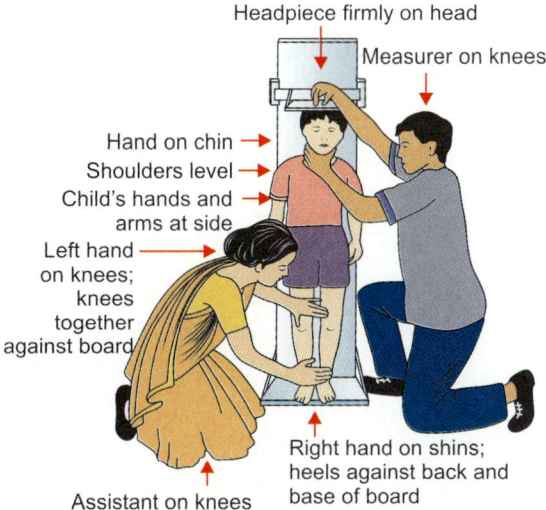

Fig. 1.5 Measurement of standing height

- Anchor the tape just above the eyebrows.
- Ensure that the tape overlies the most prominent part of the occipital prominence at the back of the head.
- The tape should be perpendicular to the long axis of the face and should be pulled firmly to compress the hair, skin, and underlying soft tissues.
- Record measurement over the parietal eminence by cross-over technique (Fig. 1.6).

Chest Circumference

- Place the infant in the lap of the mother and stand in front. The chest should be bare.
- Abduct the arms of the infant slightly to permit passage of the tape around the chest.
- Pass the tape around the chest of the infant, at the level of nipples or 4th costosternal joints.
- Lower the arm to their natural position, once the tape is snugly in place.
- Record the circumference in a horizontal plane, midway between inspiration and expiration (Fig. 1.7).

Mid-upper Arm Circumference

Mid-upper arm circumference (MUAC) is recorded for children between 6 months and 5 years of age to nearest of 0.1 cm. A mid-upper arm circumference of less than 12.5 cm indicates malnutrition.

- Palpate and mark the two important bony landmarks: ie, the acromion process and the olecranon. Forearm should be flexed while marking these points.

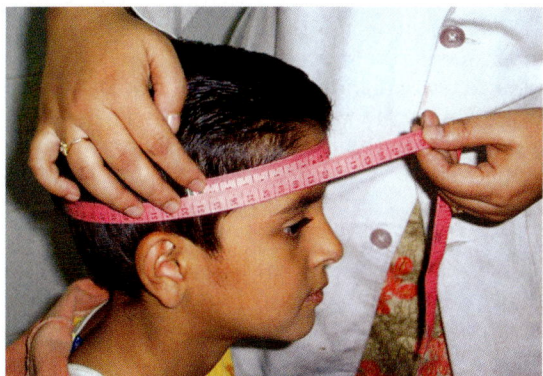

Fig. 1.6 Measurement of head circumference

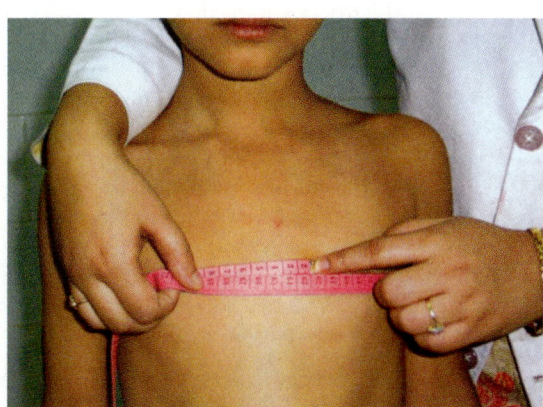

Fig. 1.7 Measurement of chest circumference

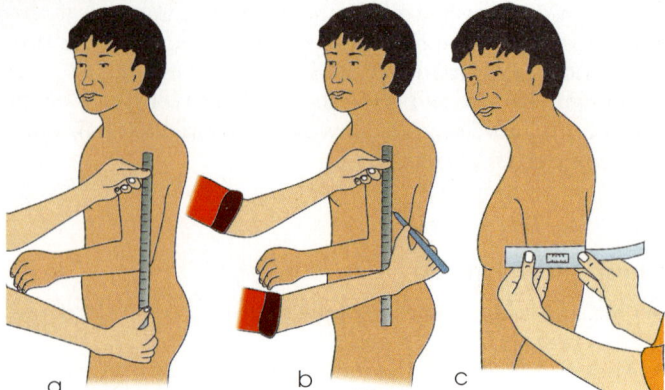

Fig. 1.8a to c (a and b) The mid-upper arm point, (b) measuring mid-arm circumference

- Mark the mid-upper arm point. It is half the distance between the acromion process and the olecranon.
- Encircle the tape around the arm, over the marked midpoint, perpendicular to the long axis of the upper arm, with arm hanging freely in a relaxed position (Fig. 1.8).
- Ensure that the tape lies flat around the arm, without compressing the skin or underlying tissue; there should be no gap or compression on the inner part of the arm.

4. Skinfold Thickness

Measurements of skinfold thickness may be useful in the estimation of muscle mass or of body fat content. The proportionate mass of subcutaneous tissue is greatest at about 9 months. It decreases steadily till about 6 years, when the increase begins again.

In clinical practice, however, measurements of triceps and subscapular skinfold thickness generally are sufficient. The thickness is expressed in mm and is taken using a skinfold caliper (*Holtain* or *Harpenden*).

5. Body Proportions

Useful body proportions that may help in understanding various growth disturbances include body mass index (BMI), sitting height for upper segment/lower segment ratio, and arm span.

Body mass index It is calculated as weight in kg/(height in m)^2 and considered as the most important parameter used for assessment of growth in adolescents and adults. For Asian adults, the normal BMI lies between 18.5 and 23. Those having a BMI of between 23 and 28 are called *overweight*. *Obesity* is defined as a BMI of more than 28. Adults with BMI of less than 18.5 are termed to be having '*chronic energy deficiency*.'

Absolute cut-off values for defining chronic energy deficiency, overweight, and obesity are not applicable for children and adolescents. Therefore, evaluation of BMI in these age groups is carried out by comparison with age-related standard percentile charts. **Obesity** is defined as BMI greater than the 95th percentile for age whereas **overweight** refers to BMI between 85th and 95th percentile.

Sitting height It denotes the upper segment length and represents 65–70% of total length in the newborn infant. After birth, limbs grow much faster than the trunk resulting in

reduction of sitting height percentage. By the time of adolescence, the upper segment almost equals with the lower segment. High upper/lower segment ratio indicates short limb dwarfism.

Arm span It is the physical measurement of the length from one end of an arm (measured at the fingertips) to the other when raised parallel to the ground at shoulder height at 180° angle. The arm span as compared to the total stature is an useful index. Usually, the difference between the two is not more than 3 cm. Longer arm span is seen in Marfan syndrome.

For detailed description of methods of anthropometry and its interpretation, refer to "*Clinical Methods in Pediatrics*" by Piyush Gupta.

6. Velocity of Physical Growth

Measurement of the velocity of growth or increment in a unit of time is a better tool for early identification of factors affecting growth. Velocity of growth can also help in predicting the ultimate adult height. The normal growth velocity curve for height is shown in Fig. 1.9. The growth velocity is maximum during the first year of life. A second growth spurt occurs during puberty. This is known as the *peak height/weight velocity*. Maximum growth velocity occurs at sexual maturity rate (SMR) stage 3–4 in girls and SMR stage 4–5 in boys. Girls achieve pubertal growth spurt about 2 years prior to boys.

7. Bone Age Assessment

Bone age is a tool to evaluate skeletal maturation which in turn depends on hormonal influences. Assessment of bone age is thus used for diagnostic evaluation of children with growth failure, and advanced or delayed puberty. In healthy children, bone age corresponds to chronological age. A discrepancy between the two suggests a defect of the endocrine system. Characteristically, hypothyroidism slows the skeletal growth; ossification is delayed and bone age is less than the chronological age.

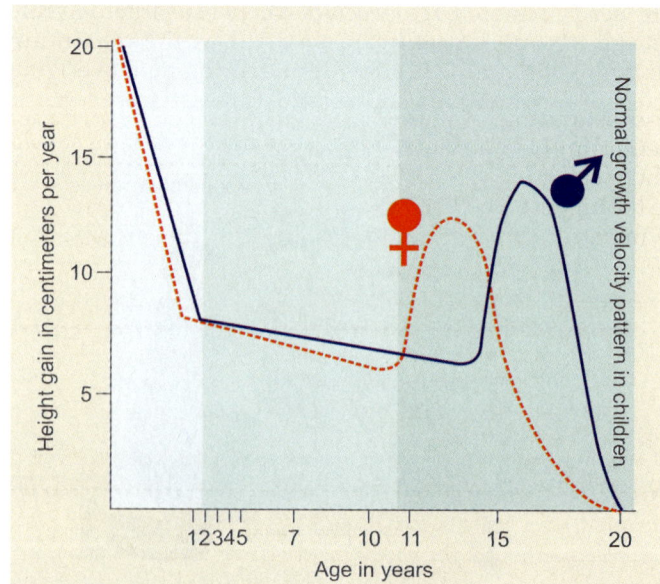

Fig. 1.9 Normal growth velocity in children (boys and girls). The figure shows that girls achieve pubertal growth spurt about 2 years prior to boys

Ossification of skeleton begins in the intrauterine period—starting first in the clavicles followed by skull, long bones, and spine. Shaft ossifies earlier than the ends of the bone. The earliest epiphyseal centers to appear are those for os calcis and talus (22–26 weeks of gestation). At the time of birth in a full term newborn, the distal epiphyses of femur (age of appearance: 31–39 weeks of gestation) and the proximal epiphyses of tibia (age of appearance: 34 weeks of gestation to 5th postnatal week) are usually present. Two carpal bones are present at 1 year; and by 6 years, epiphyses of 7 carpal bones are present except pisiform, which ossifies later during puberty.

By convention, radiograph of the left limb is taken for computing bone age. At different chronological ages, radiographs of different parts of the body are required for correct assessment. For example, in the newborn period, radiographs of foot and knee are helpful. Between 3 and 9 months, radiographs of the shoulder is taken. X-ray of hands and wrists should be obtained between 1 and 12 years of age. For children between 12 and 14 years, radiographs of elbow and hip are helpful. A serial evaluation is always much more helpful than a single radiograph. Girls are more advanced than boys in skeletal development at all ages. Bone age corresponds more closely to SMR staging than to chronological age during puberty.

The two most widely used tools to assess bone age are the Greulich-Pyle Atlas method and the Tanner-Whitehouse 2 Individual Bones method (TW2 method). It is important to note that these methods are not always comparable and cannot be considered interchangeable. Readers are advised to refer to advanced text for more details.

Greulich WW, Pyle SI. Radiographic Atlas of Skeletal Development of Hand and Wrist. Stanford, CA: Stanford University Press;1959.

Tanner JM, Whitehouse RH, Cameron N, *et al*. Assessment of Skeletal Maturity and Prediction of Adult Height (TW2 Method), 2nd edn. London: Academic Press;1983.

1.6 STATISTICAL PRINCIPLES IN ASSESSMENT OF GROWTH

1. Gaussian Distribution

If measurements of any of the growth parameters (eg, weight, height) are obtained in a large population of normal children and then arranged in a regular order starting from the lowest to the highest, a bell-shaped curve is formed (Fig. 1.10). This symmetrical curve illustrates a typical Gaussian (Normal)

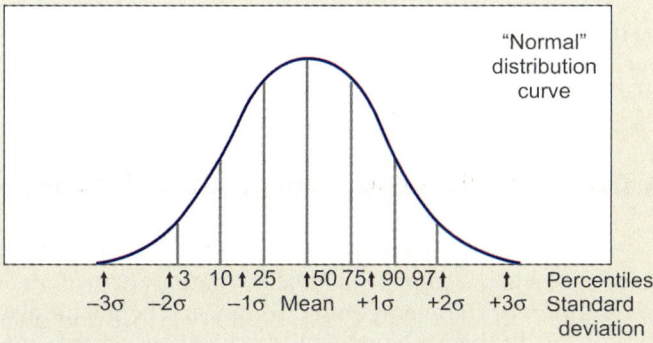

Fig. 1.10 Normal bell-shaped distribution curve

distribution, in which maximum values lie around the middle of the curve. The curve tapers off on the either side, with fewer observations at both the ends of the curve. Mean and median are equal in a Gaussian distribution.

2. Mean and Standard Deviation

Measurement of a parameter in a sample and its recording in a continuous numerical manner generates several measurements, the most important of them being mean and standard deviation (SD).
- *Mean* It is obtained by dividing the sum of all observations by the number of observations. In a Gaussian distribution, the maximum number of values cluster around the average or *mean*.
- *Standard deviation* It denotes the degree of dispersion or the scatter of observations away from the mean. It is estimated that 68.3% (approximately two-thirds) of the observations lie within 1 standard deviation (SD) above or below the mean value of the observations. Values within the range of ±2 SD include 95.4% of all values. Values beyond 2SD are unusual in a normal population. 3 SD around the mean includes 99.7% of all values.

3. Median and Percent Median

When data are arranged in ascending or descending order of magnitude, half of the observations are above and the other half below a certain point. This point or value is known as the *median*. The median thus indicates that 50% of observations are above and 50% are below this point. In a typical Gaussian distribution, the median is expected to be equivalent to the arithmetic mean. **Median, rather than the mean, is considered as the central value for most of the anthropometric parameters, since the population data has a non-Gaussian (skewed) distribution.**

4. Percentiles

Percentile indicates the position that a measurement would hold in a typical series of 100 arranged in ascending order. The median lies at the 50th percentile, on either side of which lie half the observations. Another example is the 85th percentile curve, which denotes that 15% of observa-tions are expected to be above and 84% below it.

Percentile location is used to designate where an individual stands with respect to other members of the population. The WHO growth standards show curves at 3rd, 15th, 50th, 85th and 97th percentiles, corresponding to distances from the average values. One standard deviation above or below the mean coincides with the 84th or 16th percentile curve, respectively.

Eighty percent of the weight/height measurements of healthy children at a given age are expected to lie between 10th and 90th percentiles. Further, 95% of the weight/height measurements of healthy children at a given age are expected to lie between 3rd and 97th percentile values. Thus, allowable normal range of variation in observations is between 3rd and 97th percentiles, which roughly corresponds to ±2 SD.

A healthy child normally remains and follows the same percentile curve during the entire period of his/her growth.

5. *Z* (SD)-Score

It represents the deviation of anthropometric measurement from the reference median and is calculated as follows:

$$\frac{\text{observed value} - \text{median reference value}}{\text{standard deviation (SD) of the reference population}}$$

An SD score value of +1.5 means that the difference between the present (observed) and the expected (reference median value) is 1.5 times of the standard deviation of the reference population.

A negative value of Z-score means that the observed value is less than the expected; and *vice versa*. Similarly, a positive (+) value of Z-score indicates that the observed value of the measurement/index is more than the reference median.

Usually, –1, –2, and –3 Z-scores correspond to 15.8, 2.28, and 0.13th percentiles; while 1st, 3rd, and 10th percentiles correspond to –2.33, –1.88, and –1.29 Z-scores, respectively. Thus, the 3rd percentile roughly corresponds to –2SD.

Abnormal values usually refer to measurements below –2 Z-score (2.3rd percentile) or above +2 Z-score (97.7th percentile), relative to the reference median.

1.7 GROWTH CHARTS, GROWTH REFERENCE, AND GROWTH STANDARDS

1. Growth Charts

The growth charts comprise of an X-axis that corresponds to the age in months or years; and Y axis denoting the value of the anthropometric parameter: for example; weight (kg), height (cm), body mass index (kg/m^2), etc. WHO Growth Charts are available for both percentiles and Z-score, separately.

- The *WHO percentile charts* depict 5 percentiles lines corresponding to 3rd, 15th, 50th, 85th and 97th percentiles (from below to above) (Fig. 1.11a). Any child who is below the 3rd or above the 97th centile is *likely* to be abnormal.
- The *WHO Z-score charts* display curves for median, –2Z, –3Z, 2Z, and 3Z-scores (Fig. 1.11b). Abnormal is defined as any discrepancy of more than –2Z-scores. A deviation by more than –3Z-score denotes severe malnutrition. On the charts of growth velocity, the cutoff line for defining low height velocity is below the 25th centile.

WHO growth standards for children less than 5 years have been adopted in many countries including India as the universal global standard, for monitoring growth in *under-five children*. In 2015, Indian Academy of Pediatrics published new revised growth charts for Indian children 5–18 years of age in view of the changing trend in nutritional status of older children.

2. Growth References vs Growth Standards

- *Growth standards* These represent data on how a population of children should grow, under the given optimal nutritional and health conditions.
- *Growth references* These are descriptive data that define how children in the population are growing under the best possible state of nutrition and health in a given community. They represent how children are actually growing rather than how they should be growing.

The WHO growth charts published in 2006, based on *WHO Multicenter Growth Reference Study (MGRS)* for children under the age of 5 years, are an example of growth standards. Whereas, the 2015 IAP growth charts are growth references which describe how children in India were actually growing at that point of time.

3. WHO Growth Standards

The 2006 growth curves and charts developed by World Health Organization (WHO) provide a single international standard that represents the best description of physiological growth for all children from birth to 5 years of age. These charts are based on the growth of *exclusively breastfed infants*. The second unique feature of these standards is that it is based on growth of children from many of the world's major regions: Brazil (South America), Ghana (Africa), India (Asia), Norway (Europe), Oman (the Middle East) and the USA (North America).

These standards show that all children of the world grow similarly till 5 years of age, provided the optimal environment, regardless of ethnicity and socioeconomic status. The Standards show that nutrition, environment, and healthcare are stronger factors in determining growth and development than gender or ethnic background. The WHO standards differ from other existing growth charts in a number of innovative ways.

1. WHO standards are based on longitudinally collected data as opposed to cross-sectional data in erstwhile NCHS reference (based on growth of North American Children). This is particularly useful in development of growth velocity standards.
2. WHO standards describe "how children should grow," as compared to earlier NCHS references which simply stated "how children are growing."
3. WHO standards make breastfeeding the biological "norm" and establishes the breastfed infant as the normative growth model. NCHS reference was based on the growth of artificially-fed children.
4. WHO Standards also include other growth indicators such as the skinfold thickness, and body mass index. These are useful to define obesity and overweight.
5. MGRS also provide the Windows of Achievement standards for 6 motor development milestones including sitting, standing, and walking.

WHO charts have now replaced the National Center for Health Statistics (NCHS)/Centers for Disease Control (CDC) Growth Charts for assessing the growth of children up to 5 years of age. The WHO growth charts are provided for weight-for-age (birth–5 y) (Fig. 1.11a–d); length/height-for-age (birth–5 y) (Fig. 1.12a–d); weight-for-length (birth–2 y) (Fig. 1.13a–d); and weight-for-height (2–5 y) (Fig. 1.14a–d). Corresponding tables are reproduced in the *Annexures*.

4. Growth Reference for Indian Children 5–18 Years

Even though growth occurs in a similar manner amongst under-five children throughout the world, but there do exist some regional variations amongst the pattern of growth of older children. The average adult weight and height are also different in different regions of the world because of the same reason. Thus for Indian children older than 5 years, the ideal reference standards would be the ones derived from Indian population itself.

In 2015, Indian Academy of Pediatrics (IAP) published the revised growth charts based on data collected from published studies on apparently healthy Indian children and adolescents in the past one decade. IAP recommends use of these charts as reference values for Indian children between 5 and 18 years of age. These reference curves are provided as Figs 1.15 to 1.18. We suggest using these charts as reference values for children above 5 years of age. Corresponding tables are reproduced in the *Annexures*.

5. Growth Monitoring

Growth monitoring is a screening tool used to diagnose nutritional discrepancies, chronic systemic illnesses, and endocrine disorders. Growth monitoring involves taking the same and multiple anthropometric measurements at regular intervals, approximately at the same time of the day and to see their changing trend. A single value only denotes the measurement at that point of time.

National Health Mission encourages growth monitoring of children less than 5 years of age. Children are monitored monthly during the 1st year of life, every 2 months during the 2nd year and every 3 months thereafter till 5 years of age. Weight, length, and head circumference should be measured at birth followed by measurements at the time of immunization visits at 6 weeks, 10 weeks, 14 weeks, 9 months, 15 months and 18 months of age. Between 18 months and 5 years of age, it should be monitored 6 monthly. After 5 years of age, growth can be monitored annually, especially for body mass index (BMI).

1.8 NORMAL GROWTH

1. Size at Birth

Birth weight The average birth weight of Indian infants is around 2.8 to 2.9 kg as compared to 3.4 kg in White Caucasian infants. The birth weight is influenced by the following factors:
- *Maternal nutrition:* Infants born to mothers who are short (height <145 cm), underweight (<45 kg pre-pregnancy weight), anemic (hemoglobin <8 g/dL), or hypoalbuminemic (serum albumin <2.5 g/dL) are likely to be born low birth weight, ie, less than 2.5 kg.
- Maternal infection, cigarette smoking, alcoholism or drug addiction, exposure to radiation, and living at high altitude also may lead to decreased birth weight.
- *Fetal factors:* Chromosomal anomalies, like Down syndrome and gonadal dysgenesis, are associated with low birth weight.
- Singleton babies are heavier than infants of multiple births.
- Maternal toxemia, hypertension, and cardiac disease can result in low birth weight.
- Infants of diabetic mothers are generally heavier than average.

Length of a normal full-term male infant is around 50 cm.

Head circumference at birth is 35–37 cm.

Physical proportions The head is large for body size, face is small and rounded, mandible is small, chest is rounded, and the abdomen is protuberant. Limbs are short and ratio of upper to lower segment is high (1.7:1).

2. Growth in Infancy (First year of life)

Weight A term child loses 10% of his weight during first three days of life as a result of excretion of excess extravascular fluid and possibly poor intake. The birth weight is regained by 10 days of life. Subsequently, the weight gain occurs at a rate of 25–30 g per day for the first 3 months of life. Thereafter about 400 g of weight gain occurs every month, for the remaining part of the first year. The consistent gain of weight during infancy provides a useful guide to nutritional status and health of the infant; it is not as sensitive a guide in the older child. Usually, the infant doubles his birth weight by 5 months and triples the birth weight by 1 year of age. The weight at 5 months, one year, and 2 years is approximately 6, 9, and 12 kg, respectively.

Length The most dynamic linear growth spreads over during the first two years of life. A term newborn measures 50 cm at birth, 60 cm at 3 months, 70 cm at 9 months, and 75 cm at 1 year of age.

Head growth It occurs in parallel to the rapid brain growth during this period. There is a 5–6 cm increase in head size during the first 3 months after birth and an additional 5–6 cm during the rest 9 months in the first year. Head circumference at 1 year of age is 45–47 cm. If the head growth exceeds 1 cm in 2 weeks during the first 3 months, hydrocephalus should be suspected.

Chest circumference This is less than the head circumference at birth. The two equalize by 6 months of age.

3. Growth after Infancy

Weight The weight of a child at the age of 2 years is four times and at 3 years is usually five times that of the birth weight. The child gains, on an average, about 1.5–2.5 kg per year, from the age of 2 years till onset of adolescence. During the pre-school years, between 2 and 5 years, the child gains on an average 2 kg (1.5–2.5 kg) in weight per year. Weight for age at a given age is more for boys as compared to girls. The adolescent acceleration in weight occurs earlier in girls (10–12 years) than boys (beginning 2 years later). The rapid weight gain is greatest in the year before menarche. Find below some formulae for a rough and quick calculation of expected weight between the ages of 3 months to 12 years. However, refer to the standard reference growth charts for exact values.

3–12 months	expected weight = (age in months + 9)/2
1–6 years	expected weight = 2 (age in years) + 8
7–12 years	expected weight = [7 (age in years) – 5]/2

Stature The child usually reaches a length of approximately 88–90 cm by 2 years. Height at 4 years of age is 100 cm (which is double the length at birth). The child gains on an average about 4–5 cm/year from the age of 2 years till the onset of puberty. By 13 years of age, a child triples the birth length. Adolescent spurt of growth in height corresponds closely to weight gain. The following formula can be used for a rough and quick calculation of expected height, between the ages of 2 to 12 years.

$$\text{Expected height} = (\text{age in years} \times 6) + 77$$

Head circumference It increases less rapidly during the second year of life in accordance with the decreased growth of the brain. The head circumference increases by 2 cm in the second year of life (47–49 cm by 2 year) and then at a rate of 1 cm per

Weight-for-age BOYS

Birth to 5 years (percentiles)

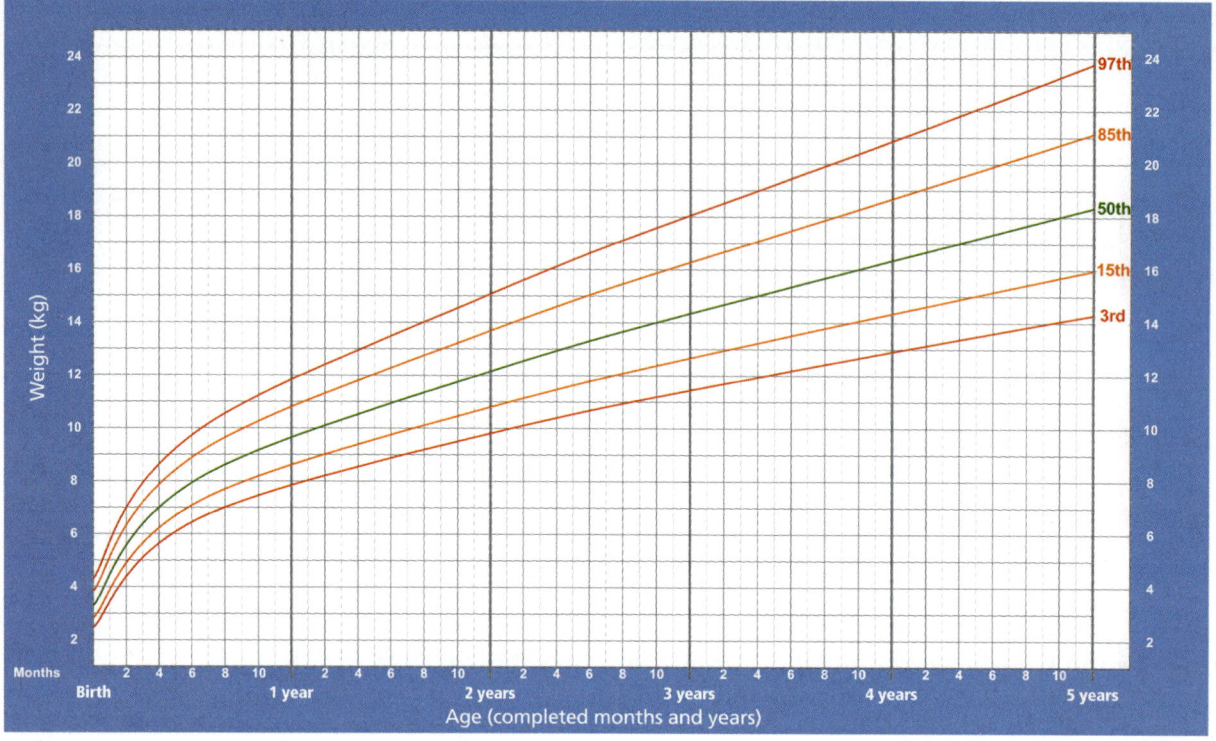

Fig. 1.11a WHO growth chart for weight-for-age for boys 0–5 years of age (percentiles)

Weight-for-age BOYS

Birth to 5 years (z-scores)

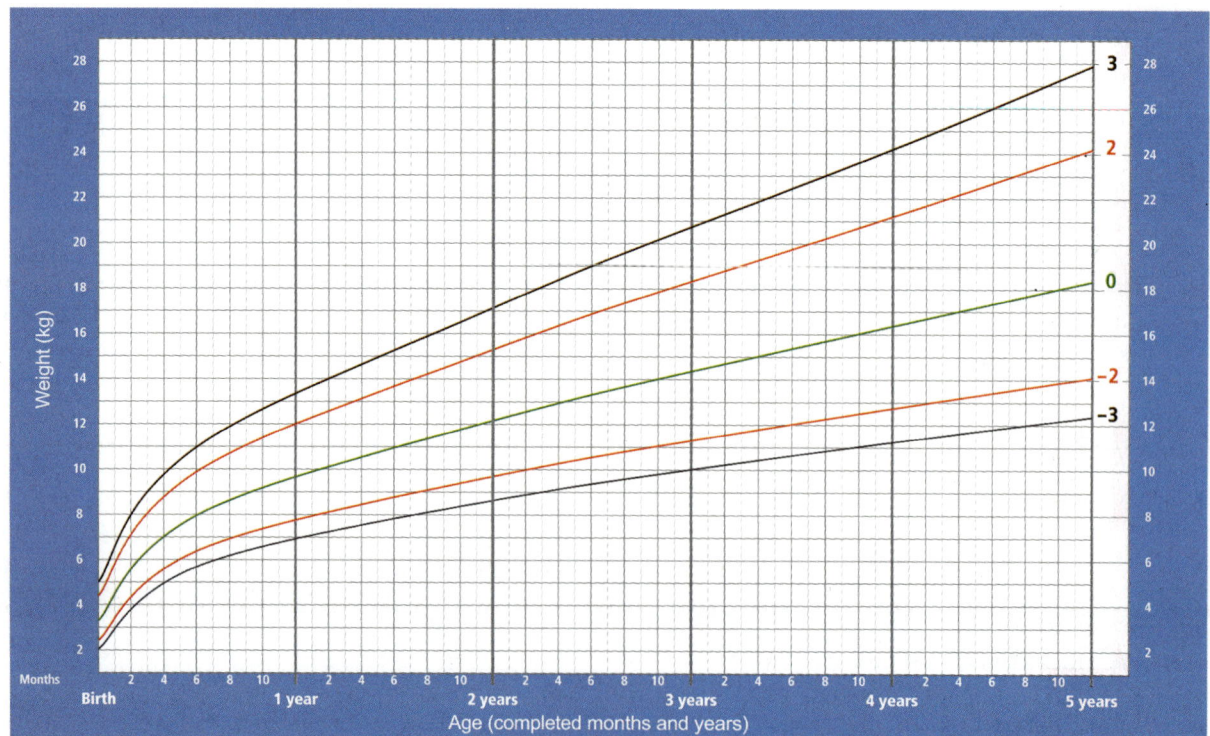

WHO Child Growth Standards

Fig. 1.11b WHO growth chart for weight-for-age for boys 0–5 years of age (Z-scores)

Weight-for-age GIRLS

Birth to 5 years (percentiles)

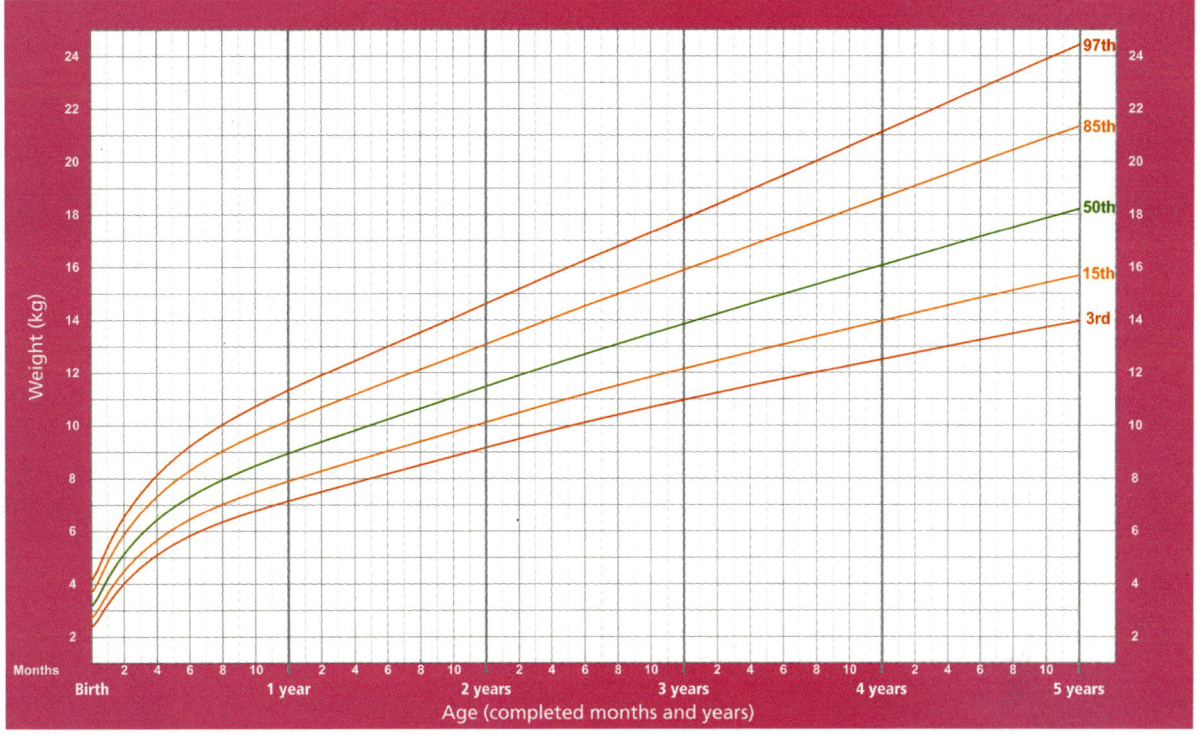

WHO Child Growth Standards

Fig. 1.11c WHO growth chart for weight-for-age for girls 0–5 years of age (percentiles)

Weight-for-age GIRLS

Birth to 5 years (z-scores)

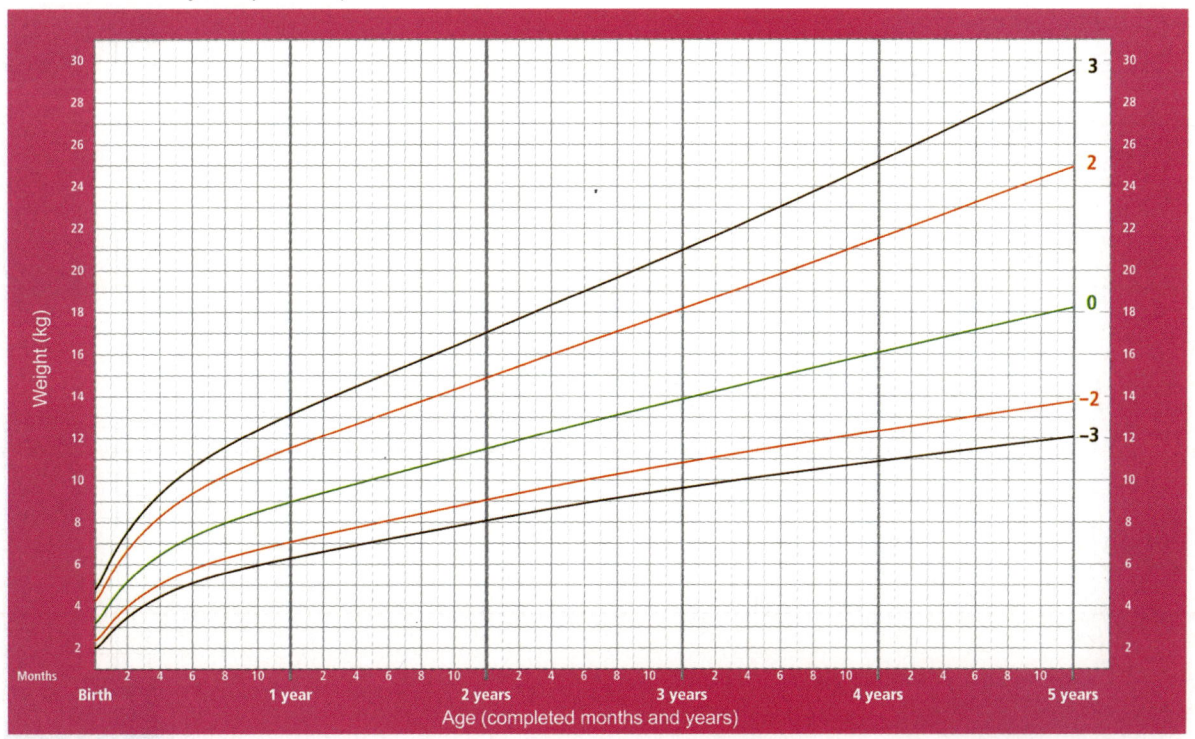

WHO Child Growth Standards

Fig. 1.11d WHO growth chart for weight-for-age for girls 0–5 years of age (Z-scores)

Length/height-for-age BOYS

Birth to 5 years (percentiles)

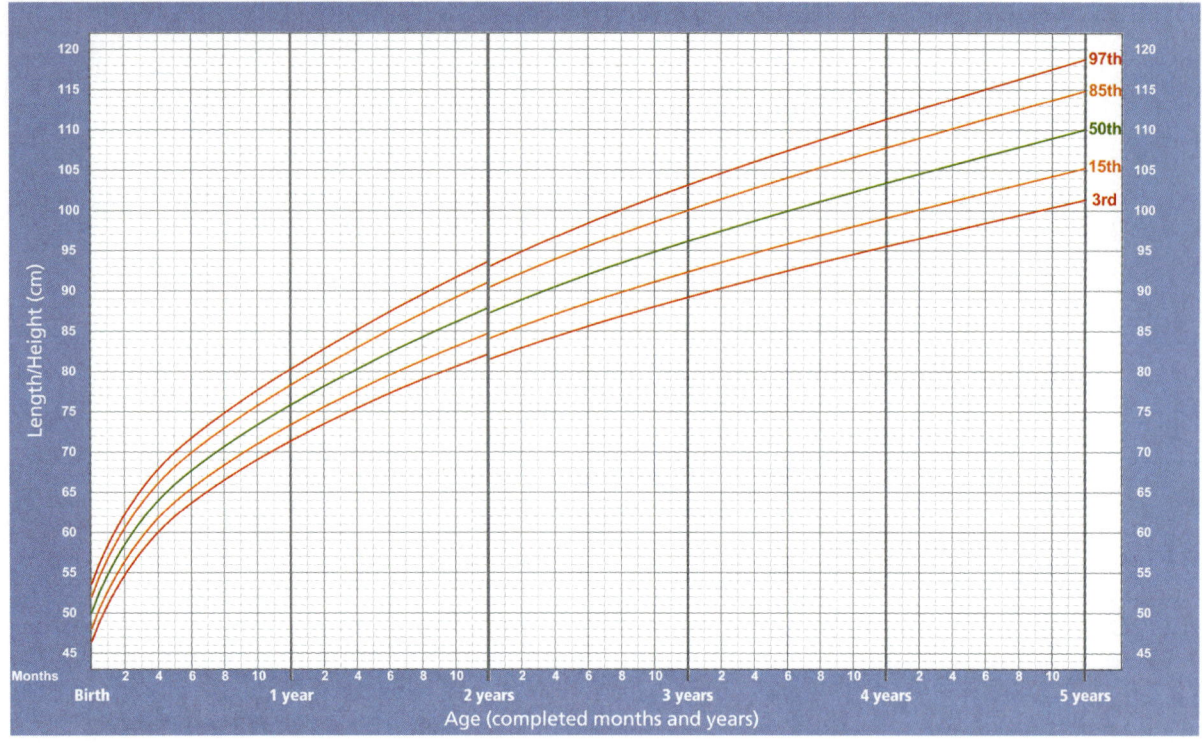

Fig. 1.12a WHO growth chart for length/height-for-age for boys 0–5 years of age (percentiles)

Length/height-for-age BOYS

Birth to 5 years (z-scores)

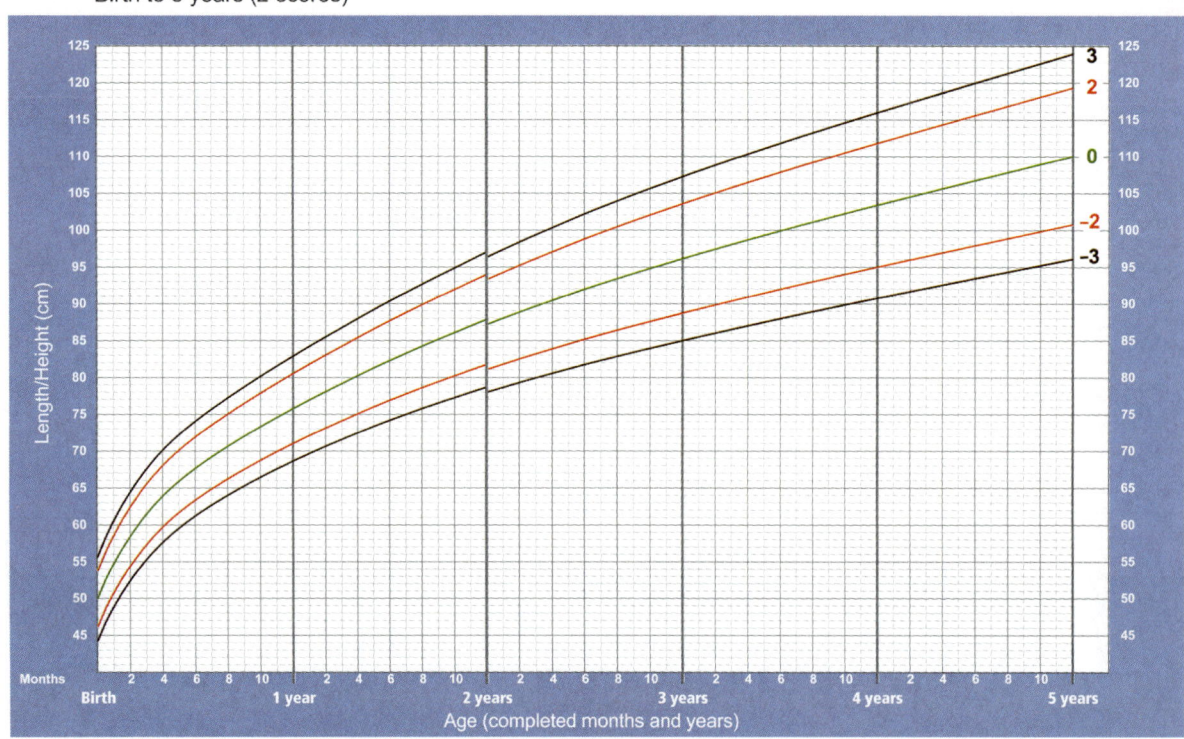

Fig. 1.12b WHO growth chart for length/height-for-age for boys 0–5 years of age (Z-scores)

Length/height-for-age GIRLS

Birth to 5 years (percentiles)

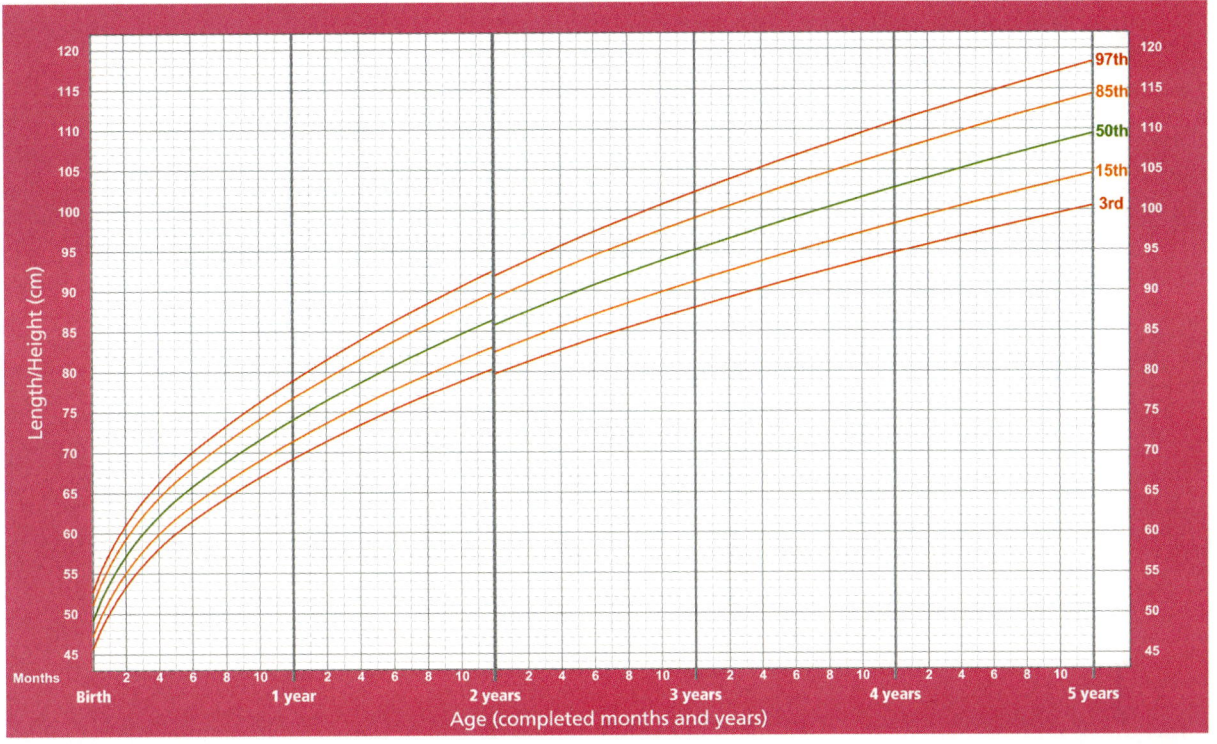

Fig. 1.12c WHO growth chart for length/height-for-age for girls 0–5 years of age (percentiles)

WHO Child Growth Standards

Length/height-for-age GIRLS

Birth to 5 years (z-scores)

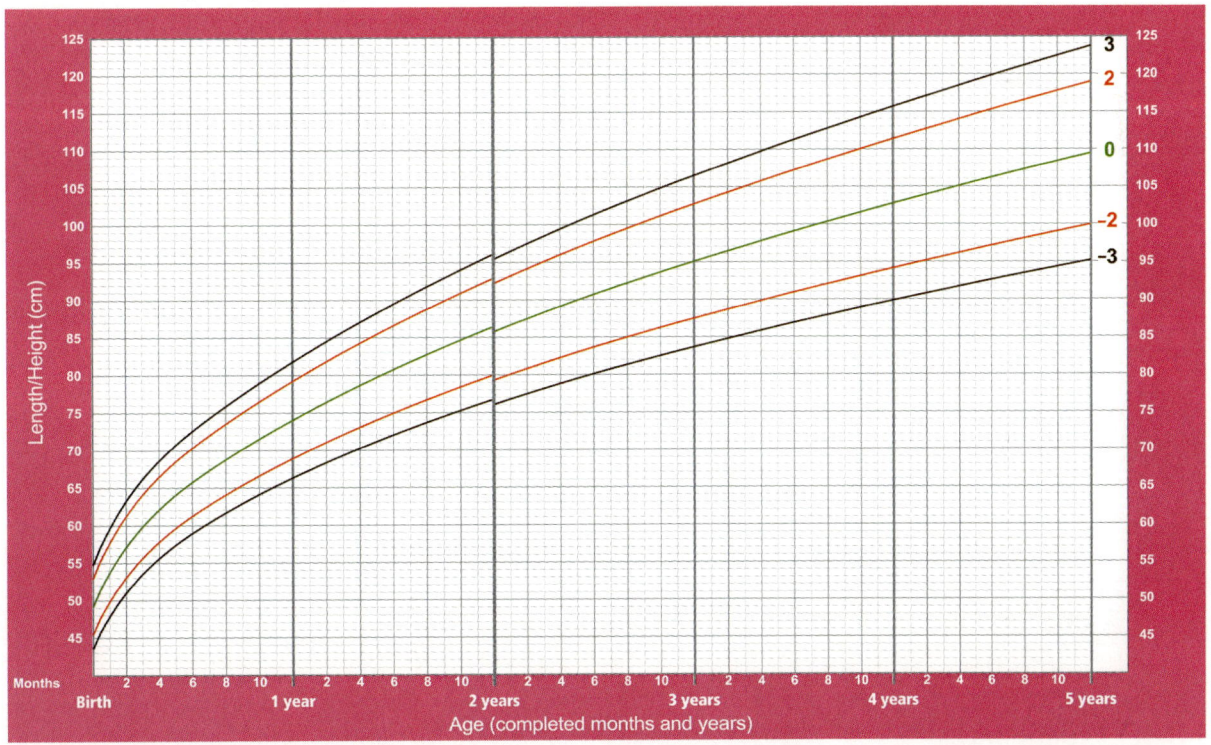

Fig. 1.12d WHO growth chart for length/height-for-age for girls 0–5 years of age (Z-scores)

WHO Child Growth Standards

Weight-for-length BOYS

Birth to 2 years (percentiles)

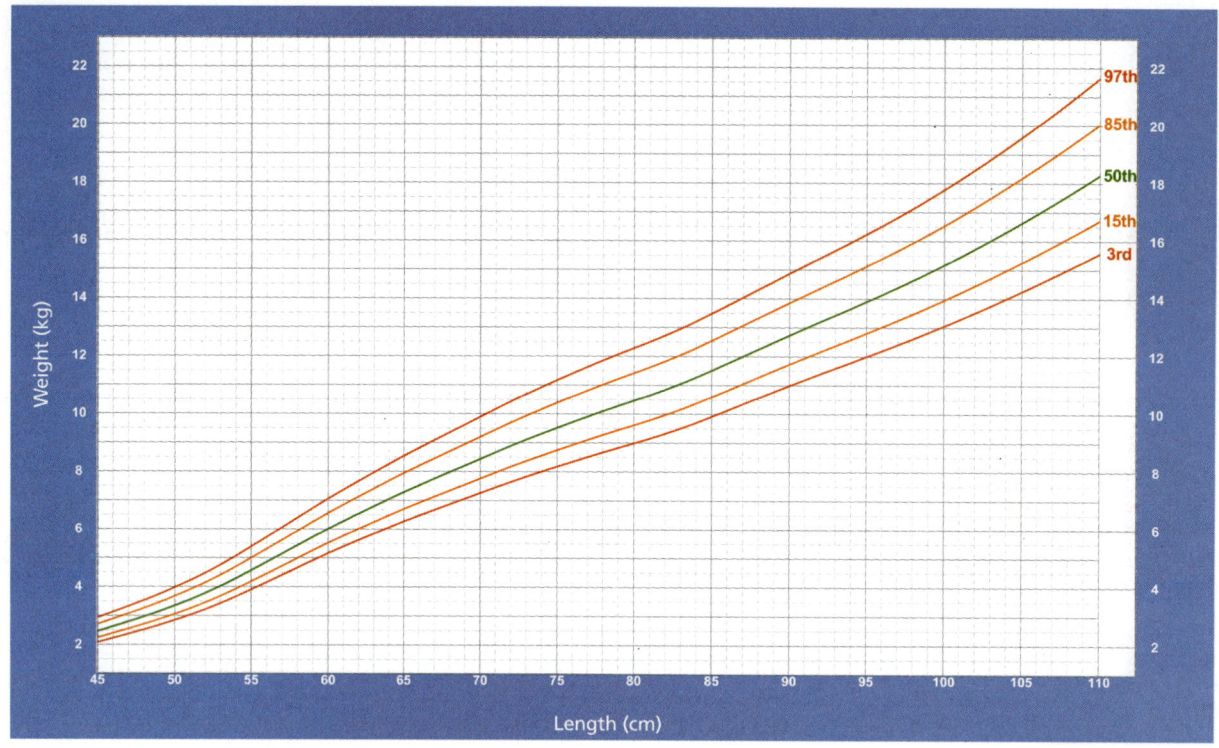

WHO Child Growth Standards

Fig. 1.13a WHO growth chart for weight-for-length for boys 0–2 years of age (percentiles)

Weight-for-length BOYS

Birth to 2 years (z-scores)

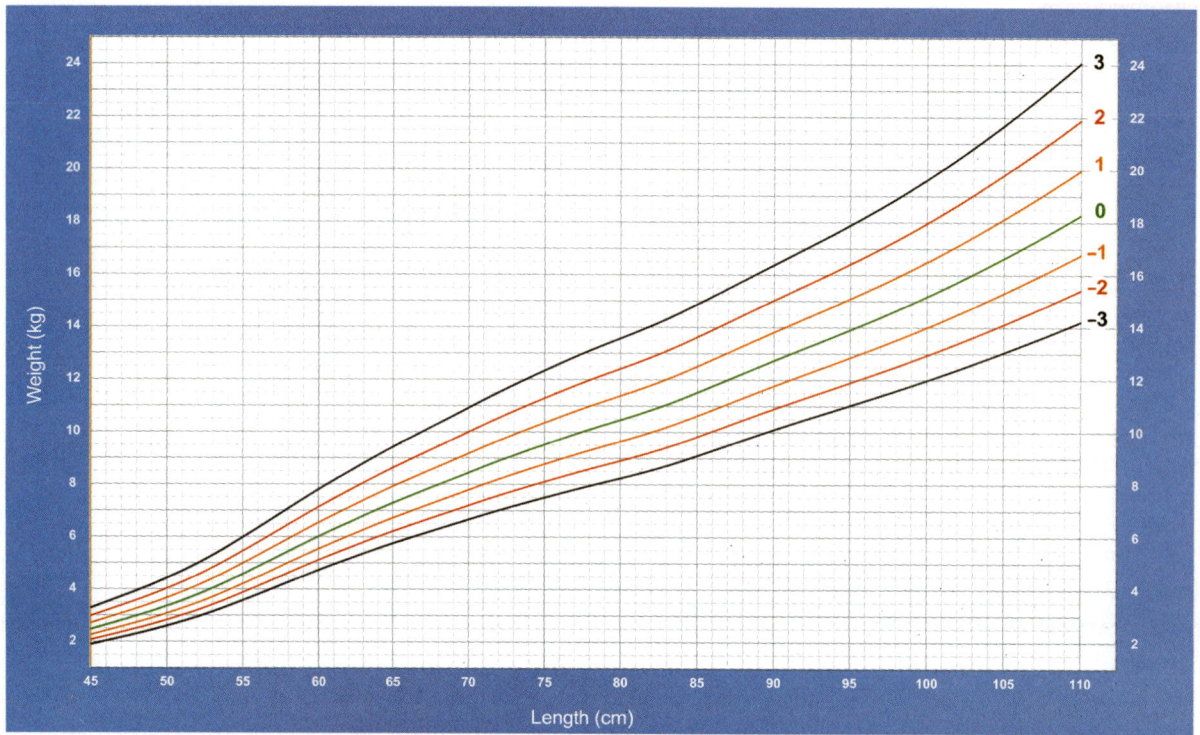

WHO Child Growth Standards

Fig. 1.13b WHO growth chart for weight-for-length for boys 0–2 years of age (Z-scores)

Weight-for-length GIRLS

Birth to 2 years (percentiles)

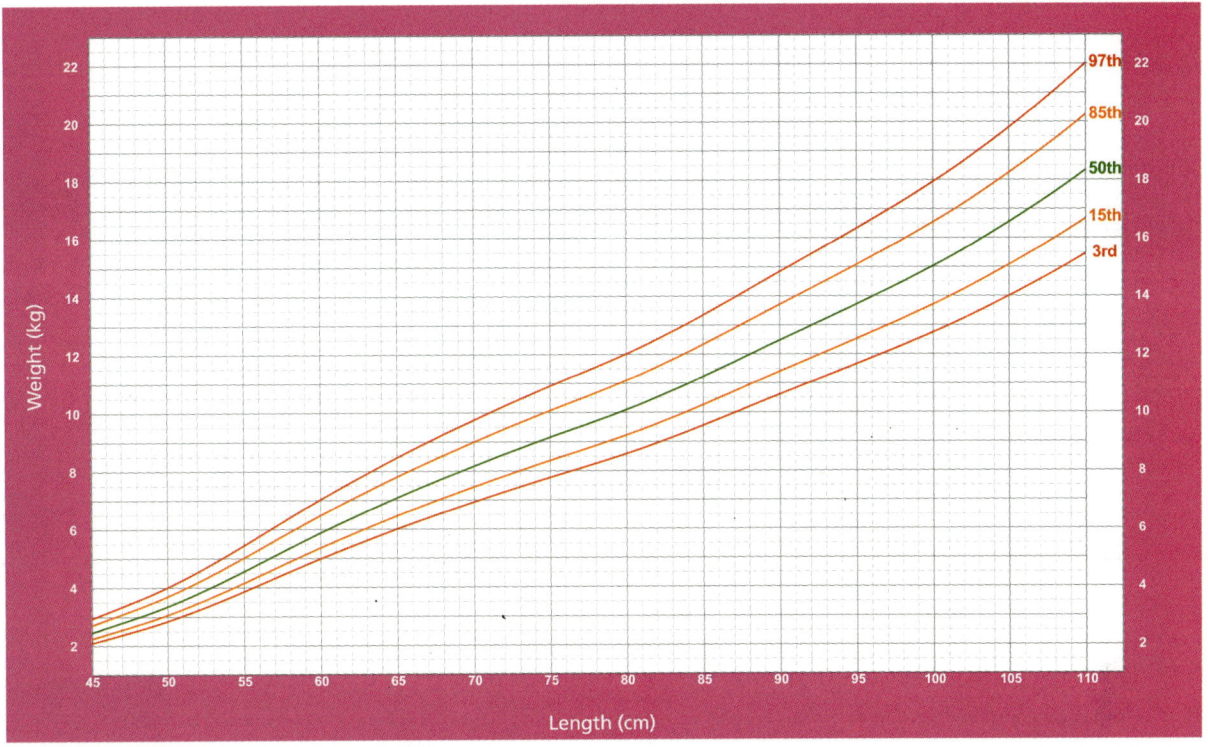

WHO Child Growth Standards

Fig. 1.13c WHO growth chart for weight-for-length for girls 0–2 years of age (percentiles)

Weight-for-length GIRLS

Birth to 2 years (z-scores)

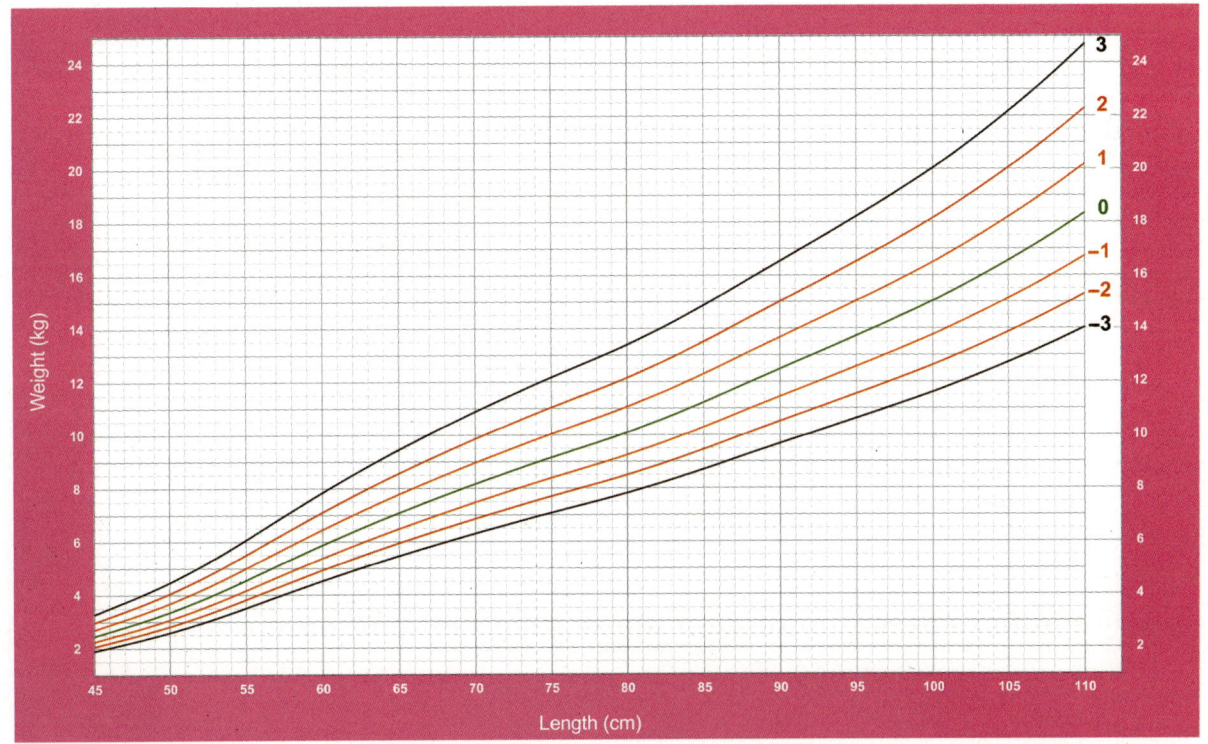

WHO Child Growth Standards

Fig. 1.13d WHO growth chart for weight-for-length for girls 0–2 years of age (Z-scores)

Weight-for-height BOYS

2 to 5 years (percentiles)

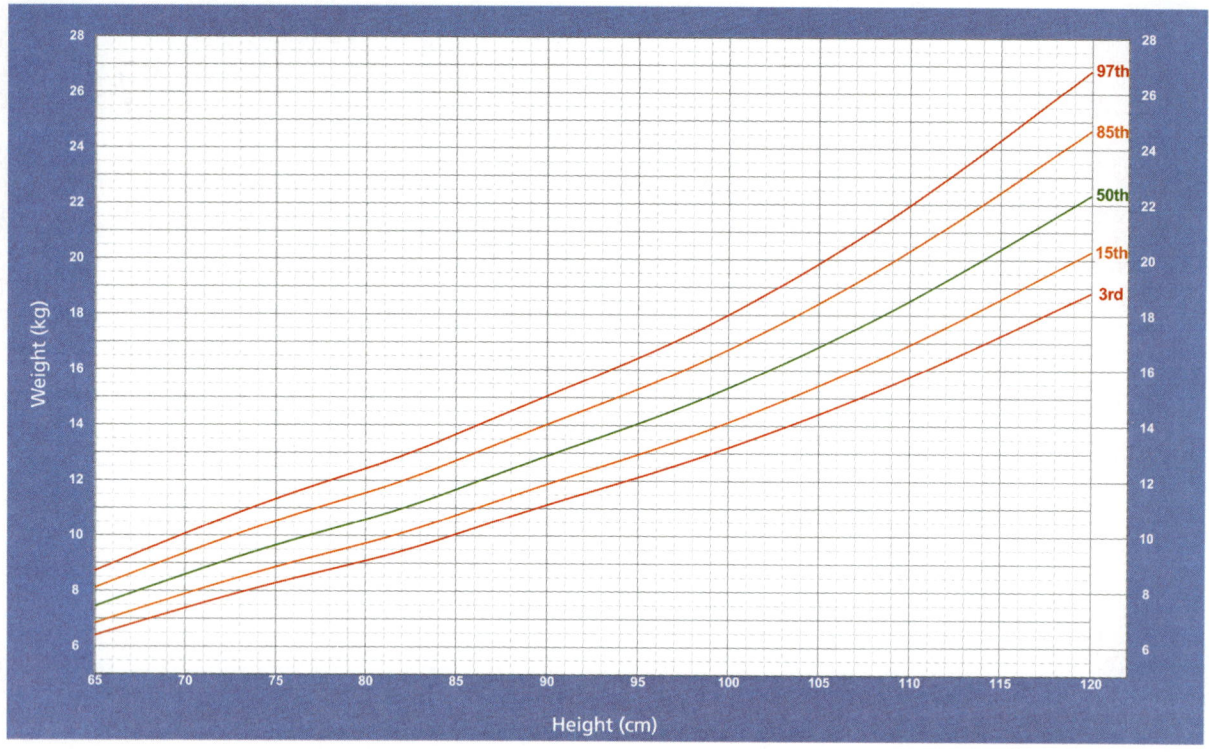

Fig 1.14a WHO growth chart for weight-for-height for boys 2–5 years of age (percentiles)

Weight-for-height BOYS

2 to 5 years (z-scores)

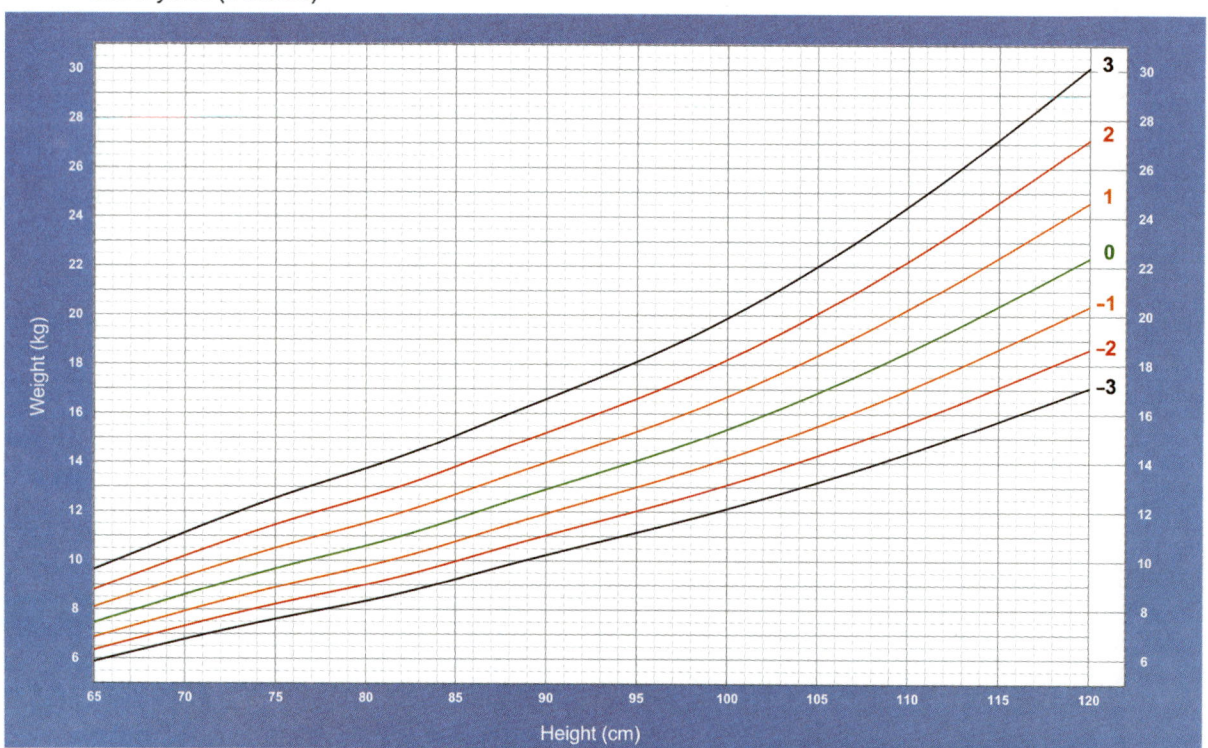

Fig. 1.14b WHO growth chart for weight-for-height for boys 2–5 years of age (*Z*-scores)

Weight-for-height GIRLS

2 to 5 years (percentiles)

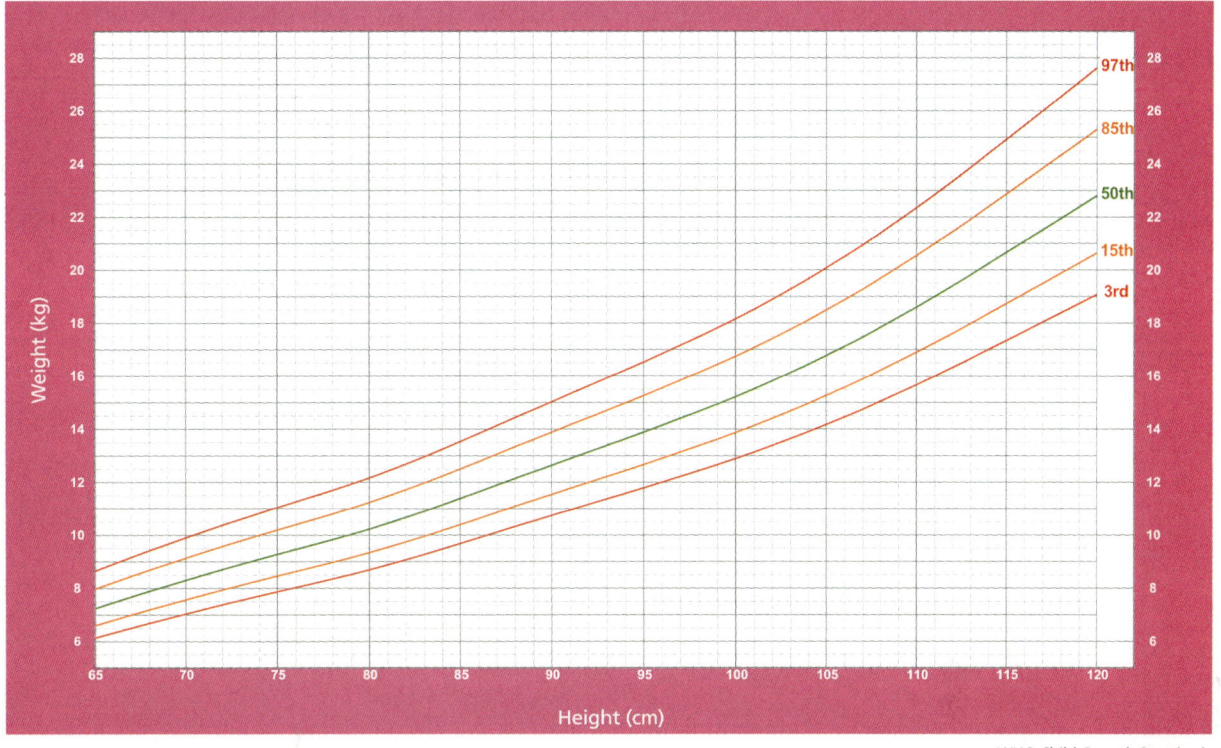

WHO Child Growth Standards

Fig. 1.14c WHO growth chart for weight-for- height for girls 2–5 years of age (percentiles)

Weight-for-height GIRLS

2 to 5 years (z-scores)

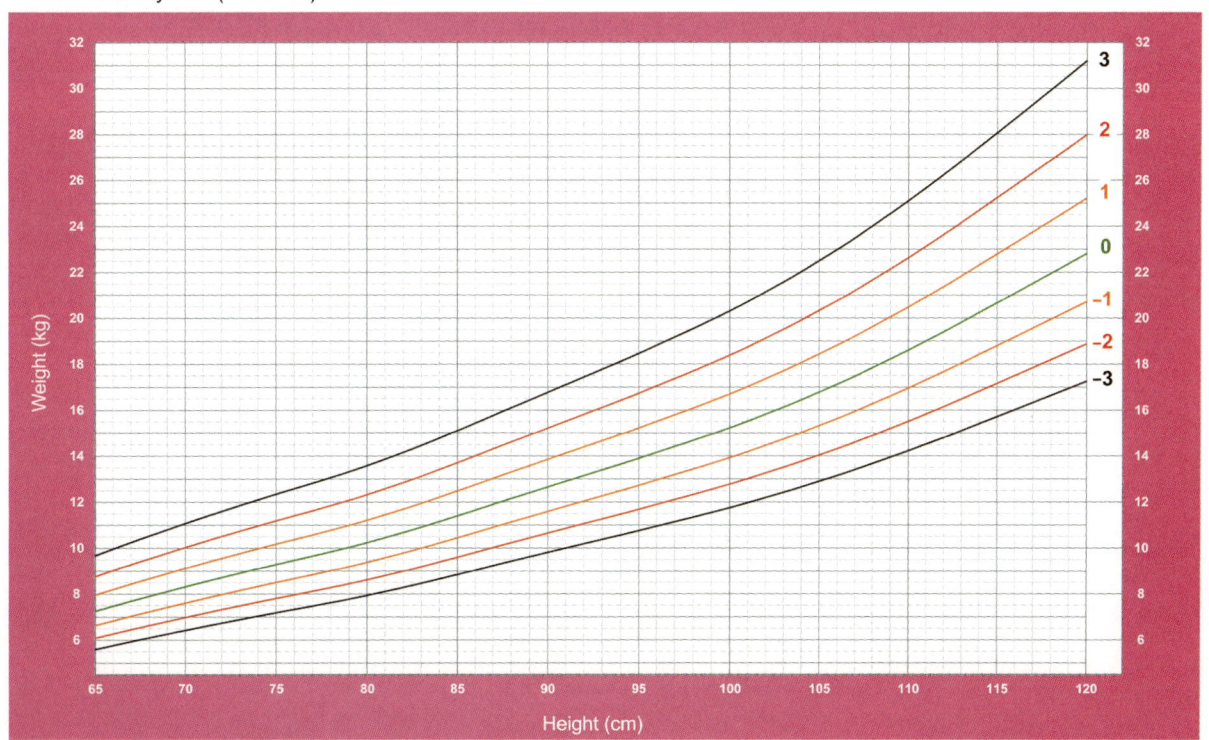

WHO Child Growth Standards

Fig. 1.14d WHO growth chart for weight-for-height for girls 2–5 years of age (Z-scores)

5 to 18 Years: IAP Boys Height and Weight Charts

Father's Height_____, Mother's Height_____, Target Height_____

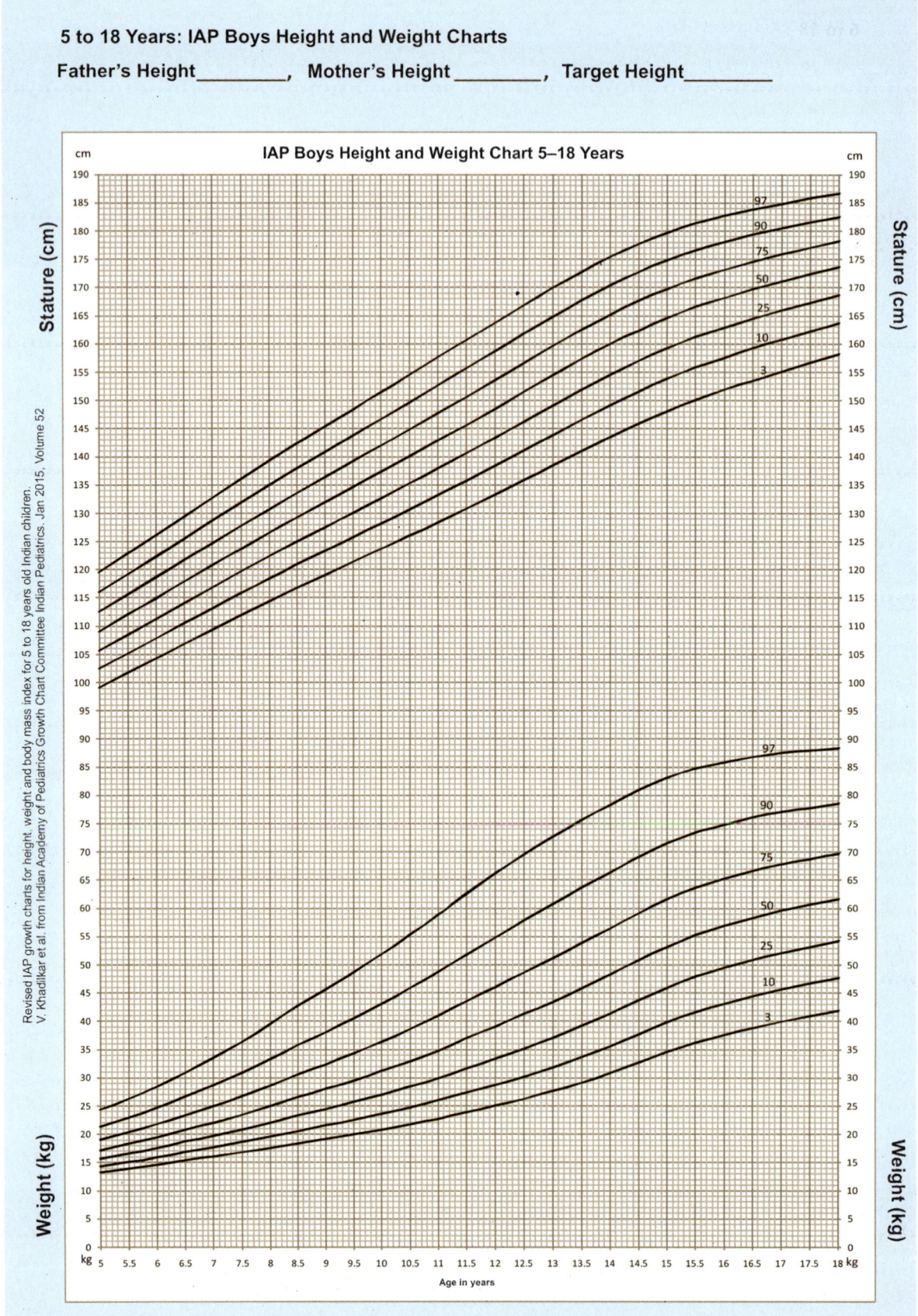

Revised IAP growth charts for height, weight and body mass index for 5 to 18 years old Indian children.
V. Khadilkar et al. from Indian Academy of Pediatrics Growth Chart Committee Indian Pediatrics, Jan 2015, Volume 52

Fig. 1.15 Indian Academy of Pediatrics (IAP) Growth Charts for height-for-age, and weight-for-age of boys (5–18 years)

5 to 18 Years: IAP Girls Height and Weight Charts

Father's Height_____ , Mother's Height_____ , Target Height_____

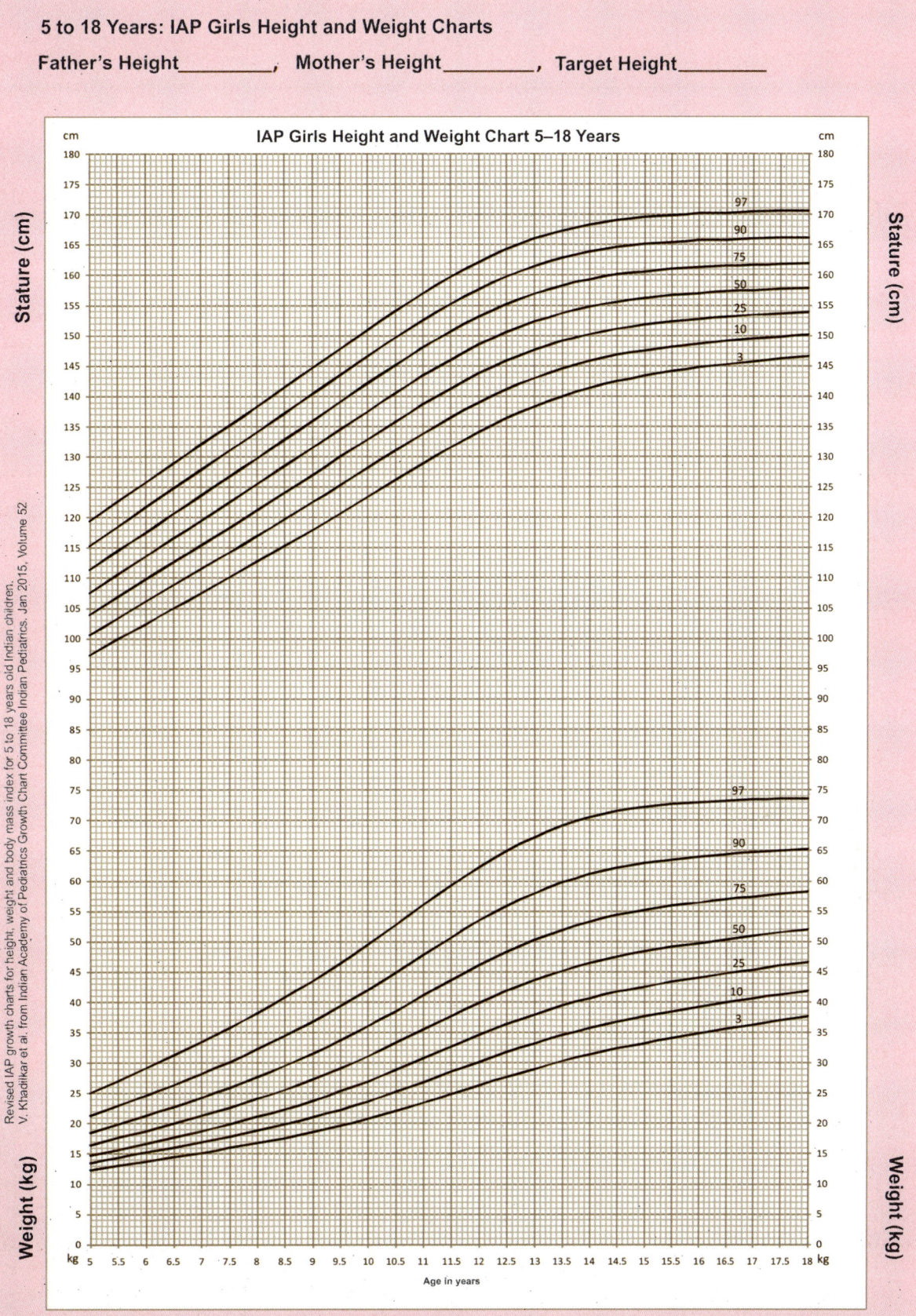

Fig. 1.16 Indian Academy of Pediatrics (IAP) Growth Charts for height-for-age and weight-for-age of girls (5–18 years)

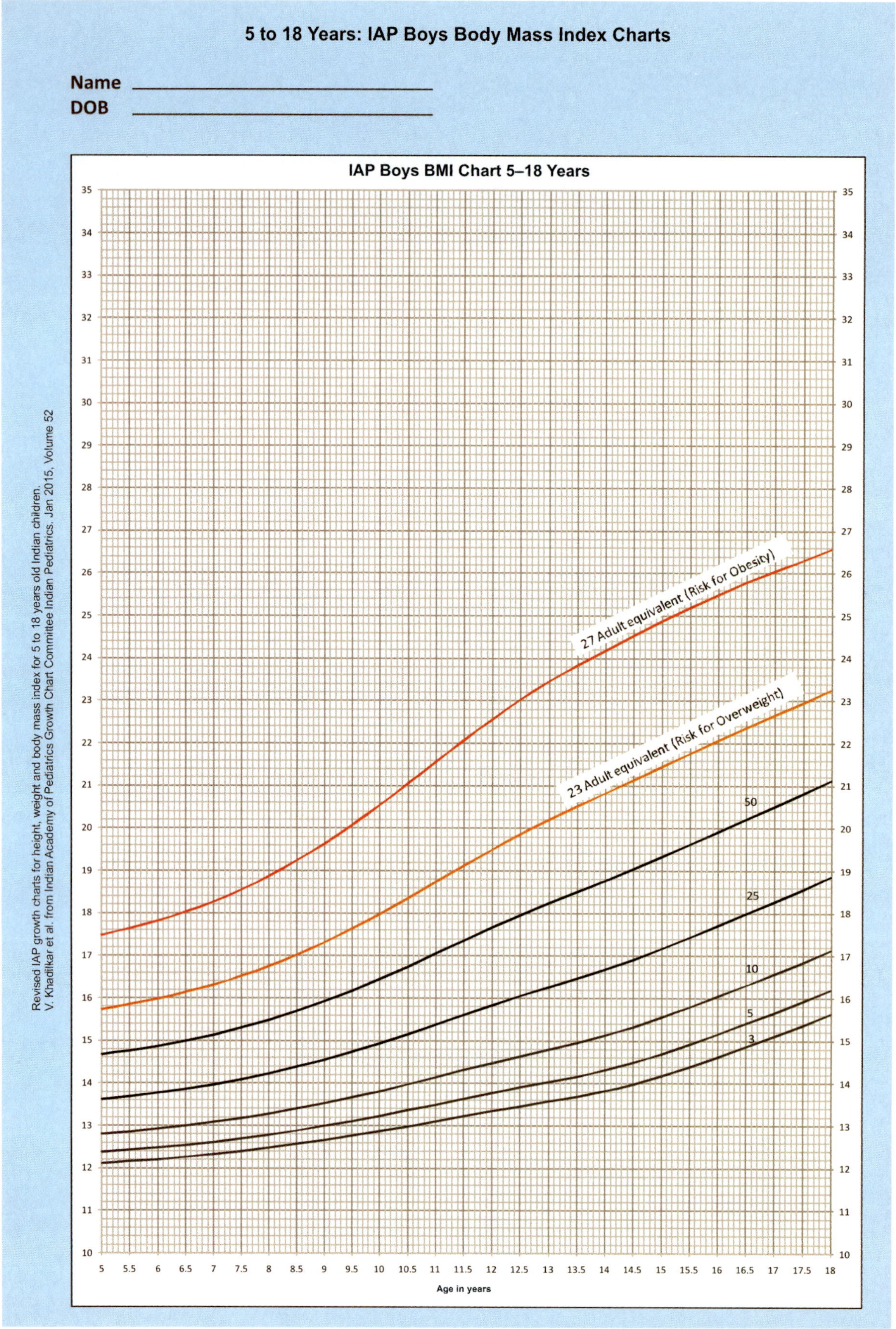

5 to 18 Years: IAP Boys Body Mass Index Charts

Name _____

DOB _____

Fig. 1.17 Indian Academy of Pediatrics (IAP) Growth Charts for body mass index (BMI) of boys (5–18 years)

5 to 18 Years: IAP Girls Body Mass Index Charts

Name _____

DOB _____

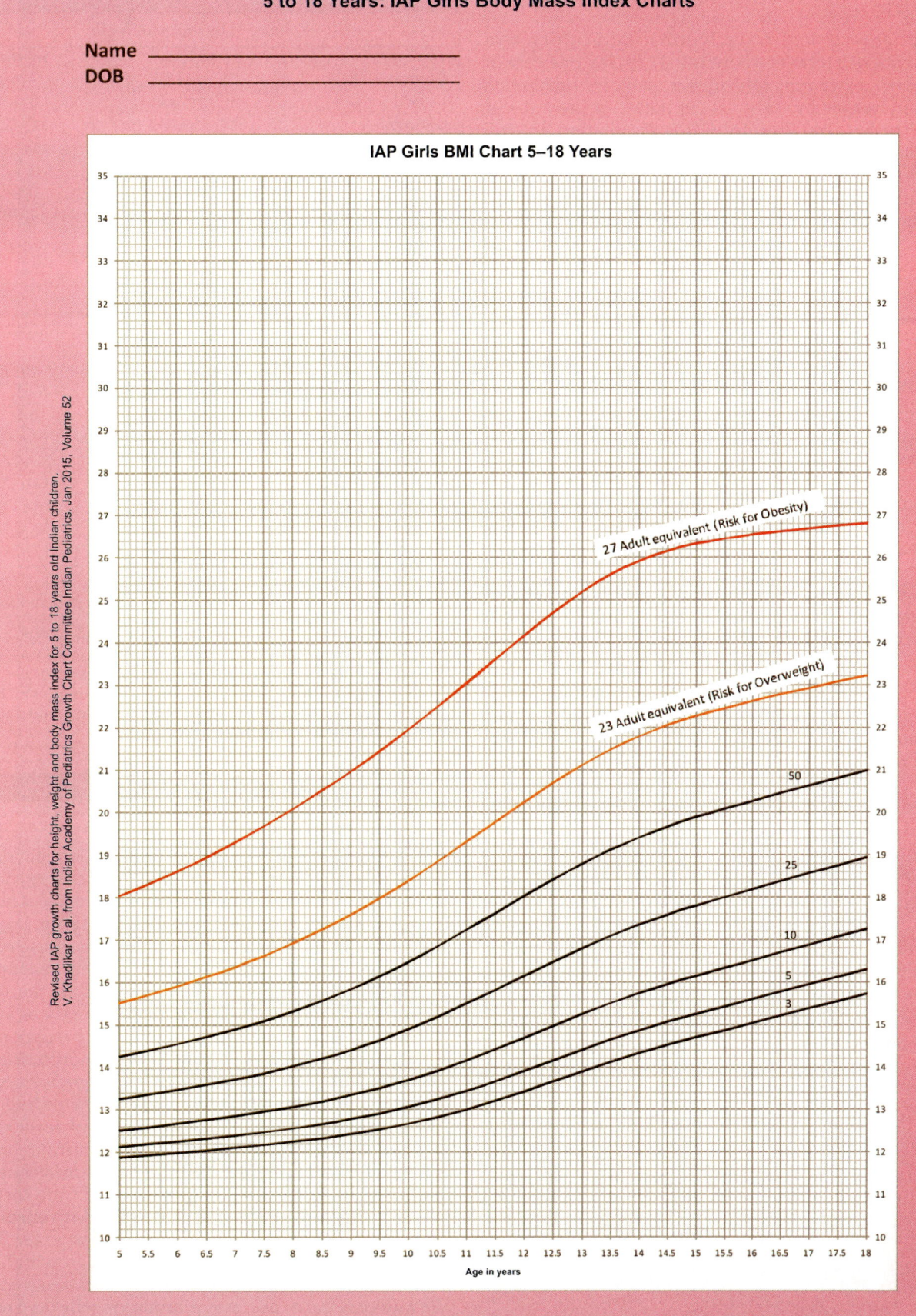

Fig. 1.18 Indian Academy of Pediatrics (IAP) Growth Charts for body mass index (BMI) of girls (5–18 years).

year from 2–5 years of age. At 12 years of age, the average head size is 52 cm.

Mid-upper arm circumference Normal mid-upper arm circumference of a term newborn is 9–11 cm. By one year of age, it grows to 16 cm. Mid-upper arm circumference (MUAC) increases by only 1.0 cm between the ages of 6 months to 5 years, therefore, it is also called an *age-independent criterion* between these ages. A child between 6 months and 5 years is termed undernourished, if the mid-arm circumference is less than 12.5 cm. Severe acute malnutrition is characterized by mid-arm circumference less than 11.5 cm (between 6 months and 5 years of age).

Velocity of growth in terms of both height and weight is most rapid during the first year of life and then falls rapidly. Weight velocity is 6 kg in the first year of life, and 2 kg/year in the preschool child, and 3 kg/year till puberty. Height velocity is 25 cm in the first year of life, 12 cm in the second year, followed by around 5–6 cm per year till puberty.

Body proportion The ratio of upper segment (crown to pubic symphysis) and the lower segment (pubic symphysis to heel) is 1.7 at birth. Thus, sitting height represents 65–70% of total length in the newborn infant. After birth, limbs grow much faster than the trunk resulting in reduction of sitting height percentage. The ratio is 1.3 at 3 years of age. The upper segment equalizes the lower segment by 8 to 10 years of age (ratio 1:1).

Arm span is less than the stature by 1–2 cm by 10 years of age. Thereafter arm span exceeds the height but the difference always stays less than 3–5 cm.

4. Eruption of Teeth

The deciduous teeth start erupting at 6 months of age and the permanent teeth at about 6 years of age. All the deciduous teeth are replaced by the permanent teeth by the age of 12 years. A child between the age of 6 and 12 years has a mixed dentition. Ages of eruption for various human teeth are provided in **Table 1.1**.

Primary dentition The lower central incisors appear between the ages of 5 and 8 months. The upper central incisors appear a month later and the lateral incisors usually within the next 3 months. The first molar teeth appear around the age of 12 to 15 months, preceding the eruption of canine teeth by 6 months, which appear between the age of 18 and 21 months. The second molars are out at the age of 21 to 24 months.

Permanent teeth erupt in the following order. 1st molar—6 years; central and lateral incisors—6 to 8 years; canines and premolars—9 to 12 years; second molars—12 years; third molars—18 years or later (Fig. 1.19)

Christoforidis A, Maniadaki I, Stanhope R. Growth hormone/insulin-like growth factor-1 axis during puberty. *Pediatr Endocrinol Rev*. 2005;3:5–10.

de Onis M, Garza C, Onyango AW, Borghi E. Comparison of the WHO child growth standards and the CDC 2000 growth charts. *J Nutr*. 2007;137:144–8.

Dunger DB, Ahmed ML, Ong KK. Effects of obesity on growth and puberty. *Best Pract Res Clin Endocrinol Metab*. 2005;19:375–90.

Fernández MA, Delchevalerie P, Van Herp M. Accuracy of MUAC in the detection of severe wasting with the new WHO growth standards. *Pediatrics*. 2010;126:e195–201.

Gupta P. *Clinical Methods in Pediatrics*. 4th edition. New Delhi: CBS Publishers;2017.

Table 1.1 Eruption of Primary and Secondary Teeth

Primary (Deciduous) Teeth		
Maxillary	Eruption	Shedding
Central incisor	7½ months	7–8 years
Lateral incisor	9 months	8–9 years
Canine	18 months	11–12 years
First molar	14 months	10–11 years
Second molar	24 months	10–12 years
Mandibular		
Central incisor	6½ months	6–7 years
Lateral incisor	7 months	7–8 years
Canine	16 months	9–11 years
First molar	12 months	10–12 years
Second molar	20 months	11–13 years
Eruption of Permanent Teeth		
	Maxillary	Mandibular
Central incisor	7–8 years	6–7 years
Lateral incisor	8–9 years	7–8 years
Canine	11–12 years	9–10 years
First premolar	10–11 years	10–12 years
Second premolar	10–12 years	11–12 years
First molar	6–7 years	6–7 years
Second molar	12–13 years	11–13 years
Third molar	17–21 years	17–21 years

Rogol AD, Roemmich JN, Clark PA. Growth at puberty. *J Adolesc Health*. 2002;31:192–200.

WHO Multicentre Growth Reference Study Group. Relationship between physical growth and motor development in the WHO Child Growth Standards. *Acta Paediatr Suppl*. 2006;450:96–101.

WHO Multicentre Growth Reference Study Group. WHO Child Growth Standards based on length/height, weight and age. *Acta Paediatr Suppl*. 2006;450:76–85.

1.9 NORMAL DEVELOPMENT

1. Laws of Development

1. *Development implies maturation of function*, interaction with environment, communication, and independence in day-to-day activity. For example, at birth, a neonate is not able to roll over, sit, approach objects voluntarily, laugh, or interact with the help of language. In due course of time, chronologically the infant acquires all these functions.

2. *Normal development requires an anatomical and functionally normal central nervous system*, peripheral nervous system, musculoskeletal system, hearing and vision, supported by suitable environment. A child with a morphologically abnormal CNS (eg, anencephaly, meningomyelocele) or damaged neurons and pathways (eg, following hypoxic or ischemic insult) is unlikely to have a normal development.

3. *Abnormal development may result from intrauterine and perinatal insults* (perinatal asphyxia, kernicterus, etc., resulting in delayed development right from birth), or disease affecting neuronal pathways and myelination in later life (trauma, meningitis, CNS hemorrhage, etc. during first 6 years of life, while the brain is still growing).

4. *Primitive reflexes are lost before voluntary functions are acquired.* Primitive reflexes are group of motor reflexes found in neonates and infants; these are protective brainstem reflexes, which develop sequentially during late fetal life.

Permanent tooth eruption chart

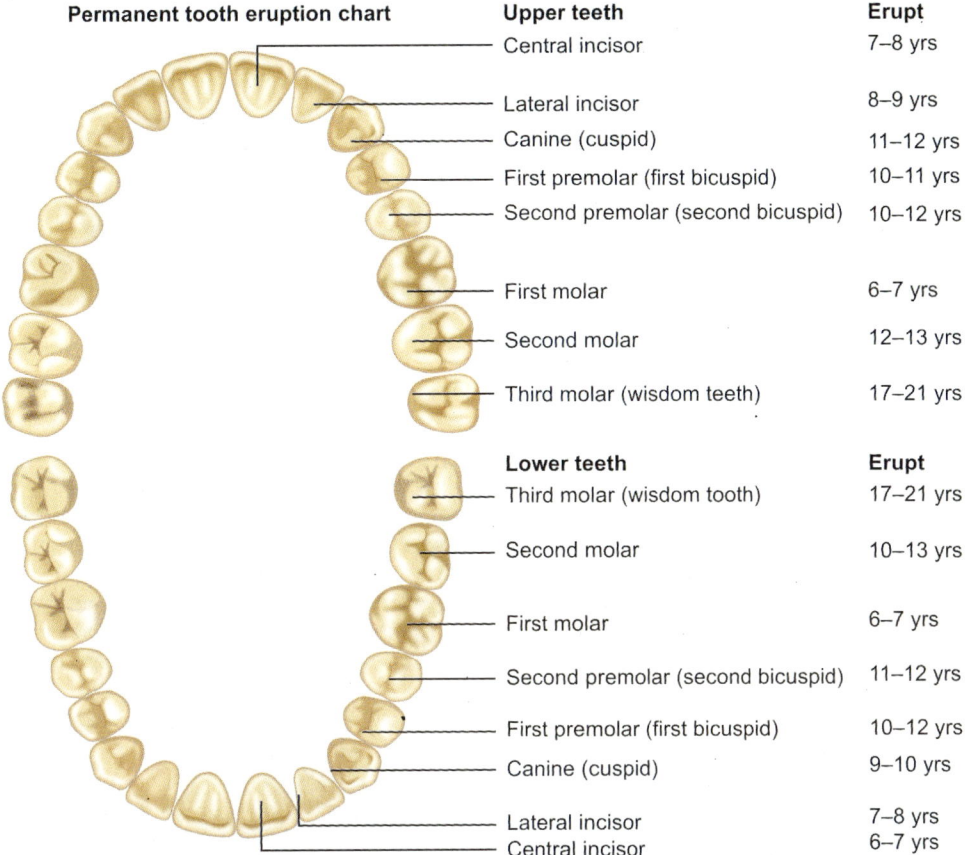

Upper teeth	Erupt
Central incisor	7–8 yrs
Lateral incisor	8–9 yrs
Canine (cuspid)	11–12 yrs
First premolar (first bicuspid)	10–11 yrs
Second premolar (second bicuspid)	10–12 yrs
First molar	6–7 yrs
Second molar	12–13 yrs
Third molar (wisdom teeth)	17–21 yrs

Lower teeth	Erupt
Third molar (wisdom tooth)	17–21 yrs
Second molar	10–13 yrs
First molar	6–7 yrs
Second premolar (second bicuspid)	11–12 yrs
First premolar (first bicuspid)	10–12 yrs
Canine (cuspid)	9–10 yrs
Lateral incisor	7–8 yrs
Central incisor	6–7 yrs

Fig. 1.19 Timing of permanent tooth eruption. Adapted from: Eruption charts (tooth eruption charts). American Dental Assosiation. Accessed From: http://www.ada.org/sections/public Resources/pdfs/chart_eruption_perm.pdf

These reflexes are essential for survival, feeding and movement while neonatal CNS is immature. For example, the Grasp reflex should be lost (by 3–4 months) before the infant can learn to reach for objects and to grasp them voluntarily (by 4–5 months). Similarly, asymmetric tonic neck reflex should be lost before a child learns to turn over in bed (think, why?).

Persistence of a primitive reflex, beyond the age at which it should have disappeared, indicates and predicts abnormal development. For example, Moro reflex should disappear by 4–6 months of age. A 6-month-old child with a positive Moro reflex is suggestive of abnormal development.

5. *Development always proceeds in a cephalocaudal manner*; ie, from head to toe. Thus, a child will learn to hold his head, followed by ability to sit and then be able to walk. This sequence will always remain the same though the age at which each function is achieved may differ within physiological range.

6. *Developmental delay* (delayed achievement of certain milestones) *should be differentiated from developmental regression* or neuroregression (loss of already acquired milestones).

2. Domains of Development

Developmental milestones in first five years of life are categorized in 5 different domains for assessment and screening purpose:

1. *Motor development Gross motor*: Pertaining to development of locomotion, general body control and specific motor skills; *Fine motor*: Pertaining to development of finer limb movements and coordination, *ie,* grasping, fine hand movements, hand-eye co-ordination.

2. *Adaptive/activity of daily living* Development of skills needed by the child to adapt to initiate new experiences and to profit by past experiences. This adaptivity includes alertness, intelligence and various forms of constructiveness and exploration. This subset majorly decides for self-help activities transforming into independent living in society in later life.

3. *Cognition/problem solving* This includes imitation, simple problem solving, puzzles, drawings that eventually transform into reading, writing, and academic skills.

4. *Personal-social development* Child's personal reaction to other persons and his adjustment to domestic life, social groups, and community conventions. This includes social behavior, feeding, sphincter control, general under-standing, play activity, and dressing.

5. *Language and speech* Development of ability to communicate; including comprehension (receptive language) as well as expression of language (expressive language includes gestures, speech, written language).

3. Developmental Milestones

Children accomplish maturation of different biological functions (level of development or milestone) at an anticipated age, with a margin of a few months on either side.

Motor Milestones

Gross motor development It involves control of the child over his body and locomotion; ie, head control, sitting, standing, walking, jumping, etc. Motor development depends on the maturation of muscular, skeletal, and nervous systems (Figs 1.20 to 1.27). Ages of attainment of important gross motor milestones are provided in **Table 1.2**.

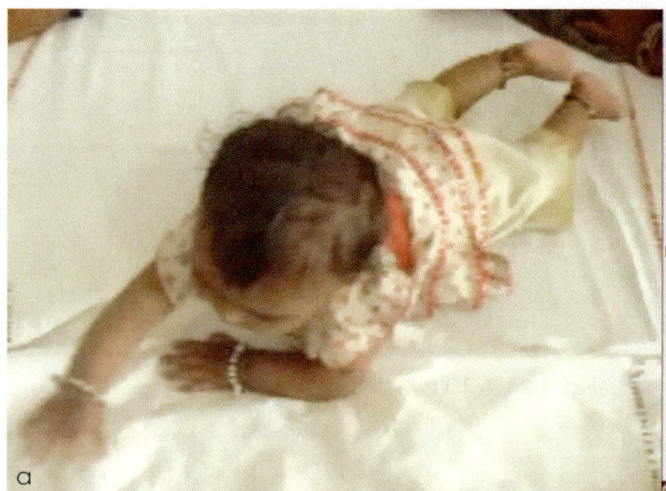

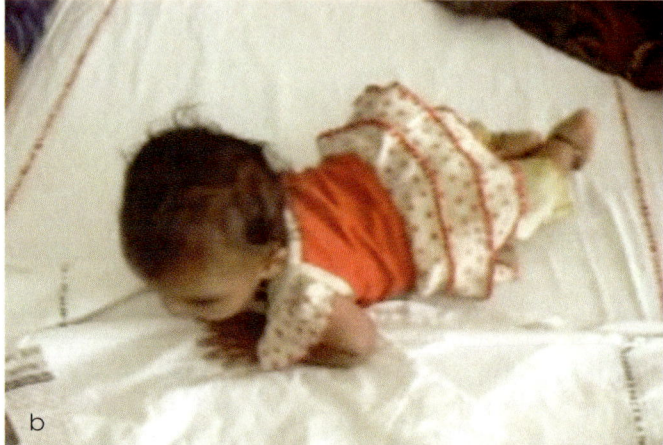

Fig. 1.22a and b An 8-month-old infant in commando crawl position moving forward to grab an object

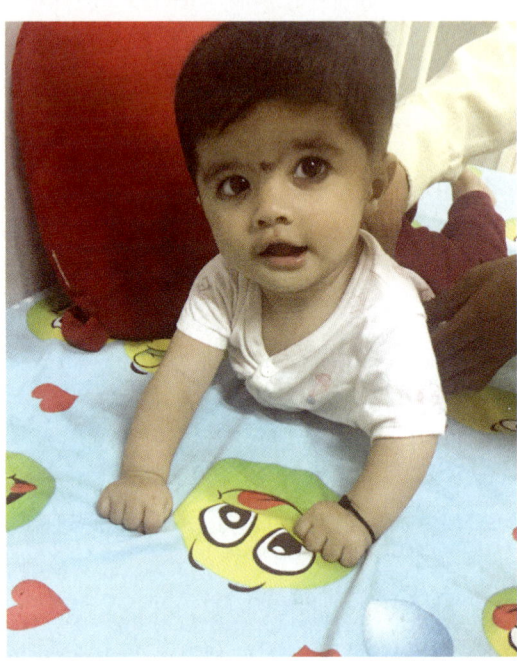

Fig. 1.20 A12-week-old infant. The child can lift the chin and shoulders bearing weight on forearms. Plane of face reaches 90° to couch, also can be noted here social smile and connect

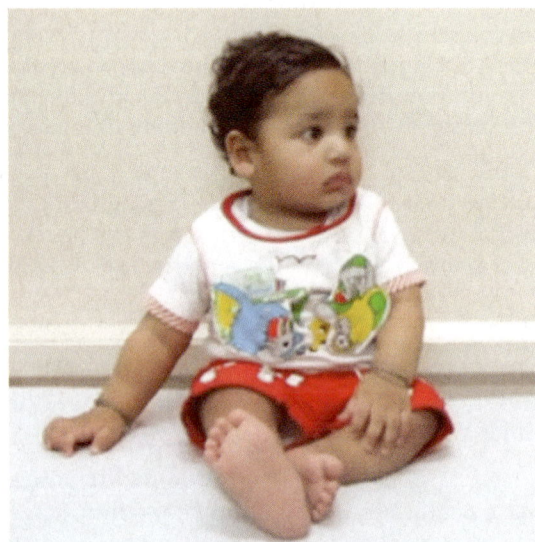

Fig. 1.21 A 6-month-old child sitting supported by hands in front or side

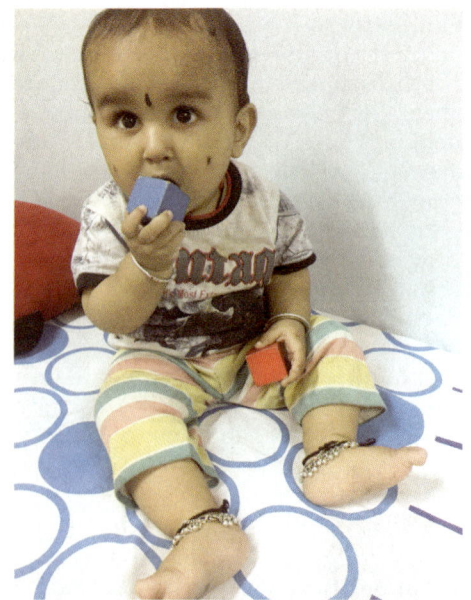

Fig. 1.23 A 9-month-old infant with stable independent sitting, mouthing from right hand and radiodigital grasp on left hand

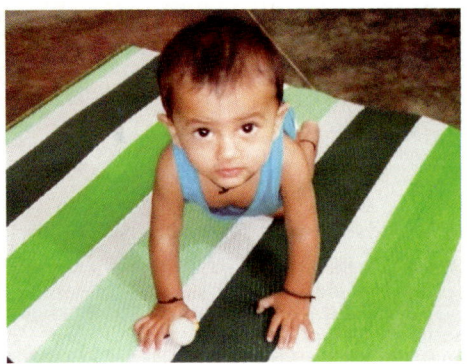

Fig. 1.24 A 10-month-old-child creeping on four

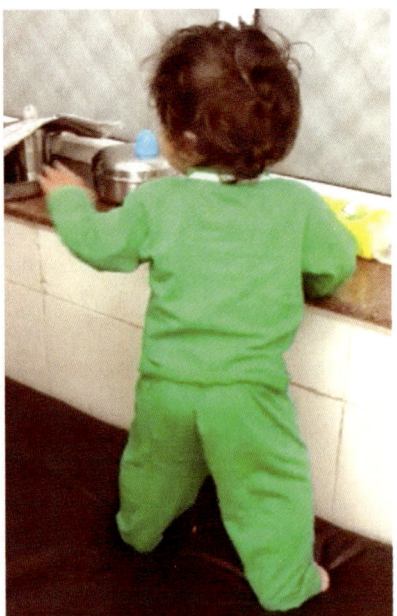

Fig. 1.25 An 11-month-old-child walking with support (cruising) able to free hands intermittently

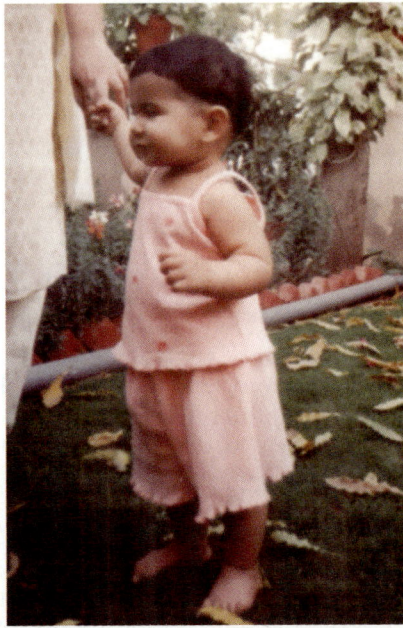

Fig. 1.26 A 12-month-old child walking with one hand held

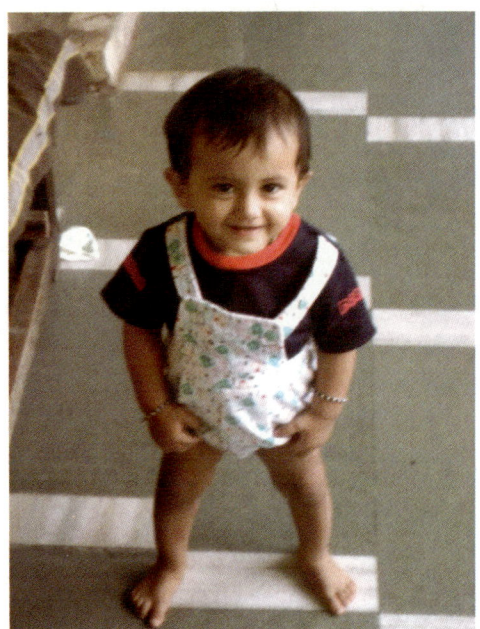

Fig. 1.27 A 13-month-old child walking independently

Table 1.2 Gross Motor Milestones: Age of Achievement	
1 month	Lifts up chin momentarily in prone position
1–3 months	Lifts and controls head in the horizontal plane and then above the horizontal plane when held in ventral suspension
3 months	Neck holding, infant lifts his head and upper part of chest on forearms in prone position
5 months	Sitting with support, head control is complete
6 months	Rolling over prone to supine, sits with support
7 months	Rolling over supine to prone
8 months	Commando crawling, sits without support
9 months	Pulls to stand, begins creeping (on four)
10 months	Walking with support, creeps well
11 months	Pivots, cruises
12 months	Walks with one hand-held, stands well
13 months	Walking without support
18 months	Runs stiffly, walks backwards
2 years	Climbing upstairs (2 feet per step)
30 months	Jumps on both feet
3 years	Climbing upstairs (1 foot per step), riding tricycle
4 years	Comes downstairs (1 foot per step), hops on one foot
5 years	Skips with both feet

Fine motor development It assesses the finer body movements and coordination. This includes coordination of eyes, hand-eye coordination, hand-mouth coordination, and skills for manipulation with hands; ie, grasping, fine hand movements (Figs 1.28 to 1.30), making a tower, writing, etc. Ages of attainment of important fine motor milestones are provided in **Table 1.3.**

Adaptive/Cognitive Milestones

Adaptive/cognitive development is the ability to learn or deal with new situations. In initial few weeks of life, infant

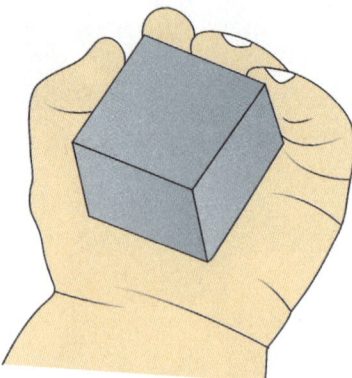

Fig. 1.28 6 months: Approaches cube with fingers and holds with palm

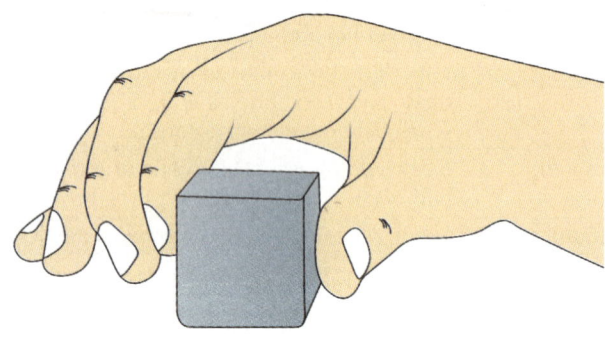

Fig. 1.29 9 months: Holds cube steady with index finger and thumb

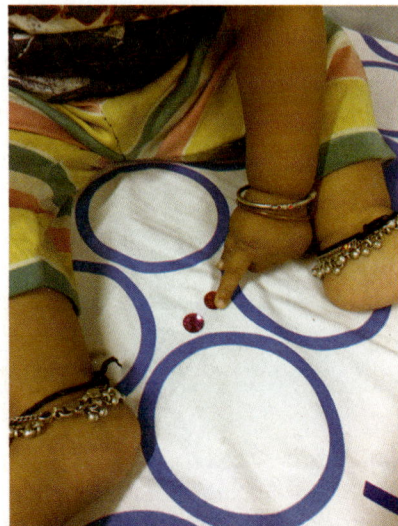

Fig. 1.30 A 9-month-old child developing pincer grasp, raking the object with index finger

Table 1.3 Fine Motor Milestones: Age of Achievement	
3 months	Opens hand spontaneously, holds objects when given in hand, inspects fingers (hand regard)
4 months	Tries to reach for objects (red ring), overshoots
5 months	Reaches (bidextrous approach) for a red cube held within reach; holds it with both hands
6 months	Unidextrous approach, transfers objects from one hand to another hand
7 months	Radial palmar grasp
8 months	Finger-thumb scissors grasp
9–10 months	Pincer grasp (holding between index finger and thumb), voluntary release (mature)
10–11 months	Mature pincer grasp (can pick a pellet neatly, using ends of his thumb and index fingers.
1 year	Tower of 2 cubes, casting, imitates scribbling
13 months	Can turn two or three pages of a book at a time
15 months	Tower of 3 cubes
18 months	Tower of 4 cubes, imitates vertical line
2 years	Tower of 6 cubes, imitates a horizontal line, imitates train, no chimney
2½ years	Tower of 8 cubes, imitates train, adds chimney
3 years	Tower of 9–10 cubes, copies a circle, imitates bridge
4 years	Copies a cross (plus sign), imitates gate
5 years	Copies multiplication sign, triangle, gate

explores the environment visually. Initially, he follows faces and then objects. After gaining better control of arms and hands, he starts batting at and then reaching for objects. At first, objects are brought to the mouth for oral exploration. Later, the infant visually examines an object held in one hand while manipulating it with the other.

With maturation of vision, infant can focus on small objects by about 5 months of age. By 1 year, the child explores objects by poking and discovering how they work. The child learns to shift attention between two objects, learns how his actions produce certain effects, and how to repeat these actions to get the same effects and later how to vary the action to produce a novel effect. These skills need combined efforts of motor skills, normal vision, hearing, coordination, and cognitive skills. Ages of attainment of important adaptive/cognitive milestones are provided in **Table 1.4.**

Personal Social Milestones

Personal social development is a very broad area that includes intellectual, moral, emotional, social, and spiritual development. Ages of attainment of important personal social milestones are provided in **Table 1.5.**

Language Milestones

Receptive language is ability to understand what is being said. *Expressive language* refers to the ability to make thoughts, ideas known to others through speech, gestures, and facial expressions. Ages of attainment of important language milestones are provided in **Table 1.6.**

Table 1.4 Adaptive/Cognitive Milestones: Age of Achievement	
4 weeks	Follows red ring by 45°
6 weeks	Follows up to 90°
8 weeks	Follows moving person
3 months	Hand regard, follows to 180°
4 months	Excited on seeing food, toys; shows pleasure by massive response
5 months	Mouthing, no hand regards
6 months	Looks for dropped toy
7 months	Observes cubes in each hand, finds partially hidden objects
8 months	Reaches for out of reach toys
10 months	Responds to 'No'
11 months	Looks at picture in book, finds toys under the cup
1 year	Mouthing and drooping stops, puts objects in and out of container
15 months	Turns 2–3 pages at a time
18 months	Turns 1 page at a time, names one common object
2 years	Points at 4–6 body parts, sorts objects
30 months	Names 1 color, matches shape/colors
3 years	Names 2 color, knows gender and age
4 years	Names 5–6 colors, right-left discrimination
5 years	Counts till 10, names 10 colors, identifies coins

Table 1.5 Personal Social Milestones: Age of Achievement	
2 months	Social smile (Fig. 1.31)
3 months	Recognizing mother
5–6 months	Smiles at mirror image
6–7 months	Enjoys peak-a-boo
8–9 months	Stranger anxiety
10 months	Waves 'bye-bye'
1 year	Helps in dressing, plays a simple ball game
18 months	Engages in domestic mimicry
2 years	Dry by day
30 months	Washes hands, brushes teeth
3 years	Dry at night, can withhold bowel movement, dresses, undresses fully if helped with buttons
4 years	Goes to toilet alone
5 years	Dressing and bathing independently

Table 1.7 provides a bird's eye view of achievement of various milestones at key ages.

4. Variations in Normal Development

There is no set age at which all children must acquire a particular milestone. One particular aspect, eg, motor development or speech, may be delayed in the child without being abnormal or retarded. Due to wide variability in the ages of attainment of different milestones, it may be difficult to draw a strict line between normal and abnormal on single assessment.

Table 1.6 Language Milestones: Age of Achievement	
1 month	Turns head to sound
3 months	Cooing
4 months	Laughs aloud, says Ah-goo
6–7 months	Speaks monosyllables (ma, ba)
8–9 months	Speaks bisyllables (mama, baba)
1 year	Speaks 2–3 words with meaning
18 months	Speaks 10 words with meaning
2 years	Can form simple sentence using 2 words
3 years	3 words sentence, 250 words vocabulary
4 years	4 words sentence, tells stories
5 years	5–8 words sentence, knows telephone number

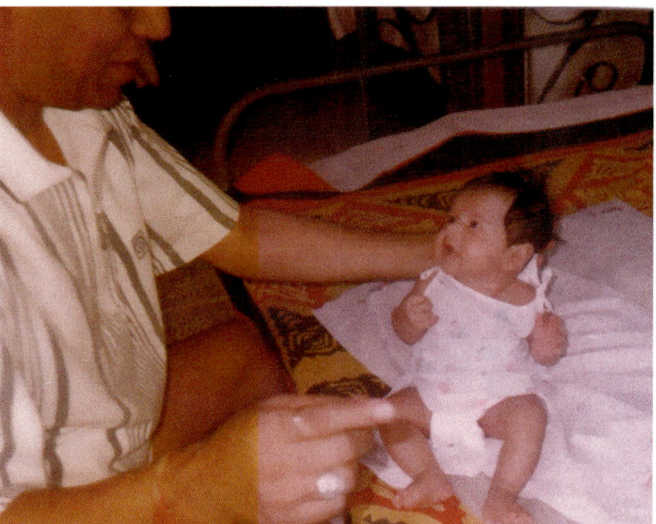

Fig. 1.31 A 6-week-old with eye contact and social smile

Children who are at borderline may ultimately turn out to be abnormal or just a variant of the normal. For correct diagnosis, one should follow these children regularly with a screening test as described in the next section.

Children who are ideal in all fields are not that common. Some are slow starters in a field and then catch up after a time-lag. Some children start well but may have a temporary cessation in development due to illness, protein energy malnutrition or other factors. Some may deteriorate after a point accounting to neurological or developmental regression. A few children with gross development delay may show unexpected improvement when placed in appropriate environment. On the other hand, there are mentally superior children whose responses are much more complex and difficult to assess.

1.10 DEVELOPMENTAL DELAY

Developmental disabilities are a group of related chronic disorders of early onset estimated to affect 5 to 10% of children. These are responsible for subsequent intellectual disability and handicaps prevalent in society.

Developmental delay It refers to a significant delay in the acquisition of milestones or skills. It is defined as

Table 1.7 A Guide to Developmental Assessment of the Child					
Age	*Gross motor*	*Fine motor/vision*	*Adaptive/congnitive*	*Language/hearing*	*Personal/social*
6 weeks	Body straight on ventral suspension	Turns to light	Follows red ring up to 90°	Startles to loud sound	Social smile
3 months	Neck holding	Tries to reach for objects, overshoots	Follows up to 180°, hand regard	Vocalization, cooing	Recognizing mother
6 months	Rolls prone to supine, sits with support	Unidextrous approach, transfers objects from hand to hand	Looks for dropped toy	Monosyllables (ma)	Smiles/vocalizes at mirror image (5–6 mo peek-a-boo (6–7 mo)
9 months	Sits unsupported (8 mo) standing with support	Assisted pincer grasp	Responds to "no" (10 mo)	Bisyllables (ma-ma)	Stranger anxiety (8–9 mo)
12 months	Walks with one hand held	2 cubes tower	Puts objects in/out of container	Speaks 2–3 words with meaning	Plays simple ball game, helps in dressing
15 months	Walks alone (13 mo)	3 cubes tower	Turns 2–3 pages at a time	Speaks 3–5 words	Indicates desire by pointing at objects
18 months	Running, walks backwards	4 cubes tower, imitates | (vertical line)	Turns 1 page at a time, names 1 object	Speaks 10–15 words	Symbolic play alone, feeds independently
2 years	Climbs upstairs (2 feet per step)	6–7 cubes tower, imitates —— (horizontal line)	Points at 4–6 body parts	2 words sentence, use 50+ words	Dry by day, parallel play
3 years	Climbs upstairs (1 foot per step), walks downstairs (2 feet per step), rides tricycle	10 cubes tower, copies ◯ (circle)	Names 2 colors, knows gender/age	3 words sentence, 250+ words vocabulary	Dry by night
4 years	Walks downstairs, (1 foot per step), hops on one foot	Copies bridge and + (plus sign)	Names 5–6 colors, discriminates right-left	4 words sentence, 250+ words vocabulary	Goes to toilet alone, plays up to with 3 other kids
5 years	Skips with both feet	Copies gate, ×, △ (cross and triangle)	Names 10 colors, identifies coins	5–8 words sentence, grammatical speech	Independent dressing and bathing

performance two standard deviations or more below the mean on age-appropriate, standardized norm referenced testing (or more than 25% from the expected rate), in one or more of five domains of development (as discussed earlier in this chapter).

Developmental quotient (DQ) It is the numeric expression of a child's developmental level as measured by dividing the developmental age by the chronologic age and multiplying by 100. Ideally, chronological age should be equal to that of developmental age and the DQ should, therefore, be 100. A child having DQ below the 2/3 or 3/4 ratio (DQ between 65 and 75) is considered at risk of developmental delay. DQ should be estimated separately for each area of development viz., motor, adaptive/cognitive, language, and personal/social.

Global developmental delay is a subset of developmental disabilities defined as significant delay in two or more of the following developmental domains: Gross/fine motor, speech/language, cognition, social/personal, and activities of daily living. This term is reserved for children below 5 years of age. Intellectual disability is the term used for older children in whom formal IQ testing is possible.

Developmental dissociation Development in one area may not necessarily run parallel to that in the other spheres.

Developmental dissociation occurs when the rates of development differ widely in different developmental domains. For example, a child with autism is grossly delayed in language, personal social spheres but may have a normal gross motor development.

Developmental deviance There is non-sequential unevenness in the achievement of milestones within one or more streams of development. It is considered normal variant. For example: Some infants are bottom shufflers and never attain creeping, still walking will be achieved within physiological period.

Developmental regression It refers to loss of previously acquired skills or milestones, and should alert to a possibility of degenerative brain disorders.

1. Early Detection of Developmental Delay

A. Developmental Screening Tests

Developmental screening refers to administration of standard and validated tests that help in early identification of children *at risk* for a developmental disorder. It is desirable for a developmental screening tool to have a specificity and sensitivity of at least 70–80%. Children who fail a screening test need close follow-up and additional diagnostic assessment.

American Academy of Pediatrics (AAP) recommends routine developmental screening at 9, 18, and 24–30 months of age using PEDS (Parents' Evaluation of Developmental Status) or ASQ (Ages and Stages Questionnaire) screening tests. ASQ takes just 15 minutes to administer and has better sensitivity/specificity. ASQ can be used to screen children between 1 month and 5.5 years of age while PEDS can evaluate children up to 8 years of age.

Several Indian adaptations and versions for development screening tests are also available: These include the Phatak's Baroda Screening Test (for children up to 30 months) and Trivandrum Development Screening Chart (TDSC) (till 2 years of age). Both these tests have been developed from the Bayley scales of infant development. TDSC can be administered within 5 minutes.

Denver Development Screening Test (DDST) had been one of the most widely accepted screening test in clinical practice, since 1967. DDST is no more recommended as a developmental screening test because of its poor sensitivity and specificity.

B. Developmental Surveillance

Surveillance refers to the process of identification of potential risk factors for abnormal development. It goes hand in hand with developmental screening and is achieved by eliciting a good history, observing the child by a close follow-up, keeping a continuous record of these findings, and attending to parents' concerns. Close continuous contact with the parents is the key for good developmental surveillance. Developmental screening supported with culturally accepted tools is considered superior to developmental surveillance.

C. Definitive Tests for Diagnosis of Developmental Delay

Children suspected to be abnormal on a screening test should undergo definitive intelligence tests. Bayley's Scale of Infant Development (BSID-II) is the most commonly used intelligence scale for children 1 month to 3 years of age. The Indian counterpart of this test is known as DASI (Developmental Assessment Scale for Indian Children) and is the most widely applied tool for definitive diagnosis of developmental delay in Indian children. These tests are based on evaluation of gross motor, fine motor, language, behavior, and visual problem solving skills.

Wechsler Intelligence Scale is used to assess intelligence in children above 6 years. In India, MISIC (Malin's Intelligence Scale for Indian Children) is used for assessment in more than 5 years old; this test is an adaptation of WISC.

2. Approach to Developmental Delay

It is difficult to diagnose developmental delay in the early weeks of life. A correct diagnosis is mainly based on a detailed history. History of prenatal and perinatal risk factors is highly relevant to mental and physical development. Also obtain history of important genetic conditions, degenerative disorders, and environmental factors that may lead to delayed development. The history must include environmental factors (child abuse, parent child relations, etc.) that may influence development. Inquire about relevant illnesses like rickets, malnutrition, and systemic disorders. Causes of abnormal development are enumerated in **Table 1.8.**

Table 1.8 Common Causes of Abnormal Development
1. Organic
a. *Maternal factors*. Exposure to teratogens (alcohol, drugs, radiation, etc.) in pregnancy, infections such as cytomegalovirus, rubella, toxoplasma, HIV, placental dysfunction, toxemia, antepartum hemorrhage, etc.
b. *Fetal factors*. Chromosomal disorders (fragile X chromosome, Down syndrome), congenital CNS malformations, extreme prematurity, metabolic disorders (hypoglycemia, galactosemia, mucoplysaccharidosis, phenylketonuria), etc.
c. *Hypothyroidism* is the most important preventable cause of mental retardation.
d. *Natal factors*. Hypoxic-ischemic insult and birth injuries, intracranial hemorrhage
e. *Postnatal causes*. Meningitis, encephalitis, malnutrition, hypoxia, kernicterus, stroke, etc.
f. *CNS disorders*. Cerebral palsy, neurocutaneous syndromes (neurofibromatosis, tuberous sclerosis) and degenerative brain diseases.
2. Environmental
The poor intelligence may be inherited or be due to psychosocial deprivation, restrictive child rearing practices and nutritional deprivation. Children living in poverty are potentially susceptible to the cultural/environmental stress.

Assessment of chronology of development and age of achievement of milestones is the next step. Ask this history from the mother or caregiver. There may be a family history of early or late motor, sphincter, or language development. Be careful to ask the developmental history in simple language and in a precise manner. When inquiring about developing a new skill, ask: (*i*) when did it develop; (*ii*) how often it is practiced; and (*iii*) what is the degree of maturity with which this skill is performed.

Additionally, the child should be subjected to complete developmental examination which is beyond the scope of this text. Interested readers may refer to *Clinical Methods in Pediatrics* by Piyush Gupta.

A. Early Diagnosis of Global Developmental Delay and Intellectual Disability

A severely disabled child exhibits global developmental delay from the very beginning and may exhibit one or more of the following features:

- Sleeps excessively, is lethargic, and has feeding difficulties.
- Does not take notice of surroundings, and social smile is delayed.
- Constantly keeps watching his hands even after 20 weeks of life (persistent hand regard).
- Mouths all objects even beyond one year of life.
- Speech is delayed.
- May have abnormal physical findings suggestive of a recognizable syndrome.
- Has delayed motor development as seen in ventral suspension, supine, or prone position.

The degree of intellectual disability (mild, moderate, or severe) affects the age of diagnosis. Infants with *severe disability* are markedly delayed with their psychomotor skills in the first year of life. Those with *moderate delay* have delayed speech and languages abilities though they may be having normal motor development. It is unusual to diagnose speech impairment, hyperactivity, or emotional disorders before the age of 3 or 4 years. *Mild intellectual and learning disabilities* can be only detected at or after school entry point. If one can diagnose developmental delay early, the intervention can reduce long-term sequelae or handicap.

B. Early Diagnosis of Cerebral Palsy

The age at which the diagnosis can be made differs according to the type of cerebral palsy. Spastic cerebral palsy can be diagnosed in the neonatal period. Ataxic and athetoid forms may not be diagnosed till 6 months to 2 years of age.

- *Spastic cerebral palsy* can be diagnosed early as the sufferers lie immobile with limbs unduly extended and clenched fists. They may have microcephaly. When held by the axilla, lower limbs are held in scissoring or abnormal extension. Tendon reflexes are exaggerated. There is hypertonia and history of seizures or a neurological insult.
- A history of hyperbilirubinemia, hypotonia, abnormal movements, etc. suggests *athetoid or dyskinetic cerebral palsy* secondary to bilirubin encephalopathy.
- The child lies totally limp with hypotonia and exaggerated reflexes in cases of *hypotonic cerebral palsy*. This is usually a transient phase in a child with evolving dyskinetic or spastic cerebral palsy. Hence this term is no longer used in recent text.

In all forms of cerebral palsy, there is delay in achieving motor milestones.

3. Visual, Speech, and Hearing Handicaps

Sensory handicaps include visual, speech, and hearing defects. They may be isolated or associated with mental or physical handicaps.

Visual Disabilities

The severity of visual handicaps varies from complete blindness to not being able to see clearly. Some children are born blind while others become blind during early or late childhood.

How to Recognize a Child with Visual Handicap

- The infant may have a white or a gray pupil.
- If by 3 months the child does not look at mother's face or object or light and does not follow them, suspect a visual handicap.
- The child does not reach for an object held in front of him/ her unless it makes a sound.
- Child is slow to begin using hands, move about, and may bump into objects while moving around.
- The child has a squint.
- The child has difficulty in seeing after sunset (night blindness).
- In school, the child cannot read clearly from the blackboard or complains of headache while reading.

Management

- Early referral must be made to an eye specialist for ascertaining the cause and extent of visual handicap. With

help and encouragement from family and community, a blind child can be made to develop early skills related to activities of daily living like feeding, bathing, dressing, and caring for self.

- Early stimulation by touch, sound, and smell is important. The child should be informed about each activity and sound to orient to his environment.
- They can be taught to identify places and landmarks and walk with the help of a stick.
- They can be sent to special schools that teach blind children to read and write.

Speech and Hearing Handicaps

A child's inability to speak properly or a speech that is not easily understood or draws attention is a speech defect. The most common cause is hearing impairment. In this sub-section, we shall be discussing the two together.

Causes

Speech impairment may occur because of deafness, intellectual disability, cleft palate, or voice disorders. Hearing handicaps are secondary to birth asphyxia, hyper-bilirubinemia, maternal infections and drugs, encephalitis, meningitis, or chronic ear infections.

How to Recognize a Child with Hearing Disorder

- *0–6 months* When an infant does not startle in response to loud clap within 3 feet or does not turn towards the source of sound, suspect a hearing defect.
- *6 months–2 years* Suspect if the child does not respond to name, voice or a sound, does not understand phrases like 'no-no' or 'bye-bye'; does not initiate simple sounds and words; does not follow simple directions; child uses gestures for needs and desires rather than speaking.
- *2–5 years* Suspect speech handicap when the child cannot understand and use simple words like go, come, me, etc., cannot carry on a simple conversation and speech is difficult to understand.
- *Schoolgoing child* A hearing or speech disability should be suspected, if the child has trouble paying attention, does not answer when called, gets confused about directions or questions, appears slow and does not do well in school.

Management

- All high-risk neonates should be screened by OAE (otoacoustic emissions) and BERA (brainstem evoked response audiometry) for timely detection of hearing impairment.
- These children should be referred to speech and hearing clinic, ENT clinic or special institutions for the handicapped for initial work up and guidance for assessment of hearing loss.
- Treatment of local ear infections can improve temporary hearing loss.
- Hearing aids may be needed to improve the level of hearing which would help in speech therapy.
- Cochlear implant is preferred for sensorineural hearing loss in children and widely used for secondary prevention of hearing handicap.
- Communication can be improved by lip reading, gesture, sign language, pictures and drawing, or finger spelling.

4. Early Stimulation

Infants who show suspect or early signs of developmental delay need to be provided opportunities that promote body control, acquisition of motor skills, language development, and psychosocial maturity. These inputs, termed *early stimulation*, include measures such as making additional efforts to make the child sit and walk, giving toys to manipulate, playing with the child, showing objects, speaking to the child, and encouraging him to speak, and prompting the child to interact with others, so as to stimulate all sensory and motor faculties.

Drotar D, Stancin T, Dworkin PH, *et al*. Selecting developmental surveillance and screening tools. *Pediatr Rev.* 2008;29:e52–8.

Elbers J, Macnab A, McLeod E, Gagnon F. The Ages and Stages Questionnaires: feasibility of use as a screening tool for children in Canada. *Can J Rural Med.* 2008;13:9–14.

Glascoe FP, Robertshaw NS. New AAP policy on detecting and addressing developmental and behavioral problems. *J Pediatr Health Care.* 2007;21:407–12.

Glascoe FP. Screening for developmental and behavioral problems. *Ment Retard Dev Disabil Res Rev.* 2005;11:173–9.

Juneja M, Mohanty M, Jain R, Ramji S. Ages and Stages questionnaire as a screening tool for developmental delay in indian children. *Indian Pediatr.* 2012;49.

Mackrides PS, Ryherd SJ. Screening for developmental delay. *Am Fam Physician.* 2011;84:544–9.

Nair MK, George B, Philip E, *et al*. Trivandrum Developmental Screening Chart. *Indian Pediatr.* 1991;28:869–72.

Poon JK, LaRosa AC, Pai GS. Developmental delay timely identification and assessment. *Indian Pediatr.* 2010;47:415–22.

Shevell M, Ashwal S, Donley D, et al. Practice parameter: Evaluation of the child with global developmental delay. *Neurology* 2003;60:367–80.

1.11 PUBERTY

Puberty is the phase in which sexual characteristics develop and capability of reproduction is attained. Deviations from the normal pubertal pattern have significant diagnostic and therapeutic implications.

PHYSIOLOGY

Puberty involves development of primary (testicular and penile growth in boys; and breast and uterine growth in girls) and secondary sexual characteristics (pubic and axillary hair growth, acne, and axillary odor). Sex hormones (estrogen in girls and testosterone in boys) are responsible for primary sexual characteristics while adrenal androgens are involved in the development of secondary sexual characteristics. These processes are distinct and under separate endocrine control as evidenced by gonadarche being controlled by gonadotropin-releasing hormone (GnRH) and adrenarche by ACTH.

Pulsatile GnRH secretion is the triggering event for gonadarche. Initially, GnRH pulses occur only during nights. This results in increase in gonadotropin levels and thereby sex hormones. Kisspeptin, a hypothalamic peptide, is the key regulator of puberty. Acting as the "on-off switch" of puberty, kisspeptin initiates GnRH pulses. The hypothalamic-pituitary-gonadal axis is under feedback control of gonadal hormones. LH secretion is inhibited by sex hormones (testosterone and estrogen)

produced by the Leydig cells and theca cells. Inhibin produced by the Sertoli cells and granulosa cells inhibits production of FSH. The trigger for adrenarche is unclear but believed to be related to increased responsiveness of zona fasiculata to ACTH.

ASSESSMENT OF SEXUAL MATURITY

Sexual maturity should be assessed in all adolescents (10–19 years) and those approaching adolescence. Sexual growth is measured in terms of (*i*) growth in genitalia, (*ii*) pubic and axillary hair, and (*iii*) breast size and contour.

Sexual growth is graded in terms of SMR (sexual maturity rating) and given a rating of 1 to 5 as suggested by Tanner. The system suggested by Tanner includes assessment of genitalia and pubic hair for boys and genitalia and breast for females. Genital and pubic hair growth is treated separately for the male because of a considerable degree of dissociation between the two. SMR 1 indicates no sexual growth (prepubescent stage) while SMR 5 denotes complete maturation.

PATTERN OF PUBERTAL DEVELOPMENT

The pattern of pubertal development in girls is different from boys **(Table 1.9)**. Maximum growth occurs during early part of puberty in girls (Tanner stage 2 and 3) compared to boys where it occurs later (Tanner stage 3 and 4).

Girls Puberty starts at the age of 10 years (range 8–12 years) and is completed in 5 years. Enlargement of breast (*thelarche*) is the first sign of sexual maturation followed by the development of pubic hair (*pubarche*) and onset of menstrual cycles (*menarche*). Menarche usually occurs 2.5 years after thelarche—usually between SMR 3 and 4—just after achieving the peak height velocity. Thus, girls gain little in height (max 5 cm) after they have achieved menarche. Tanner staging for sexual maturity rating in girls is shown in **Table 1.10**.

Boys The first sign of sexual maturation in boys is the enlargement of testes at 11.5 years (range 9–14 years). This is followed by penile enlargement and pubarche. Spermarche occurs by the age of 14 years. The testicular enlargement is best assessed by palpation in comparison with a string of plastic models of testicular shape known as the **Prader orchidometer**. The testicular volume increases from less than 4 mL in the prepubertal stage to 20–25 mL at complete maturation. Tanner staging for sexual maturity rating in boys is shown in **Table 1.11**.

Table 1.9 Pattern of Pubertal Development in Boys and Girls		
Feature	*Girls*	*Boys*
Onset	10–12 years	12–14 year
First sign	Breast development	Testicular enlargement
Peak growth	Early (Tanner 2 and 3)	Late (Tanner 3 and 4)
Sexual maturity	Menarche 14 years	Spermarche 15 years

1

Table 1.10 Tanner Staging for Sexual Maturity Rating (SMR) in Girls

Tanner stage	Breast (B)	Pubic hair (P)	
Stage 1	Prepubertal—no breast tissue	Same as abdominal hair	
Stage 2	Breast bud appears, enlargement of areola	Sparse hair along labia, minimally pigmented	
Stage 3	Further enlargement of breast and areola but contour separation between the two	Darker and coarser hair on mons pubis	
Stage 4	A secondary mound is formed by areola and papilla above the level of the breast	Adult type, but limited to mons and labia	
Stage 5	Adult breast contour with projection of papilla alone	Adult type, spreads to medial thigh	

Table 1.11 Tanner Staging for Sexual Maturity Rating (SMR) in Boys

Tanner stage	Genitalia (G)	Testicular volume	Pubic hair (P)	
Stage 1	Prepubertal	<4 mL	Same as abdominal hair	
Stage 2	Early penile growth, thinning and reddening of scrotal skin	4–10 mL	Sparse growth at the base of penis	
Stage 3	Increase in penile length, scrotal thickening and darkening	10–15 mL	Darker, coarser, curled hair: spreads to mons pubis	
Stage 4	Increase in penile length and breadth, pigmentation of scrotum	15–20 mL	Adult type, not on thighs	
Stage 5	Adult genitalia	>20 mL	Adult type, spreads to medial thigh	

1.12 ADOLESCENCE

Traditionally, adolescence is defined as the period from the onset of puberty to the termination of physical growth and sexual maturity; and achievement of adult characteristics. WHO defines *Adolescence* as the period between 10 and 19 years of age. People between 15 and 24 years are referred to as *Youth*. Adolescents and youths together constitute *Young People*. Adolescents constitute 22.8% of the total population in India.

CHANGES DURING ADOLESCENCE

Physical changes Adolescence is a rapid phase of growth and development as 50% of adult weight, more than 20% of the adult height, and 50% of the bone mass is gained during this period. Nutritional requirement increases dramatically and this period can be the last opportunity for an adolescent to catch up and realize the full growth potential. Adolescent girls are at particularly high risk of anemia, malnutrition, and micronutrient deficiency. Urban adolescents are at a higher risk of overweight and obesity. The recommended dietary allowance for Indian adolescents is shown in **Table 1.12**.

Biological changes These refer to onset of puberty which we have discussed in the previous section. Puberty primarily refers to the maturational, hormonal, and growth process that occur when the reproductive organs begin to function and secondary sexual characters develop. It is primarily due to hormonal activity under the influence of central nervous system.

Appearance of secondary sexual characters before the age of 8 years in girls and 9 years in boys, and non-appearance of secondary sexual characters by the age of 13 years in girls and 14 years in boys is considered abnormal. A girl who does not menstruate by 16 years should be thoroughly evaluated for the presence of chronic illness, malnutrition, or other conditions that may affect physical development.

Emotional and social changes Adolescents also have to cope with associated emotional changes and emerging and compelling sex urges. Bodily changes cause emotional stress and strain as well as abrupt and rapid mood swings. Hormonal changes are likely to result in thoughts pertaining to body image, sex, irritability, restlessness, anger, and tension. Sexual attraction leads to a desire to mix freely and interact with each other.

Adolescence is characterized by an emerging capacity to reason in an increasingly sophisticated manner. Because of their developmental level, adolescents have a sense of uniqueness and personal invulnerability. This sense of personal invulnerability, coupled with a desire to test and

Box 1.3 Areas of Stress in Adolescents
1. Body image
2. Sexuality conflicts
3. Scholastic pressures
4. Competitive pressures
5. Relationship with parents
6. Relationship with siblings and peers
7. Finances
8. Decision about present and future roles
9. Career planning
10. Ideological conflicts

master, and their newly emerging physical and mental capabilities, may provide one explanation for the risk-taking behaviors observed during this age. Areas of stress in adolescents are listed in **Box 1.3**.

Changes in sexual behavior Adolescence is a time of heightened feelings, arousal, urges, and sexual feelings directed towards self and others. Puberty brings with it an intensification of sex response and the beginnings of sexual behaviors, which for most will eventually lead to sexual intercourse and the possibility of procreation. Adolescents may indulge in homosexual and heterosexual acts as part of sexual experimentation. The median age of initiation of sexual activity in India is considered to be 15–16 years (NFHS-3, 2006).

Spontaneous erections, nocturnal emissions (wet dreams), and masturbation manifest in mid or early adolescence in a majority of boys. Vaginal discharge, tingling pain in the breasts, and masturbation—along with menstrual concerns—may occur in girls. Unsafe sexual behavior may end up in adolescent pregnancy, abortion, and sexually transmitted infections including HIV and AIDS.

PRIORITY HEALTH PROBLEMS

Priority health problems affecting adolescents are listed below:
1. *Intentional and unintentional injuries* Violence, depression and suicide, road traffic accidents, poisoning.
2. *Mental health problems* Depression, sadness, anxiety, other psychiatric disorders, learning disorders.
3. *Substance use and abuse* Tobacco, alcohol and other substances.
4. *Nutritional problems* Undernutrition, iron deficiency anemia, iodine deficiency, obesity, anorexia nervosa, bulimia.
5. *Sexual and reproductive health problems* Teenage pregnancy, abortion, menstrual problems, reproductive tract infections including HIV/AIDS.
6. *Endemic and chronic diseases* TB, malaria, asthma, etc.

Table 1.12 Recommended Dietary Allowance for Indian Adolescent (ICMR 2010)						
	Boys			*Girls*		
Age	10–12 y	13–15 y	16–17 y	10–12 y	13–15 y	16–17 y
Energy (kcal)	2190	2750	3020	2010	2330	2440
Protein (g)	40.0	54.3	61.5	40.4	51.9	56.5
Calcium (mg)	800	800	800	800	800	800
Iron (mg)	21	32	28	27	27	26

MULTIFACTORIAL CAUSATION OF HEALTH PROBLEMS

The cause of most of the adolescent health problems is multifactorial.

Immediate causes Studies and program experiences around the world have shown that the problems among adolescents are caused by a set of immediate causes, including:

- Inadequate education and skills;
- Poor access to health information and services;
- Unsafe and unsupportive environment—this concerns family and friends, service providers, policies and legislations and the media; and
- Exploitation and abuse.

Underlying factors These include gender-based discrimination, poverty, unemployment, urbanization and migration, social values and norms, and wars and emergencies. These factors bring about changes in values and norms, behavior and lifestyles; and lead to adolescents adapting risky behavior because of peer pressure, and temptations such as easy access to tobacco, drugs, and sex.

Risk behaviors Centers for Disease Control (CDC), Atlanta has identified 6 priority health risk behaviors in youth:

1. Behavior contributing to unintentional violent injuries
2. Tobacco use
3. Alcohol and other drug use
4. Sexual behaviors contributing to unintended pregnancy, STD and HIV infection
5. Unhealthy dietary behavior
6. Physical inactivity

It is important to develop surveillance systems to monitor the health risk behaviors of adolescents in developing countries including India. This will go a long way in describing risk behaviors, creating awareness, setting program goals, developing programs, and seeking program resources for adolescents and young people.

Dino GA, Pignataro R, Breland A, *et al*. Adolescent smoking cessation: promising strategies and evidence-based recommendations. *Adolesc Med State Art Rev*. 2011;22:614–30.

Lal S. Reaching adolescents for health and development. *Indian J Community Med*. 2001;26:167–72.

National Family Health Survey 2004–05 (NFHS-3). Mumbai: International Institute for Population Science; Mumbai: 2006.

Scott ME, Wildsmith E, Welti K. Risky adolescent sexual behaviors and reproductive health in young adulthood. *Perspect Sex Reprod Health*. 2011;43:110–8.

Secor-Turner M, Kugler K, Bearinger LH, Sieving R. A global perspective of adolescent sexual and reproductive health: context matters. *Adolesc Med State Art Rev*. 2009;20:1005–25.

Sivagurunathan C, Umadevi R, Rama R, et al. Adolescent health: present status and its related programmes in India. Are we in the right direction? *J Clin Diagn Res*. 2015; 9 LE 01–6.

Taliaferro LA, Sieving R, Brady SS, Bearinger LH. We have the evidence to enhance adolescent sexual and reproductive health—do we have the will? *Adolesc Med State Art Rev*. 2011;22:521–43.

UNFPA. Adolescent and Youth Demographics: A Brief Overview (2014). Availabel from: https://www.unfpa.org/resources/adolescent-and-youth demographics-a-brief-overview. Accessed 1 January 2018.

WHO. Broadening the Horizon: Balancing Protection and Risk for Adolescents. Geneva: World Health Organization; 2001.

WHO. Consultation on action to address adolescent health (2016). Avalable from: http://www.who.int/maternal-child-adolescent/topics/adolescence/evy. Accessed 1 January 2018.

DISORDERS OF PHYSICAL GROWTH

1.13 SHORT STATURE

DEFINITION

Short stature is defined as height below –2 Z-score or below 3rd percentile. Height below –3 Z-score or below the first percentile indicates severe short stature with a high likelihood of pathological cause. Growth velocity below 10th percentile over a year or crossing of two percentile lines between the age of 2 years and puberty are also indicative of growth failure **(Box 1.4)**.

Box 1.4 Indicators of Short Stature
Presence of any one of these:
1. Height below –2 Z-score or 3rd centile for age and gender within the population
2. Height below –2 Z-score of the mid-parental target height
3. Abnormally slow growth velocity
4. Height dropping across two major centile lines on the growth chart

DETERMINANTS OF GROWTH

Mid-parental height Height shows a marked variability between children which is dependent on their age, gender, nutrition, genetics, ethnicity and racial differences. One of the important determinants of height in children is their genetic potential which is determined by their parents' heights and is calculated as mid-parental height (MPH). A child may remain short, if he is born to shorter parents and may be diagnosed as having *familial* or *genetic short stature*.

Box 1.5 shows the formula to calculate MPH for boys and girls. MPH is marked at gender appropriate chart at 18/ 20 years. In normally growing child, height at any given age corresponds to lie within 2 standard deviation of the MPH when it is extrapolated till adult height on a growth chart.

Box 1.5 Calculation of Mid-Parental Height (MPH)
MPH (boy) = (Father's height + Mother's height + 13)/2, or = [(Father's height + Mother's height)/ 2] + 6.5
MPH (girls) = (Father's height + Mother's height – 13)/2, or = [(Father's height + Mother's height)/2] – 6.5

Nutrition The effect of nutrition on final height may be seen starting as soon as during fetal period. For example, a few babies who experience intrauterine growth retardation and are born as small for gestational age, may fail to achieve normal height in childhood and may remain short. Deficiency of both macronutrients and micronutrients like zinc and iron during growing years adversely impacts attainment of height. Malnutrition has been reported as one of the commonest causes of short stature in Indian settings. Such children show growth faltering for both weight and height which can be easily discerned on a growth chart.

Systemic diseases Chronic diseases, syndromic genetic disorders, diseases of musculoskeletal system, and those affecting the hypothalamic-pituitary axis (affecting growth hormone, etc.) are other causes of short stature.

ETIOLOGY

Physiological variants account for over two-thirds of all cases of short stature. Pathological short stature can be caused by a variety of factors related to genetics or nutrition, systemic diseases, and endocrine imbalance **(Table 1.13)**. Short stature may be *proportionate* or *disproportionate* as assessed by the ratio of upper and lower segment length.

A. Disproportionate Short Stature

Disproportionate short stature occurs as a result of abnormal skeletal growth. Either the limbs or the trunk is short. Short limb dwarfism can be further classified into rhizomelic (shortening of proximal limb segment), mesomelic (shortening of middle segments), and acromelic (shortening of the distal segments) short stature. These disorders present with severe short stature, disproportionate development of spine and limbs, and abnormal facies.

- In *short limb dysplasia*; eg, achondroplasia (Fig. 1.32), chondrodysplasia, arm span is less than height and US/LS ratio is high.
- In *short trunk anomalies*; eg, mucopolysaccharidosis, spondyloepiphyseal dysplasia, US/LS ratio is decreased and arm span exceeds the height.

B. Proportionate Short Stature

This is more common; all the body proportions are equally shortened. This may occur secondary to constitutional delay in growth, chronic infections, malabsorption, congenital heart disease, renal failure, or endocrine malfunctioning. The only exception to this rule is hypothyroidism. A child with proportionate short stature may be thin or fat. Thin and short children result due to an underlying systemic disorder; while fat and short children are likely to have an endocrine etiology.

Constitutional delay This represents a group of children with delayed maturation with preserved growth potential. This is particularly common in boys. Family history of delayed puberty is common. These children grow at a normal rate and continue to grow beyond the normal stage of growth. Final height is usually normal. Children with *familial short stature* on the other hand have normal bone age and usually end up short.

Malnutrition It is the commonest pathological cause of short stature. Growth failure is preceded by poor weight gain. This contrasts endocrine short stature where weight is usually normal. Zinc deficiency is an important rare but treatable cause of short stature.

Intrauterine growth retardation (IUGR) This might be due to genetic disorders, intrauterine infections, maternal malnutrition, and placental disorders. Most of these children achieve catch-up growth and have final height in the target height range. Around 15%, however, fail to grow normally and have adult short stature.

Systemic diseases Short stature occurs in all chronic systemic disorders and infections. Most of these conditions are readily identifiable; celiac disease, renal failure, and renal tubular acidosis might be asymptomatic and be missed.

Table 1.13 Causes of Short Stature
Normal variants
• Familial short stature   • Constitutional growth delay
Pathological short stature

• *Malnutrition:* Macronutrient or micronutrient deficiencies, small for gestational age
 • Chronic systemic diseases
   – *Gastrointestinal:* Celiac disease, chronic liver disease
   – *Cardiopulmonary:* Acyanotic and cyanotic heart disease, congestive heart failure
   – *Infections:* Tuberculosis, giardiasis, HIV
   – *Renal:* Chronic kidney disease, renal tubular acidosis, chronic pyelonephritis
   – *Hematological:* Nutritional anemia, leukemia, thalassemia
   – *Pulmonary:* Chronic asthma, bronchiectasis
   – *Storage disorders:* Mucopolysaccharidosis, glycogen storage disorders
   – *Neurological:* Cerebral palsy
 • Metabolic bone disease—Rickets
 • Endocrine causes
   – *Hypothalamic-pituitary axis:* Growth hormone deficiency, growth hormone receptor defect (Laron dwarfism)
   – *Other endocrine organs:* Hypothyroidism, Cushing syndrome, diabetes, precocious puberty
 • *Genetic syndromes:* Turner syndrome, Prader-Willi syndrome, Russell-Silver syndrome, Noonan syndrome
 • *Skeletal dysplasias:* Achondroplasia, osteogenesis imperfecta
 • Psychosocial dwarfism
 • *Drugs:* Systemic steroids, substance abuse

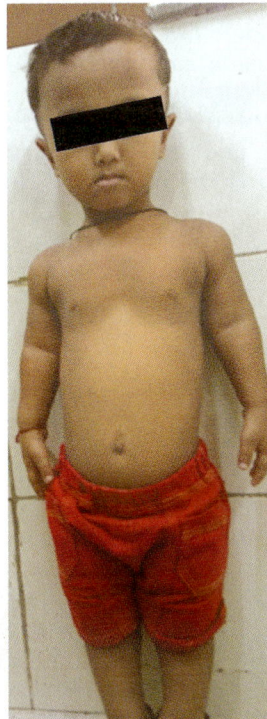

Fig. 1.32 A 6-year-old boy with achondroplasia. Note the short stature with apparent increased upper segment than lower segment

Chromosomal/genetic syndromes Down syndrome is the commonest chromosomal disorder associated with growth retardation. Turner syndrome is an important cause of short stature in girls. While classical features are easily identified, girls with mosaic forms of Turner syndrome might appear normal. Turner syndrome should be considered in all short girls.

Endocrine causes Disorders of the growth hormone are important causes of short stature and discussed in Chapter on Endocrine Disorders. These children have normal growth at birth; retardation becomes apparent around 1 year of age. Hypothyroidism, Type 1 diabetes mellitus, pseudohypoparathyroidism, and rickets are also associated with growth retardation.

Table 1.14 shows the differentiating features between various causes of short stature in children.

EVALUATION

No evaluation is required, if height is more than –2 Z-score (third percentile) or growth velocity is above 25th percentile. On the other hand, immediate evaluation is warranted, if height is below –3 Z-score (first percentile). Children with height Z-score between –2 and –3 should be followed up. Work-up is required, if growth velocity is below 25th percentile.

A summary of clinical clues to ascertain the etiology of short stature is provided in **Table 1.15**.

Step 1: History Taking

Perinatal history and birth weight should be recorded. Nutritional assessment is crucial part of evaluation of short stature. Family history of short stature or delayed puberty suggests familial short stature or constitutional short stature.

- Features of chronic infections, malabsorption, raised intracranial tension, and cardiopulmonary disorders should be enquired.
- Polyuria and polydipsia suggest diabetes insipidus, diabetes mellitus and/or renal tubular acidosis.
- Constipation, delayed milestones, lethargy, and cold intolerance pinpoint hypothyroidism.
- History of birth asphyxia, breech presentation, neonatal hypoglycemia, and prolonged jaundice is indicative of hypopituitarism.

Step 2: Growth Assessment

It involves comparison of height with population standards and parental height along with monitoring of longitudinal growth.

- Growth velocity should be measured over a period of at least 12 months. Growth velocity less than 6 cm/year from the age of 1–3 years, 5 cm/year from 4–8 years and 4 cm/year from 8 years is suggestive of growth retardation.
- Mid-parental height (MPH) should be plotted on the growth curve at around 18–20 years and the percentiles compared with current height percentiles. Plot this value of adult height prediction on the Reference growth chart of height-for-age. The percentile line nearest to this point is known as the mid-parental 50th percentile. The child's own percentile curve is expected to be between 10th and 90th percentiles (MPH ± 8.5 cm) on the MPH percentile chart.

- *Height age* The height age (HA) of the child is the age at which his/her current height would match the 50th percentile or median for that age and sex. It can be assessed on a growth chart by drawing a horizontal line from the child's current height to intersect the growth curve at 50th percentile.

Step 3: Physical Examination

Detailed anthropometric measurements (weight, weight for height, and head circumference) should be taken. Reduced weight is suggestive of nutritional growth retardation (malnutrition, systemic illness, and malabsorption) while weight is generally preserved in endocrine causes. Body proportions are helpful in identifying skeletal dysplasia.

- Increased upper segment to lower segment ratio is indicative of hypothyroidism, achondroplasia, and Turner syndrome.
- Decreased upper segment to lower segment ratio is characteristic of Morquio syndrome and spondyloepiphyseal dysplasia.
- Body proportions are normal in growth hormone deficiency.

Specific features of growth hormone deficiency, hypothyroidism, and Turner syndrome should be looked for. Rickets and anemia should prompt evaluation for malnutrition, celiac disease, or renal failure. Shortening of fourth metacarpal is present in children with Turner syndrome and pseudohypoparathyroidism. Evaluation for dysmorphism, skeletal deformities, and sexual maturity rating is essential part of examination of children with short stature.

Step 4: Investigations

1. *Skeletal age.* Estimation of skeletal age or bone age (BA) is the first investigation to be ordered in a child with short stature. It is estimated by evaluating the skeletal maturity of bones of the left hand and wrist using standard bone atlas (Greulich-Pyle atlas or Tanner-Whitehouse method). Normally, the bone age matches the chronological age (CA) of the child. In case the BA shows a delay of more than 2 standard deviations than the CA, it is called *delayed BA* as seen in pathological short stature. An understanding of the BA can help us understand the normal variant growth patterns.
   - *Familial short stature (FSS):* This variation is seen as short stature in a child who is born to short parents, thereby implying the role of genetic potential for growth. These children are short but their extrapolated height falls within the range of MPH. The general and systemic examination is normal. They have normal skeletal maturation and thus their BA matches their CA. However, as they are short, the height age is lesser than both chronological age and bone age (BA = CA > HA). This entity does not need any further investigation or treatment. It is essential to reassure and monitor their growth annually. The growth pattern of FSS is shown in Fig. 1.33.
   - *Constitutional delay in growth and puberty (CDGP)* Another variant of growth which is considered normal is 'constitutional short stature' or constitutional delay in growth and puberty. These children have normal growth potential but show poor growth in late childhood. The

Table 1.14 Differences between Various Causes of Short Stature

	Familial short stature	CDGP	Hypothyroidism	Growth hormone deficiency	Malnutrition/ chronic systemic illness
Age of onset	Short since birth	Short after infancy	Short since birth	Short since late infancy	Short since onset of disease/ nutrient deficiency
Birth weight	Low	Normal	High or normal	Normal	Normal
Family history	Present—parents are short	Present—parents have history of delay in growth	Normal	Normal	Normal
Pubertal onset	Normal	Delayed	Delayed	Delayed	Delayed
Clinical examination	Normal	Normal	Coarse facies and delayed developmental milestones	Infantile facies	Stigmata of chronic disease or vitamin deficiencies
Body proportion	Normal	Normal	Disproportionate	Normal	Normal
Height velocity	Normal	Normal	Delayed	Delayed	Delayed
Bone age (relation with CA & HA)	Normal CA = BA > HA	Delayed CA>BA=HA	Delayed CA>HA>BA	Delayed CA> HA>BA	Delayed CA>HA>BA (BA delay is lesser than in endocrine causes)
Management	Reassurance	Reassurance	Thyroid hormone	Growth hormone	Treatment of underlying cause

Footnote: BA—bone age, CA—chronological age, HA—height age, CDGP—constitutional delay in growth and puberty

Table 1.15 Clinical Clues to Etiology of Short Stature

	HISTORY
Present history	• Age of onset of growth faltering • Prior growth record • Any other associated symptoms
Specific symptoms • Polyuria • Chronic diarrhea, greasy stools • Lethargy, constipation, weight gain • Headache, visual disturbance, seizures	• Renal tubular acidosis, chronic kidney disease • Malabsorption, celiac disease • Hypothyroidism • Intracranial tumor affecting pituitary or hypothalamus
Past history disease, Birth and antenatal history	Known disorder—history of chronic systemic disorder like asthma, chronic liver chronic kidney disease, congenital heart disease • Birth weight—whether born small for gestational age • Maternal symptoms of Intrauterine infections • Maternal ill-health, maternal alcohol or tobacco use • Neonatal hypoglycemia or prolonged jaundice—GH deficiency
Dietary history	Evaluation of daily protein and calorie consumption. Also evaluate for micronutrients
Family history	Chronic systemic disorder, history of pubertal delay in parents
Social history	Psychosocial environment
	EXAMINATION
Anthropometry	Weight, height, height velocity, body proportions, head circumference
Face including skull	• Facies—syndromic or dysmorphic facies in genetic syndromes, infantile facies in growth hormone deficiency, coarse in hypothyroidism or mucopolysaccharidosis • Skull—microcephaly, craniotabes in rickets, large fontanelle in achondroplasia • Eyes—anemia, cataract in intrauterine infections, blue sclera in osteogenesis imperfecta • Ears, nose, palate—for any congenital defects in genetic syndromes • Teeth—delayed dentition in hypothyroidism and rickets, dental caries in rickets
Musculoskeletal	Limbs for deformities seen in rickets, skeletal dysplasia
Genitalia	Assess for pubertal maturation (delayed or advanced), any abnormalities in structure
Systemic	Evaluate for any underlying systemic disorder
Miscellaneous	Clubbing, skin for striae (Cushing syndrome), stigmata of Turner syndrome, goiter

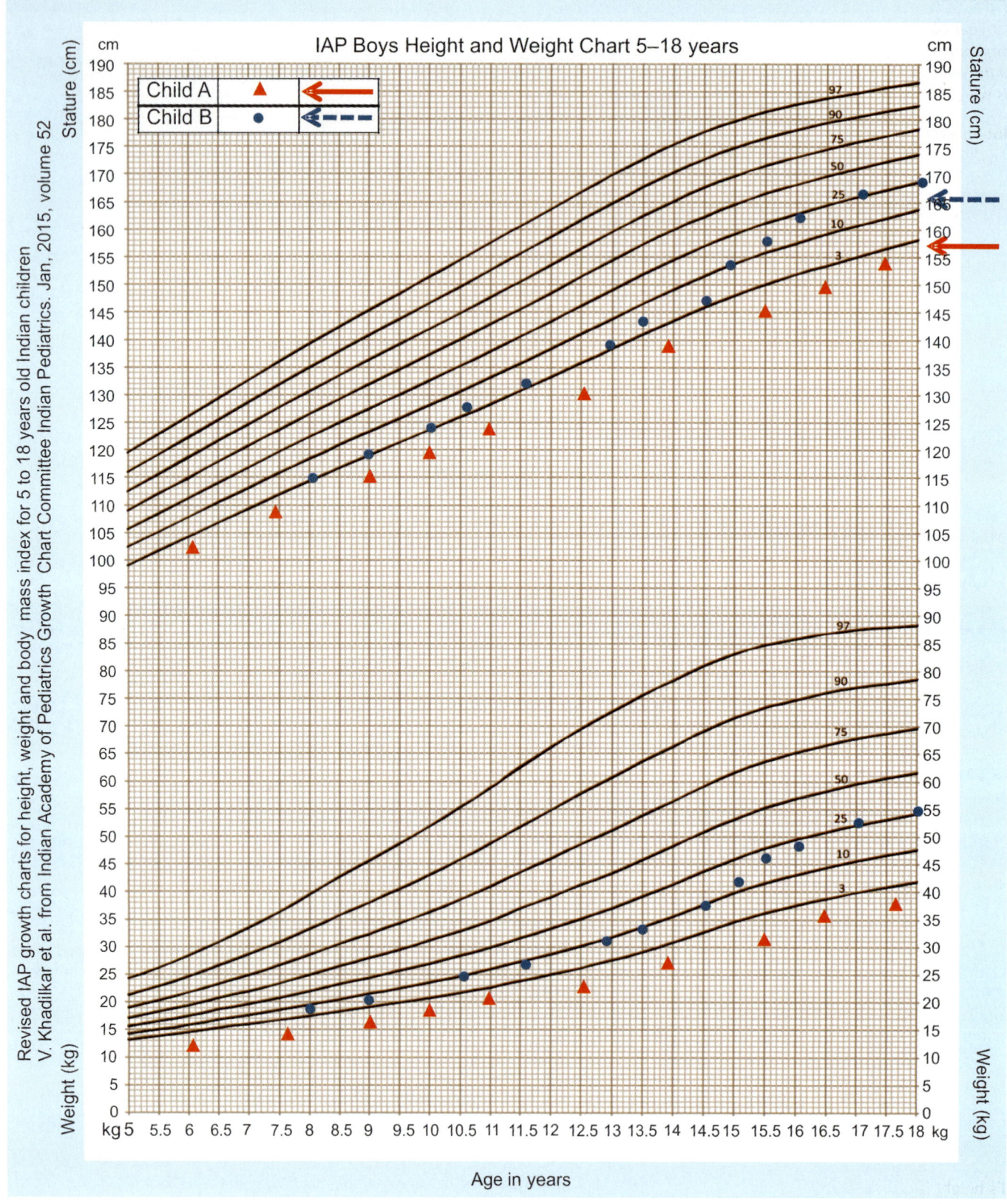

Fig. 1.33 Growth patterns in short stature. The figure above shows growth monitoring of two boys with their respective mid-parental heights marked as arrows on right. Child A has familial short stature and Child B has constitutional delay in growth and puberty. (Weight and height should be marked as small dots on growth chart; magnification and use of shapes is for better depiction only)

Case Study | Short Stature

A 9-year-old boy was brought with complaints of not growing well since early childhood. His birth weight was 2.5 kg. Mother gave some non-specific history of abdominal discomfort and frequent loose stools in early childhood, but the child was never investigated for the same. There were no other significant systemic complaints. Family history was normal, his elder brother was tall. On examination, his weight was 15 kg and height was 107 cm. Mother and father height were 153 and 158 cm, respectively.

Plot his growth on a growth chart? How will you proceed?

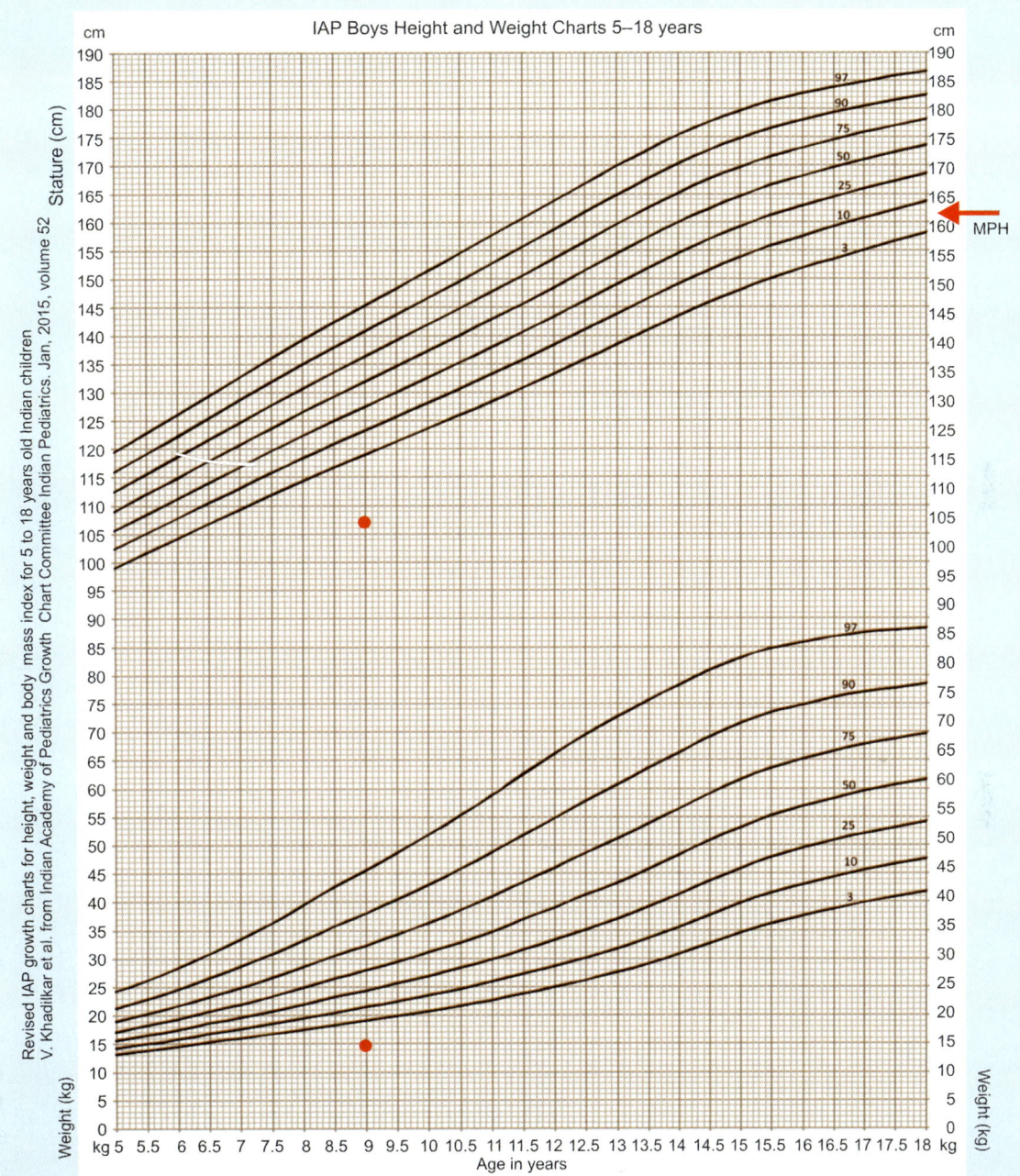

His height is grossly below his MPH (162 cm). There are no prior height records available. But with a corresponding low weight against a low height, a systemic disorder should be looked for. Next investigation to be ordered is a bone age.

His bone age was 5 years. Examination revealed clubbing, anemia, and signs of vitamin B deficiency. How will you proceed now?
Bone age is grossly delayed. Height age was 5.5 years. Therefore, diagnosis of pathological short stature is made. We will like to order the next line of screening investigations.

Case Study | **Short Stature (Contd...)**

The investigations were suggestive of celiac disease (serum tissue transglutaminase was raised). This is a malabsorption disorder which was confirmed by duodenal biopsy. The micronutrient deficiencies were a result of malabsorption. The child was shifted on gluten-free diet and started on micronutrient supplements after which he showed improvement in growth (chart shown below).

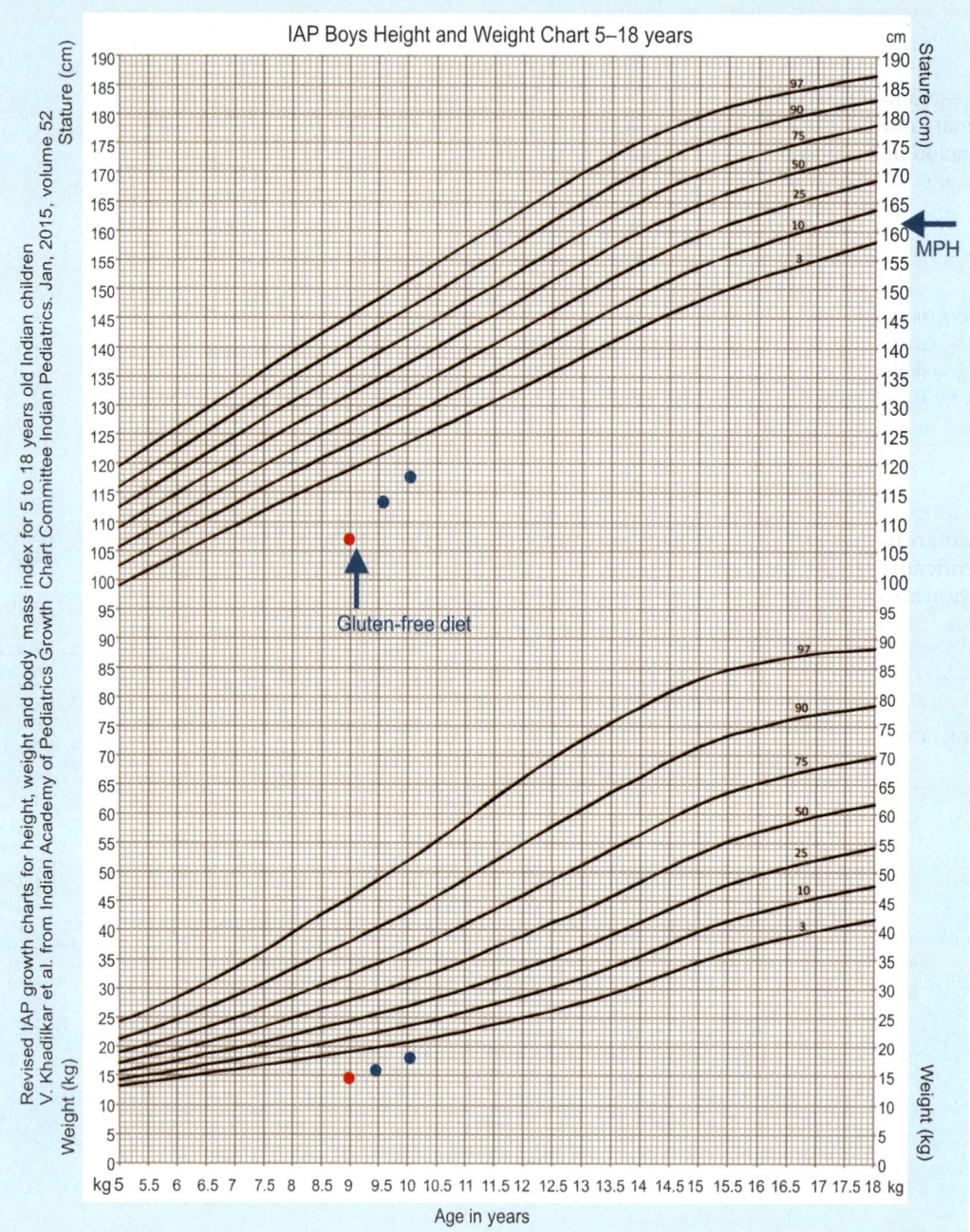

height velocity is normal. There is usually associated delay in puberty which makes poor height more discernible in peripubertal years. They need close monitoring of growth as they catch up subsequently on their height to attain final height within their MPH range. Usually, there is history of similar delay in puberty in their parents. These children have delayed BA which matches their HA. Both are less for their CA (HA = BA<CA). The growth pattern of CDGP is shown in Fig. 1.33.

2. *Laboratory investigations* A simple screening set of investigations which should be ordered initially is mentioned in **Table 1.16**. The screening set includes tests which screen for commoner causes of short stature. Further investigations, including hormonal assays, should be ordered on individual case basis according to historical and clinical cues.

Evaluate for growth hormone deficiency (GHD) Evaluate for growth hormone (GH) deficiency after other common causes

Table 1.16 Investigations in Pathological Short Stature

First line tests

- Hemoglobin, blood counts, ESR—anemia, hematological disorders, chronic inflammatory diseases
- Kidney function tests—chronic kidney disease
- Liver function tests—chronic liver disease
- Serum calcium, phosphorus—rickets
- Thyroid function test—hypothyroidism
- Serum transglutaminase—celiac disease
- Urine routine examination—diabetes, urinary tract infection
- Urine pH—renal tubular acidosis
- Chest X-ray, including bone age assessment
- Karyotype (in girls)—Turner syndrome

Specific tests (done on case to case basis)

- Infections—tuberculosis, HIV
- Serum growth hormone (GH), IGF-1 levels and GH stimulation test—growth hormone deficiency (GHD)
- Serum cortisol—Cushing syndrome
- Skeletal survey—skeletal dysplasia
- Imaging of brain including pituitary fossa—GHD
- Genetic mutations—*POU1F1, PIT1, PROP1, HESX1, SHOX*

IGF–insulin like growth factor

of growth retardation have been excluded. These children generally have infantile facies (Fig. 1.34). The extrapolated height falls significantly short of the respective MPH. The skeletal maturation also shows a significant delay than their chronological age (BA < HA < CA). Basal GH has no role in evaluating the GH–IGF axis. IGF-1 and its binding protein-3 (IGFBP-3) are screening tests for GH deficiency. Low levels should be followed by a GH stimulation test. Stimulated GH levels below 10 ng/mL are suggestive of GH deficiency. This

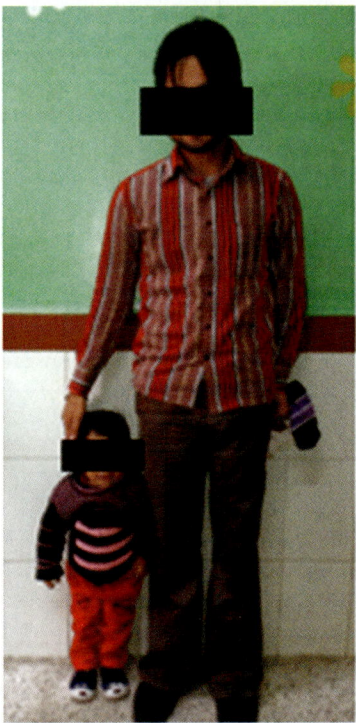

Fig. 1.34 A 4-year-old boy with growth hormone deficiency. Note how the child is short for his age

should be followed with evaluation of other pituitary hormones and brain imaging. High GH levels are suggestive of rare GH insensitivity disorders such as Laron syndrome.

Figure 1.35 shows a schematic approach to evaluate a child with short stature.

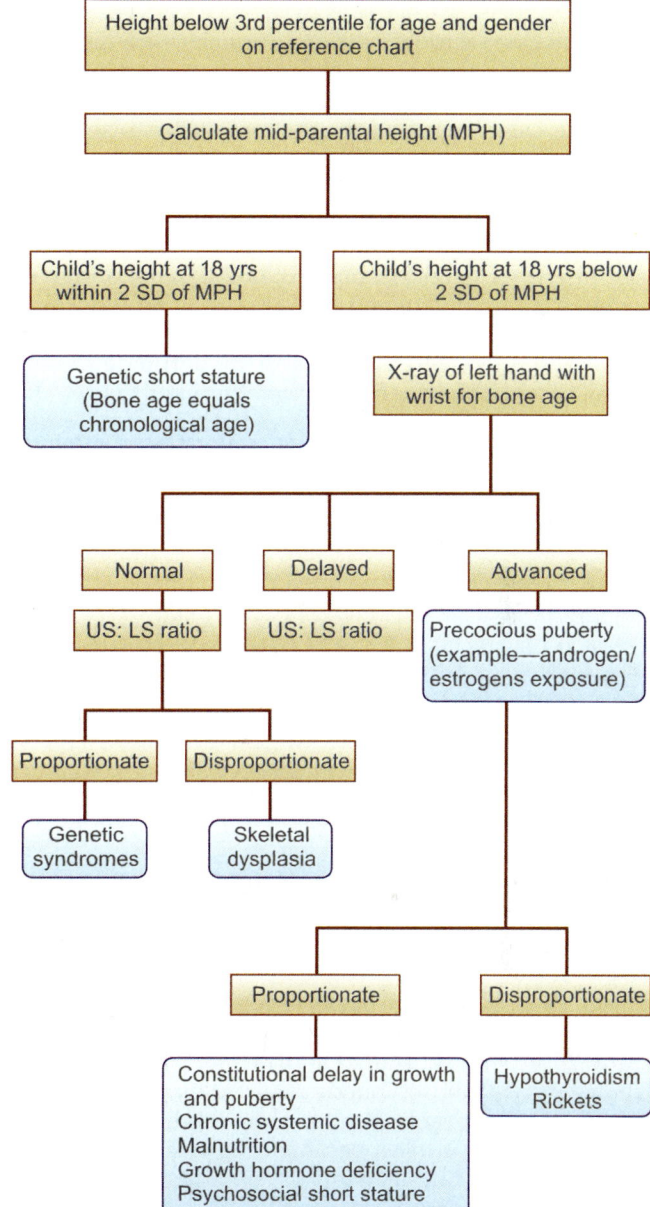

Fig. 1.35 Algorithmic approach for clinical evaluation of short stature

Treatment	**Short Stature**

Management includes treatment of underlying cause and provision of adequate nutrition intake. Patients with short stature should be advised high protein and calorie diet. They should be encouraged to increase physical activity. Iron and vitamin deficiency should be corrected. Zinc supplementation (10 mg/day for 3–6 months) has been shown to be effective in improving growth in idiopathic short stature.

Specific therapy Initiation of specific treatment is effective in restoration of growth in hypothyroidism (thyroxine), celiac disease (gluten-free diet) and renal tubular acidosis (bicarbonate). Testosterone (short course) should be given in boys with constitutional delay of puberty and growth. Treatment of genetic syndromes and skeletal dysplasia is difficult. GH, androgen, and anabolic steroids have been tried with success in some of these conditions. Bone lengthening (Ilizarov technique) has been used with variable success in a few children.

Growth hormone is highly effective in GH deficiency, Turner syndrome, chronic renal failure, small for gestational age infants, Prader-Willi syndrome, and idiopathic short stature.

TALL STATURE

A child with a height of more than 2 Z-score above the median or beyond 97th percentile is said to be abnormally tall. This may occur because of hereditary factors (if the parents are tall), cerebral gigantism, acromegaly, and chromosomal abnormality (Klinefelter syndrome). Tall stature associated with disproportionately long limbs is characteristic of Marfan syndrome and homocystinuria.

Bajpai A, Menon PSN. Growth hormone therapy. *Indian J Pediatr.* 2005;72:139–144.

Bajpai A, Sharma J, Menon PSN. Short stature. *In: Practical Pediatric Endocrinology.* New Delhi: Jaypee Brothers; 2003;3–8.

Lifshitz F, Botero D. Worrisome growth. *In:* Lifshitz F. *Pediatric Endocrinology,* 4th edition. New York: Marcel Dekker; 2003;1–47.

Patel L, Clayton PE. Normal and disordered growth. *In:* Brook CGD, Clayton PE, Brown RS. *Clinical Pediatric Endocrinology,* 5th edition. London: Blackwell Publishers; 2005;90–112.

Rosenfeld GR, Cohen P. Disorders of growth hormone/insulin like growth factor and action. *In:* Sperling MA. *Pediatric Endocrinology,* 2nd edition. Philadelphia: WB Saunders; 2002;211–88.

Yadav S, Dabas A. Short stature. *Indian J Pediatrics.* 2015;82(5):462–470.

1.14 FAILURE TO THRIVE (FTT)

The term 'failure to thrive' (FTT) is assigned to a child whose weight-for-age is below 3rd percentile or a downward change in growth that has crossed two major growth percentiles (ie, downward shifting from 75th percentile to below 25th percentile) in a short time. FTT objectively denotes growth failure. Criteria used to define FTT are listed in **Box 1.6**. For practical purpose, weight remains the commonest and simplest parameter to define FTT as it is affected first during any illness, much before stunting manifests.

Box 1.6 Diagnostic Criteria of Failure to Thrive

- Weight-for-age below 5th percentile
- Weight deceleration Serial weight monitoring shows downward trend and has crossed two major growth percentiles (ie, 75th percentile to below 25th percentile) in a short time.
- Weight-for-age less than 75% of the median
- Weight-for-length less than 75% of the median
- Length-for-age less than 5th percentile
- Body mass index less than 5th percentile

This term should not be confused with short stature as FTT describes retarded growth in height and weight, whereas short stature is diagnosed in comparison to a reference height-for-age or to one's own height over a period of time.

Besides growth deficit, FTT also results in alteration in immunity (predisposing to infections) and dysfunction in intellect, development, and behavior. Other associated complications with FTT are listed in **Box 1.7**. It is important to appreciate that FTT in itself should never be considered as a primary disease. FTT is always a manifestation of an

---

Box 1.7 Systemic Complications of Failure to Thrive

Short-term
- Hypothermia
- Hypoproteinemia
- Predisposition to infections
- Nutritional deficiencies and electrolyte imbalance

Long-term
- Neurocognitive delay
- Behavioral problems
- Short stature
- Adult onset metabolic diseases

---

underlying cause which should be investigated through proper clinical examination and relevant investigations.

ETIOLOGY

Adequacy of growth is dependent on various physiological processes in the body. The chief determinant is food intake measured in terms of both quality and quantity. Failure to thrive can result, if the child is taking less food, the food is not being properly absorbed, or nutrients and fluids are being lost excessively. The second process which can result in FTT is an underlying organic disease (renal, cardiac, gastrointestinal, respiratory) or a metabolic cause which causes increased energy expenditure, thereby creating an energy deficit. Apart from these biological causes, psychosocial or environmental deprivation, child abuse and neglect can also result in growth failure in childhood. Major organic causes of FTT are listed in **Table 1.17**. **Table 1.18** categorizes the causes of FTT based on energy balance.

Approach to Diagnosis

A child with FTT should have a detailed evaluation of the following aspects: 1. Dietary assessment; 2. Medical assessment; 3. Psychosocial assessment; and 4. Developmental assessment.

History

Ask the parents about the onset of growth failure to differentiate between congenital and acquired causes. Ask for common symptoms of possible organic disorders. An assessment of dietary intake and dietary habits is essential part of clinical history. The amount of food offered and consumed should be separately measured. Details of milk preparation, dilution, and reconstitution should be checked in an infant. Growth failure due to energy deficit is commonly seen during late infancy when the baby is shifted from breastfeeding to complementary feeding. Feeding

Table 1.17 Major Organic Causes of Failure to Thrive	
System	*Cause*
Gastrointestinal	Recurrent diarrhea (poor sanitation), Gastroesophageal reflux disease, Celiac disease, pyloric stenosis, Cleft palate/cleft lip, lactose intolerance, Hirschprung disease, milk protein intolerance, hepatitis, cirrhosis, pancreatic insufficiency, biliary disease, inflammatory bowel disease, malabsorption, food alkalines
Renal	Urinary tract infection, renal tubular acidosis, diabetes insipidus, chronic renal insufficiency
Cardiopulmonary	Cardiac diseases leading to congestive heart failure, asthma, bronchopulmonary dysplasia, cystic fibrosis, anatomic abnormalities of upper airway, obstructive sleep apnea(snoring)
Endocrine	Hypothyroidism, diabetes mellitus, adrenal insufficiency or excess, parathyroid disorders, pituitary disorders, growth hormone deficiency
Neurological	Mental retardation, cerebral hemorrhages, degenerative disorders
Infectious	Parasitic or bacterial infections of the gastrointestinal tract, Human immunodeficiency virus disease
Metabolic	Inborn errors of metabolism
Congenital	Chromosomal infections, congenital syndromes (fetal alcohol syndrome), perinatal infections
Miscellaneous	Psychosocial/environmental neglect, lead poisoning, malignancy, collagen vascular disease

Table 1.18 Causes of Failure to Thrive based on Energy Balance		
Inadequate caloric intake	*Inadequate caloric absorption*	*Excessive caloric expenditure*
Infancy • Inadequate breastmilk • Inadequate amount or improper dilution of top/formula milk • Inadequate complementary feeding • Gastroesophageal reflux disease • Cleft palate/cleft lip • Maternal factors—low education, younger age	*Infancy* • Congenital GI anomalies like duodenal atresia, malrotation of gut • Cow milk protein allergy • GI parasitic infections • Chronic liver disease • Short gut syndrome (leal resection post-surgery)	*Infancy* • Chronic systemic diseases—congenital heart disease, lung disease, renal disease, cystic fibrosis, endocrinal causes • Chronic infection like intrauterine infections, tuberculosis • Immunodeficiency—congenital or acquired (HIV) • Genetic syndromes • Inborn error of metabolism • Malignancy
Childhood • Food scarcity • Neurodevelopmental disorders which affect swallowing coordination like cerebral palsy • Gastroesophageal reflux disease • Behavioral disorders, eating disorders	*Childhood* • Food allergy • Malabsorption—celiac disease, chronic diarrhea • Inflammatory bowel disease • Inborn error of metabolism	*Childhood* • Chronic systemic illness • Chronic systemic infections • Malignancy • Inborn error of metabolism

habits should be enquired for both home and outside home settings (day-care, school). Socio-cultural environment of the child should be assessed. Family dynamics, parental education, employment, substance abuse, and cultural factors should also be assessed.

Psychosocial assessment should include evaluation of socioeconomic status; family dysfunction; and feeding problems. Child's drive for autonomy, attention seeking, gaining independence, and expressing anger or dislike by refusing food are also important causes for creating a feeding disorder. Physical or mental traumatic behavior, though seen in small percentage of cases, is an important cause of FTT. Developmental assessment should include assessment for developmental delay; and abnormalities of posture, tone, and attention and language domains. Standardized developmental assessment may be required. Any delay in two or more domains is abnormal. Mild degree of motor delay is commonly seen in children with FTT due to poor skeletal mass and muscle tone.

Clinical Examination

Obtain complete and accurate anthropometry. Serially measured values rather than a single observation are mainstay for diagnosing FTT. Anthropometry should be interpreted on age and gender specific population reference growth charts. Separate charts for preterm babies should be used to monitor their growth during infancy. Besides this, a thorough general and systemic examination should be done to search for:

• Any clue to organic disorders (facial dysmorphism, neurocutaneous markers, clubbing, etc.)
• Physical abuse (fractures, bruises, hematomas, cigarette marks, etc.)
• Markers of severe malnutrition and associated deficiencies (loss of buccal fat, edema, mucositis, corneal ulcers, etc.)
• A detailed neurological and developmental assessment using appropriate tests.
• Any abnormal behavioral pattern, response to external stimulus, etc.

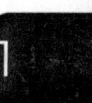

Table 1.19 Red Flag Signs in a Child with Failure to Thrive with Probable Etiology

Clinical symptoms/signs	Probable etiology
Failure to show catch up growth after calorie deficit has been corrected	Underlying systemic disorders
Global developmental delay	Syndromic causes, chromosomal disorders
Family history of un-explained sibling deaths or abortions	Chromosomal disorders, inborn errors of metabolism
Seizures	Inborn errors of metabolism, brain malformations, intra-uterine infections
Jaundice	Chronic liver disease, storage disorders
Non-diarrheal dehydration	Diabetes, adrenal insufficiency
Dysmorphic features	Chromosomal disorders
Skeletal deformities	Child abuse, distal renal tubular acidosis, metabolic bone disease
Lymphadenopathy	Tuberculosis, lymphoreticular malignancies
Clubbing	Chronic disease of liver, lung
Skin lesions	Specific patterns seen in different diseases

The red flag signs that should alert the physician towards an underlying systemic cause of FTT are highlighted in **Table 1.19**.

Laboratory Evaluation

FTT is a clinical diagnosis and most children do not need investigations. Tests are of prime importance when an organic etiology is suspected or in the presence of a red flag sign.

- Some minimal initial tests which may be performed are: hemoglobin, blood counts, urea, electrolytes, creatinine, liver function tests, total proteins, anti-endomysial bodies (to screen for celiac disease), and urinalysis.
- Other tests include sweat chloride test for cystic fibrosis in genetically predisposed population; blood pH, anion gap and urine pH for renal tubular acidosis; and stool examination in children with diarrhea or suspected malabsorption.
- Radiological assessment may be useful for determining bone age in some cases or fractures, if physical abuse is suspected.
- A karyotype may be ordered in suspected chromosomal disorder.

An algorithmic approach to management of failure to thrive is shown in Fig. 1.36.

Treatment	**Failure to Thrive**

Clinical trials have shown that there is no difference in the outcome of children who are hospitalized or managed at home. Indications of hospitalization are as follows:

- Severe malnutrition especially with life-threatening complications.

Case Study	**Failure to Thrive**

A 30-month-old girl was brought with complaints of not gaining weight for 1 year. Parents also noticed excessive urination for last three months. She used to be 'dry by day' at 2 years of age but now she is no longer continent. Recently her mother has noted a soft swelling over her scalp for last 1 month. Her dietary intake does not reveal any major deficit in intake of protein or calories.

She now weighs 9.2 kg. Her present height is 85 cm. Her birth weight was 2.8 kg. She weighed 9 kg at 18 months as recorded on her immunization chart. Examination revealed mild anemia, dry skin, and loss of subcutaneous fat. There was a 2 × 3 cm soft swelling over occipital region of scalp. Systemic examination was normal.

Interpret the anthropometry.
Her weight at birth (2.8 kg) was at 15th centile (WHO charts). She continued to follow her centile for weight till 18 months of age. Her present weight is 9.2 kg which is below the 3rd centile. Her weight has crossed two major centiles and shown a downward trend which is pathological. Her current height is just above 3rd centile. According to these measurements, she has failure to thrive.

What is the cause of FTT? Justify.
The likely case is organic. Her dietary assessment seems normal which rules out nutritional etiology.
Clinical clues in this case which suggest an organic cause are:
- Growth faltering in a previously normal growing child
- Urinary incontinence and excessive urination (other systemic symptoms)
- Positive systemic findings—scalp swelling, anemia.

The case was further worked up to find an underlying organic cause. Polyuria was documented and confirmed. Laboratory tests showed anemia (hemoglobin 9.5 g%) and high serum sodium (149 mEq/L). Needle aspirate from the scalp swelling was positive for malignant cells which were confirmed to be Langerhan cells on special stains (S-100 and CD1A). X-ray of the skull showed a bony defect. Bone marrow examination was normal.

How will you confirm the diagnosis? Outline the management.
Central diabetes insipidus was diagnosed by demonstrating a high serum osmolality and low urine osmolality, confirmed on water deprivation test. MRI brain showed absence of posterior pituitary bright spot. The patient was diagnosed as Langerhans cell histiocytosis and started on chemotherapy. She was also started on oral desmopressin for diabetes insipidus. The child gradually improved and achieved a catch up in her growth on follow-up.

- As a part of diagnostic work-up, if organic cause is suspected.
- Child unresponsive to initial management.
- Where parent neglect, abuse, or maltreatment is suspected.

FTT resolves with medical interventions. However, the management should be comprehensive and long term. A multidisciplinary and stepwise approach is most effective.

Dietary management Nutritional rehabilitation aims at: Achievement of ideal weight for height and correction of nutritional deficits; allowing catch up growth; restoration of optimal body composition; and parental education regarding

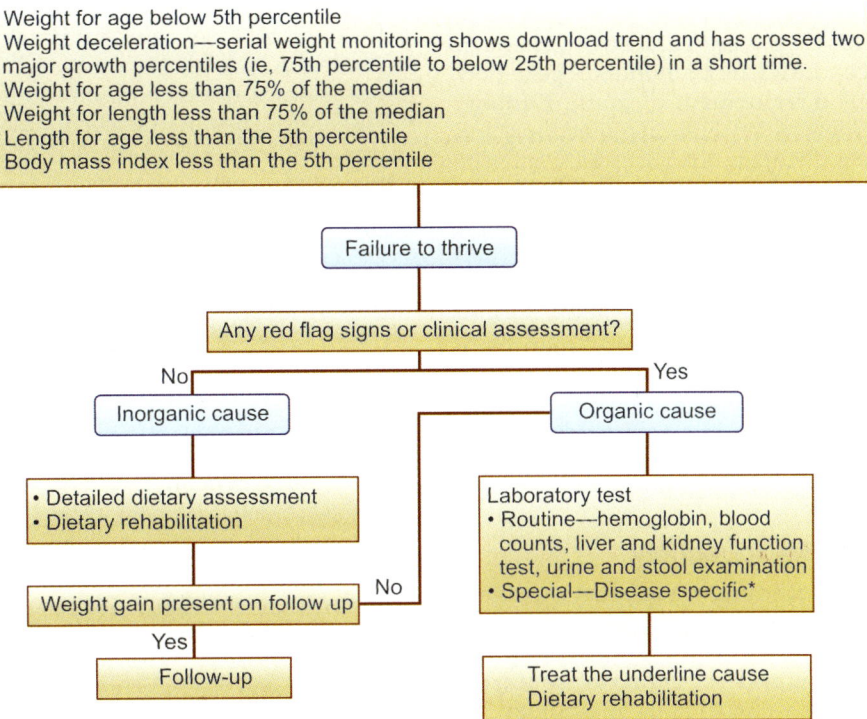

- Weight for age below 5th percentile
- Weight deceleration—serial weight monitoring shows download trend and has crossed two major growth percentiles (ie, 75th percentile to below 25th percentile) in a short time.
- Weight for age less than 75% of the median
- Weight for length less than 75% of the median
- Length for age less than the 5th percentile
- Body mass index less than the 5th percentile

Failure to thrive

Any red flag signs or clinical assessment?

No → Inorganic cause

Yes → Organic cause

- Detailed dietary assessment
- Dietary rehabilitation

Laboratory test
- Routine—hemoglobin, blood counts, liver and kidney function test, urine and stool examination
- Special—Disease specific*

Weight gain present on follow up — No

Yes → Follow-up

Treat the underline cause
Dietary rehabilitation

Investigation specific for an underlying systemic disorder

Fig. 1.36 Approach to a child with FTT

nutritional requirements and feeding of the child. Diet management of a child with FTT is similar to that of a child with severe acute malnutrition (see details in Chapter 3).

Parental education Parents should be involved in feeding actively. They should be told about their child's requirements and how they can be met. They should gain knowledge about calorie content of different food items, how to make calorie rich, simple, and appealing preparations, right techniques of feeding, and how to inculcate good feeding habits in their children. Misconceptions and food fads should be addressed carefully.

Medical management Several medical issues may be identified in children with FTT which may be primary or secondary and require specialized interventions. Special diets may be required lifelong, for example, celiac disease; or special enzyme supplements for cystic fibrosis. Drugs may be required (eg, for gastroesophageal reflux disease) or special training in neuromotor dysfunction (eg, cerebral palsy).

Psychosocial management The psychosocial aspects differ widely and hence the management cannot be generalized. A good rapport is essential for both diagnosing and managing such issues. The need for psychiatrist in cases of depression, substance abuse, and behavioral problems is unavoidable. Behavioral modifications in feeding disorders, psychotherapy, and counseling are of tremendous help. In cases where poverty is the cause of malnutrition, social relief organizations can be approached. In cases where there is severe abuse, neglect, and maltreatment; hospitalization or foster homes may be essential temporarily before the parental issues are resolved.

Developmental management This is the most difficult and unrewarding area. Studies have shown that even after aggressive nutritional rehabilitation, there are minor deficits like language skills, subnormal IQ scores, and decreased head circumference. Thus the key to neurodevelopmental management lies in prevention of severe FTT, early recognition of the condition, and management, before a permanent brain deficit occurs.

Atalay A, McCord M. Characteristics of failure to thrive in a referral population: Implications for treatment. *Clin Pediatr*. 2012;51:219–25.

Cole SZ, Lanham JS. Failure to thrive: an update. *Am Fam Physician*. 2011;83:829–34.

Daniel M, Kleis L, Cemeroglu AP. Etiology of failure to thrive in infants and toddlers referred to a pediatric endocrinology outpatient clinic. *Clin Pediatr (Phila)*. 2008;47(8):762–5.

Jaffe AC. Failure to thrive: current clinical concepts. *Pediatr Rev*. 2011;32:100–7.

Krugman SD, Dubowitz H. Failure to thrive. *Am Fam Physician*. 2003;68:879–84.

1.15 ABNORMALITIES OF HEAD SIZE AND SHAPE

MICROCEPHALY

A child is labeled as having microcephaly, if the head circumference is below –3 Z-score below the median for that age. The size of head is closely related to the size of brain. Microcephaly can result from any process that impairs the brain development, ie, cell proliferation, cell differentiation, and cell migration. There is a reduction in head size resulting from a decrease in brain volume or premature closure of sutures (craniosynostosis). Causes of microcephaly could be genetic or acquired.

Etiology

Primary microcephaly This may occur because of genetic or intrauterine disturbances during first 7 months of gestation, resulting in anomalous development of brain. Etiology includes chromosomal defects, intrauterine infections, and exposure to teratogens. Primary microcephaly may be familial or inherited in an autosomal dominant fashion with no other malformations. Most common genetic cause of microcephaly is *MCPH 1–12* gene mutation resulting in autosomal recessive primary microcephaly.

Secondary microcephaly This results primarily because of environmental disturbances during the last 2 months of gestation or in the postnatal period. Most common intrauterine cause is perinatal asphyxia. Once the child is born, insult to the growing brain can be caused by meningitis, malnutrition, hypothermia, and asphyxia.

Causes of microcephaly are summarized in **Table 1.20**.

Approach to a Case of Microcephaly

- Antenatal history (maternal drug or radiation exposure, history of fever with rash to rule out CMV) and natal history (history suggestive of perinatal asphyxia, prematurity, neonatal jaundice, neonatal seizures, meningitis) could provide valuable hints for etiology.
- Screen for co-morbidities like vision impairment, seizures, spasticity, and dystonia.
- Head circumference at birth is most crucial record to differentiate primary from secondary microcephaly.
- Look for dysmorphic features that could suggest a particular syndrome like Rubinstein-Taybi syndrome.
- Fundus evaluation for cataract, optic atrophy, chorioretinitis (congenital TORCH infection) would be useful.

Table 1.20 Causes of Microcephaly
Prenatal onset
Genetic
• Primary microcephaly (AD, AR, XLR)
• Chromosomal disorders—trisomy 21, 18, 13
• Syndromic causes (Angelman syndrome, Cornelia de Lange syndrome, Rubinstein-Taybi syndrome, Rett syndrome)
• Craniosynostosis
• Disorders of cortical development (lissencephaly, polymicrogyria, periventricular nodular heterotopias)
Nongenetic
• Maternal intake of drugs—alcohol, smoking, AED, corticosteroids
• Maternal illnesses—toxemia, diabetes, chronic renal failure, phenylketonuria,
• Intrauterine infections—CMV, rubella, toxoplasmosis, congenital Zika virus infection
Postnatal onset
• Perinatal insults (eg birth asphyxia)
• Inborn errors of metabolism—phenylketonuria, organic acidemia, congenital disorders of glycosylation, peroxisomal disorders
• Other CNS insults—encephalitis, meningitis
• HIV infection

- Presence of overriding skull sutures with premature closure of fontanel could indicate craniosynostosis.
- Obtain chromosomal analysis, if child has abnormal facies, short stature, or other stigmata of syndromic features.
- MRI brain is useful to screen for malformations of cortical development. CT scan is indicated for those with suspected craniosynostosis.
- Genetic evaluation test for determining the etiology of microcephaly includes karyotyping, fluorescent in situ hybridization (FISH) to look for subtelomeric deletion, array comparative genome hybridization (array CGH) analysis, chromosomal breakage analysis, and sequencing of selected genes.

Treatment	Microcephaly

Microcephaly is rarely reversible. Presence or absence of intellectual disability among children with microcephaly is often determined by associated structural abnormalities of the brain rather than the size of the brain alone. Genetic counseling is essential to prevent future pregnancies being affected with similar condition.

MACROCEPHALY

Macrocephaly is defined as a head circumference that is >2 Z-score above the median for that age, height, and gender. Normally, head circumference is greater by 1–2 cm in males, ranges ±2.5 cm around median and increases linearly with height. It may be caused by increased brain size (megalencephaly), or increased ventricular size (hydrocephalus).

- *Megalencephaly* is a proliferation disorder caused by metabolic CNS disease, Tay-Sachs disease, mucopolysaccharidoses), neurocutaneous syndrome (neurofibromatosis, tuberous sclerosis), or cerebral gigantism. It may also be familial or genetic. There is increase in all neural constituents of the brain.
- *Hydrocephalus* may be caused by congenital infections (toxoplasmosis, syphilis, rubella), anatomical malformations (aqueduct stenosis, Chiari malformation, Dandy-Walker malformation), or acquired secondary to CNS infection, intraventricular hemorrhage, or infarction.

Examination of ocular fundi is a must in children with macrocephaly: Cherry red spot may be seen in Tay-Sachs disease; papilledema and secondary optic atrophy may be seen in hydrocephalus. MRI brain would be useful to establish the diagnosis and to delineate the site of obstruction among patient with hydrocephalus. CT scan is associated with radiation exposure and hence may be avoided as far as possible.

Approach to diagnosis of a child with large head is shown in Fig. 1.37.

CRANIOSYNOSTOSIS

Premature closure of one or more sutures of the skull is known as craniosynostosis. This results in an abnormal shape of the head. Normally, the metopic suture closes before the age of 2 years, and sagittal and coronal sutures usually fuse in the second decade of life. Due to premature fusion,

Table 1.21 Craniosynostosis: Shapes of Skull

Suture closing prematurely	Head growth occurs in	Head growth arrested in	Resultant skull shape
Sagittal suture	AP diameter	Lateral growth	Dolicocephaly/scapocephaly
Coronal suture bilateral	Transverse diameter	AP diameter	Brachycephaly
Metopic suture		Lateral growth of forehead	Trigonocephaly
Unilateral coronal		Flat forehead on involved side	Plagiocephaly
All sutures			Oxycephaly

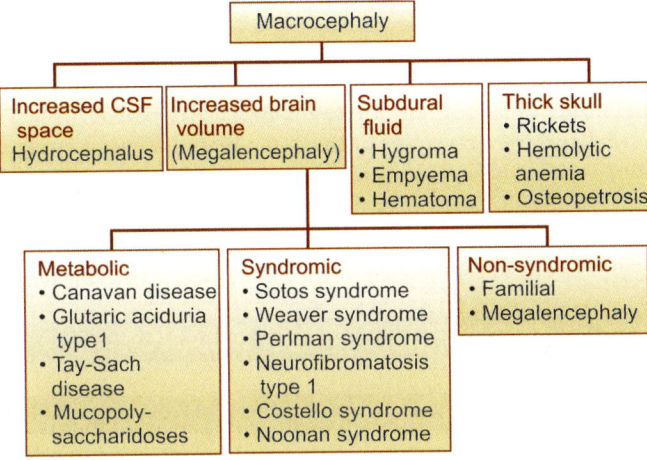

Fig. 1.37 Approach to diagnosis of a child with large head

the growth of the skull is arrested perpendicular to the fusion of the suture line; the skull continues to grow parallel to the line of fusion and results in structural abnormalities.

If only one suture closes prematurely, it is *simple craniosynostosis*. Involvement of multiple sutures indicates *complex craniosynostosis*.

Classification

Primary craniosynostosis There is an intrinsic failure of suture development due to abnormality of the mesenchymal matrix surrounding suture line; this primary defect of ossification usually presents at birth. There may be a genetic basis for the defect and it may be associated with other congenital anomalies in one-third cases. Sagittal suture is affected the most (in 60% cases), followed by coronal suture (in 25% cases). Metopic and lambdoid statures are involved in 15% and 2% cases, respectively.

Primary craniosynostosis is characteristic of Apert syndrome, Carpenter syndrome, and Crouzon disease.

Secondary craniosynostosis Premature closure of the sutures occurs because of an underlying failure of growth of the brain. Common causes include congenital hypothyroidism, microcephaly, and rickets.

Clinical Features

The skull shape is abnormal due to growth at right angles to the suture that undergoes premature fusion. The head is small in size and there is microcephaly. A prominent ridge is present along the suture that has closed prematurely. Shape of the skull is characteristic depending upon the sutures that are involved **(Table 1.21)**.

Brachycephaly is usually associated with proptosis. The common presenting symptoms include small head, intellectual disability, seizures, features of increased intracranial pressure, strabismus, optic atrophy, exophthalmos, hypertelorism, and cosmetic deformities.

Investigations

Diagnosis is confirmed by CT scan of skull with 3D reconstruction to visualize patency of suture lines. MRI brain is required to screen for corpus callosum agenesis or ventriculomegaly.

Associated Syndromes

Crouzon syndrome Autosomal dominant inheritance with variable penetrance. Maxillary hypoplasia, beak type nose, exophthalmos, strabismus, a short upper, protruding lower lip, and normal intelligence. Although the coronal sutures are usually involved, the lambdoid and, rarely, the sagittal sutures may also be affected.

Apert syndrome Autosomal dominant with high mutation rate, syndactyly, flat facies with maxillary hypoplasia, downward slanting eyes, prominent forehead, high vertex (turricephaly, acrocephaly, or tower head) and occasionally intellectual disability may be present.

Carpenter syndrome Autosomal recessive, similar to Apert syndrome with polydactyly, obesity, hypogenitalism, and intellectual disability.

Treatment	Craniosynostosis

Goals of management, apart from reduction of raised intracranial pressure, include protection of eye, nutritional support, and maintaining the airway. Most of these defects except scaphocephaly may be associated with arrested brain development and hence may require surgery early in life to maximize brain growth, reduce complications, and for cosmetic correction.

Piyush Gupta; Jaya Shankar Kaushik (*Growth, Disorders of Head Shape and Size*); Rachna Dubey (*Development*); and Aashima Dabas (*Short Stature, FTT*)

Behavioral Problems

2.1 INTRODUCTION

Behavioral disorders represent significant departures or deviations from the accepted 'normal' behavior. Common behavioral disorders include thumb-sucking, pica, breath-holding spells, and nocturnal enuresis. Up to 20% of children presenting to primary care are estimated to have behavioral and psychosocial problems. Common behavioral problems are listed below.

1. *Habit problems* Thumb-sucking, nail-biting, bruxism, tics, enuresis, encopresis, breath-holding spells, trichotillomania, and aerophagia.
2. *Eating problems* Pica, food fads, food refusal/overeating, vomiting, and anorexia.
3. *Personality problems* Shyness, timidity, fears, anger, and jealousy.
4. *Antisocial problems* Juvenile delinquency.
5. *Sleep problems* Night terrors, nightmares, somnambulism, insomnia, sleep-talking, and narcolepsy.
6. *Speech problems* Stuttering, mutism, phonation, and articulation disorders.
7. *Scholastic problems* Reading, writing or mathematical disorders, repeated failures, absenteeism, truancy, and school phobia.

ETIOLOGY

Behavioral problems are usually caused by maladjustment at home or school, in a child with precipitating factors operating during pregnancy, during delivery and in neonatal period. Some or all of the following: Faulty emotional environment, constituted by parental attitudes, siblings, neighborhood, school and mass media, play a major role. Faulty parental attitudes resulting in behavioral difficulties include rejection, overprotection, unrealistic expectations, discrimination, over criticism, over discipline, and unfavorable comparisons with sibs and peers.

Neurobehavioral disorders, eg, attention deficit hyperactivity disorder (ADHD), autism, learning disorders, on the other hand, do not have their antecedents in the child's environment but still present as problems of behavior in different social settings.

MANAGEMENT

Behavioral assessment is used to determine the precipitating events and consequences that maintain the behavioral problem. The ABC (antecedent-behavior-consequence) model and the principles of reinforcement and punishment are used for assessment and management of behavioral problem. Behavioral assessment guides *behavioral intervention*, which is designed to modify variables that trigger, maintain, or mediate problem behavior.

PROBLEMS DURING INFANCY

2.2 INFANTILE COLIC

Evening colic is characterized by the *rule of three*. The diagnosis should be considered in an infant younger than 3 months of age, who presents with intermittent episodes of abdominal pain and excessive crying for more than 3 hours per day, for more than 3 days per week, and lasting for longer than 3 weeks. The infant is otherwise well fed and healthy. Colic is a diagnosis of exclusion after ruling out less common organic causes of incessant and repetitive crying. Around 5–25% of infants in the community have colic.

ETIOLOGY

Exact cause of colic is not known. Gastrointestinal (increased gas production from colon, milk allergy, hyperperistalsis), psychosocial, and neurodevelopmental disorders have been suggested as the possible etiology. Infantile colic is more likely to occur, if the child is overactive and the parents are overanxious. These episodes could also be a manifestation of hunger, aerophagia, or overfeeding. It appears unrelated to environmental events.

CLINICAL FEATURES

Attacks usually begin suddenly with a bout of screaming in the evening. Crying is associated with motor behaviors such as flushed face, furrowed brow, and clenched fists. The legs are pulled up to the abdomen, and the infant emits a piercing, high-pitched scream. Crying is concentrated in the late afternoon and evening, occurs in prolonged bouts, and is unpredictable and spontaneous. The child cannot be soothed, even by feeding. Attacks may terminate after the infant is exhausted, or passes feces or flatus.

Typically, the paroxysms of colic start within a few weeks after birth, reach a peak by 4–6 weeks, and subside by 3–4 months of age. Differential diagnosis includes CNS abnormality or infection, gastroesophageal reflux, otitis media, urinary tract infection, foreign body in the eye, fractured bone, and child abuse.

| Treatment | **Infantile Colic** |

Treatment is limited. The physician's role is to ensure that there is no organic cause for the crying, offer balanced advice on treatments, and provide support to the family. Long-term follow-up studies have shown no difference in behavior amongst colicky and non-colicky infants. Above all, parents need reassurance that their baby is healthy and that colic is self-limited with no long-term adverse effects.

During an episode, hold the child erect or prone in the lap or on a hot water bottle. There is not much role of carminatives, suppositories or enema. Avoid drugs to reduce intestinal motility. Sedate the child. If attacks do not respond to above measures. Anticholinergic drugs have shown some benefit for the acute episode, but should be used with caution.

Feeding technique should be explained. Feed in erect position. Practice proper burping and place the child on right lateral position for about half an hour after feeding. Possible allergenic food should be identified and removed. Selected probiotics have demonstrated efficacy in infantile colic, especially in the breastfed group.

Infant should not be given undue attention. They should be nurtured in emotionally stable environment. Try to calm the anxious parents and clear their self-doubts regarding child rearing. Reduce the parental anxiety by counseling them about the nature of the problem, lack of effect of soothing, and self-remission by about 4–6 months. Encourage exclusive breastfeeding.

Revision Point

Infantile Colic

1. Infantile colic is characterized by the "rule of 3", ie excessive cry for >3 h/day for >3 times/week and lasting for >3 weeks; in a child younger than 3 months.
2. Etiology is not known.
3. There is no effective medication. Child needs to be comforted and parents need counseling.
4. Infantile colic is self-remitting and subsides spontaneously by 4–6 months of age.

2.3 FEEDING PROBLEMS

Feeding problems in the first year of life occur because of erratic feeding, oversensitive infant and parents' ignorance regarding feeding. Other parental problems leading to feeding difficulties include anxiety, depression, unwillingness to nurture, substance abuse, psychosocial stress, or other serious mental illness. Usual manifestations are underfeeding, overfeeding, spitting, regurgitation, and constipation.

UNDERFEEDING

Underfeeding occurs when either (*i*) infant is not offered sufficient quantity of feed; or (*ii*) the infant is not able to take a sufficient quantity of food even when offered. This can be caused by improper feeding techniques such as decreased frequency or duration of feeding, inadequate quantity and quality of feeding, early introduction of top feeding, nipple confusion, breast problems, improper burping, abnormal mother–infant bonding and chronic systemic illness in the infant.

Clinical features depend upon the extent and duration of underfeeding. Initially, there might be constipation, failure to sleep, irritability, and excessive crying. If underfeeding continues for prolonged period, the child fails to gain weight and may progress to have failure to thrive.

Management depends upon the condition of the child. If severe malnutrition is present, it is of utmost importance to manage fluid and electrolyte, associated infection, hypoglycemia, hypothermia, and anemia. Following this, the child should be provided adequate calories and supplemented with appropriate minerals and vitamins. Treat the underlying systemic infection and diseases, if any. Identify and treat associated psychological problems such as child abuse or neglect. Counsel the parents about feeding techniques.

OVERFEEDING

Overfeeding can be qualitative or quantitative. It is usually caused by parents' ignorance about nutritional requirement of their infants. Psychosocial problems in parents may also result in overfeeding. Unwillingness of mother to breastfeed and reliance on bottle feeding is another major factor.

Clinical features The most common clinical manifestation of overfeeding is regurgitation and vomiting. Infant may present with abdominal distension and discomfort due to delayed gastric emptying, if the diet contains too much fat or carbohydrates. It may be associated with abdominal distension or passage of excessive flatulence. Overfeeding leads to rapid and excessive weight gain, resulting in childhood obesity.

Management Proper nutritional assessment including dietary history and intake should be taken. This is to be followed by a detailed physical examination and anthropometry. On this basis, one can determine the infant's status by calculating appropriate nutritional value of the food and comparing them with actual required recommended dietary allowances. Parents should be counseled regarding daily dietary allowance, feeding technique, and types of food to be used. They should be told that healthy child does not mean obese child. Adequate and exclusive breastfeeding can overcome the problem of overfeeding.

EXCESSIVE SPITTING

It is normal in 15% of infants. It can also be associated with gastroesophageal reflux (GER) and overfeeding. Clinical manifestations depend upon severity of the problem. Failure to thrive occurs in extreme cases.

Management Reassure the parents, if their infant is gaining weight adequately and there are no underlying factors such as overfeeding, psychosocial stress and GER. Determine whether stress is present during feeding. If yes, identify its cause and manage appropriately. Provide proper counseling.

RUMINATION

This is habitual regurgitation and re-swallowing of stomach contents by increasing intra-abdominal pressure by putting finger or fist in the mouth. This disorder may be associated with gastroesophageal reflux, esophagitis, or intellectual disability. Infants with psychogenic rumination respond well, if they are held 15 minutes before and after feeding. Child with intellectual disability or global developmental delay can be managed with behavior technique such as "time out."

Campbell K, Peebles R. Eating disorders in children and adolescents: state of the art review. *Pediatrics*. 2014;134:582–92.

Kelly NR, Shank LM, Bakalar JL, Tanofsky-Kraff M. Pediatric feeding and eating disorders: current state of diagnosis and treatment. *Curr Psychiatry Rep.* 2014;16:446.

2.4 STRANGER ANXIETY

By about 6–7 months, the infant can differentiate between the primary caregivers and others. Thus at this age, they develop fear of unfamiliar people or strangers. The infant, when approached by unfamiliar person, turns away, even cry or crawls towards the primary caregiver. This is known as *stranger reaction*. It is a normal phenomenon and may last a few months or persist to peak at about 13–15 months.

But, if the infant on approaching the stranger behaves with more intense discomfort manifesting with psychological and physiological distress such as continuous crying, vomiting and refusal to socialize, then it is called as *stranger anxiety*. It might be an indication for later development of behavioral problem, especially separation anxiety disorder.

Management The infant is managed with relaxation technique such as slowly exposing them to the stranger, initially from a distance, asking them to greet and slowly advancing towards them. Reassurance of parents is required as this behavior gradually declines. But, if the behavior persists, then the child should be referred to psychiatrist to evaluate for associated anxiety disorders.

EARLY CHILDHOOD PROBLEMS

2.5 THUMB-SUCKING

It is a common, generally harmless, behavior of infancy and early childhood, and appears to be a way of securing extra self-nurturance. When persisting after age four, it is a mild to moderate health risk as it may occasionally lead to dental, dermatological, orthopedic, and psychological problems. It poses risk of malocclusion of developing dentition, and digital deformity. Some children may develop speech difficulty for consonants D and T.

A child who discards this habit initially and resumes again at 7 to 8 years, needs to be evaluated for associated psychological problems. Resumption of this habit suggests that the child is suffering from stress or insecurity.

Treatment	**Thumb-Sucking**

Indications Persistent thumb-sucking after 4–5 years age should be treated when it is associated with presence of dental problems due to the behavior. Treatment is not indicated when thumb-sucking is infrequent or it has an important function in alleviation of stress due to substantial loss (eg, parent, pet), fear (eg, surgery), or pain (eg, injury, illness), when it acts as a temporary adaptive coping strategy.

Strategies Management options are (*i*) planned ignoring; (*ii*) giving attention to more positive aspects of the child's behavior; and (*iii*) monitoring followed by rewards or incentives for sucking-free days (*positive reinforcement*). Use of bitter agents on thumbs or tying a cloth on thumb should not be considered as a first line approach.

Parental counseling Parents should be counseled regarding the self-remitting nature. Children with thumb-sucking should not be punished for this act. Punishment would only reinforce this habit. A positive feedback is helpful when the child is not sucking. Child who looks depressed should be referred for detailed psychological evaluation and management. The child should be praised and encouraged, if he tries to indulge in activities other than thumb-sucking.

Borrie FR1, Bearn DR, Innes NP, Iheozor-Ejiofor Z. Interventions for the cessation of non-nutritive sucking habits in children. *Cochrane Database Syst Rev.* 2015;(3): CD008694.

2.6 BREATH-HOLDING SPELLS

Breath-holding spells are paroxysmal self-limiting events usually consisting of multiple (three or more) episodes of the following sequence: provocation, followed by crying to a point of noiselessness and accompanying change of color, and ultimately, a loss of consciousness with an associated alteration in body tone. These episodes occur in up to 10% of healthy children between the age of 6 months and 6 years.

The episodes are involuntary in nature and occur during expiration, contrary to the terminology, which implies that the child voluntarily holds the breath in inspiration.

ETIOLOGY

Breath-holding spells are a neurobehavioral problem and categorized as a non-epileptic paroxysmal disorder. Recent research indicates that a genetically mediated dysregulation of autonomic nervous system reflexes is responsible for the spells. As no difference has been found in prevalence of behavioral problems in children with breath-holding spells and controls; the time-honored belief that these spells result from frustration due to a disciplinary conflict between parents and the child stands discounted.

CLASSIFICATION

The spells are classified according to skin color change of the child during the episode, as cyanotic, pallid, and mixed. Cyanotic episodes are commoner than pallid episodes.

- *Cyanotic* type in which the face turns blue; this is precipitated by anger or frustration.
- *Pallid* type where face is pale; usually provoked by sudden fright or pain.
- *Mixed* There is no clear distinction between cyanosis or pallor, or a conflicting history is given by the parents.

CLINICAL FEATURES

The typical age of onset is between 6 and 18 months. The frequency ranges from multiple episodes daily to as few as one per year, and gradually increases in frequency during the second year of life followed by gradual decrease to nil by 6 years.

The spell usually occurs at the initiation of a tantrum. The child holds his breath in expiration after a bout of crying. The child becomes rigid and attains opisthotonic posture. This is followed by limpness. Normal breathing and alertness is resumed within a minute.

DIFFERENTIAL DIAGNOSIS

Breath-holding spell should be differentiated from *epilepsy* and *hypercyanotic spell*.

- *Epilepsy* A breath-holding spell is predisposed by anger, frustration, or fright. The child becomes completely normal after the attack. An epileptic fit has no such predisposing factor and the child remains in a post-ictal stage, with short-lasting altered sensorium or drowsiness after the attack. Cyanosis occurs earlier in breath-holding spell but in epilepsy it occurs after the seizure. EEG is likely to be normal in majority of children with breath-holding spell.
- *Hypercyanotic spell (Tet spells)* Differentiation from hypercyanotic spells associated with cyanotic congenital heart disease can be done by the presence of physical findings (clubbing, auscultation findings, cyanosis of mucosa persisting for a long time, and no spontaneous resolution) and presence of baseline cyanosis since early infancy. In a hypercyanotic spell, the cyanosis is also present before and after the attack, while there is no cyanosis before or after a breath-holding spell.
- Child never develops neurological deficits after the breath-holding spells.

INVESTIGATIONS

Usually no laboratory tests are needed to make the diagnosis but an ECG is useful in ruling out long-QT syndrome. An EEG is not required except when clear description of attacks is not available, history of painful stimulus/crying is not present in some episodes, risk factors for epilepsy are present, or there is associated status epilepticus. Work-up for iron deficiency must be done.

Breath-Holding Spells

1. Breath-holding spells are characterized by multiple episodes of "excessive cry followed by cessation of breath" following some provocation event. They typically occur between 6 months and 5 years of age.
2. Breath-holding spells should be differentiated from hypercyanotic spells which are characteristic of congenital cyanotic heart disease.
3. Breath-holding spell is a clinical diagnosis and does not require EEG or neuroimaging.
4. Iron therapy is effective in management.

Case Study — Breath-Holding Spell

A 2½-year-old girl is brought with complaints of poorly controlled seizures since 8 months. There is one year history of sudden cry following any sudden painful stimulus, followed by cessation of respiration and fall. This is followed by tonic-clonic activity that lasts for 1–2 minutes. There is no clear-cut history of any color change during the episode. After the episode is over, the child usually gets up and is alert, though she goes off to sleep after some episodes. These episodes occur up to 3–4 times per day, though may not occur for up to a week also. An initial diagnosis of breath-holding spells had been made. However, her episode was observed by her local physician, who advised an EEG. The child was started on valproate by the physician, after the EEG was reported as abnormal (showed occasional sharp waves). The frequency of attacks is the same but tonic-clonic movements rarely occur. The parents were not satisfied with the response and wanted a second opinion. History and course were consistent with a diagnosis of breath-holding spells. The parents were counseled and anticonvulsants stopped. Investigations revealed iron deficiency that was managed by oral iron therapy. The frequency of the attacks gradually decreased and stopped completely over the next 2 years.

Learning points

1. Breath-holding spells may occasionally be followed by tonic or tonic-clonic movements. Starting anticonvulsants would not have any effect on the spells.
2. EEG is not required in the evaluation of breath-holding spells.
3. Treatment of iron-deficiency in those with breath-holding spells has been shown to reduce the frequency of the spells.

Treatment — Breath-holding Spells

- *Immediate measures* Prevent injury during the episode. Help the child to floor and have him lie flat. If loss of consciousness occurs, place the child on the side to protect against aspiration. Maintain patent oral airway but do not start CPR. Do not shake the baby, splash water or put anything in the mouth.
- *Long-term measures* There are no prophylactic medications. Iron deficiency has been reported to be associated with breath-holding spells, and treatment with oral iron (4–6 mg/kg/d) for 6–8 weeks is recommended, if documented. Such attacks can be averted by behavioral modification and strong physical stimuli before the onset of attack. Parents should also be advised to divert the attention of the child when a precipitating factor occurs.
- *Parental education* Parents should be reassured that breath-holding spell does not cause irreversible hypoxia, brain injury, epilepsy, and subsequent impairment in cognitive development. Avoid precipitating factors such as exhaustion, hunger, or injury. Do not give toys or tasks beyond the child's abilities. Avoid excessive rules and restrictions. Try to remove unnecessary frustrations.
- *Refer* If the child is less than 3 months, unconsciousness lasts for more than 1 minute, attacks are too frequent, or seizure disorder or hypercyanotic spell is suspected.

Goldman RD. Breath-holding spells in infants. *Can Fam Physician.* 2015;61:149–50.

Robinson JA, Bos JM, Etheridge SP, Ackerman MJ. breath-holding spells in children with long QT syndrome. *Congenit Heart Dis.* 2015;10:354–61.

2.7 TEMPER TANTRUM

From the age of 18 months to 3 years, the child begins to develop autonomy and starts separating from primary caregivers. At this age, they also develop *negativism*, ie, they do things opposite to what has been requested or opposite of their own desire (*oppositionalism*). And when they cannot express their autonomy, they become frustrated and angry. Some of them show their frustration and defiance with physical aggression or resistance such as biting, crying, kicking, throwing objects, hitting, and head banging. This type of physical aggressive behavior is known as *temper tantrum*.

This behavior reaches its peak point during second and third year of life and gradually subsides between 3 and 6 years as the child learns to control his negativism and complies to the requests of others.

ETIOLOGY

Noncompliant or defiant behavior is a normal part of the developmental process, particularly in the preschool-age child (and also at adolescence). The most likely function of noncompliant behavior is access to positive attention and escape/avoidance of undesirable tasks, commands or activities. Continuation of temper tantrums depends on parental response to this behavior. Inconsistent and indiscriminate use of behavioral management strategies by parents is one of the main predisposing factors of temper tantrums. Parental anger and frustration may reinforce the defiance of the non-compliant child and aggravate the problem further.

Treatment	Tempur Tantrum

- At the time of the tantrum, parents should turn away briefly (to give the child time and space to recover). The child can later be explained that such behavior is not acceptable.
- For noncompliant behavior, consequences should be provided immediately after every occurrence, and should be constant across all time periods and settings. Deviating his attention from the immediate cause and changing the environment can reduce the tantrum.
- Parents should provide ample amount of praise for positive behavior. Clear communication and consistent limit setting regarding what is acceptable and not acceptable, and frequent approval are helpful strategies.
- Parents should be calm, loving, firm and consistent; and such behavior should not allow the child to take advantage of gaining things.
- Time-out may be used (1 minute/year of age), if the behavior continues, but requires detailed instructions for effective use.

2.8 PICA

Pica is an eating disorder defined as "the repeated and chronic ingestion of non-nutritive substances including mud, plaster, charcoal, chalk, paint, earth, clay, etc. for a period of at least one month. This should be inappropriate to the developmental level of the child and should not be a part of culturally acceptable practices" (DSM5).

ETIOLOGY

The cause of pica remains unknown and a variety of nutritional, neuropsychiatric, cultural, and psychological theories are proposed. Pica is a physiological phenomenon during oral phase. Children between 18 and 24 months often try to eat non-food items and it is not considered abnormal. Persistence after two years of age needs attention and work-up for lead toxicity, iron-deficiency anemia, and parasitic infections. Although it has been thought of as a symptom of iron-deficiency, it is more commonly found in patients who are not anemic. Pica is more prevalent among children with intellectual disabilities, and those with lack of parental supervision.

COMPLICATIONS

Complications include: Inherent toxicity; intestinal obstruction (such as that occurring with trichophagia, or hair eating); excessive caloric intake (such as that occurring with starch); nutritional deprivation; parasitic infestations; and dental injury. In many cases, complications do not occur or are not recognized. It usually remits with age.

Treatment	Pica

- Pica below two years does not need any intervention.
- Children with pica are at increased risk of lead poisoning, iron-deficiency, bezoars, and parasitic infections. They should be investigated for these problems and if present, treated suitably. Deworming needs to be done, as worm infection is generally associated.
- Education, guidance and counseling of the family. The reason for parental conflict and neglect needs to be looked into, if present.
- Child should be given more affection and love. The child has to be kept occupied in other tasks and provided with environmental stimulation.
- Prevent unsupervised access to mud/chalk/paint, etc.

PROBLEMS OF THE YOUNG CHILD

2.9 ENURESIS (BEDWETTING)

Voluntary or involuntary repeated discharge of urine into clothes or bed, after a developmental age when bladder control should be established (usually 5 years), is labeled as enuresis. Bedwetting or urinary incontinence is labeled as enuresis, only if urine is being voided twice a week for at least 3 consecutive months, or if it is causing clinically significant distress in the child's life.

CLASSIFICATION

Enuresis may be primary or secondary; or nocturnal/diurnal.

A. Primary Enuresis

This is defined as repeated (at least twice a week for at least three consecutive months) passage of urine into clothes/bed during night in a child more than 5 years, who has never been dry in night. This is three times more common in boys.

- *Pathogenesis* is multifactorial and could be related to sleep disorder, genetic, psychologic causes, or reduced nocturnal secretion of antidiuretic hormone.
- Less than 3% cases have organic etiology such as obstructive uropathy or urinary tract infections.
- There might be a delay in neurological maturation to control bladder sphincter; associated with mental retardation or spinal cord abnormalities.
- Children who undergo training late (after 24 months) are prone to develop late nocturnal bladder control; recommended age to begin toilet training is around 12–18 months.
- *Physiologic factors* have been studied the most. These include some role singly or together for: Hyposecretion of arginine vasopressin (AVP), decreased responsiveness to low urine osmolality, loss of circadian rhythm of ADH secretion, altered AVP receptor function in the tubule, diminished capacity to be aroused, and altered sleep architecture.
- Around 15% of the 5-year-olds have primary enuresis; approximately 15% enuretics resolve their symptoms each year and about 5% of ten-year-old and 1% of the adolescents remain enuretic.

B. Secondary Enuresis

The child had been dry for several (at least 6) months and again starts bedwetting. In such cases, look for the underlying causes. Too enthusiastic and immature toilet training can result in secondary enuresis. Other causes include emotional stress, parent–child maladjustment, urinary tract infections, diabetes mellitus, or diabetes insipidus. Secondary enuresis is frequently associated with stressful or traumatic events.

C. Nocturnal and Diurnal Enureses

Nocturnal and diurnal enureses refer to voiding of urine during night-time and while awake, respectively. Diurnal enuresis is more common in girls, is usually due to micturition deferral (waiting till the last moment to pass urine, and then being unable to hold any longer) in the preschool child, and usually settles by age 9 years. Stress incontinence, urinary tract infection, and diabetes are the other causes of diurnal enuresis. When both diurnal and nocturnal enureses are present, abnormalities of the urinary tract or voiding disorders are likely.

Chronic constipation is an important risk factor for enuresis and encopresis occurs in about 15% of the enuretics.

EVALUATION

History and examination should be able to rule out the possibility of any underlying neurological disorder, polyuric conditions (diabetes mellitus, diabetes insipidus, chronic renal failure) and bacterial cystitis.

- Evaluation in case of primary nocturnal enuresis involves *routine urine examination* including osmolality, microscopy, sugar, and culture.
- A *frequency void chart* often helps to differentiate primary nocturnal enuresis from voiding dysfunction. The normal frequency of daytime void in a child is 4–7 times per day. A frequency of more than 8 times or at duration of less than 2 hours is considered abnormal.

- A good *ultrasonogram* on full bladder can also give a rough estimate of bladder capacity.
- *Urodynamic study* is needed to assess bladder capacity and detrusor pressures in a child who has an abnormal frequency void chart.

Treatment	Nocturnal Enuresis

Management should be aimed at completely stopping the enuresis. After establishing the diagnosis of primary nocturnal enuresis, a treatment plan should be discussed. The child's cooperation in the management plan is essential. Any serious attempt to treat the condition should begin only beyond 7–8 years of age as enuresis interferes with socialization and behavior in older children.

A. Non-pharmacological Methods

Non-pharmacological management is effective in 30% cases and consists of behavior modification, bladder strengthening exercises and alarm systems.

1. Behavioral Treatment

Behavioral treatment is the first mode of therapy for a child with enuresis without any disorder of the genitourinary tract.
- Counseling and reassurance to the family is the most essential step. They need to be assured of the benign nature of the condition, and high spontaneous resolution rate.
- Ask the parents to maintain a diary record of dry nights; reward the child for such nights.
- Parents should provide emotional support to the child, avoid criticism, and change the bed sheets without child's notice.
- Avoid punitive measures. Positive reinforcement has been shown to have a success rate of more than 85%.
- Children should have an early dinner and appropriate fluids with dinner. It is recommended to avoid any form of fluid at least 2–3 hours prior to sleep. Ask the child to void before going to sleep.
- Repeated waking to void is not helpful, though using an alarm clock to wake the child once 2–3 hours after falling asleep is indicated. Child should be fully aroused and walk unaided to the toilet to urinate.

2. Behavior Conditioning

Behavior conditioning with use of alarms is extremely effective. The alarm is either a sound or a vibratory device and rings as soon as voiding starts, and is helpful in training the child to improve bladder capacity and avoid enuresis. It requires long-term use and approximately 70% improve on this therapy. Relapse rates are lower than that with pharmacotherapy.

3. Bladder Training Exercises

Daytime bladder exercises are useful, especially in those with low functional bladder capacity. (*i*) Hold urine as long as possible during the day; (*ii*) practice repeated starting and stopping the stream at the toilet bowl; and (*iii*) practice getting up from bed and going to the bathroom at bedtime before sleep.

4. Caffeine Reduction

Some dietary products like soft drinks, cocoa and chocolates have significant amount of caffeine, which is known to have a diuretic action. Excessive consumption of these items can result in enuresis and should be avoided.

B. Drug Therapy

Medications are indicated only in children older than 6 years who fail behavioral treatment. Drugs used are (*i*) imipramine; (*ii*) desmopressin (DDAVP); and (*iii*) oxybutinin.

- *Desmopressin acetate* (DDAVP) orally or intranasally (nasal spray, 10 µg per spray) at bedtime. It acts by reducing the nocturnal urine output to a volume less than the functional bladder capacity. Start with 10 µg given at bedtime daily and increase gradually by 10 µg/per week to a maximum of 40 µg per day. If effective, it should be used for 3–6 months. Success rate is 40–60%, relapse rate 90%. Costly drug, has a fast onset of action.
- *Oxybutinin* is an anticholinergic agent that can be used in those above 6 years of age. It reduces uninhibited bladder contractions and useful in children manifesting with urgency and urge incontinence during the daytime.
- Tab *Imipramine* (25, 50 mg tabs): 6–8 yr (25 mg), 9–12 yr (50 mg), >12 yr (75 mg) once a day at bedtime. It is a tricyclic antidepressant which alters the arousal-sleep mechanism. Success rate 30–60%, relapse rate 90%. Common side effects are drowsiness, lethargy, and sleep disturbances.

The various treatment modalities available are not used exclusive of each other and often a combination works best. Failure of one form of therapy should result in substitution or addition of another. The best treatment option, if behavioral therapy fails, is the use of combination therapy with alarms and drugs simultaneously.

Nocturnal Enuresis

1. Primary nocturnal enuresis is defined as repeated passage of urine in clothes/bed during night in a child more than 5 years of age.
2. Primary enuresis needs to be differentiated from secondary enuresis, where the child had been dry for at least 6 months, before starting bedwetting.
3. Behavioral modification, bladder training exercises, use of alarm systems, and desmopressin (DDAVP) either singly or in combination are the treatment modalities.
4. Relapse rate after any treatment is high.

Caldwell PH, Nankivell G, Sureshkumar P. Simple behavioural interventions for nocturnal enuresis in children. *Cochrane Database Syst Rev.* 2013;(7):CD003637.

Roth EB, Austin PF. Evaluation and treatment of nonmonosymptomatic enuresis. *Pediatr Rev.* 2014;35:430–6.

Traisman ES. Enuresis: evaluation and treatment. *Pediatr Ann.* 2015;44:133–7.

van de Walle J, Rittig S, Bauer S, et al; American Academy of Pediatrics; European Society for Paediatric Urology; European Society for Paediatric Nephrology; International Children's Continence Society. Practical consensus guidelines for the management of enuresis. *Eur J Pediatr.* 2012;171:971–83.

2.10 STUTTERING, TICS AND NAIL BITING

STUTTERING (STAMMERING)

It is characterized by difficulty in pronouncing the initial consonants, pausing, and spasmodic repetition of same syllables. Stuttering presents usually during the preschool years (2 to 5 years) which is the stage of rapid acquisition of language. The child becomes more hesitant. Stammering aggravates, if the child is reminded or corrected when stammering. It is also exacerbated by stress or excitement, eg, while speaking in front of an audience. Stuttering is reduced or absent in low stress situations like, talking to toys or pets, singing, etc. The difficulty generally resolves spontaneously although 1% children continue to have significant stuttering.

Management Parents of young children with stuttering should be reassured for the self-regression of the problem. The child should not be teased or reprimanded when stuttering. They should be asked to recite a poem and to read loudly. The fluency of speech improves, if they are made to practice. In younger children, stuttering disappears by about six years but older children need emotional support. Specialty advice/management should be requisitioned, if it persists for longer than 6 months or appears *de novo* after 5 years of age. Speech therapy is very helpful in the management.

TICS

Tics is a habit disorder, characterized by involuntary, sudden, rapid, repetitive, non-rhythmic, stereotyped movements, or phonic productions. The range of tic symptoms is almost limitless with muscles of the face, neck, shoulder, trunk, and hands being commonly involved. Most frequently there is lip smacking, tongue thrusting, eye blinking, shoulder jerking, and twitching of fingers. Tics are exacerbated by anxiety, excitement, anger or fatigue, and they are reduced by absorbing activity or sleep. Usual age is 6 years with a peak of prevalence in pre-adolescent years.

Tics must be differentiated from seizure disorders (which are usually characterized by loss of ability to interact during the episode and amnesia for the event) and occasionally EEG may be required. Tics may be transient (ie, present for <12 months) or chronic (for >12 months). *Gilles de la Tourette syndrome* is a chronic neuropsychiatric disorder characterized by the presence of involuntary motor and phonic tics that wax and wane.

Management Parents should be counseled about spontaneous resolving nature of the disorder and behavior therapy. Relaxation exercises have proven efficacy. Medications have associated side effects and in many cases supportive management alone is effective. However, when tics are interfering with social development or school functioning, treatment is indicated. Haloperidol, pimozide and risperidone can be used. Botulinum toxin is also effective.

NAIL BITING

Nail biting, the habit of biting nails is a common oral habit, affecting around 30% of children between the age of 7 and 10 years and 45% of adolescents.

Likely etiology includes emotional insecurity, stress, imitation of family members, transference from thumb-sucking, and poorly manicured nails, etc. Complications include damage to the cuticle and nails, secondary bacterial infection, bleeding, inflammation, and dental problems.

Management should address the precipitating causes of stress and if no stressful condition is discovered, then attention should be focused on efforts to build up the child's self-confidence and esteem. Care of nails, behavioral modification, positive reinforcement, relaxation exercise, and positive emotional support will help.

Woods DW, Houghton DC. Evidence-based psychosocial treatments for pediatric body-focused repetitive behavior disorders. *J Clin Child Adolesc Psychol.* 2016;45:227–40.

Murphy TK, Lewin AB, Storch EA, Stock S; American Academy of Child and Adolescent Psychiatry (AACAP) Committee on Quality Issues (CQI). Practice parameter for the assessment and treatment of children and adolescents with tic disorders. *J Am Acad Child Adolesc Psychiatry.* 2013;52:1341–59.

2.11 MASTURBATION

Masturbation is referred to as stimulation of one's own genitals for derivation of pleasure. This phenomenon is universal from infancy to adulthood.

In toddlers, masturbation may be a manifestation of systemic problem such as abdominal pain, motor tics, epilepsy, or other unusual behavioral patterns. It may be triggered by vulvovaginitis or urethral irritation. By 8 years, 10% of girls and 30% of boys are reported to engage in this activity, increasing to 90% by adolescence.

Compulsive, intense masturbation that interrupts other activities, involves objects or is persistently public is not normative and usually signals a disturbance in some aspect of the child's emotional life. Masturbation may also be the result of an experience of sexual exploitation or an exposure to explicit sexual materials or events.

Treatment	Masturbation

- Children need counseling, modeling, and suggestions that this behavior should be private. Punishment only solidifies this behavior.
- Preschoolers and children should be provided with non-genital tactile input such as rocking and holding. Try to change the environment where such activity occurs. Any underlying cause such as sexual exploitation should be identified.
- Masturbation should be accepted as a normal aspect in a child's life. Adolescents should be counseled that such activities do not cause physical or mental harm and they should not feel guilty about it.
- Parents should be counseled regarding normal nature of this type of behavior in adolescence. About 90% of the boys and 33% of girls are engaged in such activities and it does not cause any physical or mental disturbance.
- Parents should not worry until masturbation is compulsive or results in isolation of the child from healthy interpersonal relationships.

ADOLESCENT BEHAVIORAL DISORDERS

2.12 ANOREXIA NERVOSA

This is an eating disorder occurring more commonly in adolescent girls and young women shortly after completion of puberty. The male to female ratio is 1:10 with a bimodal age distribution with one peak at 14.5 years and other at 18 years. In western countries, it occurs in 1% of all adolescent girls. The disorder is characterized by deliberate weight loss induced by the adolescent by reducing food intake, in relentless pursuit of thinness.

ETIOLOGY

Anorexia nervosa is more common in girls with excessive dependence, low self-esteem, high anxiety and affective disorder. Their families are overprotective. It is now thought to be a disorder of mood or problem in identity development. Hypothalamic abnormalities are noted in them prior to onset of weight loss. Although the fundamental cause is not clear, a complex interaction between sociocultural, biological and psychological factors contributes to its causation.

DIAGNOSTIC CRITERIA

1. Persistent restriction of energy intake leading to significantly low body weight;
2. Either an intense fear of gaining weight or of becoming fat, or persistent behavior that interferes with weight gain; and
3. Disturbance in the way one's body weight or shape is experienced.

CLINICAL MANIFESTATIONS

- Young females begin to eat less and less food, leading to profound weight loss and emaciation. Typically, there is avoidance of 'fattening foods' with or without self-induced vomiting or purging. There may be a history of excessive exercise, use of appetite suppressants, or diuretics. Physical profile of starvation is present.
- Affected girl will complain of abdominal pain and bloating of abdomen even with ingestion of small amounts of food.
- There is disorder of hypothalamic-pituitary axis, manifesting as amenorrhea.
- Weight loss more than 30% leads to lethargy, cachexia, and generalized weakness.
- There is under-nutrition of varying severity, with resulting secondary endocrine and metabolic changes and disturbance of bodily functions.
- The mortality is 10% and is due to electrolyte imbalance, cardiac arrhythmias or congestive heart failure, hypothermia, and hypotension. Bone marrow hypoplasia, constipation, esophagitis, hypophosphatemia, potassium depletion, hypochloremic alkalosis, and elevation of BUN may also be present.

Treatment	Anorexia Nervosa

Treatment involves a combined approach of (*i*) individual and family psychotherapy, (*ii*) behavioral modification, and (*iii*) nutritional rehabilitation. Those with associated depression may require antidepressants.

Role of parents is very important and they should be fully involved in their child's therapy. Psychotherapy helps children improve their self-esteem, peer relationship, and resolving parental conflicts.

The adolescent needs to be hospitalized, if there is severe malnutrition or danger of suicide is present, otherwise they can be treated in outpatient setting. Diet therapy should be instituted after explaining the problems related with starvation. Diet should be increased slowly, and weight gain is monitored. The ultimate target should be to achieve the weight and height appropriate for age.

BULIMIA NERVOSA

Bulimia nervosa is an associated disorder characterized by repeated bouts of overeating and an excessive preoccupation with the control of bodyweight, leading the patient to adopt extreme measures so as to counter the 'fattening' effects of ingested foods.

Lock J, La Via MC; American Academy of Child and Adolescent Psychiatry (AACAP) Committee on Quality Issues (CQI). Practice parameter for the assessment and treatment of children and adolescents with eating disorders. *J Am Acad Child Adolesc Psychiatry*. 2015;54:412–25.

2.13 CONDUCT DISORDERS

All children and adolescent have some disruptive behaviors while growing up. These behaviors come to attention when they become troublesome or unsettling and are experienced by a parent, teacher, clinician or other adults. When such disruptive behavior becomes repetitive, persistent (ie, at least 12 months) and threatens the rights of other people or their property, a diagnosis of conduct disorder is made.

ETIOLOGY

Conduct disorders are frequently associated with adverse family or school environments including unsatisfactory family relationship and failure at school, and is more commonly noted in boys. Examples are physical fighting, stealing, deceitfulness, lying, destruction of property, use of a weapon, robbing, physical cruelty, and repeated attempts to run from home.

PATTERNS

Two distinct groups of children and adolescents have conduct disorder:

Under-socialized These children have impairment of interpersonal relationships. They are unpopular, do not have any close friends and prefer a state of generalized social isolation. These children may lack empathy for peers and are hostile and argumentative towards adults. This form of aggressive and undersocialized behavior is persistent, typically occurring at school, at home and in the community.

Socialized Pattern of conduct disorder consists of participation in antisocial behavior (eg, criminal acts) in the context of peer groups. Interpersonal attachment binding among peers is strong but relationships with adults are inconsistent and characterized by confrontation with authority.

CLINICAL FEATURES

Antisocial behavior is characterized by a repetitive and persistent pattern of unsocial, aggressive, or defiant conduct. Such behavior should amount to major violations of age appropriate social expectations, and is thus more severe than ordinary childish mischief or adolescent rebelliousness. Isolated acts are not included. But, when a child or adolescent indulges in premeditated, purposeful, unlawful activities habitually and repeatedly, he is considered to have a conduct disorder or antisocial behavior.

Oppositional defiant disorders refer to recurrent patterns of defiant, disobedient and hostile behavior towards authority; eg, losing temper, arguing with adults, defying or refusing to comply with requests or rules of adults, annoying behavior, blaming others, and being irritable, spiteful and resentful. However, there is absence of more severe unsocial or aggressive acts that violate the law or the rights of others.

The diagnosis is usually not made unless the duration of the defiant behavior has been more than 6 months. These disorders are usually seen in children below 10 years.

Treatment	**Conduct Disorders**

These children require team approach for the management. The cause for such behavior should be sorted out first. Family members should be more loving and should be calm when dealing with such children and try to understand the root of the problems. Children should be given rehabilitation training for their behavior pattern and improve their self-esteem. If individual therapy is not effective, group therapy should be tried. Drug therapy is not of much use.

Parents should try to change the environment when conflict arises and should not use physical punishment to change their behavior pattern. They should be counseled to improve parent–child communication and for reinforcement of appropriate and healthy behavior.

2.14 JUVENILE DELINQUENCY

Juvenile delinquent is a child who commits an act considered as a crime for adults.

CAUSES

1. *Psychological* Family dispute is the major factor in the development of delinquent activity. The child learns social norms from the parents and parents guide them in development of behavior. If child abuse and neglect or dispute exists in the family, they become aggressive and violent. This also results in lack of development of emotions and attachment.

2. *Sociological* Problems in schools, educational system, environmental desolation, poverty and peer influence may lead to delinquent behavior. Schools are the primary site of formal education for all children in their most formative years. A poor academic performance leads to commission of delinquent acts.

3. *Physical* Children with minimal brain dysfunction, mental retardation, and chromosomal anomalies such as XYY are not able to control their emotions and impulse and indulge in delinquent activity.

MANAGEMENT

Management requires team approach. The family members have the primary responsibility. Social workers, psychologists, psychiatrists, pediatricians, schoolteachers and police should help these children. The child should be rehabilitated and educated for adjustment in society. These children should be provided opportunity to work and recreational facilities so as to change their behavior.

2.15 ATTENTION DEFICIT HYPERACTIVITY DISORDER

Attention deficit hyperactivity disorder (ADHD), a common childhood neurobehavioral disorder, is characterized by persistent inattention, hyperactivity, and impulsivity, for at least consecutive 6 months, starting in a child prior to 12 years of age.

ETIOLOGY

ADHD is attributable to abnormal dopamine transmission in the frontal lobes and the frontostriatal circuitry. Many children with symptoms suggestive of ADHD have neurologic or psychiatric conditions that are the cause of those symptoms or these may be coexisting with ADHD. These include sleep disorders, epilepsy, and learning disorders.

CLINICAL FEATURES

The diagnosis of ADHD is based on specific clinical criteria, given by American Psychiatric Association in 2013 and diagnostic tool based on these criteria. The criteria provide list of symptom for inattention and for hyperactive-impulsive behavior.

I. *Six or more of the following symptoms of inattention for at least 6 months:*
1. Makes careless mistakes in schoolwork, work, or other activities.
2. Has difficulty in keeping attention on tasks or play activities.
3. Does not seem to listen when spoken to directly.
4. Does not follow instructions and fails to finish schoolwork, chores, or duties in the workplace
5. Has trouble organizing activities.
6. Avoids, dislikes, or doesn't want to do things that take a lot of mental effort
7. Loses things needed for tasks and activities (eg toys, school assignments, pencils, books, or tools).
8. Easily distracted.
9. Is forgetful in daily activities.

II. *Six or more of the following symptoms of hyperactivity-impulsivity have been present for at least 6 months to an extent that is disruptive and inappropriate for developmental level:*

Hyperactivity
1. Fidgets with hands or feet or squirms in seat.
2. Gets up from seat when remaining in seat is expected.
3. Runs about or climbs when and where it is not appropriate (adolescents or adults may feel very restless).
4. Has trouble playing or enjoying leisure activities quietly.
5. Acts as if "driven by a motor" and is often "on the go"
6. Talks excessively.

Impulsivity
7. Blurts out answers before questions have been finished.
8. Has trouble waiting one's turn.
9. Interrupts or intrudes on others (eg, butts into conversations or games).

| Case Study | Hyperactive Child |

A 7-year-old male is brought to the OPD with complaints of ARI. While entering the OPD, the child is noticed pushing other children out of the way. The physician had previously noted that the child was repeatedly jumping from the bench to the ground. However, on entering the doctor's room, he is an alert, quiet child who, however, keeps getting distracted by outside noises. On inquiry, the parents agreed that the child is always very active at home and frequently engages in dangerous activities like jumping from walls, breaking household objects, running on the road among heavy traffic, etc. They also informed about similar complaints from teachers. There is a history of changing three schools due to the educational problems and taking opinion from multiple doctors, all of whom advised that child is 'hyperactive' and would grow out of the problem.

Learning points
1. As the parents have consulted many doctors previously, they did not even complain of the behavioral problem. The physician noted the child's overactivity and lack of inhibition and probed further.
2. In an unfamiliar situation, the child may in fact be not hyperactive; as in the doctor's chamber.
3. 'Growing out of hyperactivity', and not 'coping with studies' are common misconceptions among doctors, educationists, and parents.

The course of ADHD is highly variable. Symptoms may persist into adolescence or adult life; they may remit at puberty; or the hyperactivity may disappear, but the decreased attention span and impulse-control problem may persist.

EVALUATION

Routine diagnostic testing is not needed in the evaluation of a child for ADHD. Hearing and vision screening and evaluation for learning disability (especially when problems are specifically restricted to the school or during studies) should be undertaken. Hypothyroidism, hyperthyroidism, phenylketonuria and excessive lead exposure have all been reported to manifest with ADHD. Investigations for these disorders may be carried out depending on clinical findings. Imaging studies for a stable child with ADHD (without any coexisting conditions) are not indicated.

INCLEN Diagnostic Tool for ADHD (INDT-ADHD) is an Indian diagnostic tool based on DSM-IV and available in multiple Indian languages. Other diagnostic tools include Conners 3 parent and teacher rating scales, and Vanderbilt parent scale.

| Treatment | ADHD |

Treatment of ADHD is multidisciplinary involving parents, teachers, behavioral therapist, clinical psychologist, pediatrician, and social worker.
- *Behavioral and psychological treatment* involves reinforcing positive behaviors by praise or by using daily consistency charts ('star' or 'happy face' charts), providing a distraction free environment, social skills training, and adapting tasks to

ensure ease of completion (simple clear commands, addressing tasks one at a time, etc).

- *Pharmacotherapy* involves the use of *stimulant* medications [methylphenidate, norepinephrine-specific reuptake inhibitors (atomoxetine), dextroamphetamine, etc.], and nonstimulant medications (*tricyclic antidepressants*—desipramine, alpha-adrenergic agonists).
- *Nonpharmacologic therapies* like biofeedback programs are less effective than stimulants but when used with drugs, may improve social skills. Nutritional supplements or exclusion diets are not of much use.

Attention Deficit Hyperactivity Disorder

1. Persistent inattention, hyperactivity, and impulsivity for at least 6 months should alert to a possibility of attention deficit hyperactivity disorder (ADHD), starting in children before 12 years of age.
2. The diagnosis should be considered, if the problem behavior is present in at least 2 different settings, eg home, school, play, social situations, tuition, etc.
3. Behavioral management is the initial treatment modality.
4. Methylphenidate and atomoxetine are the most commonly used drugs for therapy.
5. Best success rate is achieved with a combination of behavioral and drug therapy.

Cerrillo-Urbina AJ, García-Hermoso A, Sánchez-López M, et al. The effects of physical exercise in children with attention deficit hyperactivity disorder: a systematic review and meta-analysis of randomized control trials. *Child Care Health Dev.* 2015;4179–88.

Chan E, Fogler JM, Hammerness PG. Treatment of attention-deficit/hyperactivity disorder in adolescents: a systematic review. *JAMA.* 2016;315:1997-2008.

Punja S, Shamseer L, Hartling L, et al. Amphetamines for attention deficit hyperactivity disorder (ADHD) in children and adolescents. *Cochrane Database Syst Rev.* 2016;2:CD009996.

Richardson M, Moore DA, Gwernan-Jones R, et al. Non-pharmacological interventions for attention-deficit/hyperactivity disorder (ADHD) delivered in school settings: systematic reviews of quantitative and qualitative research. *Health Technol Assess.* 2015;19:1–470.

Storebø OJ, Krogh HB, Ramstad E, et al. Methylphenidate for attention-deficit/hyperactivity disorder in children and adolescents: Cochrane systematic review with meta-analyses and trial sequential analyses of randomised clinical trials. *BMJ.* 2015 Nov 25;351:h5203.

Subcommittee on Attention-Deficit/Hyperactivity Disorder; Steering Committee on Quality Improvement and Management, Wolraich M, Brown L, Brown RT, et al. ADHD: clinical practice guideline for the diagnosis, evaluation, and treatment of attention-deficit/hyperactivity disorder in children and adolescents. *Pediatrics.* 2011;128:1007–22.

2.16 AUTISM

Autism spectrum disorders (ASD) previously also known as pervasive developmental disorders (PDD) are a continuum of associated cognitive and neurobehavioral disorders, with the following core defining features: Deficits in social communication and restricted and repetitive patterns of behavior interest and activities. Childhood autism is the commonest disorder in this spectrum.

Recently, *autism has been classified as a **disability** for purpose of availing benefits under various government schemes.

EPIDEMIOLOGY

Worldwide prevalence of autism spectrum disorder is around 6 per 1000. Cognitive functions can range from profound mental retardation to above average on IQ tests. Male to female ratio is 4:1 for milder form and 1.3:1 with severe cognitive impairment.

CLINICAL FEATURES

- The average age of diagnosis of autism is 3–6 years but can be reliably diagnosed in children as young as 2 years.
- The correct diagnosis is often delayed or missed altogether with many children diagnosed as hearing deficient, learning disabled, ADHD, or mental retardation.
- Autism characteristics observable in children younger than 3 years include: *Decreased use of non-verbal behavior* (eye-to-eye gaze, facial expressions, body postures, gestures); *lack of social or emotional reciprocity:* lack of seeking to share enjoyment, interests or achievements with other people (absent showing or pointing); and *delayed or absent language skills.*

DIAGNOSIS

A two-level approach has been recommended for diagnosis of autism in which development screening as part of routine well-child care followed by an ASD-specific screen for children with developmental delay is at level 1. Level 2 involves formal diagnostic procedures for ASD.

The modified checklist for Autism in Toddlers (M-CHAT), Pervasive Developmental Disorders Screening Test-II (PDDST-II), and Social Communication Questionnaire (for children above 4 years of age) are some of the *screening instruments.*

INCLEN Diagnostic Tool for Autism Spectrum Disorders (INDT-ASD) and Indian Scale for Assessment of Autism (ISAA) are the two DSM-IV based tools for assessment of autism. These are also approved by the Government of India for certification of the disease for disability benefits. The former is available in many Indian languages.

Childhood Autism Rating Scale II (CARS-II), Autism Diagnostic Interview-Revised (ADI-R), and Autism Diagnostic Observation Schedule-General (ADOS-G) are the other *diagnostic instruments* for ASD.

Hearing evaluation is essential both to guard against misdiagnosis and because of the presence of associated significant hearing loss.

Treatment	Autism

Management of ASD is a life-long process and requires a multi-disciplinary team. It involves speech and language therapy, special education, parent education, and pharmacotherapy for co-morbid conditions or symptoms like ADHD, anxiety, epilepsy, sleep problems, etc.

Stimulants for hyperactivity, risperidone for maladaptive behaviors, and SSRIs for rigidity/repetitive behaviors are the commonly used drugs for ASD.

Autism

1. Autism spectrum disorders (ASD) are characterized by deficits in social communications, repetitive behavior, and lack in interest and activities. The IQ is usually normal.
2. Average age of diagnosis is 3–6 years. It is important to screen for autism at 18 months for early recognition.
3. Delay in verbal/non-verbal communication is the most important early pointer to autism.
4. Management of autism is life-long, consisting of individualized multiple disciplinary approach.

Kendall T, Megnin-Viggars O, Gould N; Guideline Development Group. Management of autism in children and young people: summary of NICE and SCIE guidance. *BMJ*. 2013;347:f4865.

McGuire K, Fung LK, Hagopian L, *et al.* Irritability and problem behavior in autism spectrum disorder: a practice pathway for pediatric primary care. *Pediatrics*. 2016;137Suppl 2:S136–48.

Schaefer GB, Mendelsohn NJ; Professional Practice and Guidelines Committee. Clinical genetics evaluation in identifying the etiology of autism spectrum disorders: 2013 guideline revisions. *Genet Med*. 2013;15:399–407.

Zwaigenbaum L, Bauman ML, Choueiri R, *et al.* Early intervention for children with autism spectrum disorder under 3 years of age: recommendations for practice and research. *Pediatrics*. 2015;136Suppl 1:S60–81.

Zwaigenbaum L, Bauman ML, Fein D, *et al.* Early screening of autism spectrum disorder: recommendations for practice and research. *Pediatrics*. 2015;136Suppl 1:S41–59.

Zwaigenbaum L, Bauman ML, Stone WL, *et al.* Early identification of autism spectrum disorder: Recommendations for Practice and Research. *Pediatrics*. 2015 Oct;136Suppl 1:S10–40.

2.17 LEARNING DISORDERS

Learning disorders (previously learning disabilities) present as significant, unexpected, specific, and persistent difficulties in the acquisition and use of efficient reading (*dyslexia*), writing (*dysgraphia*), or mathematical (*dyscalculia*) abilities; despite conventional instructions, intact senses, normal intelligence, proper motivation and adequate sociocultural opportunity. The child with learning disorder is one who does not meet expectations for academic performance in school but has intelligence in the normal range.

Learning disorders constitute an invisible handicap and are an important cause of poor school performance and even dropout. The incidence of dyslexia, dyscalculia, and dysgraphia, in primary schoolchildren in India has been reported to be 2.2%, 5.5%, and 14%, respectively.

TYPOLOGY

Dyslexia (Reading Disorder)

Reading achievement is below that expected for the age and intelligence of the child. Oral reading is characterized by distortions, substitutions, or omissions. Both oral and silent reading are characterized by slowness and errors in comprehension. Children with dyslexia have a deficit at the level of the single word (ie, word recognition skills) and not in text processing ability (ie, comprehension). The cause of this deficit is due to processing problems involving language, particularly phonologic processing.

Age at diagnosis Although, symptoms of reading difficulties may occur as early as kindergarten, dyslexia is usually not diagnosed until the grade I because formal reading instructions usually begin at that age. A child with dyslexia associated with high IQ may be diagnosed still later, at around IV grade.

Dyscalculia (Mathematical Disorder)

Dyscalculia is estimated to constitute 20% of all learning disorders. It is difficult to diagnose the disorder before II/III grades (V grade or later for those with high IQ).

Dysgraphia (Disorder of Written Expression)

It consists of a combination of difficulties in the ability to compose written texts evidenced by grammatical or punctuation errors within sentences, poor paragraph organization, multiple spelling errors, and excessively poor handwriting. This diagnosis is generally not given, if there are only spelling errors or poor handwriting in the absence of other impairment in written expression. Usually, apparent by II grade and is rare when not associated with other learning disorders.

Dyscalculia and dysgraphia are commonly associated with dyslexia and they rarely occur alone.

ETIOLOGY

Learning disorders are presumed to be due to CNS (temporo-parieto-occipital) dysfunction and result from impairment in one or more processes related to perceiving, thinking, remembering or learning. Dyslexia is both familial and heritable but does not show classical Mendelian inheritance. The rate among siblings of affected persons is around 40%. Learning disorders are frequently found in association with a variety of general medical conditions (eg, lead poisoning, fetal alcohol syndrome, fragile-X syndrome).

DIAGNOSIS

Learning disorder is diagnosed when achievement on individually administered standardized tests in reading, mathematics, or written expression is <2SD than that expected for that age, schooling and level of intelligence (IQ).

Grade Level Assessment Device for Children and the **NIMHANS Index** are Indian tools for assessment of LD. The Woodcock-Johnson tests of achievement are also useful for assessment.

Currently, it is difficult to diagnose a learning disorder conclusively until the child is about 8–9 years old. Learning disorder can only be diagnosed, if the opportunity for learning is present.

Early markers of learning disorders are listed below.

1. Language delay (by 2½ years, most children should be able to put sentences together).
2. Pronunciation problems (by 3 years, others should understand what children say more than half of the time).
3. Slow vocabulary growth.
4. Difficulty rhyming words (or confusing words that sound alike).
5. Trouble learning numbers, alphabet, days of the week, colors and shapes.

6. Repeated spelling mistakes; untidy and illegible handwriting with poor sequencing.

7. Inability to perform simple mathematical calculations correctly.

8. Slow to learn the connection between letters and sounds, slow reading, confuses basic words (run, eat, want).

9. Makes consistent reading and spelling errors including letter reversal.

10. Transposes number sequences and confuses arithmetic signs.

Schoolgoing children may present with problems more commonly centred on school performance, sometimes without realizing the difficulty in one particular subject. School drop-out rate for children or adolescents with learning disorders is about 40%.

DIFFERENTIAL DIAGNOSIS

Other common reasons for poor learning ability are normal variations in academic achievement, lack of opportunity or motivation, poor teaching, and sociocultural factors. Impaired vision and hearing, ADHD, mental retardation, autistic spectrum disorder, chronic infections, anemia, parasitic infections, and emotional block are some other causes for poor school performance.

With the **Right to Education** law in force, all children with LD are mandated to be taught in regular school with additional inputs, as appropriate.

Treatment	Learning Disorder

Children with learning disabilities require early identification, timely specialized assessments, and interventions involving home, school, community and workplace settings. The interventions need to be appropriate for each individual's learning disability subtype.

- *In younger children*, the focus is on *remediation*, that includes: intensive instruction of appropriate duration provided by trained teachers. Special reading programs need to be designed. To learn to read, children must discover that spoken words can be broken down into smaller units of sound, that letters on the page represent these sounds, and that written words have the same number and sequence of sounds heard in the spoken word. Phoneme awareness also needs to be taught explicitly.

- *When the child enters the more time demanding setting of secondary school, the emphasis shifts to the important role of providing accommodations.* Accommodations include: Extra time; allow use of laptop computers with spell checkers, tape recorders; or recorded books; providing access to lecture notes; alternatives to MCQs; and separate quiet room for taking tests. Many of these remediation measures are allowed by the CBSE and many of the state examination boards.

With early identification and intervention, the prognosis is good in majority. Residua of the phonologic deficit persist, so that reading remains effortful, even for the brightest people with childhood histories of dyslexia.

Chacko A, Uderman J, Feirsen N, et al. Learning and cognitive disorders: multidiscipline treatment approaches. *Child Adolesc Psychiatr Clin N Am.* 2013;22:457–77.

Galuschka K, Ise E, Krick K, Schulte-Körne G. Effectiveness of treatment approaches for children and adolescents with reading

disabilities: a meta-analysis of randomized controlled trials. *PLoS One.* 2014;9(2):e89900.

Schulte EE. Learning disorders: How pediatricians can help. *Cleve Clin J Med.* 2015;82(11 Suppl 1):S24–8.

Tan ML, Ho JJ, Teh KH. Polyunsaturated fatty acids (PUFAs) for children with specific learning disorders. *Cochrane Database Syst Rev.* 2016;9:CD009398.

2.18 IMPACT OF ELECTRONIC MEDIA

There has been exponential advancement in the electronic media. Electronic games, interactive CD-Rom and innovations in television are among the many advances in the last decade. They may represent a mixed blessing for developing children and their parents. Both children as well as adults watch a great deal of television. Viewing peaks between the ages of 2 and 5 years. Children watch much of their television alone and 80% of their viewing is developmentally inappropriate adult fare. Numerous studies have shown that there is an increase in aggression in children immediately after viewing violent content. Research on effect of television on attention, cognition and learning is still not clear.

The new media in vogue today is Internet and computer games. The computer software intended to develop specific processing skills show great promise. Concern about internet is the exposure of child to sexually explicit material. Thus there is need for parental supervision and monitoring.

RECOMMENDATIONS FOR PARENTS

- Parents should be alert to the shows their children see. They should watch the shows their children are watching.
- Avoid using electronic media as baby-sitter.
- Limit the use of media, eg, television should not be viewed for more than 1–2 hours per day.
- Keep television, computer, etc. out of children's bedrooms.
- Turn the television off during mealtimes. Use this time to catch up and connect with each other.
- Do not turn the TV on to see 'if there is something on.'
- Do not make TV the focal point of the house.
- Parents should become media literate, thus be able to evaluate media offerings critically.
- Parents should limit their own television viewing.
- Parents should also insist for better programming for children.

2.19 SLEEP DISORDERS

Disorders of sleep are quite prevalent in childhood but infrequently recognized. They have a significant effect on the quality of life but most are easily treatable.

NORMAL SLEEP

Wakefulness and sleep can be differentiated by 27–28 weeks postconceptional age in the preterm infant. Sleep onset is facilitated by melatonin, which is released by the pineal gland and the release is modified by light intensity (bright light suppresses melatonin release and *vice-versa*). The suprachiasmatic nucleus of the hypothalamus has receptors for melatonin and is the ultimate center for the once-a-day (circadian) rhythm of sleep and wakefulness. After about 3 months of age, the physiological transition from wakefulness is first into non-rapid eye movement sleep, with rapid eye movement sleep occurring 90–140 minutes later.

- Night awakening up to 3 to 7 times is regarded normal in sleep; it often occurs following REM sleep and allows the child to change their posture, address their bladder needs. However, most children return to sleep soon without full awakening.
- Sleep requirements generally decrease with age and it varies from child to child.
- Irregular sleep patterns might result in inattentiveness, irritability, aggressiveness, and social withdrawal. The child may fall asleep in odd hours of day or during the class hours (excessive daytime sleepiness).

SLEEP DISORDERS

Primary sleep disorders are classified as, (*i*) dyssomnias, disorders accompanied by excessive sleepiness (narcolepsy), insomnia, or obstructive sleep apnea; and (*ii*) parasomnias, that manifest as unpleasant and undesirable events intruding onto sleep without altering sleep quality or quantity, eg, sleepwalking, sleep terrors, nightmares, etc. Sleepwalking and sleep terrors may occur throughout the first decade, and most subside by 10–12 years of age.

Management involves combination of lifestyle changes and pharmacotherapy. Short (20–30 min) planned daytime naps at school and another at home may improve alertness. Regular sleeping and wake-up times should be observed. Drug therapy may help.

PRINCIPLES OF SLEEP HYGIENE

Sleep is an essential part of daily routine of children. Inadequate sleep can lead to poor school performance in terms of lack of attention, memory, and concentration. The child can also develop behavioral and mood problems like irritability.

Factors that maintain a good sleep hygiene include good health, exercise, a meaningful and consistent daily schedule, a balanced diet, a bedtime environment that encourages sleep, and a pleasant, relaxing sequence of activities in the hour before bedtime.

1. Set up a routine for bedtime. Bedtime and wake-up time must be the same during school days and holidays. The differences must not be more than an hour.
2. Pre-bedtime routines should prepare the child mentally for bed. These include a warm gentle massage, warm bath, a story telling, or any other pleasurable activity.
3. Avoid vigorous activities like outdoor play, watching television, playing computers or heavy studying just before bed. Avoid heated conversations and scolding just prior to bed.
4. Bedtime food must include light snacks, a heavy meal must be avoided as it might interfere with sleep.
5. Avoid the use of caffeine-containing products like coffee, tea, chocolate beyond the evening hours.
6. The bedroom environment must be conducive to sleep. The room must be dark and quiet. Avoid bright lights in the room during the sleep hours. A small night lamp is permissible, if the child finds darkness frightening. Keep the temperature of the room comfortable for the child, it must be neither too warm nor too cold.
7. Use of bed must be restricted to sleep and ensure that the child does not use bed to eat, watch television, read or listen to radio. Flickering computers and television in the child's bedroom might distract the sleep onset in the child.
8. Ensure good exercise and physical activity for the child during the day hours which must include outdoor play activities. A good exercise promotes good sleep.

Carter KA, Hathaway NE, Lettieri CF. Common sleep disorders in children. *Am Fam Physician.* 2014;89:368–77.

Kotagal S, Chopra A. Pediatric sleep-wake disorders. *Neurol Clin.* 2012;30:1193–212.

Meltzer LJ, Plaufcan MR, Thomas JH, Mindell JA. Sleep problems and sleep disorders in pediatric primary care: treatment recommendations, persistence, and health care utilization. *J Clin Sleep Med.* 2014;10:421–6.

2.20 APPROACH TO A SUSPECTED BEHAVIORAL DISORDER

Childhood behavior is typically considered a problem when the child's behavior, or developmental stage does not match with parental expectations. Inconsistent expectations are most frequent with children under age 3, because some parents are not prepared for the frequent crying, negativism and high energy levels of normal infants and small children. An important aspect of the physician's role is to educate parents about the normal phases and behavior problems that tend to occur at each age.

EVALUATION

1. *Background history* Child's early development of the personality and behavior depends upon the environment in which he is raised. Children raised in emotionally supportive, caring and responsive environment are well adjusted. The type of family, school, community and society has a lot of influence on the overall development of behavior. Hence, it is important to take a detailed history about the place, family and society when dealing with children having behavior problem.
2. *Severity assessment* It is important to find out day-to-day activity of the child and influence on day-to-day activity by this problem. It is also important to assess severity of the problem.

3. *Identify triggers* In order to classify the severity of the problem, it is important to find out the events, nature, duration, frequency and situations that trigger the problem.

ACTION

When problem behaviors arise in children, three approaches can be considered by the physician: (*i*) identify the behavior as age-appropriate and reassure the parents; (*ii*) advise the parents to attempt to stop the unacceptable behavior and/or (*iii*) introduce a new, preferred behavior. Parents need to avoid power struggles and "no-win" situations.

Some principles related to behavioral modification are: People tend to continue a behavior when it is rewarded; they tend to stop a behavior when it is consistently ignored (extinguished) or punished; alternately rewarding and ignoring the same behavior (intermittent reinforcement) is known to prolong a behavior and make it very difficult to suppress. This is one reason, consistency is so important in changing behavior. When change is desired, parents are encouraged to limit their focus to one or two related behaviors. If too many behaviors are addressed simultaneously, the effort will be less effective.

1. Increase Appropriate Behavior

Interventions that are intended to increase the appropriate behaviors use principle of reinforcement and intervention. The reinforcement techniques are: (*i*) social reinforcement (attention, praise), (*ii*) tangible reinforcement (material objects of personal value), and (*iii*) token economy.

2. Decrease Inappropriate Behavior

Those used to decrease inappropriate behavior use the principle of punishment. The punishment techniques are: (*i*) extension, (*ii*) time out for positive reinforcement, (*iii*) response cost, and (*iv*) overcorrection.

3. Skill Development

Children are helped to develop particular skills. Skill training is encouraged in pro-social activities of children such as sharing toys, waiting for turn, asking for helps. This helps the children for joining in-group activities and resolving conflicts. The areas of skill training are: (*i*) problem solving skill, (*ii*) social skills, and (*iii*) anger coping skills.

4. Loving Attitude

Provide supportive, tender and loving care to children with behavior problems. Parents should also be great listeners to understand the exact nature of their problems. Physician should counsel the parents and family members appropriately.

Children who are taught that inappropriate behavior is not going to be tolerated and that appropriate behavior will be consistently rewarded and praised, are learning skills that will lead to lifelong discipline.

Nutritional Disorders

Nutrition is a universal factor, which affects as much as it defines—the health of all children. Nutrition has a powerful impact on maintaining health and preventing disease. The nutritional well-being of children and adolescents is both an outcome and an indicator of national development. Nutrition is also an issue of survival, health, and development for current and succeeding generations.

The increased recognition of the relevance of nutrition as a basic pillar for social and economic development has placed childhood undernutrition among the targets of the first Millennium Development Goal to "eradicate extreme poverty and hunger".

- *Macronutrients* Carbohydrates, fats, and proteins are the chief sources of energy for man, and constitute macro-nutrients.
- *Micronutrients* are nutrients required in tiny amounts, may be a few micrograms per day, and include various minerals and vitamins.

3.1 MACRONUTRIENTS

1. ENERGY

Energy is required for growth, metabolism, maintenance of body temperature, and physical activities. The factors that affect energy requirements are age, sex, type and extent of physical activity, climate, body size and composition, and physiological status such as pregnancy and lactation. Children require energy for growth, whereas pregnant and lactating mothers need additional energy for the growth of fetus, and maintaining milk secretion, respectively. Even when an individual is in a state of complete rest, energy is spent for basal metabolism.

A. Sources of Energy

Carbohydrates, fats, and proteins are the chief sources of energy for man. Of the total energy, at least 10–15% should be provided by proteins, 20–30% by fats, and 50–60% by carbohydrates. The energy obtained from food is usually expressed in terms of thermochemical kilocalories (10^3 calories), also referred to as kilocalories (kcal) or simply Calories (Cal). As per the International system of units, energy requirement of the body is mentioned in Joules [1 calorie = 4.184 Joules, one thermochemical kilocalorie (kcal or Cal) = 4184 Joules (J) or 4.184 kJ]. One gram of carbohydrate or protein provides 4 kcal or 16.7 kJ, while one gram of fat releases 9 kcal or 37.7 kJ of energy.

B. Energy Requirement for Different Ages and Groups

The energy requirement of infants, older children, and adults as recommended by Food and Agriculture Organization of the United Nations (FAO/WHO) in 2004 and adapted for Indian scenario by ICMR 2010 is presented in **Table 3.1**.

Pregnant women require additional supplements of energy giving foods for the growth of the fetus and the deposition of fat which is used during lactation to meet the additional energy needs for milk secretion. The optimal additional needs are estimated as 70–85 kcal per day during the first trimester and 350 kcal per day during the second and third trimesters. Even though malnourished mothers continue to produce good quantity of milk during lactation, additional energy is required for maintaining mother's own nutritional status so that this additional input could be utilized for breastmilk production.

During the period of lactation, additional energy requirement is 600 kcal/day during first 6 months of exclusive breastfeeding and 520 kcal/day for continued breastfeeding from 7–12 months (ICMR, 2010).

2. PROTEINS

Protein is the second most abundant substance in the body, next to water. These are made up of 20 different amino acids. The proteins differ in their arrangement and quantity of amino acids. A few amino acids can be adequately synthesized in the body (*non-essential amino acids*), while others must be supplied in the diet (*essential amino acids*).

Essential amino acids include leucine, isoleucine, lysine, methionine, phenylalanine, threonine, tryptophan, and valine. Histidine and arginine are essential during infancy because their rate of synthesis is inadequate for sustaining the growth.

A. Functions of Protein

Protein helps the child to grow, as the constituent amino acids are necessary for the synthesis of tissues in the body. Protein is essential for the formation of digestive juices, hormones, plasma proteins, enzymes, vitamins, and hemoglobin. Proteins also act as buffers to maintain acid-base equilibrium in the body. They are also a source of energy for the body.

Age	ICMR, 2010		WHO/FAO/UNU 2004	
	Boys	*Girls*	*Boys*	*Girls*
0 to 6 mo	500 (92 kcal/kg)	500 (92 kcal/kg)	80–100 kcal/kg	80–100 kcal/kg
6 to 12 mo	670 (80 kcal/kg)	670 (80 kcal/kg)	77 kcal/kg	77 kcal/kg
1–2 yr	910	830	948	865
2–3 yr	1120	1030	1129	1047
3–4 yr	1230	1150	1252	1156
4–5 yr	1290	1200	1360	1241
5–6 yr	1390	1290	1467	1330
6–7 yr	1510	1400	1573	1428
7–8 yr	1630	1510	1692	1554
8–9 yr	1750	1630	1830	1698
9–10 yr	1890	1740	1978	1854
10–11 yr	2030	1880	2150	2006
11–12 yr	2180	2010	2341	2149
12–13 yr	2370	2140	2548	2276
13–14 yr	2580	2260	2770	2379
14–15 yr	2760	2340	2990	2449
15–16 yr	2890	2390	3178	2491
16–17 yr	2980	2430	3322	2503
17–18 yr	3060	2450	3410	2503

Table 3.1 Recommended Daily Energy Requirements (kcal/d) for Children

*Assuming moderate activity

Excess protein, not used for building tissues or providing energy, is converted by the liver into fat and stored in body tissues.

B. Requirements

Protein requirements of children are given in **Table 3.2.** Indian estimates are higher as these are calculated in terms of the proteins actually present in Indian diets (cereals + legumes + milk).

- An adult eating a standard Indian predominantly vegetarian diet requires 1.0 g/kg body weight of protein daily. If the protein in the diet is obtained from animal sources like egg, meat, fish, or milk; lower intake of protein may be sufficient.
- During pregnancy (assuming 10 kg gestational weight gain), additional requirements are 1, 7, and 23 g/day of high quality protein in 1st, 2nd, and 3rd trimesters, respectively.
- During lactation, an additional daily intake of 23 g of high quality protein during the first six months and 15 g during 6–12 months is required.

C. Protein Quality

Complete Protein

A complete protein contains all of the essential amino acids in relatively the same amount as humans require for maintenance of good health and optimal growth. Protein in the food is obtained either from the animal or vegetable sources. The proteins of animal origin generally have a higher content of essential amino acids. These are,

Table 3.2 Protein Requirements of Children

Age	Requirements (g/kg/d)	
	ICMR (2010)*	*WHO/FAO/UNU 2007*
1–2 mo		1.77
2–3 mo		1.50
3–4 mo	1.16	1.36
4–5 mo		1.24
5–6 mo		1.14
6–12 mo	1.69	1.31
1–2 yr	1.47	1.14
2–3 yr	1.25	0.97
3–4 yr	1.16	0.90
4–5 yr	1.11	0.86
5–6 yr	1.09	0.85
6–9 yr	1.17	0.92
10–12 yr	1.15	0.90
13–15 yr	1.10	0.90
16–18 yr	1.05	0.85

* ICMR requirements are in terms of cereal-pulse-milk based Indian diets for children beyond six months of age.

therefore, classified as biologically complete protein. Proteins from vegetable sources are often biologically incomplete, as these usually lack one or more of the essential amino acids. However, proteins of vegetable origin may be used together in a judicious combination so that limiting essential amino acid in one of these is compensated for by an excess of that amino acid in the complementing protein. Proteins of rice and potato are considered good vegetable proteins.

Biological Value

A high quality protein should be complete as well as digestible. This is measured best by the biological value of the protein. Biological value is calculated as the fraction of absorbed nitrogen retained in the body for growth or maintenance. Egg protein is considered a *reference protein* in this context as it is complete and well digested. The biological value (BV) of egg protein is 100. Biological values of milk, rice, and fish are 75, 67, and 75, respectively. The combination of vegetable proteins may provide all the essential amino acids as in the reference protein. For example, protein from legumes is deficient in methionine whereas cereals are poor in lysine; both taken together in the diet compensate for each other.

> Report of a Joint FAO/WHO/UNU Expert Consultation. Human Energy Requirements, FAO, Food And Nutrition Technical Report Series 1, Rome, 2004. Available from: URL: http://www.fao.org/docrep/007/y5686e/y5686e00.htm. Accessed June 29, 2012.
> Report of a Joint WHO/FAO/UNU Expert Consultation: Protein and amino acid requirements in human nutrition, Technical Report Series No.935, 2007. Available from: URL: http://whqlibdoc.who.int/trs/WHO_TRS_935_eng.pdf . Accessed June 29, 2012.
> Nutrient Requirements and Recommended Dietary Allowances for Indians: A Report of the Expert Group of the Indian Council of Medical Research. Hyderabad: National Institute of Nutrition; 2010.

3. LIPIDS

Lipids are a concentrated source of energy and provide insulation to the body. These also act as carriers for fat-soluble vitamins. Fats improve the palatability of diet and delay gastric emptying. Lipids include triglycerides (fats and oils), phospholipids (lecithin), and sterols (cholesterol); each important to nutrition.

A. Triglycerides

Triglycerides are the most abundant lipids. Food lipids are 95% triglycerides. Lipids stored in the body are 99% triglycerides. These are esters of 3 molecules of fatty acids attached to glycerol. Glycerol molecule is thus similar in all triglycerides while fatty acids differ in the (*i*) length of carbon chain (short chain, medium chain, and long chain); and (*ii*) degree of unsaturation (saturated, monounsaturated, and polyunsaturated).

Saturated fatty acids These are primarily derived from animal sources (except coconut oil) and remain solid at 20–30°C. Palmitic and stearic acids are saturated fatty acids. These can be synthesized in the body from the acetate residues following catabolism of carbohydrates and protein.

Unsaturated fatty acids These are usually liquid at room temperature, and obtained from vegetables, nut, or seed sources. Unsaturated fats may be converted to solid fats by hydrogenation. *Monounsaturated fatty acids* (MUFAs), such as oleic acid, have only one point of unsaturation while *polyunsaturated fatty acids* (PUFAs) have two or more points of unsaturation. Fatty acids with one unsaturated link can also be synthesized in the body, but polyunsaturated fatty acids cannot be adequately synthesized in the body.

Two families of PUFA are important: (*a*) *omega-6 fatty acids* [linoleic acid (LA: 18:2 omega-6) and arachidonic acid (AA: 20:4 omega-6)] and (*b*) *omega-3 fatty acids* [alpha-linolenic acid (ALA: 18:3 omega-3), eicosapentaenoic acid (EPA: 20:5 omega-3) and docosahexaenoic acid (DHA: 22:6 omega-3)].

B. Essential Fatty Acids (EFA)

Polyunsaturated fatty acids are important components of cell membrane, besides being involved as inflammatory mediator precursors for prostaglandin. These should be available in the diet for maintaining good health and are referred to as *essential fatty acids*. At least 3% of energy requirement of an individual should be derived from linoleic and linolenic acids. Important essential fatty acids include linoleic acid, arachidonic acid, linolenic acid, EPA, and DHA.

EPA and DHA lower blood cholesterol and triglyceride concentrations. These may also serve as raw materials for synthesis of eicosanoids (prostaglandins, thromboxane, and leukotrienes). Eicosanoids play an important role in regulation of lipid concentration, blood pressure, immune response, and inflammatory response to injury and infection. EPA produces the series-3 prostanoids, *eg*, PG_3, thromboxane-3 (Tx_3), and PGI_3. PG_3 and Tx_3 inhibit formation of series-2 prostanoids (PG_2 and Tx_2), which favor atherogenesis. DHA is especially active in retina and cerebral cortex.

It has been shown that body can synthesize very small amounts of (*i*) arachidonic acid from ingested linoleic acid; and (*ii*) EPA and DHA from linolenic acid. But the endogenous synthesis is not enough to sustain the body demands, therefore, omega lipids have to be supplied in diet.

Normal diet with vegetable oils is usually sufficient in omega-6 lipids but may lack optimal quantity of omega-3 lipids. Omega-3, especially DHA and EPA are plentiful in fish. Conventional formula milk may contain linoleic acid and linolenic acid but is low in arachidonic acid. Arachidonic acid is plentiful in meat. Mustard oil, safflower oil, corn oil, and sunflower oil are rich in polyunsaturated essential fatty acids.

Deficiency of essential fatty acids in the diet may result in growth retardation, reproductive failure, skin disorders, increased susceptibility to infections, decreased myocardial contractility, renal hypertension, and hemolysis. Selective deficiency of omega-6 fatty acids leads to skin changes while lack of omega-3 results in neurological and visual symptoms.

C. Lecithin

Lecithin is the most important phospholipid. It is a major constituent of cell membranes. Lecithins are not essential in diet as they can be synthesized in the body by liver. Phospholipids also act as emulsifying agents.

D. Cholesterol

Cholesterol is a lipid essential for good health. It is an important constituent of cell membrane. Cholesterol deficiency does not usually occur as it can also be synthesized in the human body in the liver from carbohydrates, protein, or fat. Cholesterol can be transformed into related compounds like hormones, bile, and vitamin D. Cholesterol

Table 3.3 Composition of Circulating Lipoproteins

	Triglyceride	Phospholipid	Cholesterol	Protein
Chylomicron	80–90%	3–6%	2–7%	1–2%
HDL	5%	30%	20%	40–50%
LDL	10%	22%	45%	25%
VLDL	55–65%	15–20%	10–15%	5–10%

HDL: high density lipoprotein; LDL: low density lipoprotein; VLDL: very low density lipoprotein

is found only in animal foods including eggs, liver, kidney, cheese, and *ghee*. Essential fatty acids are essential for transport and breakdown of cholesterol. Excess cholesterol is stored and may lead to atherosclerosis.

E. Recommended Intake of Fats

Total fat intake (beyond infancy) should provide no more than 30% of daily energy intake. Saturated fats should not exceed 10% and *tras* fatty acids should not exceed 1% of total energy intake from fats. A minimum of 6% energy should be derived from PUFA (with at least 2.5% from linoleic acid and 0.5% from linolenic acid). Excess fat contributes to obesity, Type-2 diabetes, cancer, hypertension, and atherosclerosis. It is better to avoid excess of total fats, *trans* fats, saturated fats, and cholesterol, in that order of priority.

F. Circulating Lipoproteins

As soon as the dietary fat reaches the intestine, bile acids identify and emulsify them. Following emulsification, triglycerides are digested by the enzymes, resulting in production of monoglycerides and glycerol. Glycerol, short chain, and medium chain fatty acids are absorbed directly into blood at the portal vein. Monoglycerides and long chain fatty acids cannot be absorbed as such and form *micelles*. Micelles move to intestinal cells, where monoglycerides and fatty acids are reassembled into triglycerides. Triglycerides, cholesterol, and phospholipids along with some apoproteins are assembled into chylomicrons and are released into the lymphatic system. Later, chylomicrons enter the bloodstream.

Lipids in circulation are bound with proteins that serve as transport vehicles. The lipid–protein complex is called **lipoprotein.** Four main types of lipoproteins are formed differing in their size and density. These are known as chylomicrons (rich in triglycerides), high density lipoprotein (HDL), low density lipoprotein (LDL), and very low density lipoprotein (VLDL). Lipoproteins with a higher percentage of lipids have a lower density, ie, LDL and VLDL; those with a higher percentage of proteins have a higher density (HDL). Composition of these lipoproteins is depicted in **Table 3.3.**

High levels of chylomicrons and LDL are associated with a higher risk of cardiovascular diseases. HDL is a protective lipoprotein and high levels tend to protect against the heart diseases.

Cells all over the body remove fat from the passing by chylomicrons. A few remnants, that loiter for long, are removed by the liver. Liver is also an active site of lipid synthesis. The synthesized lipids are transported as VLDL to various organs that need them. The body cells remove triglycerides from the VLDL and convert them to LDL. Liver cells also have special receptors that remove LDL from circulation.

4. CARBOHYDRATES

Carbohydrates provide energy, contribute to taste and texture of foods, preserve foods, and are essential for digestion and assimilation of other foods. They also protect the proteins from being used for energy. Monosaccharides (glucose, fructose, galactose, ribose, deoxyribose) and disaccharides (sucrose, lactose, and maltose) are known as *simple carbohydrates* while polysaccharides (starch, glycogen, fiber) are referred to as *complex carbohydrates.*

Starch is a complex carbohydrate made up of thousands of glucose molecules linked together. Grains are the richest food source of starch. Other important sources of starch are legumes (beans and peas) and tubers (potato, cassava, *etc.*). Body converts all carbohydrates (except those coming from fiber) to glucose. Glucose is used as a fuel by brain and muscle tissue or converted to glycogen and stored by liver and muscles. Excess carbohydrates are converted to fat.

Carbohydrates should contribute to 50–60% of total energy intake; and preferably obtained from grains, legumes, vegetables, and fruits. Such a diet is lower in fat and energy and higher in fiber, vitamin, and minerals. These diets also contribute to lower rates of undernutrition, obesity, tooth decay, cardiovascular disease, and diabetes. Excessive carbohydrate consumption in form of concentrated sweets is associated with dental caries, obesity, and ischemic heart disease.

Lack of carbohydrates may produce ketosis, loss of energy, depression, and breakdown of body proteins.

5. FIBER

Dietary fiber is the remnant of the edible part of plants and analogous carbohydrates that are not digested or absorbed in the human small intestine. Fiber components include polysaccharides such as cellulose, hemicellulose, pectins, gums, mucilages, and non-polysaccharide lignins. Organic acids (butyric acid) and polyols (sorbitol) are also considered as part of fiber. Fibers are important because of their water-holding capacity, bile acid binding capacity, and for the growth of the normal microflora of the intestines. They also help in lowering blood cholesterol and limit glucose absorption. Fibers insoluble in water result in softening of stools and acceleration of intestinal transit time.

Major fiber-containing foods include cereals, vegetables, fruits, and dried beans. Fruits and vegetables contain more water-soluble fiber. An adequate fiber consumption can be achieved by having at least 2 servings of fruits, 3 servings of vegetables, and 6 servings of grain products per day after the age of 2 years. The recommended fiber intake of 40 g/2000 kcal can be rationalized in different groups based on recommended energy intake. High fiber intake (>60 g/day), on the other side, decreases the bioavailability of minerals and can lead to flatulence, diarrhea, and decreased appetite.

High fiber diet is advocated for chronic constipation, diabetes, obesity, and hypercholesterolemia. Low fiber diet is particularly useful in irritable bowel syndrome, chronic colitis, and partial chronic gastrointestinal obstruction.

Docosahexaenoic acid (DHA). Monograph. *Altern Med Rev.* 2009;14:391–9.

Joint FAO/WHO Expert Consultation on Fats and Fatty Acids in Human Nutrition. Interim Summary of Conclusions and Dietary Recommendation on Total Fat and Fatty Acids. Nov 10–14, 2006. Available from: http://www.fao.org/ag/agn/nutrition/docs/fats%20 and %20fatty%20 acids%. Accessed, Oct 1, 2012.

Martin SS, Blumenthal RS, Miller M. LDL cholesterol: the lower the better. *Med Clin North Am.* 2012;96:13–26.

Woodruff SJ, Hanning RM, Barr SI. Energy recommendations for normal weight, overweight and obese children and adolescents: are different equations necessary? *Obes Rev.* 2009;10:103–8.

3.2 INFANT AND YOUNG CHILD FEEDING

BREASTFEEDING (ALSO SEE SECTION 7.6)

Breastfeeding is the ideal form of infant feeding and is crucial for lifelong health and well-being. It provides unique nutritional, immunological, psychological, and child spacing benefits. Artificial feeding exposes the infant to infections and results in over a million deaths annually worldwide. Although breastfeeding is natural and physiological, the current infant feeding practices are far from optimum. As per Fourth National Family Health Survey (NFHS-4, India), only 54.9% children aged less than six months were exclusively breastfed and only 41.6% children received breastfeeding within one hour of birth. Lack of updated knowledge and training among medical and paramedical personnel, misconceptions in the community, misinformation by infant food manufacturers, and lack of community and family support to women are the main reasons for adverse infant feeding practices.

Definitions

- *Exclusive breastfeeding* Only breastmilk is given. No other food or drink, not even water, is given. Medicines, vitamins or mineral drops are permitted, if indicated. An infant should be exclusively breastfed for first 6 months of life.

- *Predominant breastfeeding* The main source of nutrition is breastmilk but the child is also receiving other fluids like water or water-based drinks such as tea or juices.

- *Partial breastfeeding (mixed feeding)* The child receives non-human milk, formula or cereal based foods (before six months) in addition to breastmilk.

Recommendations

- Breastfeeding should be initiated as soon as possible after birth; ie, within 30 minutes after normal delivery and within 1 hour after cesarean section.

- Nothing should be given to the baby before initiation of breastfeeding.
- The baby should be given exclusive breastfeeding, not even water, for first 6 months of life.
- Breastfeeding should be given, whenever baby feels hungry (*demand feeding*).
- *Complementary foods* (other foods in addition to breastmilk) should be started after 6 months of age.
- Breastfeeding should be continued with semisolid/solid foods minimum up to 2 years of age; and if possible beyond also.
- Mother and family should be motivated, educated, and supported regarding healthy feeding practices for maintaining and sustaining healthy infant feeding practices.

Nutritional composition of breastmilk, advantages of breastfeeding, and process of breastfeeding are detailed in *Section* 7.6.

Complementary Feeding

Complementary feeding implies giving the child other nutritious foods in addition to breastmilk. The literal meaning of the term *weaning* is taking the infant away from the breast and nourishment by other means. As breastmilk continues to be an important source of good quality proteins, vitamin A and C even for older infants, the use of this term has now been discarded in favor of *complementary feeding*.

Breastfeeding alone is sufficient food for first 6 months. Thereafter, concentrated energy dense complementary foods are essential to maintain an adequate velocity of growth for the infant. Care must be taken to ensure that these foods complement, and not replace the breastmilk.

The introduction of complementary feeding is a difficult period in the infant's life, because if the food supplements or substitutes are not adequate in quantity or quality, the child becomes malnourished. Also, the child is just learning to eat at this time, it is important to be patient and gentle with the child. Unhygienic feeding practices may result in enteric infections and diarrhea, further compromising the nutritional state and undermining the parents' confidence in complementary foods.

Age of Introduction

From about 6 months age onwards, there is a gap between the total energy needs and the energy provided by breastmilk. The gap increases as the child gets older. Also, by 6 months, the child's teeth begin to erupt and the biting movements begin. The tendency to push solids out of mouth also decreases. Thus 6 months is considered the correct time to begin complementary feeding as the child is ready to eat soft and starchy foods. Introduction of complementary foods before 6 months leads to displacement of breastmilk, making it difficult to meet the child's nutritional needs as other foods are nutritionally inferior to the breastmilk. Also, it exposes the child to risks of diarrhea and other infections at an earlier age. Starting complementary foods too late is also risky as it leads to non-fulfillment of nutritional gap leading to malnutrition and anemia.

Attributes of Complementary Foods

All foods provide some energy. However, the taste, consistency, and the texture of foods have important bearing on successful complementary feeding. The stomach of a young child is small. Thin foods and liquids fill it quickly. The consistency or thickness of foods makes a big difference to how well that food meets the young child's energy needs. Foods of a thick consistency help to fill the energy gap. *A food that stays easily on the spoon is just the right consistency.*

The first food the child eats should be soft, homogenous (mashed or strained), and bland in taste. When the infant has accepted soft food, different tastes should be gradually introduced with increasing thickness and varying texture. Small, chopped pieces of food can also be mixed. Apart from taste and consistency, it is imperative that the complementary food should be:

i. Culturally acceptable, in consonance with the traditional feeding practices;
ii. Adequate to provide all the nutritional requirements of the infant with respect to energy, protein, vitamins, and minerals;
iii. Locally available and inexpensive;
iv. Easily prepared at home with the existing facilities; and
v. Physiologically suitable, easily digestible, and nourishing.

DIETS FOR COMPLEMENTARY FEEDING

The complementary foods should be well balanced nutritionally and at least 8 to 10% of the energy should be obtained from proteins of good quality. Complementary foods should be prepared from cereals like rice, wheat or maize, pulses, milk, and root staples like potato. Deficiency of lysine, an essential amino acid in the protein of wheat, can be compensated, if both wheat and legumes (rich in lysine) are consumed simultaneously. Complementary foods based on vegetable protein alone may not always provide essential amino acids in a balanced proportion, comparable to the egg or milk protein. Therefore, addition of small quantities of proteins of animal origin such as milk, egg, or meat is usually sufficient to make up the deficiency of limiting amino acids, in a diet based on a mixture of a staple cereal and a legume.

Addition of vegetables and fruits will further enhance the nutritional quality of food by providing minerals like iron and vitamins. Oils, fats, and sugars increase dietary energy levels and improve taste of the food.

In most parts of India, a well cooked gruel (*Khichri, Kanji*) prepared from rice (3 parts), legume (1 part), green leafy vegetable, and some milk curd is a satisfactory complementary food. Another good complementary food is wheat gruel (*dalia*) made in milk with added sugar. Oil should be added to these foods to make them energy dense. Local variations of the complementary food may be made according to the availability of food in the region. Legumes are scarce and expensive in Sri Lanka and Maldives but fish is cheap and easily available. In some complementary foods, soyabean replaces *dals* or lentils. Commercially available complementary foods are convenient but expensive and offer no distinct advantages over the home made complementary foods.

STARTING COMPLEMENTARY FEEDING

A good regimen of complementary feeding is to start with mashed bananas, as it is easily accepted. Within 1–2 weeks the infant can be administered semolina (*suji*) cooked in milk. Both of these provide additional calories. Shortly thereafter, well-cooked and mashed lentils or peas, followed by khichri (*kanji*) are added. By 8–9 months of age, the child should be consuming most of foods (after appropriate modification) cooked in the house for adults. Infants fed on top milk require additional vitamin A and C. Boiling destroys vitamins. Animal milk is also a poor source of iron. Delayed complementary feeding and undue dependence on milk as food result in iron deficiency anemia. Soup or purees of dark green leafy vegetables are good source of iron for infants.

Frequency

When food is first introduced, a small amount should be given 1–2 times a day and slowly increased to 3–4 times daily. The approximate amount of foods required by young children in addition to breastmilk is given in **Table 3.4**. If a child is not breastfed, complementary foods should be given more frequently.

Feeding Technique

As a general principle, a single complementary food is added at a time, in small quantities. This is followed by introduction of the second complementary food after some time. The child should be fed slowly and patiently. A child should be actively encouraged to eat by paying attention, talking, playing with him, and showing pleasure. Force feeding and bribing should be avoided. As the child grows older, he should be encouraged to feed by self with fingers or spoon.

Hygienic Feeding

Careful preparation and storage of the complementary food is essential to prevent contamination. The utensils should be washed thoroughly and the hands should be washed before preparing foods and before feeding the child. Clean water and raw materials should be used to prepare foods. Foods should be kept covered to protect from dust and insects. Cooked food should preferably be freshly prepared and is not to be stored for prolonged periods, if there is no refrigeration. Unhygienic feeding practices result in infections like diarrhea which may further compromise the child's nutritional state.

Complementary Feeding: Report of the Global Consultation. Geneva: WHO; 2003.

Global strategy for infant and young child feeding. Geneva: WHO; 2003.

Infant and young child feeding: A tool for assessing national practices, policies and programmes. Geneva: WHO; 2003.

Kramer MS, Kakuma R. The optimal duration of exclusive breastfeeding: a systematic review. WHO/NHD/01.08. Geneva: WHO; 2001.

Shah D, Singh M, Gupta P, et al. Effect of sequencing of complementary feeding in relation to breastfeeding and total intake in infants. *J Pediatr Gastroenterol Nutr*. 2014;58:339–43.

World Health Organization. Feeding the non-breastfed child 6–24 month of age. Meeting report, Geneva: 8–10 March 2004. WHO/FCH/CAH/04.13.

Table 3.4 Amount and Frequency of Complementary Foods

Age	Energy needed per day in addition to breastmilk	Texture	Frequency	Amount of food an average child will usually eat at each meal
6–8 months (semisolids)	200 kcal	Start with thick porridge, well mashed foods Continue with mashed family foods, ready to eat infant mixes, well-blended porridge, kheer, well-mashed lentil with a boiled vegetable, potato and spinach puree, blended rice khichri, vermicelli khichri, sweet dalia	2–3 meals per day Depending on the child's appetite, 1–2 snacks may be offered	Start with 2–3 tablespoonful per feed, increase gradually to ½ of a 250 mL cup
9–11 months (semisolids-solid)	300 kcal	Finely chopped or mashed foods, and foods that baby can pick up: Poha with curd, potato with curd, millet khichri, upma, idli, moong dal mixture	3–4 meals per day Depending on the child's appetite, 1–2 snacks may be offered	½ of a 250 mL cup/bowl
12–23 months (solids)	550 kcal	Family foods, chopped or mashed, if necessary; roti, cheela, parantha, laddoo, biscuits, rice, dal (family food)	3–4 meals per day Depending on the child's appetite, 1–2 snacks may be offered	¾ of a 250 mL cup

Reproduced with permission. From Infant and Young Child Feeding: Model Chapter for Textbooks for Medical Students and Allied Health Professionals. WHO; 2009.

3.3 FEEDING DURING LATER CHILDHOOD

BALANCED DIET

The child should receive adequate amount of calories and protein in the diet (as per **Tables 3.1** and **3.2**), which should be prepared from the locally available, inexpensive foods. A balanced diet should provide around 50–60% of total calories from carbohydrates, preferably from complex carbohydrates, about 10–15% from proteins, and 20–30% from both visible and invisible fats. Besides macronutrients, the diet should also be rich in micronutrients such as iron, vitamins, and zinc. Intake of green leafy vegetables, fruits, and foods of animal origin (eg, milk, eggs, meat, fish) should be encouraged. Fast-foods and junk foods are to be avoided.

FOOD GROUPS

Indian Council of Medical Research (ICMR) in 2011 identified four main food groups in our diet. These are (*a*) cereals and pulses, (*b*) milk, egg, and meat products, (*c*) vegetables and fruits, and (*d*) oils, fats, nuts, and oilseeds based on their predominant nutrients. It is important to include each group in daily diet, in the recommended proportion, to fulfill the nutritional requirement of the body. Nutritive values of common food items in these groups are provided in **Tables 3.5** to **3.13**.

Foods can also be categorized according to their functions:
- *Energy-rich food* Carbohydrate-rich foods like cereals, millets, sugar, starchy vegetables, and the fat-rich foods

such as oil, ghee, butter, nuts, and oilseeds are rich in calories. Intake of these foods is a must for physical activity and maintenance of overall health, growth, and recovery from illness.
- *Body building food* Protein rich foods, eg, pulses, legumes, and nuts; milk and other dairy products, egg, meat, fish, belong to this group. This category is vital for growth spurt, maturation, and bone development.
- *Protective food* Protective food comprises of vitamin and mineral-rich food sources such as fruits and vegetables, eggs, milk, and milk products. Food material from this group is required to fight infections in children and prevent oxidative damage.

An in-depth learning about food groups allows us to comprehend the types of nutrients, and their impact on our body. This is vital not only in determining what constitutes a balanced diet, but also in assessing nutritional adequacy, as an aid for nutritional counseling, while briefing therapeutic diet to the patients, and understanding food labeling. **Table 3.14** provides calorie contents of some commonly cooked food items.

FOOD PYRAMID

The food pyramid, a valuable roadmap for healthy diet planning, rests on the concept of energy density which combines nutritional values with portion sizes to cater to different needs or situations such as, the high energy density requirement in children and elderly people, or low energy density needs in case of obesity. Since no single food offers

3

Table 3.5 Nutritive Value of Common Cereals (per 100 g of edible portion)

Name of foodstuff	Energy (kcal)	Protein (g)	Fat (g)	CHO (g)	Crude fibers (g)	Zinc (mg)	Iron (mg)	Calcium (mg)
Bajra (*Pennisetum typhoideum*)	347	11.0	5.4	61.8	11.5	2.8	6.4	27.4
Jowar (*Sorghum vulgare*)	333	10.0	1.7	67.7	10.2	2.0	4.0	27.6
Maize, dry (*Zea mays*)	333	8.8	3.8	64.8	12.2	2.3	2.5	8.9
Ragi (*Eleusine coracana*)	320	7.2	1.9	66.8	11.2	2.5	4.6	364.0
Rice, raw, milled (*Oryza sativa*)	355	7.9	0.5	78.2	2.8	1.2	0.7	7.5
Rice, puffed (*Oryza sativa*)	360	7.5	1.6	77.7	2.6	1.5	4.6	15.1
Wheat, flour, refined (*Triticum aestivum*)	350	10.4	0.8	74.3	2.8	0.9	1.8	20.5
Wheat, whole (*Triticum aestivum*)	321	10.6	1.5	64.7	11.2	2.9	4.0	39.4

Table 3.6 Nutritive Value of Commonly Consumed Pulses (per 100 g of edible portion)

Name of foodstuff	Energy (kcal)	Protein (g)	Fat (g)	CHO (g)	Crude fibers (g)	Zinc (mg)	Iron (mg)	Calcium (mg)
Bengal gram, dal (*Cicer arietinum*)	328	21.6	5.3	46.7	15.2	3.7	6.1	46.4
Black gram, dal (*Phaseolus mungo*)	323	23.1	1.7	51.0	11.9	3.0	4.7	55.7
Green gram, dal (*Phaseolus aureus*)	325	23.9	1.4	52.6	9.4	2.5	3.9	43.1
Green gram, whole (*Phaseolus aureus*)	293	22.5	1.5	46.1	17.0	2.7	6.8	150.0
Moth beans (*Vigna aconitifolia*)	307	19.8	1.8	52.1	15.1	1.9	7.9	154.0
Rajmah, red (*Phaseolus vulgaris*)	298	19.9	1.8	48.6	16.6	2.7	6.1	126.0
Soybean, white (*Glycine max*)	376	37.8	19.4	10.2	22.6	3.5	8.2	195.0

Table 3.7 Nutritive Value of Common Vegetables (per 100 g of edible portion)

Name of foodstuff	Energy (kcal)	Protein (g)	Fat (g)	CHO (g)	Crude fibers (g)	Zinc (mg)	Iron (mg)	Calcium (mg)
Roots and tubers								
Carrot, red (*Dacus carota*)	38.0	1.0	0.5	6.7	4.5	0.3	0.7	41.1
Colocasia (*Colacasia antiquorum*)	89.0	3.3	0.2	17.9	3.2	0.4	0.7	30.2
Onion big (*Allium cepa*)	48.0	1.5	0.2	9.6	2.5	0.4	0.4	21.0
Potato (big) (*Solanum tuberosum*)	70.0	1.5	0.2	14.9	1.7	0.3	0.6	9.5
Radish, round white skin (*Raphanus sativus*)	31.0	0.8	0.1	6.1	2.4	0.2	0.4	30.2
Leafy vegetables								
Bathua leaves (*Chenopodium album*)	27.6	2.5	0.4	2.6	4.0	1.0	2.7	211.0
Cabbage, green (*Brassica oleracea*)	21.4	1.4	0.1	3.3	2.8	0.2	0.4	51.8
Fenugreek leaves (*Trigonella foenum graecum*)	34.3	3.7	0.8	2.2	4.9	0.5	5.7	0.00
Lettuce (*Lactuca sativa*)	21.6	1.5	0.3	3.0	1.8	0.5	2.7	0.00
Mustard leaves (*Brassica juncea*)	30.2	3.5	0.5	2.4	3.9	0.7	2.8	0.00
Spinach (*Spinacia oleracea*)	24.2	2.1	0.6	2.1	2.4	0.5	3.0	82.3
Other vegetables								
Bitter gourd (*Momordica charantia*)	20.7	1.4	0.24	2.8	3.8	0.3	1.2	21.4
Brinjal-all varieties (*Solanum melongena*)	25.2	1.5	0.32	3.5	4.0	0.2	0.4	16.6
Cauliflower (*Brassica oleracea*)	22.8	2.2	0.44	2.0	3.2	0.3	1.0	25.2
Cucumber (*Cucumis sativus*)	19.5	0.7	0.16	3.5	2.1	0.2	0.5	16.4
French beans, country (*Phaseolus vaulgaris*)	24.2	2.5	0.26	2.7	4.4	0.5	1.3	56.0
Jackfruit, raw (*Artocarpus heterophyllus*)	26.2	2.0	0.35	3.5	7.7	0.2	0.3	45.7
Ladies fingers (*Abelmoschus esculentus*)	27.3	2.1	0.22	3.6	4.1	0.5	0.8	86.1
Pumpkin, orange (*Cucurbita maxima*)	23.0	0.8	0.16	4.00	2.6	0.1	0.4	23.1
Tinda, tender (*Praecitrullus fistulosus*)	13.8	1.0	0.17	1.9	2.0	0.2	0.4	19.7

Source: Indian Food Composition Tables. National Institute of Nutrition, Indian Council of Medical Research; 2017.

3

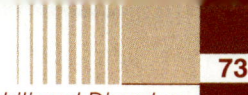

Table 3.8 Nutritive Value of Common Fruits (per 100 g of edible portion)								
Name of foodstuff	Energy (kcal)	Protein (g)	Fat (g)	CHO (g)	Crude fibers (g)	Zinc (mg)	Iron (mg)	Calcium (mg)
Apple, big (*Malus domestica*)	62.1	0.3	0.64	13.1	2.6	0.1	0.3	13.7
Banana, ripe (*Musa × paradisiaca*)	110.2	1.3	0.32	30.0	2.2	0.2	0.4	6.8
Grapes, green (*Vitis vinifera*)	56.0	0.8	0.29	12.2	1.3	0.1	0.2	11.2
Guava, white flesh (*Pasidium guajava*)	32.1	1.4	0.32	5.1	8.6	0.2	0.3	18.5
Jambu fruit, ripe (*Syzygium cumini*)	56.0	0.8	0.17	12.3	3.1	0.1	0.3	25.4
Lemon, juice (*Citrus limon*)	36.4	0.4	0.75	7.0	0	0.1	0.1	22.7
Litchi (*Nephelium litchi*)	53.5	1.0	0.26	11.4	1.3	0.2	0.8	5.8
Mango, ripe, kesar (*Mangifera indica*)	55.0	0.5	0.57	11.4	2.0	0.1	0.0	15.7
Orange, pulp (*Citrus aurantium*)	37.0	0.7	0.1	7.9	1.3	0.0	0.8	19.5
Papaya, ripe (*Carcia papaya*)	24.0	0.42	0.2	4.6	2.8	0.1	0.2	15.0
Pineapple (*Ananas comosus*)	43.0	0.52	0.2	9.4	3.5	0.1	0.3	10.9
Pomegranate (*Punica granatum*)	55.0	1.33	0.2	11.6	2.8	0.2	0.3	10.7
Tomato, ripe (*Lycopersicon esculentum*)	19.0	0.8	0.3	3.2	1.6	0.1	0.2	8.9
Watermelon (*Citrullus vulgaris*)	287.0	2.9	0.15	67.4	5.3	0.1	0.2	5.3

Table 3.9 Nutritive Value of Milk (per 100 mL)						
Name of foodstuff	Energy (kcal)	Protein (g)	Fat (g)	CHO (g)	Zinc (mg)	Iron (mg)	Calcium (mg)
Milk, whole, buffalo	107.0	3.7	6.6	8.4	0.3	0.2	121.0
Milk, whole, cow	73.0	3.3	4.5	4.9	0.3	0.2	118.0
Khoa	315.0	16.3	20.6	16.5	2.3	2.3	602.0
Paneer	257.0	18.9	14.8	12.4	2.7	0.9	476.0

Table 3.10 Nutritive Value of Egg, Meat, Fish (per 100 g of edible portion)						
Name of foodstuff	Energy (kcal)	Protein (g)	Fat (g)	Zinc (mg)	Iron (mg)	Calcium (g)
Fish and other sea foods						
Cat fish (*Tandanus tandanus*)	123	15.9	6.2	0.7	0.8	22.0
Catla (*Catla catla*)	94	17.9	2.2	0.7	1.1	43.5
Crab (*Menippe mercenaria*)	82	10.2	1.4	0.8	1.1	128.0
Crab (*Pachygrapsus sp.*)	102	19.7	2.4	2.5	1.1	199.0
Hilsa (*Tenualosa ilisha*)	258	21.8	18.5	0.6	1.2	19.8
Labster, brown (*Thenus orientalis*)	70	16.0	0.6	1.2	0.7	73.1
Oyster (*Crassostrea sp.*)	60	9.5	2.4	7.4	0.9	126.0
Pomfret, white (*Pampus argenteus*)	122	19.0	5.1	0.5	0.3	13.6
Prawns, big (*Macrobrachium rosenbergii*)	73	13.2	0.9	1.4	0.8	48.6
Rohu (*Labeo rohita*)	203	17.1	16.8	0.8	1.0	39.4
Salmon (*Salmo salar*)	172	21.0	9.9	0.5	1.0	24.3
Sardine (*Sardinella longiceps*)	152	17.9	9.0	0.9	0.8	42.3
Tuna (*Euthynuus affinis*)	112	24.5	1.4	0.7	1.6	9.8
Meat and Poultry						
Beaf, shoulder	212	20.6	14.6	4.6	2.2	6.5
Chicken, poultry, leg, skinless	382	19.4	12.6	1.8	1.3	20.5
Egg, country hen, whole, raw	168	13.1	13	1.1	1.6	50.1
Egg, poultry, whole, raw	134	13.3	9.2	1.2	1.8	49.4
Goat, chops	135	20.4	6.0	4.6	1.9	7.4
Goat, shoulder	187	20.3	11.9	4.2	1.5	6.2
Pork, shoulder	236	17.4	18.8	2.1	0.9	10.0
Turkey, breast, with skin	160	22.0	8.0	1.3	1.0	14.4

Source: Indian Food Composition Tables. National Institute of Nutrition, Indian Council of Medical Research; 2017.

Table 3.11 Nutritive Value of Nuts and Oilseeds (per 100 g of edible portion)

Name of foodstuff	Energy (kcal)	Protein (g)	Fat (g)	CHO (g)	Crude fibers (g)	Zinc (mg)	Iron (mg)	Calcium (mg)
Almond (*Prunus amygdalus*)	607	18.4	58.5	3.0	13.1	3.5	4.6	228.0
Cashewnut (*Anacardium occidentale*)	580	18.8	45.2	25.5	3.9	5.3	6.0	34.0
Coconut, kernel, dry (*Cocos nucifera*)	622	7.3	63.3	8.0	15.9	1.4	3.1	32.0
Coconut, kernel, fresh (*Cocos nucifera*)	407	3.8	41.4	6.3	10.4	0.6	1.3	8.0
Groundnut (*Arachis hypogea*)	518	23.7	39.6	17.3	10.4	3.2	3.4	54.0
Pistachio nut (*Pistacla vera*)	537	23.4	42.5	15.8	10.6	2.4	4.5	135.0
Walnut (*Juglans regia*)	669	14.9	64.3	10.1	5.4	2.9	3.2	105.0

Table 3.12 Nutritive Value of Sugar and Jaggery (per 100 g of edible portion)

Name of foodstuff	Energy (kcal)	Protein (g)	Fat (g)	CHO (g)	Zinc (mg)	Iron (mg)	Calcium (mg)
Honey Jaggery, cane (*Saccharum officinarum*)	352	1.9	0.2	84.9	0.5	4.6	107
Sugarcane, juice (*Saccharum officinarum*)	58	0.2	0.4	13.1	0.1	1.1	18

Table 3.13 Nutritive Value of Condiments and Spices (per 100 g of edible portion)

Name of foodstuff	Energy (kcal)	Protein (g)	Fat (g)	CHO (g)	Crude fibers (g)	Zinc (mg)	Iron (mg)	Calcium (mg)
Asafoetida (*Ferula assa-foetida*)	330	6.3	10.3	72.0	5.1	1.0	15.7	266.0
Cardamom, green (*Elettaria cardamomum*)	254	8.1	2.6	47.8	23.1	3.7	8.3	378.0
Chilies, red (*Capsicum annum*)	236	12.7	6.4	29.5	31.2	1.7	6.2	99.8
Cloves dry (*Syzygium aromaticum*)	186	5.9	8.4	18.7	34.5	1.1	9.4	567.0
Coriander, seeds (*Coriandrum sativum*)	268	10.7	17.5	13.0	44.8	3.9	17.6	718.0
Cumin seeds (*Cuminum cyminum*)	303	13.9	16.6	22.6	30.4	4.3	8.5	135.0
Fenugreek seeds (*Trigonella foenum graecum*)	234	25.4	5.7	10.6	47.6	3.8	8.5	135.0
Ginger fresh (*Zinziber officinale*)	55	2.2	0.9	9.0	5.4	0.4	1.9	18.9
Papper, black (*Piper nigrum*)	217	10.1	2.7	36.2	33.2	1.2	11.9	405.0
Turmeric powder (*Curcuma domestica*)	280	7.7	5.0	49.2	21.4	2.6	46.1	122.0

Source: Indian Food Composition Tables. National Institute of Nutrition, Indian Council of Medical Research; 2017.

all essential nutrients in sufficient amount, a diet can be balanced only if it consists of food from all different food groups. Not all foods in a food group contain the same nutrients. Within each food group, the food selection should be assorted or diverse to fulfill the requirements of essential ingredients.

As illustrated in Fig. 3.1, in each of the food groups, a specific number of serving is recommended and healthy choices are emphasized. For example, in the **first layer of the pyramid** (at the bottom) are the cereals and milk, advised to be taken in adequate amount, as cereals/millets are used as staple food and are major sources of most nutrients, in this category. Whole grains are emphasized; and low-fat dairy products are encouraged.

Vegetables and fruits are at the **second layer of the pyramid** and unlimited amounts of fresh or frozen forms of each are recommended. Vegetables and fruits are rich sources of minerals, vitamins, and phytonutrients. Fruits and vegetables are also rich in complex carbohydrates and fiber. Dietary fiber is important for proper bowel function, to reduce chronic constipation, and reduce plasma cholesterol. Some vegetables and fruits provide very low calories, whereas some others such as potato, sweet potato, tapioca, and yam and banana are rich in starch which provide energy in good amount. Therefore, vegetables and fruits can be used to increase or decrease calories in our diet.

The **third layer of pyramid** about the use of protein and fat dictates that it should be used in moderation. The intake of PUFA should be 8–10% of energy intake. Ideally a ratio of polyunsaturated/saturated (PUFA/SFA) fat of 0.8–1.0 is required. The intake of *trans*-fatty acids should not exceed 1% of energy intake. A combination of oils like soyabean, sesame, mustard, and sunflower should be used to achieve minor components in the diet. The use of ghee, butter, vanaspati, animal food, and processed food should be minimized. Prefer fish over meat and poultry. Use of

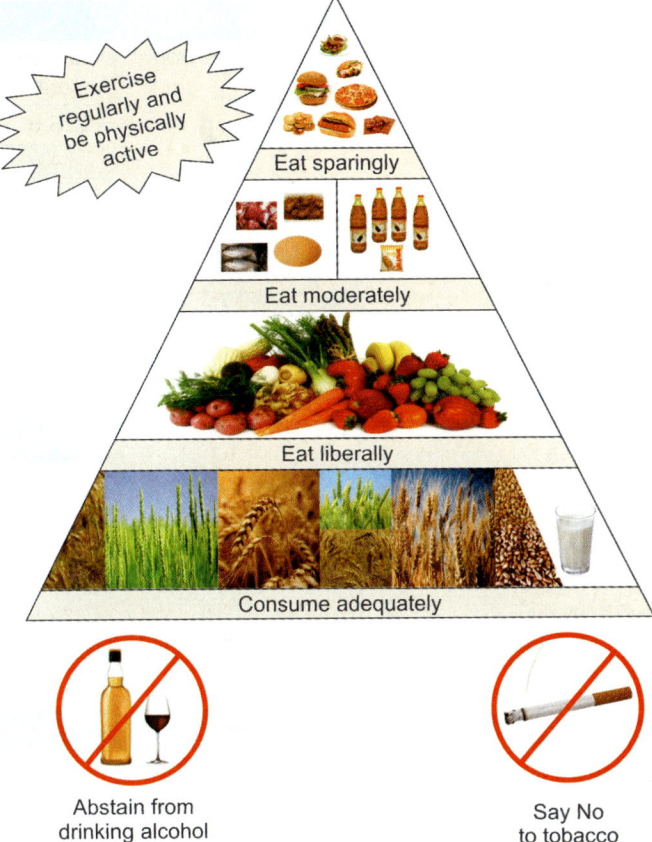

Fig. 3.1 Food pyramid (*Source:* Dietary Guidelines for Indians. 2nd ed. National Institute of Nutrition, Indian Council of Medical Research; 2011)

reheated oil and fat should be avoided. Ill effects of excess dietary fats are initiated early in life. Use of skimmed milk is advocated beyond 2 years of age. Consumption of fish, beans, and low-fat dairy products are encouraged from this layer. Increased amount of protein is needed for growing and ill children.

The **top (fourth) layer** consists of processed food and sugar that should be used as little as possible.

Food pyramid also offers the right combination of food intake to match with the physical activity. Daily physical activity from lifestyle activities throughout the day as well as planned exercise, is an important component for weight management, especially of school children and adolescents. The ICMR food pyramid also cautions against intake of alcohol and tobacco.

The dietary habits vary according to socioeconomic status, customs, and traditions. **Box 3.1** offers a few tips for developing healthy dietary habits in childhood.

My Plate

The concept of **My Plate** (Fig. 3.2) originally populated by the USDA provides a visual concept of the proportion of different food groups needed for ensuring a balanced diet. Variety is encouraged within the different food groups. This is an easy to follow food guide and helps in nutritional education of parents and children.

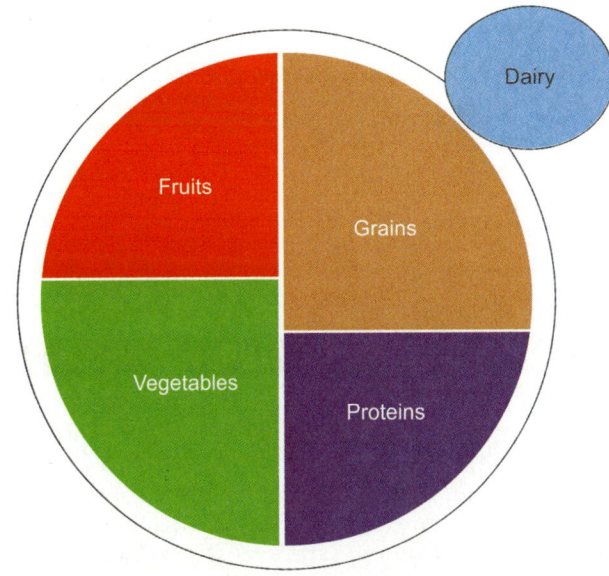

Fig. 3.2 My plate—ensures balance diet

Table 3.14 Approximate Calorific Value of Some Cooked Preparations

Preparation	Quantity for one serving	Calories (kcal)	Preparation	Quantity for one serving	Calories (kcal)
1. Cereal			**5. Savoury snacks**		
Rice	1 cup	170	*Bajjior pakora*	8 nos.	280
Phulka	1 no.	80	*Besan ka pura*	1 no.	220
Paratha	1 no.	150	Chat (*dahipakori*)	5 pieces	220
Puri	1 no.	80	Cheese balls	2 nos	250
Bread	2 slices	170	*Dahivada*	2 nos	180
Poha	1 cup	270	*Vada*	2 nos	140
Upma	1 cup	270	*Masala vada*	2 nos.	150
Idli	2 nos.	150	*Masala dosa*	1 no.	200
Dosa	1 no.	125	Pea-kachori	2 nos.	380
Khichdi	1 cup	200	Potato bonda	2 nos.	200
Wheat porridge	1 cup	220	Sago vada	2 nos.	210
Semolina porridge	1 cup	220	*Samosa*	1 no.	200
Cereal flakes with milk (corn/wheat/rice)	1 cup	220	Sandwiches (butter 2 tbsp)	2 nos.	200
			Vegetable puff	1 no.	200
2. Pulse			Pizza (cheese and tomato)	1 slice	200
Plain *dal*	½ cup	100	**6. Chutney**		
Sambar	1 cup	110	Coconut/groundnut/til	2 tbsp	120
3. Vegetable			Tomato	1 tbsp	10
With gravy	1 cup	170	Tamarind (with jaggery)	1 tbsp	60
Dry	1 cup	150	**7. Sweets and desserts**		
4. Nonvegetarian			*Besan barfi*	2 small pieces	400
Boiled egg	1 no.	90	Chikki	2 pieces	290
Omelette	1 no.	160	Fruit cake	1 piece	270
Fried egg	1 no.	160	Rice puttu	½ cup	280
Mutton curry	¾ cup	260	Sandesh	2 nos.	140
Chicken curry	¾ cup	240	Double ka meetha	½ cup	280
Fish fried	2 big pieces	190	*Halwa (kesari)*	½ cup	320
Fish cutlet	2 nos.	190	Jelly/jam	1 tbs	20
Prawn curry	¾ cup	220	Custard (caramel)	½ cup	160
Keema kofta curry	¾ cup (6 small koftas)	240	*Srikhand*	½ cup	380
			Milk chocolate	25 g	140
			Ice cream	½ cup	200

Source: Dietary Guidelines for Indians. 2nd ed. National Institute of Nutrition, Indian Council of Medical Research; 2011.

Indian Council of Medical Research. Nutrient Requirements and Recommended. Dietary Guidelines for Indians-A Manual. Hyderabad: National Institute of Nutrition, ICMR; 2011.

Indian Food Composition Tables. Hyderabad: National Institute of Nutrition, Indian Council of Medical Research; 2017.

U.S. Department of Health and Human Services and U.S. Department of Agriculture. 2015–2020 Dietary Guidelines for Americans. 8th Edition. December 2015. Available at http://health.gov/dietaryguidelines/2015/guidelines/..

World Health Organization. Diet, Nutrition and the Prevention of Chronic Diseases. WHO Technical Report Series No.916. Geneva: WHO; 2003.

3.4 PROTEIN ENERGY MALNUTRITION (PEM)

Nutritional deficiency of macronutrients is a major health problem in the developing countries. Severe acute malnutrition (SAM), often associated with infection, contributes to high child mortality in underprivileged communities. Early onset of malnutrition can also have lasting effects on growth and functional status. The magnitude of undernutrition cannot be easily calculated from the prevalence of commonly recognized clinical syndromes of malnutrition such as marasmus and kwashiorkor because these constitute only proverbial tip of the iceberg. Children with mild to moderate undernutrition are likely to remain unrecognized because clinical criteria for their diagnosis are imprecise and difficult to interpret accurately.

Assessment of nutritional status by anthropometry is the simplest and most useful tool for assessing the nutritional status of children. Weight, height, and mid-arm circumference should be compared to the reference norms for the corresponding age in the well nourished and healthy children of the community. It is difficult to define "what constitutes an appropriate and optimum body size?" Both Indian and International references for anthropometric measurements have been advocated. These include Harvard standards (UK), NCHS/CDC standards (US), and Indian Academy of Pediatrics (IAP) Growth charts (India). Reference values provided by World Health Organization (WHO) provide the most recent and widely acceptable international growth standards for comparison for under-5 children; while IAP growth charts are recommended for children 5–18 years age.

CLASSIFICATION OF PEM

PEM may be classified according to the severity, course, and the relative contributions of energy or protein deficit. Severity classifications are mainly based on anthropometric measurements: weight and height. For the purpose of these classifications, the term *'expected'* means the median (50th centile) value of the reference standard. Reference values for weight-for-age, height-for-age, and weight-for-height are given in *Annexures*.

1. Indian Academy of Pediatrics (IAP) Classification based on Weight for Age

IAP identifies a weight of more than 80% of expected for that age as normal. Grades of malnutrition are *Grade I* (71–80%), *Grade II* (61–70%), *Grade III* (51–60%) and *Grade IV* (≤50%) of expected weight for that age. Alphabet *K* is postfixed in presence of edema. For example, a male child weighing 8 kg at 2 years of age with pedal edema (50th percentile for 2 years is 12.3 kg) is classified as PEM Grade II(k) as per IAP classification.

IAP classification is simple and the cut-offs are suitable for Indian population. However, the disadvantage is that it does not take in account the child's height. The weight is also dependent on height besides the built; thus children who are short statured (not necessarily because of nutritional deprivation) are also misclassified as PEM by this classification.

2. Wellcome Trust Classification

This classification is also based on (a) deficit in body weight for age and (b) presence or absence of edema. Children weighing between 60 and 80% of their expected weight for age with edema are classified as *kwashiorkor*. Those weighing between 60 and 80% of expected without edema are known as having *undernutrition*. Those without edema and weighing less than 60% of their expected weight for age are considered to be having *marasmus. Marasmic kwashiorkor* is applied to children with edema and body weight less than 60% of expected.

3. WHO Classification

This classification is based on two anthropometric indicators (stunting and wasting) and one clinical indicator (edema).

- *Wasting* (measured by deficit in weight-for-height) indicates a deficit in tissue and fat mass and may result either from failure to gain weight or from actual weight loss. It usually signifies *acute onset malnutrition.* A child is considered wasted, if the weight for height/length is less than –2SD (Z) score or less than 80% of the expected.
- *Stunting* (deficit in height-for-age) signifies accumulated consequences of retarded growth over a prolonged period of time and generally points towards a *chronic course of malnutrition.* It may also be a residue of past malnutrition or could be due to non-nutritional disorders like genetic short stature or endocrinal disorders. The diagnosis of stunting is based on a height for age less than –2SD (Z) score or less than 90% of the expected.
- Children are classified as having *moderate malnutrition*, if they are stunted or wasted.

Table 3.15 WHO Classification for Undernutrition

	Moderate undernutrition	Severe undernutrition
Symmetrical edema *Edematous malnutrition*	No	Yes[a]
Weight for height *(measure of wasting)*	SD score[b] –2 to –3 (70–79% of expected[c]) Wasting	SD score < –3 (<70% of expected) Severe wasting
Height for age *(measure of stunting)*	SD score[b] –2 to –3 (85–89% of expected[c]) Stunting	SD score < –3 (<85% of expected) Severe stunting

[a] *This includes kwashiorkor and marasmic kwashiorkor.*

$$^b SD\ score = \frac{observed\ value - expected\ value}{standard\ deviation\ of\ reference\ population}$$

[c] *Median (50th percentile of NCHS standards).*

- Presence of edema along with stunting or wasting indicates *severe undernutrition.*
- A child with *severe wasting* (weight for height/length less than –3Z-score or less than 70% of expected) or *severe stunting* (height for age less than –3Z-score or less than 85% of expected) is also considered to have *severe malnutrition* **(Table 3.15)**.

4. Severe Acute Malnutrition (SAM)

The term severe acute malnutrition was coined by international agencies (WHO and UNICEF) to identify malnourished children at highest risk of death, and for the purpose of therapeutic feeding in the hospital or community. SAM is defined by (*a*) very low weight for height (below –3Z-scores of the median WHO growth standards), (*b*) visible severe wasting, (*c*) presence of nutritional edema, or (*d*) mid-arm circumference below 11.5 cm for children aged between 6 months and 5 years.

Moderate acute malnutrition A child who has WFH SD score between –3Z and –2Z, or mid-upper arm circumference of 11.5–12.4 cm and has no bilateral pitting edema is classified as having moderate acute malnutrition.

Prevalence

In 2014, of 667 million under-five children in the world, 159 million (23.8%) were stunted, 90 million (13.5%) underweight, and 50 million (7.5%) wasted. Among the wasted, nearly one-third were severely wasted.

India

As per National Family Health Survey (NFHS)-4 (2015-16), 35.7% of under-five children are underweight, 38.4% stunted, and 21% are wasted. Prevalence of severe wasting (weight-for-height <-3SD) is 7.5% in children below 5 years of age. WHO growth standard median was taken as normal reference value. **Figure 3.3** depicts the trends of nutritional status of children in India from 1993 to 2014. The average annual reduction rate of stunting was 2.6% between NHFS-2 and NFHS-3. It was below the target rate of 3.7%. Wasting has also declined. In 2014, Ministry of Health and Family Welfare, Government of India conducted a Rapid Survey of

Children (RSoC) and collected national and state level data. **Figure 3.4** compares the statistics of NFHS surveys with that of RSoC.

In a state-wise assessment, as per NFHS-3, undernutrition was most pronounced in Madhya Pradesh, Bihar, and Jharkhand (60%); and least evident in Mizoram, Sikkim, Manipur and Kerala (less than 20%). NFHS-4 data has been released only for a few states and hence a comparative study could not be done. The RSoC data has shown maximum wasting in Andhra Pradesh and Tamil Nadu, maximum underweight in Jharkhand, and maximum stunting in Uttar Pradesh. Minimum wasting was recorded in Sikkim, minimum underweight in Mizoram, and minimum stunting in Kerala.

Etiology

Low birth weight (LBW) Malnourished mothers have a high incidence of low birth weight and growth retarded babies with poor nutritional reserve. **Table 3.16** compares the prevalence of LBW in different countries of South Asia with United States of America. These low birth weight babies are more likely to become malnourished.

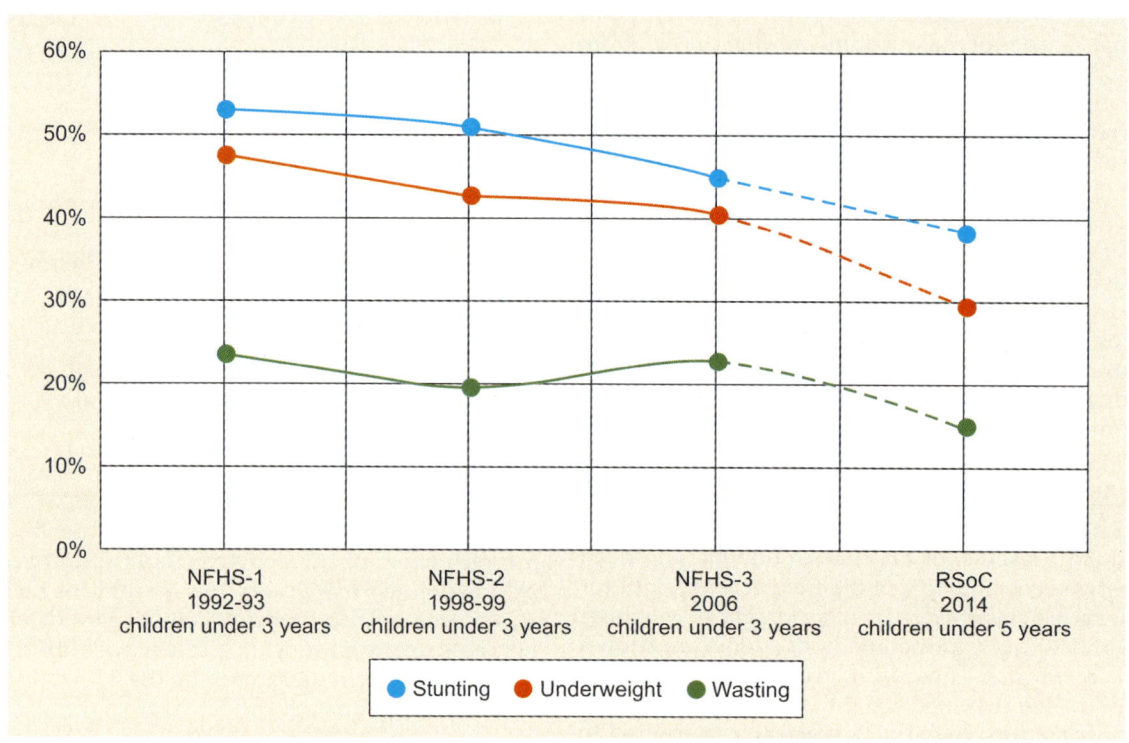

Fig. 3.3 Trends in Nutrition Status in India, 1993 to 2014.
(*Source:* India Health Report: Nutrition 2015. New Delhi, India: Public Health Foundation of India; 2015).

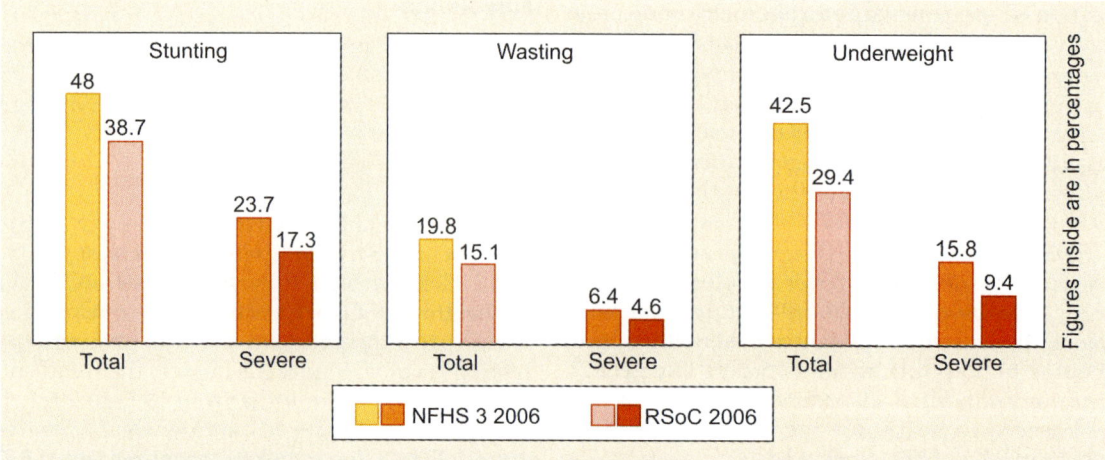

Fig. 3.4 Comparison of Prevalence of Undernutrition from two National Surveys
(*Source:* India Health Report: Nutrition 2015. New Delhi, India: Public Health Foundation of India; 2015).

Table 3.16 Prevalence of Low Birth Weight	
Country	*Low birth weight (% of total live births)*
Bangladesh	22% (2006)
Bhutan	10% (2010)
India	28% (2005)
Maldives	11% (2009)
Myanmar	9% (2009)
Nepal	18% (2011)
Pakistan	32% (2006)
Sri Lanka	17% (2006)
Thailand	11% (2010)
United States of America	8% (2010)

Source: The State of the World's Children 2017, UNICEF. Figures in parentheses indicate the pertaining year, for which latest information is available.

Feeding habits Lack of exclusive breastfeeding for first 6 months makes the child prone to early onset malnutrition. Artificial feeding is disastrous for the baby because of the poor quality of the substitute milk, excessive dilution, and use of unhygienic feeding bottles and nipples. Another major cause of malnutrition is delayed introduction of complementary feeding. According to NFHS-4 data, only 42.7% of infants aged 6–8 months receive complementary semi-solid foods as recommended.

Parents often withhold food supplements or dilute the milk during episodes of diarrhea. Affluent families may also have irrational beliefs about the nutritional needs of infants and nutritional quality of common foods. Some foods are erroneously believed to be hot or cold in nature. Prevailing dietary practices and cultural taboos are important conditioning factors leading to malnutrition.

Infections Diarrhea, pneumonia, malaria, measles, whooping cough, and tuberculosis precipitate acute malnutrition and aggravate the existing nutritional deficit. During infections, child's appetite is impaired. There may be iatrogenic restriction of food by the parents. The patient catabolizes his own tissues to produce the additional heat energy, which is lost during fever. Metabolic demands for protein during infections are higher. Protein may be lost because of tissue breakdown and in pus and exudates. Also, malnutrition may adversely affect the immune status and make the malnourished individuals more vulnerable to infections. This sets up a vicious cycle of malnutrition-infection-malnutrition.

High pressure advertising of baby foods by baby food manufacturers and social demands on the urban educated working women have encouraged early discontinuation of breastfeeding. Evaporated dry milk powders and packaged foods are expensive. An economically disadvantaged mother tends to conserve on their use and offers diluted milk formula to the infant. Unhygienic feeding practices in the preparation of milk formula result in frequent episodes of diarrhea and diminished absorption of food by the infant.

Social factors Repeated pregnancies, inadequate child spacing, food taboos, broken homes, and separation of a child from his parents are the important social factors that may play a part in etiology of PEM. Share of women and pre-school children is disproportionately less compared with the economically active male adults. Wars and civil unrest exaggerate pre-existing malnutrition in the community. Natural disasters such as floods, earthquakes, and droughts shift the precarious nutritional balance towards the negative side.

Poverty The poor cannot purchase adequate amount of food of the desired quality for meeting their and their family's nutritional requirements. This deprivation adversely affects their capacity for physical work resulting in low earning and poverty. A vicious cycle is thus set-up. In the new social milieu, competing demands for non-food expenditure on housing, clothing, and entertainment have gone up significantly often at the cost of the expenditure on food.

CLINICAL MANIFESTATIONS OF PROTEIN ENERGY MALNUTRITION

Clinical manifestations of undernutrition depend on the severity and duration of nutritional deprivation, the age of the undernourished subject, relative lack of different nutritional components of food, and the presence of associated infections. In India and many other developing countries, the major limiting factor in the diet of pre-school children is energy. Lack of protein in the diet is more often due to low food intake, rather than a qualitative defect in the diet. Nutritional marasmus and kwashiorkor are two extreme forms of malnutrition.

Marasmus

The most characteristic feature of marasmus is *visible severe wasting* of muscle and subcutaneous tissues. Child is usually alert, has an emaciated look, and has no edema (Fig. 3.5). Skin

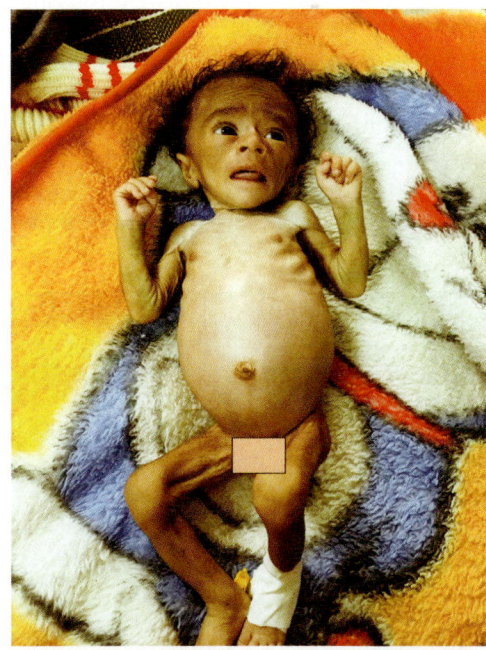

Fig. 3.5 Marasmus: An emaciated grossly wasted child without edema. (Photo Courtesy: Prof. Praveen Kumar, Lady Hardinge Medical College, New Delhi)

is thin, dry, scaly, and wrinkled with loose folds apparent over the gluteal region and thighs. Subcutaneous fat gets depleted as it is used up for providing energy. Buccal pad of fat is the last to disappear because of presence of saturated fats which are utilized after all other sources are depleted. Atrophic muscles make a contour under the thin and wrinkled skin. Bones appear prominent giving a skeleton-like look. Hair may become hypopigmented. Abdomen appears distended because of hypotonia of abdominal wall muscles. Appetite may be voracious, especially in absence of infection or without a secondary cause of malnutrition.

Kwashiorkor

Essential features of kwashiorkor include (*i*) edema of the dependent parts; (*ii*) markedly retarded growth; and (*iii*) psychomotor changes. Other features that help in making a diagnosis include skin and hair changes (Fig. 3.6), hepato-megaly, impaired appetite, and associated nutritional deficiencies. Edema and preserved subcutaneous tissues mask muscle wasting which becomes apparent when the child recovers from edema. Infections (eg, diarrhea, acute respiratory infections, skin infection) and infestations (eg, scabies, lice) are present in majority of cases.

Edema Edema is the clinical manifestation of expansion of extracellular water (ECW) volume caused by prerenal diversion of fluid from the capillary bed to extracellular space. Edema may be caused by (*i*) hypoalbuminemia; (*ii*) retention of fluid and water due to increased capillary permeability as a result of infection, potassium deficiency being a major contributing factor; and (*iii*) free radical induced damage to cell membranes.

The edema starts in the lower extremities and progresses to involve the upper limbs and the face. The face appears moon-shaped and puffy. The trunk is affected to a lesser extent, and ascites is rare unless there is a co-existent cause such as tuberculosis. In a previously malnourished child, edema is precipitated by debilitating illnesses such as measles or diarrhea. Presence of edema may mask features of severe dehydration secondary to diarrhea in a severely malnourished child.

Psychomotor changes Child with kwashiorkor is lethargic, listless, and apathetic. Play activity and interaction with others is reduced. Child resists attempts to examination by

medical personnel. Child loses appetite, and it is difficult to feed him orally in the initial phase of dietary management. Child may need nasogastric feeding for nutritional rehabilitation. Appetite improves once co-existent infection is controlled by antibiotics.

Skin changes A variety of skin changes have been described in kwashiorkor. Dry and scaly skin with cracking is apparent over large areas of trunk and limbs giving mosaic appearance. Most typical skin lesion is *crazy pavement dermatosis* which is characterized by jet black patches over flexures and pressure sites, especially of extremities (Fig. 3.7) which later exfoliate to expose raw hypopigmented or reddish skin. Peeling plaques of this dermatosis give appearance of old paint peeling off the surface, and is termed *flaky paint dermatosis*. Multiple punctate pinkish areas over the legs are seen in a few cases. Perioral lesions occur frequently which are caused by riboflavin deficiency and zinc deficiency. Deep and indolent ulcerations and fissures in flexures or over pressure points may also occur. Skin changes regress rapidly following successful dietary management of kwashiorkor.

Hair changes Hair become hypopigmented, lustreless, thin, and easily pluckable. The discoloration may be seen only in some segments, often the growing ends. During recovery, segmental discoloration (*flag sign*) is more apparent as the growing part of the hairs gets pigmented. Alternating bands of hypopigmented and normally pigmented hair are sometimes seen when there are multiple periods of nutritional deprivation and nutritional recovery.

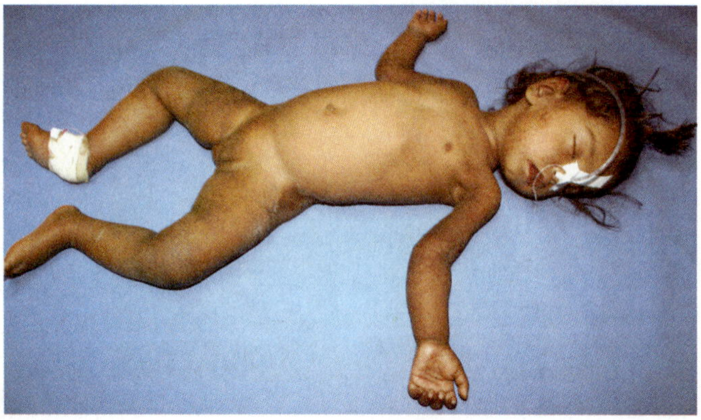

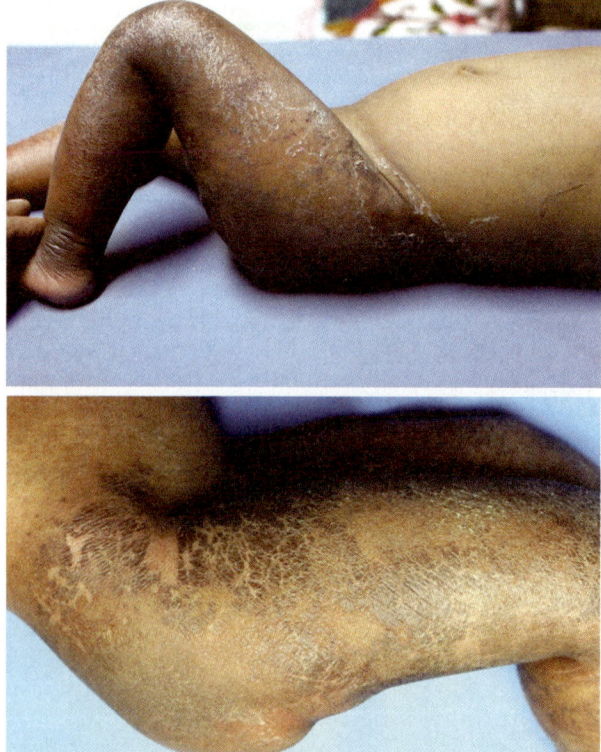

Fig. 3.7 Crazy pavement dermatosis characterized by jet black patches over flexures and pressure sites

Fig. 3.6 Kwashiorkor: Edematous malnutrition with skin changes

Pathophysiology of Kwashiorkor and Marasmus

Classical theory of protein deficiency It hypothesizes that edema in kwashiorkor is caused by hypoalbuminemia secondary to a protein deficient diet and inadequate amino acid supply. In marasmus, energy appears to be the principal lacking factor.

Gopalan's theory of dysadaptation Gopalan did not find any quantitative or qualitative differences in the protein intake of children developing kwashiorkor or marasmus. He hypothesized that the outcome of protein energy deficiency is determined not by the diet, but by the child's response to deficient nutrients. Children differ in their nutritional requirements as well as in their response to deficiency. Marasmus occurs as a result of **adaptation** to chronic nutritional deficiency via cortisol while kwashiorkor is an acute condition wherein the body fails to adapt to the nutritional stress resulting in edema and other manifestations, possibly because of inhibitory effects of dietary carbohydrates mediated by insulin.

Golden's theory of free radicals Kwashiorkor results from an imbalance between the production of free radicals and their safe disposal. Various *noxae* to which these children are exposed produce an oxidative toxic stress which leads to excess of free radical, peroxide, and carbonyl formation. These toxic products cause damage as the mechanisms for their disposal are also compromised. The free radical damage is much more in kwashiorkor than marasmus. Red cell glutathione, serum ferritin, and proportion of red cell NADP in oxidized form are, therefore, markedly different in two conditions. Free radicals cause cell membrane damage that leads to increased permeability and hence edema of kwashiorkor. Free radicals are also linked with a fatty liver and characteristic skin changes of kwashiorkor. The free radical theory may explain the whole range of manifestations of kwashiorkor whereas the protein deficiency theory just accounts for edema.

To conclude, there are numerous complex and interrelated factors that could promote the development of edema. There is no single most important factor. Hypoalbuminemia is probably the major cause followed by potassium depletion and damage by free radicals.

Changes in Body Composition and Function

A severely malnourished child undergoes various changes in structure and function of organ systems. There is a preferential loss of muscle and subcutaneous tissues which in the resting state have a low metabolic activity; while essential organs with high rate of activity, such as brain and heart, are relatively spared. Body fat and total bone mass are reduced.

Fluid and electrolytes Total body water in malnourished children is increased to 70–80% of body weight as compared to 60% in age matched well nourished controls. Greater part of this increase is constituted by extracellular fluid. Activity of the sodium pump is reduced. Cell membranes become more permeable leading to increased intracellular sodium levels and reduced total body potassium and magnesium. Fluid and sodium administration, especially in face of clinical dehydration, should be planned with caution in these children. Dehydration should preferably be corrected orally; intravenous fluids are best avoided unless there is shock.

Metabolic alterations Basal metabolic rate (BMR) is reduced by 30% and energy expenditure due to activity is very low. Heat generation and heat losses are affected so that the child may behave like a poikilotherm. These factors predispose to hypothermia.

Biochemical changes Synthesis of all proteins is reduced. Capacity of the liver to take up, metabolize, and excrete toxins is severely affected. Gluconeogenesis is impaired leading to increased risk of hypoglycemia. Plasma transferrin concentration is markedly reduced. Plasma triglycerides, cholesterol, and β-lipoproteins are reduced in kwashiorkor; they may stay normal or get reduced in marasmus. VLDL accounts for most of the triglycerides in kwashiorkor.

Other nutritional deficiencies As most nutrients are obtained from diet, PEM is frequently associated with multiple nutritional deficiencies. Anemia occurs because of deficiency of iron, vitamin B_{12}, and folic acid; hookworm infestation may also contribute. Vitamin A deficiency may result in keratomalacia. Riboflavin deficiency is also common. Scurvy may manifest as painful legs and knees, and gum bleeding. Subperiosteal hemorrhages may occur, acutely mimicking osteomyelitis. A knee radiograph may unmask subclinical scurvy. As rickets is a disease of growing bones, and PEM results in an impairment of growth, frank changes of rickets might not be apparent despite vitamin D deficiency. Changes get unmasked during recovery, if appropriate vitamin D supplementation is not given during this stage.

Immunity Severe malnutrition is a state of relative immuno-deficiency. These children are more prone to infection because of the following reasons:

- There is impaired *cell-mediated immunity* due to atrophy of thymus and lymphoid tissues. Sensitization to antigens and recognition of earlier sensitization is impaired. Infections requiring cell-mediated immunity (eg, tuberculosis) tend to be unusually severe. Delayed hypersensitivity reactions (eg, Mantoux test) are impaired.
- *Humoral immunity* is relatively less affected. Circulating antibody levels are normal or elevated because of frequent co-existence of infections. B lymphocyte level and proportion are also preserved. Antibody response to most vaccines (eg, measles, diphtheria, tetanus, poliomyelitis) is adequate. However, secretory IgA may be reduced resulting in increased severity, prolonged infectivity, and delayed recovery from infections.
- *Leukocyte count* is generally normal in severe malnutrition. Leukopenia may occur because of associated vitamin B_{12} and folic acid deficiency. Chemotaxis is impaired but phagocytosis is usually normal. There is impaired fungicidal and bactericidal capacity of leukocytes.
- *Physical barriers* against infection such as skin and mucosal membranes are breached. Skin is thin and ulcerated which is easily penetrated by microbes. Mucosae are atrophic resulting in increased risk of gastrointestinal and respiratory tract infections.

Gastrointestinal system Salivary glands atrophy. The liver shows fatty infiltration, fat initially appearing in the periportal area, later spreading towards the central hepatic vein. Pancreatic acini are atrophied and zymogen granules are reduced. Intestinal mucosa demonstrates a moderate reduction in the villus height, increase in the width of villi with a tendency to fusion at the base, and change of columnar villus epithelial into cuboidal cells. Total absorptive surface is reduced. Steatorrhea may occur. Lactose malabsorption is common. Abdominal muscles and large intestine are hypotonic resulting in protuberant abdomen. Rectal prolapse is common.

Central nervous system Growth and development of the brain are adversely affected, especially if malnutrition sets in first two years of life which is a period of rapid brain growth. Associated micronutrient deficiencies (eg, iron, thiamine, vitamin B_{12}, zinc, iodine) further impair the brain function resulting in lower developmental scores. There is impairment of sensory coordination and recognition of figures and shapes. Lag in development and intelligence (IQ) may persist even after recovery from malnutrition.

Renal impairment Glomerular filtration rate and renal plasma flow are reduced in severe PEM. Capacity of the kidneys to excrete excess acid or water is greatly affected. Urinary phosphate and sodium excretion are reduced.

Endocrine system Insulin levels are reduced and the child has glucose intolerance. Cortisol and growth hormone levels are increased.

Cardiovascular system Cardiac output and stroke volume are reduced. Blood pressure is low and renal perfusion is compromised.

3.5 MANAGEMENT OF SEVERE ACUTE MALNUTRITION (SAM)

Criteria for identifying children with SAM for treatment
(Indian Academy of Pediatrics (IAP) 2013; and WHO 2013)

1. *Between 6 months and 5 years.* Children with weight-for-height/length < –3 Z-score of the WHO growth standards or mid-upper arm circumference (MUAC) < 11.5 cm or bilateral pedal edema of nutritional origin.

2. *<6 months of age.* MUAC cannot be used as a criterion for diagnosis of SAM in children below 6 months of age. The other two criteria remain the same as above. For children with length less than 45 cm, visible severe wasting may be used to diagnose SAM.

IAP Guidelines (2013) also included visible severe wasting as one of the criteria for diagnosis of SAM; however, this may be subjective and used only when measurement of weight/length/height/MUAC is not feasible.

Criteria for hospitalization in children with SAM
1. *Between 6 months and 5 years.* A majority of children with SAM may be managed in the community, if (*i*) they are having a good appetite (judged by the presence of appetite test) (**Box 3.2**) and (*ii*) absence of complications. Those with poor appetite or complications need inpatient care (**Box 3.3**).

2. *All infants <6 months* with SAM should be managed as inpatients.

> **Box 3.2** Appetite Test
>
> *Procedure* Ask the mother to offer RUTF to the child in a quiet area gently. Child is allowed to drink water while feeding. *Interpretation* **Passed** test, if child eats eagerly. **Fails**, if refuses therapeutic food even after persistent encouragement.
>
> *RUTF: Ready to use therapeutic food*

> **Box 3.3** Criteria for Admission in a Child with SAM
>
> • Failed appetite test
> • Age <6 months
> • Presence of any of the following complications: 1. Fever (39°C) or hypothermia (<35°C); 2. Persistent vomiting; 3. Severe dehydration; 4. Edema; 5. Very weak, apathetic; 6. Hypoglycemia; 7. Severe anemia; 8. Severe pneumonia; 9. Extensive superficial infection; 10. Purpura or bleeding; and 11. Systemic infection
> • If caregiver is unable to take care of the child at home

Why Children with Severe Acute Malnutrition Need to be Treated Differently?

A child with SAM has higher risk of mortality due to several physiological changes in these children, known as *reductive adaptation*.

Reductive Adaptation

The body systems slow down to allow survival on limited calories. When a child's carbohydrate intake is insufficient, fat stores are utilized to provide energy. Later, protein is mobilized from muscles, skin, and gut. Physiological and metabolic changes also take place to conserve energy. These changes take place in an orderly progression, which is called reductive adaptation. A child with SAM conserves energy by reducing physical activity and growth; reducing basal metabolism by slowing protein turnover; reducing the functional reserve of organs; slowing the sodium and potassium pumps in cell membranes and reducing their number; and reducing inflammatory and immune responses.

Consequences of Reductive Adaptation

The functioning of every cell, organ, and system is affected and this puts the child in a very fragile state. Following is a brief description of the effects on different organs:

• The liver is less able to make glucose; so there is increased risk of hypoglycemia and hypothermia. In addition, liver is less able to excrete excess dietary protein and toxins. These changes have implications for feeding. First, long gaps without food must be avoided. This means giving frequent feeds day and night, which is a ready source of glucose. Second, we must limit protein intake to avoid stressing the liver.

• The kidneys are less able to excrete excess fluid and sodium. So, excess fluid and sodium (from feeds or rehydration fluid) can lead to fluid overload.

• The heart is smaller and weaker and has a reduced output. Any excess fluid in the circulation stresses the heart and can lead to death from heart failure. This means that fluid intake must be carefully controlled initially. Also, feeds and rehydration fluid must be low in sodium.

- The gut produces less acid and smaller amounts of enzymes. The intestinal villi are flattened, and motility is reduced. These changes cause bacterial colonization of the small bowel, damage of the mucosa, and deconjugation of bile acids. So, initially, feeds must be small to avoid exceeding the gut's functional capacity, and the composition of feeds should be such that it can easily be absorbed. Feeds should be *enteral, never parenteral*, to reduce the risk of fluid overload. Repair of the gut is also quicker, if nutrients are physically present in the lumen.
- During reductive adaptation, sodium leaks into cells due to fewer and slower pumps, leading to excess body sodium. Potassium leaks out of cells and is lost in urine, contributing to electrolyte imbalance, anorexia, fluid retention, and heart failure. So, we need to restrict sodium and provide potassium. We must also provide magnesium to help the potassium get into cells.
- Reduction in muscle mass is accompanied by loss of intracellular nutrients and smaller reserves of muscle glycogen.
- Red cell mass is also reduced, liberating iron. Conversion of harmful free iron to ferritin needs glucose and amino acids, and there may not be enough glucose available to put all the iron into safe storage. Free iron promotes the growth of pathogens and the production of free radicals which damage cell membranes. So, during initial feeding, we need to withhold iron, and provide vitamins and minerals to help mop up free radicals.

Median case fatality rate in children with SAM is very high, ie, approximately 23.5%, if these changes are not kept in mind. Reasons for high case fatality are listed in **Box 3.4**. The case fatality can be brought down to approximately 7–10% by standard case management protocol.

Box 3.4 Ten Reasons for High Mortality in Severe Acute Malnutrition

1. Inability to distinguish between acute and rehabilitation phases
2. Excessive use of intravenous fluids
3. Fluid overload due to lack of monitoring during rehydration
4. Use of diuretics for edema
5. Use of albumin for edema
6. Not keeping the child warm and euglycemic
7. Low index of suspicion for infection
8. Early use of diets high in protein and sodium
9. Failure to monitor food intake
10. Early treatment of anemia with oral iron.

Treatment | **10 Steps for Management of Severe Malnutrition**

Sequential management of SAM is depicted in Fig. 3.8. WHO describes the 10 steps of management of severe acute malnutrition. These steps are accomplished in two phases: An initial *stabilization phase* where the acute medical conditions are managed (steps 1–6); and a longer *rehabilitation phase* (steps 7–10).

- The first six steps (steps 1–6) are related to treatment of complications, and can be remembered with the mnemonic **SHIELDED.**

S —Sugar deficiency—ie, hypoglycemia
H —Hypothermia
I —Infection and septic shock
EL —ELectrolyte imbalance
DE—Dehydration
D —Deficiencies of iron, vitamins, and other micronutrients.

- Steps 7–10 are related to dietary management which can be remembered by the mnemonic **BEST** as described below:

B — Beginning of feeding
E — Energy dense feeding
S — Stimulation of emotional and sensorial development
T — Transfer to home-based diets before discharge or transfer to nutritional rehabilitation centers.

Step 1: Hypoglycemia: Treat and Prevent

Obtain blood sugar. The child may throw seizures or become unconscious due to hypoglycemia (blood sugar <54 mg/dL). If the child is unconscious, lethargic, or convulsing, administer 10% glucose 5 mL/kg intravenously. If the child is conscious, administer 50 mL 10% glucose solution orally or by nasogastric tube. Feeding should be started immediately with F-75 milk-based diet (described in step 7) and continued every 30 minutes for two hours.

If blood sugar continues to be low after two hours, give another 50 mL bolus of 10% glucose and continue feeding F-75 every 30 minute until stable. Thereafter, feeds are given every 2 hourly.

Step 2: Hypothermia: Treat and Prevent

Infants under 1 year of age and those with marasmus, extensive skin loss, or serious infections are prone to get hypothermic (rectal temperature < 35.5°C). Cover the hypothermic child with a warmed blanket and place near a heat source (not hot water bottle). Start feeding immediately with F-75. Alternatively, use *kangaroo technique* (placing the child on mother's bare chest or abdomen and covering both of them). Monitor body temperature two-hourly (half-hourly, if heater is used) until it rises to >36.5°.

For prevention of hypothermia in a severely malnourished child, give two-hourly feeding and cover with a warm blanket, specially during the night. Keep the child dry and let the child sleep with mother at night for warmth.

Step 3: Dehydration: Treat and Prevent

Evaluation of dehydration is difficult in children with severe malnutrition. Skin turgor (elasticity of skin) may be lost either due to loss of the subcutaneous fat or due to loss of extracellular water in dehydration. On the other hand, presence of edema in kwashiorkor may mask the signs of dehydration. As assessment of dehydration is difficult in malnourished children, it is suggested that all children having watery diarrhea should be assumed to have at least *some dehydration*. Presence of weak pulses and oliguria indicate *severe dehydration* or septic shock.

Treatment Do not use intravenous route to correct dehydration except in presence of shock. Give WHO low osmolarity ORS 5 mL/kg every 30 minutes for 2 hours, orally or by nasogastric tube, then 5–10 mL/kg/h for next 4–10 hours: the exact amount to be given should be determined by how much the child wants, stool loss, and vomiting. Replace the ORS doses at 4, 6, 8, and 10 hours with F-75, if rehydration is continuing at these times. ReSoMal (recommended ORS solution for malnourished children), advocated by WHO is not universally available; and,

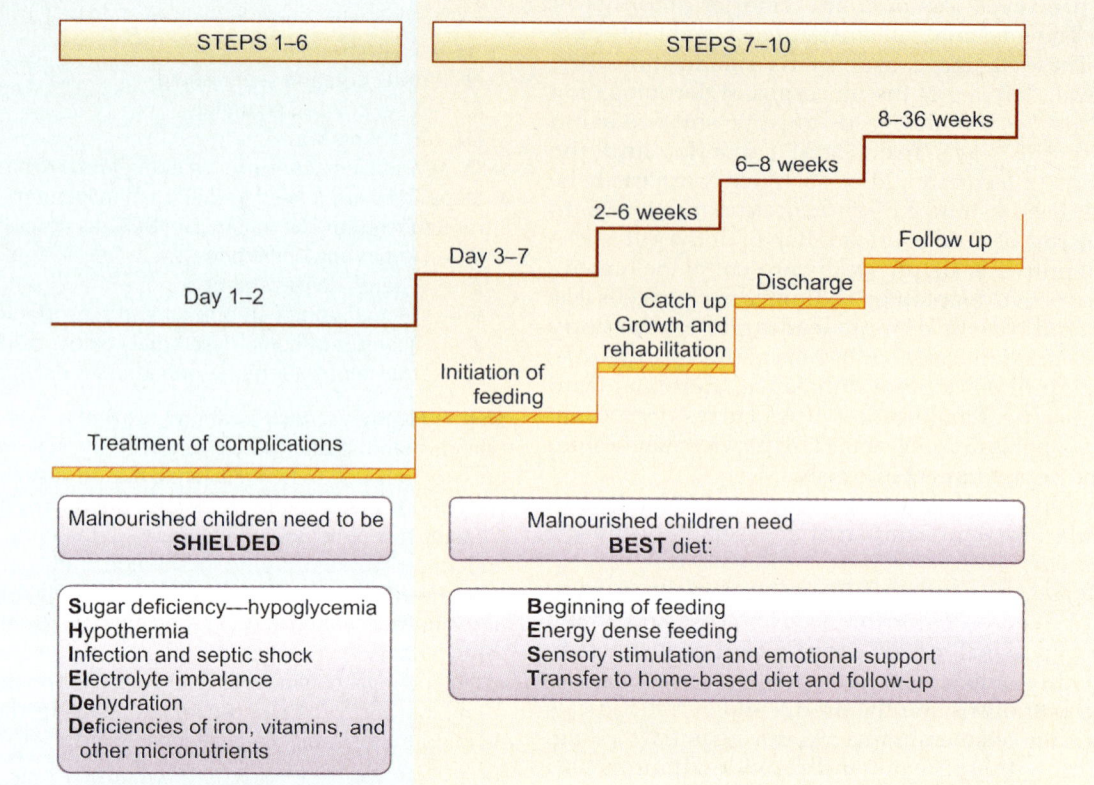

Fig. 3.8 Sequential management of severe acute malnutrition (SAM)

it can be safely replaced by the standard low osmolarity WHO ORS (glucose and sodium: 75 mMol/L each; potassium: 20 mEq/L; chloride: 65 mEq/L; and citrate: 10 mEq/L).

Return of tears, moist mouth, eyes and fontanel appearing less sunken, and improved skin turgor, may indicate rehydration. However, severely malnourished children may not show these changes even when fully rehydrated. Continuing rapid breathing and pulse during rehydration suggest coexisting infection or over hydration. Signs of excess fluid (overhydration) are increasing respiratory rate and pulse rate, increasing edema, and puffy eyelids. If these signs occur, stop fluids immediately and reassess after one hour.

Severe dehydration

Intravenous therapy should be given to children with weak pulse or oliguria to correct severe dehydration. Administer Ringer lactate or N/2 saline in 5% dextrose (15 mL/kg) over 1 hour. If the child fails to improve after the first hour of treatment (15 mL/kg), assume septic shock and manage accordingly (*see* Step 5). If there are signs of improvement (pulse volume improves, and pulse rate decreases), repeat IV fluids at 15 mL/kg over next 1 hour. Then switch to oral or nasogastric rehydration with low osmolarity ORS (100 mL/kg at the rate of 10 mL/kg/h in next 10 hours). Alternate aliquots of ORS can be replaced with starter F-75. If the child cannot be given orally due to paralytic ileus or repeated vomiting, same fluid (100 mL/kg @ 10 mL/kg/h) can be given as N/6 saline in 5% dextrose, intravenously. Maximum attempt should, however, be made to stop IV fluids and shift to feeding F-75 diet, as soon as possible.

To prevent dehydration when a child has continuing watery diarrhea, keep feeding with starter F-75 and replace approxi-

mate volume of stool losses with low osmolarity ORS. Give 50–100 mL of ORS after each watery stool. If the child is breastfed, encourage to continue breastfeeding.

Step 4: Electrolyte Imbalance: Treat and Prevent
All severely malnourished children have excess body sodium even though plasma sodium may be low. Therefore, give low sodium fluid (ie, WHO reduced osmolarity ORS) when rehydrating. Hypertonic saline should not be used even in presence of hyponatremia.

Deficiencies of potassium and magnesium are also present and may take at least two weeks to correct. Child should receive extra potassium (3–4 mMol/kg/d) and magnesium (0.4–0.6 mMol/kg/d). Prepare food without salt.

Congestive heart failure CHF may occur secondary to overhydration, severe anemia, and high sodium intake. Fluid intake must be restricted and frusemide 1 mg/kg IV is given. However, diuretics should never be given to reduce edema in a malnourished child.

Step 5: Infection: Treat and Prevent
The child should be clinically examined for the presence of infections and adequately treated. Most common sites of localised infections are skin, gastrointestinal, respiratory, and urinary tracts. Skin infections are due to *Staphylococcus aureus* or streptococci. *Candida* may cause secondary infection over exudative lesions. Skin infections can be prevented by applying barrier cream on raw areas. Perineum should be kept dry.

Osteomyelitis is generally caused by staphylococci, *H. influenzae*, or *Streptococcus*. Malaria may present with diarrhea and no fever. Always obtain blood culture, chest radiograph, peripheral smear for malarial parasite, and urine culture in a severely malnourished child before starting antimicrobials.

Preferred antibiotics In severe malnutrition, infections are often hidden. Therefore, antibiotics should be given routinely on admission. If the child appears to have no complications, give oral amoxicillin; and if the child is severely ill (apathetic, lethargic) or has complications (hypoglycemia, hypothermia, broken skin, respiratory tract infection, or urinary tract infection), administer a combination of ampicillin and gentamicin, parenterally. If the child fails to improve clinically within 48 hours, add chloramphenicol. Where specific infections are identified, give specific antibiotics as appropriate.

Continuing diarrhea Diarrhea should subside during the first week of treatment with cautious feeding. In the rehabilitation phase, loose, poorly formed stools are no cause for concern provided weight gain is satisfactory. Mucosal damage and giardiasis are the two most common causes of continuing diarrhea. Where possible, examine the stools by microscopy. Administer metronidazole (7.5 mg/kg 8-hourly for 7 days), if not already given. Rarely, diarrhea is due to lactose intolerance. Starter F-75 is a low-lactose feed. In exceptional cases, substitute milk feeds with yoghurt or a lactose-free infant formula. Reintroduce milk feeds gradually in the rehabilitation phase.

Tuberculosis If TB is strongly suspected (contacts with adult TB patient, poor growth despite good intake, chronic cough, chest infection not responding to antibiotics), perform Mantoux test (false negatives are frequent) and chest X-ray. If test is positive or there is a strong suspicion of TB, treat according to national TB guidelines.

Septic shock Shock from dehydration and sepsis are likely to coexist in severely malnourished children. They are difficult to differentiate on clinical signs alone. Children with dehydration will respond to IV fluids. Those with septic shock will not respond to initial bolus of 15 mL/kg over 1 hour. In this case, give maintenance IV fluids (4 mL/kg/h) while waiting for blood. When blood is available transfuse fresh whole blood at 10 mL/kg *slowly* over 3 hours. Broad-spectrum antibiotics are immediately initiated. Steroids and adrenaline are of no use. If facilities are available, a central venous pressure line should be inserted and the patient should be managed with vasopressors, etc. as for septic shock, in an intensive care unit.

Step 6: Micronutrient Deficiencies

All severely malnourished children should receive vitamins and minerals as follows:
- Vitamin A orally on day 1 (200,000 IU for age >12 months; 100,000 IU for 6–12 months and 50,000 IU for 0–5 months) unless there is definite evidence that a dose has been given in the last month. In presence of xerophthalmia, the same dose should be repeated on the next day and 2 weeks later. Children receiving F-75, F-100 or RUTF do not require high dose prophylactic vitamin A supplementation; they should receive 5000 IU vitamin A daily (WHO, 2013). If there is corneal clouding or ulceration, give additional eye care in form of antibiotic drops, atropine, and padding.
- Folic acid 5 mg on day 1, followed by 1 mg everyday.
- Magnesium sulfate 2 mL of 50% solution on day 1.
- Vitamin K 2.5 mg IM on day 1

- Give multivitamin supplements, zinc (2 mg/kg/d), copper (0.3 mg/kg/d), and potassium (2 mEq/kg/d) daily for at least 2 weeks.

Anemia Blood transfusion is required, if hemoglobin is less than 4 g/dL. If there is respiratory distress, transfusion can be given with hemoglobin between 4 and 6 g/dL. Give whole blood 10 mL/kg body weight slowly over 3 hours with furosemide 1 mg/kg IV at the start of the transfusion. It is particularly important that the volume of 10 mL/kg is not exceeded in severely malnourished children. If the severely anemic child has signs of cardiac failure, transfuse packed cells (5–7 mL/kg) rather than whole blood. In mild or moderate anemia, oral iron should be given for two months to replenish iron stores but this should not be started until the child has begun to gain weight (usually by the second week), as giving iron in the initial phase can make infections worse.

Step 7: Begin Cautious Feeding (0–7 days)

Start feeding after electrolyte, water imbalance and infections are brought under control. Do not force food and avoid overloading the system. Vigorous feeding may lead to heart failure and death due to (*i*) excessive dietary sodium; (*ii*) rapidly expanding ECF volume; or (*iii*) activated sodium pump secondary to increased energy supply again leading to increased ECF volume.

The essential features of feeding in the stabilization phase are as follows:
1. Small, frequent feeds of low osmolarity and low lactose;
2. Oral or nasogastric (NG) feeds (never parenteral preparations); and
3. *Calories*: 100 kcal/kg/d; *Proteins*: 1–1.5 g/kg/d; and *Fluids*: 130 mL/kg/d (100 mL/kg/d, if the child has edema.)

Route of feeding Feeds should be initiated as early as possible. If oral feeding is not possible, give nasogastric feeding. Feeding through a nasogastric tube for a few days results in a dramatic change in the behavior of the patient, who then starts accepting oral feeds after a few days. When the child is able to take fluids by mouth, they should be given frequently and in small amounts. Record the volume taken. If the child is breastfed, encourage to continue breastfeeding.

Type of feed To start with, milk-based formulas such as starter F-75 containing 75 kcal/100 mL and 0.9 g protein/100 mL *(consisting of dried full cream milk powder 35 g or fresh full-cream cow's milk 300 mL, sugar 100 g, vegetable oil 20 g; electrolyte/mineral solution 20 mL; all mixed and volume made up to 1000 mL)* will be satisfactory for most children. Give from a cup or spoon.

Amount of feed A recommended schedule in which volume is gradually increased, and feeding frequency gradually decreased is as follows:

Days	Frequency	Vol/kg/feed	Vol/kg/d
1–2	2-hourly	11 mL	130 mL
3–5	3-hourly	16 mL	130 mL
6–7+	4-hourly	22 mL	130 mL

Use the day 1 weight to calculate how much to give, even if the child loses or gains weight after admission. If the oral intake does not reach 80 kcal/kg/d (105 mL starter formula/kg), give the remaining feed by nasogastric tube. Do not exceed 100 kcal/kg/d in this phase. During this phase, diarrhea should gradually diminish and edematous children should lose weight.

Step 8: Energy Dense Feeding: Achieve Catch-up Growth

Increase in the amount of calories by giving energy dense foods is required once the child is free of complications, shows signs of recovery and the appetite returns after initiation of dietary therapy. This helps the child to restore normal weight for height.

For optimum catch-up growth of severely malnourished children, therapeutic diet should contain energy (150–220 kcal/kg/day) and protein (4–5 g/kg/d). Energy, rather than protein is the principal determinant of catch up growth rate. The type of foods used during this phase should be energy dense.

The aim should be to achieve a rapid weight gain of >10 g per kg per day.

F-100—the catch-up formula diet The recommended milk-based F-100 diet contains 100 kcal and 2.9 g protein per 100 mL. F-100 consists of dried full cream milk powder 110 g, sugar 50 g, vegetable oil 30 g; electrolyte/mineral solution 20 mL; all mixed and volume made up to 1000 mL. To change from starter to catch-up formula, replace starter F-75 with the same amount of catch-up formula F-100 for 48 hours then, increase each successive feed by 10 mL. After the transition, give frequent feeds (at least 4-hourly) of unlimited amounts of a catch-up formula to achieve caloric intakes of 150–220 kcal/kg/d and protein intakes of 4–6 g/kg/d. If the child is breastfed, encourage to continue. **Table 3.17** provides a detailed comparison of F-75 and F-100 formula diets.

Ready-to-use therapeutic foods (RUTFs) These are soft or crushable foods used in the domiciliary management of severe malnutrition. These are meant to be consumed without any modification. These are particularly useful in situations where preparation and availability of home made catch-up food is doubtful. RUTFs have a similar nutrient composition to F-100 but are not water-based, and have a longer shelf life. Most RUTFs are made of peanut paste, fats, and added micronutrients and minerals. At least half of the proteins contained in these foods should come from milk products.

The concept of community based management emerged from the observations that many children classified as severe malnutrition have preserved appetite, and thus can be managed at home with safe high energy foods. Also, the success of RUTF in emergency situations prompted the international agencies to promote its use. RUTFs are to be used in severely malnourished children older than 6 months of age when there are no medical complications and appetite is preserved. RUTF can also be used in place of F-100 in the rehabilitation phase of management of SAM.

Modified family foods can be used provided they have comparable energy and protein concentrations. These foods can be prepared from mixture of cereal flour (eg, wheat), pulses (eg, Bengal gram flour), oil or ghee and jaggery. One example of such energy dense food is *'besan panjiri'* which is prepared by mixing one part each of the above items. It provides 500 calories and 9 g of proteins per 100 g of the preparation. Other such foods can also be prepared based on the local availability and taste. Home available foods can also be used at this stage with added oil and sugar/jaggery to make the food energy dense (eg, adding oil and curd to *khichdi*, cooking *'parantha'* in place of *'chapati'* and cooking rice with jaggery and oil).

Step 9: Sensory Stimulation and Emotional Support

Severe malnutrition leads to delayed mental and behavioral development. It is important to provide tender loving care; and a cheerful, stimulating environment. Structured play therapy is essential for at least 15–30 min/day. Encourage physical activity as soon as the child is well enough. Maternal involvement is a must for ensuring complete recovery and also maintaining a good nutritional status in future also.

Step 10: Transfer to Home-based Diet and Prepare for Follow-up

As the child will be ultimately managed at home, it is necessary that the child should be shifted to the adequate quantities of home-based diets. As a general rule, the diet prescribed for the child should be such, which the family can afford to provide for the baby within its limited income, can be easily cooked at home, does not perish easily, is culturally acceptable and easily available in the local market.

Return of appetite, gain in body weight with loss of edema, disappearance of hepatomegaly, and rising serum albumin are the early signs of recovery. A child who has achieved 90% weight-for-length can be considered to have completely recovered. This may take 6–8 weeks. The child is still likely to have a low weight-for-age because of stunting.

Good feeding practices and sensory stimulation should be continued at home. Show parent or caregiver how to feed frequently with energy- and nutrient-dense foods. Advise parent/caregiver to bring child back for regular follow-up checks and immunization.

Failure to Respond to Treatment

This is characterized by inadequate weight gain during rehabilitation phase. The rate of weight gain is classified as (*i*) *Poor*: <5 g/kg/d; (*ii*) *Moderate*: 5–10 g/kg/d; and (*iii*) *Good*: >10 g/kg/d. Possible causes of poor weight gain include (*a*) inadequate feeding, (*b*) specific nutrient deficiencies, (*c*) untreated infection, (*d*) HIV/AIDS; (*e*) underlying systemic disorder; and (*f*) psychological deprivation. A child may have a primary or secondary failure to respond to treatment.

Primary failure to respond may be characterized by the following criteria:
  (*i*) Failure to regain appetite by day 4;
 (*ii*) Failure to start losing of edema by day 4;
(*iii*) Failure of disappearance of edema by day 10; or
(*iv*) Failure to gain weight at least by 5 g/kg of body weight per day by day 10 of therapy.

Secondary failure to respond is said to have occurred, if the child does not gain >5 g/kg/d body weight for 3 consecutive days any time during the rehabilitative phase.

Table 3.17 Milk-based F-75 and F-100 Diets for Severe PEM

Diets contents (per 100 mL)	F-75 Starter	F-100 Catch up
Cow's milk (mL)	30	95
Sugar (g)	9	5
Vegetable oil (g)	2	2
Water (mL)	100	100
Energy (kcal)	75	100
Protein (g)	0.9	2.9
Lactose (g)	1.2	3.8

Case Study | Approach to a Child with Severe Acute Malnutrition

An 18-month-old unimmunized girl is brought to the emergency with frequent loose stools, vomiting, and poor feeding for 7 days. The child is predominantly milk fed (half diluted buffalo's milk with bottle) in addition to some biscuits. Her weight and length are 5 kg and 68 cm, respectively. On examination, she has pallor, weak pulses, cold clammy skin, loss of skin turgor, and sunken eyes.

Q1. Assess and classify the nutritional status of this child.
Assessment The child is obviously malnourished as suggested by her weight and dietary pattern. These children have multiple medical and social problems. The following problems can be identified in this child.
1. Acute diarrhea
2. Cold clammy skin and weak pulses (severe dehydration and/or septic shock)
3. Severe malnutrition and anemia
4. Poor feeding (possibility of hypoglycemia and/or infection)
5. Faulty feeding (no semi-solids, dilution of milk, bottle feeding)
6. Lack of immunization

Classification Classify severity of malnutrition as per IAP or WHO classification. This child would be classified as *PEM Grade IV* by IAP Classification; and as *severely wasted* and *severely stunted* by WHO classification. Child's weight is 46% of the expected for age (50th percentile at 18 months is 10.8 kg)—*hence PEM IV*. Her length is 84% (<3 SD) of the expected for age (50th percentile at 18 months is 80.9 cm and –3 SD is 71.7 cm)—*hence severely stunted*. The weight for length is 64% (≤3 SD) of the expected (50th percentile for 68 cm is 7.8 kg and –3 SD is 5.5 kg)]—*hence severely wasted*. The child thus has **severe acute malnutrition**.

Classify state of dehydration In view of sunken eyes and cold clammy skin, the child is classified as having severe dehydration with shock. Alternatively, the child could be in *septic shock*. Loss of skin turgor may not be a reliable sign in severe acute malnutrition.

Q2. Outline the immediate management of this child.
• Admit the child.
• Secure intravenous line and draw samples for blood glucose, blood counts, electrolytes, blood gas, and blood culture.
• Give 25 mL (5 mL/kg) of 10% dextrose IV, if *hypoglycemic*. Give empirically, if blood sugar report is not immediately available.
• Record *temperature* and provide warmth to the child. Keep the child dry, cover with blankets and shift to a warm area.
• *Start fluids for dehydration and shock*. This child has shock which should be initially managed with intravenous fluids. The fluid management in this child would be:
  – *First hour*: 75 mL (15 mL/kg) Ringer lactate or N/2 saline in 5% dextrose intravenously. If there is improvement after 1 hour (pulse rate and respiratory rate decrease and pulse volume improves), repeat 75 mL (15 mL/kg) over next hour. If there is no improvement, consider septic shock and manage in an intensive care setting. In case of improvement, continue fluid administration as below.
  3–12 hours: Put a nasogastric tube and give WHO reduced osmolarity ORS at 50 mL/hour (10 mL/kg/hr). Replace the ORS doses at 4, 6, 8 and 10 hours with F-75 (50 mL @ 10 mL/kg).
• *Screen and treat for infections* This child is severely malnourished and has presented with diarrhea, and poor feeding. Start antibiotics immediately and continue even when no organism is identified in urine, stool, or blood culture. The starting antibiotics in this case could be Inj. ampicillin 100 mg/kg/day (4 divided doses) with gentamicin 7.5 mg/kg/day (3 divided doses). Ceftriaxone and vancomycin may be given for severe Gram-negative and Gram-positive infections, respectively. Obtain a chest X-ray and send urine and stool for culture. Screen for tuberculosis.
• Administer vitamin A 2 Lakh IU orally or 1 Lakh IU intramuscularly.
• Administer vitamin K 2.5 mg IM/IV single dose.
• Administer 2 mL of 50% magnesium sulfate IV and 5 mg of folic acid orally.
• Correct electrolyte disturbances, if any, once serum electrolytes report is available.

Q3. Present a detailed plan for dietary management for this child.
Start dietary therapy as soon as possible, if there is no abdominal distension and the bowel sounds are present. Give nasogastric feeds, if the child does not accept orally.

Begin feeding
Start F-75 diet at 130 mL/kg/day. This child will need 55 mL of F-75 every two hourly. This will provide around 100 kcal/kg/day. Continue 2 hourly F-75 for first two days. Make the feeds 3 hourly (80 mL @ 16 mL/kg/feed) from day 3 to day 5, and 4 hourly (110 mL @ 22 mL/kg/feed) from day 6. Shift to high energy F-100 diet or RUTF, if the child's appetite is good (ie, easily finishes all F-75 feeds orally).

Phase of high energy feeding
Readiness to enter this phase is signaled by a return of appetite, usually about one week after admission. When the appetite returns, feed with a cup. Replace starter F-75 with the same amount (110 mL 4 hourly) of catch-up formula F-100 for 48 hours. Increase the amount of F-100 by 10 mL in each successive feed from day 3 onwards till the intake reaches 30 mL/kg/feed (200 mL/kg/d).

| Case Study | Approach to a Child with Severe Acute Malnutrition *(Contd.)* |

Introduce solid foods as early as possible to accustom the child to home-based foods. If the child is able to accept solid home-based foods, she can be shifted to full home-cooked meal providing the desired calories. The high energy therapeutic diets should be continued till the child's weight for height is about 90% of the median.

Preparing the diet for home care

Provide diet chart to the mother which can be modified daily by the mother to provide the variety to the child's food. The diet should provide caloric intake of 150 kcal/kg of the present weight (which should have become 90% of median for that height). Use **Table 3.14** to make a diet chart.

A sample vegetarian North Indian diet for this child is depicted in **Table 3.18**. This diet is based on caloric requirement of 1050 kcal/day (150 kcal/kg) for a 7 kg child. (The weight of this child should have become 90% of median for 68 cm, ie, 7 kg by this time.) The protein and mineral content is usually adequate, if the diet is wholesome containing foods from all food categories shown in **Fig. 3.1**. If the child is unable to consume the suggested amount at one time, divide into frequent small meals. Non-vegetarian foods like egg, fish, meat, etc. can be included, if culturally acceptable.

Table 3.18 Sample Home-based Diet

Foodstuff	Calories
Morning breakfast	
1 cup (200 mL) milk + 1tsp sugar	155 (135+20)
1slice bread (big) + ½ tsp (2.5 g) butter	103 (85+18)
2 Biscuits	60
Lunch	
1 chapati	80
½ cup dal	100
½ cup vegetable (dry)	75
Evening snack	
1 Banana	90
Dinner	
1 cup khichdi	200
100 mL curd	32
Night	
1 cup milk + 1 tsp sugar	155 (135+20)
	Total = 1050 kcal

Treatment of micronutrient deficiencies (iron, vitamins, zinc)

Screen for associated micronutrient deficiency. Pallor of conjunctiva or, palm suggests *anemia*. *Zinc deficiency* is characterized by perianal rash, redness, and excoriation. Night blindness, bitot spots, or conjunctival dryness are the pointers of *vitamin A deficiency*. *Riboflavin deficiency* results in ulceration and excoriation at angle of mouth. Bleeding gums, swelling or pain in lower limbs may suggest scurvy due to *vitamin C deficiency*. Wrist widening, frontal bossing and prominent costochondral junctions are the early features of *rickets*. Clinical deficiency of any micronutrient, if present has to be treated accordingly.

This child is having anemia. Anemia in SAM is multifactorial. Provide iron (3 mg/kg/day), folic acid (0.1 mg/kg/day), vitamin B_{12} (0.1 mg/kg/day), copper (0.3 mg/kg/day) and pyridoxine (70 mg/kg/day).

This child does not have any other symptom or sign of vitamin deficiency but that does not rule out subclinical micronutrient deficiencies. Therefore, administer vitamin D 6 Lakh U orally or intramuscularly (single dose) and zinc (2 mg/kg/day) even when there is no clinical evidence of their deficiency.

Children who fail to respond to treatment should be screened for persistent diarrhea, giardiasis, shigellosis, amebiasis, otitis media, pneumonia, urinary tract infections, fungal infections, scabies, tuberculosis, helminthiasis, malaria, and HIV/AIDS. If the search proves futile, one should also look for any underlying immunological disease, inborn errors of metabolism and malignancies.

Criteria for Discharge

As per recent WHO recommendations (2013), a child with SAM should be discharged when WFH/WFL is ≥ –2 Z-score, or MUAC is ≥ 12.5 cm; and has no edema for at least 2 weeks. Ensure that all immunizations have been initiated and mother trained and counseled for care at home. For some children, earlier discharge may be considered, if effective alternative supervision is available.

Early discharge may be considered only if the following criteria are met:

- *The child* is aged >6 months; has completed antibiotic treatment; has good appetite and good weight gain; and has taken potassium/magnesium/mineral/vitamin supplement for 2 weeks (or continuing supplementation at home is possible).
- *The mother/caregiver* is not employed outside the home; is specifically trained to give appropriate feeding; has the financial resources to feed the child; lives within easy reach of the hospital for urgent readmission, if the child becomes ill; can be visited weekly; is trained to give structured play therapy; and is motivated to follow the advice given.

• *Local health workers* are trained to support home care; are specifically trained to examine the child clinically at home, to decide when to refer, to weigh the child, and give appropriate advice; and are motivated.

When children are being rehabilitated at home, it is essential to give frequent meals with a high energy and protein content. Aim for achieving at least 150 kcal/kg/d and adequate protein intake (at least 4 g/kg/d). This means feeding the child at least 5 times per day with foods that contain approximately 100 kcal and 2–3 g protein per 100 g. A practical approach would be using simple modifications of the usual home foods or by use of RUTF. Vitamin, iron and electrolyte/mineral supplements can be continued at home.

Management of Mild and Moderate Malnutrition

Children with mild and moderate malnutrition are best managed in their home and communities because it is feasible, economical and effective. Mother learns about nutritional needs of child and hygienic feeding which are important to prevent recurrence of malnutrition.

The parents are advised to increase the amount and energy density of the food consumed by the child by all available means. Child may receive initial treatment and health education from a nutritional rehabilitation center. After recovery, they should be kept under nutritional surveillance to detect and prevent deterioration in their nutritional status, as early as possible and to promote their nutrition and health by prompt remedial measures.

Give a diet chart to the mother which can be modified daily by the mother to provide the variety to the child's food. The diet should provide caloric intake of 150 kcal/kg of the present weight. For the purpose of preparing a diet chart, caloric content of various foodstuffs is given in **Table 3.5**.

Bhatnagar S, Lodha R, Choudhury P, *et al*. IAP guidelines 2006 on hospital based management of severely malnourished children. *Indian Pediatr*. 2007;44:443–61.

Community based management of severe acute malnutrition. A joint statement by the World Health Organization, World Food Programme, United Nations Standing Committee on Nutrition, United Nations Children's Fund. Geneva: World Health Organization/World Food Programme, United Nations Standing Committee on Nutrition/United Nations Children's Fund; 2007.

Dalwai S, Choudhury P, Bavdekar SB, *et al*. Consensus Statement of the Indian Academy of Pediatrics on integrated management of severe acute malnutrition. *Indian Pediatr*. 2013;50:399—404.

Management of severe malnutrition: a manual for physician and other senior healthworkers. Geneva: World Health Organization; 1999.

Ministry of Health and Family Welfare, Government of India. Operational guidelines on facility based management of children with severe acute malnutrition. National Rural Health Mission, New Delhi, India: Ministry of Health and Family Welfare; 2011.

WHO child growth standards and identification of severe acute malnutrition in infant s and children. A joint statement by the World Health Organization and the United Nations Children's Fund. Geneva: World Health Organization; 2009.

WHO Guidelines Approved by the Guidelines Review Committee. Guideline: Updates on the Management of Severe Acute Malnutrition in infants and Children. Geneva: World Health Organization; 2013.

3.6 MICRONUTRIENT DEFICIENCIES

Micronutrients are nutrients needed in tiny amounts, may be a few mg or micrograms per day and include various *vitamins* and *minerals*. They do not contribute to the energy intake but normal healthy living is not possible without them.

While deficiencies in any of the essential micronutrients can result in health problems, there are a few that are vital to intelligence, immunity, reproduction, and work capacity. They cannot be synthesized endogenously and have to be supplied in diet; eg, vitamin A, iron, iodine, zinc, and folic acid.

Extent of Problem

Micronutrient malnutrition continues to affect over 2000 million people worldwide. According to WHO estimates, over 2 million child deaths (around 20% of total) are attributable to zinc, vitamin A, and iron deficiencies. There are several reasons for such deficiencies. The population may be deficient because they have poor access to micronutrient rich food due to poverty, defective crop growing pattern, deficient soil quality, inappropriate climate, or geographical isolation. Traditional dietary fads may also hinder intake, absorption, or utilization of micronutrient rich foods.

Vitamins

Vitamins are organic compounds required in a small quantity from diet to maintain vital body functions. These serve diverse functions such as cofactors and coenzymes in enzyme systems (eg, vitamin B complex), hormones (eg, vitamin D), and antioxidants (eg, vitamin E). Vitamin deficiencies may be caused by (*i*) deficient intake (ignorance, food fads, faulty cooking methods); (*ii*) faulty absorption (malabsorption, chronic diarrhea); (*iii*) increased losses; (*iv*) poor utilization (chronic liver disease), or (*v*) greater demand. The requirement of vitamins increase in preterm babies, during postoperative stress, infections, and in some genetic metabolic disorders.

Vitamins are classified into (*i*) *water-soluble vitamins*: vitamin B complex and vitamin C; and (*ii*) *fat-soluble vitamins*: vitamin A, vitamin D, vitamin E, and vitamin K.

Minerals

These are small inorganic elements and are indestructible unlike other major nutrients and vitamins. Calcium, phosphorus, potassium, sodium, chloride, magnesium, and sulfur are known as macrominerals and are usually required in amounts more than 100 mg per day, as they are present in relatively higher amounts in body tissues.

Trace Elements

The term trace is applied to concentrations of element not exceeding 250 µg per g of matrix. The definitive feature of a nutritionally significant trace element is either its essential intervention in physiological processes or its potential toxicity when present at low concentrations in tissues, food or drinking water. A WHO expert consultation has categorized nutritionally significant trace elements into three groups: (*i*) *essential elements* such as iron, iodine, zinc, selenium, copper, molybdenum, and chromium; (*ii*) *elements which are probably essential*, ie, manganese, silicon, nickel, boron, and vanadium; and (*iii*) *potentially toxic element*, some of which may have some essential functions at low levels, ie, fluorine, lead, cadmium, mercury, arsenic, aluminum, lithium, and tin.

3

de Fátima Costa Caminha M, da Figueira MA, *et al*. Co-existence of micronutrient deficiencies in hospitalized children with severe malnutrition treated according to the WHO protocol. Trop Doct. 2011;41:230–2.

Imdad A, Bhutta ZA. Effect of preventive zinc supplementation on linear growth in children under 5 years of age in developing countries: a meta-analysis of studies for input to the lives saved tool. *BMC Public Health*. 2011;11:S22.

Imdad A, Yakoob MY, Sudfeld C, *et al*. Impact of vitamin A supplementation on infant and childhood mortality. *BMC Public Health*. 2011;11:S20.

Scrimgeour AG, Lukaski HC. Zinc and diarrheal disease: current status and future perspectives. *Curr Opin Clin Nutr Metab Care*. 2008;11:711–7.

Waddell L. The power of vitamins. *J Fam Health Care*. 2012;22:14,16–20,22–5.

3.7 VITAMIN A DEFICIENCY

Vitamin A is a subgroup of retinoids exhibiting the biological activity of retinol. Naturally occurring retinoids include retinol (vitamin A alcohol), retinyl ester (vitamin A ester), retinal (vitamin A aldehyde), and retinoic acid (vitamin A acid). Retinoic acid is the most active form of the vitamin. Vitamin A from the diet is ingested as carotene (from plant sources) and retinal (from animal sources). Out of many different carotene pigments, beta-carotene (provitamin A) yields the highest amount of retinol. The absorption of dietary beta-carotenes vary according to the source, and is generally assumed to be 50%. Absorbed vitamin A is stored in liver as retinyl palmitate. Zinc is required for mobilization of retinyl palmitate to free retinol. Retinol is transported in blood, bound to a retinol binding protein (RBP).

1 µg of retinol   = 3.33 international units (IU) of vitamin A
1 IU of vitamin A= 0.6 µg of β-carotene
60 mg of retinol = 110 mg of retinyl palmitate = 69 mg retinyl acetate = 2 lakh IU of vitamin A

Physiology

Vitamin A has essential role in vision through its aldehyde (retinal) form which is the prosthetic group on visual proteins rhodopsin and iodopsin. During low intensity light, 11-*cis* retinal in rhodopsin is converted to all-*trans* retinal which generates an electrical signal transmitted via the optic nerve to brain, resulting in night (low-intensity light) vision. Thus, deficiency of vitamin A results in night blindness.

Apart from its role in vision, vitamin A is necessary for regulation of many genes involved in cell division and differentiation. Many physiologic processes involving the fetal growth and development, reproduction, gastro-intestinal, and respiratory function, and immunity are dependent on vitamin A. Vitamin A is essential for integrity of respiratory epithelium and skin.

These effects are mediated via retinoic acid which is an important signalling molecule acting as a ligand for specific nuclear transcription factors. Carotenoids, precursors of vitamin A, are also important antioxidant defences.

Sources

Breastmilk fulfils the needs of vitamin A entirely for first 6 months of life, and continues to be an important source up to 2 years. Preformed vitamin A (retinol) is abundant in fish liver oils, liver, dairy products, and egg yolk. Vegetarian sources of vitamin A are green leafy vegetables, and yellow fruits and vegetables, where it is present as carotenoids.

Recommended Daily Allowance

Infants (0–12 months): 350 µg; children (1–6 years): 400 µg; children (7–9 years): 600 µg; adolescents and adults: 600 µg; pregnant women: 800 µg; lactating women: 950 µg. All these values are in terms of retinol equivalents (RE) (ICMR, 2010). If carotenes are the sources, the RDA in term of RE is multiplied by 8 assuming a 1:8 conversion efficiency. It is recommended that minimum 50% of retinol equivalents should be derived from animal sources to ensure adequacy in vulnerable groups.

Causes of Deficiency

Severe malnutrition is an important cause of deficiency. The requirement of vitamin A is increased in preterms, and during infections (eg, measles and respiratory tract infections) making children prone to its deficiency during these states. Chronic diarrhea, malabsorptive states, and chronic liver disease cause significant vitamin A deficiency.

Clinical Features

Subclinical deficiency Respiratory system, urinary tract, intestinal epithelium, and immune system are affected before the deficiency manifests clinically. Subclinical vitamin A deficiency contributes to an increased severity of certain infections and an increased risk of infection related mortality.

Early features Defective dark adaptation is the most characteristic early clinical feature, resulting in night blindness.

Xerophthalmia Prolonged deficiency of vitamin A in the diet results in a syndrome of xerophthalmia, especially prevalent in 6–36 months old. It is often combined with general malnutrition.

- *Xerosis of the conjunctiva* is usually the first clinical sign. Palpebral conjunctiva loses its sheen and wetness. Wrinkling appears in the conjunctiva which can be appreciated as conjunctival folds when the child moves the eyeball towards the opposite side.
- *Bitot spots* are the most characteristic feature of xerophthalmia and appear next as triangular areas on the temporal aspects of junction of cornea with sclera. The spots are made up of heaped up dry masses of conjunctival epithelium. There may be more than one spot measuring from 1–5 mm. The spots are whitish grey, look dry, non-reflective, and may have embedded wrinkles. These are present bilaterally and associated with a muddy conjunctiva. The spots may be stained black, if the mother has applied *kajal* (*surma*) in the eyes of the infant (Fig. 3.9).
- *Cornea dries up as the next step.* A dry cornea is susceptible to exposure injury and can get ulcerated easily. Ulcers are pinpoint initially and later coalesce. The ulceration spreads to involve most of the cornea. This stage is known as *keratomalacia* and is a forerunner to corneal perforation.
- Aqueous humor and iris prolapse out, that ultimately results in corneal blindness. Corneal xerosis is reversible while keratomalacia is irreversible.

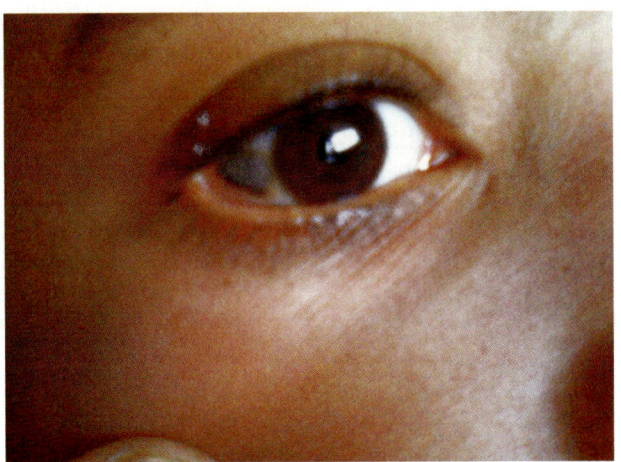

Fig. 3.9 Xerophthalmia: Bitot spot stained black with *kajal*

Table 3.19 WHO Classification of Xerophthalmia		
	Primary signs	*Secondary signs*
X1A	Conjunctival xerosis	XN Night blindness
X1B	Bitot spots	XF Fundal changes
X2	Corneal xerosis	XS Corneal scarring
X3A	Corneal ulceration (<1/3 of cornea)	
X3B	Corneal ulceration (>1/3 of cornea)	

The sequence of changes described above remains the same, through the rate of progression may be acute, subacute or chronic. Serum vitamin A level is less than 20 µg/dL.

On fundoscopy, pale yellow spots can be visualised near the course of retinal vessels and also in the periphery. Vitamin A deficiency is a common cause of preventable blindness in India. **Table 3.19** presents the WHO classification for ophthalmic manifestations of vitamin A deficiency.

Treatment	**Vitamin A Deficiency**

Xerophthalmia can progress from conjunctival xerosis to perforation very rapidly, resulting in blindness. Thus any evidence of vitamin A deficiency should be treated on priority and emergency basis.
Specific Immediately on diagnosis, oral vitamin A is administered in a dose of 50,000, 1 lakh, and 2 lakh international units in children aged <6 months, 6–12 months, and >1 year, respectively. The same dose is repeated next day and 2 weeks later. Parenteral, water-soluble vitamin A administration is recommended (in half the doses suggested above) in cases with impaired oral intake, persistent vomiting, and severe malabsorption. Oil-based injections should not be used to treat xerophthalmia.
Local treatment Antibiotic drops or ointment should be instilled three times a day to prevent secondary infection in the event of presence of corneal ulcer. Padding the eye in such cases prevents dehydration and further corneal exposure. Padding also enhances epithelial healing and reduces pain and photophobia. Mydriatics are necessary; usually atropine drops 1% or ointment is applied once a day.

Prevention

Prophylactic vitamin A (one dose of 1 lakh units of vitamin A along with measles vaccine at 9 months followed by four more doses of 2 lakh IU each at 18, 24, 30, and 36 months) may be administered in areas with high prevalence of vitamin A deficiency. Children suffering from measles and severe malnutrition should be administered oral vitamin A (1 and 2 lakh IU each for <1 year and >1 year olds, respectively), on two consecutive days. Those with persistent diarrhea and other prolonged febrile conditions are given one dose in each episode, keeping at least 1 month interval between the two doses.

Consumption of vitamin A rich food should be encouraged including locally available carotene rich foods, ie green leafy vegetables and yellow and orange vegetables and fruits like pumpkin, carrots, papaya, mango, oranges, along with cereals and pulses. Consumption of milk and milk products, egg, and liver must be promoted. Long-term prevention strategies include nutrition education for dietary diversification, horticultural interventions including home gardening, nutritional supplementation, and selective fortification for risk areas and special groups.

Vitamin A Supplementation and Child Mortality

Vitamin A supplementation has been linked with 23% reduction in child mortality in several trials in developing nations. However, these claims have been challenged. In north India, VAD (retinol <0.70 µmol/L) is common in preschool children and 2–3% die at ages 1.0–6.0 years. A large [Deworming and Enhanced Vitamin A (DEVTA)] trial in preschool children from 8,338 villages from north India contradicts the expectation from other trials that vitamin A supplementation would reduce child mortality by 20–30%, but cannot rule out some modest effect. Meta-analysis of DEVTA plus eight previous randomized trials of supplementation yielded a weighted average mortality reduction of 11% (95% CI 5–16).

HYPERVITAMINOSIS A

Acute hypervitaminosis A It causes pseudotumor cerebri manifesting as bulging fontanel, vomiting, and irritability in young infants. Older children may complain of diplopia and headache. Papilledema and cranial nerve palsies are rare. Symptoms and signs improve rapidly on withdrawing vitamin A. Acetazolamide, mannitol, or a therapeutic lumbar tap may be needed in severe cases.

Chronic hypervitaminosis A It results in skin desquamation, alopecia, hepatosplenomegaly, bone swellings, and increased intracranial tension. The shaft of long bones may show hyperostosis. Chronic toxicity usually results from intake of medicinal vitamin A over a period of several weeks. Excessive intake of vitamin A is teratogenic during first trimester of pregnancy.

3.8 VITAMIN B COMPLEX GROUP

Vitamin B complex includes: thiamine (B_1), riboflavin (B_2), niacin or pellagra preventing factor (B_3), pyridoxine (B_6), folic acid, cyanocobalamin (B_{12}), pantothenic acid, and biotin.

3

THIAMINE (VITAMIN B₁)

Thiamine diphosphate, the active form, acts as a cofactor for several enzymes involved in carbohydrate metabolism and nucleic acid synthesis. It is also required for the synthesis of acetylcholine and gamma-aminobutyric acid (GABA), essential for nerve conduction. In thiamine deficiency, utilization of pyruvic acid is decreased. Therefore, pyruvic acid and lactic acid accumulate in the tissue, and their blood levels are increased.

Sources Rice, wheat and legumes are main sources for vegetarians. Poultry and seafood are additional sources for non-vegetarians. Polishing, processing, and cooking destroy the thiamine content of cereals.

Recommended daily allowance (ICMR, 2010) 0–6 mo: 0.2 mg; 7–12 mo: 0.3 mg; 1–3 yr: 0.5 mg; 4–6 yr: 0.7 mg; 7–9 yr: 0.8 mg; 10–12 yr: male 1.1 mg, female 1.0 mg; 13–15 yr: male 1.4 mg, female 1.2 mg; 16–17 yr: male 1.5 mg, female 1.0 mg.

Deficiency

Thiamine deficiency mainfests as beriberi. *Beriberi* is characteristically associated with consumption of polished rice as a staple food. Deficiency of vitamin B₁ is also associated with severe malnutrition and chronic alcoholism.
- Initial symptoms are non-specific such as fatigue, apathy, nausea, and abdominal pain.
- *Dry beriberi* Neuritic form manifests as irritability, ataxia, tenderness of calf muscles, hypotonia, and diminished deep tendon reflexes. A pseudomeningeal form occurs in infants between 8 and 10 months of age. These children present with altered sensorium, signs of raised intracranial pressure, meningeal irritation, and neurologic deficit. This presentation is known as *Wernicke encephalopathy*. CSF shows pleocytosis and elevated proteins.
- *Wet beriberi* This manifests in apparently healthy infants between the ages of 2–4 months with cardiovascular involvement, is characterized by cardiomegaly, edema, and congestive heart failure. Cyanosis and pulmonary edema may also develop and carry a bad prognosis.
- *Laryngeal variety* presents with cough and hoarseness of voice, or aphonia.
- Mixed and atypical forms may also occur.

Treatment	**Thiamine Deficiency**

Diagnosis can be made by demonstrating decreased levels of RBC transketolase. Beriberi is treated with 3–5 mg of thiamine per day, orally, for at least 6 weeks. Parenteral preparations are needed in very sick children, including those having congestive heart failure. Treatment of dependency states requires higher doses.

Prevention
Undermilled or parboiled rice prevents thiamine deficiency. Cooking destroys as much as 25% of vitamin B₁; alternative diet preparation methods must be explored.

RIBOFLAVIN (VITAMIN B₂)

Riboflavin enzymes are involved in many oxidative enzyme systems in energy metabolism, synthesis of glycogen and erythropoiesis. Riboflavin is cardinal to cellular growth and tissue respiration. Retina also contains free riboflavin.

Sources Milk, eggs, green leafy vegetables and organ meats are good sources of riboflavin.

Recommended daily allowance 0–6 mo: 0.3 mg; 7–12 mo: 0.4 mg; 1–3 yr: 0.6 mg; 4–6 yr: 0.8 mg; 7–9 yr: 1.0 mg; 10–12 yr: male 1.3 mg, female 1.2 mg; 13–15 yr: male 1.6 mg, female 1.4 mg; 16–17 yr: male 1.8 mg, female 1.2 mg.

Deficiency

Malnutrition, malabsorption, and prolonged diarrhea are the main causes of riboflavin deficiency. Riboflavin deficiency is characterized by lesions in oral cavity, eye, and skin.
- *Oral lesions* Angular cheilosis (fissuring and cracking at the angles of mouth) and glossitis (fissuring, redness or paleness of tongue) are the predominant oral lesions seen in riboflavin deficiency.
- *Skin lesions* The dermatitis may involve the nasolabial folds (nasolabial dysbacea). Scrotal dermatitis may be frequently present.
- *Eye manifestations* include photophobia, lacrimation, itching, and circumcorneal congestion. Corneal vascularization and opacity may develop in severe cases.

Treatment	**Riboflavin Dificiency**

Diagnosis is mainly clinical, and can be confirmed by a urinary riboflavin excretion of <30 mg in 24 hours. Treatment consists of 3–10 mg riboflavin PO daily. Parenteral riboflavin may be given in cases resistant to oral therapy.

NIACIN (VITAMIN B₃)

Niacin containing cofactors, NAD and NADP, are important in many biologic reactions such as respiratory chain, DNA synthesis and repair, fatty acid synthesis, and steroid synthesis. Niacin is essential for functioning of skin, intestinal tract, and nervous system. Deficiency results in pellagra.

Niacin administration causes vasodilatation, flushing, tingling, and a sensation of warmth. In pharmacological doses, it controls blood cholesterol and lipids. Deficiency is more prevalent in maize-eating population. High leucine content of the maize is one of the major factors contributing to the development of pellagra on maize diets.

Sources Cereals, pulses, and green leafy vegetables are main sources in vegetarian diet whereas fish, meat and poultry form are main sources for non-vegetarians. Eggs and milk, though contain little niacin, are rich sources of tryptophan which can be converted to niacin.

Recommended daily allowance 0–6 mo: 710 µg/kg; 7–12 mo: 650 µg/kg; 1–3 yr: 8 mg; 4–6 yr: 11 mg; 7–9 yr: 13 mg; 10–12 yr: male 15 mg, female 13 mg; 13–15 yr: male 16 mg, female 14 mg; 16–17 yr: male 17 mg, female 14 mg. These intakes are expressed in terms of niacin equivalents (1 mg niacin equivalent = 1 mg niacin = 60 mg tryptophan).

Deficiency

Pellagra is the classical syndrome resulting from niacin deficiency. It is predominantly seen in populations where maize is the main staple food. High leucine content and low tryptophan content of the maize contribute to niacin deficiency. Severe malnutrition and anorexia nervosa are other common causes. *The classical triad of diarrhea, dermatitis, and dementia summarizes the clinical presentation of pellagra.*

Dermatitis of pellagra is characterized by symmetrical hyperpigmented scaly lesions on exposed parts such as hands (*pellagrous glove*), feet (*pellagrous boot*) and neck (*Casal necklace*). In a severely malnourished child, it is sometimes difficult to differentiate these features from dermatosis of kwashiorkor. The lesions heal promptly following administration of niacin. Neurological features include irritability, apathy, disorientation and confusion. An acute encephalopathy may develop occasionally.

Treatment	Pellagra

Pellagra is treated by administration of oral nicotinamide 50–300 mg for 2–3 weeks. Sun exposure should be avoided.

PYRIDOXINE (VITAMIN B₆)

Pyridoxine is essential for normal brain metabolism and growth of infants. Through its active coenzyme form (pyridoxal phosphate), pyridoxine plays a central role in amino acid metabolism, heme synthesis, and neurotransmitter synthesis.

Sources Liver, meat, fish, yeast, cereals, pulses, and peas are rich sources.

Recommended daily allowance 0–6 mo: 0.1 mg; 7–12 mo: 0.4 mg; 1–6 yr: 0.9 mg; 7–12 yr: 1.6 mg; 13–17 yr: 2 mg.

Deficiency

Deficiency states are unusual and are either secondary to another disease or to an inborn error of metabolism. Deficiency may lead to seizures and peripheral neuropathy. Clinical features include failure to thrive, hyperirritability, hyperacusis, microcytic hypochromic anemia, nausea and vomiting.

Pyridoxine deficiency may be seen after prolonged isoniazid, penicillamine and hydralazine therapy, and parenteral alimentation. Vitamin B₆ has been found to have a beneficial effect in nausea and vomiting of pregnancy and radiation sickness.

Subclinical deficiency can be detected by estimating urinary excretion of pyridoxic acid. In pyridoxine deficiency states, urinary excretion of xanthurenic acid increases after tryptophan loading.

Pyridoxine Dependency

Pyridoxine dependency refers to a condition characterized by increased pyridoxine requirements. Pyridoxine-dependent syndromes include pyridoxine dependent seizures, pyridoxine responsive anemia, and homocystinuria.

Pyridoxine dependency in neonates causes convulsions. Therapeutic trial with intramuscular administration of 100 mg of pyridoxine, in newborn infants not responding to usual seizure management and with a normal metabolic profile is the best method to diagnose pyridoxine-dependent seizures. This should be followed by prolonged administration of pyridoxine 10–100 mg/day orally.

COBALAMIN (VITAMIN B₁₂)

Vitamin B₁₂ plays an important role in lipid and carbohydrate metabolism, nucleic acid synthesis and protein synthesis.

Sources Vitamin B₁₂ is present only in foods of animal origin such as liver, meat, eggs and milk. Fortified cereals and milk are the main sources for vegetarian populations.

Recommended daily allowance 0.2 mg for infants and 0.2–1.0 mg for older children and adolescents.

Absorption and Transport

Vitamin B₁₂ combines with *intrinsic factor* present in the gastric juice. The vitamin B₁₂ intrinsic factor complex reaches ileum, and attaches itself to specific receptor sites on the brush border of the cells. The vitamin is absorbed from the receptor sites leaving behind the intrinsic factor. In the blood, vitamin B₁₂ is transported mainly by transcobalamin II. It is stored in the body bound to transcobalamin I.

Deficiency

Vitamin B₁₂ malabsorption occurs in blind loop syndrome and tropical sprue, Crohn disease, and intestinal tuberculosis. Vitamin B₁₂ deficiency is also seen in methylmalonic aciduria, in breastfed infants of vitamin B₁₂ deficient vegetarian mothers, and following administration of drugs such as neomycin, para-aminosalicylic acid, and colchicine. Lack of intrinsic factor in the stomach results in failure of absorption of vitamin B₁₂, and causes pernicious anemia.

Deficiency of vitamin B₁₂ impairs synthesis of DNA and causes defective myelin formation. In the bone marrow, erythropoiesis is arrested in the later stages. Bone marrow shows megaloblastic reaction. The immature forms of red blood cells, which are larger than the normal cells, enter the circulation. These cells have a short lifespan. The failure of maturation does not prevent hemoglobinization, resulting in macrocytic normochromic anemia.

Demyelination of large nerve fibers of the spinal cord, especially the long tracts and posterior columns occur. Early signs are numbness and tingling sensation in the fingers and toes. Advanced cases result in subacute combined degeneration of the cord.

Details of diagnosis and management of vitamin B₁₂ deficiency are available in Chapter 8.

BIOTIN

Biotin acts as a cofactor for enzymes needed in gluconeogenesis, fatty acid metabolism, and amino acid metabolism. It is present in a wide variety of non-vegetarian and vegetarian foods, including organ meats, fruits, nuts, cereals and legumes. Recommended dietary intake per day is as follows: 0–6 mo: 5 μg; 7–12 mo: 6 μg; 1–3 yr: 8 μg; 4–8 yr: 12 μg; 9–13 yr: 20 μg; 14–18 yr: 25 μg.

3

Deficiency

Biotin deficiency may arise from excessive intake of raw egg-white over long period. The egg-white is rich in avidin, a biotin antagonist. Prolonged parenteral alimentation, without biotin added to infusates, may also cause deficiency.

Deficiency may result in a periorificial dermatitis, anorexia, extreme lassitude, muscle pain, and alopecia. Therapeutic dose is 1–10 mg/day given orally.

FOLIC ACID

Folic acid (vitamin B$_9$) products dihydrofolate and tetra-hydrofolate are coenzymes in amino acid and nucleotide metabolism as single-carbon donors. Green leafy vegetables especially spinach and broccoli, cereals, beans, nuts, fruits and leafy vegetables are good sources of folate. Recommended daily intake is as follows: Infants (0–12 mo): 25 μg; 1–3 yr: 80 μg; 4–6 yr: 100 μg; 7–9 yr: 120 μg; 10–12 yr: 140 μg; 13–15 yr: 150 μg; 16–17 yr: 200 μg.

Deficiency

Hematological manifestation of folic acid is megaloblastic anemia (also *see* Chapter 8). Other manifestations include glossitis, growth retardation, and impaired immunity. Folic acid deficiency is also associated with increased thrombotic events, which may be related to increased homocysteine levels. Folic acid seems to be protective against development of atherosclerosis and other vascular disease by virtue of its homocysteine lowering effect.

Low maternal folate status is associated with increased incidence of neural tube defects. Folic acid is now recommended for preventing both occurrence and recurrence of these congenital disorders. It is, however, essential that all women should receive folic acid before or immediately after conception to have the desired effect. The ultimate goal of achieving better folate status in women of reproductive age group may be achieved by increasing the folate-rich food intake, supplementation, or food fortification.

- A daily intake of 400 μg of folic acid in women of reproductive age is recommended to prevent the first occurrence of neural tube defect. It is to be started before conception and continued till the end of 12th week of gestation.
- A daily intake of 4000 μg (4 mg) of folic acid, starting from one month before to 3 months after conception, is recommended in pregnant women with previously affected pregnancies, to prevent recurrence.

3.9 VITAMIN C AND SCURVY

Vitamin C (ascorbic acid) is essential for formation of collagen and intercellular matrix in teeth, bones, and capillaries. It is also involved in tyrosine metabolism, adrenal cortical functioning, and electron transport. It is a cofactor in activation of hydroxylating enzymes in oxidation processes. It also helps in transfer of iron from plasma transferrin into tissue ferritin and thus helps in storage of iron in the bone marrow, spleen, and liver.

Being a strong reducing agent, it provides protection to eyes and lungs against oxidizing agents, and reduces oxidation of low-density lipoproteins and prevents deposition of atheromatous plaques. It helps in maintenance of vascular integrity through prostacyclin (antiplatelet and vasodilatory effect).

Sources Citrus fruits and vegetables including tomatoes, cabbage, leafy greens and germinating pulses. Large quantities occur in liver and kidney but not in lean meat. Vitamin C is destroyed in cooking.

Recommended daily allowance Infants: 25 mg; older children and adolescents: 40 mg; pregnancy: 60 mg; lactation: 80 mg. Requirements are increased during fever, diarrhea, iron deficiency, and hypoproteinemia.

Deficiency of Vitamin C

Severe vitamin C deficiency causes scurvy The usual age of onset is 6 to 18 months. Severely malnourished children, and children dependent on boiled animal milk for their nutritional needs are at significant risk. Breast-fed children are protected as the breastmilk contains enough vitamin C to meet most of the requirements in the first two years of life.

Irritability, anorexia, low grade fever, fretfulness, and crying on handling are early features of scurvy. This is followed by swelling of limbs with the child assuming a frog-like position (abduction of thighs and slight flexion of knees). Child may be so reluctant to move his limbs that he appears paralysed (pseudoparalysis). After a few days of onset, swelling may show hardening because of calcification of subperiosteal hematoma. Gums are swollen and purplish which start bleeding easily. Petechiae may be seen over the skin. Orbital or conjunctival hemorrhages may also be observed. Costochondral junctions become prominent and appear sharp and angular. In rickets, prominence of costochondral junction is dome-shaped and semicircular. Scorbutic rosary is attributed to separation of epiphyses of ribs and backward displacement of sternum. Wound healing is delayed.

Differential diagnosis Other causes of pseudoparalysis such as septic arthritis, osteomyelitis, and congenital syphilis should be considered. Pseudoparalysis of scurvy may be confused with poliomyelitis.

Diagnosis

Diagnosis is based on radiological features, mainly seen at the lower end of femur and upper ends of humerus and tibia. Bone assumes a ground glass appearance with a pencil thin cortex. Metaphyses demonstrate a zone of well-calcified cartilage, referred to as white line of Frenkel. White line may also be seen in healing rickets, severe PEM, plumbism, acute leukemia, and congenital syphilis.

Epiphyseal centers of ossification are surrounded by a white ring (*Wimburger sign*) (Fig. 3.10). A zone of rarefaction or destruction appears proximal and parallel to the white line. Epiphyseal separation may occur along this line. Subperiosteal hemorrhage results in periosteal elevation. Diaphyseal fractures are rare.

Plasma ascorbic acid levels vary widely and cannot be relied upon to detect early vitamin C deficiency. Ascorbic acid content of WBC offers a sensitive estimate of its status in the body (25–40 mg/100 mg is normal). Fasting vitamin C level >0.6 mg/dL excludes scurvy. Urinary excretion of

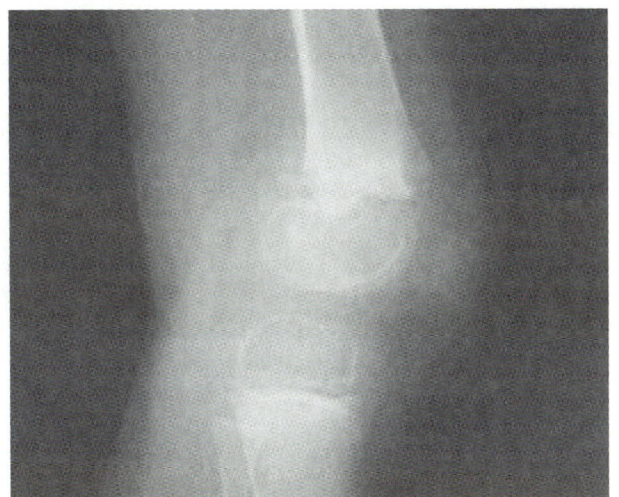

Fig. 3.10 White ring around epiphysis (Wimburger sign), and pencil thin cortex, suggestive of scurvy

vitamin C 3–5 hours after a loading dose of 11 mg/kg is more than 80% in normal subjects.

Treatment	Scurvy
Ascorbic acid 100–200 mg per day provides quick relief. Treatment should continue for three months to ensure full recovery. Vitamin C rich foods need to be given.	

3.10 VITAMIN D AND RICKETS

Cholecalciferol (vitamin D_3) and calciferol (vitamin D_2) are biologically equivalent compounds. Vitamin D_3 is synthesized in the skin on exposure of 7-dehydrocholesterol (present under normal skin) to ultraviolet rays in the sunlight. The metabolically active form of vitamin D is 1,25-$(OH)_2D_3$ which is obtained by conversion of cholecalciferol to 25-hydroxy-cholecalciferol 25-$(OH)D_3$ in the liver followed by another hydroxylation in the kidney. 1,25-$(OH)_2D_3$ is a hormone which helps in absorption of calcium and phosphorus in the gut, and promotes bone dissolution, and mineralization, thereby increasing the serum calcium and alkaline phosphatase activity. The feedback control in synthesis is mediated by parathormone which diminishes in response to elevation of serum calcium level inhibiting further synthesis of 1,25-$(OH)_2D_3$ in the kidney.

Sources Fish oils, liver, egg yolk, and fortified foods are main sources of vitamin D besides exposure to sunlight. Milk, including breastmilk, provides very less amounts of vitamin D.

Recommended daily allowance An intake of 400 IU/day is recommended for breastfed infants and 600 IU/day for older children. As breastmilk is a poor source of vitamin D, this may need to be provided by supplements, especially if exposure to sunlight is deficient.

VITAMIN D DEFICIENCY RICKETS

Vitamin D deficiency in growing children (before closure of epiphyses) leads to rickets whereas the manifestations are termed osteomalacia in adolescents and adults. The main causes of deficiency are inadequate dietary intake and lack of exposure to sunlight. Poor vitamin D content of milk and vegetarian diets contribute to deficiency of vitamin D.

Biochemical Changes

As a result of decreased absorption of calcium from the gut, there is compensatory increase in parathormone concentration to maintain blood calcium levels. Parathormone acts on osteocytes to release calcium from bones, and also reduces the excretion of calcium by kidneys. There is associated decrease in the renal tubular reabsorption of phosphate. The net result is normal serum calcium level and low serum phosphorus. An increase in the osteoblastic activity results in elevation of serum alkaline phosphatase level. In later stages, the compensatory increase in parathormone cannot sustain normal calcium level and hypocalcemia occurs.

Skeletal Changes

In rickets, there is inadequate mineralization of bone matrix at the growth plates due to increased bone resorption secondary to increased parathormone activity, and also because of low calcium and phosphorus levels in blood. Deposition of unmineralized matrix leads to widening of growth plate and metaphysis causing manifestations such as wrist widening and rachitic rosary. Bone becomes less rigid and is prone to bending, deformities, and fractures. On weight bearing, soft end of bone is compressed leading to flaring of the metaphyses.

Clinical Manifestations

Most clinical manifestations of rickets are due to bone changes related to deposition of unmineralized osteoid and softening. Craniotabes, the earliest manifestation of rickets, is the ping pong ball feeling of skull in infants on giving pressure over the occipital or parietal bones. There is enlargement and delayed closure of anterior fontanel. Frontal and parietal bossing may be evident beyond infancy. Anterior fontanel is large and its closure is delayed beyond 18 months.

There is clinically apparent widening of the wrists (Fig. 3.11). Long bones of legs get deformed when the child starts bearing weight (after one year). Anterior bowing of legs, knock knee, and coxa vera are the usual deformities. Medial malleolus of tibiae widen giving the appearance of double malleolus.

Costochondral junctions become prominent to give appearance of a rosary (*rachitic rosary*) (Fig. 3.12). There may be an increase in anteroposterior diameter of chest wall (*pigeon chest*). A horizontal depression (*Harrison's groove*) is seen along the lower border of chest, corresponding to the insertion of diaphragm. Scoliosis, kyphosis, or lordosis may occur in severe cases. Deformities of chest and softening of ribs impairs air movement and make the child more prone to respiratory tract infections.

Abdomen becomes protuberant (*pot-belly*) because of marked hypotonia of abdominal wall muscles, visceroptosis, and lumbar lordosis. Eruption of primary teeth is delayed.

Diagnosis

The diagnosis of rickets is based on typical skeletal manifestations of wrist widening, rachitic rosary or/and bow

3

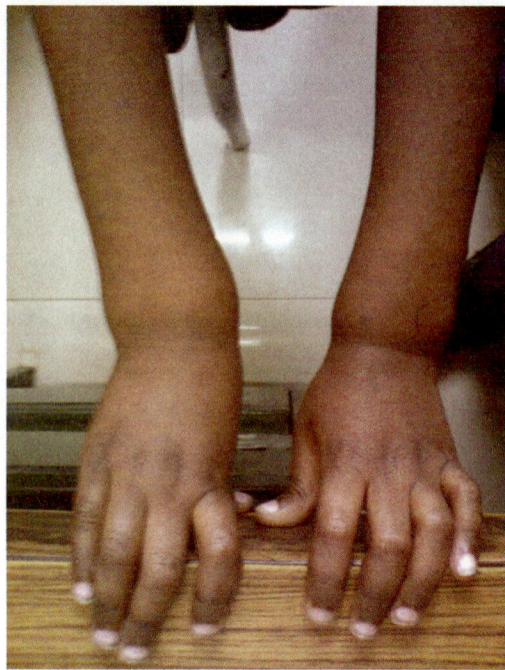

Fig. 3.11 Rickets: Widening of the wrists

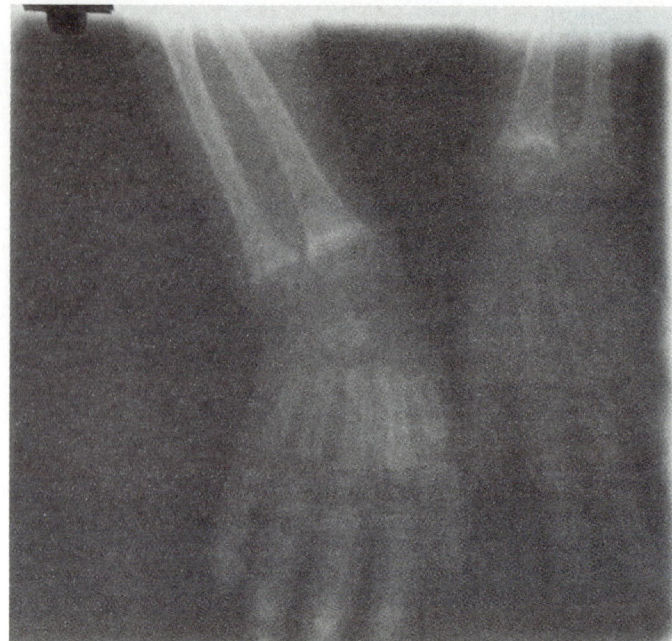

Fig. 3.13 Rickets: Early radiological changes showing cupping and fraying at lower ends of radius and ulna

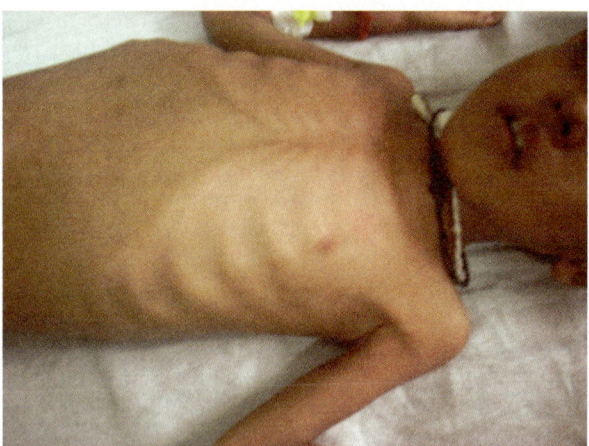

Fig. 3.12 Rachitic rosary: Costochondral junctions become prominent

legs in a child at risk of vitamin D deficiency. Radiological changes are confirmatory, and the biochemical changes help in finding the etiology of rickets.

Early radiological changes are observed in wrist at lower ends of radius and ulna (Fig. 3.13). The normally convex or flat appearing metaphyses become concave (cupping). There is widening of distal end of metaphysis with elongation of both ends (splaying). The smooth margin of metaphysis appears irregular (fraying). Rachitic rosary may be apparent as beading of costochondral junctions in the chest radiograph. In long-standing cases, the diaphysis is also rarefied due to resorption of cancellous bone.

US Endocrine Society classificaton Based on serum levels of 25(OH)D$_3$, vitamin D status is classified as follows: *Severe deficiency*: <5 ng/mL; *Deficient*: <20 ng/mL; *Sufficient*: >30 ng/mL; and *Toxic*: >150 ng/mL.

The typical biochemical changes of vitamin D deficiency rickets are low or normal serum calcium, markedly high alkaline phosphatase, and normal or low serum phosphorus. High phosphate levels are associated with renal osteodystrophy. Other evidences of gross renal damage such as high blood urea, creatinine, and low creatinine clearance are also present.

Treatment	Nutritional Rickets

The treatment regimen (Stoss regimen) is administration of a single large dose (100,000 to 600,000 international units) of vitamin D$_3$ orally or intramuscularly. Alternative regimen is administration of 1,000 to 5,000 units of vitamin D$_3$ orally for 8–12 weeks. Various regimens for treating rickets are summarised in **Table 3.20**. Healing is apparent in 3–4 weeks at the end of long bones in form of a white line of calcification. Thereafter, consumption of 400–600 units of vitamin D$_3$ per day should be encouraged. Adequate calcium and phosphorus intake should also be ensured.

If there is no response after vitamin D or if there is a family history or if biochemical changes are not typical of vitamin D deficiency, other variants of rickets should be suspected **(Table 3.21)**.

- Low phosphate level with aminoaciduria is seen in (*i*) vitamin D deficiency or malabsorption, (*ii*) hepatic disease or prolonged anticonvulsant therapy, and (*iii*) Fanconi syndrome. Glycosuria indicates Fanconi disease.
- Low phosphate level without aminoaciduria with acidic urinary pH indicates proximal renal tubular acidosis. Urinary pH is normal in familial hypophosphatemia.

Primary Hypophosphatemia (X-linked Vitamin D Resistant Rickets)

It is the most common non-nutritional form of rickets and is transmitted in X-linked dominant fashion. Defects occur in proximal tubular reabsorption of phosphate and in the

Table 3.20 Treatment Regimens for Treating Vitamin D Deficiency

Age group	Daily regimen (8–12 weeks)	Weekly regimen (8–12 weeks)	Stoss therapy	Maintenance dosage
< 1 month	1,000 IU	50,000 IU*	Not recommended	400–1,000 IU/day
1–12 months	1,000–5,000 IU	50,000 IU	1–6 lakhs units over 1–5 days oral (preferably 3 lakhs)**	400–1,000 IU/day
1–18 years	5,000 IU	50,000 IU	3–6 lakhs units over 1–5 days oral**	600–1,000 IU/day
Any age with obesity, malabsorption syndrome or those on medications affecting vitamin D status	6,000–10,000 IU/day			3,000–6,000 IU/day

*To convert (IU) to µg of calciferol, divide by 40.
** Parenteral (intramuscular) therapy—best avoided unless there is severe malabsorption or concern for compliance to oral regimens.

Table 3.21 Clinical Variants of Rickets

	Type I	Type II	Type III
	Calcium deficient	Phosphate deficient	End organ resistance to 1, 25(OH)$_2$D$_3$
Serum calcium	Normal or low	Normal	Low
Serum phosphorus	Usually low*	Low	Normal
Alkaline phosphatase	Elevated	Elevated	Elevated
Secondary hyperparathyroidism	Present	Absent	–

Causes	i. Deficiency of vitamin D
	  – dietary
	  – lack of sunlight
	  – congenital
	ii. Malabsorption of vitamin D
	iii. Liver disease
	iv. Anticonvulsant therapy
	v. Renal osteodystrophy
	vi. Vitamin D dependent rickets, type I
		i. Familial hypophosphatemia
		ii. Fanconi syndrome
		  – tyrosinosis
		  – Lowe syndrome
		  – cystinosis
		iii. Proximal renal tubular acidosis
		iv. Deficiency of phosphate or malabsorption
			Vitamin D-dependent rickets, type II

*Except in renal osteodystrophy, where alkaline phosphatase is elevated
Related conditions: Hypophosphatasia, metaphyseal dysostosis

conversion of 25(OH) D$_3$ to 1, 25(OH)$_2$D$_3$. Urinary phosphate excretion is increased. Children present at an early age with short stature, waddling gait, bowlegs, coxa vara, and genu valgum. Teeth have abnormal enamel. Serum calcium is normal or low, phosphorus is reduced, and alkaline phosphatase is elevated. Aminoaciduria, glycosuria, and bicarbonaturia are absent.

Treatment is with oral phosphate (0.5–4 g/day in 4–6 divided doses as sodium phosphate and/or phosphoric acid) along with vitamin D (dihydrotachysterol in a dose of 0.02 mg/kg daily) administration.

Vitamin D-Dependent Rickets

The condition is also known as pseudovitamin D deficiency. It occurs even when the normal daily requirements of vitamin D are being met in the diet.

Vitamin D-dependent rickets, type I is an autosomal recessive disorder, manifesting at around 3–6 months of age. Enzyme activity of 25(OH)D$_3$-1α-hydroxylase is deficient resulting in low levels of 1,25(OH)$_2$D$_3$, even in presence of hypocalcemia, hypophosphatemia, and high parathormone levels. Condition is treated with a massive dose (2 lakh to 1 million IU) of vitamin D$_2$.

Patients who fail to respond to above therapy are labeled as having *vitamin D-dependent rickets type II*. The defect lies in marked reduction of binding of 1,25(OH)$_2$D$_3$ to its nuclear receptor and defective nuclear translocation. This may be associated with short stature and alopecia.

PREVENTION OF NUTRITIONAL RICKETS

A recent study in Indian infants (Meena et al, *Indian Pediatrics* 2017) has shown that there is a significant correlation between sunlight exposure and serum vitamin D in breastfed infants at 6 months of age, independent of maternal vitamin D status. Afternoon sun exposure of 30 minutes per week for 16–18 weeks (starting from 6 weeks) over 40% exposed

3

body surface can achieve sufficient vitamin D (20 ng/mL) in infants, at 6 months of age.

Indian Academy of Pediatrics 2017 guidelines (*Indian Pediatrics. 2017;54:567–73*) recommend that all exclusively breastfed infants should receive vitamin D supplements as follows:

- For the prevention of rickets in premature infants, 400 IU of vitamin D and 150–220 mg/kg of calcium, and in neonates, 400 IU of vitamin D and 200 mg of calcium are recommended daily.
- For prevention of rickets and hypocalcemia in infants (after neonatal period) up to 1 year of age, and from 1–18 years, 400 IU and 600 IU vitamin D/day and 250–500 mg/day and 600–800 mg/day of calcium, respectively, are recommended.
- For treatment of rickets in premature neonates, infants up to 1 year and from 1–18 years, 1000 IU, 2000 IU, and 3000–6000 IU of vitamin D daily, respectively, and elemental calcium of 70–80 mg/kg/day in premature neonates and 500–800 mg daily for all children over that age are recommended. Larger doses of vitamin D may be given from 3 months to 18 years of age as 60,000 IU/week for 6 weeks.

HYPERVITAMINOSIS D

Administration of vitamin D in therapeutic doses for long periods results in toxicity. The upper limit of daily intake of vitamin D is 1000 IU for infants and 2000 IU for older children and adults. Hypercalcemia and consequent symptoms develop in overdosages. Gastrointestinal manifestations are anorexia, abdominal pain, and constipation. Renal manifestations are polyuria, nephrocalcinosis, nephrolithiasis, and renal failure. Child may have hypotonia, irritability, disorientation, convulsions, and coma. Death may occur due to cardiac arrhythmias or due to electrolyte abnormalities secondary to dehydration.

Treatment It comprises of elimination of source of excess vitamin D, and management of dehydration and electrolyte abnormalities. Oral prednisolone, calcitonin, and bisphosphonates are effective in decreasing serum calcium.

3.11 VITAMIN E (TOCOPHEROL)

Vitamin E is an antioxidant. It protects membrane phospholipids from free radical induced peroxidase damage. As an antioxidant, it is used as a free radical scavenger. It has anti-neoplastic effect and may raise the concentration of high-density lipoprotein cholesterol. Vitamin E is transported in the body by lipoprotein. Preterm newborns have low tissue stores.

Sources Nuts and polyunsaturated vegetable oils are rich sources. Seeds and whole wheat grain are good sources.

Recommended daily allowance Intake of 4–5 mg/day is considered adequate for infants. Recommended daily intake for children (1–3 years) 6 mg; children (4–8 years) 7 mg; children (9–13 years) 11 mg; and adolescents 15 mg. One mg of d-alpha-tocopherol provides 1.5 IU activity of vitamin E.

Vitamin E Deficiency

Vitamin E deficiency might be observed in low birth weight infants; it may result in anemia, reticulocytosis, thrombocytopenia, and abnormal erythrocyte metabolism. Low levels of vitamin E in premature infants are associated with hemolytic anemia, hyperbilirubinemia, and intraventricular hemorrhage. Vitamin E prophylaxis reduces the incidence of retinopathy of prematurity.

Majority of children with vitamin E deficiency have cholestatic disease with coexistent malabsorption. Clinical manifestations include loss of reflexes, ataxia of trunks and limbs, diminished proprioception, muscle weakness, ptosis, pes cavus, scoliosis, and dysarthria.

3.12 VITAMIN K

It is a cofactor of the enzyme that catalyzes one step in the formation of prothrombin. It is also needed for the generation of several blood clotting factors in the liver. Green leafy vegetables are good source of vitamin K.

Deficiency results in coagulation defects due to hypoprothrombinemia and deficiency of factor VII resulting in hemorrhagic disease of the newborn. This should be prevented by giving 1 mg of intramuscular vitamin K to the newborn at birth. Idiopathic vitamin K deficiency of infancy or acquired prothrombin complex deficiency is a bleeding disorder of infants between two weeks and two months old. In severe deficiency, 2.5 to 5 mg of aqueous vitamin K is given parenterally.

3.13 IODINE DEFICIENCY DISORDERS (IDD)

Iodine deficiency in pregnancy has long been linked to cretinism and possible fetal wastage. Recognition of this has led to highly effective programs for making iodized salt available in iodine-deficient areas. As a result, while more than two billion people live in areas that used to be iodine-deficient, it is estimated that the current burden of disease caused by iodine deficiency is only 0.2% of the global total as measured in lost disability-adjusted life years (DALYs). IDD is currently a significant public health problem in 118 countries.

Iodine deficiency disorders (IDD) refer to the wide spectrum of effects of iodine deficiency on growth and development. It includes endemic goiter, endemic cretinism, impaired mental function in children and adults with goiter, and increased stillbirths and perinatal and infant mortality. Evidence is now available that these conditions can be prevented by correction of iodine deficiency.

IODINE: ESSENTIAL TRACE ELEMENT

Iodine is an essential component of thyroid hormones. Seafoods and vegetables grown on iodine-rich soil are good sources of iodine. Soil in Himalayan regions has low iodine content due to leaching caused by deforestation. Low lying areas subject to flooding or high rainfall, such as Ganges valley in India and Bangladesh are also severely iodine deficient. In these areas, salt is being iodinated to cut down a higher incidence of IDD. Long-term intervention is achievable, however, with only dietary diversification.

Requirement A daily iodine intake of 110 µg (0–6 mo), 130 µg (7–12 mo), 120 µg (1–13 yr) and 150 µg from 14 years onwards is recommended. The intake should be increased, if there is presence of goiterogens in the diet. Cassava, maize, bamboo shoots, sweet potatoes, and millets are important goiterogens.

Clinical Features of Deficiency

Lack of iodine may result in abortion and stillbirth in the mothers and congenital anomalies, neurological and myxedematous cretinism, goiter, and psychomotor defects in the newborn. Iodine deficiency disorders may contribute to increased infant and perinatal mortality. In children, it may result in goiter, juvenile hypothyroidism, impaired mental function, and retardation of physical and sexual growth.

Endemic goiter is present when the prevalence in a defined population exceeds 10%. The differential diagnosis is established by epidemiological criteria. Clinical evidence of hypothyroidism is difficult to demonstrate. Usually TSH is elevated with low T4 and T3 levels.

Endemic cretinism occurs with an iodine intake <25 µg/day in contrast to a normal intake of 80–150 µg/d affecting up to 10% of populations living in severely iodine deficient areas. It is associated with endemic goiter and characteristic clinical features, which include deaf-mutism, squint, mental retardation, characteristic spastic or rigid neuromotor disorder (spastic diplegia), and dwarfism. Two types of endemic cretinism are described:

- *Neurological cretinism* is characterized by deaf-mutism, squint, proximal spasticity, and rigidity more in the lower extremities, disorders of stance and gait with preservation of vegetative functions, occasional signs of cerebellar or oculomotor disturbance, and severe mental deficiency.
- *Myxedematous cretinism* is characterized by retarded psychomotor development, severe short stature, coarse facial features, and myxedema without deaf-mutism. The pathogenesis of endemic cretinism is poorly understood.

Prevention and Control

Iodine deficiency disorders can be prevented by the use of iodinated salt or iodized oil. But little information is available on treatment of iodine deficiency disorders. Prolonged administration of iodine or thyroxine is effective in reducing the size of the goiter. Goiters while on treatment may shrink with appearance of nodules. Treatment of endemic cretinism may eliminate signs of hypothyroidism but neuromotor and intellectual deficiency are irreversible. Surgical removal of large goiters is useful in airway obstruction and for cosmetic reasons.

Mild and moderate IDD can be eliminated with iodized salt (20–40 parts per million). In the presence of long-standing iodine deficiency, an increase in intake, even to normal levels, may be associated with hyperthyroidism. This can be avoided by introducing the community iodine supplementation programme at an early stage of deficiency.

Severe IDD areas require administration of iodized oil (1 mL contains 480 mg of iodine), given either orally or parenterally.

One mL of oil should be dispensed to all females up to 40 years and all males up to 20 years in areas with severe IDD; repeat the dose after 3 years, if severe iodine deficiency persists.

3.14 ZINC

Zinc is vital for functioning of the immune, reproductive, neurologic, dermatologic and gastrointestinal systems. It is a constituent of metallo-enzymes such as transferases, hydrolases, ligases, isomerases and oxidoreductases which help in nucleic acid and protein synthesis and degradation. Zinc chelates with the amino acids, cysteine and histidine, forming 'zinc fingers' that are important for protein transcription.

Sources Human milk satisfies the need of an exclusively breastfed infant for first six months. Animal foods such as lean red meat of chicken, pork, beef and lamb are rich sources of zinc. Zinc is also found in nuts, whole grains, legumes and yeast. Low calcium and high protein intake promote absorption and retention of zinc. Animal proteins, including milk appear to promote zinc release and bioavailability from its phytate complex. Phytates (present in bran, whole grain cereals, and legumes) and high medicinal iron intake inhibit zinc absorption. Iron has little effect on zinc absorption from a complex meal.

Requirements A zinc intake of 2–3 mg/day is considered adequate for infants. Recommended daily intake for children is: 1–3 years: 5 mg; 4–6 years: 7 mg; 7–9 years: 8 mg; 10–12 yrs: 9 mg; 13–15: 11 mg, and 16–17 yr: 12 mg. Requirements during pregnancy and lactation are 12 mg/day.

ZINC DEFICIENCY

Recent research suggests that zinc deficiency is very common, especially among populations in South East Asia and sub-Saharan Africa. The main reasons for deficiency are: (*i*) low dietary intake of zinc-containing foods and low zinc content of soil, (*ii*) presence of inhibitors of zinc absorption in cereals and legumes, and (*iii*) high fecal losses of zinc due to recurrent episodes of diarrhea. Zinc supplementation in under-five children reduces the risk of diarrhea and pneumonia, and results in faster recovery from diarrhea. The estimated global prevalence of the zinc deciency is 31% with prevalence in South and South-East Asia being 34–73%. A study from five states of India reported the prevalence of zinc deficiency amongst children 6–60 months of age as 43.8%.

Zinc deficiency occurs in malnutrition, diarrhea (especially if recurrent or persistent), and because of inadequate consumption of zinc-rich foods. *Acrodermatitis enteropathica*, a severe zinc deficiency state, is an autosomal recessive inborn error of metabolism resulting from a defect in intestinal zinc-specific transporter gene (SCL39A4). The cutaneous manifestations of acrodermatitis enteropathica are dry, scaly, eczematous or vesicobullous lesions mainly distributed around perioral and perianal regions (Fig. 3.14); limbs may also be involved. Alopecia, severe growth retardation, chronic diarrhea, and immunodeficiency are other common features.

Milder form of zinc deficiency, as seen in malnutrition and chronic diarrhea, is characterized by stunting, anorexia,

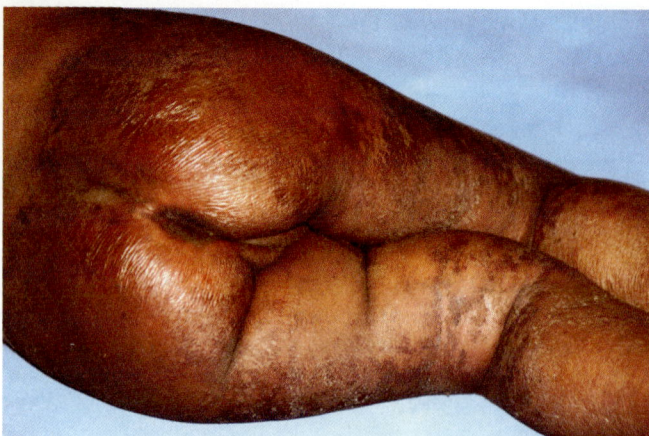

Fig. 3.14 Acrodermatitis enteropathica: Dry, scaly, and eczematous lesions around perianal region

periorificial rash, and excoriation, behavioral changes and increased susceptibility to infections, especially diarrhea and pneumonia. The typical periorificial (around mouth and anus) distribution of rash is a pointer towards zinc deficiency. In severe cases of dietary deficiencies (eg, severe malnutrition) and losses (chronic and recurrent diarrhea), the clinical features might be very similar to those seen in Acrodermatitis enteropathica.

Diagnosis

It is mainly clinical, based on typical rash in a predisposed child. Serum or plasma zinc is the best available biomarker of the risk of zinc deficiency in populations. A serum zinc cut-off of 65 µg/dL (9.9 µmol/L) is recommended for identifying zinc deficiency in populations for children aged between 2 and 10 years. The risk of zinc deficiency is considered to be of public health concern when the prevalence of low serum zinc concentrations is greater than 20%. Amongst the functional outcomes, height- or length-for-age is the parameter of choice for estimating zinc deficiency in populations.

Treatment	Zinc Deficiency

Acrodermatitis enteropathica should be treated with 50 mg (infants) or 150 mg (older children) of elemental zinc daily. Clinical deficiency secondary to malnutrition and diarrhea is treated with 2 mg/kg/day of elemental zinc, given for two weeks. Zinc supplementation is also required during acute diarrhea; daily dose of 20 mg of elemental zinc for children older than 6 months, and 10 mg for children aged 2 to 6 months should be started as soon as diarrhea starts and continued for a period of 14 days. The preventive strategies include improvement in quality and quantity of diet, improvement in zinc content of agricultural soil, food fortification, and prevention of diarrhea.

3.15 CALCIUM AND MAGNESIUM

CALCIUM

It is the most abundant mineral in the body with 99% deposited in bone and teeth. Rest is involved in blood clotting process, nerve conduction and muscle stimulation, signal response coupling, parathyroid function and vitamin D metabolism. Calcium in the body must be accompanied with magnesium, phosphorus and vitamin A, C, D and E to function optimally. Vitamin D, calcitonin, and parathyroid hormone regulate calcium metabolism.

Milk, milk products and millet like *ragi* are rich sources of calcium. Moderate fat content facilitates calcium absorption. Phytic acid (present in cereals), oxalic acid and fatty acids make calcium insoluble and, therefore, hinder its absorption.

Requirements Intake of 500 mg/day is considered adequate for infants. Recommended daily intake for children (1–9 years) is 600 mg, and for adolescents (10–19 yr) is 800 mg. During pregnancy and lactation, 1200 mg of calcium is required per day.

Deficiency Calcium deficiency may lead to (*i*) tetany (characterized by muscle cramps, numbness and tingling in limbs); (*ii*) rickets; and (*iii*) osteoporosis. Moderate deficiency may result in joint pains, heart palpitations, insomnia, and impaired growth. Calcium is helpful for cramps, growing pains, skin protection, and tooth disorders.

MAGNESIUM

Magnesium is an essential element, necessary for the synthesis of fatty acids, proteins, and cyclic-AMP. It is also involved in oxidative phosphorylation. Magnesium ion is extremely important for autonomic control of the heart. Magnesium is the most abundant mineral cation in cells, second only to potassium.

Deficiency Deficiency of magnesium may be observed in malabsorption syndrome, protein-energy malnutrition, chronic renal failure and diarrhea. Clinical manifestations include irritability, tetany and increased or decreased reflexes.

Sources and requirements Magnesium is present widely in plant foods and meat. Milk is a poor source. In the first 6 months of life, the infant requires 30 mg of magnesium; in the second 6 months the allowance is 45 mg/day. Recommended daily intake for children (1–3 years) 50 mg; children (4–6 years) 70 mg; children (7–9 years) 100 mg; adolescent males 120–195 mg and adolescent females 160–235 mg.

3.16 FREE RADICALS AND ANTIOXIDANTS

FREE RADICALS

A free radical is a molecule containing one or more unpaired electrons, formed as a result of addition or subtraction of one electron to non-radical biomolecules. Most of free radicals are formed during oxidation and thus are known as free oxygen radicals or reactive oxygen species (ROS). Oxygen derived free radicals such as superoxide (O_2^-), hydrogen peroxide (H_2O_2), and hydroxyl (OH^-) are highly unstable and reactive as these tend to generate chain reactions rendering the non-radical molecules to radical molecules.

Generation of free radicals is an integral feature of normal metabolism during mitochondrial respiratory chain, detoxification, phagocytosis, and metabolism of arachidonic acid. These are also generated in association with trauma, inflammation, and sepsis and also in response to certain drugs, chemicals, pollutants, and radiation. Free radicals have important role to play in killing of phagocytosed microorganisms, assisting detoxification process, triggering and regulating cell division, and maintenance of vascular tone via endothelium-derived relaxing factor (nitric oxide).

However, increased production and uncontrolled propagation of these reactive species result in damage and degeneration of tissues. Free radicals have been implicated in many diseases of childhood like kwashiorkor, rheumatoid arthritis, inflammatory bowel disease, cystic fibrosis, cancers, hepatic disorders (iron and copper storage disorders, autoimmune hepatitis), and neonatal disorders (retinopathy of prematurity, hypoxic ischemic encephalopathy, necrotizing enterocolitis, and bronchopulmonary dysplasia).

ANTIOXIDANTS

In the body, antioxidant defence system is present to balance the generation of free oxygen radicals. These antioxidant defences consist of intracellular antioxidants (superoxide dismutase, catalase, glutathione peroxidase); extracellular antioxidants [bilirubin, uric acid, albumin, transferrin, haptoglobin and ceruloplasmin); and membrane antioxidants (vitamin E, β-carotenes, and coenzyme Q)].

Nutritional antioxidants are β-carotenes, vitamin E, vitamin C, selenium, and many phytochemicals present in plant products. Certain drugs, like allopurinol and desferrioxamine, act as synthetic antioxidants. Antioxidants act by lysing and inactivating free radicals, separating free radicals from susceptible molecules and rapidly repairing the damage done by free radicals.

Endogenous antioxidant mechanisms can adjust their activity in relation to the changes in oxidative stress. However, exogenous antioxidant activity is mainly dependant on the individual intake of antioxidant. Even though free radical-mediated damage seems to be important in many pediatric diseases, supplementation with antioxidants does not have a definite role in disease prevention. It appears that the most effective disease prevention strategy regarding antioxidants is achieved by eating a wide variety of fruits and vegetables thereby ensuring a balance of naturally occurring antioxidants. Recommended daily allowances of naturally occurring antioxidants, like vitamins should be met in deficiency states such as malnutrition and liver disorders. Role of supplementation with antioxidant vitamins or drugs in the free radical-mediated diseases is the subject of interest in current research. Caution is to be exercised in isolated antioxidant supplementation as it can upset the balance of antioxidant defenses, which operate in an interdependent manner.

3.17 ESSENTIAL TRACE ELEMENTS

SELENIUM

Selenium is essential to the production of glutathione peroxidase, a constituent of the antioxidant defence system.

Selenium functions as an antioxidant along with vitamin E. Recent studies have shown that selenium deficiency markedly reduces the conversion of T3 from T4. Combined deficiency of iodine and selenium may, therefore, have adverse effects on neonatal growth, survival and development. Meat and seafoods are rich sources. Infants require 15–20 µg per day of selenium. Requirement of older children ranges from 20–40 µg. Adolescents require 55 µg per day.

Deficiency of selenium has resulted in *Keshan disease* (a form of cardiomyopathy endemic in China) and *Kashin-beck disease* (an endemic osteoarthritis of preadolescents, in China). Other dietary factors, such as low intake of vitamin E, protein and methionine, are also considered relevant to causation of Keshan disease. Selenium deficiency is usually associated with vitamin E deficiency. Viral infections in individuals with selenium or/and vitamin E deficiency may be associated with adverse outcome. The association between low selenium intake and high risk of cancer, cardiovascular disease, and cerebral thrombosis is being investigated.

Excessive intake of selenium is associated with *selenosis* (loss of hair and nail).

COPPER

Copper is present in enzymes amine oxidases, ferroxidases, cytochrome C oxidase, and superoxide dismutase. Copper is essential for connective tissue formation, iron metabolism, myelin production, melanin synthesis, and utilization of oxygen during cell respiration and energy utilization. Adult human body contains 80 mg of copper. Tissue copper levels range from <1 µg/g in many organs to 10 µg/g in the liver and brain. Copper in humans exists in erythrocytes (60%) and bound form (40%). Copper binding proteins include metallothionein, albumin, transcuperein, and blood clotting factor V. In plasma, about 93% of copper is bound to ceruloplasmin that also acts as an oxidant. Plasma copper ranges from 0.8–1.2 µg/mL.

Sources and requirements Good dietary sources of copper (> 2 µg/g) include seafood, organ meats, legumes, and nuts. Refined cereals, sugar, milk, and many other dairy products are low in copper. Low intake of dietary copper and high level of protein intake enhances the bioavailability of copper. Excessive intake of certain substances such as ascorbic acid, calcium, cadmium, fiber, iron, lead, sucrose, and zinc reduce the bioavailability of copper.

Human breastmilk contains 200–400 µg of copper/L. Infants require 200–220 µg of copper per day. Older children need 340–700 µg/day while 900 µg/day is sufficient for adolescents.

Deficiency state Deficiency is accompanied with anemia, neutropenia, hypopigmentation of hair and skin, vascular abnormalities, osteoporosis, metaphyseal fraying and fractures. Serum shows hypocupremia (<0.8 µg/mL of serum) and low ceruloplasmin levels. Copper intake of less than 0.4 mg per day in adults is being linked with defective immune function. Decrease levels of superoxide dismutase may provide an early indication of deficiency. Genetic defects in copper metabolism may give rise to Menkes kinky hair syndrome and Wilson disease.

MOLYBDENUM

Molybdenum is a constituent of xanthine dehydrogenase/oxidase, aldehyde oxidase, and sulfite oxidase, all of which contain a common factor, molybdopterin. Reduced activity of xanthine dehydrogenase/oxidase is associated with xanthinuria. Clinical manifestations include renal calculi and myopathy. A nutritional deficiency of molybdenum giving rise to clinical symptoms has been reported in a patient on prolonged total parenteral nutrition. In animals, diets low in molybdenum have resulted in low conception rate and increased incidence of abortion. Molybdenum deficiency has also been linked with high incidence of esophageal cancer, dental caries, and Keshan disease. A daily intake of 2–3 µg is sufficient for infants whereas older children require 17–34 µg/day. The RDA for adolescents is 43 µg.

CHROMIUM

It influences the metabolism of carbohydrate, lipid, and protein by potentiating the action of insulin. It has been suggested that biologically active form of chromium is a glucose tolerance factor, though still undocumented. Processed meats, whole grain products, pulses, and spices are the best sources of chromium. Deficiency in humans is on record only in patients on prolonged total parenteral nutrition. Inadequate status may be partially responsible for impaired glucose tolerance, hyperglycemia, glycosuria, and insulin refractoriness. The intake of 11–25 µg/day is considered adequate for children whereas adolescent males and females require 35 µg and 24 µg of chromium, respectively. Supplementation of the diet with chromium appears to improve glucose tolerance in children with protein energy malnutrition.

3.18 TRACE ELEMENTS PROBABLY ESSENTIAL

MANGANESE

Several enzymes including hydrolases, kinases, decarboxylases, and transferases may contain or get activated by manganese. Manganese deficiency has been produced in animals but not in humans. Signs of deficiency include growth impairment, skeletal anomalies, and depressed reproductive function. It has been suggested that high incidence of cartilage disorders in children in some areas may be the result of low manganese intake. Diets high in unrefined cereals, nuts, leafy vegetables, and tea are high in manganese. Indian diets high in foods of plant origin supply an average of 8.3 mg of manganese per day. The intake of 1.2 to 1.9 mg/day is considered adequate for children whereas adolescent males and females require 1.6 mg and 2.2 mg, respectively of manganese per day.

SILICON

Silicon's mode of action in animals is probably related to bone formation. The element can be detected in small areas of ossifying bone during early stages of mineralization. Silicon concentration in human arteries decreases with increasing age and atherosclerosis. Relationship of silicon to the process of aging has been suggested. Vegetarian food contains more silicon than the animal products.

NICKEL

Nickel may play a role in certain enzyme systems including urease, hydrogenase, and carbon monooxide dehydrogenase. Bread, cereals, and beverages are good sources. Hypernickelemia is defined as a serum concentration of >1.0 µg of nickel per liter. The tolerable upper intake levels for nickel are 0.2 mg/day, 0.3 mg/day, 0.6 mg/day, and 1.0 mg/day for age groups of 1–3 years, 4–8 years, 9–13 years, and 14–18 years, respectively. Excessive nickel exposure leads to contact dermatitis.

BORON

Boron affects steroid hormone metabolism in humans. Plant foods are good sources. Low boron diets in adults have been found to be associated with hypocalcemia and hypercalcitoninemia. Higher boron intake has been linked with a lower incidence of osteoporosis. The tolerable upper intake levels for boron are 3 mg/day, 6 mg/day, 11 mg/day, and 17 mg/day for age groups of 1–3 years, 4–8 years, 9–13 years, and 14–18 years, respectively.

VANADIUM

Vanadium might play a role in the regulation of sodium potassium exchange and associated enzyme system. Lower intake has been linked to cardiovascular diseases, though inconclusively.

3.19 TOXIC ELEMENTS

FLUORINE

Fluorine enters the body as dissolved in drinking water. Seafood and tea are also good sources. Fluoride is required for formation of *apatite*, the main mineral in skeletal tissues. Ingested fluoride accumulates in bones. The body and bone fluoride status depends on the quantity of fluoride in drinking water as well as its amount consumed per day. Fluoride content of water may range from <0.1 mg/L to 20 mg/L.

Fluorine is said to prevent dental caries. Excess consumption of fluoride is associated with established toxic effects. Earliest signs of toxicity are evident in teeth manifesting as mottling. Long-term exposure may lead to dental destruction. Fluoride concentration in drinking water of >1 mg/L(1 ppm) results in its accumulation in the body followed by a clinical syndrome referred to as *fluorosis.* Excess fluoride in the bones stimulates new bone formation and exostoses that may present as radiculopathy, myelopathy, and peripheral neuropathy. Secondary and tertiary hyperparathyroidisms are also described.

The tolerable upper intake levels for fluoride are 0.7 mg/day, 0.9 mg/day, 1.3 mg/day, 2.2 mg/day, and 1.0 mg/day for age groups of 0–6 mo, 7–12 mo, 1–3 years, 4–8 years, and >9 years, respectively. In parts of India where skeletal fluorosis is endemic, water fluoride usually ranges from 2–11 mg/L with total intakes between 6 and 30 mg per day. Ingestion of more than 5 mg of fluoride per day produces crippling skeletal deformities including deformities of spine and joints. Endemic genu valgum is the most common deformity observed from endemic fluorosis areas. Radio-logical features include osteosclerosis, osteoporosis, and osteomalacia, and those of secondary hyperparathyroidism.

Severe clinical form of fluoride toxicity is seen in communities whose calcium status is poor. Fluorine may interfere with calcium metabolism resulting in increased bone accretion and resorption rates. Simultaneous calcium deficiency predisposes to the osteomalacial form of skeletal fluorosis.

LEAD

Lead can be transferred transplacentally as well as through breastmilk. Children are prone to absorb more and excrete less of lead as compared to adults; also, kids have little capacity to resist accumulation of lead in the CNS and thus are more vulnerable to the adverse neurological effects at relatively lower levels of lead exposure. Blood levels of lead tend to be higher in children having concurrent iron or calcium deficiency.

Lead is widely distributed in rocks and soils. Soil lead can be inadvertently increased by poor methods of urban waste disposal and presence of road traffic. Cereals and beverages are the chief sources of lead. Mean dietary intake of children is in the range of 9–278 µg/day.

Adverse Effects

Toxic effects of lead are collectively known as **plumbism** and involve many body systems, principally resulting in nervous, hematological, and renal manifestations in children.

Neurological Lead encephalopathy occurs at a blood lead level of 80 mg/dL with early symptoms including lethargy, vomiting, irritability, loss of appetite, and later on progressing to ataxia, alteration in sensorium, coma, and death. Those who recover are left with sequelae as intellectual disability, epilepsy, and blindness. Decrements in IQ have been observed with increasing blood levels, ie, by 5, 4, and 1–2 points at corresponding blood lead levels of 50–70, 30–50, and 15–30 µg/dL, respectively.

Hematological Plumbism results in a microcytic hypochromic type of anemia with marked basophilic stippling. Anemia occurs both as a result of reduced RBC lifespan and defective heme formation. Increased fragility of the cell membrane causes increased erythrocyte destruction at an early stage. Activity of ferrochelatase is inhibited leading to an excess of protoporphyrin. Excess protoporphyrin takes place of heme in the hemoglobin molecule. Zinc is chelated at the center of the molecule at the site usually accompanied by iron. Erythrocytes containing zinc-protoporphyrin are fluorescent and can be used as biochemical markers of lead toxicity. Depressed heme synthesis increases the activity of δ-aminolevulinate synthetase, the first step in heme synthesis. This increases the circulating blood levels and urinary excretion of δ-aminolevulinic acid.

Renal Reversible renal tubular dysfunction is associated with acute exposure while chronic toxicity leads to irreversible interstitial nephropathy. Lead also reduces uric acid excretion.

Measurement of blood lead is the most useful indicator of the risk of toxic effects. It is recommended that weekly intake of lead in children should not exceed 25 µg/kg of body weight.

Diagnosis

Blood lead level (BLL) >2 µg/dL is suggestive of exposure. Levels more than 45 µg/dL require chelation therapy. Lead can also be measured in urine and hair but less reliable.

Treatment	Lead Toxicity

Chelation is required for children with lead encephalopathy or those with BLL >45 mg/dL. Chelating agents include penicillamine, BAL, 2–3-DMSA, and CaNa$_2$EDTA. Lead levels between 45 and 70 mg/dL can be treated with only DMSA; while 2 drugs are required to chelate higher lead levels. Rebound increase in BLL is common following chelation therapy because of release of lead in circulation from bones.

3.20 PREVENTION OF MICRONUTRIENT DEFICIENCY

Simple, effective, and inexpensive strategies should be adopted to stop the drain on the nation's exchequer and human resources arising out of micronutrient deficiency. A few of them are listed below.

Dietary diversification New crops to include more micronutrient-rich foods should be planned. Nutrition education should be imparted to improve the cooking and preservation methods in order to preserve micronutrient. Dietary diversification remains a sustainable long-term solution but is not very useful in communities where micronutrient deficiency is widespread requiring immediate relief.

Supplementation Micronutrients may be supplemented in a capsule, tablet, or syrup form to the suffering population as a short-term measure to reduce the deficiency quickly.

Food fortification Micronutrient is added to common food. This requires presence of an appropriate food that can be enriched. An appropriate food is one that is widely consumed by the target group, is centrally processed, and whose taste and appearance do not change with the addition of the micronutrient; examples include fortification of common salt with iodine, sugar and ghee with vitamin A, and cereals with iron.

Public health interventions aimed at preventing or correcting micronutrient deficiencies can be expected to reduce both mortality and disability substantially, especially in children. To achieve the maximum benefits, such interventions need to be done on the appropriate scale in deficient populations. Recent estimates indicate that fortification or supplementation with iron, vitamin A, and zinc are among the most cost-effective interventions available, even in areas that are very poor or have high rates of HIV infection. Public health interventions that can prevent or correct these micronutrient deficiencies merit the highest priority for national programs.

Micronutrient Interactions

At this point, it appears that the effects of iron, vitamin A, and zinc deficiencies are largely independent. However, it is also important to understand the interactions of the essential micronutrients. When provided in supplements, vitamin A may enhance iron status and zinc may increase vitamin A absorption. On the other hand, iron and zinc may interfere with the absorption of each other. Thus it should not be assumed that providing supplements with multiple micronutrients will have the same benefits as supplements with single micronutrient.

Allen L, Benoist B, Dary O, *et al*. Guidelines on Food Fortification with Micronutrients. Geneva: WHO; 2006.

Ames BN. A role for supplements in optimizing health: the metabolic tune-up. *Arch Biochem Biophys*. 2004;423:227–34.

Argo EA, Heubi JE. Fat soluble vitamin deficiency in infants and children. *Curr Opin Pediatr* 1993; 5: 562.

Arthur JR, Beckett GJ. New metabolic roles for selenium. *Proc Nut Soc*. 1994;53:616–624.

Assessment of iodine deficiency disorders and monitoring their elimination. A guide for programme managers, third edition. Geneva: WHO; 2007.

Bhaskaram P. Micronutrient malnutrition, infection, and immunity: an overview. *Nutr Rev*. 2002;60:S40–5.

Bienz D, Cori H, Hornig D. Adequate dosing of micronutrients for different age groups in the life cycle. *Food Nutr Bull*. 2003;24:S7–15.

Black MM. Micronutrient deficiencies and cognitive functioning. *J Nutr*. 2003;133:3927S–3931S.

Black MM. The evidence linking zinc deficiency with children's cognitive and motor functioning. *J Nutr*. 2003;133:1473S–6S.

Caballero B. Global patterns of child health: the role of nutrition. *Ann Nutr Metab*. 2002;46:3–7.

Darnton-Hill I, Darnton-Hill I, Nalubola R. Fortification strategies to meet micronutrient needs: successes and failures. *Proc Nutr Soc*. 2002;61:231–41.

De Benoist B, Mclean E, Egli I, *et al*. Worldwide prevalence of anaemia 1993–2005. WHO Global Database on Anaemia. Geneva: WHO; 2008.

Diaz JR, de las Cagigas A, Rodriguez R. Micronutrient deficiencies in developing and affluent countries. *Eur J Clin Nutr*. 2003;57:S70–2.

Elimination of Iodine Deficiency Disorders: A Manual for Health Workers. EMRO Technical Publications Series No. 35.WHO Regional Office for the Eastern Meditarranean; 2008.

Global prevalence of vitamin A deficiency in populations at risk:1995–2005. WHO Global Database on Vitamin A Deficiency. Geneva: WHO; 2009.

Gross R, Dwivedi A, Solomons NW. Introduction to the proceedings of the International Research on Infant Supplementation (IRIS) Initiative. *Food Nutr Bull*. 2003;24:S3–6.

Gupta H, Gupta P. Folic acid and neural tube defects. *Indian Pediatr*. 2004; 41.

Gupta P, Indrayan A. Effect of vitamin A on childhood mortality and morbidity - critical review of Indian studies. *Indian Pediatr*. 2002; 39:1099–1118.

Lutter CK, Rivera JA. Nutritional status of infants and young children and characteristics of their diets. *J Nutr*. 2003;133:2941S-9S.

Narasinga Rao BS. Anaemia and micronutrient deficiency. *Natl Med J India*. 2003;16:46–50.

National Nutrition Monitoring Bureau. NNMB Technical Report No. 22: Prevalence of Micronutrient Deficiencies. Hyderabad: National Institute of Nutrition, Indian Council of Medical Research; 2003.

Oken E, Duggan C. Update on micronutrients: iron and zinc. *Curr Opin Pediatr*. 2002;14:350–3.

Ramakrishnan U. Prevalence of micronutrient malnutrition worldwide. *Nutr Rev*. 2002;60:S46–52.

Rivera JA, Hotz C, Gonzalez-Cossio T, *et al*. The effect of micronutrient deficiencies on child growth: a review of results from community-based supplementation trials. *J Nutr*. 2003;133:4010S-4020S.

Shah D, Garg K, Choudhary P. Oxidants and anti-oxidants in pediatric nutrition and disease. *Nutrisearch*. 2001; 8: 1–8.

The state of the world's children. New York: UNICEF; 2017.

Trace elements in human nutrition and health. Report of a WHO Expert Committee. Geneva: WHO, 1996.

Vitamin A Supplements: a Guide to their Use in the Treatment and Prevention of Vitamin A Deficiency and Xerophthalmia. Second Edition. Geneva: WHO; 1997.

Vitamin and Mineral Requirements in Human Nutrition.2nd edition. Geneva: WHO; 2005.

Fluid and Electrolytes

4.1 BODY FLUIDS

Total body water (TBW) constitutes approximately 75% of body weight at birth that declines to 60% at 2 years of age. Two-thirds of body fluid is located within the cells and is termed the *intracellular fluid* (ICF). The remaining one-third of body water is *extracellular fluid* (ECF) (Fig. 4.1).

Extracellular fluid includes (*i*) *interstitial fluid* (80%), (*ii*) *plasma* (15–20%), and (iii) *transcellular fluid* (5%). Dehydration occurs because of reduction in interstitial fluid. Transcellular fluids include lymph, CSF, synovial fluid, humors of the eye, endolymph, perilymph, gastric juices, pleural, pericardial, and peritoneal fluid.

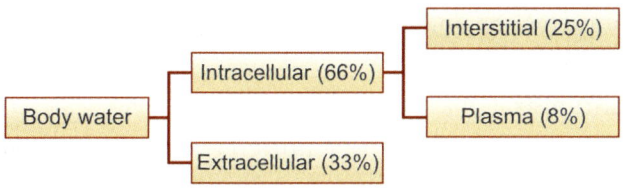

Fig. 4.1 Distribution of body water

FLUID COMPARTMENTS

Selectively permeable cell membranes separate body fluids into 3 fluid compartments. The plasma membranes of individual body cells separate intracellular fluid from interstitial fluid and endothelial cells separate interstitial fluid from plasma. The proportion of plasma at all ages is about 6% and that of transcellular water about 2–3%; whereas interstitial fluid declines from maximum at birth to about 18–20% of body weight by 2 years. Plasma along with blood cells constitutes the blood volume.

Although fluids are in constant motion between the three compartments, the volume of fluid in each compartment at any given time remains fairly constant. Osmosis is the mechanism by which water moves from one compartment to another. As a result, the concentration of the solutes (mainly electrolytes) in the compartments is a major determinant of fluid balance.

Movement across the cell membrane occurs because of osmotic pressure that is related to osmolality. Osmolality indicates number of mols in 1 kg of solution while osmolarity refers to number of mols in 1 liter of solution. Clinically, osmolarity and osmolality are often used interchangeably. Osmolality is also referred to as tonicity. In a crisis situation,

body prefers to maintain tonicity in preference over maintenance of body volume.

ELECTROLYTES

Electrolytes are substances, capable of conducting an electric current in solution. They exist as ions, namely positively charged cations (Na^+, K^+, Ca^+, etc.) and negatively charged anions (Cl^-, HCO_3^-). The total number of cations in body is equal to anions. Electrolytes have a greater effect on osmosis (water movement between compartments) than non-electrolytes because water moves to an area with a greater total number of particles in solution.

In extracellular fluid, the most abundant cation is Na^+. In the intracellular fluid, the most abundant cation is K^+. In extracellular fluid, the most abundant anion is Cl^-, while in intracellular fluid, the most abundant anions are proteins and phosphates (PO_4^-).

Milliequivalent (mEq) is the unit for measurement of electrolytes, calculated as one thousandth part of the equivalent weight. Equivalent weight of a substance is derived by dividing the atomic weight by valency. For example, equivalent weight of calcium is 20(40/2). Concentration of an electrolyte is expressed in mEq per liter (mEq/L) and can be calculated from mg/L.

Example 1: Calcium level in blood is 10 mg/dL. Converting this into mg/L, we get 100 mg/L. Divide this by equivalent weight of calcium, ie, 20 and we get 5 mEq/L.

Example 2: The 7.5% solution of sodium bicarbonate contains 7.5 g/dL, ie, 75000 mg/L. Molecular weight of sodium bicarbonate ($NaHCO_3$) is 84 (23+1+12+48). The molality of 7.5% $NaHCO_3$ is thus 75000 ÷ 84 = 892.8 mMol per liter, containing 892.8 mEq/L of sodium and 892.8 mEq/L of bicarbonate. One mL of 7.5% $NaHCO_3$ thus contains 0.89 mEq of sodium and 0.89 mEq of bicarbonate. Osmolarity of 7.5% sodium bicarbonate is thus 892.8 plus 892.8 = 1785 mOsm/L.

FLUID COMPOSITION

The distribution of body fluid is determined by the composition of electrolytes and proteins in different compartments. The composition of plasma and interstitial fluid and major cations and anions in different biological fluids are mentioned in **Tables 4.1** and **4.2**.

Despite difference in composition, it is noteworthy that all fluid compartments have similar osmolarity (290 mOsm/L).

Table 4.1 Ionic Composition of Different Fluids

Concentration (mEq/L)	Plasma	Interstitial fluid	Intracellular fluid
Sodium	135–145	144	6
Potassium	3.5–5.5	5	154
Calcium	4.25–5.25	5	—
Magnesium	1.5–2.0	5	40
Bicarbonate	20–26	27	13
Chloride	95–106	118	
Proteins (g/dL)	6–8	—	60
Phosphates	2.6–4.4	5	106
Sulfates	4	4	17

Table 4.2 Major Cations and Anions in Body Fluids

Concentration (mEq/L)	Gastric juices	Ileal fluid	Cerebrospinal fluid	Diarrheal stool	Bile	Sweat
Sodium	20–80	100–140	140	10–90	120–140	10–30
Potassium	5–20	5–15	3	10–80	5–15	3–10
Chloride	100–150	90–130	120	10–110	80–120	10–35

REGULATION OF WATER AND SODIUM BALANCE

The main source of body water is from ingested liquids and foods that have been absorbed by the gut. This water is called *preformed water*. The second source of body water is *metabolic water*, the water produced by the various chemical reactions of the body. It amounts to about 200 mL/day. For every 100 calories metabolized, the body loses about 65 mL water in urine, 40 mL by sweating, 15 mL by lungs, and about 5 mL in feces; whereas it gains 15 mL from production as a result of metabolic processes. Thus, 110 mL of water is utilized for every 100 calories metabolized.

The loss of water through sweating depends on the surface area, temperature, and environmental humidity; that from lungs on respiratory rate and humidity of inspired gases; and that in feces on the frequency and fluidity of stools.

Fluid intake is regulated by thirst. When water loss is greater than water gain, the resulting dehydration stimulates thirst. Dehydration causes decreased saliva production with dry mouth and throat. Tactile receptors in the mucosa relay nerve impulses to the thirst center of the hypothalamus, giving rise to a thirst sensation. Dehydration also increases osmotic pressure, stimulating osmoreceptors in the hypothalamus, which in turn stimulate the hypothalamic thirst center.

Dehydration decreases blood volume and thus blood pressure, causing the kidneys to activate the *renin-angiotensin system*. Angiotensin II directly stimulates the hypothalamic thirst center. As a result of these mechanisms, the sensation of thirst and the conscious desire to drink are increased. Initially, wetting the mouth and throat quenches thirst but, the major inhibition of thirst results from stretch of the stomach and a decrease in the blood osmotic pressure.

Loss of Na$^+$ (excess sweating, vomiting, diarrhea, coupled with low Na$^+$ intake or plain water intake) causes the interstitial fluid osmotic pressure to decrease, leading to increased net filtration pressure, net loss of water from the plasma, decreased blood volume, decreased blood pressure, and finally circulatory shock.

Net osmosis into the cell leads to overhydration. As a result, water intoxication occurs, producing neurological symptoms ranging from disorientation to convulsions to coma to death.

Hormones

Aldosterone, antidiuretic hormone, atrial natriuretic peptide, and renin-angiotensin system play a major role in water regulation. Action of all these hormones is ultimately reflected by increased or decreased urine output (as the case may be).

- *Antidiuretic hormone* (ADH) synthesized in hypothalamus and secreted from posterior pituitary, increases the permeability of the distal tubules and collecting ducts of the kidney to water, causing increased reabsorption of water.
- *Aldosterone* secreted from adrenal cortex in response to production of renin and angiotensin by the kidneys, increases Na$^+$ reabsorption by the distal convoluted renal tubules, leading to increased obligatory reabsorption of water.
- *Atrial natriuretic peptide* produced by right atrial myocyte in response to stretching, cause decrease in Na$^+$ reabsorption, leading to decreased obligatory reabsorption and increased water loss in the urine (diuresis). Hence, the major site of regulation of water and sodium is the kidney.

Factors regulating water and sodium are depicted in Fig. 4.2.

REGULATION OF POTASSIUM BALANCE

Potassium homeostasis is maintained both by renal and extrarenal mechanisms. High serum level of potassium

4

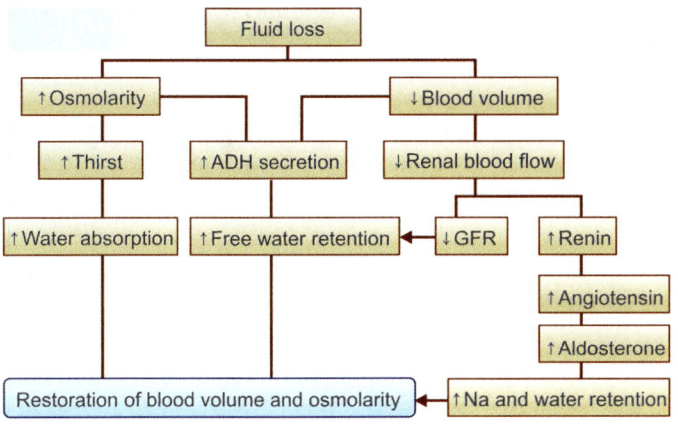

Fig. 4.2 Regulation of water and sodium balance

stimulates secretion of aldosterone, which acts upon distal convoluted tubules to reabsorb sodium; and thus only potassium is excreted. Aldosterone also promotes loss of potassium in colon, sweat, and saliva. Hyperkalemia also stimulates Na$^+$–K$^+$ ATPase pump at distal convoluted tubule resulting in sodium absorption and potassium excretion in urine.

Three factors responsible for enhanced movement of potassium into cells are alkalosis, insulin secretion, and catecholamines. Alkalosis causes efflux of H$^+$ from cells in exchange for K$^+$. Insulin increases potassium uptake by cells by directly stimulating Na$^+$–K$^+$ ATPase activity independent of cyclic-AMP. β_2-agonists act by stimulating cyclic-AMP via adenylate cyclase enzyme, which in turn activate Na$^+$–K$^+$ ATPase pump. All this results in hypokalemia.

Body Fluids

1. Total body water consists of intracellular fluid (66%) and extracellular fluid (33%).
2. ECF consists of (i) interstitial fluid (80%); (ii) plasma (15–20%), and (iii) transcellular fluid (5%).
3. Major cations in the body are sodium and potassium. While sodium is mainly in extracellular fluid, most of potassium is intracellular.
4. Major anions include chloride (extracellular), and proteins, phosphates (intracellular).
5. Aldosterone, ADH, ANP, and renin-angiotensin system hormones are responsible for water regulation.

Kaplan LJ, Kellum JA. Fluids, pH, ions and electrolytes. *Curr Opin Crit Care.* 2010;16:323–31.
Weir MR, Rolfe M. Potassium homeostasis and renin-angiotensin-aldosterone system inhibitors. *Clin J Am Soc Nephrol.* 2010;5:531–48.

4.2 FLUID THERAPY

Fluid and electrolyte therapy has three major components:
1. *Provision of maintenance requirements* These are required for normal metabolism and include insensible water loss and urinary losses. Insensible losses include losses through breathing and evaporative skin losses.
2. *Correction of pre-existing deficits* These losses, via renal or extrarenal route, should be estimated and corrected as soon and safely as possible; for example, rehydration therapy for diarrheal dehydration.
3. *Correction of ongoing losses* These losses mainly occur via the gastrointestinal tract, as in diarrhea, vomiting, etc. or removal (suction, aspiration, etc.). Replacement of such losses should be similar in type and amount to the fluid being lost.

1. MAINTENANCE FLUID THERAPY

The maintenance fluids are generally composed of a solution of water, glucose, sodium, and potassium. This solution should have a long shelf life, low cost, and compatibility with peripheral intravenous administration. The goal of maintenance fluid therapy is to prevent dehydration, electrolyte disorders, ketoacidosis, and protein degradation. Maintenance fluid usually does not provide adequate calories, protein, fat, minerals or vitamins; and children on maintenance fluid lose 0.5–1% of weight each day. Thus, maintenance fluids cannot be substituted for nutrition over long periods of time.

A. Amount of Maintenance Fluid

Under normal condition, a child requires water: 100 mL/100 kcal/day; sodium 1–3 mEq/100 kcal/day; and potassium 1–2 mEq/100 kcal/day. Holiday and Segar showed that the basal caloric requirements for children are as follows:

Body weight 0 to 10 kg	:	100 kcal/kg/day
Between 11 and 20 kg	:	1000 kcal + 50 kcal/kg/day for each kg
More than 20 kg	:	1500 kcal + 20 kcal/kg/day for each kg

For children with normal renal function and under basal metabolic conditions, provision of 50 mL for every 100 kcal consumed per day will replace the normal insensible water losses (IWL), and 66.7 mL per 100 kcal consumed per day will replace the average urinary losses. This adds up to 116.7 mL per 100 kcal consumed per day as maintenance fluids, if we ignore the minimal losses through stool. But 16.7 mL of water is produced as water of oxidation for every 100 kcal metabolized by the body. So the net requirement comes to 100 mL/100 kcal losses. Using the weight-based calculations for caloric requirements as described above, the total maintenance fluid requirements can thus be calculated as shown in **Table 4.3**.

B. Composition of Maintenance Fluid

The composition of the maintenance fluid should be such that its osmolality is close to the normal plasma osmolality of 285–295 mOsm/kg. The body also needs 3 mEq/kg of sodium, 2 mEq/kg of potassium and 2 mEq/kg of chloride per day for maintenance of normal homeostasis.

It may be a good idea to start with 0.45% (half-normal) saline with 5% dextrose and 20 mEq/L of potassium chloride (provided the child is passing adequate urine). Hypotonic fluids (such as 0.2% or 1/5 normal saline) should not be used as maintenance fluids.

Table 4.3 Estimation of Maintenance Fluid Requirements		
Body weight	*Fluid*	*Infusion rate*
Up to 10 kg	100 mL/kg/day	4 mL/kg/hr
10.1–20 kg	1000 + 50 mL/kg/day × (wt–10)	40 mL/hr + 2 mL/kg/hr × (wt–10)
20.1–30 kg	1000 + 500 + 20 mL/kg/day × (wt–20)	60 mL/hr + 1 mL/kg/hr × (wt–20)
Maximum	2400 mL per day	100 mL/hr

For obese children, calculate the fluid requirements according to the ideal body weight (wt) and not the actual weight.

2. DEFICIT THERAPY

This is best assessed by measuring acute weight loss. Weight loss occurring over a matter of hours or a few days is assumed to be due to fluid deficit, because any significant weight change attributable to nutrition would occur over several days to weeks. The deficit volume should be replenished over 4–6 hours.

If the baseline weight is not known, one has to take recourse to clinical assessment as No, Some, or Severe dehydration. When body fluids are lost, approximately 60% of that loss originates in the ECF and 40% in the ICF compartments. The more acute the dehydration, the greater is the proportion of ECF loss; and the more chronic the dehydration, the greater is the proportion of ICF loss. The loss of 1 liter of ECF means approximately 140 mEq of sodium and 100 mEq of chloride have got lost. Similarly, the loss of 1 liter of ICF implies a concomitant loss of approximately 150 mEq of potassium.

If the child can accept oral fluids, replenishment with standard WHO ORS solution over 3–6 hours is the treatment of choice. This is described at length elsewhere. However, if enteral intake is not possible, one would have to administer intravenous fluids. Assuming a 60:40 ratio of loss from the ECF and ICF, for each kilogram total body water deficit, there would be net deficit of 85 mEq of sodium, 60 mEq of potassium, and 60 mEq of chloride. Making a fluid of such precision is not actually required in clinical situations because the body's physiology is able to adjust for approximations. The maintenance requirement may be added to the deficit, and this simplifies the fluid calculation.

For a 10% fluid deficit in a 10 kg child, one would need a N/2 saline preparation with 2 mL potassium chloride added per 100 mL fluid. A total of 1250 mL over 6 hours (1000 mL deficit + 250 mL maintenance for 6 hrs) would take care of deficit and maintenance needs.

3. REPLACEMENT FLUID THERAPY

Gastrointestinal tract is a potential site of water and electrolyte loss, leading to hypokalemia and dehydration. It is often accompanied with bicarbonate loss in acute diarrhea and may cause metabolic acidosis, which may be accentuated, if volume depletion causes hypoperfusion and a concurrent lactic acidosis. Frequent emesis or massive losses from nasogastric tube in intestinal obstruction may lead to metabolic alkalosis.

The losses are to be replaced every 1–6 hours depending on rate of loss, with very rapid losses being replaced more frequently. Composition of replacement IV fluids is given in **Table 4.4.** Choice and amount of fluid are mentioned below:

- *Ongoing losses in stool* 5% dextrose in 1/4 normal saline + 15 mEq HCO_3/L + 25 mEq/L potassium.
- *Emesis and nasogastric losses* 5% dextrose in 1/2 normal saline + 10 mEq/L potassium.
- *Oliguria or anuria* Insensible fluids (400 mL/m^2/24 hr) + replace urine output mL for mL with half-normal saline.
- *Polyuria (post-obstructive diuresis, polyuric phase of renal failure, diabetes mellitus and diabetes insipidus)* Insensible fluids (400 mL/m^2/24 hr) + replace urine output mL/mL with a solution based on urinary electrolytes.
- *Third space losses and chest tube output* Isotonic fluid; Normal saline or Ringer lactate mL for mL, every 1–6 hours.

Surgical drains and chest tubes can produce measurable fluid output and should be replaced when they are significant. Third space losses are due to shift of fluid from intravascular space into interstitial space. The losses cannot be quantified. It can be massive and lead to intravascular volume depletion despite weight gain of children. Thus replacement of third space is empirical but should be anticipated. Protein losses from chest tubes drainage can be significant and occasionally require 5% albumin as replacement fluid.

4. FLUID RESUSCITATION IN SHOCK

In most children with early shock, a fluid bolus of 20 mL/kg of NS or Ringer lactate should be given rapidly. The child is reassessed to determine, if more fluid is required or other form of therapy, ie, antibiotics, vasopressors should be initiated. Children with hypovolemic shock may require and tolerate fluid boluses of 60–80 mL/kg within first 1–2 hrs of presentation. However, the risk of fluid overload must be monitored. Algorithm of fluid resuscitation is provided in Fig. 4.3.

Table 4.4 Composition of Available IV Fluid Solutions					
Fluids	*Na$^+$(mEq/L)*	*Cl$^-$(mEq/L)*	*K$^+$(mEq/L)*	*Ca^{++}(mEq/L)*	*Lactate(mEq/L)*
Normal saline (0.9% NaCl)	154	154	—	—	—
Half-normal saline (0.45% NaCl)	77	77	—	—	—
N/4 Normal saline (0.225% NaCl)	38.5	38.5	—	—	—
Ringer lactate	130	109	4	3	28

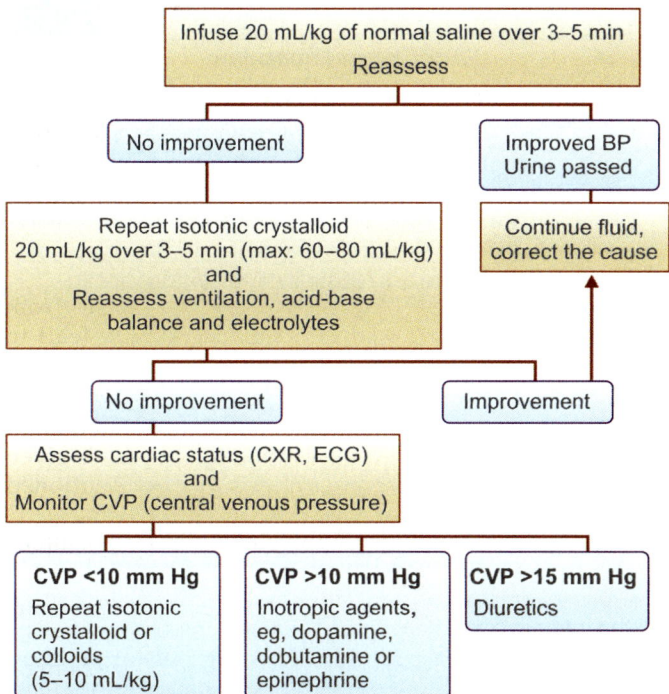

Fig. 4.3 Fluid resuscitation in shock. The initial fluid of choice should be an isotonic solution (Ringer lactate or Normal saline)

Revision Point

Fluid Therapy

1. Normally, a child requires 100 mL/kg/day of fluids (0–10 kg body weight). Additional 50 mL/kg/d is required for weight (11–20 kg) and another 20 mL/kg/d for weight >20 kg.
2. Normal plasma osmolality is 285–295 mOsm/kg. Maintenance fluid needs to be iso-osmolar. Normal saline is the first choice.
3. Deficit therapy in dehydration: Ringer lactate is the preferred solution for intravenous rehydration in diarrheal dehydration.
4. Fluid bolus of 20 mL/kg is required immediately in hypovolemic shock. This requirement may go up to 60–80 mL/kg.

Fang C, Mao J, Dai Y, *et al.* Fluid management of hypernatraemic dehydration to prevent cerebral oedema: a retrospective case control study of 97 children in China. *J Paediatr Child Health.* 2010 ;46:301–3.

Greenbaum LA. Pathophysiology of body fluids and fluid therapy. In: Behrman RE, Kliegman RM, Jenson HB (eds). *Nelson Text Book of Pediatrics* 17th edition. Philadelphia: Saunders;. 2004. p.199–202.

Moritz ML, Ayus JC. Intravenous fluid management for the acutely ill child. *Curr Opin Pediatr.* 2011;23:186–93.

Subba Rao SD, Thomas B. Electrolyte abnormalities in children admitted to pediatric intensive care unit. *Indian Pediatr.* 2000; 37:1348–53.

4.3 ACID–BASE EQUILIBRIUM

Human physiology has evolved to maintain blood pH at a value of 7.35–7.45. Disturbance in the acid direction produce "acidemia", which becomes life-threatening below 7.0. Alkalemia produces comparable morbidity at values over 7.8. The acute toxicity of acid–base derangements would primarily involve the heart and brain. Chronic acid–base disorders also produce problems such as growth retardation and osteomalacia in metabolic acidosis by the gradual dissolution of bone from the titration of bone base.

ACID, BASE, AND pH

Acid is a substance, which donates H-ion or proton. *Base* is defined as a substance that accepts a proton.

The concentration of hydrogen ions in a solution can be expressed either as nanomoles/L or pH (it is negative log of hydrogen ion concentration). Normal pH is a ratio between acid and base in the body; it can also be expressed in a complex manner by Handerson-Hasselbach equation.

Normal values of arterial blood gas
  pH   : 7.35–7.45
  HCO_3^- : 20–28 mEq/L
  $PaCO_2$: 35–45 mm Hg

BUFFER

Buffer is a substance that has the capacity to minimize pH change that an addition of an acid or base would produce. Acid–base homeostasis centers on the regulation of the HCO_3^-/CO_2 buffer system. The ratio between bicarbonate and carbonic acid is 20:1, at this ratio pH is normal. Three key features of this buffer make it ideal for this purpose:
(*a*) Highest concentrations in the body;
(*b*) pK value is 6.1, ie, near physiologic pH; and
(*c*) Independent regulation by the lungs (CO_2) or kidneys (HCO_3^-).

Since HCO_3^-/CO_2 buffer pair is the most important buffer in body, all acid–base disorders are classified as being either respiratory (too much/too little CO_2) or metabolic (too much/too little HCO_3^-). Acid–base balance is maintained when the lungs and kidney quantitatively excrete the net quantity of acid or base ingested. In this balance, systemic pH will be stable and the body buffers are preserved.

All acid or base challenges are buffered. In the ECF, this is predominantly done by the HCO_3^-/CO_2 buffer system and inside cells the major buffers are proteins and PO_4. Buffering reactions are instant and extremely effective.

COMPENSATION

If a child has severe metabolic acidosis with markedly reduced HCO_3^- levels of 5 mEq/L, the normal respiratory response will be to increase ventilation, blow off CO_2, and reduce pCO_2. Had there been no respiratory compensation, pCO_2 would remain at its normal value of 40 with a resulting pH of 6.70. The respiratory compensation therefore converts a life-threatening degree of acidosis to a tolerable level.

Respiratory disorders evoke a compensatory renal response, which will tend to correct the pH back towards normal. Metabolic disorders evoke a respiratory compensatory response.

CORRECTION

In metabolic acidosis or alkalosis, the kidney can increase net acid or base excretion to correct the primary abnormality.

4

Respiratory disorders should be corrected by normalizing lung function and ventilation.

The fall in pH directly stimulates the peripheral and eventually the central chemoreceptors, resulting in hyperventilation and a further improvement in systemic pH; the respiratory compensation also reduces pCO_2 levels. Finally, the kidney will begin to correct the disorder by increasing net acid excretion. A normal child may be able to excrete about 150 mEq/day of acid in response to an acute acid load, the adaptive response enables net acid excretion to approach 500–600 mEq/day in chronic metabolic acidosis.

RENAL REGULATION

A. Proximal Acidification

The proximal nephron is very sensitive to the ECF volume state. In general, ECF volume depletion increases electrolyte reabsorption, while ECF expansion depresses reabsorption. This seems to be true for the electrolytes handled by the Na/H exchanger. Besides increasing Na reabsorption, ECF depletion also increases H^+ secretion. This will further augment acidification and HCO_3^- reabsorption.

ECF expansion conversely depresses proximal acidification and HCO_3^- will be dumped in the urine because it will escape the proximal nephron and overwhelm the low-capacity distal system.

Proximal acidification is also increased by CO_2 and mediates the renal compensation for respiratory acidosis. Likewise, the renal response to respiratory alkalosis is mediated by a decline in proximal nephron acidification in response to the low pCO_2. Proximal acidification is also sensitive to K^+ and is increased in metabolic alkalosis with coexisting hypokalemia. PTH, angiotensin, and systemic pH also affect acidification.

B. Distal Acidification

Distal acidification is primarily thought to be regulated by aldosterone, which augments both H^+ and K^+ secretions. The distal system is also sensitive to systemic pH, pCO_2, and K^+. The electrogenicity of distal H^+ secretion makes acidification sensitive to Na^+ handling. Furosemide is also a potent stimulator of the distal system and in fact a standard test to measure net acid exretion.

Acid–base Equilibrium

1. Normal values of arterial blood gases are as follows: pH: 7.35–7.45; bicarbonate (HCO_3): 20–28 mEq/L; $PaCO_2$: 35–45 mm Hg
2. Metabolic acidosis is characterized by low pH and low bicarbonate. Common etiology includes dehydration, renal failure, and shock. Treatment consists of volume replacement and administration of bicarbonate.

Kaplan LJ, Kellum JA. Fluids, pH, ions and electrolytes. *Curr Opin Crit Care.* 2010;16:323–31.

Rabinstein AA, Bruder N. Management of hyponatremia and volume contraction. *Neurocrit Care.* 2011;15:354–60.

Weir MR, Rolfe M. Potassium homeostasis and renin-angiotensin-aldosterone system inhibitors. *Clin J Am Soc Nephrol.* 2010;5:531–48.

4.4 EVALUATION OF ACID–BASE DISORDERS

The history gives important clues to acid–base disturbances, eg, loss of base (diarrhea) or acid (emesis). You should always think about the child's known medical problems and how they might be acting to produce acid–base disorders by changing the status of ECF volume, K^+, aldosterone, etc. Physical examination should include evaluation of ECF volume by looking for edema, skin turgor, blood pressure, neck veins, crackles, ventilation, and tendon reflexes.

Arterial blood gases are essential to define acid–base abnormalities. The expected arterial blood gas abnormalities are shown in **Table 4.5**.

1. URINARY pH

Urine pH is usually acid and varies from 5–6.5. This reflects the ongoing secretion of H^+ by the kidney to excrete the daily acid load. The urine pH should always be checked in children with acid–base disorders to ascertain appropriate renal response.

With normal renal function, children with metabolic acidosis should have a very low urine pH, unless children have associated renal tubular acidosis. Likewise, the urine should be maximally alkaline after infusing HCO_3^- to produce metabolic alkalosis, unless the kidneys are the cause of the alkalosis, as in the alkalosis associated with vomiting or volume depletion.

Table 4.5 Primary Acid–base Disturbances with Responses			
Types	*Primary alteration*	*Secondary response*	*Mechanism of secondary response*
Metabolic acidosis	Decrease in plasma HCO_3^-	Decrease in $PaCO_2$	Hyperventilation
Metabolic alkalosis	Increase in plasma HCO_3^-	Increase in $PaCO_2$	Hypoventilation
Respiratory acidosis	Increase in $PaCO_2$	Increase in plasma HCO_3^-	Acid titration of tissue buffers; transient increase in acid excretion and sustained enhancement of HCO_3^- Reabsorption by kidney
Respiratory alkalosis	Decrease in $PaCO_2$	Decrease in plasma HCO_3^-	Alkaline titration of tissue buffers; Transient suppression of acid excretion; Sustained reduction in bicarbonate reabsorption by kidney

An alkaline urine pH is seen in several circumstances, ie, after meal as the "alkaline tide" from gastric acid secretion raises blood HCO₃⁻ enough to produce a urine pH around 8 due to ammonia formation and in strict vegetarians.

2. ACID–BASE NOMOGRAM

The acid–base nomogram (Fig. 4.4) illustrates the blood gas pattern that is seen when the various primary acid–base disorders are reproduced in otherwise normal children. A simple acid–base disorder will produce a blood-gas pattern that falls in the shaded areas, and these responses reflect normal buffering and compensation. Another way of judging whether the buffering and compensatory responses are appropriate is to use the rules of thumb derived from the nomogram as mentioned in **Table 4.6**.

3. ANION GAP

Serum electrolytes are essential in unraveling acid–base disorders because hypokalemia is often associated with metabolic alkalosis and it provides information about anion gap, which normally has a value of 12 ± 2 mEq/L. The gap reflects unmeasured anions, mostly the negative charge on albumin. The gap is used to differentiate metabolic acidosis caused by loss of HCO₃⁻ (normal gap) from acidosis caused by organic acids like ketoacids, lactic acid, or toxins like ethylene glycol, or methanol.

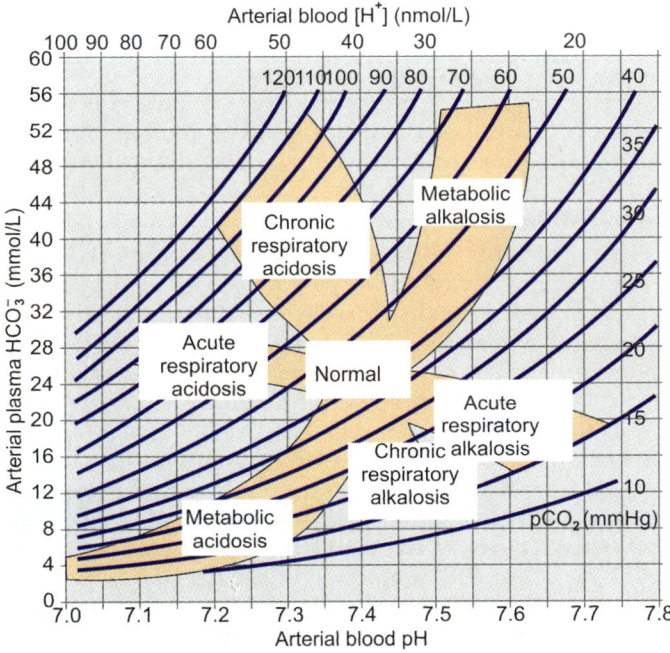

Fig. 4.4 Acid–base nomogram

Kaplan LJ, Kellum JA. Fluids, pH, ions and electrolytes. *Curr Opin Crit Care.* 2010;16:323–31.

Lawn CJ, Weir FJ, McGuire. Base administration or fluid bolus for preventing morbidity and mortality in preterm infants with metabolic acidosis. *Cochrane Database Syst Rev.* 2010;2:CD003215.

Table 4.6 Rules of Thumb for Interpretation of Acid–base Disorders

Metabolic acidosis	PaCO₂ should fall by 1.0 to 1.5 × the fall in plasma HCO₃⁻ concentration
Metabolic alkalosis	PaCO₂ should rise by 0.25 to 1.0 × the rise in plasma HCO₃⁻ concentration
Acute respiratory acidosis	Plasma HCO₃⁻ concentration should rise by about 1 mmol/L for each 10 mmHg increment in PaCO₂ (± 3 mmol per liter).
Chronic respiratory acidosis	Plasma HCO₃⁻ concentration should rise by about 4 mmol/L for each 10 mm Hg increment in PaCO₂ (± 4 mmol per liter).
Acute respiratory alkalosis	Plasma HCO₃⁻ concentration should fall by about 1 to 3 mmol/L for each 10 mm Hg decrement in the PaCO₂, usually not to less than 18 mmol/L.
Chronic respiratory alkalosis	Plasma HCO₃⁻ concentration should fall by about 2 to 5 mmol/L per 10 mm Hg decrement in PaCO₂ but usually not to less than 14 mmol/L.

4.5 ACID–BASE ABNORMALITIES

METABOLIC ACIDOSIS

Metabolic acidosis is characterized by low arterial pH, reduced plasma bicarbonate (HCO₃⁻), and compensatory hyperventilation.

Pathophysiology

Decrease in bicarbonate (HCO₃⁻) is the primary defect. This causes a respiratory response resulting in stimulation of ventilation. This causes wash-off of CO₂ through lungs. Overall, the pCO₂ will be reduced by 1–1.5 mm Hg/mEq/L fall in HCO₃⁻.

Renal response. In metabolic acidosis, the plasma HCO₃ is low and, therefore, the filtered load of HCO₃⁻ will be reduced. The renal response is distal acidification system and increase in H⁺ excretion. Because the renal excretion of phosphate is essentially stable, this increased net acid excretion is largely in the form of NH₄⁺.

Etiology

I. **Metabolic acidosis with normal anion gap** (4–12 mEq/L):
   1. *Diminished excretion of acid*: Renal tubular acidosis (RTA)
   2. *Loss of bicarbonate*: Diarrhea, use of acetazolamide.
   3. Hypoaldosteronism
II. **Metabolic acidosis with increased anion gap** (accumulation of organic acids):
   1. *Lactic acidosis*: Tissue hypoxia, liver failure, intestinal bacterial overgrowth syndrome, metformin therapy
   2. *Ketoacidosis*: Diabetes, starvation, alcohol
   3. *Inborn errors of metabolism*: Aminoacidopathies, organic acidemias
   4. Renal failure
III. **Metabolic acidosis with both increased anion and osmolar gap**
   Poisoning: Ethylene glycol, methanol, salicylates.

4

Clinical Manifestations

Acute metabolic acidosis is characterized by rapid and deep breathing (Kussmaul respiration). The fall in pH below 7 may predispose children to fatal ventricular tachyarrhythmias and may result in vasodilation, hypotension, and impaired cardiac contractility. The consequence is decreased cardiac output and persistence of shock and lactic acidosis.

Chronic metabolic acidosis is either asymptomatic or may present with anorexia, vomiting, weight loss, muscle weakness, listlessness, lethargy, and coma. Long-standing acidosis results in bone lysis and growth retardation.

Hyperchloremic Metabolic Acidosis

It represents the loss of HCO_3^- from either the kidney or the gastrointestinal tract. In either case, the HCO_3^- is lost in exchange for chloride. This results in hyperchloremia and a normal anion gap because each lost HCO_3^- is replaced by Cl^-. If for some reason the history could not be obtained, the urinary findings should clearly distinguish whether the HCO_3^- loss is from the kidney or GI tract.

With GI loss, HCO_3^- will augment both proximal and distal acidification to increase net acid excretion. This will tend to correct the acidemia, because each additional H^+ excreted returns one HCO_3^- to the blood to restore the deficit. The urine, therefore, is acidic (pH <6) with generous amounts of NH_4Cl. Urinary NH_4 can be estimated by calculating the urinary anion gap as $(Na + K) - Cl$. Because of the high concentrations of the unmeasured cation NH_4^+, the urinary anion gap is negative in children with metabolic acidosis due to acid ingestion or from GI loss of HCO_3^-. In contrast, in distal RTA, the urine is usually not as acidic (pH is > 6.0) and the anion gap is near zero or positive because of the inability to trap ammonia in the urine.

Diabetic Ketoacidosis

It represents the accumulation of beta-hydroxybutyric acid and acetoacetic acids as a result of the metabolic effects of insulin deficiency. There is increased lipolysis with release of fatty acids and the acetyl-CoA end products cannot be effectively utilized in the Krebs cycle. The acetyl-CoA is further shunted to produce the ketoacids, which accumulate because of an associated defect in utilizing these substrates. The presence of metabolic acidosis in association with hyperglycemia and an elevated anion gap suggests the diagnosis of diabetic ketoacidosis. The diagnosis should be confirmed by demonstrating "ketones" in the blood or urine using standard bedside tests.

Lactic Acidosis

This results from overproduction of lactate by muscle combined with inadequate lactate removal by the liver and kidney. The diagnosis is made by elevated serum lactate levels, negative ketone measurements, and no osmolar gap.

Renal Tubular Acidosis

Metabolic acidosis can originate from renal defects in acid secretion, resulting in renal tubular acidosis (RTA). All types of RTA produce a systemic metabolic acidosis with a normal anion gap. Serum K^+ is often high or low, depending on the type of RTA. The normal function of the renal acidification system is to first reabsorb all of the filtered HCO_3^- and then form the 50–60 mEq/day of net acid that will keep pH in balance. In RTA, one of these systems is defective.

Treatment	Metabolic Acidosis

Acidosis can be treated by the administration of HCO_3^- but correction of underlying causes is most important. The initial therapeutic goal should be to raise systemic pH to above 7.1–7.2, a level at which arrhythmias become less likely. Finally, it needs to be restored to 7.4 by correcting the base excess within 48 hours. The correction should not be aggressive in these cases, as it will produce an alkalosis.

The amount of HCO_3^- required to correct acidemia can be calculated by the following formula.

$$HCO_3^- \text{ required} = 0.3 \times \text{body weight (kg)} \times \text{standard base excess}$$

Half (50%) of the amount thus calculated is given over 1 hour and the rest over next 5 hours, intravenously. One mL of 7.5% $NaHCO_3$ solution provides 0.9 mEq of sodium and 0.9 mEq of bicarbonate.

Treat the Cause

Correct volume deficit. Administer insulin for diabetic ketoacidosis. Acidosis of renal failure and renal tubular acidosis respond to oral bicarbonate therapy (0.5–2 mEq/kg/day). Steroids may be needed for hypoaldosteronism. Drug-induced acidosis will require stopping the drug and facilitate its excretion. Treatment of lactic acidosis depends on reversing the underlying disorder and using bicarbonate therapy to keep systemic HCO_3^- levels over 10–15 mEq/L. Dichloroacetate is an experimental drug which may increase hepatic pyruvate utilization, thus consuming lactate.

METABOLIC ALKALOSIS

Metabolic alkalosis is characterized by an increase in blood HCO_3^-, high arterial pH, and compensatory hypoventilation.

Pathophysiology

Increased bicarbonate occurs most commonly due to loss of acid either from the kidney or the GI tract. It can be occasionally due to gain of base when renal function is poor and HCO_3^- excretion is compromised. Since the primary problem is metabolic, the compensation is respiratory.

The chemoreceptors respond to metabolic alkalosis by depressing ventilation. The pCO_2 will rise about 0.8 mm Hg for each mEq/L increase in HCO_3^-. The depression of alveolar ventilation will also produce hypoxemia. Potassium is almost always reduced in metabolic alkalosis. The hypokalemia can in turn contribute to the alkalosis by inducing cellular K^+ depletion. This directly stimulates proximal acidification, potentiates aldosterone effects on distal H^+ secretion, and causes immediate H^+ shifts in cells.

Clinical Manifestations

There is shallow respiration. As alkalosis becomes severe (pH >7.65), children will develop clinical features of increased neuromuscular irritability, ie, increased reflexes, tetany, carpopedal spasm, and cardiac arrhythmias. It also worsens the pre-existing hepatic encephalopathy due to shift of ammonia mass equation towards the uncharged

Interpret the ABG report of an 18-month-child weighing 10 kg, which revealed pH 7.1; PaCO₂ 39 mm Hg; PaO₂ 90 mm Hg; HCO₃ 8 mEq/L; and base excess -22.

What is the diagnosis? Justify?

The pH is less than 7.35 indicating acidosis. Serum bicarbonate is also low (<20 mEq/L). Low pH along with reduced bicarbonate indicates metabolic acidosis. The pCO_2 has remained normal indicating that there is no hyperventilation that could have resulted in a compensatory response. Thus the diagnosis is *uncompensated metabolic acidosis*. The expected CO_2 level when compensation occurs is at least 24–28 mm Hg. If the CO_2 level had been less than 24 mm Hg, the compensation would have been operating, and the diagnosis would change to compensated metabolic acidosis.

Name a few likely causes of the disorder.

Acute dehydration, shock, diabetic ketoacidosis, renal failure, and sepsis.

How will you treat the metabolic abnormality?

HCO_3 required = 0.3 x body weight (kg) x standard base excess
$$= 0.3 \times 10 \times 22 = 66 \text{ mEq.}$$
One mL of 7.5% $NaHCO_3$ solution provides 0.9 mEq (approximately 1 mEq) of bicarbonate; thus approx 66 mL of 7.5% solution of sodabicarbonate is needed. Of this 15–30 mL can be given immediately diluted in equal volume of distilled water (IV) and the remaining is given over next 5 hours.

If this child had a serum sodium of 155, how would your treatment differ.

In this case, sodium bicarbonate cannot be used to correct acidosis, because this will also provide additional sodium. This child is already having hypernatremia so more sodium can be dangerous. Such children need to be treated with THAM or peritoneal dialysis.

A 7-year-old girl presented in emergency with history of altered sensorium, polyuria and polydipsia. Her blood gas analysis revealed pH 7.26; pCO₂ 16 mm Hg; HCO₃ 7.1 mmol/L; Serum sodium 136 mEq/L; potassium 4.8 mEq/L; and chloride 101 mEq/L.

Interpret ABG report of this patient with justification.

The first thing to look in ABG is pH which is lower than normal (normal: 7.35–7.45), HCO_3^- is also less than normal (21–28 mmol/L), thus metabolic acidosis. $PaCO_2^-$ is less than normal (normal: 35–45), indicating a compensatory response in the form of hyperventilation that has resulted in washing off of CO_2. This child is thus having a *compensated metabolic acidosis*.

Calculate the anion gap in this ABG and interpret further.

Anion gap = (Sodium + potassium) – (bicarbonate + chloride) = 140.8–108.1 = 32.7. Normal value is 12 ±2 mEq/L. Thus this chid is having a 'high anion gap metabolic acidosis'. Common causes are diabetic ketoacidosis, renal failure, lactic acidosis in shock, and acidosis due to toxin.

NH_3 species, which can more readily cross the blood–brain barrier.

There is often associated hypokalemia and hypomagnesemia; due to emesis or from the hyperaldosteronism that almost always accompanies metabolic alkalosis.

Etiology

1. **Chloride responsive metabolic alkalosis** (urinary chloride <15 mEq/L):
   - *Gastric losses*: Emesis, nasogastric aspiration, chloride-losing diarrhea
   - *Diuretic therapy*: Frusemide, thiazide
   - Cystic fibrosis
2. **Chloride resistant metabolic alkalosis** (urinary chloride >20 mEq/L):
   - *With high blood pressure*: Congenital adrenal hyperplasia, renovascular disease, renin secreting tumor, Cushing syndrome, Liddle syndrome.
   - *With normal blood pressure*: Gitelman syndrome, Barter syndrome, base administration

The differential diagnosis in a child with established alkalosis is between "chloride-resistant" and "chloride-responsive" disorders. This distinction is based on whether or not the alkalosis resolves by simply giving chloride (usually as IV NaCl). The two conditions can be differentiated by measuring urinary chloride.
- In the *chloride-responsive alkalosis*, there is volume depletion (or chloride depletion) and signs of volume depletion, ie, orthostasis, decreased turgor, and low urinary Na and Cl.
- In *chloride-resistant alkalosis*, there is generally ECF volume expansion resulting in hypertension, possible edema, and generous amounts of urinary Na^+ and Cl^-.

Treatment | **Metabolic Alkalosis**

Treatment of metabolic alkalosis includes therapy of primary diseases, correction of volume depletion, and replenishing K, Cl, and Mg deficits. Oral and intravenous sodium chloride and water is recommended for chloride-responsive metabolic alkalosis but ineffective in chloride-resistant form.

In emergencies, bicarbonate levels can be directly reduced by dialysis, administration of acid (intravenous HCl, arginine HCl or oral NH_4Cl), or promotion of bicarbonate excretion in urine with the carbonic anhydrase inhibitor, acetazolamide.

In edematous children, withholding diuretics are the corrective therapy. The efficacy of treatment may be assessed by monitoring urine pH.

RESPIRATORY ACIDOSIS

Respiratory acidosis is characterized by a reduced arterial blood pH, an elevated pCO_2, and increase in plasma HCO_3^-.

Causes

1. *Pulmonary disease* Pneumonia, pneumothorax, bronchiolitis, asthma, ARDS, bronchopulmonary dysplasia, meconium aspiration syndrome, pulmonary hemorrhage, pulmonary embolism.
2. *Respiratory muscle weakness* Muscular dystrophy, hypothyroidism, malnutrition, hypokalemia, corticosteroid therapy.

4

3. *Upper airway diseases* Aspiration, laryngospasm, angioedema, vocal cord paralysis, and extrinsic and intrinsic compression of airways.
4. *Depression of CNS* Encephalitis, brain tumor, sleep apnea syndrome, stroke, HIE, increased intracranial pressure, medications (narcotic, benzodiazepines, barbiturates, anesthesia, and alcohol).
5. *Diseases of spinal cord, peripheral nerve or neuromuscular junction* GB syndrome, poliomyelitis, diaphragmatic paralysis, spinal muscular atrophy, botulinism, myasthenia gravis, spinal cord injury, aminoglycoside and organophosphates.
6. *Miscellaneous* Flail chest, cardiac arrest, kyphoscoliosis.

Pathophysiology

It can be any—acute (<24 hours) or chronic. During the *acute phase*, buffering response is present (HCO_3^- will increase about 1 mEq for every 10 mm Hg increase in CO_2) but there will be no renal response. Over the next a few days, renal acidification is stimulated by the increased pCO_2, and by about the 4th day the fully compensated picture may emerge with increase in HCO_3^-.

Clinical Manifestations

Clinical manifestations include restlessness, anxiety, headache, blurred vision, and excessive sweating. Later stages are characterized by features of CO_2 narcosis (tremor, asterixis, delirium, and drowsiness). There may be features of raised intracranial pressure, vasodilation, and shock.

Treatment	Respiratory Acidosis

Treatment of acute respiratory acidosis includes correction of underlying conditions and mechanical ventilation. The aim is to restore normal alveolar ventilation.

Bicarbonate therapy is recommended only in status asthmaticus to correct pH and to minimize ventilator settings but there are associated risk of volume overload, hypernatremia, and persistence and worsening of tissue acidosis.

In chronic respiratory acidosis, control of infections, diuretic and bronchodilator therapy, along with low flow oxygen are useful.

RESPIRATORY ALKALOSIS

Respiratory alkalosis is characterized by elevated arterial pH, low pCO_2, and a reduction in plasma HCO_3^- concentration.

Causes

With tissue hypoxia Pneumonia, pulmonary edema, ARDS, aspiration, cyanotic congenital heart disease, CHF, shock, severe anemia, CO poisoning.

Without tissue hypoxia Meningoencephalitis, brain tumor, anxiety, pain, fever, early sepsis, inappropriate mechanical ventilation, ECMO, hemodialysis.

Pathophysiology

The acute buffering response will drop HCO_3^- by about 1–3 mmol/10 mm Hg change in pCO_2. The more chronic renal response is not well developed but there is usually a small depression in renal acidification, which will lead to HCO_3^- wasting and a further decline in blood HCO_3^- so that the total change is 2–5 mmol/10 mm Hg fall in pCO_2.

Clinical Features

The clinical manifestations are due to impairment of cerebral function and cell membrane excitability and include altered sensorium, paresthesias, cramps, and carpopedal spasms. In sick children, supraventricular tachycardia and ventricular arrhythmias may also occur.

Treatment	Respiratory Alkalosis

Treatment is usually not required and management should be directed at diagnosis and correction of underlying causes. In critically sick children, rebreathing into a reservoir may partially increase pCO_2 and relieve symptoms.

Amer MB. Fuzzy-based framework for diagnosis of acid–base disorders. *Comput Biol Med*. 2011;41:737–41.

Durand P. Management of metabolic acidosis in children, inherited metabolic disorders excluded. *Arch Pediatr*. 2010;17:678–9.

Fencl V, Jabor A, Kazda A, Figge J. Diagnosis of metabolic acid–base disturbances in critically ill patients. *Am J Respir Crit Care Med*. 2000;162: 2246–51.

Gennari FJ. Pathophysiology of metabolic alkalosis: a new classification based on the centrality of stimulated collecting duct ion transport. *Am J Kidney Dis*. 2011;58:626–36.

Gunnerson K, Kellum JA. Acid–base and electrolyte analysis in critically ill patients: are we ready for the new millennium? *Curr Opin Crit Care*. 2003;9:468–73.

Kraut JA, Madias NE. Metabolic acidosis: pathophysiology, diagnosis and management. *Nature Rev Nephrol*. 2010;6:274–85.

Oh YK. Acid–base disorders in ICU patients. *Electrolyte Blood Press*. 2010;8:66–71.

Rastegar A. Attending rounds: patient with hypokalemia and metabolic acidosis. *Clin J Am Soc Nephrol*. 2011;6:2516–21.

4.6 HYPONATREMIA

Hyponatremia is defined as serum sodium concentration less than 130 mEq/L. It is the most common electrolyte abnormality encountered in pediatric practice with an incidence of 1.5% of all pediatric hospital admissions. Symptoms appear when the serum sodium concentration is less than 125 mEq/L.

Etiology

Hyponatremia can be produced by three different mechanisms: (*i*) Deficiency in sodium intake, (*ii*) excessive loss of sodium (renal or extrarenal), and (*iii*) excessive water retention.

Because the human body protects itself from hyponatremia through an intact thirst mechanism, conditions associated with alteration in thirst mechanism are more prone to hyponatremia. Hyponatremia rarely is caused by a deficient intake, except in infants fed with hypotonic fluids.

The most common cause of hyponatremia in children is diarrhea. Sodium loss also occurs via the kidneys. Diuretics are the most common culprit followed by salt-losing nephritis, mineralocorticoid deficiency, and cerebral salt-wasting syndrome. Causes are listed below:

1. *Hypervolemic hyponatremia* Congestive heart failure, cirrhosis, nephritic syndrome, acute or chronic renal failure.

2. *Hypovolemic hyponatremia due to renal loss* Diuretic excess, osmotic diuresis, salt wasting, adrenal insufficiency, proximal renal tubular acidosis, metabolic alkalosis, pseudohypoaldosteronism.
3. *Hypovolemic hyponatremia due to extrarenal loss* Vomiting, diarrhea, fistula, excessive sweating, acute pancreatitis, burns, trauma, peritonitis, effusions, ascites.
4. *Normovolemic hyponatremia* SIADH(syndrome of inappropriate secretion of ADH), acute leukemia, lymphoma, asthma, empyema, pneumonia, ligation of PDA, cystic fibrosis, meningitis, encephalitis, HIE, ventriculoperitoneal shunt, head trauma.
5. *Drugs* Chlorpropamide, vincristine, vinblastine, diuretics, clofibrate, carbamazepine, fluphenazine, amitriptyline, morphine, isoproterenol, nicotine, adenine arabinoside, colchicine, barbiturates.
6. *Endocrinal* Addison disease, hypothyroidism, congenital adrenal hyperplasia, IV fluid therapy.

Syndrome of Inappropriate ADH Secretion

Excessive antidiuretic hormone (ADH) secretion causes water retention and subsequent dilutional hyponatremia. It occurs in response to pain, nausea, vomiting, and physiologic stimuli (increased serum osmolality, decreased intravascular volume). Some drugs also can cause SIADH.

Arterial blood volume may be increased, decreased, or normal depending on the underlying clinical condition. Intravascular volume is determined by distribution of water and solute in the intracellular space and extracellular space. Fluid shifts from extracellular space into intracellular space with a subsequent decrease in arterial blood volume. This may result in hypotension. Because of this fluid shift, hyponatremia causes more pronounced hemodynamic disturbance for a particular degree of dehydration.

In children with cirrhosis, cardiac failure, or renal failure, hyponatremia may be caused by one of many mechanisms.

Pathophysiology

When serum sodium declines, the serum osmolality also decreases. This results in an osmotic gradient across the blood–brain barrier causing water to move into intracellular compartment. The resultant cerebral edema manifests as headache, nausea, vomiting, irritability, and seizures. The brain's adaptation to hyponatremia is accomplished by loss of interstitial fluid into the cerebrospinal fluid, and loss of cellular solute and organic osmolytes.

When water moves into the brain, increasing hydrostatic pressure shifts interstitial fluid into cerebrospinal fluid, which subsequently is absorbed through the arachnoid villi. The interstitial fluid is rich in sodium. The brain equilibrates the osmolar gradient by removing this fluid. In addition, intracellular potassium acts similarly with a maximal response occurring in 24 hours. If hyponatremia lasts longer, intracellular amino acids extrude to maintain the osmolar gradient. This shifting of solutes and organic osmolytes plays an important role in protecting the brain from cerebral edema. The resultant hypo-osmolar state makes the brain vulnerable to dehydration secondary to rapid correction of hyponatremia. The optimum speed of correction is not known. However, rapid correction in fully compensated chronic hyponatremia results in a demyelinating lesion in the pons known as central pontine myelinosis (CPM).

Clinical Features

Clinical manifestations vary from asymptomatic to severe neurologic dysfunctions. Neurological symptoms are predominant in hyponatremia, although cardiovascular and musculoskeletal findings are also present. Factors contributing to CNS symptoms include (*i*) rate of change in serum sodium; (*ii*) level of serum sodium; and (*iii*) duration of the elevated serum sodium level.

Early signs of CNS involvement include anorexia, headache, nausea, and emesis. Advanced signs include impaired response to verbal and painful stimuli, bizarre behavior, hallucinations, obtundation, incontinence, and respiratory insufficiency.

In late stage, children may have decorticate or decerebrate posturing, bradycardia, hypertension or hypotension, altered temperature regulation, dilated pupils, seizure, respiratory arrest, and coma. Renal failure may occur. Musculoskeletal features include weakness and muscular cramps.

Investigations

Serum sodium, osmolality, urea, creatinine, and urine osmolality should be measured. Urine sodium changes according to the type of hyponatremia.

- *Hypovolemic hyponatremia* Renal losses result in a urine sodium concentration greater than 20 mEq/L.
- *Normovolemic hyponatremia* Urine sodium is greater than 20 mEq/L.
- *Hypervolemic hyponatremia* Urine sodium concentration is less than 20 mEq/L. Extrarenal losses caused by vomiting, diarrhea, sweat, and third spacing result in a urinary sodium less than 20 mEq/L.
- If hyponatremia is caused by acute or chronic renal failure, urine sodium concentration is greater than 40 mEq/L.
- Other laboratory studies include aldosterone, cortisol, thyroid function tests, adrenocorticotropic hormone, and ADH.
- Imaging studies, such as radiograph of skull and CT scan, should be done to delineate intracranial pathology. Ultrasound may reveal an abdominal mass in individuals with bilateral adrenal hyperplasia and adrenal tumor.

Treatment	Hyponatremia

The aim of treatment is to restore circulatory adequacy with 20–30 mL/kg of normal saline or Ringer lactate. In symptomatic children, serum sodium should be rapidly raised by intravenous administration of 3% sodium chloride in a dose of 5–6 mL/kg over 10–15 minutes. If clinical improvement does not occur, administer additional bolus dose of 3–4 mL/kg.

Seizures resulting from acute water intoxication are not responsive to antiepileptic drugs; however, such seizures respond very well to 3% sodium chloride. In children with chronic hyponatremia, correction of sodium should be slow to prevent potential demyelinating lesions. Optimal rate of correction is 0.5 mEq/hour, not to exceed serum sodium of 125 mEq/L.

The amount of sodium required to raise serum sodium by a given amount can be calculated by the following formula.

$$\text{Sodium required (mEq)} = \text{Weight in kg} \times 0.6 \times (125 - \text{observed sodium})$$

4

Each milliliter of 3% sodium chloride contains approximately 0.5 mEq Na/L. Administering 1 mL/kg of 3% sodium chloride raises the serum sodium by 1.6 mEq. The current evidence suggests that it is safe to raise plasma sodium concentration in asympmtomatic children by 10–12 mEq/L on first day and 18 mEq/L over the first two days.

- In children with *hypovolemic hyponatremia*, administer 3% sodium chloride to correct hyponatremia and 0.9% sodium chloride for intravascular volume expansion.
- In children with *normovolemic* and *hypervolemic hyponatremia*, administer 3% sodium chloride to correct hyponatremia and restrict fluids (two-thirds of maintenance). Administer loop diuretics, if needed.
- Children with salt-wasting disorders (eg, salt-losing nephropathies) need sodium supplementation whereas those with SIADH and renal failure require fluid restriction.

Cerebral Pontine Myelinolysis

Clinical features include slowly progressive flaccid paralysis, cranial nerve abnormalities (dysphagia or pseudobulbar palsy), alteration of mental status (behavioral changes, depression of sensorium, lethargy), seizures, and coma. The condition is usually fatal in 3–5 weeks. MRI permits visualization of the brainstem and is sensitive to alterations in white matter. Lesions become apparent 1–2 weeks later.

Marcialis MA, Dessi A, Pintus MC, *et al.* Neonatal hyponatremia: differential diagnosis and treatment. *J Matern Fetal Neonatal Med.* 2011;24:75–9.

Rabinstein AA, Bruder N. Management of hyponatremia and volume contraction. *Neurocrit Care.* 2011;15:354–60.

Wakil A, Atkin SL. Serum sodium disorders: safe management. *Clin Med.* 2010;10:79–82.

4.7 HYPERNATREMIA

Hypernatremia is defined as serum sodium concentration of more than 150 mEq/L. It is characterized by seizures, doughy skin, dehydration; and carries high morbidity and mortality, especially during treatment.

Etiology

Hypernatremia usually occurs because of pure water depletion (diabetes insipidus), sodium excess (ORS administration), or water depletion exceeding sodium depletion (diarrhea). Important causes are listed below:

1. *Hypovolemic hypernatremia* Diarrhea, excessive perspiration, renal dysplasia, obstructive uropathy, osmotic diuresis.
2. *Normovolemic hypernatremia* Diabetes insipidus (central and nephrogenic).
3. *Hypervolemic hypernatremia* Sodium bicarbonate/NaCl administration, primary hyperaldosteronism.
4. *Drugs* Amphotericin, phenytoin, lithium, aminoglycosides, methoxyflurane.

Pathophysiology

As a result of increased extracellular sodium, plasma osmolarity increases, which results in shift of fluid from within the cells, resulting in cell desiccation. Extracellular volume remains normal at the expense of intracellular dehydration, which is responsible for the clinical manifestations of hypernatremia.

The central nervous system has special adaptive capabilities during hypernatremic episodes with water efflux from neurons during acute phases and increased intracellular concentration of electrolytes. Central nervous system problems occur, if the cellular shrinkage goes beyond a certain limit, causing thrombosis of small arteries and veins. It can also lead to rupture of blood vessels and intracranial bleed.

Chronic hypernatremia (>48 hours) Organic osmolytes start appearing inside the neurons. Some of them move inside the cells, while others are synthesized within the cell. These osmolytes were initially called idiogenic molecules and the primary function is to prevent cellular dehydration. Though the presence of organic osmolytes is considered to be protective, it causes significant problems during rehydration. Rapid rehydration results in cerebral edema by relative hypotonic fluids entering the cerebral neurons.

Clinical Manifestations

Children usually present with irritability, fever, high-pitched cry, lethargy, altered sensorium, seizures, oligoanuria, and increased muscle tone. Skin turgor is reduced and a doughy characteristic feel of the skin is present, when the severity of dehydration results in loss of 10% of body weight. Seizures can occur because of hypernatremia *per se*, however, it is more commonly seen during treatment of hypernatremia because of rapid decline in serum sodium.

Laboratory Evaluation

Serum sodium, serum osmolarity, urea, creatinine, and urinary sodium should be estimated in all cases of suspected hypernatremia:

- In euvolemic hypernatremia, urine sodium is variable.
- In hypervolemic hypernatremia, urine sodium is greater than 20 mEq/L and urine osmolarity less than 800 mOsmol/kg.
- In diabetes insipidus, urine osmolarity is usually less than 300 mOsmol/kg, which increases following desmopressin administration.

Computed tomography and MRI scan of the brain should be done to exclude intracranial tumors, granulomatous diseases (sarcoid, tuberculosis), histiocytosis, and other intracranial pathology. Ultrasound of the kidney is to be done to rule out renal diseases.

Other tests include serum aldosterone, cortisol, ADH, and ACTH to exclude associated endocrine disorders.

Treatment	Hypernatremia

The management of hypernatremia includes correction of underlying causes and the prevailing hypertonicity.

1. Correcting Hypernatremia

While correcting hypernatremia, do not reduce sodium level rapidly. The goal of correction is to decrease plasma sodium by approximately 0.5 mEq/L/h (12 mEq/L/24h). Rapid reduction of sodium level may cause cerebral edema.

- The recommended duration of correction is based on serum sodium level (145–157 mEq/L over 24 hours, 158–170 mEq/L over 48 hours, and more than 170 mEq/L over 72 hours). The rate of correction remains same at 0.5 mEq/L/h.

- The type of fluid used for correction is 5% half normal saline (N/2) and the amount of fluid is roughly 1.5 times of maintenance requirement. This is best achieved by giving deficit correction and maintenance fluids over 48–72 hours.
- Calcium may be added, depending on the serum calcium content.
- Once the child starts passing urine, potassium may be added to fluid in a dose of 20 mEq/L to facilitate water absorption into cells.
- If the serum sodium concentration is more than 180 mEq/L, peritoneal dialysis should be done using a high glucose and low sodium dialysate.

2. Replacement Fluid

The volume of replacement fluid needed to correct the water deficit is determined by the concentration of sodium in the replacement fluid. The replacement volume can be determined as follows:

$$\text{Replacement volume (L)} = \text{TBW deficit} \times (1/1 - x)$$
$$(x = \text{replacement fluid Na}/154).$$

If the child is hypotensive, correct hypotension with normal saline, Ringer lactate solution or 5% albumin, regardless of serum sodium concentration. Hyperglycemia may accompany hypernatremia. Insulin treatment is not recommended because it may increase brain idiogenic osmole content.

3. Other Modalities

- Peritoneal dialysis is indicated for renal failure, obstructive uropathy, or serum sodium level more than 180 mEq/L.
- Surgical intervention is recommended for children with renal dysplasia, medullary cystic disease, reflux nephropathy and polycystic disease.

Prognosis

Mental retardation, intracranial hemorrhage, intracerebral calcification, cerebral infarction, cerebral edema, hypocalcemia, and hyperglycemia may occur in children with hypernatremia. Children, who have recovered from hypernatremia and have recurrent history, will develop neurologic sequelae. The incidence of persistent neurologic abnormality is 11–15% consisting of intellectual deficits, seizure disorders, and spastic plegias. The overall mortality is about 10%.

Fang C, Mao J, Dai Y, *et al*. Fluid management of hypernatraemic dehydration to prevent cerebral oedema: a retrospective case control study of 97 children in China. *J Paediatr Child Health*. 2010;46:301–3.
Wakil A, Atkin SL. Serum sodium disorders: safe management. *Clin Med*. 2010;10:79–82.

4.8 HYPOKALEMIA

Hypokalemia is defined as a plasma potassium level less than 3.5 mEq/L. Clinically, it is characterized by hypotonia, muscle weakness, and cardiac arrhythmia. Most common causes are diarrhea and severe malnutrition. Prognosis is good, if treated in time.

Pathophysiology

Potassium is essential for transmission of nerve impulses, contraction of cardiac muscle, maintenance of intracellular tonicity, skeletal and smooth muscles and maintenance of normal renal function. Derangements of potassium regulation often lead to neuromuscular, gastrointestinal, and cardiac conduction abnormalities.

Acute depletion may result from diuretic therapy, primary or secondary hyperaldosteronism, diabetic ketoacidosis, severe diarrhea, vomiting, or inadequate replacement during prolonged parenteral nutrition.

Gradual potassium depletion occurs via renal excretion, through GI loss or because of low intake.

Etiology

1. *Gastrointestinal and skin losses* Vomiting, acute diarrhea, villous adenoma, excessive sweating, severe burns, nasogastric aspiration, laxative use.
2. *Decreased stores* Protein energy malnutrition.
3. *Shift from extracellular to intracellar compartment* Insulin, catecholamines therapy, alkalosis, periodic paralysis.
4. *Renal* RTA, Bartter syndrome, Gitelman syndrome, dialysis, diuretic therapy.
5. *Endocrinal* Diabetic ketoacidosis, hyperaldosteronism, Cushing syndrome, steroid therapy.
6. *Drugs* Theophylline, verapamil, high-dose penicillin, ampicillin, carbenicillin, aminoglycosides, amphotericin B and cisplatin.
7. *Miscellaneous* Hypothermia, cystic fibrosis, hypomagnesemia, acute myelogenous monomyeloblastic or lymphoblastic leukemia.

Clinical Features

Muscle weakness is characteristic and initially observed in limbs, followed by trunk and respiratory muscles. In infants, paralytic ileus and gastric dilatation are common. Life-threatening complications include acute respiratory failure from muscle paralysis and cardiac arrhythmias. Occasionally, tachycardia with irregular beats may be heard. Severe hypokalemia may manifest as bradycardia with cardiovascular collapse.

Investigations

The serum level reflects the severity of deficiency.
- Serum potassium <2 mEq/L indicates a massive loss of intracellular potassium.
- Urinary potassium less than 15 mEq/L indicates that extrarenal losses are unlikely.
- Children should also be evaluated for concurrent electrolyte abnormalities and arterial blood gases, which may affect treatment.
- ECG shows ST segment depression, T wave flattening, prolongation of QT interval and appearance of U waves (Fig. 4.5). Hyponatremia and alkalosis aggravate ECG abnormalities.
- Although ECG changes may be helpful, if present, their absence should not be taken as normal cardiac conduction. The ECG may be normal or may have only subtle findings prior to clinically significant dysrhythmias.

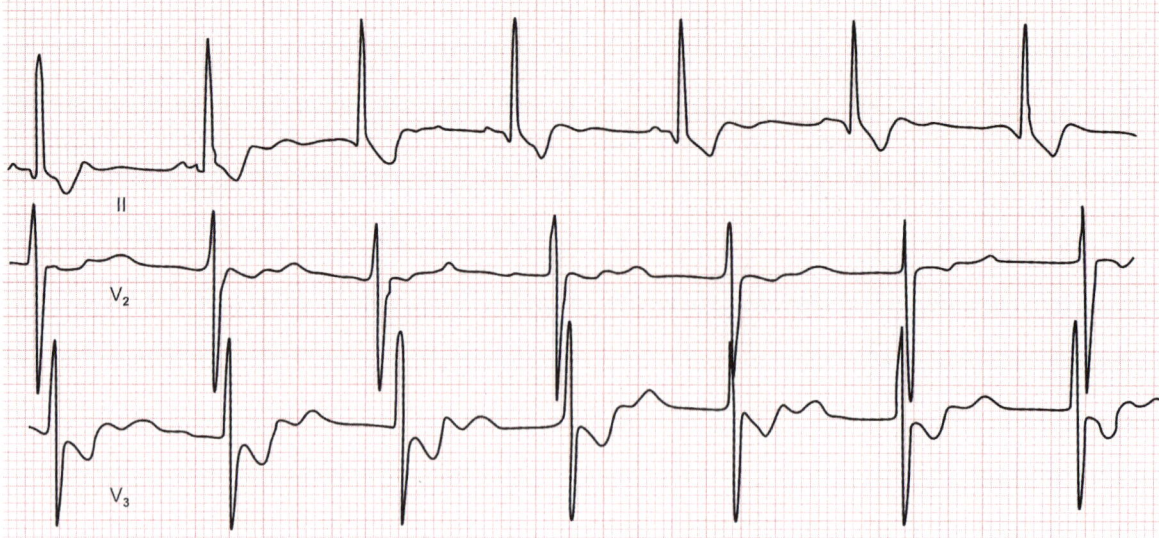

Fig. 4.5 ECG showing prominent U waves, suggesting hypokalemia

- Children should also be evaluated for Cushing syndrome, Conn syndrome, or adrenal hyperplasia, if clinical manifestations suggest the diagnosis.
- MRI of brain is indicated in children with suspected pituitary tumor as a cause of hypercortisolism.
- Abdominal ultrasound or CT should be done, if adrenal tumor or hyperplasia is suspected.

Treatment	Hypokalemia

Medical therapy is aimed at potassium supplementation and correction of underlying causes.

Transient, asymptomatic, or *mild hypokalemia* may resolve spontaneously or may be treated with enteral potassium supplements. Oral dose of potassium is 2–4 mEq/kg/day PO in divided doses to avoid gastric distress.

Symptomatic or *severe hypokalemia* should be corrected with intravenous potassium chloride (1 mL of 10% KCl contains 2 mEq of potassium). The usual dose of intravenous replacement is 0.3–0.5 mEq/kg/hour for non-critical hypokalemia. Infusion rates of 0.5 mEq/kg/h or more can be delivered in life-threatening hypokalemia, but require ECG monitoring to detect fatal ventricular arrhythmia. If a child is receiving concurrent intravenous fluids, potassium can be infused @ 40 mEq/L of fluid.

Prognosis

Mortality is rare except when hypokalemia is severe or occurs in a child with underlying heart disease requiring digoxin therapy, following cardiac surgery or when accompanied by arrhythmia. Short-term morbidity is common including ileus, cardiac dysrhythmia, and muscle weakness or cramping.

Kaplan LJ, Kellum JA. Fluids, pH, ions and electrolytes. *Curr Opin Crit Care*. 2010 ;16:323–31.

Rastegar A. Attending rounds: patientchild with hypokalemia and metabolic acidosis. *Clin J Am Soc Nephrol*. 2011;6:2516–21.

Unwin RJ, Luft FC, Shirley DG. Pathophysiology and management of hypokalemia: a clinical perspective. *Nat Rev Nephrol*. 2011;7:75–84.

4.9 HYPERKALEMIA

Hyperkalemia is defined as a serum potassium level of more than 5.5 mEq/L and characterized by tachycardia, muscular weakness, and arrhythmia. Most common etiology is impaired excretion of potassium due to renal insufficiency, that involve defects in mineralocorticoid, aldosterone, and insulin function. Sudden and rapid onset of hyperkalemia can be fatal.

Pathophysiology

Potassium is the principal intracellular cation in body and plays a key role in intracellular volume regulation. Total body potassium is approximately 53–55 mEq/kg body weight. Both animal and vegetable foods contain significant amounts of potassium and are consumed every day regardless of the type of diet. Despite the level of consumption, a balance between intake and excretion maintains plasma potassium levels within a narrow range (3.5–4.5 mEq/L). Less than 10% of potassium is excreted through sweat and stool, while kidneys excrete more than 90%.

Increased levels of aldosterone stimulate potassium secretion, while low levels inhibit potassium secretion by the cortical collecting duct. In addition, potassium levels are partly responsible for a negative feedback to the adrenal cortex, so that high levels of potassium decrease aldosterone production, while low levels increase the secretion of aldosterone.

Etiology

I. Inadequate excretion
- *Renal*: Acute or chronic renal failure, RTA type IV.
- *Adrenal failure*: Hypoaldosteronism, congenital adrenal hyperplasia (salt-losing variant), Addison disease, pseudohypoaldosteronism
- *Drugs*: Potassium sparing diuretic; acute digoxin toxicity

II. Shift of potassium from tissues
- *Metabolic acidosis*
- *Tissue injury*: Acute rhabdomyolysis, tumor lysis syndrome, burns, surgery, repeated blood transfusions
- *Drugs*: Succinylcholine, ACE inhibitors, beta blockers

Clinical Manifestations

The history of acute gastroenteritis, decreased urine output, adrenogenital syndrome, chemotherapy, crush injuries, and ingestion of potassium containing preparations should be taken in all children. Clinical findings depend on the degree of hyperkalemia and primarily related to its effects on the heart.

Children with serum potassium levels more than 8 mEq/L can present with circulatory failure and wide-complex tachycardia or ventricular fibrillation. Other symptoms include weakness of skeletal muscles that progresses to paralysis and respiratory failure. Children may complain of nausea, vomiting, and paresthesias.

Levels exceeding 8.5 mEq/L cause respiratory paralysis and cardiac arrest and are usually fatal. It causes abnormal heart and skeletal muscle function by lowering resting action potential and preventing repolarization and muscle paralysis.

Investigations

Serum urea, creatinine, uric acid, urinalysis, and urine electrolytes including potassium, and electrocardiogram (ECG) should be done in all children. The sequences of changes that occur in ECG in hyperkalemia are mentioned below and shown in Figs 4.6 and 4.7:

Serum $K^+ > 6.0$ mEq/L: T waves tall and tented
Serum K^+ 7.0–8.0 mEq/L: Prolonged PR interval, P wave may become smaller and amplification of R wave; QRS widens.
Serum $K^+ > 8.0$ mEq/L: The wide QRS merges with the T wave, thus forming a sinusoidal wave. P wave is absent.

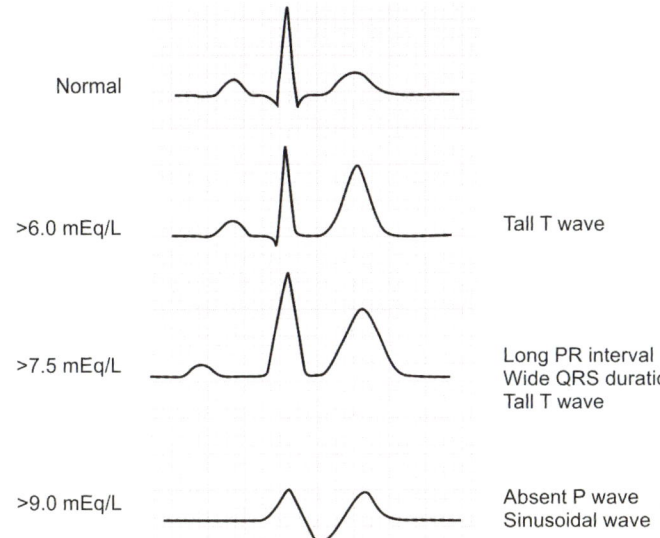

Fig. 4.6 ECG changes at various levels of serum potassium

Treatment	Hyperkalemia

The goals of management include (*i*) counteracting the deleterious electrophysiologic effects of hyperkalemia; (*ii*) shifting potassium intracellularly; (*iii*) removing excess potassium; and (*iv*) identify and, treat the cause. Various approaches to achieve these goals are tabulated in **Table 4.7**.

Mild to Moderate Hyperkalemia

- *Inhaled beta-adrenergic agents* (eg, salbutamol or terbutaline: 5–10 mg) are highly effective in lowering serum potassium for 4–6 hours. It induces the intracellular movement of potassium via the stimulation of the Na–K ATP pump. However, peak response is unclear; therefore, it is not recommended as the first line of therapy in severe hyperkalemia.
- *Insulin and glucose infusion* (0.25–0.5 g/kg, ie, 2–5 mL/kg of 10% dextrose with 0.3 U/g of regular insulin infusion over

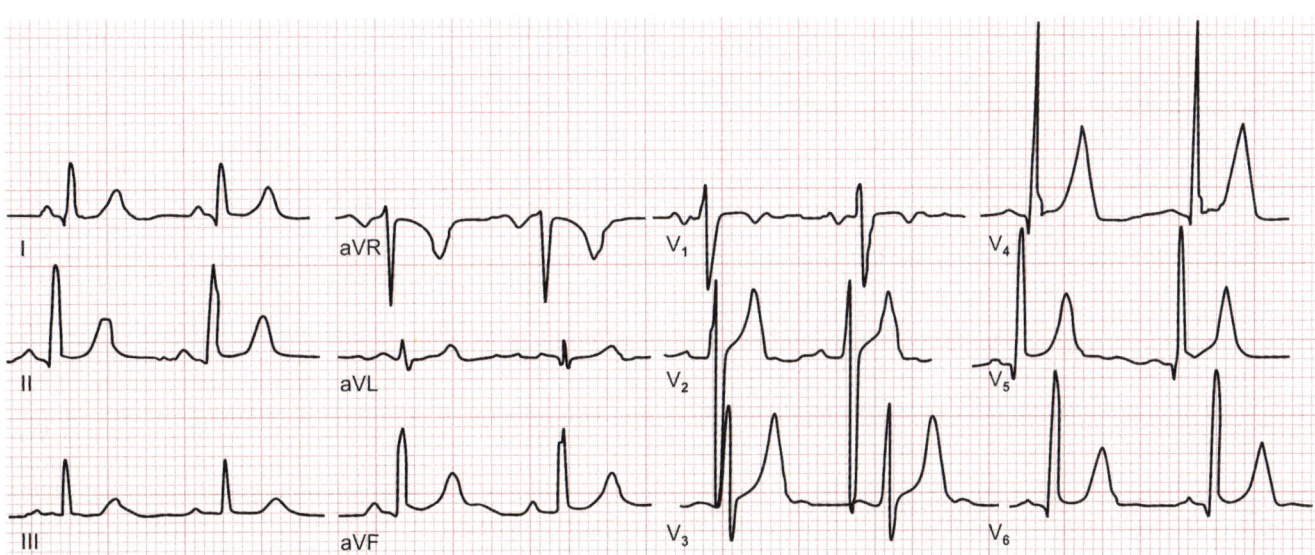

Fig. 4.7 Tall, slender T waves in leads I, II, aVF and V$_{2-6}$ in ECG

Table 4.7 Treatment of Hyperkalemia	
Goal	*Management modality*
Counteracting the dele-terious electrophysiologic effects of hyperkalemia	10% Calcium gluconate 1 mg/kg IV
Shifting potassium intracellularly	1. Beta-2 agonist nebulization 2. Insulin and glucose infusion (0.25–0.5 g/kg, ie 2–5 mL/kg of 90% dextrose with 0.3 U/g of regular insulin infusion 3. Sodium bicarbonate
Removing excess potassium	Sodium polystyrene sulfonate resin (1 g/kg orally or rectally), Peritoneal dialysis and hemodialysis
Identify and treat the cause	Surgical removal of bilateral ureteric stone, fulguration of posterior urethral valve, and surgery for PUJ obstruction

20–30 minutes) causes a transcellular shift of potassium into muscle cells, thereby temporarily lowering serum levels of potassium. Although the effect is almost immediate, it is temporary and, therefore, should be followed by therapy that actually enhances potassium clearance.

- *Sodium bicarbonate 7.5% IV* (1–2 mEq/kg over 10–30 minutes) is used as a buffer that breaks down to water and carbon dioxide after picking up free hydrogen ions, thus counteracts acidosis by raising blood pH. The role of bicarbonate therapy is questionable.

- *Sodium polystyrene sulfonate* is an exchange resin that can be used to treat mild-to-moderate hyperkalemia. Each mEq of potassium is exchanged for 1 mEq of sodium. It exchanges sodium for potassium and binds it primarily in the large intestine and decreases total body potassium. The onset of action after oral administration ranges from 2–12 hours and is longer when administered rectally.

Severe Hyperkalemia

Severe hyperkalemia requires immediate therapy consisting of IV 10% calcium gluconate (0.5–1.0 mL/kg over 1–3 minutes under cardiac monitoring) to stabilize the myocardium, rapid decrease of serum levels by alkalinization with sodium bicarbonate and a continuous IV infusion of dextrose and insulin.

Hemodialysis or peritoneal dialysis (PD) sometimes is necessary to treat severe symptomatic hyperkalemia, which is resistant to drug therapy. Rates of removal with PD are almost equal to the removal rate of Kayexalate. Continuous arteriovenous (CAVHD) or venovenous (CVVHD) hemofiltration with dialysis also has been used to remove potassium. Supportive care may include adequate intravascular volume expansion, if indicated.

Lehnhardt A, Kemper MJ. Pathogenesis, diagnosis and management of hyperkalemia. *Pediatr Nephrol*. 2011;26:377–84.

Weir MR, Rolfe M. Potassium homeostasis and renin-angiotensin-aldosterone system inhibitors. *Clin J Am Soc Nephrol*. 2010;5:531–48.

4.10 HYPOMAGNESEMIA

Magnesium (Mg) is the second most abundant intracellular cation. Almost all enzymatic processes require magnesium for activation. Approximately 60% of total body magnesium is present in bone, 38% in intracellular compartment, and only less than 2% in the extracellular fluid. Thus, serum levels of magnesium do not reflect the status of total body stores. Normal serum concentration ranges from 1.8–2.5 mEq/L (1 mEq = 12 mg elemental magnesium).

Etiology

Prolonged administration of magnesium-free parenteral fluids, prolonged nasogastric suction, infectious diarrhea, steatorrhea, inflammatory bowel disease, and gastro-intestinal neoplasms may cause hypomagnesemia. Several drugs can also cause increased urinary loss of magnesium particularly with furosemide. A congenital defect in tubular reabsorption of magnesium also has been described. Severe hypomagnesemia may occur during the recovery phase of diabetic ketoacidosis.

Clinical Manifestations

Hypomagnesemia may manifest clinically as CNS and neuromuscular hyperexcitability. Early manifestations may include painful muscle cramps, nausea, vomiting, and lethargy. At serum magnesium levels less than 1.0 mEq/L, children may have tremor, hyperactive deep-tendon reflexes, hyper-reactivity to sensory stimuli, muscular fibrillations, positive Chvostek and Trousseau signs, and carpopedal spasms progressing to tetany. Mental status changes may be present and include irritability, disorientation, depression, and psychosis. Reversible respiratory muscle failure may occur in severe hypomagnesemia.

Investigations

Laboratory analysis by atomic absorption spectro-photometry is the most specific technique available to measure total serum magnesium. Hypomagnesemia may be associated with nonspecific ECG changes such as ST segment depression, altered T waves, or loss of voltage. Severe magnesium deficiency may cause prolonged QT interval and ventricular arrhythmias.

Treatment	Hypomagnesemia

Treatment for hypomagnesemia depends on the degree of deficiency and the child's clinical symptoms and signs. Therapy can be oral for children with mild symptoms or IV for children with severe symptoms.

- If hypomagnesemia is mild (serum magnesium levels >1.2 mEq/L) and the child is asymptomatic, oral replacement is appropriate.
- In children with normal renal function, if serum magnesium levels are less than 1 mEq/kg, the therapeutic dose is approximately 4 mEq/kg of body weight. With renal impairment, reduce this dose by 50%.
- In emergent cases, ie, refractory ventricular tachycardia, 16 mEq (2 mL of a 10% solution) of magnesium sulfate may be

Dyselectrolytemia

1. Hyponatremia (serum sodium <130 mEq/L) can cause seizures and cerebral edema. It can occur in adrenal insufficiency, SIADH, and diarrhea. Symptomatic hyponatremia needs to be treated with 3% NaCl infusion.

2. Hypernatremia (serum sodium >150 mEq/L) can occur in diarrhea, diabetes insipidus, and inappropriate ORS administration. It can also present with seizures.

3. Hypernatremic dehydration needs correction slowly (over 72 hours).

4. Hypokalemia (serum potassium <3.5 mEq/L) may manifest as hypotonia, abdominal distension, and muscle weakness. Hypokalemia is a common finding in children with severe malnutrition.

5. Hyperkalemia (serum potassium >5.5 mEq/L) can be detected by ECG changes (prolonged PR internal, wide QRS, tall T waves).

6. Hypomagnesemia (serum magnesium below 1.5 mEq/L) usually accompanies hypocalcemia. Seizures are the most commonly presenting symptoms.

administered IV over 5–7 minutes then 1 mEq/kg on the first day, thereafter 0.5 mEq/kg daily during the next 3 days.

- Rapid IV administration can be life-threatening. Risks involved with IV magnesium therapy include hypermagnesemia, hypocalcemia, and hypotension.
- Continuously monitor electrolytes, deep tendon reflex, renal function, and hemodynamic parameters during replacement under high infusion rates.
- In overdose, calcium gluconate, 10–20 mL IV of 10% solution can be given as antidote for clinically significant hypermagnesemia, hypotension, hypocalcemia, and respiratory depression.

Alexander RT, Hoenderop JG, Bindels RJ. Molecular determinants of magnesium homeostasis: insights from human disease. *J Am Soc Nephrol*. 2008;19:1451–8.

Akhtar MI, Ullah H, Hamid M. Magnesium, a drug of diverse use. *J Pak Med Assoc*. 2011;61:1220–5.

Allan R, Mara N. Magnesium and the acute physician. *Acute Med*. 2012;11:3–7.

Garrison SR, Allan GM, Sekhon RK, et al. Magnesium for skeletal muscle cramps. *Cochrane Database Syst Rev*. 2012;9:CD009402.

Swaminathan K, Wilson J. Elusive cause of hypomagnesemia. *BMJ*. 2011;343 doi: 10.1136/bmj.d5087.

Rajniti Prasad, OP Mishra, and Utpal Kant Singh

Immunity and Immunization

5.1 THE IMMUNE SYSTEM

The chief function of the immune system is to prevent or limit infections by microorganisms and their products. It also plays an important role in autoimmune and malignant disorders. There are two types of immune responses, *viz.* innate and acquired; both of which have two major arms—cell-mediated immunity and antibody-mediated (humoral) immunity.

NATURAL IMMUNITY

Immunity may be either natural (innate) or acquired (adaptive). Natural immunity is offered regardless of the previous exposure to an antigen. It is nonspecific and includes host defenses such as barriers to infectious agents (such as skin and mucous membranes), cells (like natural killer cells), proteins (like the complement cascade and interferon), and other processes such as phagocytosis and inflammation **(Table 5.1)**. Natural immune response precedes acquired immune response in evolutions.

Natural immunity does not improve after exposure to the organism, in contrast to acquired immunity. In addition, natural immune processes have no memory, whereas acquired immunity is characterized by long-term memory. Phagocyte and complement are the two major components of natural immune response.

The acute-phase response, which consists of an increase in the levels of various plasma proteins, like C-reactive protein and mannose-binding protein, is also part of natural immunity. These proteins are synthesized by the liver and are nonspecific responses to microorganisms and other forms of tissue injury. The liver synthesizes these proteins in response to certain cytokines, namely, interleukin-1, interleukin-6, and tumor necrosis factor, produced by the macrophage after exposure to microorganisms. Some acute-phase proteins bind to the surface of bacteria and activate complement, which in turn kill the bacteria.

ACQUIRED IMMUNITY

Acquired or adaptive immunity occurs after exposure to an antigenic challenge, is specific and improves upon repeated exposure to the antigen. Adaptive immunity takes time to evolve and is pathogen specific. It is mediated by antibody and by T-lymphocytes, namely, helper T-cells and cytotoxic T-cells. The cells responsible for acquired immunity have long-term memory for a specific antigen. Acquired immunity can be active or passive. The relationships between the main components of natural and acquired immunity and the humoral and cell-mediated arms of the immune system are shown in **Table 5.2.**

Table 5.1 Natural Immunity	
Mechanism	*Factor*
To limit the entry of microorganism	1. Keratin layer of intact skin (mechanical barrier) 2. Fatty acids of the skin (inhibit growth of microorganisms) 3. Respiratory cilia (mucociliary clearance helps in clearing trapped organisms) 4. Normal flora of throat, colon, and vagina (inhibits colonization by pathogens) 5. Lysozyme in tears and other secretions (degrades peptidoglycan in bacterial cell wall) 6. Low pH of vagina and stomach (inhibits or kills certain pathogens) 7. Surface phagocytes, eg, alveolar macrophages

To limit the growth of microorganism in body	1. Cellular
	  • Phagocytes; eg, neutrophils, monocyte, macrophages (ingest and kill bacteria)
	  • Inflammatory mediator releasing cells (eosinophils, basophils, mast cells)
	  • Natural killer cells
	2. Molecular
	  • Complement
	  • Acute phase protein
	  • Cytokines

Table 5.2 Cell-Mediated versus Humoral Immunity

	Cell-mediated immunity	Humoral immunity
Natural immunity	Macrophages	Complement, neutrophils
Acquired immunity	Helper T-cells, cytotoxic T-cells	B-cells, plasma cells

ACTIVE AND PASSIVE IMMUNITY

Active immunity is resistance induced after contact with foreign antigens, such as microorganisms which can be acquired through clinical or subclinical infection and by immunization. In all these instances, the host actively produces an immune response consisting of antibodies and activated helper and cytotoxic T-lymphocytes. The biggest advantage of active immunity is that it is long lasting. But the disadvantage is that it has slow onset especially for the primary response **(Table 5.3)**, so may not be useful when immediate protection is needed.

Passive immunity is resistance offered by pre-formed antibodies in another host. It is conferred by maternal antibodies or immunoglobulin preparations and is short lasting. During pregnancy, IgG is transferred from mother to baby through placenta and baby receives IgA antibodies through breastmilk. In conditions like diphtheria and tetanus, to neutralize the toxins immediately, large amount of antitoxin can be made available by administration of antisera against diphtheria or tetanus. To limit the viral load from multiplication as in case of hepatitis B and rabies, pre-formed antibodies can be injected during the incubation period. In contrast to active immunity, the primary advantage is the ability to confer immediate protection, but would be short lasting.

Passive–active immunity involves giving both pre-formed antibodies to provide immediate protection and a vaccine to provide long-term protection. This approach is used selectively in the prevention of tetanus, hepatitis B, and rabies. The administered antibodies can neutralize immunogenic antigens of the vaccine and might yield sub-optimal response. To minimize the same, vaccine and the antibodies should be administered at different sites in the body.

Antigens

Antigen is any foreign particle or molecule that reacts with the antibodies, while *immunogen* is any foreign particle that triggers an immune response. Consequently, all immunogens are antigens, but not all antigens are immunogens. Although

Table 5.3 Characteristics of Active and Passive Immunity

Active immunity	Passive immunity
Mediated by antibodies and T-cells	Mediated by antibodies only
Lasts for very long duration (years)	Lasts for short duration only (months)
It has slow onset, so may not be useful for immediate protection	Protection is immediately available

terminologies of antigens and immunogens are frequently used interchangeably, there are certain important exceptions like *haptens*.

Haptens are low-molecular weight molecules that contain an antigenic determinant but which are not itself antigenic unless complexed with an immunogenic carrier. The term hapten is derived from the Greek *haptein* which means 'to fasten'. They lack the ability to bind to MHC proteins and to activate helper T-cell and also are not able to activate B-cells and, therefore, are not immunogenic. But haptens can react with specific antibodies. When haptens are bound to a "carrier" protein, they can stimulate primary or secondary response. The interaction of antigen and antibody is highly specific, and this characteristic is extensively used to identify microorganisms.

Different molecules would be able to generate varying immune responses. Following factors determine the immunogenicity of molecules.

- *Molecular size* Immunogen would be more potent, if has high molecular weight especially above 100,000. Molecules with molecular weight below 10,000 are weakly immunogenic, and very small ones such as amino acid, are non-immunogenic. Haptens are small molecules and become immunogenic only when linked to a carrier protein.
- *Chemical nature* Most naturally occurring antigens are proteins and polysaccharides. Lipids and nucleic acids are less antigenic. Their antigenicity can be enhanced by combining them with protein.
- *Structural complexity* A certain amount of chemical complexity or diversity is required for antigenicity. For example, amino acid homopolymers are less immunogenic than heteropolymers containing two or three different amino acids.
- *Foreignness* Only antigens which are recognized as 'foreign' or 'non-self' induce an immune response. The molecules recognized as "self" are not immunogenic.
- *Epitopes (antigenic determinants)* An epitope is the specific site on an antigen to which an antibody binds. For very small antigens, practically the entire chemical structure may act as a single epitope. Depending on its complexity and size, an antigen may affect production of antibodies directed at numerous epitopes. Polyclonal antibodies are mixtures of serum immunoglobulins and collectively are likely to bind to multiple epitopes on the antigen. Most antigens have *many determinants; means they are multivalent.*
- *Affinity, avidity* The antibody affinity refers to the tendency of an antibody to bind to a specific epitope at the surface of an antigen, it indicates the strength of the interaction. The avidity is the sum of the epitope-specific affinities for a given antigen and refers to cumulative strength of this affinity. It directly relates its function.
- *Genetic constitution* of the host (HLA genes) determines whether a molecule is immunogenic. Different strains of the same species of animal may respond differently to the same antigen.
- *Adjuvants* Adjuvant is a component of a vaccine that increases specific immune responses to an antigen. Adjuvants are particularly added for vaccines containing inactivated microorganisms or their products (eg, hepatitis B, diphtheria, and tetanus toxoids). They facilitate the activation of T-helper (CD-4) lymphocytes that helps to

5

induce an exaggerated immune response. More than one adjuvant may be present in a single vaccine. Despite rapid progress made in the field of developing new adjuvants to increase immunogenicity of existing and newer vaccines, only aluminum hydroxide and aluminum or calcium phosphates have been used routinely in human vaccines. A few recently approved novel adjuvants include emulsion-based and cytokines-containing substances.

- *Toll-like receptors (TLRs)* They are single membrane-spanning non-catalytic receptors that recognize structurally conserved molecules derived from microbes. Once microbes have breached physical barriers such as the skin or intestinal tract mucosa, they are recognized by TLRs which activate immune cell responses. They act as the principal sensors of infection in mammals.

Age and Immune Response

Humans are vulnerable to infections at extremes of the age. Neonates have less effective B-cell, T-cell, and neutrophil functions. Preterm infants may also have low concentrations of immunoglobulins. Both preterm and term infants have quantitative and qualitative defects of the complement system. In newborns, antibodies are provided primarily by the transfer of maternal IgG across the placenta which gradually decreases and little remains by 3–6 months of age, and the risk of infection in the child is high.

Early life immune responses are characterized by age-dependent limitations of the magnitude of responses to all vaccines. Antibody responses to most polysaccharide antigens are not elicited during the first 2 years of life, which is likely to reflect numerous factors including slow maturation of the spleen marginal zone, limited expression of CD21 on B-cells, and limited availability of the complement factors. Although this may be circumvented in part by the use of glycoconjugate vaccines, even the most potent glycoconjugate vaccines elicit markedly lower primary IgG responses in young infants. Although maternal antibodies interfere with the induction of infant antibody responses, they may allow a certain degree of priming, ie, of induction of memory B-cells.

Colostrum also contains antibodies, especially secretory IgA, which can protect the newborn against various respiratory and gastrointestinal infections. The fetus can mount an IgM response to certain (probably T-cell-independent) antigens.

5.2 IMMUNE RESPONSE

BASIS OF THE IMMUNE RESPONSE

The specific reactivity induced in a host by an antigenic stimulus is known as immune response. Blood cell precursors originate mainly in the fetal liver and yolk sac during embryonic period. During postnatal life, the stem cells reside in the bone marrow. Stem cells differentiate into cells of the erythroid, myeloid, or lymphoid series. Mainly lymphoid cells are capable of responding to immunologic stimuli and they evolve into two main lymphocyte populations: T-cells and B-cells. The ratio of T-cells to B-cells is approximately 3:1.

- T-cell precursors differentiate into immunocompetent T-cells within the thymus that are responsible for cell-mediated immunity.
- B-cell precursors do not pass through thymus; these differentiate into immune competent B-cells in the bone marrow. These are primarily responsible for humoral or antibody-mediated immunity.
- Prevention of infection may only be achieved by vaccine-induced antibodies, whereas disease attenuation and protection against complications may be supported by T-cells even in the absence of specific antibodies.

CELL-MEDIATED IMMUNITY

T-cells

T-cells are broadly classified as regulatory and effector cells based on their functions. T-cells are categorized into four types: helper T-cells, suppressor T-cells, cytotoxic T-cells, and memory cells based on their surface markers, targe-cells, and their functions. The regulatory functions are mediated primarily by helper (CD4-positive) T-cells, which produce interleukins while the effector functions are carried out primarily by cytotoxic (CD8-positive) T-cells. T-cells constitute 65–80% of the circulating pool of small lymphocytes. The lifespan of T-cells is long (months or years). In association with antigen receptors, all T-cells have CD3 proteins on their surface.

CD4 Lymphocytes

Helper or regulatory functions of CD4 lymphocytes are to help B-cells develop into antibody-producing plasma cells, to help CD8 T-cells to become activated cytotoxic T-cells and to help macrophages affect delayed hypersensitivity. Under the effect of cytokines, helper T-cells differentiate into Th-1 and Th-2 cells. Th-1 cells help the delayed hypersensitivity response by producing IL-2 and gamma interferon, whereas Th-2 cells perform the B-cell helper function by producing IL-4 and IL-5. Interleukin-12 (IL-12), produced by macrophages, keeps regulation on the balance between Th-1 and Th-2 cells. IL-12 increases the number of Th-1 cells, thereby enhancing host defenses against organisms that are controlled by a delayed hypersensitivity response (**Table 5.4**). Gamma interferon is another important regulator which inhibits the production of Th-2 cells. CD4 cells make up about 65% of peripheral T-cells and predominate in the thymic medulla, tonsils, and blood.

Table 5.4 Comparison of Th-1 Cells and Th-2 Cells	
Th-1 cells	*Th-2 cells*
Secrete IL-2, IL-3, IFN-gamma, TNF-alfa and beta	Secrete IL-4, IL-5, IL-6, IL-10, IL-13
Support activation and differentiation of B-cells	Support activation and differentiation of B-cells
Provide support to cytotoxic T-cells (CD8+ T-cells) and macrophages	Inhibitory influences on cytotoxic T-cells (CD8+ T-cells)
Helps elimination of intracellular pathogens (eg, viruses)	Helps elimination of extracellular pathogens (eg, helminths)

5

CD8 Lymphocytes

CD8 lymphocytes perform cytotoxic or effector functions. They can kill and lyse target cells carrying new or foreign antigen like virus-infected, allograft cells, and tumor. They kill by inducing apoptosis or by the release of perforins, which destroy cell membranes. CD8 cells predominate in human bone marrow and gut lymphoid tissue and constitute about 35% of peripheral T-cells.

Memory T-cells

After the initial exposure to a microbe or other foreign material, memory T (and B) cells provide host defense by ability to respond rapidly and vigorously for many years. This phenomenon of immunological memory is antigen specific.

Natural Killer Cells

They are important part of innate host defense. They kill virus-infected cells and tumor cells by secreting cytotoxins (perforins and granzymes) similar to those of cytotoxic T-lymphocytes. They are active without prior exposure to the virus, are not enhanced by exposure, and are not specific for any virus, and for the same reason they are called "natural" killer cells.

Cytokines

Cytokines are the molecules (glycopeptides) which are produced by appropriately stimulated lymphocytes (lymphokines) or monocytes (monokines) and mediate immune cell activity. There are many different types of cytokines, eg, interferons that make cells more resistant to subsequent viral infections. Cytokines include interleukins 1 to 10, interferons, tumor necrosis factors (TNFs), and colony-stimulating factors. The major source of IL-1 is macrophage which activates helper T-cells while IL-2 is produced by Th-1 subset of helper T-cells and has a role in activating helper and cytotoxic T-cells. Gamma interferon stimulates phagocytosis.

Others

Macrophages and polymorphonuclear cells are the other important components of the cell-mediated arm. Macrophages have three main functions: Phagocytosis, antigen presentation, and cytokine production (IL-1, TNF-α). As discussed earlier, polymorphonuclear cells play a major role by the process of phagocytosis.

HUMORAL IMMUNITY

Humoral immunity—also called as *antibody-mediated immunity*—is the principal defense mechanism against extracellular microbes and their toxins, against certain infections in which virulence is related to polysaccharide capsules (like pneumococci, meningococci, *Haemophilus influenzae*), and for certain viral infections. B-lymphocytes secrete antibodies that act by neutralization, complement activation, or by promoting opsonophagocytosis which results in early reduction of pathogen load and clearance of extracellular pathogens.

B-cells

B-cells constitute about 30% of the circulating pool of small lymphocytes, and their lifespan is short; ie, days or weeks. Unlike T-cells, they do not require thymus for maturation.

They differentiate into plasma cells and produce antibodies and they act as antigen-presenting cells (APCs).

Immunoglobulins

There are five different types of immunoglobulins: IgG, IgM, IgA, IgD, and IgE. IgG forms the major component (75%) of immunoglobulins and is the only immunoglobulin which can be transferred transplacentally. The properties of immunoglobulins are shown in **Table 5.5.**

Table 5.5 Important Functions of Immunoglobulins	
Immunoglobulin	*Major functions/properties*
IgM	Has a marked antibacterial activity. Does not cross the placenta. Produced in the primary response to an antigen. Fixes complement.
IgA	Secretory IgA found in mucous membranes and secretions and prevents attachment of bacteria and viruses to mucous membranes. Does not fix complement.
IgG	Predominant antibody in the secondary response. Makes phagocytosis of bacteria easier by opsonization. Enhances bacterial killing by fixing complement. Crosses the placenta and provides passive immunity to newborn. Neutralizes bacterial toxins and viruses.
IgD	Found on the surface of many B-cells as well as in serum, but the function is uncertain.
IgE	Upon exposure to allergen mediates immediate (anaphylactic) hypersensitivity by causing release of mediators from mast cells and basophils. Participates in the host defense against helminth infections.

Basis of Humoral Immune Response

The antibody response to an initial antigenic stimulus differs qualitatively and quantitatively from the response to subsequent stimuli with the same antigen. The former is called as *primary immune response* while the later the *secondary immune response*.

Primary Response

When host is exposed to the antigen for the first time, there is a considerable lag period in eliciting antibodies in the plasma. The lag period is typically 7–10 days but can be longer depending on the nature and dose of the antigen and the route of administration. The primary response is slow, sluggish, and short-lived and the titers of antibodies are low that do not persist for long. A small clone of B-cells and plasma cells specific for the antigen is formed. The first antibodies to appear are IgM followed by IgG or IgA. The serum antibody concentration continues to rise for several weeks, then declines and may drop to very low levels. IgM levels decline earlier than IgG levels.

5

Secondary Response

When the host gets exposed to the antigen to which he already had been exposed previously, there is a prompt, powerful and prolonged antibody response. The lag period is only 3–5 days, antibody levels are higher than the primary response (Fig. 5.1). After the first contact, antigen-specific "memory cells" persist which proliferate to form a large clone of specific B-cells and plasma cells, which mediate the secondary antibody response. During the secondary response, the amount of IgM produced is similar but much larger amount of IgG antibody is produced and the level also persists much longer than in the primary response.

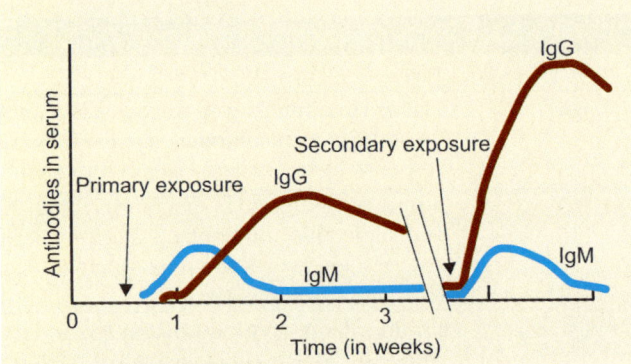

Fig. 5.1 Primary and secondary immune response

COMPLEMENT SYSTEM

The 'complement' refers to a system of factors that are present in normal serum. They are activated by antigen–antibody interaction and mediate a number of biologically significant consequences. Complement proteins are synthesized mainly by the liver. Complements are heat-labile; ie, they are inactivated by heating serum at 56°C for 30 minutes.

Main effects of complements are: (1) they cause lysis of cells such as bacteria, allografts and tumor cells; (2) cause opsonization, ie, enhancement of phagocytosis; and (3) generate mediators that participate in inflammation and attract neutrophils.

Activation

There are two pathways: the classic pathway and the alternative pathway by which the sequential activation of complement components occurs. While we are infected with the microorganism for the first time, the alternative pathway is more important as the antibody required to trigger the classical pathway is not present. Both pathways lead to the production of C3b, the central molecule of the complement cascade. C3b combines with other complement components to generate C5 convertase. This enzyme leads to the production of the membrane attack complex, and it opsonizes bacteria as phagocytes have receptors for C3b on their surface. Classic pathway is activated by antigen-antibody complexes while the alternative pathway is activated by many unrelated cell surface substances, eg, bacterial lipopolysaccharides (endotoxin), fungal cell walls, and viral envelopes.

Biologic Effects of Complement

Complement mediates immunological membrane damage (cytolysis), amplifies the inflammatory response, and participates in the pathogenesis of certain hypersensitivity reactions. It also exhibits antiviral property and promotes phagocytosis. It also interacts with coagulation, fibrinolytic and kininogenic systems of the blood.

- *Opsonization* In the presence of C3b, viruses, antigen–antibody complexes and cells are phagocytized in much better way. This is because many phagocytes have C3b receptors on their surface.
- *Cytolysis* Insertion of the membrane attack complex of complement (C5b6789) into the cell membrane leads to killing or lysis of many types of cells.
- *Enhancement of antibody production* Antibody production is greatly enhanced by binding of C3b to its receptors on the surface of activated B-cells compared to activation of B-cells by antigen alone. Patients with deficiency of C3b have significantly less antibody production compared to normal individuals.
- *Immune adherence* Complement bound to antigen-antibody complexes adheres to erythrocytes or to nonprimate platelets. This reaction is called as immune adherence, which contributes defense against pathogenic microorganisms since such adherent particles are rapidly phagocytized.
- *Chemotaxis* Certain complements like C5a and the C5,6,7 complex cause chemotaxis and attract neutrophils.
- *Anaphylatoxin* C3a, C4a, and C5a cause release of mediators like histamine by causing degranulation of mast cells.

AUTOIMMUNITY

Our immune system is able to discriminate between self and foreign antigens. It does not react against antigens of self's tissues. Self-tissues may also be damaged, if the immune regulatory mechanisms fail. Number of foreign proteins derived from various microbes or drugs can induce autoimmunity. Evidence also suggests the possible role of genetic factors in autoimmunity.

IMMUNOLOGICAL TOLERANCE

Immunological tolerance or non-reactivity to antigens means there is absence of potential immune response following exposure to antigen. This can be induced by immuno-suppressive drugs, irradiation, or by administration of anti-lymphocyte serum. The mechanisms that break immuno-logical tolerance may be important in the pathogenesis of autoimmune disease.

5.3 VACCINATION AND IMMUNIZATION

VACCINATION

The terms vaccine and vaccination are derived from *vacca*, the Latin term for cow. Vaccine was the term used by Edward Jenner to describe material used (ie, cowpox virus) to produce immunity to smallpox. The term vaccination was used by Louis Pasteur in the 19th century to include the physical act of administering any vaccine or toxoid. The classical definition of vaccine is given below. It is followed by a definition of various other products in use today for inducing or enhancing immunity.

Immunobiologicals

Antigenic substances (eg, vaccines and toxoids) or antibody-containing preparations (eg, globulins and antitoxins) from human or animal donors. These products are used for active or passive immunization or therapy and include vaccines, toxoids, immunoglobulins, antitoxins and monoclonal antibodies.

Vaccine

A suspension of live (usually attenuated) or inactivated microorganisms (eg, bacteria or viruses) or fractions thereof administered to induce immunity and prevent infectious disease or its sequels. Some vaccines contain highly defined antigens (eg, the polysaccharide of *Haemophilus influenzae* type b or the surface antigen of hepatitis B); others have antigens that are complex or incompletely defined (eg, *Bordetella pertussis* antigens or live-attenuated viruses).

Toxoid is a modified bacterial toxin that has been rendered nontoxic, but retains the ability to stimulate the formation of antibodies to the toxin.

Immune Globulin

A sterile solution containing antibodies, usually obtained from human blood. It is obtained by cold ethanol fractionation of large pools of blood plasma and contains 15–18% protein. Intended for intramuscular administration, immune globulin is primarily indicated for routine maintenance of immunity among certain immunodeficient persons and for passive protection against measles and hepatitis A.

Hyperimmune Globulin (Specific)

Special preparations obtained from blood plasma from donor pools preselected for high antibody content against a specific antigen (eg, hepatitis B immune globulin, varicella-zoster immune globulin, rabies immune globulin, tetanus immune globulin, vaccinia immune globulin, cytomegalovirus immune globulin, botulism immune globulin).

Others

Monoclonal antibody An antibody product prepared from a single lymphocyte clone, which contains only antibody against a single antigen.

Antitoxin A solution of antibodies against a toxin. Antitoxin can be derived from either human (eg, tetanus immune globulin) or animal (usually equine) sources (eg, diphtheria and botulism antitoxin). Antitoxins are used to confer passive immunity and for treatment.

IMMUNIZATION

It denotes the process of inducing or providing immunity by administering an immunobiological. Immunization can be *active* or *passive*.

- *Active immunization* is the production of antibody or other immune responses through administration of a vaccine or toxoid.
- *Passive immunization* implies acquisition of temporary immunity by the administration of preformed antibodies.

Vaccination and immunization are not synonymous because the administration of an immunobiological cannot be equated automatically with development of adequate immunity.

Seroconversion Change from antibody negative state to antibody positive state, in serum.

Seroprotection A state of protection from disease due to the presence of a certain detectable level of antibodies in serum.

Immunogenicity A vaccine is said to be immunogenic, if it is able to evoke an immune response in the body. This response could be cellular, humoral, or both. Most importantly, immunogenicity does not necessarily imply protection from the disease.

Active Immunization

Active immunization involves the administration of all or a part of a microorganism or a modified product of that microorganism to evoke an immunologic response to protect that individual from that disease. There are two basic types of vaccines—live-attenuated and inactivated (killed). The characteristics of live-attenuated vaccines are different from those of killed vaccines and these characteristics ultimately determine that how the vaccine is to be used. Different types of vaccines are shown in **Table 5.6**.

Live-Attenuated Vaccines

Live-attenuated vaccines are produced by modifying a disease producing (wild) bacteria or virus in a laboratory by repeated culturing. The examples of live-attenuated vaccines are measles, mumps, rubella, varicella, oral polio vaccine, rotavirus vaccine, BCG vaccine. The live-attenuated vaccines have the following characteristics:
- The vaccine virus or bacteria must grow (replicate) in the vaccinated child to produce an immune response.
- The immune response produced is similar to that produced by a natural infection.

Table 5.6 Types of Vaccines	
Types of antigen	*Vaccine*
Live-attenuated bacterial	BCG, Oral typhoid
Live-attenuated viral	OPV, measles, MMR, varicella, yellow fever
Killed, bacterial	Pertussis, whole cell typhoid
Inactivated viral	Inactivated polio, hepatitis A, rabies
Toxoid	DT, TT, Td
Capsular polysaccharide	Hib, pneumococcal, meningococcal, typhoid Vi
Viral subunit (recombinant)	Hepatitis B
Bacterial subunit	Acellular pertussis

- Though live-attenuated vaccines replicate in the host, they usually do not cause the disease as such that can occur with the wild form of the organism.
- These vaccines are extremely sensitive to heat and light and hence must be handled and stored carefully. These are also sensitive to circulating maternal antibodies.
- Although active infection (with active viral replication) ensues after vaccine administration, usually little or no adverse reaction occurs. Very rarely, live-attenuated vaccine virus could revert to its original virulent disease producing form.
- Live vaccines are contraindicated in children with significant immune suppression.

Inactivated/Killed Vaccines

Inactivated vaccines are produced by growing the bacteria or virus in culture media and then inactivating it with either heat and/or chemicals (usually formalin). The vaccines for some viruses and most bacteria are inactivated (killed) or are subunit (purified components) preparations or are conjugated chemically to immune biologically active proteins (eg, tetanus toxoid). Inactivated vaccines have the following characteristics:

- Inactivated vaccines cannot cause an infection but they still stimulate a protective immune response.
- These vaccines are less affected by circulating antibody than the live vaccines.
- As the organisms in the inactivated (killed) vaccines cannot replicate (grow), these vaccines require multiple doses.
- The antibody titers tend to diminish with time and as a result some inactivated vaccines require periodic supplemental doses to boost the antibody titers.

Currently available inactivated vaccines are either whole cell vaccines such as inactivated polio vaccine (IPV), pertussis, hepatitis A, whole cell typhoid or subunit vaccines (hepatitis B, acellular pertussis) or toxoids (diphtheria and tetanus) or polysaccharide antigen vaccine.

Passive Immunization

Passive immunization is accomplished with the administration of preformed antibodies contained in the immunoglobulins.

Immunoglobulins

Immunoglobulins are derived from the pooled plasma of the adults by an alcohol fractionation procedure and are the agents used for passive immunization of the person. The immunoglobulins consist primarily of immunoglobulin (IgG) with trace amount of IgA and IgM and are not known to transmit HIV, hepatotropic or other infectious disease agent. Large number of donors are used to ensure inclusion of a broad-spectrum of antibodies.

Immunoglobulin (IG) and specific hyperimmune IG are recommended for intramuscular administration. A few of the indications for the use of immunoglobulin for passive prophylaxis are as follows:

- Replacement therapy in congenital or acquired immune deficiency disorders.
- Prevention of complications of the disease in a high-risk child, such as those of leukemia, who can develop potentially life-threatening complications when exposed to diseases such as measles or varicella.
- When the time does not permit the adequate protection by active immunization alone in post-exposure situations involving rabies, hepatitis B, tetanus, and measles.

Antibodies of animal origin (animal antisera) are now used decreasingly as they pose risk of reactions to the recipient. The use of such products should be limited strictly to certain indications for which specific IG preparations of human origin are not available (such as diphtheria and botulism).

Immune Response to Vaccination

Primary Response

Primary responses are those observed after the first injection of a vaccine, as opposed to secondary responses, which are observed when injections are repeated. In brief, after the first injection of the vaccine, there are three distinct periods:

- *Latency period* It occurs between the injection of the vaccine and the appearance of the serum antibodies. This period varies, ranging from 24 hours to 2 weeks depending on the development of the individual's immune system as well as on the nature, the form and the dose of the antigen used.
- *Growth period* As soon as the latency period is over, the antibody level increases exponentially, reaching its maximum within a lapse of time varying from 4 days to 4 weeks. This period is approximately 3 weeks for tetanus or diphtheria toxoids, and 2 weeks for microbial vaccines. The production of IgM antibodies usually precedes that of IgG. The antibody level may remain at a high, plateau level for several days, and then they decrease.
- *Period of decline* After reaching the maximum concentration, the antibody level declines, rapidly at first, then slowly. The period of decline varies in length—it depends both on the rate of synthesis and breakdown of the antibodies, and on their quality and quantity. IgA and IgM decline more rapidly than IgG.

Secondary Response

Reintroduction of the same antigen after a suitable period of time triggers a response of the secondary type characterized both by the rapid appearance of specific antibodies and by the large number of antibodies secreted; these are mostly IgG from the outset. The peak antibody level is reached in a few days. The growth phase remains exponential; but its development is more rapid, whereas the period of decline is longer. Furthermore, a temporary decrease in the antibody level is observed, followed by a further rise, if the second injection is given before the antibodies induced by the first injection have disappeared. This means that a second antigenic stimulation occurring very shortly after the first one may be ineffective due to the elimination of the antigen by the serum antibodies, which are still highly concentrated. The secondary antibodies persist for a longer period of time, and sometimes indefinitely.

The importance of the secondary response is due to the presence of a population of lymphocytes endowed with a "memory", which are stimulated by the immunogenic molecule and are differentiated into antibody-secreting cells. Both T- and B-cells have an immunological memory. The intensity of the secondary response is greatest during subsequent stimulation, when the doses of antigen are increased. Immunological memory persists for a long time in man, even when the serum concentration of antibodies has dropped below the detectable threshold. It depends on the quality and quantity of the antigen inoculated, and, as already noted, on the periodicity of the stimulation.

Maternal Antibodies and Immune Response

The immune globulins present in the blood at birth are transplacentally transferred IgG of maternal origin, mostly composed of antiviral and antibacterial antibodies, which play a major protective role during the first months of life. These antibodies disappear in some infants as early as at 5 months, whereas in others, a low level may persist until the age of 9 months or more. The age at which immunization is planned must, therefore, take into account the disappearance of passive antibodies of maternal origin, especially in the case of the live-attenuated vaccines (measles, rubella or mumps). Presence of maternal antibodies interferes with the infant's own immune production of antibodies in response to an antigenic challenge.

Herd Immunity and Herd Effect

Herd immunity is the proportion of immune individuals in a population. Individuals may acquire immunity following a disease or immunization against that disease. For example, all those who have had chickenpox plus those who have acquired immunity because of varicella immunization shall constitute the immune individuals in a given population.

Herd effect is the protection offered to unvaccinated members when good proportion (usually more than 85%) of the population is vaccinated. Herd effect is due to reduced carriage of the causative microorganism by the vaccinated cohort and thus is seen only with vaccines against those diseases where humans are the only source (there is no herd effect for tetanus). An effective vaccine is a prerequisite for good herd effect.

Vaccine Immunogenicity, Efficacy, and Effectiveness

Vaccine immunogenicity is the ability of a vaccine to induce antibodies which may or may not be protective. The protective threshold for most vaccines is defined.

Vaccine efficacy is the ability of the vaccine to protect an individual under experimental conditions. It can be assessed through clinical trials, cohort studies or case control studies. It is calculated as:

$$VE = \frac{\text{Disease in unvaccinated} - \text{disease in vaccinated}}{\text{Disease in unvaccinated}}$$

Vaccine effectiveness is the ability of the vaccine to protect the community under programmatic conditions. Vaccine effectiveness is a combination of vaccine efficacy, coverage, and herd effect.

Adverse Event Following Immunization (AEFI)

AEFI is defined as an untoward event that occurs after a vaccination that might be caused by the vaccine product or vaccination process. It includes events that are:

1. *Vaccine-induced* These are caused by the intrinsic characteristic of the vaccine preparation and the individual response of the vaccine: These events would not have occurred without vaccination (eg, BCG adenitis, DPT-induced encephalopathy, vaccine-associated paralytic poliomyelitis);
2. *Vaccine-potentiated* The events would have occurred anyway, but were precipitated by the vaccination (eg, first febrile seizure in a predisposed child);
3. *Programmatic error* The event was caused by technical errors in vaccine preparation, handling, or administration (eg, toxic shock syndrome due to staphylococcal contamination of measles vaccine); or
4. *Coincidental* The event was associated temporally with vaccination by chance or caused by underlying illness. Special studies are needed to determine, if an adverse event is a reaction to the vaccine or the result of another cause.

A history of any past allergic reactions must be enquired in a potential vaccine recipient and any child with a history of severe allergic reaction to any constituent of the vaccine should not be given that vaccine. As the occurrence of anaphylaxis cannot be predicted, the vaccinee should be observed for 15 minutes after vaccine administration and resuscitation equipment and essential drugs should be kept ready.

EPI VACCINES

5.4 BCG VACCINE

Since its development in 1921, Bacillus Calmette–Guérin (BCG) vaccine has remained the sole weapon in the immunological armamentarium against tuberculosis. BCG vaccine is named after a French bacteriologist Leon Charles Albert Calmette and a veterinarian Camille Guerin who are credited with development of BCG strain. BCG is a live-attenuated vaccine. The BCG parent strain developed by Calmette and Guerin from the Pasteur Institute in Lille was obtained from a primary strain of *Mycobacterium bovis*. In India, the BCG was produced from Danish 1331 strain at Guindy (Tamil Nadu). Other strains prevalent worldwide are Glaxo, Tokyo, and Pasteur strains. These strains differ in their morphological and biochemical characteristics as well as immunogenic and reactogenic potential.

Characteristics

BCG vaccine is a live-attenuated vaccine and contains 0.1 to 0.4 million bacilli per dose. BCG vaccine is supplied as lyophilized (freeze-dried) powder in multi-dose, vacuum-sealed, dark-colored ampoules as the vaccine is light and heat sensitive and deteriorates rapidly on exposure to ultraviolet rays. The ampoule needs to be opened carefully by gradually filing at the junction of the neck and the body of the ampoule so the air does not rush in causing the spillage. Normal saline is supplied as the diluent for the vaccine and the reconstituted vaccine must be used within 4 hours of its reconstitution. Freeze-dried vaccine can be stored at 2–8°C for up to 1 year.

Protective Efficacy

BCG vaccine is currently being used in over 100 countries with the objective of preventing disseminated and other life-threatening manifestations of *M. tuberculosis* infection in infants and young children. However, BCG immunization does not prevent infection with *M. tuberculosis*. The various BCG vaccines used throughout the world differ in composition and efficacy. Other factors affecting the vaccine efficacy are endemicity of the disease, heavy bacillary load during primary infection, nutritional status, constant contact with open TB case and concomitant HIV disease. Earlier reports on efficacy of BCG vaccines reported wide variability with studies reporting 0 to 80 % protection. However, recent analysis of the efficacy of BCG vaccines report that BCG vaccine has relatively high protective efficacy (approximately 80%) against meningeal and miliary tuberculosis in children but no protection against primary infection. A meta-analysis of various studies of BCG efficacy concluded that BCG vaccine significantly reduced the risk of active tuberculosis cases and deaths. The protective efficacy against pulmonary tuberculosis differs significantly depending on the factors discussed above and averages around 50%.

Administration

The vaccine provides cell-mediated immunity which is adequate in newborns and it is recommended to give BCG at birth or soon thereafter and for any unimmunized individual recommended till 5 years of age. For all ages, the recommended dose is 0.1 mL. The vaccine is given intra-dermally on left deltoid region just above its insertion for the sake of convenience and uniformity using tuberculin syringe and a 26G needle. Local antiseptics are not necessary before vaccinating. This vaccination with BCG is followed by a development of scar at injection site within 8–12 weeks.

Phenomena Seen after Vaccination

Day 0: Wheal of 5–8 mm develops at the site of injection, which subsides in 20–30 min.

2–3 weeks: Papule develops.

3–6 weeks: Papule increases in size up to 4–8 mm.

6–12 weeks: Papule breaks into a shallow ulcer, healing occurs spontaneously leaving behind a permanent, tiny 4–8 mm, round papery thin scar.

If no local reaction is seen in the local site at the end of 12 weeks, the vaccine should be repeated. Routine tuberculin test is not necessary prior to administration of the second dose.

Adverse Effects

The adverse reactions and the complications of BCG vaccine are rare. Local ulceration and regional lymphadenitis are major but occasional complications of the vaccine. These events usually resolve spontaneously and medical treatment does not seem to reduce the frequency of suppuration in BCG adenitis. Osteitis and disseminated BCG disease are extremely infrequent in immunocompetent patients. BCG should not be given to child with immunosuppression and symptomatic HIV infection.

Other Uses

Apart from tuberculosis, BCG vaccine offers some protection against leprosy. BCG has also been used as an immune modulating agent in diseases like nephrotic syndrome and urinary bladder cancer.

5.5 VACCINES FOR DIPHTHERIA, PERTUSSIS, AND TETANUS

Diphtheria and tetanus are potentially fatal childhood diseases, which used to cause tremendous childhood mortality in the pre-vaccination era while pertussis causes prolonged respiratory morbidity in children. Widespread immunization with DPT vaccine has resulted in decline in incidence of these diseases.

Composition

Vaccines against these diseases are available as *monovalent* (TT; tetanus only), *bivalent* (DT-pediatric, dT-adult; diphtheria and tetanus) and *trivalent* (DPT; diphtheria, pertussis and tetanus) preparations. The trivalent vaccine is available in two forms; DTwP containing the *whole* cell pertussis vaccine and DTaP containing the *acellular* pertussis vaccine. Each dose of DPT vaccine contains diphtheria toxoid 25 Lf, tetanus toxoid as 5–25 Lf and pertussis as >4 IU of formalin inactivated *Bordetella pertussis* cells. DTaP (acellular pertussis) vaccine contains 4 purified inactivated pertussis antigens (pertussis toxin, filamentous hemagglutinin, fimbrial agglutinogen, and pertactin).

Immunity to diphtheria is conferred by antibodies produced against the exotoxin of *Corynebacterium diphtheriae*; antitoxin levels of 0.1 IU/mL are essential to provide clinical immunity. Diphtheria vaccines contain modified bacterial toxin (toxoid), adsorbed with aluminum hydroxide which acts as adjuvant and improves the immunogenicity of the vaccine.

Schedule of Administration

DPT vaccine is indicated for universal and routine immunization in infants. Three primary doses are to be given at 6, 10, 14 weeks of age, separated by a minimum interval of four weeks. For the child whose immunization schedule is resumed after deferral or interruption of the recommended schedule, the next dose in the sequence should be given, regardless of the interval since the last dose—that is, the schedule is not reinitiated. The first booster is recommended at 16–24 months and second booster at 4½ –5 years of age. DwPT or DaPT can be used only up to 7 years, thereafter dT should be used. These vaccines are available in ready to use form and dose is 0.5 mL given intramuscular in anterolateral thigh. These vaccines are stored at 2–8°C and should never be frozen. If frozen accidentally, the vaccine should be discarded.

The primary doses of DPT are given as pentavalent vaccine (combination of DPT + Hib + HBV) at 6, 10, 14 weeks, under UIP.

Efficacy

The vaccine efficacy after completing three doses of primary immunization is 80%, 70–80% and 100% for diphtheria, pertussis and tetanus, respectively. The whole cell vaccine (DTwP) and the currently available acellular vaccine (DTaP) have similar efficacy against clinical or culture confirmed pertussis. The protection offered against all the disease components decreases over a period requiring booster dosages.

Adverse Reactions

The adverse reactions observed after DPT can either be *mild* or *severe*. Mild reactions to DPT vaccines most commonly include redness, edema, induration, tenderness and sterile abscess at injection site. Drowsiness, fretfulness, vomiting, crying, and slight to moderate fever are also seen. These manifestations occur within several hours of the injection and subside spontaneously. Local and febrile adverse reactions are less common and less severe with acellular than with whole cell pertussis vaccine.

Contraindication

The contraindications and the precautions to further DPT vaccination are shown in **Table 5.7**. These events, previously considered as contraindications, are to be taken as precautions and decision for further vaccination to be taken as per the risk benefit ratio. Incidence of encephalopathy is 0–10 cases per million and shock like state is 1 in 30,000 cases. The absolute contraindications to pertussis-containing vaccine (DTaP or DTwP) are (*i*) immediate anaphylactic reaction; and (*ii*) progressive encephalopathy within 7 days of vaccination. In anaphylaxis, further immunization with any DPT vaccine is contraindicated. For those with encephalopathy, all pertussis vaccines are contraindicated. Instead, DT may be used. A child who has recovered from diphtheria or tetanus must be actively immunized because amount of toxin responsible for these diseases in humans does not elicit protective immunity.

Table 5.7 Contraindications and Precautions to Further DPT Vaccination

Contraindications
- An immediate anaphylactic reaction
- Encephalopathy occurring within 7 days following DPT

Precautions
- Temperature of >40.5° C within 48 hours not due to other identifiable cause
- Collapse/shock-like state (hypotonic-hyporesponsive episode within 48 hours)
- Persistent, inconsolable crying lasting >3 hours occurring within 48 hours
- Convulsions with/without fever occurring within 3 days

TETANUS TOXOID (TT) VACCINE

Despite the availability of effective vaccine since 1923, tetanus remains a major health problem in developing world causing significant morbidity and mortality. Tetanus toxoid vaccine is prepared by chemically inactivating tetanus toxin called "toxoid", which evokes immune response but do not cause disease. It is available as monovalent vaccine as tetanus toxoid or a combination vaccine as DPT. Two types of tetanus

toxoid are available, which are adsorbed toxoid (aluminum salt precipitated) and fluid toxoid. Adsorbed toxoid has higher rate of seroconversion and provides more persistent level of antibodies.

Under national immunization policy, tetanus immunization is recommended as combination with DPT vaccine at 6, 10, 14 weeks of age and with boosters doses at 18 months and 5 years. Further doses of TT (tetanus toxoid) are recommended at 10 and 16 years of age (preferably Td) and then every 10 years (ideally Td). Two doses of TT are recommended during early pregnancy 1 month apart and the second dose at least 2 weeks before delivery. Single dose will suffice for subsequent pregnancies, if these happen to be within the next 5 years. For primarily unimmunized school age and above children, 2 primary doses 1 month apart will suffice.

Tetanus toxoid is given 0.5 mL intramuscularly and is stored at 2–8°C and not to be frozen. Adverse reactions associated with this vaccine are pain, swelling at local site, low-grade fever and very rarely may cause severe allergic reaction. The only contraindication is severe allergy to a vaccine component or prior dose. A child who has recovered from tetanus must be actively immunized because the amount of toxin responsible for disease in humans does not elicit protective immunity. Tetanus antitoxin levels of >0.1 IU per mL are considered protective. Tetanus toxoid is recommended for HIV infected children irrespective of presence of symptomatology.

Tdap VACCINE

Tdap, a new product available recently, contains standard quantity tetanus toxoid and reduced quantity diphtheria and acellular pertussis vaccine (Tdap) instead of Td. The standard strength DTwP and DTaP vaccines cannot be used for vaccination of children 7 years and above due to increased reactogenicity.

In children who have received all three primary and the two booster doses of DTwP/DTaP, Tdap should be administered as a single dose at the age of 10–12 years. Catch up vaccination is recommended till the age of 18 years. A single dose of Tdap may also be used as replacement for Td/TT booster in adults of any age, if they have not received Tdap in the past. Earlier it was recommended to observe a gap of 2–5 years between Tdap and previous TT/Td vaccines to decrease local adverse reactions.

5.6 POLIO VACCINES

Poliomyelitis is a viral disease caused by poliovirus, of which 3 serotypes are known: 1, 2 and 3. The disease mainly affects children under the age of five years, and vaccination is the only available method of prophylaxis. Two types of vaccines are available against poliomyelitis: Live-attenuated oral polio vaccine (OPV) and inactivated polio vaccine (IPV).

TYPES OF VACCINES

A. Live-Attenuated Oral Poliovirus Vaccine (OPV)

This vaccine, developed by Albert Sabin, was licensed in 1961. The wild poliovirus is attenuated by repeated passages on non-optimal tissue culture. The Sabin strains are then cultured on monkey kidney cells (vero cells) to produce large quantities of the vaccine. The oral polio vaccine contains 10^5 to 10^6 median cell culture infectious doses of all three types of polio virus derived from the original Sabin strain. This vaccine is given orally, and to be effective, the virus needs to multiply in the gastrointestinal tract. Vaccine consists of 1 million particles of each of the three serotypes with magnesium chloride as the stabilizing agent.

B. Enhanced Inactivated Poliovirus Vaccine (eIPV)

The first effective IPV vaccine, a killed virus vaccine, was developed by Johan Salk, in 1955. It is prepared by formalin inactivation of wild type poliovirus strain by Salk method; ie, 1:1000 formalin treatment for 12–14 days at 37°C. It contains 40, 8, 32 D antigen units of the type 1, 2, and 3 viruses, respectively. New production techniques include seed strains grown in vero cells or human diploid cells grown in micro-carrier cultivation systems. It is a highly effective trivalent vaccine.

Protective Efficacy

After OPV vaccination, the serological response to the vaccine is similar to a natural infection. After three doses, the seroconversion rate is 73% for type 1, 90% for type 2 and 70% for type 3. OPV provides a state of local resistance in the gastrointestinal tract, based on mucosal immunity. This gastrointestinal resistance results in a significantly decreased number of successful implantations (challenge), a shorter period of virus excretion upon re-infection challenge, and lower titers of virus excreted. Studies have reported protective effects against paralytic poliomyelitis and interruption of wild poliovirus circulation. The persistence of protective effects lasts nearly 10 years, even if antibodies are at very low levels or undetectable. Studies conducted in developing countries, however, report that seroconversion rates even after multiple doses of OPV are lower than that reported from developed countries, particularly against type 1 virus. The reasons proposed for this difference include high prevalence of non-polio enteroviruses in gut and high incidence of malnutrition and diarrhea in children in developing countries, temperature variations often in temperate climate, and improper storage.

Enhanced IPV, on the other hand, induces the development of neutralizing antibody against all three poliovirus serotypes in virtually 90–95% after second dose and 99% of the vaccinees after the third dose. IPV produces excellent humoral immunity, as well as local pharyngeal and possible intestinal immunity and thus offers herd protection. The relative benefit of mucosal immunity induced by OPV compared with that of eIPV remains controversial. The secretory antibody response after OPV administration is greater, both in titer and in frequency, than after eIPV administration. Consistent with its ability to induce greater secretory antibody response, OPV is also more effective than eIPV in preventing and limiting intestinal infection following oral challenge. However, eIPV also provides herd immunity, although less than that of OPV, by inhibition of pharyngeal infection by poliovirus in vaccinees; furthermore, intestinal excretion, although not eliminated, is greatly reduced. IPV can be also combined with DTwP and Hib as a pentavalent vaccine.

Administration and Schedule

OPV is given orally while IPV is given by intramuscular route in a dose of 0.5 mL. OPV is required to be stored at outreach facility at 2–8°C. It can, however, be stored for 1–2 years at –20°C. IPV is stable for long periods at 4–8°C.

Primary Doses

Three doses of OPV are administered in most immunization schedules, at an interval of 4–8 weeks. The vaccine is given at the same visit as the DPT vaccine for the sake of convenience; hence most countries follow schedule 6, 10, 14 weeks or 2, 4, 6 months although the latter is immuno-logically preferable. However, in India, due to logistics reasons, primary doses are administered at 6, 10, 14 weeks only.

Zero Dose

In India, hospital-born children are also administered another dose, immediately or within 14 days of birth (zero dose). This additional early (zero) dose of polio vaccine (OPV or IPV) has been noted to enhance seroconversion and protect babies who subsequently receive three conventional doses. This is the basis of the concept of zero dose of OPV in India. Zero OPV should be given either at birth or within 14 days and not beyond, if not received previously. Even preterm infants mount good immune response to zero dose, though titers of antibodies is low against type-3 poliovirus.

Further Doses

Fourth dose of OPV is administered at the same time as the booster DPT dose; ie, first booster between 16 and 18 months; and the fifth dose (OPV-5) at 5 years of age. In addition, the child should also receive the pulse-polio doses administered on National Immunization Days (NIDs and sNIDs).

Countries using IPV usually use four doses, of which the first two are administered 8 weeks apart followed by a third dose anywhere between 6 and 18 months of age. A late booster dose at entry to school (fourth dose) is also used in some countries. Countries that use IPV will have to take into account local epidemiological factors before deciding the age at vaccination.

Intradermal IPV

Subsequent to the polio eradication in India, many states in India have included two intradermal doses of IPV (at 6 weeks with first DPT; and at 14 weeks along with the 3rd dose of DPT vaccine). Additionally as a polio end game strategy, and as a preparation for switch over, trivalent oral polio vaccine has been replaced by a bivalent oral polio vaccine bOPV (type I and III) in routine immunization program to reduce the incidence of vaccine-associated paralytic poliomyelitis.

Adverse Effect

Vaccine-associated Paralytic Poliomyelitis (VAPP)

The most significant adverse effect associated with administration of oral polio vaccine is vaccine-associated paralytic poliomyelitis (VAPP). The overall risk is estimated at 1 case per 2.5 million doses (distribution), or 1 case per 1.5 million OPV recipients. In these cases, the live-attenuated poliovirus contained in OPV, while replicating in the intestinal tract of recipients, regains its neurovirulence. The reverted virus might reach the CNS and spread like the wild poliovirus. Strains produced during intestinal replication carry sufficient neurovirulence to cause predictable rates of paralysis in recipients and contacts. The risk of VAPP is higher with the first dose that "takes" with P2 virus and in patients with B-cell immunodeficiency.

The risk is higher for the first dose: 1 case per 750,000 first OPV doses administered. In India, 50 cases of VAPP per year are documented, 50% of which are type 2. The clinical features of this illness are identical to those of natural paralytic poliomyelitis due to the wild virus.

Circulating Vaccine-Derived Poliovirus

Vaccine-derived polioviruses (VDPVs) are rare strains of poliovirus that have genetically mutated from the strain contained in the OPV. The ability to circulate determines whether neurovirulent vaccine-derived viruses may cause outbreaks of VAPP; hence the term 'circulating vaccine-derived polioviruses' (cVDPV) has been coined. Clearly cVDPVs are de-attenuated and wild-like. They have intermediate degrees of virulence and transmissibility, compared to wild and vaccine strains.

If a population is seriously under-immunized, there are enough susceptible children for the excreted vaccine-derived polioviruses to begin circulating in the community. The lower the population immunity, the longer these viruses survive. The longer they survive, the more they replicate, change, and exchange genetic material with other enteroviruses as they spread through a community.

There are three types of vaccine-derived poliovirus:
1. Circulating vaccine-derived poliovirus (cVDPV)
2. Immunodeficiency-related vaccine-derived poliovirus (iVDPV)
3. Ambiguous vaccine-derived poliovirus (aVDPV).

Enhanced IPV vaccine contains killed poliovirus, and thus it never causes cVAPP or formation of cVDPV strains. There are no significant side effects induced by the eIPV, although allergy to one of the vaccine components or reaction to a previous dose may be observed.

Contraindications

Oral polio vaccine is contraindicated in situations where immunity is unpredictable or definitely compromised; such as HIV positive children, those suffering from lympho-reticular malignancies and immune dysfunction. OPV is also contraindicated to household contacts of such persons since there is the risk of acquiring the virus through the secretions of vaccinated contacts. Pregnancy is also a relative contraindication to use of OPV. In all such situations, IPV remains the preferred vaccine. Mild diarrhea is not a contraindication for OPV administration. Repeat dose of OPV should be given, if the child vomits within 10 minutes of administration.

5.7 MEASLES VACCINE

Measles is an extremely contagious viral disease with a high burden of childhood morbidity and mortality in developing countries. Since the 1960s, an effective live-attenuated vaccine has been available. Measles vaccine is available in monovalent (measles only) formulation and in combination as MMR vaccine. Measles vaccine is a live-attenuated vaccine developed from Edmonston Zagreb strain grown in human diploid cells or purified chick embryo cells. Many other strains cultivated by different laboratories are Schwartz, Moraten, Leningrad-4, and Shanghai-191 strains. Each dose of measles vaccine contains 1000 $TCID_{50}$.

Age at Administration

Measles vaccine is most immunogenic when administered after the disappearance of transplacentally derived maternal antibodies as they interfere with vaccine uptake. These antibodies fade away from infant's blood over a varying period of time, ranging from 6–12 months. But considering high chance of acquiring measles and complication related with it, WHO–EPI advocates routine vaccination with measles at completed 9 months of age. National Immunization Schedule of India also recommends measles vaccine administration at 9 months of age. However, during an outbreak, infants as young as 6 months can be vaccinated and a booster measles vaccine has to be given at 12–15 months.

In view of about 15% cases of primary vaccine failures with the first dose of the vaccine, an additional dose of measles vaccine preferably as MMR vaccine at the age of 15 months is required for durable and possibly lifelong protection against measles.

Protective Efficacy

The efficacy of measles vaccines is 85–90% when given at 9–11 months of age in Indian context due to persistence of measles maternal antibodies in 5 to 10% of children of this age group. The data for western countries reports sero-conversion rates in the range of 95 to 98%. Efficacy can be affected by factors like maternal antibodies, intercurrent illnesses, immune status, presence of malnutrition, and maintenance of cold chain.

Vaccine Characteristics

The dose of measles vaccine is 0.5 mL to be given subcutaneously at upper arm/anterolateral thigh. Measles is heat-labile lyophilized vaccine, should be stored at 2–8°C. It must be protected from ultraviolet light. The vaccine reconstituted with sterile water should be keep in refrigerator and to be used within 4–6 hours of reconstitution.

Adverse Effects

Measles vaccine is remarkably safe vaccine; side effects are a few and generally mild, which may include mild fever, local pain, and transient maculopapular rash, observed within 5–12 days of immunization in 5–15% vaccine recipients. Adverse events such as thrombocytopenia, encephalitis/encephalopathy, Guillain-Barre syndrome and serious allergic reactions such as anaphylaxis are extremely rare. Toxic shock syndrome is a dreaded complication due to contamination of measles vaccine with *Staphylococcus aureus*.

Contraindications

Measles vaccine is contraindicated in children with HIV infection and low CD4 count. Those receiving immunosuppressive medication should receive live vaccines at least

5

1 month before starting drug therapy. Measles vaccine should not be given during pregnancy or those having history of anaphylactic reaction following administration of either topical or systemic neomycin.

Measles vaccine can be safely administered on the same setting along with any other vaccine.

Second Dose of Measles Vaccine

Vaccine immunogenicity and efficacy are best when the vaccine is administered beyond the age of 12 months. However, in India, a significant proportion of measles cases occur below the age of 12 months. Hence, in order to achieve the best balance between these competing demands of early protection and high seroconversion, completed 9 months of age has been recommended as the appropriate age for measles vaccination in India. A second dose of measles vaccine should be introduced in UIP at the time of first DPT booster (at 18 months) in states with more than 80% coverage with the first dose of measles vaccine.

Following the NTAGI recommendations, routine immunization for measles now should include administration of 2 doses of MR (measles/rubella) vaccine instead of single component measles vaccine with first dose at 9 months and 2nd dose with DPT booster at the age of 16–24 months. Thus, MR vaccine would be introduced in the routine immunization and would replace single component measles vaccine given at 9–12 months of age and 16–24 months of the age.

NON-EPI VACCINES

5.8 MMR VACCINE

Measles, mumps and rubella (MMR) vaccine is a live-attenuated vaccine. Each dose of this vaccine contains approximately 1000 $TCID_{50}$ of measles, 5000 $TCID_{50}$ of mumps and 1000 $TCID_{50}$ of rubella virus. In addition, each dose also contains small amounts of additives such as neomycin, sorbitol and hydrolyzed gelatin. The strains currently used in India are:

i. Edmonston-Zagreb strain grown on human diploid cell culture for measles virus vaccine.
ii. L-Zagreb strain grown in chick embryo cell culture for mumps. A new MMR vaccine containing less reactogenic Jeryl Lynn mumps strain is also commercially available.
iii. Strain RA 27/3 grown in human diploid cell culture for rubella.

Protective Efficacy

Single dose of MMR vaccine has 95% efficacy in preventing mumps and rubella. The duration of vaccine-induced immunity is probably lifelong in most vaccine recipients.

For prevention of mumps, the MMR vaccine is recommended to be given at 15 months of age. For prevention of rubella and congenital rubella syndrome, double-pronged approach is required. All adolescent girls also need to be vaccinated with MMR vaccine, if they have not received it earlier.

MMR can also be given as early as 12 months of age but not before the first birthday. A second dose of MMR vaccine is recommended at 4–6 years of age to produce immunity in those who failed to respond to first dose. The route of vaccine administration is by subcutaneous route either at upper arm or anterolateral thigh.

Adverse Effects

MMR vaccine is very safe. Most adverse reactions following MMR vaccine such as fever, rash and local pain are transient and short lived and occur in 5–15% of vaccine recipients. Lymphadenopathy and arthralgia/arthritis are rare adverse events. MMR vaccine does not cause autism, or inflammatory bowel disease.

Contraindications

MMR and component vaccines should not be administered during pregnancy due to the risks to the fetus from the live virus vaccines. Children who have experienced a severe allergic reaction following a prior dose of MMR vaccine or a vaccine component (gelatin, neomycin) should also not be vaccinated with MMR vaccine.

5.9 HEPATITIS B VACCINE

THE VACCINE

The availability of genetically engineered preparations revolutionized the scope of hepatitis B immunization. Hepatitis B virus (HBV) vaccine is a recombinant DNA vaccine antigen incorporated in the genetic material of the yeast (*Saccharomyces cerevisiae*) which then begins to produce the surface antigen. This method nullifies the risk of transmission of infection from inadvertent contamination and guarantees almost limitless supply of antigen.

Protective Efficacy

Administration of 3 doses of HBV vaccine in different schedules results in a high degree of seroconversion. Over 95% of vaccinated individuals develop protective level of antibodies (more than 10 mIU/mL) which is believed to confer life-long immunity against hepatitis B infection. Routine booster doses are not recommended for immuno-competent children and adults.

Administration and Schedule

HBV vaccine should be given intramuscularly in antero-lateral thigh in infants and deltoid in older children and adults. Injection into gluteal region elicits decreased immune response and thus must always be avoided. The pediatric dose of vaccine is 10 µg and adult dose is 20 µg per dose. Larger vaccine doses (40 µg) are needed to induce protective antibody in high proportion of children on hemodialysis and with immunocompromised status.

HBV vaccine may be given in any of the following schedule:

1. Birth (0), 1 month, and 6 months
2. Birth (0), 6 weeks, and 6 months
3. Birth (0), 6 weeks, and 14 weeks
4. 6, 10, and 14 weeks

Immunologically, 0, 1, and 6 months schedule of HBV immunization is most widely used and proven to be ideal with high antibody titer at the end of immunization series.

However, the other two schedules due to operational feasibility allow HBV vaccine to be given during the same visit for routine DPT/OPV vaccination. In India, UIP follows the 6, 10, 14 weeks schedule. Additional birth dose is also recommended for institutional deliveries within 24 hours of birth (zero dose). This can be given at the same time when zero dose of OPV is being given. If the mother is HBsAg positive, the baby should receive Hepatitis B immunoglobulin (HBIG) within 12 hours of birth along with first dose of HBV vaccine using two separate syringes at different injection sites.

Adverse Effects

The adverse effects of HBV vaccine include fever, headache and soreness at injection site. These symptoms are usually mild, transient and do not last beyond three days. Anaphylaxis is uncommon. There is no scientific evidence of association of HBV vaccine with SIDS, diabetes mellitus or multiple sclerosis. The only absolute contraindication to HBV vaccine is the occurrence of anaphylaxis to a previous dose or an allergy to vaccine component but is extremely rare. Pregnancy and lactation are not contraindications to immunization.

5.10 HAEMOPHILUS INFLUENZAE B (Hib) VACCINE

Infections due to *Haemophilus influenzae* type b (Hib) are one of the common causes of invasive bacterial infections including meningitis, pneumonia, and bacteremia in children less than 5 years of age. Mass immunization with Hib vaccine has led to virtual elimination of Hib disease from UK and USA. WHO recommends inclusion of Hib vaccine in routine infant immunization programs in view of its demonstrated safety and efficacy. The estimated incidence of Hib infections in India is 50–60 per 1 lac children less than 5 years of age and 30–45% cases of pyogenic meningitis and 8–12% pneumonia in children are due to Hib infection.

The Vaccine

Hib vaccine is a conjugate vaccine consisting of Hib capsular polysaccharide (polyribosylribitol phosphate) covalently linked to a carrier protein directly or *via* an intervening spacer molecule. This process of conjugation changes the polysaccharide antigen from a T-cell independent to T-cell dependent antigen and greatly improves the immunogenicity. Thus Hib vaccine is effective from the age of 6 weeks onwards, induces IgG antibodies leading to boosting effect with better short- and long-term immunity, and leads to herd effect.

The conjugate Hib vaccines differ from one another on the size of PRP molecule, the type of carrier protein, the type of linkage between PRP and carrier protein and the presence or absence of an adjuvant in the vaccine. These include (*i*) diphtheria toxoid (PRP-D), (*ii*) diphtheria toxoid-like carrier protein (PRP-HbOC) (*iii*) tetanus toxoid (PRP-T) and (*iv*) meningococcal outer membrane protein (PRP-OMP).

Protective Efficacy

Hib conjugate vaccines are very immunogenic and high antibody titers are observed following PRP–T and HbOC vaccines. PRP-OMP is less immunogenic at the end of schedule and hence has been withdrawn. PRP-D is least immunogenic of all Hib vaccines and hence is not recommended for primary series but only as booster dose. These conjugate vaccines do not interfere with the immunogenicity of other simultaneously administered vaccines. The first dose of vaccine gives 71%, second dose 89% and third dose 95 to 100% vaccine efficacy.

Schedule

Routine vaccination with Hib vaccine is started at 6 weeks of age, and three primary doses of vaccine are given intramuscularly at an interval of 4 weeks. Thus Hib vaccine can be given along with DPT vaccine at 6, 10 and 14 weeks. However, a time lag of 8 weeks between any two doses is ideal. For a child between 6 and 12 months, two primary doses are given at 6 to 8 weeks interval. For a child 12 to 15 months only one primary dose is given. All these children are given a booster dose between 15 and 18 months of age. Hib vaccine is stored at 2–8°C.

Adverse Effects

The adverse effects are uncommon and are mild such as local pain, tenderness and fever. There are no absolute contraindications except for hypersensitivity to vaccine components.

5.11 PNEUMOCOCCAL VACCINES

Streptococcus pneumoniae is one of the most important causes of pneumonia, meningitis, febrile bacteremia, otitis media, sinusitis and bronchitis. An estimated 1 million under-five children succumb to these diseases every year. Of 90 serotypes of pneumococci, about 20 are responsible for more than 80% of invasive pneumococcal disease in all age groups while only 13 are responsible for 70–75% of global disease burden in children. The common serotypes responsible for invasive disease in under-five children in India include 1, 4, 5, 6, 7, 14 and 19.

Currently, two types of vaccine are available: (*i*) a 23-valent unconjugated polysaccharide vaccine (PPV-23); and (*ii*) a 13-valent polysaccharide-protein conjugated vaccine (PCV 13) and a 10-valent conjugate vaccine (PCV 10) in combination with non-typeable *Haemophilus influenzae* vaccine. The 23-valent vaccine is for older children and adults and is not immunogenic in less than 2 years of age, while PCV 13 can also be used in infants and toddlers below 2 years of age.

PNEUMOCOCCAL POLYSACCHARIDE VACCINE (PPV-23)

This vaccine is composed of purified preparations of pneumococcal capsular polysaccharides (PPV23) and is capable of preventing 88% of invasive disease (pneumonia, meningitis and bacteremia) caused by *S. pneumoniae*. Each dose of 0.5 mL contains 25 µg of polysaccharide of each of 23 serotypes contained in vaccine. As this vaccine is an unconjugated polysaccharide vaccine, this vaccine is poorly immunogenic in children below two years of age who suffer from the maximum morbidity and it does not result in immunological memory. The vaccine is administered either intramuscular or subcutaneously.

5

The vaccine is useful for high-risk children above the age of 2 years including those with underlying chronic/systemic diseases like diabetes, cardiovascular diseases, HIV infection, sickle cell disease, asplenia, and nephrotic syndrome. These children should simultaneously also receive monthly penicillin prophylaxis.

Revaccination with a single dose is recommended after 5 years. Mild local reactions may be seen in 30–50% of vaccine recipients and systemic reactions are uncommon.

PNEUMOCOCCAL CONJUGATE VACCINE (PCV–13 AND PCV-10)

The drawbacks of pneumococcal polysaccharide vaccine led to the development of pneumococcal conjugate vaccine. Conjugation of the polysaccharide antigen to a protein carrier (cross-reactive variant of diphtheria toxin) increases the immunogenicity of the vaccine by converting it to a T-cell dependent antigen. The vaccine contains aluminum phosphate as an adjuvant.

The 13-valent conjugate vaccine contains the serotypes 1, 3, 4, 5, 6A, 6B, 7F, 9V, 14, 18C, 19A, 19F, and 23F, whereas PCV10 also contains all these subtypes except 3, 6A, and 19A.

- The vaccine is used in a 3-dose schedule in infancy at an interval of 4 to 8 weeks followed by a booster dose at 12–15 months of age.
- Unvaccinated children 7 months of age and older do not require a full series of four doses: Children between 7 and 11 months need two doses of vaccine at 4 weeks interval followed by booster between 12 and 15 months.
- Children between 12 and 23 months should receive two doses of vaccine 8 weeks apart.
- Previously unvaccinated healthy children from 24–59 months should receive at least one dose of PCV 13 or PCV 10.
- Conjugate 13 valent vaccine can be used as a catch-up vaccine in a single dose in children even beyond 5 years of age who have not received this vaccine earlier.

The newer PCVs have protective efficacy ranging from 80 to 99% against invasive pneumococcal disease caused by the serotypes contained in the vaccines. Revaccination or further doses after age appropriate primary series with PCV 13/10 is not currently recommended. The common side effects include injection site soreness, malaise, and low-grade fever.

Replacement Disease

While introduction of pneumococcal vaccine on a large scale will reduce the nasal carriage of vaccine serotypes, it is possible that these are replaced by non-vaccine serotypes and finally the overall nasopharyngeal carriage of pneumococci remains the same. Thus, theoretically, benefit from reducing disease caused by vaccine serotypes may be partially offset by an increase in the disease caused by non-vaccine serotypes of pneumococci and *H. influenzae*. However, replacement disease is NOT expected to increase the overall burden of pneumococcal disease.

5.12 TYPHOID VACCINES

There are three types of vaccine against typhoid fever: (*i*) parenteral killed whole cell vaccine; (*ii*) polysaccharide subunit vaccine (Vi antigen); and (*iii*) Vi conjugate vaccine. Typhoid vaccine is not included in the National Immunization program, at present.

PARENTERAL KILLED VACCINE

This is a heat-killed phenol preserved vaccine, which has been used in India for a long time. This is a trivalent vaccine containing bacterial cell wall endotoxins of *S.typhi*, *S. paratyphi* A and *S. paratyphi* B (TAB vaccine). Due to frequently associated side effects, this vaccine has fallen out of favor and is not currently being manufactured in India. This vaccine is protective through the induction of antibodies against the cell wall somatic O antigen and flagellar H antigen. Unlike the other typhoid vaccines, the vaccine is effective even in young children from the age of 6 months upwards.

The vaccine efficacy has been observed to range between 50 and 70% and the primary vaccination requires two doses 0.5 mL each given subcutaneously at an interval of 4–6 weeks. Children between the ages of 6 months and 10 years should receive half the dose. Revaccination is to be given once every 3 years.

Vi POLYSACCHARIDE VACCINE

This typhoid vaccine consists of purified antigenic fraction of Vi antigen of *S. typhi*. It is extracted from the capsule strain of *S. typhi* Ty2 and the process of purification and extraction preserves the Vi antigen. Each dose of vaccine contains 25 μg of purified polysaccharide in 0.5 mL of phenolic isotonic buffer. As the vaccine is a polysaccharide vaccine, it is not effective in children below 2 years of age and has no immune memory.

The biological marker is anti-Vi antibodies and 1 μg/mL is proposed as the serologic correlate of protection. The vaccine does not interfere with the interpretation of the Widal test. Efficacy drops over time and the cumulative efficacy at 3 years against culture confirmed typhoid fever is reported as 55%. To maintain protection, revaccination should be done once every 3 years.

The vaccine needs to be given subcutaneously or intramuscularly in a dose of 0.5 mL to children above 2 years of age. Adverse effects are mild which include fever, local pain and erythema at injection site. There are no contra-indications to its use other than prior severe reaction to vaccine components.

Vi CONJUGATE TYPHOID VACCINES

The limitations of the currently available typhoid vaccines, eg, non-effectiveness below the age of 2 years, limited efficacy of around 60%, T-cell independent response which lacks immune memory, lack of booster effect, and no protection against paratyphoid fever, strongly indicate the need of effective Vi conjugate vaccines.

A new Vi polysaccharide conjugate typhoid vaccine using tetanus toxoid as a carrier protein is now available for infants and children. This vaccine is recommended to be used between the ages of 9 and 12 months (minimum age >6 months). An interval of at least 4 weeks with measles/MMR vaccine should be maintained while administering this

5

vaccine. The vaccine should be followed by a second (booster) dose at 24 months of age for long-term protection.

5.13 VARICELLA VACCINE

Varicella vaccine is a live-attenuated viral vaccine derived from the Oka strain of varicella-zoster virus (VZV). The varicella vaccines may vary by their passage numbers in human diploid cells, virus contents (between 1000 and 10000 PFU), presence of trace antibiotics to ensure sterility and stabilizers. The minimum infectious dose of the vaccine virus content should be 1000 PFU per dose.

Varicella vaccine is highly immunogenic and more than 95% of immunized healthy children between the ages of 12 months and 12 years develop seroconversion after a single dose of varicella vaccine. In children 13 years of age and older, seroconversion rates are 78 to 82% after one dose and 99% after second dose. The immunity induced in vaccine recipients appears to be long lasting, though exact duration of protection is not known.

Although varicella vaccine prevents varicella, breakthrough varicella infections may occur in 15% of vaccinated children who have seroconverted following vaccination. Most cases of breakthrough infections are milder than infections that occur in unvaccinated children.

Administration

Varicella vaccine is a lyophilized product and must be reconstituted with its diluent before its use. It should be stored at –15°C and should be used within 30 minutes of reconstitution. The vaccine is administered subcutaneously either in the upper arm or the anterolateral thigh. The vaccine is recommended to be used in a 2 dose schedule, with the first dose administered at 15 months of age and followed by the 2nd dose between the age of 4 and 6 years. However, the 2nd dose can be given anytime, 3 months after the first dose. There is some evidence that varicella vaccine may be effective in preventing varicella or modifying the severity of the disease, if given within 3 to 5 days after exposure to a case of varicella.

Adverse Effects

Varicella vaccine is safe and side effects reported are mild and transient. These may include fever, minor injection site reactions, vaccine-associated rash. Systemic adverse events are uncommon. Varicella vaccine should not be given in moderate and severe illness, immunocompromized children, leukemia, HIV infection, children on corticosteroid therapy and households with potential contact with immuno-compromised people and pregnancy. It is recommended that pregnancy should be avoided for four weeks following the vaccine. The vaccine can be given safely with all other routine childhood immunizations without any risk of reduced efficacy and lower tolerability. The vaccine is not recommended for universal immunization in India at present.

Current Status

Routine childhood immunization against varicella is considered in countries where (*i*) this disease is a relatively important public health problem; (*ii*) the vaccine is affordable; and (*iii*) high (85–90%) and sustained vaccine coverage can be achieved.

Varicella is still not among the priority vaccine preventable diseases in developing countries including India, where other vaccine preventable diseases cause significantly greater morbidity and mortality. The vaccine is costly and not affordable by the masses. Due to lack of resources, presently it is not possible to achieve high varicella vaccination coverage. Childhood immunization with lower coverage could shift the epidemiology of the disease and increase the number of severe cases in adolescents and adults. Therefore, routine childhood immunization with varicella vaccine in India is not recommended at present.

The vaccine, however, may be used freely in adolescents and adults who have not had natural disease previously. Those at increased risk of contracting or spreading the infection should be vaccinated on priority basis. Vaccination of adolescents and adults will protect at risk individuals but will not disturb the general epidemiology of the disease.

Passive Prophylaxis

Varicella-zoster immunoglobulin (VZIG) is used for passive prophylaxis in children without evidence of immunity to varicella and who are at high risk for the severe disease and/ or its complications. It has to be given intramuscularly in a dose of 125 units for every 10 kg of body weight. The indications include (*i*) immunocompromised children; (*ii*) neonates whose mothers have varicella 5 days before to 2 days after delivery; and (*iii*) susceptible pregnant women.

5.14 RABIES VACCINES

Vaccine Characteristics

Since transmission of rabies virus is almost exclusively through the bite of an infected animal and since the incubation period is relatively long, post-exposure prophylaxis is possible. Three types of vaccine are currently available: (*i*) derived from rabies virus grown in human diploid cell (HDC vaccine), (*ii*) derived from virus grown in purified chick embryo cells (PCEC vaccine), and (*iii*) derived from purified vero cells (PVR vaccine). All these vaccines are virtually free from the risk of neuroparalytic reactions and are extremely effective.

All these vaccines are lyophilized products and must be reconstituted before use. The potency of cell culture vaccines is assessed using a National Institute of Health Test and the WHO requirement is a potency of at least 2.5 IU per intramuscular dose. Considered as gold standard in the treatment of rabies prevention, these vaccines satisfy all criteria of potency, immunogenicity, safety and convenience of use. With reference to efficacy, failures are rare (1 in one million) in post-exposure prophylaxis, which is almost always due to severe bites on or near head or inappropriate administration of vaccine.

There are no contraindications to the use of these vaccines for post-exposure prophylaxis. Pregnancy is not a contra-indication to the post-exposure prophylaxis. The vaccines are well tolerated and allergic reactions are uncommon in children.

5

Post-Exposure Prophylaxis

After the completion of wound care, concurrent use of immunoprophylaxis should begin as soon as possible after exposure, ideally within 24 hours. Rabies vaccine is administered intramuscularly on the anterolateral thigh or on deltoid on days 0, 3, 7, 14 and 30 as per *Essen protocol* with day 0 being the day of commencement of post-exposure vaccination. A sixth dose on day 90 is optional and should be given to patients with severe debility or those who are immunocompromised. The dose of vaccine remains same for adults and children as 1.0 mL for PCEC and HDCV vaccines and 0.5 mL per dose for PVR vaccine. The vaccine must never be given on gluteal region. Several other schedules for rabies immunization such as *Zagreb schedule* (2 – 1 – 1; two doses on day 1 on each thigh followed by second and third dose on day 7 and 21, respectively) and/or an intradermal route have been recommended for the reasons of cost and availability of vaccines, but are not routinely practiced.

Rabies Immunoglobulin

Rabies immunoglobulin (RIG) is to be administered in all category III exposures **(Table 5.8)**. RIG is also indicated, if the bite of an infected animal is on head, neck, hands or genitalia.

Inject equine antirabies immunoglobulin (ERIG) 40 IU/kg body weight, or human antirabies immunoglobulin (HRIG) 20 IU/kg. Always use HRIG in multiple severe exposures. The dose is injected on day 0, in and around the wound site. Remainder, if any should be injected by deep injection into anterolateral thigh. RIG should not be administered later than day 7 after the bite.

Intradermal Schedules for Post-Exposure Prophylaxis

The following two regimens are recommended: (*i*) 8 site intradermal (8-0-4-0-1-1): 0.1 mL per dose. On day 0, give 8 intradermal injections (both upper arms, both thighs, both suprascapulars, and both lower abdomen); one injection at 4 sites on day 7 (both upper arms, both thighs); and one single injection on upper arm on day 30 and 90, each. (*ii*) 2 site intradermal schedule (2-2-2-0-2): One intradermal injection at 2 sites on days 0, 3, 7, and 28. While the first schedule is applicable to HDCV and PCEC vaccines, the later schedule can be followed with PVR or PCEC vaccines.

Local Treatment of the Wound

Immediate washing/flushing for a minimum of 15 minutes with soap/detergent and water, or water alone is recommended. Ethanol 70%, iodine, or povidone-iodine can be applied after washing. Avoid suturing. If suture needs to be applied, inject RIG before suturing.

Pre-Exposure Prophylaxis

Cell culture rabies vaccine is also suitable for pre-exposure prophylaxis to people at risk of exposure to rabies such as laboratory staff, animal handlers, etc. The schedule is 1 mL of vaccine, 3 doses on days 0, 7 and 28. Vaccine is to be given IM on anterolateral thigh only, never in the gluteal region. It can also be given 0.1 mL intradermal on days 0, 7 and 21/28.

In the event of a new exposure to a previously vaccinated child, 2 boosters should be administered on day 0 and 3, following the bite, along with wound treatment. RIG is not indicated.

5.15 JAPANESE ENCEPHALITIS VACCINES

The types of available JE vaccines are: (*i*) Mouse brain-derived, inactivated Nakayama strain vaccine; (*ii*) Cell culture-derived inactivated vaccine; (*iii*) Cell culture-derived live-attenuated vaccine; and (*iv*) Newer JE vaccines. JE vaccines are recommended in UIP immunization schedule for children living in districts highly endemic for JE.

MOUSE BRAIN INACTIVATED VACCINE

Mouse brain inactivated vaccine is produced in India at Central Research Institute, Kasauli and the commercially available vaccine is imported. Thiomersal is added as a preservative for the vaccine. The vaccine is given in 3 doses of 0.5 mL (1–3 years) or 1 mL (>3 yr) each subcutaneously given on 0, 7 and 30 days. A booster dose is recommended after one year and subsequently at three years intervals. The vaccine is stable at 4°C for at least 1 year. The protective efficacy is 90–95%. Adverse events include fever, malaise, local tenderness, and redness in 20% of vaccine recipients. The vaccine should be given to pregnant woman, only if clearly indicated as no specific information is available on the safety of JE vaccine in pregnancy. The disadvantages of this vaccine include its limited duration of protection, need for multiple doses, and high cost.

CELL CULTURE-DERIVED KILLED VACCINE

Cell culture-derived *killed vaccine* also offers 85% protection, is inexpensive and has a high viral yield. Two doses of this vaccine, given 4 weeks apart, have achieved 94–100% seroconversion. It is less reactogenic as compared to mouse brain vaccine. In view of rare cases of fatal encephalitis and hypersensitivity following vaccination with mouse brain

Category	Exposure	Type	Schedule
I	Touch, lick on intact skin	None	None
II	Nibbling of uncovered skin, minor scratch, abrasions without bleeding	Minor	Start vaccine*
III	Single/multiple transdermal bites/scratches, licks on broken skin, contamination of mucous membrane with saliva	Major	Rabies immune globulin + vaccine*

Table 5.8 Categorization of Wound Following Dog-bite

*Stop if animal remains healthy for 10 days or is proved to be negative by laboratory tests

vaccine, WHO recommends that the cell culture-derived live vaccines should replace it altogether.

LIVE-ATTENUATED VACCINE

A live-attenuated vaccine (SA 14–14–2) has been developed and tested in China. Live vaccine offers long-term protection (single dose followed by a booster 1 year later). This live vaccine constitutes to over 50% of global production of JE vaccine. Initial studies done on this vaccine have shown an efficacy of 80% with one dose and 98% with two doses. The vaccine is given in a dose of 0.5 mL for all ages by subcutaneous route. The vaccine has been used under public health program by Government of India since 2006, and currently this is the only JE vaccine available in India.

NEWER JE VACCINES

Cost, efficacy and safety concerns led to the development of a live-attenuated virus vaccine (SA14-14-2) and more recently, a number of JE vaccines are in development, some are licensed and some are approaching licensure. These include inactivated whole virus, chimeric vaccine, genetically engineered and DNA vaccines. The following three new JE vaccines though not yet available in India but are available in some parts of the world:
1. Chimeric vaccine (IMOJEV by Sanofi Pasteur)
2. Inactivated SA-14-14-2 vaccine (IC51) (IXIARO by Intercel)
3. Inactivated vero cell-derived JE vaccine (Beijing-1 JE strain by Biken and Kaketsuken, Japan)

5.16 MENINGOCOCCAL VACCINES

Routine immunization against meningococcal disease is not recommended. A quadrivalent vaccine containing 50 µg each of purified bacterial polysaccharide antigen from serogroups A, C, Y and W135 is available. In India, epidemics are usually caused by type A or C while endemic cases are mainly due to Type B. No vaccine is available from protection against Group B disease. Group A antigen is immunogenic in children over 3 months of age and Group C over 2 years of age.

Type of Vaccines

Vaccines are available as (*i*) polysaccharide unconjugated; or (*ii*) conjugated vaccines. Unconjugated vaccines are not immunogenic in children below 2 years of age and do not induce immunological memory. These are either bivalent (A and C) or tetravalent (A, C, Y, W 135). Polysaccharide-protein conjugate meningococcal vaccines are also immunogenic in infants.

Conjugated meningococcal vaccines are now available in India. These are effective in infants and younger childen and are approved for use from the age of 9 months onwards.

Administration

A single subcutaneous injection of 0.5 mL is recommended for high-risk children with asplenia and complement deficiencies. During an outbreak, immunization may be recommended to persons at risk. The vaccine is indicated for use (as an adjunct to chemoprophylaxis) in close contacts of patients with disease, in immune deficiency conditions

and travel to high endemicity belt in African Continent. The vaccine is mandatory for Haj pilgrims and residential students in some universities abroad.

Protective Efficacy

Meningococcal vaccines are safe and induce protective antibodies in adults and children over the age of two years. However, like other polysaccharide vaccines, it does not produce immunological memory and repeated doses are required for long-term protection. In children over two years, a single dose is recommended. For children who are first immunized at the age of less than 4 years, who remain at high risk of infection, revaccination may be indicated after 2 to 3 years and after 5 years for older chiidren and adults.

Adverse Events

The adverse events are mild and primarily include pain and redness at injection site lasting for one to two days.

5.17 HEPATITIS A VACCINE

Hepatitis A vaccination is recommended for children who are at increased risk for infection and for those wishing to obtain immunity. Two categories of hepatitis A vaccines, inactivated and live-attenuated vaccines, are currently available in Indian market.

INACTIVATED VACCINE

Inactivated hepatitis A vaccine is derived from HM 175/GBM strains and grown on MRC5 human diploid cell lines. It is formalin inactivated and adjuvenated with aluminum hydroxide. The vaccine is stored at 2–8° C. The vaccine does not contain thiomersal.

Administration

The vaccine is administered IM in children older than 12 months of age in a two dose schedule, given 6 months apart. Seroconversion rates range from 90–100% after 2 doses. Booster is not recommended at present.

Hepatitis A virus (HAV) vaccine is recommended for use in children older than two years, some countries recommend its use beyond one year of age. The standard pediatric dose is 720 EU (0.5 mL) and adult dose (>13 years) 1440 EU (1.0 mL).

Protective Efficacy

HAV vaccine is highly effective and immunogenic in children and adolescents, when administered in the recommended dosages and schedules. Protective antibody titers are seen within 4 weeks of first dose and one month after the last dose. There is some evidence that higher doses generate protective antibody levels more rapidly. Although the geometric mean titer (GMT) of antibodies produced after vaccination is lower than those produced by natural infection, they are sufficiently high to provide lifelong immunity following the two doses schedule of HAV vaccine.

Adverse Events

HAV vaccine is a safe vaccine with a few side effects such as fever and pain at injection site that are mild and transient.

Recently, a live-attenuated HAV vaccine has become commercially available in our country, which has been developed and used in China. This vaccine is injected subcutaneously in a dose of 1.0 mL.

LIVE-ATTENUATED VACCINE

A live-attenuated HAV vaccine is now commercially available in India. It was developed and being used in China since 1990. This vaccine is derived from the H2 strain of the virus attenuated after serial passage in human diploid cell (KMB 17 cell line). This vaccine is injected subcutaneously in a dose of 1.0 mL. Immunogenicity studies with single dose show seroconversion rates of more than 98% two months after vaccination and persistence of protective antibodies in more than 80% of vaccinees at 10 years follow-up. IAP committee on immunization recommends one dose of this vaccine after the age of 12 months.

5.18 CHOLERA VACCINES

PARENTERAL CHOLERA VACCINE

The currently available parenteral cholera vaccine is composed of 10^9 phenol killed *V. cholerae* O1 organisms (Inaba, Ogawa, and Eltor biotypes). The protection offered by this vaccine is modest (50–60%) and short lived (3–6 months). The vaccine is neither effective during cholera outbreaks nor interrupts the transmission of *V. cholerae* in the community. The vaccine was recommended to be given in two doses at an interval of 7–28 days, subcutaneously or intramuscularly. Adverse effects were common and included fever, malaise, headache, local pain, and induration. The vaccine is contraindicated in infants below 6 months of age and the adverse events profile often precludes its use in pregnant women.

In view of low potency, poor efficacy and poor protection for individual as well as for the community, a need for newer vaccine is being felt. Immunity to cholera is serotype specific with a stronger response to Ogawa and Inaba antigens and is antibacterial than antitoxin.

ORAL CHOLERA VACCINES

Overall three oral cholera vaccines have been developed which are safe, immunogenic and effective: Namely, (*i*) killed bacterial vaccine, (*ii*) live, genetically engineered mutants deleted of cholera toxin (CtxB) genes, and (*iii*) avirulent vectors genetically engineered to express protective cholera antigens. B subunits of cholera toxin have been used as adjuvant in some of the newer cholera vaccines.

Oral Inactivated Vaccine

This consists of killed whole cell *V. cholerae* O1 with purified recombinant B subunit of cholera toxoid (WC/rBS). The protective efficacy is 85–90% when two doses are administered 1 week apart. Duration of protection lasts for 6 months, among all age groups. The vaccine does not provide protection against cholera caused by *V. cholerae* O139. This vaccine is now manufactured and licensed in India for children above 14 monthsage.

A variant of WC/rBS vaccine has been developed, that does not contain the recombinant B subunit. Its efficacy in Vietnam is shown to be 66%.

Live-Attenuated Vaccine

CVD 103HgR vaccine is a live-attenuated oral cholera vaccine. It consists of genetically modified *Vibrio cholerae* O1 strain (CVD 103-HgR). This vaccine appears to be safe and immunogenic and efficacious in children >2 years of age. A single dose confers 95% and 65% protection against the Classical and El tor biotypes, respectively.

Genetic Vaccine

In this approach, the genes controlling the expression of Inaba O antigen are cloned into a plasmid and introduced into the Ty21a typhoid vaccine strain. The hybrid vaccine strain Ex 645 appears to be well tolerated and immunogenic.

5.19 ROTAVIRUS VACCINES

Rotavirus is a common cause of diarrhea and almost all children get infected by the age of 5 years. The first rotavirus vaccine was licensed in USA in 1998 but subsequently withdrawn in October 1999 due to an increased incidence of intussusception following the administration of vaccine.

Two types of rotavirus vaccine are now available in India.
1. Live oral rotavirus vaccine developed from human and bovine parent rotavirus strains. Each dose of this vaccine contains approximately 2×10^6 infectious units of each reassortant strains.
2. Another rotavirus vaccine (live-attenuated human (G1P 8) monovalent vaccine.

Both these vaccines are found to be safe and highly efficacious. The immunization and dosage recommended for use in USA is a three-dose schedule at 2, 4, and 6 months. WHO now recommends introduction of rotavirus vaccines into routine immunization programs as part of a comprehensive strategy to control diarrheal diseases. The vaccines are proven to be safe and effective, and where introduced have resulted in dramatically lower rates of diarrhea-related hospitalization and death of children. They are also shown to be cost-effective. The vaccine has been introduced initially in four States under routine immunization program in Andhra Pradesh, Haryana, Himachal Pradesh and Odisha and would be expanded to the entire country in a phased manner.

5.20 INFLUENZA VACCINES

Inactivated influenza viral vaccine comprises of current strains of type A and type B viruses for parenteral use in humans. Immunity following infection by one strain may not protect fully against subsequent antigenic variants. Thus the influenza vaccine has to be regularly updated each year to match the circulating strains that are most likely to cause the next epidemic. WHO gives the annual recommendations on the influenza vaccine composition. The protective efficacy of the vaccine is shown to be 70 to 90% to prevent laboratory-confirmed illness.

The vaccine is recommended for children older than 6 months by intramuscular route in anterolateral thigh/

deltoid muscle. The dose of vaccine is 0.25 mL for children aged between 6 and 36 months and 0.5 mL for older children and adults. Previously unvaccinated children should receive 2 doses at an interval of 4 weeks. Annual vaccination is recommended for children belonging to high risk groups including those with chronic systemic disease, hemoglobinopathy, immunosuppression, and household contacts. A few vaccine recipients may develop short-lasting local and transient systemic reactions such as fever, malaise and myalgia.

A live-attenuated cold adapted trivalent influenza virus vaccine (nasal spray) has been shown to be effective in children. The vaccine has been currently approved for use in children above 5 years of age. Children between 5 and 8 years of age receiving influenza vaccine for first time should receive two doses by intranasal route given at least 6 weeks apart.

5.21 COMBINATION VACCINES

A combination vaccine consists of two or more separate immunogens that have been physically combined in a single preparation. Certain combination vaccines, such as DTP, DT, MMR, trivalent oral polio vaccine (OPV), are available and are in use for many years. More recently, licensed combination vaccines incorporate newer components such as Hib, acellular pertussis, or hepatitis B virus antigen.

The prerequisites for combining two or more different antigens into a single vaccine are: (*a*) The combination should not decrease purity, potency and safety of or efficacy of any of the individual component; and (*b*) The combination vaccine should not be inferior with respect to any of its individual components.

Advantages

The benefits of combination vaccine are listed below:
- Reduced number of injections
- Reduced pain and anxiety to the child and parent
- Reduced number of visits and better compliance
- Successful implementation of immunization program
- Reduced burden and logistics
- Reduced burden on cold chain
- Reduced packaging, handling and transportation

Disadvantages

- Combination of different antigens into one vaccine may lead to chemical incompatibility or immunologic interference that may be difficult to overcome.
- The process of production of combination vaccines is different from that of mixing two vaccines in a single vaccine vial.
- Different vaccine schedules may cause certain degree of uncertainty and confusion.
- Combination product must fit into immunization schedule without much compromise in the recommended age and interval of individual vaccines.
- Rarely the occurrence of an adverse event following combination vaccine can cause uncertainty over the specific cause of antigenic reaction.

Considering these factors, only licensed combination vaccines should be used. Additionally, separate vaccines should not be combined at the time of administration unless approved by regulatory authority. Several examples of newer combination vaccines include DPT with Hib/HBV, DTaP with Hib, DTaP with Hib/HBV/IPV, hepatitis A and B vaccines and MMR with varicella.

5.22 NEWER VACCINES

Various vaccines including those for dengue fever, malaria, HIV, chikungunya, hepatitis C, hepatitis E, Epstein-Barr virus, enterovirus, respiratory syncytial virus, parainfluenza virus are under various phases of clinical trials. Therapeutic vaccines are being investigated against cancers, rheumatoid arthritis, multiple sclerosis, Alzheimer disease, and type I diabetes.

DENGUE VACCINE

There are various challenges in the development of vaccines against dengue fever, like prevalence of four different serotypes, lack of animal model, and poor growth of dengue virus in cell culture. Various vaccine technologies have been tried for development of dengue vaccines including live-attenuated vaccine, inactivated virus vaccine, recombinant subunit vaccines or from virus-like peptides (VLPs), plasmids, or viral vectors.

Dengvaxia (CYD-TDV), the first dengue vaccine, was initially licensed in four countries—Mexico, Brazil, El Salvador and Philippines. It is a live recombinant tetravalent vaccine that has been evaluated as a 3-dose series on a 0/6/12 month schedule in phase III clinical studies. It has been registered for use in individuals 9–45 years of age living in endemic areas. This dengue vaccine is showing promising results.

There are five additional vaccine candidates under evaluation in clinical trials, including other live-attenuated vaccines, as well as subunit, DNA and purified inactivated vaccine candidates. Additional technological approaches, such as virus-vectored and VLP-based vaccines, are under evaluation in preclinical studies.

MALARIA VACCINE

Despite years of research, an effective Malaria vaccine still eludes the scientific community. It is difficult to formulate an effective vaccine against malaria due to complex life cycle of parasite and involvement of two host organisms. The vaccines can be broadly grouped into pre-erythrocyte vaccines, blood stage vaccines, and transmission blocking vaccines. Most of the research is for vaccine against *P. falciparum*. Only one vaccine candidate RTS, S/AS01 is showing positive results and is under phase III human trials.

HIV VACCINE

The main obstacle in development of vaccine is the peculiarity of the virus which dampens the immune system, disease process may be slowed down but complete eradication is not achieved. HIV isolates are highly variable with a vast genetic divergence so vaccine needs to be broad enough to map all the variability. Various vaccines like whole-inactivated vaccines, live-attenuated vaccine, virus-like peptides (VLPs), recombinant vaccines, subunit vaccines and DNA vaccines are under evaluation. None of them is approved for clinical use.

5.23 IMMUNIZATION SCHEDULE

Immunization schedules are the basic framework for the delivery of vaccines and immunization to the individuals and the community. A well-planned immunization schedule should be epidemiologically relevant, immunologically effective, operationally feasible and socially acceptable. Various factors that need to be considered for planning the immunization schedule, include (*i*) epidemiology of the disease; (*ii*) age specific morbidity and mortality; (*iii*) vaccine effectiveness; (*iv*) risks of vaccine-related adverse events; (*v*) cost-effectiveness; and (*vi*) health care infrastructure.

Vaccines for universal immunization are recommended at the youngest age at which a significant risk of disease and its complication exists and at which a protective immunological response can be expected. Logistics and operational feasibility of administering the vaccine at appropriate age without much increase in the cost and number of visits and requirement of the manpower are also important determinants of any immunization schedule.

NATIONAL IMMUNIZATION SCHEDULE, INDIA

In 1974, the expanded program of immunization (EPI) was launched globally by WHO with the goal of reducing morbidity and mortality from six target diseases: Tuberculosis, poliomyelitis, diphtheria, pertussis, tetanus and measles by providing immunization services for all children less than 5 years of age and pregnant women. The vaccines included were BCG, DPT, OPV, measles and tetanus toxoid.

In India, the EPI was launched in 1978, but the coverage of the program remained very low. In view of this—a revised strategy, Universal Immunization Program (UIP) was launched in 1985 to achieve target immunization goals in a phased and planned manner. The UIP targeted infants below 1 year of age against target diseases as well as pregnant women who were to be immunized against tetanus. The aim was to achieve 100% coverage of all pregnant women and at least 85% coverage of infants. The National Immunization Schedule of India is shown in **Table 5.9**. The schedule was devised to protect infants and children from 6 major vaccine, preventable diseases namely tuberculosis, diphtheria, pertussis, tetanus, poliomyelitis and measles.

The epidemiological patterns of the diseases are often different in different countries and thus the immunization schedule of one country often differs from another. Besides, the childhood immunization being a dynamic process, the disease patterns and the immunization needs can change in future as more information on diseases becomes available and the development of newer vaccines continues to take place. One of the examples is of hepatitis B vaccine (HBV) which though not administered universally in India, has been recommended by WHO to be included under national immunization program. A few states in India—Delhi, Puducherry, Goa, and Sikkim, have already introduced the MMR vaccine over the last few years. Other vaccines that have been used in state-specific programs include typhoid vaccine in Delhi.

Table 5.9 National Immunization Schedule	
Age	*Vaccine*
Birth	BCG, OPV (0), Hep B (0)
6 weeks	DPT (1), OPV (1), Hep B (1), Hib (1)*, IPV (intradermal)
10 weeks	DPT (2), OPV (2), Hep B (2), Hib (2)*
14 weeks	DPT (3), OPV (3), Hep B (3), Hib (3)*, IPV (intradermal)
9–12 months	Measles vaccine (1)
16–24 months	Measles vaccine (2)**
18–24 months	DPT (booster 1) (OPV (4)
5 years	DPT (booster 1)
10 years	TT
16 years	TT

In addition, Japanese encephalitis (JE) vaccination is provided in endemic districts, in a two dose schedule (1st dose: 9–12 mo age; 2nd dose 16–24 mo age).

*Hib (given as pentavalent vaccine containing Hib + DPT + Hep B) in selected states.

**Second dose of measles vaccine can also be given as MMR (measles, mumps, rubella) vaccine

IAP IMMUNIZATION SCHEDULE

The Indian Academy of Pediatrics (IAP) has suggested certain modifications and addition of vaccines in the current national immunization schedules, for use on individual level by pediatrician. IAP endorses the use of national immunization schedule, but in view of data available on vaccine preventable diseases (VPDs) and the availability of several vaccines, IAP recommends the use of vaccines for hepatitis A, *Haemophilus influenzae* type b, MMR, typhoid, pneumococcal, varicella, HPV, and rotavirus vaccine. The revised IAP schedule is provided in **Table 5.10**.

5.24 COLD CHAIN

The term cold chain is used to denote a chain of personnel, equipment, and processes which are utilized for maintaining the potency and effectiveness of vaccines by keeping them at recommended temperatures during transportation, distribution, and storage from the site of manufacture to the point of their actual use.

The cold chain plays a crucial role in the immunization process because vaccines are sensitive to heat and light and improper cold chain maintenance can irreversibly affect their potency and efficacy. The maintenance of cold chain alone accounts for approximately 14% of the total costs of immunization per year. The vital components of cold chain include the following;
- Proper monitoring, maintenance, handling and storage of vaccines;
- Transport and storage equipment; and
- Trained personnel.

HEAT SENSITIVE VACCINES

Vaccines are biological products and, therefore, vulnerable to the extreme temperature change. All the vaccines are

Table 5.10 IAP Immunization Schedule	
Age	*Vaccine*
Birth	BCG, OPV0, Hep B1
6 weeks	DPT 1, IPV 1, Hib 1, Hep B2, rotavirus 1, PCV 1
10 weeks	DPT 2, IPV 2, Hib 2, rotavirus 2, PCV 2
14 weeks	DPT 3, IPV 3, Hib 3, rotavirus 3, PCV 3
6 months	Hep B 3, OPV 1
9 months	OPV 2, MMR 1
9–12 months	Typhoid conjugate vaccine
12 months	Hep A1
15 months	MMR 2, varicella 1, PCV booster 1
16–18 months	DPT booster 1, IPV booster 1, Hib booster 1
18 months	Hep A2
2 years	Typhoid booster 1
4.5 to 6 years	DPT booster 2, OPV 3, varicella 2, typhoid booster 2
10 to 12 years	Tdap/ Td, HPV 3 doses at 0,1,6 mo (for girls only)
16 years	Td# / TT

Polio: All doses of IPV may be replaced with OPV, if former is unaffordable or unavailable; additional doses of OPV on all SIAs.

Vaccines recommended for high-risk children: Influenza vaccine; meningococcal vaccine; Japanese encephalitis vaccine; cholera vaccine; rabies vaccine; yellow fever vaccine; pneumococcal polysaccharide vaccine (PPSV 23)

High-risk category of children: Congenital or acquired immunodeficiency (including HIV infection); chronic cardiac, pulmonary (including asthma if treated with prolonged high-dose oral corticosteroids), hematologic, renal (including nephrotic syndrome), liver disease and diabetes mellitus; and children on long-term steroids, salicylates, immunosuppressive or radiation therapy.

sensitive to heat to some extent but some are more sensitive than others. Repeated exposure to high temperatures has a cumulative damaging effect on vaccine potency. The commonly used vaccines can be ranked according to their sensitivity to heat as shown in Fig. 5.2. The vaccines sensitive to freezing are shown in Fig. 5.3.

- Vaccines such as BCG, measles, MMR and rubella are both light- and heat-sensitive. These vaccines are supplied in vials made up of dark-brown glass, which protects them against damage from light. Care must be taken to cover and protect them from strong light at all times.
- The diluents must never be frozen and need to be stored between 2° and 8°Celsius.
- Vaccines containing aluminum-based adjuvants (DPT, DT, TT) are adversely affected by freezing temperatures. If these vaccines are accidentally frozen, they should not be used, and discarded.

STRUCTURE OF COLD CHAIN

The structure of cold chain consists of two aspects, which are complementary to each other.

a. *Fixed component* Walk in coolers, ice-lined refrigerators (ILR), deep freezers, and refrigerators.

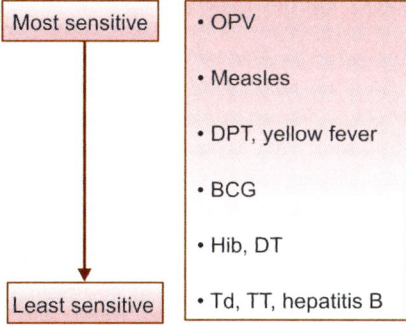

Fig. 5.2 Heat sensitivity of vaccines

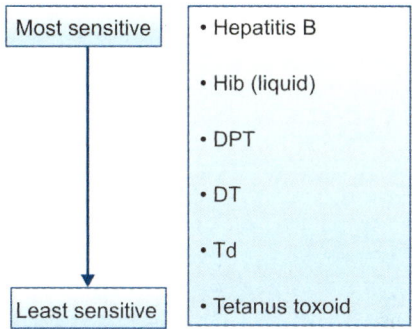

Fig. 5.3 Vaccine sensitivity to cold

b. The *mobile component* of the chain represented by isothermal boxes and ice boxes. These make it possible to transport the vaccines to health units and are effective for outreach services, the only requirement being that the vaccines are properly packed with the required number of frozen ice packs.

At the higher levels of cold chain; ie, national and regional, OPV must be kept frozen between –15° and –25° Celsius. Freeze-dried vaccines (BCG, measles, MMR, yellow fever) may also be kept frozen at –15° to –25° Celsius but it is neither essential nor recommended. All the vaccines at other levels of cold chain should be stored between +2° and +8° Celsius.

Care of Vaccines in Refrigerator

With the use of refrigerators for vaccine storage, the following guidelines must be followed:

- Refrigerator must be at least 10 cm away from the wall to allow proper air circulation.
- Ice packs to be kept in freezer compartment and water-filled bottles in the shelves.
- Store vaccine boxes or trays with spaces in between to allow air circulation inside the refrigerator.
- No vaccines should be stored in door compartment.
- Voltage control, and periodic defrosting (when the ice layer in freezer is more than 5 mm) are important maintenance issues.
- Vaccines should be used on the first in and first out basis.
- Temperature log should be done twice daily.

5

VACCINE VIAL MONITORS (VVM)

The vaccine vial monitor (VVM) is an indicator device applied to the each vial of vaccine and helps decide the potency of the vaccine at the time of its use. The VVM is a small square of heat sensitive material, which on exposure to heat becomes darker in color, thus giving a visual indicator of the usability of the particular vaccine vial of oral polio vaccine. Combined effects of time and temperature cause the VVM to change the color gradually from the light to dark and the outer colored circle is used as a reference to compare the color of VVM (Fig. 5.4). VVMs were first introduced on the vials of OPV in 1996. WHO and UNICEF have issued a policy statement in 1999 stating the value of VVM and recommend that agencies purchasing the vaccines request manufacturer to supply all the vaccines with VVM meeting WHO specifications.

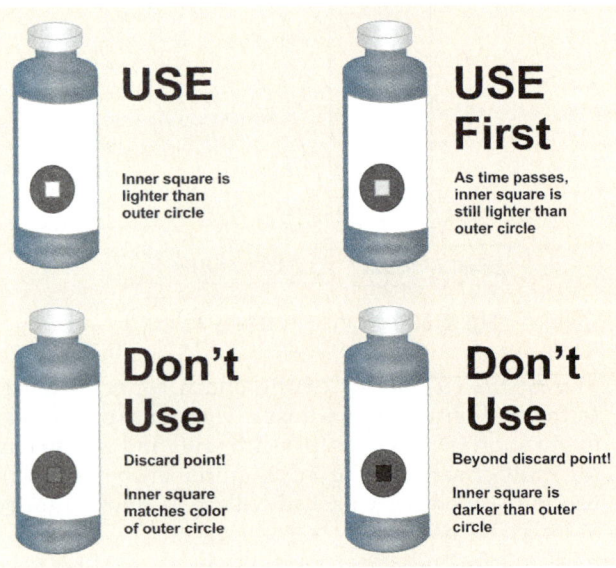

Fig 5.4 Vaccine vial monitor

5.25 VACCINE ADMINISTRATION

Infection Control and Sterile Techniques

The administration of vaccines should observe appropriate steps and precautions to minimize infection.
- The hands should be cleansed either with an alcohol-based waterless antiseptic hand rub or washed with soap and water between each patient contact.
- The needle and syringes used for injection must be sterile and disposable to minimize the risk of contamination and a separate needle and syringe should be used for each injection.
- The changing of needle between drawing the vaccine from the vial and injecting it into the recipient is not necessary.
- The vaccines should never be mixed in the same syringe unless specifically licensed for such use.

Route and Site of Administration

The vaccines should always be administered by their recommended route and at appropriate site. Deviation from the recommended route might reduce vaccine efficacy and/ or increase local side effects. The routes of administration for childhood vaccines are intradermal (BCG), subcutaneous (measles, MMR), intramuscular (DPT, TT, typhoid), oral (OPV), and intranasal (influenza).

The method of administration is partly determined by the presence of adjuvants in some vaccines and such vaccines should be given intramuscularly to avoid local irritation, inflammation and granuloma formation. Adjuvants are the agents (mostly aluminum salts), which are distinct from the antigen and enhance the immunogenicity of the vaccines. The common vaccines that contain adjuvant include DPT, DT, TT, Hib, HBV vaccines.

The subcutaneous injections are administered at a 45° angle usually in the thigh in infants and in the upper outer triceps area for children older than 12 months, using a 5/8 inch 23 to 25-gauge needle. The intramuscular injections are given at a 90° angle preferably into the anterolateral aspect of the thigh (infants < 12 months) as it provides a large muscle mass. The gluteal region should not be used for vaccine administration due to the potential risk of injury to sciatic nerve and a decreased immunogenic response to the vaccine. The deltoid muscle should be used for intramuscular injection, if the muscle mass is adequate in children older than 12 months.

A 23 to 25 gauge needle with a length of 0.6–1 inch is appropriate for intramuscular vaccines in infants and children. Separate sites should be used, if multiple vaccines are to be given during the same visit. If two vaccines are to be given in the same limb, these should be separated from each other by at least one inch, so that any local reaction can be differentiated.

Non-Standard Practices

The recommendation for the dosage, site and route of administration of immunobiologicals must be observed as any deviations from these recommendations can result in the inadequate protection of the vaccine recipient. A few of the examples of such practices include the gluteal/intradermal administration of HBV vaccine, which results in substantially lower immunogenicity of the vaccine. Similarly, the doses of rabies vaccine given in gluteal region should not be counted as valid doses and should be repeated. The usage of reduced dosages given at multiple immunization visits that equal a full dose or using smaller divided doses is also not recommended.

Injection Safety

WHO estimates that at least 50% of world's 12 billion injections administered each year are unsafe—posing serious health risk to recipients, health workers and the public. Unsafe injection practices can cause local infections like abscess and nerve injury and result in transmission of number of infections such as HBV, HCV and HIV. Improving the safety of injection is an important component of universal precautions. The essential steps for a safe injection include:
- Preparation with clean hands in a clean area.
- Medication to be drawn in from a sterile vial
- Use of sterile equipment at an appropriate site
- Immediate discarding of needles and syringes to prevent needle stick injuries, in labeled puncture-proof containers located in the same room where the vaccines are administered. Needles should not be recapped before being placed in the container for appropriate disposal.

Timing and Spacing Issues

While immunizing children, it is important to follow certain guidelines to derive the maximum benefit from the vaccines and to minimize the cost and the risk associated with vaccination. Optimal response to a vaccine depends upon multiple factors including the nature of the vaccine and the age and immune status of the recipient.

Spacing of Multiple Doses

The vaccines should be given as closely as possible to the recommended immunization schedule. Inactivated vaccines do not interfere with the immune response to other inactivated or live vaccines. An inactivated vaccine can be administered either simultaneously or any time before or after a different inactivated or live vaccine.

There should be an at least 4-week interval between the live injected vaccines (measles, MMR, varicella), if they are not administered on the same day. This is important to eliminate or reduce the interference from the vaccine given first on the vaccine given later. The dose of vaccine given too close to each other could reduce the efficacy of the vaccine. The recommended minimum interval for DPT and OPV vaccines in primary immunization is four weeks.

Simultaneous Administration

Most of the childhood vaccines can be safely and effectively be given simultaneously (during the same visit but not combined in the same syringe). Simultaneous administration of vaccines can improve the vaccine compliance and result in significant improvement of immunization rates in children. Simultaneous administration of most widely used live and inactivated vaccines does not result in decreased antibody response or an increased rate of adverse reactions. The rates of adverse reactions seen after the use of combination vaccines are similar to those seen after the most reactogenic component, if given separately. Unless the vaccines have been approved for mixing, individual vaccines should not be mixed together in the same syringe.

Spacing with Immunoglobulins

The presence of circulating antibody; eg, immunoglobulins may reduce to eliminate an immune response to the vaccine antigen. Inactivated vaccines are not affected by immunoglobulins and thus can be given before, after or at the same time as the immunoglobulins.

Blood (whole blood, packed cells, plasma) and other antibody containing blood products can inhibit the immune response to measles and rubella vaccines for three to four months. The effect of blood and immune globulin preparations on the response to mumps and varicella vaccines is unknown; however, commercial immune globulin preparations contain antibodies to these viruses. The length of time that interference with injectable live-virus vaccine (other than yellow fever) can persist after the antibody-containing product is a function of the amount of antigen-specific antibody contained in the product. Therefore, after an antibody-containing product is received, live vaccines (other than yellow fever, oral Ty21a typhoid, LAIV, zoster, and rotavirus) should be delayed until the passive antibody has degraded.

Interference can occur, if administering an antibody containing product becomes necessary after giving measles or MMR or MMRV vaccine. If the interval between administering any of these vaccines and subsequent administration of immunoglobulin is less than 14 days, the vaccination should be repeated after an interval of 3 to 6 months unless a serologic testing indicates an immune response. Response to oral polio vaccine, yellow fever vaccine and oral typhoid vaccine is not affected by antibody-containing product and thus these vaccines can be given simultaneously with blood products or separated by any interval.

5.26 IMMUNIZATION IN SPECIAL SITUATIONS

PRETERM BABIES

In the majority of preterm and low birth weight babies, immunizations should be carried out at the same chronological age and according to the same schedule and precautions as for full term infants and children. The full recommended doses of the vaccines should be used and divided or reduced doses are not recommended.

Decreased seroconversion rates might occur among certain preterm babies who are less than 2.0 kg at birth, after hepatitis B vaccine. However, if the mother is HBsAg positive and those with unknown HBsAg status, their babies should receive HBV vaccine and hepatitis B immunoglobulin (HBIg) prophylaxis within 12 hours of birth for immediate protection. The babies weighing less than 2.0 kg born to HBsAg negative mothers should receive the first dose of HBV vaccine at one month of age. All other EPI vaccines evoke satisfactory immune response in stable preterm/low birth weights who are otherwise stable.

LAPSED IMMUNIZATIONS

Due to persistence of immunologic memory, longer than routinely recommended intervals between the doses do not impair the immunologic response, to live and attenuated vaccines that need more than one dose to achieve primary immunity. Similarly delayed administration of booster doses does not adversely affect the antibody response to vaccines. The interruption of the recommended primary series or an extended and delayed interval for boosters does not need re-initiation of entire vaccination series.

UNKNOWN IMMUNIZATION STATUS

Such children should always be considered as being susceptible to the disease and age appropriate immunizations should be administered. There is nothing to suggest that the administration of polio vaccine, hepatitis B vaccine, MMR, Hib or varicella vaccine to already immune recipients is harmful. Td rather than DPT should be given to children who have unknown status and are above 7 years age. **Table 5.11** shows immunization for a child who has unknown/unimmunized status.

Missed opportunities for immunization are defined as situations when a child visits a health facility and is not immunized. Minor illnesses, such as fever, respiratory infections and diarrhea and malnutrition, should not be considered as contraindications to immunization.

Table 5.11 Immunization Schedule for Unimmunized Child

Age	Below 7 years	More than 7 years
First visit	BCG*, OPV*, DPT, HBV	Td, HBV
Second visit (1 month later)	DPT, OPV*, HBV	Td, HBV
Third visit (1 month later)	Measles or MMR, typhoid vaccine	MMR, typhoid vaccine
Fourth visit (6 months after 1st visit)	DPT/HBV	HBV

BCG/OPV recommended up to 5 years of age.

IMMUNIZATION OF ADOLESCENTS

The adolescents represent an important additional target group for immunization. Adolescents may not have received vaccines due to earlier unavailability of a few vaccines and they present unique challenges for immunization due to their life style and other social issues. Such visits for immunization provide opportunities for:
- Ensuring immunization for those adolescents not previously vaccinated with HBV vaccine, varicella vaccine or second dose of MMR vaccine.
- Administering a booster dose of Td vaccine.
- Administering other vaccines that may be recommended for certain adolescents and providing other recommended preventive and counseling services. The schedule for adolescent immunization is shown in **Table 5.12**.

CHILDREN WITH IMMUNE DEFICIENCY OR DYSFUNCTION

These conditions can be primary (such as inherited disorders of T- and B-cell dysfunction, phagocytic function or complement function) or may be secondary (malignancy, HIV infection, steroids/other immunosuppressive therapy and organ transplants). Primary and secondary immunodeficiencies might display a combination of deficits of both cellular and humoral immunity. The determination of immunocompetence in such children is important.
- Incidence or severity of certain diseases is higher and thus inactivated influenza and pneumococcal vaccines are recommended.
- Most of such children should not receive live viral/bacterial vaccines due to risk of serious disseminated disease caused by the vaccine strain. BCG, OPV, measles, MMR, oral typhoid and varicella vaccine should not be used.
- Toxoid and killed vaccines can be used safely in these children since they pose no threat.

- Vaccine efficacy is important consideration for such children. Due to their inability to mount adequate immune response, the vaccine efficacy may remain suboptimal. Specific serum antibodies need to be measured to evaluate immune response.
- Transmission of vaccine virus (such as OPV) from a household contact to immunocompromised host can occur and hence injectable poliovaccine (IPV) should be used for children living in the same house.

CHILDREN ON STEROID THERAPY

Children who are receiving 2 mg/kg/day or 20 mg/day of prednisolone or its equivalent are considered immuno-suppressed. Live vaccines should not be given to these children; killed/inactivated vaccines and toxoids are safe.

Corticosteroid therapy is not a contraindication to administering live vaccines, if the administration is short term (<2 weeks), a low to moderate dose (<20 mg prednisolone per day), long term alternate day therapy and for steroids given by topical, inhaled or intra-articular routes. Children who have received steroid therapy in high doses for more than two weeks should be vaccinated one month after stopping the treatment, as it is believed that the immune function would have returned to normal by then.

HIV INFECTION

Children infected by HIV are vulnerable to severe, recurrent, or unusual infections by vaccine preventable pathogens. The efficacy and safety of vaccines depends on the degree of immunodeficiency. In general, in early life, most vaccines are safe and efficacious as the immune system is relatively well preserved. The duration of protection may be compromised as there is impairment of memory response with immune attrition. Efficacy and safety are significantly lower in advanced disease. Consideration should be given

Table 5.12 Immunization Schedule for Adolescents

Vaccine	Age
Tdap/Td*	One dose at 11–12 years
HPV#	Three doses at 11–12 years
MMR vaccine	One dose, if not given earlier
Hepatitis B vaccine	Three doses 0, 1, 6 months, if not given earlier
Typhoid vaccine	V_i polysaccharide vaccine once every three years
Varicella vaccine	Two doses (4–8 weeks interval), if not given earlier
Hepatitis A vaccine	Two doses at 0 and 6 months, if not given earlier

*Tdap preferred to Td, followed by repeat Td every 10 years (Tdap to be used once only)
#Only females, three doses at 0, 1 or 2 (depending on the vaccine used) and 6 months

Table 5.13 Recommendations for Immunization of HIV Infected Children

Vaccine	Asymptomatic	Symptomatic
BCG	Yes (at birth)	No
DTwP/DTaP/TT/Td/Tdap	Yes as per routine schedule at 6 wk, 10 wk, 14 wk, 18 mo and 5 years	
Polio vaccines	IPV at 6, 10, 14 weeks, 15–18 months and 5 years. If indicated IPV to household contacts. If IPV is not affordable, OPV should be given*	
Measles vaccine	Yes at 9 months	Yes if CD4 count ≥15%
MMR vaccine	Yes, at 15 mo and 5 yr	Yes if CD4 count ≥15%
Hepatitis B	Yes, at 0, 1, 6 months	Yes, four doses, double dose, check for seroconversion, regular boosters
Hib	Yes, as per routine schedule at 6 wk, 10 wk, 14 wk, and 18 mo	
Pneumococcal vaccines (PCV and PPV 23)	Yes, as per routine schedule at 6 wk, 10 wk, 14 wk, and 15 mo	
Inactivated influenza vaccine	Yes as per routine schedule beginning at 6 mo, revaccination every year	
Rotavirus vaccine	Insufficient data to recommend	
Hepatitis A vaccine	Yes	Yes, check for seroconversion, boosters if needed
Varicella vaccine	Yes, two doses at 4–12 weeks interval	Yes, if CD4 count >15%, two doses at 4–12 weeks interval
Vi typhoid vaccine	Yes as per routine schedule at 2 years and every 3 years	
HPV vaccine	Yes (females only) as per routine schedule 3 doses at 0, 1–2, and 6 mo at 10 years	

* OPV has been found to be generally safe in HIV infected especially in early stages

to re-administering childhood immunizations to such children when their immune status has improved following anti-retroviral therapy. Vaccination of a baby born to an HIV positive mother but with an indeterminate HIV status should be as per the normal schedule. **Table 5.13** summarizes IAP recommendations for vaccination of HIV infected children.

CHILDREN WITH SPLENECTOMY

Children with anatomic or functional asplenia (such as sickle cell disease) are at an increased risk of infections with encapsulated organisms especially with *S. pneumoniae*, *N. meningitidis*, and *Haemophilus influenzae b*. Vaccines against these organisms should be considered at least two weeks before elective splenectomy, if possible. If these vaccines are not administered before surgery, they should be given as soon as the child's condition stabilizes after the surgery.

CHILDREN ON IMMUNOSUPPRESSIVE DRUGS

Whenever feasible, all indicated vaccines should be provided before the initiation of chemotherapy with immuno-suppressive drugs and radiation. Children with leukemia, solid tumors, or organ transplants are considered to be immunodeficient. Live vaccines should not be given for at least 3 months after such immunosuppressive treatment while inactivated vaccines given during chemotherapy might need to be repeated after immune competence is regained.

23-valent pneumococcal polysaccharide vaccine. WHO position paper.*Wkly Epidemiol Rec*. 2008;83:373–84.

Cholera vaccines: WHO position paper.*Wkly Epidemiol Rec*. 2010;85:117–28.

Global Programme for Vaccines and Immunization (GPV). The WHO position paper on Haemophilusinfluenzae type b conjugate vaccines. *Wkly Epidemiol Rec*. 1998;73:64–8.

Human papillomavirus vaccines. WHO position paper.*Wkly Epidemiol Rec*. 2009;84:118–31.

IAP Committee on Immunization. Consensus Recommendations on Immunization and IAP Immunization Timetable 2012. *Indian Pediatr*. 2012; 49:549–64.

Measles vaccines: WHO position paper.*Wkly Epidemiol Rec*. 2009;84:349–60.

Meningococcal vaccines: WHO position paper, November 2011.*Wkly Epidemiol Rec*. 2011;86:521–39.

Pertussis vaccines: WHO position paper.*Wkly Epidemiol Rec*. 2010; 85:385–400.

Pneumococcal conjugate vaccine for childhood immunization—WHO position paper.*Wkly Epidemiol Rec*. 2007;82:93–104.

Pneumococcal vaccines. WHO position paper.*Wkly Epidemiol Rec*. 1999 Jun;74:177–83.

Polio vaccines and polio immunization in the pre-eradication era: WHO position paper.*Wkly Epidemiol Rec*. 2010;85:213–28.

Rabies vaccines. WHO position paper.*Wkly Epidemiol Rec*. 2007;82:425–35.

Rubella vaccines: WHO position paper.*Wkly Epidemiol Rec*. 2011 86:301–16.

Typhoid vaccines: WHO position paper.*Wkly Epidemiol Rec*. 2008;83:49–59.

Varicella vaccines. WHO position paper.*Wkly Epidemiol Rec*. 1998;73:241–8.

Vashishtha VM, Ajay K, Thacker N. FAQs on Vaccine and Immunization Practices. New Delhi: Jaypee Brothers; 2011.

WHO.Pertussis vaccines—WHO position paper.*Wkly Epidemiol Rec*. 2005 ;80:31–9.

World Health Organization. WHO position paper on Haemophilusinfluenzae type b conjugate vaccines.(Replaces WHO position paper on Hib vaccines previously published in the Weekly Epidemiological Record.*Wkly Epidemiol Rec*. 2006;81:445–52.

World Health Organization.BCG vaccine. WHO position paper.*Wkly Epidemiol Rec*. 2004;79:27–38.

World Health Organization.Yellow fever vaccine. WHO position paper.*Wkly Epidemiol Rec*. 2003;78:349–59.

Yewale V, Choudhury P, Thacker N. IAP Guide Book on Immunization, IAP Committee on Immunization 2009–11.

Niranjan Shendurnikar and Pareshkumar A Thakkar

5

Infections and Infestations

Infections are defined as invasion of the body with organisms which have a potential to cause disease. Most of the hospitalizations and deaths due to childhood infections occur in developing countries; where it is estimated that 5 groups of illnesses: Acute respiratory infections (ARI), diarrheal illnesses, malaria, measles and other vaccine-preventable diseases, and congenital infections (principally HIV), cause deaths of millions of children every year.

Apart from community-acquired infections, children are also vulnerable to nosocomial infections in traditionally open wards and modern intensive care units. Another major threat is the increasing incidence of resistance to antimicrobials for common infections, due to irrational use of antibiotics.

6.1 FEVER

Fever is a condition in which the body's temperature is elevated as a result of the body's thermostat (ie, hypo-thalamus) being reset to a higher than usual temperature. Fever occurs in response to a variety of insults, infection being the most common. Fever is induced by pyrogens. Bacteria, fungi, viruses, malignancies, connective tissue disorders, certain drugs, and trauma may endogenously stimulate production of pyrogens.

- Common *endogenous pyrogens* include interleukin-1 (IL-1), tumor necrosis factor (TNF) and interferon. Other endogenous pyrogens include IL-6, IL-11, leukemia inhibitory factor (LIF), ciliary neurotropic factor (CNTF) and oncostatin-M.

- *Exogenous pyrogens* include the bacterial cell wall component lipopolysaccharide (LPS), enterotoxins, and exotoxins. Exogenous pyrogens can induce production of endogenous pyrogens via activation of Toll signaling, and both endogenous and exogenous pyrogens stimulate the synthesis of prostaglandins (PG). Prostaglandin E_2 (PGE_2) is the ultimate endogenous pyrogen. It resets the temperature of the hypothalamus. Aspirin acts as an antipyretic by inhibiting cyclo-oxygenase (COX) 1 and 2, the rate limiting enzyme in PGE_2 synthesis. Ibuprofen is also a COX-inhibitor.

Definition of Fever

Body (rectal) temperature normally fluctuates between 36.6 °C in the morning and 37.9 °C in the evening. Because of the normal variation in body temperature, there is no single value that can be used as cut-off to define fever. However, a clinically significant fever is generally defined as a rectal temperature of 100.4°F (38°C) or higher. This is equivalent to an oral temperature of 99.5°F (37.5°C), and axillary (armpit) temperature of 99°F (37.2°C).

Fever above 41.5°C (107°F) is called *hyperpyrexia* and warrants aggressive antipyretic therapy because of risk of irreversible organ damage. Usual underlying etiology of hyperpyrexia includes meningitis, pneumonia, bacteremia, and heatstroke in tropical climates. Acetaminophen (paracetamol), non-steroidal anti-inflammatory drugs (NSAIDs) and steroids are effective antipyretics.

Fever may be beneficial in the sense that it increases host defense mechanisms, augments immunological functions, and suppresses growth of some microbes. However, there is no overwhelming evidence against use of antipyretic therapy for fever in children. Fever in children increases the risk of febrile seizure and should, therefore, be cautiously handled.

Initial Assessment

Before proceeding to identifying the etiology of fever, it is essential to clinically assess the child for vital signs and severity of illness. This includes assessing the general look and behavior of the patient, measurement of temperature, heart rate, respiratory rate, capillary refill time, blood pressure and pulse oximetry. Watch the patient for any evidence of cyanosis or dehydration (in form of dry mucosa, decreased skin turgor and bulging or depressed fontanel). The criteria to define tachycardia, tachypnea, and hypotension are shown in **Table 6.1**.

- All children with cardiopulmonary compromise should be provided with immediate life-saving resuscitative procedures to ensure earliest restoration of airway, breathing and circulation.
- SpO_2 less than 94% is considered hypoxia. It should be aggressively managed with oxygen and respiratory support, if needed.
- Capillary refill time of more than 3 seconds suggests poor perfusion and demands immediate intervention in form of isotonic fluids and ionotropes.

In children older than 6 months, do not use height of body temperature alone to identify those with serious illness. One should not also use the duration of fever to predict the likelihood of serious illness. Besides, in neonates, fever may or may not be present during systemic infections. They may alternatively present with hypothermia.

Table 6.1 Cut-off values for Heart Rate, Respiratory Rate and Blood Pressure		
Tachycardia	*Tachypnea*	*Hypotension (1–10 years)*
<12 months: >160 beats/min	<2 months: >60 breaths/min	<1 year: SBP<70 mm Hg
12–24 months: >150 beats/min	2–12 months: >50 breaths/min	1–10 years: SBP <(70 + age*2)
2–5 years: >140 beats/min	1–5 years: >40 breaths/min	>10 years: SBP<90 mm Hg

Etiology of Fever

The commonest cause of fever in children is a viral infection. In viral infection, fever is usually short-lived and signs are usually more generalized than those with bacterial infection. Common viral and bacterial illnesses like colds, gastroenteritis, ear infections, croup, and bronchiolitis are the most likely illnesses known to cause short fevers. The classical signs of an upper respiratory tract infection are coryza, inflamed tympanic membranes, fever or tonsillitis. Bacterial tonsillitis and otitis media are difficult to differentiate from viral causes, but a bacterial otitis media is more likely to be unilateral. Viral infections usually resolve within a week of onset. Persistence of fever for a longer period demands thorough investigation. The term 'fever of unknown origin' has been used to denote fever persisting for more than 21 days.

Evaluation of a Febrile Child

A good history and thorough examination are essential for the early diagnosis of fever in childhood. The history should include questions regarding characteristics of fever (onset, intensity, duration, and type of fever—continuous, remittent or intermittent); localizing symptoms of fever; vaccination; past history of any significant illnesses such as congenital heart disease or tuberculosis; and family history of members with fever; and recent history of contact with infectious disease.

Ask about any other symptom that the child is having. This will give an important clue in localizing the disease to a particular system. Examination should take note of the following:

1. *General condition* whether alert, active, playful, irritable, lethargic, or comatose?
2. *Rash*. If present, appeared on which day of fever? Describe: Macular, papular, maculopapular, vesicular, or pustular.
3. Examination for pallor, icterus, clubbing, edema.
4. Examination of eyes for conjunctivitis and ears for suppurative otitis media.
5. *Throat examination* for tonsillar enlargement (tonsillitis), pharyngeal membrane (for diphtheria).
6. Examination of *neck*, axillae and inguinal region for lymphadenopathy.
7. Palpation of *abdomen* for hepatosplenomegaly or other abdominal masses or tenderness.
8. Examination of genitalia for any swelling, pain, or redness.
9. Examination of *chest* for any abnormal chest signs.
10. Examination of *bones and joints* for swelling or tenderness.
11. *Cardiovascular system* examination for murmurs.
12. Rule out *neck rigidity* and other *meningeal signs*.

Once an appropriate history has been taken and examination performed, the next steps are to (*i*) localize the fever to a particular organ system by presenting complaints; and to (*ii*) identify the probable etiology of fever, depending upon its duration, and clinical examination.

A. Localizing the Focus of Fever

Every effort should be made to delineate the system involved, based on following localizing symptoms.

Exanthematous fevers: Rash, mucosal erythema, nodules, pustules, maculopapular rash.

Upper respiratory tract: Cough, cold, coryza, throat pain, difficulty in swallowing, earache, hoarse voice, stridor, regional lymphadenopathy.

Lower respiratory tract: Cough, difficult and fast breathing, wheezing, chest pain, sputum production.

Urinary tract: *Upper*: Vomiting, abdominal pain, diarrhea; *Lower*: burning micturition, frequency, urgency, hematuria.

Gastrointestinal and hematological systems: Pallor, rash, bleeding from any site, petechiae, ecchymosis, lymph node enlargement, joint or bone pains, lump in abdomen.

CNS involvement: Vomiting, nausea, headache, altered sensorium, seizures, abnormal movements, abnormality of tone, opisthotonus, neck rigidity, irritability, and photophobia.

Hepatobiliary system: Jaundice, abdominal distension, diarrhea, and vomiting.

Cardiovascular system: Dyspnea, palpitation, chest pain, pedal edema, prominent neck veins, and cough.

Musculoskeletal system: Joint swelling, pain or limited movements in a muscle group, or joint.

B. Identify the Etiology of Fever

Short duration Fevers

Fever of less than 2 weeks duration is usually infectious in origin, and due to viruses, bacteria or protozoa. Many of these patients recover completely, even before a precise diagnosis is made or treatment is given. These children may present with or without localizing manifestations. Localizing symptoms can give a clue as to the etiology of fever, as detailed in **Table 6.2**.

Prolonged Fever

Fever lasting for more than 2 weeks requires a different approach. Infections still remain the most important cause of prolonged fever; however, non-infectious causes are also responsible. Common causes of prolonged fever are listed below:

1. *Infections* Tuberculosis, urinary tract infections, HIV, chronic fungal infections, etc.

6

Table 6.2 Determining Etiology of Fever based on Presenting Features

Cough and coryza	Viral fever
Rash	Exanthematous illnesses like measles, rubella, chickenpox, erythema infectiosum, roseola infantum, herpes simplex; or other illnesses like meningococcemia, dengue, Henoch-Schönlein purpura, leukemia, and Kawasaki disease
Ear pain	Acute suppurative otitis media (ASOM)
Skin boils	Abscess, pustules, cellulitis, impetigo
Fast breathing and cough	Pneumonia, bronchiolitis, pleural effusion, tuberculosis
Joint swelling	Septic arthritis, rheumatic fever, tubercular arthritis, connective tissue diseases
Vomiting	Gastritis, gastroenteritis, viral hepatitis, meningitis, enteric fever
Diarrhea	Gastroenteritis, enteric fever, dysentery
Urinary frequency, burning micturition, or crying during micturition	Urinary tract infection
Chills or pallor or jaundice	Malaria, hepatobiliary involvement
Altered sensorium	Meningoencephalitis (bacterial, viral, tubercular), cerebral malaria, enteric encephalopathy, brain abscess
Abdominal pain	Gastroenteritis, appendicitis, liver abscess, hepatitis, cholecystitis

2. *Inflammatory disorders* Rheumatoid arthritis, systemic lupus erythematosus, Kawasaki disease, and other connective tissue disorders including polyarteritis nodosa, Behcet disease, Wegener granulomatosis.
3. *Malignancies* Lymphoma (including Hodgkin disease), leukemia, hepatoblastoma, Wilms tumor, neuroblastoma, brain tumors, etc.
4. *Endocrine causes* Thyrotoxicosis, diabetes insipidus.
5. *Hematological and immune deficiency disorders* Spherocytosis, agranulocytosis, hemolytic anemia; disorders of T or B cells; disorders of phagocytosis.
6. *Neurologic disorders* Familial dysautonomia, hypothalamic and third ventricle lesions; anhidrotic ectodermal dysplasia.
7. *Miscellaneous causes* Drug fever, periodic fever, factitious fever.

Table 6.3 provides a detailed list of common causes of fever associated with hepatosplenomegaly, rash, or lymphadenopathy. When fever has been persistent for a week, and no cause has been found, serious consideration should be given to hospital admission to confirm pyrexia and initiate investigations.

Treatment   **Fever**

The primary objective of treating a child with fever is to improve the comfort of the child. The primary focus should not be on normalization of body temperature; though this is acceptable as a secondary outcome following measures taken to make the child (and parents) comfortable.

There are two major methods of antipyresis:

1. *Non-pharmacological* Environmental measures, fluids, and hydrotherapy; and
2. *Pharmacological* Antipyretics.

Non-pharmacological Antipyresis

Non-pharmacological methods include environmental modifications, increased fluid intake, and sponging or hydrotherapy.

Table 6.3 Etiology of Fever with Rash, Lymphadenopathy, and Hepatosplenomegaly

1. Fever with Hepatosplenomegaly
A. *Infectious causes*
   Malaria, enteric fever, kala-azar, tuberculosis, infectious mononucleosis, brucellosis, echinococcosis, TORCH infection, dengue, septicemia, and infective endocarditis.
B. *Malignancies*
   Leukemias, lymphomas, histiocytosis, infantile hemangio-endothelioma, hepatoblastoma, and metastases.
C. *Connective tissue diseases*
   Systemic lupus erythematosus (SLE); systemic juvenile rheumatoid arthritis (JRA), sarcoidosis, scleroderma, and rheumatic fever
D. *Chronic hepatitis/chronic liver disease*
   Autoimmune hepatitis, chronic hepatitis B/C, and Wilson disease.

2. Fever with Rash
A. *Infectious causes*
   Meningococcemia, dengue, measles, rubella, varicella, roseola infantum, erythema infectiosum, herpes simplex, and lupus vulgaris.
B. *Malignancies*
   Leukemia and histiocytosis
C. *Vasculitis*
   Henoch-Schönlein purpura, Kawasaki disease, rheumatic fever, systemic JRA, and SLE

3. Fever with Lymphadenopathy and/or hepatosplenomegaly
• Suppurative lymphadenitis (bacterial, often accompanying pharyngitis, tonsillitis, dental infections, scalp infections)
• Tuberculosis
• Lymphoma (Hodgkin and non-Hodgkin lymphomas)
• Histiocytosis
• Acute lymphoblastic leukemia (ALL)
• HIV infection
• Connective tissue disorders such as systemic JRA or sarcoidosis
• Kawasaki disease

A. *Environmental measures*

Environmental measures include placing the child in cool and airy environment (21–22°C) which enhances heat loss by convection. Minimal clothing, ie, dressing the child in only one layer of clothing is advocated as this further enhances heat loss. Some theories even support a gentle body massage to dilate the cutaneous blood vessels which further increases heat dissipation.

B. *Hydration*

As fever increases, the metabolic loss of the body also needs to be compensated. For each 1°C rise of temperature above 37.2°C, there is an increase in insensible water loss of 7 mL/kg body weight/day. Hence extra fluid intake is advised in febrile patients. For each 1°C of increase in temperature, a 12% increase in fluid intake is recommended.

C. *Sponging or hydrotherapy*

It is considered the mainstay of non-pharmacological antipyresis. External cooling lowers the temperature of febrile patients by evaporation, conduction and convection. Evaporation is rated as the most effective physical mean of promoting heat loss in febrile children because it has the least capacity to induce shivering. External cooling acts by impairing the overwhelming effect or mechanisms that have been evoked by elevated thermoregulatory set point; rather than by lowering the elevated set point. The capacity of external cooling to lower core temperature is limited because it induces both cutaneous vasoconstriction and shivering. Therefore, unless concomitant antipyretic therapy or other pharmacological methods are used to abolish shivering, external cooling is vigorously opposed in febrile patients by thermoregulatory mechanisms endeavoring to maintain elevated temperature.

Sponging should be done by continuous wiping of the body with tepid water (28–30°C) from head to toe for 15–20 minutes. Sponging action ensures that water film is constantly moving thus maximizing heat conduction. Tepid sponging acts by conduction of heat from skin to cooler water.

Studies indicate that use of hydrotherapy alone is clearly inferior for reduction of fever for periods longer than 30 minutes after initiation of treatment. However, external cooling could still be of value, if it potentiates activity of antipyretics.

Results of randomized trials comparing the combination of antipyretics and physical methods with antipyretics alone have provided mixed results. In 4 out of 7 such studies, the combination treatment was superior to use of antipyretics alone for reduction of temperature during first 30 minutes of initiation of therapy and overall. In three other studies, both modes of treatment were equally effective in lowering temperature. It is recommended to administer antipyretic drugs at least 30 minutes before sponging.

However, main disadvantage of hydrotherapy as compared to use of drugs is patient discomfort and shivering. Shivering not only impedes cooling during fever but also imposes considerable metabolic burden. Studies in volunteers have shown that shivering increases the oxygen consumption, respiratory minute volume, respiratory quotient, increase in percentage of carbon dioxide in exhaled air during exposure to cold and increase in mean arterial pressure. Perhaps in febrile patients with cardiovascular disease, external cooling can cause coronary artery vasoconstriction by cold press or response and thus decrease coronary perfusion. Sponging, though rapid in reduction of temperature, has an ill sustained effect.

Indications for immediate sponging with lukewarm water include the following: (*i*) febrile delirium; (*ii*) febrile seizure; or (*iii*) fever >41.1°C. Paracetamol should be given 30 minutes prior to sponging. Heatstroke requires cold water sponging. An absorbent towel should be soaked, rinsed and placed on the legs, trunk and forehead in order to reduce the body temperature. Hydrotherapy should be continued till the body temperature comes down to 38°C.

Pharmacological Antipyresis

Commonly available antipyretics are aspirin, paracetamol, indomethacin, mefenemic acid, and ibuprofen. Aspirin was the first antipyretic used in children. However, after reports of its association with causation of Reye's syndrome, aspirin is not recommended in children.

Mechanism of action

Paracetamol, aspirin and other NSIADs all seem to block conversion of arachidonic acid to PGE_2 by inhibiting COX, the enzyme that catalyses rate limiting step from arachidonic acid of prostacyclin H_2 the precursor of all PG isomers. Paracetamol and NSAIDs differ with respect to their relative potencies as inhibitors of peripheral and central nervous system COX. Paracetamol is nearly as effective as aspirin and 10% as effective as indomethacin in inhibiting central COX but only 5% as effective as aspirin and 0.02% as effective as indomethacin in inhibiting peripheral COX. Brain COX is more sensitive to inhibition by paracetamol than spleen COX and thus the relatively weak action of paracetamol against peripheral COX accounts for its poor anti-inflammatory response.

Available drugs

Paracetamol It is clearly established as the most commonly used standard antipyretic and analgesic. The recommended dose is 15 mg/kg at 4–6 hourly intervals not exceeding 60 mg/kg/day. Compared to 10 mg/kg, the dose of 15 mg/kg maintains lower temperature for longer time and is more effective in decreasing the mean temperature from baseline. Paracetamol reduces the temperature by 2–3°F after 2 hours of intake. The rate of fall of temperature is directly related to the initial temperature. Greater the initial temperature, greater is the fall after drug intake and *vice versa*. Hence drug administration in low grade temperature may not lead to any significant fall. On the other hand, antipyretic treatment in high grade fevers (>104°F) would result in reduction of temperature by 2°F, thus failing to touch the baseline.

Ibuprofen It belongs to propionic acid group of NSAIDs. Efficacy of paracetamol and ibuprofen has been compared in a number of studies, with variable results. Some studies have shown greater antipyretic effect with 10 mg/kg of ibuprofen as compared to 15 mg/kg of paracetamol. Ibuprofen has the advantage of longer duration of antipyresis (8 hours) as compared to paracetamol (4 hours).

Ibuprofen can also be used as a first-line antipyretic. Recent evidence indicates that there is no difference in the safety and effectiveness of paracetamol and ibuprofen in the care of a generally healthy child with fever. There is evidence that combining these 2 drugs is more effective than using them alone. However, this should not be followed as a routine because of associated risk of inappropriate dosages. The practice of alternating ibuprofen and paracetamol has limited value.

Choice of antipyretic

With extensive commercial claims and counterclaims about the antipyretics drugs, the decision regarding the use of antipyretic should be based on personal experience, scientific data regarding efficacy, safety, duration of effect and cost. Aspirin and paracetamol are equally effective at similar doses. Ibuprofen is also efficacious and has longer duration of action. In therapeutic dosages, aspirin is more toxic and causes considerable gastritis, gastrointestinal bleeding, impaired platelet function, diminished urinary excretion of sodium, Reye's syndrome and blunted immune response. These side effects are known to occur less frequently with ibuprofen and none with paracetamol. Paracetamol can be used in children with asthma, with sensitivity to aspirin or ibuprofen, coagulation disorders, peptic ulcer or reflux esophagitis. No association has been seen with the use of acetaminophen and development of Reye's syndrome in children or adolescents who have influenza or chickenpox. Thus, paracetamol is considered to be the safest antipyretic in children at therapeutic dosages.

Parental Education

As fever is so common and causes considerable parental anxiety and concern, parents should be counseled adequately. Most parents suffer from so-called fever phobia and hence parental education will be an important step towards decreasing this. Fever issues such as what is fever, what is high grade fever, are all fever harmful and should be treated, which fever should be treated and how, when should a doctor be consulted need to be addressed. Parents should be told that fever is a protective response of body and helps to fight the disease.

The facts that (*i*) *fever per se is just a symptom of underlying illness and not a disease itself;* and (*ii*) *underlying disease and not thermometer is to be treated* should be highlighted. Low fevers in absence of associated risks are harmless and should be left untreated. Medicines should be used only when indicated. Aspirin use for control of fever should be discouraged in children. Febrile children should be advised to drink plenty of water and wear as little as possible. The fact that febrile seizures occur in minority of children and are benign and do not cause any permanent brain damage or epilepsy should be told to parents to prevent unnecessary panic. In children who have a past history of such seizure, close monitoring is required. Parents should be told about the danger signs of fever and when to consult a doctor. This will prevent unnecessary phone calls and outpatient attendance.

Fever Management Guidelines

Recently new guidelines on management of fever in children have been released. A summary of these are highlighted in **Boxes 6.1–6.3.**

HEAT HYPERPYREXIA

Heat hyperpyrexia is not an unusual cause of fever in tropical countries where ambient temperature may go as high as 45°C. Heat hyperpyrexia may occur even without exposure of the child to the direct sunlight. The predisposing factors include high temperature and humidity in the environment,

---

Box 6.1 NICE (National Institute for Care and Health Excellence) Guidelines, 2013

- For infants less than 4 weeks, body temperature should be measured in axilla with an electronic thermometer. For children 4 weeks to 5 years, electronic thermometer in axilla or infrared tympanic thermometer should be used.
- Forehead chemical thermometers are not recommended due to poor reliability.
- Antipyretic agents do not prevent febrile convulsions and hence not to be used specifically for this purpose
- Use antipyretics only till child appears distressed.
- Tepid sponging is not recommended for treatment of fever.
- Children with fever should not be underdressed or overwrapped.

Source: Fever in under 5s: assessment and initial management. National Institute for Care and Health Excellence. NICE 2013

Box 6.2 Italian Pediatric Society Guidelines 2017

- For infants less than 4 weeks, body temperature should be measured in axilla with an electronic thermometer. For children 4 weeks to 5 years, electronic thermometer in axilla or infrared tympanic thermometer should be used.
- Use of paracetamol/ibuprofen is not recommended prophylactically to reduce the incidence of fever and local reactions in children undergoing vaccination.
- Combined or alternating use of paracetamol/ibuprofen is not recommended.
- Ibuprofen is not recommended in chickenpox/Kawasaki disease.
- Preventive use of Ibuprofen is not recommended in prevention of febrile seizure.
- Paracetamol/ibuprofen is contraindicated in known case of NSAID induced asthma but not in other febrile children with asthma.

Source: Chiappini E, Veturini E, Principi N et al. 2016 Update of the Italian Pediatric Society Guidelines for Management of Fever in Children. J Pediatr 2017.

Box 6.3 Consensus Guidelines on Febrile Child Presenting to the Emergency Department in India 2017

- Rectal temperature is the preferred method of temperature determination in very young children.
- Temporal artery and tympanic membrane thermometer can be used for quick access of temperature.
- Evaluation and management of well looking child is based on defined age groups: neonate (<28 days), young infant (29–90 days), old infant and young child (91 days–2 years) and children >2 years
- In patients with fever without localization, chest X-ray is mandatory for neonates whereas in young infants, chest X-ray is indicated, if temperature >102.2°F, leukocyte count >20,000/mm^3 or respiratory distress is present.

Source: Mahajan P, Batra P, Thakur N et al. Consensus Guidelines on Evaluation and Management of the Febrile Child Presenting to the Emergency Department in India. Indian Pediatr. 2017

---

unsuitable clothing, dehydration and debilitating illness, such as malaria, pneumonia, measles and renal disorders. Invariably, heat hyperpyrexia is associated with cessation of sweating. Children with ectodermal dysplasia and absence of sweat glands are more prone to develop episodes of heat hyperpyrexia.

The onset of high fever may be quite sudden. The rectal temperature may exceed 42°C to 43°C. The skin appears hot and dry (without sweating). Tachycardia and tachypnea are present. The loss of consciousness occurs early. The patient may develop peripheral circulatory failure and hemorrhages. Headache, faintness, abdominal discomfort and delirium are usually complained of. The liver and kidney failure may complicate heat hyperpyrexia.

Treatment	Heat Hyperpyrexia

When the temperature exceeds 41°C, body of the child below the neck should be immersed in the cold water without further delay to prevent irreversible brain damage. The parents should be reassured that this seemingly drastic measures will not induce shock. Ice cold bath does not cause significant vasoconstriction. The rectal temperature should be recorded continuously and the hydrotherapy should be discontinued as the temperature falls below 38°C.

Fever

1. Fever is defined as rectal temperature of 100.4°F or higher.
2. The height and duration of fever should not be considered criteria to judge the severity of the illness.
3. Paracetamol 15 mg/kg/dose is the optimal symptomatic treatment for fever.
4. Combined or alternating use of paracetamol and ibuprofen should be avoided.

Bartfai T, Conti B. Fever. *Scientific World Journal.* 2010;10:490–503.

Chiappini E, veturini E, Principi, N et al. 2016 Update of the Italian Pediatric Society Guidelines for Management of Fever in Children. *J Pediatr* 2017;180:177–83.

Cunha BA. Fever myths and misconceptions: the beneficial effects of fever as a critical component of host defenses against infection. *Heart Lung.* 2012; 41:99–101.

Fever in under 5s: assessment and initial management. National Institute for Care and Health Excellence. NICE 2013. Available at nice.org.uk/guidance/cg160. Accessed on 20 June 2016.

Gupta H, Shah D, Gupta P, Sharma KK. Role of paracetamol in treatment of childhood Fever: a double-blind randomized placebo controlled trial. *Indian Pediatr.* 2007;44:903–11.

Hay AD, Redmond NM, Costelloe C, *et al.* Paracetamol and ibuprofen for the treatment of fever in children: the PITCH randomised controlled trial. *Health Technol Assess.* 2009;1–163.

Hoover L. AAP reports on the use of antipyretics for Fever in children. *Am Fam Physician.* 2012 ;85:518–9.

Kiekkas P. Peak fever: helpful or harmful? *Heart Lung.* 2011;40:272–3.

McIntyre J. Management of fever in children. *Arch Dis Child.* 2011;96:1173–4.

Mahajan P, Batra P, Thakur N, et al. Consensus Guidelines on Evaluation and Management of the Febrile Child Presenting to the Emergency Department in India. *Indian Pediatr.* 2017.

Sarkar R, Mishra K, Garg VK. Fever with rash in a child in India. *Indian J Dermatol Venereol Leprol.* 2012;78:251–62.

Sherman JM, Sood SK. Current challenges in the diagnosis and management of fever. *Curr Opin Pediatr.* 2012;24:400–6.

Section on Clinical Pharmacology and Therapeutics; Committee on Drugs, Sullivan JE, Farrar HC. Fever and antipyretic use in children. *Pediatrics.* 2011;127:580–7.

Walsh A. Available evidence does not support routine administration of antipyretics to reduce duration of fever or illness. *Evid Based Nurs.* 2011;14:58–9.

Young PJ, Saxena MK, Beasley RW. Fever and antipyresis in infection. *Med J Aust.* 2011;195:458–9.

6.2 FEVER WITHOUT FOCUS

Fever without focus refers to fever, not presenting with any other symptom-complex. It is further categorized as "fever without localizing sign" and "fever of unknown origin".

Fever without localizing signs or fever without a source is defined as fever for less than a week without adequate explanation after a thorough history and physical examination. This should be differentiated from **fever of unknown origin (FUO)** defined as fever (rectal temperature >38.3°C) of more than 3 weeks duration documented by a health care provider, for which the specific diagnosis could not be established even after 1 week of admission and investigation in a hospital setting. The recent literature has shown the duration of FUO to vary from 1 week to 3 weeks in different settings.

1. Fever without Localizing Signs

These children are represented by short duration fever (< 7 days), having no symptoms or signs that could indicate involvement of a particular system or a probable etiology. These children represent an important group because of higher risk of occult bacteremia and serious bacterial infections (range 5–20%). Therefore, it may sometimes become essential to start specific and empirical treatment without establishing an etiological diagnosis.

Approach to a child with fever without localizing signs will primarily depend upon his/her age; as the risk of occult bacteremia, risk of severe bacterial infection, and common etiological diagnosis are different for newborn, young infants (1–3 months), and children (3 months–3 years).

A. Neonates and Fever without Localizing Signs

Newborns having a fever without any localizing signs are the most tricky to evaluate. Evaluation should start with consideration of possibility of dehydration fever, especially in tropical climate. Such infants would usually respond to increased fluid intake and control of environmental temperature.

Serious bacterial infection (SBI) should be considered a possibility even in an apparently otherwise healthy neonate with fever, if there is no response to these measures. SBI include meningitis, pneumonia, urinary tract infection, osteomyelitis, septic arthritis, and occult bacteremia. In India, *H. influenzae* B and *Streptococcus* are still considered as important causes of SBI, besides *Klebsiella, Staphylococcus aureus,* and *E. coli.* In recent times, the incidence of SBI caused by *H. influenzae* and *Streptococcus* has come down due to vaccination against these infections. Malaria, scrub typhus, dengue, and chikungunya should also be considered as strong possibilities in endemic areas.

All febrile neonates without focus should be hospitalized. Initial management should consist of environmental cooling and frequent breastfeeding. Non-responders should be subjected to sepsis screen (blood counts, urine microscopy, blood culture, urine culture, chest X-ray, and peripheral smear for malarial parasite, peripheral blood smear for band forms, toxic granules, vacuolization, and immature/total neurtophil ratio, rickettsial, dengue and chikungunya serology in endemic cases). Cerebrospinal fluid examination should also be done in children who appear lethargic or fail to breastfeed. Empirical antibiotics should be started. Cefotaxime 150–200 mg/kg or ceftriaxone 100 mg/kg/d is the initial agent of choice. Ampicillin (50–100 mg/kg/d IM or IV q 12 h) should be added in infants below 4 weeks of age, to cover *Listeria* and enterococci.

B. Fever in Young Infants between 1 and 3 months of Age

Febrile infants ≤3 months with diminished spontaneous activity, lethargy, respiratory compromise (tachypnea, chest retraction and grunting), diminished muscle tone, mottled cool extremities, irritability, and weak sucking are at high risk. They must be evaluated for sepsis by complete blood count, lumbar puncture, blood culture, urinalysis, urine culture and chest radiograph. *Haemophilus influenzae, E. coli,* pneumococcus, enterococci and *Neisseria meningitidis* infections are a major cause of bacterial infections at this age.

Infants 1–3 months of age with fever who appear well and had been previously healthy, and have a normal physical examination, can be categorized as at 'low-risk' or 'high-risk' for serious bacterial infections by certain investigations. Several criteria are available to classify them into one of these two categories.

As per *Rochester criteria,* well-looking infants are at low risk if they have a white blood cell count 5000–15000 per mm^3, a band count of <1500 cells per mm^3, and a normal urine (<10 white blood cells per high power field), and normal stool (<5 pus cells per high power field) microscopy. Such infants can be watched safely without starting antibiotics, till the reports of blood and urine culture are available.

C. Fever without Focus in 3 months to 3-year-old

Viral infections are responsible for majority of children having non-localizing fever in this age group. However, serious bacterial infection can also occur due to *Streptococcus pneumoniae, Neisseria,* and *Haemophilus influenzae.* Risk factors for occult bacteremia in these children include rectal temperature >39°C, WBC counts >15000/mm^3, raised ESR, and raised C-reactive protein. Rectal temperature >40°C and WBC count >25000/mm^3 indicate a higher probability of serious bacterial infection. Management options are detailed in Fig. 6.1.

Infants with moderate to high-risk factors should be treated with ceftriaxone (50–80 mg/kg/day in one or two divided doses IV or IM). Infants who do not satisfy the above criteria for low-risk should be started on injection ceftriaxone.

2. Fever of Unknown Origin (FUO)

Definition

Fever of unknown origin (FUO) is defined as fever (rectal temperature >38°C) of more than 3 weeks duration documented by a health care provider, for which the specific

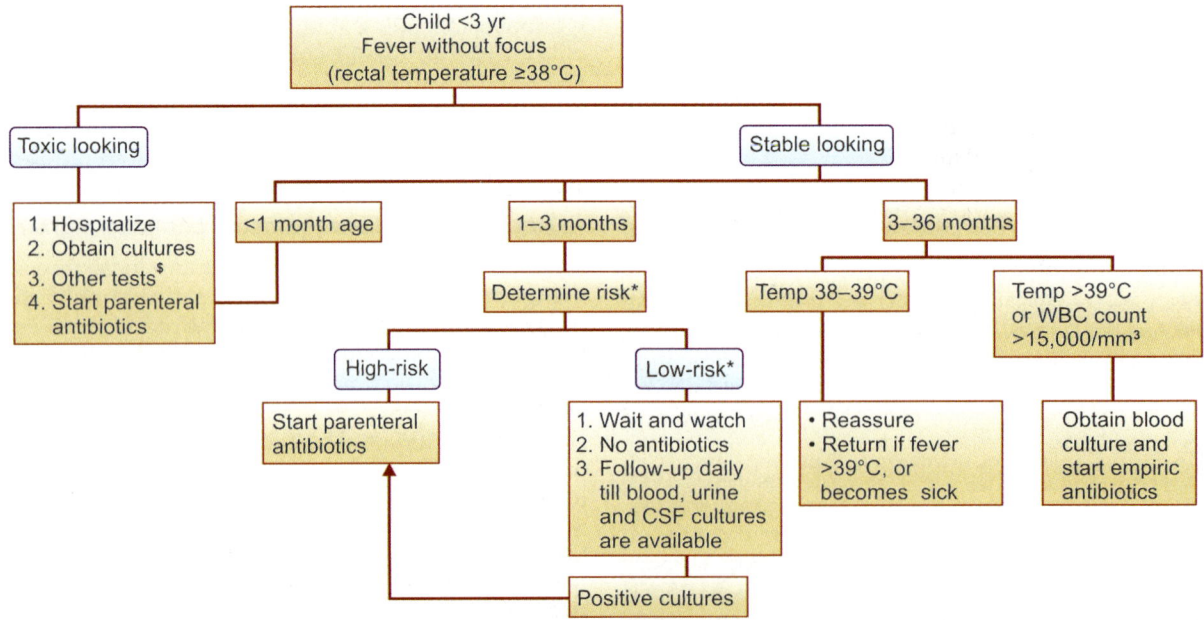

*Determine risk based on history, examination, and laboratory studies:

Low risk: Normal history and physical examination; WBC 5000–15000/mm^3; band cell <1500/mm^3
urine pus cells <10/hpf; stool pus cells <5/hpf; normal chest radiograph; and CSF <8 lymphocytes/mm^3

$Other tests include WBC count; urine and stool microscopy; chest X-ray; CSF Gram stain.
Cultures include that of blood, urine, and CSF.

Fig. 6.1 Management of fever without focus in young children

diagnosis could not be established even after 1 week of admission and investigation in a hospital setting.

Nosocomial or health care-associated FUO refers to hospitalized children receiving acute care in whom infection or fever were absent on admission but in whom a fever of 38.0°C or more occurs on several occasions, for at least a week.

Neutropenic FUO is defined as multiple readings of more than 38°C in a child with absolute neutrophil count <500 per cubic mm, after at least 3 days of investigations including at least 48 hours of incubation of cultures.

Human immunodeficiency virus associated FUO This is defined as temperature more than or equal to 38.3°C or (≥101°F) on several occasions over a period of 4 weeks for outpatients or more than 3 days for hospitalized patients with HIV infection when appropriate investigations for 3 days, including 2 days incubation of cultures, reveal no source.

Etiology

FUO in children is usually due to infection, connective tissue or autoimmune diseases. Malignancies should also be considered in the differential diagnosis. Drug fever is another differential diagnosis in a child receiving certain drug for a long time.

In a 2011 systematic review of 18 studies of FUO including 1338 children (<18 years of age), the most common causes of FUO were as follows:

- *Infection*—51% of cases; 59% of infections were bacterial; the most common bacterial infections were tuberculosis and typhoid fever in resource-poor countries
- No diagnosis or resolution before diagnosis—23% of cases
- *Rheumatologic disease*—9% of cases, most commonly juvenile idiopathic arthritis and SLE
- *Neoplastic disorder*—6% of cases, most commonly leukemia and lymphoma

Other causes included Kawasaki disease, inflammatory bowel disease, factitious fever, hemophagocytic lympho-histiocytosis, immunodeficiency, familial Mediterranean fever, non-specified autoimmune diseases, and drugs.

Infections Epidemiologically relevant infections must be considered first in differential diagnosis. Pulmonary or extra-pulmonary tuberculosis, typhoid and paratyphoid fevers, malaria and kala-azar, amebic hepatitis and amebic liver abscess, and subacute bacterial endocarditis should always be excluded by appropriate clinical, laboratory and radiological evaluation.

Other common infectious causes of FUO include hidden abscesses; especially in liver, urinary tract, pelvic viscera, ovaries, retroperitoneum, lungs, pleural cavity, media-stinum, subdiaphragmatic region, bones and brain. Urinary tract infections, infections of bone and joints, spirochetal and chlamydial infections, infectious mononucleosis, CMV infection or hepatitis and fungal diseases such as candidiasis, histoplasmosis, coccidioidomycosis, and cryptococcosis also result in prolonged undiagnosed fever.

Rickettsial infections (eg, typhus, Q fever), brucellosis, leptospirosis and relapsing fever are rare but should be considered in differential diagnosis, if epidemiologically relevant. Nosocomial infections with unusual organisms, eg, anaerobic bacilli, should be considered in differential diagnosis of patient who had received various antibiotics, especially aminoglycosides, for several days in the hospital.

Malignancies such as Hodgkin disease, non-Hodgkin lymphoma, leukemia, aleukemia, preleukemia, neuro-blastoma, and central nervous system tumors may also result in FUO.

Autoimmune diseases that should be considered in the differential diagnosis of FUO include systemic onset juvenile idiopathic arthritis (JIA), systemic lupus erythematosus, Still disease, polyarteritis nodosa, mixed connective tissue disorders, rheumatic fever, vasculitis and drug fever.

Granulomatous disorders including sarcoidosis, inflam-matory bowel disease, and hypertriglyceridemia can also present as FUO.

Other causes of FUO include various neurological, hematological, genetic and miscellaneous disorders as already detailed under causes of prolonged fever. Several metabolic abnormalities, such as diabetes insipidus or mellitus and hyperthyroidism, may also not be diagnosed early.

Factitious fever should be a possibility, if fever persists for more than 6 months without diagnosis.

Investigations

Evaluation of Fever

Before starting to investigate, it is essential to document fever and observe the type of fever. The onset, type and character of fever and the course of illness should be evaluated clinically to arrive at the possible diagnosis. Hodgkin disease has a typical *Pel-Ebstein* type of fever (3–10 days cycles of febrile and afebrile periods). Fever with chills and rigors suggests malaria, urinary tract infection, abscesses or nosocomial infections.

Clinical Examination

Detailed history-taking and a frequently repeated physical examination remain the most important clinical tools for diagnosis. History of any skin rash, nature of medications, travel to an endemic area, exposure to certain animals and heavy metals are especially important. While examining the child, particular attention should be paid to evaluation of skin, fundus, throat, lymph nodes, genitalia and sinuses. Detailed eye inspection including that of cornea, conjunctiva, orbit, uveal tract and retina may point towards many infectious, collagen vascular, malignant or metabolic disorders (for details, see chapter on Ophthalmology: Ocular Manifestations of Systemic Diseases).

Laboratory Tests

Appropriate laboratory investigations such as total leukocyte count, differential leukocyte count, peripheral blood smear examination for malaria and filaria (night blood) are routinely performed. Similarly, simple serological tests for typhoid, brucellosis, leishmaniasis, rickettsiosis, toxo-plasmosis and amebiasis, and bacteriological culture of blood for *Salmonella* and *Brucella* should be undertaken.

6

Repeated microscopic examination and cultures of blood, urine, throat, sputum, stool for bacterial and fungal infections should be carried out at periodic intervals. If specifically indicated, cultures of bone marrow, cerebrospinal fluid, gastric aspirate, lymph node aspirate and liver aspirate for aerobic and anaerobic bacteria, mycobacteriae and fungi may prove to be invaluable. Serology should also be repeated to look for any rising antibody titer. Modern molecular diagnostic techniques, eg, polymerase chain reaction (PCR), are now available for diagnosis of several infectious agents. A variety of seroimmunological tests for detection of various autoantibodies are now available to rule out various autoimmune disorders.

Procedures

Radiograph of the chest, barium studies of gastrointestinal tract, ultrasonography, whole body CT scan, radionuclide scans and magnetic resonance imaging (MRI) are the important non-invasive diagnostic procedures, that may be required for diagnosis. Imaging studies, particularly of central nervous system, abdomen, pelvis and heart, may supply substantial clues. Lymphangiography can be resorted to, for demonstrating retroperitoneal, iliac and periaortic lymph nodes.

Endoscopic evaluation of respiratory, genitourinary and gastrointestinal tracts may help. Skin tests are not much useful except the PPD test for *Mycobacterium*. Biopsies of lymph node, liver, and bone marrow are routinely carried out in prolonged undiagnosed fevers. If indicated, skin, pleura, muscle, kidneys, etc. can also be biopsied.

Fever without Focus

1. Fever without localizing signs or fever without a source is defined as fever for ≤1 week without adequate explanation after a thorough history and physical examination.
2. Fever of unknown origin (FUO) is defined as fever (rectal temperature >38.3°C) of more than 3 weeks duration documented by a health care provider, for which the specific diagnosis could not be established even after 1 week of admission and investigation in a hospital setting.
3. The most common causes of FUO in developing countries are typhoid and tuberculosis.

Bonadio WA. Evaluation, treatment and therapy for febrile infants younger than 3 months of age. *Curr opin Pediatr*. 1992;4:745–50.

Chow A, Robinson JL. Fever of unknown origin. A systematic review. *World J Pediatr*. 2011;7:5–10.

Harris JA. Managing fever without a source in young children: the debate continues. *Am Fam Physician*. 2007;75:1774, 1776.

Machado BM, Cardoso DM, de Paulis M, Escobar AM, Gilio AE. Fever without source: evaluation of a guideline. *J Pediatr*. 2009;85:426–32.

Sur DK, Bukont EL. Evaluating fever of unidentifiable source in young children. *Am Fam Physician*. 2007;75:1805–11.

Varghese GM, Trowbridge P, Doherty T. Investigating and managing pyrexia of unknown origin in adults. *BMJ*. 2010;341:C5470.

6.3 CHICKENPOX (VARICELLA)

Chickenpox is a highly infectious disease caused by primary infection of varicella-zoster virus. The illness is characterized by an exanthematous vesicular rash with a centripetal distribution. The rash typically begins as maculopapular lesion on first day of fever. The course is usually benign and lasts for about 7 days. Chickenpox infections give lifelong immunity. However, varicella-zoster virus can remain latent and can recur years later as herpes zoster (shingles). Primary disease is vaccine-preventable.

Epidemiology

Varicella-zoster virus is an enveloped DNA virus that is transmitted from person-to-person by direct contact, droplet, airborne spread, or fomites. Only 1 serotype is known. Man is the only reservoir. Infectivity is maximum during prodromal period and completely wanes when eruptions become crusted. Crusts from chickenpox lesions do not contain live virus. Period of infectivity ranges from 48 hours prior to appearance of rash, up to 3–7 days after the rash appears. Varicella virus is transmitted to 65–86% of susceptible household contacts. This secondary attack rate is lower in a school setting. Subclinical varicella is almost non-existent.

Pathogenesis

Airborne virus enters the oropharynx through inhalation by droplet infection. Primary seeding occurs in tonsillar tissue and mucosa of the upper respiratory tract. Virus replication for initial 10 days is followed by primary viremia that spreads the virus to reticuloendothelial system. No clinical symptoms occur. Skin lesions appear only during the secondary viremic phase that lasts for 3–7 days. Infectious virus is carried to vesicular fluid and also back to respiratory mucosa, from where it is shed, transmitting infection to susceptible contacts. The virus may be transported to the dorsal root of spinal cord, where a latent infection is established. Reactivation of this focus at a later stage results in herpes zoster.

Clinical Features

Chickenpox occurs at all ages (including neonates) with peak incidence between 2 and 8 years. The median incubation period is 14–16 days (range 10–21 d). The disease ushers in with fever and malaise. Prodromal symptoms also include headache, sore throat, and backache. The rash appears within 24 hours of the onset of prodrome. At times, prodromal symptoms may be absent and the illness may straightaway begin with a rash.

Fever is usually moderate, usually between 102° and 103°F, but may rise to 106°F. Fever usually resolves after 3–4 days of appearance of rash.

Evolution of the Rash

The rash begins as crops of macules, which evolve into papules and then vesicles. The vesicles are initially filled with clear fluid that soon becomes cloudy. The vesicles persist for 3 to 4 days, become pustular and then form crust. The vesicles may be round, oval, elliptical or irregular, often surrounded by red areola. The lesions first appear over face, scalp, or trunk; and then spread to whole body. Palms and soles are spared. The lesions measure 5–10 mm in diameter. New lesions may keep occurring for 1 week. Most children have >250 lesions. Lesions of different stages; ie, macules, papules, vesicles, and scabs can be seen simultaneously. Lesions tend to be more abundant on covered than exposed parts of the body. By the time of vesicle formation, there is excessive itching. Vesicles may also be observed over conjunctiva, palate, tongue, and buccal mucous membranes.

Vesicles dry up within 1–2 days, starting from the center, forming crusts and scabs. Scabs fall off in 10–20 days. Underlying skin becomes hypo- or hyperpigmented that stays for days to weeks. Permanent scarring is unusual.

Complications

Bacterial infections Secondary skin infection due to group A Streptococcus and *Staphylococcus aureus* results in cellulitis, erysipelas, and skin abscesses. Bacteremic spread may lead to pneumonia, osteomyelitis, and septic arthritis.

Neurological complications Neurological complications occur towards the end of first week of illness as the rash reaches maturity. The most common manifestation is a pure cerebellar ataxia which has an excellent prognosis. Meningoencephalitis is a dreaded complication with 5–25% mortality. Acute disseminated encephalomyelitis (ADEM) is a rare form of post-varicella encephalitis with cerebral demyelination. It presents with cranial nerve involvement, long tract signs, and convulsions. Transverse myelitis, acute infantile hemiplegia, and Guillain-Barré syndrome are the other neurological complications. Chronic neurological sequelae are rare.

Pneumonitis Varicella pneumonia appears 3–5 days after the onset of rash. These children present with acute respiratory distress and hemoptysis and diffuse nodular infiltration in chest radiograph.

Others Myocarditis, pericarditis, endocarditis, hepatitis, glomerulonephritis, appendicitis, keratoconjunctivitis, arthritis, thrombocytopenia, and purpura fulminans are the other notable complications. Immunocompromized children, adolescents, and pregnant women are at increased risk of severe disease. Children with AIDS can develop chronic chickenpox lasting for months.

Congenital Varicella

If the mother contacts chickenpox in the first trimester, there is 2% risk of the baby developing congenital varicella embryopathy. The child may be born with multiple malformations, including cicatricial scarring of the limbs, cortical atrophy, limb hypoplasia, digital defects, retinitis, and cataract.

Varicella Neonatorum

If the maternal rash appears less than 5 days before delivery or up to 2 days after delivery, there is 17–30% risk that the baby will receive a large inoculum without maternal antibody. Such babies are at a very high risk of disseminated disease with death (fatality rate can be as high as 30%, if not treated in time) from pneumonitis, and should be protected at birth by giving varicella-zoster immunoglobulin (VZIG).

Neonatal varicella may still occur in 50% of these, despite VZIG administration, however, the disease is mild. If symptoms develop, the baby should receive intravenous acyclovir (10 mg/kg q 8h).

Diagnosis

The diagnosis of varicella is essentially clinical and routine laboratory investigations are not essential. Rapid laboratory diagnosis can be made by electron microscopy or by immunofluorescence. VZV can be identified quickly by direct fluorescence assay of cells from cutaneous lesions or by polymerase chain reaction amplification testing. Although multinucleated giant cells (Tzanck smear) can be detected with non-specific strains, they do not help to differentiate between varicella virus and herpes simplex virus infections, and have poor sensitivity. IgG antibodies to varicella-zoster virus can be detected by several methods and a 4-fold rise in antibody titer is also confirmatory of acute infection. Leucopenia is typical during the first 72 hours; followed by lymphocytosis. Liver enzymes are also mildly elevated.

Treatment	Chickenpox

Supportive therapy

No treatment is usually required and bed rest is unnecessary except in ill children. Paracetamol will control prodromal symptoms and fever. Aspirin should not be given because of the risk of Reye syndrome. Calamine lotion will normally soothe pruritus; if not, an antihistaminic should be tried. If the enanthem is severe, careful oral toilet is needed. Lesions on the conjunctiva should be protected from secondary infection.

Specific therapy

Acyclovir therapy is not recommended routinely for treatment of uncomplicated chickenpox in the otherwise healthy child because of marginal benefit, cost of the drug and low risk of complications of the disease. Oral acyclovir to healthy children within 24 h of onset of rash decreases the duration of rash by 1 day and number of new lesions by only 25%.

Indications for acyclovir in varicella infection are as follows:
i. Chronic cutaneous or pulmonary disorders;
ii. Those receiving short term, intermittent or aerosolized corticosteroids;
iii. Those receiving long-term salicylate therapy;
iv. Immunocompromized patients including those with HIV infection and malignancies; and
v. Disseminated varicella infection including pneumonia, encephalitis, severe hepatitis, or thrombocytopenia.

Intravenous acyclovir therapy is indicated for severe disease and for varicella in immunocompromized patients. Intravenous acyclovir (10 mg/kg q 8 hr IV) initiated within 72 h of development of initial symptoms decreases the progression of the disease in high-risk patients. The treatment is continued for 7 to 10 days. Oral acyclovir (20 mg/kg/dose) given as 4 doses/day for 5 days should be used for the other indications mentioned above. Treatment should be initiated as early as possible, within 24 h of rash. Foscarnet is the only available drug for acyclovir resistant varicella.

Cloxacillin can be used to treat skin infections. More severe sepsis will require appropriate antibacterial chemotherapy which should be guided by swabbing of the affected lesions and by cultures of the blood and of any pus.

Breakthrough Varicella

Varicella vaccine administered as a 1-dose regimen to healthy children offers 85% protection (range 44–100%). Vaccinated children can thus suffer from varicella. Breakthrough varicella is defined as varicella occurring in a child who was vaccinated at least 42 days prior to eruption of the rash with one dose of varicella vaccine, and caused by wild type varicella virus. Rash occurring between 14 and 42 days after vaccination can also be due to vaccine strains.

Breakthrough varicella is usually a mild disease. It is predominated by a maculopapular rash; vesicles are less frequent. Number of lesions is less than 50. These children are less likely to transmit the disease to others; ie, the secondary attack rate of breakthrough varicella is lower than classical varicella. Recipients of 2-dose varicella vaccine are less likely to have breakthrough varicella as compared to those having received 1 dose only.

Prevention

Active Immunization

Two doses of live virus vaccine (administered at 15–18 mo, and 4–6 y) are recommended by the Indian Academy of Pediatrics to prevent varicella in healthy children. Protective efficacy of 2-dose regimen is 98–100%. Varicella vaccine should not be given within 4 weeks of MMR vaccination; however, both can be given simultaneously.

Postexposure Prophylaxis

Varicella vaccine, if given within 3–5 days of exposure, can prevent or modify the disease in household contacts. Chemoprophylaxis with acyclovir is not an established mode of prevention.

Varicella-zoster immunoglobulin (VZIG) is recommended for newborns whose mothers have varicella 5 days before to 2 days after delivery. Other susceptible high risk contacts (pregnant women, immunocompromised children, and hospitalized, premature infants born <28 wk or <1000 g birth weight) should also be given VZIG.

VZIG is given as 125 IU/10 kg with a maximum dose of 625 IU. Minimum dose is 62.5 IU for less than or equal to 2 kg and 125 IU for 2–10 kg. Varicella vaccination should be given almost 5 months after VZIG administration.

Revision Point

Varicella

1. The rash typically begins as maculopapular lesion on first day of fever, as crops of macules, which evolve into papules and then vesicles.
2. If the maternal rash appears less than 5 days before delivery or up to 2 days after delivery, the baby should be protected by giving VZIG.
3. For all postexposure prophylaxis, administration of VZIG should be as soon as possible, ideally within 4 days for maximum efficacy, but maximum within next 10 days.
4. The most common complication of varicella is a pure cerebellar ataxia which has an excellent prognosis.
5. First dose of varicella vaccine should be given between 15 and 18 months and second dose between 4 and 6 years.

Committee on Infectious Diseases. Policy statement—Prevention of varicella: update of recommendations for use of quadrivalent and monovalent varicella vaccines in children. *Pediatrics*. 2011;128:630–2.

Javed S, Javed SA, Tyring SK. Varicella vaccines. *Curr Opin Infect Dis*. 2012;25:135–40.

Cohen A, Moschopoulos P, Stiehm RE, Koren G. Congenital varicella syndrome: the evidence for secondary prevention with varicella-zoster immune globulin. *CMAJ*. 2011;183:204–8.

Gilden D, Mahalingam R, Nagel MA, *et al*. Review: The neurobiology of varicella zoster virus infection. *Neuropathol Appl Neurobiol*. 2011;37:441–63.

Mubareka S, Leung V, Aoki FY, *et al*. Famciclovir: a focus on efficacy and safety. *Expert Opin Drug Saf*. 2010;9:643–58.

Partridge DG, McKendrick MW. The treatment of varicella-zoster virus infection and its complications. *Expert Opin Pharmacother*. 2009;10:797–812.

Smith CK, Arvin AM. Varicella in the fetus and newborn. *Semin Fetal Neonatal Med*. 2009;14:209–17.

6.4 MEASLES

Measles is a highly contagious disease caused by a virus belonging to the Paramyxoviridae family. The illness is characterized by fever, upper respiratory symptoms, a pathognomonic enanthem (ie, Koplik spots), followed by an erythematous maculopapular rash starting between 3 and 7 days after onset of fever. The rash heals leaving a browny pigmentation. The entire course of uncomplicated measles lasts for about 7–10 days. Serious and fatal complications include pneumonia, diarrhea, and encephalitis. Infection confers lifelong immunity.

Measles has the greatest incidence in children under 2 years of age, especially in developing nations. However, no age is exempt. More than 80% of cases occur in under-fives. Both sexes are equally affected; however, complication rates are higher in males.

The Problem

Measles remains the leading killer among vaccine-preventable diseases, mainly attacking the undernourished children. Before the vaccine became available in 1960s, measles used to kill between 7 and 8 million children per year and cause 135 million episodes per year worldwide. It still accounts for 25 million cases and more than half a million deaths each year, majority of these occurring in the developing world. These deaths represent 50 to 60% of deaths due to all vaccine-preventable diseases.

The disease burden has been high in India, despite availability of an effective vaccine. This is because of inadequate coverage under routine immunization (83%, UNICEF data), and non-availability of a second opportunity for measles vaccination. With introduction of second dose of measles-containing vaccine in the National Immunization program, and increasing coverage, there is a hope to control measles morbidity and mortality in near future.

Etiology

Measles is caused by an RNA virus classified as morbillivirus. The virus is composed of an outer envelope and internal helical nucleocapsid. Envelope contains proteins F, H and M, and has spikes on its surface. The virus is rapidly inactivated by heat and ultraviolet rays. Man is the only natural host and source of measles virus. Carrier state does not exist.

Transmission

Spread of infection Measles spreads from the infected person to a normal individual by the respiratory route or conjunctivae. Transmission mainly occurs through large droplet or small droplet aerosols. Sometimes large droplets or direct person-to-person contact may also spread the disease. As measles virus is highly contagious, a 5% susceptible population is sufficient to sustain periodic outbreaks in otherwise highly vaccinated populations.

Period of communicability Infection is spread from the secretions of nose and throat usually 4 days before and 5 days after the appearance of rash.

Immunity

An attack of measles makes the individual immune for whole life against subsequent infections. Serum antibodies to viral hemagglutinin, hemolysin, and complement are observed following an infection. Hemagglutinin inhibiting and neutralizing antibodies appear after two weeks, peak at 4–6 weeks, and decrease over a year, but persist lifelong. Children with defective cell-mediated responses are more prone to die from progressive measles infection. Acute measles results in a temporary defect in neutrophil motility. T, B, and null lymphocytes are reduced. Interferon response appears after 10 days and coincides with recovery from acute infection.

Transplacental immunity Measles antibodies are transferred from mother to fetus, which protect the infant for first 6–9 months of life. These antibodies may interfere with live-attenuated measles vaccination.

Pathogenesis

Measles virus is spread by aerosol and enters the susceptible host by the respiratory route. Initial infection and viral replication occurs locally in tracheal and bronchial epithelial cells. This leads to primary viremia (day 2–3) that infects local lymphatic tissues, perhaps carried by pulmonary macrophages. Following the amplification of measles virus in regional lymph nodes, a predominantly cell-associated viremia disseminates the virus to various organs prior to the appearance of rash.

This secondary viremia (day 5–7) is responsible for systemic symptoms. Two types of giant cells are seen in measles: Warthin-Finkeldey cells of reticuloendothelial system and epithelial giant cells of respiratory and other epithelia. In individuals with deficiencies in cellular immunity, the virus causes a progressive and often fatal-giant cell pneumonia. Measles causes an immunosuppression marked by decrease in delayed-type hypersensitivity, interleukin-12 production, and antigen-specific lympho-proliferative responses that persist for weeks to months after the acute infection. Immunosuppression may predispose individuals to severe bacterial infection, particularly bronchopneumonia, a major cause of measles-related mortality among younger children.

Clinical Features

Incubation period The incubation period from exposure to onset of symptoms ranges from 8–12 days.

Prodromal phase Measles is marked by an acute onset of moderate grade fever. It is associated with cough, coryza, rhinitis, conjunctivitis, malaise, and anorexia. Fever is almost continuous, exceeds 101°F and persists for at least 1 week.

Enanthematous phase On the second or third day of fever, Koplik spots appear on the buccal mucosa. These appear as bluish-gray specks or "grains of sand" on a red base at the level of premolars. They may also occur on lips, palate, conjunctivae, gums, and vagina. These spots begin 1–2 days before the onset of rash and start fading or sloughing as the exanthematous rash appears.

Exanthematous phase The rash appears on 4th day. It begins on the face and neck, near the hairline; it then proceeds to the trunk, extremities, palms, and soles and lasts for about 5 days. Patients appear most ill during the first or second day of the rash. The rash is erythematous and maculopapular. It blanches on pressure during the initial 2–3 days. In later stage, the rash does not blanch and starts darkening.

Rash may be absent in patients with underlying deficiencies in cellular immunity. Children with partial immunity develop a *'modified measles'* that is a milder illness with less severe symptoms and shorter duration of fever and rash. *Hemorrhagic measles* is a severe form characterized by generalized bleeding, altered sensorium, convulsions, coma, and a high fatality rate.

Generalized lymphadenopathy, mild hepatomegaly, and appendicitis may occur because of generalized involvement of lymphoid tissue.

Recovery phase The rash starts disappearing after 5 days in the sequence in which it had appeared, leaving behind desquamated areas, that spares the palms and soles. Fever subsides 5–7 days after appearance of rash.

Differential Diagnosis

Measles need to be differentiated from other causes of fever with maculopapular rash, including rubella, infectious mononucleosis, roseola, fifth disease, group A streptococcal infection, meningococcemia, dengue fever, rickettsial infections, mycoplasma infections, and Kawasaki disease. Koplik spots, if present, are pathognomonic of measles. However, they are present in 50–70% children only and rest may still pose a diagnostic challenge.

Rubella is a milder disease with a characteristic post-occipital lymphadenopathy. Infectious mononucleosis should be suspected, if there is generalized lympha-denopathy and hepatosplenomegaly. Children with dengue fever have a rash that is confluent and also involves palms and soles. Meningococcal and streptococcal rashes are characterized by petechiae, purpura, associated with a generalized toxic look. Rash of roseola infantum (caused by herpesvirus-6) typically starts from trunk and is associated with periorbital edema. Fifth disease caused by human parvovirus B 19 (HPV 19) is characterized by an erythematous rash on the cheeks, giving these children a typical *'slapped cheek'* appearance.

Diagnosis

The diagnosis of measles is primarily clinical and routine laboratory investigations are not essential. According to

6

WHO, *measles is clinically diagnosed in a person presenting with fever and maculopapular rash (non-vesicular) and cough, coryza, or conjunctivitis.* White cell count is usually low with relative lymphocytosis. ESR and CRP are not elevated. Serologic confirmation requires demonstration of IgM antibodies in serum. These last for almost a month after an acute infection. A fourfold rise in IgG titer between exanthematous and convalescent samples collected 2–4 weeks later is also diagnostic. The virus can be isolated from respiratory secretions, blood, and urine during the prodromal, enanthematous, and exanthematous phases.

Complications

Mortality

Mortality from measles is often the result of complications that follow the derangement in immune system and respiratory mucosa. Malnutrition, underlying malignancy or immunodeficiency, and low serum retinol (vitamin A) levels predispose to a more severe and complicated disease course. The most common cause of death from measles is pneumonia. Case fatality rate is highest in under-five children.

Morbidity

Pneumonia Pneumonia is the most common complication in Indian context, whereas otitis media is most common in western countries. Laryngotracheobronchitis, bronchiolitis, sinusitis, mastoiditis, retropharyngeal abscess, and tracheitis are other respiratory complications of measles. Primary tuberculosis may flare up following measles.

Pneumonia may be caused either by the measles virus itself (measles pneumonia) or because of superimposed bacterial infection by *Staphylococcus aureus, Streptococcus pneumoniae, Haemophilus influenzae*, or gram-negative bacilli including *Klebsiella, E.coli*, and *Pseudomonas*.

Encephalitis Approximately 1 in every 1000 patients with measles develops encephalitis. As thought earlier, it is not due to the measles virus *per se*. Encephalitis following measles is now considered to be a post-infection and immune-mediated disorder. Usual symptoms include altered sensorium and seizures. The onset occurs in the first week of illness. Approximately one-third develop long-term sequelae. Case fatality rate of measles encephalitis ranges from 10–20%.

Subacute sclerosing panencephalitis (SSPE) This is a degenerative CNS disease that can result from a persistent measles infection. The mean incubation period for SSPE is approximately 10.8 years (range 7–13 years). SSPE is characterized by behavioral and intellectual deterioration, followed by myoclonic epilepsy. The disease is progressive in nature finally leading to extrapyramidal symptoms in form of dystonia and rigidity. Dementia, coma, and death follow. There is no definitive cure.

Diarrhea and dysentery Gastrointestinal epithelium is characterized by giant cell formation, manifesting as diarrhea and vomiting. This may get prolonged as persistent diarrhea, especially in malnourished children. Appendicitis may occur due to lymphoid tissue blocking its lumens. Rare complications include hepatitis and ileocolitis.

Others Myocarditis, Stevens-Johnson syndrome, bacteremia, cellulitis, acute glomerulonephritis, and consumption coagulopathy are other complications of measles. Measles can precipitate edematous malnutrition.

Treatment	Measles

Treatment is by and large supportive and symptomatic.

WHO and UNICEF recommend *administration of two doses of vitamin A* supplements given 24 hours apart, to all children diagnosed with measles, in communities where measles related mortality is more than 1%. There is evidence that administration of vitamin A reduces severity of and mortality due to measles by 50%. Giving vitamin A at the time of diagnosis can help prevent eye damage and blindness.

Fever is controlled by paracetamol and hydrotherapy. Moderate degree of cough need not be suppressed. Cough helps in clearing of mucus from the lungs. Very irritating cough may be relieved by saline nebulization.

The child is given adequate amount of fluids orally. If there is vomiting, fluids are given intravenously. Nutrition should be maintained by a good high protein diet. Appropriate antibiotics should only be reserved for secondary bacterial pneumonia. Body and oral hygiene are important. Child should be given a bath daily.

Prevention

The Vaccine

Live-attenuated measles virus is used as the vaccine. The most popular strains of vaccine-viruses, namely *Schwartz, Moraten* and *Edmonston-Zagreb* were derived by further attenuation from the *Edmonston B* strain, which itself was attenuated from the *Edmonston A* strain. Many vaccines are available, either as monovalent vaccine or in combination with rubella, mumps or varicella (MMR or MMRV). The protective response to each component of these antigens, in a combination vaccine, remains unaltered.

The vaccine is given subcutaneously. Its shelf-life is at least one year at 4–8° C. The minimum recommended potency is 1000 median cell culture infectious doses of virus. Diluents must not be frozen. After reconstitution, its potency drops rapidly and loses all potency after 1 hour at 37°C. Moreover, several cases of staphylococcal toxic shock syndrome with high mortality have occurred in India after giving reconstituted measles vaccine stored for one or more days. For these two reasons, reconstituted vaccine should be used within 4–6 hours. Left over doses must be discarded.

Age at Vaccination

Residual maternal antibody in the infant's serum neutralizes the immunogenic property of the vaccine, and it should be offered at an age when most infants would have lost these antibodies. Therefore, in developing countries, the recommended minimum age is 9 months. Eighty-five to ninety-five percent of those vaccinated at the age of 9 months, develop antibodies in adequate titer. Second dose is to be given between 16 and 24 months.

Adverse Events

Depending upon the strain of vaccine-virus, 10 to 20% of vaccinees may develop mild to moderate fever about 6–8 days after receiving measles vaccine. It lasts for 1–3 days, and is not associated with malaise. One to five percent of children may develop a few red spots on the trunk during this period. Treatment for primary tuberculosis is not a contraindication. Since measles vaccine does not seem to aggravate primary tuberculosis, screening is not necessary before immunization.

Measles Vaccine as Aerosol

The *Edmonston-Zagreb* strain of vaccine-virus grown in human diploid cells has been successfully administered as an aerosol to immunize infants against measles. By utilizing the respiratory route, it is hoped to avoid neutralization by any maternal IgG antibodies that may be present. Hence, it is possible to successfully immunize children as young as 4–6 months. In a recent trial conducted in India, it was observed that the aerosolized vaccine was safe and resulted in 85% seroconversion between 9 and 12 months of age, but it was slightly inferior to the subcutaneous vaccine.

Contraindications

These include pregnancy, history of anaphylactic reactions to egg protein, history of anaphylaxis to neomycin, significantly immunocompromised states such as leukemia, administration of anti-metabolites, radiations or corticosteroids, and recent administration of immunoglobulin within last three months. Symptomatic and asymptomatic HIV infection is *not* a contraindication for measles vaccination because of risk of severe life-threatening measles in children with HIV infection.

Interestingly, immunization with live measles vaccine within 72 hours of exposure to a case of measles may modify the illness and provide protection in certain cases. Therefore, measles exposure is not a contraindication for active immunization. Rather in school-based outbreaks, it should be the measure of choice.

Passive Immunization

Exposure to measles may necessitate administration of immunoglobulin (IG) in a susceptible person. Immuno-globulin has to be given within 6 days of exposure in a dose of 0.25 mL/kg body weight, intramuscularly. Immunoglobulin administration is justified for children who are less than 1 year old, immunocompromised, and for pregnant women.

Measles Control and Elimination

Second Opportunity for Measles Immunization

Since 2000, WHO and UNICEF have recommended that in addition to achieving high coverage with the first dose of measles vaccine, countries should ensure a second opportunity for measles immunization for all children. The second opportunity for immunization represents another opportunity for immunization for children who missed a first dose in the routine program and for children who failed to develop immunity after their first dose.

Action Plan for India

National Technical Advisory Group of the Government of India has recommended two doses of MR (measles-rubella) vaccine, first at 9 months and second at 16–24 months of age.

Measles

1. Measles is a highly contagious acute viral illness lasting for 7–10 days that confers lifelong immunity against further episodes. It is the leading cause of death amongst all the vaccine-preventable diseases.
2. The virus spreads by the respiratory route or conjunctivae. Period of infectivity is usually 4 days before and 5 days after the onset of rash.
3. Measles is characterized by a generalized maculo-papular rash lasting more than or equal to 3 days; temperature of more than or equal to 38.3°C (101°F) and presence of cough, coryza, or conjunctivitis. Koplik spots, if present, are pathognomonic of measles.
4. Common complications include pneumonia, diarrhea, and encephalitis.
5. Uncomplicated measles generally resolves on its own within 7–10 days. Treatment is mainly symptomatic. Vitamin A should be given to all children diagnosed with measles.
6. WHO and UNICEF recommend administration of two doses of measles containing vaccine to ensure adequate protection against the disease.

This is now incorporated in the National Immunization Schedule. Indian Academy of Pediatrics recommends 3 doses of MMR vaccines at 9 months, 16–24 months, and at 4–6 years.

Global Strategy

In April 2012, the partners (WHO, UNICEF, CDC, UN) of the **Measles Initiative** introduced a global plan to tackle measles and rubella jointly by using a combined measles-rubella vaccine. The goal of this **Measles-Rubella Initiative** is to reduce measles deaths worldwide by 95% by 2015; and to eliminate measles and rubella in at least 5 of 6 WHO regions by 2020.

Measles can be eradicated because man is the only reservoir of the virus, the disease occurs due to only one serotype, and an effective vaccine is available.

Allam MF. Measles vaccination. *J Prev Med Hyg*. 2009;50:201–5.

Griffin DE. Measles virus-induced suppression of immune responses. *Immunol Rev*. 2010;236:176–89.

Kabra SK, Lodha R, Hilton DJ. Antibiotics for preventing complications in children with measles. *Cochrane Database Syst Rev*. 2008;CD001477.

Low N, Bavdekar A, Jeyaseelan L, et al. A randomized controlled trial of an aerosolized vaccine against measles. *N Engl J Med*. 2015;372:1519–29.

Moss WJ, Griffin DE. Measles.*Lancet*. 2012;379:153–64.

Moss WJ. Measles control and the prospect of eradication. *Curr Trop Microbiol Immunol*. 2009;330:173–89.

Sudfeld CR, Halsey NA. Measles case fatality ratio in India a review of community based studies. *Indian Pediatr*. 2009;46:983–9.

Uzicanin A, Zimmerman L. Field effectiveness of live attenuated measles-containing vaccines: a review of published literature. *J Infect Dis*. 2011;204:S133–48.

Vaidya SR. Commitment of measles elimination by 2020: challenges in India. *Indian Pediatr*. 2015;52:103–6.

Verma R, Khanna P, Bairwa M, *et al*. Introduction of a second dose of measles in national immunization program in India: a major step towards eradication. *Hum Vaccin*. 2011;7:1109–11.

6.5 MUMPS

Mumps is a self-limiting, vaccine-preventable, acute viral infection of the parotid and other salivary glands. It is characterized by fever, and bilateral tender swelling of salivary glands. Aseptic meningitis is the most common sequel.

The annual global incidence of mumps is 100–1000 per 100,000 population with epidemic peaks every two to five years. Natural infection with mumps virus confers lifelong protection.

Etiology

Mumps is caused by the mumps virus belonging to paramyxovirus group. It is an RNA virus and contains hemolysin, neuraminidase and hemagglutinin. The virus can be obtained from the saliva swab of the infected patients 7 days before and 7 days after the onset of salivary gland swelling. There is only one serotype of the virus.

Epidemiology

Transmission Man is the only known host. Virus is transmitted through saliva or by respiratory droplets. The virus may also be found in urine and cerebrospinal fluid. Subclinical infections are very common. These may transmit the infection to susceptible persons. The disease is most likely to transmit from 2 days before to 5 days after appearance of parotitis. Carrier state does not exist.

Host factors Mumps is commonly a disease of children with peak incidence in 5–15 years. Infantile period is protected because of the presence of transplacental antibodies. Mumps occurring in adults produces more severe disease. Mumps infection during early pregnancy increases the risk of abortion.

Pathogenesis

The virus enters human body through the inhalational route and seeds the epithelium of upper respiratory tract, where it replicates. Absorption of virus in host cell is facilitated by HN (hemagglutinin-neuraminidase) surface glycoprotein, while F (fusion) glycoprotein mediates viral penetration into the cell. This is followed by regional lymphoid invasion and viremia. Mumps virus selectively targets the salivary glands, central nervous system, pancreas, testes, heart, liver, kidneys, thyroid, and joints. The virus evokes a lymphocytic response in infected tissue, with ultimate necrosis of the salivary epithelium. Mumps virus enters the central nervous system via the choroid plexus. Cerebrospinal fluid is also characterized by a lymphocytic response. Focal ischemic infarcts are observed in the testis.

Clinical Features

Incubation period The incubation period varies from 12–25 days with a median 16–18 days.

Prodromal symptoms Initial symptoms consist of fever, malaise, headache, vomiting, and nausea. Fever is mild to moderate. Appetite is impaired.

Presenting features The disease can vary from a mild upper respiratory illness to viremia with widespread systemic involvement. The most common presentation is a parotitis that occurs in 30–40% of affected children. Other reported sites of infection are the testes, pancreas, eyes, ovaries, central nervous system, joints, and kidneys. Infection with mumps virus is asymptomatic in 20–30% of cases.

Parotitis Classic mumps is characterized by enlargement of the parotid and other salivary glands; parotitis is bilateral in three-quarters of cases; and other salivary glands are involved in 10% of cases. Swelling of parotid is preceded by pain near the ear lobe and also difficulty in swallowing and chewing. Swelling initially appears on one side of the cheek. Within 72 hours, it becomes bilateral. Swelling results in obliteration of the angle of the jaw and lifting of the ipsilateral ear lobe, upward and outward. The swelling increases in size for 3–4 days. Disease may remain unilateral in 30% cases. Lymphatic obstruction in facial and neck planes may result in local edema, extending up to sternum.

Recovery Fever subsides within 3–5 days. Parotid swelling starts receding after 5 days. It may take 10–14 days for the swelling to subside completely.

Complications

Aseptic meningitis Aseptic meningitis is the most common complication of mumps. It occurs in up to 10% of all children with mumps, more often in males. Asymptomatic pleocytosis in CSF occurs in 50% of all children with mumps. Symptomatic meningitis occurs in 15% cases, characterized by severe headache aggravated by movement, photophobia, and neck stiffness due to spasm of the spinal muscles.

Mumps meningitis is a benign condition that appears within a few days of parotid swelling, although some meningitis patients do not have any parotid swelling. Patients recover within 7 days without complications, but require hospitalization during the course of the illness. Death due to mumps is exceedingly rare, and is mostly caused by mumps encephalitis.

Meningoencephalitis Encephalitis, though less common than meningitis, can occur before, with, or after appearance of parotid swelling. *Early onset encephalitis* occurs within 1–2 weeks of onset of swelling and is due to mumps infection of the brain. *Late onset encephalitis* is an immune-mediated demyelinating condition.

Other neurological manifestations of mumps include cerebellar ataxia, ADEM, cranial nerve involvement (facial and auditory), transverse myelitis, and Guillain-Barre syndrome. Although most patients recover without prolonged sequelae, the mortality rate is reported to be up to 1.4%.

Orchitis, epididymitis, and oophoritis Epididymo-orchitis occurs in about 25% of postpubertal adolescents who contact mumps. Testicular atrophy occurs in about one-third of them, but sterility is rare. In postpubertal adolescent girls, mastitis and oophoritis can occur.

Pancreatitis Pancreatitis is seen in about 4% of patients with mumps. There is evidence suggesting that mumps virus can infect human pancreatic beta cells, and may trigger the onset of insulin-dependent diabetes mellitus in some individuals. Additional rare complications include nephritis, arthritis, thrombocytopenic purpura, mastitis, thyroiditis, and keratouveitis.

Differential Diagnosis

A parotid swelling needs to be differentiated from an enlarged cervical lymph node. For this, draw an imaginary line bisecting the long axis of the ear to the angle of jaw. A cervical lymph node usually lies posterior to this imaginary line, while a parotid swelling overlies this line.

Differential diagnoses of a parotid swelling include suppurative parotitis caused by *Staphylococcus aureus*, which is usually unilateral and is extremely painful. There may be a pus discharge from Stenson duct. Parotitis can also be caused by other viruses including parainfluenza, influenza, HIV, Epstein-Barr, and cytomegaloviruses.

Non-infective parotitis is caused by collagen vascular disorders (SLE, Sjögren syndrome), malignancies (leukemia, lymphoma), and obstruction of Stenson duct due to calculus.

Diagnosis

Diagnosis is primarily clinical. According to WHO, *clinical diagnosis of mumps is made in presence of acute onset of unilateral/bilateral, tender, self-limited swelling of the parotid or other salivary gland, lasting 2 or more days and without any other apparent cause.* Laboratory investigations are usually not required. Mumps virus can be isolated from nasopharyngeal swabs, urine, blood, and fluid from buccal cavity typically from 7 days before up until 9 days after the onset of parotitis. Mumps infection can be confirmed by demonstrating significant (4-fold) rise in mumps-specific immunoglobulin G (IgG) antibody between acute and convalescent titers or a positive mumps immunoglobulin M (IgM). IgG titer can be detected by complement fixation, hemagglutination inhibition, or enzyme immunoassay. Polymerase chain reaction (PCR) can be used to detect viral antigen. Lymphocytosis or leukopenia may be present. Serum amylase level may be elevated. CNS infections usually exhibit a lymphocytic pleocytosis in cerebrospinal fluid, with hypoglycorrhachia.

Treatment	**Mumps**

No specific treatment is available for mumps. Supportive care and outpatient follow-up is indicated for uncomplicated infections. Fever should be treated with paracetamol. Adequate hydration should be maintained. Warm salt water gargles, soft foods, and extra fluids may also help relieve symptoms. Children are advised to suck on lozenges that stimulate the salivary secretions and reduces the swelling earlier.

Complications due to mumps should be treated based on presentation. Management of complicated mumps infection should include testicular ultrasonography for orchitis, ice-packs applied to scrotal area for swelling, scrotal support and anti-inflammatory agents, intravenous hydration for severe pancreatitis, and symptomatic management for meningitis or encephalitis. Classic mumps with no major complications can be managed on an outpatient basis with supportive care and good follow-up.

Prevention and Control

Care of Contacts

Children should not be allowed to go to school for 10 days after the onset of parotid swelling. Mumps immune globulin has no role. As with measles, mumps vaccine can be given after exposure to provide protection against future exposures. If the disease develops in such contacts, who have been given mumps vaccine following exposure, no additional risk or reactions are conferred on the individuals.

Active Immunization

A live-attenuated preparation of mumps vaccine is available as a part of combined MMR vaccine. A single dose confers lifelong immunity and 98% seroconversion. In developing countries, the priority for mumps prophylaxis is low. Most commonly, the vaccine consists of the Jeryl-Lynn strain. Other strains in use are Leningrad-3 (erstwhile Soviet states); Urabe (Japan, France, Italy), L-Zagreb (Croatia, India, Slovenia), and Rubini (Switzerland). All vaccines offer more than 90% seroconversion. The ideal age for vaccinating children is 15–18 months. The vaccine is administered in a dose of 0.5 mL subcutaneously (as MMR). MMR can be given to individuals who are already immune to one or more component viruses of the vaccine. The mumps component is still not a part of National schedule in India. A few states are giving it as part of MMR vaccine at 15–18 months. IAP recommends 3 doses of MMR vaccine (9 months, 16–24 months, and 4–6 years).

Adverse events Adverse events to mumps vaccine are rare. Aseptic meningitis is reported in 0.1–100 per 100,000 vaccinees.

Contraindications These include pregnancy, history of anaphylactic reaction to egg, persons with immuno-deficiency disorders or those receiving immunosuppressives and persons who have received immunoglobulins or blood transfusion recently in the past three months. For such patients, who cannot be vaccinated, it is advisable to vaccinate their close susceptible contacts. Vaccine-virus is not transmitted by immunized persons.

Global Efforts

By 2015, a total of 121 countries or regions had included vaccination against mumps in their national immunization programs, mostly as MMR vaccine. Most countries in Africa and south-east Asia region have not adopted this strategy and the incidence of mumps remains high in these areas.

Mumps Control

Mumps can be controlled through high (more than 90%) routine coverage with an effective mumps-containing vaccine administered at 12–18 months of age. Lower immunization coverage (< 80%) fails to interrupt circulation of the mumps virus in the community and results in an epidemiological shift with increase in the number of cases in adults. Strategies for elimination are outlined below:

1. Achieving high (more than 90%) coverage with a first dose of mumps-containing vaccine at the age of 12–18 months.

2. Ensuring a second opportunity for immunization; if coverage with the first dose is less than 80%.

3. Conducting catch-up immunization of susceptible cohorts; the target age group should be that in which susceptibility to mumps is highest.

Mumps

1. Mumps is a self-limiting, acute viral illness causing inflammation of parotid and other salivary glands. Natural infection confers lifelong protection.

2. Meningoencephalitis is the most important complication of mumps infection.

3. The differential diagnosis includes cervical lymphadenopathy, suppurative (bacterial) parotitis, viral parotitis, and non-infective parotitis caused by collagen vascular disorders, malignancies, and salivary gland calculus.

4. The management is mainly supportive. Spontaneous recovery occurs in 2 weeks.

5. The disease can be prevented by administration of the mumps vaccine, available as a component of MMR vaccine.

Cascarini L, McGurk M. Epidemiology of salivary gland infections. *Oral Maxillofac Surg Clin North Am.* 2009;21:353–7.

Hviid A, Rubin S, Mühlemann K. Mumps. *Lancet.* 2008;371:932–44.

Irani DN. Aseptic meningitis and viral myelitis. *Neurol Clin.* 2008;26:635–55.

Kutty PK, Kyaw MH, Dayan GH, *et al.* Guidance for isolation precautions for mumps in the United States:a review of the scientific basis for policy change. *Clin Infect Dis.* 2010;50:1619–28.

MacDonald N, Hatchette T, Elkout L, *et al.* Mumps is back: why is mumps eradication not working? *Adv Exp Med Biol.* 2011;697:197–220.

Senanayake SN. Mumps: a resurgent disease with protean manifestations. *Med J Aust.* 2008;189:456–9.

Sällberg M. Oral viral infections of children. *Periodontol 2000.* 2009;49:87–95.

Vaidya SR, Hamde VS. Is it right time to introduce mumps vaccine in India's universal immunization program? *Indian Pediatr.* 2016;53:469–73.

6.6 RUBELLA

Rubella in children is a mild disease characterized by mild fever, rash and lymphadenopathy. Most of the times, the infection may pass off unnoticed. The primary infection *per se* does not result in significant mortality or morbidity. However, if a pregnant woman is infected with rubella virus, serious consequences can occur in her fetus. The infant may be born with **congenital rubella syndrome** with multisystem involvement (brain, heart, eyes and ears). Congenital rubella is the most important cause of preventable deafness in children. It is estimated that more than 46,000 cases occur in south-east Asian countries alone every year.

The risk of fetal infection is 50% or higher, if the mother acquires infection during first four weeks of gestation. It declines to about 25% between 23 and 26 weeks and then rises again to 70% for rubella infections acquired during the latter part of pregnancy.

Maternal rubella infection during the phase of embryogenesis; ie, the first trimester results in congenital defects in up to 90% of the offspring. The risk is reduced to 25% at 15–16 weeks. Fetal rubella infection beyond 16 weeks of intrauterine gestation does not result in congenital defects.

Epidemiology

Rubella virus is an RNA virus and can be isolated from the nasopharynx, throat, urine and cerebrospinal fluid, during the acute illness. Man is the only source of infection.

Rubella is mainly a disease of children, though it affects all age groups. Transmission occurs by droplet spread and the virus enters the host by respiratory route. Postnatal rubella is infective from 7 days before to 14 days (median 5 days) after the appearance of rash. Natural infection confers lifelong immunity. Subclinical infections are common. Transplacental protection remains for 6–9 months.

Transplacental spread of virus results in congenital rubella. Affected infants may continue to shed virus in nasopharyngeal secretions and urine for a year or more following birth.

Pathology

Rubella virus enters the human host by respiratory route, lodges in local epithelium, replicates, and also spreads to regional lymph nodes. This is followed by a viremic phase lasting for 2 weeks.

Fetal infection occurs by transplacental spread. The virus replicates extensively in the fetus and persists in the neonate and even in infant, resulting in widespread tissue damage, primarily in brain, heart, and auditory nerve. The exact mechanism of cellular injury is not clear, but ischemia, chromosomal breaks, and mitotic arrests could have some role.

Clinical Features

A. Postnatal Infection

Incubation period is 14–21 days. Half of the infections are subclinical and asymptomatic. It is difficult to differentiate this illness from other viral fevers of the childhood. Sore throat and fever herald the onset of disease. Suboccipital, posterior auricular, and anterior cervical lymph nodes enlarge by 7th day. A macular rash appears within 24 hours after the onset of fever. It first appears on face and neck and spreads centrifugally to involve the whole body.

On the first day of appearance of exanthema, small pink-colored ring lesions and petechiae also appear on the soft palate. These are known as *Forchheimer spots* and are pathognomonic of rubella infection. The rash lasts for 3 days and then fades away without any residual pigmentation or desquamation.

Postnatal rubella needs to be differentiated from other exanthematous fevers including measles, roseola, erythema infectiosum, and infectious mononucleosis, on the basis of their typical clinical features.

Complications occur rarely, and include encephalitis, thrombocytopenia, arthritis, and a progressive rubella panencephalitis (similar to SSPE associated with measles), myocarditis, and infective polyneuritis.

B. Congenital Rubella Syndrome

Fetal infection with rubella during the first trimester may lead to abortion in 10% and stillbirth in 4% of pregnancies.

The rest are born with congenital rubella syndrome: most common manifestations in the affected newborn include: (*i*) microcephaly, (*ii*) deafness, (*iii*) cardiac anomalies (patent ductus arteriosus, pulmonary stenosis, or septal defects), (*iv*) mental retardation, (*v*) congenital cataract, (*vi*) hepato-splenomegaly; and (*viii*) thrombocytopenia. Infants are born small for gestational age. Uncommon manifestations include extramedullary hematopoiesis, dermal erythropoiesis, and meningoencephalitis.

Late onset disease The infected infant may be asymptomatic in the neonatal period and develop evidence of congenital rubella syndrome subsequently. Late onset manifestations include (*i*) diabetes mellitus, (*ii*) thyroid dysfunction, (*iii*) psychomotor defects, and (*iv*) ocular abnormalities.

The newborn infant can shed virus up to the age of 18 months and serve as an important source of infection to other pregnant mothers. There is no treatment and prognosis is generally poor.

Diagnosis

Presence of rubella IgM or a fourfold rise in rubella IgG titer from paired acute and convalescent sera provide evidence of ongoing or recent rubella infection. Viral isolation is not routinely used for diagnosis.

Prevention

Active Immunization

Childhood rubella is too benign a disease to warrant routine prophylaxis. Immunization is intended solely to prevent congenital rubella syndrome. Two possible approaches are: (a) either to selectively immunize adolescent girls and/or women of childbearing age; or (b) to achieve universal immunization of infants and young children of both sexes.

  i. The *first approach of adolescent immunization* will result in a decrease in the incidence of congenital rubella syndrome (CRS). However, elimination of CRS cannot be achieved with this strategy, because it would require every susceptible woman to be effectively immunized. Unvaccinated girls who refuse vaccination will still be exposed to circulating rubella virus in male population and children.
  ii. The *second approach of childhood immunization* will reduce the circulation of virus. However, pregnant women will still continue to be exposed to rubella in adults.

It is now realized that combining in universal immunization of infants and children with vaccination of adolescent girls and adult women is the most effective approach to eliminate rubella and congenital rubella syndrome.

The Vaccine

Most of the currently-licensed vaccines are based on the live-attenuated RA27/3 strain of rubella virus, propagated in human diploid cells. The RA27/3 vaccine can be stored at 4°C for at least five years. Each dose of this vaccine, which is given by the subcutaneous route, contains a defined number of active virus particles (>1000 TCID 50). Other attenuated rubella vaccine strains, such as the Matsuba, DCRB 19, Takahashi, Matsuura and TO-336 strains are used primarily in Japan; the BRD-2 strain is used in China. Efficacy ranges from 95–100%.

As the vaccine consists of live-attenuated virus, it should be given only after maternal antibodies have disappeared; the recommended minimum age is 9 months. Vaccine-induced immunity is generally lifelong. The vaccine is often combined with measles and mumps vaccine. Adverse reactions to rubella vaccine include lymphadenopathy, arthralgia and transient skin rash, all of which are self-limiting.

Contraindications Pregnancy is an absolute contraindication for rubella vaccination. Like measles and mumps, rubella vaccine cannot be administered, if there is a history of immunoglobulin administration or blood transfusion in last three months. Immunocompromized states (except HIV infection) are also contraindications for rubella vaccination. After puberty, immunization should be advised only after estimation of hemagglutination inhibition antibody titer and if pregnancy can be effectively avoided for at least 8 weeks.

Postexposure Prophylaxis

If a pregnant mother is suspected of having been exposed to possible rubella during early pregnancy, HI antibody titer in the blood should be obtained immediately and after three to six weeks interval, irrespective of the occurrence of any rash. A fourfold or greater increase in HI antibody titer indicates rubella infection. If the infection is confirmed, medical termination of pregnancy should be advised.

Surveillance

Methods for surveillance of congenital rubella syndrome include hospital record review, deaf/blind surveys, clinician reporting, and active search for cases with congenital rubella syndrome after outbreaks of acquired rubella. Serological surveillance among antenatal women can be used to monitor the impact of the immunization program.

Indian Initiative

As per WHO recommendations, the National Technical Advisory Group on Immunization (NTAGI) in India recommended the inclusion of rubella vaccination in Universal Immunization Program (UIP), in February 2014. In accordance with the NTAGI recommendations, GOI has decided to introduce a **Rubella Initiative** as a part of the nationwide measles rubella (MR) campaign in two stages—the first stage would be targeted to cover a wide age range of children and adolescents aged 9 months to 15 years with the MR vaccine. This would be followed by the second stage that would entail inclusion of measles-rubella (MR) vaccine in the routine immunization programs in a two-dose schedule at 9–12 months and at 16–24 months of age. These campaigns, by vaccinating all young people between 9 months and 15 years, would rapidly interrupt the spread of rubella virus. As part of this initiative, mass vaccination campaigns for children and adolescents aged 9 months–15 years, with MR vaccine have been planned in the country in four phases from July 2015 to March 2017. Under the initiative, approximately 224, 488, 808 children in India are targeted to be vaccinated, as per WHO estimates. MR vaccine was chosen over MMR, given the comparatively lower cost of the vaccine and a less significant mumps disease burden in the country.

Rubella

1. Rubella is a mild viral illness characterized by mild fever, rash, arthralgia, and lymphadenopathy.
2. Fetal rubella infection occurs due to transplacental spreads from infected mothers.
3. Congenital rubella syndrome is characterized by a triad of sensorineural deafness, ophthalmologic, and cardiac abnormalities.
4. Rubella can be eliminated by active immunization.

Bedford H, Tookey P. Rubella and the MMR vaccine. *Nurs Times.* 2006;102:55–7.

Best JM. Rubella. *Semin Fetal Neonatal Med.* 2007;12:182–92.

Dewan P, Gupta P. Burden of congenital rubella syndrome in India: A systematic review. *Indian Pediatr.* 2012;49:377–99.

Elliman D, Bedford H. MMR: where are we now? *Arch Dis Child.* 2007;92:1055–7

Freij BJ, South MA, Sever JL. Maternal rubella and the congenital rubella syndrome. *Clin Perinatol.* 1988;15:247–57.

Marin M, Broder KR, Temte JL, *et al.* Centers for Disease Control and Prevention (CDC). Use of combination measles, mumps, rubella, and varicella vaccine: recommendations of the Advisory Committee on Immunization Practices (ACIP). *MMWR Recomm Rep.* 2010;59:1–12.

Morice A, Ulloa-Gutierrez R, Avila-Agüero ML. Congenital rubella syndrome: progress and future challenges. *Expert Rev Vaccines.* 2009;8:323–31.

6.7 VIRAL HEPATITIS

Viral hepatitis may be defined as the infection of liver caused by various hepatitis viruses. At least seven distinct types of the viruses are recognized based on viral, immunologic and epidemiological considerations, namely hepatitis A, B, C, D, E, F, and G. Of these, hepatitis A, B, C and E are public health concerns. Hepatitis A and E are transmitted by orofecal route and hepatitis B and C have a parenteral transmission.

Of the four types, diseases caused by hepatitis A and B are vaccine-preventable. There is no vaccine for hepatitis C. Food and water hygiene is all that is required to prevent transmission of hepatitis E.

HEPATITIS A

Hepatitis A virus (HAV) infection is common all over the world, the annual incidence being 10 to 15 per 100,000 population. Prevalence of anti-HAV antibodies in the general population varies from 15–100% in different parts of the world. An estimated 1.5 million clinical cases of hepatitis A occur each year. In young children, HAV infection is usually asymptomatic whereas symptomatic disease occurs more commonly among adults. Infection with hepatitis A virus induces lifelong immunity.

Etiology

Hepatitis A virus (HAV) is an RNA virus, 27 nm in diameter and is classified as picornavirus. It has hepatitis A antigen on its surface. The virus is relatively resistant to heat, acid and solvents but cannot survive boiling (>5 minutes), autoclaving (>30 minutes at 121 °C) and chlorination (1.5–2.5 mg/L for 15 minutes). In infected persons, HAV multiplies in liver and gets excreted in bile to stools.

All the known HAV isolates belong to one serotype and six (I–VI) genotypes. Type III is most common in India.

Epidemiology

Age Infections may occur in susceptible individuals at all ages. Most infants are protected by maternal antibody during the early months of life. In young children below six years of age, infections tend to be mild or asymptomatic, with only 10% developing jaundice. Among older children and adolescents, infection usually causes clinical disease, with jaundice occurring in more than 70% of cases. The disease severity increases with advancing age.

Reservoir Man is the only known reservoir. The infection is maintained in the community by the infected cases, who may be ill or asymptomatic.

Mode of infection The disease spreads through fecal-oral route by close contact between person-to-person. Contaminated food and water also serve as vehicles of infection.

Period of infectivity Feces are infectious from 2 weeks before to 1 week after the onset of jaundice, peak excretion occurring during the late incubation and the early prodromal phase. Viremia is usually evident from the second to sixth week after exposure. The blood and urine may be infective in the early stage of the disease.

Environment factors In temperate zones, epidemic waves have been observed with peaks in late autumn and early winter. In many tropical countries like India, the reported peak of disease tends to occur during the rainy season with low incidence in dry periods.

The patterns of disease vary considerably from population-to-population, and depend upon the standard of hygiene and sanitation. In developing countries like India, infection is acquired early in life; while in the developed countries, the pattern of reported cases has shifted from early childhood to older ages, paralleling improvements in socioeconomic and hygienic conditions.

Pathogenesis

Histologically, liver cell damage is most marked in the centrilobular region. Damage to the hepatocytes is mediated by a cell-mediated immune response. Circulating antibodies help in limiting the dissemination of infection. The virus *per se* is not cytopathic.

Clinical Features

Incubation period is 15 to 50 days.

Presenting illness Infection may be inapparent (asymptomatic, normal liver enzymes), subclinical (asymptomatic, elevated liver enzymes), anicteric (symptomatic, no jaundice) or icteric. Children <6 years mostly have anicteric/subclinical infection.

Prodromal phase The usual presentation is of vomiting, nausea, pain in abdomen, and loss of appetite. A mild to moderate grade fever is usually associated. History of passage of dark yellow urine may be obtained. This phase lasts for almost 1 week.

Case Study | Viral Hepatitis

A 5-year-old boy presented with high grade fever with nausea, vomiting, loss of appetite, malaise, and dull aching pain in abdomen for 4–5 days. The child was also passing high-colored urine for 3 days.

What is your broad hypothesis? Enumerate the differential diagnosis you would consider?

This is an acute illness, most probably of infective etiology, involving the gastrointestinal, hepatobiliary, or urinary tract, as the symptoms pertain to the abdomen. High-colored urine may indicate presence of urobilinogen or bile pigments (because of hepatitis), RBCs (UTI, cystitis), or hemoglobin (hemolysis). The differential diagnoses will thus include viral hepatitis, enteric fever, dengue fever, UTI, and malaria.

On examination, icterus was present. Vitals were stable. Pulse, BP were maintained. There was no rash. Liver was palpable 3 cm below the costal margin, soft in consistency, smooth surface, tender to touch, and moving well with respiration. The liver span was 12 cm. Spleen was not palpable.

Now, what relevant investigations you would order?

Because of icterus and tender hepatomegaly, my first suspicion will be of hepatitis. I will examine the urine to confirm presence of bile pigments and urobilinogen and to rule out hematuria and hemoglobinuria. I will order liver function tests to look at direct and indirect bilirubin levels and liver enzymes (AST and ALT) which are raised in hepatitis. I would also send IgM typhidot and blood culture for typhoid as enteric hepatitis is also a common entity. I will also obtain a complete blood count, peripheral smear for malarial parasite, and dengue serology.

Icteric phase Clinical jaundice becomes apparent. Sclera and skin show icterus which may last for 1 to 4 weeks. Liver is enlarged and tender. Spleen is palpable in 10% cases. Fever usually subsides as the jaundice appears.

Recovery phase Child starts improving 1–2 weeks after onset of jaundice. Fever subsides in one week. Appetite returns back to normal by second week and jaundice starts abating. In young children, hepatitis is usually subclinical, jaundice is uncommon and recovery occurs as a rule. Fulminant hepatitis occurs in only 0.1 to 0.35% cases. Mortality is less than 1%. Carrier state is unusual.

HAV does not result in chronic infection or chronic liver disease. Relapses are known.

Diagnosis

The virus can be isolated from the stool in the acute phase. The diagnosis can also be made by the demonstration of IgM antibodies to HAV (IgM anti-HAV) in serum. These antibodies usually disappear in 4–6 months, but may persist longer. IgG-anti-HAV appear later in the course of illness and persist for life. Liver enzyme levels are very high in the first week of illness. The transaminase levels remain elevated for 1 to 3 weeks.

Complications

Occasionally, HAV infection may result in fulminant hepatitis and death. Atypical manifestations include cholestasis, relapsing hepatitis A (10%), autoimmune hepatitis or extrahepatic manifestations.

Treatment | Viral Hepatitis A

There is no specific antiviral therapy. Treatment is mainly supportive. Rest is recommended and good nutritious diet is advised. There is no evidence for restricting fats in the diet. All hepatotoxic drugs should be avoided. Paracetamol for fever should be given only when the child is uncomfortable because of high temperature. Prognosis is excellent and complete recovery is the rule.

Prevention

A. Care of the Case

Enteric precautions are to be observed in the acute phase of the disease. These include proper washing of the hands before eating and after defecation, safe disposal of excreta and emphasizing on good personal hygiene. Children suffering from hepatitis A should not be allowed to attend school for at least one week after the onset of clinical symptoms.

B. Passive Immunization

Pooled immunoglobulin given intramuscularly in a dose of 0.02 mL/kg of 16% solution protects the close personal contacts and household members, if administered within 2 weeks of the exposure to a patient. The efficacy lasts for six months.

Immunoprophylaxis is also recommended for exposed immunocompromized hosts, and those with chronic liver disease. Postexposure prophylaxis is not indicated for non-household healthy contacts.

C. Active Immunization

Hepatitis A virus has been successfully propagated in cell culture and in continuous cell strains of primate origin, paving the way for the preparation of hepatitis A vaccine. It is a formalin-inactivated, alum-adjuvenated whole cell vaccine. Several inactivated or live-attenuated vaccines against hepatitis A have been developed, but only two inactivated hepatitis A vaccines are currently available internationally. All vaccines are similar in terms of efficacy and side effect profile. Two doses of the vaccine are given parenterally 6–12 months apart. The efficacy is reported to be more than 90%. The current vaccines are well tolerated and no serious adverse events are reported. Duration of protection is likely to be at least 20 years, and possibly lifelong.

Candidates for vaccination include travelers to areas of high endemicity, children identified in high-risk situations, drug abusers, homosexuals, and food handlers. Pregnancy is an absolute contraindication.

HEPATITIS B

Magnitude of the Problem

Global

More than two billion people worldwide have been infected with hepatitis B virus and out of them 350 million are chronically infected. Every year, 1 million hepatitis B carriers are dying of hepatocellular carcinoma or cirrhosis. The prevalence of hepatitis B surface antigen (HBsAg) varies widely in different parts of the world (Fig. 6.2).

India

HBV infection is a major public health problem in India with HBsAg prevalence rate of 1.3–12.7% in children below 15 years of age. Out of total 43 million estimated HBV carriers in India, 10% are highly infectious. Those with chronic HBV infection are at risk for morbidity and mortality associated with cirrhosis and hepatocellular carcinoma. The major mode of transmission is mother to child and by blood-borne transmission. Hepatitis B may cause either acute, persistent, or chronic active infections.

Etiology

Hepatitis B virus (HBV) is a DNA-containing double-shelled virus, 42 nm in diameter. It is the most infectious of the hepatitis viruses. The virus can survive in a dried state up to a period of 7 days. Overall, there are 10 genotypes of HBV with genotype D being the most common in India.

Antigens and antibodies Hepatitis B surface antigen (HBsAg), also known as the Australia antigen, is found on the surface of the virus. Its detection in the serum is diagnostic of active HBV infection. Core of the virus manifests hepatitis B core antigen (HBcAg) specificity. The 'e' antigen (HBeAg) is an integral part of the core of HBV and serves as a marker of active viral replication and thus is associated with high infectivity.

Antibody to hepatitis B surface antigen (anti-HBs) is diagnostic of previous HBV infection or immunization conferring immunity against HBV. Antibody to hepatitis B core antigen (anti-HBc) appears during acute HBV infection and persists in chronic HBV carriers, but not in individuals who recover from infection. Its persistence indicates continuation of HBV replication. Antibody to the 'e' antigen (anti-HBe) appears with the reduction of acute infection. Its presence in chronic carriers is associated with relatively low infectivity and a good prognosis.

Epidemiology

Host characteristics Two different patterns are recognized.
- *In populations with a high prevalence of HBV*, infection is usually acquired early in life; the highest infection and carrier rates are seen among children and young adults. The carrier rates decline with increasing age, as does the prevalence of specific antibody.
- *In population where HBV is relatively uncommon*, the majority of infection and the peak prevalence of HBsAg and of specific antibody are observed in the age group of 15–29 years.

Reservoir Man is the only reservoir. Any individual who is HBsAg positive for 6 months or who is IgM anti-HBc negative and HBsAg positive is called a *chronic HBV carrier*. These are the primary reservoirs of infection. About 10% of patients may become carriers. This state may last from a few years to the lifetime of the person. The carrier may be asymptomatic or rarely may have active liver disease. Besides liver, the virus may also replicate in spleen, lymphocytes, kidneys, and pancreas.

Mode of Spread

Infection can occur from children-to-children; children-to-adults; adult-to-adult; and mother-to-her offspring. The virus is transmitted through blood, blood products, semen,

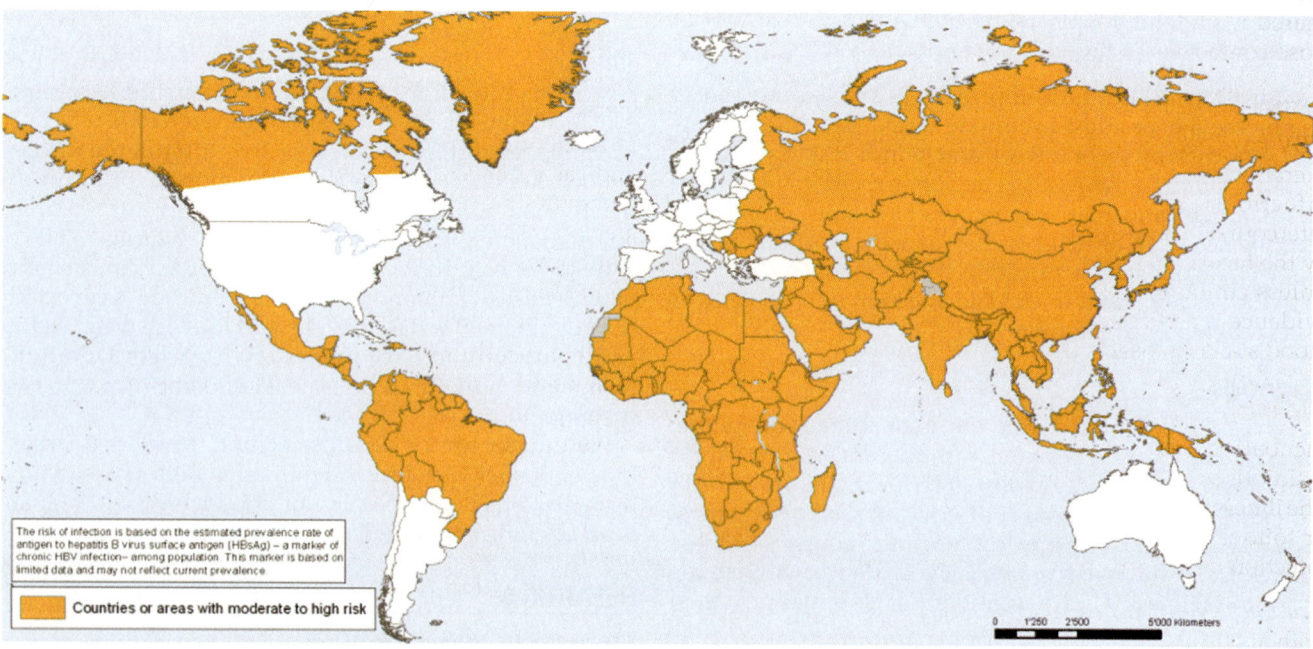

The risk of infection is based on the estimated prevalence rate of antigen to hepatitis B virus surface antigen (HBsAg) – a marker of chronic HBV infection– among population. This marker is based on limited data and may not reflect current prevalence

▮ Countries or areas with moderate to high risk

The boundaries and names shown and the designations used on this map do not imply the expression of any opinion whatsoever on the part of the World Health Organization concerning the legal status of any country, territory, city or area or of its authorities, or concerning the delimitation of its frontiers or boundaries. Dotted and dashed lines on maps represent approximate border lines for which there may not yet be full agreement

Data Source: World Health Organization/CDC
Map Production: Public Health Information and Geographic Information Systems (GIS)
World Health Organization

Fig. 6.2 Hepatitis B, countries at risk 2012 (Reproduced with permission from WHO)

and vaginal fluids. *Vertical transmission* occurs as a result of transmission from mother-to-her neonate, while *horizontal transmission* occurs mainly by sexual contact, both heterosexual and homosexual.

Mother to Child Transmission

Transmission from HBV carrier mothers to their babies appear to be the single most important factor responsible for childhood hepatitis B infection and chronic carrier state of HBV. Most infections appear to occur at birth, as result of a leak of maternal blood into the baby's circulation, or ingestion or accidental inoculation of blood. It is also transmitted through breast milk. Although HBV can infect the fetus *in utero*, this rarely happens.

The risk of infection depends upon the proportion of HBeAg positive carrier mothers, which may be as high as 40% in some countries. Infants born to HBV carrier mothers, who are also HBeAg positive, have a risk as high as 60–90% of acquiring the HBV infection during the perinatal period. Within 9 months of birth, as many as 90% of infected infants become chronic carriers of HBsAg. However, if the mother is HBsAg positive but HBeAg negative or anti-HBe positive, the infant has only 2–15% chance of becoming infected. Other factors associated are virus load, HBV-DNA levels, social status, type of delivery, etc. Presence of anti-HBe reduces the risk of transmission.

Blood-borne Transmission

Hepatitis B has traditionally been a hazard of blood transfusion, the use of shared syringes, and exposure to infected blood. Transmission can occur in the family setting and tends to be related to the degree of crowding in the household and the closeness of the relationship between the individual and the case or carrier. It may occur in adolescents as a result of accidental, percutaneous inoculation following the use of shared razors, toothbrushes, bath brushes, or towels or by close contact.

Sexual Transmission

HBV has been detected in a variety of blood secretions and excretions, including saliva, semen, and vaginal fluid, thus infection may be transmitted by kissing or by sexual intercourse. Hepatitis B does not appear to be transmitted by the fecal-oral route, and urine is probably not infectious unless contaminated with blood. There is no convincing evidence that airborne infections or mosquitoes and other blood sucking insects transmit the disease.

Clinical Features

Incubation period varies from 45 to 160 days, the onset is insidious with loss of appetite, nausea, vomiting and fever. The illness may be asymptomatic with minimal liver damage or follow an acute or chronic course. Chronic hepatitis B infection occurs in 10–20% cases.

Acute hepatitis Clinical course is same as that of hepatitis A. Both anicteric and icteric manifestations are known. Spleen is palpable in 15% children. Complications and fulminant hepatitis are much more common. Extrahepatic manifestations are characteristic and include aplastic anemia, arthritis, rash, urticaria, glomerulonephritis, pleural effusion, myocarditis, Coombs positive hemolytic anemia, and pericarditis. Recovery usually occurs in 2–3 weeks.

Chronic hepatitis In 1–5 years follow-up of patients hospitalized with acute hepatitis B infection, 10% go onto become persistent HBsAg positive; 70% of carriers have chronic persistent hepatitis and 30% develop chronic active hepatitis.

Chronically infected persons are at increased risk for developing chronic liver disease (cirrhosis, chronic active hepatitis) or primary hepatocellular carcinoma. Carrier state occurs in 6–10% of older children and adults, who acquire HBV infection. In perinatal transmission, 90% of affected individuals tend to become carriers.

Fulminant hepatitis Fulminant and subfulminant viral hepatitis (FVH, SVH) are defined as acute viral hepatitis complicated by development of hepatic failure and encephalopathy within 2 weeks and from 2 weeks to 3 months after the onset of jaundice, respectively. Principal symptoms are encephalopathy, cerebral edema, coagulopathy, hypotension, renal dysfunction, hypoglycemia, pancreatitis, and infection.

Mortality of fulminant and subfulminant hepatitis is about 80%. Hepatitis B appears to be most common viral infection leading to FVH, accounting for 35 to 70% of viral related causes; the incidence of FVH in patients with acute hepatitis B is 0.1 to 0.5%.

Laboratory Investigations

White blood cells are normal with relative lymphocytosis. Peripheral smear may show mild hemolysis. SGPT is markedly elevated with a peak in the first week of illness. Alkaline phosphatase is normal or mildly elevated.

HBsAg appears early in the disease and disappears soon. There may be a short window period after the infection when HBsAg may not be detected. In chronic carriers, HBsAg may persist longer than 6 months or even indefinitely. Anti-HBs is usually present soon after onset of jaundice and then persists indefinitely. It indicates good immunity.

Antibodies to HBcAg appear during convalescence. It indicates that the person had a recent or past infection but does not signify immunization. HBeAg suggests an infected person with increased risk of transmitting HBV. Presence of antibodies to surface antigen (anti-HBsAg) and 'e' antigen (anti-HBeAg) provides additional information regarding the stage of hepatitis B infection **(Table 6.4)**.

Hepatocellular carcinoma in chronic carriers can be diagnosed early by serial periodic monitoring of serum α-fetoprotein. A value of more than 100 µg/mL should act as a warning.

Treatment	Hepatitis B

Acute Hepatitis
Prolonged bed rest should be avoided and early ambulation is preferred. No specific dietary restrictions need to be imposed except in hepatic failure. Food selection is dictated by the taste and tolerance to particular foods. Corticosteroid, exchange transfusion, and hemodialysis are not beneficial, even in fulminant hepatitis.

Table 6.4 Serological Markers in Different Stages of Hepatitis B Infection

	HBsAg	HBeAg	Anti-HBsAg	Anti-HBeAg	Anti-HBcAg IgG
Acute infection	+	+	–	–	+
Chronic infection	+	+	–	–	+++
Recent HBV infection, cured	–	–	++	+	++
Past HBV infection, cured	–	–	±	–	±
Healthy carrier	+	–	–	+*	+++
Recent HBV vaccination	–	–	++	–	–

Presence of antibody to the 'e' antigen (Anti-HBeAg) in chronic carriers is associated with relatively low infectivity and a good prognosis.

Chronic Hepatitis

Treatment is aimed at reducing the viral replication to an undetectable level of hepatitis B virus DNA in the serum and development of anti-HBe. Treatment is indicated in a chronic disease with evidence of ongoing inflammation (serum ALT more than twice the normal). Children with low serum HBV DNA titer are most likely to respond.

Interferon and lamivudine are the two drugs that have been used maximally in children. Adefovir, a purine analog, is licensed for use in children above 12 years of age.

- *Interferon-α-2b* Recombinant α-interferon has an established role in treatment of chronic active hepatitis B. The drug is administered in a dose of 5–10 million units per m², subcutaneously thrice a week for 4–6 months. In less advanced chronic liver disease, use of interferon promotes clearance of HBeAg and HBsAg, especially in children without cirrhosis who are more than 2 years old, have abnormal ALT level, and have intermediate to low HBV DNA level.
- *Lamivudine* (3 mg/kg/d for 1 year), though recommended in adults, has limited use in children. Lamivudine monotherapy is associated with selection of mutations in the HBV polymerase. HBeAg clearance rate is noticed to be 34%.

Prevention and Control

A. Interrupting Transmission

This can be achieved by preventing entry of infectious material into the body of a susceptible person from a hepatitis B patient or HBV carrier. This can be accomplished by simple precautions while dealing with people, who are known or presumed to be infectious.

Within health care setting, transmission can be prevented by following universal precautions. All blood and blood-contaminated material should be handled carefully. Instruments including needles and syringes should be cleaned and disinfected or sterilized before reuse.

Outside the health care setting practices such as nose or ear piercing or scarification may transmit HBV, if proper precautions are not taken. Simple heating of the instruments over a flame would eliminate the risk of HBV infection.

B. Passive Immunization

Conventional immune globulin is not recommended for passive immunization against HBV infection. Hepatitis B immunoglobulin (HBIG) has been shown to be effective in pre- and post-exposure prophylaxis. General use of HBIG for long-term prophylaxis is not recommended because of its limited availability, high cost, and risk of complication

due to long-term, repeated use. The main indication for the use of hepatitis B immunoglobulin is for postexposure prophylaxis such as accidental inoculation with HBV-positive material, newborns of HBV carrier mothers, and sexual contacts of hepatitis B carriers.

HBIG must be given as soon as possible after an accidental inoculation (ideally within 6 hours and not later than 48 hours) since the efficacy of HBIG in preventing the disease and the development of a carrier state rapidly decreases with time.

Administration of hepatitis B immunoglobulin at birth and repeated during the first year of life prevents the development of the persistent carrier state in infants born to HBV carrier mothers. Neonates born to virus carrier mothers should be given human anti-hepatitis B immunoglobulin (HBIG) (0.5 mL IM, to be given within 24 hours of birth) and three doses of the vaccine at 0, 1, and 6 months of age. This is followed by post-vaccine testing for HBsAg and anti-HBs at 9–15 months of age. Administer a second complete series of hepatitis B vaccine, if the child is negative for both HBsAg and anti-HBs.

C. Active Immunization

It is the most important method of achieving widespread prevention of hepatitis B. Two types of vaccines are currently available.

- *Plasma-derived Hepatitis B vaccine* It is a subunit vaccine containing surface antigen (HBsAg), which is prepared from pooled plasma of HBV carriers who are HIV negative. HBV surface antigen particles are harvested, purified and residual virus is inactivated. The vaccine is safe, effective and has been widely used.
- *Recombinant HBV vaccine* It is a genetically engineered vaccine, which is prepared in a vector into which gene of HBsAg has been introduced.

Both vaccines are highly immunogenic, with seroconversion rates of 96% reported after 3 doses. The vaccine is given parenterally in the deltoid or in the anterolateral aspect of the thigh. The response to gluteal injection is not optimal. Dose of 10 µg is required for children less than 10 years; and 20 µg is required for adults and children over 10 years of age. Immunocompromised patients should receive twice the recommended dose.

Infants born to HbsAg negative women should receive the vaccine at 0–2 months, 1–4 months and 6–18 months of age (AAP recommendation). In a highly endemic area to raise the immunity faster, the vaccination can also be done at 0, 1 and 2 months with a booster at 12 months. Indian Academy of Pediatrics recommends hepatitis B vaccination of all children with any of the following schedules: (a) 0,6 and 14 weeks; (b) 0,1 and 6 months; and (c) 6, 10 and 14 weeks; after birth. The vaccine can be given concurrently with DPT and OPV administration.

Hepatitis B vaccine is a part of the National Immunization Schedule of India, and given at 6, 10, 14 weeks of age. Newborns delivered at institutions also get an additional '0' dose at birth.

HEPATITIS C

Hepatitis C virus is a single-stranded RNA virus, mainly transmitted through transfusions of blood and blood products; it may be transmitted sexually also. Perinatal transmission is also known in 5–20% of infected mothers. Risk of transfusion-transmitted hepatitis C has been eliminated in industrialized countries through anti-HCV screening techniques. Traditional practices such as circumcision, tattooing, and scarification with contaminated instruments can also spread HCV infection. Intravenous drug users who share needles are also at high risk of infection.

Clinical Features

Incubation period varies from 2 to 24 weeks (average 7–9 weeks). The clinical illness with insidious onset of jaundice and malaise appears mild compared with hepatitis B and may even be asymptomatic. Only 25% cases are icteric. Extrahepatic manifestations similar to that seen in HBV hepatitis may be observed. Chronic HCV infection may also be a common cause of porphyria cutanea tarda.

Persistent HCV infection develops in 85% of patients after the onset of acute hepatitis C. Chronic infection with HCV tends to persist in 50–70% of infected individuals. These chronically infected individuals are at a considerable higher risk (10–20%) of developing chronic liver disease, cirrhosis, and hepatocellular carcinoma. Chronic HCV infection can also be associated with small vessel vasculitis.

Diagnosis

Diagnosis is based on detection of antibodies to hepatitis C virus infection, ie, anti-HCV. However, these antibodies may be absent during an acute infection. Anti-HCV is usually present concomitantly along with the hepatitis C virus. Presence of anti-HCV does not denote immunity. Both false positives and false negatives are known with this test. PCR for detection of HCV RNA is the gold standard for confirmation of recent or perinatal hepatitis C infection. HCV genotype determination is an essential prerequisite for predicting the response to therapy.

Treatment	Hepatitis C

Genotype 1 responds poorly to treatment, while Genotypes 2 and 3 respond better. Treatment is directed to achieve a sustained viral response (SVR) defined as a viremia-free state for at least 6 months after stopping medications.

Interferon-α-2b, ribavirin, and peginterferon are the 3 drugs licensed for use in children above 3 years of age for treating hepatitis C infection. Interferon-α-2b therapy has demonstrated up to 50% SVR in children with genotype 1. Response is better

in genotypes 2, 3 and children older than 12 years. Demonstration of ongoing hepatic inflammation on liver biopsy is a necessary prerequisite for initiating therapy. Treatment is usually given for 48 weeks.

Prevention

There is no vaccine and prevention is difficult, particularly in developing countries where it is most common.

i. Screening of all blood products for HCV is strongly recommended.
ii. Health care worker should stick to universal precautions—cleaning and disinfecting instruments, machines and surfaces that are routinely touched, sharing articles between individuals should be avoided, frequent handwashing and the systematic use of gloves.
iii. Health education programs are needed to inform the general public and health care workers about the risk of transmitting infections with unsterile equipment.
iv. Surveillance on a global basis needs to be strengthened to improve knowledge of the transmission of the virus.
v. Pooled immunoglobulin does not confer passive immunity. For a number of technical reasons, the development of a vaccine to prevent HCV infection is also unlikely for many years.

HEPATITIS DELTA VIRUS (HDV-Delta Agent)

This is a 35–37 nm defective RNA fragment and delta protein antigen. It cannot cause disease alone, but requires hepatitis B as a helper virus, which is coated on it. Infection with Delta virus in persons already infected with acute or chronic HBV may get a fulminant illness. Chronic asymptomatic carriers of HBV are particularly at risk of developing Delta hepatitis and subsequent chronic liver disease and cirrhosis. It is transmitted by blood products or through mucous membranes inoculation. Incubation period is 2 to 8 weeks. Hepatitis D co-infection with hepatitis B increases the likelihood of development of fulminant hepatitis.

Anti-HDV antibody can be demonstrated. Association with both IgM anti-HBc and HBs antigen indicate co-infection with HBV. Patients superinfected with HDV are positive for HBsAg and anti-HDV antibody but negative for anti-HBc IgM. Hepatitis B vaccine also protects against HDV infection.

HEPATITIS E

Hepatitis E virus (HEV) is a single-stranded RNA virus, transmitted primarily by a fecal-oral route. Highest prevalence of HEV infection is reported from India. It is essentially a waterborne disease.

HEV is extremely sensitive to high salt concentrations. Transmission occurs by feco-oral route. The infection is mainly transmitted by contaminated water or food supplies contaminated by feces, although person-to-person spread by the fecal-oral route is also likely. Man is the natural host for HEV, there is only 1 serotype.

Disease severity is higher in pregnant women and adults compared with children. Mainly young adults, aged 15–40, are affected by acute hepatitis E. Hot climate favors the infection. Hepatitis E outbreaks or even sporadic cases are rare in temperate climates.

6

Clinical Features

Incubation period varies between 15 and 60 days with a median of 40 days. Acute illness is associated with icterus, loss of appetite, fever and malaise, followed by recovery. Course of illness and manifestations are similar to hepatitis caused by hepatitis A virus. Recovery is almost always complete. The virus does not lead to chronic disease or carrier state.

HEV has an inclination to induce a fulminant form of the acute disease (the mortality ranges between 0.5% and 4%) particularly in pregnant women, up to 20% of whom may develop fulminant hepatitis E, with a mortality that reaches about 80%. The importance of intrauterine death and high perinatal morbidity and mortality is currently under investigation.

Diagnosis and Treatment

Diagnosis of acute hepatitis E infection is made by the anti-HEV IgM antibodies in serum. IgG anti-HEV appear a few days after the IgM response, persist for long (>14 yrs) and provide protection against subsequent infections with hepatitis E.

There is no specific treatment, merely supportive measures exist.

Prevention

Usually elementary food hygiene precautions are recommended. Prevention of fecal contamination of drinking water supplies, and provision for safe disposal of human excreta are important public health measures. A recombinant hepatitis E vaccine is available for adults.

Passive immunoprophylaxis in the form of immunoglobulins is not effective.

Revision Point

Viral Hepatitis

1. Viral hepatitis implies inflammation of the liver caused by one of the five hepatotropic viruses, A to E. Hepatitis A and E are transmitted by orofecal route while B,C,D have a parenteral transmission.
2. Viral hepatitis is often associated with yellow discoloration of eyes and urine and elevated serum levels of liver enzymes, ie, alanine aminotransferase (ALT) and aspartate aminotransferase (AST), though a subset can be asymptomatic.
3. Hepatitis B can be transmitted from an infected mother to her infant at birth.
4. Most patients with viral hepatitis improve spontaneously. Only a few children with acute viral hepatitis progress to liver failure.
5. HBV or HCV infection may progress to chronic hepatitis.

Dentinger CM. Emerging infections: hepatitis A. *Am J Nurs.* 2009;109:29–33.

Giacchino R, Cappelli B. Treatment of viral hepatitis B in children. *Expert Opin Pharmacother.* 2010;11:889–903.

Heller S, Valencia-Mayoral P. Treatment of viral hepatitis in children. *Arch Med Res.* 2007;38:702–10.

Indolfi G, Resti M. Perinatal transmission of hepatitis C virus infection. *J Med Virol.* 2009;81:836–43.

Lai M, Liaw YF. Chronic hepatitis B: past, present, and future. *Clin Liver Dis.* 2010;14:531–46.

Liu JP, Nikolova D, Fei Y. Immunoglobulins for preventing hepatitis A. *Cochrane Database Syst Rev.* 2009;2.

Mohan N, González-Peralta RP, Fujisawa T, *et al.* Chronic hepatitis C virus infection in children. *J Pediatr Gastroenterol Nutr.* 2010;50:123–31.

Porto AF, Tormey L, Lim JK. Management of chronic hepatitis C infection in children. *Curr Opin Pediatr.* 2012;24:113–20.

Shah U, Kelly D, Chang MH, *et al.* Management of chronic hepatitis B in children. *J Pediatr Gastroenterol Nutr.* 2009;48:399–404.

Teshale EH, Hu DJ, Holmberg SD. The two faces of hepatitis E virus. *Clin Infect Dis.* 2011;51:328–34.

Yeung LT, Roberts EA. Current issues in the management of paediatric viral hepatitis. *Liver Int.* 2010;30:5–18.

Zein NN. Hepatitis C in children: recent advances. *Curr Opin Pediatr.* 2007;19:570–4.

6.8 INFECTIOUS MONONUCLEOSIS

Infectious mononucleosis is a clinical syndrome of multisystem involvement primarily caused by Epstein-Barr virus infection and characterized by high grade fever, pharyngotonsillitis, and generalized lymphadenopathy. Cytomegalovirus, hepatitis virus, adenovirus, toxoplasma, and rubella virus can also cause similar illness.

Epidemiology

Epstein-Barr virus infections are ubiquitous in nature and affect almost everybody, at one age or other. Subclinical infections are extremely common, especially in under-five children. Primary infection occurs in early childhood. Most of the infectious episodes are passed off as viral fever. Typical clinical manifestations are apparent only in older children and adolescents.

The virus is transmitted by close contact with oral secretions such as kissing; and continues to be excreted in saliva for at least 6 months after the primary infection.

Pathogenesis

Epstein-Barr virus, after entering the host through oral secretions, infects the epithelial cell of pharynx and starts replicating. This is followed by viremia and involvement of reticuloendothelial system including lymph nodes, liver, and spleen. Epstein-Barr virus has a typical affinity for B cell. Infection of B lymphocytes evokes a concomitant increase in CD8 (cytotoxic T lymphocytes) count and reversal of CD4/CD8 ratio. Increased population of CD8 T lymphocytes is aimed to counter the infected B cell population. CD8 cell spillage into the peripheral circulation manifests as presence of *'atypical large lymphocytes'* in peripheral blood smear examination. The virus remains in the host, even after the acute infection subsides; shedding through oral secretion also continues, though intermittently. Reactivation is usually asymptomatic.

Epstein-Barr virus is an oncogenic virus and has been implicated in virus associated hemophagocytic syndrome, hairy leukoplakia, nasopharyngeal carcinoma, Burkitt lymphoma, and Hodgkin disease.

Clinical Features

The incubation period is 4–6 weeks. As stated above, most infections in under-five children are asymptomatic. Older children and adolescents present with fever, malaise, fatigue, sore throat, and abdominal pain. Examination reveals marked pharyngotonsillitis, generalized tender lymphadenopathy, and moderate hepatosplenomegaly. This may be accompanied by a macular rash that is precipitated or aggravated by administration of ampicillin. Another notable finding is periorbital edema.

Lymphadenopathy is more marked in the cervical chain. Epitrochlear lymph node enlargement is almost pathognomonic of infectious mononucleosis. The acute disease is self-limiting and lasts for 4–6 weeks. Fever subsides in about 7–10 days; non-specific symptoms may take longer to resolve. Complications are listed in **Table 6.5**.

Differential Diagnosis

Infectious mononucleosis is often misdiagnosed as acute streptococcal pharyngitis and treated as such. It is clinically difficult to distinguish Ebstein-Barr infection from streptococcal or other viral infection. Generalized lymphadenopathy and failure to respond to antibiotics after 2–3 days in a child being treated for streptococcal sore throat should alert to a possibility of infectious mononucleosis.

Laboratory Investigations

There is marked leukocytosis with lymphocytic predominance. Presence of 'atypical' large lymphocytes' in the peripheral blood smear is the hallmark of infectious mononucleosis. These are mature CD8 T-lymphocytes. Atypical lymphocytes, however, are not unique to Epstein-Barr infections, and can also be documented in other infections including those by cytomegalovirus, rubella, *Toxoplasma*, *Mycoplasma*, hepatitis virus, mumps virus, *Plasmodium falciparum* and *Salmonella typhi*. Other laboratory abnormalities include thrombocytopenia and elevated hepatic enzymes.

Paul-Bunnell test This test detects heterophile IgM antibodies produced in infectious mononucleosis that agglutinate sheep red cells. These antibodies may persist in the peripheral blood for as long as 2 years. Both false-positive and false-negative results are known. Thus, for confirmation of diagnosis, Epstein-Barr specific antibody needs to be documented. Acute infection can be detected by presence of IgM antibodies to viral capsid antigen (VCA) of Epstein-Barr virus.

Table 6.5 Complications of Infectious Mononucleosis

System	Complication
Respiratory	Pneumonia, severe airway obstruction
Neurological	Convulsions, aseptic meningitis, transverse myelitis, and Guillain-Barre syndrome
Hematological	Immune hemolytic anemia of cold antibody type, thrombocytopenia, aplastic anemia, and hemorrhage
Splenic rupture	Rupture of rapidly enlarging spleen may follow minor trauma
Others	Myocarditis, hepatitis, glomerulonephritis, orchitis

Treatment — Infectious Mononucleosis

There is no specific drug therapy for infectious mononucleosis and the treatment by and large remains supportive. Corticosteroids (prednisolone 1–2 mg/kg/day for 7 days, and tapered over next 1 week) may be helpful in treatment of severe complications; eg, airway obstruction, severe bleeding due to thrombocytopenia, severe anemia due to autoimmune hemolytic anemia, and meningoencephalitis.

Revision Point — Infectious Mononucleosis

1. Infectious mononucleosis is mostly caused by Epstein-Barr virus and characterized by high grade fever, sore throat, fatigue, palatal petechiae, lymphadenopathy (posterior cervical or axillary), and splenomegaly.
2. Relative lymphocytosis (>50% lymphocytes) including 10% atypical lymphocytes or at least 20% atypical lymphocytes; or a positive heterophile antibody test favors the diagnosis.
3. Good supportive care is the mainstay of treatment, and includes antipyretics or analgesics, adequate hydration, gargling or lozenges, and bed rest.
4. Steroids may be used for life-threatening complications like airway obstruction or bleeding or CNS manifestations.
5. No vaccine is available to prevent this infection.

Bravender T. Epstein-Barr virus, cytomegalovirus, and infectious mononucleosis. *Adolesc Med State Art Rev*. 2010;21:251–64.
Hurt C, Tammaro D. Diagnostic evaluation of mononucleosis-like illnesses. *Am J Med*. 2007;120:911.
Luzuriaga K, Sullivan JL. Infectious mononucleosis. *N Engl J Med*. 2010;362:1993–2000.

6.9 INFLUENZA

Influenza, more frequently called as "the flu" among general population, is a highly contagious disease caused by influenza virus. Influenza viruses are responsible for a wide spectrum of respiratory illnesses causing significant morbidity and mortality in children.

Owing to its great propensity to change its genetic constitution, influenza viruses are responsible for many pandemics that have occurred worldwide resulting in approximately 3–5 million cases of severe illness and about 250,000 to 500,000 deaths. Influenza virus mainly affects preschool children at time of epidemics.

Etiology

Influenza viruses are negative-sense, single-strand RNA viruses belonging to family Orthomyxoviridae. They are mainly of three types: Type A, Type B, and Type C. Type A viruses are the most common and most virulent human pathogens and responsible for causing the most severe disease. Type C infections are milder.

Influenza viral RNA has 8 genetic elements but hemagglutinin (H) and neuraminidase (N) are most important antigens that help in attachment, replication, and subsequent release of the virus. There are total 16 types of H proteins and 9 types of N proteins. H 1, 2 and 3, and N 1 and

2 are the common types in humans, which in different combinations lead to different strains of virus, with 144 combinations possible. Most common influenza virus strains are H1N1, H2N2, H3N2, and H5N1.

One of most characteristic feature of influenza virus is its tendency to mutate. Antigenic variations are due to either minor changes (antigenic drift) or major changes (antigenic shift).

- *Antigenic drift* These are small changes in genetic makeup of influenza virus as they replicate. New strains of virus thus formed are different from parent virus but still related to them and cross protection is thus present. These changes may accumulate over a period of time to result into another form that may be completely different from origin virus and no cross-immunity existing for them.
- *Antigenic shift* These are sudden major changes in virus structure due to genetic re-assortment of segments coming from two different species. It is largely a feature of type A influenza virus. Antigenic shift are far less common than antigenic drift in influenza virus.

Transmission

Spread of influenza virus is mainly through air droplet route. Shedding of virus over fomites can also result in spread of virus. Shedding of virus is maximum on day 2 of illness and it continues for up to two weeks. Children are more infectious as compared to adults and start shedding virus before symptoms start. Virus is inactivated by heating it to 56°C (133°F) for approximately 60 minutes, and by acids (at pH <2).

Pathogenesis

The virus attaches to epithelial cells of nose, trachea, and bronchi. Viral replication occurs but viremia does not occur as hemagglutinin of avirulent virus strains is cleaved by proteases of respiratory epithelium cells only. But hemagglutinin of highly virulent strains (like H5N1) can be cleaved by a wide variety of proteases, subsequently leading to spread of virus to deeper lung tissues and other body parts. Other possible explanation of mechanism of symptomatology of influenza is inhibition of adrenocorticotropic hormone (ACTH) resulting in decreased cortisol levels. Common symptoms of the flu such as fever, headache, and fatigue result because of release of large amounts of pro-inflammatory cytokines and chemokines like interferon and tumor necrosis factor, from influenza-infected cells.

Clinical Features

Incubation period of influenza is 1–4 days with average of 2 days. Around one-third of people with influenza are asymptomatic. Symptoms vary in their severity ranging from mild to lethal. Symptoms are acute in onset. Fever and cough the most common symptoms. Fever is sudden in onset usually preceded by chills ranging from 38 to 39°C with severe myalgia, headache, fatigue, nasal congestion, rhinitis, sore throat, nonproductive cough, cervical lymphadenopathy, conjunctivitis. Infants and young children present more often with conjunctivitis, rhinitis and severe gastrointestinal symptoms when compared to adults. Flu can be differentiated from common cold by the presence of high grade fever and extreme fatigue.

Complications

Seasonal flu is relatively benign and self-limiting condition. It may rarely result in various complications like viral pneumonia, secondary bacterial pneumonia, sinus infections, and worsening of asthma or heart failure.

Diagnosis

Due to similarity of symptoms between influenza and other upper respiratory tract infections, clinical diagnosis of influenza is challenging. Various samples needed for isolation of virus are nasopharyngeal swab, nasal wash/swab, endotracheal aspirate, or bronchoalveolar lavage.

Diagnostic tools available for the diagnosis of influenza are as follows:

1. Viral culture of nasopharyngeal and/or throat samples
2. Hemagglutination inhibition techniques
3. Immunofluorescence assay
4. ELISA and other rapid influenza diagnostic tests (RIDTs).

Rapid diagnostic tests have a sensitivity of 50–75% and specificity of 90–95% when compared with viral culture.

Treatment	Influenza

Treatment for pediatric influenza is mainly symptomatic. Antipyretics, analgesics, and adequate oral fluids are mainstay of therapy. Aspirin should be avoided because of possibility to cause Reye syndrome. Neuraminidase inhibitors (oseltamivir and zanamivir) and M2 protein inhibitors (adamantane ineffective against influenza B viruses) are the two classes of drugs available for treatment of influenza. They reduce the severity and duration of illness, if used appropriately but are not recommended for seasonal flu. Antibiotics are only to be used for secondary infection, and are of no use in treatment of influenza *per se.*

Prevention

Infection control Frequent handwashing and wearing a surgical mask is protective.

Vaccination World Health Organization recommends yearly vaccination for high-risk populations such as children, the elderly, health care workers, and people with asthma, diabetes, heart disease, and immunocompromised status. The vaccine provides immunity against three or four types of influenza virus strains of type A and B virus but not type C. Each year a new vaccine is launched due to evolution of newer strain of virus. Two types of vaccines are available in market (*a*) killed trivalent vaccine to be given intramuscularly (recommended for people >6-month-old); and (*b*) live-attenuated intranasal vaccine (recommended >2 years age group).

Vaccines can lead to influenza-like symptoms though of lesser severity and lesser duration. Children <9 years of age need two doses of intranasal vaccine 6 months apart whereas older children and adult require only one dose. Rarely reported severe adverse effect of vaccine is a severe form of anaphylactic reaction. One in a million chance of developing Guillain–Barré syndrome due to vaccination has been reported.

Table 6.6 Recommended Dose of Oseltamivir for treatment of H1N1		
Weight	*Recommended dose for treatment (5 days)*	*Recommended dose for chemoprophylaxis (10 days)*
<15 kg	30 mg BD	30 mg OD
15–23 kg	45 mg BD	45 mg OD
23–40 kg	60 mg BD	60 mg OD
>40 kg	75 mg BD	75 mg OD
Recommended dose in infants is as follows:		
Age in months	*Recommended dose for treatment (for 5 days)*	*Recommended dose for chemoprophylaxis (10 days)*
<3 months	3 mg/kg/dose BD	Not recommended
3–5 months	3 mg/kg/dose BD	3 mg/kg/dose OD
6–11 months	3 mg/kg/dose BD	3 mg/kg/dose OD

SWINE FLU (H1N1 INFLUENZA)

A special mention should be made of H1N1 swine flu that was responsible for the most recent pandemic of influenza. WHO definitions for H1N1 influenza are given in **Box 6.4**.

Presenting signs and symptoms of swine flu are similar to other influenza virus illnesses. These include chilly sensation, fever, cough, headache, sore throat, prostration, nasal stuffiness, vomiting and diarrhea, conjunctivitis, myalgia, lymphadenopathy, with tendency to progress to severe and lethal form causing chest pain, breathing difficulty, shock, severe pneumonia, encephalitis, encephalopathy, depression of myocardium, and multi-organ dysfunction. Disease is more troublesome in newborns and young children. Virus can be diagnosed by culture of throat swab specimen or detection of viral DNA through ELISA, IHA, immunofluorescence, or PCR.

Children with H1N1 infections need to be treated with oseltamivir (**Table 6.6**). Duration of treatment is for 5 days.

Box 6.4 Case Definitions of H1N1 Influenza

- *Suspect* Patient who has acute febrile respiratory illness within 7 days of contact with a confirmed case of swine flu or who resides in a community with confirmed cases of swine flu or within 7 days of travel to a community with confirmed cases of H1NI.
- *Probable case* Patient who has acute febrile respiratory illness who is positive for influenza A by RDT but negative for H1 and H3 by influenza RT-PCR.
- *Confirmed case* Patient who has acute febrile respiratory illness who is positive for influenza by either RT-PCR or viral culture or four fold rise of H1N1 virus specific antibodies.

6.10 POLIOMYELITIS

Poliomyelitis, often called polio or infantile paralysis, is an acute viral infectious disease caused by poliovirus with three distinct serotypes; ie, 1, 2, and 3. Poliovirus spreads from person-to-person, primarily *via* the fecal-oral route. Although around 90% of poliovirus infections have no symptoms at all, affected individuals can exhibit a range of symptoms, if the virus enters the bloodstream. In less than 1% of cases, the virus enters the central nervous system, preferentially infecting and destroying motor neurons, leading to muscle weakness and acute flaccid paralysis. *Spinal polio* is the most common form, characterized by asymmetric paralysis that most often involves the legs.

Historical Perspective

Polio was one of the most dreaded childhood diseases of the 20th century. Polio epidemics had crippled thousands of people, mostly young children; the disease has caused paralysis and death for much of human history. By 1910, much of the world experienced a dramatic increase in polio cases and frequent epidemics became regular events, primarily in cities during the summer months. These epidemics which left thousands of children and adults paralyzed provided the impetus for the development of a vaccine. The polio vaccines developed by Jonas Salk in 1952 and Albert Sabin in 1962 are credited with reducing the annual number of polio cases from many hundreds of thousands to around a thousand. In 1988, the World Health Organization initiated the Global Polio Eradication Initiative to eradicate poliomyelitis; at that time, it was endemic in 125 countries. The worldwide campaign to eradicate polio continues today, as do efforts to prevent transmission of the disease into polio-free areas.

Poliomyelitis Eradication

Following the widespread use of poliovirus vaccine in the mid-1950s, the incidence of poliomyelitis declined dramatically in many industrialized countries. A global effort to eradicate polio began in 1988, led by the World Health Organization, UNICEF, and The Rotary Foundation. These efforts have reduced the number of annual diagnosed cases by 99%; from an estimated 350,000 cases from 125 countries in 1988, to only 650 cases in 2011. Should eradication be successful, it will represent only the second time mankind has ever completely eliminated a disease. The first such disease was smallpox, officially eradicated in 1979.

A number of eradication milestones have already been reached, and several regions of the world have been certified polio-free. The Americas were declared polio-free in 1994. In 2000 polio was officially eradicated in 36 Western Pacific countries, including China and Australia. Europe was declared polio-free in 2002. Today, polio remains endemic in only three countries: Nigeria, Pakistan, and Afghanistan.

Poliomyelitis in India

The year 2011 earned the unique distinction, when only 1 case of poliomyelitis occurred in India, following which no case has been reported from the entire country till date. India was removed from the list of endemic countries in February,

6

2012. On 27 March 2014, the WHO South-East Asia region was certified polio-free.

Transmission of Poliovirus

Poliovirus infects and causes disease in humans alone. All 3 serotypes of poliovirus (1, 2, 3) are extremely virulent and produce the same disease symptoms. Type 1 is the most commonly encountered form, and the one most closely associated with paralysis.

Poliovirus prefers to inhabit the gastrointestinal tract. It is highly contagious and spreads easily from human-to-human contact. In endemic areas, wild polioviruses can infect virtually the entire human population. It is seasonal in temperate climates, with peak transmission occurring in summer and autumn. These seasonal differences are far less pronounced in tropical areas.

Virus particles are excreted in the feces for several weeks following initial infection. The disease is transmitted primarily via the fecal-oral route, by ingesting contaminated food or water. Factors that increase the risk of polio infection or affect the severity of the disease include immune deficiency, malnutrition, tonsillectomy, physical activity immediately following the onset of paralysis, and skeletal muscle injury due to injection of vaccines, or therapeutic agents.

Pathogenesis

Poliovirus enters the body through the mouth, infecting the first cells it comes in contact in the pharynx and intestinal mucosa. Poliovirus replicates within gastrointestinal cells for about a week, from where it spreads to the tonsils, the intestinal lymph nodes including the M cells of Peyer's patches, and the deep cervical and mesenteric lymph nodes, where it multiplies abundantly. The virus is subsequently absorbed into the bloodstream resulting in widespread viremia. Poliovirus can survive and multiply within the blood and lymphatics for long periods of time. This sustained replication causes a major viremia, and leads to the development of minor influenza-like symptoms. Rarely, this may progress and the virus may invade the central nervous system, provoking a local inflammatory response. In around 1% of infections, poliovirus spreads along certain nerve fiber pathways, preferentially replicating in and destroying motor neurons within the spinal cord, brainstem, or motor cortex. This leads to the development of paralytic poliomyelitis.

Most commonly affected areas are the anterior horns of spinal cord, cranial nerve nuclei, vital centers in the medulla, and cerebellar nuclei and vermis. Cerebellar involvement is rare. White matter of the spinal cord and the non-motor part of cerebral cortex are usually spared.

Immunity

Individuals who are exposed to the virus, either through infection or by immunization with polio vaccine, develop immunity. In immune individuals, IgA antibodies against poliovirus are present in the tonsils and gastrointestinal tract and are able to block virus replication; IgG and IgM antibodies against poliovirus can prevent the spread of the virus to motor neurons of the central nervous system. Infection or vaccination with one serotype of poliovirus does not provide immunity against the other serotypes, and full immunity requires exposure to each serotype.

Clinical Features

The incubation period ranges from 6–20 days (range 3–35 days). In most people with a normal immune system, a poliovirus infection is asymptomatic. The estimated ratio of symptomatic to asymptomatic infection ranges between 1:100 (0.1–1%). Symptomatic infection results in 2 patterns: A minor illness which does not involve the central nervous system (CNS), sometimes called *abortive poliomyelitis*, and a major illness involving the CNS, which may be paralytic or non-paralytic. In children, non-paralytic meningitis is the most likely consequence of CNS involvement, and paralysis occurs in only 1 in 1000 cases. Paralysis rates also vary depending on the serotype of the infecting poliovirus; the highest rates of paralysis (1 in 200) are associated with poliovirus type 1, the lowest rates (1 in 2,000) are associated with type 2 (Fig. 6.3).

Minor (abortive) illness This may include respiratory tract infection (sore throat and fever), gastrointestinal disturbances (nausea, vomiting, abdominal pain, constipation or, rarely, diarrhea), and influenza-like illnesses.

Non-paralytic illness This is characterized by aseptic meningitis, with symptoms of headache, pain in neck, back, abdomen and extremities. Other symptoms include fever, vomiting, lethargy, and irritability.

Paralytic Polio

Approximately 1 in 200 to 1 in 1000 cases progress to paralytic disease, in which the muscles become weak, floppy and poorly-controlled, and finally completely paralyzed; this condition is known as acute flaccid paralysis. The paralysis is asymmetrical and characterized by weakness, pain, and loss of superficial and deep tendon reflexes. Paralysis generally develops 1–10 days after early symptoms begin, progresses for 2–3 days, and is usually complete by the time the fever subsides. Depending on the site of paralysis, paralytic poliomyelitis is classified as spinal, bulbar, or bulbospinal. Encephalitis, an infection of the brain tissue itself, can occur in rare cases and is usually restricted to infants. It is characterized by confusion, changes in mental status, headaches, fever, and less commonly seizures and spastic paralysis.

- *Spinal poliomyelitis* Spinal polio is the most common form of paralytic poliomyelitis; characterized by asymmetrical

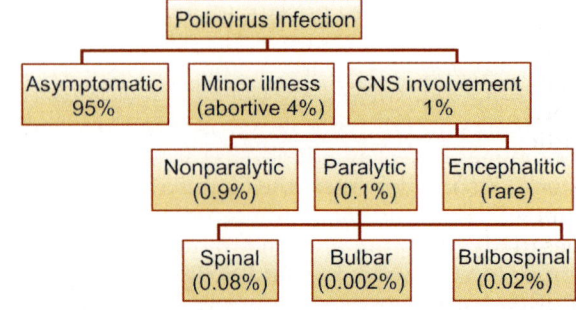

Fig. 6.3 Clinical presentation of poliovirus infection in children

motor weakness of limbs. Deep tendon reflexes are usually absent or diminished; sensation in the paralyzed limbs is not affected. Paralysis is often more severe proximally (where the limb joins the body) than distally (the fingertips and toes). Autonomic involvement may result in constipation or urinary retention. Involvement of diaphragm and intercostal muscles may cause respiratory difficulty.

- *Bulbar poliomyelitis* Involvement of cranial nerves within the bulbar region of the brainstem results in difficulty in breathing, speaking and swallowing. Cranial nerves affected are the glossopharyngeal nerve, the vagus nerve, and the accessory nerve, which controls upper neck movement. Due to the effect on swallowing, secretions of mucus may build up causing airway obstruction.

  Other signs and symptoms include facial weakness, diplopia and abnormal respiratory rate, depth, and rhythm, which may lead to respiratory arrest. Pulmonary edema and shock are also possible, and may be fatal.

- *Bulbospinal poliomyelitis* These children have both bulbar and spinal symptoms. The virus affects the upper part of the cervical spinal cord (C3 through C5). Phrenic nerve is the most critical nerve to be involved, which drives the diaphragm to inflate the lungs. Paralysis of the diaphragm resulting in respiratory depression and respiratory failure can be fatal.

Diagnosis

Paralytic poliomyelitis may be clinically suspected in individuals experiencing acute onset of flaccid paralysis in one or more limbs with decreased or absent tendon reflexes in the affected limbs that cannot be attributed to another apparent cause, and without sensory or cognitive loss. Differential diagnosis of acute flaccid paralysis is discussed in Chapter on Neurological Disorders.

Laboratory diagnosis is based on recovery of poliovirus from a stool sample. Analysis of the cerebrospinal fluid reveals mild lymphocytosis and a mildly elevated protein level.

Prognosis

Patients with abortive polio infections recover completely. In those that develop only aseptic meningitis, the symptoms can be expected to persist for 2 to 10 days, followed by complete recovery.

Spinal polio If the affected nerve cells are completely destroyed, paralysis will be permanent; cells that are not destroyed but loose function temporarily may recover within four to six weeks after onset. About 50% of children with spinal polio recover fully; 25% recover with mild disability, and the remaining 25% are left with severe disability. The degree of both acute paralysis and residual paralysis is likely to be proportional to the degree of viremia, and inversely proportional to the degree of immunity.

Poliomyelitis with respiratory involvement Overall, 5–10% of patients with paralytic polio die due to the paralysis of muscles used for breathing. The mortality rate varies by age: 2–5% of children and up to 15–30% of adults will die. Bulbar polio often causes death, if respiratory support is not provided; with support, its mortality rate ranges from 25 to 75%, depending on the age of the patient. When positive pressure ventilation is available, the mortality can be reduced to 15%.

Management

No specific treatment exists for acute poliomyelitis except supportive care, which may help to ensure survival, modify the disability, and improve the outcome. Supportive measures include analgesics for pain, moderate exercise and a nutritious diet. Treatment of polio often requires long-term rehabilitation, including physical therapy, braces, corrective shoes and, in some cases, orthopedic surgery.

Acute phase All patients should be placed on bed rest in an isolation unit. Monitor vital signs carefully; focus especially on the swallowing function, vital capacity, pulse, and blood pressure in anticipation of respiratory or circulatory complications. Children who develop respiratory failure because of depression of the brain stem respiratory center, in addition to paralysis of the intercostal and diaphragmatic muscles, may require immediate positive pressure ventilation and/or tracheotomy in the respiratory intensive care unit.

Physical therapy During the phase of acute myalgia, active massage or intramuscular injections should be avoided. Active physiotherapy must be started after the phase of myalgia is over.

Physical therapy plays an important role in rehabilitation for patients with poliomyelitis. Patients with muscle paralysis benefit from frequent (*i*) passive range of motion (PROM); and (*ii*) splinting of joints to prevent contracture and joint ankylosis. Chest physiotherapy helps those with bulbar involvement to prevent atelectasis. Frequent repositioning of the paralyzed children helps prevent bedsores.

Occupational therapy Children with paralysis of the extremities may benefit from hand or arm splints, knee or trochanter rolls, a footboard, or multipurpose boots to prevent foot drop, ulcers, and other deformities. Hot packs also are helpful to relieve the muscle pain.

Speech therapy Children with cranial nerve involvement may develop swallowing dysfunction. To protect the airway and prevent aspiration pneumonia, a speech therapist needs to be involved early to perform an evaluation of the safety of swallowing. Decisions on the appropriate consistency of oral foods and use of various strategies/techniques greatly reduce the risk of aspiration.

Recreational therapy Patients may attend leisure activities to reduce stress and learn how to get involved in group activities. In severe cases of contracture from limb immobilization, the patient may benefit from orthopedic surgery to release the contracture and restore limb function.

Polio-free Region

Before a WHO region can be certified polio-free, three conditions must be satisfied: (*a*) at least three years of zero polio cases due to wild poliovirus; (*b*) excellent certification standard surveillance; (*c*) each country must illustrate the capacity to detect, report and respond to "imported" polio cases. Laboratory stocks must be contained and safe management of the wild virus in Inactivated Polio Vaccine (IPV) manufacturing sites must be assured before the world can be certified polio-free.

Acute Flaccid Paralysis Surveillance

The key to poliomyelitis eradication is active surveillance of cases of acute flaccid paralysis (AFP). There are four steps in the surveillance (*a*) finding and reporting children with AFP, (*b*) transporting stool samples in reverse cold chain, (*c*) isolation and identifying poliovirus, and (*d*) to determine the origin of the poliovirus strain. In addition, environmental surveillance is carried out by testing sewage sample for the isolation of polio virus. International spread of poliovirus is identified by examination of sewage sample especially from countries declared free from polio.

Surveillance indicators Certain minimum standards required to be maintained for certification of standard and adequate AFP surveillance are given in **Table 6.7**. In 2016, a total of 106283 cases of AFP were reported, globally.

Vaccine-Associated Paralytic Poliomyelitis (VAPP)

OPV has one rare but significant side effect—vaccine-associated poliomyelitis. The risk is about 1 case for every 2.2 to 2.5 million doses.

The danger of OPV was particularly highlighted by outbreaks of vaccine-associated paralytic polio which occurred in areas that were previously polio-free: Madagascar (four cases in 2002), Hispaniola (22 cases in 2000–2001), the Philippines (three cases in 2001) and, upon

Table 6.7 Minimum Standards Required for Adequate AFP Surveillance

Indicators	Minimum level for certification of standard surveillance
Completeness of reporting	At least 80% of the expected reporting of AFP either weekly or monthly data should be received on time and from the representative geographical area of the country.
Sensitivity of the surveillance	Minimum of 1 case of AFP/1000,000 population in <15 yrs age. For higher sensitivity, two cases/1000,000 is required
Completeness of case investigation	All AFP cases should have full clinical and virological investigations with minimum of 805 of stool specimen of adequate amount collected at an interval of 24 hrs within 14 days of onset of AFP and sent to the laboratory in reverse cold chain
Completeness of follow up	At least 80% of AFP cases should have follow-up for residual paralysis after 60 days of onset.
Laboratory performance	All stool specimens must be processed in a WHO accredited laboratory within global polio laboratory network (GPLN)

retrospective analysis, Egypt (at least 32 cases in 1988). To avoid the risk of VAPP, many countries in Western Europe and North America, as well as Australia, New Zealand, and Guam have now switched to using the killed polio vaccine (IPV). Several other countries in Eastern Europe, Middle East as well as Bermuda are using a combination of both OPV and IPV. In the remaining endemic regions of South Asia and Africa, OPV remains the vaccine of choice on account of its ease of administration and effectiveness. Very rarely, the virus in the vaccine may genetically change and start to circulate among a population. These viruses are known as circulating vaccine-derived polioviruses (cVDPV).

Cessation of OPV

In 2003, a WHO consultation on circulating vaccine-derived polioviruses (cVDPVs) concluded that routine use of OPV must be discontinued. The consultation recommended that a strategy be developed for safely stopping OPV use as soon as possible after interruption of transmission, when population immunity is expected to be high and before surveillance sensitivity has started to decline. The objective of containment is to minimize the possibility that poliovirus will be reintroduced into the community.

Rationale Vaccine-derived polioviruses (VDPVs) can, on rare occasions, establish endemic or epidemic transmission, making continued use of OPV incompatible with polio eradication. Continued use of OPV after interruption of wPV (wild poliovirus) transmission can cause paralytic disease caused by: (*i*) cases of vaccine-associated paralytic poliomyelitis (VAPP); (*ii*) outbreaks due to cVDPVs; and (*iii*) long-term excretion of vaccine-derived poliovirus among individuals with primary immunodeficiency disorders (iVDPVs). In addition, there is a risk of paralytic cases caused by wPV from unintentional release from laboratory or manufacturing site; or intentional release due to an act of bioterrorism or biological warfare.

Advantage Discontinuation of OPV should eliminate cases of VAPP, substantially decrease and then eliminate the risks of outbreaks caused by cVDPVs, and prevent poliovirus exposure among immunodeficient individuals born after OPV cessation.

Implications for IPV With OPV no longer a viable option for routine use in the future (probably 2–3 years after interrupting wPV transmission), the only vaccine that may be considered for this purpose would be IPV. However, based on currently available information, WHO does not recommend universal IPV for routine immunization after OPV cessation, because of its cost and logistic constraints.

Coordinated OPV cessation To minimize the risk of emergence of (and exposure to) cVDPVs during the period following OPV cessation, all countries will need to stop the use of OPV during a relatively short period of time (a few weeks) everywhere, and all must institute mechanisms to ensure that OPV from throughout the health system has been recalled and destroyed. There must be agreement that no country will again use OPV, unless specifically endorsed by the international community for control of an outbreak.

THE GLOBAL POLIO ERADICATION INITIATIVE (GPEI)

In 1988, the 41st World Health Assembly, consisting of delegates from 166 member states, launched a global initiative to eradicate polio by the end of the year 2000. The Global Polio Eradication Initiative is spearheaded by national governments, WHO, Rotary International, the United States Centers for Disease Control and Prevention and the United Nations Children's Fund (UNICEF). The partnership supporting the Global Polio Eradication Initiative includes international agencies, bilateral donors, non-governmental organizations, foundations, and the private sector.

The Polio Eradication and Endgame Strategic Plan 2013–2018 is a comprehensive, long-term strategy that addresses what is needed to deliver a polio-free world by 2018. The first objective is to stop all wPV transmission by the end of 2014 and any new outbreaks due to a cVDPV within 120 days of confirmation of the index case. This plan addresses the eradication of all polio disease, whether caused by wild poliovirus or circulating vaccine-derived poliovirus. Major elements of this plan include:

- Trivalent OPV to be discontinued by 2015/2016 and switched to bivalent OPV.
- Six months before this switch, every child should receive at least one dose of IPV with third dose of DPT at 14 weeks of age in all OPV using countries.
- By 2019, there shall be complete cessation of OPV.
- At least one dose of IPV will be given to each child till 2024.

End Game

Trivalent OPV has been discontinued and switch to bivalent OPV was achieved in April 2016 from all over the world to prevent circulating vaccine derived poliovirus (cVDPV). Six months before this switch, every child should have received at least one dose of inactivated polio vaccine dose with third dose of DPT at 14 weeks of age in all countries of the world who were using OPV. This strategy shall prevent circulating VDPV by augmenting the immunity induced by earlier doses of trivalent OPV. By 2019, there shall be complete cessation of OPV and at least one dose of IPV will be given to each child till 2024.

Poliomyelitis

1. Poliomyelitis is an important wild virus disease on the verge of eradication. It is now endemic in only three countries of the world. India is now polio-free.
2. Paralytic poliomyelitis presents as AFP (acute flaccid paralysis) which is asymmetrical in nature.
3. The important differential diagnosis of poliomyelitis includes Guillain-Barre syndrome, transverse myelitis, and traumatic neuritis.
4. Vaccine-associated paralytic poliomyelitis (VAPP) and VDPV are the two major threats in the ultimate eradication of poliomyelitis.
5. Oral live polio vaccine and inactivated (killed) polio vaccines are two excellent vaccines available for prevention of poliomyelitis. Intelligent use of both these vaccines is required to eradicate this once considered dreaded disease.

Adams T. Global eradication of poliomyelitis: Is the end of the campaign in sight? *J Paediatr Child Health.* 2010 Feb 16.

Bompart F. Vaccination strategies for the last stages of global polio eradication. *Indian Pediatr.* 2005;42:163–9.

Centers for Disease Control and Prevention (CDC). Progress toward interruption of wild poliovirus transmission-worldwide, 2008. *MMWR Morb Mortal Wkly Rep.* 2009;58:308-12.

Centers for Disease Control and Prevention (CDC). Progress Toward Poliomyelitis Eradication—India, January 2004-May 2005. *MMWR Morb Mortal Wkly Rep.* 2005;54:655–9.

Chowdhary R, Dhole TN. Interrupting wild poliovirus transmission using oral poliovirus vaccine: environmental surveillance in high-risks area of India. *J Med Virol.* 2008;80:1477–88.

Cochi SL, Kew O. Polio today: are we on the verge of global eradication? *JAMA.* 2008;300:839–41.

Conclusions and recommendations of the Advisory Committee on Poliomyelitis Eradication, November 2008. *Wkly Epidemiol Rec.* 2009;84:17–28.

Duclos P, Okwo-Bele JM, Gacic-Dobo M, Cherian T. Global immunization: status, progress, challenges and future. *BMC Int Health Hum Rights.* 2009;9:S2.

Dutta A. Epidemiology of poliomyelitis—options and update. *Vaccine.* 2008;26:5767–73.

Eurosurveillance editorial team. Polio situation worldwide in 2008-update on the progress towards global eradication. *Euro Surveill.* 2009;14;pii:19178.

Francis PT. Non-polio AFP rate and polio eradication. *Indian Pediatr.* 2008;45:422–3.

John TJ. Who benefits from global certification of polio eradication? *Indian J Med Res.* 2004;120: 431–3.

John TJ, Vashishtha VM. Eradication of vaccine polioviruses: why, when & how? *Indian J Med Res.* 2009;130:491–4.

Minor P. Vaccine-derived poliovirus (VDPV): Impact on poliomyelitis eradication. *Vaccine.* 2009;27:2649–52.

Monovalent Oral Polio Vaccine: Gates Foundation Funds New Polio Vaccine to Accelerate Eradication Efforts. *Indian J Med Sci.* 2005;59:46–7.

Paul Y. Polio eradication in India: have we reached the dead end? *Vaccine.* 2010;28:1661–2.

Phadke A, Kale A. The mirage of polio eradication. *Natl Med J India.* 2004;17:282.

Polio Eradication Committee; Indian Academy of Pediatrics, Vashishtha VM, Kalra A, John TJ, Thacker N, Agarwal RK. Recommendations of 2nd National Consultative Meeting of Indian Academy of Pediatrics (IAP) on polio eradication and improvement of routine immunization. *Indian Pediatr.* 2008;45:367–78.

Progress towards global poliomyelitis eradication: Preparation for the oral poliovirus vaccine cessation era. *Wkly Epidemiol Rec.* 2004;79:349–56.

Progress towards poliomyelitis eradication in India, January 2004 to May 2005. *WER.* 2005;80: 233–240.

Progress towards poliomyelitis eradication in India, January 2007-May 2009. *Wkly Epidemiol Rec.* 2009;84:281–287.

Roberts L. Polio eradication. Rethinking the polio endgame. *Science.* 2009;323:705.

Sathyamala C, Mittal O, Dasgupta R, et al. Polio Eradication Initiative in India: Deconstructing the GPEI. *Int J Health Serv.* 2005;35:361–83.

Steinglass R. Global eradication of polio. *JAMA.* 2009;301:161–162.

Sutter RW, Jafari H, Aylward B. IAP Recommendations on Polio Eradication and Improvement of Routine Immunization. *Indian Pediatr.* 2008;45:353–355.

Tulchinsky TH. Polio eradication: End-stage challenges. *Bull WHO.* 2005;83:160.

6.11 DENGUE

Dengue infections are characterized by an acute febrile illness, usually seen in the tropics and Africa, and caused by 4 closely related virus serotypes of the genus Flavivirus, family Flaviviridae. Dengue virus is transmitted to humans by *Aedes aegypti* mosquito. The disease is characterized by a

6

biphasic fever, and may be associated with hemorrhagic manifestations. In 10–20% cases, the patient develops shock because of plasma leakage into the third space.

Dengue is recognized as the most important mosquito-transmitted viral disease in terms of morbidity and mortality. Worldwide, children younger than 15 years comprise 90% of patients with dengue fever.

Clinical Spectrum

Dengue virus infection may be asymptomatic, lead to a benign illness, or may present as a serious illness with severe manifestations.

Traditionally, symptomatic dengue virus infections in children were categorized into 3 groups: (*i*) undifferentiated dengue fever; (*ii*) dengue fever; and (*iii*) dengue hemorrhagic fever (DHF), further subclassified as without or with shock; ie, dengue shock syndrome (DSS). Case definitions were available for each of the diagnoses.

However, it was being realized that this classification was at times difficult to apply in clinical settings, was not able to categorize all patients with dengue, and was missing out cases with severe dengue.

The WHO classification in 2009 categorized children with dengue fever into 2 broad groups; ie, (*i*) dengue fever; and (*ii*) Severe dengue. The first group; ie, dengue fever is further categorized as being with or without presence of *Warning signs.* Figure 6.4 depicts the suggested dengue case classification and levels of severity according to the new guidelines. It is important to note that even patients without warning signs can develop severe dengue!

- *Non-severe manifestations* consist of a biphasic fever, generalized bodyache, rash, and a positive *tourniquet test.* These may or may not be associated with warning signs.
- *Warning signs* should be detected by close observation of the patient, so as to institute early and aggressive therapy. These include (*i*) abdominal pain or tenderness; (*ii*) persistent vomiting; (*iii*) clinical fluid accumulation

(edema, pleural effusion, ascites); (*iv*) mucosal bleeds; (*v*) hepatomegaly by >2 cm; and (*vi*) hemoconcentration as evidenced by increasing hematocrit with concomitant and rapid fall in platelet count.

- *Severe manifestations* include (*i*) severe hemorrhage; (*ii*) profound shock; and (*iii*) multisystem involvement. Presence of any one of these 3 criteria is sufficient for making a diagnosis of severe dengue infection.

Expanded dengue syndrome is a term introduced in 2011 which refers to unusual and severe involvement of liver, kidney, brain, or heart in association with dengue.

National Vector Borne Disease Control Program (NVBDCP) Nomenclature

Recently, the National Vector Borne Disease Control program has accepted the revised WHO classification for Dengue as shown in Fig. 6.5. There may be asymptomatic subjects who may be tested positive for dengue. Among symptomatic patients, they can be classified into three categories—mild, moderate, and severe dengue.

Etiology

Dengue fever is caused by a virus which has at least 4 serotypes (1, 2, 3, and 4). These are antigenically very similar but do not offer a complete cross-protection after infection by any one of them. Infections in human by a serotype will produce lifelong immunity against reinfection by the same serotype. Subsequent infection (secondary infection) by another serotype results in Severe dengue.

Epidemiology

A. Vector

The most common vector is a mosquito, *Aedes aegypti.* Female mosquito bites the man during daytime. After feeding on a person with viremia, the female mosquito can transmit dengue immediately or after a period of 10–14 days (extrinsic

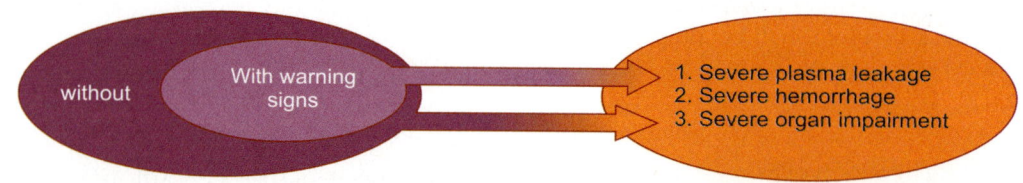

Criteria for dengue ± warning signs		Criteria for severe dengue

Probable dengue
Fever and 2 of the following criteria:
• Nausea, vomiting
• Rash
• Aches and pains
• Tourniquet test positive
• Leukopenia
• Any warning sign
 	
Laboratory-confirmed dengue
(important when no sign of plasma leakage)
	Warning signs*
	• Abdominal pain or tenderness
	• Persistent vomiting
	• Clinical fluid accumulation
	• Mucosal bleed
	• Lethargy, restlessness
	• Liver enlargement >2 cm
	• *Laboratory*
	  Increase in hematocrit (HCT)
	  concurrent with rapid decrease
	  in platelet count
	
	* *require strict observation and
	  medical intervention*
		**1. *Severe plasma leakage
		    leading to:***
		• Shock (DSS)
		• Fluid accumulation with
		  respiratory distress
		
		2. *Severe bleeding*
		as evaluated by clinician
		
		3. *Severe organ involvement*
		• Liver: AST or ALT≥1000 IU
		• CNS: Impaired consciousness
		• Heart and other organs

ALT = alanine aminotransferase; AST = aspartate aminotransferase; CNS = central nervous system; DSS = dengue shock syndrome

Fig. 6.4 Suggested dengue case classification and levels of severity (Reproduced with Permission from: Handbook for Clinical Management of Dengue. WHO; 2012. Available from http://whqlibdoc.who.int/publications/2009/9789241547871_eng.pdf.)

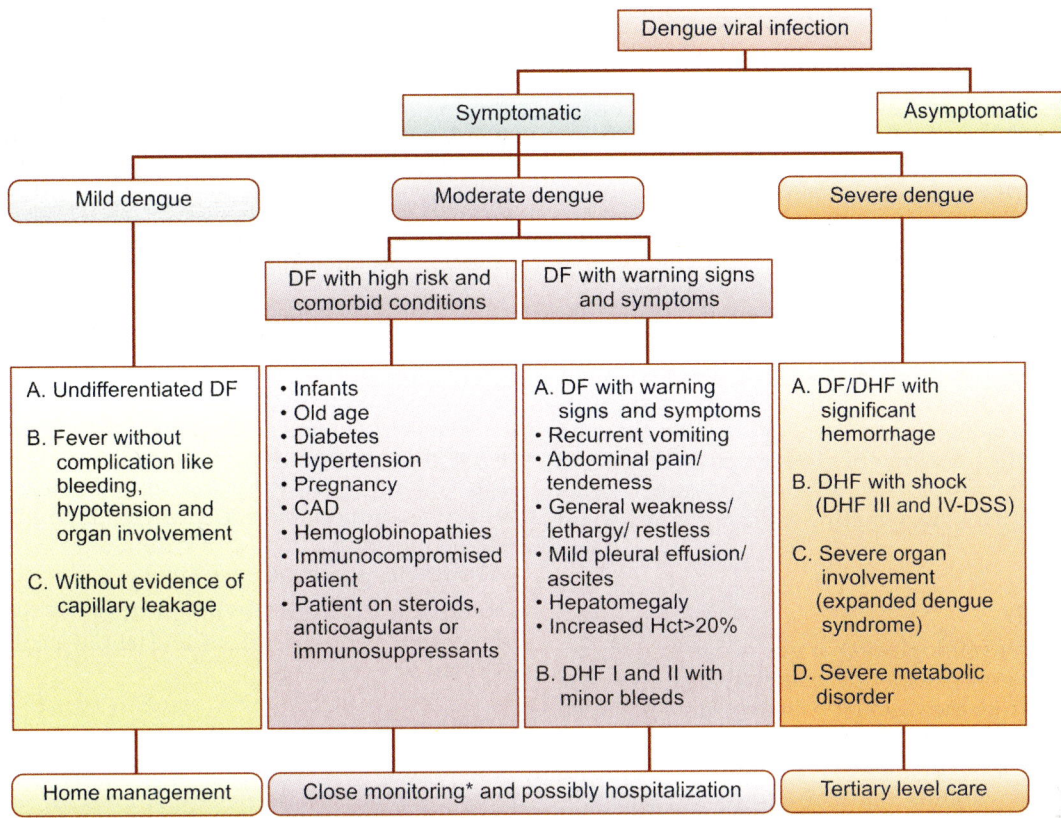

Fig. 6.5 Classification of dengue, WHO, 2015. (Source: National guidelines for clinical management of dengue fever. Available at URL: http://nvbdcp.gov.in/Doc/Dengue-National-Guidelines-2014.pdf. Accessed on 12th Oct 2016)

incubation period). The extrinsic incubation period is a critical factor in successful transmission of the disease. A lower environmental temperature increases the extrinsic incubation period, which in turn, decreases the transmission. Once the mosquito becomes infective, it remains so till it dies.

The flight range of an adult *A. aegypti* mosquito is not more than 25–50 m in an urban environment. However, the vector can be transported by water, land, and air travel contributing to the transmission. For dengue transmission, the number of infected female mosquitoes per house is important. Usually this number is small, and in an Indian epidemic it was observed to be just 1 per household. The minimum vector density, below which the dengue transmission ceases, is still unknown. The *A. aegypti* mosquito breeding is not necessarily related to the ambient temperature. The mosquito has been found at altitudes as high as 2,200 m above sea level. Vectors must survive longer than the sum of the initial non-feeding period after birth (usually 2 days) and the extrinsic incubation period to be able to infect another human. Longevity under natural conditions ranges from 8.5 days to a maximum of 42 days.

B. Host

People at all ages are susceptible to dengue. Severe dengue occurs at high frequency in (*a*) infants; and (*b*) children having experienced a previous dengue infection. The first attack gives only temporary and partial protection against the other three virus types and subsequent infections with other serotypes are possible. Non-severe dengue occurs in children and adults at equal frequency. Bronchial asthma and AIDS are significantly associated with Severe dengue.

C. Environmental Factors

In many tropical countries, a positive association between rainfall or larval density and dengue incidence has been documented. However, dengue epidemics have also been recorded in those areas where rainfall is unusually low. The transmission occurs, only if the ambient temperature is above 16°C. Therefore, the transmission tends to decline when winter approaches. This is due to prolongation of extrinsic incubation period beyond the longevity of mosquito.

D. Transmission Risk Factors

When a member of a household is infected with dengue, other family members are at risk. Dengue spread is facilitated in any vector-infested place where people congregate, such as schools, temples, cinema halls, offices, hospitals, factories, etc.

In utero transmission. Dengue infection of pregnant women may result in passive transfer of anti-dengue IgG to the fetus or a congenital infection. These infants with maternal antibody are at a higher risk of developing Severe dengue.

Pathogenesis

Dengue virus infects the peripheral blood mononuclear cells within a few days of infective mosquito bite. Two patterns of immune response follow: *Primary* and *secondary* (*anamnestic*). Persons never previously infected with a flavivirus, nor immunized with a flavivirus vaccine (*eg*, yellow fever, Japanese encephalitis), mount a primary IgM antibody response when infected with dengue virus, appearing within 2–3 days of defervescence and peaking at 2 weeks after the onset of symptoms. Anti-dengue IgG appears afterwards. Individuals with immunity due to previous flavivirus infection or immunization mount a secondary (anamnestic) antibody response when infected with dengue virus. In secondary flavivirus infections, which account for most cases of Severe dengue, the dominant immunoglobulin is IgG; the levels of IgM being much lower.

Antibody against a strain of dengue virus does not protect from a different strain of virus. Rather, it may increase its capacity to multiply in human monocytes. The infected monocytes result in activation of cross reactive CD4+ and CD8+ cytotoxic lymphocytes. Cytotoxic lymphocytes mediate release of cytokines resulting in plasma leakage and hemorrhage.

Pathophysiology

Two main pathophysiological changes occur in dengue. These are (*i*) increased vascular permeability that gives rise to loss of plasma from the vascular compartment leading to hemoconcentration, low pulse pressure, and other signs of shock; and (*ii*) disorder in the hemostasis involving thrombocytopenia, vascular changes, and coagulopathy.

Secondary dengue infection results in formation of immune complexes and activation of complement system. TNF-α, interferon, and interleukin-2 are elevated, and C1q, C3–C8, are depressed. As a result, vasoactive amines are released from the platelets. These cause massive release of water, electrolytes and plasma proteins from the blood vessels and lead to hypovolemic shock. Increased vascular permeability is mediated through the nitric oxide pathway.

Platelet defects are both quantitative and qualitative. Thus, a patient with a normal platelet count may still have a prolonged bleeding time. Maculopapular and petechial rashes are present. In these lesions, dengue antigen, IgM and complement (C3) have been observed.

Clinical Features

Dengue infections have a wide clinical presentation. Following an incubation period of 3–7 days, the illness is characterized by 3 distinct phases, in that chronological order: (*i*) febrile phase, (*ii*) critical phase, and (*iii*) phase of recovery.

A. Febrile Phase

This phase is characterized by a high grade fever up to 104°F, abrupt in onset. Fever remains at the peak for 48–72 hours before it starts declining. It is accompanied with non-specific constitutional symptoms such as generalized myalgia, bodyache, anorexia, nausea, vomiting, and headache. Parents may notice an erythematous rash, especially over the extremities. There may be flushing of skin with compromised cutaneous circulation (Fig. 6.6). Some children may have associated sore throat, or arthralgia. These features, by themselves, are, however, not sufficient enough to arrive at a diagnosis of dengue fever.

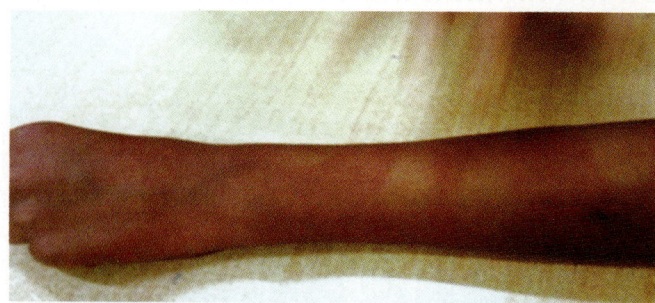

Fig. 6.6 Cutaneous flushing of forearm with blanching on applying pressure

Dengue should be strongly suspected, if above features are associated with mild hemorrhagic manifestations including petechial hemorrhages, mucosal bleeds, or a positive tourniquet test. Presence of tender hepatomegaly (without obvious icterus) strongly favors possibility of dengue infection.

The febrile phase lasts for 2–3 days.

Complications High fever in this phase can cause dehydration, febrile delirium, and febrile seizures in children less than 5 years of age.

B. Critical Phase

Onset of the critical phase is closely linked to the time of defervescence that occurs by 3rd day of illness. Not all children with dengue infection enter this phase. Many children improve progressively after defervescence (non-severe dengue).

All children in defervescence phase need to be closely monitored for the *warning signs* as described earlier. Those manifesting with one or more of these signs are likely to enter the critical phase.

Critical phase is characterized by an increase in capillary permeability, initially presenting as rising hematocrit. This is preceded by a fall in the platelet count. Increased capillary permeability results in leakage of plasma into the third space. Clinically, this manifests as polyserositis; ie, with fluid accumulation in body spaces–pleural effusion and ascites. Plasma leakage from the intravascular compartment into the third space results in hemoconcentration in the vascular bed, reflected by a rising hematocrit. Increase in hematocrit is directly proportional to the volume of plasma lost from the vascular compartment.

Epigastric discomfort, tenderness at right costal margin, and generalized abdominal pain are common. Liver becomes palpable. Petechiae may be present over extremities, axillae, face and palate.

Leakage of a significant volume of plasma leads to hypovolemia, hypoperfusion, and shock. Hypoperfusion may result in multiple end-organ impairment, metabolic acidosis, and disseminated intravascular coagulation. Consumption coagulopathy results in hemorrhage that may cause a fall in hematocrit. End organ impairment manifests with hepatitis, myocarditis, or encephalitis. Children developing profound shock, severe hemorrhage, or multisystem involvement are at higher risk of mortality and thus are said to having *Severe dengue infection*. These children need aggressive management.

This phase lasts for 48 hours.

C. Recovery Phase (plasma reabsorption phase)

Plasma starts coming back to the intravascular compartment, provided the patient survives the critical phase of plasma leakage and shock. Onset of this phase is characterized by an improvement in general well-being and appetite. Urine output improves, and pain abdomen subsides. Though this is the phase of improvement, child should be monitored carefully for hypervolemia. Reabsorption of leaked plasma plus administration of excess intravenous fluid may result in fluid overload, pulmonary edema, and congestive heart failure, manifesting as dyspnea, tachycardia, and raised jugular venous pressure. Cardiovascular manifestations (bradycardia, arrhythmias) are also reported during this phase.

Hematocrit value either normalizes or may show a decline below normal. Platelet count starts improving.

This phase lasts for 48–72 hours. Thus, most patients with dengue fever run a typical course of disease lasting from 7–10 days (Fig. 6.7).

Severe Dengue

Children and adolescents with severe dengue have a more protracted course and recovery may take 10–14 days. Dengue

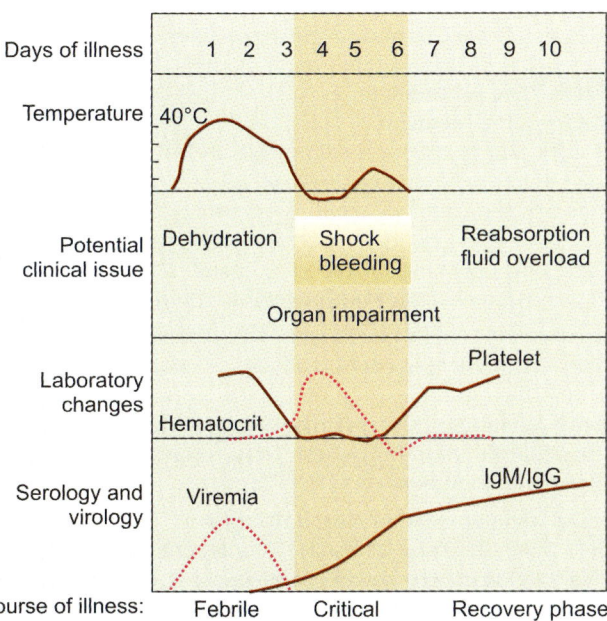

Fig. 6.7 The course of dengue illness (Reproduced with Permission from: Handbook for Clinical Management of Dengue. WHO; 2012)

shock is characterized by a narrow pulse pressure <20 mm Hg, cold extremities, delayed capillary refill time, weak pulse, and tachycardia. Skin becomes cool, blotchy, congested. Major bleeding can occur from gastrointestinal tract or brain. Organ impairment manifests as hepatic failure, renal failure, myocarditis, or encephalopathy.

Laboratory Studies

Hematological Tests

The clinical diagnosis is corroborated by raised hematocrit and thrombocytopenia.

- A hematocrit level rise of greater than 20% is a sign of hemoconcentration and precedes shock. The hematocrit level should be monitored at least every 24 hours to facilitate early recognition of Warning signs and every 3–4 hours in Severe dengue.
- Thrombocytopenia has been demonstrated in up to 50% of children with dengue. Platelet counts of less than 100,000 cells/μL indicates onset of Critical phase and typically occur before defervescence and the onset of shock. The platelet count should also be monitored at least every 24 hours initially. Leukopenia, often with lymphopenia, is observed near the end of the febrile phase of illness. Lymphocytosis, with atypical lymphocytes, commonly develops before defervescence or shock.

Biochemical Profile

Prothrombin time is prolonged. Activated partial thromboplastin time is prolonged. Low fibrinogen and elevated fibrin degradation product levels are signs of disseminated intravascular coagulation. Hyponatremia is the most common electrolyte abnormality in Critical phase. Metabolic acidosis and elevated blood urea is observed in those with shock. SGPT levels elevated. Low serum albumin levels are a sign of hemoconcentration.

Serodiagnosis

Serum specimens should be sent to the laboratory for serodiagnosis, PCR, and viral isolation. Because the signs and symptoms of dengue fever are nonspecific, attempting laboratory confirmation of dengue infection is important. Serodiagnosis is based on (*i*) detection of viral non-structural protein (NS1) during initial illness; (*ii*) detection of IgM antibodies to dengue; or (*iii*) 4-fold rise in dengue IgG in paired samples. **Table 6.8** outlines the desired timing of these tests for confirming the diagnosis.

Table 6.8 Diagnostic Tests for Dengue Fever		
Diagnostic method	*Timing of test (after disease onset)*	*Validity*
Virus isolation (culture)	1–5 d	++++
Genome detection (PCR)	1–5 d	++++
Antigen detection (NS1)	1–5 d	+++
Antibody detection (IgM)*	After 5 d	++
IgG (paired sera)	acute sera 1–5 d; convalescent sera after 15 d	+

*IgM positivity rates: by 3–5 d (50%), 5–7 d (80%), 10 d (90%). IgG appear after 1–2 weeks and may persist for life. IgM appears between 3 and 10 days and disappears by 2–3 months.

6

A 10-year-old boy arrived in emergency room with complaints of high grade continuous fever accompanied with chills and rigors, myalgia, and loss of appetite for 4 days. The child had also developed non-itchy erythematous macular rashes on whole body involving the palms and soles, since morning. He also complained of pain abdomen and vomiting. The mother noticed that from past one hour, the child's limbs were cold to touch.

What are the other points you will like to ask in history?
In a child presenting with fever, rash, abdominal symptoms, and cold extremities indicating impaired perfusion, think of dengue fever, typhoid fever, and meningococcemia. Ask for history of bleeding from any site, altered sensorium, abnormal body movements, neck pain, any preceding history of sore throat or pain, presence of similar symptoms in other family members/neighborhood.

There was no complaint of bleeding from any site. Neurological status was normal. There was history of similar illness in the locality, being diagnosed as dengue fever. Examination revealed temperature of 104.5°F, RR—34/min, HR—112/min, BP—86/52 mm Hg, and erythematous blanchable macular rashes all over body mainly distributed over extremities. Abdomen was distended. Tenderness was noted in right hypochondrium over a palpable liver 2 cm below right subcostal margin. Rest of systemic examination was well within normal range.

Discuss the differential diagnosis for this patient?
A febrile patient with rashes all over body on fourth day of fever with cold extremities alarms us towards possibility of dengue fever with shock. Other similar cases in the neighborhood support the diagnosis. Other possible differential for this patient can be meningococcemia, enteric fever, rickettsial fever, severe sepsis with shock, or algid malaria.

How will you confirm the diagnosis?
The most useful diagnostic test for dengue fever on day 4 of fever, will be documentation of NS1 antigen. This antigen can be demonstrated in serum from day 2 onwards. IgM antibodies against virus appear only on 4–5 days of fever, and may be negative in this child.

How will you manage this child?
This child is having cold extremities and hypotension which indicate shock. The illness will be classified as *severe dengue*. The child needs to be hospitalized and immediately started on IV fluids, to expand the intravascular volume. Initial fluid should consist of normal saline bolus @10–20 mL/kg over 1 hour. Further management will depend on response to initial therapy.

Laboratory criteria for definitive diagnosis include one or more of the following:
1. Isolation of the dengue virus from serum, plasma, leukocytes, or autopsy samples.
2. Demonstration of NS1, a glycoprotein induced by the virus between 1 and 4 days of illness, has a high sensitivity and specificity.
3. Demonstration of a 4-fold or greater change in reciprocal immunoglobulin G (IgG); or presence of immunoglobulin M (IgM) antibody titers to one or more dengue virus antigens in paired serum samples.

3. Demonstration of dengue virus antigen in autopsy tissue via immunohistochemistry or immunofluorescence or in serum samples via enzyme immunoassay.
4. Detection of viral genomic sequences in autopsy tissue, serum, or cerebral spinal fluid (CSF) samples via polymerase chain reaction (PCR).

Treatment	**Dengue Fever**

The mainstay of treatment is supportive therapy. Increased oral fluid intake is recommended to prevent dehydration. Supplementation with intravenous fluids may be necessary to prevent dehydration and significant hemoconcentration. Fever is managed with paracetamol. Aspirin and non-steroidal anti-inflammatory drugs should be avoided as these drugs may worsen the bleeding tendency associated with some of these infections. Shock is managed with isotonic fluids. Packed cell transfusion is indicated in refractory shock or if there is significant bleeding.

Patients with known or suspected dengue fever should have their platelet count and hematocrit measured daily from the third day of illness until 1–2 days after defervescence. Patients with a rising hematocrit level or falling platelet count should be monitored more frequently.

Management of dengue illness can be discussed in 3 steps:
Step 1: Overall assessment
Step 2: Diagnosis and severity assessment
Step 3: Categorizing into mild, moderate, or severe dengue and treating accordingly.

A. Overall Assessment
History and examination Emphasis in history should be on assessment of Warning signs. Physical examination should concentrate on hemodynamic assessment, so as to determine the presence and extent of shock, confirming or detecting the warning signs; and checking for bleeding manifestations, abdominal tenderness, mental state and hydration. Tourniquet test is a must.

Investigations Initial investigations should include a hematocrit, WBC count, platelet count, and tests to confirm the diagnosis, as described in the section on laboratory diagnosis. In Critical phase, additional tests need to be done and include liver function test, renal function test, chest X-ray, serum electrolytes, and ultrasound abdomen.

B. Deciding on need of Hospitalization
Determine the phase of disease (febrile, critical, recovery) and severity (non-severe, severe) of dengue, as per criteria outlined earlier. The child will need admission, if any of the following criteria is fulfilled
  i. Presence of any of warning signs;
 ii. Signs and symptoms of hypotension;
iii. Bleeding from any site;
 iv. Renal, hepatic, or CNS involvement;
  v. Pleural effusion or ascites;
 vi. Rising hematocrit; and
vii. Platelet count <50,000/mm^3.

C. Categorize Patients in Mild, Moderate, or Severe Dengue (Table 6.9)
This step is aimed to place the patient in an appropriate group (A, B, or C) to decide on future course of action, as follows:
Mild—Patients, who may be sent home
Moderate—Patients need close monitoring or hospitalization
Severe—Patients requiring tertiary level care

Table 6.9 Treatment of Dengue		
Category	*Patient characteristics*	*Treatment*
Mild	Accepting orally, passing urine adequately and no warning signs*	**Home therapy** • Increased oral fluids, paracetamol
Moderate	Warning signs* present High risk-infants, old age, pregnancy, Co-morbid conditions**	**Hospitalize** • Monitor hematocrit, platelets, vitals • Intravenous fluids: titrated as per hematocrit • If worsens, manage as severe dengue
Severe	Severe bleeding Severe shock Severe organ dysfunction: hepatic, CNS, heart, kidney Severe metabolic disorder	**Intensive care** • Monitor hematocrit, platelets, vitals • Treatment of shock: normal saline bolus • Blood transfusion for severe bleeding or clinical worsening. Judicious use of platelets • Supportive treatment for organ failure • Watch for signs of fluid overload, and treat, if detected (oxygen, frusemide)

*Warning signs: Abdominal pain, persistent vomiting, mucosal bleed, hepatomegaly, clinical fluid accumulation, lethargy, hemoconcentration, thrombocytopenia
**Comorbid conditions include hypertension, diabetes, thyroid illness, renal disease, hemoglobinopathy, hepatitis, heart disease

1. Mild Dengue: Home Management

All children who are tolerating oral fluids, passing urine at least once in 6 hours, and not having any of the warning sign can be sent home. Following management needs to be advised:
- Encourage fluid intake; can give ORS, fruit juice, etc.
- Paracetamol (15 mg/kg/dose), if the child is uncomfortable because of fever. Avoid aspirin, ibuprofen, mefenamic acid, and nimesulide.
- Monitor at home for fluid intake, urine output, fever, obvious bleeding, and altered sensorium.
- Bring back if any of the above is present or the child develops any of the warning signs.

2. Moderate Dengue: Hospital Management

Presence of warning sign should place the patient in Group B. Other indications for hospitalization have been outlined above. Management plan is as follows:
- Obtain baseline hematocrit
- Start isotonic IV fluids (normal saline or ringer lactate) @ 5–7 mL/kg/hour for 1–2 hours
- Reassess hematocrit and clinical status
  - If improving, decrease to 3 mL/kg/h for another 2–4 h and then continue within 1.5 mL/kg/h for 2–4 h
  - If clinical status worsens or hematocrit rises, increase rate of fluids to 10 mL/kg/h for 1–2 hours
- Reassess clinical status, repeat HCT and review fluid infusion rates, till the child is better
  - If the child improves, maintain minimum IV fluids @ 0.5 mL/kg/h for 24–28 h. Stop fluids when child demands and accepts adequate oral fluids, and food
  - Those who worsen or develop profound shock, bleeding or multisystem involvement, manage as in Fig. 6.8.

3. Severe Dengue: Emergency treatment

Emergency treatment is required in children with severe dengue or those in critical phase, as follows:
- Obtain hematocrit, blood count, and other organ function tests, as indicated.
- *Compensated shock* This stage is characterized by low SBP, narrow pulse pressure (<20 mm Hg), and rise in hematocrit (>20%). In these children, fluid resuscitation is started at 10–20 mL/kg/hour over one hour, and further directed as per Fig. 6.9.
- *Hypotensive shock* Administer isotonic fluid bolus 20 mL/kg in 15 minutes. For further management, follow the algorithm depicted in Fig. 6.10. Colloids may be needed in refractory shock.
- *Hemorrhagic complications* Suspect severe bleeding, if there is an unexplained fall in hematocrit, refractory shock not responding to 40–60 mL/kg of fluid, and persistent or worsening metabolic acidosis. Packed cell transfusion 10 mL/kg over 2–3 hours can be life-saving in these children.
- *Monitoring* This essentially remains the basic prerequisite for treating children with severe dengue, in an emergency setting.
  - Monitor vital signs and peripheral perfusion 1–4 hourly unless patient is out of critical phase. Monitor hematocrit before and after fluid replacement, then 6–12 hourly.
  - Monitor blood glucose and other organ dysfunction both clinically and biochemically.
  - A typical monitoring chart for dengue fever should record the following: Body temperature, heart rate, blood pressure, pulse volume, capillary refill time, abdominal pain, appetite, vomiting and bleeding.

Role of Platelets

There is not much evidence for platelet transfusion or fresh frozen plasma for severe bleeding. Platelet transfusions should not be used prophylactically. Its use has neither shown to prevent progression to severe bleeding nor does it shorten the bleeding time and may instead be associated with severe side effects. Platelet transfusion should be restricted to cases with severe bleeding or when platelet counts are below 10,000/cubic mm. Platelets obtained by single donor apheresis are preferred as they raise the platelet count by 30,000–50,000 as compared to random donor platelets which result in rise by 5,000–10,000 per unit.

Treatment of Fluid Overload

A patient with dengue can have fluid overload due to excessive or rapidly transfused IV fluids, use of hypotonic fluids, and inappropriate use of fresh frozen plasma or platelets. Another

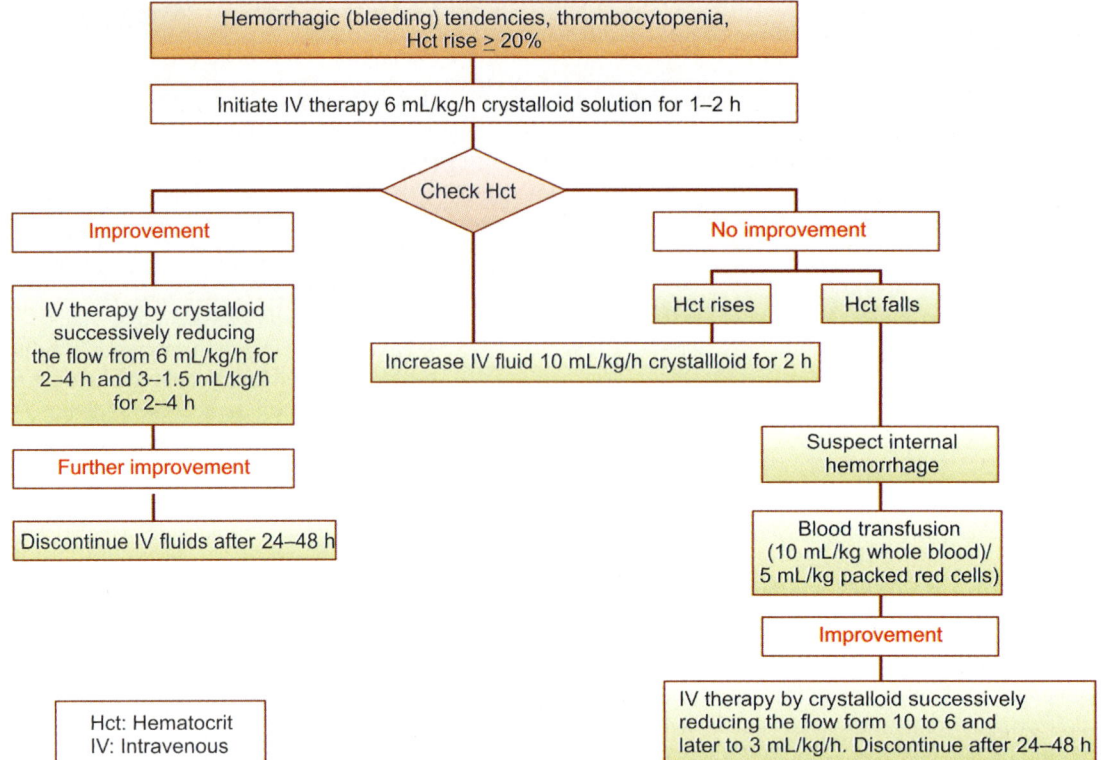

Fig. 6.8 Management of moderate dengue. (Source: National guidelines for clinical management of dengue fever. WHO, 2015. Available at URL: http://nvbdcp.gov.in/Doc/Dengue-National-Guidelines-2014.pdf. Accessed on 1st Feb 2018)

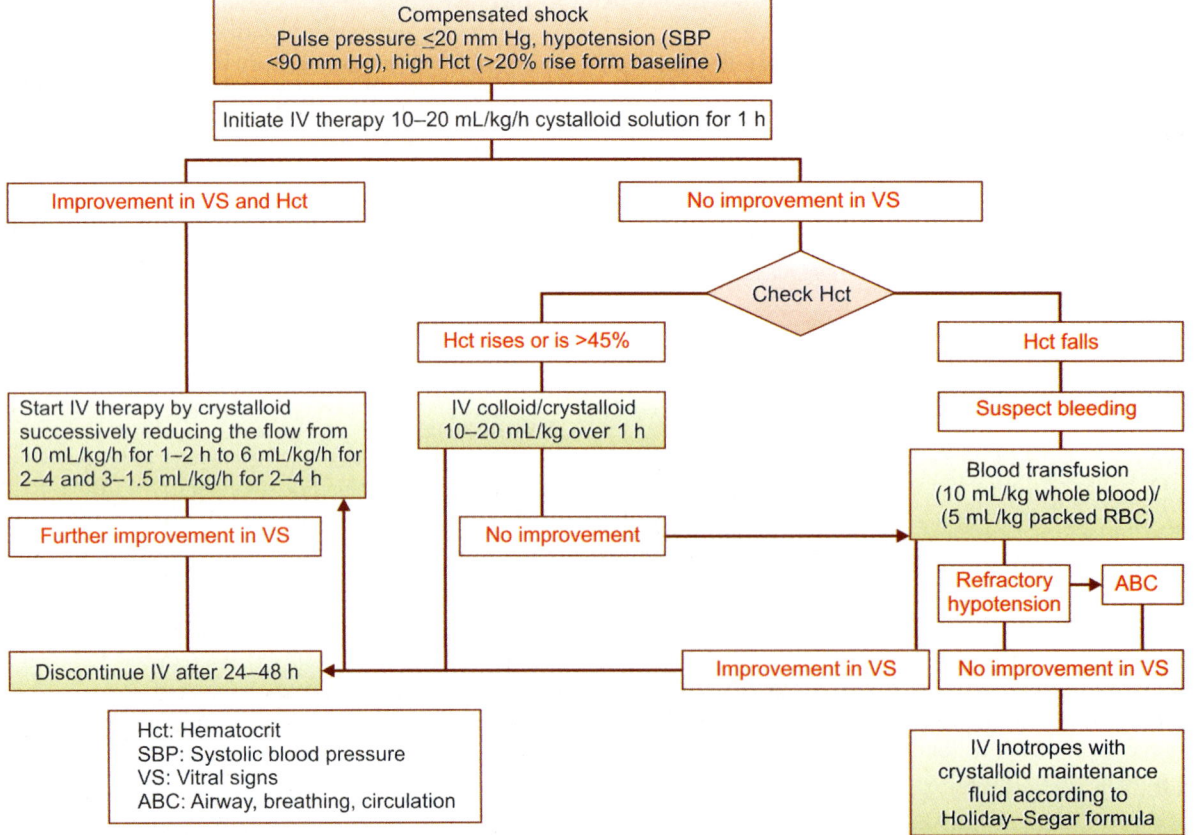

Fig. 6.9 Algorithm for fluid management in compensated shock. (Source: National guidelines for clinical management of dengue fever. WHO, 2015. Available at URL: http://nvbdcp.gov.in/Doc/Dengue-National-Guidelines-2014.pdf. Accessed on 1st Feb 2018)

6

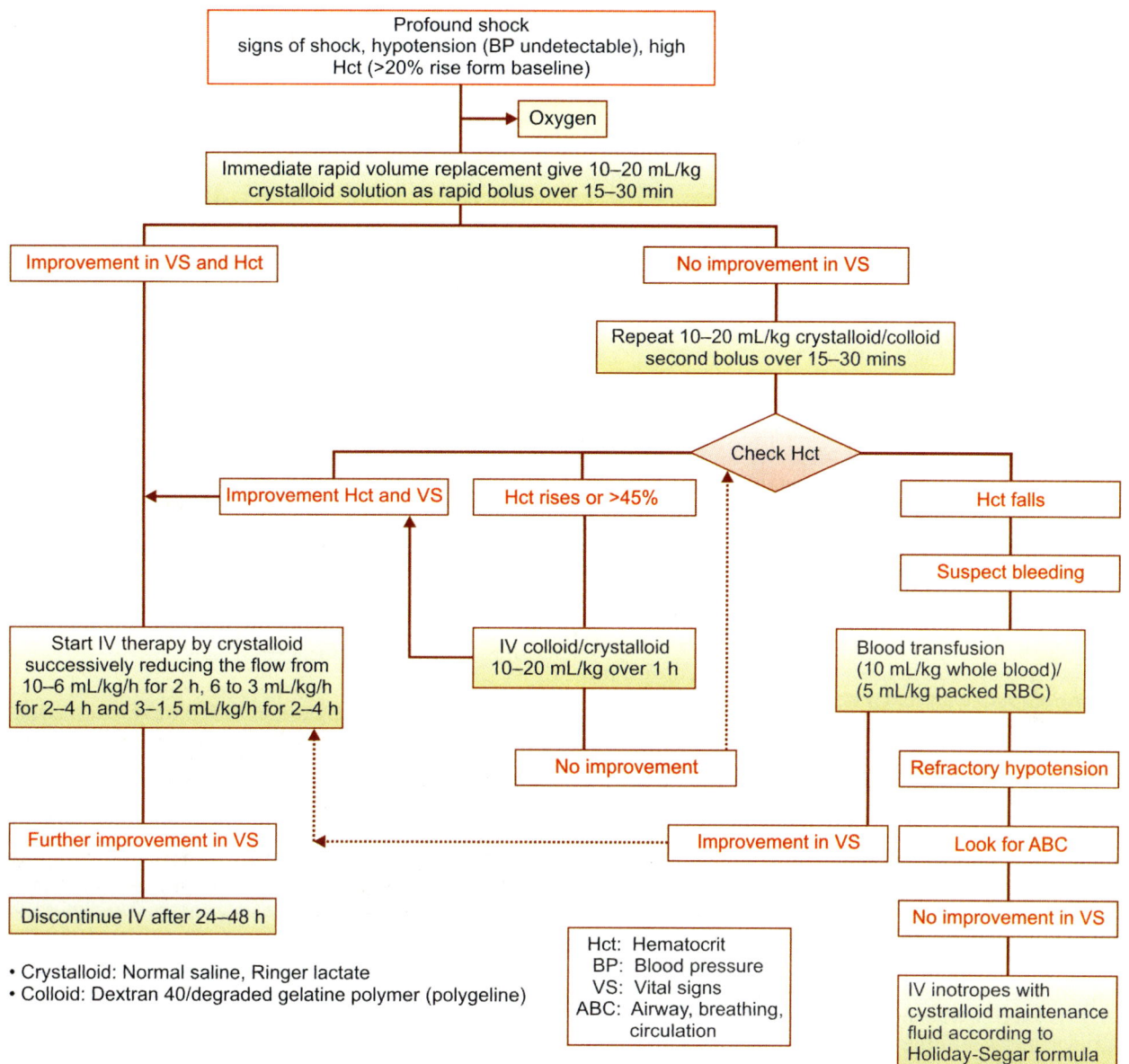

Fig. 6.10 Algorithm for fluid management in hypotensive decompensated shock. (Source: National guidelines for clinical management of dengue fever. WHO, 2015. Available at URL: http://nvbdcp.gov.in/Doc/Dengue-National-Guidelines-2014.pdf. Accessed on 5th Feb 2018)

important reason is continuation of IV fluids even during the phase of plasma reabsorption and recovery.

These children may present with features of pulmonary edema or congestive heart failure. Following management is suggested.

- Oxygen therapy
- Discontinuation/reduction of IV fluids.
- Frusemide 0.1–0.5 mg/kg/dose once or twice daily, maintaining serum potassium.
- Look for occult hemorrhage and transfuse packed cells.

Criteria for Discharge

Patient should be discharged only if he has been afebrile for at least 24 hours, passing urine normally, having improved appetite, has no respiratory distress, has a stable hematocrit and platelet count is more than 50,000/cu mm.

Prevention and Control

Aedes aegypti should be the main target of surveillance and control.

1. Surveillance

Mainly two indices are used for measuring the vector density. There are (*a*) *House index*; and (*b*) *Breteau index*. House index is defined as the percentage of houses positive for the larvae; and Brateau index as the number of containers positive for the larvae per 100 houses. These indices measure larval infestation rather than adult mosquito density.

2. Long-term Vector Control

Adequate water supply is a must. Sprays of larvicides are recommended in high-risk localities. All objects that may collect water (old tyres, broken jars, empty tins and bottles)

6

should be disposed off. Water should be changed routinely in water coolers, flower vases, and overhead tanks. Coolers, if not in use, should be drained and mopped dry. Large tanks with taps should be kept covered. Management of roof tops, porticos and sunshades to be encouraged. Health education should be provided regularly in schools and through mass media. Sensitize and involve the community for detection of *Aedes* breeding places and their elimination.

3. Biological and Chemical Control

Use of larvivorous fishes in ornamental tanks, fountains, or biocides can kill the larval stages. Use chemical larvicides like 'Abate' in big breeding containers. Aerosol space spray during daytime may be another option in high density areas.

In recent years, interest in mosquito-killing (entomo-pathogenic) fungi is reviving, mainly due to continuous and increasing levels of insecticide resistance and increasing global risk of mosquito-borne diseases. Particular focus is on species belonging to the genera *Lagenidium*, *Coelomomyces*, *Entomophthora*, *Culicinomyces*, *Beauveria*, and *Metarhizium*.

4. Vaccine Development

Development of a multivalent vaccine against all four serotypes seems necessary. Progress in vaccine development is slow because these viruses grow poorly in cell culture and there is no acceptable animal model for dengue illness.

Two live-attenuated tetravalent dengue vaccines were developed by passages of wild type strains of dengue viruses in cell culture, in Thailand and USA, respectively. Trials have shown 100% vaccine-induced immune responses to all four serotypes in the first vaccine. The second live-attenuated tetravalent vaccine induced 63% seroconversion to all four dengue serotypes.

Several research groups are successfully exploring an infectious clone technology for the development of a dengue vaccine. The ChimeriVaxTM system, originally developed to construct JE vaccine, has now been applied to dengue viruses. This vaccine was shown to be safe and immunogenic in a monkey study. Another approach is based on the use of a dengue type 4 mutant containing a deletion for the construction of a dengue chimeric vaccine. Phase I clinical trials of a deletion mutant carried out in adult humans showed good safety and immunogenicity.

Bhatt S, Gething PW, Brady OJ, et al. The global distribution and burden of dengue. *Nature*. 2013;496:504–7.

Chakravarti A, Arora R, Luxemburger C. Fifty years of dengue in India. *Trans R Soc Trop Med Hyg*. 2012; 106(5):273–82

Dengue haemorrhagic fever. Diagnosis, treatment, prevention and control. World Health Organization, 1997. Available at URL: *http://apps.who.int/iris/bitstream/10665/41988/1/9241545003_eng.pdf*. Accessed on 05th May 2015.

Ghosh A, Dar L. Dengue vaccines: challenges, development, current status and prospects. *Indian J Med Microbiol*. 2015; 33(1):3–15.

Guidelines for integrated vector management for control of dengue/dengue haemorrhagic fever. National Vector Borne Disease Control Programme, Directorate General of Health Services, Ministry of Health & Family Welfare. Available at URL: *http://nvbdcp.gov.in/Doc/dengue_1_.%20Director_Desk%20DGHS%20meeting%20OCT%2006.pdf*. Accessed on 12th Aug 2017.

Gupta N, Srivastava S, Jain A, Chaturvedi UC. Dengue in India. *Indian J Med Research*. 2012; 136: 373–90.

Dengue

1. Dengue is an acute viral illness caused by four viruses 1 to 4; and spread by *Aedes* mosquito.
2. Clinical presentation consists of a biphasic fever, myalgia, arthralgia, and hemorrhagic manifestations, lasting over 3–7 days. The most vulnerable stage is soon after defervescence (critical phase) characterized by increased capillary permeability.
3. Increased capillary permeability and coagulopathy are major pathogenic abnormalities.
4. Thrombocytopenia occurs both due to bone marrow suppression and immune-mediated destruction.
5. Serological diagnosis is possible by detecting non-structural (NS) antigen 1 between 2 and 5 days, detection of IgM antibodies between 5 and 10 days, or fourfold rise in IgG antibodies after 7–10 days.
6. Children with warning signs should be hospitalized. Those with severe shock, severe bleeding, and organ involvement need management in intensive care unit (ICU) setting.
7. Fluid therapy is the mainstay of treatment. Crystalloid is the fluid of choice during resuscitation. Best guide to fluid therapy is hematocrit.

Kaushik A, Pineda C, Kest H. Diagnosis and management of dengue fever in children. *Pediatr Rev*. 2010;31:e28–35.

National guidelines for clinical management of dengue fever. WHO, 2015. Available at URL: *http://nvbdcp.gov.in/Doc/Dengue-National-Guidelines-2014.pdf*. Accessed on 12 Aug 2017.

6.12 ACQUIRED IMMUNODEFICIENCY SYNDROME (AIDS)

In 1982, a clinical entity characterized by profound loss of immune functions associated with a depletion of CD4+ helper T-lymphocytes, formally designated acquired immunodeficiency syndrome (AIDS) was recognized. This syndrome is caused by infection with the human immunodeficiency virus (HIV).

In India, with 27 million pregnancies annually, and an estimated overall HIV prevalence of 0.4% in antenatal women, it is estimated that there are 65,000 HIV-infected pregnant women annually. About 25,000 HIV infections occur annually in Indian children and about 5,000 HIV-infected Indian children progress to AIDS annually. *It is estimated that about 115,000 children are living with HIV in India.* One out of every 25 HIV-infected children worldwide lives in India.

HIV (Human Immunodeficiency Virus)

HIV is an enveloped RNA virus, approximately 120 nm in diameter, and belongs to the lentivirus subfamily of the retrovirus family. Two serotypes, namely HIV 1 and 2, have been recognized; the former is more virulent and more infectious. HIV-2 infection is limited to West Africa.

The virion of HIV includes reverse transcriptase enzyme. The genome of HIV contains *gag, pol, env* genes which are present in all members of retroviridae family. There are 6 additional genes viz, *tat, rev, vif, vpr (R), nef, vpu*, all of which have regulatory functions. Various proteins are encoded by these genes. The important ones include glycoprotein gp120 (surface protein essential for virus binding), gp41 (envelope protein) and p24 (core protein).

HIV is a labile virus inactivated by heat (56° C for 30 min), ether, acetone, 20% ethanol, 0.2% sodium hypochlorite, and 1% glutaraldehyde. HIV is relatively resistant to ionizing radiation and ultraviolet light. Inactivation procedures employed in the preparation of viral vaccines from human plasma (eg, hepatitis B vaccine) completely destroy the infectivity of HIV.

Mode of Transmission

The transmission of HIV virus in adults occurs principally through sexual intercourse, needle sticks, contaminated blood and blood products. This *'horizontal transmission'*, however, accounts for only 10–15% cases of AIDS in children. Majority (90%) of pediatric HIV infections are acquired by *'vertical transmission"* from an infected mother to her offspring. Mother-to-child transmission may occur in utero (*intrauterine transmission*), during labor and delivery (*intrapartum transmission*) and also through breastfeeding (*postpartum transmission*). HIV is not transmitted by food, water, mosquitoes or casual contact (eg, social kissing, shaking hands and hugging) or through exposure of body fluids like tears, feces, or saliva unless they contain visible blood. **Table 6.10** depicts the risk of HIV transmission through different routes of exposure.

The rate of vertical transmission ranges from 10–45% (intrauterine: 5–10%; intrapartum: 10–15%; postpartum: 5–20%). The factors which increase the rate of mother-to-child transmission include high levels of viremia, advanced maternal HIV disease, low maternal CD4 counts, maternal p24 antigenemia, placental membrane inflammation, high CD8 counts, premature infants, first born twin, lack of anti-viral therapy to infected pregnant woman, and increasing duration of breastfeeding. The risk of transmission with mixed feeding, *ie*, breastmilk and replacement feeds combined is even higher.

Pathogenesis

Whatever the portal of entry for HIV, the gut-associated lymphoid tissue (GALT) plays a major role in HIV replication. The CD4+ helper T-lymphocytes in the GALT are targeted within days of infection with HIV and there is a specific decline in the CD4+ helper T-cells (hall mark of AIDS), resulting in inversion of the normal CD4/CD8 T-cell ratio and dysregulation of B-cell antibody production. Early decline of CD4+ cells is noticed 1–3 weeks after infection, associated with

viremia. The destruction of CD4+ lymphocytes in the gut mucosa makes it leaky allowing the passage of pathogens across gut mucosa. A vigorous cellular and humoral response (immune activation) follows, evoked by CD8+ cytotoxic T-cells, natural killer cells, and antibody dependent cell mediated cytotoxicity, resulting in decline of viremia. Then follows the long asymptomatic period of clinical latency. As time passes, there is a steady decline in the number of CD4+ T-cells. While some CD4 cells are lost due to direct viral cytopathic effect, a majority of CD4 cells are lost due to immune activation and also due to apoptosis of infected cells.

Following the latent period, immune responses to certain antigens begin to decline (immunosenescence), and the host fails to adequately respond to opportunistic infections and normally harmless commensal organisms, especially when the CD4+ cell counts fall below about 200–400 per mL. Because the defect preferentially affects cellular immunity, the infections tend to be nonbacterial (fungal, viral). Chronic immune activation and inflammation due to repeated infections accounts for most of the non-AIDS morbidity and mortality in HIV-infected individuals. Death usually follows due to infection, malignancy, or cachexia.

About 5–15% of HIV-infected individuals do not experience clinical or immunological progression despite a long duration of infection in the absence of highly active antiretroviral therapy (HAART); these are known as *long-term non-progressors* (LTNP). They have good CD4 counts and low viral loads. About <1% of HIV-infected individuals have undetectable viral loads (<50 copies/mL) in the absence of HAART; these are designated as *elite controllers* (EC).

Laboratory Diagnosis

Laboratory diagnosis is necessary to determine, if HIV infection has occurred and also to detect immunodeficiency, particularly the reduction of circulating T helper cells (CD4). Diagnosis of HIV infection in infants can be particularly challenging as vertical transmission accounts for nearly 80% of pediatric HIV infection and infants born to HIV-infected mothers carry maternal IgG antibodies which may persist for up to 12–15 months after birth. Therefore, serological diagnosis of HIV infection based on IgG antibodies is not reliable in children <18 months age.

Figure 6.11 depicts the timing for detection of antigen and antibodies following exposure to HIV which aids the

Table 6.10 HIV Transmission Risk Depending upon the Route of Exposure	
Exposure route	*Risk of HIV transmission*
Blood transfusion	90–95%
Perinatal	10–40%
Sexual intercourse	0.1–10%
Injecting drugs	0.67%
Needle stick	0.3%
Mucous membrane (splash to eyes, oronasal)	0.09%

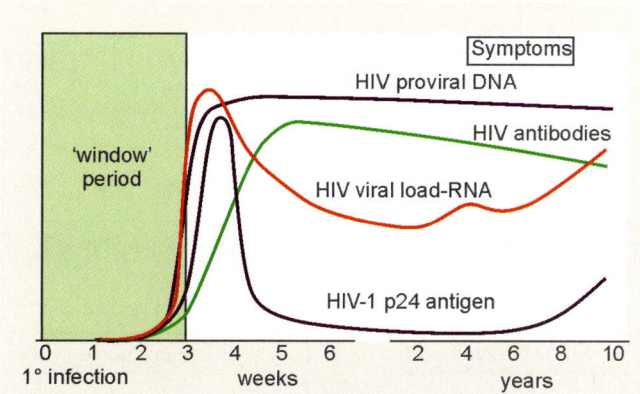

Fig. 6.11 Detection of antigen and antibodies following exposure to HIV

understanding of laboratory tests to be ordered to facilitate early diagnosis of HIV.

Diagnosis of HIV in Children <18 Months of Age (Figs 6.12 and 6.13)

Tests which may be suitable in children <18 months age for detecting HIV infection include:

1. *Viral culture* HIV culture is technically difficult, expensive, and time-consuming.

2. *Detection of HIV proviral DNA or RNA by polymerase chain reaction (PCR)* PCR is the most preferred test for detecting HIV infection in infants (sensitivity 99.3%, specificity 99.6%). The sensitivity at birth is low, increasing to 95% at 4 weeks, and 99% at 6 months of age.

3. *HIV antigen detecting tests* Detection of p24 antigen is easy, specific and cheap but has a lower sensitivity.

According to National AIDS Control Organization (NACO) guidelines, in a non-breastfed infant, the first HIV PCR should be done at 6 weeks age. If this is negative, confirm with a second PCR test at 6 months. If the test is positive, start ART and repeat immediately for confirmation. In a breastfed infant, HIV PCR is recommended at 6 weeks of age as well as 6–8 weeks after cessation of breastfeeding. A report of 'HIV positive' is given when 2 PCR tests are positive, and a report of 'HIV negative' is given when 2 PCR tests are negative, with at least one test done at or after 4–6 months of age.

The results of HIV PCR need to be confirmed by other serological tests at 18 months of age using 3 rapid tests, irrespective of the first test (PCR) results.

Diagnosis of HIV in Children >18 Months of Age

Infection is diagnosed by the detection of anti-HIV IgG. The enzyme-linked immunosorbent assay (ELISA) is used for screening (99.5% sensitivity, 99% specificity). Rapid ELISA (fourth generation ELISA) can yield results within 1–2 days. The results of ELISA test should be confirmed by Western Blot test (more sensitive) or a repeat HIV ELISA test by a different kit. In western blot test, the various viral antigens are separated using protein electrophoresis and antibodies are detected against various antigens. It is considered positive, if at least 2 out of 3 bands (p24, gp41, gp120/160) are positive. Cost is the major limitation.

Two positive HIV antibody tests (done sequentially) in a child more than 18 months of age indicate HIV infection. Recently, a diagnostic algorithm of a 4th generation HIV-1 or HIV-2 antigen/antibody combination immunoassay followed by a 2nd generation HIV-1 or 2 antibody differentiation assay has gained acceptance for HIV diagnosis.

Case Definition

HIV Infected

- *A child less than 18 months of age* who is HIV seropositive or born to HIV-infected mother and has positive results on two separate determinations (cord blood excluded) from one or more of the following tests: (*i*) HIV culture, (*ii*) HIV specific PCR, and (*iii*) HIV antigen (p24).

- *A child 18 months of age or older* born to HIV-infected mother or infected by blood, blood products or other known modes of transmission, who is HIV-antibody positive by

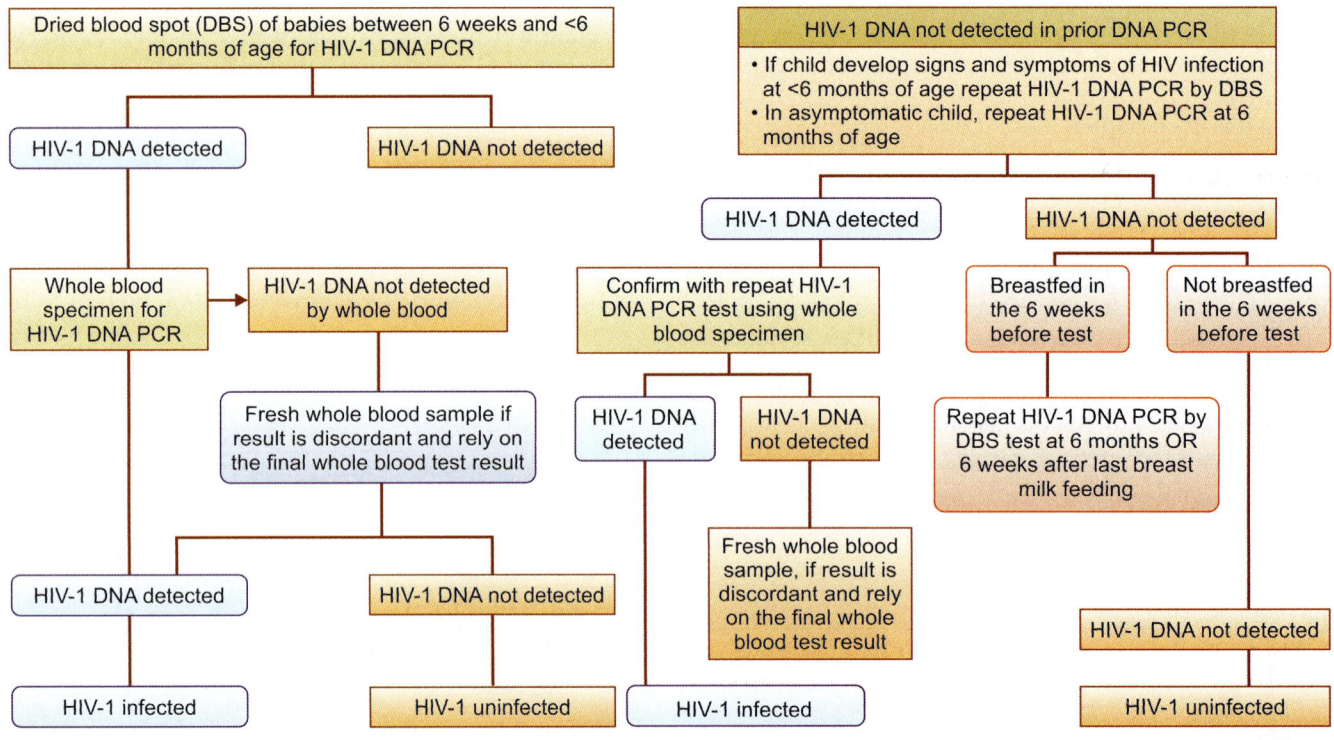

Establish definitive diagnosis at 18 months by HIV antibody test

Fig. 6.12 Diagnostic algorithm for an HIV-exposed infant less than 6 months age

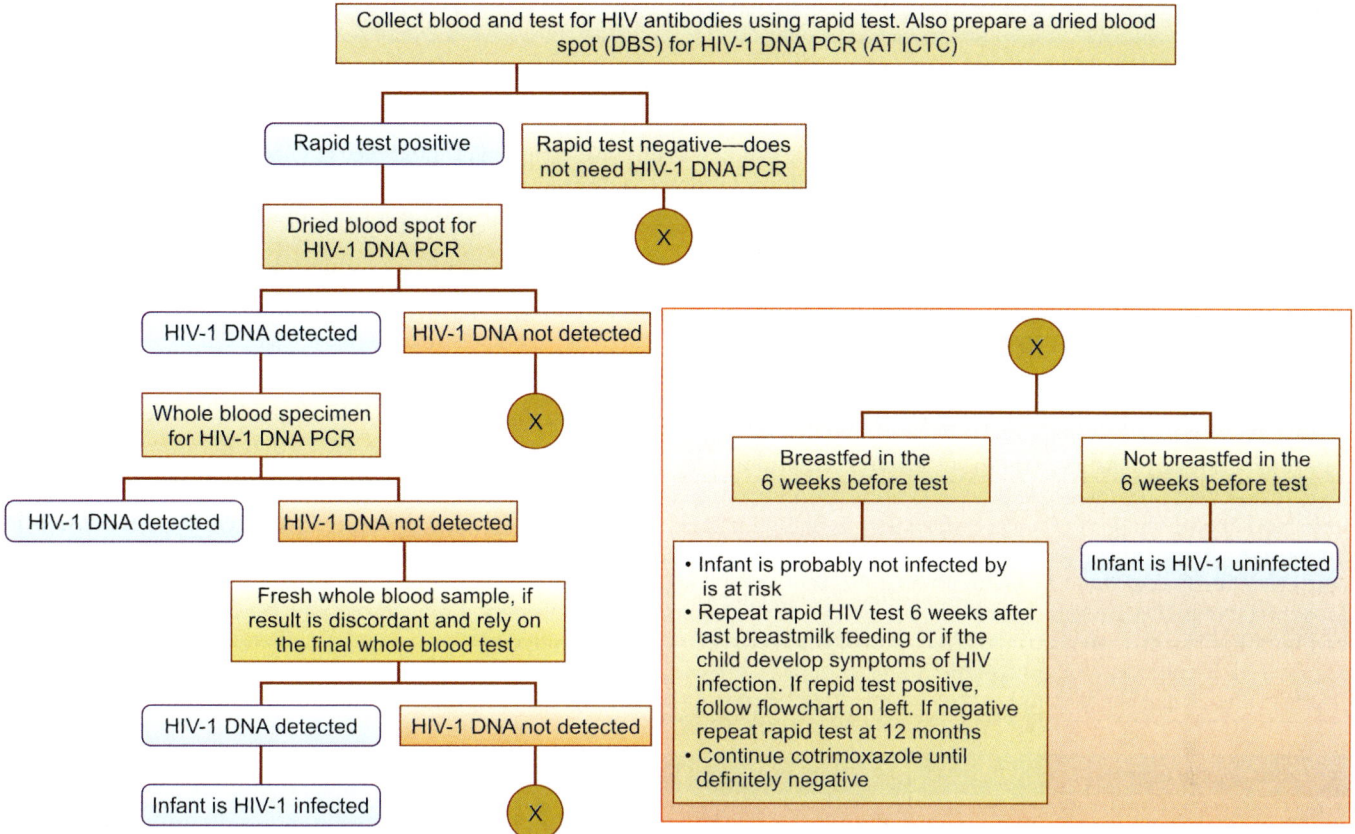

Fig. 6.13 Diagnostic algorithm for an HIV-exposed infant 6–18 months of age

being repeatedly reactive in ELISA and confirmatory test positive (*eg*, western blot, immunofluorescence assay) OR meets any of the criteria as above is labeled as HIV infected.

Perinatally Exposed

A child who does not meet the criteria above but who is HIV seropositive by ELISA and confirmatory test and is less than 18 months of age at the time of the test OR has unknown antibody status, but was born to a mother known to be infected with HIV.

Seroreverter

A child who is born to an HIV-infected mother and who has been documented as HIV antibody negative (ie, two or more negative ELISA tests performed at 6–18 months of age or one negative ELISA test after 18 months of age) and has had no other laboratory evidence of infection and has not had an AIDS-defining condition.

Pediatric AIDS Classification

The pediatric AIDS case definition was initially formulated in 1983 and was revised in 1987, 1994, and most recently in 2006 **(Table 6.11)**.

Immunological Classification

Use of CD4 counts to assess HIV-associated immuno-suppression in children is not free from problems, since (a)

normal CD4 counts are higher in infants and younger children than adults and decline over the first a few years of life, and (b) children may develop opportunistic infection at higher CD4 levels than do adults. Nevertheless, CD4 levels are apparently useful to assess the immunologic status of HIV-infected children. Since CD4 percent rather than absolute CD4 counts is subject to minimal variability, statistical analysis has been used to establish CD4 percent boundaries that best correlate with CD4 absolute count range in the immunologic category classification **(Table 6.12)**. These classifications help to determine the severity of HIV disease clinically and also simplify treatment of HIV.

Clinical Course of Vertically Acquired Infection

At birth, HIV-infected infants are generally asymptomatic, even if no ART is started. In the absence of ART, the median age at onset of symptoms is about 3 years; though some children remain asymptomatic for >5 years and with appropriate ART, may survive up to adulthood. The clinical disease in children may appear in two forms: (a) rapidly progressive or (b) slow progressive forms; observed in 80% and 20% infected children, respectively.

Rapid progression Onset of symptoms sets in from 3–4 months of age and if untreated such children die by 6–9 months age. Opportunistic infections and CNS manifestations are more common in these children. *Pneumocystis jirovecii* pneumonia is the presenting illness in 40% children. The rest usually

6

Table 6.11 WHO Clinical Staging of HIV/AIDS for Children (2006)
Clinical Stage 1 (Asymptomatic) Asymptomatic; Persistent generalized lymphadenopathy.
Clinical Stage 2 (Mild symptoms) Unexplained persistent hepatosplenomegaly; pruritic papular eruptions; fungal nail infection; angular chelitis; linear gingival erythema; extensive wart virus infection; extensive molluscum contagiosum; recurrent oral ulceration; unexplained persistent parotid enlargement; herpes zoster; and recurrent or chronic upper respiratory tract infections (otitis media, otorrhea, sinusitis, tonsillitis).
Clinical Stage 3 (Advanced symptoms) Unexplained moderate malnutrition or wasting not responding to standard treatment; unexplained persistent diarrhea ($\geq$14 days); unexplained persistent fever (>37.5°C intermittent or constant, >1 month duration); persistent oral candidiasis after 6–8 weeks of life; oral hairy leukoplakia; acute necrotising gingivitis or periodontitis; lymph node tuberculosis; pulmonary tuberculosis; severe recurrent bacterial pneumonia; symptomatic lymphoid interstitial pneumonia; chronic HIV-associated lung disease including bronchiectasis; unexplained anemia (< 8 g/dL), neutropenia (<0.5×10^9 per liter) and chronic thrombocytopenia (<50×10^9 per liter).
Clinical Stage 4 (Severe symptoms) Unexplained severe wasting, stunting or severe malnutrition not responding to standard therapy; *Pneumocystis carinii* pneumonia; recurrent severe presumed bacterial infections (eg, empyema, pyomyositis, bone or joint infection, meningitis, but excluding pneumonia); chronic herpes simplex infection (orolabial/cutaneous >1 month duration; visceral); extrapulmonary tuberculosis; Kaposi sarcoma; esophageal candidiasis or *Candida* of tracheobronchial tree or lungs; toxoplasmosis of CNS in children >1 month age; HIV encephalopathy; CMV retinitis or CMV infection in any organ in children >1 month age; extrapulmonary cryptococcosis including meningitis; disseminated endemic mycosis (extrapulmonary histoplasmosis, coccidioidomycosis, penicilliosis; chronic cryptosporidiosis; disseminated non-tuberculous mycobacterial infection; acquired HIV-associated rectal fistula; chronic isosporiasis; cerebral or B-cell non-Hodgkin's lymphoma; progressive multifocal leukoencephalopathy; and symptomatic HIV-associated nephropathy or cardiomyopathy.

Table 6.12 Age Specific CD4 Counts and Percent of Total Lymphocytes						
Immunologic category *	\<12 months		Age of child 1–5 years		6–12 years	
	cells/µL	percent	cells/µL	percent	cells/µL	percent
1. No evidence of suppression	$\geq$1500	$\geq$25	$\geq$1000	$\geq$25	$\geq$500	$\geq$25
2. Moderate suppression	750–1499	15–24	500–999	15–24	200–499	15–24
3. Severe suppression	<750	<15	<500	<15	<200	<15

* If CD4 counts and CD4 percent indicate different classification categories, the child should be classified into more severe category.

present with lymphadenopathy, hepatosplenomegaly, growth failure, encephalopathy or *Candida* infection. Prognosis is poor and death is inevitable by the age of 5 years, median survival time being 24.8 months. These children are usually those who were infected in the intra-uterine period. Age at presentation less than one year, *Pneumocystis* pneumonia, and CD4 count <750 per µL are associated with poor prognosis.

Slow progressors These children may present as late as 8 years of life and the chief presenting feature is lymphocytic interstitial pneumonia (LIP) in the majority of affected children. LIP is defined as reticulonodular pulmonary infiltrates persisting for >2 months with or without local lymphadenopathy. LIP is associated with low viral loads and, therefore, carries a better prognosis than PCP. Growth failure, fever, diarrhea, and secondary infections occur after infancy. Older children may have delayed puberty and subtle cognitive dysfunction.

End stage HIV disease (WHO stage 4) Such children have extremely low CD4 counts and are plagued by severe opportunistic infections. They have poor appetite, weight loss and severe wasting accompanied by growth failure, chronic diarrhea, and bone marrow failure.

Treatment   HIV/AIDS

There is no specific treatment either for HIV infection or for the immunodeficiency caused by it. Currently available therapy neither eradicates the virus nor offers a definitive cure. It can only suppress viral replication and modify course of the disease. A combination of antiretroviral drugs is preferred to mono-therapy. Early specific diagnosis and aggressive antimicrobial treatment of intercurrent infections prolong the life of the affected child.

Antiretroviral Therapy (ART)

These drugs inhibit viral multiplication and help to decrease the viral load in HIV-infected patients. These drugs can be categorized into 3 major groups:

1. *Nucleoside reverse transcriptase inhibitors (NRTIs)*
NRTIs like zidovudine (AZT), didanosine (DDI), zalcitabine (DDC), lamivudine (3TC), stavudine (d4T), abacavir (ABC), and emtricitabine (FTC), inhibit the enzyme reverse transcriptase and are active against HIV-1 and HIV-2. These are all prodrugs and need to be activated by undergoing intracellular phosphorylation. These drugs compete with normal nucleoside triphosphates and get incorporated into the growing proviral DNA chain; incorporation of abnormal nucleoside inhibits further viral

multiplication. Dual NRTI is the backbone of ART. Tenofovir and adefovir are nucleotide RTIs with similar mechanism of action as NRTIs.

2. Non-nucleoside reverse transcriptase inhibitors (NNRTIs)

These are active drugs which inhibit HIV-1 reverse transcriptase enzyme by binding to it which renders the enzyme inactive. These drugs, if used alone, lead to drug resistance and hence used in combination with NRTIs. There are 3 NNRTI drugs at present, namely, nevirapine (NVP), delavirdine (DLV), and efavirenz (EFV).

3. Protease inhibitors (PIs)

These drugs inhibit the protease enzyme by binding to its active site and prevent cleavage of precursor polyproteins at the late stage of viral replication. These are active against both HIV-1 and HIV-2. Drug resistance to PIs is virtually unknown. Available PIs include ritonavir (RTV), saquinavir (SQV), nelfinavir (NFV), amprenavir (APV), lopinavir/ritonavir (LPV/r), indinavir (IDV), darunavir, atazanavir, fosamprenavir (FPV), and tipranavir. These drugs are used as second line ART in the event of resistance to first line ART.

Newer antiretroviral drugs

These drugs have been developed as salvage regime in patients who have failed standard therapeutic regimens.

Entry inhibitors Enfurvirtide (T-20) inhibits viral binding and its fusion to target cells. It may be used in children >6 years but needs subcutaneous administration twice daily.

CCR5 co-receptor antagonist Maraviroc binds to CCR5 co-receptor of CD4 cells thereby preventing viral entry. Its use in children <16 years is not recommended.

Integrase inhibitors Raltegravir and elvitegravir act on the integrase enzyme thereby preventing incorporation of viral DNA into human genome. Their use in children <16 years is not recommended.

Pharmcokinetic enhancer Cobicistat has been included to boost the effect of other ART drugs like elvitegravir as it inhibits its hepatic metabolims. It also increases absorption of tenofovir, darunavir, and atazanavir.

Table 6.13 depicts the dosages of commonly used ART drugs in children and their adverse effects.

Table 6.13 Common Antiretroviral Drugs and their Dosages in Children				
Category	*Drug*	*Recommended dose*	*Maximum tolerated dose (mg)*	*Common adverse effects*
Nucleoside reverse transcriptase inhibitors (NRTIs)	Zidovudine (AZT)	3 mo–12 y: 160 mg/m²/dose q 8h PO >12 y: 200 mg/dose TID or 300 mg/dose BID	600	Anemia, granulocytopenia, nausea, headache, hepatitis, myopathy, seizures, rash, myositis, macrocytosis. Do not use with stavudine. Caution in renal/hepatic impairment
	Lamivudine (3TC)	3 mo–12 y: 4 mg/kg/dose BID. Adolescents <50 kg: 2 mg/kg/dose BID >50 kg: 150 mg/dose BID	300	Headache, nausea, diarrhea, rash, pancreatitis, peripheral neuropathy, raised liver enzymes, decreased neutrophil counts
	Abacavir (ABC)	8 mg/kg/dose PO BID	600	Fatal hypersensitivity reactions, fever, rash, nausea, diarrhea, abdominal pain
	Didanosine (ddI)	180 mg/m²	400	Headache, diarrhea, nausea, abdominal pain, peripheral neuropathy, hyperuricemia, pancreatitis, electrolyte abnormalities, raised liver enzymes, myalgia, rash. Administer empty stomach
	Stavudine (d4T)	2 mg/kg	80	Headache, GI discomfort, peripheral neuropathy, pancreatitis, elevated liver enzymes, lactic acidosis, rash. Adjust dose in renal failure
Nucleotide RTIs (NRTIs)	Tenofovir (TDF)	8 mg/kg/dose once daily. Not to be used below 2 years age. Use cautiously in <12 years age.	300	Lactic acidosis, severe liver damage, renal toxicity, osteopenia
Non-nucleoside RTIs (NNRTIs)	Nevirapine (NVP)	Start with 120 mg/m²/dose OD × 14 days, then increase to 120 mg/m²/dose BID PO, if no rash or other side effects	400	Hepatitis, rash, Stevens-Johnson syndrome, sedation, headache, GI discomfort
	Efavirenz (EFV)	15 mg/kg	600	Dizziness, sedation, insomnia, hallucinations, euphoria, transient rash, hepatitis
Protease inhibitors (PIs)	Nelfinavir (NFV)	110–150 mg/kg	2500	Hyperglycemia, lipodystrophy, hyperlipidemia, osteoporosis, diabetes, bleeding tendency
	Lopinavir/ Ritonavir (LPV/r)	460/115 mg/m²	800/ 200	
	Ritonavir (RTV)	700 mg/m²	1200	

6

Indications for Starting ART

ART once started not only has to be taken lifelong, but also has to be taken strictly as per schedule. It is necessary to counsel parents and children for long-term adherence to therapy.

The recent National AIDS Control Organization (NACO) guidelines recommend treatment in all infected children irrespective of clinical, virological, and immunological criteria.

Choice of ART

Triple combination therapy is recommended for treatment; monotherapy or dual therapy is not recommended to treat HIV infection. Dual NRTI is needed in addition to an NNRTI. Zidovudine (or abacavir in children with hemoglobin less than 9 g/dL) in combination with lamivudine are the NRTI backbones of choice in most children, while nevirapine is the most commonly used NNRTI. Efavirenz (an NNRTI) should be substituted for nevirapine in children >3 years old who are receiving antitubercular drugs, since the hepatotoxic effects of rifampicin and nevirapine are additive.

Table 6.14 provides a list of various alternatives of antiretroviral therapy in children, as recommended by NACO in 2014. Consider a brief period of hospitalization at start of therapy in selected circumstances, for patient education and to assess tolerability of medications chosen. Choose the simplest regimen possible, reducing dosing frequency and number of pills. Choose a regimen with dosing requirements that best conform to the daily and weekly routines and variations in patient and family activities. Choose the drugs with the fewest side effects; inform patient regarding medication side effects; anticipate and treat side effects.

Treatment of HIV in Special Situations

Treatment for opportunistic infections must be started before initiating ART.

Children exposed previously to ARV WHO recommends that in children exposed to maternal ART or infant ART or other ARTs used to prevent parent to child transmission (PPTCT), antiretroviral therapy should be started with lopinavir/ritonavir (LPV/r) + 2 NRTIs. For others, start ART with EFV + 2 NRTIs. The preferred dual NRTI combination is AZT + 3TC or ABC + 3TC. Combinations of zidovudine + stavudine, stavudine + didanosine, tenofovir + didanosine, and atazanavir + indinavir are not recommended.

Children with anemia/neutropenia In children with anemia (hemoglobin <7.5 g/dL) or severe neutropenia (<500 cells/mm^3), zidovudine must be avoided. In children with hepatitis B or C coinfection, the preferred NRTI combination is tenofovir and emtricitabine.

Treatment of HIV in children having TB Any child with active TB must be first initiated on antituberculous therapy and ART should be started as soon as tolerated usually 2 weeks after start of TB therapy, irrespective of CD4 count and clinical stage. Dose of nevirapine and protease inhibitors may need to be increased by 25–30% as rifampicin can decrease their concentration by induction of P450 enzyme.

Presumptive diagnosis of HIB injection in infants Sometimes, the final confirmation of HIV diagnosis in infants may be delayed and the infant presents to the hospital in a very sick condition. In such cases, ART could be started pending the availability of confirmed reports, provided the infant has been shown to be HIV antibody-positive and is symptomatic with ≥2 of the following: (a) oral thrush, (b) severe pneumonia and (c) severe sepsis OR the infant presents with any AIDS-indicator(s) like penumocystis pneumonia, cryptococcal meningitis, severe wasting or severe malnutrition, Kaposi sarcoma, extrapulmonary tuberculosis.

Monitoring

- Baseline pre-ART clinical staging, immune status, and HIV RNA viral load must be determined as far as possible. Additional essential investigations include baseline liver function tests, kidney function tests, lipid profile, and complete hemogram.
- Monitor adherence to therapy at each visit, and in between visits by telephone or letter as needed.
- Provide ongoing support and encouragement.
- Provide access to support groups or one-on-one counseling for patients with depression or drug use issues that are known to decrease adherence.

The aim should be to achieve >95% adherence with medication doses. Response to therapy is monitored by HIV copy number and CD4 lymphocyte count (3–12 monthly). Maximum response occurs within 12–16 weeks.

Table 6.14 Antiretroviral Regimens for Initial Therapy in Children (NACO 2014)

Children ≤3 years	
Hemoglobin ≥9 g/dL AND not on antituberculous therapy	Zidovudine + lamivudine + lopinavir/ritonavir
Hemoglobin <9 g/dL AND not on antituberculous therapy	Abacavir + lamivudine + lopinavir/ritonavir
Hemoglobin ≥9 g/dL AND on rifampicin containing anti-tuberculous therapy	Zidovudine + lamivudine + lopinavir/ritonavir* *For children below 10 kg:* Zidovudine + lamivudine + abacavir
Hemoglobin <9 g/dL AND on rifampicin containing anti-tuberculous therapy	Abacavir + lamivudine + lopinavir/ritonavir* *For children below 10 kg:* Stavudine + lamivudine + abacavir
Those having contraindication/intolerance to zidovudine and abacavir	Stavudine-based ART
Children ≥3 years	
Hemoglobin ≥9 g/dL	Zidovudine + lamivudine + efavirenz
Hemoglobin ≤9 g/dL	Abacavir + lamivudine + efavirenz
Those having contraindication/intolerance to zidovudine and abacavir	Stavudine-based ART

In children weighing >35 kg or ≥12 years age, Tenofovir-based regimens can be given.
*Super-boosting with Ritonavir is needed.

Treatment Failure

Suboptimal adherence, inadequate drug levels, pre-existing drug resistance and inadequate potency of ART drugs can lead to treatment failure. The diagnostic criteria for treatment failure may be clinical, immunological or virological.

Clinical Failure

- Recurrent, persistent or new HIV-related illness after receiving at least 3 months on ART. However, symptoms of opportunistic infections occurring concomitant with rise in CD4 counts within 3 months of starting ARV is not clinical failure but instead recognized as an entity IRIS (immune reconstitution syndrome), OR
- Decline of growth rate or development of encephalopathy or neuroregression is also regarded as clinical failure.

Immunological Failure

- Failure to increase age-related CD4 despite adequate trial of ART for 24 months, OR
- Developing or returning to the age-specific CD4 thresholds after 2 years of ART in a treatment-adherent child, *viz*, CD4 $<200/mm^3$ or % CD4 <10% in child aged 2–5 years and CD4 $<100/mm^3$ in child aged >5 years.
- *For children >5 y age* CD4 counts below pre-therapy baseline or drop in CD4 counts more than 50% from peak post-therapy levels.

Virological Failure

- Inability of viral load to decrease below undetectable levels within 6 months of starting ART, OR
- Repeated detection of virus (at least 3 times from lowest viral load level) in plasma after initial suppression to undetectable levels.
  Failure of ART is an indication to test for ART resistance by genotypic and phenotypic assays.

HIV and Opportunistic Infections (OIs)

In the pre-antiretroviral era and before development of potent combination highly active antiretroviral treatment (HAART) regimens, opportunistic infections (OIs) were the primary cause of death in HIV-infected children. Current HAART regimens suppress viral replication, provide significant immune reconstitution, and have resulted in a substantial and dramatic decrease in AIDS-related OIs and deaths in both adults and children.

A. Etiology

- *Bacterial infections* Recurrent bacterial infections are the commonest OIs in HIV-infected children. Common bacterial pathogens include *Streptococcus pneumoniae*, *Salmonella*, *Staphylococcus*, *Enterococcus*, *Pseudomonas*, and *Haemophilus influenzae*. Treatment of these infections is similar to those in HIV free children.
- *Viral infections* Common viral infections include herpes simplex (HSV), herpes zoster (HZV), hepatitis B, C and cytomegalovirus (CMV). HSV1 may cause recurrent gingivostomatitis as well as encephalitis while HSV2 can cause perirectal disease. Disseminated chickenpox may occur in HIV-infected children. Children with CD4 counts <50 cells/mm^3 are predisposed to disseminated cytomegalovirus infection including chorioretinitis, pneumonitis, hepatitis, bone marrow suppression, encephalitis, and colitis. CMV infection may be treated with ganciclovir or foscarnet given for 14–21 days. Extensive molluscum contagiosum can be seen in advanced HIV disease. About 10% of all HIV-infected children may have co-infection with hepatitis B. Progression to liver cirrhosis or hepatocellular carcinoma is faster in HIV co-infection. To prevent hepatitis B co-infection, all HIV-infected infants should receive hepatitis B vaccination.

- *Fungal infection* Common fungal pathogens in HIV-infected children include *Candida, Cryptococcus and Pneumocystis jirovecii*. Oral thrush or candidiasis in a child >6 months age can be a marker of HIV infection. Cryptococcus infection can present with meningitis in HIV-infected children while *Pneumocystis jirovecii* can present with pneumonia, both being AIDS defining illnesses.
- *Parasitic infections* Common parasitic pathogens include *Toxoplasma, Cryptospora, Microspora, Isospora,* and *Giardia*.

B. Role of HAART in reducing OIs

Studies in adults and children have demonstrated that HAART reduces the incidence of OIs and improves survival, independent of the use of OI antimicrobial prophylaxis. HAART can improve or resolve certain OIs, such as cryptosporidiosis or microsporidiosis infection, for which effective specific treatments are not available. However, potent HAART does not replace the need for OI prophylaxis in children with severe immune suppression. Additionally, initiation of HAART in persons with an acute or latent OI can lead to IRIS, an exaggerated inflammatory reaction that can clinically worsen disease and require use of anti-inflammatory drugs.

C. Prevention of OIs

Primary prophylaxis for Pneumocystis jirovecii pneumonia and toxoplasmosis Prophylaxis with trimethoprim-sulphamethoxazole (cotrimoxazole) is recommended for all HIV-exposed infants born to mothers living with HIV commencing at 4–6 weeks of age (or at first encounter with healthcare system) and continued until HIV infection can be excluded. For children below 5 years of age, initiation of cotrimoxazole prophylaxis is recommended irrespective of clinical or immunological staging. For children >5 years, prophylaxis is recommended, if CD4 <350 cells/mm^3 or if clinical condition warrants (WHO clinical stages 2, 3 or 4 for HIV disease). Prophylaxis (5 mg/kg trimethoprim, OD) should continue until the age of 5 years. Prophylaxis can be stopped in children older than 5 years, if immune restoration (WHO stage 1 or 2 and CD4 >350 cells/mm^3 on 2 occasion at least 3 months apart) has been documented for >6 months duration.

Primary prophylaxis against Mycobacterium avium-intracellulare complex (*MAC*) Children with advanced immunosuppression need prophylaxis against MAC with oral azithromycin 20 mg/kg, once weekly OR clarithromycin 7.5 mg/kg bid PO.

Primary prophylaxis against Mycobacterium tuberculosis Children with HIV more than 1 year age should be started on isoniazid prophylaxis (10 mg/kd/d) for 6 months after excluding active tuberculosis. Those with tuberculosis must be continued on oral isoniazid for additional 6 months after completing the antitubercular therapy, along with pyridoxine 25 mg PO daily.

Primary prophylaxis for CMV infection. Ganciclovir can be given in severely immunosuppressed children. Annual fundoscopy is recommended to detect CMV retinitis.

Primary prophylaxis for serious bacterial infections Intravenous immunoglobulin (IVIG) (400 mg/kg every 4 weeks) can prevent recurrent serious bacterial infections for symptomatic patients who have suffered from at least two documented serious bacterial infections within 1 year; have laboratory-documented inability to make antigen-specific antibodies; or in those who have hypogammaglobulinemia.

Secondary prophylaxis Secondary prophylaxis is recommended for CMV retinitis with ganciclovir, toxoplasmosis with sulfadiazine-pyrimethamine with folinic acid, *Cryptococcus neoformans* infection with fluconazole, histoplasmosis with itraconazole, and penicilliosis with itraconazole.

Immunization in HIV-infected

Children with symptomatic HIV infection should not ideally be given live vaccines like oral polio vaccine, BCG or intranasal influenza vaccines. Triple antigen (DPT), hepatitis B, inactivated polio vaccine (IPV), and typhoid vaccine, can be administered. Due to issues of safety in severely immunocompromised children, varicella and MMR vaccines should be considered for HIV-infected children who are not severely immunocompromised (ie, age-specific CD4 > 15%). Children with asymptomatic HIV infection should receive BCG in addition to the vaccines mentioned above.

Prevention of HIV Infection

Prevention of parent-to-child transmission of HIV (PPTCT) or prevention of mother-to-child transmission of HIV (PMTCT)

In the absence of intervention, the transmission rate of HIV from mother-to-child varies from 10 to 45%. Other than intrauterine and intrapartum transmission, breastfeeding assumes an important route of transmission in developing countries as the risk of transmission increases to 20–35% (with breastfeeding for 6 months) and up to 30–45% (with breastfeeding for 18–24 months). With effective interventions, this risk may be decreased to less than 2%.

NACO recommends that all HIV positive pregnant women including those presenting in labor and breastfeeding women with HIV should be initiated on a triple ART (tenofovir, lamivudine and efavirenz) irrespective of clinical, immunological and feeding option, for preventing mother-to-child transmission risk and should continue lifelong ART. The duration of nevirapine (NVP) to infant should be minimum 6 weeks but more if ART to mother was started in late pregnancy, during or after delivery and has not been on adequate period of ART as to be effective to achieve optimal viral suppression (which is at least 24 weeks), then the infant NVP should be increased to 12 weeks. This recommendation on extended NVP duration applies to infants of breastfeeding women only and not those on exclusive replacement feeding. Cesarean section should be performed in mother for obstetric indications only. **Table 6.15** depicts the dosage of NVP for the infant as per 2014 recommendations.

Choice of Feeding

The increased risk of HIV transmission by continued breastfeeding is about 10–15%. The risk is higher, if there is increased viral load in breast milk, nipple lesions, mastitis, breastfeeding for longer than 15 months (up to 45%), and mixed feeding. Exclusive breastfeeding for 6 months is associated with 3–4 times decreased risk of transmission compared to non-exclusive breastfeeding.

In India, experience has shown that exclusive replacement feeding (ERF) for infants has not been feasible for the majority of HIV-infected families. Infants on replacement feeding have more health problems such as diarrhea, respiratory infections and a high risk of death compared to infants on exclusive breastfeeding. This high risk of health problems and death of infants on replacement feeding may negate the advantage of decreased risk of transmission of HIV. Helping the HIV-infected mother/families choose the best option of infant feeding, which will ensure the best chance of infant survival, is the priority. Mixed feeding must be totally avoided.

National guidelines on feeding for HIV-exposed and infected infants <6 months old recommend that all HIV-infected pregnant women should be informed about infant feeding options, *viz* exclusive breastfeeding or exclusive replacement feeding. Breastfeeding is the preferred choice in developing countries as it maximizes the chances of infant survival. NACO proposes exclusive breastfeeding for first 6 months and continued breastfeeding till 12 months. Only in situations where breastfeeding is not possible (maternal death, severe maternal sickness) or individual mother's informed choice, then replacement feeding may be considered; only if criteria given in **Table 6.16** for replacement feeding are met.

WHO recommends that mothers living with HIV should breastfeed for at least 12 months and may continue for 24 months or longer, while on ART. Even a shorter duration of breastfeeding is better than not breastfeeding at all.

Table 6.15 Nevirapine (NVP) Prophylaxis for the Infant for PMTCT		
Birth weight (g)	*NVP daily dose (mg)*	*Duration*
<2000 g	2 mg/kg PO once daily	Up to 6 weeks* irrespective of exclusive breastfeeding or exclusive replacement feeding
2000–2500 g	10 mg PO once daily	
>2500 g	15 mg PO once daily	

*12 weeks where duration of ART for mother during pregnancy is <24 weeks

Other Preventive Strategies

Horizontal transmission (via blood, blood derivatives and needle) can be and should be prevented by stringent donor screening and sterilization of injection equipment. Accidental transmission from infected children to health care professionals must also be prevented by the blood and body fluid precautions as instituted in the situation of hepatitis B virus carrier patients. Extraordinary isolation procedures are unwarranted.

Postexposure prophylaxis is indicated for accidental contact with HIV contaminated blood or body fluids. The

---

Revision Point

HIV

1. HIV infection is transmitted by horizontal route (blood transfusion, contact with infected body fluids, needle stick injury, sexual intercourse) or vertical route (mother-to-child).
2. HIV infection can weaken the immune system and lead to acquired immunodeficiency syndrome (AIDS), if an HIV-infected person develops a CDC-defined AIDS indicator illness (like tuberculosis, cytomegalovirus retinitis, *Pneumocystis jirovecii* pneumonia, histoplasmosis, toxoplasmosis of brain, candidiasis of esophagus/bronchi/trachea/lungs, severe unexplained wasting/stunting/severe malnutrition, cryptococcosis, lymphoma, *Mycobacterium avium* complex or *M. kansasii*, disseminated or extrapulmonary, etc.) or the CD4 T cell count drops below a certain age-dependent cut-off.
3. The diagnosis of HIV-infection in a child below 18 months' age can be made by detection of viral DNA or RNA by PCR test, HIV antigen detection or viral culture. A positive virological test needs to be confirmed by a second virological test. Positive HIV antibody testing is not recommended for definitive or confirmatory diagnosis of HIV infection in children until 18 months of age.
4. In children older than 18 months, HIV antibody tests (rapid or laboratory-based ELISA) can be used for establishing the diagnosis, in addition to virological test for HIV or its components (HIV-RNA or HIV-DNA or ultrasensitive p24 antigen test). A positive antibody test needs to be confirmed by a second HIV antibody test (rapid or laboratory-based ELISA).
5. All HIV-infected children need to be started on triple antiretroviral therapy, irrespective of immunological or clinical staging of HIV infection.
6. HIV-exposed baby is initiated on cotrimoxazole prophylaxis at 6 weeks' age and is tested for HIV DNA PCR at 6 weeks by DBS (dry blood spot) collection. If the DBS sample is positive for HIV DNA PCR, then a repeat DBS sample is tested for HIV DNA PCR.
7. Prevention of parent-to-child transmission of HIV infection can be done by starting the newly born on nevirapine prophylaxis. Additionally, all pregnant women need to be given lifelong antiretroviral therapy.
8. National AIDS Control Organization proposes exclusive breastfeeding for first 6 months and continued breastfeeding till 12 months in HIV-exposed infants.

Table 6.16 Criteria for Replacement Feeding in HIV Exposed Infants

1. Availability of **safe water and adequate sanitation** at the household and community level
2. The mother or other caregiver can reliably **afford** to provide sufficient replacement feeding (milk), to support normal growth and development of the infant.
3. The mother or caregiver can **prepare replacement feeding frequently enough in a clean manner** to minimse the risk of diarrhea or malnutrition in the infant
4. The mother or caregiver can **exclusively give replacement feeding in the first six months**. This will eliminate increased transmission risk due to mixed feeding.
5. **Family is supportive** of this practice
6. **Access to comprehensive child health services** for the mother or caregiver.

---

recommended regimen is TFV+3TC+EFV for 28 days duration. In case of intolerance to EFV, a PI like LPV/r can be substituted for EFV. The first dose should preferably be given within 2 hours of exposure and subsequently taken at bed time. A non-fatty food should be taken for dinner to maximize absorption.

Counseling and Support

Counseling and psychotherapeutic support are necessary for the older children and parents. Physicians, nurses and other staff should be informed of the real nature of this disease so that panic may be avoided. Patients and parents should be treated humanely and with dignity and ethical principles appropriate for the profession.

National AIDS Control Organization 2014. Pediatric ART Guidelines. Available from: *http://naco.gov.in/upload/2014%20mslns/CST/Pediatric_14-03-2014.pdf*. Accessed March 6, 2015.

World Health Organization. Early Detection of HIV Infection in Infants and Children. Available from: *http://www.who.int/hiv/paediatric/EarlydiagnostictestingforHIV Ver_Final_May07.pdf*. Accessed March 5, 2015.

World Health Organization. Global Update on HIV Treatment 2013. Avaiable from: *http://www.who.int/hiv/pub/progressreports/update2013/en*. Accessed February 28, 2015.

World Health Organization. March 2014 Supplement to the 2013 Consolidated Guidelines on the use of Antiretroviral Drugs for Treating and Preventing HIV Infection 2014. Available from: *http://www.who.int/hiv/pub/guidelines/arv2013/arvs2013-supplement march2014/en*. Accessed March 26, 2015.

6.13 DIPHTHERIA

Diphtheria is an acute infectious disease caused by a toxin produced by the Gram-positive bacillus *Corynebacterium diphtheriae*. Infection may result in an asymptomatic carrier state; or clinical disease. The illness is characterized by moderate fever and sore throat; adherent membrane of the tonsils, pharynx, or nose; and severe toxemia.

The Problem Statement

Diphtheria used to be a leading cause of death in children until the introduction of a vaccine 50 years back. WHO estimates that there are about 100,000 cases and up to 8,000

6

deaths every year worldwide. In the last decade, epidemics were reported in Russia, Ukraine and other countries of the former USSR. The epidemics began in 1990 and since then have spread to 15 countries. The death rate was as high as 50% among children under two years in Turkmenistan. These epidemics are largely due to decreasing immunization coverage among infants and children, waning immunity to diphtheria in adults, and an irregular supply of vaccines.

Diphtheria is endemic in India. Exact figures on prevalence are not available, but of late, the incidence has shown a decline mainly due to widespread vaccination coverage of under-fives.

Etiology

The infection is caused by *Corynebacterium diphtheriae*, also known as Klebs-Loeffler bacilli.

Corynebacterium diphtheriae secretes a potent exotoxin. This exotoxin is the major determinant of pathogenicity of the organism. The toxin causes reversible early cardiac damage and late neurological lesions. Diphtheria toxin is lethal to man in a dose of 130 µg/kg body weight.

Both toxigenic and non-toxigenic strains of *Corynebacterium diphtheriae* are capable of causing disease; however, cardiac and neurological sequels are observed following infection with toxigenic strains only.

Epidemiology

Eighty percent of cases occur in individuals less than 15 years of age. Both sexes are equally affected. Diphtheria occurs more often in the autumn and winter months. Transplacental immunity acquired from the mother protects the offspring during first 8–10 weeks of life. Infection can occur in immunized, partially immunized, or unimmunized individuals.

Mode of Spread

Diphtheria is acquired by contact with a carrier or a person with the disease. Bacteria are transmitted by airborne droplet liberated during coughing, sneezing, or talking. Fomites and dust may at times serve as mode of transmission of infection. Bacteria may enter the host through respiratory tract, abraded skin, eyes, genitalia, middle ear or umbilicus in the neonate. Once infected, the patient remains infective to others till the virulent bacilli are present in the lesions, usually for a period of 2–4 weeks.

Carriers For every case of clinical diphtheria, there exist 20 asymptomatic carriers in the community. The organism is carried in nose or throat. The carrier state may be temporary or chronic.

Pathogenesis

Diphtheria is a rapidly developing, acute, febrile infection which involves both local and systemic pathology. The primary local lesion develops in the upper respiratory tract and involves necrotic injury to epithelial cells. As a result of this injury, blood plasma leaks into the area and a fibrin network forms which is interlaced with rapidly-growing *C. diphtheriae* cells. This membranous network covers the site of the local lesion and is referred to as the pseudomembrane. The membrane is adherent to underlying tissues.

The diphtheria bacilli do not tend to invade tissues below or away from the surface epithelial cells at the site of the local lesion. At this site, they produce the toxin that is absorbed and disseminated through lymph channels and blood to the susceptible tissues of the body. Degenerative changes in these tissues, which include heart, muscle, peripheral nerves, adrenals, kidneys, liver and spleen, result in the systemic pathology of the disease.

The pathogenicity of *Corynebacterium diphtheriae* thus includes two distinct phenomena:

- *Invasion of the local tissues of the throat*, which requires colonization and subsequent bacterial proliferation. Not much is known about the adherence mechanisms of *C. diphtheriae*; and
- *Toxigenesis* (*bacterial production of the toxin*). The diphtheria toxin causes the death of eukaryotic cells and tissues by inhibiting protein synthesis in the cells.

Although the toxin is responsible for the lethal symptoms of the disease, the virulence of *C. diphtheriae* cannot be attributed to toxigenicity alone, since a distinct invasive phase apparently precedes toxigenesis. Diphtheria toxin may also play an essential role in the colonization process.

Clinical Features

Incubation period is 2–5 days (range 1–10 d).

Onset of symptoms is acute with moderate fever (39°C) and nonspecific symptoms, often resembling viral upper respiratory infection. Fever is associated with chills, malaise, weakness, prostration, sore throat, and headache. Further symptoms depend on the site of involvement:

- *Nasal diphtheria* is characterized by a serosanguineous or seropurulent nasal discharge.
- *Tonsillar diphtheria* manifests with dysphagia, sore throat, and cervical lymph node enlargement.
- *Laryngeal diphtheria* should be suspected, if the child presents with cough, hoarse voice, inspiratory stridor, and dyspnea.

Examination reveals general toxic and ill-looking anxious child, who has difficulty in breathing. Typical hallmark of the disease is presence of a thick, gray, and leathery membrane covering the affected area; ie, tonsils, soft palate, oropharynx, nasopharynx, uvula, or laryngeal walls and folds. Attempt at scraping the pseudomembrane causes bleeding of the underlying mucosa.

Pharynx shows marked congestion and edema. Regional lymph nodes of the neck are involved. Extensive anterior and submandibular cervical lymphadenopathy imparts a *bull's neck* appearance. The child may hold the head in extension. It can be associated with dysphonia.

Presence of the membrane over larynx results in respiratory obstruction that may manifest itself as stridor, wheezing, cyanosis, accessory muscle use, and retractions. Untreated, it may progress to respiratory failure.

Complications

Exotoxin of diphtheria typically affects the heart, nerves, and kidneys. Cardiac toxicity typically occurs after 1–2 weeks of illness following improvement in the pharyngeal phase of the disease, and manifests as myocarditis or arrhythmia. Neurological toxicity involves both cranial and peripheral nerves and symptoms may appear as early as in the beginning of 2nd week of illness. A latent period of up to 3 months is also described. Renal complications consist of tubular necrosis and proteinuria.

Cardiac complications Myocarditis is seen in as many as 60% of patients (especially if previously unimmunized). It can present acutely with congestive heart failure, circulatory collapse, or in a more subtle way with progressive dyspnea, diminished heart sounds, cardiac dilatation, and weakness. Atrioventricular blocks, ST-T wave changes, and various dysrhythmias may be seen.

Neurologic toxicity is proportional to the severity of the pharyngeal infection. Most patients with severe disease develop neuropathy. Deficits include regurgitation of swallowed fluids due to paralysis of the soft palate and posterior pharyngeal wall; oculomotor and ciliary paralysis accounting for cranial neuropathies; and dysfunction of facial, pharyngeal, or laryngeal nerves.

Peripheral neuritis develops anywhere from 10 days to 3 months after the onset of pharyngeal disease. It manifests itself initially as a motor defect of the proximal muscle groups in the extremities. The weakness is usually symmetrical and simulates Guillain-Barre syndrome. Various degrees of dysfunction exist, ranging from diminished deep tendon reflexes to complete motor paralysis. Occasionally, a glove-and-stocking neuropathy pattern can be observed. All nerve damage due to diphtheria eventually resolves.

Cutaneous Diphtheria

Cutaneous diphtheria begins as a painful lesion resembling an erythematous pustule, which breaks down to form an ulcer covered with a gray membrane. The lesion usually develops at a site of previous trauma or a primary dermatologic disease. It follows an indolent course, typically lasting weeks to months. Occasionally, it may cause respiratory diphtheria.

Treatment	**Diphtheria**

If diphtheria is strongly suspected, specific treatment with *antitoxin* and *antibiotics* should be initiated immediately while bacteriological investigations are still pending. Antitoxin therapy is the mainstay of treatment. Antibiotic therapy is required to eradicate the organism and prevent spread. Mechanical airway obstruction and myocarditis are the main causes of death in toxigenic disease and careful supportive management is required.

1. Diphtheria Antitoxin

Diphtheria antitoxin is hyperimmune serum produced in horses. Antitoxin will only neutralize circulating toxin that is not yet bound to tissue, thus prompt administration is critical. Delayed administration increases the risk of late effects such as myocarditis and neuritis. Before antitoxin is administered, the patient should be tested for sensitivity to horse serum and if necessary, desensitized. The dose of antitoxin to be administered depends upon the site and extent of the diphtheritic membrane, the degree of toxicity and the duration of illness. **Table 6.17** indicates the suggested dose range for various clinical situations.

Table 6.17 Dosage of Antitoxin for Diphtheria

Type of diphtheria	Dosage (units)	Route
Nasal	10000–20000	IM/IV
Tonsillar	15000–25000	IM/IV
Pharyngeal or laryngeal	20000–40000	IM/IV
Combined types or delayed diagnosis	40000–60000	IV
Severe diphtheria with respiratory obstruction or bull-neck	40000–100000	IV or part IV and part IM

IV: intravenous; IM: intramuscular.

If acute anaphylaxis develops, intravenous epinephrine (0.2 to 0.5 mL of 1:1000 solution) be administered immediately by intravenous injection. Antitoxin is probably of no value for cutaneous disease, although some centers advocate 20,000 to 40,000 units of antitoxin because toxic sequels have been reported. Vigorous cleaning of the wound with soap and water and administration of antibiotics is recommended.

2. Antibiotics

Antibiotic treatment is necessary to eliminate the organism and prevent spread; it is not a substitute for antitoxin treatment. The antibiotics of choice are erythromycin or penicillin. The recommended dose regimens are as follows:

Penicillin, preferably crystalline penicillin (100,000–150,000 units/kg/d q 6h) IV or intramuscular procaine penicillin G (25000–50000 units per kg per day) in two divided doses or parenteral erythromycin (40–50 mg/kg/day, max 2 grams) are the initial therapeutic options. One can shift to oral administration of erythromycin (40–50 mg/kg/day in 4 divided doses) or oral penicillin V (125–250 mg four times daily) when the patients is able to swallow. Antibiotic treatment should be continued for 14 days.

3. Treatment of carriers

Carriers should be treated with erythromycin 40 mg/kg/day for 7–10 days or a single intramuscular dose of benzathine penicillin (0.6 megaunits for <30 kg weight and 1.2 megaunits for >30 kg). Cultures should be obtained after two weeks. If positive, give an additional course of erythromycin for ten days. Antitoxin is not recommended for asymptomatic carriers. Antitoxin is not recommended for asymptomatic carriers.

Unimmunized carriers should receive a full schedule of active immunization. Previously immunized carriers should receive a booster dose if the previous dose was received more than a year ago.

Prevention

Better control of diphtheria depends on high immunization coverage, prompt recognition and management of diphtheria cases, and rapid identification and effective management of close contacts to prevent further spread of outbreaks.

1. Isolation of the Patient

Communicability in untreated persons usually lasts for two weeks. If treated adequately, communicability lasts for less than four days. The patient should be isolated until this period is over or two cultures from nose and throat are negative.

2. Care of the Contacts

The management of close contacts depends on whether the contact can be kept under surveillance for minimum 7 days or not. Management is given in Fig. 6.14. There is no role of prophylactic diphtheria antitoxin in unimmunized close contacts. *Schick test*, previously recommended to assess the presence of circulating antibody to exotoxin and immune status of the individual with respect to diphtheria, is no longer in current use.

3. Active Immunization

The aim is to immunize the infant before the effect of transplacental acquired immunity against diphtheria is over. The vaccine currently in use is a toxoid, and available as DPT vaccine. Immunization does not eliminate *C. diphtheriae* in skin or nasopharynx.

Primary immunization consists of three doses at an interval of 4–6 weeks, starting from 6 weeks after birth. First booster is given at 18 months and a second booster at five years. Subsequent boosters are not necessary in India where *C. diphtheriae* infection is common. In case primary immunization is to be carried out in adult or older child, the adult type of toxoid (Td) containing less quantities of antigen should be employed. The Td preparation contains not more than 2 Lf of diphtheria toxoid per dose as compared to 25 Lf in DPT preparation.

All patients suffering from diphtheria should undergo active immunization because the attack of disease, by itself, may not confer immunity against subsequent infections. The immunization coverage with 3 doses of DPT vaccine in infants is still far from satisfactory in India as compared to rest of the world.

Replace TT with Td

In the light of recent diphtheria outbreaks affecting older children and younger adults in developing countries and the

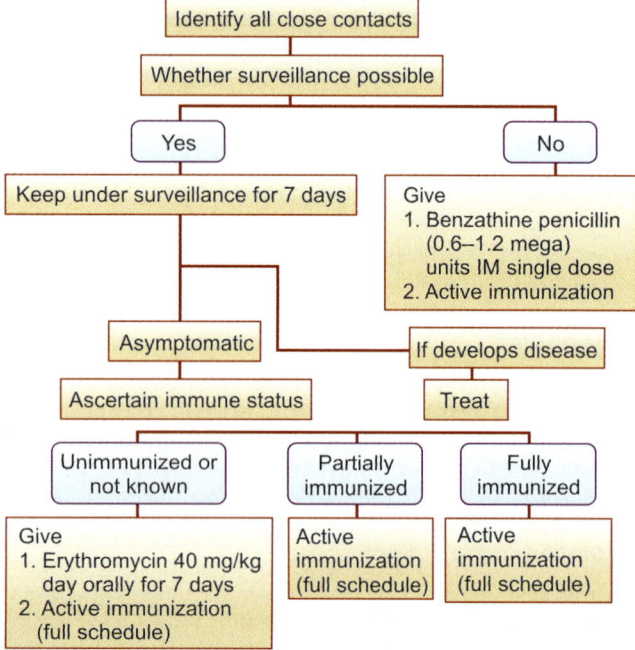

Fig. 6.14 Care of contacts of a patient with diphtheria

Diphtheria

1. Diphtheria is a potentially fatal disease caused by exotoxin producing bacteria *C. diphtheriae*.
2. Presence of pseudomembrane on the affected site is pathognomonic of the disease.
3. Diphtheria may have various clinical presentations, namely nasal, pharyngeal and tonsillar, laryngeal, cutaneous, ophthalmic or genital.
4. Pharyngeal diphtheria is commonest and these patients have a high likelihood of developing respiratory failure.
5. Myocarditis, neuritis, and renal failure are potential complications.
6. Diagnosis is established by isolation of organism in special culture media.
7. Patients need to be started with antitoxin on the basis of clinical diagnosis as soon as possible.
8. Main role of antibiotics, ie, crystalline penicillin and erythromycin is to prevent further transmission of the disease.
9. Carriers and close contacts should be managed as per the standard protocols.
10. Primary immunization with diphtheria toxin is a must for prevention.

resurgence of the disease in industrialized countries, it has become clear that periodic administration of booster doses of diphtheria toxoid are needed to ensure long-lasting protection of all individuals against diphtheria. It has, therefore, been recommended to replace TT with Td in a phased manner. As a first priority, TT should be replaced by Td in all countries that have had DTP-3 coverage of 70% or more for 5–7 years. Where boosters of DT are given at school age, replacing the first dose of DT with Td simplifies delivery programmatically.

Centers for Disease Control and Prevention (CDC). Updated recommendations for use of tetanus toxoid, reduced diphtheria toxoid and acellular pertussis vaccine (Tdap) in pregnant women and persons who have or anticipate having close contact with an infant aged <12 months. Advisory Committee on Immunization Practices (ACIP), 2011. *MMWR Morb Mortal Wkly Rep.* 2011;60:1424–6.

Efstratiou A, Engler KH, Mazurova IK, *et al.* Current approaches to the laboratory diagnosis of diphtheria. *J Infect Dis.* 2000;181:S138–45.

6.14 PERTUSSIS (WHOOPING COUGH)

Whooping cough is a highly communicable illness caused by a coccobacillus *Bordetella pertussis*. The illness affects all ages, but the effects and course is more pronounced in infants and young children. The disease is characterized by paroxysmal bouts of cough lasting for almost a month.

Etiology

Bordetella pertussis is a Gram-negative coccobacillus which colonized ciliated epithelium. The pathogenic effects are mediated through various antigens or their products produced by the organism. *Bordetella pertussis* has 2 major antigens, ie, FHA or filamentous hemagglutinin antigen and

LPF or lymphocytosis producing factor. *Bordetella pertussis* also produces several toxins, of which pertussis toxin (PT) is the most important virulence factor. It also acts as a mediator for attachment to respiratory cells. Filamentous hemagglutinin also mediates attachment of *B. pertussis* to respiratory epithelium. Both PT and hemagglutinin produce protective antibodies that prevent clinical disease. Therefore, any vaccine aiming to prevent pertussis should contain both these antigens.

B. pertussis also produces tracheal toxin (TCT), adenylate cyclase toxin (ACT), dermonecrotic toxin (DNT), and several agglutinogens. TCT disturbs mucociliary clearance and damages the epithelium. Adenylate cyclase toxin and PT inhibit phagocytic functions. TCT, DNT, and ACT contribute to local damage while PT is primarily responsible for systemic manifestations. Pertussis is not a single toxin disease like diphtheria and tetanus.

Epidemiology

Age Pertussis is typically a disease of young children. A significant epidemiological shift has been observed in many industrialized countries, indicating a higher incidence of pertussis among previously vaccinated schoolchildren, adolescents and adults. Even neonates can be affected as immunity to pertussis is not transmitted transplacentally.

Sex There is a female predilection for pertussis.

Nutritional status Incidence of pertussis as well as mortality due to pertussis is more in children whose body weight is less than 60% of the expected weight.

Environment Whooping cough is more common in winter and spring. Overcrowding, poor socioeconomic status, and low level of parental education are related with higher mortality.

Mode of Spread

Man is the only known host of *B. pertussis*. Transmission occurs directly *via* respiratory secretions. Bacteria are spread by droplets discharged from the nose or throat of an infected person, usually in close contact. Pertussis is highly contagious during the first week of illness with a secondary attack rate of almost 100% in susceptible contacts. Communicability then decreases rapidly, but may persist up to 21 days. Fomites do not constitute a major route of transmission.

Adults with overt or subclinical infection are important sources of infection for young children. People with asymptomatic infection are less likely to transmit the disease than individuals with symptomatic infection. Asymptomatic chronic carriers of *Bordetella pertussis* are uncommon.

Clinical Features

The incubation period ranges from 7 to 14 days. Natural history is classically described in 3 phases; ie, (*a*) Catarrhal phase; (*b*) Paroxysmal phase; and (*c*) Convalescent phase.

During the *catarrhal phase*, the disease is usually indistinguishable from cough and cold, sometimes with mild fever. After about 10 days, the cough worsens and the disease progresses into *paroxysmal phase* with bouts of coughing; the child's face becomes congested passing from red to blue

during bouts. The classical whoop occurs due to a rescue inspiration at the end of coughing. Post-tussive vomiting may occur. This phase may continue for about 2 weeks without improvement. If there are no complications, the disease progresses to *convalescent phase* which may last for up to 3 months. In clinical practice, the paroxysmal and convalescent phases may be considered as one. Relapses back to paroxysmal coughing are common. The disease is also known as 'cough of 100 days.' The cough is exhaustive and scaring for the child and family.

The disease may have an atypical presentation in infants younger than 3 months of age. The whoop may be absent in babies who may lack strength to mount paroxysms. These children are at high risk and the disease can present as serious respiratory infection or a cough proceeding to apneic attacks. Also, young infants are especially vulnerable since protective antibodies in childhood decline in adults and hence, there is little passive protection of the newborn by maternal antibodies.

Complications

Complications are related to pressure effects resulting from paroxysms or occur because of respiratory or neurological involvement.

- *Pressure effects* lead to venous congestion causing subconjunctival hemorrhages, skin petechiae, nose bleeds and hemoptysis. Intracranial hemorrhage is rare. Raised intracranial pressure due to incessant cough may also enlarge a number of hernias. Persistent coughing may result in increased intrathoracic pressure. Resultant barotrauma can cause air leak; ie, pneumothorax.
- *Secondary infection* in lungs may occur and should be suspected in any child with high temperature. Atelectasis, interstitial pneumonia, and bronchiectasis are other reported respiratory complications. Pertussis can flare up a pre-existing focus of tuberculosis in lungs, especially in malnourished children.
- *Neurological sequelae* are the most serious complication. They may be toxin-mediated or the sequelae of hypoxia. CNS manifestations include loss of consciousness, convulsions, or encephalopathy which may lead to brain damage, handicap or death. Neurological complications occur in 3–5% and can also manifest as motor deficits, visual and auditory loss, and aphasia.

Case Definition

Whooping cough should be *suspected* whenever there is a history of severe cough lasting for 2 weeks or more. This definition has 84–92% sensitivity and 3–90% specificity, during outbreaks.

Whooping cough is *probable*, if any of the following exist in a suspected case:
- Prolonged coughing followed by a period of apnea and cyanosis, or in older children paroxysms of coughing followed by vomiting, or a typical breath intake and 'whoop', or subconjunctival hemorrhages;
- Exposure to a suspect case in the previous 3 weeks;
- Epidemic of whooping cough in the area; or
- Lymphocytosis of $15000/mm^3$ or more.

A probable case is *confirmed*, if there is laboratory evidence of *B. pertussis* from the culture or immunofluorescence of nasopharyngeal secretions. The nasopharyngeal diagnosis is provided by a pernasal sample which requires a special cotton swab on a long flexible wand. The swab needs to be placed in a culture medium such as Stuarts, and, though storage overnight in a refrigerator is permissible, rapid transport to the laboratory for planting improves the chance of positive result.

Differential Diagnosis

Other causes of protracted cough include those caused by adenovirus, RSV, enterovirus, influenza virus, parainfluenza virus and *Mycoplasma*.

Investigations

Recovery of the organism is easier at early stages of illness. A positive culture on Bordet-Gengou medium is the gold standard of diagnosis. Peripheral smear shows absolute lymphocytosis. Direct immunofluorescent assay (DFA) of nasopharyngeal aspirate has variable sensitivity and specificity. It should be emphasized that no single serologic test is highly specific and sensitive. Newer serological methods include PCR and ELISA techniques for detection of pertussis toxin and filamentous hemagglutinin.

Treatment	Pertussis

A. Antibiotics

Once in the paroxysmal phase, drug therapy makes little impact on the course of the illness. An antibiotic (erythromycin is highly effective) should always be given to render the sufferer noninfectious and prevent the spread of disease. This is normally achieved after 5 days of erythromycin; however, treatment is best continued for 2 weeks as a few individuals remain culture positive even after 1 week of antibiotics. Azithromycin is the drug of choice for neonatal pertussis.

- Erythromycin is given in a dose of 40 mg/kg/d orally, in 4 divided doses for 2 weeks. The newer macrolides (eg, azithromycin, clarithromycin), are potential alternatives for patients who cannot tolerate erythromycin.
- Azithromycin is typically administered in doses of 10–12 mg/kg/d PO once a day for 5 days.
- Clarithromycin is administered at 15–20 mg/kg/d PO in 2 divided doses, not to exceed 1 g/d for 5–7 d.
- Trimethoprim-sulfamethoxazole (trimethoprim 8 mg/kg/d and sulfamethoxazole 40 mg/kg/d) in 2 divided doses is another antibiotic option.

B. Supportive Treatment

Adjunct therapy should center on 5 principles of care:
1. Avoid provoking paroxysms of coughing;
2. Comforting during paroxysms;
3. Clearing away mucus and vomit during paroxysms to prevent inhalation;
4. Early recognition and treatment of complications; and
5. Maintaining good hydration and reasonable nutrition.

Humidification of the air diminishes the viscosity of mucus and the affected child can bring it out more easily. Mild sedation should be done to allay anxiety. Salbutamol has no role in preventing incidence or reducing the severity of paroxysms.

C. Care of Contacts

The Committee on Infectious Diseases of the American Academy of Pediatrics currently recommends promptly treating all household and other close contacts (eg, children and staff at daycare centers) with erythromycin to limit secondary transmission. This is regardless of the age or immunization status of contacts. A 14-day course of oral erythromycin (40–50 mg/kg/d in 4 divided doses) is recommended for close contacts. Some experts prefer the estolate preparation in young infants because of more effective absorption, which may lead to decreased dosing and less frequent dosing intervals.

Prevention

Natural disease does not provide lifelong immunity. Similarly, pertussis vaccination protects the individual for a maximum period of 10–20 years. However, universal immunization of children with pertussis vaccine is essential for control of pertussis. Since protective antibodies against this disease do not cross the placenta, early immunization is desired. The National Immunization Schedule of India advocates pertussis vaccination as DPT at 6, 10, and 14 weeks of age. This is to be followed by 2 boosters at 18–24 months and at 5 years of age.

It is generally believed that pertussis vaccine should not be given to children above 5 to 6 years. There is no scientific basis for this and in countries where adult pertussis occurs, adult immunization has never caused unusual problems. In developing countries also, pertussis is commonly occurring after 5 years of age; thus a booster at 5 years is required.

Pertussis vaccine has limited impact on the circulation of *B. pertussis* even in countries with high vaccination coverage. Non-immunized children and adults may serve as reservoirs for the infection and occasionally transmit *B. pertussis* to unimmunized young infants.

Acellular Pertussis Vaccine

Studies have indicated that DPT with a whole cell pertussis (wP) component is responsible for frequent reactions. These reactions are both unpleasant and at times dangerous. This led to the development of acellular pertussis vaccine in the year 1981 in Japan. The acellular vaccine predominantly contains PT as the essential component, and different amounts of filamentous hemagglutinin (FHA), pertactin (PRN), and fimbrial hemagglutinins 1, 2 and 3 (FIM 1, 2, 3). Recent studies have demonstrated a better efficacy of whole cell vaccine for primary immunization, as compared to acellular vaccine.

Indian Academy of Pediatrics (IAP) recommends use of whole cell pertussis vaccine for primary immunization. Academy also recommends use of Tdap during each pregnancy to protect very young infants, thus urging Government to take initiatives for making the same available and set national guidelines. WHO also recommends continuation of the whole cell pertussis vaccine in countries with limited resources.

Future research will be concentrated on the development of a genetically engineered product, which carries the additional advantage of reduction in the number of required dosages for primary immunization.

Pertussis

1. Pertussis, caused by *Bordetella pertussis,* is a toxin-mediated disease, presenting as a typical whooping cough. The illness usually lasts for 3 months.
2. Diagnosis is established by isolation of organism on Bordet-Gengou medium.
3. Management is mostly supportive, targeted towards comforting the patient and monitoring for complications.
4. Azithromycin is effective, if given in the first week of illness.
5. Immunization with 3 doses and 2 boosters of DPT vaccine prevents pertussis with 70–90% efficacy.

Cherry JD, Grimprel E, Guiso N, *et al.* Defining pertussis epidemiology: clinical, microbiologic and serologic perspectives. *Pediatr Infect Dis J.* 2005;24:S25–34.

Heininger U. Pertussis: what the pediatric infectious disease specialist should know. *Pediatr Infect Dis J.* 2012;31:78–9.

Langley JM, Halperin SA, Boucher FD, Smith B; Pediatric Investigators Collaborative Network on Infections in Canada (PICNIC). Azithromycin is as effective as and better tolerated than erythromycin estolate for the treatment of pertussis. *Pediatrics.* 2004;114:e96–101.

Mathew JL. Acellular pertussis vaccines pertinent issues. *Indian Pediatr.* 2008;45:727–9.

WHO. Pertussis vaccines: WHO position paper—recommendations. *Vaccine.* 2011;29:2355–6.

Yeh SH. Pertussis: persistent pathogen, imperfect vaccines. *Expert Rev Vaccines.* 2003;2:113–27.

6.15 TETANUS

Tetanus is caused by an anaerobic bacteria, *Clostridium tetani* which produces a neurotoxin called tetanospasmin. The disease is characterized by generalized muscle rigidity and spasms, lockjaw, and opisthotonus and carries a significant morbidity and mortality. Majority of cases are reported from developing countries; with 50% of these occurring in neonates. Mortality is 30–50% even with optimal treatment.

India has been declared free from neonatal and maternal tetanus on May 15, 2015. *Elimination of neonatal tetanus is defined as less than one case in 1000 live births in every district across the country.* Maternal tetanus is considered eliminated once neonatal tetanus elimination has been achieved. Nagaland was the last state in India to achieve neonatal and maternal tetanus elimination.

Etiology

Clostridium tetani is a Gram-positive, anaerobic, motile, rod-shaped bacteria. The organism bears spores at its terminal end giving it a typical drumstick appearance. While the bacillus is an obligate anaerobe, its spores remain viable at ambient oxygen concentrations. The spores are highly resistant to extremes in temperature and humidity, and can survive indefinitely. Spores are ubiquitous in soil and in the feces of many animals and of humans.

Mode of Spread

Tetanus organism or spores may enter the body through a puncture wound, or laceration, following an acute injury. Recent surgery also accounts for several cases. Non-acute etiologies include chronic wounds, IV drug use, and complications of diabetes. Other etiologies include otitis media (*otogenic tetanus*), intranasal foreign bodies, corneal abrasions/ulcers/foreign bodies, dental procedures, injections, abortion, childbirth and burns. Neonatal tetanus follows infection of the umbilical stump of a newborn delivered to an unimmunized mother. Lack of immunization is the greatest risk factor for contracting tetanus. Tetanus is not transmitted from man-to-man by direct spread.

Pathogenesis

Spores of *Clostridium* are carried into the wounds along with soil, dirt, or dust. The spores may not germinate immediately due to unfavorable tissue conditions. They may activate well after the wound has healed, which may account for the cases of tetanus that have no identifiable source. When conditions such as gross contamination or tissue injury favor anaerobic proliferation, the spores germinate into mature bacilli, which then form the toxins *tetanolysin* and *tetanospasmin*.

Tetanolysin has an uncertain role in clinical tetanus; it may contribute to an anaerobic environment by damaging viable tissue. *Tetanospasmin* is primarily responsible for the clinical manifestations of tetanus. Tetanospasmin is highly lethal with 1 mg of toxin being enough to kill 6,40,000 mice. It enters peripheral nerves and travels via the axonal retrograde transport system to the central nervous system. Tetanospasmin then enters presynaptic neurons and disables neurotransmitter release, most importantly, the inhibitory neurotransmitters gamma-aminobutyric acid (GABA) and glycine. This results in a disinhibition of end-organ neurons, such as motor neurons and those of the autonomic nervous system. This accounts for the muscle spasms characteristic of tetanus and for the autonomic instability seen with severe tetanus.

Recovery involves synthesis of new presynaptic components and their transport to the distal axon. This accounts for the typical 2–3 week period before clinical improvement begins.

Clinical Features

The median incubation period is 7 days; 73% of patients develop their first symptom between 4 and 14 days after an injury. The rapidity of incubation and onset correlates with the severity of disease. There are 4 clinical forms of tetanus representing the extent and location of neurons involved: Generalized, local, cephalic, and neonatal.

1. Generalized Tetanus

The initial symptom is trismus (*lockjaw*) secondary to masseter muscle spasm in 50–75% of cases. *Risus sardonicus,* the "ironical smile of tetanus", can occur due to facial muscle contraction. Nuchal rigidity and dysphagia may also be initial complaints. As the disease spreads, generalized muscle spasms occur, either spontaneously or to minor stimuli such as touch or noise. Opisthotonus, a tonic contraction very similar to decorticate posturing, is classically described with tetanus. Severe spasms can result in vertebral fractures, long bone fractures, and detachment of tendons from their insertions. Unfortunately for the patient, mental status is not affected and spasms are felt with severe pain. In the acute phase, death may result from acute respiratory failure due to diaphragmatic paralysis and/or laryngeal spasms. With intensive medical intervention, including paralysis and mechanical ventilation, such deaths can be averted.

In patients surviving beyond the acute phase, autonomic instability is the major cause of death, with a fatality rate of 11–28%. Autonomic instability occurs several days after the onset of generalized spasms and manifests as labile hypertension, tachycardia, and pyrexia. Arrhythmias and myocardial infarction are the most common fatal events. The exact mechanism of this syndrome is unclear but likely involves disinhibition of the sympathetic nervous system.

2. Local Tetanus

Only a particular muscle group, which is close to the site of injury, is involved. The rigidity may linger for weeks to months and often self-resolves without sequelae. What appears to be localized tetanus may instead be the first symptom of generalized tetanus. Case-fatality rate is 1%.

3. Cephalic Tetanus

Injury to face, eyes, ears, neck, following tonsillectomy or dental extraction may result in isolated involvement of cranial nerves, known as cephalic tetanus. Cephalic tetanus uniquely results in cranial nerve palsies and muscle spasms. The seventh cranial nerve is most often involved, followed by the 6th, 3rd, 4th, and 12th in decreasing order of frequency. Cephalic tetanus also presents with trismus, but in 42% of cases, cranial nerve deficits precede the onset of trismus. In such cases, cephalic tetanus is easily misdiagnosed. With its predilection for the 7th cranial nerve, it commonly mimics Bell's palsy. Head trauma and otitis media are commonly cited etiologies. About two-thirds of the patients progress to generalized tetanus and the overall mortality is 15–30%.

4. Neonatal Tetanus

This is a generalized tetanus that occurs in the newborn around the first week of life. It occurs characteristically in a newborn of an unimmunized mother, where the umbilical cord was cut by unsterile and unconventional means. Symptoms begin with non-specific irritability and poor feeding, and rapidly progress to generalized spasms. The portal of entry of spores is the freshly cut umbilical cord.

The risk of contracting neonatal tetanus is directly related to the cleanliness of delivery conditions and to maternal immunization, since passive transfer of maternal immunoglobulins is protective. Mortality is very high (50–100%) due to the high load of toxin per kg body weight in neonates.

Diagnosis

The diagnosis of tetanus is clinical. There are no laboratory tests which can diagnose or rule-out tetanus. Fortunately, the presentation of tetanus is so characteristic that a presumptive diagnosis can be made in most cases. The differential diagnoses are discussed below:

- Trismus can be caused by *peritonsillar or odontogenic abscesses* and *dystonic reactions*. These can be ruled-out by history and examination.

- *Strychnine poisoning* can closely resemble generalized tetanus; strychnine disables glycine release like tetanospasmin, but does not affect GABA release. A strychnine level should be sent for all suspected cases of tetanus.
- *Hypocalcemia* causing tetany is another mimic, which can easily be ruled out.
- Other entities that cause diffuse muscle spasms, such as seizures, *toxidromes*, and encephalopathy are accompanied by changes in mental status.
- Processes that affect muscles locally, such as *myopathies* or *neuropathies*, tend to cause weakness rather than spasm and rigidity. In addition, neuropathies are associated with sensory deficits, which is not a feature of tetanus.
- Cephalic tetanus without trismus can be easily mistaken for *Bell's palsy*, *CNS tumor*, or *stroke*; with the inevitable appearance of trismus and muscle spasm, the diagnosis becomes clear.
- Neonatal tetanus initially presents much like a host of other disorders, including infectious, toxic and *metabolic etiology*. However, once generalized spasms begin, the diagnosis is obvious.

As an aid in clinical diagnosis, a bedside "spatula test" for tetanus has been described. A spatula is inserted into the pharynx. If the patient gags and tries to expel the spatula, the test is negative for tetanus; if the patient bites the spatula due to reflex masseter spasm, the test is positive for tetanus.

Treatment	Tetanus

Treatment strategies involve 3 management principles:
1. Organisms present in the body should be destroyed to prevent further toxin release.
2. Toxin present in the body, outside the CNS should be neutralized.
3. The effects of toxin already in the CNS should be minimized.

Neutralization of unbound toxin Human tetanus immune globulin 3000–6000 units is given intramuscularly.

Removal of the source of infection Where present, obvious wounds should be surgically debrided. Antibiotics are administered to eradicate clostridia.

- *Penicillin* has been widely used for many years but is a GABA antagonist and associated with convulsions.
- *Metronidazole* is probably the antibiotic of choice. It is safe and comparative studies with penicillin suggest equally good results.

A. Control of Rigidity and Spasms

It is best achieved by a combination of avoidance of unnecessary stimulation and sedation with a benzodiazepine. Benzodiazepines augment GABA agonism by inhibiting an endogenous inhibitor at the GABA receptor. Diazepam may be given by various routes, is cheap and widely used, and doses as high as 100 mg per hour have been used. Midazolam has been used with less apparent accumulation.

Additional sedation may be provided by anticonvulsants, particularly phenobarbitone (which further enhances GABAergic activity) and phenothiazines, usually chlorpromazine. Propofol has been used for sedation with rapid recovery on stopping the infusion.

When sedation alone is inadequate, neuromuscular blocking agents and intermittent positive pressure ventilation may be required for a prolonged period. Pancuronium (long-acting), vecuronium (short-acting), and intrathecal baclofen have been used.

B. Control of Autonomic Dysfunction

Sudden cardiac death can occur due to autonomic dysfunction in severe tetanus. The cause remains unclear but plausible explanations include sudden loss of sympathetic drive, catecholamine-induced cardiac damage, and increased parasympathetic tone or 'storms'.

Benzodiazepines, anticonvulsants, and morphine are beneficial for controlling the automonic dysfunction. Morphine is particularly useful as cardiovascular stability may occur without cardiac compromise. Proposed mechanisms of action include replacement of endogenous opioids, reduction in reflex sympathetic activity and release of histamine. Phenothiazines, particularly chlorpromazine, is another useful sedative; anticholinergic and α-adrenergic antagonism may contribute to cardiovascular stability.

Other drugs that have been used to control autonomic dysfunction include a combination of *alpha- and beta-adrenergic receptor blocking agents*. The α_2-adrenergic agonist clonidine has been used orally or parenterally, with variable success. Acting centrally, it reduces sympathetic outflow, thus, reducing arterial pressure, heart rate, and catecholamine release from the adrenal medulla. Peripherally, it inhibits the release of norepinephrine from pre-junctional nerve endings. Other useful effects include marked sedation and anxiolysis.

Magnesium sulfate has been used both in artificially ventilated patients to reduce autonomic disturbance and in non-ventilated patients to control spasms. Magnesium is a presynaptic neuromuscular blocker, blocks catecholamine release from nerves and adrenal medulla, reduces receptor responsiveness to released catecholamines, is an anticonvulsant and a vasodilator. Hypotension and bradyarrhythmia may occur. It is, therefore, mandatory to maintain levels in the therapeutic range.

C. Supportive Intensive Care Treatment

Nutrition should be established as early as possible. Enteral nutrition is associated with a lower incidence of complications and is cheaper than parenteral nutrition. Percutaneous gastrostomy may avoid the complications associated with nasogastric tube feeding and is easily performed on the intensive care unit under sedation.

Prevention

A. Primary Immunization

Infants Tetanus immunization should be started at the age of 6 weeks along with diphtheria and pertussis immuni-

zation. Three doses of DPT are recommended, 4–6 weeks apart. First booster is given at 18 months and the second at the school entry point. Thereafter a booster of tetanus toxoid is advocated at every 10-year interval.

Older children and adults If not vaccinated before, primary immunization consists of two doses of adsorbed tetanus toxoid (TT) given intramuscularly at an interval of 4–8 weeks. A booster is given one year thereafter.

B. Prevention of Neonatal Tetanus

Aseptic delivery The delivery should be conducted by a trained birth attendant, umbilical cord should be cut with a sterile blade, and application of extraneous and indigenous substances on the umbilical stump should be actively discouraged.

Maternal active immunization Tetanus toxoid should be administered to all pregnant women. According to the National Schedule on Immunization, two doses of tetanus toxoid are recommended between 20 and 36 weeks of pregnancy, given a month apart. In previously immunized women, a single dose given at around 32–34 weeks is considered sufficient.

C. Prevention of Tetanus following Injury

Care of the wound Any wound, abrasion, etc., should be thoroughly cleaned with water immediately, if nothing else is available. Foreign bodies and debris in the wound should be removed. Soil, dirt, necrotic tissue should not be allowed to remain at the injury site.

Immunization The need for immunization is determined by the state, extent, cleanliness of the wound and previous immune status **(Table 6.18)**. In case of minor clean wounds, passive immunization is not required. Active immunization is offered only in previously unimmunized or partially immunized individuals, or if the last dose of booster was given earlier than 10 years. Severe or contaminated wounds in previously immunized individuals do not require either active or passive immunization provided the individual has received a booster of tetanus toxoid in the last 5 years.

In previously immunized (where the last dose was given more than 10 years ago) and unimmunized individuals, one dose of toxoid is given shortly after the injury, followed by completion according to primary immunization schedule.

Passive immunization It is provided with tetanus immune globulin (TIG), given intramuscularly within 3 days of injury. A single intramuscular dose of 5000 units is sufficient to neutralize systemic toxin, but total dose of 3000 to 6000 units

Immune status	Completed primary immunization*		Unimmunized, partially immunized or unknown status**	
	TIG	TT	TIG	TT
Minor wounds	Not required	Not required	Not required	Required
Wounds that are contaminated or severe	Not required	Not required	Required	Required

Table 6.18 Guidelines for Tetanus Immunization Following Injury

TT: tetanus toxoid; TIG: tetanus immune globulin. *Completed primary immunization – having received 3 doses of tetanus toxoid or a booster within last 10 years. **All others who have not completed primary immunization.

6

is also recommended. TIG does not cross the blood–CSF barrier. If TIG is not available, equine-derived or bovine-derived tetanus antitoxin (TAT) is used. The usual dose of TAT is 50,000 to 1,00,000 units with half given intramuscularly and rest intravenously, is sufficient for toxin neutralization. Active immunization can be given alongside passive immunization. However, the injection of globulin and toxoid should be given in separate syringes at two different sites.

Elimination of Maternal and Neonatal Tetanus (MNTE)

World Health Organization (WHO) added tetanus toxoid vaccine in its Expanded Program on Immunization (EPI) in the year 1974. Almost 15 years later, by 1989, only a quarter (27%) of pregnant females were receiving the standard doses of tetanus toxoid. Year 1990 was initially set as target by WHO to achieve the goal of neonatal tetanus elimination, defined as less than one case per 1000 live births per year in all districts of a country; it was later extended to 1995. By the end of 1999, there were 57 countries that had yet not achieved this goal.

In the year 2000, WHO, United Nations Children's Fund (UNICEF) and United Nations Population Fund (UNFPA) partnered to re-launch their efforts to achieve the goal of neonatal tetanus elimination. As neonatal tetanus depends mainly on tetanus immunization of the mother during pregnancy, the goal of elimination of maternal tetanus was also added to this initiative which was rechristened "Maternal and Neonatal Tetanus Elimination Program" (MNTE), and year 2005 was set as the cut-off year to achieve this goal. However, 19 countries are yet to achieve this goal. India was one of the last a few countries to be declared free of maternal and neonatal tetanus on 15th May, 2015.

The strategies recommended to achieve and maintain the goal of MNT elimination include strengthening of routine immunization, surveillance, implementation of supplementary immunization activities (SIAs) targeting women of child-bearing age with three doses of properly spaced injections with tetanus toxoid in selected high-risk areas, and the promotion of clean deliveries.

Revision Point

Tetanus

1. Tetanus is caused by an anaerobic bacteria, *Clostridium tetani* which produces a neurotoxin called tetanospasmin.
2. The disease is characterized by generalized muscle rigidity and spasms, lockjaw, and opisthotonus and carries a significant morbidity, and mortality. Difficulty in swallowing, restlessness, irritability, and headache are early manifestations.
3. Laryngeal and respiratory muscle spasms can lead to airway obstruction and asphyxia.
4. Neonatal tetanus manifests within 3–12 days of birth.
5. Diagnosis is mainly clinical.
6. Human tetanus immunoglobulin (TIG) is recommended to be given immediately. Penicillin is the antibiotic of choice.
7. The average mortality is 45–55%. For neonatal tetanus, the mortality is 60–70%.
8. Active immunization is the best method to prevent tetanus.

Brook I. Current concepts in the management of Clostridium tetani infection. *Expert Rev Anti Infect Ther.* 2008;6:327–36.

Gibson K, Bonaventure Uwineza J, Kiviri W, *et al.* Tetanus in developing countries: a case series and review. *Can J Anaesth.* 2009;56:307–15.

Roper MH, Vandelaer JH, Gasse FL. Maternal and neonatal tetanus. *Lancet.* 2007 ;370:1947–59.

WHO. Maternal and Neonatal Tetanus (MNT) elimination. http://www.who.int/immunization_monitoring/diseases/MNTE_initiative/en/index4.html. Accessed 2 June, 2012.

6.16 TYPHOID FEVER

Typhoid fever is a severe multisystemic infection caused by *Salmonella Typhi*. Similar illness can be caused by related but less virulent *Salmonella paratyphi* (paratyphoid fever). Enteric fever is a collective term and refers to all illnesses caused by these organisms. The disease is characterized in endemic areas by the classic prolonged high grade fever, sustained toxemia, gastrointestinal symptoms and splenomegaly. Enteric fever is potentially fatal, if untreated.

Epidemiology

S. Typhi and *S. paratyphi* infections occur worldwide but primarily in developing nations where sanitary conditions are poor. Typhoid and paratyphoid fevers are endemic in Asia (especially the Indian subcontinent), Africa, Latin America, the Caribbean, and Oceania. Typhoid fever affects 13–17 million people yearly and kills an estimated 600,000. In endemic areas, children aged 5–19 years are at the highest risk of infection. However, children between 1 and 5 years are also susceptible. This age group is at highest risk of morbidity and mortality because of waning passively acquired maternal antibody and lack of acquired immunity.

In young children, the clinical syndrome is often a nonspecific febrile illness that is not recognized as typhoid fever. Early antibiotic therapy has transformed a previously life-threatening illness of several weeks duration with an overall mortality rate approaching 20% into a short-term febrile illness with negligible mortality.

Etiology

Salmonella Typhi is a Gram-negative, motile bacillus. It has three antigens, namely (*a*) somatic cell wall O antigen, a lipopolysaccharide, (*b*) flagellar H antigen, and (*c*) Vi (virulence) antigen, a polysaccharide capsular antigen, which is T-cell independent. Vi antigen also interferes with phagocytosis by preventing binding of C_3 to the surface of the bacterium. Systemic immunity to typhoid can be achieved through induction of antibodies to either O and H antigen or Vi polysaccharide antigen. *S. Typhi* can survive at extremely low freezing temperature and drying, and, therefore, can be transmitted through ice, frozen foods, and dust.

Mode of Spread

S. Typhi is excreted in the feces of infected persons. A person with active typhoid fever may also spread the organism through urine, respiratory secretions or vomitus. The food can be contaminated by flies which carry the bacilli from feces of an infected or carrier individual. Contaminated water or unpasteurized milk are the other sources of infection.

Reservoir Man is the only true reservoir of *Salmonella Typhi*. Carrier state can occur in convalescent patients (temporary carriers excrete the bacilli for 6–8 weeks). *Chronic carrier* is defined as an individual who continues to excrete the organism in feces for 3 months or longer. This state develops in 3–5% of individuals having suffered from *S. Typhi* infection. Chronic carrier state is less frequent in children and more often observed in females. In certain cases, carrier state persists lifelong. The bacilli are carried in the gall-bladder of a carrier. These carriers serve as a major source of infection to the community.

Environmental factors Transmission of *S. Typhi* is dependent on a multitude of *environmental, social, and cultural factors*. Cases occur more frequently during summer and rainy season, peaking with the onset of monsoons. Proper and adequate supply of potable water, proper excreta disposal system, hygienic personal and food habits, practicing of strict hand washing, pasteurization of milk, and health awareness are instrumental in preventing its transmission. Low socio-economic groups who may not have access to the above mentioned facilities are more prone to suffer from typhoid fever.

Pathogenesis

Children are typically infected with *S. Typhi* and *S. paratyphi* through contaminated food and beverages. Infective dose is 10^5 to 10^8 organisms. After ingestion by the host, the bacteria invade through the gut and multiply within the mononuclear phagocytic cells in the liver, spleen, lymph nodes, and Peyer's patches of the ileum. The infected macrophage provides *Salmonella* a vehicle safe from other elements of the immune system and in which it can multiply and travel. It passes through the mesenteric lymph nodes into the thoracic duct and the lymphatics beyond to seed the reticuloendothelial tissues—liver, spleen, bone marrow, and lymph nodes. In these, it multiplies until some critical density is reached.

From blood or from the liver via bile ducts, it infects the gallbladder and re-enters the gastrointestinal tract in the bile, spreading to other hosts via stool. In addition, it occasionally invades the urinary tract and spreads via urine. After primary intestinal infection, further seeding of the Peyer's patches occurs through infected bile. They may become hyperplastic and necrotic with infiltration of mononuclear cells and neutrophils, forming ulcers that may bleed through eroded blood vessels or perforate the bowel wall, causing peritonitis. The host induces cytokines such as interferon alpha, interleukin (IL)-12, and tumor necrosis factor-alpha, which recruit macrophages and cause the high fever of the disease. Probability of clinically evident disease is more with a higher number of infecting particles, reduced gastric acidity, and possession of Vi antigen by the bacteria.

Clinical Features

Salmonella Typhi infection can be asymptomatic, subclinical, or present with the classical illness, as described below.

Incubation Period

The incubation period of typhoid fever varies with the size of the infecting dose and averages 7–14 (range, 3–60) days. In paratyphoid infection, the incubation period ranges from 1–10 days. During the incubation period, 10–20% of patients have transient diarrhea (enterocolitis) that usually resolves before the onset of the full-fledged disease. As bacteremia develops, the incubation period ends. Patients often experience chills, diaphoresis, anorexia, dry cough, a dull frontal headache, and myalgia before the onset of a high fever. About 20–40% of patients present with abdominal pain.

Classical Typhoid Fever

The classic manifestations of enteric fever include fever, toxemia, delirium, abdominal pain, constipation, and hepatosplenomegaly.

First week Fever occurs in 75–85% of patients in the first week and is often initially remittent but becomes steady. The individual's temperature often rises to as high as 103–104°F (39–40°C) by the beginning of second week. Constipation often develops early and is likely due to obstruction at the ileocecal valve by swollen Peyer's patches. It may last for the entire duration of illness. At approximately the end of the first week of illness, some patients develop bacterial emboli to the skin known as *rose spots*. Rose spots constitute a subtle, extremely sparse (often ≤5 spots), salmon-colored, blanching, truncal, maculopapular rash with 1- to 4-cm lesions that generally resolve within 2–5 days. They are uncommon in dark-skinned individuals. Relative bradycardia and a dicrotic pulse are also common during this stage of illness.

During the *second week* of illness, the child may look toxic-appearing, anorexic and apathetic with sustained fever and significant weight loss. The abdomen is slightly distended, often with a tympanic note. Spleen becomes palpable by 7th day of illness. The patient may have a thready pulse, tachypnea, conjunctivitis, crackles over the lung bases and may enter into a *typhoid state* of apathy, confusion, and even psychosis.

Some individuals may produce liquid, foul, green-yellow diarrhea (pea soup diarrhea). Rare complications of enteric fever include pancreatitis, meningitis, orchitis, and osteomyelitis.

Untreated, the patient may die or recover in 3–4 weeks. Mortality is 10% in untreated cases, and less than 1% in those treated. Death ensues from overwhelming toxemia, myocarditis, intestinal hemorrhage, or perforation due to necrotic Peyer's patches.

Complications

Intestinal perforation and hemorrhage may occur in <1% subjects during the 2nd week of illness. The presentation can be in the form of frank blood in stools, abdominal distension, acute abdominal emergency, peritonitis, abdominal guarding, rigidity, and shock. Other common complications are hepatitis, cholecystitis, cholangitis, bronchitis and encephalopathy. Uncommon complications include myocarditis, transverse myelitis, Guillain-Barré syndrome, cerebellar ataxia, osteomyelitis, arthritis, pancreatitis, nephritic syndrome, parotitis, orchitis, etc.

Differential Diagnosis

During the initial one week, typhoid fever needs to be differentiated from common febrile illness that present without localizing signs such as viral fever, malaria, and dengue fever. Once spleen appears, other differential diagnoses that need consideration include malaria, hepatitis, infectious mononucleosis, rickettsial disease, leptospirosis, and brucellosis. Undiagnosed enteric fever beyond 2 weeks will need to be differentiated from tuberculosis, leukemia, and collagen vascular diseases.

Laboratory Diagnosis

Hematology Blood counts usually show a normal or low normal leukocyte count. There is always a moderate neutropenia leading to relative lymphocytosis. Thrombocytopenia and proteinuria may be observed.

Blood culture remains the gold standard for diagnosis of typhoid fever. It is positive in more than 75% patients during the first week of illness. Bone marrow cultures are highly sensitive (90%) for diagnosis of typhoid fever. In some children with negative bone marrow cultures, duodenal string cultures have been positive. Stool and urine cultures may also reveal *Salmonella* after 2 weeks of the illness.

Serology The Widal agglutination test measures antibodies against the somatic (O) antigen, and the flagellar (H) antigens of salmonellae. These antibodies are usually detectable only by the end of first week of illness, and rise progressively during the course of illness. Widal test is said to be positive, if antibody titer to "O" antigen is >1:160 after 7 days of onset of illness; or it demonstrates a 4-fold rise between the paired sera, collected in the first week, and then at least 2 weeks later. Widal test is of no diagnostic utility on a single sample, if obtained in first week of illness or in areas of endemicity. The somatic antigen O is common for both typhi and paratyphi, while H antigen is specific for *S. Typhi, paratyphi* A, and *paratyphi* B.

Treatment	Typhoid Fever

A. General Supportive Therapy

General supportive measures like use of antipyretics, maintenance of hydration, appropriate nutrition and prompt recognition and treatment of complications are extremely important for a favorable outcome. The child should continue to have normal diet and no food should be restricted. In areas of endemic disease, 90% or more of typhoid cases can be managed at home with proper oral antibiotics and good nursing care. Close follow-up is necessary to look for development of complications or failure to respond to therapy.

Patients with persistent vomiting, inability to take oral feed, severe diarrhea and abdominal distension usually require parenteral antibiotic therapy preferably in a hospital.

B. Antimicrobial Therapy

Chloramphenicol (50–75 mg/kg/day in 4 divided doses given for 14–21 days) has been the standard treatment for enteric fever in children. Ampicillin (100–200 mg/kg/day in 4 divided doses), amoxicillin (100 mg/kg/day in 4 divided doses), cotrimoxazole (6–8 mg/kg of trimethoprim/day) and furazolidone (10 mg/kg/day), each given for 14 days have also been used with equivocal results. This therapy can still be used for uncomplicated typhoid fever sensitive to these drugs.

Since 1990, use of chloramphenicol has been associated with drug resistance, high relapse rate, high rate of continued and chronic carriage, bone marrow toxicity, and high mortality. This has resulted in the decreasing trends of its usage. At the same time, number of culture positive cases of typhoid fever resistant to multiple conventional anti-typhoid drugs are being reported with increasing frequency from all over the world.

Multidrug resistant *Salmonella typhi* (MDRST) refers to strains, resistant to all the 3 drugs in first line treatment, ie, chloramphenicol, ampicillin, and cotrimoxazole. Fluoroquinolones (ciprofloxacin, ofloxacin, gatifloxacin) emerged as effective drug for enteric fever caused by MDRST. The dosage is 20 mg/kg in two divided doses at 12 h interval orally or 10 mg/kg/day q 12 h IV. The temperature comes down in 4 to 5 (range of 3 to 10) days. Treatment should be continued for 7–10 days. Fluoroquinolones, such as ciprofloxacin, are effective but their frequent use in children is not yet cleared officially except when the benefits far exceed the possible risk to the growing cartilage.

However, many children with MDRST typhoid fever also fail to respond to quinolones, taking a very long time to attain defervescence, and continued constitutional discomfort. These cases show *in vitro* resistance to nalidixic acid. Nalidixic acid is also a quinolone. Though not used in treatment of enteric fever, resistance to nalidixic acid by *S. Typhi* is considered a surrogate marker of resistance to other quinolones that are used for treating enteric fever; eg, ciprofloxacin and ofloxacin. These strains are now known as nalidixic acid resistant *Salmonella Typhi* (NARST).

In children with quinolone and resistant *Salmonella typhi* infection, 3rd generation cephalosporins are the initial drug of choice. Of the oral third generation cephalosporins, cefixime and cefpodoxime proxetil are used. Of parenteral preparations—ceftriaxone, cefotaxime, and cefoperazone are used—ceftriaxone being the most convenient.

Current Guidelines

Uncomplicated typhoid fever Oral third generation cephalosporin; eg, cefixime (20 mg/kg/day × 10–14 days) should be the drug of choice as empiric therapy. If by 5 days, there is no clinical improvement and the culture report is inconclusive, add a second line drug; eg, azithromycin (8–10 mg/kg/day × 7 days).

Severe typhoid fever The drug of choice is parenteral third generation cephalosporin; eg, ceftriaxone 60–75 mg/kg/d for 10–14 days. Azithromycin 20 mg/kg/day for 7 days should be added, if there is no response in 5–7 days.

Steroids Corticosteroid therapy is indicated in children with altered mental state or shock. Dexamethasone in a dose of 3 mg/kg is administered stat followed by another 8 doses of 1 mg/kg at six hourly intervals. Prolonged therapy with steroids increases the relapse rate.

Prevention

Active Immunization

Two safe and efficacious typhoid vaccines, the injectable Vi polysaccharide and the oral Ty21a, had been licensed but the oral vaccine due to its own limitation has not been used widely in the developing countries and is not available in India. Currently, the new, improved typhoid conjugate vaccines are being tested and recently marketed in India.

The Vi vaccine does not elicit adequate immune responses in children aged below 2 years. Conjugate vaccines are available now for those below 2 years of age. Detailed discussion on typhoid vaccines is available in Chapter 5.

| Case Study | Typhoid Fever—Continuous fever of 1–2 weeks with abdominal symptoms and splenomegaly |

A 7-year-old boy was brought to the emergency room with continuous, high grade fever for 10 days. Mother also complained of lethargy and anorexia for last 5 days. This was associated with non-bilious and non-projectile vomiting for last two days. There was no history of dark yellow urine, rash, urinary complaints, abdominal distension, or any other localizing symptoms.

Outline the specific clues you will look for in the physical examination.
Our patient is a 7-year-boy with complaints of prolonged fever, lethargy, and vomiting, so we will first look for vitals (HR, RR, BP, CFT) degree of fever, consciousness level, any signs of dehydration, icterus, edema, lymphadenopathy, rash, and signs of raised intracranial pressure (ICP). We also need to examine the abdomen for any distension, hepatosplenomegaly or other intra-abdominal lump/mass, shifting dullness, and bowel sounds.

Examination revealed a normal built, toxic looking child, with temperature 104°F, RR — 28/min, HR — 98/min , BP — 98/64 mm Hg. The pulse volume was normal, and CFT was <3 seconds. There was no dehydration, icterus, edema, rash, lymphadenopathy, or signs of raised ICP. Abdomen was slightly distended. Liver was palpable 3 cm below right costal margin and spleen was palpable 2 cm below left costal margin. Both liver and spleen were soft and non-tender. Liver span was 9 cm. Bowel sounds were sluggish.

Summarize the case and discuss the differential diagnosis.
A 7-year-old boy presented with high grade fever for 10 days with vomiting, toxic appearance, lethargy, mild hepatosplenomegaly, and without any other systemic or neurological signs.
Differential diagnosis will include enteric fever, malaria, dengue fever, UTI, and viral hepatitis (anicteric).
- Fever of more than one week with vomiting, toxic look, lethargy, and mild hepatosplenomegaly is in favor of *enteric fever*.
- Prolonged fever, vomiting, toxic look, lethargy, mild hepatosplenomegaly can all be seen in *malaria*. However, continuous nature of fever is not that common in malaria.
- Absence of rash, edema, shock, and bleeding rules out *dengue fever* to some extent. In second week of illness, dengue fever either recovers or has lead to some complication.
- *Anicteric viral hepatitis* can present with fever, and lethargy. However, fever usually subsides in one week and spleen is generally not palpable. A non-tender liver does not favor viral hepatitis. Absence of urinary symptoms keeps possibility of *UTI* little lower but you should keep in mind that upper UTI can present with high grade fever and vomiting without any urinary symptoms. Hepatosplenomegaly in this child does not favor the diagnosis of UTI.
Other less common but important differential diagnoses are infectious mononucleosis, sepsis, leptospirosis, brucellosis, rickettsial diseases, and kala-azar (in endemic areas).

Outline the investigations needed to make a final diagnosis, in order of importance.
Initially we will order blood culture, widal test, peripheral smear for malarial parasite (PS-MP), rapid malarial antigen (RMA), complete blood counts, kidney and liver function tests, urine microscopy and culture, and abdominal ultrasonography.

Investigations revealed total leukocyte count of 4800 per mm^3, $N_{32} L_{60} E_2 M_6$, platelet count of 1.4 lakhs per mm^3, negative RMA and PS MP, widal agglutination test T_H 1:320 T_O 1:320. Urine albumin was 1+ and microscopy was WNL. Liver enzymes were not elevated. Blood culture results were not available in 48 hours. USG abdomen revealed a few mesenteric lymph nodes with largest measuring 7 mm (which can be normal). Liver and spleen echotexture was normal. A relative neutropenia and positive widal test suggest the diagnosis of enteric fever.

Outline the specific antibiotic therapy for this patient.
We can start with oral antibiotics, if the vomiting can be controlled with antiemetic. However, the child will need to be given intravenous antibiotics, if vomiting persists. Cefixime (15–20 mg/kg/d x 10 days) is the drug of choice for oral therapy. Ceftriaxone (75 –100 mg/kg/day divided in two equal doses for 10 days) is preferred for parenteral therapy.

After 4 days of treatment with IV ceftriaxone, patient was still febrile. Toxic look had disappeared, vitals were stable and vomiting had subsided. What will you do now?
In enteric fever, the fever usually takes 4–5 days to resolve. Our patient is showing signs of improvement (nontoxic look, no vomiting, vitals stable, return of appetite), thus we will continue same treatment. The second drug (azithromycin 20 mg/kg/d) will need to be added, only if the fever does not subside after completing 7 days of IV ceftriaxone. Also, by this time, blood culture and sensitivity report should be available that can guide further therapy.

Sanitation Measures

Typhoid fever cannot be controlled by immunization alone. The prime importance should be given to proper sanitation methods for food handling and preparation, safe water supply, proper sewage disposal, strict hand washing, and adequate maintenance of personal and food hygiene. It is important to make the community aware of the potential hazards of using contaminated food or water. Health education regarding importance of good hygiene should be imparted.

Arjyal A, Basnyat B, Koirala S, *et al*. Gatifloxacin versus chloramphenicol for uncomplicated enteric fever: an open-label, randomised, controlled trial. *Lancet Infect Dis*. 2011;11:445–54.

Effa EE, Lassi ZS, Critchley JA, *et al*. Fluoroquinolones for treating typhoid and paratyphoid fever (enteric fever).*Cochrane Database Syst Rev*. 2011;10:CD004530.

Fraser A, Goldberg E, Acosta CJ, *et al*. Vaccines for preventing typhoid fever. *Cochrane Database Syst Rev*. 2007;3:CD001261.

Ochiai RL, Acosta CJ, Danovaro-Holliday MC, *et al*; Domi Typhoid Study Group. A study of typhoid fever in five Asian countries: disease burden and implications for controls. *Bull World Health Organ*. 2008;86:260–8.

Typhoid Fever

1. Typhoid fever is a severe multisystemic infection caused by *Salmonella Typhi*. Similar illness can be caused by related but less virulent *Salmonella paratyphi* (paratyphoid fever).
2. Enteric fever is characterized in endemic areas by the classic prolonged high grade fever, sustained toxemia, gastrointestinal symptoms and splenomegaly.
3. Complications of typhoid are seen in 10–15% with intestinal perforation and bleeding being the most serious.
4. Blood is the gold standard for diagnosis. Widal test is positive from 2nd week onwards.
5. Third generation cephalosporins are the first-line treatment. Azithromycin can be added for non-responders (after a week).

Poulos C, Riewpaiboon A, Stewart JF, *et al*; DOMI Typhoid COI Study Group. Cost of illness due to typhoid fever in five Asian countries. *Trop Med Int Health*. 2011;16:314–23.

Thaver D, Zaidi AK, Critchley J, *et al*. A comparison of fluoro-quinolones versus other antibiotics for treating enteric fever: meta-analysis. *BMJ*. 2009;338:b1865.

Verma M, Parashar Y, Singh, *et al*. Current pattern of enteric fever: a prospective clinical and microbiological study. *J Indian Med Assoc*. 2007;105:582,584,586.

6.17 LEPTOSPIROSIS

Leptospirosis is a zoonosis caused by *Leptospira* species of organisms. Humans are accidental hosts and get infected from contaminated water. The route of entry is cuts and abrasions on the skin or mucous membrane. The clinical syndrome ranges from an asymptomatic infection to the severe icteric leptospirosis (Weil syndrome). It is seen in tropical and subtropical countries and the incidence increases during the monsoon season and after heavy rainfall.

Epidemiology

Leptospirosis has a world-wide distribution. However, it is more commonly reported from tropical and subtropical countries where the climate is warm and soil is moist. In the Indian subcontinent, incidence of leptospirosis is known to increase during the monsoon season and after heavy rainfall. Epidemics have been reported from the states of Gujarat, Karnataka, Maharashtra, Odisha, and Andaman and Nicobar islands. Leptospirosis is being increasingly reported from the low-lying slums of Mumbai city since the year 2000 because of frequent flooding of these areas during monsoon season and heavy rainfall. States have been classified as those with high prevalence, moderate prevalence, and low prevalence **(Table 6.19)**.

Etiology

Leptospira are aerobic spiral bacteria (spirochetes). *Leptospira interrogans* is the only pathogenic strain. More than 23 serogroups and as many as two hundred serovars have been identified—each of these is believed to cause a different clinical syndrome.

Leptospira remain viable in moist soil or water for weeks and months. This is the reason why even though leptospirosis has a world-wide distribution; it is more prevalent in regions with warm climate such as tropical and subtropical countries. During heavy rainfall, flooding occurs in low-lying areas where people are likely to come in contact with contaminated water—resulting in increased risk for infection with leptospira.

Rodents and rats (*R. norvegicus, Musculu*) are the chief reservoirs. Apart from these, cattle, buffaloes, sheep, goat, pigs, and dogs are also known to harbor the leptospira organisms.

Pathogenesis

Urine, amniotic fluid, placental tissue and other body fluids of infected animals are usually the source of infection. Humans are accidental host. People working as agricultural laborers, live-stock farmers, sugarcane field workers, sewer workers, and abattoir workers are at greater risk. Certain recreational activities like wading, swimming (especially being submerged in or swallowing contaminated water), and boating in contaminated water during flooding or heavy rainfall can also expose the individuals to infection from leptospira.

The leptospira gain entry to the blood through cuts and abrasions on the skin or mucous membrane. The organisms can enter the human body through direct contact with urine or infected tissue of animals. Indirect access can take place when contaminated food or milk of infected cows or goat is ingested or when air polluted with droplets of infected urine is inhaled. Rarely, bite from an infected animal can result in entry of the leptospira into human blood. Direct transmission from man-to-man is extremely rare because low pH of human urine deters the survival of leptospira.

Clinical Features

Incubation period It is usually 10 days (range 4–20 days).

As many as 90% cases of leptospirosis infection are self-limited. It has a typical biphasic presentation where the initial acute phase with septicemia lasts for a week during which leptospira can be isolated from the blood, urine, and other body fluids. This phase is followed by immune-mediated phase during which the organisms disappear from the bloodstream but the antibodies appear. Despite presence of

Table 6.19 Prevalence of Leptospirosis in Animal Reservoirs in India		
Prevalence	*State*	*Animal species*
High	Tamil Nadu, Kerala, Andaman	Cattle, buffalo, sheep, goats, pigs.
Moderate	Maharashtra, UP, MP, Gujarat, Karnataka	Cattle, buffalo, sheep, pigs, dogs, horses
Rarely reported	Punjab, J&K, Rajasthan, Northeast region, Himachal Pradesh	Cattle, sheep

*based on isolation and serology (Source WHO, 2006)

antibodies, leptospira can be found in urine and aqueous humor. At times, these two phases are separated by an interval of 3–4 days during which patient is afebrile. Usually, each of these phases lasts for a period of less than a week to several months.

About 10% of the patients develop a more severe form where jaundice develops followed by renal failure, hemorrhagic manifestations, pneumonitis, cardiac arrhythmias, and circulatory collapse. This form of the disease can be fatal. Usually, a serovar-specific immunity develops after an infection with leptospira.

The clinical syndrome of leptospirosis is divided into following two forms: Anicteric leptospirosis and icteric leptospirosis (Weil syndrome).

A. Anicteric Leptospirosis

The initial anicteric form is further categorized into (*a*) septicemic phase; and (*b*) immune-mediated phase.

- *Septicemic phase* It is characterized by abrupt onset of fever with chills, headache, malaise, nausea, vomiting, and debilitating myalgia. Bradycardia and hypotension can be observed at times but circulatory collapse is extremely rare. Myalgia is typically seen in extremities and lumbosacral spine. Conjunctival suffusion with photophobia not accompanied by chemosis or purulent exudates is a typical feature. Abdominal pain, hepatosplenomegaly, and generalized lymphadenopathy can be observed. Rash, seen in 10% of the cases, usually lasts for 24 hours. Mostly, it is a truncal, erythematous, and maculopapular. Rarely, rash can be urticarial, petechial, or purpuric. Uncommon manifestations include pneumonitis, arthritis, carditis, and orchitis.
- *Immune-mediated phase* Followed by a brief asymptomatic period, there is recurrence of fever, aseptic meningitis, and uveitis. Almost 80% of the affected children have an abnormal CSF profile but only 50% of them present with meningeal signs. Uveitis can be unilateral or bilateral. Most of these children recover spontaneously.

B. Icteric Leptospirosis (Weil Syndrome)

This is a more severe form of leptospirosis which affects adults more often than children. It is seen in about 10% of the total cases. Initial phase presents similar to anicteric form but the second phase is distinctive, characterized by multi-organ involvement. Hepatic and renal dysfunction associated with hemorrhagic phenomenon and circulatory collapse are the usual features. Hepatic dysfunction manifests as upper abdominal pain, hyperbilirubinemia (not due to hepatocellular necrosis), and elevated liver enzymes. Hemorrhagic phenomenon manifests as multiple episodes of epistaxis, hemoptysis, GI bleed, and adrenal hemorrhage. Cardiovascular collapse is a feature. EKG can be abnormal but congestive heart failure is rare. Thrombocytopenia is seen in 50% of the cases. Mortality in this form of leptospirosis is 5–15%.

5. Diagnosis

Serology is the most commonly used method for diagnosis. ELISA for specific IgM antibodies and IgM-specific Dot ELISA are recommended. A 2–4-fold rise in titer is suggestive of infection. However, these tests become positive after fifth day of onset of illness. Other diagnostic tests include slide agglutination, Dri-Dot assay, LEPTO Dipstick, latex agglutination, compliment fixation, IFA and hemagglutination. **Microscopic agglutination test (MAT)** is a reference method used for epidemiological research purposes. It is done by using antigen suspensions of servovars of leptospira.

Isolation of leptospira in Ellinghausen-McCullough-Johnson-Harris (EMJH) culture medium is limited to research laboratories. Demonstration of organisms in body fluids by phase-contrast or dark-field microscopy is also possible even though it is less sensitive.

Table 6.20 outlines the modified Faine's criteria for diagnosis of leptospirosis.

Table 6.20 The Modified Faine's Criteria for Diagnosis of Leptospirosis					
Clinical data (Part A)		*Epidemiological factors (Part B)*		*Bacteriological and laboratory findings (Part C)*	
Headache	2	Rainfall	5	Isolation of leptospira in culture-diagnosis certain	
Fever	2	Contact with contaminated environment	4	**Positive serology**	
Temperature >39°C	2	Animal contact	1	Elisa IgM positive*	15
Conjunctival suffusion	4	**Total**	**10**	SAT—Positive*	15
Meningism	4			MAT—Single high titer*	15
Muscle pain	4			MAT—Rising titer/ seroconversion (paired sera)	25
Conjunctival suffusion + meningism + muscle pain	10			**Total**	
Jaundice	1				
Albuminuria/nitrogen retention	2				
Total score					
		Presumptive diagnosis of leptospirosis is made of Part A or Part A and Part B score: 26 or more Parts A, B, C (Total): 25 or more A score between 20 and 25 suggests leptospirosis as a possible diagnosis			

Abbreviations: MAT, Microscopic agglutination test: SAT, Slide agglutination test
*Any one of the tests only should be scored

Treatment — Leptospirosis

Usually, leptospirosis responds to oral amoxicillin, azithromycin, cefixime, or doxycycline given for a week. Use of antibiotics before the seventh day of illness reduces the length of hospitalization period. Intravenous penicillin is reserved for very sick patients with meningitis, myocarditis, hemorrhagic manifestations, hepatic and renal dysfunction. Ceftriaxone and cefotaxime are other intravenous alternates.

Prevention and Control

Immunization of the animals can prevent the clinical manifestations than can be attributed to the infecting serovars contained in the vaccine. Reservoir control programs may be undertaken in endemic areas. Swimmers are advised not to immerse or swallow water while swimming in fresh-water bodies that are likely to be contaminated. Use of protective clothing, boots and gloves must be encouraged for those people whose occupation exposes them for infection from leptospira.

Prophylactic treatment with antibiotics can be considered for people at high risk for a brief period. Doxycycline 200 mg once a week is recommended for adults as prophylaxis. However, its use in children is not established.

Rodent control measures like food source removal, harborage removal, use of rodent traps and repellants and rodent baiting are recommended in areas endemic to leptospirosis.

Case Study | Leptospirosis

A 6-year-old boy is brought with history of fever, nausea, vomiting, headache, and bodyache for 5 days. He often gets wet in rain since the rainy season has commenced and frequently plays in ponds with friends. There is history of similar illness in neighborhood. On physical examination, he is febrile, has conjunctival suffusion, has excruciating calf tenderness, and meningismus.

What is the diagnosis?

The clinical findings of fever, conjunctival suffusion, calf tenderness and meningism are classical features of leptospirosis. The epidemiological setting also suggests leptospirosis.

Which test can be done to confirm the diagnosis?

ELISA for leptospira IgM is the appropriate test. This test becomes positive after fifth day of illness.

What are the possible complications, if not treated in time?

Weil syndrome is the severe form of leptospirosis. It is characterized by multiorgan involvement. Patients can have hemorrhagic phenomenon, circulatory collapse, hepatic dysfunction, and renal failure.

Abela-Ridder B, Sikkema R, Hartskeer lRA. Estimating the burden of human leptospirosis. *Int J Antimicrob Agents.* 2010;36Suppl 1:S5–7.

Brett-Major DM, Coldren R. Antibiotics for leptospirosis. *Cochrane Database Syst Rev.* 2012 Feb 15;2:CD008264.

Guerra MA. Leptospirosis: public health perspectives. *Biologicals.* 2013;41:295–7.

Haake DA, Levett PN. Leptospirosis in humans. *Curr Top Microbiol Immunol.* 2015;387:65–97.

Hartskeerl RA, Collares-Pereira M, Ellis WA. Emergence, control and re-emerging leptospirosis: dynamics of infection in the changing world. *Clin Microbiol Infect.* 2011;17:494–501.

Hotez PJ, Bottazzi ME, Strych U, *et al.* Neglected tropical diseases among the Association of Southeast Asian Nations (ASEAN): overview and update. *PLoS Negl Trop Dis.* 2015;9:e0003575.

Picardeau M, Bertherat E, Jancloes M, *et al.* Rapid tests for diagnosis of leptospirosis: current tools and emerging technologies. *Diagn Microbiol Infect Dis.* 2014;78:1–8.

Ricaldi JN, Swancutt MA, Matthias MA. Current trends in translational research in leptospirosis. *Curr Opin Infect Dis.* 2013;26:399–403.

Sakundarno M, Bertolatti D, Maycock B, *et al.* Risk factors for leptospirosis infection in humans and implications for public health intervention in Indonesia and the Asia-Pacific region. *Asia Pac J Public Health.* 2014;26:15–32.

Verma AK, Kumar A, Dhama K, *et al.* Leptospirosis-persistence of a dilemma: an overview with particular emphasis on trends and recent advances in vaccines and vaccination strategies. *Pak J Biol Sci.* 2012;15:954–63.

Wasiński B, Dutkiewicz J. Leptospirosis—current risk factors connected with human activity and the environment. *Ann Agric Environ Med.* 2013;20:239–44.

6.18 MALARIA

Malaria (*mal*–foul; *aria*–air) is one of the most important parasitic diseases of humans. It is associated with high morbidity and mortality, accounting for nearly 1.5 to 2.5 million deaths all over the world every year. More than half of these deaths occur in children under 5 years of age. In recent years, there has been a resurgence of malaria due to increasing drug resistance, environmental changes, population migration, and inconsistent national malaria control programs.

Etiology

Malaria is caused by *Plasmodium,* an obligate intracellular protozoon. Five species of *Plasmodium* are responsible for disease in humans:
- *P. falciparum*—malignant tertian malaria
- *P. vivax*—benign tertian malaria
- *P. ovale*—ovale malaria
- *P. malariae*—quartan malaria, and
- *P. knowlesi*—fifth human malaria parasite

P. falciparum accounts for nearly all deaths and severe disease due to malaria. In India, most cases of malaria are caused by *P.vivax* (60–65%) and *P. falciparum* (35–40%). *P. malariae* accounts for only 1% of cases, mainly from a few districts of Karnataka (Hasan and Tumkur). *P. ovale* is very occasionally reported. *P. knowlesi*, a causative agent of simian malaria, has been reported from forested areas of Southeast Asia. No case is yet reported from India.

Mode of Spread

Transmission Malaria is spread to humans during the bite of an infected female anopheline mosquito. Female mosquitoes require blood meal to produce eggs. Male mosquitoes do not suck blood but feed on plant juices. Rarely, malaria may be transmitted by blood transfusion, transplacentally (congenital malaria), or through contaminated needles.

Vector Malaria is spread from person-to-person by mosquitoes belonging to genus *Anopheles.* A. *culicifacies* and A. *stephensi* are important vectors in India. The former is more active in rural areas, and later in urban areas. *A. minimus* is an efficient vector in North-East India. Transmission of malaria is directly proportional to the density of the vector.

Environment The transmission of malaria is profoundly influenced by climate. Malaria is common during rainy season because stagnant water and high humidity favor mosquito breeding and survival. Edges of streams, water-tanks, pits, cisterns, and overhead tanks are favored breeding sites of the mosquito. Irrigation schemes, dams, deforestation, urbanization, floods and agricultural practices can influence mosquito populations and alter patterns of malaria transmission. Malaria is uncommon at altitudes 2000 m above sea-level.

Life Cycle of Malarial Parasite (Fig. 6.15)

Infection with malaria begins when *sporozoites*, the infective stage of the parasite, are inoculated into subcutaneous capillaries as female mosquito takes a blood meal. Sporozoites are carried rapidly via the bloodstream to the liver where they begin a period of asexual reproduction. Salient characteristics of malaria parasites are given in **Table 6.21**.

Pre-erythrocytic (exoerythrocytic) schizogony (hepatic or tissue phase). In liver cells, *sporozoites* multiply asexually over a period of 6–15 days to form thousands of merozoites in a *hepatic* or *tissue schizont*. The swollen hepatocyte finally ruptures, releasing *merozoites* into bloodstream. These merozoites invade erythrocytes but cannot reinfect hepatocytes or start a fresh cycle of pre-erythrocytic schizogony. This phase is asymptomatic.

In *P. vivax* and *P. ovale* infections, intrahepatic sporozoites do not develop immediately but remain dormant in liver for

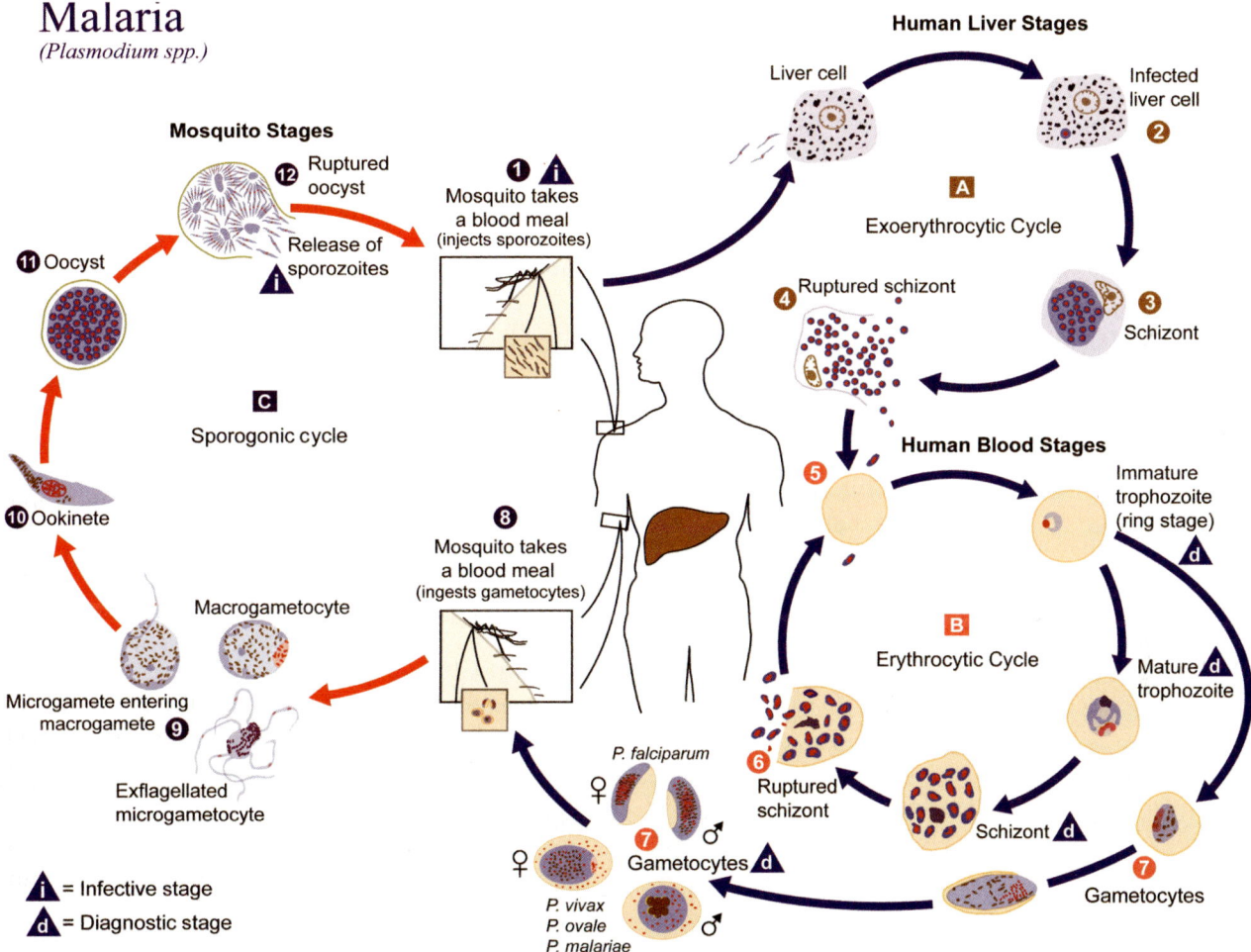

Fig. 6.15 Life cycle of malaria. The malaria parasite life cycle involves two hosts. During a blood meal, a malaria infected female *Anopheles* mosquito inoculates sporozoites into the human host (1). Sporozoites infect liver cells (2) and mature into schizonts (3), which rupture and release merozoites (4). (Of note, in *P. vivax* and *P. ovale*, a dormant stage (hypnozoites) can persist in the liver and cause relapses by invading the bloodstream weeks, or even years later.) After this initial replication in the liver (exoerythrocytic schizogony (A)), the parasites undergo asexual multiplication in the erythrocytes (erythrocytic schizogony (B)). Merozoites infect red blood cells (5). The ring stage trophozoites mature into schizonts, which rupture releasing merozoites (6). Some parasites differentiate into sexual erythrocytic stages (gametocytes) (7). Blood stage parasites are responsible for the clinical manifestations of the disease. The gametocytes, male (microgametocytes) and female (macrogametocytes), are ingested by an *Anopheles* mosquito during a blood meal (8). The parasites' multiplication in the mosquito is known as the sporogonic cycle (C). While in the mosquito's stomach, the microgametes penetrate the macrogametes generating zygotes (9). The zygotes in turn become motile and elongated (ookinetes) (10) which invade the midgut wall of the mosquito where they develop into oocysts (11). The oocysts grow, rupture, and release sporozoites (i), which make their way to the mosquito's salivary glands. Inoculation of the sporozoites (12) into a new human host perpetuates the malaria life cycle. (*Source: Public Image Health Library. CDC - DPDx/ Alexander J. da Silva, PhD, Melanie Moser*)

Table 6.21 Salient Characteristics of Malaria Parasites

Characteristic	P. falciparum	P. vivax	P. ovale	P. malariae
Exoerythrocytic cycle (days)	5.5	8	9	15
Erythrocytic cycle (hours)	48	48	48	72
No. of merozoites per hepatic schizont	40,000	10,000	15,000	2,000
Persistent exoerythrocytic cycle	No	Yes	Yes	No
Relapses	No	Yes	Yes	No
Recrudescence	Yes	Yes	Yes	Yes
Red cells parasitized	All	Reticulocytes	Reticulocytes	Old

a period ranging from weeks to years before reproduction begins. These "sleeping" forms, or *hypnozoites*, are responsible for **relapses** with these two species. Relapses can occur from *P. vivax* till 2–4 years. On the other hand, *P. falciparum* and *P. malariae* do not form hypnozoites in liver, and, therefore, relapses do not occur in infections with these species. However, **recrudescence** of infection can occur due to persistent erythrocytic forms. Recrudescence from *P. malariae* has been reported up to 5 years after the primary infection.

Erythrocytic schizogony Merozoites, released from ruptured hepatocyte, enter into the bloodstream and rapidly invade erythrocytes. Attachment is mediated by specific erythrocyte surface receptors, for example Duffy blood group antigen for *P. vivax* and glycophorins for *P. falciparum*. *P. vivax* and *P. ovale* primarily invade immature erythrocytes. *P. malariae* invades mature erythrocytes only, limiting parasitemia (number of infected erythrocytes) to less than 2%. In contrast, *P. falciparum* invades both mature and immature erythrocytes and parasitemia can be as high as 60%. Inside the red blood cells, malarial parasites are known as *trophozoites*. During early phase of development (<12 hours), the young trophozoites appear as *"ring forms"*. Approximately 36 hours after merozoite invasion, repeated nuclear division occurs (*merogony*) and erythrocyte bursts to release 6 to 32 daughter merozoites. These invade uninfected erythrocytes and cycle is repeated until it is contained by the host's immunity, antimalarial drugs, or a combination of both.

After a period of erythrocytic schizogony, some parasites differentiate into sexual forms known as *microgametocytes* (male) and *macrogametocytes* (female). These usually appear within 3 to 15 days of the onset of symptoms and are not associated with any illness. Further development of the parasite takes place in the mosquito.

Sexual development When a female mosquito takes a blood meal on an infected person, gametocytes are ingested which undergo further development in the stomach (midgut) of the mosquito (sporogony). The development of malarial parasite in mosquito culminates in the formation of sporozoites, the infected form which migrate to the salivary gland of the mosquito. The female mosquito is now infective and ready to transmit infection to humans at the next bite.

Clinical Correlates

Clinical manifestations of malaria are related to the red cell destruction and the host's response to this phenomenon. The periodicity of malarial paroxysm depends on the duration of erythrocytic cycle of the parasite. Paroxysms occur every 48 hours (*tertian*) in *P. vivax*, *P. ovale* and *P. falciparum* infections and every 72 hours (*quartan*) in *P. malariae* infection. Generally, it requires 5 to 7 days before a sufficient number of schizonts rupture at the same time and infection becomes synchronized. Therefore, malarial paroxysms are absent in the beginning of the disease. Often, in patients with asynchronous infections where more than one brood of parasites is developing in the blood at different times, periodicity is not found and fever may occur daily (quotidian). This is particularly true for *P. falciparum* infections where fever may never regularize to a tertian or subtertian (every 36 hours) pattern.

IMMUNE RESPONSE TO MALARIA PARASITE

Immune response in malaria is complex and not completely understood. Immunity against malaria develops gradually, is incomplete at best, and is not lifelong. Malarial parasite can elude host immune system by its ability to express antigens on the erythrocyte surface that change during the infection (*antigenic diversity*). This has also hampered the efforts to develop effective vaccine against malaria.

In endemic regions, newborns and young infants are protected against malaria by antibodies acquired transplacentally and through breastmilk, and high levels of fetal hemoglobin (HbF) which retards the development of the parasite.

Pathophysiology

The pathophysiology of malaria is complex and results from interaction between malarial parasite and human host. Only blood-stage parasites are involved in the pathogenesis and clinical manifestations of malaria; exoerythrocytic stages, gametocytes and sporozoites do not induce pathophysiological changes.

Cytokines In response to rupture of infected erythrocytes, proinflammatory cytokines like tumor necrosis factor (TNF) and interleukins (IL-1, IL-6, IL-8) are produced by the cells of macrophage-monocyte system. Cytokines are responsible for many clinical manifestations of malaria, particularly fever and malaise.

Cytoadherence, sequestration, and rosetting. These phenomena are essential to the pathogenesis of falciparum malaria.
• After 24 to 36 hours of merozoite invasion, infected erythrocytes become sticky and adhere to venular and

capillary endothelium. This is known as *cytoadherence*. The stickiness of erythrocytes is due to the appearance of knob-like projections consisting of histidine-rich protein (HRP).

- *Sequestration* refers to the disappearance of infected erythrocytes containing mature forms of *P. falciparum* from circulation. This is the reason why the mature forms of *P. falciparum* are rarely found in the peripheral blood and the degree of parasitemia may be greatly underestimated.
- Erythrocytes containing mature forms of *P. falciparum* also adhere to uninfected erythrocytes, a process known as *rosetting*. This is particularly prominent in cerebral malaria. Rosetting may promote cytoadherence by reducing blood flow.

The net effect of these events is impaired microcirculation and dysfunction of various organ systems.

CLINICAL FEATURES

The incubation period (time from sporozoite inoculation to the onset of fever) ranges from 9 to 40 days (shortest for *P. falciparum*, longest for *P. malariae*). It can be prolonged by partial immunity and chemoprophylaxis. The clinical features of malaria range from an asymptomatic infection to life-threatening illness. Manifestations are determined by the immune status of the host which, in turn, is determined by previous exposure to malaria.

- *In stable high transmission settings* where people are continuously exposed to a fairly constant rate of malarial inoculations and where inoculation rates are high, partial immunity to the clinical disease is acquired early in childhood. This situation prevails in much of sub-Saharan Africa and parts of Oceania. In such circumstances, severe malaria is confined to young children and becomes infrequent with increasing age.
- *With unstable malaria transmission pattern* which prevails in much of Asia and Latin America, the inoculation rates (number of bites by mosquitoes carrying infected sporozoites) fluctuate widely over seasons and years. This prevents development of immunity. In such situations, severe malaria can affect both children and adults.

A. Uncomplicated Malaria

It is defined as symptomatic infection without signs of severity and/or evidence of organ dysfunction (described under severe malaria). The clinical picture of uncomplicated malaria is common to all 4 species. It must be understood that there are no distinctive features of malaria in children. Fever may not follow any definite pattern and may be irregular, continuous, remittent, or intermittent in nature. Typical malarial paroxysms consisting of fever spikes, chills, and rigors occurring at regular intervals are uncommon, particularly in children below 5 years of age. The initial symptoms of malaria are nonspecific and similar to the symptoms of a viral illness. They include anorexia, malaise, irritability, headache, myalgia, and slight fever. As infection continues, the child may develop high fever, headache, vomiting, diarrhea, pallor with or without jaundice.

The classical malarial paroxysm, though uncommon in children, occurs more commonly with *P. vivax* and *P. ovale* infections than with other species, and consists of three successive stages, namely, the *cold stage*, the *hot stage* and the *sweating stage*. Cold stage is characterized by sudden rise of temperature; feeling of intense cold (*chills*) prompting the need for warmth or cover, and shivering with or without teeth chattering (*rigors*). There is peripheral vasoconstriction and gooseflesh. The rigors usually last 10 to 30 minutes but may last up to 90 minutes. The hot stage follows—the patient feels hot and fever becomes high grade. There is severe headache, myalgia, vomiting, tachypnea, palpitation, delirium and prostration. The hot stage lasts 2–6 hours. It is followed by the sweating stage, which is characterized by drenching sweats and rapid fall in temperature. Defervescence usually takes 2–3 hours. The entire paroxysm may last 8 to 12 hours. In between paroxysms, the patient appears well.

There are a few findings in uncomplicated malaria. Spleen becomes palpable towards the end of first week of illness; it is soft and occasionally tender. The liver may be enlarged, soft and sometimes tender. There may be anemia and slight jaundice. Absence of lymphadenopathy and skin rash are useful negative findings in malaria. Without effective treatment for *P. falciparum,* severe malaria may develop rapidly.

B. Severe Malaria

It is defined as acute malaria with signs of severity and/or evidence of vital organ dysfunction. Almost all severe morbidity and mortality in malaria are caused by *P. falciparum.* The high virulence of *P. falciparum* is attributed to its tendency to produce high parasitemia, cytoadherence, sequestration, and rosetting capacity, and antimalarial drug resistance.

Severe malaria is defined as occurrence of one or more of the following in the presence of *P. falciparum* asexual parasitemia. The features include (*i*) impaired consciousness, (*ii*) prostration; (*iii*) severe anemia (hemoglobin <5 g/dL or hematocrit <15%), (*iv*) acute renal failure, (*v*) jaundice, (*vi*) hypoglycemia (blood glucose <40 mg/dL), (*vii*) shock, (*viii*) disseminated intravascular coagulation, (*ix*) repeated convulsions (>2 episodes a day), (*x*) acidemia, (*xi*) pulmonary edema, and (*xii*) hyperparasitemia (>10%). Untreated severe malaria is almost always fatal. Even with treatment, the mortality remains unacceptably high (15–20%).

Although *P. vivax* is known to be a benign malaria, rarely it can cause severe disease with life-threatening end-organ involvement, similar to *P. falciparum* malaria.

1. Cerebral Malaria

This is the most dreaded complication of *P. falciparum* infection. Very rarely, *P. vivax* infection can also cause cerebral malaria.

Clinical manifestations The onset is generally sudden but may be gradual. The child has high fever for a few days followed by coma and seizures. There may be pallor, jaundice, or splenomegaly. However, their absence does not exclude cerebral malaria.

Cerebral malaria is a diffuse, symmetric encephalopathy. Focal signs are rare. Neurological signs are variable and include deep coma (Glasgow Coma Scale <11), variable muscle tone and tendon reflexes, absent abdominal reflexes, upgoing plantar in half the patients, opisthotonus, and decerebrate or decorticate posturing. Meningeal signs and cranial nerve abnormalities are absent. Papilledema is rare but retinal hemorrhages are found in 15% of cases. Disconjugate gaze is common.

Pathology Cerebral malaria is characterized by blockage of capillaries and venules with erythrocytes containing *P. falciparum*. Cerebral edema does not occur in cerebral malaria and anti-edema agents like mannitol and steroids are not useful in this condition. The exact cause of coma is not clear. It may be related to cytokine-induced production of nitric oxide, which is a potent inhibitor of neurotransmission. Cerebrospinal fluid is generally normal. Some patients may have slight pleocytosis and moderate elevation of protein while glucose remains normal.

Prognosis Untreated cerebral malaria is fatal. With appropriate therapy, the mortality rate is 15% in children, 20% in adults and up to 50% in pregnant women. Recovery is fast and generally complete. Most children regain consciousness within 24–48 hours. Neurological sequels in the form of hemiparesis, ataxia, cortical blindness, mental retardation and aphasia are seen more in children (10%) than in adults (3%).

2. Anemia

Life-threatening anemia can develop rapidly in malaria. It may lead to high output cardiac failure and sudden death. Anemia in malaria is more severe than expected from the destruction of parasitized erythrocytes. Other contributing mechanisms include destruction of unparasitized erythrocytes by immune mechanisms, dyserythropoiesis, increased splenic clearance of parasitized as well as unparasitized erythrocytes, and hemolysis associated with blackwater fever. At times, malarial anemia is superimposed on pre-existing nutritional anemia. Anemia is normocytic, normochromic, and reticulocyte count is low or normal.

3. Blackwater Fever

This is characterized by sudden and massive, intravascular hemolysis and the passage of 'coca-cola' colored urine due to hemoglobinuria. In severe cases, renal failure may develop. Blackwater urine can occur in three situations: (*i*) when G-6-PD deficient patients are given oxidant drugs regardless of whether they have malaria or not; (*ii*) when patients of G-6-PD deficiency develop malaria and receive quinine; and (*iii*) when patients with normal G-6-PD levels receive quinine. The mechanism of quinine-induced hemolysis is not known as it is not an oxidant drug. Probably hypersensitivity to quinine is responsible for hemolysis.

4. Hypoglycemia

It is the most common biochemical abnormality in severe malaria, observed in 30% of children with cerebral malaria. Factors responsible for hypoglycemia include cytokine-induced suppression of gluconeogenesis and increased glucose consumption caused by fever, anaerobic glycolysis, infection, and malarial parasites. This is further aggravated by quinine-stimulated pancreatic insulin secretion. Pregnant women appear to be especially susceptible to quinine-induced hypoglycemia. It is not possible to detect hypoglycemia clinically as the manifestations are indistinguishable from severe malaria. Therefore, frequent blood glucose monitoring is recommended in sick children. Quinine-stimulated hypoglycemia can be prevented by giving quinine infusion slowly over 4 hours in 5% or 10% dextrose solutions.

5. Algid Malaria

Majority of patients with severe malaria remain well perfused and warm, but some develop shock with cold extremities. This is known as algid malaria (*algid*—cold). This may result from secondary Gram-negative bacteremia and hypovolemia (dehydration and, rarely hemorrhage). Patients with severe malaria are vulnerable to bacterial infections due to transient immunosuppression.

6. Other Features

Renal failure, pulmonary edema, jaundice, DIC and metabolic acidosis are other important manifestations of severe malaria. Renal failure is caused by acute tubular necrosis following obstruction of renal microvasculature by sequestrated erythrocytes. Glomerulonephritis is very rare. Pulmonary edema occurs due to increased pulmonary capillary permeability, a finding not observed in others vascular beds. It is sometimes precipitated by excessive parenteral fluid therapy. Jaundice occurs due to hemolysis, hepatic dysfunction, and cholestasis. Frank hepatic failure suggests concomitant viral hepatitis or another diagnosis. DIC is caused by the activation of coagulation cascade by the parasitized erythrocytes and cytokines. Metabolic acidosis is attributed to anaerobic glycolysis, failure of liver and kidney to clear lactate, and lactate production by the parasite.

C. Congenital Malaria

Congenital malaria can be caused by the first four species of malaria parasite. It usually occurs in a non-immune mother. Symptomatic congenital malaria is rare in areas with stable malaria transmission pattern, probably due to transplacental transfer of protective maternal IgG antibodies. In endemic areas, it is an important cause of abortion, stillbirths, premature births and intrauterine growth restriction. Placenta may be black in color due to malaria pigment and parasites may be seen in tissue sections, although the maternal blood smear may be negative. Maternal treatment is inadequate to cure the fetus. The incubation period ranges from 2 to 8 weeks. Clinical manifestations include fever, irritability, failure to thrive, pallor, jaundice, and hepatosplenomegaly. Because there are no exoerythrocytic stages in congenital *P. vivax* and *P. ovale* infections, radical cure with primaquine is not required.

D. Chronic Complications of Malaria

Repeated malarial infections can cause chronic complications like tropical splenomegaly syndrome, nephrotic syndrome (*P. malariae*), endemic Burkitt's lymphoma, and endomyocardial fibrosis.

Tropical splenomegaly syndrome. It is also known as hyper-reactive malarial splenomegaly. It is considered to be an aberrant immunological response to repeated malarial infection. All the four species of *Plasmodium* can be associated with this condition. Constant stimulation of the reticuloendothelial system by circulating antigen–antibody complexes results in the enlargement of liver and spleen.

The essential features are residence in a malaria endemic area, massive splenomegaly, mild to moderate hepatomegaly, elevated serum IgG and IgM malarial antibody levels, and hepatic sinusoidal lymphocytosis with Kupffer cell hyperplasia. There may be anemia, leucopenia, and thrombocytopenia. Low grade fever may be present. Most children have growth retardation. Parasites are absent in the peripheral blood. Therapy consists of prolonged antimalarial chemoprophylaxis (chloroquin and/or proguanil) for at least one year. Chemoprophylaxis acts by removing the antigenic stimulus from repeated malarial infections, thus permitting the patient's immune system to return to normal. Response is generally seen within 3 months. There is no role of splenectomy.

E. Relapse and Recrudescence

Relapse results from persistence of parasites (hypnozoites) in the liver and their subsequent release into circulation. Only *P. vivax* and *P. ovale* produce hypnozoites and thus are capable of relapsing. Relapse occurs in approximately half of those infected in Southeast Asia; the frequency is lower in Indian subcontinent (15–20%) and may occur as long as 5 years after initial infection.

Relapses are not seen in *P. falciparum* and *P. malariae* infections as there is no persistent exoerythrocytic stage (hypnozoites) in these infections. However, they may give rise to repeated episodes of parasitemia called recrudescence; either by long-term persistence of erythrocytic stages (eg, within a sequestration site) or the continuation of erythrocytic schizogony at low levels for a prolonged period. Recrudescence can also occur following *P.vivax* and *P.ovale* infections. The main importance of differentiating relapse from recrudescence is that, whereas recrudescence is amenable to standard chemotherapy, relapse requires a specific treatment with primaquine (*radical cure*) to eradicate the infection.

LABORATORY DIAGNOSIS

The diagnosis of malaria is based on clinical criteria (clinical diagnosis) supplemented by the detection of parasites in the blood (parasitological or confirmatory diagnosis). Clinical diagnosis alone has very low specificity and in many areas parasitological diagnosis is not currently available. The decision to provide antimalarial treatment in these settings must be based on the prior probability of the illness being malaria. One needs to weigh the risk of withholding antimalarial treatment from a patient with malaria against the risk associated with antimalarial treatment when given to a patient who does not have malaria.

A. Parasitological Diagnosis

1. Peripheral Blood Smear

This is the gold standard for making the diagnosis of malaria. Both thick and thin smears should be prepared. Thick smear is used for the parasite detection while thin smear is used for species identification. Thick film is 20–40 times more sensitive than thin film as it contains more blood. Thick film can detect as little as 0.001% parasitemia (~50 parasites/μL) and is the only way to quantitate parasitemia. The timing of blood smears with fever spikes is less important than repeating it 2–3 times a day for making a diagnosis. It should be kept in mind that a single negative smear does not exclude malaria and repeated smears should be obtained in a strongly suspected case. The main problem with microscopic diagnosis is that it is time consuming and requires a skilled person.

P. falciparum can be recognized in peripheral smear by ring forms and crescent-shaped gametocytes, intense parasitemia (≥2%), and multiple infection in a single erythrocyte. Other species of parasite have all stages in peripheral blood. Even in the absence of parasitemia the diagnosis of acute malaria can be suspected by, the presence of malaria pigment (*hemozoin*) in monocytes or neutrophils.

Alternate diagnostic methods are used, if the laboratory does not have sufficient expertise in detecting malarial parasite in the peripheral blood smear.

2. Rapid Diagnostic Tests (RDTs)

These are immunochromatographic tests that detect parasite-specific antigens in a blood sample. RDTs are available in different formats such as dipsticks, cassettes or cards in which a colored line shows that plasmodial antigens have been detected. RDTs are simple to perform and interpret, and do not require electricity, special equipment or skilled personnel. Current tests are based on the detection of histidine-rich protein 2 (HRP2), which is specific for *P. falciparum*, pan-specific or species-specific parasite lactate-dehydrogenase (pLDH) [eg, OptiMal], or other pan-specific antigens such as aldolase. With the different tests that are currently available, the procedure may involve 2 to 6 steps and take 5 to 30 minutes. National Vector-borne Disease Control Program supplies RDT kits for detection of *P. falciparum* in areas where microscopy is not feasible within 24 hours of sample collection.

High temperature and humidity in the field settings may affect test performance leading to unpredictable sensitivity. Sensitivity for *P. falciparum* ranges from comparable to good microscopy (>90% at 100–500 parasites/μL of blood) to very poor (40–50%). Sensitivity is generally lower for other species particularly at parasite densities <500/μL. Therefore, negative RDT should not preclude treatment in a strongly suspected case, especially in severe clinical disease. One drawback of this method is that HRP2 antigen levels remain elevated for weeks after parasite clearance, thus giving false-positive results. Further, RDTs do not quantitate *P. falciparum* parasitemia.

3. Other Methods

Quantitative buffy coat (QBC) method Unlike mature erythrocytes, malarial parasites contain DNA that can be stained with acridine orange and easily visualized by fluorescence microscopy. This method is faster and more sensitive than routine microscopy but species identification is less accurate.

Polymerase chain reaction Although the test is sensitive and specific, it has limited utility due to non-availability in most places. It has the potential to identify genes which confer drug resistance.

6

Serology Antimalarial antibodies are of little diagnostic help in endemic areas since their levels remain elevated for months to years after an attack.

Histidine-rich protein 2 of P. falciparum (PfHRP2) is a water-soluble protein that is produced by the asexual stages and gametocytes of *P. falciparum,* expressed on the red cell membrane surface, and shown to remain in the blood for at least 28 days after the initiation of antimalarial therapy. Several RDTs targeting PfHRP2 have been developed.

Plasmodium aldolase is an enzyme of the parasite glycolytic pathway expressed by the blood stages of *P. falciparum* as well as the non-falciparum malaria parasites. Monoclonal antibodies against *Plasmodium* aldolase are pan-specific in their reaction and have been used in a combined 'P.f/P.v' immunochromatographic test that targets the pan-malarial antigen (PMA) along with PfHRP2.

Parasite lactate dehydrogenase (pLDH) is a soluble glycolytic enzyme produced by the asexual and sexual stages of the live parasites and it is present in and released from the parasite-infected erythrocytes. It has been found in all 4 human malaria species, and different isomers of pLDH for each of the 4 species exist. With pLDH as the target, a quantitative immunocapture assay, a qualitative immuno-chromatographic dipstick assay using monoclonal antibodies, an immunodot assay, and a dipstick assay using polyclonal antibodies have been developed.

B. The Choice between RDT and Microscopy

The choice between RDTs and microscopy depends on local circumstances, including the skills available, the usefulness of microscopy for other diseases found in the area, and the case-load. Where the case-load of fever patients is high, microscopy is likely to be less expensive than RDTs. Microscopy has further advantages in that it can be used for speciation and quantification of parasites, and identification of other causes of fever. However, in places where most malaria patients are treated outside the health services, for example, in the home or by private providers; microscopy is generally not feasible in such circumstances, but RDTs may be. The following conclusions and recommendations are based on evidence summarized by recent WHO consultations.

- In *areas of low to moderate transmission*, prompt parasitological confirmation of the diagnosis is recommended before treatment is started. This should be achieved through microscopy or, where not available, RDTs.

- In *areas of high stable malaria transmission*, the prior probability of fever in a child being caused by malaria is high. Children under 5 years of age should, therefore, be treated on the basis of a clinical diagnosis of malaria. In older children and adults including in pregnant women, a parasitological diagnosis is recommended before treatment is started.

- In *all suspected cases of severe malaria*, a parasitological confirmation of the diagnosis of malaria is recommended. In the absence of or a delay in obtaining parasitological diagnosis, patients should be treated for severe malaria, on clinical grounds.

Treatment	**Malaria**

Early diagnosis and treatment of cases of malaria aims at:
  i. Complete cure;
 ii. Prevention of progression of uncomplicated malaria to severe disease;
iii. Prevention of deaths;
 iv. Interruption of transmission; and
  v. Minimizing risk of selection and spread of drug resistant parasites.

Antimalarial drugs

There are 2 broad categories of antimalarials:

- *Schizonticidal drugs* are used for clinical and parasitological cure. These are chloroquine, amodiaquin, quinine, quinidine, pyremethamine, proguanil, sulfadoxine and pyremethamine, mefloquine, halofantrine, and artemisinine.

- *Gametocidal drugs* act on hypnozoites and gametocytes, and prevent relapses. These include primaquine and 8-amodiaquins.

In the past, chloroquine was effective in nearly all cases of malaria. Emergence of chloroquine-resistant species has now necessitated the use of alternate drugs.

A. Newer Antimalarial Drugs

Artemisinin derivatives Artemisinin or *quinghaosu* (pronounced as 'ching-how-soo') is extracted from the leaves of the Chinese herb *Artemisia annua*. The drug acts on late stage ring parasites and trophozoites. Artesunate, artemether and artemotil (arteether) are the available derivatives. They clear parasitemia more rapidly than any other antimalarial drug, and are remarkably well tolerated. The only significant adverse effect is type I hypersensitivity reactions manifesting as urticaria. These drugs also reduce the gametocytes carriage and thus the transmissibility of malaria. However, their use may be associated with a high recrudescence rate (10%) after monotherapy, so they are usually combined with other antimalarials for clinical treatment. Also monotherapy is discouraged to protect them from resistance. Artesunate has better pharmacokinetic properties than other artemisinin derivatives as it is water soluble and can be given by IV or IM route. Studies in children demonstrate equal efficacy of quinine, artesunate and artemether. Artemether is administered IM as it is formulated in oil, and may have erratic absorption in severely ill patients. Unlike quinine, artemisinin derivatives do not need dosage adjustment in renal or hepatic impairment or produce hypoglycemia. Artesunate solution should be prepared freshly for each administration and should not be stored. Dose-dependent neurotoxicity affecting brainstem nuclei in animals has not been observed in humans.

Mefloquine It is used for the treatment of uncomplicated chloroquine-resistant malaria. Mefloquine should not be used as a monotherapy for the treatment of severe malaria. For the treatment of falciparum infection, mefloquine in combination with artemisinin derivatives is used in a dose of 25 mg/kg. For *P. vivax* malaria, the dose is 15 mg/kg stat. The elimination half-life is 14 to 28 days. It destroys early trophozoites. Only oral formulation is available. Gastrointestinal side effects-like nausea and vomiting occur in 10 to 15% of patients. The dose should be repeated, if the patient vomits within one hour. Less frequent side effects include nightmares, ataxia, suicidal tendencies, anxiety neurosis, hallucinations, psychosis, seizures, and altered

Table 6.22 Antimalarial Chemotherapy for Uncomplicated Malaria
A. ***Chloroquine-sensitive malaria*** *   Chloroquine 10 mg/kg on first and second day and 5 mg/kg on third day. Repeat the dose if child vomits within 30 minutes.

B. ***Chloroquine-resistant malaria*** * (mostly *P. falciparum*, rarely *P. vivax*)
   1. *First-line antimalarial combinations (3-day regimen)*
      Artemisinin combination therapy (ACT)
     i. Artemether-lumefantrine (most preferred)
       OR
     ii. Artesunate + mefloquine
       OR
     iii. Artesunate + amodiaquine
       OR
     iv. Artesunate + sulfadoxine -pyrimethamine (not preferred due to increasing resistance to S-P)
   2. *Second-line antimalarial combinations* (to be used when first-line antimalarial combinations fail) (7-day regimen)
     i. Artesunate + clindamycin or doxycycline or tetracycline
         OR
     ii. Quinine + clindamycin or doxycycline or tetracycline
   3. *Single drug treatment* (unsuitable for *P. falciparum*; may consider for *P. vivax*)
     i. Mefloquine 15 mg base/kg as a single dose
         OR
     ii. Quinine 10 mg salt/kg three times a day for 7 days
         OR
     iii. Sulfadoxine –pyrimethamine as a single dose (no longer recommended)

* To achieve radical cure in P. vivax malaria, primaquine should be given 0.25 mg base/kg, once a day for 14 days in low malaria-transmission regions after excluding G6PD deficiency. For falciparum malaria, a single dose of primaquine (0.75 mg/kg) is given for gametocidal action.

sensorium. Splitting the 25 mg/kg dose into two parts (15 mg and 10 mg/kg) and giving at an interval of 6–24 hours increases absorption and improves tolerability. The drug is not recommended for persons involved with activity requiring fine coordination and special performance (eg, airplane crews, operators of dangerous equipment).

B. Treating Uncomplicated Malaria
Children with uncomplicated malaria are treated with oral drugs (**Table 6.22**). Parasitological confirmation of diagnosis, either by light microscopy or rapid diagnostic tests, is required before starting treatment in uncomplicated malaria. Chloroquine remains the drug of choice in sensitive regions. WHO recommends combinations of antimalarials for the treatment of uncomplicated falciparum malaria acquired in chloroquine-resistant regions. In India, resistance to chloroquine has been reported from all regions.

Artemisinin combination therapy (ACT)
Antimalarial combination therapy refers to the simultaneous use of two or more blood schizonticidal drugs with independent modes of action. The purpose of combination therapy is to improve therapeutic efficacy and to delay the emergence of resistance to single antimalarial drugs. When one of the partner drugs is the artemisinin derivative it is known as *artemisinin combination therapy (ACT)*.

Artemisinin derivatives are effective against all antimalarial parasites. In mixed malarial infections, ACTs are also the treatment of choice. The duration of artemisinin therapy is variable depending on whether the partner drug is rapidly or slowly eliminated. When used in combination with rapidly eliminated drugs (tetracycline, doxycycline, clindamycin) artemisinin compounds are given for 7 days but when given in

combination with slowly eliminated drugs (lumefantrine, mefloquine, amodiaquine, sulfadoxine-pyrimethamine), a 3-day course suffices. Artemether-lumefantrine (AL) is available as co-formulated tablets and suspension. It should be emphasized that AL should be taken with milk or fatty meal to increase absorption from gut. Inadequate fat intake may cause low blood levels, with resultant treatment failure.

In 3-day course, the dose of artesunate is 4 mg/kg once a day. In 7-day course, the dose is 2 mg/kg once a day. The dosing schedules of artemether-lumefantrine and artesunate-mefloquine are given in **Tables 6.23** and **6.24**, respectively.

Table 6.23 Dosing Schedule for Artemether-Lumefantrine							
Weight (kg)	*Age (years)*	Dose of artemether(mg) and timing					
		0 hr	*8 hr*	*24 hr*	*36 hr*	*48 hr*	*60 hr*
5–14	<3	20	20	20	20	20	20
15–24	3–8	40	40	40	40	40	40
25–34	9–14	60	60	60	60	60	60
>34	>14	80	80	80	80	80	80

Table 6.24 Dosing Schedule for Artesunate + Mefloquine						
Age	*Dose in mg (no. of tablets)*					
	Artesunate (50 mg)			*Mefloquine (250 mg)*		
	Day 1	*Day 2*	*Day 3*	*Day 1*	*Day 2*	*Day 3*
5–11 mo	25 (1/2)	25	25	–	125 (1/2)	
1–6 yrs	50 (1)	50	50	–	250 (1)	
7–13 yrs	100 (2)	100	100	–	500 (2)	250 (1)
>13 yrs	200 (4)	200	200	–	1000 (4)	500 (2)

6

Table 6.25 Antimalarial Chemotherapy for Severe Malaria
1. Artesunate* weight >20 kg: 2.4 mg/kg IV or IM on admission (0 hour), then at 12 hours, 24 hours, and then once daily for 6 days (total 7 d)   Weight <20 kg: 3.0 mg/kg   OR
2. Artemether* 3.2 mg/kg IM on admission followed by 1.6 mg/kg IM daily for 6 days (total 7 d)   OR
3. Quinine 20 mg salt/kg (loading dose)** diluted in 10 mL/kg of 5–10% dextrose IV over 4 hours, followed 8 hours after starting the loading dose with 10 mg salt/kg (maintenance dose)*** over 4 hours 8 hourly, until the child can swallow oral quinine*** 10 mg/kg three times daily to complete 7 days of treatment

*   *Following initial improvement when patient starts taking orally, add doxycycline 3.5 mg/kg once a day for 7 days except for children below 8 years where add clindamycin 10 mg/kg 2 times a day for 7 days.*

** *Loading dose should be omitted, if the patient has received quinine or mefloquine in last 24 hours.*

****If parenteral therapy is needed for more than 48 hours-reduce the maintenance dose of quinine by one-half to one-third (5–7 mg salt/kg/dose) to avoid accumulation.*

C. Treatment of Severe Malaria

Severe malaria is a medical emergency and is treated with parenteral drugs (**Table 6.25**). Delay in treatment raises mortality significantly. Therefore, when faced with a critically sick child having an illness compatible with severe malaria and no alternative diagnosis, antimalarial treatment must be started even before the diagnosis is confirmed. It is important to remember that a single negative smear or a negative RDT does not exclude malaria.

Artemisinin derivatives and quinine are the mainstay of treatment because of their activity against chloroquine-resistant *P. falciparum*. Recently, artemisinin derivatives are being used increasingly due to reported resistance to quinine. Artemisinin derivatives are easier to administer and are marginally superior to quinine in reducing mortality in severe malaria only in areas where there is quinine resistance as seen in various clinical trials. Death from severe malaria often occurs within hours of admission to hospital, and so it is essential that therapeutic concentrations of antimalarials are achieved as soon as possible.

With loading dose of quinine, effective blood levels are attained by the end of 4-hour infusion. Without loading dose, therapeutic levels may not be reached in the first 12 hours of therapy, an unacceptable delay in the treatment of severe malaria. Quinine may be given intramuscularly (IM), if intravenous infusion is not possible. For IM administration, quinine should be diluted with normal saline to concentrations of 60–100 mg/ml, and first dose should be split 10 mg/kg to each thigh. Therapeutic drug levels are similar for both routes of administration. However, IV route is preferred as quinine IM may be erratically absorbed in severe malaria particularly in patients with shock. Quinine should be given slowly by infusion and never by IV bolus injection as lethal hypotension may occur. Following initial parenteral treatment, once the patient starts accepting orally, the same drug (quinine or artesunate or artemether) is continued orally to complete a full 7-day course of treatment. In addition, the patient is also given doxycycline or clindamycin for 7 days. Recently, artemisinin combination therapy (ACT), artesunate plus amodiaquine or artemether plus lumefantrine, has also been proposed following parenteral treatment.

D. Supportive Therapy

Fluid and electrolyte requirements should be individualized. Dehydration and shock should be corrected. Septicemia may complicate severe malaria in children. Therefore, cover these children with broad-spectrum antibiotic, such as ceftriaxone after taking blood culture. Avoid overhydration as it may precipitate pulmonary edema. In cerebral malaria, the fluids should be restricted to two-thirds of usual maintenance requirements. Packed red cells are transfused for severe anemia. Fever is controlled by paracetamol and tepid sponging. Acid-base disturbances should be corrected. Blood sugar should be checked 3 or 4 times or day to detect hypoglycemia. Exchange transfusion may be beneficial, if parasitemia exceeds 5%. Renal failure is managed appropriately. Seizures are controlled with diazepam and phenobarbitone or phenytoin. Prophylactic anticonvulsants are not recommended. There is no role of steroids, heparin, low molecular weight dextrans, prostacycline, deferoxamine, pentoxyfylline, and anti-TNF-α monoclonal antibodies in the treatment of cerebral malaria. The role of mannitol in cerebral malaria is uncertain. Some authorities advocate mannitol, only if there is definite evidence of raised intracranial pressure such as strongly positive Macewan sign, unequal pupils, papilledema and deepening coma. With appropriate therapy, patients show signs of clinical and laboratory improvement within 48–72 hours.

Treatment of Relapse and Recrudescence

Relapsing malaria (*P. vivax* and *P. ovale*) is treated with a standard course of chloroquine or ACT (outlined under uncomplicated malaria) followed by primaquine 0.25 mg/kg orally per day for 14 days (radical cure). Primaquine should be taken with food to minimize abdominal discomfort. G-6-PD screening test should be performed before starting this drug. In severe G-6-PD deficiency, primaquine should not be given as it can lead to severe hemolysis. In mild to moderate G-6-PD deficiency, primaquine 0.75 mg/kg once a week for 8 weeks can be given with a minimal risk of hemolysis. *P. vivax* and *P. ovale* infections acquired congenitally or through blood transfusion do not produce relapses as they lack exoerythrocytic (hepatic) cycle. In high transmission settings, radical cure is generally considered unnecessary as the risk of reinfection is high.

Treatment Failure

It is defined as failure of fever and parasitemia to resolve or recur during a follow-up period of ≥28 days. Failure to respond within 3 days is referred to as *early treatment failure* and that between 4 and 28 days as *late treatment failure*. The treatment failure could be clinical or based on non-resolution of parasitemia. Absence of parasitemia on day 28 is labeled as *adequate clinical and parasitological response* (ACPR).

It is important to know that although drug resistance may lead to treatment failure, not all treatment failures are caused by drug resistance.

Treatment failure can also occur due to incorrect dosing, poor compliance, poor drug quality, incorrect drug administration in the home and reduced drug absorption due to individual variation in bioavailability. In a clinically suspected case, it should be confirmed by blood smear examination.

- HRP2-based tests should not be used to document treatment failure as they remain positive for weeks even after effective therapy.

- In falciparum malaria, treatment failure within 2 weeks of receiving a therapy is due to recrudescence and should be treated with a second-line antimalarials. Failure after 2 weeks could be due to recrudescence or new infection, and can be retreated with the first-line ACT. However, mefloquine should not be reused within 28 days of first treatment due to higher risk of neuropsychiatric disturbances (seizures, encephalopathy, psychosis).

- In *P. vivax* malaria, treatment failure within 16 days of starting treatment of the primary infection suggests recrudescence due to chloroquine-resistant parasites. Treatment failure between days 17 and 28 may be either a

---

| Case Study | **Malaria—Intermittent Fever of Short Duration (less than 1 week) with Splenomegaly** |

A 7-year-old girl presented with intermittent high grade fever accompanied with chills and rigors for 5 days. Fever used to get relieved with excessive perspiration. The child was relatively better in between fever episodes. Examination revealed temp of 104°F, RR—34/min, HR—112/min, BP—108/64 mm Hg. There was mild pallor, no icterus, no rash, no edema, no lymphadenopathy. Examination of the abdomen revealed a soft, non-tender liver 2 cm palpable below the right costal margin (liver span 7.0 cm) and palpable spleen 2 cm (soft, non-tender) below left costal margin. There was no evidence of free fluid in abdomen. Other systemic examination was normal.

What are the differential diagnoses in this child?

Common differential diagnoses for short duration fever (of less than 7 days) with mild hepatosplenomegaly without any other localizing signs or symptoms are (a) uncomplicated malaria, (b) infectious mononucleosis, (c) viral hepatitis, and (d) dengue fever. Enteric fever is another possibility, but splenomegaly in enteric fever usually appears in the second week of illness. Here it was present on 5th day of fever.

- *Malaria* Points in favor include intermittent fever with characteristic hot and cold cycle (relief of fever with excessive perspiration), relative well-being of child in between fever episodes, and presence of hepatosplenomegaly. Tertian and quotidian fever, ie, fever every third day as in *P. vivax* and fever every day (as in *P. falciparum*) are not characteristic of malaria in children.
- *Infectious mononucleosis* Intermittent fever with hepatosplenomegaly are in favor. Absence of sore throat, lymphadenopathy, rash, and toxic appearance are against the diagnosis.
- *Viral hepatitis* Fever is usually low grade and icterus is usually present. This may be early phase of illness and icterus may be late finding or this may be a case of anicteric hepatitis. A child with hepatitis also remains anorexic, and is not well in between fever episodes (points against).
- *Dengue fever* Fever in dengue is usually biphasic and not continuous. Absence of myalgia, bone pains, rash, edema, bleeding manifestations, and shock are also against the diagnosis.
- *Urinary tract infection (UTI)* Absence of urinary complaints like frequency, urgency, dysuria are against UTI. However, fever may be the sole presentation of upper UTI.

Outline the investigations to confirm your diagnosis?

Peripheral blood smear examination for detection of malarial parasite is the gold standard test for diagnosis of malaria. Rapid diagnostic tests (RDTs) for malarial antigen are indicated, if peripheral blood smear is negative but suspicion of malaria is high. Investigations to rule out other possibilities include complete blood counts, peripheral smear for atypical lymphocytes, blood culture, liver enzymes, and urine microscopy and culture.

Peripheral smear revealed large-sized RBCs containing ring form and trophozoites of malarial parasite. Large chromatin dots, ameboid cytoplasm with Schuffner dots suggested P. vivax infection. Hb was 8.2 g/dL, leukocyte count 6100/mm³, and platelet count was 54000/mm.³ Liver function and urine examination were normal.

What is your final diagnosis? Name the drug of choice for treatment.

This is a case of *uncomplicated malaria* (absence of neurological manifestations, anemia, coagulopathy, hematuria, metabolic and electrolyte abnormalities, shock, respiratory problems, jaundice classifies above patient as uncomplicated malaria caused by *P. vivax*)

Drug of choice will be oral chloroquine (25 mg/kg to be given over a period of three days).

As relapse is common in vivax malaria (due to presence of hypnozoites/sleeping forms), the child will also need to be treated with primaquine 0.25 mg/kg/day for 14 days (after ruling out G-6-PD deficiency), since primaquine can trigger hemolytic anemia in G6PD deficient individual.

The fever did not respond even after three days of chloroquine?

Ensure that the compliance was good and the child was receiving the correct dose. Consider chloroquine-resistant vivax malaria or mixed infection of more than one species of *Plasmodium*. Treat the child with ACT combination therapy (artemether + lumefantrine is most preferred combination).

recrudescence or a relapse. Beyond 28 days, any recurrence suggests a relapse.

- Chloroquine-resistant *P. vivax* infection is treated with quinine for 7 days, or mefloquine (15 mg/kg) as a single dose, or amodiaquine 10 mg/kg once a day for 3 days, or with ACTs as outlined in **Table 6.22**.
- Avoid the use of sulfadoxine-pyrimethamine as parasite has developed resistance to this combination in many areas.

Malaria Vaccines

Despite intensive efforts, no malaria vaccine is available. Current research is focused on three developmental stages of the malarial parasite the sporozoite, the merozoite, and the gamete. Sporozoite vaccine would prevent infection, merozoite vaccine would prevent the invasion of erythrocytes by merozoites; and gametocyte vaccine would block transmission of infection by blocking the parasite development in mosquito. The major hurdles in the development of malaria vaccine are the complex life cycle of parasite expressing a variety of antigens at different stages, antigenic variation which enables parasite to evade the host's immune response, and poor understanding of immune response in malaria.

Malaria

1. In India, most cases of malaria are caused by *P. vivax* (60–65%) and *P. falciparum* (35–40%).
2. Malaria is spread to humans during the bite of an infected female anopheline mosquito.
3. Typical malarial paroxysms consisting of fever spikes, chills, and rigors occurring at regular intervals are uncommon in children below 5 years of age.
4. Microscopy is the gold standard of diagnosis; rapid diagnostic tests (RDTs) are reserved for areas without skilled microscopist.
5. For uncomplicated *P. vivax* malaria, chloroquine is the drug of choice.
6. All cases of falciparum and complicated malaria should be treated with artemisinine combination therapy (ACT).
7. Mosquito control is the most effective way to prevent malaria.

Bejon P, Berkley JA, Mwangi T, et al. Defining childhood severe falciparum malaria for intervention studies. *PLoS Med*. 2007(8):e251.

Coll O, Menendez C, Botet F, *et al*. World Association of Perinatal Medicine Perinatal Infections Working Group.Treatment and prevention of malaria in pregnancy and newborn. *J Perinat Med*. 2008;36:15–29.

Eisele TP, Larsen D, Steketee RW. Protective efficacy of interventions for preventing malaria mortality in children in Plasmodium falciparum endemic areas. *Int J Epidemiol*. 2010;39:88–101.

Garner P, Gelband H, Graves P; EditorialBoard, Cochrane Infectious Diseases Group. Systematic reviews in malaria: global policies need global reviews. *Infect Dis Clin North Am*. 2009;23:387–404.

Infectious Diseases Chapter, Indian Academy of Pediatrics. Management of malaria in children: update 2008. *Indian Pediatr*. 2008;45:731–5.

Makanga M, Bassat Q, Falade CO, *et al*. Efficacy and safety of artemether-lumefantrine in the treatment of acute, uncomplicated *Plasmodium falciparum* malaria: a pooled analysis. *Am J Trop Med Hyg*. 2011;85:793–804.

Mathew JL. Artemisinin derivatives versus quinine for severe malaria in children: a systematic review and meta-analysis. *Indian Pediatr*. 2010;47:423–8.

Musila N, Opiyo N, English M. Treatment of African children with severemalaria - towards evidence-informed clinical practice using GRADE. *Malar J*. 2011;10:201.

Okoromah CA, Afolabi BB, Wall EC. Mannitol and other osmotic diuretics as adjuncts for treating cerebral malaria. *Cochrane Database Syst Rev*. 2011;4:CD004615.

Sharma S, Pathak S. Malaria vaccine: a current perspective. *J Vector Borne Dis*. 2008;45:1–20.

Sinclair D, Donegan S, Lalloo DG. Artesunate versus quinine for treating severe malaria. *Cochrane Database Syst Rev*. 2011;3:CD005967.

Thwing J, Eisele TP, Steketee RW. Protective efficacy of malaria case management and intermittent preventive treatment for preventing malaria mortality in children: A systematic review for the Lives Saved Tool. *BMC Public Health*.2011;11:S14.

6.19 VISCERAL LEISHMANIASIS (KALA-AZAR)

Leishmaniasis is caused by parasites of the genus *Leishmania* which are transmitted to humans by female sandflies of the genus *Phlebotomus*. There are three major clinical forms of leishmaniasis: Visceral leishmaniasis, cutaneous leishmaniasis, and mucocutaneous leishmaniasis. In India, only visceral and cutaneous forms of leishmaniasis occur. The term kala-azar (*Kala*—black; *Azar*—sickness) for this disease denotes hyperpigmentation seen in patients with visceral leishmaniasis. Infection may be asymptomatic.

The disease is world-wide in distribution and occurs on all continents except Australia and Antarctica. In India, kala-azar is most often reported from Bihar, West Bengal, Jharkhand and Eastern UP. Of the 1–3 lakh cases reported annually in India, 90% occur in Bihar alone.

Etiology

There are at least 30 species of *Leishmania*. Visceral leishmaniasis in the Indian subcontinent is most often caused by *L. donovani*.

Parasites are present in the human host as *amastigotes*, which are nonflagellated, round or oval in shape (**Leishman-Donovan bodies**), and as flagellated *promastigotes* in the sandfly and in the culture medium. Amastigotes live and multiply in the cells of the mononuclear phagocyte system which includes blood monocytes, macrophages, histiocytes, Kupffer cells and reticuloendothelial cells in spleen and lymphoid tissue.

Epidemiology

Vector *Phlebotomus argentipes* (sandfly) is the only vector responsible for Indian kala-azar. It breeds in cattle sheds, and eggs are laid above the water-line during seasonal floods. Sandflies are small insects, about one-fourth of a mosquito. Life cycle lasts for more than a month; however, duration depends on temperature and other ecological conditions. They prefer high relative humidity, warm temperature, high subsoil water and abundance of vegetation. These are ecologically sensitive insects, fragile and cannot withstand desiccation. The sandfly is a light-avoiding mosquito.

Parasite load is measured by an index known as average parasite density (APD). APD depends on the number of parasites per high power field in a stained smear of spleen:

Grade	Average parasite density
6+	100 parasites per high power field
5+	10–100 parasites per high power field
4+	1–10 parasites per high power field
3+	1–10 parasites per 10 high power fields
2+	1–10 parasites per 100 high power fields
1+	1–10 parasites per 1000 high power fields
0	No parasites per 1000 high power fields

Host Indian kala-azar primarily affects adults and children below 10 years of age, sparing infants. Mostly poor socio-economic groups of population primarily living in rural areas are affected.

Environment The conditions that permit outbreaks of kala-azar include a heavy rainfall, increased relative humidity, high ambient environmental temperature, plenty of vegetation and subsoil water. Rural areas lying within 600 feet above sea level are more susceptible. Primitive housing and low standards of hygiene increase the risk of transmission. Infection rate is usually highest among the people living at the edge of foci (forest or desert) close to zoonotic cycle.

Mode of Spread

Transmission Female sandflies feeding on infected persons ingest parasitized cells. Amastigotes transform into promastigotes, which develop and multiply in the insect's gut and migrate to the proboscis (salivary glands). The female sandfly becomes infective to man after an external incubation period of 6–9 days, ready to transmit infection to the human. Infection occurs when an infected female sandfly bites a person and injects parasites into the human host. Male sandflies feed on fruit juices and do not suck blood. Rarely, visceral leishmaniasis can be transmitted by blood transfusion, sexual intercourse, accidental needle prick, or congenitally.

Reservoir Man appears to be the only reservoir of infection for visceral leishmaniasis in India. However, in other geographical areas, dogs, cats, jackals, and rodents, also act as reservoirs.

Pathogenesis

Following the bite of an infected sandfly, promastigotes enter reticuloendothelial cells, transform into amastigotes and multiply. Parasites spread hematogenously within macrophages to the liver, spleen, bone marrow and lymphoid tissue. The protective immune response in visceral leishmaniasis is primarily cell mediated (CMI) which results in subclinical infection and spontaneous cure in many cases. Failure of CMI to develop leads to the clinical syndrome of visceral leishmaniasis. Anti-leishmanial antibodies are not protective in nature. Defective CMI correlates with increased

suppressor cell activity and decreased production of interferon-gamma, interleukin-1 and interleukin-2 by mononuclear cells. The *leishmanin skin test* (*Montenegro test*) detects delayed-type hypersensitivity to leishmanial antigens. The test is negative during active disease and becomes positive 3–6 months after recovery. For every case of visceral leishmaniasis, there are about 30 subclinical infections. Malnutrition and HIV predispose to clinical disease.

Clinical Features

The *incubation period* is generally 2 to 8 months, although it may be as long as 2 years.

The onset is insidious in most cases. The typical manifestations of kala-azar consisting of prolonged fever (>2 weeks), weight loss, abdominal discomfort, emaciation, pallor, marked splenomegaly and moderate hepatomegaly generally appear a few months after the onset of illness. However, a more rapid clinical course over 1–2 months has been observed in some patients. Fever may not follow any definite pattern. It may be high or low grade, remittent, intermittent or continuous. The *'double-rise'* of temperature in a day (*double quotidian*), although characteristic, is an uncommon finding. The patient does not appear 'toxic'.

Splenic enlargement is seen in nearly all cases. It is huge, firm, smooth and nontender unless there has been a recent infarct. Moderate hepatomegaly is seen in over 80% of cases. Unlike African visceral leishmaniasis, lymphadenopathy is infrequent in kala-azar. Hyperpigmentation of skin is characteristic and occurs in late stages of disease, affecting the face, hands and upper trunk.

Pancytopenia is common. Anemia is attributed to autoimmune hemolysis, hypersplenism, ineffective erythropoiesis, co-existing nutritional deficiencies, and gastrointestinal blood loss. Progressive emaciation occurs in all cases. Cough and diarrhea are common. Appetite is generally well maintained. There may be petechial hemorrhages, epistaxis and gum bleeding. Pedal edema may occur due to hypoalbuminemia. Jaundice is uncommon. DIC and cirrhosis of liver are rare complications of visceral leishmaniasis. Diminished cell-mediated immunity may account for the high incidence of secondary infections, mainly pneumonia, septicemia, measles, tuberculosis, dysentery, otitis media and cancrum oris. Without treatment, death occurs within 2 years in 80–90% of patients, usually from secondary infection or gastrointestinal hemorrhage.

Recently, visceral leishmaniasis has been recognized as an opportunistic infection in HIV infected persons. It may also result from reactivation of subclinical infection in HIV infected individuals. The presentation may be atypical with prominent gastrointestinal tract involvement and absence of hepatosplenomegaly.

Post kala-azar dermal leishmaniasis (PKDL) This is sequel to infection with *L. donovani*. Up to 20% of patients of Indian kala-azar may develop PKDL, 1–10 years after successful treatment of VL. Hypopigmented macules and papules appear over chin, lips, neck, extensor surfaces of the arms, trunk, and legs, sparing the scalp, palms, soles, axillae and perineum. There may be nodular skin lesions. Clinically, PKDL may be confused with lepromatous leprosy, but

6

peripheral nerves are spared. Skin lesions may persist for up to 20 years, and such patients may act as chronic reservoir of infection.

Differential Diagnosis

The differential diagnosis for visceral leishmaniasis includes all conditions which present with prolonged fever and hepatosplenomegaly such as, malaria, tropical splenomegaly syndrome, lymphoma, and leukemia, tuberculosis, schistosomiasis, portal hypertension, brucellosis, etc.

Laboratory Diagnosis

A. Demonstration of Parasites

Identification of parasites in tissue specimens (LD bodies) or by culture on *Novy-McNeal-Nicolle* (NNN) medium provides a definitive diagnosis of VL. The positivity rate is highest for splenic aspirate (>95%), followed by bone marrow or liver (85%), buffy coat (70%) and African lymph node (65%). Splenic aspiration is safe in experienced hands but is contraindicated if the prothrombin time exceeds control value by 5 seconds or more, or platelet count is below 40,000/mm³. Under these circumstances, bone marrow aspiration can be performed safely, although the yield rate is slightly low. Recently, PCR has been successfully employed to detect parasites in tissue specimens.

B. Serological Tests

Antibodies are readily detectable by several methods. These include enzyme immunoassay, indirect immunofluorescence, and direct agglutination tests. In general, serological tests have sensitivity>90% but with lower specificity.

A dipstick ELISA using recombinant K39 (rK39) antigen has shown a sensitivity and specificity close to 100%. The test is rapid, easy to perform, and much less invasive compared to splenic or bone marrow aspiration. Since, it remains positive for long periods, it is of no use in cases of relapse or reinfection. In micro ELISA format, titers to rK39 decrease following successful therapy and tend to rise in cases of relapse, thus making it useful to recognize treatment failures.

Another latex agglutination-based antigen detection test in urine has been developed (KAtex) which is highly specific, unfortunately its sensitivity is low, but it turns negative at the end of successful therapy.

Napier's aldehyde test was used in past for the diagnosis of kala-azar. The test has very low sensitivity and specificity and is no longer in use.

Treatment	Kala-azar

Antimonials Until now the pentavalent antimonials were the drug of choice for the therapy of visceral leishmaniasis. However, increasing resistance to these compounds in India, particularly in Bihar, has led to frequent treatment failures. Therefore, antimonials are not used as first-line agent in Bihar. However, it is still effective against visceral leishmaniasis in other parts of India, although resistant cases have been reported from these areas. The main reason for employing this agent is easy

availability and low cost. Sodium antimony gluconate (sodium stibogluconate) containing 100 mg antimony (stibium) per mL or meglumine containing 85 mg antimony per mL are equal in efficacy and toxicity when used in equivalent doses. IM injections are painful and better avoided. IV injections should be diluted 1:10 with 5% dextrose and infused slowly over 20 minutes. Adverse effects include vomiting, fatigue, arthralgia, myalgia, abdominal pain, elevated serum transaminases, lipase and amylase levels, bone marrow depression, and ECG abnormalities, including non-specific ST and T-wave changes and T-wave flattening or inversion. Weekly ECG monitoring is recommended during therapy. Rarely, there may be prolongation of QTc interval.

Pentamidine has been used in cases unresponsive to antimony compounds. However, resistance to this agent is now common and its use is associated with serious side effects like hypotension, hypoglycemia, renal damage, injection abscess, and diabetes. Because of these drawbacks, it is no longer preferred at present.

Amphotericin B desoxycholate is 400 times more potent than antimony compounds against *Leishmania*. The main side effects include fever, chills, thrombophlebitis, hypokalemia, and renal failure. Liposomal amphotericin B is very safe and effective drug. It is the drug of choice for antimony-resistant kala-azar. Compared to conventional amphotericin, its concentration in reticuloendothelial cells is 10 times more, and toxicity 10 times less. The drug is costly. The cure rate is less in patients co-infected with HIV.

Paromomycin is an aminoglycoside with good activity against *Leishmania,* in doses of 15 mg of paromomycin sulfate (11 mg/kg base) intramuscularly for 21 days.

Miltefosine, originally developed as an antineoplastic drug, has demonstrated a cure rate of more than 90% in visceral leishmaniasis. It was the first oral drug active against *Leishmania*. Gastrointestinal side effects are frequent but mild in nature. Miltefosine is contraindicated in pregnancy and in women of child-bearing age, unless women use appropriate contraception.

Sitamaquine is another oral drug undergoing phase 3 trials. *Aminosidine*, an aminoglycoside similar to paromomycin, has also been found to be effective.

Current Treatment Guidelines

Currently liposomal amphotericin B is the drug of choice for the treatment of visceral leishmaniasis in regions with widespread resistance to antimony compounds. Even a single dose infusion of liposomal amphotericin B has shown cure rates equivalent to conventional amphotericin B infusions (15 alternate-day infusions). There is ever growing threat of development of resistance in parasites, and thus combination therapy is being tested now. A combination of drugs, including liposomal amphotericin B (single dose), miltefosine (7 days), and paromomycin (10 days) have been used successfully. Research is also being carried out on newer delivery systems of amphotericin B, such as nanoparticles and cochleates to improve drug efficacy.

In addition to specific therapy, patients may require broad spectrum antibiotics for intercurrent infection, packed RBCs, and nutritional care. The treatment options for visceral leishmaniasis are summarized in **Table 6.26**.

Table 6.26 Treatment of Visceral Leishmaniasis

Drug	Dose and duration
Liposomal amphotericin B. Drug of first choice in antimony-resistant cases.	3 mg/kg IV on days 1–5, and again on day 10
Amphotericin B desoxycholate	0.5–1.0 mg/kg IV on alternate days for 4 weeks
Miltefosine	2.5 mg/kg/day orally in 1–2 doses orally for 4–6 weeks
Paromomycin sulfate	15 mg/kg (11mg/kg base) IM for 28 days
Pentamidine	4 mg/kg IV or IM three times a week for 8 weeks
Sodium antimony gluconate (sodium stibogluconate) or meglumine antimoniate. Drug resistance is common	20 mg/kg once a day IV or IM for 30 days

Response to Treatment

Fever, spleen size, hemoglobin, blood cell counts, serum albumin, and body weight are useful indicators of progress. In most patients, the fever subsides within 7 days, blood counts and hemoglobin levels rise, the patient feels better, and spleen becomes smaller within 2 weeks. Parasitological cure should be documented at the end of therapy by splenic or bone marrow aspiration. As relapses are common in this disease, patient should be followed for at least 6 months before a long-term definite cure is pronounced. The spleen may take 6 months to 1 year to regress completely. Relapse is suggested by an increase of spleen size, a fall in hemoglobin levels and should be confirmed by the demonstration of parasites.

Prevention and Control

Early diagnosis, complete treatment and vector control are the main components of the control program. Spread of the disease is prevented by controlling the source of infection and eradicating the vector. All infected patients should be identified and treated intensively. Patients with post-kala-azar dermal leishmaniasis are a rich reservoir of infection and pose a special public health problem.

Revision Point

Kala-azar

1. Kala-azar is caused by parasites of the genus *Leishmania* which are transmitted to humans by female sandflies of the genus *Phlebotomus*.
2. The typical manifestations consist of high fever often with rigors, abdominal discomfort, emaciation, pallor, marked splenomegaly, and moderate hepatomegaly. There is no lymphadenopathy.
3. Diagnosis is based on demonstration of amastigotes in bone marrow or splenic aspirates. K39 antigen-based rapid diagnostic tests are increasingly being used for the diagnosis of Kala-azar.
4. Liposomal amphotericin B or multidrug therapy are preferred treatment.

Croft SL, Olliaro P. Leishmaniasis chemotherapy—challenges and opportunities. *Clin Microbiol Infect.* 2011;17:1478–83.

Malaviya P, Singh RP, Singh SP, *et al*. Monitoring drug effectiveness in kala-azar in Bihar, India: cost and feasibility of periodic random surveys vs. a health service-based reporting system. *Trop Med Int Health.* 2011;16:1159–66.

Mondal S, Bhattacharya P, Ali N. Current diagnosis and treatment of visceral leishmaniasis. *Expert Rev Anti Infect Ther.* 2010;8:919–44.

Singh UK, Prasad R, Jaiswal BP, *et al*. Amphotericin B therapy in children with visceral leishmaniasis: daily vs. alternate day, a randomized trial. *J Trop Pediatr.* 2010;56:321–4.

Srivastava P, Dayama A, Mehrotra S, *et al*. Diagnosis of visceral leishmaniasis. *Trans R Soc Trop Med Hyg.* 2011;105:1–6.

Sundar S, Chakravarty J, Agarwal D, *et al*. Single-dose liposomal amphotericin B for visceral leishmaniasis in India. *N Engl J Med.* 2010;362:504–12.

Sundar S, Chakravarty J. Antimony toxicity. *Int J Environ Res Public Health.*2010;7:4267–77.

Sundar S, Agrawal N, Arora R, *et al*. Short-course paromomycin treatment of visceral leishmaniasis in India: 14-day vs 21-daytreatment. *Clin Infect Dis.* 2009;49:914–8.

6.20 COMMON INTESTINAL PARASITES

Intestinal parasites are of two main types, *viz*, single-cell protozoa and multicellular metazoan called helminths (worms). These are usually transmitted by feco-oral route. Rarely, they may enter the human body by penetrating through skin or sexual route. In their adult form, the helminths cannot multiply in the human body, while protozoa can multiply inside the human body.

- Common intestinal protozoa include *Giardia, Entamoeba, Cryptosporidium, Isospora* and *Cyclospora*.
- Helminths may be classified as *nematodes* (roundworms), *trematodes* (flatworms), and *cestodes* (tapeworms). Common intestinal helminths are listed in **Table 6.27.**

Parasites can live within the intestines for years without causing any symptoms or manifest with abdominal pain, diarrhea, dysentery, weight loss, malabsorption, rash or perianal itching, nausea, vomiting, bloating, belching, vaginitis, or passage of worms in stool. Uncommon symptoms may include joint pain, chest pain, cough, memory loss or mental symptoms, and organ infiltration.

6.21 AMEBIASIS

Amebiasis is caused by the protozoa *Entamoeba histolytica*, and usually presents with dysentery or diarrhea. The ameba may spread to various organs, the commonest being the liver where it manifests as amebic liver abscess. *E. histolytica* can be differentiated antigenically and by molecular methods from *E. dispar* which is non-pathogenic and responsible only for asymptomatic infection.

Table 6.27 Common Intestinal Parasitic Infections and Infestations
PROTOZOA
Entamoeba histolytica*, E. dispar*, Giardia lamblia, Cryptosporidium parvum, Isospora belli, and *Cysclospora*
HELMINTHS
Nematodes (soil transmitted helminths)
Type 1: Direct transmission by infective ova: *Enterobius vermicularis*, Trichuris trichiura**
Type 2: Ova infective after development in soil: *Ascaris lumbricoides*
Type 3: Penetration of skin: *Ancylostoma duodenale, Necator americanus,* and *Strongyloides stercoralis*
Trematodes
Fasciolopsis buski, Echinostoma sp., and *Heterophyses heterophyes*
Cestodes
Taenia saginata (beef tapeworm), and *Taenia solium* (pork tapeworm)

*Except these parasites (which inhabit the large intestine), and all others inhabit small intestine.

Epidemiology

E. histolytica has a worldwide distribution, and is endemic in developing countries due to low socioeconomic conditions. It is the third leading cause of parasitic death in the world after malaria and schistosomiasis. It is estimated that approximately 10% of the world's population; ie, 600 million people are infected, with an annual mortality of 40,000–110,000.

Prevalence rates vary widely with the population studied, from around 1% in the industrialized nations to 50–80% in the tropics. The exact number of persons infected by pathogenic strains is still not clear but from the data available from a few such reports, the asymptomatic carriage seems to predominate with a prevalence of 10% and only 1% for pathogenic strains. In India, the prevalence rates vary from 5–50% depending upon the population and geographical region.

Etiology

E. histolytica exists in nature in two forms: Cyst or a trophozoite (Fig. 6.16). Cysts (10–18 μm) are oval or round, asymmetrical with four nuclei. They are easily destroyed by most disinfectants and by heating to 55°C but may survive chlorination of water and in water at low temperature. Cyst is the infective stage of the parasite. Asymptomatic human cyst carriers are the principal reservoir of infection. There is no animal reservoir.

Mode of Spread

The infection is transmitted by ingestion of food or water contaminated with fecal material containing cysts of *Entamoeba.* The source of contamination may be the food handlers or flies. Cysts can remain viable and infective in water and feces for several days. Sexual transmission is also reported.

Young, immunocompromsed and malnourished children, and those receiving steroids are at a higher risk of severe *E. histolytica* infection. Other factors contributing to increased transmission include low socioeconomic status, overcrowding, lack of safe water supply, and poor sanitation.

Pathogenesis

Following ingestion, cyst hatches in the small intestine to produce 8 trophozoites. Trophozoites colonize and invade the colonic mucosa where they multiply and spread laterally underneath the intestinal epithelium producing characteristic 'flask-shaped or teardrop ulcers'. These lesions are commonly found in cecum, transverse colon, and sigmoid colon. There is little local inflammatory response. Some ameba trophozoites become cyst and are passed in the stool to survive for weeks in a moist environment. On the other hand, some trophozoites invade the intestinal mucosa and spread *via* bloodstream to the liver, lung, and brain.

Extraintestinal complications They arise from spread of infection through portal circulation. Amebic liver abscess develops because of toxin release and hepatocyte damage. It is seen more frequently in the right lobe of the liver (posterosuperior part); 5–20% have abscess in the left lobe. Single liver abscess is found in 95% of instances. Its contents are chocolate-colored and viscid (described as anchovy-sauce appearance), usually sterile, and contain no neutrophils. Amebae are located at the periphery of abscess. The abscess may regress, rupture or disseminate. Transdiaphragmatic rupture of liver abscess into the pleural space may result in amebic empyema and pulmonary amebiasis. The abscess may also rupture into the peritoneum (2–5%), or pericardial cavity (<1%).

Clinical Features

E. histolytica infection is asymptomatic in 90% of patients. About 4–10% of persons infected with *E. histolytica* develop amebic colitis; while <1% develop disseminated disease, including amebic liver abscess.

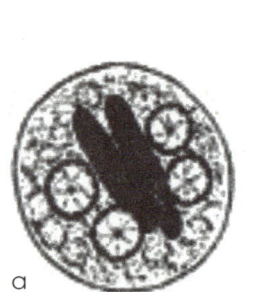
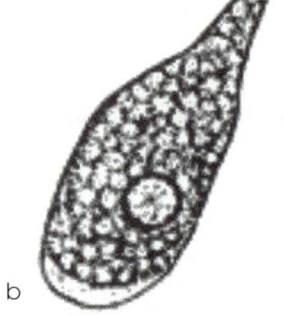

Fig. 6.16 *Entamoeba histolytica:* (a) cyst; (b) trophozoite

Intestinal disease (*amebic colitis*) Incubation period for symptomatic disease varies from 2 weeks to months. Acute intestinal amebiasis presents with colicky abdominal pain, tenesmus, and frequent loose stools containing mucus and blood. The stool may be positive for occult blood. Fever is seen in only one-third of patients and constitutional symptoms are rare. Examination may reveal diffuse tenderness in the cecal or rectosigmoid junction areas. The course of illness may be protracted lasting for weeks or even months. Rarely, a reactive collection of edematous granulation and fibrous tissue called an ameboma can grow into the lumen, causing pain, obstruction and, possibly, intussusception. Chronic amebiasis presents with intermittent diarrhea which is often followed by constipation due to spasm of the large intestines, fatigue and weight loss. Toxic megacolon, pneumatosis coli (intramural air), and peritonitis can also occur. Acute amebic dysentery should be differentiated from that caused by *Shigella, Salmonella, Campylobacter, E. coli* and *Yersinia*.

Amebic liver abscess develops in <1% of infected persons, often months to years after exposure. A past history of amebic dysentery is forthcoming in only 20% of patients and only 10% have concomitant intestinal symptoms. The child presents with high fever with chills and rigors, abdominal pain, distension and tender hepatomegaly, and appears toxic. Pain in the upper abdomen is intense and radiates to the shoulder. Jaundice is uncommon and observed in only 10–15% cases.

Abscess may rupture into pleural space, peritoneum, and pericardium, requiring emergency drainage. Mortality in children in ruptured abscess can be up to 25%.

Investigations

The amebic liver abscess needs to be differentiated from pyogenic liver abscess, hepatoma, and hydatid cyst of the liver.

Parasite detection Microscopic examination of formed stool for cysts; or diarrheal stool for trophozoites is necessary for the diagnosis of intestinal infection with *E. histolytica*. Diarrheal stools must be examined within one hour of collection to look for motility of trophozoites. Stool microscopy cannot distinguish *E. histolytica* from *E. dispar* infection, unless phagocytosed erythrocytes are seen in trophzoites (seen in *E. histolytica*). Stool antigen testing may also distinguish the two species.

A complete examination of stool for cysts includes wet-mount in saline, an iodine-stained wet mount and a fixed trichrome-stained preparation. These preparations not only delineate cyst morphology but also distinguish bacillary from amebic dysentery. At least 3 stool specimens taken on consecutive days should be examined to exclude amebic infection of the intestines, since excretion of cysts may be intermittent. However, detection of amebic cysts, even with associated gastrointestinal symptoms does not necessarily indicate acute infection.

Stool contains plenty of erythrocytes but a few leukocytes in patients with amebic colitis unlike bacillary dysentery where the inflammatory cells especially polymorphonuclear cells are replete.

Sigmoidoscopy followed by aspiration of mucosal lesions or biopsy is valuable in symptomatic sick patients, where other tests fail to provide conclusive evidence. It is difficult to demonstrate the amebae in the liver aspirate.

Liver aspirate The aspirate is usually sterile on culture. Trophozoites may be present in the aspirate and can be demonstrated only from the wall of the abscess.

Serology In extraintestinal amebiasis and invasive amebiasis, antibody detection by ELISA is the most sensitive test. Indirect hemagglutination (IHA) test may be done for invasive intestinal disease or liver abscess. IHA is usually negative in asymptomatic carriers. Serological response as detected by CIE or ELISA becomes negative 6–12 months after infection. IHA, on the other hand, may stay positive for as long as 10 years following complete recovery.

Radiology Chest radiograph in case of a liver abscess shows elevated diaphragm and pleural reaction on the right side in a child with liver abscess. Ultrasound, CT, MRI, or isotope scan can localize the exact site of abscess.

Others Leukocytosis, anemia, high ESR, and elevated alkaline phosphatase are common in amebic liver abscess. There is no eosinophilia in invasive disease.

Treatment	Amebiasis

Due to the possibility of its invasive nature and severe extraintestinal manifestations, all children with *E. histolytica* infection, whether symptomatic or not, should be treated.
- *Luminal amebicides*, such as diloxanide furoate and diiodoquinol act on only those organisms that are present in the intestinal lumen.
- *Tissue amebicides*, such as metronidazole, tinidazole, chloroquine, and dehydroemetin are effective in the treatment of invasive amebiasis but are less effective for luminal clearance.

A combination of a luminal and a tissue amebicide is thus advocated for complete parasite clearance in invasive disease. Metronidazole is the most popular drug for management of both intestinal and extraintestinal forms of amebiasis and till date, there is no evidence of resistance against this agent.

Invasive amebiasis (both intestinal and extraintestinal) should be treated initially with a tissue amebicide like (a) oral metronidazole 35–50 mg/kg/day in three divided doses for 7–10 days; or (b) tinidazole 50 mg/kg/day once daily for 3–5 days. Tinidazole is as efficacious as metronidazole but the treatment duration is shorter with fewer adverse effects. Following this, all children should be given a course of luminal amebicide: (a) Diloxanide furoate 20 mg/kg/day in three divided doses for 7 days; or (b) paromomycin 25–35 mg/kg/day in three divided doses for 7 days; or (c) iodoquinol 30–40 mg/kg/day in 3 divided doses for 20 days. Either of paromomycin, diloxanide furoate or iodoquinol may be used to treat asymptomatic carriers, given in the regimen same as for invasive disease. Reinfection is quite common, even after complete cure.
- For cases of *fulminant amebic colitis*, therapy with dehydroemetine, 1 mg/kg/day subcutaneously or IM, may be instituted. Broad-spectrum antibiotics may also be needed.
- Intestinal perforation or ruptured amebic liver abscess or toxic megacolon may warrant surgical intervention.

Amebic liver abscess It should also be treated with the same regime as advocated for invasive amebiasis, above. Image-guided aspiration is indicated in (*i*) large abscess; (*ii*) left lobe abscess; (*iii*) impending rupture of abscess; or (*iv*) failure to improve after 4–6 days of treatment with amebicidal drugs. Percutaneous drainage of abscess under USG guidance is preferred over open surgical drainage. Chloroquine may be a useful additive drug as it concentrates in liver. Abscess cavity resolves slowly over a period of several months.

Prevention

Prevention involves avoiding fecal contamination of food and water and adopting good handwashing technique. Boiling and purification of drinking water by filtration are important preventive measures. The use of night soil (human feces) for fertilization of crops should be avoided. No prophylactic drug or vaccine is a available. No prophylactic drug or vaccine is available.

Revision Point Amebiasis and Giardiasis

1. Amebiasis (caused by *E. histolytica*) and giardiasis (caused by *Giardia lamblia*) are spread by fecal-oral route.
2. Clinical spectrum may vary from asymptomatic cyst carriers, explosive diarrhea, dysentery, subacute protracted course with GI symptoms, to persistent diarrhea.
3. Diagnosis is by stool microscopy of at least three samples.
4. Treatment of choice for amebiasis is metronidazole; while for giardiasis, tinidazole, or nitazoxamide are the drugs of choice.
5. *E. histolytica* may spread hematogenously to result in liver abscess.

Bercu TE, Petri WA, Behm JW. Amebic colitis: new insights into pathogenesis and treatment. *Curr Gastroenterol Rep.* 2007;9:429–33.

Hughes MA, Petri WA Jr. Amebic liver abscess. *Infect Dis Clin North Am.* 2000;14:565–82.

Pritt BS, Clark CG. Amebiasis. *Mayo Clin Proc.* 2008;83:1154–9.

Stanley SL Jr. Amoebiasis. *Lancet.* 2003;361:1025–34.

Stauffer W, Ravdin JI. Entamoeba histolytica: an update. *Curr Opin Infect Dis.* 2003;16:479–85.

Ximénez C, Morán P, Rojas L, *et al.* Reassessment of the epidemiology of amebiasis: state of the art. *Infect Genet Evol.* 2009;9:1023–32.

6.22 GIARDIASIS

Giardia lamblia (also known as *G. intestinalis* or *G. duodenalis*) is an important flagellated protozoan enteropathogen of humans. It affects 2.5 million people annually, and is the most common parasite infection of humans worldwide. The clinical manifestations range from asymptomatic carrier state to acute and persistent diarrhea, and malabsorption syndrome. Children appear to be more severely affected than adults. Humoral immunodeficiency (such as X-linked agammaglobulinemia and common variable immune deficiency) are associated with chronic *Giardia* infection. Malnourished and children with cystic fibrosis are particularly predisposed to giardiasis. Breast milk contains glycoconjugates and secretory IgA that provide protection against giardiasis.

Etiology

The parasite exists in the form of trophozoites (10–20 μm × 5–15 μm) or cysts (8–10 μm) (Fig. 6.17). Trophozoites colonize the proximal small intestine. Cysts are excreted in the feces; these are the infective stage of the parasite.

Reservoir Man and contaminated water supply remain the major reservoirs of *Giardia*.

Mode of Spread

Giardiasis is spread by fecal-oral contamination, the prevalence being higher in populations with poor sanitation, close contact, and oral-anal sexual practices. The disease is commonly water-borne because *Giardia* is resistant to the chlorine levels in normal tap water. Boiling may inactivate the cyst. Food-borne transmission is rare but can occur with ingestion of raw or undercooked foods.

The life cycle of *Giardia* consists of two stages: The fecal-orally transmitted cyst and the disease-causing trophozoite. Cysts are passed in a host's feces, remaining viable in a moist environment for months. Ingestion of at least 10 to 25 cysts can cause infection in humans. When a new host consumes a cyst, the host's acidic stomach environment stimulates excystation. Each cyst produces two trophozoites. These trophozoites migrate to the duodenum and proximal jejunum, where they attach to the mucosal wall by means of a ventral adhesive disk and replicate by binary fission.

Pathogenesis

Growth of trophozoites is promoted by bile, glucose and relative hypoxia. The trophozoites colonize the duodenum and proximal jejunum of the host. Each trophozoite has 4 pairs of flagellae and 2 nuclei. The trophozoites carry a ventral disk on its concave surface which enables their attachment to the intestinal wall. The powerful sucking disk of the trophozoite causes mechanical irritation and damage to the microvilli of the small bowel mucosa resulting in

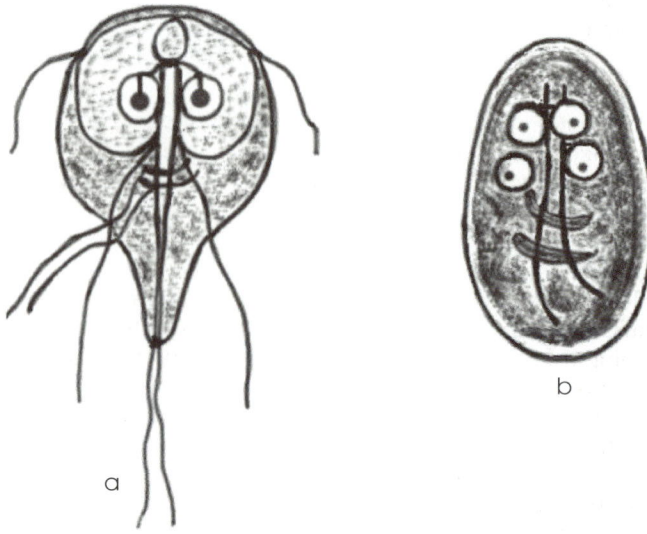

Fig. 6.17 *Giardia lamblia:* (a) trophozoite; (b) cyst.

deficiency of brush border enzyme activities. As the detached trophozoites pass through the intestine, they undergo encystations to form oval cysts containing 4 nuclei. Cysts pass in stools of infected persons and can remain viable for up to 2 months in soil. Unlike amebiasis, there are no invasive or locally destructive lesions.

Parenchymal involvement of the pancreas has been incriminated for the reported steatorrhea and decreased trypsin activity. In other cases, fat malabsorption observed in giardiasis is attributed to bacterial overgrowth in the duodenum and upper jejunum and bile salt deconjugation liberating free bile acids. Immunological studies have shown decreased levels of secretory IgA in duodenal aspirates and depressed T cell function.

Clinical Features

Asymptomatic carriage is the most common form of infection.

In symptomatic cases, incubation period after ingestion of cysts is 1–2 weeks.

In acute infections, there may be a sudden onset of explosive watery (non-bloody) foul smelling diarrhea along with abdominal distension, flatulence, nausea, anorexia and epigastric cramps. There is no blood or mucus in stools. The illness may last three or four days and is usually self-limiting in normal immunocompetent children.

Some infections may have a *subacute onset* with a protracted course, with persistent or recurrent mild to moderate symptoms such as brief episodes of loose foul smelling stools accompanied by flatus and abdominal distension. Between exacerbations, the stools are mushy or there may be constipation. Abnormal stool pattern may alternate with normal bowel movements. Symptoms last for 2–4 weeks.

Thirty to fifty percent children develop *persistent diarrhea*. Children with chronic giardiasis show lactose malabsorption, steatorrhea, iron deficiency anemia, and failure to thrive. Unlike *E. histolytica* infection, there is no extraintestinal spread of infection. Chronic giardiasis can cause growth failure and stunting. Repeated *Giardia* infections can lead to congnitive impairment.

Rarely, patients with giardiasis also present with reactive arthritis or asymmetric synovitis, usually of the lower extremities. Rashes and urticaria may be present as part of a hypersensitivity reaction.

Investigations

Diagnosis is made by examining diarrheal stools for trophozoites or cysts. At least 3 specimens of stools collected on alternate days (detection rate 90%) are examined microscopically, because the multiplication and passage of the giardial cysts is often intermittent. Sensitivity of a single stool examination is only 50%. Stool does not contain blood or leukocytes. Trophozoites are usually seen only in watery diarrhea but can also be detected by endoscopic brush cytology or intestinal biopsy. A duodenal aspirate or biopsy may yield high concentration of *Giardia*. Biopsy of the duodenum is not routinely recommended but may be done in patients with clinically suspected giardiasis, negative stool tests, negative duodenal fluid aspirate, absent secretory IgA level, hypogammaglobulinemia or chlorhydria. Another test may be recommended, if the microscopic examination of stool is negative, *viz*, the "String test". A weighted piece of string is swallowed till it reaches the duodenum. The trophozoites adhere to the string and may be visualized microscopically after withdrawal of the string.

Stool enzyme immunoassay or direct immunofluorescence tests for *Giardia* are the preferred tests for diagnosis. Blood cell counts are normal. There is no eosinophilia as there is no tissue invasion.

Treatment	Giardiasis

All symptomatic cases—acute and persistent diarrhea, failure to thrive and malabsorption syndrome require drug treatment. Asymptomatic cyst carriers require no therapy except for control of outbreaks. The drug of choice may be tinidazole or nitazoxanide. Tinidazole has very high efficacy (>90%) and need for only a single-dose therapy, while nitazoxanide has fewer side effects. A cheaper alternative may be metronidazole. Second line alternatives include furazolidone, albendazole, and quinacrine. The treatment of giardiasis is given in **Table 6.28.**

Table 6.28 Treatment of Giardiasis	
First-line therapy	
Tinidazole	>3 y, 50 mg/kg, single dose, oral
Nitazoxanide	1–3 y: 100 mg BD for 3 days, oral
	4–11 y: 200 mg BD for 3 days, oral
	>12 y: 500 mg BD for 3 days, oral
Metronidazole	15 mg/kg/day in 3 divided doses for 5–7 days
Second-line therapy	
Albendazole	>6 y: 400 mg once a day for 5 days
Furazolidone	6 mg/kg/day in four divided doses for 10 days
Quinacrine	6 mg/kg/day in three divided doses for 5 days

Paromomycin is not indicated for treating giardiasis in children.

Ganesh R, Arvind Kumar R, Suresh N, *et al*. Chronic abdominal pain in children. *Natl Med J India*. 2010;23:94–9.

Kappagoda S, Singh U, Blackburn BG. Antiparasitic therapy. *Mayo Clin Proc*. 2011;86:561–83.

Tejman-Yarden N, Eckmann L. New approaches to the treatment of giardiasis. *Curr Opin Infect Dis*. 2011;24:451–6.

6.23 CRYPTOSPORIDIOSIS

Cryptosporidium parvum causes cryptosporidiosis, primarily presenting as watery diarrhea. Children <2 years and immunocompromised children, especially AIDS and HIV-infected children are prone to this infection. The parasite is resistant to chlorination.

The infection is acquired by feco-oral route through ingestion of oocysts. The oocysts excyst in the small intestine where the sporozoites are released. Each oocyst releases 4 sporozoites. Sporozoites invade the jejunum.

Clinical features The infection presents with non-bloody watery diarrhea following an incubation period of 2–12 days. Vomiting may be seen in more than 80% of infected children. Fever occurs in about 50% of infected children. In immunocompetent persons, the disease is self-limiting, though oocysts may be shed for months. In immunocompromised patients, severe constitutional symptoms and affection of the biliary tract and pancreas may occur.

Diagnosis Infection is detected by microscopic examination of stool using modified acid-fast staining wherein the oocysts appear as small, spherical bodies (2–6 µm). At least 3 stool samples should be examined as shedding of oocysts is intermittent. However, ELISA is the investigation of choice. Biopsy of the intestine may reveal *Cryptosporidium* organisms in the microvillus border especially in the jejunum. Histopathology of the intestine reveals villus atrophy, epithelial flattening and inflammation of the lamina propria.

Treatment	Cryptosporidiosis

Treatment includes adequate rehydration along with nitazoxanide given for 3 days duration. The dose is as follows: 1–3y: 100 mg BD, PO; 4–11y: 200 mg BD, PO; and ≥12 y: 500 mg BD, PO.

Cabada MM, White AC Jr. Treatment of cryptosporidiosis: do we know what we think we know? *Curr Opin Infect Dis*. 2010;23:494–9.

Collinet-Adler S, Ward HD. Cryptosporidiosis: environmental, therapeutic, and preventive challenges. *Eur J Clin Microbiol Infect Dis*. 2010;29:927–35.

Singh BB, Sharma R, Sharma JK, *et al*. Parasitic zoonoses in India: an overview. *Rev Sci Tech*. 2010;29:629–37.

6.24 ASCARIASIS

(*Ascaris lumbricoides*: Roundworm)

Ascariasis is the most common human helminthic infection, infecting about 1.3 billion and causing 60,000 deaths annually. Infection is most prevalent in tropical and subtropical climates due to lack of sanitary facilities or the use of human feces as fertilizer. Preschool children are most vulnerable to infection due to their hand to mouth behavior. Infection may also be acquired through ingestion of contaminated fruits and vegetables. Most infected individuals are asymptomatic due to low worm load. Clinical manifestations occur due to pulmonary hypersensitivity and intestinal complications.

Pathogenesis

Ascaris lumbricoides causes the disease. Infection is acquired through ingestion of embryonated eggs. Larvae hatch in the small intestine, invade the intestinal mucosa, migrate to the lungs *via* the venous circulation, break into the alveoli, ascend through bronchi and trachea, and return via swallowing to the small intestine, where they develop into adult worms. After an interval of 2–3 months, female worms start producing eggs. A gravid female can produce up to 200,000 eggs a day, which pass with the feces. Under favorable environmental conditions, eggs embryonate and become infective after 5–10 days. Ascaris eggs are remarkably resistant to environmental stresses and can remain infective for several years.

The lifespan of adult worms is 1–2 years. Man is the only reservoir of infection.

Clinical Features

Symptoms may be produced by migration of larvae through lungs (*pulmonary ascariasis*) or the presence of adult worms in the intestine (*intestinal ascariasis*).

Pulmonary ascariasis presents as Loeffler's syndrome; characterized by fever, cough, dyspnea, wheeze, urticaria, eosinophilia, and lung infiltrates. Pulmonary ascariasis should be differentiated from other causes of Loeffler's syndrome, namely, visceral larva migrans caused by *Toxocara canis* or hookworm, schistosomiasis, pulmonary aspergillosis, and tropical pulmonary eosinophilia.

Intestinal manifestations of ascariasis result because of adult worms; and include abdominal distension, vomiting, vague abdominal discomfort and irritability. The child may pass adult worms in the vomitus or feces. In heavy worm infestation, small bowel obstruction can occur due to a mass of entangled worms. Occasionally worms migrate to aberrant sites such as biliary and pancreatic ducts, where they can cause cholecystitis, cholangitis, pancreatitis, and rarely intrahepatic abscess.

Complications Worms can also pass across the intestinal wall and cause peritonitis. As parasites compete with host for nutrients, heavy worm infestation may be associated with poor growth and nutritional deficiencies in young children.

Diagnosis

The diagnosis is established by identification of characteristic eggs in stool samples by microscopy. The eggs are round or oval (45–70 µm × 35–50 µm), brownish, with a thick mamillated covering. Occasionally, adult worm in feces or vomitus can be recognized by its large size and smooth cream colored surface. Blood eosinophilia which is prominent during early migratory phase (pulmonary ascariasis), decreases to minimal levels in established infection. Ultrasound can identify worms in pancreaticobiliary ducts. Occasionally, worms can be incidentally diagnosed on contrast studies of the gastrointestinal tract, appearing as *string shadows* due to barium in the alimentary canal of the worms, or as linear filling defects outlined by contrast media.

Treatment	Ascariasis

Adult worms in the gastrointestinal tract can be killed by single dose albendazole (400 mg, PO, for all ages), or mebendazole (100 mg BD for 3 days or 500 mg PO, single dose for all ages). Single dose of pyrantel pamoate (11 mg/kg) or ivermectin (150–200 µg/kg) is also effective. Nitazoxanide given for 3 days may be as effective as single dose albendazole. Piperazine citrate (75 mg/kg/day, 2 days) is recommended in heavy infestations at risk of intestinal obstruction, intestinal obstruction and biliary infestation. Severe obstruction may require surgery.

Re-infections can occur in endemic areas in more than 80% of the population.

6.25 HOOKWORM INFESTATION

(*Ancylostoma duodenale, Necator americanus*)

Hookworm infestation is one of the most prevalent helminthic diseases, affecting more than 500 million humans and causing iron deficiency anemia. Infection is more common in rural areas of tropical and subtropical regions. Most infected persons are asymptomatic. Hookworm disease develops when worm load is high. Two species of hookworm, *Ancylostoma duodenale* and *Necator americanus* are found exclusively in humans while less common zoonotic species *A. cannium*, *A. braziliense* and *A. ceylanicum* may affect humans.

Pathogenesis

Filariform larva is the infective stage of the parasite. Infection occurs when larvae in soil penetrate the skin (*N. americanus* and *A. duodenale*) or when they are ingested through contaminated food and water (*A. duodenale*). Following skin penetration, larvae reach lungs *via* systemic circulation, break into the alveoli, ascend through bronchi and trachea, and are swallowed to reach the small intestine, where they develop into mature worms. Orally ingested infective larvae may either undergo extraintestinal migration or remain in the intestine to develop into mature worms. Adult worms inhabit jejunum, measure 1 cm in length, and use buccal teeth (*A. duodenale*) or cutting plates (*N. americanus*) to attach to the bowel mucosa and suck blood. *A. duodenale* sucks blood at the rate of 0.15 mL per worm per day. Additional 0.05 mL blood is lost as hemorrhage from the abandoned feeding site. Blood loss is less for *N. americanus*.

Adult hookworms produce thousands of eggs daily which pass into soil where rhabditiform larvae are released which mature into the filariform larvae. Ova fail to develop into larva, if it gets dried, or the surrounding temperature drops below 13°C. The lifespan of adult worms ranges from 1–5 years. Man is the only reservoir.

Clinical Features

Symptoms due to larvae appear 1–2 weeks after infections and those due to ova appear after 42–45 days of infection.

Infective larvae may produce a pruritic maculopapular eruption known as *ground itch* at the site of skin penetration. Larvae migrating through lungs may also cause transient lung infiltration, but this is less common than with *Ascaris*. Non-specific complaints like abdominal pain, anorexia, and diarrhea have also been attributed to the hookworm infection.

Chronic blood loss due to hookworm infection causes iron deficiency anemia and occasionally, hypoproteinemia. Only heavily infected children become symptomatic. Children with light infections have minimal blood loss and, thus, may have hookworm infection but not hookworm disease. Sometimes children may develop a yellow-green pallor known as 'chlorosis.' *A. duodenale* infection during infancy may be associated with diarrhea, malaria, failure to thrive, and severe anemia.

Diagnosis

The diagnosis is established by identifying the characteristic oval hookworm eggs in the feces. Eggs of the two species are indistinguishable. Blood examination reveals microcytic hypochromic anemia, occasionally with eosinophila. Hypoalbuminemia may be seen in heavy infections.

Case Study	Hookworm Infestation

Mother of an 8-yr-old boy presented with chief complaint that her child appears to be pale than before. This was associated with history of pain in the abdomen and loose stools over the last 4–5 months. There was no history of fever, red-colored urine, yellowish discoloration of eyes, abdominal distension, rash, petechiae, bleeding from any site, or black-colored foul smelling stools. There was no history of blood transfusion in the child or any other family member. Dietary history was appropriate for age.

On examination, there was moderate pallor over conjunctiva, palms, and soles. There was no icterus, edema, or significant lymphadenopathy. Abdominal examination revealed no hepatosplenomegaly. Rest of the systemic examination was normal.

Q. Summarize your impression of this child.

This child presented with moderate pallor of insidious onset without any evidence of bleeding, fever, jaundice, and/or hepatosplenomegaly. This ruled out involvement of reticuloendothelial or hepatobiliary system. Pain abdomen and abnormal bowel habits point towards an abdominal cause of anemia. It is possible that the child was having occult bleeding from the GI tract. Nutritional deficiency of iron leading to anemia was unlikely since dietary intake was reported to be normal.

Q. How will you investigate this child?

Firstly, I would like to examine the peripheral smear to identify the morphology of RBCs and look for any abnormal cells. I will also get the hemoglobin level and blood counts. Secondly, to look for blood loss from GIT, I will order a stool occult blood test.

Blood examination revealed following: Hb 7.0 g/dL, microcytic hypochromic RBC and no features of hemolysis. WBC and platelet counts were normal. Stool for occult blood was positive.

Q. On further questioning, you realize that child belongs to a rural area and spends quite some time walking barefoot in the fields. Does that change/modify your diagnosis. How will you confirm it?

A strong possibility exists for hookworm infestation, which typically presents with anemia (without fever or RES involvement) in a physically active child. A stool microscopic examination should be done for at least 3 days, consecutively, for ova/cyst of *Ankylostoma duodenale* or *Necator americanus*. Stool examination for ova/cyst by Lugol Iodine preparation showed eggs of *Ancyclostoma duodenale*. Clinical presentation (age of the child, rural residence, anemia, abdominal complaints); peripheral smear findings (microcytic hypochromic anemia, normal WBC and platelets counts); and presence of occult blood in stool support the diagnosis of hookworm infestation.

Treatment	Hookworm

Eradication of worms is achieved with albendazole (400 mg, PO, single dose, for all ages), or mebendazole (100 mg, PO, twice a day for 3 days). Pyrantel pamoate orally (11 mg /kg once daily for 3 days) is also effective. Anemia is treated with oral iron therapy. Severe anemia may require a packed cell transfusion.

6

6.26 ENTEROBIASIS

(*Pinworm or Threadworm: Enterobius vermicularis*)

Enterobius vermicularis is a small (1 cm long), white, thread-like nematode that lives in the cecum, appendix, ileum and ascending colon. Eggs are not usually liberated in the gut. Rather, gravid females migrate at night into the perianal region and release up to 15,000 eggs there. The egg becomes infective within 6 hours. Perianal scratching causes transfer of eggs to finger nails. Infection occurs when eggs are ingested. Eggs take 35–60 days to develop into adult worms. The larvae hatch and mature within the intestine. The adult worm lives for about 2 months.

Pathogenesis

Man is the only reservoir. Larvae enter the human body by oral route. Transmission occurs by any of the following methods:

  i. Most commonly from perianal region to the mouth.
  ii. By ingestion of viable eggs present in soiled bed linen and other contaminated objects.
  iii. Via mouth or nose from contaminated eggs in dust.
  iv. Retroinfection. Eggs hatch near anus and larvae migrate up the bowel.

Pinworm can infect all age groups, but prevalence is highest in 5–14 years old children. Worm burden tends to be higher in younger age group. There appears to be no sex predilection. Pinworm usually affects all members of the family as it is easily transmitted from one child or person to a new host. The infection is common in lower socioeconomic regions where personal hygiene is poor. Ova usually contaminate the area beneath the fingernails. The lack of proper hygiene favors the transmission.

Clinical Features

Perianal itching, especially in night is the most common complaint. The exact cause of itching is not known but is believed to be due to migration of worm in the perianal region. Pruritus ani may be associated with anorexia, weight loss, irritability, and enuresis.

Itching also leads to restless sleep, irritability, and enuresis. Complications include ectopic lesions such as vulvitis. Rarely, the worm may migrate to ear, nose, liver, kidney, and lungs.

Diagnosis

Direct visualization of the adult worm or microscopic detection of eggs confirms the diagnosis, but only 5% of infected persons have eggs in their stool. The "*cellophane tape test*" can serve as a quick way to clinch the diagnosis. This test consists of touching tape to the perianal area several times, removing it, and examining the tape under direct microscopy for eggs. The test should be conducted right after awakening on at least 3 consecutive days. This technique can increase the test's sensitivity to roughly 90%.

Treatment	Enterobiasis

Infected persons and their family members should be treated with a single oral dose of mebendazole (100 mg PO for all ages) or albendazole (400 mg, PO) and repeated after 2 weeks again to achieve a cure rate of 90–100%. Single dose of pyrantel pamoate (11 mg/kg), or ivermectin (150–200 µg/kg) are also highly effective.

Pinworm infection may be difficult to eradicate due to repeated autoinfection. Maintenance of personal hygiene remains the key to prevent autoinfections. Morning bath and frequent change of underclothing are important.

6.27 TRICHURIASIS

(*Whipworm: Trichuris trichiura*)

The normal habitat of *Trichuris trichiura* is the cecum, ascending colon, and appendix. Adult worms measures 3–5 cm in length. The anterior three-fourths portion of the worm is threaded into superficial mucosa and the short posterior part is free in the lumen of the gut. Infection is transmitted directly by ingestion of embryonated eggs in contaminated food, water and hands or indirectly through flies and other insects. Larva escapes from the eggs in small intestine moving down to lodge in cecum. The average lifespan of the adult worm is up to one year. Infection is most common in the 5–15 years of age.

Incubation period is usually 60 days. Infection is asymptomatic in most cases due to low worm load. Adult worms suck approximately 0.005 mL blood per worm per day that is not sufficient enough to cause significant anemia. Heavy worm loads are associated with dysentery, anemia, rectal prolapse, epigastric pain, abdominal distension,

---

Case Study	Enterobius Infestation

A 3-yr-old girl was brought to pediatric outpatient department with chief complaint of excessive itching in the periurethral area. There was no history of fever, burning micturition or increase in itching during or after micturition. There was no history of foul smelling vaginal discharge, constipation, or history of similar illness in the family. The itching typically increased during night time. On examination, child had poor personal hygiene. Vitals and systemic examination were normal. Local examination revealed erythema in perianal and periurethral area with scratch marks. There was no rash or vaginal discharge.

Q. Enumerate causes of periurethral itching. What is the likely possibility in this case and how will you confirm the diagnosis?

It may be difficult for a small child to localize the symptoms to periurethral or perianal area. Therefore, causes for localized itching in periurethral area could be: 1) Urinary tract infection (UTI), 2) vaginitis, 3) anal fissure, and 4) pinworm infestation.

Absence of fever, burning micturition, and normal urine culture and microscopy examination will rule out UTI. Absence of foul smelling vaginal discharge rules out vaginitis. No history of constipation or hard stools with excessive straining rules out anal fissure. Scabies is also less likely, since there is no rash and no family history of itching.

Pinworm infestation appears to be most probable diagnosis, with a history of poor personal hygiene and excessive itching during night. Cellophane test is the investigation of choice. Cellophane test was done for 3 consecutive days. On two days, it revealed eggs of *Enterobius vermicularis*. Child was given albendazole and mother was counseled to maintain personal hygiene.

hypoproteinemia, and growth retardation. Trichuriasis frequently co-exists with amebiasis, roundworm or hookworm infestation.

Diagnosis is made by identification of characteristic 'barrel-shaped eggs' in the feces. Blood eosinophilia is minimal. Mebendazole (100 mg twice a day for three days or 500 mg single dose, PO, for all ages) is recommended and associated with a cure rate of 70–90%. A single dose of albendazole (400 mg) or ivermectin (150–200 µg/kg) is an effective alternative.

Brooker S, Clements AC, Bundy DA. Global epidemiology, ecology and control of soil transmitted helminth infections. *Adv Parasitol*. 2006;62:221–61.

Jex AR, Lim YA, Bethony JM, *et al*. Soil-transmitted helminths of humans in Southeast Asia—towards integrated control. *Adv Parasitol*. 2011;74:231–65.

Jia TW, Melville S, Utzinger J, *et al*. Soil-transmitted helminth reinfection after drug treatment: a systematic review and meta-analysis. *PLoS Negl Trop Dis*. 2012;6:e1621.

Keiser J, Utzinger J. The drugs we have and the drugs we need against major helminth infections. *Adv Parasitol*. 2010;73:197–230.

Keiser J, Utzinger J. Efficacy of current drugs against soil-transmitted helminth infections: systematic review and meta-analysis. *JAMA*. 2008;299:1937–48.

Knopp S, Steinmann P, Keiser J, *et al*. Nematode infections: soil-transmitted helminths and Trichinella. *Infect Dis Clin North Am*. 2012;26:341–58.

Knopp S, Mgeni AF, Khamis IS, *et al*. Diagnosis of soil-transmitted helminths in the era of preventive chemotherapy: effect of multiple stool sampling and use of different diagnostic techniques. *PLoSNegl Trop Dis*. 2008;2:e331.

Mascarini-Serra L. Prevention of soil-transmitted helminth infection. *J Glob Infect Dis*. 2011;3:175–82.

Moncayo AL, Vaca M, Amorim L, *et al*. Impact of long-term treatment with ivermectin on the prevalence and intensity of soil-transmitted helminth infections. *PLoSNegl Trop Dis*. 2008;2:e293.

Sarinas PS, Chitkara RK. Ascariasis and hookworm. *Semin Respir Infect*. 1997;12:130–7.

Steinmann P, Utzinger J, Du ZW, *et al*. Efficacy of single-dose and triple-dose albendazole and mebendazole against soil-transmitted helminths and *Taenia* spp.: a randomized controlled trial. *PLoS One*. 2011;6:e25003.

Ziegelbauer K, Speich B, Mäusezahl D, *et al*. Effect of sanitation on soil-transmitted helminth infection: systematic review and meta-analysis. *PLoS Med*. 2012;9:e1001162.

6.28 *TAENIA SOLIUM* AND *TAENIA SAGINATA*

These worms are also known as the pork tapeworm (*T. solium*) and beef tapeworm (*T. saginata*), reflecting the principal intermediate hosts for each of them. Man is the only definitive host for both the parasites. *Taenia solium* consists of a scolex with suckers and hooks, by which it attaches to the intestinal wall. Hooks are absent in *T. saginata*. Usually only one adult worm is found in the intestine which may live for up to 25 years.

Intermediate stage of *Taenia solium* is known as cysticercus. Cystricercus, on its own can also infect humans. The resultant disease—cysticercosis—can practically involve almost any part of the body.

Pathogenesis

Infection with adult tapeworm (taeniasis) is acquired by ingestion of undercooked pork and beef, containing infectious cysticerci. Human cysticercosis, on the other hand, is acquired by consumption of food and water contaminated

---

Case Study Neurocysticercosis

An 8-year-old boy was brought to pediatric emergency with right sided focal seizures lasting for more than 5 minutes. This episode was aborted with intravenous lorazepam after checking for airway, breathing, and circulation. This episode was not preceded or associated with fever, altered sensorium, behavioral abnormalities, headache, vomiting, rash, blurring of vision, or neck stiffness. There was no past history of seizures. On examination, vitals and blood pressure were normal. Child was oriented to time, place, and person. General physical examination was normal. Neurological examination was normal. Systemic examination was also normal.

Q. What is the likely diagnosis?

Seizures lasting for more than 5 minutes are labeled as status epilepticus. The most common cause of a focal seizure, in an otherwise normal child (without any neurodevelopmental or systemic manifestations), in our setting is an irritative lesion in the brain—most likely neurocysticercosis or tuberculoma. Absence of fever, altered sensorium, and meningeal signs rules out meningitis or encephalitis. Also there was no focal neurological deficit, blood pressure was normal, and bilateral pupils were reacting to light equally; so possibility of stroke involving thrombus or hemorrhage is also less likely. At present, this episode cannot be labeled as epilepsy, since that is defined as more than 1 episode of seizures, at least 24 h apart.

Q. How will you confirm your diagnosis?

I would like to get a neuroimaging done, preferably MRI of brain. MRI T2 and FLAIR images reveal a ring enhancing lesion with surrounding edema. This was associated with an eccentrically placed scolex of cysticercosis within the lesion. These findings are consistent with neurocysticercosis. Tuberculosis was ruled out by doing a chest X-ray and Mantoux test.

Q. How will you treat this child?

I would like to start the child on an anti-epileptic agent, preferably carbamazepine (to be continued for at least 2 years, from the date of last seizure activity) along with oral steroids (prednisolone 2 mg/kg/d orally x initial 3 days) to reduce the pericystic edema. After 3 days of administering steroids, I would prescribe albendazole (10 mg/kg/day PO) for 28 days.

---

with eggs of *T. solium*. Therefore, cysticercosis may occur in persons who do not eat pork. Infection can also arise by autoinfection, if eggs reflux from intestine into the stomach from reverse peristalsis. Persons infected with an adult *T. solium* may also infect themselves with the eggs by the fecal-oral route.

Clinical Features

Most infections with adult worms are asymptomatic. Some children may develop nonspecific complaints like nausea, pain in abdomen, and diarrhea. Carriers have an increased risk of developing cysticercosis by repeated autoinfection. Rarely, adult worms can cause intestinal obstruction, cholangitis, appendicitis, and pancreatitis.

Cysticercosis

Infection with the intermediate stage (larvae) of *T. solium* results in cysticercosis. The intermediate stage of beef

6

tapeworm is noninfectious to humans. Neurocysticercosis is the most common parasitic infection of the CNS and may account for as high as 20–50% cases of unprovoked seizures. Following ingestion, eggs develop into larvae in the small intestine. Larvae migrate across the intestinal wall and are carried to the target organs by bloodstream. The common target organs for cysticerci are brain, muscle and subcutaneous tissue. The larvae mature into cysticerci in about two months. The size of cysticerci varies from 2 mm to 2 cm. Clinical manifestations depend on the location, number and size of cysts in the brain and host inflammatory response. Viable cysts generally do not elicit a strong response. On the other hand, degenerating cysts provoke a vigorous host response. Most cysts remain viable for 5–10 years. Neurocysticercosis may manifest as partial or generalized seizure, raised intracranial tension, focal neurological deficits, or disturbances in consciousness or behavior.

Diagnosis

The diagnosis of taeniasis is established by the demonstration of eggs or proglottids in the stools. Patients may pass motile segments of worms through anus. Diagnosis of neurocysticercosis is made by MRI of brain. Details of diagnosis and management of neurocysticercosis are discussed in Chapter on Neurological Disorders.

Treatment	Taeniasis

Treatment of taeniasis is similar for both infestations. A single dose of niclosamide (50 mg/kg) or praziquantel (25 mg/kg) is effective. Purgation is not essential.

Cysticercosis needs to be treated with albendazole (15 mg/kg twice daily) for 15–30 days or praziquental 50–100 mg 3 times a day for 30 days.

Flisser A, Avila G, Maravilla P, *et al*. Taenia solium: current understanding of laboratory animal models of taeniosis. *Parasitology*. 2010;137:347–57.

Silva CV, Costa-Cruz JM. A glance at Taenia saginata infection, diagnosis, vaccine, biological control and treatment. *Infect Disord Drug Targets*. 2010;10:313–21.

6.29 ECHINOCOCCOSIS (HYDATID DISEASE)

(*E. granulosus* and *E. multilocularis*)
Human echinococcosis is caused by larval stages of *E. granulosus* or *E. multilocularis,* and is characterized by production of unilocular or multilocular cystic disease of lung and liver. Clinical manifestations are also known as *hydatid disease* or *hydatidosis*.

Pathogenesis

The adult parasite is a small tapeworm (0.5 cm length) with 2–6 segments. Dog is the definitive host while sheep, cattle and goats act as intermediate hosts for *E. granulosus*. Man serves as an accidental host. Adult worm lives in the intestine of dog. Eggs from the adult worm are released in the feces of the dog and contaminate the water and soil, and also the coats of dogs. Humans are infected by consuming food or water contaminated with eggs or by direct contact with infected dogs.

Larvae hatch in the human intestines, penetrate mucosa, and are carried to the target organs. Liver and lungs are the principal target organs, where larvae develop into characteristic *hydatid cysts*. Lung cysts are more common in children whereas liver cysts are more common in adults.

A cyst has two walls; an outer membrane and an inner germinal layer. Inner aspect of the germinal layer harbors daughter cysts. The fluid in a hepatic cyst appears clear and watery. After treatment, it may become thick and bile stained. The cyst keeps on expanding over years at the rate of 1 cm per year. Life cycle of *E. multilocularis* is the same except that rodents and mice serve as intermediate hosts.

Clinical Features

Symptoms occur due to mass effect of the cyst and are related to the organ in which they occur. Liver cysts present with abdominal pain and a palpable mass. Lung cyst may present with chest pain, hemoptysis and breathlessness. There may be passage of cysts in the urine (hydatiduria) and hematuria following hydatid disease of the kidneys. Rupture or leakage from a hydatid cyst may cause fever, itching, rash, anaphylaxis, and dissemination of infectious scolices. Hydatid cysts have been reported from almost all body organs. Central nervous system, subcutaneous tissue, bone, heart and eyes are the other frequently involved organs.

Diagnosis

Diagnosis is made by ultrasonography and CT scan. Ultrasound can reveal the internal membranes of cyst, floating echogenic cyst material (hydatid sand) and daughter cysts within the parent cyst. These findings are of value in differentiating hydatid cyst from simple cysts of liver. Diagnostic aspiration is generally contraindicated because of risk of infection and anaphylaxis. Antibody detection by ELISA is more sensitive but less specific.

Treatment	Hydatid Disease

PAIR This is the preferred therapy in most cases; and consists of ultrasound or CT-guided **P**ercutaneous **A**spiration, **I**nstillation of hypertonic saline or another scolicidal agent, and **R**easpiration (PAIR) after 15 minutes. The chances of spillage with PAIR are minimal. Albendazole is given both before and after percutaneous drainage of hydatid cysts, to achieve better cyst-reduction. It is started at least 1 week prior and continued up to 4 weeks after the procedure. Results of PAIR plus albendazole are similar to surgical removal of the cyst; with less adverse effects.

Medical therapy consists of albendazole 15 mg/kg/day in two divided doses for 1–6 months. The efficacy rate is 40–60%. Albendazole therapy is quite safe. Most common side effects are elevated levels of hepatic enzymes and abdominal pain. Rarely, there may be headache, abdominal distension, and alopecia. The response to medical therapy is monitored by serial ultrasonography. Successful therapy is indicated by change in size and shape of the cyst, increase in echogenicity, and separation of membranes from the capsule (*water lily sign*).

Surgical removal can be contemplated for (*i*) a large liver cyst with multiple daughter cyst; (*ii*) solitary superficial liver cysts; (*iii*) infected cyst; and (*iv*) cyst in lung, brain, bone, and kidneys.

Hydatid Disease

1. Hydatid disease is a zoonoses caused by tapeworm, *Echinococcus granulosus* and *Echinococcus multilocularis*.
2. Man is an accidental host and gets infected by the fecal-oral route while coming in contact with infected dogs and sheep.
3. Hydatid disease can cause cysts in almost any organ of the body. Liver and lungs are the most commonly affected organs.
4. Diagnosis is by ultrasound or CT.
5. Surgery is the mainstay of treatment for most cysts. Medical treatment is a necessary adjunct of surgical treatment and can be used as the sole modality for simple, isolated cysts.
6. PAIR has shown better results in hydatid cysts of the liver and other intra-abdominal organs.

Kern P. Clinical features and treatment of alveolar echinococcosis. *Curr Opin Infect Dis*. 2010;23:505–12.

Mandal S, Mandal MD. Human cystic echinococcosis: epidemiologic, zoonotic, clinical, diagnostic and therapeutic aspects. *Asian Pac J Trop Med*. 2012;5:253–60.

Nabi MS, Waseem T. Pulmonary hydatid disease: what is the optimal surgical strategy? *Int J Surg*. 2010;8:612–6.

Nasseri-Moghaddam S, Abrishami A, Taefi A, *et al.* Percutaneous needle aspiration, injection, and re-aspiration with or without benzimidazole coverage for uncomplicated hepatic hydatid cysts. *Cochrane Database Syst Rev*. 2011;1:CD003623.

Nunnari G, Pinzone MR, Gruttadauria S, *et al.* Hepatic echinococcosis: clinical and therapeutic aspects. *World J Gastroenterol*. 2012;18:1448–58.

6.30 RICKETTSIAL INFECTIONS

Rickettsia comprises a group of microorganisms that phylogenetically occupy a position between bacteria and viruses. These are arthropod-borne organisms belonging to the genus Rickettsia within the family Rickettsiaceae in the order Rickettsiales, Proteobacteria.

It is a zoonotic disease transmitted to man by arthropods e.g. lice, flea, tick, and mite. The reservoir hosts for these arthropods are humans, rodents, dogs, cattle, etc.

It is increasingly realised that rickettsial infections are under-diagnosed and they substantially contribute to the burden of preventable acute febrile illness all over the world. The greatest challenge to the clinician is the diagnostic dilemma posed by these infections early in their clinical course, when antimicrobial therapy is most effective.

The usual presentation of rickettsial fever is the classic triad of fever, headache, and rash. Yet many times the early signs and symptoms are notoriously nonspecific or mimic viral illnesses. This makes early diagnosis difficult. Delayed diagnosis and treatment can lead to severe illness, complications and death.

CLASSIFICATION OF RICKETTSIAL INFECTIONS

Based on the serological reactions, the Rickettsia is divided into "spotted fever" and "typhus" groups. The outer membrane protein A is detected in spotted fever group but not in typhus group (**Table 6.29**). More than 20 types of spotted fever varieties are described depending upon the geographical area where these are prevalent.

Among the major groups of rickettsioses, commonly reported diseases in India are scrub typhus, Indian tick typhus, murine typhus, and Q fever.

A. Scrub Typhus

Scrub typhus, also known as 'tsutsugamushi disease', is an acute, febrile infectious disease caused by *Orientia tsutsugamushi*. It is a zoonotic disease where humans are accidental hosts. Some species of trombiculid mites known as 'chiggers' (*Leptotrombidium deliense*) are known to transmit scrub typhus to rodents and humans. The humans acquire

Table 6.29 Classification of Rickettsial Infections				
Biogroup	*Disease*	*Vector*	*Host*	*Organism*
Spotted fever (SFG) (tick-borne)	Rocky mountain spotted fever (RMSF)	Tick	Dogs and rodents	*Rickettsia rickettsii*
	Rickettsialpox	Mite	Mice	*Rickettsia akari*
	Indian tick typhus /Mediterranean spotted fever (MSF)	Tick	Dogs and rodents	*Rickettsia conorii*
Typhus (insect-borne)	Epidemic louse-borne typhus	Louse	Human	*Rickettsia prowazekii*
	Brill-Zinsser disease (recrudescent typhus)	Louse	Human	*Rickettsia prowazekii*
	Endemic/murine flea-borne typhus	Flea	Rats	*Rickettsia typhi*
Scrub typhus (ST) (mite-borne)	Scrub typhus	Chigger (mites)	Rodents	*Orientia tsutsugamushi*
Miscellaneous	Ehrlichiosis and anaplasmosis	Tick	Deer, dogs and rodents	*Ehrlichia, Anaplasma*
	TIBOLA (tick-borne lymphadeno-pathy)	Tick	Wild boar	*Rickettsia slovaca*
	DEBONEL	Tick	Wild boar	*Rickettsia slovaca*
	Q fever	Nil	Cattle, sheep, goat	*Coxiella burnetii*

Abbreviation: DEBONEL: dermacentor-borne necrosis-eschar-lymphadenopathy

6

the disease when an infected chigger bites on the skin—leaving behind a characteristic black eschar.

Misdiagnosis and under-reporting of scrub typhus is common because of the non-specific nature of the clinical features and also because of the fact that the characteristic eschar is detected in as few as 40% of the cases. In addition, most of the districts in India which are endemic to scrub typhus lack diagnostic facilities. It is estimated that one million new cases surface annually and about one billion people are at risk for scrub typhus in India. Mortality varies from 0–30%.

B. Indian Tick Typhus (ITT)

R. conorii is presumed to cause Indian tick typhus. Various genera of ticks (e.g. *Rhipicephalus, Ixodes, Boophilus, and Haemaphysalis*) have been incriminated as vectors. Pet animals such as dogs and some rodents can be affected by ticks and these being the reservoirs, constitute an important link in the disease cycle. In view of close physical proximity, these animals expose humans to infection from rickettsial organisms.

Indian tick typhus (ITT) is prevalent in districts of Maharashtra, Karnataka, and Tamil Nadu. The disease bears many graphically descriptive names. For instance, *kankapya* meaning cut earlobe refers to autoamputation of the earlobes as a result of vascular endarteritis. *Bibtya* which means leopard refers to the rashes of spotted fever which remind one of the spots on a leopard skin. *Motha Govar* which means 'big measles' refers to the fact that rash of ITT is larger in comparison with the rash seen in measles. In Karnataka, it is known as *Unni Jwara* referring to its origin from ticks.

Clinical manifestations of ITT are less severe when compared to Rocky mountain spotted fever. Rash in Indian tick typhus is papular and eschar is rarely seen at the bite-site.

C. Epidemic Typhus

Epidemic typhus is a potentially lethal exhanthematous disease caused by the bacterium *Rickettsia prowazekii,* and transmitted by the human louse. Louse-bite and the ensuing scratch results in inoculation of *Rickettsia prowazekii* into the bloodstream. Since louse infestation is directly related to bad personal hygiene and overcrowding, there is a greater chance of spread of epidemic typhus in those areas that are affected by natural and man-made disasters like wars, famines and floods.

In India, epidemic typhus is known to occur among sub-Himalayan population and also in West Bengal, Himachal Pradesh, and Uttarakhand.

D. Q Fever

Q fever is caused by *Coxiella burnetii* and is highly contagious. It is prevalent all over the world. Delhi, Haryana, Punjab, and Rajasthan are affected more than the southern peninsula. Persons who come in close contact with domesticated animals like cattle, sheep, and goats are at greater risk. As per the serological surveys, overall prevalence rate of Q fever among human population is highest (18.6%) in Rajasthan.

Natural reservoirs are ticks, sheep, goat, and some wild animals. The infected animals contaminate the soil with these causative agents through their excreta and urine. Infected cows and sheep create infected aerosols while giving birth to their young ones because their placenta contains the infectious agent. Many domesticated animals like camels, horses, and sheep can act as maintenance hosts.

Unlike other rickettsial infections, Q fever is not transmitted to humans through an arthropod. Transmission of agent takes place when humans inhale dust from the soil which is already contaminated by the feces and urine of infected reservoir animals. The causative agents can gain access to the human body through skin abrasions or conjunctiva or when contaminated food materials like meat or milk products are ingested. Inhalation is regarded as the most important mode of transmission of Q fever.

MAGNITUDE OF THE PROBLEM

Scrub typhus It is the commonest occurring rickettsial infection in India. It has been reported from Delhi, Himachal Pradesh, Maharashtra, Jammu and Kashmir, Haryana, Karnataka and Tamil Nadu.

Spotted fever Megaw first observed spotted fever in the year 1917 in the foothills of Himalayas. Indian tick typhus (ITT) is widely prevalent in many districts of Maharashtra, Karnataka, and Tamil Nadu.

Q fever It is prevalent in Delhi, Rajasthan, Haryana, Punjab and many other parts of the country.

Endemic typhus It has been reported from the hills of Shimla, Jabalpur, Pune, Mumbai, and the Kashmir valley.

ETIOLOGY

A. Agent

Rickettsia are Gram-negative and non-spore forming bacteria. These are highly pleomorphic. These are obligate, intracellular micro-organisms seen as rods (1–4 microns), cocci (0.1 micron) and thread-like (10 microns). After invading the host cell, these organisms replicate by binary fission and metabolize host-derived glutamate through aerobic respiration and citric acid cycle (TCA). Rickettsiae possess major antigens such as lipopolysaccharides, lipoproteins and outer membrane proteins (ompA, ompB) on surface cell antigen (SCA). The Weil-Felix test, initially developed as a diagnostic test for rickettsioses, was based on the antigenic cross-reactions among rickettsial antigens, mostly lipopolysaccharide (LPS), and *Proteus vulgaris* strains OX19 and OX2, and *Proteus mirabilis* OXK.

B. Vector and Hosts

Natural hosts and vectors for rickettsial organisms are the ticks, fleas, mites and louse. Man is an accidental host. Infected ticks transmit the organisms to their progeny through transovarian route and trans-stadial passage.

Children aged between 5 and 15 years and male children tend to suffer more from a particularly severe form of rickettsial infection with fatal outcome. Patients with diabetes mellitus are more prone for severe form of the disease. Glucose-6-phosphate dehydrogenase (G6PD) deficiency is associated with a fulminant form of spotted fever.

C. Reservoir

Rodents and dogs serve as reservoir hosts for the vectors of rickettsial organisms. They bring the infected vectors into contact with the environment shared by the humans and expose them to infection. The reservoir and hosts themselves can develop rickettsial disease.

D. Transmission

Ticks regurgitate the infected saliva during feeding and transmit the microorganisms to their mammalian hosts that include humans.

PATHOGENESIS

Inoculation of rickettsial organisms into the dermis of the skin of the victims takes place when an infected tick bites or when feces of lice or fleas are deposited on damaged skin.

Once inoculated into the dermis, the rickettsial organisms spread through bloodstream and infect and adhere to the cells of endothelium. These organisms damage the integrity of endothelium through release of cytokines, resulting in leakage of fluid and platelet aggregation. The aggregation of platelets leads to focal occlusive endarteritis, micro-infarctions and the typical 'Typhus nodules of Wolbach' in brain, skin, skeletal muscle, cardiac muscle, liver, lungs, and kidneys. Venous thrombosis and gangrene of the extremities may result. Increased vascular permeability leads to interstitial edema, loss of blood volume, hypoalbuminemia, decreased osmotic pressure, and hypotension. Disseminated intravascular coagulation is rare.

CLINICAL FEATURES

Rickettsial infections have a wide range of presentations. They may manifest as a mild self-limiting febrile illness or a life-threatening condition requiring intensive care.

Incubation phase Incubation period varies from 2–14 days. At times, it may be as long as 28 days. Usually, diligent questioning may elicit history of a tick-bite prior to illness. At times, history of close contact with an infected or a vector-carrying pet animal such as a dog may be forth-coming. Sometimes, history of travel to and from an endemic area or presence of a similar febrile illness in a family member is available.

Prodromal phase Early in the disease course, the symptoms are non-specific. The affected patient presents with fever, headache, restlessness, myalgia, and anorexia. Pain and tenderness in calf muscles is common. Nausea, vomiting, diarrhea, and abdominal cramps are common during early phase of the disease.

Rash Typical rash of rickettsial fever does not appear until 2–3 days after the onset of symptoms. To begin with, rash is discrete. The maculopapular or pale, rose-red, blanching macules appear typically on extremities such as ankles, wrists, legs, and forearms. Later in the course, the rash spreads rapidly to involve the entire body including the palms and soles (Fig. 6.18). The rash tends to be become more petechial after several days. It can even be hemorrhagic with palpable purpura (Fig. 6.19). In a particularly severe form of the disease, the petechiae may enlarge into ecchymosis and show areas of necrosis within.

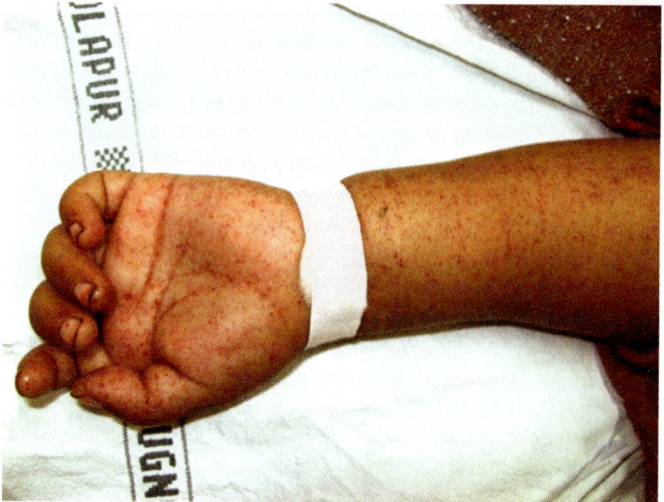

Fig. 6.18 Purpuric rash over palm

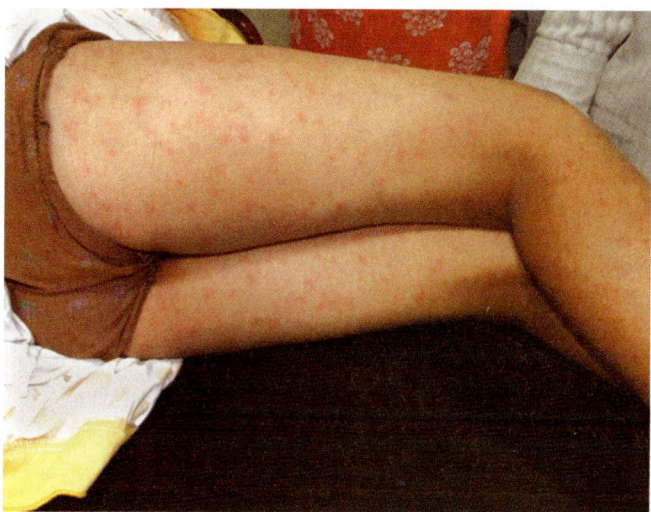

Fig. 6.19 Palpable purpura over legs

Systemic involvement Severe vaso-occlusive disease of the small-sized arteries due to endarteritis and thrombosis, though infrequent, may result in gangrene of the toes, digits, (Fig. 6.20) ear-lobes (Fig. 6.21), and sometimes entire limbs. Painless eschar, *the tache noire* may be seen at the site of initial tick-bite. Regional lymphadenopathy may also be detected. Edema over dorsum of hand and feet or generalized edema may be seen. Neurological manifestations include confusion and lethargy during initial phase and stupor, delirium and coma as the disease progresses. At times, seizures are also observed. Onset of coma and seizures usually denotes fatal outcome. Pulmonary involvement results in non-cardiogenic pulmonary edema, interstitial pneumonitis and respiratory distress syndrome. Myocarditis, acute renal failure and hepatitis are seen in more severe form of the disease.

COMPLICATIONS

- Non-cardiogenic pulmonary edema from pulmonary microvascular leakage
- Cerebral edema and meningoencephalitis

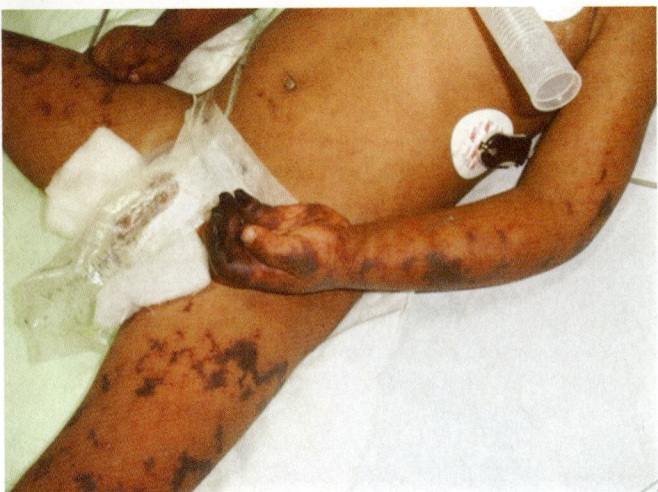

Fig. 6.20 Gangrene of digits

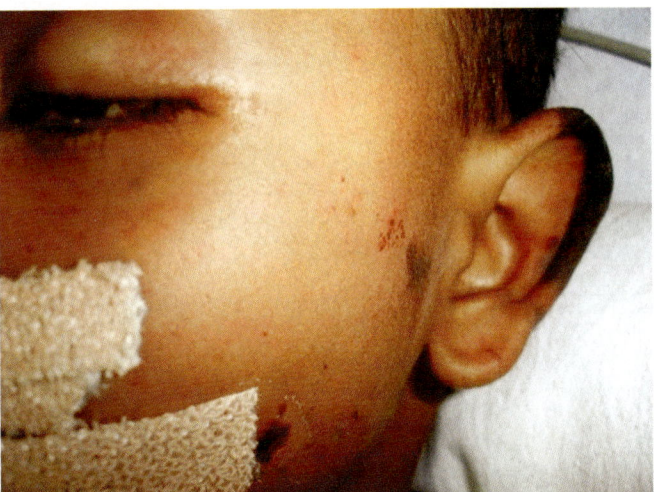

Fig. 6.21 Gangrene of earlobe

- Multiorgan damage due to microvascular occlusion, resulting in hypoperfusion, ischemia, and acute renal failure
- Paraparesis, motor dysfunction, hearing loss, peripheral neuropathy, language disorder, bladder and bowel incontinence, learning disabilities and behavioral problems

Scrub Typhus

The bite of a chigger (a family of mites) is painless. However, it may cause a localized itch. The bites may be seen usually on groins, axillae, genitalia and neck. In about 10–40% of the patients, an eschar is seen at the bite-site. The illness begins suddenly with shaking chills, severe headache and fever. Conjunctivitis and acute enlargement of the lymph nodes may be seen. A spotted rash on the trunk is seen in 40–60% of cases. Rash may be difficult to appreciate in dark skin patient and it may be transient.

Muscular pain and tenderness (myalgia) associated with colicky abdominal pain may be present. In about one-third of the patients, onset of fever is accompanied by loss of hearing. This is a useful clue for diagnosis. However, this loss of hearing must be differentiated from the transient loss of hearing due to nasal congestion which is also a common feature in scrub typhus. Sensorineural hearing loss was documented by audiometry in Thai patients. It resolved after treatment. Cough associated with soft infiltrates on a chest radiograph is a common feature in patients afflicted with scrub typhus infection.

Hemorrhage and intravascular coagulation are noticed in scrub typhus caused by more virulent strains of *O. tsutsugamushi*. In such cases, complications include atypical pneumonia, ARDS, myocarditis, and disseminated intravascular coagulation (DIC).

Q Fever

Q fever is an acute febrile illness which presents as fever coupled with chills, generalized malaise, and severe headache. The clinical picture resembles viral pneumonia or influenza rather than typhus fever. The infection can lead to pneumonia, hepatitis, encephalitis, or endocarditis.

Epidemic Typhus

Fever, headache, drowsiness, and maculopapular rash are the usual initial features. Signs of scratching on the skin are typically seen. Maculopapular rash is seen in 10–30% of the patients and appears first on back, chest, and abdomen but quickly spreads to the palms and soles. Involvement of central nervous system manifests as meningeal irritation, headache, drowsiness, seizures, and coma in severe, untreated patients. Involvement of cardiovascular and respiratory system causes myocarditis, interstitial pneumonia, and bronchiolitis. Thrombocytopenia, jaundice, and abnormal liver function tests are noticed whenever hepatobiliary system is affected.

Brill-Zinsser disease which occurs as a result of reactivation of a previous infection is usually a milder type of illness with fever and a light rash. A full-blown epidemic typhus can be fatal, if not diagnosed early and treated judiciously.

DIAGNOSIS OF RICKETTSIAL INFECTIONS

Diagnosis of rickettsial disease should be suspected in every febrile patient with the clinical features outlined in **Box 6.5**. Indian Council of Medical Research (ICMR) in 2015 has provided case-definitions for use in the country, to diagnose rickettsial infections (**Box 6.6**).

One should not wait for confirmation of rickettsial infection and treatment should be started on clinical and epidemiological clues to avoid morbidity or mortality due to delay in diagnosis.

Laboratory Diagnosis

Weil-Felix test Similarity of Proteus antigens OX 19, OX 2, OX K with rickettsial antigens is principle of this heterophile antibody agglutination test. The test is usually positive after 5–7 days and 1:80 or rising titers are suggestive of rickettsial infections. This test has low sensitivity and specificity due to which its use has been discouraged in evidence-based practice. However, since it shows good correlation with IgM by indirect immunofluorescent assay (IFA) and since it is easily available in many cities and laboratories, it has been a popular screening test and a useful diagnostic tool in the

---

Box 6.5 Clues for Clinical Diagnosis of Rickettsial Infections

1. Patient hailing from an area which is endemic to rickettsial infections.
2. A definitive history of a tick-bite and/or contact with animals like dogs, rodents, and cattle.
3. Clinical triad of fever, rash, and headache (irritability in younger children).
4. Maculopapular rash extending over palms and soles, purpuric and necrotic rash, presence of eschar.
5. Gangrene of digits, toes, earlobes.
6. Edematous swelling of the body, hands, and feet associated with hepatosplenomegaly, lymphadenopathy.
7. Fever and rash associated with convulsions and change in sensorium.
8. Fever which is unresponsive to usual antibiotics.

Box 6.6 Case Definitions (ICMR 2015) for Rickettsial Diseases

Suspected Case

Any undifferentiated fever without focus for more than 5 days should be suspected as case of rickettsial infection. Presence of eschar suggests scrub typhus, even if duration of fever is less than 5 days. Differential diagnosis of dengue, malaria, pneumonia, leptospirosis, enteric fever, meningococcemia, measles, enteroviral exanthems and uncommon causes like toxic shock syndrome, rubella, parvoviral infection, ITP, TTP, HUS, and hepatitis should be considered.

Probable Case

Positive Weil Felix test with titers >80 or fourfold rise in titers or positive Elisa test with OD > 0.5 for IgM antibodies.

Confirmed Case

Positive rickettsial DNA detection in blood or eschar, by PCR or rising antibody titer in sera by indirect immunofluorescent assay (IFA)/ indirect immmunoperoxidase assay (IPA).

---

developing countries. Single titer of >1:320 or fourfold rise of titer in paired sera is highly suggestive and specific. A high titer of only OX K antigen is fairly suggestive of *O. tsutsugamushi* infection, scrub typhus or murine typhus. Similarly, high titers of OX 2 suggest spotted fever infection and high OX 19 titers indicate typhus group, RMSF.

Enzyme-linked immunosorbent assay (ELISA) IgM ELISA is one of the more sensitive tests which is available at a few selected laboratories and some tertiary care hospitals in developing world. Its sensitivity and specificity reaches almost 90%. A significant IgM titer is seen at end of 6–7 days suggestive of acute infection, IgG antibodies appear after 2–3 weeks.

Polymerase chain reaction (PCR) Rickettsial DNA can be detected by PCR, from blood or eschar sample. This is the most definitive test for diagnosis of rickettsemia and can be positive within first week itself of the illness.

Immunofluorescent assay (IFA) Indirect immunofluorescent assay (IFA) is considered as gold standard test for diagnosis of rickettsial fever. Antibody titers IgM >1:640 and IgG >1:254 suggest acute infection, while IgG >64 but <124 is suggestive of past infection. The antibody titers rise after 5–7 days of the infection and peak at third week. These tests are available

Case Study Rickettsial Infection

A farmer from a remote village brought his 4-year-old son with history of fever for 7 days, maculopapular rash, and leg pain. Fever was not relieved by antipyretics and antibiotics as prescribed by the local doctor. Rash appeared on the extremities and later spread to involve the entire body including palms and soles.

On physical examination, the child was conscious but irritable, pale and had sick look. Fever was 103°F. Heart rate was 130/min, respiration was regular, BP 100/70 mm Hg and oxygen saturation was 94%. Rash was generalized, discrete, and maculopapular. Liver was enlarged 5 cm below costal margin and was firm. Spleen was palpable 2 cm below the costal margin. Other systems were normal on examination.

Investigations revealed Hb 10 g/dL, WBC 6,700 per mm³ (P_{54} L_{44} E_2), and platelets 4,23,000 per mm³; Urine routine: Normal; Dengue NS1, IgM negative.

What are the differential diagnoses?

Measles, dengue, scarlet fever, viral exanthem like roseola, drug fever, and rickettsial infections are the differential diagnoses.

- The classical prodrome of measles that includes cough, cold, running nose and congestion of eyes is absent.
- Fever persisting beyond 7 days, negative serology, and absence of leucopenia and thrombocytopenia rule out dengue fever.
- In scarlet fever, rash appears earlier and throat congestion is prominent.
- Rash in roseola appears when fever subsides.
- There is no history of specific drug ingestion to cause drug fever and the character of rash does not support the diagnosis of drug fever.

The diagnosis is, therefore rickettsial fever. Rickettsial fever is a classic triad of fever, headache, and rash. Rash usually appears 2–3 days after the onset of fever. Initially, rash is discrete pale, or rose red, blanching and macular or maculopapular in nature. Characteristically it starts on the extremities and spreads rapidly to involve the entire body. History of contact with animals, tick bite, stay in crowded area, and rapid defervescence with doxycycline would go in favor of rickettsial infection.

What diagnostic tests will you advise?

Weil-Felix test and Rickettsia IgM by ELISA are the available diagnostic tests.

at select advanced centers and are utilized for research purpose.

Indirect immunoperoxidase assay (IPA) This test is also a standard test, comparable with IFA but available at only a few research centers.

Treatment **Rickettsial Diseases**

ICMR has issued guidelines for treating rickettsial diseases, in 2015. Rickettsial infections respond dramatically well to treatment. The drugs are easily available and are not expensive. Tetracycline, doxycycline, and chloramphenicol are the drugs advocated for the treatment of rickettsial fever. Though these drugs are routinely used, limited evidence and data are available from randomized controlled trials.

At primary level, the health care provider needs to recognize the severity of the disease. If the patients come with complications to primary health facility and treating physician considers it as rickettsial infection, treatment with doxycycline should be initiated before referring the patient. In cases with fever of duration of 5 days or more when malaria, dengue and typhoid have been ruled out, following drugs should be administered when scrub typhus is considered likely.

- Doxycycline in the dose of 4.5 mg/kg body weight/day in two divided doses for children below 45 kg for 3–5 days after defervescence of fever, OR
- Azithromycin in the single dose of 10 mg/kg body weight for 5 days, OR
- Chloramphenicol: 50–100 mg /kg/day 6 hourly for 3–5 days after defervescence of fever

Doxycycline and/or chloramphenicol resistant strains have been seen in Southeast Asia. These strains are sensitive to azithromycin.

PREVENTION

Tick-borne typhus No effective vaccine is available. Tick infested areas should be avoided. Daily inspection for tick bites is important. Tick removal and prevention of infestation of dogs will reduce transmission of rickettsia. Health education and awareness of people about ticks and means of personal protection should be emphasized.

Scrub typhus No effective vaccine is available against scrub typhus. Use insecticides for vector control, and removal of scrub vegetation from the camp sites. Chigger-bites can be reduced by wearing protective clothes and using insect repellents.

Doxycycline and chloramphenicol may be used for chemoprophylaxis. A single dose of doxycycline is equally effective given weekly for 6 weeks after exposure. A single dose of chloramphenicol or tetracycline PO can also be used every 5 days for one month.

Q fever Pasteurization of milk constitutes an effective way of inactivating the causative agent of Q fever. Maintaining sanitized cattle sheds, adequate disinfection and sanitary disposal of animal excreta are other modes of prophylaxis.

Epidemic typhus Delousing is the most important preventive measure and has controlled epidemic of this infection effectively. Although protective vaccines have been developed, they have not been widely used.

Murine typhus It can be effectively prevented through flea control measures on pets, especially domesticated cats. No vaccine is available against murine typhus currently.

Ajantha GS, Patil SS, Chitharagi VB, Kulkarni RD. Rickettsiosis: A cause of acute febrile illness and value of Weil-Felix test. *Indian J Public Health*. 2013;57:182–3.

Aung AK, Spelman DW, Murray RJ, Graves S. Rickettsial infections in Southeast Asia: implications for local populace and febrile returned travellers. *Am J Trop Med Hyg*. 2014; 91:451–60.

Kulkarni A, Vaidya S, Kulkarni P, *et al*. Rickettsial disease-an experience. *Pediatr Infect Dis*. 2009;1:118–24.

Kulkarni A. Childhood Rickettsiosis. *Indian J Pediatr*. 2011;78:81–7.

Mahajan SK. Rickettsial Diseases. *J Assoc Physicians India*. 2012; 60:37–45.

Rahi M, Gupte MD, Bhargava A, Varghese GM, Arora R. DHR-ICMR Guidelines for diagnosis and management of Rickettsial diseases in India. *Indian J Med Res*. 2015; 141:417–22.

Rathi N, Rathi A. Rickettsial infections: Indian perspective. *Indian Pediatr*. 2010; 47:157–64.

Rathi NB, Rathi AN, Goodman MH. Rickettsial Diseases in Central India: Proposed Clinical Scoring System for Early Detection of Spotted Fever. *Indian Pediatr*. 2011;48:867–71.

Todar K. Rickettsial Diseases, including Typhus and Rocky Mountain Spotted Fever. *In*: Todar's Online Text Book of Bacteriology. From: http://textbook of bacteriology.net/Rickettsia_2.h. Accessed July 30, 2015.

Walker DH. Rickettsiae and rickettsial infections: current state of knowledge. *Clin Infect Dis*. 2007; 45 Suppl 1: S39–44

Woods CR. Rocky Mountain spotted fever in children. *Pediatr Clin North Am*. 2013;60:455–70.

6 Piyush Gupta, Kausalya Raghuraman, Sriram Krishnamurthy; Pooja Dewan (HIV); Nidhi Bedi (Fever); Ashok Kumar (*Malaria, Kala-azar*); Atul A Kulkarni (Leptospirosis and Rickettsial diseases); Vanny Arora (Influenza); and Abhishek Jain (Parasitology)

Newborn Infant

7.1 DEFINITIONS

Newborn Product of conception with signs of life, between birth and 28 days of age.

A. Definitions for Weight and Gestational Age

Term A newborn delivered between 37 and 41 weeks of gestation, irrespective of birth weight.
- *Early term* 37–38 weeks of gestation
- *Full term* 39–40 weeks of gestation
- *Late term* 41 weeks of gestation

Preterm A newborn delivered before 37 weeks of gestation.

Late preterm A newborn delivered between 34 and 36 weeks of gestation.

Moderate preterm A newborn delivered at or after 32 weeks gestation.

Very preterm A newborn delivered between 28 and <32 weeks gestation.

Extremely preterm A newborn delivered before 28 weeks gestation.

Post-term A newborn delivered at 42 weeks or more.

Low birth weight (LBW) Birth weight <2500 g, irrespective of the duration of gestation.

Very low birth weight (VLBW) A newborn weighing less than 1500 g at birth.

Extremely low birth weight (ELBW) A newborn weighing less than 1000 g at birth.

Appropriate for gestational age (AGA) A newborn weighing between 10th and 90th percentile for that gestational age.

Small for gestational age (SGA) Neonates with birth weight less than 10th percentile for that gestational age. Also known as intrauterine growth restricted (IUGR) or small-for-date (SFD).

Large for gestational age (LGA) Birth weight >90th percentile for gestational age, also known as large-for-date (LFD).

B. Definitions for Fetal Deaths

Fetal death Death of a fetus prior to complete expulsion from mother not showing any sign of life after separation.

Early fetal death Death at a gestational age <22 weeks or weighing <500 g or crown-heel length <25 cm.

Intermediate fetal death Death at a gestational age 22–27 weeks or weighing 500–999 g or crown-heel length between 25 and 35 cm.

Late fetal death Death at a gestational age ≥28 weeks or weighing ≥1000 g or crown-heel length ≥35 cm. The body may be fresh or macerated.

C. Definitions for Neonatal Deaths

Neonatal death Death occurring within 28 days of life.
First day death Death occurring within 24 hours of age.
Early neonatal death Death occurring within 7 days of life (168 hours).
Late neonatal death Death occurring between 7 and 28 days of life.

D. Age

Chronological age Age calculated from the date of birth.
Gestational age Calculated from the first day of last menstrual period till the date of birth in completed weeks.
Post-menstrual age Gestational age plus chronological age.

E. Mortality Rates

Neonatal mortality rate Newborns dying before 28 days of life per 1000 live births per year.

Perinatal mortality rate (PMR) Late fetal deaths plus neonates dying within 7 days of birth per 1000 total births per year.

7.2 FETUS AND TRANSITION TO NEWBORN

Most dramatic events in growth and development occur before birth. Major events of somatic and neurologic developments are summarized below.

Somatic Development

A. Embryonic Period

- Implantation begins by 6 days postconceptional age and blastocyst is formed.
- By 2 weeks, implantation is complete and uteroplacental circulation begins, and embryo has two distinct layers—endoderm and ectoderm.
- By 3rd week, third primary germ layer mesoderm appears along with primitive neural tube and heart begins to pump.
- By the end of 8th week, the embryonic period becomes complete; the rudiments of all major organ systems have developed.

- An average embryo weighs 9 g and has a crown–rump length of 5 cm.

B. Fetal Period

- Fetal period starts from 9th week. There is increase in cell number and size and structural remodeling of several organ systems.
- By 12 weeks, the gender of the external genitals becomes clearly distinguishable.
- By 20–24 weeks, primitive alveoli form and surfactant production begins.
- At the end of 2nd trimester, fetus weighs 1000 g and is 35 cm long.

C. Neurologic Development

- During the 3rd week, a neural plate appears on the ectodermal surface of trilaminar embryo.
- By the end of 5th week, the three main subdivisions of forebrain, midbrain and hindbrain are evident.
- Myelination begins at midgestation and continues to several years postnatal.

Perinatal Physiology

The transition from life *in utero* to life outside the womb involves dramatic changes in physiology and function. These are discussed below.

A. Cardiovascular Transition

- *In the fetal circulation*, right and left ventricles exist in a parallel circuit, as opposed to the series circuit of a newborn.
- In fetus, placenta acts as an organ of gas and metabolic exchange.
- Fetal circulation is marked by right-to-left shunting of blood through a patent ductus arteriosus (connecting the pulmonary artery to the aorta) and foramen ovale (connecting the right and left atria).
- *In fetus,* shunting is encouraged by high pulmonary arteriolar resistance and relatively low resistance to blood flow in the systemic (including placental) circulation.
- About 90 to 95% of the right heart output bypasses the lungs and goes directly to the systemic circulation.
- The fetal ductus arteriosus is kept open by low fetal systemic PaO_2 (about 25 mm Hg) along with locally produced prostaglandins.
- *At birth,* profound changes in this system occur after the first few breaths, resulting in increased pulmonary blood flow and closure of the foramen ovale. Pulmonary arteriolar resistance drops acutely as a result of vasodilation caused by lung expansion and increased PaO_2.
- *Soon after birth*, systemic resistance becomes higher than pulmonary resistance, a reversal from the fetal state. Therefore, the direction of blood flow through the patent ductus arteriosus reverses, creating left-to-right shunting of blood (called transitional circulation). This state lasts from moments after birth (when the pulmonary blood flow increases and functional closure of the foramen ovale occurs) until about 24 to 72 hours of age, when the ductus arteriosus usually closes.

- Once the ductus arteriosus closes, an adult-type circulation exists. The two ventricles now pump in series, and there are no major shunts between the pulmonary and systemic circulations.

B. Pulmonary Maturation

- *Fetal lungs* develop throughout gestation, and fairly well-developed alveoli are present by the 25th week.
- Fetal alveoli are filled with fluid which is actively secreted by pulmonary epithelium.
- For normal gas exchange to occur at birth, pulmonary alveolar fluid and interstitial fluid must be cleared promptly.
- Surfactant is secreted by type II pneumocytes. It reduces high surface tension, which would otherwise cause atelectasis and increase the work of breathing.
- Before 34 to 35 weeks gestation, surfactant is often not produced in sufficient quantities and respiratory distress syndrome develops in preterm infants born below this gestation.

C. Renal Function

- At birth, renal function is generally reduced, particularly in premature infants.
- By the age 1 to 2 years, glomerular filtration rate, urea clearance, and maximum tubular clearances reach adult levels.

D. Bilirubin Metabolism

- Aged or damaged fetal RBCs are removed from the circulation by reticuloendothelial cells, which convert heme to bilirubin.
- This bilirubin, bound with albumin, is transported to the liver, where it is transferred into hepatocytes.
- The enzyme glucuronyl transferase then conjugates the bilirubin with uridine diphosphoglucuronic acid (UDPGA) to form bilirubin mono- and diglucuronide (conjugated bilirubin), which is secreted actively into the bile ducts.
- The enzyme β-glucuronidase, present in the small-bowel luminal brush border, is released into the intestinal lumen, where it deconjugates bilirubin glucuronide; free (unconjugated) bilirubin is then reabsorbed from the intestinal tract and re-enters the systemic circulation.
- Fetal bilirubin is cleared from the circulation by placental transfer into the mother's plasma following a concentration gradient. The maternal liver then conjugates and excretes the fetal bilirubin.
- At birth, the placenta is "lost," and although the neonate's liver continues to take up, conjugate, and excrete bilirubin into bile so it can be eliminated in the stool, the neonate lacks proper intestinal bacteria for oxidizing bilirubin to urobilinogen in the gut; consequently, unaltered bilirubin remains in the stool, imparting a typical bright-yellow color.
- Additionally, the neonate's gastrointestinal tract (like that of the fetus) contains β-glucuronidase, which deconjugates some of the bilirubin.
- The unconjugated bilirubin is reabsorbed and returned to the circulation from the intestinal lumen (enterohepatic circulation of bilirubin), contributing to physiologic jaundice.

E. Hemoglobin

- *In utero*, RBC production is controlled exclusively by fetal erythropoietin produced in the liver; maternal erythropoietin does not cross the placenta.
- About 55 to 90% of fetal RBCs contain fetal hemoglobin, which has high oxygen affinity. As a result, a high oxygen concentration gradient is maintained across the placenta, resulting in abundant oxygen transfer from the maternal to the fetal circulation.
- *The transition from fetal to adult hemoglobin* begins before birth; at delivery, the site of erythropoietin production shifts from the liver to the kidney.
- The abrupt increase in PaO_2 from about 25 to 30 mm Hg in the fetus to 90 to 95 mm Hg in the neonate after delivery causes serum erythropoietin to fall, and RBC production ceases causing physiologic anemia.

F. Endocrine Homeostasis

- *The fetus* depends completely on the maternal supply of glucose via the placenta.
- Most glycogen is stored in liver during the later part of the 3rd trimester.
- *The neonate's* glucose supply terminates when the umbilical cord is cut; concurrently, levels of circulating epinephrine, and glucagon surge, while insulin levels decline.
- These changes stimulate gluconeogenesis and mobilization of hepatic glycogen stores.
- In healthy, term neonates, glucose levels reach a nadir 30 to 90 min after birth, after which neonates are typically able to maintain normal glucose homeostasis.
- Infants at highest risk for neonatal hypoglycemia include those with reduced glycogen stores (small-for-gestational-age and premature infants), critically ill infants with increased glucose catabolism, and infants of diabetic mothers.

G. Immunologic Maturity

- At birth, most immune mechanisms are not fully functional, more so with increasing prematurity. Thus, all neonates and young infants are immunodeficient relative to adults and are at increased risk for overwhelming infection.
- Neutrophils and monocytes have reduced chemotaxis and phagocytosis in neonates, especially in babies born prematurely. B cells are present in fetal bone marrow, blood, liver, and spleen by the 12th week of gestation. By about the 14th weeks of gestation, the thymus is functioning and producing lymphocytes. Thymus is most active during fetal development and in early postnatal life. Trace amounts of IgM and IgG can be detected by the 20th week and IgA by the 30th weeks; because the fetus is normally in an antigen-free environment, only small amounts of immunoglobulin (predominantly IgM) are produced *in utero*.
- Elevated levels of cord serum IgM indicate *in utero* antigen challenge, usually from congenital infection. Maternal IgM does not cross placenta due to its large size.
- Almost all IgG in the fetus is actively transferred through placenta from mother. After 22 weeks gestation, placental transfer of IgG increases to reach maternal levels or greater

at term. Preterm babies have lower IgG levels. The passive transfer of maternal immunity from transplacental IgG and secretory IgA and antimicrobial factors in breastmilk (eg, IgG, secretory IgA, WBCs, complement proteins, lysozyme, and lactoferrin) compensate for the neonate's immature immune system and confer immunity to many bacteria and viruses. Protective immune factors in breast-milk coat the GI and upper respiratory tracts via mucosa-associated lymphoid tissue and prevent invasion of mucous membranes by respiratory and enteric pathogens.

Revision Point

Fetal Neonatal Transition

1. Fetal growth is influenced by genetic potential, intrauterine environment, transplacental supply of nutrients, and maternal exposure to environmental agents.
2. The most significant transition at birth is from placenta dependent gas exchange to lung dependent gas exchange. This is facilitated by fetal lung fluid clearing in late gestation and with onset of labor. Pulmonary flow increases and pulmonary vasculature resistance decreases gradually.
3. Circulatory adaptation results in a shift from a *parallel* fetal circulation to a circulation in *series* with closure of shunts at the levels of ductus arteriosus and foramen ovale.
4. Metabolic adaptation involves gluconeogenetic and glycogenolytic mechanism to maintain euglycemia soon after birth till adequate feeding is established. These are impaired in preterm and growth-retarded infants which predispose them to increased risk of hypoglycemia.

Ballard RA. Fetal development. *In*: Taeusch HW, Ballard RA, Gleason CA (Eds.). *Avery's Diseases of the Newborn*. 8th ed. Philadelphia: Saunders; 2005. p. 23–70.

Levene MI, Tudehope DI, Thearle MJ (eds.). *Essentials of Neonatal Medicine*. 3rd ed. Oxford: Blackwell Science; 2009. p. 1–15.

7.3 NEONATAL RESUSCITATION

The word resuscitation is derived from the Latin word *'resuscitaire'* meaning 'to rouse again'. According to WHO estimates, around 10% of approximately 120 million babies born every year worldwide need resuscitation. It is also estimated that birth asphyxia or perinatal asphyxia accounts for about 1 million (20%) of 5 million neonatal deaths that occur globally each year.

Although the vast majority of newly born infants do not require any intervention at birth to breathe, approximately 10% of the newborns require some assistance to begin breathing at birth, and about 1% require extensive resuscitative measures. Current guidelines on neonatal resuscitation were jointly released in 2015 by the American Heart Association (AHA) and the American Academy of Pediatrics (AAP).

Physiology of Asphyxia

When babies become asphyxiated (either *in utero* or after delivery), they undergo a well-defined sequence of events, ie, primary apnea followed by secondary apnea (Fig. 7.1).

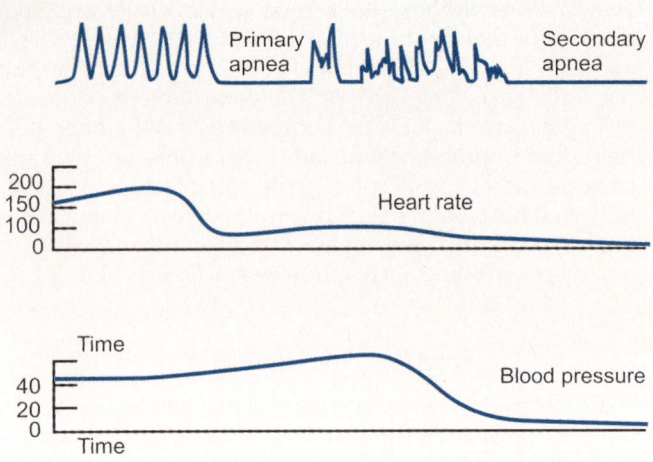

Fig. 7.1 Primary and secondary apnea

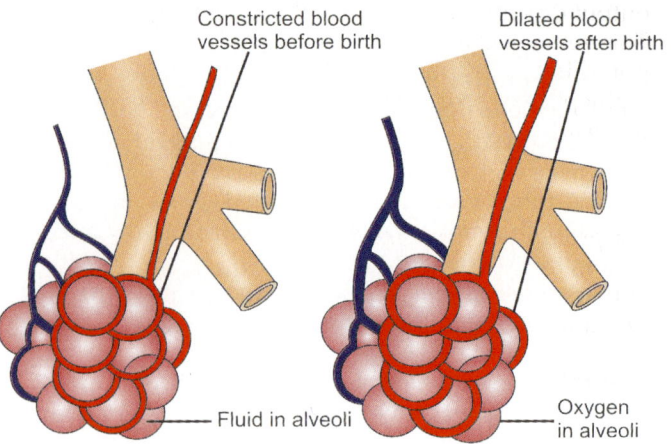

Fig. 7.2 Changes in pulmonary circulation at birth

A. Primary Apnea

- When an infant is deprived of oxygen, an initial brief period of rapid breathing occurs.
- If the asphyxia continues, the respiratory movements cease, the heart rate begins to fall, neuromuscular tone gradually diminishes, and the infant enters a period of apnea known as primary apnea.
- In most instances, physical stimulation such as drying or flicking the newborn's feet will induce breathing.

B. Secondary Apnea

- If the asphyxia continues, the infant develops deep gasping respirations, the heart rate continues to decrease, the blood pressure begins to fall, and the infant becomes nearly flaccid. The respirations become weak and weaker until the infant takes a last gasp and enters a period of apnea called secondary apnea.
- During secondary apnea, the baby is unresponsive to stimulation and will not resume respiratory efforts spontaneously unless positive pressure ventilation is initiated.

It is important to note that as a result of fetal hypoxia, the infant may go through primary apnea and into secondary apnea while *in utero*. Thus an infant may be born in either primary or secondary apnea. In a clinical setting, the two are difficult to distinguish from one another. In both instances, the infant is not breathing and the heart rate may be below 100 beats per minute. However, response to physical stimulation may help differentiate the two entities. Primary apnea will abort following physical stimulation, while secondary apnea will not.

Lungs and the Circulation

During intrauterine life, the lungs do not play a role in gas exchange because the placenta supplies the fetus with oxygen and removes carbon dioxide. The fetal lungs are expanded *in utero* but the potential air spaces are filled with fluid rather than air. Furthermore, the arterioles that perfuse the fetal lungs are constricted due to low partial pressure of oxygen in the fetus. Before birth, most of the blood from the right side of heart cannot go to lungs due to high pulmonary vascular resistance. Rather, blood takes the path of lower

resistance through the ductus arteriosus into the descending aorta. At the time of birth, several changes need to take place for the lungs to take over the vital function of supplying the body with oxygen (Fig. 7.2).

Normal Transition at Birth

At birth, as the infant takes the first few breaths, several changes occur whereby the lungs take over the lifelong function of respiration.

- The lung fluid is absorbed from the alveoli;
- Lungs get filled with air;
- Blood flow increases in the pulmonary circulation due to relaxation of pulmonary arterioles brought about by increased oxygen concentration in the alveoli;
- As oxygen tension increases in blood, the ductus arteriosus begins to constrict;
- Blood previously shunted through ductus arteriosus now goes to the lungs from where it carries oxygen to different body parts and body turns pink.

Apnea at Birth

When an infant has not taken an initial breath, it can be assumed that no expansion of alveoli has occurred and the lungs remain filled with fluid. When providing artificial ventilation to such an infant, additional pressure is often required to begin the process of expanding alveoli and clearing lung fluid.

Weak Respiratory Efforts

Shallow, ineffective respiration may occur in premature infants or in infants who are depressed as a result of asphyxia, maternal drugs, anesthesia, or other causes. These gasping, irregular respirations may be insufficient to properly expand the lungs.

Cardiac Function and Circulation

In addition to the vasoconstriction of the pulmonary blood vessels, arterioles in the bowels, kidneys, muscles and skin also constrict early in asphyxia. The resulting redistribution of blood flow helps preserve function by preferentially supplying oxygen and substrate to the heart and brain. As asphyxia is prolonged, myocardial function and cardiac output deteriorate, and blood flow to all organs is reduced. This sets the stage for progressive organ damage. At this point, it may be necessary to provide cardiac stimulants (epinephrine, dopamine) and volume expanders to support the heart and circulation.

Preparation for Resuscitation

For prompt, effective intervention to take place, two major factors must be given proper attention. These include (*i*) anticipating the need for resuscitation; and (*ii*) adequate preparation of both equipment and personnel.

A. Anticipation

A newborn depressed at birth may come as a surprise. But in many cases delivery of a depressed or asphyxiated infant can be anticipated on the basis of the antepartum and intrapartum histories. Maternal and fetal risk factors that can predict birth asphyxia include the following: (*i*) Pregnancy-induced hypertension, (*ii*) eclampsia, (*iii*) meconium-stained amniotic fluid, (*iv*) prolapsed cord, (*v*) prolonged/obstructed labor, (*vi*) breech or other abnormal presentations, (*vii*) difficult, operative or traumatic delivery, (*viii*) poly-/oligohydramnios, (*ix*) Rh isoimmunization, (*x*) prolonged rupture of membranes, (*xi*) maternal sedation, analgesia or anesthesia, (*xii*) preterm/post-term birth, multiple births, (*xiii*) maternal medical illnesses, or bad obstetric history, (*xiv*) evidence of fetal distress in the form of fetal heart rate <100 or >160 or irregular decrease or absence of fetal movements, and (*xv*) presence of congenital anomaly.

But it should always be kept in mind that up to half of newborns who require resuscitation have no identifiable risk factors at birth. Therefore, while attending a delivery, one should always be prepared for resuscitation.

B. Adequate preparation

Even with screening of cases through review of the antepartum and intrapartum histories, there will be many occasions when the birth of a depressed infant would not be expected. To allow for such situations, the equipment listed in **Table 7.1** should be available for any delivery.

Resuscitation procedure should be undertaken with full aseptic precautions. Universal precautions against HIV infection should also be observed.

Apgar Score

Apgar score provides useful information about the condition of the baby after birth. The score includes 5 signs, and each sign is awarded a value of 0, 1, or 2. All the values are then

Table 7.1 Equipment for Neonatal Resuscitation
I **Suction equipment**
• Mucus aspirator
• Low pressure (<100 mm Hg) mechanical suction
• Suction catheters, 10F or 12F
• Feeding tube 6F and 10 mL syringe
II **Equipment for positive pressure ventilation**
• Bag and mask equipment
• Face masks, normal and premature sizes
• Oxygen with flow meter and tubing
• Flow controlled pressure limited mechanical devices (eg, T-piece resuscitator) (optional)
• Laryngeal mask airway (LMA)
III **Intubation equipment**
• Laryngoscope with straight blades, [(No. 00) (extremely preterm), 0 (preterm), and No.1 (term)]
• Extra bulbs and batteries for laryngoscope
• Endotracheal tubes: 2.5. 3.0, 3.5, 4.0 mm internal diameter
• Stylet (optional)
• Scissors and adhesive tape
IV **Medications**
• Epinephrine
• Normal saline
V **Miscellaneous**
• Clock with seconds' hand
• Linen, shoulder roll
• Radiant warmer
• Stethoscope
• Syringes 1, 2, 5, 10, 20, 50 mL
• Gauze
• Umbilical catheters 3.5F, 5F
• Three-way stopcocks
• Gloves
• Nasogastric tubes 5F, 6F, 8F

added and the final sum becomes the Apgar score. Apgar scores should be assigned at 1 and 5 minutes after birth. When the five-minute Apgar score is < 7, additional scoring is done every 5 minutes for up to 20 minutes. Apgar score is recorded as in **Table 7.2.**

Apgar score cannot be used as a guide to start resuscitation because the score is not assigned until 60 seconds after birth; while on the other hand, the decision to provide positive pressure ventilation has to be taken within 30 seconds after birth. Despite limitations, Apgar score is a simple clinical tool to assess the condition of the baby at birth and to know how the newborn is responding during transition.

Table 7.2 Apgar Score			
Sign	0	1	2
Respiratory effort	Absent	Gasping	Good crying
Heart rate	Absent	≤100	>100
Color	Blue or pale	Pink body, blue extremities	Completely pink
Muscle tone	Limp	Some flexion of extremities	Active motion
Reflex irritability*	No response	Grimace	Cry or active withdrawal

* *Assessed by inserting catheter into nose*

Cord clamping should be delayed for at least 30 to 60 seconds for most vigorous term and preterm newborns. There is insufficient evidence to recommend delayed cord clamping for newborns who require resuscitation at birth.

Resuscitation Procedures

This flow diagram shown in Fig. 7.3 describes resuscitation procedures. The diagram begins with the birth of the baby. Each resuscitation step is shown in a block. Below each block is a decision point to decide for proceeding to the next step.

Neonatal resuscitation algorithm — 2015 update

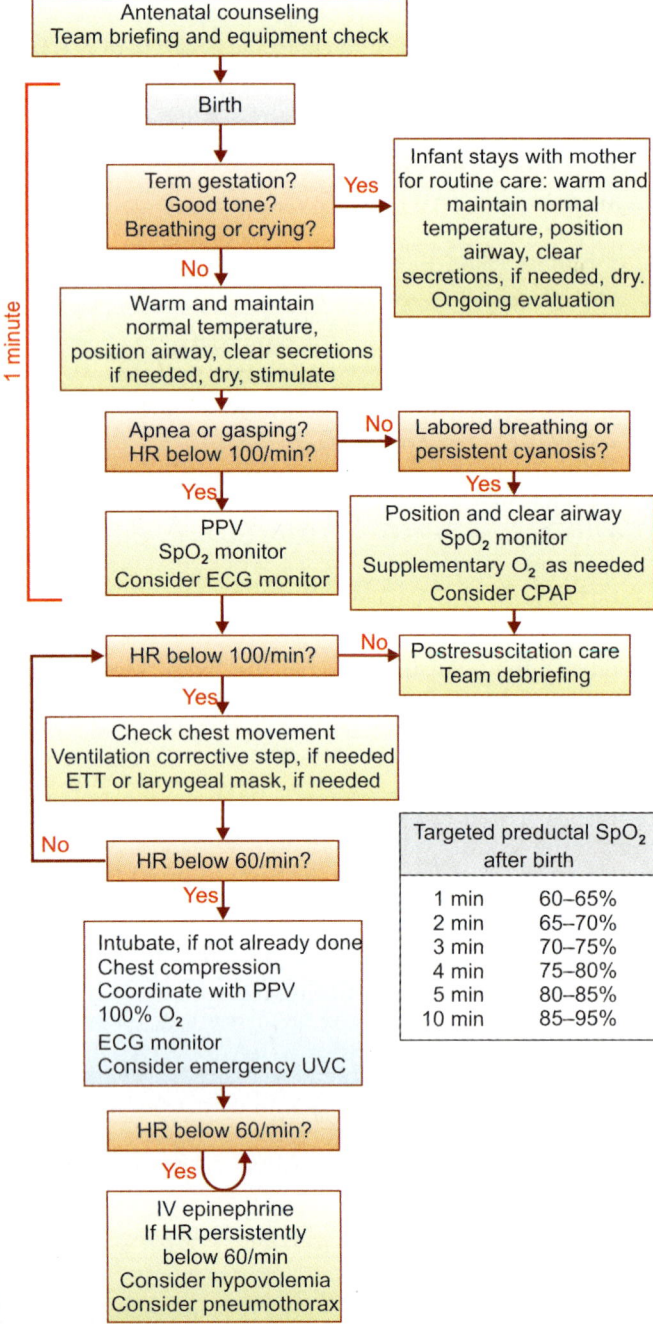

Fig. 7.3 Neonatal resuscitation algorithm

Those newly born infants who do not require resuscitation can generally be identified by a rapid assessment of the following three characteristics:
1. Term gestation?
2. Good muscle tone?
3. Crying or breathing?

If the answer to all three of these questions is 'yes' the baby does not require resuscitation and need not be separated from the mother. The baby should be dried, placed skin-to-skin with the mother, and covered with dry linen to maintain temperature. Observation of breathing, activity, and color should be ongoing.

If the answer to any of these assessment questions is "no," the infant should receive 1 or more of the following 4 categories of action in sequence:
A. Initial steps in stabilization (provide warmth, position, clear airway, dry, stimulate, reposition)
B. Ventilation
C. Chest compressions
D. Administration of epinephrine and/or volume expansion

1. Initial Steps of Resuscitation

A. Provide Warmth

The baby should be kept under radiant warmer to minimize heat loss (Fig. 7.4). Do not cover baby with blanket; this will prevent radiant heat from reaching the baby. Very low-birth-weight (<1500 g) preterm babies are likely to become hypothermic despite the use of traditional techniques for decreasing heat loss. For this reason, additional warming techniques are recommended (eg, prewarming the delivery room to 26°C, covering the baby in plastic wrapping or heat-resistant plastic, and placing the baby on an exothermic mattress.

The infant's temperature must be monitored closely because of risk of hyperthermia when these techniques are used in combination. Other techniques for maintaining temperature during stabilization of the baby in the delivery

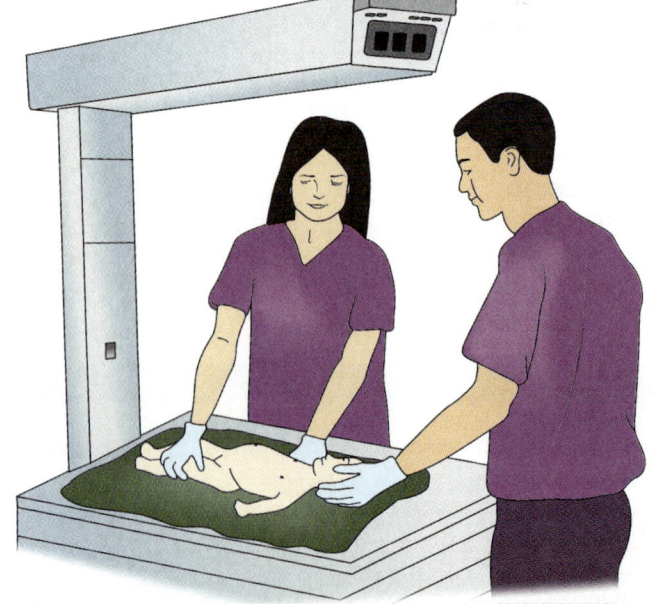

Fig. 7.4 Provision of warmth under radiant warmer

room include prewarming the linen, drying and swaddling, placing the baby skin-to-skin with the mother, and covering both with a blanket; these are also recommended. All resuscitation procedures, including endotracheal intubation, chest compression, and insertion of intravenous lines, can be performed with these temperature-controlling interventions in place.

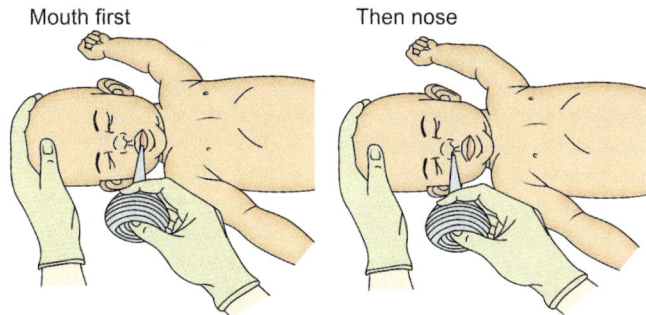

Fig. 7.6 Clearing the airway

NRP 2015: New Recommendation on Thermoregulation

1. Temperature of newly born non-asphyxiated infants be maintained between 36.5°C and 37.5°C after birth during resuscitation or stabilization.
2. For newborns <32 weeks' gestation, it is recommended to cover the newborn with food-grade plastic wrap or bag and use a thermal mattress.

B. Position by Slightly Extending the Neck

The baby should be positioned on her back, with the neck slightly extended in the sniffing position (Fig. 7.5). This permits unrestricted air entry to lungs. To help maintain the correct position, use a rolled blanket or towel under the shoulders elevating them ½ to 1 inch off the mattress.

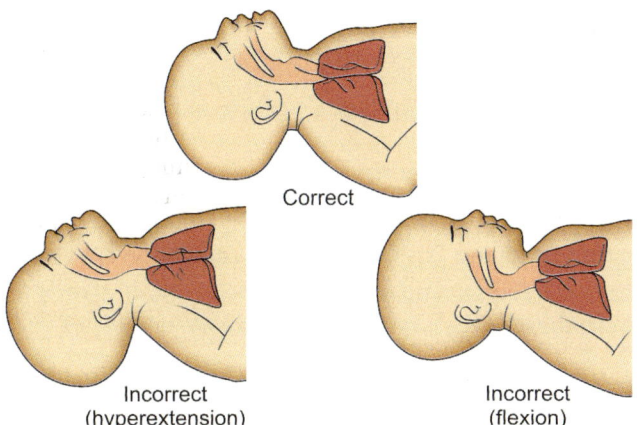

Fig. 7.5 Position by slightly extending the neck

C. Clear the Airway

The method of clearing the airway depends on whether the amniotic fluid is *clear* or *meconium stained*.

- *Clear amniotic fluid* There is no need of vigorous suction in the absence of obvious nasal or oral secretions. Vigorous suctioning of the nasopharynx can cause bradycardia. Suctioning should be reserved for babies who have obvious obstruction to spontaneous breathing or who require positive-pressure ventilation. Mouth should be suctioned first followed by nose (Fig. 7.6).
- *Meconium-stained amniotic fluid* In the presence of meconium-stained liquor, first suction mouth and posterior pharynx using 12 F or 14 F suction catheter. Direct

---

NRP 2015: New Recommendation on Meconium

Non-vigorous newborns born through meconium-stained amniotic fluid do not require routine intubation and tracheal suctioning.

---

suctioning from trachea is no longer recommended in NRP 2015 guidelines.

D. Dry, Stimulate to Breathe, and Reposition

Once the airway is clear of secretions, immediately dry the baby to prevent heat loss. Use prewarmed clean sheets to dry the baby from head to toe (Fig. 7.7). Remove wet linen from baby, otherwise heat loss will continue. Ensure correct position of the baby by repositioning.

E. Tactile Stimulation

Both suctioning and drying will stimulate the newborn to breathe. If baby is not breathing, or has weak respiratory efforts, providing tactile stimulation may help to induce breathing. Two safe methods of providing tactile stimulation are: (*i*) flicking or slapping the soles of the feet; or (*ii*) gently rubbing the baby's back, trunk, or extremities (Fig. 7.8). Tactile stimulation should not be given more than twice. Newborns in primary apnea will respond to this brief tactile stimulation. If a baby fails to respond, it implies secondary apnea; positive pressure ventilation should be started without delay.

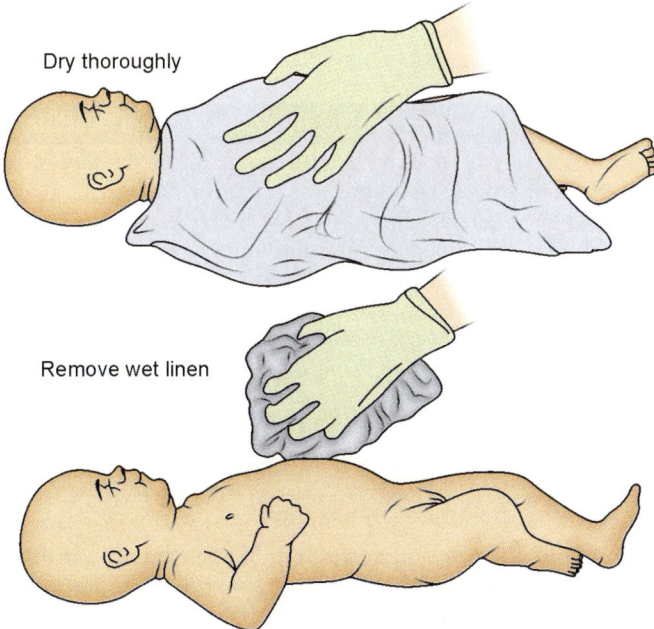

Fig. 7.7 Drying during initial steps

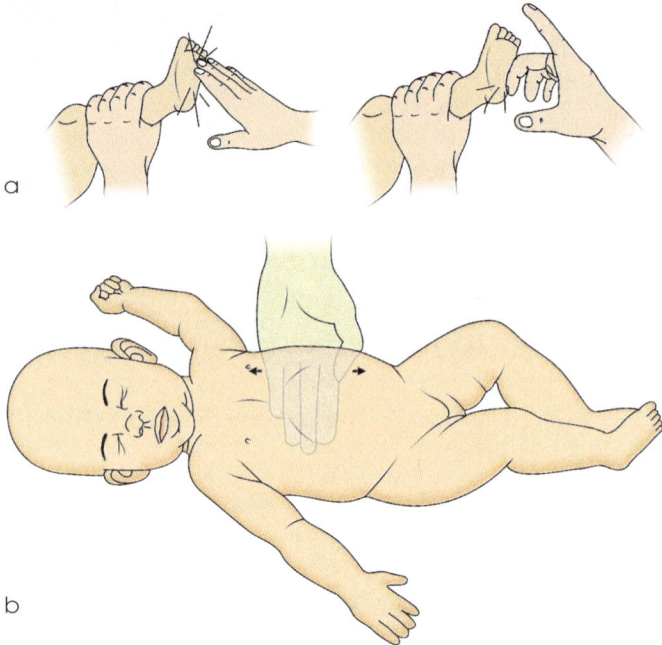

a

b

Fig. 7.8 Tactile stimulation by (a) flicking the sole, or (b) rubbing the back

F. Evaluation of Initial Steps

Approximately 60 seconds (**The Golden Minute**) are allotted for completing the initial steps, reevaluating, and beginning ventilation, if required (Fig. 7.3). The decision to progress beyond the initial steps is determined by simultaneous assessment of 2 vital characteristics: Respirations (apnea, gasping, or labored or unlabored breathing) and heart rate (whether greater than or less than 100 beats per minute).

Once positive pressure ventilation or supplementary oxygen administration is begun, assessment should consist of simultaneous evaluation of 3 vital characteristics: Heart rate, respirations, and the state of oxygenation, the latter optimally determined by a pulse oximeter. The most sensitive indicator of a successful response to each step is an increase in heart rate.

> **NRP 2015: New Recommendation on Assessment of Heart Rate**
> 1. Initial assessment of the heart rate should be made with a stethoscope. Umbilical cord base pulsations are less accurate and may underestimate the true heart rate.
> 2. Use of a pulse oximeter sensor with ECG leads or cardiac monitor to assess the heart rate is recommended.
> 3. An electronic cardiac monitor is the preferred method for accurate assessment of heart rate during PPV or chest compressions.
> 4. Use of a 3-lead electronic cardiac monitor (ECG) for continuous display of baby's heart rate is recommended for preterm babies.

G. Use of Supplementary Oxygen

In term infants receiving resuscitation at birth with positive-pressure ventilation, it is best to begin with room air rather than 100% oxygen. If, despite effective ventilation, there is no increase in heart rate or if oxygenation (guided by oximetry) remains unacceptable, use of a higher concentra-

tion of oxygen should be considered. Because many preterm babies of <32 weeks gestation will not reach target saturations in room air, blended oxygen and air should be given, ideally guided by pulse oximetry. Both hyperoxemia and hypoxemia should be avoided. If a blend of oxygen and air is not available, resuscitation should be initiated with room air.

> **NRP 2015: New Recommendation on Oxygen Management**
> 1. PPV of newborns ≥35 weeks' gestation begins with room air (21% oxygen).
> 2. PPV of newborns <35 weeks' gestation may begin with 21–30% oxygen.
> 3. Oxygen concentration should be increased, if heart rate is falling.
> 4. At the beginning of chest compression, 100% oxygen should be provided.
> 5. Free-flow oxygen administration may begin at 30% with blender.
> 6. If newborn has labored breathing, early trial of CPAP is recommended.

2. Positive Pressure Ventilation

Ventilation is the most effective step in neonatal resuscitation.

Indications

After completion of initial steps, positive pressure ventilation is indicated:
(i) If the newborn is apneic or gasping; or
(ii) If the heart rate is <100 bpm.

Method of giving Positive Pressure Ventilation (PPV)

- PPV can be given by self-inflating bag, flow-inflating bag (anesthesia bag), laryngeal mask airway, or with a T-piece resuscitator.
- Self-inflating bag is most commonly used device (Fig. 7.9). It is easier to use, does not require a compressed gas source in order to inflate, and is portable.
- The size of bag for neonatal use ranges from 240 to 500 mL.

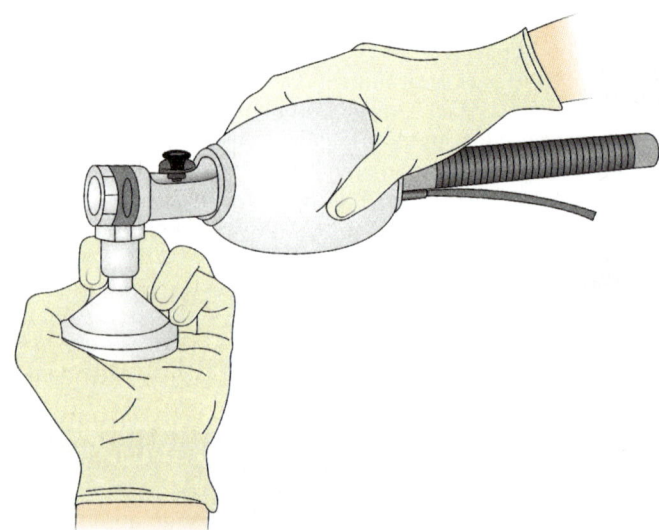

Fig. 7.9 Self-inflating bag and checking it before application

- The bag has a site for attaching oxygen reservoir.
- The bag also possesses a safety device—a pressure release valve (pop-off valve). It opens at 30 to 40 cm H_2O. This valve opens up, if ventilatory pressures greater than 30 to 40 cm H_2O are generated during resuscitation. This prevents barotrauma to the baby's lungs.
- Mask should be of correct size and is different for term (size 1) and preterm (size 0 and 00) babies. A correct size mask covers the chin, the mouth and the nose but not the eyes (Fig. 7.10).
- A tight seal between mask and face is essential to achieve positive pressure to inflate the lungs.
- Bag and mask ventilation is carried out at a rate of 40 to 60 breaths per minute.
- There should be easy rise and fall of chest with each breath.
- Improvement in baby's condition is indicated by increasing heart rate (achieve or maintain a heart rate >100 bpm), improving color, spontaneous breathing, and improving muscle tone.
- Failure to improve may be due to inadequate seal, blocked airway, or not enough pressure being applied.
- If still there is no improvement after taking corrective measures, PPV through endotracheal tube is required.
- During bag and mask ventilation, air may cause stomach distension, preventing full expansion of lungs.
- If bag and mask ventilation is given for more than a few minutes, insert an orogastric tube to decompress the stomach, and leave the uncapped tube in stomach to act as a vent for stomach gas during resuscitation.
- Average initial peak inflating pressures of 30 cm H_2O in term babies and 20–25 cm H_2O in preterm babies are generally enough for successful ventilation.
- *Laryngeal mask airway* (LMA) (Fig. 7.11) that fits over the laryngeal inlet should be considered during resuscitation of the newborn, if face mask ventilation is ineffective and

> **NRP 2015: New Recommendation on Positive-Pressure Ventilation**
>
> 1. If PPV is required for resuscitation of a preterm newborn, it is preferable to use a device that can provide positive end expiratory pressure (PEEP). To initiate, a PEEP of 5 cm H_2O is recommended.
> 2. During PPV, ventilation corrective steps are administered until the chest moves with ventilation. Insert an alternative airway (ET tube or laryngeal mask).
> 3. For preterm infants, consider using CPAP immediately after birth as an alternative to routine intubation and prophylactic surfactant administration.

tracheal intubation is unsuccessful. It is considered as an alternative to a face mask for positive-pressure ventilation among newborns weighing >2000 g or delivered at ≥34 weeks' gestation.

3. Endotracheal Tube Placement

Endotracheal intubation (Fig. 7.12) may be indicated at several points during neonatal resuscitation:

  i. If bag-mask ventilation is ineffective or prolonged (>2 min);
 ii. When chest compressions are performed;
iii. When endotracheal administration of medications is desired; and
 iv. For special resuscitation circumstances, such as congenital diaphragmatic hernia or extremely low birth weight (<1000 g).

The time taken for endotracheal intubation depends on the skill and experience of the available providers. If it is not possible to insert the tube within 20 seconds, remove the laryngoscope, provide bag and mask ventilation, and then try again. Selection of proper size of endotracheal tube and correct suction catheter sizes is summarized in **Table 7.3**.

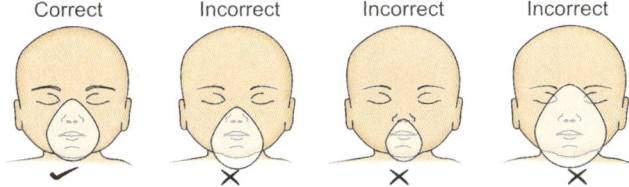

Fig. 7.10 Application of mask correctly (mask should cover nose, mouth and chin)

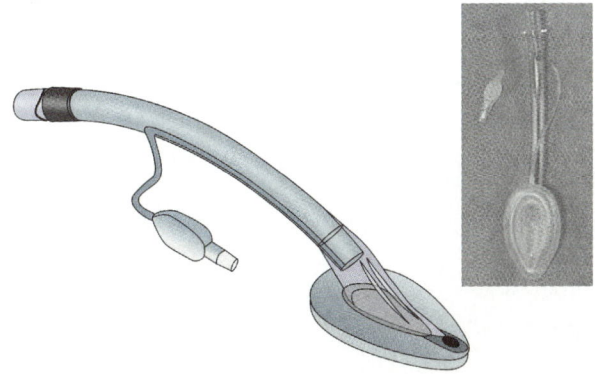

Fig. 7.11 Laryngeal mask airway

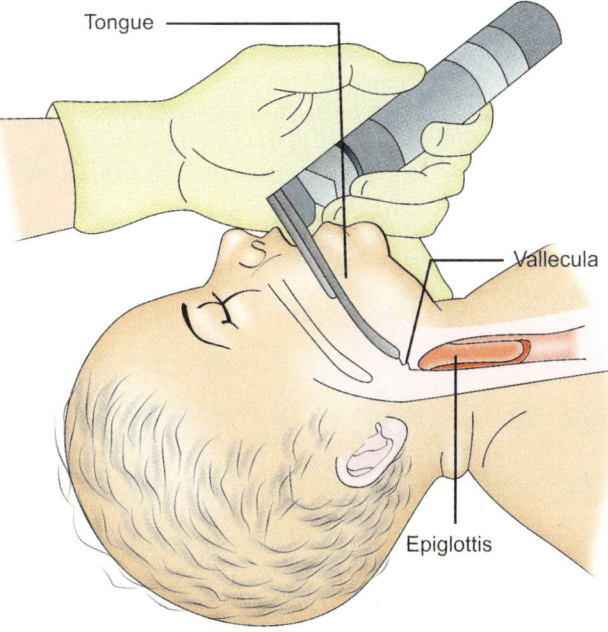

Fig. 7.12 Endotracheal tube placement

7

Table 7.3 Appropriate Endotracheal Tube Size		
Birth weight	Endotracheal tube size (mm of internal diameter)	Suction catheter size
< 1000 g	2.5	5–6
1000–2000 g	3.0	6
2000–3000 g	3.5	8
>3000 g	4.0	8

Indicators of Proper Tube Placement

- After endotracheal intubation and administration of intermittent positive pressure, a prompt increase in heart rate is the best indicator that the tube is in the trachea and providing effective ventilation.
- Symmetrical and bilateral chest movements and equal breath sounds in both the axillae.
- Exhaled CO_2 detection is effective for confirmation of endotracheal tube placement in infants, including very low birth weight infants. A positive test result (detection of exhaled CO_2) in patients with adequate cardiac output confirms placement of the endotracheal tube within the trachea, whereas a negative test result (ie, no CO_2 detected) strongly suggests esophageal intubation. Poor or absent pulmonary blood flow may give false-negative results (ie, no CO_2 detected despite tube placement in the trachea), but endotracheal tube placement is correctly identified in nearly all patients who are not in cardiac arrest.
- Presence of condensed humidified gas during exhalation signifies correct placement.

Endotracheal tube placement must be assessed visually during intubation and by confirmatory methods after intubation, if the heart rate remains low and is not rising. Except for intubation to remove meconium, exhaled CO_2 detection is the recommended method of confirmation.

4. Chest Compressions

Indication

Heart rate <60 beats per minute despite 30 seconds of positive pressure ventilation.

Rescuers should ensure that assisted ventilation is being delivered optimally before starting chest compressions. This will help in circulation with an oxygenated blood.

Technique

Compressions should be delivered on the lower third of the sternum to a depth of approximately one-third of the anterior-posterior diameter of the chest. Two techniques (Fig. 7.13) have been described:

- *2-finger technique* Compression with 2 fingers with a second hand supporting the back.
- *2-thumb-encircling hands technique* Compression with 2 thumbs with fingers encircling the chest and supporting the back.

The 2-thumb-encircling hands technique is preferred for performing chest compressions in newly born infants, because this technique may generate higher peak systolic and coronary perfusion pressure than the 2-finger technique.

Compressions and ventilations should be coordinated to avoid simultaneous delivery. The chest should be permitted to fully re-expand during relaxation, but the rescuer's thumbs should not leave the chest. There should be a 3:1 ratio of compressions to ventilations with 90 compressions and 30 breaths to achieve approximately 120 events per minute to maximize ventilation at an achievable rate (Fig. 7.14).

Evaluation

Heart rate should be reassessed every 30 seconds.

NRP 2015: New Recommendation on Chest Compressions

1. Intubation is strongly recommended prior to beginning chest compressions. If intubation is not feasible, a laryngeal mask may be used.
2. Chest compressions are to be administered with the two-thumb technique.
3. 100% oxygen should be added.
4. Chest compressions should continue for 60 seconds prior to checking a heart rate.

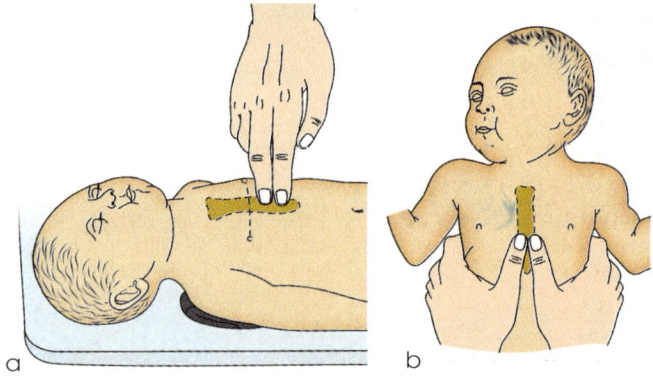

Fig. 7.13 Methods of chest compression: (a) 2-finger technique (left); (b) 2-thumb technique

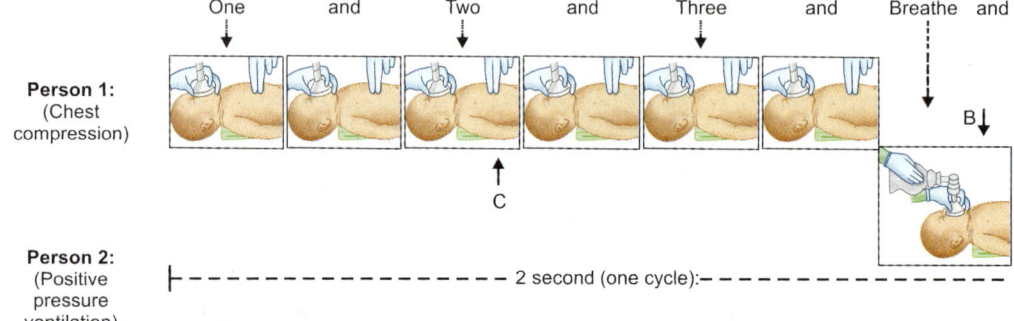

Fig. 7.14 Coordination between positive pressure ventilation and chest compression. C–chest compression; B–breathing

- *Heart rate more than 100 per minute* Stop chest compressions and gradually discontinue PPV, if baby is breathing spontaneously.
- *Heart rate 60–100 per minute* Stop chest compressions and continue PPV at 40 to 60 breaths per minute.
- *Heart rate less than 60 per minute* Intubate the baby, if not already done and give epinephrine.

5. Medications

Drugs are rarely indicated in resuscitation of the newly born infant. Bradycardia in the newborn infant is usually the result of inadequate lung inflation or profound hypoxemia, and establishing adequate ventilation is the most important step to correct it. Umbilical vein is the best intravenous route at birth (Fig. 7.15). Peripheral veins are difficult to cannulate during resuscitation.

Indications

If the heart rate remains <60 beats per minute despite adequate ventilation and chest compressions, administration of epinephrine or volume expansion, or both, may be indicated. Only 2 drugs are needed for resuscitation in the labor room **(Table 7.4)**.

Table 7.4 Doses of Drugs for Resuscitation		
Drug	*Dose*	*Formulation*
Epinephrine	0.01–0.03 mg/kg or 0.1–0.3 mL/kg	1:10,000 dilution
Volume expander	10 mL/kg	Normal saline or whole blood in presence of blood loss

Epinephrine

Epinephrine is a cardiac stimulant. It increases the strength and rate of cardiac contractions and produces peripheral vasoconstriction, which may increase blood flow through the coronary arteries and to the brain. After giving epinephrine, the heart rate should increase to more than 60 bpm within 30 seconds of administration. If this does not happen, epinephrine may be repeated twice every 3 to 5 minutes. Ensure that baby is getting PPV and chest compressions during medication use.

To make 1:10000 concentration solution, mix 1 mL of epinephrine (1:1000) with 9 mL of normal saline. IV bolus of

epinephrine should be followed by 0.5 to 1 mL flush of normal saline to ensure that the drug has reached the blood. If the endotracheal route is used, consider giving a higher dose (0.3 to 1 mL/kg). The bolus dose remains same as the first dose.

Volume Expansion

Consider volume expansion when blood loss is suspected or the infant appears to be in shock (pale skin, poor perfusion, weak pulse) and has not responded adequately to other resuscitative measures. Normal saline is the solution of choice for volume expansion in the delivery room. The recommended dose is 10 mL/kg over 5 to 10 minutes, which may need to be repeated. When resuscitating premature infants, care should be taken to avoid giving volume expanders too rapidly. Rapid infusions of large volumes can contribute to intraventricular hemorrhage.

There is no role of sodium bicarbonate, aminophylline, steroids, calcium gluconate, and respiratory stimulants such as nikethamide during delivery room resuscitation. They are not only ineffective but also harmful.

NRP 2015: New Recommendation on Medication
1. The recommended solution for treating hypovolemia is normal saline.
2. Ringer lactate is no longer recommended.
3. All medications and fluids that can be infused into a umbilical venous catheter.

6. Post-Resuscitation Management

Following resuscitation, the baby is transferred to neonatal intensive care unit (NICU) for close monitoring and anticipatory care.

- *Maintenance of temperature* Normothermia should be maintained and hyperthermia should be avoided.
- *Therapeutic hypothermia* Newly born infants born at or near term (≥ 36 weeks gestational age) with evolving moderate to severe hypoxic-ischemic encephalopathy should be offered therapeutic hypothermia (33.5°C to 34.5°C). It reduces mortality and improves neurodevelopmental outcome of asphyxiated infants. The treatment should commence within 6 hours following birth, continued for 72 hours, and then slow rewarming is done over at least 4 hours. There may be some associated adverse effects, such as thrombocytopenia and increased need for inotropic support.
- *Glucose* Intravenous glucose infusion should be considered as soon as possible after resuscitation, with the goal of avoiding hypoglycemia which may further potentiate brain damage.

7. Discontinuing Resuscitative Efforts

Infants without signs of life (no heart beat and no respiratory effort) after 10 minutes of resuscitation show either a very high mortality or severe neurodevelopmental disability. After 10 minutes of continuous and adequate resuscitative efforts, discontinuation of resuscitation is justified, if there are no signs of life.

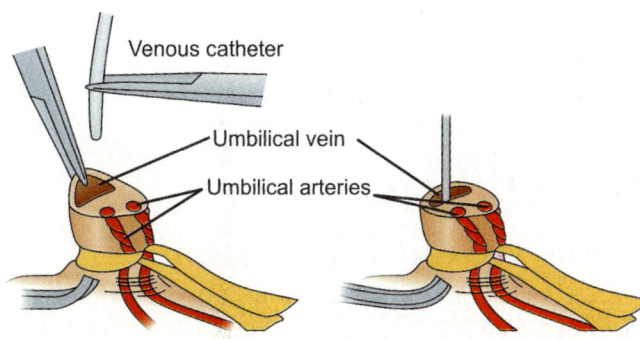

Fig. 7.15 Umbilical venous catheterization

Resuscitation

Revision Point

1. All neonates at birth must be provided essential newborn care.
2. Essential newborn care includes drying of baby, delayed cord clamping, skin-to-skin care, early initiation of breastfeeding, cord and eye care, vitamin K, and weighing all newborns.
3. Neonatal resuscitation in the delivery room is indicated in babies who do breathe adequately at birth.
4. The steps of resuscitation include initial steps, PPV, chest compressions, and medications.
5. For preterms, <32 weeks, additional care include wrapping in polythene plastic, providing CPAP, and considering surfactant therapy in those with respiratory distress.

Kattwinkel J, Perlman JM, Aziz K, *et al*. Special Report_Neonatal Resuscitation: 2010 American Heart Association Guidelines for Cardiopulmonary Resuscitation and Emergency Cardiovascular Care. *Pediatrics*. 2010;126:e1399–1415.

Perlman JM, Wyllie J, Kattwinkel J, *et al*. International Consensus on Cardiopulmonary Resuscitation and Emergency Cardiovascular Care Science with Treatment Recommendations. Part 11. Neonatal resuscitation. *Circulation*. 2010;122:S516–38.

7.4 NORMAL NEWBORN

Before examining a baby, obtain information on current pregnancy, perinatal history, past obstetric history, drug and radiation exposure and family history, as given below.

Maternal History

Age; height; pre-pregnancy weight; socioeconomic status; gravida and parity; details of antenatal care including 2 doses of tetanus toxoid vaccination, and iron and folic acid supplementation during pregnancy; blood group; chronic medical diseases like diabetes, hypertension, renal disease, cardiac disease, thyroid disease, bleeding disorders; infections, especially tuberculosis, UTI, TORCH, HIV/AIDS and other sexually transmitted diseases; and infertility and treatment received, if any.

Past obstetric history Abortions/stillbirth/neonatal deaths; prematurity/postmaturity; malformations; jaundice.

Current Pregnancy

Ask about fever, skin rash, lymphadenopathy; toxemia, pregnancy-induced hypertension (PIH); gestational diabetes; anemia; infection; antepartum hemorrhage; multiple pregnancy; cervical incompetence; trauma; polyhydra-mnios/oligohydramnios; glucocorticoids administration; results of any fetal testing (eg, ultrasound examination, TORCH screen, fetal monitoring, anti-D titer, blood sugar, amniocentesis, biophysical profile, Doppler velocimetry, genetic testing).

Drug history Medications, drug abuse, alcohol, tobacco, radiation exposure.

Perinatal History

Fever; foul-smelling discharge; meconium-stained liquor; cord accidents–prolapse, knot, rupture, cord around neck; bleeding; fetal distress; presentation; onset of labor; rupture of membranes; duration of labor; precipitate labor; cephalopelvic disproportion; fever; fetal monitoring— continuous electronic fetal monitoring, fetal scalp pH; amniotic fluid (blood, meconium, volume); anesthesia; method of delivery; Apgar score; resuscitation details; initial delivery room assessment (asphyxia, trauma, anomalies, temperature, infection); placental examination: Size, infarcts, calcifications, abnormal cord insertion.

Family history History of perinatal deaths; metabolic/ inherited disorders (eg, hemophilia, cystic fibrosis); and other disorders.

Routine Physical Examination of the Neonate

The first routine examination is important for any newborn. The baby should be unclothed and kept under a radiant warmer to prevent hypothermia during examination. If a radiant warmer is not available, the baby should be examined in mother's lap. Examiner's hands should be clean, dry and warm before touching the baby. One should always be gentle while examining newborn infants.

A general appraisal of a newborn allows one to assess quickly whether any major anomalies are present, whether jaundice or meconium staining is present, and whether the infant is having trouble making the adjustment to breathing in room air. Maximum information in newborn examination can be gained by thorough inspection only. At the initial examination, attention should be directed to determine the following:

- Whether the infant has made a successful transition from fetal life to room air breathing?
- To what extent gestation, labor, delivery, maternal analgesics, or anesthetics have affected the neonate?
- Whether there are any signs of illness?
- Whether any congenital anomalies are present?

1. Skin

Color

Skin color is an important marker of cardiorespiratory function. The epidermis of a newborn (especially a premature infant) is thin and the oxygenated capillary blood makes it pink. Good color means an overall reddish-pink hue, except for possible cyanosis of the hands and feet (acrocyanosis) which is normal immediately after birth.

Abnormal color (pale, blue, icteric), temperature (hypo-/ hyperthermia) and mottling (indicating poor circulatory status) should be noted in all babies. Jaundice should be looked for in daylight.

Infants of diabetic mothers and premature infants are pinker than average, and postmature infants are paler. Newborn with polycythemia may have unusually red color. Blood loss or shock may cause pale appearance, or ashen gray color. Mottled skin appearance may be due to circulatory insufficiency or hypothermia.

Capillary Filling/Refilling Time (CFT/CRT)

This is a useful method for assessment of circulatory status and early detection of shock in newborns. It is tested by blanching the skin overlying the upper part of sternum (Fig. 7.16). Moderate pressure (enough to blanch the skin) is

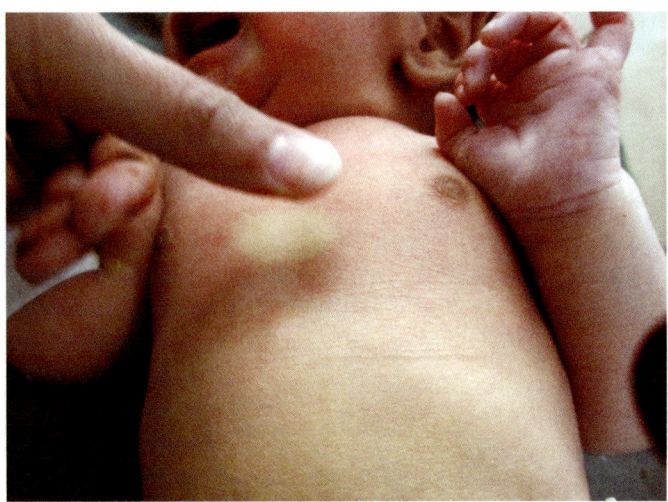

Fig. 7.16 Capillary refill time. Blanching after pressure regains color in less than 3 seconds

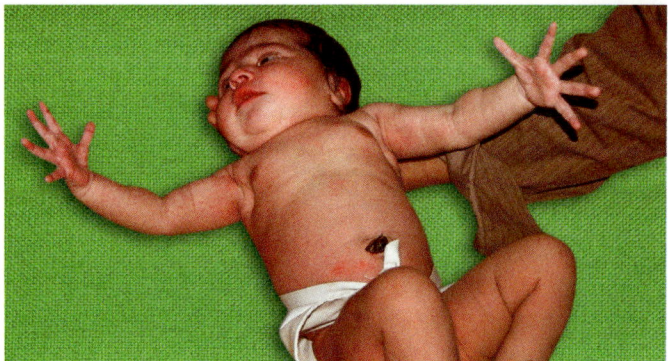

Fig. 7.17 Moro reflex. Note: bilateral abduction of shoulders, extension at elbows, and opening of hands

applied for 5 seconds by the index finger of the examiner; followed by release and simultaneous observation for return of normal color in the blanched area. The pink color should return immediately. A delay of >3 seconds is indicative of poor tissue perfusion and shock. Two persons are needed to perform the test—one for doing the procedure and other person for recording the time using stop watch or wrist watch.

Alternatively, one can do this alone by counting loudly one-thousand-one; one-thousand-two; one-thousand-three; one-thousand-four; one-thousand-five while pressing over the sternum. This will approximate 5 seconds. Then release the pressure and start counting again one-thousand-one; one-thousand-two; one-thousand-three. If blanch disappears before saying one-thousand-three, CFT is normal. If it persists, CFT is prolonged.

CFT should not be tested on peripheral body parts such as palms and soles as it may be falsely prolonged due to low temperature of distal parts.

2. Activity, Tone and Reflexes

Look for symmetry of movement and posturing, body tone, and response to being handled and disturbed (ie, crying appropriately and quieting appropriately). Also note the amplitude and pitch of the cry. Elicit the following neonatal reflexes:

Moro Reflex

Moro reflex is elicited by sudden drop of the infant's head and trunk from an angle of 30° with the bed with immediate support by the examiner's hand. The response consists of symmetrical abduction at shoulders, extension at elbow joints, opening of hands, followed by flexion and adduction of upper extremities (Fig. 7.17).

An *asymmetric response* may indicate a fractured clavicle or humerus, brachial plexus injury, or a hemiparesis. Absence of Moro reflex suggests significant CNS insult, such as developmental anomaly, asphyxia, infection, metabolic disturbance, or intracranial hemorrhage. Moro reflex appears by 28 weeks of gestation but the arms tend to fall backwards during the adduction phase due to weakness of anti-gravity muscles. It is fully developed by term age. It disappears by 4 to 5 months of age. Persistence beyond 6 months signifies brain damage.

Rooting and Sucking Reflex

Touching the upper lip laterally will cause most infants to turn toward the touch and open their mouths; more hungry and vigorous the infant, the more intense is the rooting response. Placing a clean finger in the mouth 2–3 cm deep will initiate a vigorous rhythmic sucking response. These reflexes are present at birth and disappear by 3–4 months of age.

Palmar and Plantar Grasp

Examiner's finger is placed against the ulnar border of the palm of hand. The baby will close fingers over examiner's finger. This reflex is present at birth and disappears by 3–4 months of age. For eliciting the plantar grasp, examiner's finger is placed against the soles of feet near the bases of toes. The baby will close toes over examiner's finger. This reflex is present at birth and disappears by 10 months of age.

Stepping and Placing Reflex

Infant is held in a standing position with both feet on flat surface. The baby takes alternate steps. This reflex appears by 28 weeks of gestation and disappears by 2–3 months of age. To elicit the placing reflex, the dorsum of the baby's foot is touched against the edge of the table. The baby lifts his leg as if to step up a ladder. This reflex appears by 1st week of age and disappears by 6–8 weeks.

Asymmetric Tonic Neck Reflex

With the infant supine, turn the head to one side. There is extension of arm on the ipsilateral side (towards face) and flexion on the contralateral side. The reflex disappears by 2–3 months of age. Persistence suggests brain damage.

3. Head, Neck, Mouth, and Eye

- *Size of the head* The average head circumference is 25 cm at 28 weeks, 28 cm at 32 weeks, 32 cm at 36 weeks, and 33–36 cm at 40 weeks of gestation.
- *Scalp* The infant's scalp should be inspected for cuts or bruises due to forceps application, operative delivery, or fetal monitor leads.

- *Swellings* Check for caput succedaneum, cephal-hematoma, and encephalocele. Cephalhematoma may not become full-blown until the third or fourth day.
- *Molding* The degree of molding of the skull bones should be noted. Usually, molding subsides within 5 days.
- *Fontanels* Normal size of anterior fontanel is 3 × 3 cm and posterior fontanel should be closed at birth. Very large fontanels reflect a delay in bone ossification and may be associated with hydrocephalus, hypothyroidism, trisomy syndromes, intrauterine malnutrition, hypophosphatasia, rickets, and osteogenesis imperfecta. Very small fontanel could be due to molding, microcephaly, or cranio-synostosis. Abnormal tension should be noted when the infant is raised to the semi-sitting position and not crying.
- *Ears* Note size, shape, position, and presence of auditory canals as well as preauricular sinus, pits or skin tags.
- *Face* Look for dysmorphic features such as hypertelorism, epicanthal fold, microphthalmia, depressed bridge of nose, micrognathia, asymmetry of face on crying due to 7th nerve palsy or congenital absence of depressor anguli oris muscle, upward slanting of eyes due to trisomy 21, etc.

Neck

Neck appears relatively short in neonates. It should be checked for cystic hygroma, goiter, and sternomastoid tumor. Sternomastoid tumor presents as firm swelling and torticollis at about 2 weeks of age. Neck has limited rotation towards the side of lesion. It is not a true tumor; the swelling is due to intramuscular hematoma and fibrosis. Treatment consists of passive exercises.

Mouth

Mouth should be examined to exclude soft and hard palate clefts, congenital (present at birth) or neonatal (eruption after birth) teeth, oral thrush (candidiasis), and ranula (cyst of sublingual salivary gland). Tongue-tie or ankyloglossia refers to abnormally short lingual frenulum that may restrict the tongue movement. Severe tongue-tie is recognized by the inability of the baby to protrude tongue over the gums. It is extremely rare.

Eyes

Newborns usually keep their eyes closed due to photophobia. No attempt should be made to forcefully open the eyes; doing so will produce crying and result in tighter eye closure. Eye opening can be aided by holding the baby upright and rocking gently forward and backward. Inspect eyes for purulent discharge, subconjunctival hemorrhages, cataract, coloboma, corneal haziness, and glaucoma.

4. Respiration and Lungs

Respiratory rate of a normal newborn is usually 40–60 breaths per minute. Breathing may be irregular in newborns. Periodic breathing characterized by fast respirations followed by pause of 5–10 seconds may be present. In a warm infant, there should not be any expiratory grunting and little or no flaring of the nostrils. Mild subcostal and intercostal retractions are common in normal babies, more so in premature babies because of their compliant chest wall. Neonatal breath sounds are harsh and have broncho-

vesicular character because of better transmission of large airway sounds across the thin chest wall. Chest percussion is best avoided in neonates as it rarely provides any meaningful information, and baby may not tolerate the procedure well.

5. Heart

The examiner should observe the rate, rhythm, quality of the heart sounds, and the presence or absence of murmurs. The heart rate is normally 120–160 beats per minute. It varies with changes in the infant's activity, increasing when she is crying, active, or breathing rather rapidly. Heart rate decreases when the baby is quiet and breathing slowly. An occasional term or postmature infant may, at rest, have a heart rate below 100.

Murmurs do not mean much because a newborn can have extremely serious heart anomalies without any murmurs. On the other hand, a closing ductus arteriosus may cause a very loud and worrisome murmur, though transient. The femoral pulses should be felt, although often they are weak in the first day or two. If there is doubt about the femoral pulses by time of discharge, the blood pressure in the upper and lower extremities should be checked (to rule out coarctation of aorta). Preductal (right wrist) and postductal (lower limb) oxygen saturation should be evaluated by pulse oximetry to rule out persistent pulmonary hypertension where a difference of 5–10% will be present between pre- and postductal measurements.

6. Abdomen

The edge of the liver is occasionally seen, and intestinal patterning is easily visible due to thin abdominal musculature. Asymmetry due to congenital anomalies or masses often is first appreciated by observation. When palpating the abdomen, start with gentle pressure or stroking, moving from lower to upper quadrants to reveal the edges of the liver or spleen. The normal newborn liver extends 2.0–2.5 cm below the costal margin. The spleen tip may be palpable in a normal newborn.

Male genitalia. Boys almost invariably have marked phimosis. The scrotum is often quite large, hydrocele is not uncommon, but unless it is communicating types, it will disappear in time without being the forerunner of an inguinal hernia.

Female genitalia. Occasionally, a mucosal tag from the wall of the vagina is noted. A discharge from the vagina, usually creamy white in color, is commonly found and, on occasion, replaced after the second day by menstrual like withdrawal bleeding.

Anus and rectum. Anus and rectum should be checked carefully for patency, position, and size (normal diameter is 10 mm).

7. Extremities and Spine

Common problems include syndactyly, polydactyly, talipes equinovarus (club feet), and developmental dysplasia of hip. Mild tibial bowing is also normal. Diminished movement of an arm is suggestive of Erb palsy or a fracture of a clavicle or humerus.

Barlow Test

To examine for hip dislocation, infant is placed on his back with hip and thighs flexed. The examiner places the middle finger of each hand on the greater trochanter and thumb of each hand on the inner thigh opposite the lesser trochanter. One hip is tested at a time, with stabilization of pelvis with other hand. The hip to be tested is flexed, adducted and pushed posteriorly. If the hip is dislocable, it can be readily felt during the maneuver.

Ortolani Maneuver

This maneuver reduces a recently dislocated hip. The test is done by flexing and abducting the thigh and at the same time femoral head is pushed anteriorly. If it is possible to achieve reduction, relocation of femoral head will be felt as a "clunk", not an audible click. After 6–8 weeks, reduction is not possible due to development of soft tissue contractures. The "clunk" of reduction should not be confused with audible clicks which may occur due to breaking of surface tension across the hip joint and snapping of gluteal muscles.

Examination of Back

The back, especially the lower lumbar and sacral areas, should be examined for pilonidal sinus tracts and small soft midline swellings that might indicate a small meningocele or other anomaly. Look for tufts of hair, hemangioma, or pigmented nevus which may suggest a tethered cord.

Assessment of Gestational Age

Reliable history of maternal LMP and early ultrasound in first trimester are the best means of determining the gestational age. In the presence of uncertain LMP and unavailability of first trimester ultrasound, gestational age can be estimated by various methods. Presently the most favored method is the New Ballard Score, also known as the Expanded Ballard Score **(Table 7.5)**. The score includes 6 parameters related to *neuromuscular maturity* and 6 parameters related to *physical maturity*. However, even with this method, there may be error in assessment of gestational age by 1 to 2 weeks.

Examination at Discharge

At discharge, the infant should be re-examined for the following:

- *Feeding* Adequacy of breastfeeding, vomiting, abdominal distension, degree of weight loss
- *Cord* Infection
- *Infection* Signs of sepsis
- *Skin* Jaundice, pyoderma
- *Heart* Murmur, cyanosis, femoral pulsess
- *Lungs* Any sign of respiratory distress
- *CNS* Fullness of fontanels, sutures, activity
- *Abdomen* Any masses, stools, urine output
- *Follow-up* Next date of visit should be fixed

CARE OF NORMAL NEWBORN

The events during first few minutes of life have an immense bearing on the immediate and long-term outcome of the infant. The aims of neonatal care at birth are directed at establishment of breathing; prevention of hypothermia; establishment of breastfeeding; prevention of infection; and identification of at risk neonates.

We shall discuss the care of normal newborn under the following 4 subheads: Preparation before delivery; immediate care at birth; care after birth; and essential postnatal care.

A. Preparation before Delivery

1. Select a clean well-lighted, warm and well-ventilated room for delivery.
2. Keep enough linen which has been washed and sun-dried for use at the time of delivery for the baby.
3. Ensure that disposable delivery kit is available with the family for use at the time of delivery. If not, ensure that a new blade is available for cutting the cord at birth.
4. For a hospital delivery, ensure availability of all equipment.
5. Ensure that the birth is attended by trained health personnel.
6. Follow the 'five cleans' to prevent infection in the newborn—clean surface, clean hands, clean cord tie, clean blade and clean (dry) cord care.

B. Immediate Care at Birth

Cord clamping should be delayed for at least one minute in babies who do not require resuscitation. This improves their iron status during infancy and preterm babies also benefit from this approach by improved blood pressure and lower incidence of intraventricular hemorrhage. However, these babies are more likely to receive phototherapy for hyperbilirubinemia due to higher blood volume. Cord clamping should not be delayed in babies requiring resuscitation.

Routine Care

Over 90% of the newborns do not require any active resuscitation. Routine care is sufficient for them. Efforts are directed to prevent hypothermia and attention is focused on the airways so that they are cleared off any secretions and kept patent. The overhead radiant warmer of the resuscitation trolley should be turned on 20 minutes before the birth of the baby. The baby should be received in a pre-warmed linen. After thorough drying, the baby should be positioned on the back or side. If there are secretions, the mouth should be suctioned first followed by suctioning of the nose using 10 F catheter. The suction force should be gentle and intermittent using a maximum suction pressure of 100 mm Hg. Suctioning should not be more than 5 seconds at a time to avoid vagal mediated bradycardia.

These steps usually take around 20–30 seconds and by this time most babies are vigorously crying, actively moving and are pink in color. Centrally cyanosed babies require free flow of oxygen with the help of tube and mask. If the baby is not crying by this time and she is gasping or having no breathing efforts give one or two flicks or gentle slaps over the soles to stimulate breathing. Prolonged stimulation should not be done as it delays the resuscitation of the baby. Details of further resuscitation has been discussed in section on neonatal resuscitation.

7

Table 7.5 New Ballard Score. Estimation of Gestational Age

Parameters for Physical Maturity

			Score				
	−1	0	1	2	3	4	5
Skin	Sticky, friable transparent	Gelatinous, red, translucent	Smooth, pink, visible veins	Superficial peeling, &/or rash, a few veins	Cracking pale areas, rare veins	Parchment deep cracking, no vessels	Feathery cracked wrinkled
Lanugo	None	Sparse	Abundant	Thinning	Bald areas	Mostly bald	
Breast	Imperceptible	Barely perceptible	Flat areola, no bud	Stippled areola, 1 mm bud	Raised areola, 3 mm bud	Full areola, 5 mm bud	
Genitals male	Scrotum flat smooth	Scrotum empty, faint rugae	Testes in upper canal, rare rugae	Testes descending, a few rugae	Testes down, good rugae	Testes pendulous, deep rugae	
Genitals female	Clitoris prominent, labia flat	Clitoris prominent, small labia minora	Clitoris prominent, enlarging minora	Majora and minora equally prominent	Majora large, minora small	Majora covers clitoris & minora	
Plantar surface	Heel-toe length 40–50 mm: −1 <40 mm: −2	Heel-toe > 50 mm, no crease	Faint red marks	Anterior transverse crease only	Creases anterior two-thirds	Creases over entire sole	
Eye and ear	Lids fused loosely: −1 tightly: −2	Lids open, pinna flat, stays folded	Slightly curved, pinna soft with slow recoil	Well-curved, pinna soft with ready recoil	Formed and firm with instant recoil	Thick cartilage, ear stiff	

Parameters for Neuromuscular Maturity

Posture	Wrists, arms, hips and legs and legs straight	Wrists bent and legs slightly bent	Elbows, hips, and legs bent	Elbows, hips and drawn bent to 90°	Elbows & legs bent and drawn close to body	
Square window (wrist)	> 90°	90°	60°	45°	30°	0°
Arm recoil		180°	140–180°	110–140°	90–110°	< 90°
Popliteal angle	180°	160°	140°	120°	110°	90°	< 90°
Scarf sign	Elbow beyond opposite axillary line	Elbow to opposite axillary line	Elbow to opposite midclavicular line	Elbow to midline	Elbow to axillary line	Elbow does not reach axillary line
Heel to ear	Leg straight, heel reaches ear	Leg straight, toes reach chin	Knee slightly bent, heel reaches 140° from prone	Knee bent, heel reaches 120° from prone	Knee bent to 90° heel reaches 90° from prone	Knee bent, heel reaches 45° from prone

New Ballard Score = Sum total of points for each parameter

Correlation of score with Gestational Age

Score	Week	Score	Week	Score	Week	Score	Week
−10	20	5	26	20	32	35	38
−5	22	10	28	25	34	40	40
0	24	15	30	30	36	45	42
						50	44

C. Care after Birth

Prevent Hypothermia

After having ensured that the baby has established effective breathing, it is essential that all efforts are made to prevent the occurrence of hypothermia. The baby is received in prewarmed linen. She should be placed under a radiant warmer or any heat source during the procedure of resuscitation.

Prevent Infection

Separate sterile delivery kit should be available for each baby to prevent cross-infection. The umbilical cord should be tied using two sterile ligatures or rubber band or a disposable clamp. The clamp or ligature should be applied at least 2–3 cm beyond the base of the cord to avoid inadvertent incision of gut contained in minor exomphalos. Do not apply anything over the cord.

Rule Out Congenital Anomalies

Quick but thorough clinical screening is essential to identify any life-threatening congenital anomalies and birth injuries. The infant should be examined for location and patency of all the orifices. Choanal atresia is excluded by inserting a catheter through both nostrils. Anorectal malformation can be excluded by visual examination of the perineum. Examine the umbilical stump for the number of vessels. Normally, there are two arteries and one vein. A single umbilical artery occurs in about 1% of newborns and may be associated with other congenital malformations such as tracheoesophageal fistula and genitourinary anomalies.

Others

Vitamin K 0.5 mg below 1 kg and 1.0 mg above 1 kg should be administered intramuscularly using a 26-gauge needle on anterolateral aspect of mid-thigh to all babies. A baby should have an identification tag applied mentioning mother's name and date and time of birth before being shifted out of labor room.

D. Essential Postnatal Care

1. Practice rooming-in. Mother and baby should be kept in the same bed. Baby should be well clothed and room should be kept warm.
2. Care of the umbilical stump:
   - It should be clean and dry.
   - The tie should be tight.
   - There should be no bleeding.
   - It should be left open without any dressing.
3. The baby should be cleaned off blood, mucus, and meconium before handing over to the mother. There is no need to remove vernix caseosa as it protects the skin of the baby. Bathing is discouraged during hospital stay for fear of hypothermia and risk of infection. The skin should be checked especially at the creases for development of any pyoderma. The baby should have good suckling at breast. If suckling is poor, ensure correct positioning and attachment to breast.
4. The baby should be checked for crying well and having no breathing difficulty. If the baby develops breathing difficulty or any other danger signals, she should be referred to appropriate healthcare facility.
5. The mother should be advised regarding the immunization schedule (BCG, OPV, and hepatitis B zero dose at birth).
6. Each baby should be followed up in the well baby clinic for assessment of growth and development, early diagnosis and management of illnesses and health education of parents. Follow-up should coincide with immunization schedule as far as practicable.

E. Advice at Discharge of a Normal Newborn

1. Exclusive breastfeeding for 6 months—day and night.
2. Prevention of hypothermia: Appropriate clothing/wrapping of the baby according to climate and rooming-in and kangaroo mother care (KMC) for low birth weight babies.
3. Prevention of infection: To use clean clothings/beddings and handwashing with soap and water before touching the baby.
4. Keep the cord stump dry and clean.
5. Vaccination as per National Immunization Schedule.
6. To identify danger signs early and contact a health personal.
7. To attend follow-up/well baby clinic for monitoring of growth and development.

Normal Variations of Newborns

- *Milia* These are superficial epidermal inclusion cysts. These are pearly white or pale yellow papules or cysts, 1–2 mm in diameter, and are found over nose, chin, forehead and cheeks. They disappear spontaneously in a few weeks requiring no treatment.
- *Sebaceous gland hyperplasia* The lesions are similar in distribution to milia, but are smaller (pinpointed), more numerous, and more yellow. They represent hyperplastic sebaceous glands due to maternal androgen stimulation, and disappear within a few weeks.
- *Blue-gray macule of infancy* Commonly known as mongolian spots. *The* lesions are bluish or slate-gray macular lesions with indistinct margins. They are due to accumulation of melanocytes within the dermis. They occur most commonly on lumbosacral area and buttocks but may be found on the trunk and extremities. The lesions may be single or multiple, and are not palpable or elevated. They are much more common in Asians (80%) than in Caucasians (10%). These are benign lesions and gradually fade by 1 to 2 years of age. These lesions have no relationship with trisomy 21. Malignant change has never been reported.
- *Erythema toxicum* It is a benign, self-limited eruption, probably secondary to the exposure to different allergens after birth, characterized by small papules or pustules or rarely vesicles with intense surrounding erythema. At times, blotchy erythema is the only manifestation. The lesions appear on day 1 or 2 of age and are usually located on trunk but may be found on extremities and face. Palms and soles are spared. Erythema toxicum is found in 50% of term newborns; and is less common in preterm babies. The lesions should not be confused with pyoderma; the differentiating feature being intense erythema surrounding pustules in erythema toxicum. The scrapings

from skin lesions show eosinophils, as opposed to neutrophils in pyoderma. No treatment is required and eruptions disappear by 7 to 10 days.

- *Peeling skin* Dry skin with peeling and exaggerated transverse skin creases is seen in post-term and some term babies, especially. Parents need only reassurance.
- *Cutis marmorata* It is characterized by an evanescent, lacy, reticulated, red or blue marbled cutaneous vascular pattern over the extremities. It occurs due to accentuated physiological vasomotor response to cold, and disappears with increasing age.
- *Harlequin color change* It is an interesting phenomenon seen in neonates. When the baby is placed on side, the body appears divided longitudinally into paler upper half and a red dependent half. By reversing the position of body, the color pattern may also reverse. It reflects an imbalance in the autonomic vascular regulatory mechanism, and disappears spontaneously.
- *Acne neonatorum* Typical acne lesions may be seen over the forehead, nose and cheeks at birth in term babies. They occur due to transplacental passage of maternal androgens to the fetus. The skin lesions disappear spontaneously within the next couple of days.
- *Sucking blisters* These are thought to arise from vigorous sucking on the affected part in utero. Common sites are radial aspect of forearm, thumb, index finger and even great toe. They resolve without sequelae.
- *Epstein's pearls* These are milia that occur in oral mucosa. The lesions are opaque and white and usually are found on the palate, along the midpalatine raphe and at the junction of hard and soft palates.
- *Sacral dimple* A dimple in the midline of the sacrococcygeal region should not be confused with a pilonidal sinus. It is of no clinical significance.
- *Umbilical hernia* It is due to incomplete closure or weakness of umbilical ring. It presents as soft swelling that protrudes during crying or straining. Most umbilical hernias disappear by 1 year of age. There is no role of strapping with coin. Surgery is indicated, if it causes strangulation any time or if it persists beyond 2 to 3 years of age.
- *Umbilical granuloma* Normally when umbilical stump falls off, epithelium grows over the raw area and healing is complete. Delayed epithelialization results in formation of granulomatous tissue at the umbilicus. It presents as dull red or pink papule, and there may be mucoid or mucopurulent discharge. Careful application of silver nitrate to the lesion, avoiding contact with surrounding skin, twice a week is curative. Umbilical granuloma should be differentiated from umbilical polyp which is bright red in appearance and has a mucoid discharge. It represents persistence of all or part of the omphalomesenteric duct or urachus. Treatment is surgical excision of the entire omphalomesenteric or urachal remnant.
- *Hymenal tags* Mucosal tags at the margin of hymen are seen in two-thirds of female infants.

MINOR NEONATAL PROBLEMS

Regurgitation and Vomiting

Regurgitation refers to return of small amount of swallowed milk during or shortly after feeding. Vomiting, on the other hand, is more complete emptying of stomach contents and arises due to forceful contractions of abdominal musculature. Regurgitation is a normal finding and the baby remains otherwise healthy. Regurgitation can be lessened by burping the baby after feeding and by placing him/her in right lateral position after feeding. Occasional episode of vomiting is also quite common in newborn babies. Vomiting is more common in bottlefed babies due to aerophagia and overfeeding.

Persistent vomiting may indicate intestinal obstruction, septicemia, intracranial pathology or a metabolic disorder. Intestinal pathology is suggested, if vomiting is bile-stained, projectile or associated with visible peristalsis, abdominal distention and failure to pass meconium.

Failure to Pass Meconium

Most babies usually pass meconium within 24 hours of age and urine by 48 hours of age. Premature babies may have slight delay in the passage of meconium due to reduced gut motility. Occasionally, high anal sphincter tone may delay the passage of meconium. In this case, baby will pass meconium after insertion of rectal catheter or thermometer.

- *Failure to pass* meconium is seen in imperforate anus.
- *Delayed passage* of meconium is seen in congenital hypothyroidism, Hirschsprung disease and meconium ileus due to cystic fibrosis.

Breastfed babies usually pass up to 10–15 stools a day which are yellow in color, and slightly loose in consistency. Sometimes, baby may pass stool during or after each feeding. This is known as gastrocolic reflex. This is a normal phenomenon and mother should be reassured that this causes no harm to the baby and will disappear after a few weeks.

Failure to Pass Urine

Fetus voids urine regularly *in utero* after 12 weeks of gestation. Most babies pass urine by 48 hours of age. The most common cause of non-passage of urine by 48 hours is that the baby might have passed urine at birth without being noticed. Inadequate feeding may account for delayed passage of urine. Ensuring proper feeding will result in the passage of urine in a few hours time. Infants with delayed passage of urine should be investigated for obstructive uropathy and agenesis of kidneys.

A baby can pass urine 8 to 10 times a day, or even more frequently. It is light colored. Some babies may cry before or during passing urine due to discomfort of full bladder. This should not be interpreted as indicative of urinary tract infection.

Hiccups, Sneezing and Yawning

These are normal physiological phenomena. Some parents may be upset by these symptoms. Baby appears comfortable. Reassure the parents about the benign nature of these symptoms.

Excessive Crying

In the first few weeks, most newborn babies sleep during daytime and remain active and awake for extended periods

Case Study   Normal Newborn

You receive a call for attending a delivery in your hospital.

Q1. How will you proceed for the resuscitation of this baby?
- Switch on the radiant warmer at least 20 minutes before delivery.
- Note down relevant details of maternal history and investigations.
- Check whether all the equipment are in working order including bag and mask, laryngoscope, suction machine, oxygen source, etc.
- *As soon as the baby is born, ask 3 questions*:
  A. Is the baby of term gestation?
  B. Is the baby crying or breathing?
  C. Is the baby having good muscle tone?
- If the answer to all the questions is yes, baby requires no resuscitation and needs routine care only. If the answer to any one of the questions is no, baby requires resuscitation.

The baby is a full term girl. She cried immediately after birth and is moving limbs actively.

Q2. Outline the management.

Receive the baby in a prewarmed sheet. Put the baby prone on mother's abdomen with head turned to one side or place under radiant warmer. Gently wipe out excess secretions from mouth and nose with a sterile gauze piece. If copious secretions are present, suction mouth and then nose using disposable mucus extractor. Dry thoroughly, including head; and discard wet linen. Assign APGAR score at 1 and 5 minutes. Cut cord about 1 inch from the base. Tie the cord using disposable cord clamp/sterile rubber band.

Assess respiratory rate and breathing efforts, heart rate and color. Do a general inspection from head to toe for detection of any abnormality. Auscultate chest for bilateral air entry and precordium for murmurs. Palpate abdomen for any mass. Look for any congenital malformation. Record weight, length and head circumference.

Put identification bracelet on the baby. Clothe the baby appropriately. Give inj. vitamin K 1 mg IM stat in anterolateral aspect of thigh. Keep mother and baby together (rooming-in). Start breastfeeding within ½ to 1 hour of birth.

Q3. When should you visit the baby next? What should you ensure at this stage?

The next visit should be made at 4–6 hours. Look for temperature; ensure that the hands and feet are warm to touch. Assess whether breastfeeding is going on well. Check the cord for bleeding. Look for any danger signs such as respiratory distress, refusal to feed, excessive irritability/lethargy, hypothermia, cyanosis, bleeding from any site.

Q4. When will you discharge this baby? What advice will you give?

Baby can be discharged from hospital at 48–72 hours of age provided both mother and baby are well. Baby is immunized with BCG, and received zero dose OPV and hepatitis B before discharge.

Perform a complete clinical examination and record weight before discharge. Advise regarding temperature maintenance, hygiene, exclusive breastfeeding, and immunization. Explain danger signs to the mother and when to seek help. Call baby for follow-up after 1 week and then arrange follow-up visits coinciding with immunization schedule. Assess growth and development in follow-up visits.

Continue exclusive breastfeeding till 6 months of age.

during night. This is normal *in utero* behavioral pattern which continues for some time after birth. There are many reasons for excessive crying in newborn infants. Sometimes the cause may not be obvious. Crying may be due to hunger, wet nappy, exposure to cold, loud noise or excessive light, nasal blockage. Bottle feeding may also be a source of excessive crying due to overfeeding or aerophagia. Sometimes overclothing may also distress the baby. Breastfed babies are generally more calm and quiet and cry less often as compared to topfed babies.

More serious causes of excessive crying include septicemia, meningitis, hypoxic-ischemic encephalopathy, painful conditions such as cellulitis, birth trauma, osteomyelitis, metabolic disorders, infants of drug addicted mothers, etc.

Caput Succedaneum

Caput succedaneum is a serosanguineous, subcutaneous, *extraperiosteal* fluid collection with poorly defined margins. The swelling pits on pressure. It is caused by the pressure of the presenting part against the dilating cervix. Caput succedaneum extends across the midline and over suture lines, is non-fluctuant and is associated with head molding. It does not usually cause complications and usually resolves over the first few days. Management consists of observation only.

Cephalhematoma

Cephalhematoma is a *subperiosteal* collection of blood secondary to rupture of subperiosteal veins between the skull and the periosteum. It does not cross the suture lines. The swelling is cystic or fluctuant in nature. Most commonly parietal, cephalhematoma may occasionally be observed over the occipital bone.

Complications The hemorrhage may be severe enough to cause anemia and rarely hypotension. Another complication is hyperbilirubinemia due to extravasated blood which may require phototherapy and rarely exchange transfusion. Sometimes, cephalhematoma may get infected. Occasionally, cephalhematoma may be associated with linear skull fracture.

Treatment	Cephalhematoma

Resolution generally occurs over 2–8 weeks, occasionally with residual calcification. No laboratory studies are usually necessary. In the absence of neurological features, X-ray skull or CT scanning is not indicated. Management consists of observation only. Parents should be advised not to massage the swelling. Transfusion for anemia, hypovolemia, or both is necessary, if blood accumulation is significant. Aspiration is not required for resolution and is likely to increase the risk of infection. Aspiration is indicated only when it is infected or if it is contributing to severe hyperbilirubinemia necessitating exchange transfusion.

Disorders due to Transplacental Passage of Maternal Hormones

Mastitis Neonatorum

This refers to enlargement/engorgement of one or both breasts in neonates of both sexes. It commonly presents by one week of age and may last for a few weeks. It is a painless swelling, without any erythema or tenderness. It results from the action of maternally transmitted progesterone and estrogens on breast tissue due to lack of metabolism by immature liver. No intervention is needed. Local massage, fomentation and temptation to express the milk should not be done.

Vaginal Bleeding

It mimics menstrual-like withdrawal bleeding in female babies. It is usually seen on day 3 or 4 of age. The bleeding is mild and lasts 2–3 days only. No intervention is required except local cleaning and parental reassurance.

Revision Point	Normal Newborn

1. Assessment of a newborn requires detailed antenatal, natal and postnatal history.
2. Examination of a newborn should be done in a warm room with warm hands.
3. Umbilical cord should be left dry; no applications should be made in a healthy cord.
4. *Kangaroo mother care* should be encouraged in the 1st week.
5. Newborn babies should be discharged only if they are breastfeeding well, have no major illness, and have been immunized.
6. During hospital stay and at discharge, communicate with parents and extended family regards care of the infant at home.

Mucoid Vaginal Secretions

It is a common problem in female babies who may present with thin grayish-white mucoid vaginal secretions. No treatment is required and secretions should be gently cleaned.

Margolis PA, Stevens R, Bordley WC, *et al*. From concept to application: the impact of a community-wide intervention to improve the delivery of preventive services to children. *Pediatrics*. 2001;108:E42.

National Neonatology Forum and UNICEF. Facility based care of sick neonate ay referral health facility. *Comprehensive Newborn Care Initiative*. New Delhi: 2011.

World Health Organization. *Essential Newborn Care*. Geneva: WHO; 2010.

7.5 TEMPERATURE MAINTENANCE

Hypothermia is an important cause of morbidity and mortality in newborns, particularly in preterm, low birth weight babies. Neonates are more prone to hypothermia because of high surface area to mass ratio, thin vascular skin, lack of insulating subcutaneous fat, and inability to shiver. All these handicaps are worse in preterm low birth weight (LBW) infants which makes them most susceptible to hypothermia.

THERMOREGULATION

Thermoregulation is the ability to balance heat production and heat loss in order to maintain body temperature within a certain "normal" range. Thermoregulation is controlled by the hypothalamus. Thermal stimuli providing information to the hypothalamus are derived from the body's skin and deep thermal receptors and from thermal receptors in the preoptic area of the hypothalamus.

Fetal temperature is 0.3–0.5°C higher compared to the mother due to higher metabolic rate in the fetus. Like other functions such as gas exchange and excretion of metabolic waste products, fetus is entirely dependent on mother for heat dissipation. Approximately 85% of fetal heat loss occurs through umbilical circulation and remaining through fetal skin to amnion. The temperature difference between mother and fetus is known as *heat clamp* which is maintained even when the mother is febrile. At birth, the transition from intrauterine to extrauterine life presents a very different thermal environment which is 10–12°C lower; this challenges the infant's thermoregulatory abilities.

Mechanisms of Heat Loss after Birth

A neonate loses heat by the following mechanisms (Fig. 7.18):
- *Evaporation* Heat loss occurs due to evaporation of water from skin. Quantum of heat loss depends on relative humidity of surroundings, air turbulence, and environmental temperature. The newly born baby is most susceptible to hypothermia due to evaporation of amniotic fluid from skin surface.
- *Conduction* Heat loss occurs from skin to cold objects in direct contact with the baby, eg, mattress, cold cloth, tray, etc.
- *Convection* Neonate loses heat to a colder surrounding through air flow. The degree of heat loss largely depends

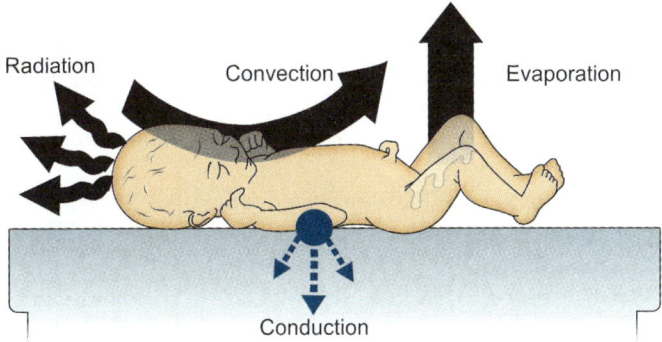

Fig. 7.18 Mechanisms of heat loss after birth

on the temperature and speed of the surrounding air; eg, it is facilitated by open windows, fans, and cold oxygen.
- *Radiation* Heat dissipates to colder surroundings by infrared electromagnetic radiation.

Heat Production: Non-Shivering and Shivering Thermogenesis

When an animal is acutely exposed to a 'low' environmental temperature, it needs extra heat to compensate for the increased heat loss in order to defend its core body temperature. In a human neonate, thermogenic response begins within minutes of birth. There are two heat production modalities in humans: (1) as a result of increased cellular metabolic activity; and (2) extra heat production via non-shivering and shivering thermogenesis.

Non-shivering thermogenesis is the primary source of heat production in newborn infants; shivering thermogenesis is insignificant as neonatal muscles are relatively immature. The main organ responsible for non-shivering thermogenesis is *brown adipose tissue* (brown fat) that works as an electric blanket to the body.

Brown adipose tissue (BAT) in human infants is mainly deposited after 28 weeks gestation, and principally found around scapulae, kidneys, adrenals, neck, and axillae. In full term infants, brown fat constitutes 1–2% of body weight. BAT contains plenty of mitochondria, is richly supplied by blood vessels and extensively innervated by sympathetic nervous system. Stimulation of sympathetic innervation to brown adipose tissue releases norepinephrine, which acts via $\alpha 3$ receptors to increase lipolysis. Increased fatty acid oxidation in the mitochondria increases heat production. This is mediated by the presence of uncoupling protein (UCP-1) in mitochondria of brown adipose tissue that uncouples oxidative phosphorylation, producing heat. Blood circulating through the brown fat becomes warm and through circulation carries heat to other body parts. Preterm and IUGR infants have poor reserves of BAT, making them prone to hypothermia.

Thermoneutral Environment

It is defined as a narrow range of environmental temperatures within which the baby can maintain normal body temperature with minimal metabolic rate and minimal oxygen consumption. Within this range, the infant is in thermal equilibrium (thermoneutrality) with the environment. This range of temperature varies according to the weight and gestational age of the baby. Smaller, preterm babies have higher thermoneutral temperature requirement compared to larger, term babies. Other factors which influence thermoneutral environment are postnatal age, clothing, air currents, and humidity. **Table 7.6** provides the recommended thermoneutral temperatures for neonates, categorized as per their birthweight, gestational age, and post-conceptional age.

Recording of Temperature

Low reading thermometers (records between 30°C and 40°C) should be used in the newborns to record temperature and detect hypothermia.

Axillary temperature Temperature is recorded by placing the tip of the bulb of the thermometer against the roof of dry axilla. Baby's arm is held close to the body to keep the thermometer in place. The temperature is read after 3 minutes. It is a safe method of recording temperature as it has lesser risk of cross-infection and injury compared to rectal temperature recording.

Rectal temperature Rectal temperature is recorded by inserting the bulb of the thermometer in the rectum in a direction backwards and downwards to a depth of 3 cm in a

Table 7.6 Neutral Thermal Environmental Temperatures		
	Temperature	
Age and weight	*At start (°c)*	*Range (°C)*
Day 1		
Under 1200 g	34.0–35.0	34.0–35.4
1200–1500 g	33.8–34.0	33.3–34.4
1500–2500 g	32.8–33.4	31.8–33.8
Over 2500 g		
(and >36 wk gestation)	32.4–32.9	31.0–33.8
Day 2–3		
Under 1200 g	34.0	34.0–35.0
1200–1500 g	33.5	33.0–34.2
1500–2500 g	32.4	31.2–33.6
Over 2500 g		
(and >36 wk gestation)	31.7–32.1	30.1–33.5
72–96 hours		
Under 1200 g	34.0	34.0–35.0
1200–1500 g	33.5	33.0–34.0
1500–2500 g	32.2	31.1–33.2
Over 2500 g		
(and >36 wk gestation)	31.3	29.8–32.8
4–14 days		
Under 1500 g	33.5	32.6–34.0
1500–2500 g	32.1	31.0–33.2
Over 2500 g		
(and >36 wk gestation)	30.4	29.0–31.2
2–3 weeks		
Under 1500 g	33.1	32.2–34.0
1500–2500 g	31.7	30.5–33.0
3–4 weeks		
Under 1500 g	32.6	31.6–33.6
1500–2500 g	31.4	30.0–32.7

term baby and 2 cm in a preterm baby. The tip of the rectal thermometer is rounded to avoid any injury to the rectum. The temperature is read after 2 minutes. It is not used for routine monitoring as the procedure is inconvenient, and caries the risk of infection and trauma.

Human touch method It is an easy, noninvasive, and convenient method to detect hypothermia even at home. The mother/health professional can feel the hands and feet of baby and compare it with abdominal temperature. Abdominal temperature represents core temperature and is reliable in the diagnosis of hypothermia.

- If hands/feet and abdomen both are warm, it indicates that the baby is in thermal comfort.
- Cold hands/feet and warm abdomen indicate that the baby is in cold stress.
- If hands/feet and abdomen both are cold, it indicates moderate to severe hypothermia.

It has the drawback of underestimating hypothermia. However, the sensitivity of this method can be improved by training.

Liquid crystal thermometry-thermospot This is a simple device to record temperature of a baby on continuous basis in both hospital and community settings. It consists of 12 mm liquid crystal temperature dot that is placed on newborn's skin, medial to and just above the axilla. It turns green, if the baby is normothermic and black, if the baby is hypothermic.

HYPOTHERMIA

Definitions

Normal temperature : 36.5–37.5°C.
Cold stress : 36–36.4°C
Moderate hypothermia: between 32 and 36 °C
Severe hypothermia : less than 32°C.

Signs and Symptoms

During early stages of hypothermia, a neonate feels cold to the touch, is restless, irritable or lethargic. As the condition worsens, the neonate develops tachypnea or apnea, cyanosis or mottling, refusal to feed, bradycardia, hypoglycemia, and metabolic acidosis. There may be coagulation defects, acute renal failure and necrotizing enterocolitis, and ultimately death.

Metabolic Consequences

- Hypoxemia from increased oxygen consumption
- Hypoglycemia from increased glucose metabolism
- Metabolic acidosis secondary to anaerobic metabolism
- Inhibition of surfactant production related to acidosis
- Decreased pulmonary blood flow related to pulmonary vasoconstriction in response to decreased body temperature
- Increased pulmonary vascular resistance compromises the delivery of oxygen at the cell level.

Prevention

1. Warm Chain

Warm chain is a set of 10 interlinked procedures carried out to ensure thermal stability in a newborn. These procedures prevent heat loss and promote heat gain. The 10 points of warm chain are:

1. Warm delivery room (>25°C).
2. Warm resuscitation corner (>28°C).
3. Immediate drying of baby (including head) and removing wet linen.
4. Skin-to-skin contact between baby and the mother.
5. Breastfeeding.
6. Postponement of bathing.
7. Appropriate clothing and bedding.
8. Rooming-in of the mother and baby together.
9. Warm transportation.
10. Training/awareness of healthcare providers about significance of prevention of heat loss and maintenance of body temperature in newborns.

A. *Prevent Hypothermia in the Delivery Room*

1. Delivery room temperature should be >25°C.
2. Term newborns delivered normally can be put directly over the mother's abdomen immediately after delivery in prone position. Routine care can be provided in this posture and the mother–infant pair can be covered together.
3. If it is not possible or baby is delivered by cesarean section, newborn should be dried immediately to prevent evaporative heat loss, wrapped in prewarmed towel and kept well covered. Head should be thoroughly dried as it has a large surface area and kept covered.
4. Preterm babies can be put inside food grade, heat resistant plastic bags immediately after delivery even before drying or can be kept under radiant warmer. All resuscitative measures should be done under radiant warmer.

B. *Prevent Hypothermia in Postnatal Ward*

1. Baby should share the same bed as the mother.
2. Bathing should be avoided during hospital stay.
3. Baby should be clothed adequately including head and extremities.

C. *Prevent Hypothermia at the Home/Hospital or during Transport*

2. Kangaroo Mother Care (KMC)

KMC involves skin-to-skin contact between mother and her newborn to keep baby warm. It is an alternative to expensive incubators and radiant heat warmers which may not be available or affordable in resource-poor settings. KMC is given in home or in hospital to a hemodynamically stable LBW baby or during transport of a sick baby to hospital.

Method of giving KMC

The baby is placed naked, with a nappy, semi-upright inside mother's clothing against the bare skin over the chest in frog leg posture. Mother should wear a loose blouse or gown with a wrap tied at the waist to hold the baby in position (Fig. 7.19). Head of the baby is covered with a cap. Baby suckles at breast as often as she wants, but at least every 2 hours. Mother should lie propped up so that the baby stays upright. KMC can be continued as long as mother is comfortable. Kangaroo mother care can also be provided by the father or some other family member.

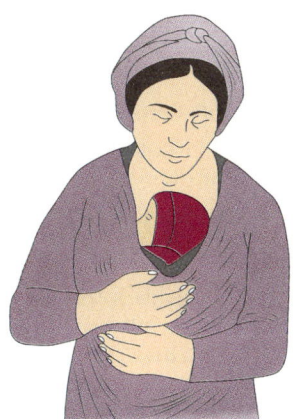

Fig. 7.19 Method of giving kangaroo mother care

Advantages

 i. Maintenance of temperature of the baby;
 ii. Facilitation of breastfeeding;
 iii. Better cardiorespiratory stability;
 iv. Fewer apneic episodes;
 v. More alertness and less activity resulting in more weight gain;
 vi. Lower infection rate;
 vii. Improvement of mother infant bonding;
viii. Early discharge from NICU; and
 ix. Improved survival in low-resource settings.

3. Other Measures to Prevent Heat Loss

Polyethylene and polyurethane bags and wraps have been used to prevent heat loss in the newborn. Application of topical agents such as paraffin, corn oil, sunflower oil, or safflower oil results in better thermoregulation in newborns. However, care should be taken to limit environmental exposure during massage.

Treatment	Hypothermia

Various methods like skin-to-skin contact, prewarmed mattress, or a radiant warmer can be used to warm the baby. The method selected will depend on the severity of hypothermia and availability of staff and equipment.
Cold stress (between 36 and 36.4°C) Can be managed by skin-to-skin contact or placing under a radiant warmer
Moderate (between 32.0 and 35.9°C) to severe (<32.0°C) hypothermia Baby should be kept naked under a radiant warmer over a prewarmed towel. The ambient temperature should be 28 ±2°C. Extremely low birth weight babies can also be kept in air heated humidified incubators (air temperature 35–36°C) or on a thermostatically controlled heated mattress set at 37–38°C. Skin-to-skin contact in a warm room and a warm bed may be used, if a radiant warmer is not available immediately. Re-warming should be continued till the temperature reaches the normal range. The baby should be monitored every 15–30 minutes. Hot water bottles should not be used. In addition to these, the following measures should be taken simultaneously:
• Monitor blood glucose
• Start 10% dextrose IV and maintain blood glucose >45 mg/dL
• Give oxygen inhalation

• Give vitamin K, if not given before
• Screen for associated sepsis and start antibiotics, if indicated
• Treat other complications
• Provide nutritional support by oral or gavage (orogastric) feeding

HYPERTHERMIA

When the newborn is in an environment that is too hot, the baby's temperature can rise above 37.5° C. This is known as hyperthermia.

Hyperthermia should not be confused with fever, which is a raised body temperature in response to infection with microorganisms or other sources of inflammation. However, it is not possible to distinguish between fever and hyper-thermia by measuring the body temperature or by clinical signs, and when the newborn has a raised temperature it is important to consider both causes. Infection should always be suspected first, unless there are very obvious external reasons. Some of the common causes of hyperthermia are wrapping the baby in too many layers of clothes, especially in hot, humid climates; leaving a baby in direct sunlight; putting a newborn baby too close to a fire or room heater, etc.

Dehydration fever is little understood entity which presents on day 3–4 of age. Other than raised body temperature, baby continues to be active and feeding well. It generally subsides in 24–48 hours. Relative dehydration due to inadequate feeding may be causative factor.

Treatment	Hyperthermia

The baby should be moved away from the source of heat, and undressed partially or fully, if necessary. It is important that the baby be breastfed more frequently to replace fluids. Every hyperthermic baby should be examined for infection. When hyperthermia is severe, i.e. body temperature is above 40°C, the baby can be given a bath with tepid water. If it is possible to measure the water temperature, it should be about 2°C lower than the baby's body temperature. Cold water should not be used.

Temperature Maintenance

1. Neonates are prone to hypothermia due to limited capacity of thermal regulation, large body surface area, and less subcutaneous fat.
2. Preterm, LBW, and asphyxiated newborns are at higher risk of hypothermia.
3. Temperature of a newborn should be maintained between 36.5 and 37.5°C.
4. Temperature between 36.0 and 37.5°C indicates cold stress. Abdomen will be warm to touch while soles will be cold.
5. Temperature below 36.0°C indicates hypothermia. Both abdomen and soles will be cold to touch. Place the child under a radiant warmer.
6. Warm chain (the 10 steps) is to be maintained for prevention of hypothermia in newborn.

Knobel R, Holditch-Davis D. Thermoregulation and heat loss prevention after birth and during neonatal intensive-care unit stabilization of extremely low birthweight infants. *Adv Neonatal Care.* 2010; 10:S7–14.

McCall EM, Alderdice F, Halliday HL, Jenkins JG, Vohra S. Interventions to prevent hypothermia at birth in preterm and/or low birthweight infants. *Cochrane Database Syst Rev.* 2010; (3):CD004210.

National Neonatology Forum and UNICEF. Facility based care of sick neonate ay referral health facility. *Comprehensive Newborn Care Initiative.* New Delhi:2010.

7.6 BREASTFEEDING

Breastfeeding is of fundamental importance for survival and well-being of children. It is estimated that over 1 million children die each year from infections and malnutrition because they are not adequately breastfed. It is not only a source of best food for the young child but also provides numerous other benefits such as protection from infection, better brain development, and protection from many life-style disorders including hypertension, diabetes, and atherosclerosis.

Early initiation and exclusive breastfeeding for the first 6 months of life helps ensure young children the best possible start to life. Breastfeeding fosters emotional security and affection, with a lifelong impact on psychosocial development.

Composition of Human Milk

Protein in Breastmilk

There are broadly two classes of proteins present in milk: (*a*) whey (acid-soluble) proteins, and (*b*) casein (acid-precipitable curd). Human milk is whey predominant (whey-casein ratio of 60:40 in mature milk) which makes it easily digestible. Cow's milk is casein predominant (whey-casein ratio of 20:80).

Human milk is considered to be the highest quality protein source for infants. The major whey proteins in breastmilk are α-lactalbumin, lactoferrin, and secretory IgA. Breastmilk is also a rich source of taurine and cysteine which are important neurotransmitters essential for the development of brain and retina. Taurine also helps in conjugation of bile acids. The protein content of preterm milk is higher than term milk which is in keeping with the higher protein requirements of these babies.

Fat in Breastmilk

Nearly 50% of energy in human milk is derived from fat. Fat is the most variable constituent of human milk. Maternal diet influences the fat content of milk. Fat content becomes higher in the latter portion of the breastfeeding (*hindmilk*) which may help to satiate the infant at the end of feeding. Human milk is rich in long chain fatty acids including essential fatty acids and medium chain triglycerides. Long chain fatty acids (eg, docosahexaenoic acid) present in human milk may influence brain structure and function. This may partly help explain better cognitive functioning of breastfed babies. Fat in human milk is better absorbed than in cow's milk.

Carbohydrate in Breastmilk

Nearly all the carbohydrate in human milk is lactose. It accounts for 40% of the energy content of milk. Galactose, an important component of galactocerebroside, is essential for brain growth. It also facilitates absorption of calcium.

Vitamins and Minerals in Breastmilk

Breastmilk is sufficient in vitamins A, C, D, and B complex. Vitamin K content of human milk is less. This can cause vitamin K deficiency bleeding. However, it can be easily prevented by giving 0.5 to 1.0 mg of vitamin K intramuscularly after birth. Though the iron content of breastmilk is low (0.03 mg/dL), its bioavailability is high (50%). Calcium-phosphorus ratio is optimal in human milk (>2) than in cow's milk **(Table 7.7)**.

Table 7.7 Differences between Human Milk and Cow's Milk

	Human milk	*Cow's milk*
Protein (g/dL)	1.1	3.3
Fat (g/dL)	4.2	3.8
Carbohydrate (g/dL)	7.4	4.8
Energy (kcal/dL)	67.0	67.0
Water (g/dL)	87.0	87.0
Calcium (mg/dL)	35.0	120.0
Phosphorus (mg/dL)	15.0	90.0

Others

Bile salt-stimulated lipase facilitates the complete digestion of fat once the milk has reached the small intestine. Epidermal growth factor stimulates maturation of the infant's intestine, so that it is better able to digest and absorb nutrients, and is less easily infected or sensitized to foreign proteins.

Advantages of Breastfeeding

1. Protection from Infection

Breastfeeding is crucial to child survival in developing countries. It affords protection against diarrhea, pneumonia and other infectious diseases by virtue of its anti-infective properties. The risk of death in breastfed infants from diarrhea and pneumonia is 14 and 4 times less, respectively, than in artificially fed infants.

Anti-infective factors in human milk
   i. Immunoglobulins: IgA, IgG, IgM
   ii. Cells: Macrophages, lymphocytes
   iii. Complements: C3, C4
   iv. Lysozymes
   v. Lactoperoxidase
   vi. Lipids (antiviral and anti-staphylococcal)
   vii. Iron binding proteins: Lactoferrin
   viii. Bile salt-stimulated lipase (anti-protozoal)
   ix. Interferon
   x. Growth factor for *Lactobacillus bifidus*

2. Intelligence

Studies show improved scores of cognitive function on average 8 points higher among children who were breastfed compared with those who were formula fed. This may be due to unique composition of breastmilk, better mother–infant bonding, and lower infectious morbidity and thus better brain growth in these children.

3. Economic Benefits

Breastmilk is much cheaper than animal milk or powdered milk. All it costs is the extra food needed by the lactating mother. In a way, breastfeeding contributes to national economy as in its absence; young infants would require alternative resources for feeding.

4. Psychological Benefits

Breastfeeding helps form a close, loving relationship between the mother and the baby. Close contact soon after birth helps this relationship to develop. This process is called bonding. There is better parent–child adjustment and fewer behavior disorders in these children. Child abuse is also less common.

5. Miscellaneous

Breastfeeding provides some protection against allergic disorders such as atopic eczema and asthma. The incidence of sudden infant death syndrome (SIDS) is less in breastfed children. Human milk reduces the incidence of necrotizing enterocolitis (NEC) in preterm babies.

The beneficial effects of breastfeeding may extend to later life. There is compelling evidence to suggest that breastfeeding reduces the incidence of atherosclerosis, non-insulin-dependent diabetes mellitus, obesity, hypertension and certain cancers later in life.

6. Benefits to the Mother

Breastfeeding helps stop uterine bleeding after delivery and better postpartal involution of the uterus. Both these effects are mediated through the action of oxytocin on the uterus. Breastfeeding also helps in birth spacing due to lactational amenorrhea. The effect is mediated through prolactin-induced ovulation suppression. Lactational amenorrhea also preserves maternal iron stores. Breastfeeding mothers are less likely to develop the cancers of the breast and ovaries.

In addition, breastfeeding is highly convenient to the mother and is always readily available at right temperature, thus saving her time. It can be practiced whenever and wherever human milk is required. No fuel is needed to prepare the feed and boil the bottles/utensils, and thus it saves energy and is eco-friendly.

Anatomy and Physiology of Breast

Breast Anatomy

The breast structure includes the nipple and areola, mammary tissue, supporting connective tissue and fat, blood and lymphatic vessels, and nerves.

The Mammary Tissue

This tissue includes the alveoli, which are small sacs, made of milk-secreting cells, and the ducts that carry the milk to the outside. Between feeds, milk collects in the lumen of the alveoli and ducts. The alveoli are surrounded by a basket of *myoepithelial* or muscle cells which contract and make the milk flow towards the nipple through lactiferous ducts. These ducts widen to form lactiferous sinuses before they open into the tip of the nipple. The sinuses which store small quantities of milk lie below the areola (Fig. 7.20).

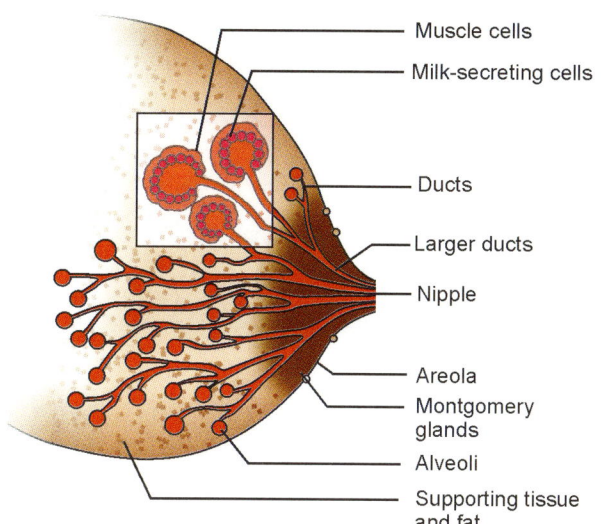

Fig. 7.20 Anatomy of the breast

Nipple and Areola

The nipple has an average of nine milk ducts passing to the outside, and also muscle fibers and nerves. The nipple is surrounded by the circular pigmented *areola*, in which are located *Montgomery glands*. These glands secrete an oily fluid that protects the skin of the nipple and areola during lactation, and produce the mother's individual scent that attracts her baby to the breast.

During pregnancy, the breast tissues undergo hypertrophy and hyperplasia under the influence of maternal and placental hormones. Milk synthesis is inhibited by estrogens and progesterone at this stage. At delivery, the inhibiting influence is removed and milk production is stimulated by prolactin released in response to suckling. The ducts beneath the areola fill with milk and become wider during a feed, when the oxytocin reflex is active.

Milk Production and Secretion

Milk is produced as a result of the interaction between hormones and reflexes. During pregnancy, the glandular tissue is stimulated to produce milk due to various hormonal influences. Two hormones come into play during lactation. They are *prolactin* and *oxytocin* which help in production and ejection of milk, respectively.

1. Prolactin Reflex or Milk Producing Reflex

Prolactin is produced by the anterior pituitary gland and is responsible for milk synthesis by the mammary gland cells. When a baby suckles at breast, sensory impulses from nipple are carried by nerves to the anterior pituitary which makes prolactin (Fig. 7.21). Through blood, prolactin reaches the breast and induces mammary epithelial cells to secrete milk. Therefore, frequent suckling and emptying of the breast is the best stimulus for milk production. There is diurnal variation in prolactin levels, with higher prolactin release in night-time. Therefore, night-time breastfeeding improves milk output and sustains breastfeeding.

2. Oxytocin Reflex or Let Down Reflex

This reflex is also known as *milk ejection reflex* or *draught reflex*. Oxytocin is released from posterior pituitary in response to

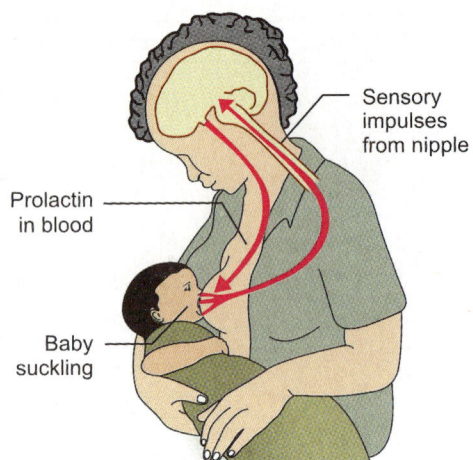

Fig. 7.21 Prolactin reflex

suckling at breast. Oxytocin causes contraction of myoepithelial cells surrounding the alveoli. This causes milk to flow from alveoli, ducts and lactiferous sinuses towards the nipple. Sometimes the reflex is so strong that milk can come out from other breast when the baby is suckling at one breast. There are many factors which can influence this reflex. (Fig. 7.22). If a mother thinks lovingly of her baby, or if she hears him crying, the reflex becomes active and she may feel pressure in her breasts and milk may start flowing from the breast. On the other hand, the reflex is inhibited, if the mother is anxious, depressed or lacks confidence.

3. Feeding Reflexes in the Baby

Rooting reflex When the mother's nipple touches the baby's cheek, the baby turns in the direction of the nipple, opens his mouth. This can be demonstrated by touching the baby's cheek with a finger (Fig. 7.23a).

Suckling reflex This reflex is essential for successful lactation. A baby reflexly suckles at the nipple and areola placed in his mouth. The tongue presses the nipple and areola against the palate squeezing the underlying sinuses by compressing and stretching the nipple between the tongue and palate,

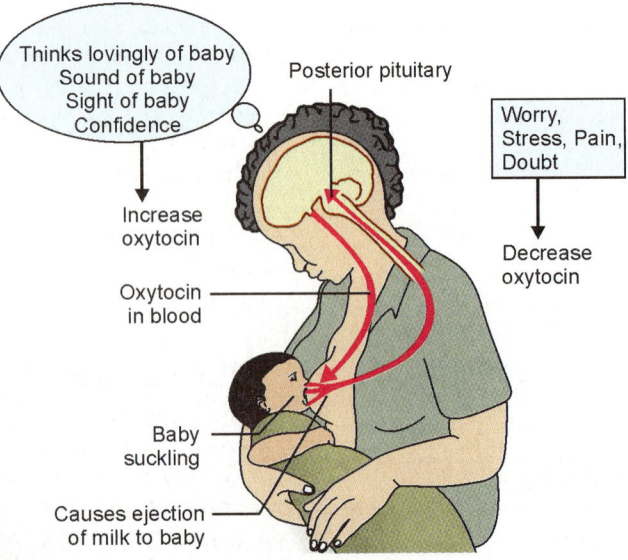

Fig. 7.22 Oxytocin reflex

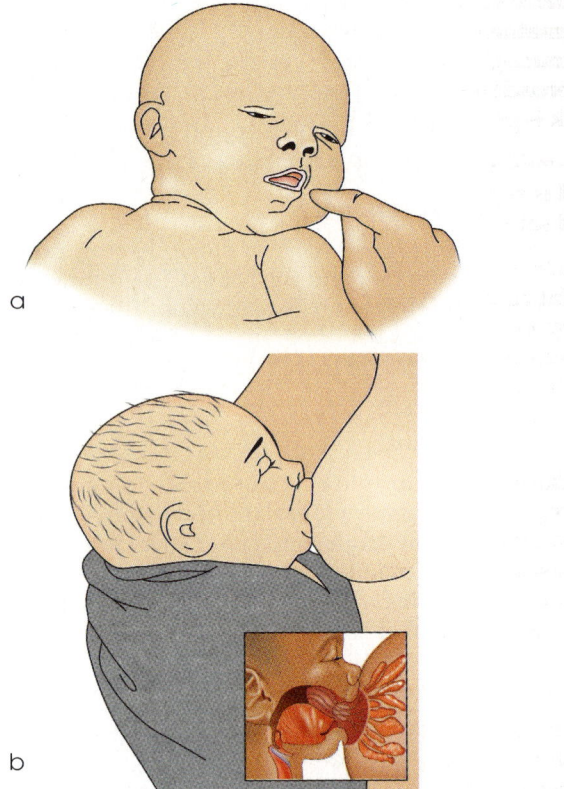

Fig. 7.23 (a) Rooting reflex; (b) Suckling reflex

thus milking the lactiferous sinuses (Fig. 7.23b). Hence, for effective suckling not only the nipple but a part of the areola should also be in the baby's mouth. If the baby suckles only at the nipple, milk is not ejected, baby does not get sufficient milk, suckles more vigorously resulting in sore nipples.

Swallowing reflex A baby swallows the milk suckled into the mouth. This reflex develops earlier than the suckling reflex, so that a baby who can suckle effectively at the breast will always be able to swallow the milk.

Types of Breastmilk

The composition of breastmilk varies at different stages after birth to suit the needs of the baby.

Colostrum is the breastmilk produced in the first 5 days after delivery. It is yellow, thick and very rich in immuno-globulins, especially secretory IgA. Though secreted only in small quantities, it has high protein content and is most suited for the needs of the baby. The social practice of discarding colostrum in some communities must be condemned as it deprives newborn of life-sustaining fluid. Feeding colostrums, a rich source of anti-infective factors, to a baby soon after birth has been called the "first oral immunization".

Transitional milk is produced between 5th and 10th day of lactation. The immunoglobulin and protein content decreases, while the fat and sugar content increases.

Mature milk follows transitional milk. It is thinner and watery but contains all the nutrients essential for optimal growth of the baby.

Preterm milk is the breastmilk of a mother who delivers prematurely. It contains more proteins, sodium, iron, and immunoglobulins that are needed by her preterm baby. It approaches term milk in composition after 4–6 weeks. Term milk is produced by mothers who deliver at term gestation.

Foremilk is the milk secreted at the start of a feed. It is watery and is rich in proteins, sugar, vitamins, minerals and water and satisfies the baby's thirst.

Hindmilk comes later towards the end of a feed and is richer in fat content and provides more energy and satisfies the baby's hunger. For optimum growth, the baby needs both foremilk and hindmilk. The baby should, therefore, be allowed to empty one breast before being offered the other breast.

Exclusive breastfeeding implies giving a baby no other food or drink including water other than breastfeeding with the exception of syrup/drops of vitamins, minerals and medicines (expressed breastmilk is permitted). Exclusive breastfeeding should be continued for first 6 months of life. Since breastmilk is 90% water, additional water is not necessary even in summer.

Successful Breastfeeding

Motivation and support to the mother are the most important factors for successful breastfeeding. The following steps must be practiced for initiation and continuation of successful breastfeeding.

1. *Motivate* Mother should be motivated right from the antenatal period. Her breasts should be examined and she should be informed about the benefits of breastfeeding.
2. *Start early* The baby must be put to the breast within 30 minutes of birth. Babies born by cesarean section should be put to the breast within 4 hours or earlier after birth.
3. *Rooming in* Since suckling is the best stimulus for milk production, babies should be roomed-in with mother and fed on demand till the baby is satisfied. One breast must be emptied out fully before the second is offered, so that the baby receives both foremilk and hindmilk.
4. *Frequency* Frequent suckling helps to stimulate milk production. It also prevents engorgement of breasts. The baby should be fed whenever hungry. Initially, some babies feed at short intervals of 1 to 2 hours. Later the babies settle into a more relaxed routine of feeding every 2 to 3 hours.
5. *Prelacteal feeds* This refers to giving small quantities of fluids such as water, glucose water, tea, honey, etc. as the first feed to the baby. This harmful practice must be condemned as it deprives baby of colostrum, delays initiation of breastfeeding, and also exposes the baby to the risk of infection.
6. *Avoid bottle feeds* No bottle feed should ever be given. It causes nipple confusion and interferes with suckling at the breast. It is also a potent source of infection. Bottle-feeding also undermines mother's confidence in breastfeeding.
7. *Feeding from both breasts* When the baby releases one breast the other breast is offered. If the baby is still hungry, he/she will feed on the other breast. Alternate breasts should be offered first at each feed. This ensures complete emptying of both the breasts. The baby should be allowed to feed till satisfied.
8. *Duration/continuation of breastfeeding* A baby should be exclusively breastfed for the first 6 months. Supplementary feeds given to the baby before six months reduce milk production and also lead to infection and poor weight gain in the baby.
9. *Cost of lactation* Nursing mother needs only 600 calories extra for maintaining her lactation, which amounts to additional home-made food and fluids.
10. *Cleaning the breasts* There is no need to wash the breasts before or after a feed as frequent washing removes the natural oil from the nipple and predisposes to fissures in the nipple. The mother should wash her breasts during her daily bath.
11. *Complementary feeds* A baby should be given additional food after 6 months. Breastfeeding should be continued for at least two years; and also beyond, if feasible.

Technique of Breastfeeding

Positioning

Both mother and baby should be in comfortable position for proper breastfeeding. Mother can feed either in lying down or in sitting position. Baby should be supported so that the head, neck and back are in the same plane. The entire baby should face the mother. The baby will have easy access to the breast, if the baby's abdomen touches the mother's abdomen (Fig. 7.24).

Attachment

After proper positioning, the baby's cheek is touched (rooting reflex), the baby will open the mouth. The baby is then quickly brought on the breast, so that the nipple and most of the areola is within the baby's mouth (Fig. 7.25). As the baby is well positioned, the mother will feel no pain while feeding.

Signs of Good Attachment

1. Baby's chin touches mother's breast
2. Baby's mouth wide open

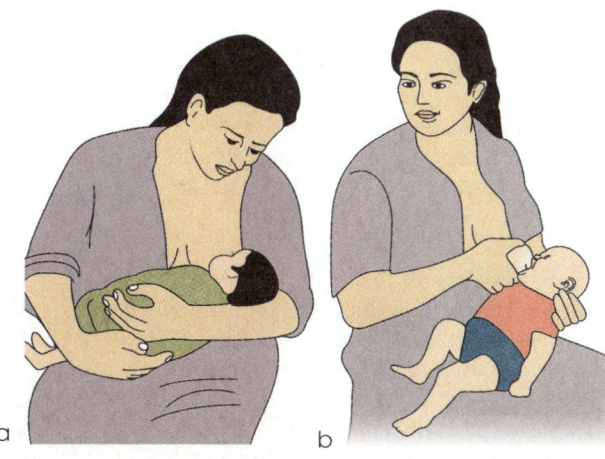

Fig. 7.24 (a) Proper positioning; (b) Improper positioning

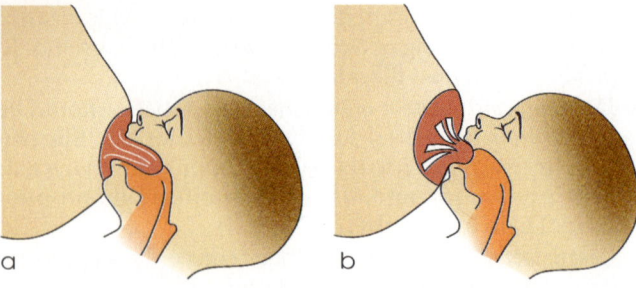

Fig. 7.25 (a) Proper attachment; (b) Improper attachment

3. Majority of areola inside baby's mouth, with more areola visible above than below baby's mouth
4. Lower lip turned outwards, and
5. Rounded cheeks.

PROBLEMS IN BREASTFEEDING

Not Enough Milk

Almost all mothers can produce enough breastmilk for one or even two babies. Perceived milk insufficiency is one of the important reasons for not initiating breastfeeding, terminating it prematurely, or introducing complementary feeding before it is needed. True lactational failure is very uncommon.

If the baby is nursing and sleeping well and gaining weight adequately, the mother needs reassurance that her baby is getting sufficient milk. Some infants are "light sleepers" and cry frequently. This may be misinterpreted by the mother as infant not getting enough milk.

Management consists of counseling the mother to put baby to breast frequently, making sure the baby is attached well to breast and building mother's confidence. Galactogogues like metoclopramide and chlorpromazine are of limited value in increasing milk output.

Retracted Nipples

Severely retracted nipples may cause difficulty in breastfeeding. Holding the nipple from sides and pulling it out several times a day will help make it normal. One can also use a plastic syringe for treatment of inverted nipples (Fig. 7.26). The nozzle end of 10 mL plastic syringe is cut (step 1). The plunger is withdrawn from its usual position and inserted through the cut end (step 2). The open end of the syringe is kept over the nipple and areola and negative suction is applied by pulling out the plunger (step 3). The nipple becomes protractile after a few attempts.

It is important to remember that the syringe method should be practiced by mother herself and not some other person who can apply excessive suction causing severe discomfort to mother.

Breast Engorgement, Mastitis, and Sore Nipples

Breast engorgement presents as painful and hard breasts. *Management* includes frequent suckling by the baby, hot fomentation, and analgesics for pain relief. Mastitis is managed by antibiotics, analgesics, and hot fomentation. Mother should continue breastfeeding from the affected side. Sore nipples are managed by proper suckling, positioning, and applying hindmilk on nipple and areola. If the suckling

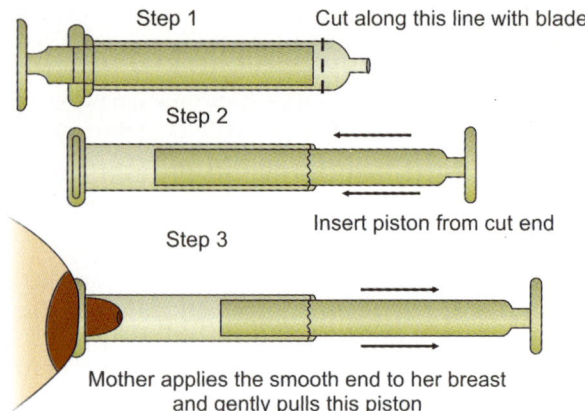

Fig. 7.26 Syringe method for treating retracted nipples

is impossible, the milk can be expressed out manually for a day or so. Do not apply ointments or antiseptics onto the nipples. Exposing the nipples to air, avoiding soap, and frequently changing breast pads are helpful.

Breast Abscess

If congested engorged breast, infected cracked nipple, blocked duct or mastitis are not treated in the early stages, then an infected breast segment may form a breast abscess. The mother complains of high grade fever, severe pain and localized redness. She should be treated with analgesics and antibiotics. The abscess must be incised and drained.

Breastfeeding must be continued. If it is not possible to breastfeed on affected breast due to pain, gently express the milk and start breastfeeding on affected breast as soon as possible.

Expressed Breastmilk

If a mother is not in a position to feed her baby (eg, ill mother, preterm baby, working mother, etc.), she should express her milk in a clean, wide-mouthed container; and this milk should be fed to her baby. Expressed breast milk can be stored at room temperature for 4 hours, in a refrigerator for 24 hours and in a freezer at –20°C for 3 months.

Method of Milk Expression

- Hands must be washed before starting the procedure.
- The mother should lean forward, supporting the breast over the cup or bowl.
- With thumb above and first finger below the nipple at the areola, the breast should be pressed in towards the ribcage.
- Then the thumb and finger should be brought together, producing squeezing movements behind the nipple (Fig. 7.27).
- The breast should be released and the procedure repeated till milk starts to drip or flow.
- The areola should be pressed to the left and right of the nipple in the same way, to make sure that milk is expressed from all sectors of the breast.

THE BABY FRIENDLY HOSPITAL INITIATIVE (BFHI)

BFHI is the World Health Organization's primary intervention strategy for strengthening the capacity of national health

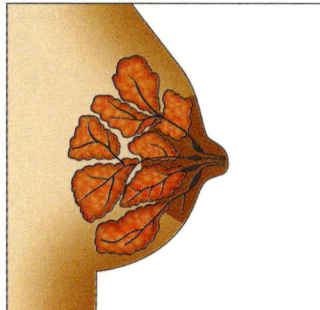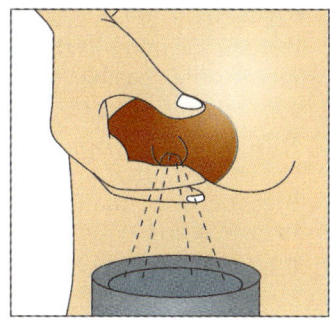

Fig. 7.27 Manual expression of breastmilk

systems to protect and support breastfeeding. A baby friendly hospital (BFH) is a health care facility where the practitioners who provide care for women and babies adopt practices that aim to protect, promote and support **exclusive breastfeeding** from birth.

The 2 Goals of BFHI

1. To transform facilities providing maternity services and care for newborn infants through implementation of the "10 Steps to Successful Breastfeeding".
2. To end the practice of distribution of free and low-cost supplies of breastmilk substitutes to hospitals and health care facilities.

10 Steps to Successful Breastfeeding

Every facility providing maternity services and care for newborn infants should:

1. Have a written breastfeeding policy that is routinely communicated to all health care staff.
2. Train all health care staff in skills necessary to implement this policy.
3. Inform all pregnant women about the benefits and management of breastfeeding.
4. Help mothers initiate breastfeeding within half-hour of normal delivery.
5. Show mothers how to breastfeed and how to maintain lactation, even if they should be separated from their infants.
6. Give newborn infants no food or drink other than breastmilk, unless medically indicated.
7. Practice rooming-in. It allows mothers and infants to remain together for 24 hours a day.
8. Encourage breastfeeding on demand.
9. Give no artificial teats or pacifiers (also called dummies or soothers) to breastfeeding infants.
10. Foster the establishment of breastfeeding support groups and refer mothers to them on discharge from the hospital or clinic.

Contraindications to Breastfeeding

- *Neonatal conditions* Galactosemia or phenylketonuria in the baby.
- *Maternal conditions* Psychosis (untreated) in the mother, or if the mother is receiving cancer chemotherapy, antithyroid drugs, (carbimazole, methimazole), ergotamine, MAO inhibitors, lithium, gold salts, or radioactive pharmaceuticals (^{125}I, ^{131}I, ^{69}Ga).

Maternal infections, such as hepatitis B or open tuberculosis, do not contraindicate breastfeeding, provided the baby is given immunoprophylaxis (hepatitis B vaccine + hepatitis B immunoglobulin) soon after birth in case of maternal hepatitis; and chemoprophylaxis (INH + rifampicin) in case of maternal tuberculosis. Mother should be treated for tuberculosis as per national guidelines.

NACO 2013 RECOMMENDATIONS ON HIV AND INFANT FEEDING

1. *Ensuring mothers and babies receive the care they need*

   Mothers known to be HIV-infected should be provided with lifelong antiretroviral therapy and intrapartum antiretroviral prophylaxis to reduce antenatal or intrapartum HIV infection and transmission through breastfeeding. Babies exposed to HIV infection should receive daily oral nevirapine prophylaxis from birth to 6 weeks.

2. *Which breastfeeding practices and for how long?*

   Mothers known to be HIV-infected (and whose infants are HIV uninfected or of unknown HIV status) should exclusively breastfeed their infants for the first 6 months of life, introducing appropriate complementary foods thereafter, and continue breastfeeding for the first 12 months of life. Breastfeeding should only stop once a nutritionally adequate and safe diet without breastmilk can be provided. If an HIV-infected mother takes appropriate antiretroviral therapy and intrapartum retroviral prophylaxis, and the baby is on nevirapine prophylaxis, the risk of transmission through breastmilk is minimal.

3. *When mother decides to stop breastfeeding…*

   Mothers known to be HIV-infected who decide to stop breastfeeding at any time should stop gradually within one month. Stopping breastfeeding abruptly is not advisable.

4. *What to feed infants when mothers stop breastfeeding*

   When mothers known to be HIV-infected decide to stop breastfeeding at any time, infants should be provided with safe and adequate replacement feeds to enable normal growth and development. If the mother opts against breastfeeding or is extremely sick or expired, the baby should be fed exclusively with formula feed (exclusive replacement feeding), maintaining hygiene. Mixed feeding and animal milk feeding should be avoided.

5. *Conditions needed to safely formula feed*

   Mothers known to be HIV-infected should only give commercial infant formula milk as a replacement feed to their HIV-uninfected infants or infants who are of unknown HIV status, when following conditions are met:

   - Safe water and sanitation are assured at the household level and in the community;
   - The mother, or other caregiver can reliably provide sufficient infant formula milk to support normal growth and development of the infant;
   - The mother or caregiver can prepare it cleanly and frequently enough so that it is safe and carries a low risk of diarrhea and malnutrition;

Breastfeeding

1. Breastmilk is the most optimum nutrition for the newborn babies and young infants.
2. Breastfeeding must be initiated within 1 hour of birth.
3. Every infant should receive exclusive breastfeeding for 6 months. Complementary feeding should be started at 6 months of age and breastfeeding continued till at least 2 years of age.
4. Good attachment on the breast, good sucking by the baby and frequent feeding (at least 8 times in 24 hours) are essential for successful lactation.
5. Breastfeeding has been established before discharge from the health facility.
6. Expressed breastmilk can be provided to low birth weight babies and those newborns who cannot suck well.

- The mother or caregiver can, in the first 6 months, exclusively give infant formula milk;
- The family is supportive of this practice; and
- The mother or caregiver can access health care that offers comprehensive child health services.

These descriptions are intended to give simpler and more explicit meaning to the concepts represented by AFASS (acceptable, feasible, affordable, sustainable and safe).

6. *When the infant is HIV infected*

If infants and young children are known to be HIV-infected, mothers are strongly encouraged to exclusively breastfeed for the first six months of life and continue breastfeeding as per the recommendations for the general population, which is up to two years or beyond.

HIV and Infant feeding, Geneva: WHO 2010.

Infant and Young Child Feeding, Geneva: WHO; 2009.

Updated Guidelines for Prevention of Parent to Child Transmission (PPTCT) of HIV using Multi Drug Anti-retroviral Regimen in India. National AIDS Control Organization (NACO); New Delhi: December, 2013.

7.7 HIGH-RISK NEWBORN AND DANGER SIGNS

High-risk newborns are those who need special attention and close observation because of presence of certain adverse factors. Health care personnel and parents should be aware of these situations and be prepared for the associated difficulties. Factors associated with high-risk neonates are listed in **Table 7.8**.

Table 7.8 Factors Associated with High-risk Newborn	
Maternal conditions	*Associated risk for fetus or neonate*
1. Age at delivery	
• Over 35 years	Chromosomal abnormalities, macrosomia, intrauterine growth restriction (IUGR), blood loss (abruption, placenta previa)
• Teenage pregnancy	IUGR, prematurity, child abuse/neglect (mother herself may be abused)
2. Personal factors	
• Poverty	Prematurity, infection, IUGR
• Lack of antenatal care	Prematurity, IUGR
• Smoking	IUGR, increased perinatal mortality
• Drug, alcohol abuse	IUGR, fetal alcohol syndrome, withdrawal syndrome, sudden infant death syndrome (SIDS), child abuse/neglect
• Poor nutritional status	LBW/IUGR
• Trauma (acute, chronic)	Fetal demise, prematurity
3. Medical history	
• Diabetes mellitus macrosomia/birth injury	Congenital anomalies, stillbirth, respiratory distress syndrome (RDS), hypoglycemia,
• Thyroid disease	Goiter, hypothyroidism, hyperthyroidism, IUGR, stillbirth, prematurity
• Renal disease	IUGR, stillbirth, prematurity
• Urinary tract infection	Prematurity, sepsis
• Heart, lung disease	IUGR, stillbirth, prematurity
• Hypertension (chronic or pre-eclampsia)	IUGR, stillbirth, asphyxia, prematurity
• Anemia	IUGR, stillbirth, asphyxia, prematurity, hydrops
• Isoimmunization (Rh, ABO, minor blood groups)	Stillbirth, anemia, jaundice, hydrops
4. Obstetric history	
• Past history of infant with prematurity, jaundice, RDS, or anomalies	Same with current pregnancy

Table 7.8 Factors Associated with High-risk Newborn *(Contd.)*

Maternal conditions	Associated risk for fetus or neonate
• Maternal medications	IUGR, congenital anomalies
• Bleeding in early pregnancy	Stillbirth, prematurity
• Hyperthermia	Fetal demise, fetal anomalies, stillbirth
• Bleeding in third trimester	Infection/sepsis
• Premature rupture of membranes, fever, infection	Infection, prematurity

5. Fetal conditions

• Multiple gestation	Twin-twin transfusion syndrome, IUGR, asphyxia, birth trauma
• Intrauterine growth restriction (IUGR)	Fetal demise, congenital anomalies, asphyxia, hypoglycemia, polycythemia
• Macrosomia	Congenital anomalies, birth trauma, hypoglycemia
• Abnormal fetal position	Congenital anomalies, birth trauma, hemorrhage
• Abnormality of fetal heart rate or rhythm	Hydrops, asphyxia, congestive heart failure, heart block
• Decreased activity	Fetal demise, asphyxia
• Polyhydramnios	Anencephaly, other central nervous system (CNS) disorders, neuromuscular disorders, problems with swallowing (eg, esophageal atresia), diaphragmatic hernia, omphalocele, gastroschisis, trisomy, tumors, hydrops, isoimmunization, anemia, cardiac failure, intrauterine infection, maternal diabetes
• Oligohydramnios	IUGR, placental insufficiency, postmaturity, fetal demise, intrapartum distress, renal agenesis, pulmonary hypoplasia

6. Conditions of labor and delivery

• Premature labor	Respiratory distress syndrome (RDS)
• Labor occurring 2 weeks or more after term	Stillbirth, asphyxia, meconium aspiration
• Maternal fever	Infection/sepsis
• Maternal hypotension	Stillbirth, asphyxia
• Rapid labor	Birth trauma, intracranial hemorrhage
• Long labor	Stillbirth, asphyxia, birth trauma
• Abnormal presentation	Birth trauma, asphyxia
• Uterine tetany	Asphyxia
• Meconium-stained amniotic fluid	Stillbirth, asphyxia, meconium aspiration syndrome, persistent pulmonary hypertension
• Prolapsed cord	Asphyxia, intracranial hemorrhage
• Cesarean section	RDS, retained fetal lung fluid/transient tachypnea, blood loss
• Obstetric analgesia and anesthesia	Respiratory depression, hypotension, hypothermia
• Placental anomalies	
a. Small placenta	IUGR
b. Large placenta	Hydrops, maternal diabetes
c. Torn placenta	Blood loss
d. Vasa previa	Blood loss

7. Immediate neonatal conditions

• Prematurity	RDS, other consequences of prematurity (discussed in Low Birth Weight chapter)
• Low birth weight/IUGR	
• Foul smell of amniotic fluid or membranes	Infection
• Low 5-minute Apgar score	Prolonged transition (especially respiratory)
• Birth weight >4 kg	Perinatal asphyxia, trauma, hypoglycemia, RDS
• Absent/delayed cry	Perinatal asphyxia
• Congenital malformations	Risk depends on organ-system involved

DANGER SIGNS IN NEONATES

Danger signs are the clinical features which may suggest that the neonate is sick and needs early referral to an appropriate health care facility. Parents and health workers should be aware of these signs so that there is no undue delay in seeking care. Some of the common danger signs are enumerated below:

- Failure to pass meconium within 24 hours
- Failure to pass urine within 48 hours
- Lethargy/poor feeding
- Respiratory distress—fast breathing, retraction, grunting
- Abnormal color—pallor/cyanosis/jaundice
- Jaundice within 24 hours or persisting beyond 14 days
- Hypothermia/hyperthermia
- Abnormal movements (seizures)
- Persistent vomiting
- Diarrhea
- Abdominal distension
- Bleeding from any site
- Poor weight gain/weight loss

Management of High-Risk Neonates

- Anticipate the need of resuscitation, a skilled team should be present for delivery.
- The cord blood and placenta should be saved after delivery.
- Observation for at least 72 h after delivery for development of complications.
- Admission to the neonatal unit at earliest suspicion and provision of appropriate management.
- Transfer to higher facility, if necessary.
- At discharge, parents should be made aware of the possible danger signs.
  Long-term follow-up for high-risk newborns is discussed later.

Browne JV. Developmental care for high-risk newborns: emerging science, clinical application, and continuity from newborn intensive care unit to community. *Clin Perinatol.* 2011; 38:719–29.
  Moddemann D, Shea S. The developmental paediatrician and neonatal follow-up. *Paediatr Child Health.* 2006; 11:295.
  National Neonatology Forum and UNICEF. Facility based care of sick neonate ay referral health facility. *Comprehensive newborn care initiative.* New Delhi; 2010.

7.8 LOW BIRTH WEIGHT (LBW)

Birth weight less than 2500 g irrespective of gestational age is defined as low birth weight (LBW). Every year, more than 30% neonates in India are delivered with low birth weight. These babies require additional care and resources as approximately 75% of neonatal deaths and 50% of infant deaths occur in LBW infants.

LBW babies are prone to malnutrition, recurrent infections, and neurodevelopment handicaps. There is evidence to suggest that LBW infants are more likely to develop diabetes mellitus, obesity, hypertension, and coronary artery disease in later life. Low birth weight, therefore, is a key risk factor of adverse outcome throughout life.

Types of LBW

A newborn baby may be LBW due to birth before 37 weeks of gestation (preterm LBW) or more commonly, born at term gestation but LBW due to intrauterine growth restriction (IUGR) (term LBW). Two-thirds of LBW neonates in our country are term babies. At times, an LBW neonate may be both preterm and having intrauterine growth restriction.

Symmetric and Asymmetric IUGR

IUGR babies are further categorized on the basis of having symmetric or asymmetric intrauterine growth restriction.

- *Symmetrical* IUGR occurs early in pregnancy (first trimester) and is often associated with diseases that reduce fetal cell number, such as chromosomal, genetic, teratogenic and infectious etiologies. There is proportionate reduction in head circumference, length and weight. These infants are also known as hypoplastic IUGR.

- *Asymmetric* IUGR is of late onset and is associated with poor maternal nutritional status or maternal conditions that impair fetal growth in third trimester. Growth restriction is due to reduction in the size of cells, while the number of cells remains unaffected. Thus these infants have the potential to grow near-normal with optimum nutrition and medical care. Most of the IUGR infants in our country are asymmetric in type.

Ponderal index (PI) can be used to differentiate between the symmetrical and asymmetrical babies with IUGR. Ponderal index is calculated as follows: [(weight in gram/ length in cm^3) x 100]. The index is less than 2 in asymmetric IUGR and more than 2 in symmetric IUGR (>2.5 in term appropriate for gestational age newborns).

Etiology of LBW

LBW is multifactorial in etiology. Several responsible factors are listed:

1. Poor nutritional status of the mother (pre-pregnancy weight less than 40 kg; height less than 145 cm, body mass index (BMI) <18.5;
2. Poor weight gain during pregnancy;
3. Maternal anemia and trace element deficiency;
4. Maternal infections including TORCH and other intrauterine infections;
5. Chronic maternal diseases of heart, kidneys, lungs, or liver;
6. Multiple pregnancy, frequent pregnancies, short inter-pregnancy interval, and teenage pregnancy;
7. Maternal hypertension, pregnancy induced hypertension (PIH);
8. Heavy physical work particularly in third trimester;
9. Lack of antenatal care, postmaturity; and
10. Tobacco use, alcohol or drug addiction in mother.

Most of the above factors can cause preterm delivery as well as growth restriction. Additional causes of preterm birth include cervical incompetence, previous preterm delivery, premature rupture of membranes, maternal genital tract colonization, chorioamnionitis, and uterine anomalies such as bicornuate uterus.

Preterm LBW versus Term IUGR LBW

There are differences in the physical characteristics of term LBW and preterm LBW newborns (Fig. 7.28). They are summarized in **Table 7.9**. Preterm baby is diagnosed on the basis of period of gestation calculated from the first day of last menstrual period of the mother. If it is less than 37 weeks, the baby is preterm.

Ultrasonography is very useful in estimating gestational age during antenatal period. In first trimester, crown-rump length accurately predicts gestational age while in second and third trimesters, measurement of biparietal diameter (BPD) and fetal femur length best predict gestational age.

A. Problems of Term-IUGR LBW Neonates

- Perinatal asphyxia
- Hypothermia, hypoglycemia, hypocalcemia
- Meconium aspiration syndrome
- Persistent pulmonary hypertension of newborn
- Pulmonary hemorrhage
- Polycythemia/hyperviscosity
- Poor postnatal growth
- Infection
- Higher incidence of degenerative diseases, such as diabetes mellitus, hypertension and atherosclerosis later in life.

B. Problems of Preterm LBW Neonates

- Perinatal asphyxia
- *Respiratory*: Respiratory distress syndrome (RDS), apneic spells, congenital pneumonia, bronchopulmonary dysplasia (late complication)

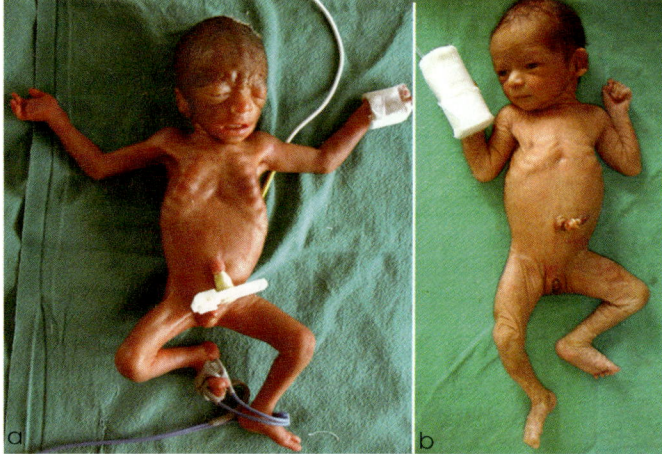

Fig. 7.28 (a) Preterm low birth weight; (b) Term low birth weight

- *Cardiovascular*: Patent ductus arteriosus, hypotension
- *Central nervous system*: Periventricular/intraventricular hemorrhage, periventricular leucomalacia, neuro-developmental handicaps
- *Gastrointestinal and hepatobiliary*: Feeding intolerance, gastroesophageal reflux, necrotizing enterocolitis, indirect hyperbilirubinemia, cholestatic jaundice
- *Thermoregulation*: Hypo-/hyperthermia
- *Immunologic*: Repeated infections
- *Nutrition*: Poor growth
- *Metabolic*: Hypo-/hyperglycemia, hypocalcemia, metabolic bone disease of prematurity
- *Renal*: Late metabolic acidosis, electrolyte imbalance

Table 7.9 Differences between Preterm and Term IUGR Newborns

Characteristic	Preterm	Term IUGR
Appearance	Small baby with extended limbs and less activity and alertness	Small body size, emaciated or marasmic look with loose folds of skin, extremities well flexed, active and alert
Behavior	Sleepy most of the time	Alert/hyperalert appearance
Skin	Red, gelatinous, translucent	Pink, pale, opaque, rough, dry, wrinkled, peeling
Lanugo	Abundant	Mostly absent
Ear		
Pinna	Poorly developed	Well developed
Cartilage	Poorly formed	Well formed
Curvature	Poorly developed	Well developed
Recoil	Poor	Good
Sole creases	Absent or only in anterior third	Present all over the sole
Areola with breast nodule	Areola poorly formed and depigmented, nodule barely palpable	Well formed pigmented areola, palpable firm nodule
Genitalia—male		
Scrotum	Small sized, smooth surface	Pendulous, bigger in size
Rugae	Absent	Present
Median raphe	Absent	Present
Color	Pink	Darkly pigmented
Testes	Undescended	Descended
Genitalia—female		
Labia	Labia minora not covered with majora	Labia minora well covered with majora
Clitoris	Enlarged	Small
Muscle tone	Less	Good
Abdomen	Normal in appearance	May be scaphoid

7

- *Hematologic*: Anemia, disseminated intravascular coagulation, vitamin K deficiency bleeding
- *Skin*: High transepidermal water loss, skin abrasions
- *Eye*: Retinopathy of prematurity, myopia, strabismus
- *Ear*: Hearing impairment

Treatment	Low Birth Weight

A. Care at Delivery

- The baby may require resuscitation and admission to the NICU. Therefore, delivery should take place in a hospital with facilities for neonatal care. *In utero* transport is far more safe than transport of a sick baby after birth.
- Delivery should be attended by health professionals skilled in neonatal resuscitation.
- Not all babies require hospital care. An otherwise healthy LBW newborn with a birth weight of 1800 g or above or gestation of 34 weeks or more can be managed at home with assistance from a health worker.
- Indications for admission:
  i. Birth weight less than 1800 g;
  ii. Gestation less than 34 weeks;
  iii. Not able to take feeds from the breast or by cup (irrespective of birth weight and gestation); or
  iv. Sick neonate (irrespective of the birth weight or gestation).

B. Maintenance of Temperature

LBW babies are prone to hypothermia due to large surface area, poor insulation due to decreased subcutaneous fat, large evaporative heat loss due to thin skin, and less heat production due to poor stores of brown adipose tissue. A hypothermic baby has increased oxygen demand and may develop hypoglycemia, apnea, acidosis, hypoxemia, bleeding diathesis, respiratory failure, shock and eventually death.

- *Rooming-in* The temperature can be maintained at home or hospital by keeping mother and baby together in the same bed under a single blanket.
- *Kangaroo mother care (KMC)* is a low tech readily available alternative to radiant heat warmers and incubators to keep babies warm. There are other benefits of KMC such as enhanced breastfeeding, better bonding between mother and baby, better weight gain, and reduced risk of sepsis. For all these reasons, KMC needs to be widely popularized and practiced in resource-limited settings.
- *The baby should be clothed well* At least two or three layers of clothes are generally required. If the room is not warm enough, woolen sweater should also be put on. Feet should be covered with socks, hands with mittens and head with a cap. Further, the room where an LBW baby is kept should be warmed using electrical heater, especially in winter months. The baby should not be kept directly in front of electrical heater. This may produce thermal injury.
- *Monitor temperature* If the baby is maintaining normal body temperature, both trunk and soles/palms should be warm to touch and pink in color. In early stages of hypothermia, the trunk is warm but the soles and palms are cold to touch and bluish in appearance. The mother should be educated and trained in the touch technique to detect hypothermia in the early stages. This condition, known as cold stress, can be managed by providing KMC and keeping the room warm.
- *In the hospital*, apart from the above methods, overhead radiant warmer or incubator may be used to keep the baby

warm. Regular monitoring of axillary temperature should be carried out in all sick babies.

C. Intravenous (IV) Fluids

Sick LBW babies who cannot be given oral or gavage (tube) feeding should be given intravenous fluids. Fluid requirement of LBW babies are summarized in **Table 7.10**. Key points to remember are:

- On day 1, the fluid requirements range from 60–80 mL/kg.
- The daily increment in fluid volume is around 15 mL/kg till day 7 by which time a baby should be getting around 150 mL/kg/day.
- Initiate fluid therapy with plain 10% dextrose. For newborns weighing below 1 kg, 5% dextrose is preferred to avoid hyperglycemia.
- Sodium (3 mEq/kg/day) and potassium (2 mEq/kg/day) are added after 48 hours by which time most babies will pass urine. Isolyte-P is a readymade electrolyte containing solution which can be used after 48 hours of age.
- For administering intravenous fluids to the neonate, a small volume infusion set/syringe pump should be used. Fluid therapy should be carefully monitored. Too rapid infusion may result in pulmonary edema or even death in a small baby.

D. Nutrition

Nutrition is an essential part of the care of LBW newborns. Their little reserves of fat and carbohydrate are rapidly depleted unless provided sufficient nutrients. Inability to take oral feeds and limited feeding tolerance of these infants make feeding a challenging task.

The method of feeding depends on the birth weight, gestation, postnatal age, and presence or absence of sickness and vigor (feeding effort) of the baby. The options include breastfeeding, cup feeding or tube feeding (nasogastric/orogastric). Details follow:

- Always use breastmilk to feed an LBW baby. Mother's milk is best suited to meet the requirements of the individual baby.
- *Babies weighing >1800 g or >34 weeks. Start directly on breastfeeding*. If the sucking effort is weak, give expressed breastmilk with cup. Even for babies who appear to take breastfeed satisfactorily, it is desirable to give them expressed breastmilk with cup at the end of breastfeeding in order to ensure adequate milk intake.
- *Newborns weighing between 1500 and 1800 g (32–34 weeks). Try cup feeding*. If it is unsuccessful, give tube feeding and try cup feeding again after 3 to 5 days.

Table 7.10 Fluid Requirements (Intravenous or Oral) of Neonates (mL/kg body weight/day)*		
Day of life	*Birth weight*	
	>1500 g	*≤1500 g*
1	60	80
2	75	95
3	90	110
4	105	125
5	120	140
6	135	155
7 onward	150	170

Orally increase up to 180–200 mL/kg/day by 7–10 days.

- *For newborns weighing between 1200 and 1500 g (30–32 weeks). Begin tube feeding* (preferably orogastric) and introduce cup feeding after 3 to 5 days and breastfeeding after 1 to 2 weeks as tolerated.
- *Newborns weighing less than 1200 g. Only IV fluids are given initially.* Start tube feeding after 1 to 3 days and shift to cup feeding after 1–3 weeks and breastfeeding after 4 to 6 weeks.
- Feedings are given 2–3 hourly.

Prefeed Aspiration

For tubefed babies, prefeed aspiration of stomach contents need not be done routinely before each feed for diagnosis of feeding intolerance. It is better to measure baseline abdominal girth. If prefeed abdominal girth increases by 2 cm or more from baseline, gastric contents should be aspirated and its volume and color noted.

- If the aspirate is milky and volume is less than 25% of previous feed and baby is otherwise stable, continue feeding.
- If the aspirate is milky and volume is 25–50% of previous feed and baby is otherwise stable, miss that feed and again check for the next feed.
- If the aspirate is bilious/hemorrhagic or the baby is looking sick, stop feeding and consider the possibilities of paralytic ileus, infection, hypokalemia or early necrotizing enterocolitis.

The guidelines for feeding LBW infants are summarized in Table 7.11.

Trophic Feeding

Trophic feedings are defined as giving very small volumes of feeds (up to *24 mL/kg/day*) every 4 to 6 hours for the purpose of gut maturation rather than nutrient delivery. Trophic feeds are indicated when clinical condition of the newborn precludes normal volume enteral feeding.

In the past, these newborns would have remained nil per orally for a few days. Keeping a newborn baby nil orally for a few days can produce intestinal changes including involution of gut villi, mucosal thinning and loss of intestinal enzymes. Trophic feeding prevents these changes.

Trophic feeds can be started on the first day in newborns who are hemodynamically stable. Benefits of trophic feedings (gut priming) include less feeding intolerance, earlier progression to full enteral feedings, and improved weight gain. It is best to start trophic feedings with breastmilk.

Assessing Adequacy of Feeding

Adequacy of nutrition can be judged by assessing growth of a LBW baby. Weight should be recorded daily and head and length measurements should be taken weekly.

All newborns lose weight in the first week of age. Term newborns may lose 5–10% of their birth weight while preterm newborns may lose up to 10–15% of their birth weight. All newborns should regain birth weight by 10 to 14 days of age and should gain weight at a rate of about 10–15 g/kg/day. IUGR infants may not lose much weight and may start gaining weight early. A baby should gain at least 125 g each week. Poor weight gain may indicate inadequate intake, cold stress, infection, anemia, or other systemic disorders.

Adequately breastfed baby will pass light colored urine at least 6–8 times a day. If a baby is passing urine <6 times a day and the urine is concentrated, ie, dark yellow in color, it indicates that the baby is not getting enough breastmilk.

Supplements

All LBW babies should receive intramuscular vitamin K 0.5 mg at birth to prevent vitamin K deficiency bleeding. Human milk fortifiers should be added in breastmilk (3–4 sachets/day) in very low birth weight neonates when full enteral feeding is achieved and continued till they achieve a weight of 2 kg. Vitamin D (400 IU/day) and iron (2 mg/kg/day) are added from 2 weeks of age when full enteral feeding is achieved and continued till one year of age.

E. Prevention of Infection

LBW babies are prone to develop infections; and mortality due to sepsis is high. Following measures are helpful in preventing infections:

- Ensure exclusive breastfeeding and avoid prelacteal feeds.
- Handwashing by the health professionals, mother and family members before touching the baby.
- For cup-feeding, mother should wash her hands before expressing the milk into a clean cup. Cup should be cleaned by washing with soap and water and then putting it in boiling water for five minutes. Alternatively cup can be cleaned by pouring boiling water into the cup and leaving it there for a few minutes.
- Keep the umbilical stump dry. Do not apply anything over it.
- Avoiding unnecessary handling of the baby by multiple persons.

F. Immunization

LBW infants should be immunized at the same chronological age as term appropriately grown infants and according to the national immunization schedule. LBW does not increase the incidence of vaccine-related adverse events, and the dose should not be reduced for any vaccine.

Table 7.11 Guidelines for Feeding of LBW Infants				
	Age categories of neonates			
Birth weight (g) Gestation (wk)	*<1200* *<30*	*1200–1500* *30–32*	*1500–1800* *32–34*	*>1800* *>34*
Initial	Intravenous fluids Try gavage feeds, if not sick	Tube feeding	Cup-feeding	Breastfeeding. If unsatis-factory, give cup feeds
After 1–3 days	Tube feeding	Cup-feeding	Cup-feeding	Breast + Cup-feeding
Later (1–2 wk)	Cup-feeding	Breast + Cup-feeding	Breast + Cup-feeding	Breast + Cup-feeding
After some more time (4–6 wk)	Breast + Cup-feeding	Breast + Cup-feeding	Breast + Cup-feeding	Breast + Cup-feeding

Modified from Teaching Aids on Newborn Care. National Neonatology Forum, India

Low Birth Weight (LBW)

1. In India, 7.5 million LBW infants (<2500 g) are born every year and account for 40% of the total of 20 million LBW babies born globally.
2. Newborn infant can be LBW because of intrauterine growth restriction (IUGR) or prematurity.
3. Poor maternal nutrition is the principle risk factor for LBW.
4. The major immediate complications encountered in LBW are difficult resuscitation, respiratory distress syndrome, apnea, hypotension, hypothermia, hypoglycemia, necrotizing enterocolitis, intracranial hemorrhage, feeding difficulties, and vulnerability to infections and iatrogenic complications.
5. Breastmilk remains the choice of feeding in LBW along with mineral and vitamin supplements.
6. Nearly three-fourths of neonatal deaths and half of infant deaths occur amongst LBW infants.

Outcome of LBW Babies

Outcome of LBW newborns is determined by birth weight, gestational age, underlying etiology, extent and timing of intrauterine growth restriction, immediate postnatal complications, and catch-up growth.

• For similar birth weight, preterm newborns perform worse than IUGR newborns in the immediate postnatal period, due to greater immaturity of their organ systems.
• Compared to appropriately grown newborns, IUGR babies experience higher morbidity and mortality.
• Asymmetric IUGR infants have more favorable outcome than symmetric IUGR infants due to better potential for growth.
• Overall, former IUGR infants remain shorter (less height) and lighter (less weight) compared to their normal siblings.
• Recent studies suggest that certain diseases like diabetes mellitus, insulin resistance, obesity and cardiovascular disease are more common in adults who were IUGR/LBW at birth. These pathologies may be a consequence of 'programming' in which an insult occurring at a critical stage of human development may result in a long-lasting effect on the structure and function of the organism (*Barker's hypothesis*). Mechanisms underlying these morbidities are poorly understood.

Jobe AH."Miracle" extremely low birth weight neonates: examples of developmental plasticity. *Obstet Gynecol*. 2010;116:1184–90.

National Neonatology Forum and UNICEF. Facility based care of sick neonate ay referral health facility. New Delhi: *Comprehensive Newborn Care Initiative*; 2010.

Shankaran S, Fanaroff AA, Wright LL, *et al*. Risk factors for early death among extremely low-birth-weight infants. *Am J Obstet Gynecol*. 2002;186:796–802.

7.9 PERINATAL ASPHYXIA AND HYPOXIC-ISCHEMIC ENCEPHALOPATHY

Perinatal asphyxia is the second most common cause of neonatal death after infections and is the leading cause of neurodevelopmental disability in children. The term perinatal asphyxia is preferred to birth asphyxia as asphyxial injury may occur before, during, or after birth.

Hypoxic-ischemic encephalopathy (HIE) refers to the characteristic neurological manifestations in term and near-term newborns which develop soon after birth following perinatal asphyxia. HIE occurs at a rate of approximately 3–5 cases per 1,000 full-term live births, half of which progress to moderate to severe HIE.

Definition

Perinatal asphyxia may be defined as hypoxic insult to the fetus severe enough to cause metabolic acidosis, neonatal encephalopathy, and multiorgan system dysfunction. The National Neonatology Forum of India has defined asphyxia as "gasping or ineffective breathing or lack of breathing at one minute of life". The essential criteria for diagnosing perinatal asphyxia as outlined by the American Academy of Pediatrics (AAP) are as follows:

i. Umbilical artery metabolic or mixed acidemia with pH <7.0;
ii. 5-minute apgar score of ≤ 3;
iii. Neonatal encephalopathy manifesting as seizures, hypotonia or coma in the immediate neonatal period; and
iv. Evidence of multiorgan system dysfunction.

Etiology

Perinatal asphyxia is multifactorial in origin. In most cases (>90%), the asphyxia insult occurs during the antepartum or intrapartum period. Postpartum insult is responsible for the remaining cases of perinatal asphyxia.

A. Prepartum Insult

Placental insufficiency during the antepartum or intra-partum periods results in an inability to provide oxygen and remove carbon dioxide and hydrogen ion from the fetus leading to perinatal asphyxia. Causes of placental insufficiency include:

i. *Impaired maternal oxygenation* as in maternal hypoxia due to anemia, pulmonary, cardiac, or neurologic disease in the mother.
ii. *Decreased blood flow from the mother to the placenta* as in maternal infection, shock, dehydration and hypotension.
iii. *Decreased blood flow from the placenta to the fetus* as in placental abruption, cord prolapse, cord entanglement, true knot, cord compression, and abnormality of the umbilical vessels.
iv. *Impaired gas exchange across placenta or fetal tissues* as in maternal hypertension, vascular disease, diabetes, drug abuse, postmaturity, placental calcification, infarct, or fibrosis, etc.
v. *Increased fetal oxygen requirement* as in fetal anemia, fetal infection, or intrauterine growth restriction.

B. Postpartum Causes

Postpartum insults occur secondary to pulmonary, cardio-vascular, or neurologic insufficiency during immediate postpartum period.

Pathophysiology

Perinatal asphyxia results in lack of oxygen (hypoxia) and lack of perfusion (ischemia) to various organs. The most vulnerable organ to be affected by hypoxic-ischemic injury is brain, as neonatal brain has very high requirements for oxygen and baseline blood flow. Hypoxic insult to the fetus initiates *diving seal reflex*, causing shunting of blood to brain, heart and adrenals and away from lungs, gut, kidneys, liver, spleen and skin, in an attempt to maintain perfusion to more vital organs.

Biochemically, hypoxia impairs cerebral oxidative metabolism, resulting in increase in lactate, fall in pH (acidosis), and decrease in ATP levels. Acidosis causes myocardial depression and reduced cardiac output. During prolonged hypoxia, hypotension develops and cerebral blood flow is compromised, and a combined hypoxic and ischemic insult leads to further failure of oxidative phosphorylation. Energy failure impairs ion pumps, leading to accumulation of Na^+, Cl^-, H_2O, and Ca^{++} intracellularly; and K^+ and neurotoxic excitatory amino acids—glutamate and aspartate, extracellularly. Reperfusion of previously ischemic tissues provokes generation of oxygen free radicals which further produce neuronal damage.

Pathologically, brain damage occurs mainly in cerebral cortex and basal ganglia in term newborns. In preterm newborns, the insult predominantly involves periventricular white matter.

Clinical Features

Clinical manifestations and course vary depending on the severity of hypoxic-ischemic insult. The clinical picture is described as mild, moderate and severe as given in **Table 7.12.**

Mild hypoxic-ischemic Encephalopathy

Transient abnormalities are observed, such as poor feeding, irritability, or excessive crying or sleepiness. Muscle tone may be slightly increased and deep tendon reflexes may be brisk.

Moderate Hypoxic-ischemic Encephalopathy

The infant is lethargic, with significant hypotonia, and diminished deep tendon reflexes. The grasp, Moro, and sucking reflexes may be sluggish or absent and the baby may develop occasional periods of apnea. Seizures may occur within the first 24 hours of life, most commonly within first 12 hours.

Severe Hypoxic-ischemic Encephalopathy

The baby becomes comatosed and may not respond to any physical stimulus. Breathing becomes irregular, and she may require ventilatory support. Tone is decreased and deep tendon reflexes are depressed. Neonatal reflexes (eg, sucking, swallowing, grasp, Moro) are absent. Disturbances of ocular motion, such as a skewed deviation of the eyes, nystagmus, bobbing, and loss of "doll's eye" (ie, conjugate) movements may be revealed by cranial nerve examination. Pupils may be dilated, fixed, or poorly reactive to light.

Seizures occur in up to 50% newborns with HIE and may be subtle, tonic, or clonic. Anterior fontanel may be full or bulging due to cerebral edema. Irregularities of heart rate and blood pressure (BP) are common during the period of reperfusion injury, as is death from cardiorespiratory failure. These neonates would eventually die or have permanent neurologic sequelae.

Organ System Involvement

In addition to brain, perinatal asphyxia may affect kidneys, heart, lungs, intestine and liver. Organ systems involved following a hypoxic-ischemic events include the following:

* *Renal* After brain, kidney is the next most commonly affected organ in perinatal asphyxia. Hypoxic-ischemic insults lead to acute tubular necrosis with oliguria.
* *Heart* Reduced myocardial contractility, severe hypotension, passive cardiac dilatation, and tricuspid regurgitation.
* *Lungs* Respiratory distress due to pulmonary edema, hemorrhage and pulmonary hypertension.
* *Liver* Deranged liver function, hyperammonemia, and coagulopathy.
* *Gastrointestinal system* Poor peristalsis, delayed gastric emptying, and necrotizing enterocolitis.
* *Hematologic* Increased nucleated RBCs, neutropenia or neutrophilia, thrombocytopenia, and coagulopathy.

Investigations

There are no confirmatory laboratory tests to diagnose perinatal asphyxia. Tests are helpful to assess the severity of brain injury and to monitor the functional status of systemic organs.

Table 7.12 Grading of Neonatal Hypoxic-Ischemic Encephalopathy			
	Grade I (mild)	*Grade II (moderate)*	*Grade III (severe)*
Conscious level	Irritable/hyperalert	Lethargic	Comatose
Tone	Either[a] mildly abnormal (hypo/hyper)	Moderately abnormal (hypotonic or dissociated)	Severely abnormal (hypotonia)
Suck	Or[b] abnormal	Poor	Absent
Primitive reflexes	Exaggerated	Depressed	Absent
Seizures	Absent	Present	Present
Brainstem reflexes	Normal	Normal	Impaired
Respiration	Tachypneic	Occasional apneas	Severe apnea

(Adapted from Fenichel)
The features in bold must be described to meet the minimum requirements for each grade. Features not in bold may be present but are not required to make the syndrome assignment. [a/b]: *Either abnormal tone or abnormal suck should accompany altered conscious level to assign grade I.*

- *Blood glucose* Should be monitored frequently. Both hypoglycemia (blood glucose <45 mg/dL) and hyper-glycemia (blood glucose >125 mg/dL) are to be avoided.
- *Serum electrolytes* Daily assessment of serum electrolytes, especially calcium, is valuable until the infant's status improves. Markedly low serum sodium, potassium, and chloride levels in the presence of reduced urine flow and excessive weight gain may indicate acute tubular damage particularly during the initial 2–3 days of life.
- *Renal function tests* Blood urea, and serum creatinine.
- *Liver function tests* To assess the degree of hypoxic–ischemic injury.
- *Coagulation* Prothrombin time and partial thrombo-plastin time.
- *Blood gas monitoring* To assess acid-base status; and to avoid hyperoxia, hypoxia as well as hypercapnia and hypocapnia.
- *Neuroimaging* Neuroimaging is helpful in demonstrating diffuse or focal brain injury and predicting long-term outcome. Cranial ultrasound has better predictive ability in preterm infants while cranial CT is more useful in term infants. MRI is the imaging modality of choice for the diagnosis and follow-up of infants with moderate-to-severe HIE. MRI can reveal specific patterns of brain injury in both preterm and term neonates which may not be demonstrated by other imaging modalities.
- *EEG* It is a valuable tool in predicting outcome. Burst suppression, low voltage, or electrocerebral inactivity are associated with poor outcome.

Treatment — Perinatal Asphyxia

The management of perinatal asphyxia is essentially supportive. Initial resuscitation and stabilization are important for prevention of perinatal asphyxia and HIE. A normal metabolic state including glucose, calcium and acid-base balance should be maintained.

A. Supportive Therapy

1. *IV fluids* An intravenous line should be started with 10% dextrose at 60 mL/kg/day.
2. *Perfusion and blood pressure* Hypotension is common in infants with HIE and is due to myocardial dysfunction, capillary leak syndrome, and hypovolemia. It should be promptly treated. A systemic mean arterial BP of at least 45 to 50 mm Hg is desirable for term infants, 35–40 mm Hg for infants weighing 1000–2000 g and 30–35 mm for infants <1000 g to maintain cerebral perfusion. Vasopressor agents like dobutamine or dopamine should be used judiciously, if BP is low.
3. *Maintenance of temperature* Temperature should be maintained in the normal range of 36.5–37.5°C. Recent studies suggest that therapeutic hypothermia is associated with reduction in mortality and disability in survivors. Modest hypothermia (33–34°C) may be beneficial by virtue of preventing energy depletion, inhibiting glutamate release and inhibiting apoptosis. Hyperthermia is also detrimental as it increases the metabolic and energy expenditure and induces neuronal injury.
4. *Glucose* Blood glucose level should be kept at 75–100 mg/dL to provide adequate substrate for the brain. If the baby is hypoglycemic, a bolus of 2 mL/kg of 10% dextrose should be administered followed by a continuous glucose infusion at a rate of 6 mg/kg/minute.
5. *Calcium* Calcium level should be kept in the normal range (9–11 mg/dL). Hypocalcemia is a common metabolic alteration in the HIE. A subnormal serum Ca^{++} level may compromise cardiac contractility and may cause seizures. Hypercalcemia should be avoided as it can enhance neuronal injury.

B. Anticonvulsants

Seizures should be controlled to avoid further brain injury. Phenobarbitone is used in a loading dose 20 mg/kg slowly at the rate of 1 mg/kg/min intravenously. The maintenance dose is started 12-hour later in a dose of 5 mg/kg/day in two divided doses. One should always be vigilant for respiratory depression, cardiovascular compromise, and hypotension during administration of phenobarbitone. If seizures persist, phenytoin may be administered as a second drug.

Before starting anticonvulsants, one should ascertain that metabolic derangements that may complicate asphyxia and cause seizures (hypoglycemia, hypocalcemia, hyponatremia) have been taken care of.

If seizures persist, a benzodiazepine, eg, lorazepam 0.05 to 0.10 mg/kg/dose intravenously may be given as the third drug.

When the infant's condition has been stable for 3 to 4 days, all anticonvulsants are weaned except phenobarbitone. If seizures have resolved, neurologic findings are normal and EEG is normal, anticonvulsants are stopped by 14 days of life. If anything is abnormal, anticonvulsants are continued for 1 to 3 months. If the neurologic findings are normal with no recurrent seizures, phenobarbitone is tapered over 2 weeks.

C. Cerebroprotective Interventions

Brain-sparing or cerebroprotective interventions are being studied for improving the outcome of perinatal asphyxia. These include therapeutic hypothermia, free radical scavengers, antagonists of excitotoxic amino acids, calcium channel blockers, etc.

Cerebral edema is an uncommon complication of HIE. Patent sutures and fontanels in newborns offer protection against rise in intracranial pressure in HIE. Therefore, drugs like mannitol, steroids, and furosemide used in past are no longer recommended.

D. Monitoring

Early detection of complication by clinical and biochemical monitoring and prompt management is essential to prevent extension of cerebral injury.

Regular clinical assessment should be made by recording respiratory rate, heart rate, capillary filling time, blood pressure, temperature and oxygen saturation. Urine output should be monitored. Biochemical monitoring consists of estimation of blood sugar by dextrostix, hematocrit, serum electrolytes (Na, K), serum calcium, BUN, creatinine, blood gases, and pH.

Oxygenation should be kept in the normal range by monitoring transcutaneous or arterial PaO_2 or percent oxygen saturation (SpO_2) by pulse oximetry. PaO_2 should be maintained between 60 and 80 mm Hg and SpO_2 should be maintained between 90 and 94%. Hypoxia should be treated with O_2 and, if required, ventilation. Hyperoxia should always be avoided. CO_2 levels should be kept in the normal range by maintaining $PaCO_2$ between 35 and 45 mm Hg.

Perinatal Asphyxia and HIE

1. Perinatal asphyxia is the second most common cause of neonatal death after infections.
2. Hypoxic-ischemic encephalopathy (HIE) refers to the characteristic neurological manifestations which develop following perinatal asphyxia.
3. Brain damage occurs mainly in cerebral cortex and basal ganglia in term newborns. In preterm newborns, the insult predominantly involves periventricular white matter.
4. Seizures occur in up to 50% newborns with HIE and are mostly subtle.
5. Sarnat staging is used for grading the severity of HIE.
6. Therapeutic hypothermia is the most promising neuroprotective intervention to date for infants with moderate to severe HIE.
7. The mortality is 20%; and 30% of survivors have neuro-developmental sequelae including cerebral palsy and intellectual disability.

Prognosis

The mortality is 20%; and 30% of survivors have neuro-developmental sequelae. Long-term handicaps include developmental delay, cerebral palsy, microcephaly, seizures, blindness, deafness; and problems with cognition, memory, fine motor skills, and behavior.

Predictors of poor outcome The presence of one or more of the following features is associated with poor outcome: Failure to establish respiration by 5 minutes of life; apgar score of 3 or less at 5 minutes; onset of seizures within 12 hours; refractory seizures; stage III HIE; persistent oliguria (<1 mL/kg/h) for the first 36 hours of life; inability to establish oral feeds by 1 week; abnormal EEG and failure to normalize by day 7; and abnormal CT, MRI in post-asphyxial period.

Azzopardi DV, Strohm B, Edwards AD; TOBY Study Group. Moderate hypothermia to treat perinatal asphyxial encephalopathy. *N Engl J Med*. 2009;361:1349–58.

Cilio MR, Ferriero DM. Synergistic neuroprotective therapies with hypothermia. *Semin Fetal Neonatal Med*. 2010;15:293–8.

Iwata O, Iwata S. Filling the evidence gap: How can we improve the outcome of neonatal encephalopathy in the next 10 years? *Brain Dev*. 2011;33:221–8.

7.10 BIRTH INJURIES

Injuries to the infant that result from mechanical forces (ie, compression, traction) during the birth process are categorized as birth trauma. Significant birth injury occurs in 6–8 newborns per 1000 live births. In general, larger infants are more susceptible to birth trauma.

Factors Predisposing to Injury

Primigravida; cephalopelvic disproportion, small maternal stature, maternal pelvic anomalies; fetal macrosomia (large-for-date infants, especially infants weighing more than 4500 g); prolonged or precipitate labor; deep transverse arrest of descent of presenting part of the fetus; oligohydramnios; abnormal presentation (breech); use of midcavity forceps or vacuum extraction; versions and extractions; very low birth weight infant or extreme prematurity; multiple gestation; large fetal head; and fetal anomalies.

Types of Injuries

The following injuries can be encountered during birth trauma:

1. *Soft tissue injuries* Abrasions, ecchymosis, lacerations, subcutaneous fat necrosis
2. *Skull* Caput succedaneum, cephalhematoma, linear fractures
3. *Face* Subconjunctival hemorrhage, retinal hemorrhage
4. *Nerve injuries* Brachial plexus injury, cranial nerve and spinal cord injuries
5. *Musculoskeletal injuries* Clavicular fractures, fractures of long bones, sternocleidomastoid injury
6. *Intra-abdominal injuries* Liver hematoma, splenic hematoma, adrenal hemorrhage, renal hemorrhage

A. Soft Tissue Injuries

Abrasions and lacerations occur because of scalpel cuts during cesarean section or instrumental delivery (ie, vacuum, forceps). Infection remains a risk, but most of them heal uneventfully. Management consists of careful cleaning, application of antibiotic ointment, and surgical suturing, if necessary. Other common injuries, such as caput succedaneum and cephalhematoma, are discussed elsewhere.

B. Nerve Injuries

Brachial plexus injury occurs most commonly in large babies, frequently with shoulder dystocia or breech delivery. Incidence for brachial plexus injury is 0.5–2.0 per 1000 live births. Most cases are of Erb palsy. Entire brachial plexus involvement occurs in 10% of cases.

- *Duchenne-Erb palsy* (lesion in C5–C6) is the most common type of brachial plexus injury and is associated with lack of shoulder motion. The involved extremity lies adducted, prone, and internally rotated with flexion of the wrist and fingers in the characteristic waiter's tip posture. Moro, biceps, and radial reflexes are absent on the affected side. Grasp reflex is usually present.
- *Klumpke paralysis* (C7–8, T1) is rare and results in weakness of the intrinsic muscles of the hand; grasp reflex is absent. If cervical sympathetic fibers of the first thoracic spinal nerve are involved, this will lead to ipsilateral Horner syndrome.

Treatment	Erb/Klumpke Paralysis

X-ray of shoulder and upper arm should be done to rule out bony injuries. Diaphragmatic palsy should be excluded. Management is expectant. "Statue of liberty" splinting should be avoided due to the risk of contractures in the shoulder girdle. Physiotherapy with passive movements should be started within 7–10 days, when the postinjury neuritis has resolved. Prognosis depends on the extent of injury, whether nerve roots are intact (excellent outcome) or avulsed (guarded outcome). Significant clinical improvement within 2 weeks means normal or near-normal function will be eventually restored. Most babies recover fully

7

by 3 months. Surgery is recommended in those with poor biceps function at 3 months after electromyography and nerve conduction studies.

Cranial nerve and spinal cord injuries result from hyperextension, traction, and overstretching with simultaneous rotation; they may range from localized neuropraxia to complete nerve or cord transection.

C. Clavicular Fracture

Clavicle is the most frequently fractured bone in the neonate during birth. It is an unpredictable unavoidable complication of normal birth. Some correlation with birth weight, midforceps delivery, and shoulder dystocia exists. The infant may present with pseudoparalysis. Examination may reveal crepitus, palpable bony irregularity, and sternocleidomastoid muscle spasm. Radiographic studies confirm the fracture. Healing usually occurs in 7–10 days. In order to decrease pain, arm motion may be limited by pinning the infant's sleeve to the shirt. Assess other associated injury to the spine, brachial plexus, or humerus.

Uhing MR. Management of birth injuries. *Pediatr Clin North Am.* 2004;51:1169–86.

7.11 NEONATAL SEPSIS

Definition

Neonatal sepsis is a clinical syndrome characterized by systemic signs of infection in association with a positive blood culture in the first month (28 days) of life. It encompasses various infections of the newborn such as pneumonia, septicemia, meningitis, arthritis, osteomyelitis, urinary tract infections (UTIs), etc. Newborn babies are highly vulnerable to infection due to immaturity of their immune defense mechanisms.

Incidence

World Health Organization estimates that 1 million deaths per year are due to neonatal sepsis and 42% of these deaths occur in first week of life. The incidence of neonatal sepsis in India is estimated to be 38/1000 live births in tertiary care hospitals as compared to 1–5/1000 in West. Sepsis is also the most common cause of neonatal mortality in India, accounting for 30–50% of neonatal deaths in the community. The higher incidence of infection may be due to increased prevalence of maternal genital tract infections, unhygienic delivery practices, high proportion of low birth weight babies, and poor infant feeding and rearing practices.

Classification

Depending on the age of onset, two patterns of the disease have been recognized:

Early Onset Sepsis (EOS)

The signs and symptoms of sepsis appear within first 72 hours of birth. The source of pathogens is the maternal genital tract or the delivery area. Respiratory distress due to congenital (intrauterine) pneumonia is the predominant manifestation of early onset sepsis. Risk factors for development of EOS include:

Obstetric Risk Factors

i. Prolonged (>18 hours) rupture of membranes;
ii. Clinical chorioamnionitis defined as intrapartum maternal fever (>37.8°C) with two or more features: fetal tachycardia (>160/min), uterine tenderness, malodorous vaginal discharge or maternal leukocytosis (>15,000 leukocytes/dL);
iii. Multiple ($\geq$ 3) per vaginum examinations in 24 hours; and
iv. Maternal Group B Streptococcus colonization.

Neonatal Risk Factors

i. *Very low birth weight (<1500 g) and prematurity (<35 weeks of gestation)* The incidence of septicemia is 10 to 20 times more in very low birth weight babies than in average birth weight babies. This is primarily due to poor host defense mechanisms in these infants.
ii. *Male sex* Male babies are at higher risk of developing infection, suggesting the possibility of sex-linked factor in host susceptibility.

Late Onset Sepsis (LOS)

The signs and symptoms of sepsis appear after 72 hours of age. The pathogens are acquired from community or hospital (nosocomial). Late onset sepsis commonly presents as septicemia, pneumonia or meningitis. Risk factors of LOS include:

- Very low birth weight;
- Lack of breastfeeding;
- Indiscriminate use of antibiotics: It encourages development of resistant organisms;
- Frequent handling;
- Presence of central venous catheters;
- Delayed enteral feeding;
- Prolonged hyperalimentation;
- Mechanical ventilation;
- Improper hand washing techniques; and
- Unhygienic infant feeding and rearing practices.

Etiology

Predominant causes of neonatal sepsis in India are Gram-negative organisms like *Klebsiella pneumoniae, Escherichia coli, Acinetobacter baumannii, Pseudomonas, Citrobactor,* etc. Gram-positive organisms, eg, *Staphylococcus aureus, Staphylococcus albus* and *Enterobacter* sp. are less frequent. In contrast to Western countries where Group B Streptococcus (GBS) is a predominant pathogen responsible for neonatal sepsis, it is isolated in very a few cases in India. *Candida* sp. (*C. albicans, C. tropicalis,* etc.) can also cause late onset sepsis in very low birth weight neonates exposed to broad-spectrum antibiotics.

Clinical Manifestations

The clinical picture of neonatal sepsis is highly variable. The signs and symptoms may be minimal, subtle, or nonspecific. This may cause delay in diagnosis with serious consequences. The early features of septicemia are lethargy, sluggishness, poor feeding, poor cry, irritability, hypothermia, and loss of or inadequate weight gain.

There should be high index of suspicion of sepsis. Otherwise diagnosis can be easily missed. Sometimes the baby does not "look well", appears off color, and is less alert/

active. This may be an important clue to diagnosis. Parents are very perceptive and concerned about the subtle changes in the behavior and activity of their infants and their concerns should not be easily dismissed. A baby requires careful observation and meticulous examination for the following systemic manifestations:

- *Respiratory*: Tachypnea, apnea, retractions, grunting and cyanosis;
- *Cardiac*: Tachycardia, and shock in late stages;
- *GIT*: Vomiting, diarrhea and abdominal distension, hepatosplenomegaly;
- *Renal*: Oliguria due to renal failure;
- *CNS*: Excessive irritability, full fontanel, seizures, staring look, hypotonia/hypertonia, apneic spells. It is uncommon to find neck rigidity in neonatal meningitis;
- *Hematologic*: Pallor, disseminated intravascular coagulation, icterus, bleeding spots;
- *Skin*: Impetigo, cellulitis, sclerema, bleeds, petechial spots;
- *Miscellaneous* Metabolic acidosis, hypoglycemia.

Investigations

A. Direct Evidence of Infection

1. *Blood Culture*

The diagnosis of septicemia can be made reliably only by recovery of the organism from blood culture or other normally sterile body fluids. It is the gold standard test for confirming neonatal septicemia. Blood culture should always be obtained before starting antibiotics. One-two mL of blood is sufficient for culture as neonates have high degree of bacteremia. The ratio of blood to culture medium should be 1:10. All blood cultures should be observed for at least 48 hours before declaring them negative. It is now possible to detect bacterial growth within 12–24 h by using newer bacteriological techniques such as BACTEC and BACT ALERT.

2. *Lumbar Puncture*

Meningitis may co-exist without any clinical signs. Therefore, lumbar puncture should be performed on all cases of suspected sepsis. The interpretation of CSF findings is problematic in neonates because of higher cell count (up to 32 cells per mm^3 with 60% of these cells being polymorphs) and increased protein levels (120–150 mg/dL) as normal values.

CSF samples should be cultured immediately to avoid loss of viability of organisms. Gram stain should also be done. Apart from culture and Gram stain, other parameters to be evaluated are: Total WBC count, neutrophil count, glucose and protein. Traditionally, the following cut-offs have been used: >30 cells, more than 60% of polymorphs, glucose less than 50% of blood glucose, protein more than 150 mg/dL in term babies and 180 mg/dL in preterm babies.

It is important to remember that CSF WBC and glucose rapidly fall with time, giving spurious results. If the LP is traumatic, the CSF should be sent for Gram stain and culture. If the neonate is too sick, lumbar puncture should be deferred, until stabilization is achieved.

B. Indirect Evidence of Infection

1. *Sepsis Screen*

Sepsis screen refers to a combination of several tests in an attempt to improve the diagnosis of neonatal sepsis early in the course of illness. In general, sepsis screen has shown little increase in positive predictive value (if a test is abnormal, disease is present), although negative predictive value (if a test is normal, disease is absent) has improved remarkably. The main value of this screen lies in excluding infection rather than confirming the diagnosis of infection. If repeat screen is still negative 12–24 h later, then infection can be excluded confidently. A sepsis screen consists of:

- Total leukocyte count <5000/mm^3
- Absolute neutrophil count <1800/mm^3
- Immature (band cells + myelocytes + metamyelocytes) to total neutrophils ratio >0.2;
- Raised µESR (>15 mm/h); and
- Raised C-reactive protein (CRP) (>10 mg/L).

If two or more tests are positive in a neonate with maternal risk factors then it is reasonable to initiate antibiotic therapy after taking blood culture.

Complete blood count Leucopenia (<5000/mm^3) is more common than leukocytosis (>25,000/mm^3) in neonatal sepsis. Neutropenia (<1800/mm^3) is considered to be a better predictor of septicemia. However, certain conditions like birth asphyxia, and toxemia of pregnancy may be associated with neutropenia in the neonate.

Apart from these, thrombocytopenia (platelet count <1,00,000/mm^3) and presence of Dohle bodies (aggregates, of rough endoplasmic reticulum), toxic granulation (eosinophilic granules in the cytoplasm), and vacuolization in neutrophils can also be taken as additional parameters to diagnose sepsis.

Acute phase reactants In the presence of inflammation due to infection, hepatocytes under the influence of interleukin (IL)-1, rapidly synthesize certain proteins. These are known as acute phase reactants. These include: C-reactive protein (CRP), fibrinogen, haptoglobin, etc.

The levels of certain proteins such as, prealbumin, fibronectin and transferrin, decrease in response to infection. These are known as negative reactants. CRP has a sensitivity of 87% and specificity of 83% in predicting infection. Serial changes in CRP levels are more useful in diagnosing infection and in assessing response to therapy.

2. *Cytokines and Other Markers*

Cytokines are being studied for their potential usefulness in diagnosing neonatal septicemia. Two such cytokines are tumor necrosis factor (TNF) and interleukin-6 (IL-6). The levels increase early in the course of illness. Other potential markers of infection include serum fibronectin, soluble CD14 and procalcitonin. Recently, polymerase chain reaction (PCR) has been successfully employed in the diagnosis of neonatal septicemia.

C. Other Investigations

Chest X-ray, blood glucose, urea, creatinine, electrolytes, arterial blood gases, and coagulation studies provide useful information for determining supportive management.

Problems in Diagnosis

No laboratory test can rapidly confirm or exclude neonatal sepsis. Therefore, one must use one's clinical judgment

7

taking into account maternal/neonatal risk factors and infant's condition. Since neonatal sepsis can progress rapidly in a matter of a few hours, it is justified to start antibiotics in symptomatic babies before diagnostic results are available. For asymptomatic babies with maternal or obstetric risk factors for infection, antibiotics are started, if two or more tests in sepsis screen are positive. The subsequent duration of antibiotic therapy is based on the clinical course and the results of laboratory tests.

Treatment	Neonatal Sepsis

A. Specific Therapy

Antibiotics are the mainstay of therapy. These should be started after the diagnostic studies are complete. It is not always essential to wait for the results of laboratory tests before starting antibiotics.

Choice of antibiotics This is based on the knowledge of the prevalent organisms responsible for septicemia and their antibiotic sensitivity. A combination of ampicillin and an aminoglycoside (gentamicin or amikacin) is a good choice for early onset septicemia and late onset community-acquired infections. If there is associated meningitis, the preferred combination is ampicillin and cefotaxime. For community-acquired septicemia of staphylococcal origin, cloxacillin and an aminoglycoside is preferred. If there is concern regarding methicillin-resistant *Staphylococcus aureus* (MRSA), use vancomycin instead of cloxacillin. **Table 7.13** details the dosages of antibiotic in neonates.

Aminoglycosides The choice is based on sensitivity pattern, cost, safety profile and efficacy record. Where resistant organisms are unlikely, gentamicin is preferred choice because of its low cost. For resistant organisms, amikacin is selected. Netilmicin has got highest antistaphylococcal activity but has the disadvantage of high cost. Tobramycin has very good activity against *Pseudomonas.*

Third generation cephalosporins Cefotaxime, ceftriaxone and ceftazidime have good activity against Gram-negative bacilli. Compared to aminoglycosides, they are more safe, do not require monitoring of serum concentrations, and have better penetration through meninges. For these reasons, they are preferred, especially if there is associated meningitis. Only ceftazidime has antipseudomonal activity. Although third generation cephalosporins have only modest activity against *Staphylococcus aureus,* cefotaxime has better antistaphylococcal coverage than other third generation cephalosporins. Ceftriaxone has the potential to displace bilirubin from albumin. For this reason, ceftriaxone is not used in newborn babies for treating septicemia.

The duration of antibiotic therapy is 10–14 days for septicemia, 14–21 days for meningitis and at least 28 days for osteomyelitis/arthritis. Intrathecal or intraventricular instillation of antibiotics for neonatal meningitis is not beneficial, and may, in fact, be harmful due to release of bacterial products due to very rapid bacterial killing, resulting in exuberant host inflammatory response with further tissue damage.

B. Supportive Therapy

- Temperature maintenance—set temperature at 36.5°C.
- *Circulation* If perfusion is poor as evidenced by capillary refill time (CRT) of more than 3 seconds—infuse normal saline 10 mL/kg over 20–30 minutes. Repeat the same dose 1–2 times, if perfusion continues to be poor. Start dopamine at the dose of 5–10 µg/kg/min, if CRT is still prolonged.
- *Respiration* Maintain an oxygen saturation of 88–94%.
- Correction of hypoglycemia, hypocalcemia, and metabolic acidosis.
- Management of renal failure.
- Control of seizures with phenobarbitone.
- Fresh frozen plasma or platelets or packed RBCs for DIC.
- Vitamin K, if not received before or having active bleeding.
- Assisted ventilation for respiratory failure.
- Phototherapy and exchange transfusion, if required, for severe hyperbilirubinemia.
- *Nutrition* If baby is hemodynamically unstable, start total parenteral nutrition. As soon as stability is achieved, start orogastric feeding and gradually shift to breastfeeding. Mother must be advised to express her breastmilk frequently during the period the baby is kept nil orally.

C. Adjunctive Therapy

Exchange transfusion Exchange transfusion may be beneficial in septic neonates presenting with DIC, sclerema, and significant hyperbilirubinemia. It helps by removing bacteria and bacterial toxins, providing immune factors like immunoglobulins, neutrophils and macrophages and by improving tissue perfusion. However, this modality has procedure-related morbidity and mortality, especially in very sick infants and, therefore, has limited scope in management of neonatal septicemia.

Intravenous immunoglobulin (IVIG) A recent clinical trial has confirmed that IVIG is not beneficial in neonatal septicemia. *Other therapies* such as granulocyte-colony stimulating factor (G-CSF), granulocyte macrophage-colony stimulating factor (GM-CSF), activated protein C, and pentoxifylline are still under evaluation for the treatment of neonatal sepsis.

Outcome and Prognosis

Mortality due to neonatal septicemia ranges from 15–40%. Early onset septicemia, low birth weight, disseminated

Antibiotic	Dose	Frequency		Route
		<7 days age	*>7 days age*	
Ampicillin	50–100* mg/kg/dose	12 hrly	8 hrly	IV
Cloxacillin	50 mg/kg/ dose	12 hrly	8 hrly	IV
Gentamicin	5 mg/kg/dose	24 hrly	24 hrly	IV
Amikacin	15 mg/kg/dose	24 hrly	24 hrly	IV
Cefotaxime	50 mg/kg/ dose	12 hrly	8 hrly	IV

Table 7.13 Dose of Antibiotics for Neonatal Sepsis

* Higher dose is given in meningitis

7

intravascular coagulation, meningitis, shock, sclerema, and multiorgan failure carry poor prognosis.

NEONATAL TETANUS

Neonatal tetanus is characterized by onset of lock jaw and muscular spasms 5–7 days after birth in infants born to mothers who are not protected against tetanus during pregnancy. These newborns are generally delivered at home under unhygienic conditions and their cords are cut with unsterile blades or scissors which are potential sources of *Clostridium tetani*. Cultural practice of applying cowdung to umbilical stump also promotes the contamination of umbilical stump with *Clostridium*.

Clinical Features

The onset occurs commonly between 5 and 15 days of age. There is no sex or seasonal predilection. The initial features include excessive irritability, refusal to feed (due to trismus), and stiffness of limbs. Tonic muscle spasms appear soon thereafter.

Muscle spasms are precipitated by touch, sound, or bright light. During spasms, the baby can be apneic and cyanosed. Muscle spasms and rigidity are less marked in low birth weight infants. Frequent muscle spasms lead to fever. Respiratory and laryngeal muscle spasms can cause upper airway obstruction and asphyxiation. Muscle rigidity can progress to opisthotonic posturing. There may be tachycardia and tachypnea. Bronchopneumonia resulting from aspiration is a common complication and cause of death.

The diagnosis is essentially clinical.

Treatment	Neonatal Tetanus

1. *General measures* Since any stimulus can precipitate spasms, the infant is managed in a quiet room with minimal handling. Initially it is not possible to feed the infant orally, therefore, intravenous fluids are given to maintain fluid and electrolyte balance. Oxygen is required as frequent spasms lead to hypoxemia.
2. *Antibiotics* Crystalline penicillin is given in a dose of 1 lac units/kg/day for 10 days to eradicate the vegetative forms of *C. tetani,* the source of tetanus toxin.
3. *Antitoxin* It neutralizes circulating toxin. The toxin already bound to tissues remains unaffected. Two types of preparations are available. (*i*) tetanus immune globulin (TIG), and (*ii*) tetanus antitoxin (TAT).
   - TIG is derived from humans. A single dose of 500 units is administered intramuscularly. There is no need to infiltrate it around the umbilicus. TIG does not cross blood–brain barrier. Intrathecal use of TIG is still experimental and its role is not well established. There is no need to repeat the dose as it has long half-life.
   - TAT is derived from equines. Though it is cheaper but it has a shorter half-life and is associated with adverse effects like serum sickness and hypersensitivity and is no longer preferred. The recommended dose is 5000 units, half the dose is given intravenously and rest is given intramuscularly.
4. *Control of muscle spasms* Various drugs have been used to control muscle spasms. These include diazepam, chlorpromazine, magnesium sulfate, baclofen, dantrolene,

and barbiturates. Diazepam is commonly used in a dose of 0.3 mg/kg intravenously every 3–6 hours. Doses as high as 20–40 mg/kg/day as continuous IV infusions have been used to control spasm in some cases. Therapy is generally required for 2–6 weeks; the dose may be tapered as muscle spasms and rigidity subside. Intractable muscle spasms are managed by neuromuscular blockade and mechanical ventilation.

5. *Respiratory care* Meticulous nursing care is imperative. Gentle suctioning of oropharyngeal secretions is done. Although tracheotomy need not be considered a routine procedure, it should be done prior to the development of severe asphyxia.

Prognosis

Mortality is about 60%. Bad prognostic signs include (i) onset in the first week of life; (*ii*) interval between lock-jaw (trismus) and onset of muscle spasms less than 48 hours; (*iii*) high fever; and (*iv*) tachycardia.

Recovery is almost complete. An attack of tetanus does not confer immunity so active immunization following recovery is a must.

Prevention

Universal immunization of pregnant mothers between 16 and 36 weeks of pregnancy with 2 doses of tetanus toxoid can prevent neonatal tetanus. The second dose should be given at least 4 weeks before the expected date of delivery.

Additionally, sterile delivery practices need to be emphasized; such as: Conducting the delivery in a clean room, sterile gloves to be worn while conducting delivery, cutting the umbilical cord with sterile equipment, sterile cord ties are to be used to tie the cord, not to apply anything over umbilical stump. These are also known as following **5 cleans**: Clean surface, clean hands, clean blade, clean cord, and clean cord tie.

SUPERFICIAL INFECTIONS

Pyoderma

- It is characterized by pustules, are most commonly found in axillae, groin, neck and periumbilical area.
- *Staphylococcus aureus* is the causative bacteria.
- Diagnosis can be confirmed by Gram staining of the pus aspirated from the pustules, which reveals neutrophils and Gram-positive cocci.
- A few small lesions in a healthy term infant can be treated with topical mupirocin alone. Multiple big lesions in a healthy neonate necessitate oral antibiotics like cefadroxil or amoxicillin-clavulenate combination (for 5–7 days). Big lesions should be pricked with a sterile needle, and cleaned with betadine solution.
- In more extensive lesions, septicemia or lesions in a preterm infant, detailed sepsis screen including blood culture should be sent and the baby should be treated with intravenous cloxacillin and aminoglycosides (or antibiotics as per sensitivity pattern) for 7–10 days.

Omphalitis

- Omphalitis is characterized by erythema or induration of the periumbilical area along with purulent discharge from

Case Study	Newborn with Sepsis and Meningitis

A 5-day-old male baby (weight 1550 g) is brought to the neonatal unit with complaints of multiple pustules on the back, umbilical discharge and excessive irritability. The baby was born at 34 weeks and the birthweight was 1700 g. The axillary temperature is 37.2 °C, extremities are warm, RR is 52/min without retractions and grunting. Bilateral air entry in the chest is equal and there is no cyanosis. Heart rate is 148/min. Color is pink, CRT is 5 sec. Blood sugar is 65 mg/dL. There are no signs of bleeding from any site. Anterior fontanel is tense and bulging.

Q1. What is your diagnosis? Justify.

Diagnosis: Preterm LBW with late-onset sepsis, pyoderma, umbilical sepsis, meningitis, and shock. Presentation of disease after 72 hours of age suggests a late onset disease. Prolonged CRT beyond 3 sec is suggestive of shock. Excessive irritability and bulging anterior fontanel point to a CNS problem: Could be meningitis or intracranial bleed. However, other evidence of infection (pustules, umbilical discharge) favors an infective cause such as meningitis. This child needs to have a complete septic workup including blood counts, blood culture, chest X-ray, and a lumbar puncture. Neuroimaging (ultrasound/CT of cranium) should also be obtained.

Q2. How will you manage this baby?
- Child is having a normal temperature which needs to be maintained.
- *Management of shock* should be the first priority. Infuse Normal saline bolus 10 mL/kg over 20 minutes, and reassess for the need of second bolus.
- Start *maintenance IV fluids*. On day 5 of life, the normal requirement is 120 mL/kg of Isolyte P per day, ie, 204 mL given as 68 mL 8 hourly IV.
- *Medications* to be given on priority will include (*a*) Injection vitamin K 1 mg IM, if not received before; and (*b*) IV antibiotics. The antibiotics should be chosen so as to cover staphylococcal infections (*S. aureus* is the most common cause of umbilical sepsis and pustules), and Gram-negative infections (*Klebsiella, E. coli, Proteus* are the usual cause of neonatal meningitis). First-line drugs will consist of a combination of cloxacillin (50 mg/kg/dose 8 hourly) and cefotaxime (50 mg/kg/dose 8 hourly). It there is no response in 48 hours, change antibiotics according to the culture reports.
- *Feeding* will depend on clinical improvement and feeding readiness of the baby. Tube feeding or cup feeding can be offered to the child, once he stabilizes.
- *Monitor* the temperature, respiration, color, and CRT.
- *Communicate* with caregivers. Inform parents about the baby's condition and stay in touch.

Lumbar puncture revealed a turbid CSF, with 480 cells/mm³, 90% polymorphs, protein 180 mg/dL and CSF glucose 24 mg/dL with corresponding blood glucose 75 mg/dL. CRP is positive. After 4 hours of your treatment, the child developed repeated episodes of multifocal clonic seizures.

Q3. Outline further management of this child.

Since the blood glucose is normal, hypoglycemia is unlikely to be the cause of seizures. Obtain serum calcium. Control the seizures by administration of phenobarbitone 20 mg/kg IV over 20 minutes. Continue maintenance phenobarbitone 3–5 mg/kg/day in two divided doses, after 24 h. Since meningitis is established, continue IV antibiotics for 2–3 weeks. Repeat vitamin K 1 mg IM every week for the duration of antibiotics. Stop phenobarbitone 5–7 days after the last episode of seizure. Monitor head circumference weekly for hydrocephalus. Discuss with parents the progress of the baby. Plan the first follow up after 1 week of discharge and next two visits every fortnight, and then coincide subsequent visits with immunization schedule. Advise regarding exclusive breastfeeding, prevention of infection, temperature maintenance, immunization, danger sign evaluation and early care seeking. Assess growth and development in each follow-up visit.

the umbilical stump. Causative organisms include both Gram-positive and Gram-negative species.
- Omphalitis may spread to cause abdominal wall cellulitis or septicemia. Management consists of a full sepsis screen including blood culture and oral/parenteral cloxacillin and aminoglycosides (or antibiotics as per sensitivity pattern) for 7–10 days.

Conjunctivitis (Ophthalmia Neonatorum)

Conjunctivitis is characterized by inflammation of the conjunctiva within the first month of life. Inflammation can be caused by a local irritant (chemical conjunctivitis) or by bacteria (*Neisseria gonorrhoeae, Chlamydia trachomatis*, staphylococci, streptococci, and Gram-negative sp.) and herpes simplex virus.

- *Chemical conjunctivitis* It is most commonly seen with silver nitrate prophylaxis, requires no specific treatment, and usually resolves within 48 hours.
- *Gonococcal conjunctivitis* It is presents with chemosis, lid edema, and purulent exudate beginning 1 to 4 days after birth. There may be clouding of cornea or panophthalmitis with loss of vision. The disease is generally bilateral. In suspected cases, the infant should receive single dose of ceftriaxone 25 to 50 mg/kg IV or IM (not to exceed 125 mg) at birth.
- *Chlamydial conjunctivitis* It presents with variable degrees of inflammation, eye discharge, and eyelid swelling 5 to 14 days after birth. It is treated with erythromycin (50 mg/kg/day in 4 divided doses) for 14 days. Only topical treatment alone is not adequate, and is unnecessary when systemic therapy is given.

Neonatal Sepsis

1. Sepsis is among the top three causes of neonatal deaths.
2. Major pathogens causing infections in neonates in developing countries are *Klebsiella pneumoniae, Staphylococcus aureus, E. coli, and Pseudomonas.*
3. Neonatal sepsis presents with nonspecific and subtle features, which often overlap with common non-infectious conditions.
4. Blood cultures should be obtained in every suspected case prior to start of antibiotics.
5. A combination of ampicillin and an aminoglycoside (gentamicin or amikacin) is a good choice for early onset septicemia and late onset community-acquired infections.
6. If there is associated meningitis, the preferred combination is ampicillin and cefotaxime.
7. Hand hygiene is the single most important preventive measure for sepsis.

- Other bacterial infections can be treated with local ophthalmic ointments, such as erythromycin or gentamicin.

INIS Collaborative Group, Brocklehurst P, Farrell B, *et al.* Treatment of neonatal sepsis with intravenous immune globulin. *N Engl J Med.* 2011;365:1201–11.

National Neonatology Forum and UNICEF. Facility based care of sick neonate ay referral health facility. New Delhi.: *Comprehensive Newborn Care Initiative.* 2010

National Neonatology Forum. *Evidence based clinical practice guidelines.* New Delhi; 2010.

7.12 RESPIRATORY DISTRESS IN NEWBORN

Respiratory distress in the neonate is defined as presence of any one of the following features: (*i*) Respiratory rate >60/min; (*ii*) subcostal or intercostal retractions; and (*iii*) expiratory grunt. Cyanosis may or may not be present.

Etiology

The etiology of respiratory distress in newborn depends on the age of onset of symptoms, gestational age, maternal factors and feeding and infant care practices. The causes of respiratory distress in neonates are summarized in **Table 7.14.**

RESPIRATORY DISTRESS SYNDROME (RDS)

RDS is characterized by onset of respiratory distress in a preterm newborn soon after birth. The incidence is inversely related to the gestational age. Approximately 50% of newborns delivered at 26 to 28 weeks of gestation develop RDS, whereas the disease becomes infrequent after 34 weeks, affecting less than 5%.

Pathophysiology

RDS is caused by deficiency of the surfactant in the lungs. Pulmonary surfactant is synthesized and secreted by type II epithelial cells in alveolus. The major constituents of surfactant are (*i*) dipalmitoyl phosphatidylcholine (lecithin)

Table 7.14 Causes of Respiratory Distress in Neonates

Category	Cause
Respiratory	Respiratory distress syndrome, transient tachypnea of the newborn, meconium aspiration syndrome, pneumonia, sepsis, pneumothorax and other air-leak syndromes, pulmonary hemorrhage, pulmonary hypoplasia, congenital deficiency of surfactant proteins B or C
Cardiac	Congestive heart failure from any cause, eg, patent ductus arteriosus (PDA) in a preterm baby or transposition of great arteries (TGA), etc.
Neurologic	Perinatal asphyxia, intracranial hemorrhage, birth trauma
Hematologic	Polycythemia, severe anemia
GIT	Necrotizing enterocolitis, abdominal distension from any cause
Surgical causes	Tracheoesophageal fistula, diaphragmatic hernia, bilateral choanal atresia, congenital lobar emphysema, cystic adenomatoid malformation of the lung
Miscellaneous	Septicemia, hypothermia, hypoglycemia, hemorrhage, metabolic acidosis, shock

and phosphatidylglycerol, (*ii*) apoproteins (surfactant proteins A, B, C, D), and (*iii*) cholesterol.

Surfactant synthesis begins at 20 to 24 weeks of gestation. Mature levels of surfactant are usually present after 34 weeks. Surfactant diminishes the surface tension of the water film that lines alveoli, thereby decreasing the tendency of alveoli to collapse at the end of expiration. With surfactant deficiency, the lungs become diffusely atelectatic (collapsed), triggering inflammation and pulmonary edema. Because blood passing through the atelectatic portions of lung is not oxygenated (due to right to left intrapulmonary shunt), the infant becomes hypoxemic. Lung compliance is decreased, thereby increasing the work of breathing. In severe cases, the diaphragm and intercostal muscles fatigue, and CO_2 retention and respiratory acidosis develop. Pathogenesis of RDS is summarized in Fig. 7.29.

Risk Factors

Besides prematurity, other risk factors include multifetal pregnancies, maternal diabetes, Cesarean section, asphyxia and hypothermia. Risk decreases with fetal growth restriction, pre-eclampsia or eclampsia, maternal hypertension, prolonged rupture of membranes, maternal opiate addiction, and antenatal corticosteroid use.

Histopathology

Lungs appear deep purplish red and are liver-like in consistency. Microscopically, there is diffuse atelectasis, pulmonary edema, pulmonary vascular congestion, hemorrhage, and evidence of injury to respiratory epithelium. *Hyaline membranes*, a characteristic feature of RDS, consist of acidophilic, homogeneous or granular membranes, lining the alveoli, alveolar ducts and respiratory

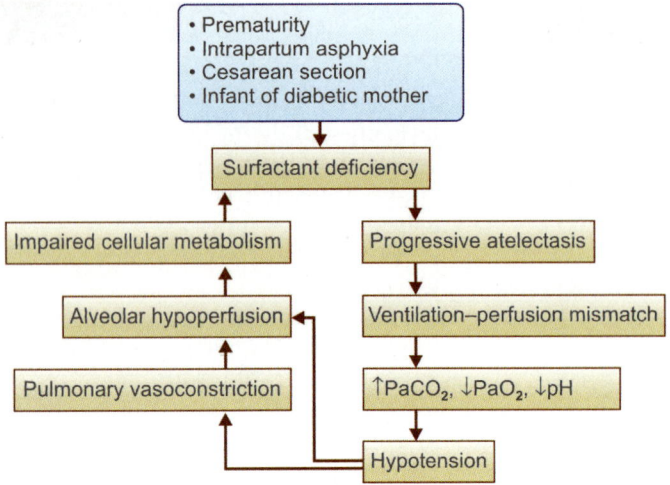

Fig. 7.29 Pathogenesis of respiratory distress syndrome (RDS)

bronchioles. Hyaline membranes may not be seen, if a baby dies within 6–8 hours of birth. Although, hyaline membranes are characteristic of RDS but they are not pathognomonic and may be seen in other conditions such as pneumonia.

Clinical Manifestations

Tachypnea (respiratory rate >60/minute) appears immediately or within six hours after delivery. This is often associated with chest retractions and flaring of alae nasi. Another characteristic feature of RDS is the *expiratory grunt*. This sound is produced due to exhalation against a partially closed glottis, due to an attempt by the baby to maintain some alveolar volume. Expiratory grunt may also be heard in severe pneumonia. Cyanosis appears, as hypoxia ensues. Atelectasis and respiratory failure are characterized by lethargy, irregular breathing, and apnea.

Assessment of the Severity of Respiratory Distress

The severity of RD can be judged clinically by the respiratory score (Downe Score) **(Table 7.15)**. The score is used in babies who are breathing spontaneously, including those receiving continuous positive airway pressure (CPAP). A score of <5 indicates mild RD, a score of 5 to 8 moderate RD, and a score of >8 severe RD.

Diagnosis

Diagnosis of RDS is made, if a preterm baby develops respiratory distress within 6 hours of age, with characteristic radiological findings with or without hypoxia and hyper-

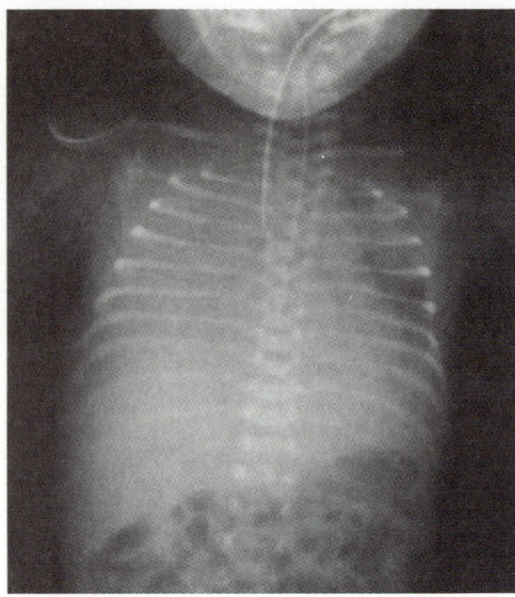

Fig. 7.30 X-ray of respiratory distress syndrome showing diffuse haziness, air bronchogram, and blurring of heart borders and diaphragm. This diffuse haziness gives a gound glass appearance, also known as white-out lungs

carbia in arterial blood gas (ABG) analysis. Radiological features include fine reticulogranular pattern in both the lung fields, reduced lung volume, air bronchograms, blurring of heart borders and margins of diaphragm, and complete white out of lungs (ground glass appearance) in late stages (Fig. 7.30).

Assessment of Fetal Lung Maturity

RDS can be anticipated prenatally using tests of fetal lung maturity, which measure surfactant levels in the amniotic fluid. The amniotic fluid can be obtained by amniocentesis or collected from the vagina (if membranes have ruptured). Risk of RDS is low when lecithin/sphingomyelin ratio in the amniotic fluid is >2. Exceptions include infants of diabetic mothers, perinatal asphyxia, and Rh hemolytic disease where despite L/S ratio above 2, the baby may still develop RDS.

Postnatally, lung maturity can be assessed by the *Shake test* on gastric aspirate. One mL of amniotic fluid or gastric aspirate of the baby is mixed with 1 mL of absolute alcohol in a test tube. The test tube is shaken for 15 seconds and allowed to stand for 15 minutes. The amount of air bubbles at the meniscus is noted and graded as follows:

+   : 1/3rd of meniscus has bubbles

++   : 2/3rd of meniscus has bubbles

+++   : One row along the circumference of meniscus has bubbles

++++ : More than one row of bubbles

The risk of hyaline membrane disease is minimal, if the test is more than ++.

Differential diagnosis includes early onset sepsis, transient tachypnea of the newborn, persistent pulmonary hypertension, meconium aspiration syndrome, pulmonary edema, and congenital cardiopulmonary anomalies.

Table 7.15 Repiratory Distress Score (Downe Score)			
Score	*0*	*1*	*2*
Respiratory rate	40 to 60/min.	60 to 80/min.	> 80/min
Oxygen requirement	None	≤50%	>50%
Retractions	None	Mild to moderate	Severe
Grunting	None	With stimulation	At rest
Breath sounds	Normal	Decreased	Barely heard

Treatment — Hyaline Membrane Disease

1. *Antenatal corticosteroids* RDS can be prevented by using antenatal corticosteroids to pregnant women between 24 and 34 weeks of gestation with threatened preterm labor. A complete course consists of two doses of betamethasone (12 mg IM) at 24 hourly interval or four doses of dexamethasone (6 mg IM) at 12 hourly interval. Betamethasone is more effective and safe than dexamethasone. Multiple courses of steroids are not recommended due to fear of brain damage to the fetus.

2. *Maintenance of temperature* The baby should be kept under servo-controlled radiant warmer with a set temperature of 36.5°C. Baby should be placed prone to prevent collapse of chest wall. Excessive handling should be avoided.

3. *Oxygen* Target oxygen saturations (SpO_2) in the range of 88–95%. Oxygen therapy must be monitored by pulse oximeter to avoid hypoxia or hyperoxia, as both are harmful to the baby.

4. *IV fluids* 10% dextrose should be started at 60–80 mL/kg/day. Sodium and potassium are added on day 3 once adequate diuresis is achieved. Monitoring of urine output, body weight and serum electrolytes should be done and fluids are adjusted accordingly. Excessive fluid intake is harmful and may lead to patent ductus arteriosus (PDA) and bronchopulmonary dysplasia (BPD).

5. *Surfactant replacement therapy (SRT)* reduces the mortality and complication rates of RDS, and shortens the duration of mechanical ventilation. Surfactant is instilled directly into the lungs through endotracheal tube. In symptomatic babies, early rescue therapy (within 2 hours) is better than delayed therapy (more than 2 hours). Prophylactic SRT, within 15–20 minutes of birth and before the onset of significant respiratory distress, is indicated for newborns under 26 weeks' gestation and in older preterm babies requiring intubation in delivery room for stabilization. Natural surfactants, bovine or porcine, are better than synthetic preparations. The dose is 100–200 mg/kg. Single dose is sufficient for most infants. Dose may be repeated 6 to 12 hours later, if significant respiratory distress persists. There is a dramatic response to surfactant replacement. Ventilatory requirements come down immediately.

6. *Ventilation* Once the baby develops RDS, therapeutic options depend on the severity of the disease. Along with supportive management, mild disease is managed with oxygen supplementation by hood; moderate disease requires CPAP; and severe disease needs mechanical ventilation.

   a. *Continuous positive airway pressure (CPAP)* CPAP is simple, safe, effective, cheap, and noninvasive alternative to mechanical ventilation to provide initial respiratory support in RDS. In CPAP, a continuous distending pressure of 6–8 cm H_2O is given through nasal prongs. It works by preventing alveolar atelectasis, thereby reducing work of breathing. CPAP is utilized in spontaneously breathing babies. Intractable apnea is a contraindication for CPAP. Regular monitoring of ABG is essential. A PaO_2 <50 mm Hg and/or a $PaCO_2$ >60 mm Hg indicate CPAP failure and need for mechanical ventilation. Early CPAP diminishes the need of mechanical ventilation and its attendant complications. One newer approach successfully employed to avoid mechanical ventilation in newborns with RDS is **INSURE**—intubation, surfactant and extubation to CPAP.

   b. *Mechanical ventilation* This is a life-saving but invasive therapy which has greatly improved the outcome of respiratory distress. Mechanical ventilation should be considered when baby has moderate to severe respiratory distress, CPAP fails to maintain blood gases within normal range, or there is intractable apnea. Many types of ventilators are available to provide respiratory support. In newborns, time-cycled, pressure-limited, continuous flow ventilators are most frequently used conventional ventilators. Synchronized intermittent mandatory ventilation (SIMV), which synchronizes with the newborn's own repiratory effort, is the most commonly used mode of ventilation. The main complication of mechanical ventilation is ventilator-induced lung injury (VILI) including air leaks and BPD. VILI can be reduced by using lowest inspiratory pressures and oxygen concentrations to maintain adequate gas exchange (PaO_2 >50 mm Hg; $PaCO_2$ <55 mm Hg). High-frequency oscillatory ventilation (breath rate >150/minute) may be useful when conventional ventilation fails.

7. *Hemodynamic support* Hypotension is common in preterm newborns with RDS. On day one, the acceptable lower limit of mean arterial pressure (MAP) approximates gestational age in weeks. After day 3, most babies under 26 weeks' gestation have MAP >30 mm Hg. In the absence of blood pressure measurement, capillary refill time (CRT) may be used to assess circulatory status. Prolonged CRT (>3 sec) is treated by infusing normal saline bolus 10 mL/kg slowly over 20 to 30 minutes followed by dopamine infusion @ 5 to 10 µg/kg/min, if needed.

8. *Nutrition* Trophic feeding may be started in a hemodynamically stable newborn as early as day 2–3 of age. Use expressed breastmilk at a volume of 10–20 mL/kg/day every 4 hours and advance as tolerated. If feeding is not possible/indicated, begin total parenteral nutrition.

9. *Antibiotics* It is virtually impossible to differentiate intrauterine pneumonia from RDS. Therefore, ampicillin and gentamicin should be started after obtaining blood culture and sepsis screen.

10. *Monitoring* Along with monitoring of vitals, biochemical monitoring of blood glucose and sodium, potassium and calcium is necessary.

Prognosis

Acute complications include air leaks (pneumothorax, pneumomediastinum, pulmonary interstitial emphysema); PDA, intracranial hemorrhage, and infection. Long-term complications are retinopathy of prematurity, BPD, neurodevelopmental impairments, and other complications of prematurity. Antenatal steroids, surfactant replacement therapy, CPAP, mechanical ventilation, and good supportive care have reduced mortality of RDS to less than 10%.

PNEUMONIA

Pneumonia is an important cause of respiratory distress and mortality in newborns. It may present soon after birth as a

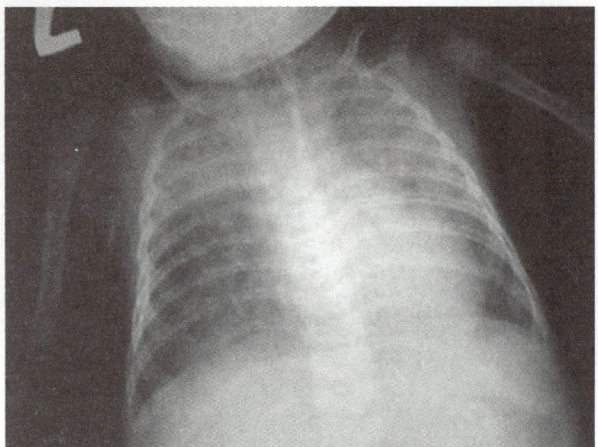

Fig. 7.31 X-ray showing bilateral diffuse haziness suggestive of pneumonia, more so in upper zones

part of early onset sepsis (congenital or intrauterine pneumonia), or later in the neonatal period as a more localized disease. Since pneumonia shares the same risk factors, causative organisms, and clinical manifestations with neonatal sepsis, its diagnosis and management are discussed under sepsis. Radiological features of pneumonia are shown in Fig. 7.31.

MECONIUM ASPIRATION SYNDROME

Meconium aspiration syndrome (MAS) is characterized by respiratory distress soon after birth in a term or post-term newborn delivered through *meconium-stained amniotic fluid (MSAF), whose symptoms cannot be explained otherwise.* MSAF occurs in 10–15% of total live births. Meconium aspiration syndrome develops in 5–10% of newborns delivered through MSAF.

Etiopathogenesis

Fetal distress (eg, from hypoxia caused by umbilical cord compression or placental insufficiency or from infection)

may cause the fetus to pass meconium into the amniotic fluid before delivery. In the presence of fetal distress, gasping by the fetus can lead to the aspiration of meconium before, during, or immediately after delivery. Aspirated meconium blocks airways and causes release of cytokines and other vasoactive substances, resulting in pulmonary hypertension. The net effect is ventilation-perfusion mismatch and arterial hypoxemia. The pathogenesis of MAS is summarized in Fig. 7.32.

Clinical Manifestations

These include tachypnea (respiratory rate >60/minute) appearing soon after delivery, nasal flaring, chest retractions, cyanosis or desaturation, bilateral crepitations, barrel-shaped chest due to air trapping; and greenish yellow staining of the umbilical cord, nail beds, or skin.

Chest X-ray findings include patchy infiltrates, coarse streaking of lung fields, areas of hyperinflation and atelectasis, flattening of diaphragm, and air leaks (Fig. 7.33).

Treatment	Meconium Aspiration Syndrome

- *Management in delivery room* Direct intratracheal suctioning is indicated in a non-vigorous newborn delivered through MSAF immediately after delivery (detailed in resuscitation section), followed by other resuscitative measures as per need.
- *Supportive management* like maintenance of temperature, intravenous fluids, oxygen inhalation, oral or parenteral nutrition, inotropic support for shock.
- *Antibiotics* (usually ampicillin and an aminoglycoside), if risk factors for sepsis are present.
- *Regular monitoring* of pulse oximetry and arterial blood gas analysis (ABG).
- *Mechanical ventilation* It is required, if there is severe hypoxemia (PaO_2<50 mm Hg) and/or hypercarbia ($PaCO_2$ >60 mm Hg).
- *Other therapies* Since surfactant may be inhibited by meconium, surfactant replacement therapy may be considered, if baby's condition does not improve. Sildenafil, magnesium

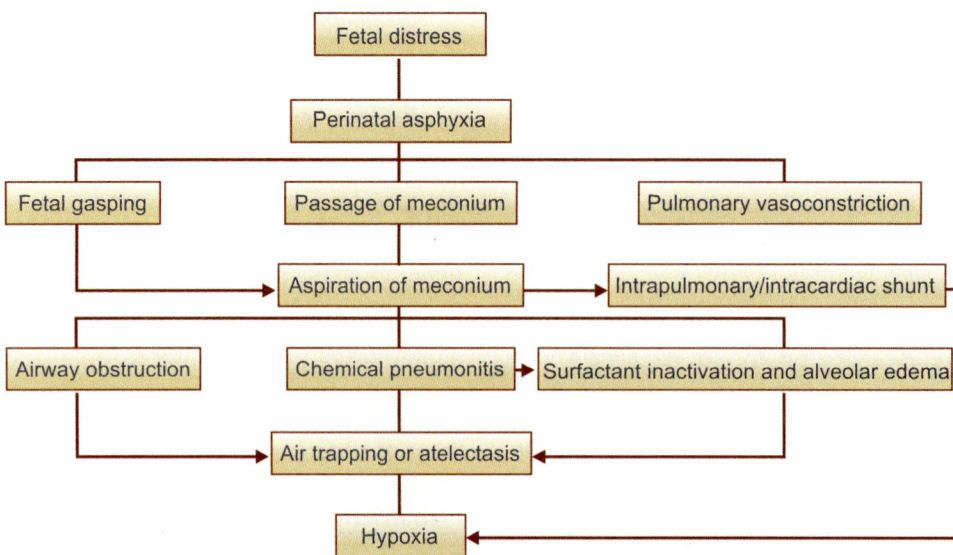

Fig. 7.32 Pathogenesis of meconium aspiration syndrome (MAS)

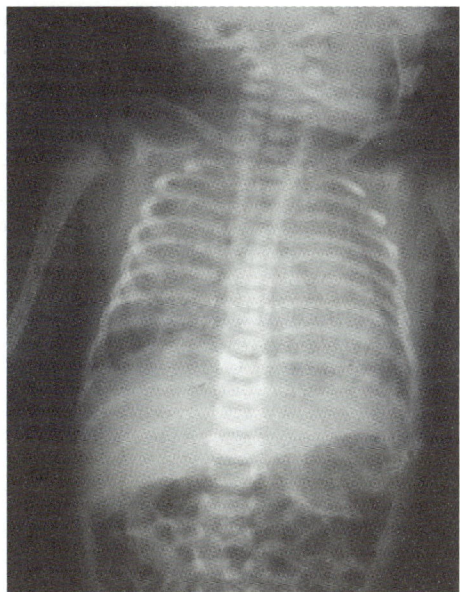

Fig. 7.33 Chest X-ray showing bilateral patchy infiltrates in meconium aspiration syndrome

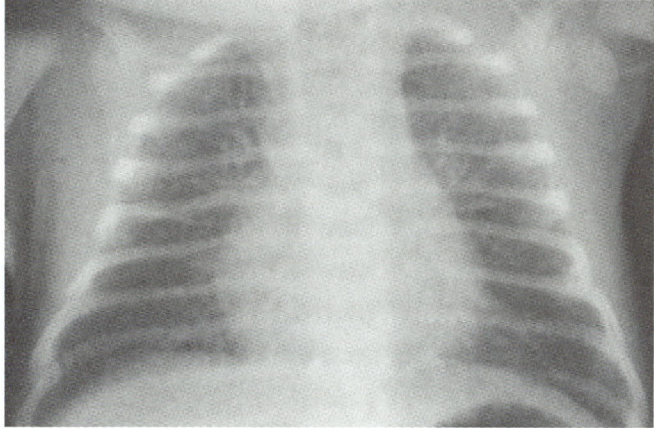

Fig. 7.34 Chest X-ray showing streaky perihilar markings with fluids in the interlobar fissures. Suggesting transient tachypnea of newborn

sulfate, or inhaled nitric oxide (iNO) therapy may be considered for persistent pulmonary hypertension of the newborn (PPHN).

- Extracorporeal membrane oxygenation (ECMO) is indicated in intractable respiratory failure.

TRANSIENT TACHYPNEA OF THE NEWBORN (WET LUNG SYNDROME)

Transient tachypnea of the newborn (TTN), also known as wet lung syndrome, is respiratory distress caused by delayed resorption of fetal lung fluid. TTN usually affects term and late preterm infants (34–36 weeks) delivered by cesarean section without labor. But it can also occur following vaginal delivery. Maternal diabetes and asthma are also risk factors for TTN.

Pathophysiology

Alveolar epithelium secretes fetal lung fluid which is required for normal lung growth and development *in utero*. At the time of birth, under the influence of hormones and other chemicals, alveolar epithelium changes from secretory mode to absorptive mode, leading to absorption of lung fluid from alveoli to the interstitium and then to pulmonary capillaries and lung lymphatics. Delay in clearance of fetal lung fluid results in transient pulmonary edema that characterizes TTN.

Diagnosis

Rapid respirations, grunting, and retractions begin soon after delivery, and cyanosis may occasionally develop. Chest X-ray shows normal or hyperinflated lungs with streaky perihilar markings with fluids in the interlobar fissures (Fig. 7.34). Rapid recovery within 2 to 3 days helps differentiate it from other causes of respiratory distress in newborn. In severe cases, baby may need respiratory support in the form of continuous positive airway pressure and

occasionally even mechanical ventilation. TTN is a diagnosis of exclusion and other causes of respiratory distress must be ruled out.

Treatment	**Transient Tachypnea of the Newborn**

Supportive management should be provided as discussed in RDS. TTN is a self-limited disease and the outcome is good.

PULMONARY AIR-LEAK SYNDROMES

Air-leak syndromes include pneumothorax, pulmonary interstitial emphysema, pneumomediastinum, pneumopericardium, pneumoperitoneum, and subcutaneous emphysema.

Etiology

The most common cause is delivery room resuscitation or mechanical ventilation. Other causes are pneumonia, meconium aspiration syndrome, RDS, and use of CPAP. Occasionally, air leaks can occur in normal neonates, probably because large negative intrathoracic forces are created when the neonate starts breathing, occasionally disrupt alveolar epithelium, which allows air to move from the alveoli into extra-alveolar soft tissues or spaces.

Air leak is more common and severe in infants with lung disease, who are at risk because of poor lung compliance and the need for high airway pressures (eg, in respiratory distress) or because of air trapping (eg, meconium aspiration syndrome), which leads to alveolar overdistension and rupture.

Management

Diagnosis is suspected clinically due to sudden deterioration or because of fall in oxygen saturation status and is confirmed by X-ray (Fig. 7.35). Transillumination of chest with a fiberoptic probe (increased transillumination on the affected side) can also aid in bedside diagnosis of pneumothorax. Breath sounds may not be diminished and chest percussion is rarely helpful/performed in a critically sick baby. *Treatment* is chest tube drainage under water seal in symptomatic pneumothorax.

7

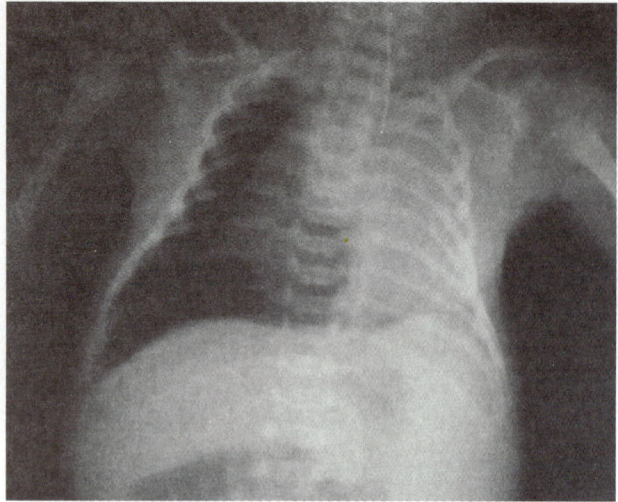

Fig. 7.35 Chest X-ray of tension pneumothorax right side

SURGICAL CAUSES OF NEONATAL RESPIRATORY DISTRESS

Etiology

I. Common obstructive lesions of the newborn airway

- *Nose, oral cavity and pharynx* Bilateral choanal atresia; macroglossia, Pierre Robin syndrome; neoplasm-like lymphangioma, teratoma, or cyst.
- *Larynx* Laryngomalacia, bilateral vocal cord palsy, subglottic stenosis, cysts and laryngoceles, webs, lymphangioma, teratoma, and cystic hygroma.
- *Tracheobronchial tree* Tracheomalacia, bronchomalacia, vascular anomalies, tracheoesophageal fistula, webs, mediastinal masses like bronchogenic cysts or teratomas.

II. Common conditions causing pulmonary compression

- Congenital diaphragmatic hernia
- Pneumothorax, congenital lobar emphysema, congenital cystic adenomatoid malformation (CCAM)
- Eventration of diaphragm, pleural effusions (especially chylothorax)
- Congenital lung cysts

TRACHEOESOPHAGEAL FISTULA (TEF)

Tracheoesophageal fistula is a congenital communication between the trachea and esophagus. Approximately 17–70% of children with TEFs have associated developmental anomalies like Down syndrome, duodenal atresia, and cardiovascular defects. As per Gross classification, there are 5 types of TEF with type C, blind upper esophageal pouch and lower esophageal pouch communicating with the trachea, being the most common type (Fig. 7.36).

Clinical Features

Neonates with TEF usually develop copious, fine white frothy bubbles of mucus in the mouth and nose. Secretions recur despite suctioning. Infants may develop rattling respiration and episodes of coughing and choking in association with cyanosis. Symptoms worsen during feeding in the presence of a TEF.

Diagnosis

Fetal diagnosis Esophageal atresia in the fetus should be suspected in presence of maternal polyhydramnios. Absence of stomach gas on prenatal ultrasound is another indication of esophageal atresia.

Diagnosis in the neonate is confirmed when an orogastric tube cannot be passed beyond 10 cm. Plain chest radiographs may reveal tracheal compression and deviation. Absence of a gastric bubble indicates esophageal atresia without a TEF or esophageal atresia with a proximal TEF. X-ray is usually done after putting an orogastric tube and pushing around 10 mL of air; coiling of the tube within dilated blind pouch of esophagus can be seen.

Treatment	Tracheoesophageal Fistula
The baby should be kept nil orally and given intravenous fluids. The baby is nursed supine or in semi-upright position with frequent suctioning of esophageal pouch to avoid aspiration of secretions. Surgical repair is undertaken at the earliest.	

CONGENITAL DIAPHRAGMATIC HERNIA (CDH)

The incidence is 1 in 4000 live births. Herniation of abdominal visceral contents through the posterolateral foramen of Bochdalek (more common) or the anterior foramen of Morgagni (rare) leads to diaphragmatic hernia. Maldevelopment of the post-hepatic mesenchymal plate and closure of pleuroperitoneal canal, which is crucial for normal diaphragmatic development, results in CDH. Presence of abdominal viscera in the chest during fetal life also prevents normal development of the lungs. Defect is more common on the left side.

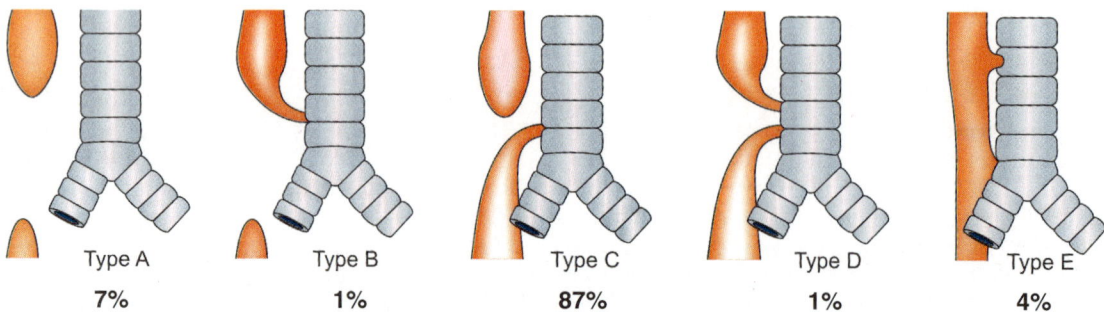

Type A	Type B	Type C	Type D	Type E
7%	1%	87%	1%	4%

Fig. 7.36 Types of tracheoesophageal fistula with incidence

Clinical Features

Cyanosis, tachypnea, grunting, and retraction are commonly seen soon after birth. On physical examination, the abdomen is scaphoid, the anteroposterior diameter of the chest is increased, mediastinal shift may be noted, breath sounds are absent on the affected side, and bowel sounds may be heard in chest.

Diagnosis

Prenatal diagnosis can be made on ultrasonography. There may be maternal polyhydramnios. The advantage of prenatal diagnosis is that baby can be delivered in a center where surgery can be done. Postnatal diagnosis is made from the chest radiograph which shows air-filled bowel loops in the chest cavity with non-visualization of diaphragmatic margin, mediastinal shift, and a relative paucity of abdominal gas (Fig. 7.37). Findings can be confirmed on ultrasonography/CT scan.

Treatment	Congenital Diaphragmatic Hernia

Bag and mask ventilation is contraindicated in babies with known or suspected diaphragmatic hernia as it causes bowel distension and increases the mediastinal shift further which affects the contralateral lung and also compromises cardiac function. If needed, use bag and endotracheal tube to provide ventilation in these babies.

After admission in NICU, baby is given supportive care. Mechanical ventilation should be done with low inspiratory

Case Study	Newborn with Respiratory Distress

A 34-week male baby delivered by cesarean section developed fast breathing soon after birth and was brought to the neonatal unit. There is a history of premature rupture of membrane 24 h before delivery. The birth weight of the baby is 1500 g. On examination, the axillary temperature is 37.2°C, respiratory rate is 82/min with moderate retractions and intermittent grunting. Bilateral air entry in the chest is poor and there is no cyanosis. Heart rate is 148/min. Capillary refill time (CRT) is 2 sec. Blood sugar is 55 mg/dL.

Q1. What is the likely diagnosis? What is minimal diagnostic work-up?

Early-onset sepsis with intrauterine pneumonia is the most likely diagnosis due to presence of maternal risk factor for infection. Other differential diagnoses include respiratory distress syndrome (RDS) and transient tachypnea of newborn (TTN).

We will like to obtain a chest X-ray and do a septic screen including total blood counts, C-reactive protein, and blood culture. If facilities are available, arterial blood gas should also be done. A shake test can be done on the gastric aspirate to see for lung maturity. This could help in ruling out respiratory distress syndrome.

Q2. How will you manage this baby?

National Neonatology Forum (NNF) of India has popularized the abbreviation **TABC-FM-FM-CF** to deal with all aspects of care in a sick newborn admitted to a health care facility. This approach simplifies care of a sick baby and ensures comprehensive management, including stabilization, medications, monitoring, communication, and follow-up advice. Let us manage this baby step by step by following this approach:

- **T:** *Temperature*: Nurse the baby prone under radiant warmer
- **A:** *Airway*: Ensure open airway
- **B:** *Breathing*: Provide oxygen by hood (2–4 L/min) or nasal cannula. Monitor oxygen saturation by attaching to a pulse oximeter. Consider CPAP/ventilation, if the child fails to maintain SpO_2 between 90 and 94%.
- **C:** *Circulation*: No need of fluid bolus as CRT is normal (<3s).
- **F:** *Fluids*: Baby should be given intravenous fluids as feeding is not possible due to illness. Fluid requirement on day 1 in a preterm child = 80 mL/kg of 10% dextrose = 80 x 1.5=120 mL that can be given as 40 mL 8 hourly IV.
- **M:** *Medications*: Injection vitamin K 1 mg IM, if not received before. Start first-line antibiotics after taking sample for blood culture. [ampicillin (50 mg/kg/dose 8 hourly) and gentamicin (2.5 mg/kg/dose 12 hourly)].
- **F:** *Feeding* should not be started initially as the baby is sick.
- **M:** *Monitor*: RR, HR, CRT, temperature, SpO_2, and urine output.
- **C:** *Communication*: Inform parents what is wrong with the baby and what you are doing. Update them frequently on the progress of the baby.
- **F:** *Follow-up*: This point will be covered at the time of discharge

After 24 hours, baby is stable, CRP is positive and total WBC count is 4800/cu mm. Chest X-ray showed bilateral diffuse infiltrates suggestive of intrauterine pneumonia. SpO₂ is 92% with oxygen 2 L/min. Sepsis work-up suggests infection. Final confirmation awaits blood culture report.

Q3. How will you proceed further?

Investigations have confirmed the presence of pneumonia, so the antibiotics will be continued for 10 days. Initiate breastfeeding as soon as respiratory distress settles down (RR <60/min, no retractions or grunting). Advise regarding temperature maintenance, exclusive breastfeeding.

F: *Follow-up*: Advise first follow-up after 1 week and then fortnightly for two more visits. Subsequently, follow-up visits should coincide with immunization schedule. Assess growth and development and treat medical problems as they arise.

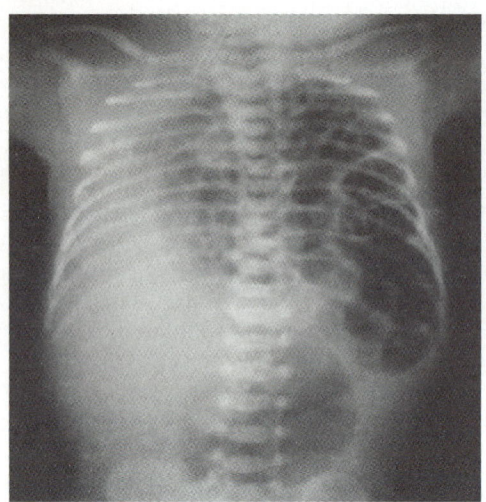

Fig. 7.37 Chest X-ray showing air-filled bowel loops in the left chest cavity with non-visualization of left dome of diaphragm and mediastinal shift to the right; suggestive of left-sided diaphragmatic hernia

pressures to avoid rupture of contralateral lung. Ionotropic support may be needed to maintain blood pressure and peripheral circulation. PPHN may require sildenafil or inhaled nitric oxide therapy. Some babies may require high frequency oscillatory ventilation and extracorporeal membrane oxygenation (ECMO) to maintain life.

Respiratory Distress Syndrome

1. Respiratory distress in newborn can be because of respiratory, metabolic, cardiac, CNS, or surgical causes.
2. It is important to assess severity of respiratory distress by using a respiratory distress score.
3. Common causes include RDS in preterm neonates and MAS and pneumonia in term neonates.
4. Surgical causes must be ruled out as these are correctible by surgical intervention.
5. Hyaline membrane disease is the most important cause of respiratory distress in preterm neonates. The clinical features are related to surfactant deficiency and manifest as tachypnea, intercostal retractions and grunt.
6. Surfactant should be used as early rescue in infants who need intubation and those who continue to need more than 30–35% oxygen in spite of adequate CPAP support.
7. Early CPAP support is the mainstay of treatment for HMD.
8. Antenatal steroids are highly cost-effective in decreasing the incidence of HMD and its complications. They must be given to all women with threatened preterm delivery from 24 to 34 weeks of gestation.
9. Amnioinfusion and tracheal suction after birth are no longer recommended as strategies for prevention of meconium aspiration syndrome.
   ECMO must be considered in select cases of refractory hypoxic respiratory failure.

After initial stabilization, definitive treatment is surgical repair. Severe cases diagnosed antenatally have been successfully managed with EXIT procedure (*ex-utero* intrapartum treatment). EXIT involves maternal laparotomy, partial delivery of fetus through the uterine opening, fetal intubation followed by either complete delivery or immediate institution of ECMO.

Eventration of the Diaphragm

It results from maldevelopment of the diaphragm muscle which is replaced by a thin membranous structure. It usually presents in older children but in newborns it may be difficult to differentiate from CDH. The treatment consists of diaphragmatic plication which can be carried out either by thoracotomy or laparotomy.

Davis PG, Morley CJ, Owen LS. Non-invasive respiratory support of preterm neonates with respiratory distress: continuous positive airway pressure and nasal intermittent positive pressure ventilation. *Semin Fetal Neonatal Med*. 2009;14:14–20.

Liu J, Shi Y, Dong JY, Zheng T, *et al*. Clinical characteristics, diagnosis and management of respiratory distress syndrome in full-term neonates. *Chin Med J* (Engl). 2010;123:2640–4.

National Neonatology Forum and UNICEF. Facility based care of sick neonate ay referral health facility. *Comprehensive Newborn Care Initiative*. New Delhi 2010.

7.13 APNEA IN NEWBORN

Apnea in the newborn is defined as cessation of breathing for longer than 20 seconds; or of shorter duration, if accompanied by bradycardia, or oxygen desaturation.

Pathogenesis

Apneic spells are common in preterm newborns. More immature the baby, higher is the risk of apnea. Up to one-fourth of preterm infants below 34 weeks gestation have at least one episode of apnea.

Apnea of prematurity arises due to physiologic immaturity of respiratory control mechanisms. Possible mechanisms include developmental immaturity of brainstem respiratory center, altered chemoreceptor response to hypoxia and hypercarbia, and intrinsic instability of upper airway muscles leading to airway obstruction.

Apnea of prematurity generally begins 24 hours after birth and no later than day 7 of life. Apnea that develops after 1 week of age signifies an underlying illness other than apnea of prematurity, such as infection, hypothermia, hypoglycemia, PDA, and intraventricular hemorrhage.

Classification

Apnea of prematurity is classified as: (*i*) Central; (*ii*) obstructive; or (*iii*) mixed.

- *Central apnea* is defined as the cessation of both airflow and inspiratory efforts. It is caused by immaturity of medullary respiratory control centers; insufficient neural impulses from the respiratory centers in the medulla reach the respiratory muscles, and the infant stops breathing.
- *Obstructive apnea* is the cessation of airflow in the presence of continued inspiratory efforts. It is caused by obstructed airflow or neck flexion causing opposition of hypopharyngeal soft tissues, nasal occlusion, or reflex laryngospasm.

• *Mixed apnea* contains elements of both central and obstructive apnea. Most apneic spells are mixed in origin.

Periodic Breathing

Apneic spells should be differentiated from periodic breathing which is a normal developmental characteristic of neonatal breathing.

Periodic breathing is characterized by alternation between regular breathing for 10 to 15 seconds and apneic pauses of 3 to 10 seconds. It is common in preterm babies but is also seen in term neonates and young infants. In most cases, periodic breathing accounts for 2–6% of the breathing time in healthy term neonates and as much as 25% of the breathing time in preterm neonates. There is no associated change in heart rate or color. Periodic breathing diminishes over 6–8 weeks of age. It is attributed to immaturity of respiratory control mechanism in newborns. It requires no treatment and has no prognostic significance.

Etiology of Apnea

Important secondary causes of neonatal apnea are mentioned below:

a. *Infection*: Septicemia, meningitis, pneumonia
b. *Central nervous system*: Intracranial bleed, perinatal asphyxia, seizures
c. *Respiratory*: Respiratory distress syndrome, obstructive airway disorders
d. *Metabolic*: Hypoglycemia, hypocalcemia
e. *GIT*: Necrotizing enterocolitis, gastroesophageal reflux
f. *CVS*: Patent ductus arteriosus, congestive heart failure
g. *Developmental*: Apnea of prematurity
h. *Others*: Hypothermia, hyperthermia, anemia, drug-induced depression, polycythemia.

Evaluation

Evaluation should include a thorough history and physical examination to rule out the causes outlined above, determination of blood glucose and calcium, arterial blood gases, sepsis work-up and other investigations based on probable etiology. Pulse oximetry may be helpful for measuring the severity and duration of oxygen desaturation.

Treatment	**Neonatal Apnea**

1. Gentle tactile stimulation by flicking the soles of feet or rubbing the trunk with hand may abort apneic spell.
2. Nurse the baby in prone position. This stabilizes the chest wall and may reduce apnea.
3. Avoid vigorous pharyngeal suction to prevent vagal stimulation.
4. Maintain temperature
5. Ensure normoglycemia (blood sugar >45 mg/dL and normocalcemia (serum calcium >7 mg/dL).
6. Supplemental oxygen, if there is hypoxia. Maintain oxygen saturation between 88 and 95%.
7. *Pharmacotherapy* Drugs are indicated, if apneic episodes occur more than 2 to 3 times or bag and mask ventilation is required.
    i. Methylxanthines (caffeine and aminophylline) are the mainstay of therapy for apnea of prematurity. They act by stimulating respiratory center, antagonism of adenosine

that can produce respiratory depression, and improving diaphragmatic contractility.
    • *Caffeine citrate:* The loading dose of caffeine is 20 mg/kg of caffeine citrate (10 mg/kg of caffeine base) orally or intravenously over 30 minutes, followed by maintenance dose of 5–8 mg/kg (2.5–5 mg/kg of caffeine base) once a day, beginning 24 hours after the loading dose.
    • *Aminophylline:* The dose of aminophylline is 5–6 mg/kg IV infusion over 20 minutes as loading dose followed by 1.5–2 mg/kg IV every 8 hours as maintenance therapy, beginning 12 hours after loading dose.
    • Caffeine is preferred over aminophylline as it has lesser side effects and can be administered as once daily dose.
    • Methylxanthines are discontinued at 34 to 36 weeks of gestation, if no apneic spells have occurred for 5 to 7 days.
    ii. Doxapram is central and peripheral stimulant. It is used when methylxanthines fail. Side effects, such as 'gasping syndrome', preclude its routine use.
8. Investigate and treat the underlying cause, if one is identified.
9. Packed red cell transfusion, to maintain hemoglobin >10 g/dL.
10. If baby does not respond to tactile stimulation, use bag and mask ventilation to resuscitate the baby.
11. Continuous positive airway pressure (CPAP): CPAP is useful in obstructive or mixed apnea. It splints the airway and thereby prevents obstruction. CPAP is indicated when drug therapy fails.
12. *Mechanical ventilation* Intractable apnea not responding to above measures should be managed with mechanical ventilation.
13. *Discharge* Otherwise healthy preterm neonates should be apnea-free at least for 7 days before discharge.

Abu-Shaweesh JM, Martin RJ. Neonatal apnea: what's new? *Pediatr Pulmonol*. 2008;43:937–44.
Mathew OP. Apnea of prematurity: pathogenesis and management strategies. *J Perinatol*. 2011;31:302–10.
Zhao J, Gonzalez F, Mu D. Apnea of prematurity: from cause to treatment. *Eur J Pediatr*. 2011;170:1097–105.

7.14 NEONATAL JAUNDICE

Physiological jaundice occurs in nearly two-thirds of newborns, with excellent outcome. However, in 3–5% of newborns, serum bilirubin levels can exceed physiological limits, raising concerns of brain damage.

Bilirubin Metabolism

Bilirubin is derived from the breakdown of heme proteins in the reticuloendothelial system. Three-fourths of the bilirubin come from destruction of senescent erythrocytes. The remaining 25%, known as early labeled bilirubin, is derived from hemoglobin released by ineffective erythropoiesis in bone marrow, and other heme-containing proteins in tissues such as myoglobin, cytochromes, catalase, peroxidase, and from free heme. One gram of hemoglobin gives rise to 34 mg of bilirubin. The normal term newborn produces about 6–10 mg/kg/day of bilirubin, in comparison to 3 to 4 mg/kg/day in the adult. Bilirubin metabolism is summarized as follows (also see Fig . 7.38).

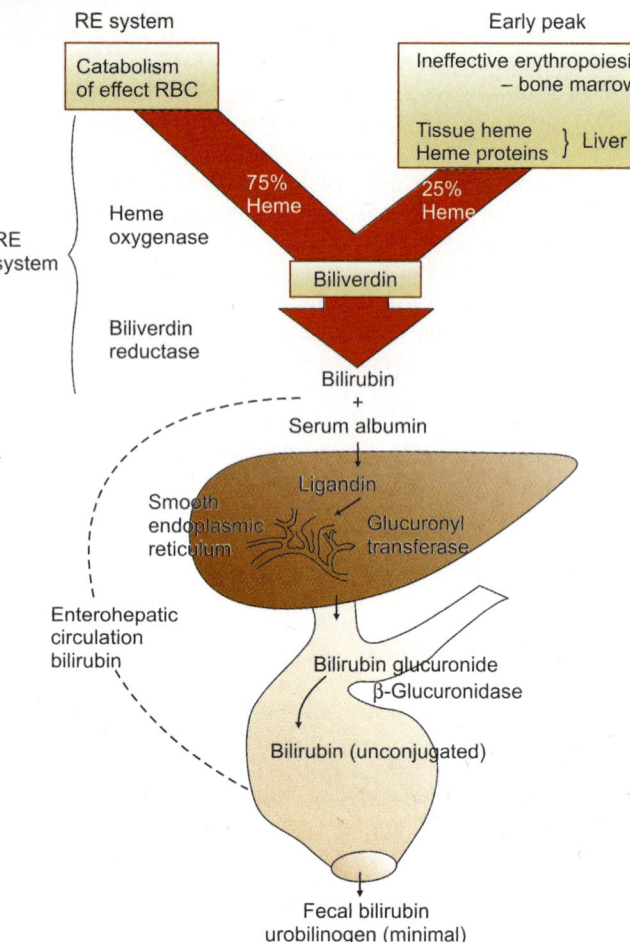

Fig. 7.38 Metabolism of bilirubin

- Bilirubin is bound to albumin for transport in the blood. This bound bilirubin does not enter the central nervous system and is nontoxic.
- Upon reaching the liver, bilirubin enters the liver cell and gets bound to ligandin which helps to transport it to smooth endoplasmic reticulum, the site of conjugation in hepatocyte.
- Uridine diphosphate glucuronyl transferase 1 A1 (UGT1A1) enzyme causes conjugation with glucuronic acid to produce mono- and di-glucuronides which are water soluble, and are excreted in bile.
- The conjugated bilirubin is transported with the bile to the gut. The sterile newborn gut contains beta-glucuronidase, an enzyme which converts bilirubin glucuronide into unconjugated bilirubin. Unconjugated bilirubin gets reabsorbed into the circulation; this is called enterohepatic circulation.
- With frequent feeding, early colonization of gut occurs. These bacteria reduce bilirubin glucuronide into stercobilinogen which is excreted in stool, thus preventing the enterohepatic circulation.

Physiological Mechanisms of Neonatal Jaundice

Neonatal jaundice occurs due to the following mechanisms:

I. *Increased bilirubin production*
- Higher erythrocyte mass

- Shorter RBC lifespan (90 days vs 120 days)
- Increased ineffective erythropoiesis
- Increased turnover of nonhemoglobin heme proteins

II. *Reduced hepatic metabolism*
- Defective uptake
- Defective conjugation

III. *Increased enterohepatic circulation* due to high levels of intestinal β-glucuronidase, paucity of intestinal bacteria, and decreased gut motility.

Clinical Assessment of Jaundice

In newborns, the jaundice is detected by blanching the skin with finger, revealing the yellow staining of skin and subcutaneous tissues. The baby should be examined preferably in daylight for better appreciation of jaundice.

Jaundice is seen first in the face at serum bilirubin levels of 5 to 6 mg/dL and then progresses in a cephalocaudal manner to the trunk and extremities. In adults, sclera appears icteric when serum bilirubin exceeds 2 mg/dL. It is difficult to detect jaundice in eyes of a newborn as unlike adults, neonates keep their eyes shut because of physiological photophobia.

Kramer described the approximate serum bilirubin level with the level of skin discoloration which can be used as a rough guide to the level of jaundice (Fig. 7.39). Once palms and soles are distinctly yellow stained, serum bilirubin exceeds 15 mg/dL. After phototherapy is started, skin gets bleached and it becomes difficult to assess jaundice clinically.

Transcutaneous Bilirubinometry

This is a noninvasive method to assess serum bilirubin levels. The device measures the intensity of yellow staining of skin and subcutaneous tissues and the value is displayed as either

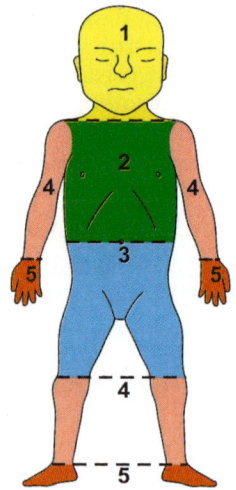

Area of body	Level	Range of bilirubin (mg/dL)
Face	1	5–6
Chest	2	6–10
Abdomen and thigh	3	10–12
Legs	4	12–15
Palms/soles	5	>15

Fig. 7.39 Cephalocaudal progression of jaundice (Kramer's rule)

transcutaneous bilirubin index or a bilirubin value which correlate reasonably well with serum bilirubin levels. There is no trauma to the baby and repeated measurements can be done. It is a good screening method.

PHYSIOLOGICAL JAUNDICE

This is defined as jaundice in healthy babies during the first a few days of life due to physiological reasons. It appears on second or third day of life, rises at a rate less than 5 mg/dL/day; peaks at 4 to 5 days of age; and spontaneously disappears by 10–14 days of life. It is always indirect reacting hyperbilirubinemia and serum bilirubin levels do not exceed 15 mg/dL. Apart from jaundice, these neonates have no other problem. Term infants with physiological jaundice do not require any treatment and outcome is excellent.

PATHOLOGICAL JAUNDICE

Neonatal jaundice is considered pathological, if it appears on day 1 of age; persists beyond 2 weeks; total serum bilirubin levels exceed 15 mg/dL or conjugated serum bilirubin is >2 mg/dL or >20% of total bilirubin; rise in serum bilirubin level is more than 0.5 mg/dL/hour; or associated with signs of illness.

Causes of Jaundice

I. Jaundice appearing within 24 hours of age
   i. Hemolytic disease of newborn: Rh, ABO and minor group incompatibility
   ii. Intrauterine infections
   iii. G6PD deficiency
   iv. Hereditary spherocytosis
   v. Crigler-Najjar syndrome
   vi. Alpha-thalassemia
II. Jaundice appearing between 24 and 72 hours of life
   i. Physiological
   ii. Septicemia
   iii. Polycythemia
   iv. *Concealed hemorrhages:* Cephalhematoma, subarachnoid bleed, intraventricular hemorrhage.
III. Jaundice appearing after 72 hours
   i. Septicemia
   ii. Idiopathic jaundice
   iii. Hypothyroidism
   iv. Metabolic disorders

Common causes of pathological jaundice in India include blood group incompatibilities, infections, idiopathic jaundice (breastmilk jaundice), G6PD deficiency, bruising, and cephalhematoma.

BREASTMILK JAUNDICE

Breastmilk jaundice is a misnomer since no factor in breastmilk has consistently been shown to be causative of jaundice in neonates and this terminology should be better avoided. It is more appropriate to term this condition as idiopathic jaundice. Labeling the condition as breastmilk jaundice may undermine the efforts to promote breastfeeding.

Diagnosis

Breastmilk jaundice is suspected in an otherwise healthy exclusively breastfed neonate whose physiological (unconjugated) jaundice fails to decline after first week of birth, and persists beyond two weeks of birth. The exact cause is not known. Male gender, East Asian ancestry, and genetic mutations are likely to play a role.

Management

Phototherapy is indicated, if serum bilirubin exceeds 20 mg/dL, and exchange transfusion, if serum bilirubin reaches 25–30 mg/dL. Some people advocate stopping breastfeeding for 48 hours, if serum bilirubin levels are approaching 25 mg/dL. Temporary interruption of breastfeeding may be followed by fall in serum bilirubin values. With re-introduction of breastmilk, there may be some rise in serum bilirubin levels but does not reach the previous high levels. However, in majority of cases the jaundice can be managed without need of stopping breastfeeding.

BILIRUBIN ENCEPHALOPATHY

Unconjugated bilirubin is neurotoxic. Conjugated bilirubin does not cause brain damage. Severe unconjugated hyperbilirubinemia can result in neuronal damage. Acute bilirubin encephalopathy refers to clinical manifestations of bilirubin toxicity in the neonatal period. The term kernicterus is reserved for the chronic and permanent sequelae of bilirubin toxicity. This condition is characterized by yellow staining of the basal ganglia and brainstem nuclei, and involves diffuse neuronal damage.

Predisposing Factors

The risk of bilirubin toxicity depends on serum bilirubin levels, gestational age, underlying cause of jaundice and other comorbid conditions. Factors predisposing to bilirubin toxicity include acidosis, birth asphyxia, hypercarbia, hypoglycemia, pyogenic meningitis, intracranial hemorrhage and drugs displacing bilirubin from albumin (eg, ceftriaxone, diazepam).

Factors other than serum bilirubin levels such as asphyxia, hypercarbia, sepsis, etc. may be involved in producing brain injury in jaundiced preterm newborns. Thus bilirubin toxicity in preterm newborns may be a function of their overall clinical status rather than serum bilirubin levels *per se.*

What is the highest bilirubin value that is safe?

There is no single value of serum bilirubin which is considered safe for all neonates. In term neonates with hemolytic disease, kernicterus rarely occurs with bilirubin levels lower than 20 mg/dL. In case of nonhemolytic jaundice, serum bilirubin levels up to 25 mg/dL are generally considered safe in otherwise healthy term newborns. However, in premature babies, brain damage may occur at lower bilirubin levels, so called "low bilirubin kernicterus".

Clinical Features

Early phase (first 1–2 days) Poor sucking, hypotonia, lethargy, high-pitched cry, loss of Moro reflex.

7

Intermediate phase (3–7 days) Hypertonia, opisthotonus, retrocollis, fever, seizures, bulging of anterior fontanel. Many babies die in this phase. Most survivors develop chronic sequelae.

Advanced phase (>1 week) Pronounced opisthotonus (hypotonia may replace hypertonia after 1 week of age), apnea, seizures, coma, and death.

Chronic phase (first year) Hypotonia, brisk tendon reflexes, delayed development

After first year Choreoathetosis, tremors, upward gaze palsy, sensorineural hearing loss, dental dysplasia, and mental retardation

Workup for Pathological Jaundice

1. *Review maternal and perinatal history* Age of onset of jaundice; any other sign of illness; color of urine and feces; previous sibling with jaundice for blood group incompatibility; maternal illness during pregnancy; traumatic delivery, delayed cord clamping, oxytocin use; birth asphyxia, delayed feeding, delay in meconium passage; feeding status of the baby; difficulty in breastfeeding.
2. *Physical examination* Excessive weight loss (>10% of body weight); signs of dehydration; bruising, cephalhematoma; prematurity; small for gestation; polycythemia; pallor: hemolysis; petechiae: sepsis, TORCH infections; hepato-splenomegaly: features of acute bilirubin encephalopathy.
3. *Laboratory tests* Total serum bilirubin; direct and indirect; blood group and Rh of mother and baby; direct Coomb's test; hematocrit; reticulocyte count; peripheral smear for RBC morphology, evidence of hemolysis; sepsis screen; thyroid profile, G6PD assay, TORCH titres, if indicated.

Prediction of Severe Hyperbilirubinemia

Predischarge serum bilirubin or transcutaneous bilirubin plotted on an hour-specific bilirubin nomogram is useful in identifying newborns at high risk for developing significant hyperbilirubinemia. Risk factors for development of severe hyperbilirubinemia in infants of 35 or more weeks' gestation can be classified as *major* or *minor*:

Major Risk Factors

- Predischarge total serum bilirubin (TSB) or transcutaneous bilirubin (TcB) level in the high-risk zone (Fig. 7.40)
- Jaundice observed in the first 24 hours
- Blood group incompatibility with positive direct antiglobulin test, other known hemolytic disease (eg, G6PD deficiency)
- Elevated end tidal carbonmonoxide content in exhaled air (ETCO$_2$)
- Gestational age 35–36 weeks
- Previous sibling received phototherapy
- Cephalohematoma or significant bruising
- Exclusive breastfeeding, particularly if nursing is not going well and weight loss is excessive.

Minor Risk Factors

- Predischarge TSB or TcB level in the high intermediate-risk zone (Fig. 7.40)
- Gestational age 37–38 weeks
- Jaundice observed before discharge
- Previous sibling with jaundice
- Macrosomic infant of a diabetic mother
- Maternal age ≥25 years
- Male gender

Decreased risk (these factors are associated with decreased risk of significant jaundice, listed in order of decreasing importance)

- TSB or TcB level in the low-risk zone (Fig. 7.40)
- Gestational age ≥41 weeks
- Discharge from hospital after 72 hours

Treatment	Hyperbilirubinemia

The aim of therapy is to maintain serum bilirubin levels within safe range and thus prevent brain damage. This is achieved by phototherapy and/or exchange transfusion. In addition, any co-

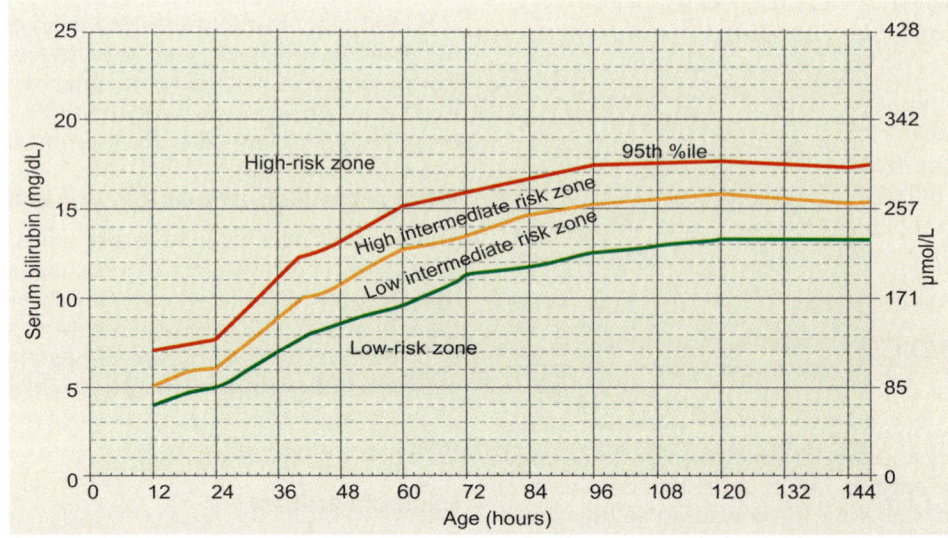

Fig. 7.40 Nomogram for designation of risk in newborns at 35 or more weeks gestational age

morbid condition or a treatable etiology needs to be specifically addressed.

Phototherapy

A. Mechanism of Action

Phototherapy converts toxic water insoluble unconjugated bilirubin to nontoxic water-soluble photoisomers which can be excreted in bile and urine without the need for hepatic conjugation. There are two types of reactions: Configurational isomerization and structural isomerization.

- In *configurational isomerization*, native isomers of bilirubin, 4Z, 15Z is converted to **4Z, 15E** isomer which can be excreted by the liver without the need for conjugation. This is a reversible reaction.
- In *structural isomerization*, the native bilirubin molecule is converted to lumirubin which can be readily excreted in bile and urine. This is an irreversible reaction. Structural isomerization mainly accounts for phototherapy-induced reduction in serum bilirubin levels.

In addition to photoisomerization reactions, photooxidation can also occur during phototherapy but it has minor contribution to the effects of phototherapy. The most effective light spectrum for phototherapy is 420–480 nm. There is no role of prophylactic phototherapy.

B. Technique of giving Phototherapy

Various phototherapy devices used include fluorescent tubes (CFL), light-emitting diodes (LED), halogen lamps and fiberoptic systems (biliblanket). Fluorescent tubes are most commonly used. These could be cool-white or special blue tube lights.

- Baby is placed under phototherapy naked except for eye patches to shield eyes from intense light. There is no need to cover the genitalia in male infants.
- The distance between the baby and phototherapy lights should be around 30 cm. Shorter distance can lead to overheating.
- Turn the baby sideways every 2–3 hours for maximal skin exposure.
- Monitor skin temperature as baby can develop hypo- or hyperthermia.
- Phototherapy is given continuously except breaks for breastfeeding.
- Offer breastfeeding frequently. Generally, there is no need to give extra fluids in breastfed babies as increasing the frequency of breastfeeding will meet the requirement.

C. Side Effects

- Increased insensible water loss can cause dehydration. Increasing the frequency of breastfeeding will take care of this problem.
- Loose green stools: No treatment is needed.
- Skin rashes: Harmless, no need to discontinue phototherapy.
- Bronze baby syndrome: Occurs, if baby has conjugated hyperbilirubinemia.
- Hypo- or hyperthermia: Monitor temperature frequently.

The guidelines for phototherapy for the management of hyperbilirubinemia in neonates more than 35 weeks are detailed in Fig. 7.41.

Exchange Transfusion

It is the most effective method to reduce serum bilirubin levels. However, the procedure has inherent risks to the baby. Complications include infection; metabolic disturbances; hypoglycemia, hypocalcemia; bleeding; necrotizing enterocolitis; volume overload; and thrombosis/embolic phenomenon.

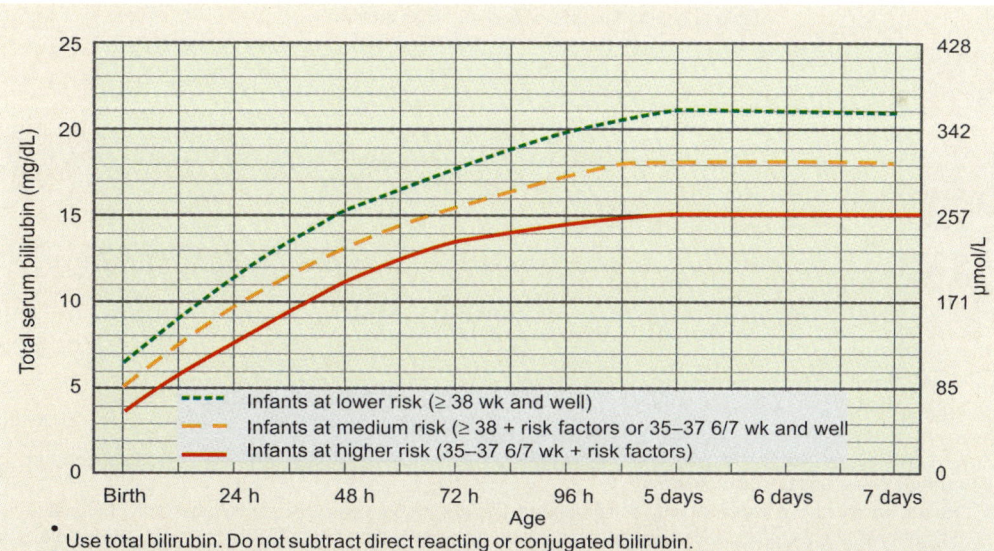

- Use total bilirubin. Do not subtract direct reacting or conjugated bilirubin.
- Risk factors = isoimmune hemolytic disease, G6PD deficiency, asphyxia, significant lethargy, temperature instability, sepsis, acidosis, or albumin < 3.0 g/dL (if measured).
- For well infants 35–37 6/7 wk can adjust TSB levels for intervention around the medium risk line. It is an option to intervene at lower TSB levels for infants closer to 35 wks and at higher TSB levels for those closer to 37 6/7 wk.
- It is an option to provide conventional phototherapy in hospital or at home at TSB levels 2–3 mg/dL (35–50 mmol/L) below those shown but home phototherapy should not be used in any infant with risk factors.

Fig. 7.41 Guidelines for phototherapy in hospitalized infants of 35 or more weeks' gestation. (Practice Guideline, American Academy of Pediatrics, 2004)

A. *Choice of Blood*
- *For ABO incompatibility*: O Rh compatible blood cross-matched against mother and infant. One may use type O packed red cells re-suspended in AB plasma to ensure that no anti-A or anti-B antibodies are present.
- *For Rh isoimmunization*: O negative blood crossmatched against mother and infant.

B. *Indications*

I. At birth
- Hydrops fetalis due to Rh hemolytic disease
- Cord blood bilirubin >4.5 mg/dL
- Cord blood hemoglobin <11 g/dL

II. After birth
- Rise in bilirubin values more than 1 mg/dL/hour despite phototherapy
- Serum bilirubin levels >20 mg/dL in hemolytic jaundice
- Serum bilirubin levels >25–30 mg/dL in non-hemolytic jaundice
- Clinical suspicion of acute bilirubin encephalopathy

C. *Mechanism*

Exchange transfusion removes bilirubin, antibodies, sensitized RBCs and corrects anemia. Normally double volume exchange transfusion is carried out (normal blood volume 80 mL/kg). This replaces 87% of infant's blood volume and serum bilirubin levels decline by 50%. The guidelines for exchange transfusion in neonates more than 35 weeks are detailed in Fig. 7.42.

Management of hyperbilirubinemia in low birth weight babies is described in **Table 7.16**.

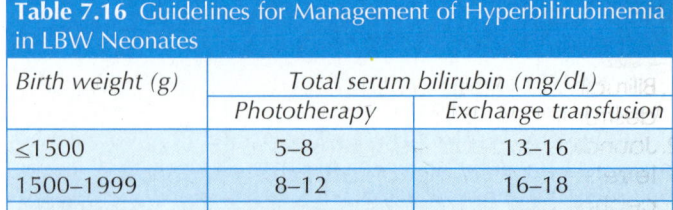

Table 7.16 Guidelines for Management of Hyperbilirubinemia in LBW Neonates

Birth weight (g)	Total serum bilirubin (mg/dL)	
	Phototherapy	Exchange transfusion
≤1500	5–8	13–16
1500–1999	8–12	16–18
2000–2499	11–14	18–20

Pharmacological Therapy for Unconjugated Hyperbilirubinemia

1. *Intravenous immunoglobulin* It is effective in preventing immune-mediated hemolysis due to Rh and ABO hemolytic disease. The dose is 0.5–1.0 g/kg intravenously over 2–4 hours. It inhibits hemolysis by blocking Fc receptors on reticuloendothelial cells, thereby preventing them from taking up and lysing antibody-coated RBCs. It has no role in nonimmune-mediated hemolysis or nonhemolytic jaundice.

2. *Metalloprotoporphyrins* Such as tin and zinc protoporphyrins can reduce bilirubin levels by inhibiting heme oxygenase, enzyme necessary for the conversion of heme to biliverdin. These agents are still experimental, and more data is needed on efficacy and safety.

3. *Inhibitors of enterohepatic circulation* These agents include charcoal, agar, and cholestyramine. The efficacy is doubtful.

4. *Phenobarbitone* It is an inducer of hepatic microsomal enzymes and increases bilirubin conjugation and excretion. However, it is not used due to its side effects and late onset of action.

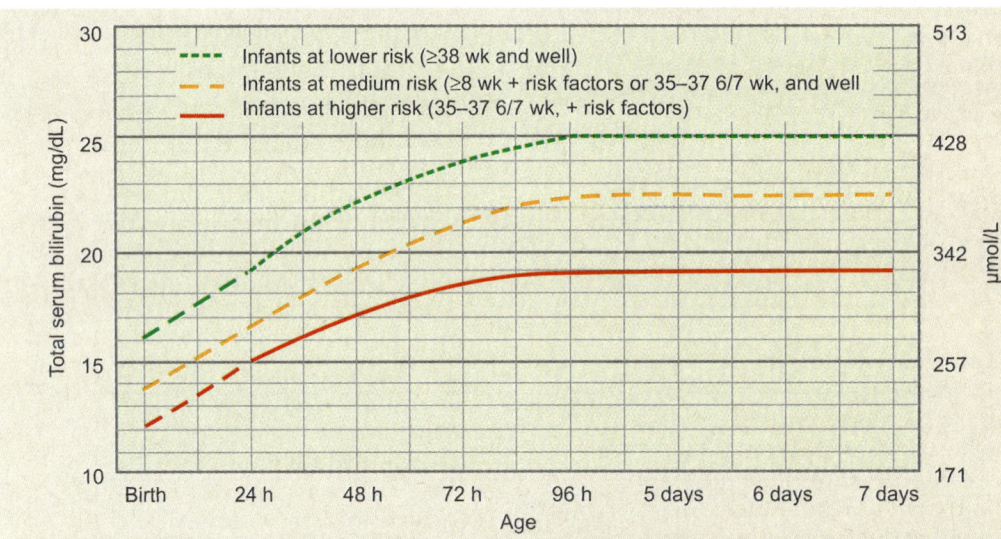

- The dashed lines for the first 24 hours indicate uncertainly due to a wide range of clinical circumstances and a range of responses to phototherapy.
- Immediate exchange transfusion is recommended, if infant shows signs of acute bilirubin encephalopathy (hypertonia, arching, retrocollis, opisthotonus, fever, high-pitched cry) or if TSB is ≥5 mg/dL (85 µmol/L) above these lines.
- Risk factors—isoimmune hemolytic disease, G6PD deficiency, asphyxia, significant lethargy, temperature instability, sepsis, acidosis.
- Measure serum albumin and calculate B/A ratio (see legend).
- Use total bilirubin. Do not subtract direct reacting or conjugated bilirubin.
- If infant is well and 35–37 6/7 wk (median risk) can individualize TSB levels for exchange based on actual gestational age.

Fig. 7.42 Guidelines for exchange transfusion in infants 35 or more weeks' gestation. (Practice Guideline, American Academy of Pediatrics, 2004)

Revision Point

Neonatal Hyperbilirubinemia

1. Bilirubin is derived from the breakdown of heme from destruction of RBCs.
2. Jaundice appears first on the face at serum bilirubin levels of 5 to 6 mg/dL and then progresses in a cephalocaudal manner to the trunk and extremities. Staining of palms and soles indicates serum bilirubin >15 mg/dL and considered a danger sign.
3. Neonatal jaundice is considered pathological, if it appears on day 1 of age; persists beyond 2 weeks; total serum bilirubin levels exceed 15 mg/dL or conjugated serum bilirubin is >2 mg/dL or >20% of total bilirubin; rise in serum bilirubin level is more than 0.5 mg/dL/hour; or associated with signs of illness.
4. Unconjugated bilirubin is neurotoxic. Severe unconjugated hyperbilirubinemia can result in neuronal damage (kernicterus/bilirubin encephalopathy). Conjugated bilirubin does not cause brain damage.
5. Phototherapy forms the backbone of effective management of unconjugated hyperbilirubinemia.

Is there any beneficial role of bilirubin?

It has been recognized that bilirubin has antioxidant properties. Newborn babies have inadequately developed antioxidant defenses. Bilirubin may serve as a transient antioxidant in the first a few days of life before antioxidant defense mechanisms mature. This may explain near universal elevation of bilirubin levels in neonate.

American Academy of Pediatrics Subcommittee on Hyperbilirubinemia. Management of hyperbilirubinemia in the newborn infant 35 or more weeks of gestation. *Pediatrics*. 2004;114:297–316.

Moerschel SK, Cianciaruso LB, Tracy LR. A practical approach to neonatal jaundice. *Am Fam Physician*. 2008;77:1255–62.

National Neonatology Forum and UNICEF. Facility based care of sick neonate ay referral health facility. *Comprehensive Newborn Care Initiative*. New Delhi:2010.

7.15 NEONATAL SEIZURES

Seizures are the most common neurological emergency in newborns with an incidence ranging from 1–5 per 1000 live births. Neonatal age is the period of highest incidence of seizures in life. Newborn babies are more prone to seizures due to immaturity of brain. Seizures are more common in preterm newborns than in term babies. Most cases of neonatal seizures are either due to underlying cerebral insult or secondary to a systemic disorder. Idiopathic seizures are rare in neonates.

Pathophysiology

Seizures occur when a large group of neurons undergo excessive, synchronized depolarization. Depolarization can result from excessive excitatory amino acid release (eg, glutamate) or deficient inhibitory neurotransmitter, e.g. gamma-aminobutyric acid (GABA). Another potential mechanism is disruption of ATP-dependent resting membrane potentials, which causes a flow of sodium into the neuron and potassium out of the neuron.

Etiology

1. *Hypoxic-ischemic encephalopathy* (HIE) is the most common cause of neonatal seizures, constituting 50–65% of all cases. Most seizures (50–65%) due to HIE start within 12 hours, remaining have an onset within 24–48 hours, and are subtle in nature. Such seizures may be severe and difficult to treat, but they tend to subside after about 5 to 7 days even without treatment.
2. *Ischemic stroke* is more likely in neonates with polycythemia or with thrombophilia due to a genetic disorder but may also occur without any risk factors. Stroke typically occurs in the middle cerebral artery distribution or watershed zones. Seizures resulting from stroke tend to be focal.
3. *Infections* such as meningitis and sepsis may cause seizures.
4. *Hypoglycemia* (blood glucose <45 mg/dL) should be suspected in neonates whose mothers have diabetes, who are small for gestational age, or who have hypoxia-ischemia or other stresses. Prolonged or recurrent hypoglycemia may cause permanent brain damage.
5. *Hypocalcemia* (serum total Ca level <7.0 mg/dL or ionic Ca level <4 mg/dL) is an important cause of seizures in newborns. It may be early onset (first 3 days of life) or late onset (after 3 days of age, usually 1 week). *Early onset hypocalcemia* is associated with prematurity and complications of birth. *Late onset hypocalcemia* is seen in neonates fed with high-phosphate milk, such as cow's milk or in very low birth weight neonates with associated metabolic bone disease of prematurity.
6. *Intracranial hemorrhage,* including subarachnoid, intracerebral, and intraventricular hemorrhage, may cause seizures. Intraventricular hemorrhage, which occurs in premature infants, results from bleeding in the germinal matrix.
7. *Hypernatremia or hyponatremia* (serum Na >150 mEq/L or <125 mEq/L) may cause seizures.
8. *Hypomagnesemia* is a rare cause of seizures, which may occur when the serum magnesium level is <1.4 mEq/L. Hypomagnesemia often occurs with hypocalcemia and should be considered in neonates with hypocalcemia, if seizures continue after adequate calcium therapy.
9. *Inborn errors of metabolism* (eg, amino or organic aciduria) can cause neonatal seizures. Rarely, pyridoxine deficiency or dependency causes seizures.
10. *Other causes* include CNS malformations, maternal substance abuse (eg, cocaine, heroin, diazepam), familial, kernicterus, etc.

Classification of Neonatal Seizures

The clinical manifestations of seizures in neonates differ from those seen in older children. Due to immaturity of brain, generalized seizures rarely occur in neonates. Relatively advanced development of limbic system may account for predominance of subtle seizures in neonates. During the neonatal period, any unusual repetitive or stereotypic movement may represent a seizure. Alterations in autonomic functions such as blood pressure or heart rate may also represent seizure activity. Apnea may also be a manifestation of seizure in neonates. Classification of neonatal seizures is summarized as follows.

1. *Subtle seizure* Most common seizure type. *Eye signs*—staring, deviation, blinking, etc. *Buccal-oral-lingual*: chewing, sucking, lip smacking; *Limbs*—cycling, swimming, rowing; *Systemic*—apnea. Heart rate may help to decide whether apnea represents a seizure phenomenon or not. In epileptic apnea, there is tachycardia, as opposed to bradycardia seen in nonepileptic apnea. It may be difficult to differentiate subtle seizures from extremes of normal behavior. Many subtle seizures are thought to arise from the basal ganglia as a result of diminished cortical inhibition. Further depression of the cortex with anticonvulsants may not alter these seizures.

2. *Clonic seizure* These consist of rhythmic movements of muscle groups in a focal distribution, which consist of a rapid flexion phase followed by a slower extensor movement. Clonic seizures may be focal or multifocal. These usually involve one limb or one side of the body jerking rhythmically at 1–4 times per second. Most common etiology is a metabolic abnormality: hypoglycemia or hypocalcemia; may be a clue to an underlying focal neuropathology, eg, hemorrhage or cerebral infarction. Prognosis is good.

3. *Tonic seizure* Sustained flexion or extension of axial or appendicular muscle groups involving limbs or trunk or deviation of the head. It may mimic decerebrate or decorticate posturing. May be focal or generalized. Background EEG patterns tend to have multifocal or generalized voltage depression. These are indicative of severe neocortical dysfunction or damage and are often difficult to treat with anticonvulsants.

4. *Myoclonic seizure* These consist of rapid, isolated jerks which can be generalized, multifocal or focal in an axial or appendicular distribution lacking the slow return phase of the clonic movement complex. EEG background activity tends to be low-voltage, slow-wave activity or a burst suppression pattern with focal sharp waves. Myoclonic seizures reflect injury at multiple levels of the neuraxis from the spinal cord, brainstem to cortical regions. These can also occur in a very severe form of encephalopathy and are associated with poor long-term outcome. Another cause is drug withdrawal (especially opiates). If it occurs during sleep, then it is probably "benign neonatal sleep myoclonus".

It is important to distinguish seizures from jitteriness. *Jitteriness* or *tremulousness* consists of symmetrical rapid movements of the hands and feet, is stimulus sensitive, and may be initiated by sudden movement or noise. It can be abolished by holding the extremity or repositioning the baby, a feature which helps differentiate it from seizures. There are no associated eye movements and EEG is normal.

Investigations

Evaluation begins with a detailed history and a physical examination.

- *Biochemical evaluation* Investigations include measurement of plasma glucose, Na, K, Cl, HCO_3, Ca, and Mg; and lumbar puncture for CSF analysis (cell count and differential, glucose, protein) and culture. The need for other metabolic tests (eg, arterial pH, blood gases, serum bilirubin, urine amino or organic acids) or tests for commonly abused drugs depends on clinical suspicion.

- *Electroencephalogram* EEG (waking and sleep) is essential, especially when it is difficult to determine whether the neonate is having seizures; EEG is also helpful for monitoring response to treatment.

- *Neuroimaging* Most infants should have a cranial CT because it can detect intracranial bleeding and some brain malformations. Cranial ultrasonography may detect intraventricular bleeding but not subarachnoid bleeding; it may be preferred as a bedside test for very sick infants who cannot be moved to radiology. Diffusion-weighted MRI may detect ischemic tissue within a few hours but is usually done after the 2nd day to look for parenchymal damage.

Treatment	Neonatal Seizures

The first step in treatment is to identify the potentially treatable cause. The steps of management are outlined below:

1. Stabilize and monitor temperature, airway, breathing, circulation, and oxygenation.

2. Identify and treat metabolic disorders. Send samples for blood sugar, calcium, and ABG immediately and proceed accordingly. If laboratory facility is not available, give a trial of dextrose and calcium empirically before starting anticonvulsants:
   - *Hypoglycemia (blood glucose <45 mg/dL)* 10% dextrose 2 mL/kg, followed by continuous infusion at the rate of 6 mg/kg/min.
   - *Hypocalcemia (serum calcium <7 mg/dL)* 10% calcium gluconate 2 mL/kg under cardiac monitoring. Add calcium gluconate in IV fluid (5–8 mL/kg/day) in documented hypocalcemia.
   - *Hypomagnesemia* 50% magnesium sulfate 0.2 mL/kg IM.

3. If seizures persist, administer phenobarbitone 20 mg/kg slow IV. Phenobarbitone can be repeated in aliquots of 5–10 mg/kg/dose every 30 minutes up to a total loading dose of 40 mg/kg, if seizures are not controlled. Maintenance dose is 5 mg/kg/day in two divided doses, beginning 24 hours later. There is a danger of respiratory depression beyond 20 mg/kg loading dose

4. If seizures persist, administer phenytoin 20 mg/kg slow IV loading dose followed by 5 mg/kg as maintenance dose, beginning 24 hours later.

5. *Lorazepam* 0.05 mg/kg IV to terminate ongoing seizures.

6. If seizures persist, a trial of pyridoxine 50–100 mg slowly may be given IV. In pyridoxine dependency/deficiency, there is a dramatic response to pyridoxine.

Duration of Antiepileptic Therapy

Unlike older children and adults, anticonvulsants are not used for a long period in neonates. Most experts suggest early termination of seizure medications, to minimize side effects and because neonatal seizures typically abate within days, independent of the therapeutic intervention, and have a low risk of early recurrence.

Monotherapy is the most appropriate strategy to control seizures. Attempts should be made to stop all anti-epileptic drugs and discharge the baby to only oral phenobarbitone at 3–5 mg/kg/day. The natural history of seizures due to various etiologies may be used to guide duration of therapy.

For seizures due to moderate hypoxic-ischemic brain injury, subarachnoid hemorrhage, or treatable and reversible metabolic disorders, medical therapy can be discontinued early, preferably within 7 days of seizure treatment or prior to discharge.

If neurological examination is persistently abnormal at discharge, AED is continued and the baby is reassessed at 1 month. If the baby is normal on examination and seizure free at 1 month, AED is discontinued over 2 weeks. If neurological assessment is not normal, or infant has a history of status epilepticus, an EEG is obtained. If EEG is not overtly paroxysmal, AED is tapered and stopped. If EEG is overtly abnormal, the infant is reassessed in the same manner at 3 months and then 3 monthly till 1 year of age.

Prognosis

The outcome depends on the underlying etiology of seizures. In late onset hypocalcemia, prognosis is excellent with normal outcome in 100% of the babies. Subarachnoid hemorrhage also carries favorable prognosis (90% normal). About 50% of neonates with seizures due to perinatal asphyxia, meningitis, hypoglycemia and early hypocalcemia develop normally. Neonatal seizures due to cerebral dysgenesis carry uniformly bad prognosis.

Neonatal Seizures

1. Common causes of neonatal seizures include HIE, ischemia, hypoglycemia, hypocalcemia, CNS infections, dyselectrolytemia, and metabolic errors.

2. Neonatal seizures are classified as subtle, clonic, tonic, or myoclonic. They may be unifocal or multifocal.

3. Phenobarbitone is the first drug of choice in treatment of neonatal seizures.

4. Early stopping (48–72 hours) of antiepileptic drug is now advised as to prevent long-term side effects.

5. Long-term prognosis of babies with neonatal seizures strongly depends on gestation age, etiology, and interictal EEG pattern.

6. Parental counseling and regular neurodevelopmental screening has to be done in babies with neonatal seizures till the age of 2 years to prevent long-term abnormal neurological outcome.

Hahn J, Olson D. Etiology of neonatal seizures. *NeoReviews.* 2004;5:327–35.
Volpe JJ. Neonatal seizures. In: *Neurology of the Newborn.* 4th ed. Philadelphia: Saunders; 2001:178–214.

7.16 BLEEDING NEWBORN

Hemostasis in the Newborn

- *Clotting factors* The concentrations of most of the clotting factors, especially vitamin K dependent factors (II, VII, IX and X) and contact factors (XI, XII, pre-kallikrein and high molecular weight kininogen) are reduced in term newborns compared to older children and adults. The levels are even lower in the premature infants. Only factors V, VIIIc and XIII are present in concentrations approaching those of adult levels. Coagulation proteins do not cross the placental barrier. Fetus starts synthesizing coagulation factors by 10 weeks of intrauterine life.

- *Platelets* Platelet numbers are similar in premature, term infants and adults, though their function may be somewhat impaired. Megakaryocytes are seen in yolk sac by 5 weeks of gestation and in liver and spleen by 10 weeks. Platelets first appear in circulation by 5 weeks.

- *Antithrombin* III, plasminogen and protein C levels are also low in the neonates, especially in the premature infants.

Causes of Neonatal Bleeding

Bleeding could result from disorders of platelets, coagulation proteins, and disruption of vascular integrity.

I. Coagulation disorders
  A. *Congenital deficiencies*
   - X-linked recessive: Hemophilia A (factor VIII) and hemophilia B (factor IX)
   - Autosomal recessive (rare): Factors V, VII, X, XI, XII, XIII, afibrinogenemia
  B. *Acquired deficiencies*
   - Vitamin K deficiency bleeding (also known as hemorrhagic disease of newborn)
   - Disseminated intravascular coagulation
   - Liver disorders

II. Platelet disorders
  A. *Thrombocytopenia* (platelet count $<150 \times 10^9/L$):
   - Decreased platelet production: Congenital infections (eg, CMV, rubella), certain syndromes (eg, thrombocytopenia absent radius, Fanconi syndrome), Wiskott-Aldrich syndrome.
   - Increased platelet consumption, eg, sepsis and disseminated intravascular coagulation, maternal autoimmune disease (eg, ITP, SLE), neonatal alloimmune thrombocytopenia, maternal thiazide intake, IUGR with toxemia of pregnancy, necrotizing enterocolitis, heparin-induced thrombocytopenia.
  B. *Impaired platelet function* is rare in the newborn except for decreased platelet adhesivenesss associated with indomethacin therapy; and von Willebrand disease.

III. Combined platelet and coagulation factor disorders
   - Disseminated intravascular coagulation (DIC)
   - Hepatic dysfunction due to shock, infection, neonatal hepatitis

IV. Disorders of vascular integrity
   - Hemangiomas or vascular malformations, which may rupture and directly bleed, or sequester platelets and secondarily cause bleeding.

Clinical Manifestations

Signs and symptoms vary with the cause of bleeding, magnitude of blood loss and the underlying disease. Signs of abnormal bleeding tendency include petechiae, excessive bruising, prolonged bleeding from puncture sites, umbilical oozing, gastrointestinal bleeding, hematuria, pulmonary hemorrhage, subgaleal hemorrhage and intracranial hemorrhage. When blood loss is large, the infant may present with signs of hypovolemia (pallor, weak pulses, tachycardia, hypotension, metabolic acidosis).

Evaluation of Bleeding Neonate

A. History

Family history of bleeding diathesis, maternal medications (aspirin, phenytoin, thiazides, hydralazine), information about pregnancy and delivery, and any illness, medication, anomalies, or procedures done to the infant.

B. Physical Examination

The clinical appearance of a bleeding neonate as 'sick looking' or 'well looking' is helpful in differential diagnosis.

- *Sick neonate* Consider infection, DIC, asphyxia, NEC, liver disease, renal vein thrombosis.
- *Well neonate* Consider vitamin K deficiency bleeding, immune thrombocytopenia, inherited clotting factor deficiencies.
- Petechiae, small ecchymosis or mucosal bleeding suggest a platelet disorder.
- Large bruises or hematomas or prolonged bleeding from venipuncure sites indicate DIC, vitamin K deficiency bleeding, liver disease or inherited clotting factor defects.
- Hepatosplenomegaly, growth restriction, microcephaly, retinal findings suggest intrauterine infection.
- Deformity and shortening of forearms suggest absence of radii—TAR syndrome.
- Hemangiomas point to Kasabach-Merritt syndrome.

C. Laboratory Tests

- *Peripheral blood smear* To find out number and size of platelets and the presence of fragmented RBCs as seen in DIC. The presence of large platelets (megathrombocytes) points to immune destruction of platelets.
- *Platelet count* Significant bleeding from thrombocytopenia is associated with platelet counts below 20000 to 30000/mm^3. Depending on platelet count, thrombocytopenia is defined as mild (100000–150000/mm^3), moderate (50000–100000 mm^3), and severe (<50000 mm^3). Depending on the age of onset, thrombocytopenia is defined as

early onset (within the first 72 hours of life) or late onset (after 72 hours of age). Approach to thrombocytopenia is depicted in Fig. 7.43 and **Table 7.17**.

- Prothrombin time (PT)
- Partial thromboplastin time (PTT)
- *Fibrin degradation products (FDP)* Elevated levels suggest disseminated intravascular coagulation.
- *D-dimer test* D-dimers are produced from the action of plasma on fibrin clot. Normal values are less than 0.5 μg/mL. Elevated levels are observed in DIC and deep vein thrombosis.
- *Apt test* Differentiates fetal blood from maternal blood. The test should be performed when a possibility of swallowed maternal blood is kept in an otherwise healthy baby with hematemesis or malena soon after birth.
- *Maternal platelet count* Low in neonatal autoimmune thrombocytopenia while it is normal in neonatal alloimmune thrombocytopenia.

VITAMIN K DEFICIENCY BLEEDING

Etiology

Vitamin K deficiency bleeding is also known as *hemorrhagic disease of the newborn*. Incidence is 1 in 200 to 400 neonates not given vitamin K prophylaxis. Vitamin K is required for the activity of clotting factors II, VII, IX and X. It acts by creating calcium-binding sites in these proteins by carboxylating glutamic acid residues. Other vitamin K dependent proteins are proteins C, S, Z and osteocalcin.

Neonates are vulnerable to vitamin K deficiency bleeding due to poor transplacental passage of vitamin K from mother to fetus and inadequate hepatic vitamin K stores. This is further aggravated by low vitamin K content of breastmilk

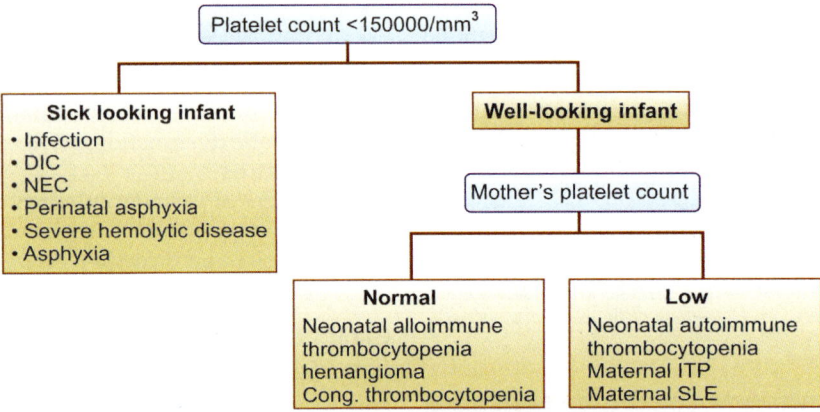

Fig. 7.43 Approach to the diagnosis of thrombocytopenia in a newborn

Table 7.17 Approach to the Diagnosis of Bleeding Neonate with Normal Platelet Count			
Condition	*Appearance*	*Prothrombin time*	*PTT*
Vitamin K deficiency bleeding	Well	↑	↑
Hemophilia	Well	N	↑
von Willebrand disorder	Well	N	N or ↑
Platelet function disorder	Well	N	N
Hepatic disease	Sick	↑	↑

and absence of bacterial flora in intestine responsible for vitamin K synthesis.

Clinical Features

Clinically, vitamin K deficiency bleeding presents as prolonged bleeding from multiple sites in an otherwise well baby. Three patterns are described:

- *Early hemorrhagic disease* It presents within first 24 hours of life. Clinical features include cephalhematoma, intracranial, intrathoracic and intra-abdominal hemorrhages. It is associated with maternal drug use, eg, warfarin, anticonvulsants, salicylates and antituberculous drugs. These drugs interfere with vitamin K stores or function.

- *Classical hemorrhagic disease* This is the most common type of vitamin K deficiency bleeding. It presents between 1 and 7 days of age, most commonly on day 2nd and 3rd day of life. Clinically, it manifests as bleeding from umbilicus and puncture sites and gastrointestinal hemorrhage (hematemesis or hematochezia/malena). Intracranial hemorrhage may also occur but is rare.

- *Late or delayed hemorrhagic disease* Manifests after 1 week of age, usually between 2 and 16 weeks of life. This is rare in infants who have received parenteral vitamin K at birth. Intracranial hemorrhage is the most dreaded complication. Predisposing factors include chronic diarrhea, cholestatic liver disease, malabsorption syndromes, cystic fibrosis, etc.

Diagnosis

Vitamin K deficiency bleeding should be suspected in a bleeding neonate who is otherwise well looking and not sick. There is prolonged bleeding from multiple sites and absence of petechial and purpuric spots in the skin.

Laboratory tests reveal a normal platelet count and prolongation of PT and PTT. Thrombin time (TT), fibrinogen and FDP levels are normal. Serum vitamin K levels are difficult to measure. However, in vitamin K deficiency, the levels of precursor proteins—PIVKA (proteins induced in vitamin K absence)—are elevated. This can be used as a sensitive indicator of vitamin K deficiency.

Treatment	Hemorrhagic Disease of Newborn

Vitamin K_1 1–5 mg slow IV stops bleeding in a few hours. If there is active bleeding, the baby should also be given 10 mL/kg of fresh frozen plasma.

Prevention

Administer 0.5 mg or 1 mg of vitamin K_1 intramuscularly to neonates weighing less than or more than 1 kg, respectively at birth to all infants. This practice has virtually eliminated the problem of hemorrhagic disease of the newborn. Intramuscular route is both safe and effective way to prevent this disorder. There is no evidence that IM vitamin K at birth is associated with increased risk of childhood malignancies, as was reported earlier. Oral vitamin K is not effective in preventing late disease.

Infants on broad-spectrum antibiotics for more than 2 weeks should receive weekly vitamin K (0.5 mg). Mothers receiving phenytoin or phenobarbitone should be given

Vitamin K_1 10 mg IM 24 hours prior to delivery to prevent early hemorrhagic disease.

DISSEMINATED INTRAVASCULAR COAGULATION (DIC)

DIC is characterized by diffuse, inappropriate activation of clotting system throughout the vascular space. Bleeding results from depletion of clotting factors and platelets. Septicemia is the most common cause. Other etiologic factors include perinatal asphyxia, hypothermia, acidosis, shock, and severe Rh hemolytic disease.

Infants with DIC are sick with multiorgan failure. Bruising, petechiae, bleeding from puncture sites, mucosal bleeding, pulmonary and gastrointestinal hemorrhages are common. Laboratory evaluation shows thrombocytopenia, and prolongation of PT and PTT. Peripheral smear shows red cell fragments. Fibrinogen levels are decreased, and fibrin degradation products or D-dimers are elevated.

Treat the underlying cause (eg, sepsis); provide fluid and ionotropic support to correct cardiovascular collapse; administer vitamin K_1, 1 mg slow IV; and consider replacement therapy with platelets, FFP, or packed RBCs, as per need. Exchange transfusion with fresh blood may be planned, if bleeding persists.

NEONATAL ALLOIMMUNE (ISOIMMUNE) THROMBOCYTOPENIA

This condition is analogous to Rh hemolytic disease. Fetal platelets possess an antigen which is lacking in mother. When these platelets cross the placenta into maternal circulation, mother develops antibodies against fetal platelets. Transplacental passage of antiplatelet IgG antibodies causes destruction of fetal/neonatal platelets. Most cases of neonatal alloimmune thrombocytopenia are caused by antibodies directed against human platelet antigen Ia (HPA-I).

Presentation Neonatal alloimmune thrombocytopenia presents as severe thrombocytopenia on day one of life. Baby's platelet count is low but maternal platelet count is normal. Neuroimaging should be done in all newborns to exclude intracranial hemorrhage.

Management consists of transfusion of compatible antigen-negative platelets and exchange transfusion to remove pathological antibody and intravenous immunoglobulin (IVIG). Recent studies show that random-donor platelets are also effective. Methylprednisolone may be useful in cases not responding to random-donor platelets and IVIG, and when antigen-negative platelets are not available.

Prevention In high-risk pregnancies (previous history of severely affected neonate), prenatal therapy includes weekly IVIG to mother with or without steroids or repeated intrauterine transfusion of compatible antigen negative platelets to the fetus. The route of delivery is determined by fetal platelet count obtained by percutaneous umbilical blood sampling. If the fetal platelet count is less than 50000/mm^3, delivery by cesarean section is recommended.

NEONATAL AUTOIMMUNE THROMBOCYTOPENIA

Clinical and laboratory features are similar to alloimmune thrombocytopenia, except that the maternal platelet count is low. Autoimmune thrombocytopenia in the neonate is usually secondary to maternal ITP or SLE. Therapeutic options include intravenous immunoglobulin and platelet transfusion.

Chalmers EA. Neonatal coagulation problems. *Arch Dis Child Fetal Neonatal Ed.* 2004;89:F475–8.

Kenet G, Chan AK, Soucie JM, et al. Bleeding disorders in neonates. *Haemophilia.* 2010;16:168–75.

Strauss T, Sidlik-Muskatel R, Kenet G. Developmental hemostasis: primary hemostasis and evaluation of platelet function in neonates. *Semin Fetal Neonatal Med.* 2011;16:301–4.

7.17 INFANT OF DIABETIC MOTHER

Diabetes has long been associated with maternal and perinatal morbidity and mortality. Approximately 6% of pregnancies are complicated by maternal diabetes mellitus (80% of which are gestational).

Fetal Effects of Maternal Hyperglycemia

Glucose and amino acids can traverse the placental membrane. On the other hand, insulin is unable to cross from maternal to fetal circulation. The fetus is subjected to high levels of glucose during times of maternal hyperglycemia. The fetus responds to hyperglycemia with pancreatic beta-cell hyperplasia and increased insulin levels. The combination of hyperglycemia and insulin, in the presence of increased fetal amino acids, increases fat and glycogen stores, resulting in increase body weight associated with hepatosplenomegaly and cardiomegaly, without an increase in head circumference (macrosomia) (Fig. 7.44).

Elevated insulin levels may inhibit the maturational effect of cortisol on the lung, including the production of surfactant from type 2 pneumocytes. This puts the fetus at risk for developing respiratory distress syndrome after birth.

Moreover, poor glycemic control during embryogenesis can result in a 4- to 8-fold increase in congenital malfor-mations, like cardiac defects, CNS defects (including anencephaly and spina bifida), genitourinary and limb defects.

Neonatal Complications

1. *Macrosomia*: Premature birth; difficult delivery; perinatal asphyxia; birth trauma.
2. *Intrauterine growth retardation:* It occurs, if maternal diabetes is complicated by microvascular disease.
3. *Metabolic*: Hypoglycemia; hypocalcemia; and hypo-magnesemia.
4. *Pulmonary*: Respiratory distress syndrome; and transient tachypnea of the newborn.
5. *Hematologic*: Polycythemia; hyperbilirubinemia; thrombocytopenia; arterial/venous thrombosis.
6. *Cardiac*: Asymmetric septal hypertrophy; cardio-myopathy.
7. *CNS*: Spina bifida, anencephaly, caudal regression syndrome.
8. *GIT*: Small left colon syndrome, duodenal or anorectal atresia.

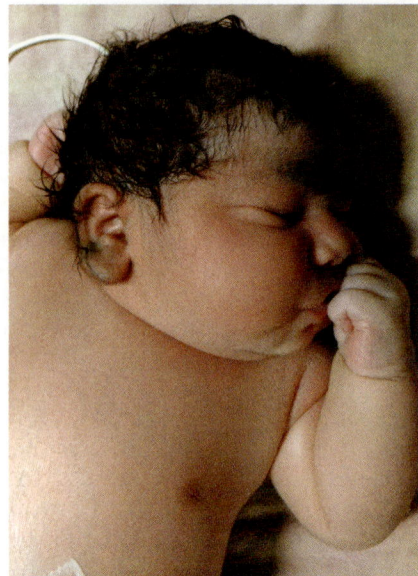

Fig. 7.44 Infant of diabetic mother. Note chubby facies and hairy pinna

9. *Renal*: Renal agenesis
10. *Others*: Poor feeding

Treatment	Infant of Diabetic Mother

A. Management at Delivery

Macrosomia leads to increased risks of shoulder dystocia, clavicular fracture, brachial plexus injury, facial nerve injury, cephalhematoma, perinatal asphyxia and neonatal mortality at delivery. Tight glucose control during pregnancy will prevent these complications.

B. Management of Hypoglycemia

Hypoglycemia is a major problem in infant of diabetic mothers (IDM). *In clinically stable newborn with normal blood glucose values (>45 mg/dL)*, start breastfeeding within ½ hour of birth and continue feeding every 2–3 hours. Screening for and treatment of hypoglycemia should be instituted early. Blood glucose levels are checked at 1, 3, 6, 12, 24, 36, and 48 hours. Hypoglycemia (blood glucose <45 mg/dL) may be symptomatic

Revision Point

Infant of Diabetic Mother (IDM)

1. Poor glycemic control in pregnancy is associated with increased risk of adverse fetal and neonatal outcomes.
2. Fetal macrosomia is associated with increased risk of perinatal asphyxia, birth trauma, neonatal hypo-glycemia, polycythemia and asymmetrical septal hypertrophy.
3. All IDMs must be carefully examined for malformations and monitored for respiratory distress, hypoglycemia, hypocalcemia and polycythemia.
4. All IDMs with respiratory distress must undergo a chest skiagram and echocardiography (to exclude cardiac malformation and asymmetric septal hypertrophy).
5. Only symptomatic IDMs need to manage in NICU, the others can be managed in a well baby area with adequate monitoring.

or asymptomatic. Depending on blood glucose levels and clinical condition of the newborn, the baby is managed as discussed in the next chapter on hypoglycemia:

All babies born to diabetic mothers should be closely observed for other problems and managed accordingly.

Hay WW Jr. Care of the Infant of the Diabetic Mother. Curr Diab Rep. 2011 Epub Nov 19.

Walsh JM, Mahony R, Byrne J, Foley M, McAuliffe FM. The association of maternal and fetal glucose homeostasis with fetal adiposity and birthweight. Eur J Obstet Gynecol Reprod Biol. 2011;159:338–41.

7.18 NEONATAL HYPOGLYCEMIA

Hypoglycemia is the most common metabolic disorder of newborn infants. Even asymptomatic hypoglycemia can cause brain damage. Anticipation, prevention, and early treatment are essential to reduce morbidity and mortality, and long-term neurodevelopmental sequelae.

Definition

Hypoglycemia is defined as a blood glucose level of less than 45 mg/dL (2.2 mmol/L) in all newborns irrespective of birth weight or gestational age.

Neonates at Risk

- Preterm and low birth weight (LBW) neonates especially those weighing less than 2.0 kg
- Post-term infants
- Infants of diabetic mother
- Any sick neonate requiring intensive care such as perinatal asphyxia, hypothermia, poor and/or delayed feeding, sepsis, shock, respiratory distress syndrome, meconium aspiration syndrome, and polycythemia. Hypoglycemia can occur any time during the course of illness.
- Infants whose mothers received treatment with beta-adrenergic drugs or oral hypoglycemic agents
- Congenital syndrome such as Beckwith-Wiedemann syndrome
- Inborn errors of metabolism

Symptoms of Hypoglycemia

Infants with low blood glucose concentrations may remain *asymptomatic*. In these at-risk infants, hypoglycemia is usually detected by routine screening of blood glucose.

In *symptomatic* infants, signs of hypoglycemia are nonspecific and reflect responses of the nervous system to glucose deprivation. The common symptoms include the following: Jitteriness or irritability; lethargy, limpness; weak- or high-pitched cry; poor feeding, vomiting; hypothermia; poor respiratory effort or apnea, tachypnea; dusky color or cyanosis; seizures, and coma.

Screening for Hypoglycemia

Capillary blood glucose can be estimated at bedside by a glucometer as a point of care screening. However, it should be remembered that glucometers are not sensitive to detect very low glucose concentrations. In cases of very low glucose concentrations, laboratory confirmation is necessary. Newborns at risk of hypoglycemia should be screened at 2 h, 6 h, 12 h, 24 h, 36 h, 48 h and, if indicated at 72 h of age.

Asymptomatic hypoglycemia and blood glucose concentration between 25–45 mg/dL.

Give a breastfeed and repeat blood glucose after 1 hour.

Symptomatic neonate or blood glucose is <25 mg/dL

Establish an IV line and give a bolus of 2 mL/kg body weight of 10% glucose IV slowly over 1 minute.

- Start infusion of dextrose-containing fluid at the daily maintenance volume according to the neonate's age to provide a glucose infusion rate (GIR) of 6 mg/kg/min.
- Check blood glucose 30 minutes after starting the infusion of glucose or any change in GIR.
- If the blood glucose remains below 45 mg/dL, GIR is increased in steps of 2 mg/kg/min to a maximum of 12 mg/kg/min.
- If hypoglycemia continues even after reaching a GIR of 12 mg/kg/min, start hydrocortisone 5 mg/kg/day IV in two divided doses for 24 to 48 hours.
- Once the blood glucose levels remain above 45 mg/dL for over 24 hours, begin tapering GIR in steps of 2 mg/kg/min every 6 hours ensuring blood glucose levels above 45 mg/dL before changing GIR. If blood sugar drops below 45 mg/dl any time, go back to the previous GIR.
- Begin breastfeeding. If the baby cannot be breastfed, give expressed breastmilk using katori spoon and/or paladai.
- As the baby's ability to feed improves, slowly decrease (over a 2–3 day period) the volume of IV fluids while increasing the volume of oral feeds. Do not discontinue the glucose infusion abruptly to prevent rebound hypoglycemia.

Refractory Hypoglycemia

It is defined as failure to maintain normal blood sugar levels despite a glucose infusion of 12 mg/kg/min or when stabilization is not achieved by 7 days of therapy. Important causes are as follows:

1. *Endocrine disorders* Congenital hypopituitarism, adrenal insufficiency, hypothyroidism, hypothalamic deficiency, glucagon deficiency, epinephrine deficiency.
2. *Hyperinsulinemic states* They are islet cell hyperplasia, hyperfunction, focal/diffuse hyperinsulinism, Beckwith-Wiedemann syndrome, and insulin-producing tumors.

Revision Point

Neonatal Hypoglycemia

1. Hypoglycemia in newborns is defined as blood glucose <45 mg/dL.
2. Preterm, IUGR, LBW babies, infants of diabetic mother; and neonates with sepsis, asphyxia, hypothermia, RDS are predisposed to hypoglycemia.
3. Asymptomatic hypoglycemic infants can be given a breastfeed and reassessed after 1 hour.
4. Symptomatic infants or those with blood glucose <25 mg/dL should be administered glucose infusion @ 6 mg/kg/min, which can be gradually increased to 12 mg/kg/min. if still no response, steroids may be tried.
5. Prolonged neonatal hypoglycemia can lead to permanent brain damage.

3. *Inborn errors of metabolism*
   a. Defects in carbohydrate metabolism, eg, fructose intolerance, galactosemia, glycogen storage disorders
   b. Defects in amino acid metabolism, eg, maple syrup urine disease
   c. Mitochondrial disorders
   d. Fatty acid oxidation defect

Adamkin DH, Polin R. Neonatal hypoglycemia: is 60 the new 40? The questions remain the same. *J Perinatol.* 2016;36:10–2.

Arsenault D, Brenn M, Kim S, *et al.* American Society for Parenteral and Enteral Nutrition Board of Directors. Clinical Guidelines: hyperglycemia and hypoglycemia in the neonate receiving parenteral nutrition. *JPEN J Parenter Enteral Nutr.* 2012;36:81–95.

Gregory KE. New approaches to care of the infant with hypoglycemia. *J Perinat Neonatal Nurs.* 2016;34:284–7.

Hawdon JM. Best practice guidelines: Neonatal hypoglycaemia. *Early Hum Dev.* 2010;86:261.

Thompson-Branch A, Havranek T. Neonatal hypoglycemia. *Pediatr Rev.* 2017;38:147–57.

7.19 NEONATAL HYPOCALCEMIA

Hypocalcemia is defined as total serum calcium <7 mg/dL (1.75 mmol/L) or ionized fraction <4 mg/dL (1 mmol/L).

Classification

Neonatal hypocalcemia is classified as *early-onset* and *late-onset* depending on the age of manifestation. Common causes of hypocalcemia are summarized in **Table 7.18**.

- Early-onset hypocalcemia is defined as hypocalcemia occurring *within first three days* after birth.
- Late-onset hypocalcemia develops *after third day of life*, usually manifested at the end of the first week.

Clinical Features

Most infants with early-onset hypocalcemia are asymptomatic and are identified by routine screening. Infants with late-onset hypocalcemia usually present with signs of hypocalcemia including severe neuromuscular irritability, jitteriness, or seizures. Seizures may be multifocal or focal clonic in nature. These neonates can rarely present with laryngospasm, bronchospasm, or pylorospasm.

Table 7.18 Causes of Hypocalcemia in Neonates
A. Early hypocalcemia
1. Preterm and intrauterine growth restriction (IUGR)
2. Infants of diabetic mother (IDM)
3. Perinatal asphyxia
4. Hypoparathyroidism
5. Maternal hyperparathyroidism
6. CATCH-22 and DiGeorge syndrome
7. Hypomagnesemia
B. Late hypocalcemia
1. Excess phosphate intake by feeding with cow's milk or cow's milk-based formula
2. Bicarbonate or lipid infusion
3. Phototherapy
4. Acute kidney injury
5. Maternal vitamin D deficiency

Treatment	**Neonatal Hypocalcemia**

Asymptomatic hypocalcemia

Most infants with early-onset hypocalcemia recover with nutritional support alone. Adequate calcium intake should be ensured by initiating early feedings. For neonates on parenteral nutrition, calcium is supplemented as 50 mg/kg/day of elemental calcium (10% calcium gluconate solution) given as a continuous infusion.

Symptomatic hypocalcemia

Most infants with late-onset hypocalcemia are symptomatic and require treatment with 10% calcium gluconate 1–2 mL/kg intravenously. The solution is diluted with equal amount of 5% dextrose and infused slowly over 5 to 10 minutes strictly under heart rate monitoring. Infusion should be stopped at earliest sign of bradycardia. The dose can be repeated in 10 minutes, if no response occurs. After acute therapy, maintenance calcium should be started. Infusion sites are monitored regularly for any extravasation which may result in necrosis and subcutaneous calcifications. After initial management, treatment should be directed against the underlying disease causing hypocalcemia.

Revision Point

Neonatal Hypocalcemia

1. Neonatal hypocalcemia is defined as total serum calcium <7 mg/dL or ionized fraction <4 mg/dL (1 mmol/L).
2. Hypocalcemia is early-onset (0–3 d of life) or late-onset (after 3d).
3. Most children are asymptomatic. Multifocal clonic seizure is the most important clinical manifestation.
4. Hypocalcemia should be treated with parenteral calcium gluconate infusion.

Cho WI, Yu HW, Chung HR, Shin CH, Yang SW, *et al.* Clinical and laboratory characteristics of neonatal hypocalcemia. *Ann Pediatr Endocrinol Metab.* 2015;20:86–91.

Jain A, Agarwal R, Sankar MJ, Deorari A, Paul VK. Hypocalcemia in the newborn. *Indian J Pediatr.* 2010;77:1123–8.

Levy-Shraga Y, Dallalzadeh K, Stern K, *et al.* The many etiologies of neonatal hypocalcemic seizures. *Pediatr Emerg Care.* 2015;31:197–201.

Thomas TC, Smith JM, White PC, Adhikari S. Transient neonatal hypocalcemia: presentation and outcomes. *Pediatrics.* 2012;129:e1461–7.

7.20 NEONATAL SHOCK

Shock or circulatory failure in neonates is defined as a dynamic and unstable pathophysiological state characterized by inadequate tissue perfusion leading to tissue hypoxia. It is manifested by features of tissue hypoperfusion, hypotension, and metabolic acidosis.

Shock and hypotension are not synonymous as hypotension is a late feature of neonatal shock. Shock is often reversible initially, but if it is not recognized and treated immediately, prolonged hypoxemia leads to irreversible end-organ dysfunction and finally death.

Blood Pressure in Neonates

It is difficult to assess blood pressure in neonates. Non-invasive blood pressure monitors are commonly used to determine systolic, diastolic and mean arterial pressure (diastolic pressure + 1/3rd pulse pressure). There is a wide variability in normal blood pressure values in neonates, particularly in extremely preterm newborns. Mean arterial pressure depends on gestational age at birth as well as postnatal age. Moreover, there is no standard definition of hypotension in neonates. As a rough estimate for initial few days after birth, mean arterial pressure corresponds to the gestational weeks at birth.

Etiology

Neonatal shock can be classified as hypovolemic, distributive, cardiogenic, and obstructive shock. Most of the time, circulatory failure in neonatal shock occurs secondary to the combination of more than one factor as listed above.

Hypovolemic shock It occurs due to insufficient circulating blood volume most commonly due to hemorrhage. Common causes of hypovolemic shock include: Fetomaternal hemorrhage, twin-to-twin transfusion, acute hemorrhage from umbilical cord rupture (vasa previa, velamentous cord), slippage of umbilical cord ligature, massive internal bleeding, eg, subgaleal hematoma, gastrointestinal bleeding, intracranial bleeding or pulmonary hemorrhage, or third space fluid loss in volvulus, necrotizing enterocolitis, intestinal perforation, etc.

Distributive shock It occurs in cases with severe reduction of systemic vascular resistance due to impairment of vascular tone leading to a maldistribution of blood flow within the microcirculation resulting in tissue hypoperfusion. Common causes of neonatal distributive shock are extremely prematurity, sepsis, and adrenal insufficiency.

Cardiogenic shock It occurs due to cardiac dysfunction causing a decrease in cardiac output and inadequate pulmonary blood flow. Common causes of neonatal cardiogenic shock include:
- *Myocardial injury and dysfunction* Perinatal asphyxia, severe sepsis, and chronic fetal hypoxemia.
- *Congenital heart disease* Hypoplastic left heart syndrome, critical aortic valve stenosis, coarctation of the aorta, interrupted aortic arch, total anomalous pulmonary venous connection.
- *Cardiac arrhythmias* Complete congenital heart block due to maternal SLE, supraventricular or ventricular tachycardia, myocarditis, congenital cardiomyopathy.

Obstructive shock This is a rare cause of circulatory failure in neonates and occurs when extracardiac diseases lead to decreased cardiac output. Common causes of neonatal obstructive shock include: Severe pulmonary hypertension, pulmonary embolism, tension pneumothorax, and pericardial tamponade.

Clinical Manifestations

Clinical presentations of neonatal shock include:
- Signs of poor peripheral perfusion—cool extremities, acrocyanosis, pallor, mottling
- Tachycardia
- Delayed capillary refill time >3 seconds
- *Hypotension*—Hypotension is generally a late feature of neonatal shock.

- Metabolic acidosis with elevated levels of lactate
- Features of end-organ changes in the brain, kidney, respiratory, and gastrointestinal system.

Laboratory Investigations

The common laboratory features characteristic of neonatal shock are as follows:
- Metabolic acidosis with a decrease in serum bicarbonate levels and an increase in lactate levels
- Anemia in hemorrhagic hypovolemic shock or secondary to sepsis
- Prolonged prothrombin time, INR and partial thromboplastin time and decreased platelets. Decreased platelets in association with tests can occur with consumptive coagulopathy
- Hypoglycemia
- Increased blood urea and serum creatinine levels
- Hyperkalemia
- Increased serum bilirubin levels and elevated liver enzymes.

Treatment	Neonatal Shock

1. **Initial stabilization** Temperature maintenance, assessment and stabilization of the airway and respiration, including administration of supplemental oxygen and/or respiratory support including mechanical ventilation.
2. **Fluid therapy** Secure vascular access should be established as early as possible with necessary blood sampling for diagnostic evaluation and fluid resuscitation. Initial fluid resuscitation is done with normal saline bolus of 10 mL/kg over 20 minutes, which can be repeated only after reevaluation. Excessive fluid administration in preterm infants is associated with an increased risk of intraventricular hemorrhage, opening of ductus arteriosus, and bronchopulmonary dysplasia.
3. **Vasopressors** These are recommended in distributive shock after initial fluid resuscitation, and in cardiogenic shock with myocardial depression. Commonly used vasoactive agents include dopamine (first-line), dobutamine (second-line), and epinephrine. Dobutamine can be used as a first-line agent in neonates with cardiogenic shock. Epinephrine is added as the third-line agent. To begin with, dopamine and dobutamine are started at a rate of 10 µg/kg/min and gradually stepped up to 15–20 µg/kg/min depending on clinical response. Epinephrine is started at a rate of 0.1 µg/kg/min and increased up to a maximum of 1 µg/kg/min.
4. **Hydrocortisone** For all neonates with septic shock or preterm neonates with vasomotor instability, hydrocortisone can be added at a dose of 1 mg/kg eight hourly till the condition stabilizes.
5. Appropriate **antibiotics** should be added in neonates with sepsis along with other supportive management.

Bhat BV, Plakkal N. Management of shock in neonates. *Indian J Pediatr.* 2015;82(10):923–9.

Gupta S, Donn SM. Neonatal hypotension: dopamine or dobutamine? Semin Fetal Neonatal Med. 2014;19:54–9.

Ibrahim CP. Hypotension in preterm infants. *Indian Pediatr.* 2008;45:285–94.

Seri I. Inotrope, lusitrope, and pressor use in neonates. *J Perinatol.* 2005;25Suppl 2:S28–30.

7.21 CONGENITAL MALFORMATIONS

The term 'congenital malformations' is used to describe developmental defects that are present at birth. Approximately 3% of all live births have a detectable malformation and 15–20% of stillborn babies have a major malformation. The causes of congenital malformations may be genetic or environmental. However, many common congenital malformations are caused by the interaction of genetic and environmental factors (multifactorial inheritance), and in a substantial proportion, no cause can be identified.

Classification

Congenital malformations can be classified based on their severity, ie, their medical or social consequences, their pathogenesis or clinical presentation, ie, whether they involve single or multiple systems.

A. Classification based on Severity

1. *Major Malformations*

These are congenital malformations that have medical or social consequences for the affected child. About 2–3% of children are born with a major malformation that is evident at birth, such as cleft lip and palate, neural tube defects and anorectal malformations. A similar number of children are born with a major malformation that only becomes evident later in life, such as atrial septal defect, polymicrogyria or hemivertebrae.

2. *Minor Malformations*

Congenital malformations that have no significant health or social implications for the affected child are called 'minor malformations'. Congenital malformations classified as minor, represent distinct departures from normal development, occurring in 4% or less of the population. Examples include up- or downslanting palpebral fissures, high-arched or narrow palate, single palmar crease, etc. Their importance lies in the fact that infants with one or more minor malformations may also have a major malformation. Multiple minor malformations can provide clues to the diagnosis of multiple congenital malformation syndromes and they may also be a marker for a chromosomal aberration.

3. *Common Variants*

These are structural/anatomical changes that represent one end of the spectrum of normal development rather than congenital malformations. They are also called 'phenotypic variants'. They are seen in more than 4% of the population and like minor malformations they can serve as indicators of altered morphogenesis and clues to patterns of malformation. Examples include broad forehead, Brushfield spots, bulbous nasal tip, smooth philtrum, absent ear lobules, sacral dimple, and sandal gap.

B. Classification based on Pathogenesis

1. *Deformation*

This describes a congenital malformation that results from an aberrant mechanical force distorting normally developing structures. The defect can be an abnormality of form, shape or position of part of the body. Deformations result in loss of body symmetry. The mechanical forces responsible are usually external (eg, constraint within an unusual shaped uterus or uterine fibroid compressing the growing fetus), but they are occasionally internal (eg, in the case of fetal edema). Deformations occur in approximately 2% of newborns and include talipes deformities, plagiocephaly and developmental dysplasia of the hip.

2. *Disruption*

These are congenital malformations that result from destructive processes that alter a structure after it has formed normally. They can lead to loss or division of body parts, abnormal fusion of body parts, or alterations in shape. For example, an amniotic band following amnion rupture may cut across the scalp, face or digits of the fetus, penetrating the skin, soft tissue and bone.

3. *Malformation*

Congenital malformations that result from failure or inadequate completion of normal developmental processes are called 'malformations'. Such intrinsic anomalies may be limited to a single anatomic region, involve an entire organ system, or produce a malformation syndrome affecting a number of different body systems.

4. *Dysplasia*

This term refers to abnormal cellular organization or function within a specific tissue type throughout the body, resulting in apparent structural changes. Dysplasias can be thought of as disorders of histogenesis. Examples include metabolic disorders such as the storage diseases, the skeletal dysplasias, the ectodermal dysplasias and tissue hamartoma.

C. Classification based on Clinical Presentation

Congenital malformations can also be classified depending on whether they involve single or multiple systems and the relationship between the components of multiple-system defects.

1. *Syndrome*

This term is derived from Greek, literally meaning 'running together'. Syndrome refers to a constellation of congenital malformations that consistently occur together and usually have a common specific etiology, eg, Down syndrome, Turner syndrome, Apert syndrome, Noonan syndrome.

2. *Association*

Multiple congenital abnormalities that are associated in a non-random fashion but in which the link among the various component abnormalities is not strong enough or consistent enough to justify definition as a syndrome are termed 'associations'. In addition, the component abnormalities of associations have no common specific etiology, eg, VATER/VACTERL association.

3. *Sequence*

A pattern of multiple malformations that can be shown on developmental and embryologic grounds to be the result of a cascade of seemingly unrelated consequences, proceeding from one primary defect is called a 'sequence', eg, Potter sequence, Pierre-Robin sequence.

4. Complex

This is an infrequently used term that implies the existence of several 'developmental fields' in the embryo. A developmental field is a part of the embryo in which the developmental processes were controlled and coordinated in a spatially ordered, temporally synchronized and epimorphically hierarchical manner. Any deleterious influence that acts on a developmental field can cause abnormalities in adjacent structures that might be of different embryologic origins but share the same geographic location at a particular point during development. Examples include hemifacial microsomia, holoprosencephaly with cyclopia, Poland anomaly, etc.

Genetic Causes of Congenital Malformations

It has been estimated that genetic factors account for about 25% of all congenital malformations, and nearly 85% of all those with a known cause. Genetic causes of congenital malformation include chromosomal aberrations, mutations in single genes (single gene defects) and the interaction of both environmental and genetic factors (multifactorial disorders). Synergistic interaction of environmental factors with particular variations (polymorphisms) in single genes is increasingly being reported in the causation of single congenital malformation such as cleft lip and palate.

Multifactorial Inheritance

Many common congenital malformations such as neural tube defects, cleft lip and/or palate, ventricular septal defect, congenital hypertrophic pyloric stenosis, hypospadias and congenital talipes have a familial distribution consistent with multifactorial inheritance. The recurrence risks used for genetic counseling of families with multifactorial congenital malformations are determined empirically and are based on the frequency of the congenital malformations in the general population, the genetic distance of the person seeking genetic advice from the affected individual (ie, first, second- or third-degree relative), and the severity of the malformation in the affected individual.

Environmental Causes of Congenital Malformations

Environmental factors can be wholly or partially responsible for some congenital malformations. These factors may be inherent in the maternal environment (eg, acetylcholine receptor antibodies in a mother with myasthenia giving rise to congenital contractures in the fetus), or may be extraneous agents such as drugs taken by the mother or maternal infections in the early antenatal period. Environmental factors are responsible for approximately 10% of congenital malformations.

Any agent or factor to which *in utero* fetal exposure produces a permanent alteration in the form or function of the offspring is thought to be a teratogen. The effects of a teratogen are dependent on several different factors such as timing of exposure in relation to the stage of development and its dose. Teratogens produce their effects by causing cell death, by altering tissue growth and by interfering with cellular differentiation.

A. Drugs/Medications

Exposure of the developing embryo to drugs can result in a variety of congenital malformations. Teratogenic drugs include alcohol, many anticonvulsant agents such as phenytoin, sodium valproate and carbamazepine, lithium, which is used in the treatment of bipolar disorder, vitamin A and its analogues such as etretinate, angiotensin-converting enzyme inhibitors such as captopril and enalapril, the antithyroid agent carbimazole and thalidomide, which is undergoing resurgence in its clinical applications.

B. Maternal Disorders

Some maternal medical conditions can result in congenital malformations in the baby, if poorly controlled prior to conception. Examples include maternal diabetes mellitus and maternal phenylketonuria. Maternal hyperthermia in the antenatal period may also be associated with an increased incidence of congenital malformations in the baby.

C. Physical Agents

The importance of antenatal exposure to physical agents such as X-rays and other ionizing radiation as a cause of congenital malformations is unclear. The effects of antenatal exposure to ionizing radiation depend on the gestational age at exposure and the dose of radiation absorbed by the fetus. The developing embryo appears to be very sensitive to the teratogenic effects of ionizing radiation from the end of the second week to the eighth week post-conception. The developing brain is also sensitive to radiation exposure between the 8th and 15th weeks of gestation. Several studies have shown that antenatal exposure to high doses of ionizing radiation (more than 1.0 gray) can be associated with microcephaly and reduced growth of fetal organs.

Diagnostic radiological procedures in pregnant women associated with exposure to less than 0.05 gray of radiation are not thought to be associated with an increased risk of congenital malformations or growth retardation in their babies.

Brent RL. Environmental causes of human congenital malformations: the pediatrician's role in dealing with these complex clinical problems caused by a multiplicity of environmental and genetic factors. *Pediatrics*. 2004;113:957-68.

Falk MJ, Robin NH. The primary care physician's approach to congenital anomalies. Prim Care. 2004;31:605–19

Hennekam RC. A newborn with unusual morphology: some practical aspects. *Semin Fetal Neonatal Med*. 2011;16:109–13.

7.22 TRANSPORT OF A SICK NEWBORN

Transporting a sick neonate to a health care facility is a difficult task in India due to limitations such as lack of well-organized transport services, long geographical distances, and virtual lack of linkage between peripheral and tertiary level hospitals. The problem is further compounded by poor infrastructure, and poverty and ignorance of parents.

During transport, a baby struggles not only with illness and physiological immaturity but also with other factors such as noise, vibrations, sudden jerks, and temperature variation which can further compromise the already sick baby. As a consequence, large number of newborns die en route while being transported to the health care facility.

If the birth of a high-risk neonate is anticipated, it is far better to safely transport the baby *in utero* rather than shift a sick baby to a hospital after birth under hostile conditions. Nevertheless, if transport of a sick baby becomes necessary, it is important to understand the principles of neonatal transport and practical issues involved to optimize the outcome.

Neonatal transport encompasses not only transfer from community to the health care facility, but also transfer between two hospitals, or transport even within the different sectors of the same hospital such as radiology and pediatric surgery services. Transport also includes transfer of a baby back to community hospital or home from higher health care facility. The rules and requirements of transport remain the same regardless of the level of transport.

Principles of Safe and Stable Transport

A. Prepare Well before Transport

1. *Assess* Carefully assess the condition of the baby before transport. Transport only if there is a definite indication. Referring a newborn for a minor problem unnecessarily stresses the baby and the parents and brings bad name to the doctor.

2. *Communicate* Explain to parents the condition of the baby and the reasons for referral well before taking the decision to transport. Give them enough time to organize and arrange for the journey. It should not come as a surprise to parents to immediately shift the sick baby to a hospital. Tell them where to go and whom to contact in the hospital. If possible, the institution/facility where the referral is being made should also be informed telephonically beforehand, so that they are also well prepared to receive the baby.

3. *Correct hypothermia before transport* Other than the illness itself, hypothermia is a major killer of babies during transport. Therefore, correction and prevention of hypothermia is crucial for the well-being of the baby. If the baby is hypothermic (temperature <36.5°C), normalize the temperature before transport. Take measures to keep baby warm during transport as mentioned below.

4. *Stabilize the baby before transport*
   a. Clear the airway of secretions
   b. Resuscitate and oxygenate, if required
   c. Give a feed, if the baby is able to suckle
   d. Put an IV line and start 10% dextrose or maintenance IV fluid with Isolyte P, if indicated. Secure IV cannula properly.
   e. Give medications including antibiotics, if indicated
   f. Administer injection vitamin K, if not given before
   g. Make sure that neck is not flexed during transport

5. *Documentation* A proper referral note should be written which includes relevant history including maternal and birth details, present condition of the baby, need for referral and treatment given along with dosage, and reports of investigations, X-rays, etc. If the baby is having severe jaundice, or jaundice appeared on day 1 of life,

send 2 to 3 mL of maternal blood in double oxalate vial for further work up and management.

6. *Encourage mother to accompany the baby* As far as possible, mother should accompany the baby for breastfeeding, providing KMC and other supportive care to the baby on the way. If it is not possible for mother to accompany the baby, father or some other close relative should go with the baby.

7. *Arrange for trained health care provider to accompany on the way* A doctor/nurse/trained dai/health worker should accompany the baby to provide care to the baby during transport.

8. *Provide bag and mask, mucus extractor, and portable O_2 cylinder.*

B. Care during Transport

The accompanying person should be explained to ensure the following:

1. *Ensure warm feet and warm transport* During transport, baby is likely to become hypothermic due to cold environment and air turbulence. Maintaining thermal stability is crucial for baby's survival. Baby's hands and feet should remain warm to touch during transport. If the baby passes urine or stool, wipe her promptly and remove the wet linen. During transportation, warmth can be ensured by following:
   - *Skin to skin care* (kangaroo mother care) This is the most effective, safe and convenient method to maintain temperature during transport.
   - *Covering the baby* Cover the baby fully with clothes (or cotton) including the head and the limbs. Nurse the baby next to the mother or another adult during transport.
   - *Improvised containers* Different workers have used thermocol box, basket, padded pouch, plastic covering, etc. for ensuring temperature stability during transport. The ideal mode of transport is transport incubator but this is rarely available. The use of rubber hot water bottle is fraught with considerable danger due to accidental burns to the baby, if the bottle is not wrapped properly or remains in contact with baby's body. It is, therefore, best avoided. But if no other means of providing warmth is available, this method may be employed, making sure that the hot water bottle is wrapped in 4-layered clothing.

2. *Ensure an open airway*
   - Keep the neck of the baby in slight extension
   - Do not cover the baby's mouth and nose
   - Gently wipe the secretions from the nose and the mouth with a cotton or cloth covered finger.
   - Attendants can be trained to use mucus extractor to remove secretions from mouth.

3. *Check breathing* Watch baby's breathing. If the baby stops breathing, provide tactile stimulation by rubbing the back or flicking the soles. Accompanying health worker can use bag and mask ventilation in the event of apnea not responding to tactile stimulation.

4. *Provide feeds* If baby is in a position to suckle on the breast, she should be offered breastfeeds. If she can take cup-

Revision Point

Transport of Neonates

1. Infants requiring advance medical and/or nursing care exceeding what is available in their current settings will need transfer to a higher health facility.
2. Prior stabilization and adequate care during transport is essential to avoid hypoglycemia, acidosis and mortality.
3. Neonatal transport programs require appropriate referral systems, management structures and trained transport personnel.
4. The key components of neonatal transport are human resources, vehicles and equipment, communication, family support and documentation.

feeding, expressed breastmilk can be provided carefully. If the distance is long, a nasogastric catheter may be inserted and gavage feeding given. In that case, the amount and interval of feed should be specified. If the baby is on IV fluids, the measured volume set should contain no more fluid than is needed for the duration of journey.

In recent years, although neonatal care has improved in many government and private hospitals, neonatal transport has not kept pace with it. There is an urgent need to improve the neonatal transport facilities in the country to optimize the outcome of these newborns.

Harrison C, McKechnie L. How comfortable is neonatal transport? *Acta Paediatr.* 2011. Epub Sep 13.

Kempley S. Neonatal transport-where next? *Early Hum Dev.* 2009;85:475.

National Neonatology Forum and UNICEF. Facility based care of sick neonate ay referral health facility. *Comprehensive Newborn Care Initiative.* New Delhi; 2010.

7.23 FOLLOW-UP OF HIGH-RISK NEONATES

With the improvement in the quality of neonatal care in India, more and more sick neonates including extremely low birth weight (ELBW) ones are surviving today. Unfortunately, the incidence of long-term morbidities and adverse outcome such as blindness, deafness, cognitive and learning disabilities, and behavioral problems still continues to be high in the survivors. Timely and appropriate intervention are, therefore, of utmost importance to prevent or modify most of these disabilities. All neonatal health care facilities should have a structured follow-up program involving a multidisciplinary team.

Objectives

The objective of follow-up is to provide a continuum of specialized care to high-risk neonates (**Table 7.19**) and to identify early deviation of growth, development, or behavior from normal and provide support and interventions as indicated. Prior to discharge, a detailed medical and neurological assessment, neurosonogram, and screening for retinopathy of prematurity (ROP) and hearing loss should be initiated. A psychosocial assessment of the family should also be done. The neonate "at-risk" of neurodevelopmental disability must be identified before discharge from birth admission.

Table 7.19 High-risk Neonates Who Need Regular Follow-up

- Very low birth weight (<1500 g)
- Gestational age at birth <32 weeks
- Small for date (<3rd centile) or large for date (>97th centile)
- Major morbidities in postnatal period:
  - Perinatal asphyxia with hypoxic-ischemic encephalopathy
  - Neonatal sepsis/meningitis
  - Respiratory distress syndrome
  - Meconium aspiration syndrome
  - Shock requiring inotropic/vasopressor support
  - Acute kidney injury
  - Seizures
  - Intraventricular hemorrhage
  - Periventricular leukomalacia
  - Chronic lung disease
  - Congenital cardiac conditions
- Persistent hypoglycemia or hypocalcemia
- Mechanical ventilation for more than 24 hours
- Bilirubin encephalopathy
- Necrotizing enterocolitis
- Surgical conditions like diaphragmatic hernia, tracheo-esophageal fistula, intestinal obstruction, etc.
- Major malformations
- Infants born to HIV-positive mothers
- Inborn errors of metabolism/other genetic disorders

Follow-up Team

Regular follow-up program requires a multi-disciplinary team approach involving a team consisting of primary care neonatologist/pediatrician, pediatric neurologist, developmental therapist, radiologist, ophthalmologist, audiologist, physiotherapist, cardiologist, orthopedician social worker, and dietician.

Management

1. Early intervention program (early stimulation) must be started in the NICU once the neonate is medically stable.
2. Timely specific intervention must be ensured after detection of deviation of neurodevelopment from normal.

NEONATAL GROWTH CHARTS FOR FOLLOW-UP

Common growth charts used in different Indian set ups to assess fetal and postnatal growth include Fenton and Olsen charts. None of these charts meet the Indian standards of fetal and neonatal growth, as data of both of these charts are derived from the neonates of developed countries. To complement the WHO Multicenter Growth Reference Study (MGRS), the International Fetal and Newborn Growth Consortium for the 21st century (INTERGROWTH-21st) developed similar standards for fetuses, newborn infants, and the postnatal growth of preterm infants. Primary data were collected from a population-based sample of healthy pregnant women and their babies in eight countries including India. INTERGROWTH-21st included newborn standards for birth weight, length, and head circumference. It is the first international standards for fetal growth, and newborn size at birth as per gestational age and sex. In absence of any exclusive Indian data, we can use these charts in Indian NICUs. Separate charts are available for boys and girls for newborn size at birth (33 to 43 weeks). Postnatal growth charts for preterm neonates from 27th to 64th weeks are also available (*see* **Annexures**).

Doyle LW, Anderson PJ, Battin M, *et al*. Long term follow up of high risk children: WHO, why and how? *BMC Pediatr*. 2014;14:279.

Villar J, Cheikh Ismail L, Victora CG, Ohuma EO, *et al*. International standards for newborn weight, length, and head circumference by gestational age and sex: the Newborn Cross-Sectional Study of the INTERGROWTH-21st Project. *Lancet*. 2014;384:857–68.

Villar J, Giuliani F, Fenton TR, Ohuma EO, *et al*. INTERGROWTH-21st Consortium. INTERGROWTH-21st very preterm size at birth reference charts. *Lancet*. 2016;387:844–5.

Walker K, Holland AJ, Halliday R, Badawi N. Which high-risk infants should we follow-up and how should we do it? *J Paediatr Child Health*. 2012;48:789–93.

7

Ashok Kumar and Sriparna Basu

Hematological Disorders

8.1 COMPONENTS AND PHYSIOLOGY OF BLOOD

Red blood cells (RBCs) or erythrocytes, white blood cells (WBCs) or leukocytes, and platelets or thrombocytes, constitute the cellular part of blood. The plasma is the river in which the blood cells travel. It carries not only the blood cells but also dissolved gases (carbon dioxide and oxygen), nutrients (like sugars, amino acids, fats, and minerals), waste products (like lactic acid, and urea), antibodies, clotting proteins (called clotting factors), chemical messengers such as hormones, and proteins including enzymes that help maintain the body's fluid balance. Blood also serves to maintain normal body temperature and body's pH balance (normally between 7.35 to 7.45; range 6.8–7.45).

HEMATOPOIESIS

All the blood cells develop from a population of hematopoietic stem cells (HSCs) that have the potential to differentiate into any of the blood cells. These stem cells differentiate into progenitor cells which under the influence of various hematopoietic growth factors mature into erythrocytes, platelets, monocytes, macrophages, lymphocytes, neutrophils, eosinophils, and basophils (Fig. 8.1).

- *Erythropoiesis* leads to differentiation of a progenitor cell into a red blood cell under the influence of erythropoietin (EPO). Normoblasts and reticulocytes are different stages in the process of maturation. In the process the red cell size decreases, the nucleus is extruded, and hemoglobinization of the cell takes place.
- *Lymphopoiesis* is the process of maturation of progenitor cells into lymphocytes.
- *Granulopoiesis* is the process of maturation of myeloblasts into different types of granulocytes, ie, basophils, neutrophils, and eosinophils under the influence of GM-CSF (granulocyte and monocyte colony stimulating factor), G-CSF, and M-CSF.

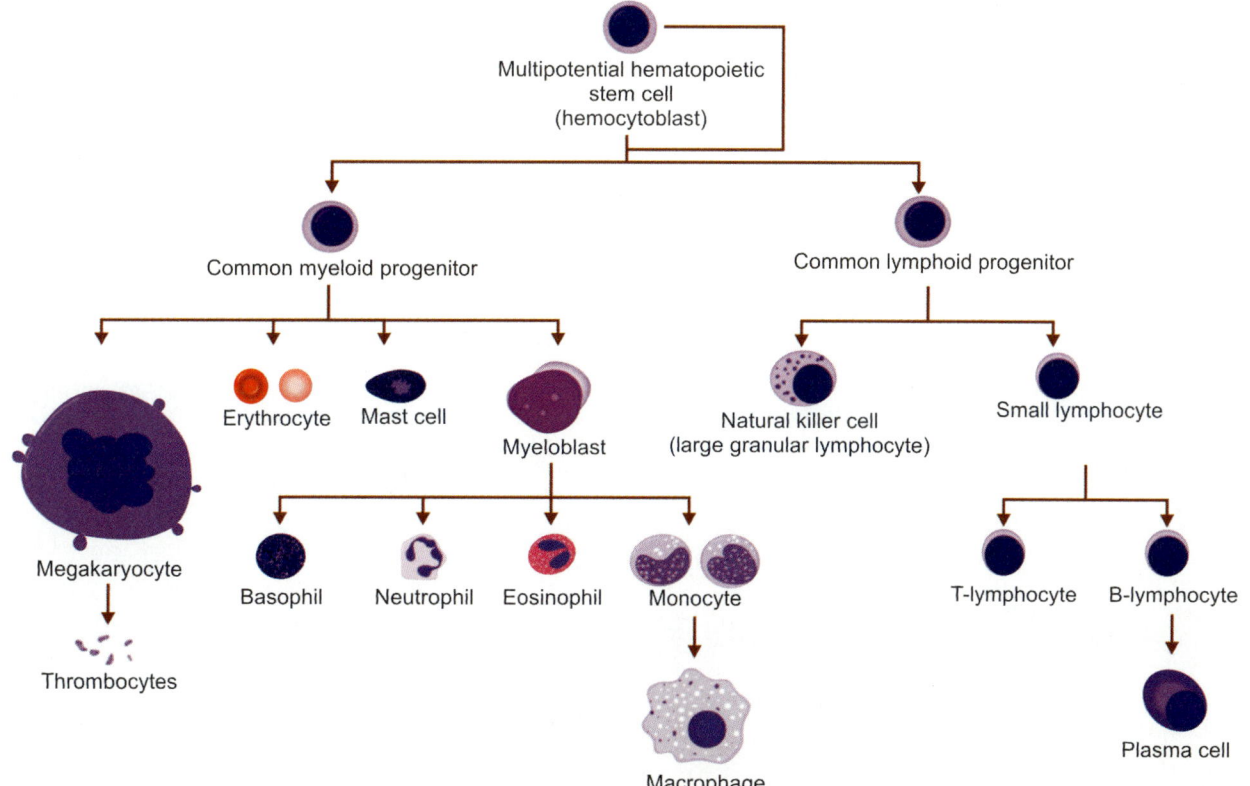

Fig. 8.1 Hematopoiesis

- *Monocytopoiesis* is the process of maturation of myeloblasts into monocytes. The monocytes further mature as macrophages.
- *Megakaryocytopoiesis* is the hematopoiesis of platelets. Thrombopoietin is the growth factor responsible for regulating the maturation of megakaryocytes into mature platelets (thrombopoiesis).

Once the progenitor cells have differentiated into mature cells they are released into the blood.

LOCATION OF HEMATOPOIESIS

These cells are produced in the body at different sites depending upon the stage of life. Hematopoiesis starts by the 2nd week of gestation in the yolk sac; this function is gradually taken over by the liver. The spleen and lymph nodes also starts contributing to a lesser extent. By the fifth month of gestation the bone marrow becomes active; and from 7th month of gestation onwards it remains the main site of hematopoiesis.

In children, hematopoiesis occurs in the marrow of the long bones such as the femur and tibia. In adults, it occurs mainly in the medulla of flat bones like pelvis, cranium, vertebrae, and sternum. Maturation and some proliferation of lymphoid cells occurs in lymph nodes, spleen and thymus. Sometimes, liver, thymus, and spleen may resume their hematopoietic function (extramedullary hematopoiesis), if necessary.

Revision Point **Components and Physiology of Blood**

1. Blood comprises 55% plasma and 45% as cellular components (99% erythrocytes and 1% as leucocytes and thrombocytes).
2. Leucocytes can be categorized as agranulocytes (lymphocytes and monocytes) and granulocytes (neutrophils, basophils and eosinophils).
3. Hematopoiesis starts by the 2nd week of gestation in the yolk sac and this function is gradually taken over by the liver. By the fifth month of gestation, the bone marrow becomes active; and from 7th month of gestation onwards it remains the main site of hematopoiesis.

Normal Values

Hematological parameters including hemoglobin, total leukocyte count, differential counts, red blood indices such as mean corpuscular volume, etc. vary with age **(Table 8.1)**.

8.2 ANEMIA

Anemia is defined as a reduction in the red cell mass or blood hemoglobin concentration 2 standard deviations below the expected values for age and sex. The WHO cut-off values of hemoglobin for defining anemia in children are as follows:
- 6 months to 6 years: hemoglobin < 11 g/dL
- 6 to 14 years: hemoglobin <12 g/dL

Severity Severe anemia is hemoglobin level below 7 g/dL while that between 7 and 10 g/dL indicates moderate anemia. Hemoglobin levels <13.5 g/dL in a neonate indicate anemia.

ETIOLOGY

Normal RBC values represent a balance between RBC synthesis and their destruction. Usually RBCs circulate in the blood for about 120 days before they are sequestered in the spleen. Hence, anemia may occur when there is (a) excessive RBC loss (as occurs with hemorrhage), (b) premature RBC destruction (hemolysis), or (c) insufficient RBC production. However, anemia may be physiological in children aged 2–3 months (physiological anemia of infancy). Likewise, transient erythroblastopenia in children may occur in children aged 3 months to 6 years, especially following viral infections. These conditions usually do not warrant much treatment and are not a cause for concern. **Table 8.2** enlists the etiology of anemia.

PHYSIOLOGY OF ANEMIA

Anemia leads to decreased oxygen carrying capacity of the blood, which causes signs and symptoms depending upon the severity of anemia. In response to a decrease in hemoglobin levels, the body tries to increase the red cell production by secreting more erythropoietin. Erythropoietin stimulates the bone marrow, which becomes more active and hypercellular resulting in the release of more immature red cells into the peripheral circulation. This results in increased number of nucleated red blood cells (normoblasts) and reticulocytes in the peripheral blood.

Age	Hb(g/dL) mean	PCV(%) mean	R/C(%) mean	MCV(fL) lower limit	TLC(/mm³) range	N(%) mean	L(%) mean
Cord blood	17	55	5	110	9,000–30,000	60	30
2 wks	16	50	1	90	5,000–21,000	40	65
3 mo	12	35	1	77	6,000–18,000	30	50
6 mo–6 y	12	37	1	70	6,000–15,000	45	50
7–14 y	13	38	1	80	4,000–13,000	55	40
>14 y girls boys	14 16	42 48	1.5	80	5,000–10,000	55	35

Table 8.1 Hematological Values in Different Age Groups

Hb—hemoglobin, PCV—packed cell volume, R/C—reticulocyte count, MCV—mean corpuscular volume, TLC—total leucocyte count, N—neutrophil, L—lymphocyte

Table 8.2 Etiology of Anemia

Mechanism of anemia	Clinical condition
Blood loss	• Acute: Hemorrhage • Chronic: Worm infestation, cow's milk allergy
Decreased production of RBCs	• Deficiency of iron, vitamin B_{12}, folic acid, zinc or other micronutrients • Aplasia or hypoplasia of bone marrow (aplastic anemia) • Impaired erythropoietin production as in chronic kidney failure, hypothyroidism, or hypopituitarism • Infiltration of the bone marrow as in leukemias, storage disorders • Chronic inflammatory conditions (lupus, rheumatic illness), chronic infections (tuberculosis)

Increased RBC destruction (hemolytic anemia)	• Corpuscular defects
	  – RBC membrane defects (spherocytosis, elliptocytosis)
	  – RBC enzyme defects [pyruvate kinase deficiency, glucose-6-phosphatase deficiency (G6PD)]
	  – Hemoglobin defects (thalassemia, sickle cell anemia)
	• Extracorpuscular defects
	  – Immune (autoimmune hemolytic anemia, lupus, etc.)
	  – Nonimmune (fragmentation hemolysis, hypersplenism, infections like malaria, Gram-negative sepsis, leishmaniasis, clostridia, toxoplasmosis, cytomegalovirus)

The body also compensates for the decreased oxygen carrying capacity of blood by increasing the cardiac output. This is achieved by increasing the stroke volume, heart rate, and shunting of blood towards vital organs. All this leads to a high output state and a flow ejection systolic murmur can be heard in chronic cases. The body also tries to increase the oxygen delivery to tissues by shifting the oxygen dissociation curve to right. However, compensatory mechanisms become insufficient with progress of anemia and the child becomes symptomatic.

SYMPTOMS AND SIGNS

Anemia manifests as pallor, fatigue, loss of appetite, irritability, tachypnea, dyspnea, tachycardia and finally the child develops congestive cardiac failure. The most important sign is pallor, which is visible in the palpebral conjunctiva, lips, tongue, nails, palms, and soles.

A simple way to grade the severity of anemia is palmar pallor. If palms are pale but creases are pink, it indicates moderate anemia. If creases are also pale, it usually means severe anemia. A rapid fall in hemoglobin results in more severe symptoms at a higher hemoglobin level than a slow gradual fall in hemoglobin level because there is not sufficient time for the compensatory mechanisms to operate fully.

MORPHOLOGICAL CLASSIFICATION OF ANEMIA

A peripheral smear examination is needed for classifying anemia according to the morphology of red blood cells. The important things to be observed are the size of the red blood cell and pattern of staining. Other important features that also need attention are shape of RBC, any inclusion bodies, morphology, and number of leukocytes and the platelets (Table 8.3).

A. Microcytic Anemia

The mean corpuscular volume (MCV) is less than the lower limit of normal for age. After 6 months of age, MCV <83 fL is considered microcytosis. This is also associated with decrease in mean corpuscular hemoglobin (MCH) and decrease in mean corpuscular hemoglobin concentration (MCHC) also called hypochromia. In this type of anemia there is defect in the RBC formation mainly affecting the hemoglobin synthesis; other cellular components are spared. The important causes of microcytic anemia are listed below.

I. Iron Deficiency Anemia

a. During infancy
  i. Nutritional
  ii. Post-hemorrhagic
b. Older children
  i. Nutritional
  ii. Post-hemorrhagic

II. Ineffective Erythropoiesis

a. Thalassemia
b. Pyridoxine responsive anemia
c. Dyserythropoietic anemia
d. Lead poisoning

B. Macrocytic Anemia

The MCV of red blood cells in patients with macrocytic anemia is more than the upper limit of normal for that age. In children >6 month of age, MCV >97 fL, is defined as macrocytosis. The defect lies in the DNA synthesis instead of hemoglobin synthesis and therefore also affects other cell lines. The red blood cells are usually normochromic, ie, MCH and MCHC are normal. It is usually associated with a megaloblastic bone marrow, ie, the erythroid precursors are also larger in size than normal. However, macrocytosis is not synonymous with megaloblastosis as a macrocytic peripheral blood picture may be associated with a normoblastic bone marrow picture. Important causes of macrocytic anemia are listed below.

I. Megaloblastic Erythropoiesis

a. Nutritional
  i. Vitamin B_{12} deficiency (breastfed infants of anemic mothers)

8

Table 8.3 Specific Red Cell Morphologic Abnormalities

Abnormality	Description	Causes
Target cells	Abnormal form of RBC appear to have a dark center (a central, hemoglobinized area) surrounded by a white ring (an area of relative pallor), followed by dark outer (peripheral) second ring containing a band of hemoglobin like a shooting target with bull's eye	Alpha and beta thalassemia, hemoglobin C disease, hemoglobin E (homozygous or heterozygous), autosplenectomy caused by sickle cell anemia, liver disease, post-splenectomy, LCAT (lecithin cholesterol acyltransferase) deficiency
Spherocytes	Sphere-shaped RBCs rather than bi-concave disk-shaped with decreased surface/volume ratio, raised MCHC	Hereditary spherocytosis, immune hemolytic anemia, fragmentation of RBCs (microangiopathy, burns)
Acanthocytes (spur cells)	RBCs with 5–10 spicules of varying length with wide bases	Liver disease, DIC, post-splenectomy, vitamin E deficiency, abetalipoproteinemia
Echinocytes (Burr cells)	RBCs with 10–30 spicules evenly distributed over RBC surface caused by alteration in intracellular or extracellular environment	Artifact, uremia, dehydration, liver disease, immediately following RBC transfusion, pyruvate kinase deficiency
Schistocytes (helmet cells)	Helmet or triangular shaped RBCs or fragmented RBCs	Disseminated intravascular coagulation (DIC), severe hemolytic anemia, microangiopathic hemolytic anemia, hemolytic uremic syndrome (HUS), burns, purpura fulminans, renal vein thrombosis
Elliptocytes	Elliptical RBCs, normochromic	Hereditary elliptocytosis, iron deficiency, sickle cell disease, thalassemia major, megaloblastic anemia, leukoerythroblastic reaction, malaria
Tear drop cells	Shape of drop, usually microcytic, often hypochromic	Newborn, thalassemia major, myeloproliferative disorders
Nucleated RBCs	Immature RBCs not normally seen in peripheral blood beyond neonatal period	Neonate (up to 7 days of life), intense bone marrow stimulation as in hemolytic anemias, acute bleeding, hypoxia, postsplenectomy, leuko-erythroblastic reaction, megaloblastic anemia
Basophilic stippling	Coarse/fine punctate basophilic inclusions (aggregates of ribosomal RNA)	Hemolytic anemia, iron deficiency anemia, lead poisoning
Howell-Jolly bodies	Small, well-defined, round, densely stained inclusions, eccentric in location, 1 μm in diameter	Postsplenectomy, newborn, megaloblastic anemia, dyserythropoietic anemia

   ii. Folate deficiency
   iii. Kwashiorkor
b. Toxic
   i. Drug induced: Antifolate compounds (eg, methotrexate, trimethoprim), anticonvulsant (eg, phenytoin).
c. Malabsorption
   i. Pernicious anemia
   ii. Post-gastrectomy, ileal resection
   iii. HIV enteropathy
d. Increased demands including hemolysis, leukemia.

II. Non-megaloblastic Erythropoiesis

a. *Chronic hemolytic anemia* Peripheral smear shows macrocytic erythrocytes due to relative folate deficiency resulting from increased compensatory erythropoiesis.
b. Liver diseases
c. Hypothyroidism
d. Diamond-Blackfan syndrome

C. Normocytic Anemia

The MCV is within normal limits along with the MCH and MCHC so the RBCs are also normochromic.

I. Impaired Cell Production (reticulocyte count is low)

a. Leukocytes and platelets are normal
   i. Physiological anemia of infancy
   ii. Infections
   iii. Pure red cell aplasia
b. Leukocytes and platelets are normal or decreased
   i. Chronic renal and liver disease
   ii. Hypothyroidism
c. Leukocytes and platelets are reduced
   i. *Aplastic anemia:* Hereditary, idiopathic
   ii. *Myeloproliferative disorders:* Leukemia

II. Acute Hemolysis (reticulocyte count is high)

CLINICAL APPROACH TO ANEMIA

Relevant history like the age of onset, progression, blood loss, jaundice, bleeding tendency, blood transfusion, and family history are very important and will give some clue to the cause. A detailed examination from head to toe is important especially regarding the degree of pallor, icterus, petechiae, ecchymotic patches, presence of lymphadenopathy,

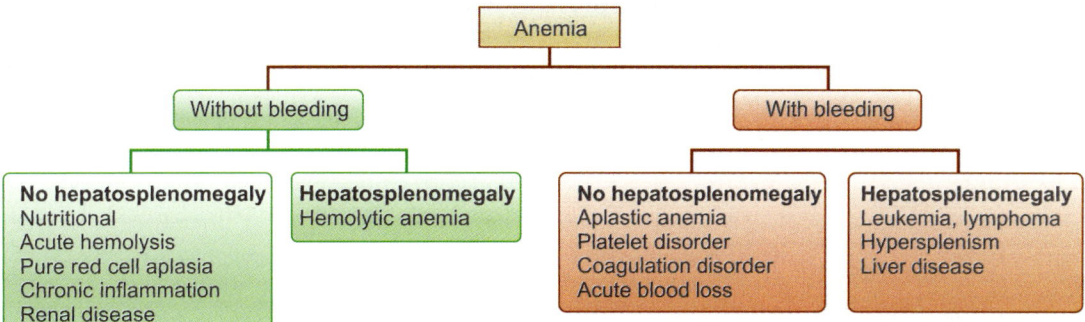

Fig. 8.2 Clinical approach to anemia

enlarged liver and spleen, and bony tenderness. Association of anemia with bleeding and the presence or absence of hepatosplenomegaly are important in making a differential diagnosis (Fig. 8.2).

1. *Age of onset* Nutritional anemias usually manifest between 6 months to 3 years of age. Alpha-thalassemia presents with anemia or hydrops *in utero* or just after birth. Beta-thalassemia usually presents after 6 months of age when fetal hemoglobin (HbF) starts decreasing. A congenital bone marrow hypoplasia will present at or soon after birth. Anemia in a neonate will mostly be due to hemorrhage, hemolysis (usually with indirect hyperbilirubinemia) or rarely due to failure of RBC production (pure red cell aplasia or Diamond-Blackfan syndrome).

2. *Family history of blood transfusions indicates an inherited* cause such as thalassemia, enzyme defects (G6PD deficiency), or membrane defects (hereditary spherocytosis).

3. Repeated history of blood transfusions usually indicates a non-nutritional anemia such as hemoglobinopathy, thalassemia, or bone marrow hypofunction.

4. *Community* G6PD deficiency is more common in *Parsis* and *Sindhis*. Thalassemia is seen more in *Punjabis* and *Sindhis*. Sickle cell anemia is more common in Madhya Pradesh, Tamil Nadu, Kerala, and Andhra Pradesh. Hemoglobin E beta-thalassemia is mostly seen in Indians residing in North Eastern states, West Bengal, Odisha, and Andaman and Nicobar.

5. *Dietary history* A child with predominantly milk-based diet with minimal or no complimentary feeding is more likely to suffer from nutritional anemia. History of pica suggests an iron deficiency anemia. A child on goat's milk is predisposed to folic acid deficiency due to its poor folate content.

6. *History of passage of worms, blood in stools or melena* for a long time leads to chronic blood loss and anemia.

7. *History of skin bleeds (petechiae or ecchymosis) or bleeding from any other sites* This suggests a platelet or a hepatic involvement. Chronic liver disease could be a cause of anemia that will also affect the coagulation factors and lead to bleeding manifestations. Skin bleeds associated with anemia suggests hypoplasia or infiltration of the bone marrow.

8. *History of fever* with sudden appearance of pallor suggests malaria.

9. *Facies* A typical hemolytic facies is characteristic of thalassemia.

10. *Jaundice* Presence of mild jaundice without passage of high colored urine indicates a process of hemolysis whereas the presence of conjugated hyperbilirubinemia indicates primary hepatic pathology.

11. *Malnutrition and wasting* may be associated with nutritional anemia.

12. *Hepatosplenomegaly* Presence of significant hepato-splenomegaly with lymphadenopathy is highly suggestive of malignancy (leukemia and lymphoma). Significant hepatosplenomegaly without lymphadeno-pathy suggests hemolytic anemia, eg, thalassemia, or infective pathology (malaria). HIV/AIDS should also be ruled out in presence of hepatosplenomegaly.

13. *Presence of associated anomalies like* skeletal deformities, hyperpigmentation, hypopigmentation, renal anomalies, eye and ear malformations, etc. point towards a possibility of inherited pancytopenia such as Fanconi anemia or dyskeratosis congenita or Diamond-Blackfan syndrome.

LABORATORY APPROACH TO ANEMIA

1. *Hemoglobin* Estimation of hemoglobin to confirm anemia, and assess its severity to decide for the need of packed red blood cell transfusion.

2. *Red blood cell indices* Hematocrit (packed cell volume), mean corpuscular volume (MCV), mean corpuscular hemoglobin (MCH), mean corpuscular hemoglobin concentration (MCHC), and red cell distribution width (RDW) are helpful in indicating the type of anemia (Fig. 8.3). RDW indicates the variation in red blood cell size. Increased RDW indicates presence of anisocytosis as seen in iron deficiency anemia and folate/vitamin B_{12} deficiency. A normal RDW (12–14%) indicates not much variation in size of the red blood cells as in thalassemia, anemia of chronic disease, hemorrhage, hereditary spherocytosis, and aplastic anemia. RDW when used together with MCV can aid in diagnosing the cause of anemia.

3. *Reticulocyte count* Number of reticulocytes in the blood reflects the bone marrow activity and is expressed as the percentage of the total red blood cell count. If the bone marrow is hyperactive as in cases of hemolytic anemia or following hemorrhage, the reticulocyte count increases. The reticulocyte count is decreased in patients with bone marrow hypoplasia or aplasia, malignancies, and infections.

Anemia *per se* results in increased bone marrow activity to compensate for decreased hemoglobin, leading to falsely high reticulocyte count. Therefore, correction

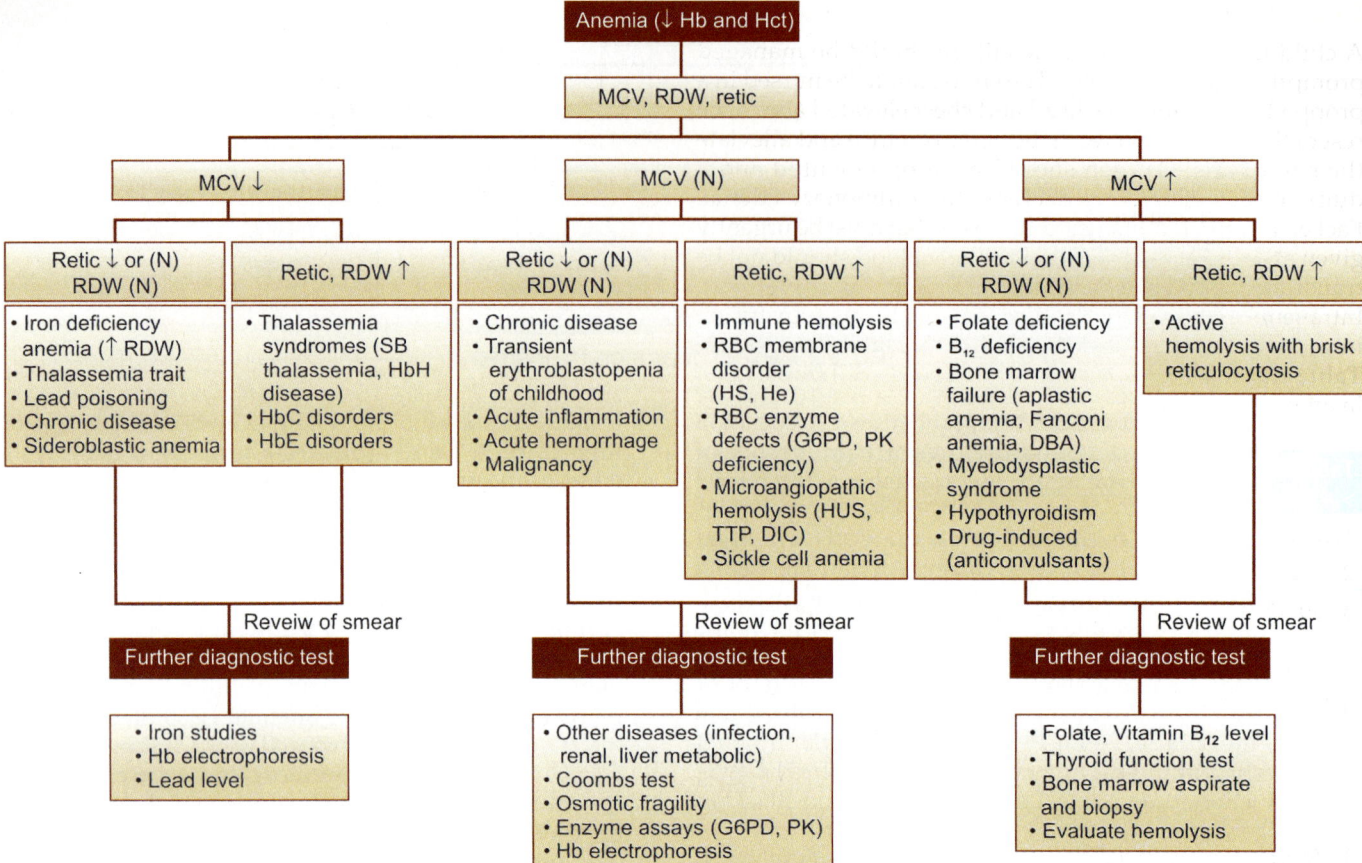

Fig. 8.3 Laboratory approach to anemia. Hb: Hemoglobin; Hct: Hematocrit; MCV: Mean corpuscular volume; RDW: Red cell distribution width; Retic: Reticulocyte count

should be made for the existing severity of anemia. This is done as follows:

$$\text{Corrected reticulocyte count} = \frac{\text{Actual reticulocyte count} \times \text{packed cell volume (PCV)}}{0.45 \text{ (normal PCV)}}$$

4. *Bone marrow* Bone marrow examination is very helpful in making a diagnosis as many times, the peripheral blood examination may not reveal the true picture. A peripheral pancytopenia may not be associated with bone marrow aplasia suggesting an alternate diagnosis. Similarly, a peripheral macrocytic picture may not be associated with megaloblastosis in bone marrow suggesting towards a diagnosis other than vitamin B_{12} or folic acid deficiency. Bone marrow examination can be diagnostic in aplastic anemia and leukemia. It is important to ascertain the cellularity and the myeloid to erythroid ratio (M:E ratio) in marrow.

The ratio of myeloid to erythroid precursors in bone marrow normally varies from 2:1 to 4:1. An increased M:E ratio may suggest infections or chronic myeloid leukemia. Erythroid hyperplasia is seen in hemolytic anemia, megaloblastic anemia, and hypersplenism (decreased M:E ratio). The various bone marrow erythroid series are as follows:

- *Normoblastic:* Iron deficiency anemia, infection, malignancy, renal disease, connective tissue disorders, hemolytic anemia.

- *Megaloblastic:* Vitamin B_{12} deficiency, folate deficiency, congenital/acquired disorders in DNA synthesis, drug-induced (methotrexate, phenytoin)
- *Sideroblastic:* Hereditary (X-linked, autosomal recessive, mitochondrial disorders, DIDMOAD, Pearson syndrome), drugs (isoniazid, linezolid, cycloserine, chloramphenicol), pyridoxine deficiency, lead poisoning, copper deficiency. The bone marrow produces ringed sideroblasts rather than healthy RBCs. Bone marrow shows erythroid hyperplasia with maturation arrest.
5. *Other investigations* Specific investigations for etiological diagnosis include serum iron studies, serum folate and vitamin B_{12} levels for deficiency anemias; and hemoglobin electrophoresis for hemoglobinopathies and thalassemia.

GENERAL MANAGEMENT

All children should be regularly dewormed as hookworm infestation is a very common cause of anemia especially in children from lower socioeconomic strata. For nutritional anemia, specific supplementation needs to be started once the diagnosis is made. Apart from medication, proper dietary advice needs to be given regarding which food is rich in the deficient nutrient. All children with fever in the endemic zone for malaria should be treated with antimalarials unless there is some other known cause for fever.

Emergency Management

A child in congestive cardiac failure should be managed promptly and aggressively. The child should be nursed in a propped-up position, ie, head and chest elevated above the rest of the body, to decrease the venous return and alleviate the symptoms. Oxygen should be supplemented and a diuretic administered to decrease the pulmonary edema. Packed red blood transfusion 10–15 mL/kg must be urgently given at a rate of 3–5 mL/kg/h. Whole blood should not be transfused as it increases the chances of fluid overload. Intravenous furosemide should be given during transfusion in a dose of 1–2 mg/kg to avoid circulatory overload. **Table 8.4** enlists the indications for packed cell transfusion in anemia in children.

Table 8.4 Indications of Packed Red Cell Transfusion in Children > 4 months
1. Blood loss >15 of total blood volume
2. Hb <13 g/dL: Severe cardiopulmonary disease
3. Hb <8 g/dL: Severe infection, perioperative period, marrow failure, symptomatic chronic anemia, signs of hypoxia, congestive cardiac failure
4. Hb <4 g/dL

Anemia

1. Anemia is a reduction in the red cell mass or blood hemoglobin concentration, 2 standard deviations below the expected values for age and sex. The WHO cut-off values of hemoglobin for defining anemia in children are <11g/dL in children aged 6 months to 6 years, and <12 g/dL in children aged 6 to 14 years.

2. Anemia may occur when there is (a) excessive RBC loss (as occurs with hemorrhage), (b) premature RBC destruction (hemolysis), or (c) insufficient RBC production.

3. A peripheral smear examination is essential for classifying anemia according to the morphology of RBCs (size, pattern of staining, shape, any inclusion bodies, morphology and number of leucocytes and the platelets).

4. The most common cause of microcytic anemia (MCV <83 fL) in children is iron deficiency anemia. The most common cause of macrocytic anemia (MCV >97 fL) is nutritional anemia (folate or vitamin B_{12} deficiency).

5. In all children with anemia, a corrected reticulocyte count must be computed because anemia may lead to falsely high reticulocyte count. Reticulocyte count increases in cases of hemolytic anemia or following hemorrhage, and decreases in patients with bone marrow hypoplasia or aplasia, malignancies, and infections.

6. The ratio of myeloid to erythroid precursors in bone marrow normally varies from 2:1 to 4:1. An increased M:E ratio may suggest infections or chronic myeloid leukemia. Erythroid hyperplasia is seen in hemolytic anemia, megaloblastic anemia, and hypersplenism (decreased M:E ratio).

Brown RG. Determining the cause of anemia. General approach, with emphasis on microcytic hypochromic anemias. *Postgrad Med.* 1991;89:161–4, 167–70.

Ford J. Red blood cell morphology. *Int J Lab Hematol.* 2013;35:351–7.

Janus J, Moerschel SK. Evaluation of anemia in children. *Am Fam Physician.* 2010;81:1462–71.

Lacroix J, Demaret P, Tucci M. Red blood cell transfusion: decision making in pediatric intensive care units. *Semin Perinatol.* 2012;36:225–31.

Wallerstein RO Jr. Laboratory evaluation of anemia. *West J Med.* 1987;146:443–51.

8.3 BONE MARROW FAILURE

Bone marrow failure is a disorder of the hematopoietic stem cell which may present as isolated failure to produce one cell line (single cytopenia: Anemia, leukopenia, or thrombocytopenia), two cell lines (bicytopenia) or all the three cell lines (pancytopenia due to hypoplastic or aplastic marrow). The bone marrow failure could be congenital or acquired.

ETIOLOGY

The etiology of bone marrow failure could be:

1. A decrease in or damage to the hematopoietic stem cells and their microenvironment, resulting in hypoplastic or aplastic bone marrow.
2. Maturation defects, eg, vitamin B_{12} or folate deficiency.
3. Differentiation defects, eg, myelodysplasia, congenital dyserythropoietic anemia.

Table 8.5 lists the causes of bone marrow failure.

APLASTIC ANEMIA

Aplastic anemia is the commonest form of bone marrow failure. It is characterized by the presence of anemia, leukopenia, and thrombocytopenia (pancytopenia), resulting from physiological and anatomical failure of the bone marrow.

Diagnostic Challenges

Pancytopenia in the peripheral blood picture is not synonymous with aplastic anemia. Myelodysplastic anemia also can cause pancytopenia. Myelophthisic anemia may result from marrow destruction because of tumor invasion or granulomas. Likewise, hypersplenism may cause pancytopenia but bone marrow examination will reveal a hyperactive marrow. Bone marrow examination is thus warranted in every case of pancytopenia to make a diagnosis.

In aplastic anemia, the hematopoietic tissue in the bone marrow is replaced by fat cells resulting in decrease in the mature cells to be released into the blood. Scattered islands of hematopoiesis may be seen with evidence of erythroid prominence with megaloblastic changes.

The diagnostic criteria for aplastic anemia include hypocellular bone marrow with no abnormal cells and no fibrosis. Additionally, at least 2 among the following are essential for the diagnosis: Hb <10 g/dL, platelet count <50 × 10^9/L, and absolute neutrophil count <1.5 × 10^9/L.

Etiology

The etiology be congenital or acquired. The incriminating factor may act by causing destruction of hematopoietic

Table 8.5 Causes of Bone Marrow Failure
Failure of all three cell lines (hypoplastic/aplastic anemia)
A. *Congenital*
• Fanconi anemia
• Dyskeratosis congenita
• Dubowitz syndrome
• Aplastic anemia with constitutional chromosomal abnormalities: Down syndrome, Dubowitz syndrome, Seckel syndrome
B. *Acquired*
• Idiopathic
• Secondary/Acquired
– Drugs: Anticancer drugs, chloramphenicol, antiepileptics
– Infections: CMV, hepatitis B and C virus, HIV, EBV
– Radiation, radiotherapy
– Paroxysmal nocturnal hemoglobinuria (PNH)
Failure of single cell line (single cytopenia)
Red blood cells
A. *Congenital*
• Pure red cell aplasia (Diamond-Blackfan syndrome)
• Congenital dyserythropoietic syndrome
• AASE syndrome
B. *Acquired*
• Idiopathic: Transient erythroblastopenia of childhood
• Secondary
– Drugs
– Infection: Parvovirus
– Malnutrition
– Thymoma
– Hematological disorders: Chronic hemolytic anemia, iron deficiency anemia, folate or B_{12} deficiency
White blood cells
• Shwachman-Diamond syndrome
• Infantile genetic agranulocytosis (Kostmann disease)
• Reticular dysgenesis
Platelets
Congenital amegakaryocytic thrombocytopenia

progenitors, destroying the bone marrow microenvironment, or may act through an immune-mediated pathway. The causes of aplastic anemia are listed in **Table 8.5**.

ACQUIRED APLASTIC ANEMIA

Etiology

Majority of the cases of acquired childhood aplastic anemia are idiopathic where no cause is identified. The most probable cause is immunological injury due to activated T-cells and cytokines, which act on the marrow progenitor cells and suppress them. Drugs are the next most common causes of acquired aplastic anemia. A genetic predisposition seen in some children make them prone to bone marrow aplasia.

Drug-induced Aplasia

Anticancer drugs and radiation cause bone marrow suppression in exposed patients. This suppression is predictable, dose-related, and reversible. Some drugs, which are normally tolerated well in most people, may lead to bone marrow suppression in certain genetically predisposed people, which is not related to dose or duration of therapy (idiosyncratic reaction), which is more severe and irreversible. It can be seen with some commonly used drugs such as chloramphenicol, phenytoin, chlorpromazine, carbamazepine, sulphonamides, quinacrine, cimetidine and oxyphenylbutazone. Chemicals like DDT, benzene, aromatic hydrocarbons, heavy metals like arsenic and gold can also induce aplasia of the bone marrow.

Infections

Common viral infections leading to aplastic anemia include infection with parvovirus B19, Epstein-Barr virus, hepatitis B, C, and D viruses, measles, mumps, and cytomegalovirus.

Paroxysmal Nocturnal Hemoglobinuria

Paroxysmal nocturnal hemoglobinuria (PNH) is caused by a mutation in the hematopoietic stem cells which results in production of red blood cells deficient in certain surface proteins that protect normal red blood cells from destruction by the complement system proteins. PNH may be primary or occur in a patient with hypoplastic or aplastic anemia.

Clinical Presentation

The course of aplastic anemia is usually insidious and progressive with manifestation due to decrease in all the three cell lines.

1. *Anemia* Decrease in the red blood cells leads to gradual fall in hemoglobin and symptoms like weakness, loss of appetite and lethargy. Gradually there is severe anemia that may lead to congestive cardiac failure. Anemia is usually severe and persistent needing repeated packed red blood cell transfusions.
2. *Leukopenia* This manifests as fever because decrease in leukocytes makes the patient prone to infections. Fever may or may not have an identifiable cause or localizing sign and symptom and patients present with pyrexia of unknown origin. The patient may present with repeated episodes of infections.
3. *Thrombocytopenia* This manifests as bleeding from different sites like mucocutaneous bleeds such as petechiae or ecchymosis, subconjunctival hemorrhage (Fig. 8.4), epistaxis, gum bleeds, gastrointestinal bleed, hematuria, and rarely intracranial hemorrhage. Hemorrhage and infection are the main causes of death in aplastic anemia.

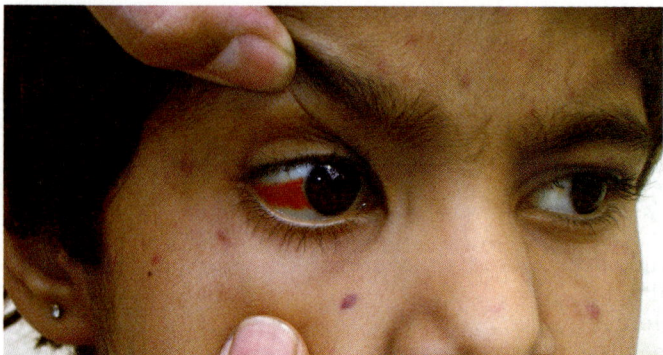

Fig. 8.4 Subconjunctival hemorrhage

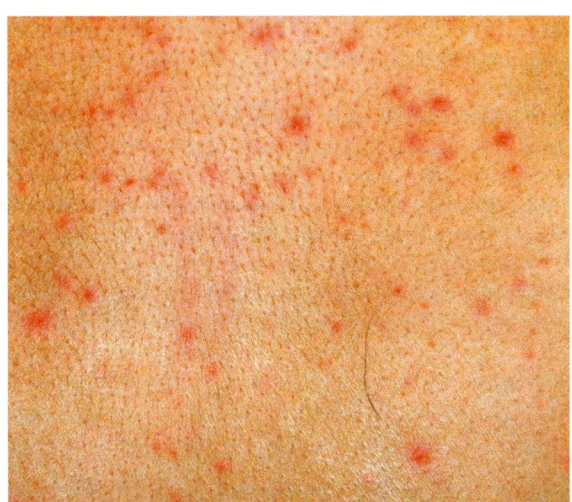

Fig. 8.5 Cutaneous bleeding

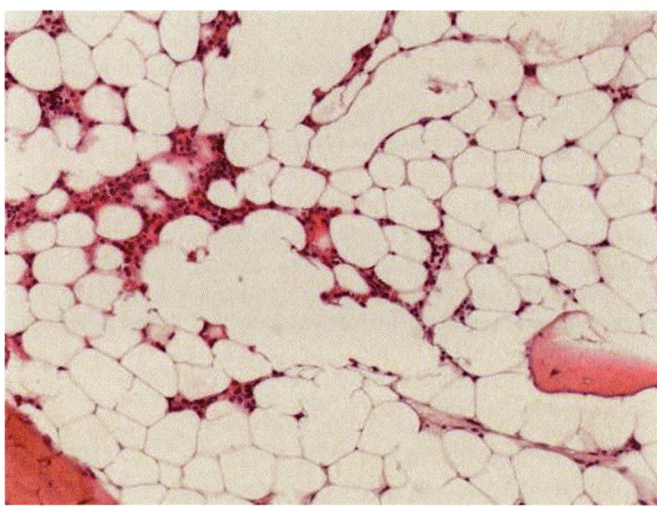

Fig. 8.6 Bone marrow picture in aplastic anemia shows hypocellularity and fat cells

On examination, there is moderate to severe pallor. The child looks sick and toxic. Petechiae or ecchymotic patches may be visible on the skin (Fig. 8.5). There is no jaundice, lymphadenopathy, and hepatosplenomegaly.

Diagnosis

Peripheral smear shows pancytopenia, the red blood cells are usually normocytic and normochromic but may be macrocytic. All the leukocyte series are decreased in number but neutrophils are worst affected (granulocytopenia, often <1500/mm^3). The platelets are markedly reduced in number. The reticulocyte count is decreased, especially when seen in context to the degree of anemia. Hemoglobin levels vary and are usually less than 7g/dL.

Bone marrow aspiration or biopsy is diagnostic. Sometimes the bone marrow aspiration may end up as a dry tap as most of the marrow tissue is replaced by fat. A bone marrow biopsy should be done in these cases and is of immense importance. The involvement of bone marrow is heterogeneous and proportion of fat cells increase and hematopoietic tissue decreases ranging from moderate reduction to complete absence (Fig. 8.6).

Severity

Based on the marrow and blood smear examination, aplastic anemia is classified as severe when absolute neutrophil count is <500/mm^3, platelet count <20,000/mm^3, corrected reticulocyte count <1% and bone marrow has <25% cellularity (Camitta criteria).

Aplastic anemia is moderate in severity when absolute neutrophil count is between 500 and 1500/mm^3, platelet count is between 20,000 and 1,00,000/mm^3, and reticulocyte count is <1%.

Prognosis

Idiopathic aplastic anemia, granulocyte count >500/mm^3, platelet count >20000/mm^3, retained cellular marrow elements, younger age, and absence of hemorrhagic manifestations and infections, are associated with a favorable prognosis.

Treatment	Acquired Aplastic Anemia

1. Supportive care

Remove the incriminating agent as the first step. Treatment of infections and blood component (packed cell and platelet) transfusions are the mainstay of the supportive management. Mortality usually results from excessive bleeding or fulminant infection.

Blood component therapy

Transfusions should be avoided in patients in whom hematopoietic stem cell transplant is being planned. Repeated transfusions can cause sensitization of the patient to blood and blood products and increase the chances of rejection of the graft and graft versus host disease. There is also risk of transmission of infections like hepatitis B, C, and HIV.

The aim of transfusion should not be to attain normal values but to alleviate the complications. Hemoglobin of 7–8 g/dL is acceptable. A prophylactic platelet transfusion is warranted only at levels of <20000/mm^3 to avoid bleeding into vital organs. One unit of platelet concentrate (whole blood derived platelets) per square meter will raise the platelet count by 10,000/mm^3. Transfusion of one unit of platelet concentrate per ten kg of body weight should raise the platelet count by 50,000/uL. Transfused platelets have a short lifespan and will need to be redosed within 3–4 days if given for prophylaxis. A platelet count of >20,000/mm^3 without any bleeding need not be treated with platelet transfusion. However, drugs that impair platelet function like aspirin should be avoided.

Intramuscular injections should be avoided and followed by application of ice-packs to injection sites. Children should avoid injury by refraining from contact sports as well as by brushing teeth with a soft brush.

Treat infections

Infections need to be treated promptly and aggressively (third generation cephalosporins and aminoglycosides). Attempts should be made to identify the infection and isolate the causative organism. Use antibiotics and antifungal agents, if required. Prophylactic use of antibiotics to prevent infections has no role.

2. Definitive treatment

Different options are available depending upon the feasibility and the affordability.

Hematopoietic stem cell transplant (HSCT)

It is the treatment of choice for patients with severe aplastic anemia who have a HLA-matched sibling donor. It provides complete cure but is not feasible in majority due to the lack of availability of compatible stem cell donor, exorbitant costs involved, and because very few centers have the required expertise and facilities. The survival rate in children may be as good as 80%. Best results are obtained if the age is less, patient has received minimum or no blood product transfusions, and does not develop infection during or after HSCT.

Immunotherapy

Immunotherapy is the treatment of choice in all those children who are not eligible for HSCT because of any reason. Available immunomodulators include: (i) cyclosporin A, (ii) antithymocytic globulin (ATG), or anti-lymphocyte globulin (ALG), and (iii) methylprednisolone. They may be used alone or in combination.

- Cyclosporin is given orally for at least 3 months. It is started at a dose of 8 mg/kg/day for 14 days; the dose is increased to 15 mg/kg/day for the next 14 days. Thereafter, the dose is titrated according to the clinical response and serum drug levels.
- ATG and ALG are polyclonal antibodies against the lymphocytic antigen and therefore act as an inhibitor of T-cell suppression of the bone marrow. These are given intravenously (20–40 mg/kg/day) for 4–8 days.
- Methylprednisolone is given orally or intravenously in a dose of 5 mg/kg/day for 8 days, followed by 1 mg/kg/day for the next 5 days. It is then tapered over the next week.

All these agents cause immunosuppression and the cost is much less than that of HSCT. However, these drugs are still not affordable for many patients. The response rates when ATG is used alone are around 50%. About 25% of patients may respond to steroids alone. However, when combination of cyclosporin A, ATG (or ALG), and methylprednisolone is used there may be complete or partial remission in about 60–70% patients.

Other modes

Cyclophosphamide, androgenic steroids, or other steroids like prednisolone have been used in children who are unable to afford HSCT and immunotherapy as detailed above. Recombinant human GM-CSF (8–32 µg/kg/day) given IV along with cyclosporin A or ALG has also shown some promise but the results are transient.

CONSTITUTIONAL (INHERITED) APLASTIC ANEMIA

These disorders are inherited as autosomal dominant, autosomal recessive, or X-linked disorders. All these patients are at risk for malignant transformation.

Fanconi Anemia

Fanconi anemia (FA) is the commonest constitutional aplastic disorder with autosomal recessive inheritance. The mutant gene responsible leads to chromosomal fragility and genomic instability. FA occurs in about 1 per 130,000 births, with a slightly higher frequency in Ashkenazi Jews in Israel and Afrikaners in South Africa.

Clinical features The manifestations of bone marrow aplasia may occur anytime in the first decade, mean age of presentation is 6–8 years. Characteristic physical abnormalities include skin changes (hyperpigmentation of the trunk and neck along with café au lait spots and vitiligo), short stature, limb anomalies (absent radius, abnormal thumbs, congenital dislocation of hip), hypogonadal changes in boys, and renal and ear abnormalities. Some children may have characteristic facies consisting of microcephaly, small eyes with epicanthic folds, and abnormal ears. The bone marrow aplasia progresses with age and most cases ultimately develop severe aplasia. These patients are prone to develop myelodysplastic syndrome (MDS) and acute myeloid leukemia (AML) with time.

Laboratory investigations Macrocytic anemia, decreased reticulocyte count, increased serum erythropoietin levels, and increased fetal hemoglobin characterize Fanconi anemia. Bone marrow biopsy reveals hypoplasia. Characteristic chromosomal breaks and rearrangements including exchanges and endoduplications induced by diepoxybutane (DEB) or mitomycin C are diagnostic.

Treatment	Inherited Aplastic Anemia

Only cure is hematopoietic stem cell transplantation (HSCT) without which majority of the children die before completion of second decade. Nearly, 50% children may respond to androgen therapy (nandrolone decanoate, oxymethalone), though there is a risk of developing hepatoma on prolonged use.

DIAMOND-BLACKFAN ANEMIA (CONGENITAL PURE RED CELL APLASIA)

This is also known as congenital pure red cell aplasia, and inherited in an autosomal dominant or autosomal recessive manner. There is isolated erythroid hypoplasia presenting in early infancy.

Clinical features Anemia is associated with congenital eye anomalies (strabismus, blue sclera, hypertelorism, glaucoma, cataract, and epicanthal folds), deformities of ribs and fingers (abnormalities of thumbs: Absent, bifid, malformed or triphalangeal), renal anomalies, and craniofacial dysmorphism (wide set eyes, thick upper lip, webbed neck and intelligent expression). Profound anemia sets in the second and third month of life.

Laboratory investigations Anemia and reticulocytopenia appear in early infancy with normal platelet and leukocyte counts. The red blood cells are macrocytic with increased fetal hemoglobin (HbF). There is increased activity of 'i' antigen and increase in adenosine deaminase activity in erythrocytes. Bone marrow shows decreased erythroid precursors with other cell line precursors being intact.

Treatment	Diamond-Blackfan Anemia

Corticosteroids are effective in 70–80% of the patients. Hemoglobin is restored to normal levels after 4–6 weeks of therapy with prednisolone (2 mg/kg/day given in three or four divided doses), following which the dose is gradually reduced. Long-term side effects may force the steroids to be withdrawn.

Hematopoietic stem cell transplant (HSCT) provides cure for the disease. Repeated packed red blood cell transfusions are the only option if HSCT or steroid treatment is not feasible.

Prognosis Long-term survival is good with median survival up to fourth and fifth decades of life.

CONGENITAL DYSERYTHROPOIETIC ANEMIA

Congenital dyserythropoietic anemia (CDA) is a group of disorders characterized by ineffective erythropoiesis and specific bone marrow abnormalities (increased multi-nucleated red cell precursors). There are four major types of CDA: Type I, type II, type III and type IV.

Clinical features These include chronic mild anemia, hepatosplenomegaly, mild jaundice, and hemochromatosis.

Laboratory investigations There is mild to severe anemia with macrocytic/normocytic RBCs with reticulocyte count ranging from 1 to 5%. Bone marrow reveals megaloblastoid or bi-/multinucleated normoblasts. Bone marrow iron may be increased. Red cell lifespan is reduced.

Treatment Repeated blood transfusions are needed to treat the anemia. Splenectomy may be needed in severe cases. Desferrioxamine may be useful to treat iron overload. HSCT is the specific treatment.

SHWACHMAN-DIAMOND SYNDROME

This autosomal recessive syndrome is characterized by anemia and steatorrhea due to fatty infiltration of the pancreas. Bone marrow aplasia manifests towards the

Case Study	Aplastic Anemia

A 10-year-old girl was brought to the emergency department with complaints of fever of one month, and passing black-colored stools for five days. The mother also noticed that the child had been pale, listless and was tired easily for the past one month. Examination revealed severe pallor, ecchymotic patches over body, with no lymphadenopathy or bony tenderness. There was no hepatosplenomegaly. Laboratory examination revealed: Hemoglobin 3.2 g/dL, total leukocyte count 2,300 cells/mm³, platelet count 20,000/mm³. Peripheral smear showed macrocytic RBCs, leucopenia and thrombocytopenia.

What is the differential diagnosis?
The following possibilities need to be considered in a child presenting with pancytopenia without hepatosplenomegaly or lymphadenopathy: Aplastic anemia, megaloblastic anemia, paroxysmal nocturnal hemoglobinuria (PNH), and autoimmune disorders. A bone marrow biopsy is needed to distinguish aplastic anemia from megaloblastic anemia. Additionally, ham test or sucrose hydrolysis test and flow cytometry can be done to evaluate for PNH. Other tests include liver function tests, serology for hepatitis/HIV, reticulocyte count, anti-neutrophil antibody, and Coombs test. Acquired aplastic anemia must be distinguished from inherited bone marrow failure syndromes by doing a chromosome breakage study (preferably at least a few weeks after blood transfusion). Transient bone marrow suppression can occur following viral illnesses but mostly will recover spontaneously.

second half of first decade with anemia and infections secondary to neutropenia. Majority of the children have short stature. Apart from neutropenia, immune deficiency and neutrophilic dysfunction also coexist. Delayed skeletal maturation and metaphyseal dysplasia are frequently observed.

Treatment includes enzyme replacement and fat-soluble vitamin supplementation. Bone marrow aplasia can be cured by HSCT. Severe neutropenia responds to G-CSF.

DYSKERATOSIS CONGENITA

This X-linked recessive disorder is a rare form of ectodermal dysplasia, cutaneous hyperpigmentation of face, neck, shoulders and short stature, along with pancytopenia, without skeletal or renal lesions. Nails are dystrophic and there is early loss of teeth. HSCT is the treatment of choice and androgens and steroids have limited role.

 Revision Point

Bone Marrow Failure

1. Bone marrow failure is a disorder of the hematopoietic stem cell. It may present as single cytopenia, bicytopenia, or pancytopenia.

2. Common mechanisms of bone marrow failure include damage to the hematopoietic stem cells (hypoplastic or aplastic bone marrow), hematopoietic cell maturation defects (megaloblastic anemia), and hematopoietic cell differentiation defects (eg, myelodysplasia, congenital dyserythropoietic anemia).

3. Pancytopenia in the peripheral blood picture is not synonymous with aplastic anemia. Bone marrow examination is warranted in every case of pancytopenia to exclude other causes like hypersplenism, infections, leukemia, etc.

4. Aplastic anemia should be considered in a child presenting with pancytopenia without hepatosplenomegaly or lymphadenopathy. The diagnostic criteria for aplastic anemia include hypocellular bone marrow with no abnormal cells and no fibrosis, and at least 2 among the following: Hb <10 g/dL, platelet count <50 × 10⁹/L, and absolute neutrophil count <1.5 × 10⁹/L.

5. Treatment of aplastic anemia includes adequate supportive care (blood transfusion, treatment of infections), and definite treatment (hematopoietic stem cell transplant, immunotherapy). Anabolic steroids and androgens have a role to play in treatment of inherited aplastic anemia.

Barone A, Lucarelli A, Onofrillo D, et al. Marrow Failure Study Group of the Pediatric Haemato-Oncology Italian Association. Diagnosis and management of acquired aplastic anemia in childhood. Guidelines from the Marrow Failure Study Group of the Pediatric Haemato-Oncology Italian Association (AIEOP). *Blood Cells Mol Dis.* 2015;55:40–7.

Guinan EC, Shimammura A. Acquired and inherited aplastic anemia syndromes. In: Greer JP, Foester J, Rodgers GM, Paraskevas F, Glader B. Wintrobe's Clinical Hematology, 11th edition. Philadelphia: Lippincott Williams & Wilkins; 2004. p.1397–1438.

Korthof ET, Békássy AN, Hussein AA. Management of acquired aplastic anemia in children. *Bone Marrow Transplant.* 2013;48:191–5.

Marsh JC, Ball SE, Cavenagh J, et al. British Committee for Standards in Haematology. Guidelines for the diagnosis and management of aplastic anaemia. *Br J Haematol.* 2009;147:43–70.

Niemeyer CM, Baumann I. Classification of childhood aplastic anemia and myelodysplastic syndrome. Hematology *Am Soc Hematol Educ Program.* 2011;2011:84–89.

8.4 IRON DEFICIENCY ANEMIA

Nutritional deficiency of iron is the most common cause of anemia in children. The most vulnerable age is 6 to 24 months. The rapid growth seen in children increases the demand of iron substantially for hemoglobin synthesis and any deficiency in the diet leads to anemia.

Apart from nutritional deficiency, other factors that may lead to iron deficiency anemia (IDA) are (i) poor iron body stores at birth as seen in preterm infants and due to iron deficiency in the mother; (ii) worm infestations; and (iii) impaired absorption from intestine as seen in celiac disease. IDA may also be seen in children from good socioeconomic strata due to food fads and unhealthy eating practices. Excessive phytates in diet can impair iron absorption. Chronic blood loss due to peptic ulcer, Meckel diverticulum, gastrointestinal polyps or hemangiomas, and irritable bowel disease can also cause of iron deficiency. In infants, cow milk allergy may lead to occult gastrointestinal blood loss. In developing countries, infestation with hookworm, *Trichuris trichiura*, *Plasmodium* parasite, and *H. pylori* can contribute to blood loss.

In the initial stages of iron deficiency, the body stores of iron are mobilized for hemoglobin synthesis. When the stores are all used up, the hemoglobin synthesis is decreased, and the affected child becomes pale and symptomatic.

IRON METABOLISM

Stores

Iron is present in the body in 3 forms: Hemoglobin, plasma iron, and tissue iron. Hemoglobin iron constitutes a major part of body iron which gets released into plasma when the RBCs get lysed. The plasma iron is reutilized for synthesis of hemoglobin. The tissue iron is present as ferritin and hemosiderin in liver, spleen, and bone marrow; and myoglobin in muscles and cellular enzymes. Of the available storage forms, ferritin is normally predominant.

Serum ferritin levels vary with age and sex and body iron stores. It may be falsely elevated in conditions like infection, inflammation, malignancy and liver disease even in the presence of iron deficiency. Iron, when absorbed by the mucosal cells, binds to form ferritin which is released as and when required into the plasma. This ferritin stored in the mucosal cells gets excreted when the mucosal cells are exfoliated once in 2–3 days.

Transport

Iron is carried from the intestines to the tissue stores, from storage sites to bone marrow, and from one storage site to another with the help of transferrin. The transferrin present in the serum can bind to a maximum of 40–80 mol/L of iron. This is known as the total iron binding capacity (TIBC).

Percentage of total transferrin present in the serum to which iron is bound is called percentage saturation of transferrin. Under normal conditions, 33% of transferrin is bound to iron and rest is free.

Transferrin carries iron to the site of storage as well as utilization. When it reaches the desired site, transferrin attaches itself to the transferrin receptors and iron is released into the cells.

Absorption

Absorption of iron mainly takes place in the duodenum and the proximal jejunum. This mechanism can be up or down regulated through a feedback system depending upon the iron stores. Iron is best absorbed when taken on an empty stomach with water or fruit juice about one hour before or 2 hours after meals. The bioavailability of iron through normal diet is 10%. Phytates in diet interfere with absorption of dietary iron. The body absorbs iron from animal sources (such as meats), ie, heme iron, better than iron from plant sources, ie, non-heme iron.

Requirements

1 mg/day of iron should be absorbed by the body to meet the physiological demands of iron. Since, only 10% of dietary iron is ultimately absorbed, 10–15 mg/day iron is needed.

Causes of Iron Deficiency

Iron deficiency results whenever there is an imbalance between supply and demand. Three major reasons for a negative balance are (i) increased physiological demands of iron; (ii) pathological blood loss; and (iii) inadequate intake of iron. Main reasons are given below:

1. *Decreased intake*
2. *Increased demand* Prematurity, twins, multiple gestation, infancy, adolescence, cyanotic congenital heart disease.
3. *Chronic blood loss* Worm infestation (hookworm, *Trichuris trichiura*), *Plasmodium* infections, esophageal varices, cow's milk protein intolerance, hemorrhoids, rectal polyp, and peptic ulcer.
4. *Impaired absorption* Celiac disease, inflammatory bowel disease, post-gastrectomy, and severe prolonged diarrhea impair iron absorption. Intake of large amounts of antacids or a diet rich in phytates also decrease absorption of dietary iron. Large amounts of tea or coffee consumed with a meal (the polyphenols bind the iron) can impair absorption of iron.

Increased Demand

A child born with normal iron stores (200–300 mg at birth) can meet the increased physiological demand till 4–6 months of age. Iron deficiency results, if the body stores are poor at the time of birth because of prematurity, low birth weight, or perinatal hemorrhage from cord, fetofetal, or fetomaternal hemorrhage. Children have higher growth rates and so demand is always high and they are at risk of iron deficiency anemia especially during later half of infancy till 24 months or by 6–8 weeks of age in a premature baby. Adolescent girls are especially prone to IDA due to adolescent growth spurt (increased demand) and menstrual losses (chronic blood loss).

Inadequate Intake

It is the commonest cause of IDA especially in developing countries like India. Inappropriate dietary practices result in a negative iron balance. Babies who remain on predominant milk diet are prone to IDA. Breastmilk as well as cow milk, are poor sources of dietary iron (1 mg/L). Though, bioavailability of breastmilk iron is 2–3 times more than that from cow milk, both are inadequate to meet the nutritional dietary needs of the body. Infants in whom appropriate complementary feeding is not started by 6 months age, may develop iron deficiency.

Chronic Blood Loss

It also causes depletion of the body iron stores, eg, abnormal bleeding from gut as in worm infestation, esophageal varices, hemorrhoids, cow milk protein intolerance, and Meckel diverticulum.

CLINICAL FEATURES

The manifestations are insidious in onset. The child may stop eating well, becomes irritable, gets tired easily and becomes lethargic. There is failure to thrive. Pallor and paleness of body gradually increases in severity. If the pallor is not severe, the parents may not notice paleness of the body at all. There may be other associated signs of malnutrition and vitamin deficiencies. The child may just lose interest in studies or the school performance may go down. Some children with iron deficiency anemia have a history of pica (craving for non-edible things like chalk, mud, paper, etc.) and pagophagia (desire to eat ice). There may be history of dyspnea on exertion.

On examination, the most striking finding is pallor of varying degree. Iron deficiency leads to certain epithelial tissue changes especially if deficiency is long standing. The fingernails become thin, brittle and lusterless and flat (platynychia) or even spoon shaped (koilonychias, Fig. 8.7). There is atrophy of the tongue papillae resulting in a smooth looking tongue. Tachycardia may be present along with

cardiomegaly and a functional systolic murmur due to hyperdynamic circulation. If the child is in congestive cardiac failure; pedal edema, increased jugular venous pressure, congestive hepatomegaly, and basal crepitations in the chest can be documented.

The nutritional status of the child may vary. In India, most of these children are malnourished with multivitamin deficiency. But the nutritional status may be normal or some children may even be obese.

LABORATORY FINDINGS

1. *Assessment for type and severity of anemia* A peripheral smear will show microcytic and hypochromic anemia when the hemoglobin level is below 10 g/dL (Fig. 8.8). Red blood cell indices can confirm this; MCV <83 fL, MCH <27 pg, MCHC <30%. Other cells lines are usually not affected. Thrombocytosis is frequently seen in IDA, though severe IDA is associated with thrombocytopenia.

2. *Assessment of iron status* Serum iron, serum ferritin, and percent saturation of transferrin, are reduced to <10 μmol/L, <12 ng/mL, and <16%, respectively. Total iron binding capacity (TIBC) and free erythroid porphyrin (FEP) on the contrary increase (TIBC >350 μg/dL, FEP >40 mg/dL,) as now more transferrin and porphyrin are free.

The sequence of events is usually as follows: Decreased serum ferritin → decreased serum iron → decreased % saturation of transferring → increased TIBC → increased FEP → microcytic hypochromic anemia → increased red cell distribution width (RDW).

DIFFERENTIAL DIAGNOSIS

Although microcytic hypochromic anemia is usually caused by iron deficiency anemia, several other conditions may have similar peripheral blood picture. The most common alternative causes include α- and β-thalassemia and hemoglobinopathies, including hemoglobin E and C.

- Iron studies and red cell distribution width are normal in microcytic hypochromic anemia secondary to thalassemia trait.
- The anemia of chronic disease is usually normocytic but can be microcytic sometimes.

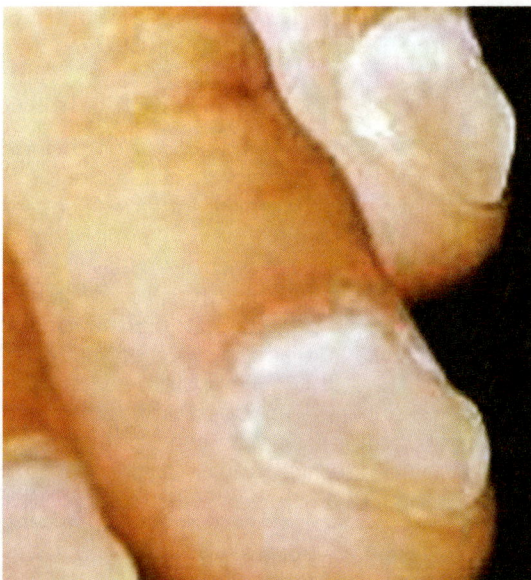

Fig. 8.7 Koilonychia seen in iron deficiency anemia

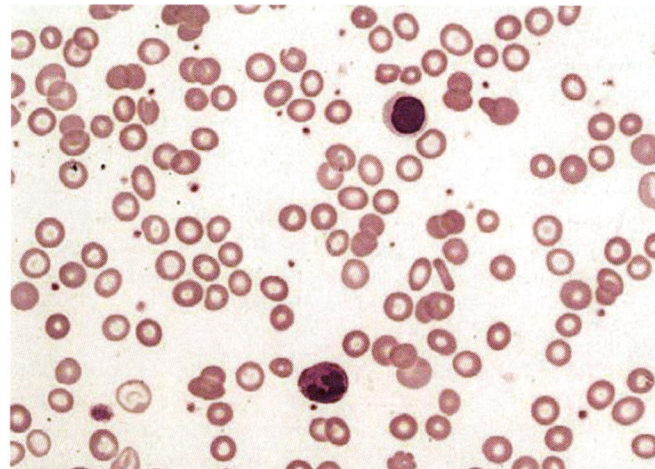

Fig. 8.8 Peripheral smear showing microcytic hypochromic RBCs in a child with iron deficiency anemia

8

- Serum iron is also low in anemia of chronic diseases, but associated with normal or increased serum ferritin, and decreased total iron binding capacity.
- Lead poisoning can also cause microcytic anemia, but more commonly IDA leads to pica which results in lead intoxication.
- Other disorders associated with microcytic anemia include: Sickle cell thalassemia, hemoglobin SC disease, lead poisoning, chronic infections, copper deficiency, hereditary orotic aciduria, sideroblastic anemia, malignancy, hypo- or atransferrinemia, and congenital defect of iron transport to red cells.

Treatment	Iron Deficiency Anemia

1. Iron supplementation

Oral iron supplementation is administered at the dose of 3–6 mg/kg/day of elemental iron. The expected rise in the hemoglobin is 1.5 g/dL/week. To achieve best results, iron preparations should be given on empty stomach.

The elemental iron content in the various chemical oral iron preparations commonly available is: Ferrous fumarate (33%), ferrous lactate (19%), anhydrous ferrous sulfate (37%), exsiccated ferrous sulfate (30%), ferrous carbonate (16%), ferrous succinate (23%), ferrous gluconate (12%) and ferric ammonium citrate (15.5%). Ferric compounds should be avoided as these are heavily chelated and so poorly absorbed.

The intake of oral iron is associated with side effects like metallic taste, constipation or loose stools, nausea, vomiting, staining of teeth, and dark-colored stools. Ferrous sulfate has the best iron absorption but the incidence of gastrointestinal side-effects is greater compared to other iron preparations like ferrous fumarate, ferrous lactate and ferrous glucobionate. Simultaneous intake of vitamin C enhances iron absorption, when given empty stomach or in between meals. The phytates in cereals and phosphates in milk impair iron absorption. The supplementation should continue for at least 8 weeks after the hemoglobin levels have returned to normal to replenish the depleted body stores.

The first sign of improvement is an increase in the activity and appetite. A rise in the reticulocyte count indicating the bone marrow response can be demonstrated after 2–3 days of supplementation; it peaks at day 5–7 of therapy. A rise of hemoglobin is seen by the end of the first week. The iron stores are replenished after 2–3 months of therapy.

Failure of response should be investigated by looking for following causes: (i) inadequate dose; (ii) poor compliance; (iii) malabsorption; (iv) wrong diagnosis; (v) continuing blood loss especially occult gastrointestinal bleeding; (vi) concurrent folate or vitamin B_{12} deficiency, and (vii) concurrent infection.

2. Blood transfusion

Transfusion of packed red blood cells is needed if the anemia is severe (Hb <4 g/dL), or the child is in congestive cardiac failure, or there is associated superimposed severe infection which can interfere with the response to supplementation.

3. Diet

Apart from therapeutic interventions the child's diet needs to be modified. Diet rich in iron should be advised. Sources rich in iron include animal products liver, meat, egg yolk, green vegetables, and fruits. Jaggery is rich in iron. Cooking food in iron utensils can increase the iron content of the food. Milk is a poor source of iron. Inhibitors of iron absorption like phytates

(vegetarian diet), phosphates and tea should be restricted in diet, while vitamin C which facilitates iron absorption should be included.

4. Identity and treat the underlying cause

Hookworm infestation, chronic infection, or celiac disease, or any other underlying cause of anemia needs to be treated.

PREVENTION

To prevent IDA, supplementary foods rich in iron should be initiated as soon as complementary feeding is started, preferably at 6 months of age. Pulses, green leafy vegetables and beans must be included in diet. Vulnerable groups like preterm low birth weight infants need to be supplemented with iron in a dose of 2–4 mg/kg/day starting from 4 to 6 weeks age. Diet of girls attaining menarche should be fortified with iron. Iron supplements are also necessary during adolescence for preventing anemia of puberty. Hookworm infestation should be curbed by regularly deworming children every 6 months and by encouraging them to not walk bare feet.

Weekly Iron and Folic Acid (IFA) Supplementation (WIFS) Program

Government of India has implemented the Weekly Iron and Folic Acid Supplementation (WIFS) program since January 2013, under the National Rural Health Mission (NRHM) in government/ aided and municipal schools (nationwide) and aaganwadi centers across all states in India to combat anemia amongst adolescents. Weekly prophylactic supplementation of iron is as effective as daily supplementation.

Iron Fortification

The Government of India is implementing fortification of common salt with iron to control IDA in community. The National Institute of Nutrition has successfully fortified the common salt with iron (ferrous sulfate: 3.2 g, sodium acid sulfate: 5 g, orthophosphoric acid: 3.2 g in one kg of common salt).

 Revision Point

Iron Deficiency Anemia (IDA)

1. Nutritional deficiency of iron is the most common cause of anemia in children.
2. A child with IDA manifests with pallor, nail changes like koilonychias and platynychia, bald tongue, pica, and irritability. Laboratory diagnosis includes presence of microcytic hypochromic RBCs on peripheral smear with low reticulocyte count and raised RDW. Serum iron, serum ferritin, and percent saturation of transferrin, are reduced to <10 µmol/L, <12 ng/mL, and <16%, respectively. TIBC is increased (>350 µg/dL).
3. Common differential diagnosis of microcytic hypochromic anemia includes IDA, thalassemia trait, hemoglobinopathies, sideroblastic anemia, copper deficiency, and anemia of chronic disease.
4. Treatment of IDA includes deforming, oral iron supplementation and dietary modification (dietary sources of iron include animal products liver, meat, egg yolk, green vegetables, fruits, and jaggery).

Lokeshwar MR, Mehta M, Mehta N, Shelke P, Babar N. Prevention of iron deficiency anemia (IDA): How far have we reached? *Indian J Pediatr.* 2011;78:593–602.

Zimmerman MB, Hurrell RF. Nutritional iron deficiency. *Lancet.* 2007;370:511–20.

8.5 MEGALOBLASTIC ANEMIA

Megaloblastic anemia is characterized by ineffective erythropoiesis associated with macrocytic anemia (MCV >97 fL) in the peripheral smear and megaloblasts in the bone marrow. Deficiency of vitamin B_{12} and folic acid are the most common causes in children. Deficiency of vitamin B_{12} and/or folic acid results in defective DNA synthesis leading to cytological and functional abnormalities in peripheral blood and bone marrow.

Megaloblasts are abnormal nucleated red blood cell precursors, which are larger than normal. They result in abnormal mature red blood cells, which are also larger in size known as macrocytes (Fig. 8.9). There is an asynchrony between nuclear and cytoplasmic maturation. The nuclear maturation is delayed. There is an increased erythrocyte production but early cell death. The maturation of myeloid and platelet precursors is also affected. There is an associated thrombocytopenia and leukopenia. Neutrophils are characteristically hyperlobated (>5 lobes).

ETIOLOGY OF MEGALOBLASTOSIS

i. Vitamin B_{12} deficiency
ii. Folate deficiency
iii. *Disorders of DNA synthesis*
  - *Congenital* Orotic aciduria, thiamine-responsive megaloblastic anemia, congenital familial megaloblastic anemia, congenital dyserythropoietic anemia, Lesch-Nyhan syndrome.
  - *Acquired* Liver disease, sideroblastic anemia, leukemia, aplastic anemia, DiGuglielmo disease, and refractory megaloblastic anemia.
iv. *Drug-induced* Methotrexate, 6-mercaptopurine, azathioprine, thioguanine, 5-fluorouracil, valproate, lithium, pyrazinamide, cytosine arabinoside, hydroxyurea, phenytoin, and nitrous oxide.

A. Vitamin B_{12} Deficiency

Vitamin B_{12} (cobalamin/extrinsic factor) acts as a cell coenzyme in chemical reactions affecting the synthesis of DNA and plays a crucial role in cell metabolism. Humans obtain vitamin B_{12} third hand, either by eating animals that have ingested the bacteria that synthesize cobalamin or by eating animal products like milk, cheese, and eggs. Cobalamin binds to the intrinsic factor derived from parietal cells and this complex is endocytosed by the ileal cells after which it is further activated to methylcobalamin and adenosylcobalamin.

The recommended daily allowance of vitamin B_{12} is 1–2 μg. It plays a significant role in hematopoiesis and maintenance of the integrity of nervous system.

- Foods rich in vitamin B_{12} are mostly of animal origin, eg, meat, heart, liver, kidney and eggs. A little amount is present in milk and cheese.

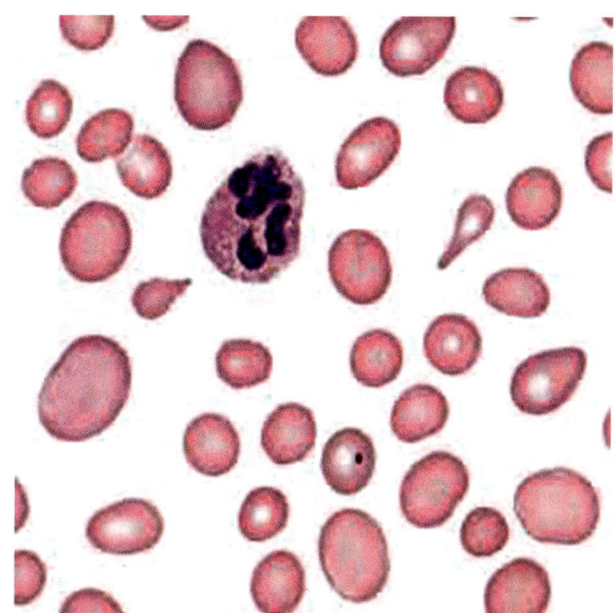

Fig. 8.9 Macrocytic RBCs in peripheral blood smear from a child with megaloblastic anemia

- Vitamin B_{12} is absorbed effectively in the stomach and to a lesser extent in the small intestine.
- Vitamin B_{12} is largely stored in the liver in the form of adenosylcobalamin.

Causes of Vitamin B_{12} Deficiency

1. *Inadequate dietary intake (<1 mg/day)* Nutritional deficiency is the most common cause of vitamin B_{12} deficiency. Vegetarians and malnutrition are commonly associated with vitamin B_{12} deficiency.
2. *Defective vitamin B_{12} absorption*
   - Failure to secrete intrinsic factor: Pernicious anemia (intrinsic factor deficiency), gastric mucosal disease (post-gastrectomy, corrosives).
   - Failure of intestinal absorption (malabsorption syndromes), abnormal intrinsic factor, abnormal ileal uptake, ingestion of EDTA and phytates, small-bowel bacterial overgrowth, *Diphyllobothrium latum* infestation
3. *Defective B_{12} transport* Deficiency of transcobalamin I and II.
4. *Disorders of vitamin B_{12} metabolism* Specific inability to form adenosylcobalamin (vitamin B_{12} responsive methylmalonic aciduria), defect in methylmalonyl CoA mutase apoenzyme (vitamin B_{12} non-responsive methylmalonic aciduria), failure to form both adenosylcobalamin and methylcobalamin (methylmalonic aciduria), abnormality of N5-methyltetrahydrofolate homocysteine methyltransferase apoenzyme.

B. Folic Acid Deficiency

Folic acid also plays a crucial role in cellular metabolism. But contrary to vitamin B_{12}, it is present in abundance in plants. Rich sources are liver, kidneys, and green leafy vegetables. The vitamin gets destroyed on cooking or heating (boiling can lead to 40% loss of dietary folate). Milk is not a good source of folic acid. Goat milk is particularly deficient in folate. Inadequate intake is the commonest cause of folic acid

8

deficiency. Folic acid is a labile vitamin and gets destroyed during cooking. The absorption of folic acid occurs throughout the small intestine. Recommended daily allowance of folic acid is 100–250 µg/day.

Absorption of folic acid can be impaired in chronic diarrhea, celiac disease, and anticonvulsant therapy with phenytoin and phenobarbitone. Methotrexate, pyrimethamine, and trimethoprim also have antifolic acid activity. Secondary folic acid deficiency can be precipitated by increased demand as in hemolytic anemia, inflammatory diseases, leukemia, and lymphoma.

The metabolism of folate and vitamin B_{12} is interlinked. Folate and vitamin B_{12} are involved in the DNA synthesis and in addition vitamin B_{12} has a role in myelin synthesis, hence a deficiency of vitamin B_{12} also produces neurological manifestations in addition to features of macrocytic anemia.

Clinical Manifestations

The deficiency is mostly seen in children <5 years of age with median age of presentation being 1.5 to 2 years. Inadequate dietary intake is the most common cause because of vegetarian and predominantly milk-based diet in young children, both of which are poor in vitamin B_{12} and folic acid.

The clinical features of vitamin B_{12} and folate deficiency are identical, difference being in the neurological dysfunction, which occurs with vitamin B_{12} deficiency. Folate deficiency has a rapid evolution (weeks or months) and is usually associated with signs of other vitamin deficiencies. Vitamin B_{12} has a slow onset (years) and is usually a purer deficiency state because of the usual specificity of cobalamin malabsorption. The most important clinical finding is anemia with its associated symptoms. Some children have a characteristic hyperpigmentation of the hands, feet, or face, and presence of glossitis (beefy red tongue). Vitamin B_{12} deficiency also leads to peripheral neuropathy, and subacute combined degeneration of spinal cord. These children can present with neurological symptoms such as paresthesias, sensory deficits, hypotonia, seizures, and developmental delay. Neurological features may present without any anemia.

DIAGNOSIS

Peripheral Smear

The red blood cells are macrocytic (Fig. 8.9) and normochromic. This may be associated with presence of hypersegmented neutrophils (>5 lobes) (Fig. 8.10). There may also be associated neutropenia and thrombocytopenia, which are usually symptomless. Reticulocyte count is decreased. Howell-Jolly bodies may be seen (Fig. 8.11).

Macrocytic anemia of vitamin B_{12} and folic acid deficiency is characterized by increased red cell width (RDW). A normal RDW should alert to other causes of macrocytic anemia; such as hemolytic anemia, post-hemorrhagic anemia, acute leukemia, aplastic anemia, liver disease, bone marrow infiltration, and hypothyroidism.

Bone Marrow

The marrow smear demonstrates megaloblastic changes in all the stages of red cells (Fig. 8.12). The marrow is hypercellular with erythroid hyperplasia and M:E ratio of

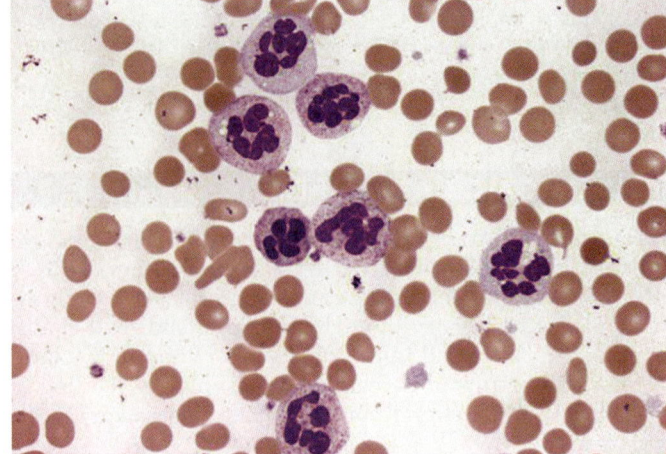

Fig. 8.10 Hypersegmented neutrophils in peripheral blood smear of megaloblastic anemia

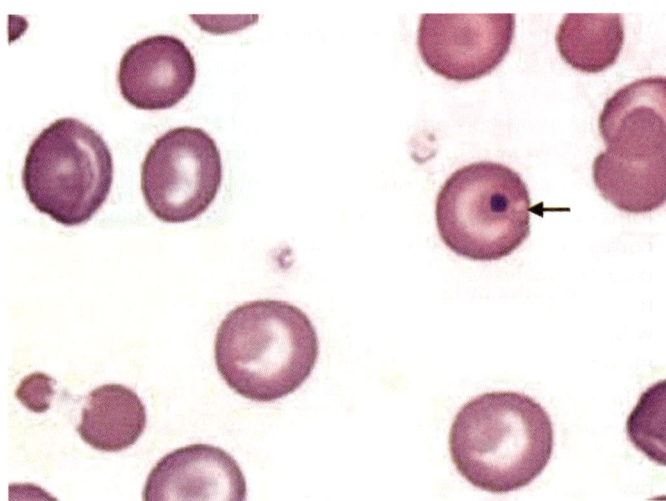

Fig. 8.11 Howell-Jolly bodies

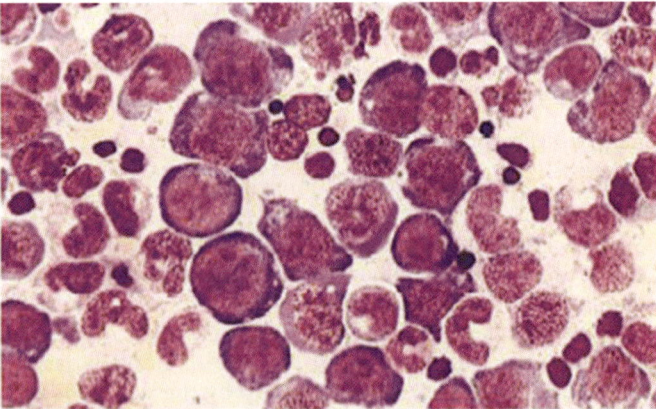

Fig. 8.12 Megaloblastic red cell precursors in bone marrow

1:1. The leukocyte precursors are also abnormal and large in size. Macrocytosis is not synonymous with megaloblastosis. Macrocytic anemia with a normoblastic marrow is suggestive of other causes of macrocytosis, as outlined above.

Serum Levels

Serum levels of folic acid and vitamin B_{12} can be assessed to confirm the deficiency. Normal levels of folic acid are 5–20 ng/mL. Red cell folate level (74–640 ng/mL) is a better indicator of the folate stores and it is decreased in case of megaloblastic anemia due to folate deficiency. Serum B_{12} levels < 200 pg/mL are suggestive of cobalamin deficiency.

Schilling Urinary Excretion Test

Where vitamin B_{12} deficiency is suspected to be due to intrinsic factor deficiency (pernicious anemia) or intestinal malabsorption of vitamin B_{12}, Schilling urinary excretion test should be performed. Following an overnight fast, 1000 µg of non-radioactive vitamin B_{12} is given intramuscularly to saturate the B_{12}-binding sites. Thereafter, 0.5–2 µg of radioactive vitamin B_{12} is given orally. The urine passed thereafter is collected for the next 24 hours. Normal subjects excrete 10–35% of the administered dose; those with vitamin B_{12} deficiency due to lack of intrinsic factor or intestinal malabsorption excrete less than 3%.

Treatment — Megaloblastic Anemia

Folic acid is orally supplemented in the dose of 0.5–1 mg/day for at least 4–6 weeks followed by 0.5 mg/day. Vitamin B_{12} is supplemented in doses of 0.1–1 mg/day orally or parenterally for 2 weeks followed by 0.1–0.2mg/dose every month till correction of anemia. In case of neurological manifestations or doubtful absorption, parenteral administration of vitamin B_{12} is recommended. In case of pernicious anemia, lifelong treatment with parenteral vitamin B_{12} administered monthly (1 mg intramuscular) is needed. Dietary advice is important apart from supplementation.

Response to treatment in vitamin B_{12} deficiency
Administration of either vitamin B_{12} or folate influences manifestations of vitamin B_{12} deficiency. Symptoms improve within a day with a sense of well-being. However, administration of folate alone is dangerous in cases of vitamin B_{12} deficiency resulting in megaloblastic anemia as the neurological manifestations do not improve but in fact may worsen. Vitamin B_{12} administration results in the reversion of erythropoiesis to normoblastic from megaloblastic, glossitis heal, and neurological symptoms improve.

Response to treatment in folate deficiency
Folate deficiency responds completely to folic acid administration. Vitamin B_{12} may cause partial remission of anemia.

Symptomatic and supportive treatment
Blood transfusions may be needed to tide over initial crisis if the patient is in congestive heart failure. Other conditions like achlorhydria and fish tapeworm infestation may need specific management. Celiac sprue may need gluten-free diet apart from vitamin replacement. Broad spectrum antibiotics may be needed in tropical sprue.

Follow-up

It is needed to detect relapse or development of gastric carcinoma or intestinal lymphoma.

Chandra J. Megaloblastic anemia: Back in focus. *Indian J Pediatr.* 2010;77:795–9.

A 5-year-old boy was brought to the outpatient department by his mother. She noticed that the child had been listless and tired easily for the past 3 months. She also noticed that the child had been complaining of perianal itching and has passed small worms in his stools on several occasions. Dietary history of the child revealed that he was a vegetarian. He consumed about half a liter of cow's milk everyday. Examination revealed moderate pallor with no lymphadenopathy. The child's weight was 15 kg and height was 111 cm. Other systemic examination was non-contributory.

Laboratory examination revealed: Hemoglobin 9 g/dL, total leucocyte count 4,300 cells/mm³, platelet count 200,000/mm³. Peripheral smear showed hypochromic red blood cells with presence of both microcytes and macrocytes. Stool microscopy showed ova of hookworm. The child was started on oral iron preparation at 15 mg/day. After 3 months of treatment, the child showed no clinical improvement.

What is the diagnosis?
The child is suffering from "Dimorphic anemia with hookworm infestation". The presence of both microcytes and macrocytes on the peripheral smear was suggestive of dimorphic anemia due to combined deficiency of iron and folic acid in diet. The child was a vegetarian and had been consuming mainly cow milk which is a poor source of iron, vitamin B_{12}, and folic acid. High concentration of phytates, calcium salts and fiber in vegetarian diet also leads to impaired absorption of dietary iron. Hookworm infestation leads to occult blood loss in stools which further predisposes to iron deficiency.

Pallor is the most common sign. Symptoms include lassitude, fatigability, anorexia, and failure to thrive. Mild splenomegaly is seen in only 15% of cases. Bald tongue and koilonychias may be seen in iron deficiency anemia while hyperpigmented extensor surfaces characterize megaloblastic anemia due to vitamin B_{12} or folate deficiency.

What was wrong with his treatment?
The child was misdiagnosed as iron deficiency anemia and started on only iron supplementation. In addition, the dose of iron prescribed was inadequate to treat anemia. Iron should be given in a dose of 3 mg/kg/day for a period of about 3 months instead of 1 mg/kg/day that was prescribed for him in this case. He should have also been given folic acid in a dose of 2–5 mg/d to correct the folate deficiency. In addition at least 1 µg of vitamin B_{12} should be given to ensure adequate hematological response. He should also have been dewormed with antihelminthics to reduce the occult blood loss because of hookworm infestation. Dietary modification in the forming of increasing intake of animal products liver, meat, egg yolk, green vegetables, fruits, and jaggery should be asserted to correct the underlying deficiency of iron. Green leafy vegetables and sprouted pulses can help provide dietary folate.

Chandra J, Jain V, Narayan S, Sharma S, Singh V, Kapoor AK, Batra S. Folate and cobalamin deficiency in megaloblastic anemia in children. *Indian Pediatr.* 2002;39:453–7.

Rosenblatt DS, Whitehead VM. Cobalamin and folate deficiency: acquired and hereditary disorders in children. *Semin Hematol.* 1999;36:19–34.

Whitehead VM. Acquired and inherited disorders of cobalamin and folate in children. *Br J Haematol.* 2006;134:125–36.

Megaloblastic Anemia

1. Megaloblastic anemia is characterized by ineffective erythropoiesis associated with macrocytic anemia (MCV >97 fL) and hypersegmented neutrophils in the peripheral blood smear and megaloblasts in the bone marrow. Deficiency of vitamin B_{12} and folic acid are the most common causes of megaloblastic anemia in children.

2. Vitamin B_{12} deficiency is commonly seen in vegetarians as its sources are mostly of animal origin (eg, meat, heart, liver, kidney and eggs). Pernicious anemia (intrinsic factor deficiency), gastric mucosal disease (post-gastrectomy, corrosives), and malabsorption (eg, small bowel bacterial overgrowth, *Diphyllobothrium latum* infestation) are other common causes of vitamin B_{12} deficiency.

3. Folate deficiency can occur due to over-cooking, poor intestinal absorption (chronic diarrhea, celiac disease), anticonvulsant therapy (phenytoin), drug-induced (methotrexate, pyrimethamine, and trimethoprim) and in conditions with increased demand (eg, hemolytic anemia).

4. Serum levels of folic acid and vitamin B_{12} can be assessed to confirm the deficiency. Normal levels of folic acid are 5–20 ng/mL. Red cell folate level (74–640 ng/mL) is a better indicator of the folate stores and it is decreased in case of megaloblastic anemia due to folate deficiency. Serum B_{12} levels <200 pg/mL are suggestive of cobalamin deficiency.

5. Schilling urinary excretion test can help to diagnose vitamin B_{12} deficiency due to intrinsic factor deficiency (pernicious anemia) or intestinal malabsorption.

6. Clinical manifestations of vitamin B_{12} and folate deficiency are nearly identical (pallor, hyperpigmented extensors, glossitis) except that neurological manifestations are more common with vitamin B_{12} deficiency.

8.6 HEMOLYTIC ANEMIA

All red blood cells are destroyed once their lifespan of 90–120 days is over. But in certain conditions the cells get lysed earlier; the lifespan of RBCs is reduced leading to increased red blood cell destruction (hemolysis). There is compensatory bone marrow hyperplasia, which increases the red cell production manifold to maintain normal hemoglobin levels. Hemolytic anemia results when this bone marrow hyperplasia is unable to keep up the hemoglobin levels to normal.

Bone marrow hyperplasia also leads to increased release of immature red cells in the blood, elevating the reticulocyte count. Erythropoietin-induced erythroid hyperplasia leads to expansion of medullary spaces. Extramedullary erythropoiesis also starts in the liver and spleen leading to hepatosplenomegaly.

Common causes of hemolytic anemia are listed below.

I. Intracorpuscular Defects (within RBC)

1. *Membrane defects* Hereditary spherocytosis, hereditary elliptocytosis, hereditary stomatocytosis.

2. *Hemoglobin defects* Thalassemia, sickle cell anemia, other hemoglobinopathies (HbC, HbD, HbE, HbH, HbM).

3. *Enzyme defects* Glucose-6-phosphate dehydrogenase deficiency, pyruvate kinase deficiency.

4. *Congenital dyserythropoietic anemia (CDA)* Types I–IV.

II. Extracorpuscular Defects (outside RBC)

1. *Immune mechanism* Autoimmune hemolytic anemia, incompatible blood transfusion, hemolytic disease of the newborn and drug-induced.

2. *Non-immune mechanism* Hemolytic uremic syndrome, disseminated intravascular coagulation, and paroxysmal nocturnal hemoglobinuria.

3. *Others* Drug-induced infection (malaria, *Salmonella*, leishmaniasis, clostridial infections, Gram-positive infections), burns, lead poisoning, hypersplenism, Wilson disease, and lead poisoning.

CHARACTERISTICS OF HEMOLYTIC ANEMIA

Peripheral Blood Film

Red cells are microcytic hypochromic in thalassemia; or they can be normocytic and normochromic. The red cell distribution width is normal. There is presence of spherocytes, schistocytes, teardrop cells, and Heinz body formation. Reticulocytosis is prominent with the reticulocyte count increasing to 5–20% against a normal of 0.5 to 2%. Nucleated red blood cells (normoblasts) are also seen commonly in the peripheral blood.

Bone Marrow

It is generally unremarkable except for erythroid hyperplasia. The myeloid erythroid ratio of 3–4:1 reduces to 1:1.

Skeletal Changes

In hereditary hemolytic anemia, the marrow hyperplasia causes bony changes that are evident on an X-ray. Changes are most marked in thalassemia major but less marked in sickle cell disease. There is widening of the diploic spaces with medulla getting less dense and development of trabeculae giving the typical hair-on-end appearance. Widening of the marrow cavity and decreased density of the medulla is evident in tubular bones of the extremities.

Biochemical Evidence of Hemolysis

A mild to moderate rise in unconjugated bilirubin in a child with anemia suggests hemolytic anemia. The excess breakdown of heme leads to increased production of bilirubin; liver is not able to conjugate all this bilirubin and the unconjugated component accumulates in the blood. Absence of jaundice or hyperbilirubinemia does not rule out hemolytic anemia. The levels of hemopexin and haptoglobin, which bind with free heme and hemoglobin respectively, are reduced. Plasma lactate dehydrogenase is moderately elevated.

Evidence of Intravascular Hemolysis

Presence of free hemoglobin and methemoglobin in blood and detection of hemoglobin and hemosiderin in urine indicates intravascular hemolysis which is seen in conditions like incompatible blood transfusion, black water fever, and paroxysmal nocturnal hemoglobinuria.

POINTERS TO THE DIAGNOSIS OF HEMOLYTIC ANEMIA

1. A family history of repeated blood transfusion or death due to severe anemia or gallstones suggests a congenital hemolytic anemia.
2. A long-standing anemia with multiple transfusions suggests a chronic hemolytic anemia.
3. Non-response to iron therapy in a child with microcytic, hypochromic anemia suggests thalassemia minor.
4. Jaundice without dark yellow urine suggests un-conjugated hyperbilirubinemia due to excessive hemolysis.

Case Study	Hemolytic Anemia

A mother brings her 10-month-old girl child to the emergency with increasing pallor and difficulty in feeding for last 1 month. There was no history of fever, swelling over the body, bleeding from any site, or jaundice. The baby had been started on appropriate complementary feeds at 6 months of age. Examination revealed marked pallor, no lymphadenopathy or petechial rash. Systemic examination revealed HR =180/m, RR = ejection systolic murmur over the precordium with marked tachycardia, abdominal examination = liver palpable 5 cm below costal margin with moderate splenomegaly.

Laboratory investigations revealed Hb 3 g/dL, TLC 4500/mm³, platelet count: 500,000/mm³. Peripheral smear showed microcytic hypochromic red cells with target cells and tear drop cells, reticulocyte count 20%. Serum iron 96 µg/dL, TIBC 250 µg/dL. Hemoglobin electrophoresis suggests beta-thalassemia major.

Outline the expected abnormalities on hemoglobin electrophoresis in β-thalassemia.
Beta-thalassemia occurs due to impaired production of beta chains in the hemoglobin. The genes for beta chain production are present on the short arm of chromosome 11. The presence of β thal° gene results in absent beta chains while presence of β thal+ gene results in decreased beta chains. Hemolysis occurs due to imbalance in production of α and β chains. Since β chain synthesis is impaired, the excess of α chains produces α-tetramers which get precipitated in red cells. Hemoglobin electrophoresis reveals raised fetal hemoglobin ($\alpha_2\gamma_2$), and HbA₂ ($\alpha_2\delta_2$) and decreased HbA ($\alpha_2\beta_2$).

What are the major sites of extramedullary hematopoiesis?
The liver and spleen are the chief sites of extramedullary hematopoiesis in children with thalassemia.

Describe in brief the options for chelation therapy in this child.
Deferoxamine (DFX), Deferiprone (DFP), and Deferasirox (ICL-670) are the commonly used iron chelating agents in thalassemia. DFX is administered as continuous subcutaneous infusion in a dose of 25–50 mg/kg/d over a period of 8–12 hours during night using microinfusion pumps (5–6 nights/week). Vitamin C should be administered prior to DFX administration to facilitate iron excretion. DFP is given orally in a dose of 75–100 mg/kg/d in 2–3 divided doses. Deferasirox can be given orally in a daily dose of 20–40 mg/kg. It has a half-life of 8 to 16 hours thereby allowing once a day dosing.

5. A hemolytic facies characterized by frontal bossing, depressed nasal bridge, maxillary prominence, prominent malar eminences and malformed teeth is seen typically in thalassemia (Fig. 8.13).
6. Hepatosplenomegaly is almost universal in children with hemolytic anemia because of the extramedullary hematopoiesis.
7. Platelets and coagulation factors are not affected.
8. *Peripheral smear* RBCs are microcytic and hypochromic in thalassemia; and normocytic or macrocytic and normochromic in acute hemolysis. Hemolysis in peripheral smear is evidenced by presence of tear drop cells, fragmented RBCs, increased number of reticulocytes, nucleated RBCs, and characteristic cell morphology like spherocytes and elliptocytes (Fig. 8.14).
9. Reticulocyte count is increased.
10. Osmotic fragility of RBCs is increased in hereditary spherocytosis, ie, they demonstrate an enhanced tendency

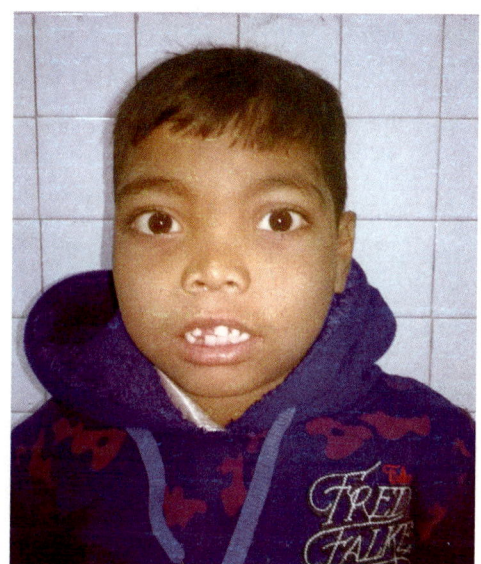

Fig. 8.13 Hemolytic facies

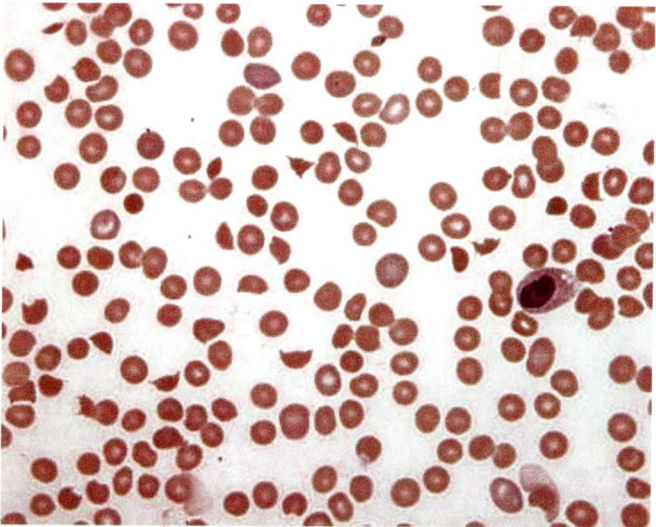

Fig. 8.14 Peripheral blood smear in a child with hemolytic anemia showing spherocytes, helmet cells, and fragmented cells

to lyse in hypotonic saline. The spherocytes swell in presence of hypotonic saline and get lysed more easily than normal biconcave cells. In contrast, in thalassemia, the osmotic fragility of RBCs is decreased.

11. Red cell width (RDW) is normal.
12. *Hemoglobin electrophoresis:* Detects presence of abnormal hemoglobins like HbS, HbH or HbE or variation in different types of hemoglobin, ie, HbA_1, HbA_2 and HbF as in thalassemia.
13. Special investigations like sickling test, G6PD levels, Coombs test, etc. are required according to the disease being suspected.

Laboratory Evidence of Hemolysis

I. Evidence of increased hemoglobin breakdown
  a. Unconjugated hyperbilirubinemia
  b. ↓ Haptoglobin, hemopexin
  c. ↑ Plasma lactate dehydrogenase
II. Evidence of intravascular hemolysis
  a. Hemoglobinemia
  b. Hemoglobinuria
  c. Methemoglobinemia
III. Evidence of erythroid hyperplasia
  a. ↑ Reticulocyte count, nucleated RBCs
  b. M:E ratio changes from 3–4:1 to 1:1
  c. Bone marrow biopsy showing hypercellularity with sheets of erythroid cells.

GENERAL MANAGEMENT

Packed Red Cell Transfusions

Repeated regular packed red cell transfusions are the mainstay of the treatment in most congenital hemolytic anemias. The frequency of transfusion depends upon the severity of the disease. Ideal would be to transfuse irradiated or washed packed cells to minimize the risk of transmission of infection and prevent the development of antibodies against antigen on leukocytes and platelets. Leukocytes can also be filtered out at the time of transfusion by using microfilters. As washing or irradiation of red cells is very expensive and not easily available, leukocytes filters (Fig. 8.15) are commonly used to prevent transfusing WBCs along with RBCs. Leukodepletion is more important in these children because of the need of repeated and lifelong transfusions.

Iron Chelation

Because of excessive continuing hemolysis and repeated transfusions these children are in the state of iron overload which tends to pose problems apart from the existing problem of anemia. The extra iron gets deposited and affects the functioning of heart, liver and endocrine organs. So the proper iron chelation therapy is mandatory in the children with requirement of repeated blood transfusions. This is discussed in detail later in this chapter.

Naegel RL. Hemoglobins: Normal and abnormal. In: Nathan DG, Orkin SH, Ginsburg D, Look AT. Nathan And Oski's Hematology of Infancy and Childhood, 6th edition. Philadelphia: Saunders; 2003, p. 743–89.

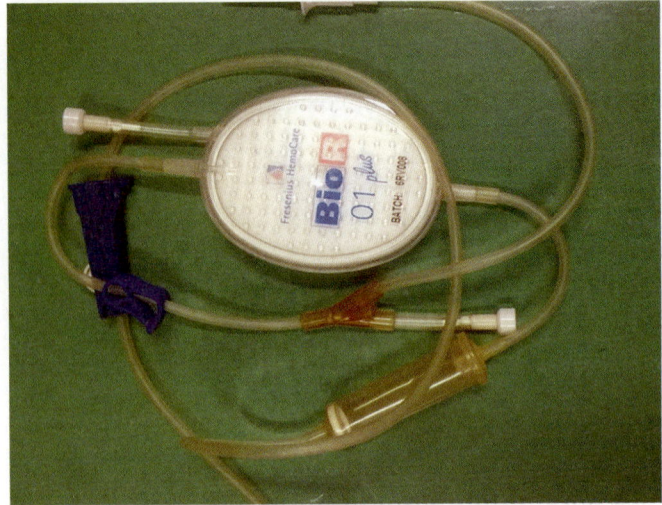

Fig. 8.15 Leukodepleting filters

Revision Point

Hemolytic Anemia

1. Hemolytic anemia is characterized by a reduction in the lifespan of the circulating RBCs (normal red cell lifespan 90–120 days).
2. Bone marrow hyperplasia in hemolytic anemias leads to increased release of immature nucleated RBCs and reticulocytes in peripheral blood. Erythroid hyperplasia leads to expansion of medullary spaces and extramedullary erythropoiesis in the liver and spleen leading to hepatosplenomegaly.
3. Hemolytic anemia may be due to defects in the RBCs (intracorpuscular defects: Hemoglobinopathies, red cell enzyme defects, RBC membrane defects, CDA) or outside the RBCs (extracorpuscular: Immune-mediated, drug-induced infections, metabolic conditions like Wilson disease, DIC, hemolytic uremic syndrome, etc.).
4. Presence of free hemoglobin and methemoglobin in blood and detection of hemoglobin and hemosiderin in urine indicates intravascular hemolysis which is seen in conditions like incompatible blood transfusion, black water fever, and paroxysmal nocturnal hemoglobinuria.
5. Chronic hemolytic anemias are characterized by characteristic hemolytic facies, mild jaundice, hepatosplenomegaly, and history of regular blood transfusions.

Segel SB. Definitions and classification of hemolytic anemia. In: Kliegman RM, Stanton BF, St. Geme JW III, Schor NF, Behrman RE. Nelson Textbook of Pediatrics, 19th edition. Philadelphia: Saunders, Elsevier; 2011, p.1659–83.

8.7 HEMOGLOBIN AND ITS DISORDERS

NORMAL HEMOGLOBIN

Normal hemoglobin (Hb) is a protein consisting of two pairs of polypeptide chains to each of which haem is attached. The different types of hemoglobin differ in the globin chains.

Hemoglobin A (HbA) consists of two alpha (α) and two beta (β) chains and comprises 97% of adult hemoglobin. HbA$_2$ has two alpha and two delta (δ) chains and is the minor hemoglobin; normal values are up to 3.5% in adults. HbF or fetal hemoglobin comprises two α (alpha) and two γ (gamma) chains and is the major hemoglobin in the fetal and neonatal period comprising 70–90% of the total hemoglobin in a term child. It falls rapidly thereafter to 25% at 4 weeks and ~5% at 6 months. HbF is less than 1% in adults. HbA$_2$ is increased in most β-thalassemia traits but decreased in iron deficiency anemia. HbF is elevated in many hemoglobin defects.

DEFECTS OF HEMOGLOBIN

Defects of hemoglobin can be categorized into two groups:
- Hemoglobinopathies in which there is production of structurally abnormal hemoglobin due to abnormalities of the formation of globins moiety, eg, HbS (sickle cell disease), HbC, HbD, or HbE disease.
- Thalassemias in which there is reduced rate of production of normal hemoglobin due to absent or decreased synthesis of the globin chains, eg, α- and β-thalassemia.

Hemoglobinopathies thus refer to qualitative defect of hemoglobin (resulting in abnormal or variant hemoglobin, while thalassemia is a result of quantitative defects of hemoglobin.

Hemoglobinopathies

Abnormal hemoglobin arises due to some genetic defect affecting the synthesis of a specific pair of polypeptide chain. The common abnormal hemoglobins are HbS, HbC, HbE and HbD. These are all β chain variant hemoglobins, in which there is defect in the synthesis of β chains.

Thalassemia

Thalassemias are genetic group of disorders in which there is decreased synthesis of one or more types of polypeptide chains and are autosomal recessive in inheritance. The Hb in which the affected globin and polypeptide chain is incorporated is reduced. α and β are the two main types of globin chains used. Thalassemia can be categorized as (i) α-thalassemia in which production of α chains are reduced, (ii) beta-thalassemia in which β chains are reduced.

Alpha-thalassemia occurs most often in people from Southeast Asia, the Middle East, China, and in those of African descent. Beta-thalassemias occur most often in people of Mediterranean origin. To a lesser extent, Chinese, other Asians, and African Americans can be affected. Thalassemia is one of the commonest genetic hematological disorders in India with over 10,000 children of thalassemia major born each year. It is more common in north-west India. The case rate can be as high as 5–15% in some ethnic groups of north India (*Punjabis, Sindhis*).

8.8 BETA-THALASSEMIA

A genetic mutation leads to decreased rate of synthesis of β chain. The main hemoglobin beyond 6 months of age is adult hemoglobin A (HbA). Therefore, there is a decrease in amount of HbA (α2, β2) in the affected children. A decrease in the β chains triggers a compensatory increase in production of fetal hemoglobin and δ chains. This leads to an increase in HbF (α2, γ2) or HbA$_2$ (α2, δ2). The excess of uncombined α chains results in their accumulation and precipitation to form tetramers (α4) in the RBCs and normoblasts. These intracytoplasmic inclusions lead to increased destruction of normoblasts and RBCs in the marrow, rendering the erythropoiesis as ineffective. As a result, the maturation and function of RBCs is affected and hemolysis occurs.

A complete absence of beta chain synthesis is known as β-thalassemia and an incomplete suppression is known as β^+-thalassemia. Based on the clinical severity, thalassemia is categorized as thalassemia major, minor, and intermedia.

BETA-THALASSEMIA MAJOR (COOLEY ANEMIA)

This is the most severe form of the disease resulting from a complete or major suppression of β chain synthesis. This is a homogenous form of the disease (β^0, β^0).

Clinical Features

Age at Presentation

Newborns with beta-thalassemia major are asymptomatic at birth. The high level of fetal hemoglobin at birth, which does not require the chains, protects these children till 4–6 months of age. The clinical features of thalassemia major start manifesting only after 6 months of age.

Signs and Symptoms

Anemia is the first and most prominent manifestation. There is associated failure to thrive and anorexia. Anemia becomes severe if regular blood transfusions are not given. There is hepatosplenomegaly due to extramedullary hematopoiesis; and spleen progressively increases in size. Mild jaundice may be present. Gradually there is development of typical hemolytic facies.

These children have increased susceptibility to bacterial and viral infections including respiratory tract infections, gastroenteritis, cutaneous abscesses and leg ulcers. Because of the frequent need for blood transfusions, blood-borne infections are a major problem, but the routine screening of

---

Revision Point

Hemoglobin and its Disorders

1. Normal hemoglobin (Hb) is a protein consisting of two pairs of polypeptide chains to each of which haem is attached. The different types of hemoglobin differ in the globin chains. Hemoglobin A (HbA) consists of two alpha (α) and two beta (β) chains, HbA$_2$ has two alpha and two delta (δ) chains, and HbF or fetal hemoglobin comprises two α and two γ (gamma) chains.
2. Normal adult hemoglobin comprises 97% HbA, up to 3.5% HbA$_2$ and <1% HbF. HbA$_2$ is increased in β-thalassemia trait (minor) but decreased in iron deficiency anemia. HbF is elevated in many hemoglobin defects like thalassemia major.
3. Hemoglobinopathies occur when there is production of structurally abnormal hemoglobin molecules due to abnormalities of the formation of globins moiety, eg, HbS (sickle cell disease), HbC, HbD or HbE disease.

blood and blood products for HIV, hepatitis B and hepatitis C has significantly brought down the incidence of these infections. Psychosomatic changes like depression, poor self-esteem, and poor school performance frequently accompany this chronic disease.

Skeletal Changes

Skeletal changes occur due to extramedullary erythropoiesis and include widening of medullary spaces, thinning of cortical bone and resorption of cancellous bone resulting in decreased bone density and rarefaction. The typical hair-on-end appearance on skull radiographs (Fig. 8.16) results from accentuated vertical trabeculae between the inner and outer tables of the skull because of excessive bone marrow hyperplasia. It can be seen by the time the child is 2–3 years of age.

Natural History

These children are transfusion dependent and require packed red cell transfusion every 3–4 weeks. Untreated children may not survive beyond 3–4 years of age. All the complications and manifestations depend on how regular the transfusions are; and how well the child is chelated to prevent the iron overload.

Children on irregular transfusions or those on regular transfusion but poor chelation have more complications. These children usually die in the 2nd decade of life due to cardiac complications. The ongoing endogenous hemolysis as well as repeated red cell transfusions lead to release of excess of iron which gets deposited in heart, liver, kidney, pancreas, and endocrine glands affecting their function. Compromise of cardiac and endocrine functions results in hypothyroidism, gonadal failure, hypoparathyroidism, and diabetes mellitus. There is delayed puberty and bronze discoloration of the skin because of iron overload.

Children who receive regular transfusions and proper chelation therapy have significantly prolonged survival and better quality of life. In the last two decades, with the advent of blood component therapy and improved chelation therapy, thalassemia major has evolved from an invariably fatal genetic disorder into a chronic disease that permits normal or at least prolonged survival.

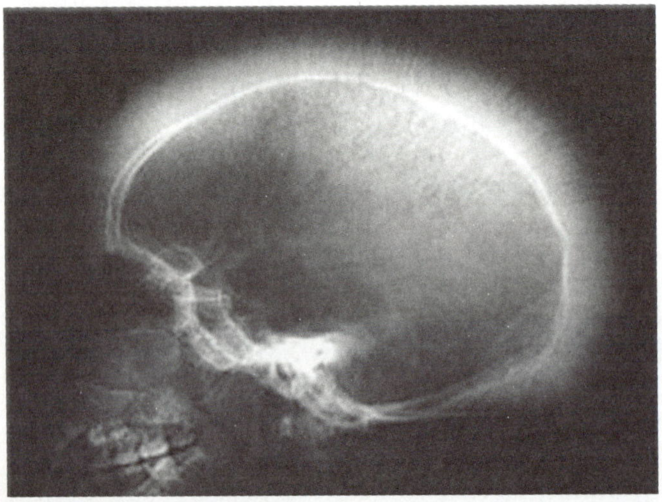

Laboratory Investigations

Peripheral Blood Picture

The RBCs are microcytic and hypochromic with marked anisocytosis and poikilocytosis. Target cells and tear drop cells are seen. Reticulocytes and nucleated RBCs are increased. Heinz bodies, which represent inclusions within RBCs consisting of denatured hemoglobin (Hb), may also be seen in the peripheral blood when stained with supravital stains (bromocresol green or new methylene blue). Howell-Jolly bodies, basophilic nuclear remnants, or remnants of DNA, may be seen in the cytoplasm of RBCs. Granular cytoplasmic inclusion bodies representing the alpha chains are visible in normoblasts or reticulocytes. Pappenheimer bodies, erythrocytic inclusions containing iron that are usually located at the periphery of the cell and stain with Prussian blue, may be seen in multi-transfused thalassemic. The white cells and platelets are normal unless there is hypersplenism which leads to leukopenia and thrombocytopenia.

Bone Marrow

Examination of the bone marrow is usually not indicated in a suspected case of thalassemia. Marrow shows erythroid hyperplasia with a little effect on WBCs and platelets. Staining for iron deposits (Prussian blue staining) reveal increased hemosiderin deposits in bone marrow.

Biochemical Indicators

Serum bilirubin Bilirubin levels are mildly elevated due to hemolysis and production of bilirubin along with compromised function of the liver due to iron deposition.

Indicators of iron overload Serum ferritin levels are raised (normal levels: 10–200 ng/mL). Total iron binding capacity is reduced (normal: 250–400 µg/dL) and % saturation of transferrin is increased (normal: 20–45%).

Hemoglobin electrophoresis Hemoglobin electrophoresis at alkaline pH can enable quantification of HbA_2 and HbF. At birth, HbF is the predominant hemoglobin amounting to 95–98% of the total hemoglobin. HbA_2 amounts to ~2% and adult hemoglobin HbA is in traces **(Table 8.6)**. Hb electrophoresis of the parents may establish them as carriers (raised HbA_2, up to 5%) and thereby provide supportive evidence to diagnose thalassemia in the child. It will also help the parents to plan future pregnancy and plan antenatal diagnosis in case of the next child. Figure 8.17 illustrates the inheritance pattern in beta-thalassemia.

High performance liquid chromatography This technique achieves accurate diagnosis of hemoglobinopathies and thalassemia. It achieves good separation and quantification of HbF and HbA_2.

Treatment	Beta-Thalassemia

1. Packed red blood cell transfusion
Repeated lifelong transfusions are the backbone of the treatment. The aim is to maintain hemoglobin of 10–12 g/dL. Most children

Fig. 8.16 Hair-on-end appearance seen in skull radiographs in chronic hemolytic anemias

Table 8.6 Hemoglobin Electrophoresis Profile of Beta-thalassemia

Type	Hemoglobin (%)		
	HbA	HbA$_2$	HbF
β-thalassemia minor	90–95	3.5–7.0	1–5
β-thalassemia major			
β$^+$	10–90	1–4	10–90
β^0	0	1–2	98

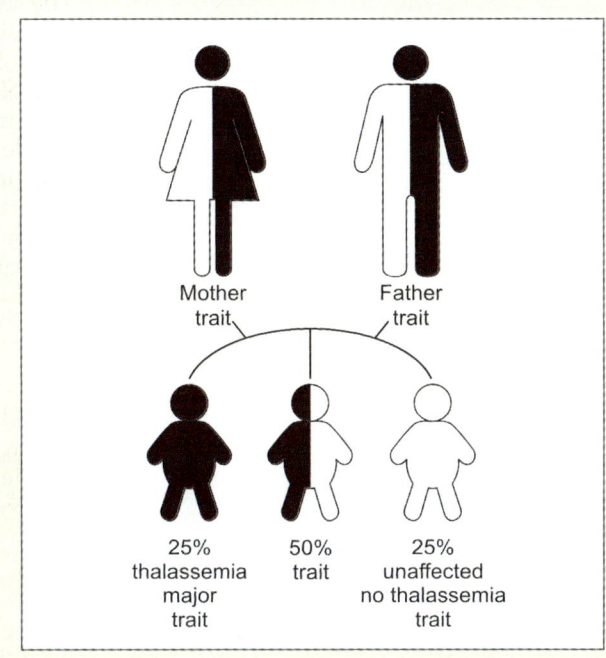

Fig. 8.17 Genetics of beta-thalassemia major

require a transfusion at every 3–4 weeks interval. Ideally, washed RBCS should be transfused to reduce the side effects of transfusion. Otherwise, bedside leukofilters should be used. The main problem of repeated transfusions is risk of transmission of hepatitis B, HIV, hepatitis C infections and iron overload. Increased absorption of iron from gut due to chronic anemia, and ongoing hemolysis both add to the state of iron overload.

2. Chelation therapy

Apart from repeated transfusions to take care of symptoms due to chronic anemia, adequate chelation is essential to prevent transfusion related hemosiderosis. Serum ferritin level is a useful marker for screening and assessing the iron stores but ideal is to measure the iron stores in the liver by doing a liver biopsy.

When to start?

Chelation therapy should be started when serum ferritin levels rise above 1000 ng/mL and hepatic iron concentration exceeds 3.2 mg/g of dry weight. The chelators bind with iron allowing its excretion in urine and stool. All the thalassemic patients on chelators should be periodically monitored for serum ferritin levels and liver biopsy or MRI assessment of iron overload. Serum ferritin levels should be maintained between 1000 and 2000 ng/mL.

Choice of Chelating Agent

- *Deferoxamine* (DFO) It was the first iron chelator used and is very effective but has a disadvantage that it has to be administered subcutaneously with a pump over 10–12 hours, 5–6 days in a week. It is given in a dose of 25–50 mg/kg/day through a microinfusion pump which is strapped to the child's body. This agent is excreted in bile and urine, resulting in red discoloration. It readily chelates iron from ferritin and hemosiderin, but not from transferrin. This is an ototoxic drug and also affects the retina. It also affects the linear growth with evidence of cartilaginous dysplasia of long bones and spine.
- *Deferiprone* (L1) It is taken orally and so compliance is better. It is given 2–3 times per day at a dose of 75–100 mg/kg/day. Adverse effects include arthropathy, agranulocytosis, and hepatotoxicity. Patients on deferiprone should be monitored for complete blood count every 2–3 weeks and for liver functions every month. Using DFO in combination with L1 increases the quantity of iron excreted from the body (additive effect). Using DFO 2–5 days per week with L1 can lead to negative iron balance in most patients.
- *Deferasirox* (ICL-670) It is an effective oral iron chelator that needs to be given in the dose of 20–30 mg/kg/day once daily. Adverse effects include gastrointestinal disturbances like nausea, vomiting, diarrhea, abdominal, pain and skin rash. The adverse effects are usually mild and transient and resolve even if treatment is continued.

3. Curative therapy

Allogenic hematopoietic stem cell transplantation (HSCT) is the only permanent cure. It is expensive and available at few centers. Availability of a matched HLA donor is another limiting factor. HSCT is cost effective if compared to the cost of lifelong transfusions, chelation therapy, and treatment of other complication apart from the psychological trauma. Best results after stem cell transplantation are expected in younger children who have mild or no hepatomegaly, minimal hepatic fibrosis, and good iron chelation. Role of gene therapy is under research.

4. Splenectomy

Splenectomy is indicated for hypersplenism or when the requirement of blood exceeds 200–250 mL/kg/year. It should be avoided before 4–5 years of age. Children should be vaccinated against encapsulated bacteria like pneumococcus, *H. influenzae* b, and *N. meningitidis* before splenectomy and started on antibiotic prophylaxis for at least 2 years after splenectomy or till 6 years of age, whichever is later. In an ideal situation, prophylaxis should be given lifelong. All thalassemic children should be vaccinated with hepatitis B, pneumococcal, typhoid and *H. influenzae* vaccine before splenectomy.

5. Newer therapies

Therapies under investigation are the induction of fetal hemoglobin with pharmacologic compounds and stem cell gene therapy.

8

6. Diet and nutrition

Folic acid, 1 mg should be given daily to prevent folate deficiency. Drinking tea may help to reduce iron absorption through the intestinal tract. Vitamin C may improve iron excretion in patients receiving iron chelation.

GENETIC COUNSELING

Carrier Detection

Carrier detection should be attempted in parents of affected children (retrospective diagnosis) and those belonging to high-risk communities (prospective screening programs). As the mode of inheritance is autosomal recessive, if both the parents have thalassemia trait, the risk of having an affected child with thalassemia major is 25%, chances of an unaffected child would be 25% and that of having a child with thalassemia trait would be 50%.

The target population for screening would include couples in high-risk communities at the time of marriage, pre-conception, or early pregnancy. Carrier detection is done by hematological tests followed by mutation detection by DNA analysis. Beta-thalassemia is characterized by a mutation in the beta globin (HBB) gene located on the short arm of chromosome 11. More than 200 disease-causing mutations have been so far identified; majority are single nucleotide substitutions, deletions, or insertions of oligonucleotides leading to frameshift. The five common mutations: IVS-1-5(G → C), IVS 1-1 (G → T), Codon 41/42 (-TCTT), Codon 8/9 and the 619 bp deletion account for over 90% of the mutations in beta-thalassemia patients. IVS-1-5 (G → C) is the most common beta-thalassemia allele in the Indian population. *Sindhis* and *Lohanas* especially from Gujarat show high prevalence of the 619 bp deletion mutation. A classic case of thalassemia trait will have an elevation of the RBC count, decrease in the MCV (<78 fl) and MCH (<27 pg), a normal RDW and Mentzer index (MCV/RBC) below 13.

NESTROFT: Screening Test

If the facility for automated cell counter is not available, then naked eye single tube red cell osmotic fragility test (NESTROFT) is highly sensitive for mass screening and detection of thalassemia carrier. NESTROFT is performed using 2 mL of 0.36% buffered saline solution in a tube (10 cm × 1 cm diameter) and 2 mL distilled water taken in another tube. A drop of blood is added to each tube and they are left undisturbed for half an hour at room temperature. Both the tubes are then shaken and held against a white paper on which a thin black line is drawn. The line is clearly visible through the contents of the tube containing distilled water. If the line is similarly visible through the contents of the tube with the buffered saline, the test is considered negative. If the line is not clearly visible, the test was considered positive. A positive test indicates lowered red cell osmotic fragility, suggestive of thalassemia trait. Measurement of HbA$_2$ levels (>3.5%) is also used for carrier detection.

Prenatal Diagnosis

Prenatal diagnosis is done in the first trimester of pregnancy by chorionic villous sampling (8–10 weeks of gestation) and analysis of fetal DNA by PCR based methods. Information

A 14-year-old girl was started on oral iron therapy as her blood counts indicated iron deficiency anemia, with MCV of 75 fL, Hb 10 g/dL, Hct 33%, and RBC 5.8 × 1012/L. She had complaints of fatigue and lethargy. But 3 weeks later her laboratory results were virtually the same.

Which inherited hematological condition can show a clinical picture similar to iron deficiency anemia?

The case illustrates problem in the management of patients with microcytic anemia. In this case the girl was offered a trial of oral iron supplementation based on her red cell indices and iron profile was not ordered. However, failure to respond should make the physician consider thalassemia trait which can present with mild to moderate lifelong microcytic hypochromic anemia. Such patients may be asymptomatic or may become symptomatic during pregnancy, adolescence (menstrual losses), or during illnesses which could worsen anemia.

What laboratory test can aid the differentiation of this condition from IDA?

Thalassemia trait can be confirmed by performing hemoglobin electrophoresis as HbA$_2$ will be raised (5–8%) in such cases. Moreover, unlike IDA, these patients have high RBC counts with normal RDW.

should be provided about the mode of transmission, available tests for antenatal diagnosis, carrier detection and their reliability and treatment options to the parents. Explanatory booklets are very useful. Emphasis should be laid on details of fetal testing, ie, sampling procedure, risk to the fetus, failure and misdiagnosis. The predicted natural course of the disease based on the genotype should be discussed.

Detection of the carrier state in the parents and early detection of the disease in the fetus will help the parents in handling the situation and decide about the fate of the unborn child. Finally, the information regarding risks to their relatives should be given with recommendation to inform them so that they can choose to take the test as well.

THALASSEMIA INTERMEDIA

Severity of the disease lies in-between the major and minor thalassemia. It does not fit into the clearly defined major and minor thalassemia. It includes a range of mutations in different thalassemia genes resulting in a milder defect in globin chain synthesis and so a milder clinical picture.

The children have microcytic, hypochromic anemia which is less severe (7 g/dL) and these children are not transfusion dependent. They need packed red cell transfusion occasionally. The splenomegaly is moderate and all the features and complications are less severe. Hemoglobin electrophoresis reveals increased fetal hemoglobin (10–90%), decreased adult hemoglobin (10–90%), and normal HbA$_2$.

THALASSEMIA MINOR

This is the mildest variety and a heterozygous form in which there is only mild to moderate suppression of the globin chain. There is compensatory increase in the delta (δ) chains. These children usually remain undiagnosed as anemia is mild (~10 g/dL) and may never require a transfusion. They may be picked up on a routine hematological examination. The spleen may be normal in size and the complications and features of thalassemia major and intermedia are not seen. They lead normal lives and life expectancy is normal. They are usually treated for iron deficiency anemia but failure of the hemoglobin to rise despite iron supplementation should raise the suspicion of thalassemia minor.

Microcytosis is more marked in thalassemia minor and anisocytosis is more marked in iron-deficiency anemia (RDW is increased in IDA and normal in thalassemia trait). The two conditions may also be differentiated based on red cell counts which are decreased in IDA and increased in thalassemia trait. Serum iron profile will be normal in thalassemia minor and Hb electrophoresis reveals elevated HbA_2 (3.5–7%), a near normal HbF (1–5%) and HbA (90–95%).

ALPHA-THALASSEMIA

This is a disorder where there is absence or deficiency of alpha (α) globin chains. Since the α chain is essential for all the three types of hemoglobin, ie, fetal, adult, and A_2, the levels of all these are decreased. There is a resultant excess of uncombined β and γ chains. The excess of β chains form tetramers ($\beta4$) known as HbH and γ chains form Hb Bart ($\gamma4$). HbH is beta tetramer and is milder variant. Hb Bart is gamma tetramer and is more severe and fatal. The alpha-thalassemias have a high incidence in Asian, Filipinos and Saudi Arabian populations. It is seen in 4 different clinical variants **(Table 8.7)**.

Hydrops fetalis is the most severe form characterized by a total absence of alpha chain synthesis. Hemoglobin A is absent and instead only hemoglobin Bart, a high oxygen affinity hemoglobin, is formed. Hemoglobin Bart holds onto oxygen and resists delivering oxygen to the tissues and the resultant anemia is severe and usually leads to stillbirth or spontaneous abortion.

Hemoglobin H disease is the next most severe condition wherein scant hemoglobin A is produced and a new hemoglobin H is formed, which represents 5 to 40% on alkaline electrophoresis. Individuals with hemoglobin H disease have lifelong anemia with variable splenomegaly and bone changes.

Alpha-thalassemia trait (two-gene deletion state) and the silent carrier (one gene deletion state) are relatively asymptomatic conditions.

Revision Point

Beta-Thalassemia

1. Hemoglobin A (HbA): Two globin alpha chains and two globin beta chains ($\alpha_2 \beta_2$)
2. Hemoglobin F (HbF): Two globin alpha chains and two globin gamma chains ($\alpha_2 \beta_2$)
3. Hemoglobin A_2 (HbA_2): Two globin alpha chains and two globin delta chains ($\alpha_2 \beta_2$)
4. Thalassemias are hereditary (autosomal recessive) hemolytic anemias in which there is reduced rate of production of normal adult hemoglobin (HbA) due to absent or decreased synthesis of the α or β globin chains. Imbalances of globin chains cause hemolysis and impair erythropoiesis.
5. Alpha thalassemia is characterized by a reduced production of α chains and β-thalassemia have reduced β chain production.
6. Alpha thalassemia is less common. Silent carriers of alpha-thalassemia and persons with alpha thalassemia trait are asymptomatic. Alpha-thalassemia intermedia, or hemoglobin H disease, causes hemolytic anemia. Alpha-thalassemia major with hemoglobin Bart usually results in fatal hydrops fetalis.
7. Beta-thalassemia major is a severe transfusion-dependent anemia and necessitates regular iron chelation therapy (subcutaneous desferrioxamine injections, or oral deferiprone, or oral deferasirox) to remove iron introduced in excess with transfusions. Hematopoietic stem cell transplantation (HSCT) is the only permanent cure for beta-thalassemia major.
8. Thalassemia intermedia is suspected in individuals who present at a later age with similar but milder clinical findings. Individuals with thalassemia intermedia require episodic blood transfusion but may later require frequent blood transfusions.
9. Thalassemia minor is the mildest variety and a heterozygous form in which there is only mild to moderate suppression of the β globin chain. There is compensatory increase in the delta (δ) chains with consequently increased HbA_2 on electrophoresis.
10. Prenatal diagnosis of beta-thalassemia major can be done in the first trimester of pregnancy by chorionic villous sampling (8–10 weeks of gestation) and analysis of fetal DNA by PCR based methods.

Table 8.7 Clinical Classification of Alpha-thalassemia		
Condition	*Genotype*	*Clinical features*
Silent carrier	$\alpha\alpha/\alpha$_	Clinically and hematologically normal
Thalassemia trait	$\alpha\alpha/$_ _ α_/α_	Microcytosis, hypochromia, mild anemia
HbH disease	_ _/α_	Moderate to severe microcytic hypochromic chronic hemolytic anemia, mild jaundice, moderate hepatosplenomegaly
Hb Bart/Hydrops fetalis syndrome	_ _/_ _	Severe anemia, generalized anasarca, ascites, hepatosplenomegaly, skeletal and cardiovascular abnormalities, fatal at birth

8

Ho PJ, Tay L, Lindeman R, et al. Australian guidelines for the assessment of iron overload and iron chelation in transfusion-dependent thalassaemia major, sickle cell disease and other congenital anaemias. *Intern Med J.* 2011;41:516–24.

Origa R, Galanello R. Pathophysiology of β-thalassemia. *Pediatr Endocrinol Rev.* 2011;8 Suppl 2: 263–70.

Panigrahi I, Vaidya PC, Bansal D, Marwaha RK. Efficacy of deferasirox in North Indian β-thalassemia patients. A preliminary report. *J Pediatr Hematol Oncol.* 2012;34:51–3.

Roberts D, Brunskill S, Doree C, et al. Oral deferiprone for iron chelation in people with thalassemia. *Cochrane Database System Rev.* 2007;3:DOI:10.1002/14651858.CD004839.pub2.

Vanorden HE, Hagemann TM. Deferasirox—an oral agent for chronic iron overload. *Ann Pharmacother.* 2006;40:1110–7.

Viprakasit V, Lee-Lee C, Chong QT, Lin KH, Khuhapinant A. Iron chelation therapy in the management of thalassemia: the Asian perspectives. *Int J Hematol.* 2009;90:435–45.

8.9 SICKLE CELL DISEASE

Sickle cell hemoglobinopathy is a group of hereditary disorders in which the red cells contains an abnormal hemoglobin, ie, HbS. This hemoglobin consists of two alpha and two beta chains, however, the β chain in HbS contains valine instead of glutamic acid in the 6th position from N terminal end.

This hemoglobinopathy may manifest as (i) sickle cell trait (heterozygous state, AS); (ii) sickle cell disease (homozygous state, SS), or (iii) in compound heterozygous states for HbS with hemoglobins C, D, E, or other structural variants and the combination of the sickle cell gene with different forms of thalassemia. Sickle cell disease is more common in central India (Madhya Pradesh and Maharashtra). It is also seen in African populations near areas endemic for malaria including Central and West Africa, and some parts of the Mediterranean and Asia.

PATHOPHYSIOLOGY

The HbS is less soluble compared to HbA when it is in the deoxygenated state leading to sickling (assuming a crescent shape) of the red blood cells. The cells assume a normal shape in the oxygenated state. The sickling can also be precipitated by dehydration, fever, and acidosis. This phenomenon of sickling of RBCs has two major effects:

- Sickled cells are rigid and distorted; they lead to sluggish blood flow and blockage of capillaries causing ischemia and infarction. Infarction can occur in any organ including liver, spleen, bones and brain.
- Repeated sickling-unsickling of the cells makes the RBCs fragile leading to excessive hemolysis.

CLINICAL FEATURES

Most of the children present after 6 months of age because till that age the presence of fetal hemoglobin prevents sickling of cells. Varying degree of anemia is seen due to RBC lysis. All the children have hepatosplenomegaly initially but the spleen undergoes recurrent infarction and atrophies with time and by 7–8 years most of the children do not have a palpable spleen. This is also referred to as autosplenectomy. There may be mild jaundice. These children have growth retardation and delayed puberty. Other features are detailed below:

Infections All children with sickle cell disease are prone to infections especially by encapsulated bacteria such as pneumococcus or *H. influenzae* b because of functional asplenia and defective opsonization. Bacterial sepsis is the one of the most common causes of morbidity and death in these children.

Hand and foot syndrome (dactylitis) This is due to micro-infarction of the medulla of the carpal and tarsal bones symmetrically due to vaso-occlusive crisis. This leads to swollen and tender dorsum of hands and feet. This is an extremely painful condition.

Vaso-occlusive episodes These extremely painful episodes may affect any part of the body involving the chest, abdomen, and extremities more commonly. A stressful condition like physical stress, dehydration, hypoxia, exposure to cold, etc. can precipitate these painful episodes due to compromised blood flow leading to ischemia.

Splenic sequestration This is characterized by acute pooling of blood in the spleen, hypovolemia, shock and sudden increase in the splenic size. This is a potentially fatal condition.

Aplastic crisis This is precipitated by parvovirus B19 infection which causes erythroid hypoplasia and reticulocytopenia.

Hyperhemolytic crisis During painful crises there may be a marked increase in the rate of hemolysis with a fall in the hemoglobin level.

Other features These include chronic leg ulcers, gallstones, neurological complications like stroke and seizures, priapism, pulmonary complication, renal and retinal involvement, and the skeletal changes secondary to chronic erythroid hyperplasia.

LABORATORY INVESTIGATIONS

Peripheral Smear

It reveals varying degree of anisocytosis and poikilocytosis. Typical sickle-shaped cells may be present but are not universal (Fig. 8.18). Reticulocytes are increased in number and may go up to 10–20%.

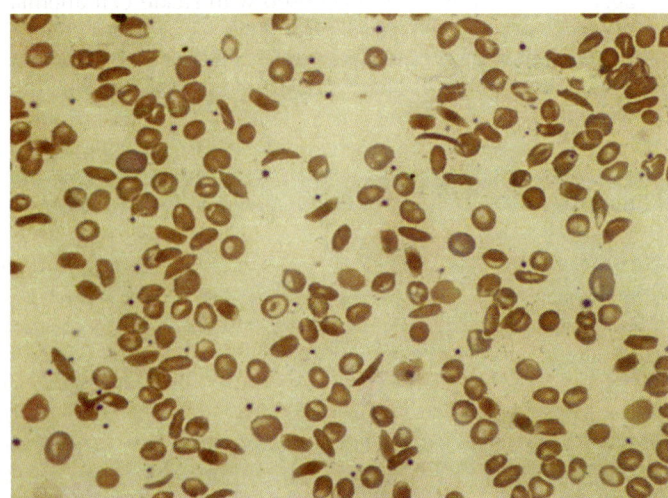

Fig. 8.18 Peripheral blood smear showing sickle cell RBCs

Sickle Test

This test demonstrates the tendency of RBCs to 'sickle' in hypoxic state. Sickling occurs because of distortion of red cells containing HbS, which undergoes polymerization. When HbS gets deoxygenated, it undergoes a pronounced decrease in solubility. Deoxy HbS polymers in the cells exist as highly ordered fiber aggregates which fill the cell and distort it into the classic sickle shape. This is demonstrated by adding sodium metabisulphite to the blood of the patient following which the RBCs rapidly change to sickle shape.

Sickle Solubility Test

The solubility test is the most common screening test for sickle cell or presence of HbS. When anticoagulated blood is mixed with a reducing agent like sodium dithionite, the red cells will lyse due to the presence of saponin and the hemoglobin in the red cells will be released. If HbS is present, it will give a cloudy or turbid appearance to the solution due to poor solubility. If HbS is not present, the solution will appear clear. The solubility test cannot differentiate sickle cell disease (HbSS) from sickle cell trait (HbAS).

Hemoglobin Electrophoresis

Definite diagnosis can be made only on hemoglobin electrophoresis that reveals the presence of HbS. The typical pattern is as follows:

	HbS	HbF	HbA$_1$	HbA$_2$
Sickle cell disease	70–90%	10–30%	-	-
Sickle cell trait	30–40%	<2%	50–60%	1–3%
Normal	-	<1%	95–98%	1–3%

Treatment	**Sickle Cell Anemia**

Treatment is by and large supportive.
1. *Transfusion* Anemia and all the other complications in these patients need specific management. Packed red cell transfusions are required to treat chronic anemia. An urgent blood transfusion may be required in conditions like splenic sequestration and aplastic crisis.
2. *Infections need to be identified early and managed aggressively* All children diagnosed with sickle cell anemia should be started on penicillin prophylaxis (oral penicillin V 125 mg BD) to prevent *S. pneumoniae* infection till at least 5 years of age. After 5 years of age the dose of oral penicillin V is 250 mg BD. If compliance is considered to be a problem, monthly injections of 600,000 units of benzathine penicillin IM can be used. However, these injections are painful, and the effectiveness of the injection for the later half of the month is questionable. Amoxicillin 20 mg/kg/day is an alternative to penicillin. For patients who are allergic to penicillin, erythromycin 125 mg twice daily is given to children younger than 5 years of age, and erythromycin 250 mg twice daily is given to children 5 years of age or older. Children older than 5 years may discontinue their penicillin prophylaxis provided they have not had previous pneumococcal infection or functional asplenia. Prevention of infection by encapsulated bacteria can be done by immunizing the child with pneumococcal and meningococcal vaccine.

3. *Management of pain* Analgesics and psychological support are required. Severe pain may warrant hospitalization and narcotic analgesics.
4. Dehydration should be prevented and managed aggressively by intravenous fluids.
5. Stem cell transplant can provide cure for some children.
6. Hydroxyurea, 5-azacytidine, and butyrates have been used to stimulate HbF production and decrease the levels of HbS.
7. Red cell HbS concentration reducing agents like nifedipine, verapamil and DDAVP have been used.

SCREENING OF POPULATION

Screening procedures for adults include the dithionite solubility, a solubility test based on the principle that hemoglobin S precipitates in high molarity buffered phosphate solutions. The end point is easy to read as a turbid solution in the presence of hemoglobin S and a clear solution if hemoglobin S is not present.

Neonatal screening involves collection of newborn blood samples by heel prick onto a dried filter paper. The samples are then analyzed by hemoglobin electrophoresis at either alkaline or acid pH or both, isoelectric focusing, or high-performance liquid chromatography. If electrophoretic techniques are used, two bands, hemoglobin F and hemoglobin S, will be seen in patients with sickle cell anemia because hemoglobin F is predominant in neonates. The healthy neonate will show two bands at hemoglobin A and hemoglobin F, while the individual with sickle cell trait will show three bands: One at F, one at A, and one at S.

Revision Point

Sickle Cell Disease

1. Sickle cell hemoglobin (HbS) results from an autosomal recessively inherited mutation in which the 17th nucleotide of the beta globin gene is changed from thymine to adenine, and the amino acid glutamic acid is replaced by valine at position 6 in the beta globin chain.
2. Sickle solubility test can be used as a screening test for detecting HbS.
3. Hemoglobin electrophoresis is needed to confirm the diagnosis of sickle cell disease (no HbA, 80–95% HbSS, and 2–20% HbF).
4. Sickle cells have a reduced deformability and are easily destroyed, causing occlusion of the micro-circulation and a chronic hemolytic anemia.
5. Clinical severity of sickle cell disease is very variable. Some have few complications and remain largely asymptomatic; majority have intermediate forms; and a few have severe complications (vaso-occlusive crisis, aplastic crisis, sepsis, acute chest syndrome, splenic sequestration, stroke, and priapism).

Inati A. Recent advances in improving the management of sickle cell disease. *Blood Rev.* 2009;23 Suppl 1:S9–13.

Kavanagh PL, Sprinz PG, Vinci SR, Bauchner H, Wang CJ. Management of children with sickle cell disease: a comprehensive review of the literature. *Pediatrics.* 2011; 128: 1552–74.

Patra PK, Chauhan VS, Khodiar PK, Dalla AR, Serjeant GR. Screening for the sickle cell gene in Chhattisgarh state, India: an approach to a major public health problem. *J Community Genet.* 2011; 2: 147–51.

8.10 RBC MEMBRANE DEFECTS

HEREDITARY SPHEROCYTOSIS

Hereditary spherocytosis is an autosomal (autosomal dominant inheritance in 75% and autosomal recessive in 25%) defect of the red cell membrane, resulting in chronic hemolytic anemia. The disease is characterized by anemia, mid icterus, moderate splenomegaly, and presence of microspherocytes in the peripheral smear.

Pathophysiology

There is a molecular defect of spectrin protein which is a major component of the cytoskeleton responsible for RBC shape. Deficiency of spectrin results in change of RBC shape from biconcave to spherical. A spherical RBC is more rigid and cannot be deformed easily; it is thus prone to hemolysis while passing through the spleen. This is associated with an increased permeability to sodium and increased glycolysis by the cell.

Clinical Features

The age of presentation depends upon the severity of the disease. It may present in the neonatal period as hyperbilirubinemia and anemia warranting phototherapy or exchange transfusion.

It may also present later in life as mild to moderate anemia, moderate splenomegaly, mild jaundice, fatigue and asymptomatic gallstones. Complications of bone marrow hyperplasia evident in the skeletal system are less marked than β-thalassemia major. They are also prone to aplastic crisis resulting from parvovirus infection like sickle cell disease.

Many children may go undetected and remain asymptomatic till adulthood.

Laboratory Diagnosis

- Peripheral smear shows anemia with microspherocytosis.
- Reticulocyte count is increased. MCV is normal but the MCHC may be raised.
- Osmotic fragility of the red cells is increased, due to increased permeability of the cell membrane to sodium, leading to increased absorption sodium and water when exposed to hypotonic saline. The spherical cells swell up and lyse more readily than the normal concave cells. However, increased osmotic fragility is not pathognomonic of hereditary spherocytosis and can be seen in other hemolytic anemias as well.
- Serum bilirubin levels are mildly elevated.

Treatment	Hereditary Spherocytosis

Packed red cell transfusion may occasionally be required. Regular transfusions are not required.

Splenectomy is warranted only in symptomatic patients. As the spleen is the site for lysis of cells, the anemia and associated symptoms improve following splenectomy. The reticulocyte count goes down and there is almost a complete and sustained remission of the disease.

All modalities to prevent infection as described earlier should be adopted before and after splenectomy. Folic acid is supplemented to prevent megaloblastic erythropoiesis.

RBC Membrane Defects

1. Red cell membrane disorders are inherited diseases due to mutations in various membrane or skeletal proteins, resulting in decreased red cell deformability, reduced lifespan and premature removal of the erythrocytes from the circulation.
2. The red cell membrane disorders include hereditary spherocytosis (HS), hereditary elliptocytosis, hereditary ovalocytosis, and hereditary stomatocytosis.
3. Hemolytic anemia in HS can range from compensated to severe, sometimes requiring exchange transfusion at birth and/or repeated blood transfusions, variable jaundice, splenomegaly, and cholelithiasis.
4. Osmotic fragility test is used for screening patients with HS as the osmotic fragility of the red cells is increased in HS.

HEREDITARY ELLIPTOCYTOSIS

It is a genetically determined, uncommon RBC disorder that varies markedly in severity and is characterized by elliptical red cells in the peripheral smear. The disorder is transmitted as an autosomal dominant trait. Clinical symptoms vary from asymptomatic carrier state to severe hemolytic anemia. Members of the same family may show different clinical severity and an individual's frequency and severity of symptoms may change with time.

Other rare disorders of RBC membrane are ovalocytosis, pyropoikilocytosis, xerocytosis, and acanthocytosis.

Bolton-Maggs PH, Langer JC, Iolascon A, Tittensor P, King MJ. Guidelines for the diagnosis and management of hereditary spherocytosis—2011 update. *Br J Haematol*. 2012;156:37–49.

Guitton C, Garçon L, Cynober T, et al. Hereditary spherocytosis: guidelines for the diagnosis and management in children. *Arch Pediatr*. 2009;16:556–8.

Guitton C, Garçon L, Cynober T, Gauthier F, Tchernia G, Delaunay J, et al. Hereditary spherocytosis: guidelines for the diagnosis and management in children. *Arch Pediatr*. 2008;15:1464–73.

8.11 RBC ENZYME DEFECTS

There are two pathways in a RBC to utilize glucose, namely (*i*) the anerobic Embden-Mayerhof pathway and (*ii*) the oxidative hexose monophosphate (HMP) shunt pathway. If any of the pathways is affected, the ATP production decreases and the RBC lifespan reduces. Deficiency of pyruvate kinase enzyme is the major disorder of glycolytic pathway while deficiency of enzyme glucose-6-phosphate dehydrogenase is the most common defect in the HMP pathway.

The enzyme defect ultimately leads to Na$^+$ impaired ATP synthesis and hence impaired membrane function of transportation. The cells become rigid and prone for lysis. The RBC morphology is preserved, the osmotic fragility is not increased, and splenectomy does not offer much relief to these children.

GLUCOSE-6-PHOSPHATE DEHYDROGENASE DEFICIENCY

Glucose-6-phosphate dehydrogenase (G6PD) deficiency is the most common RBC enzyme defect, inherited as an

X-linked recessive disorder. In hemizygous male or homozygous female, the G6PD activity is <5% of normal. Heterozygous females have moderate activity of G6PD as some cells have normal activity and others are deficient. These girls are asymptomatic on exposure to oxidant drugs.

Clinical manifestations depend on the severity of the deficiency of the enzyme. There are more than 400 variants of G6PD. There are five known genotypes: Two are normal and three are abnormal with varying amounts of hemolysis. The disease is more common in blacks than whites and amongst males. People of the Mediterranean region are particularly affected. Neonatal screening for G6PD deficiency is routinely done in some countries.

Severity Classification

The severity of hemolysis depends upon the precipitating factor or drug, the dose, and severity of the enzyme deficiency **(Table 8.8)**.

Type I It is the mildest type and commonly seen in American blacks (G6PDA–). These patients have hemolysis only in strong antioxidant exposures and do not usually have associated neonatal hyperbilirubinemia.

Type II They have moderately severe syndrome and favism is quite common. This variety is seen in people of Mediterranean origin (G6PDB– and G6PD canton). Neonatal hyperbilirubinemia is quite common.

Type III These patients suffer from non-spherocytic hemolytic anemia even without oxidant exposure and neonatal jaundice is severe. It is seen in North Americans and Europeans.

Pathophysiology

G6PD is needed to protect the RBCs from oxidant damage as it converts the oxidized glutathione to reduced form which protects the RBCs. In the absence of G6PD, the RBCs become susceptible to oxidant damage and hemolysis.

Clinical Features

Four clinical conditions are associated with G6PD deficiency: (*i*) drug-induced acute hemolytic anemia, (*ii*) favism, (*iii*) neonatal jaundice, and (*iv*) congenital non-spherocytic anemia.

The enzyme deficiency is characterized by acute hemolytic episodes (in an otherwise normal individual), precipitated by infections, drugs with oxidant properties, severe stress and some foods (like fava beans). Individuals with G6PD deficiency are resistant to *P. falciparum* infection. Chronic anemia is seen in individuals with a severe deficiency of the enzyme.

Drug-induced Acute Hemolysis

Common drugs that cause hemolysis in patients with G6PD deficiency include the following: Chloroquine, primaquine, nitrofurantoin, dapsone, acetyl salicylic acid, nalidixic acid, methylene blue, rasburicase, sulphamethoxazole, and sulphasalazine. The hemolysis starts 2–3 days after exposure to the incriminating agent and is usually self-limiting even if the drug is continued as new RBCs are released into the patients blood everyday, which have sufficient G6PD levels. The older cells are more easily destroyed and younger cells are resistant. Once all the older cells have been destroyed and are replaced the younger cells the hemolysis stops on its own. There is sudden appearance of pallor, jaundice and hemoglobinuria (cola-colored urine) due to intravascular hemolysis. Spleen may become palpable. The LDH and reticulocytes are increased, while the anemia is normochromic and normocytic.

Favism

Favism is usually found in individuals of the G6PD Mediterranean or Canton type. A few hours after ingesting fava beans, the individual develops irritability, fever, nausea, and abdominal pain. The patient can develop gross hemoglobinuria after 2–3 days.

Neonatal Jaundice

Neonatal jaundice (NNJ) related to G6PD deficiency occurs within 2 to 3 days after birth. In contrast to hemolytic disease of the newborn, patients with G6PD show more jaundice than anemia which gets exaggerated by vitamin K administration or some inciting drugs.

Non-spherocytic Congenital Hemolytic Anemia

These patients have a history of neonatal jaundice complicated by gallstones, enlarged spleen, or both and may be investigated for jaundice or gallstones in their adult life. The anemia varies in severity from minimum to transfusion dependent and is due to chronic extravascular hemolysis. Splenectomy may be considered in these patients.

Laboratory Diagnosis

Peripheral blood picture is normal in-between episodes of hemolysis. During hemolysis there may be basophilic

Table 8.8 Classes of Glucose-6-Phosphate Enzyme Variants

Class	Level of deficiency	Enzyme activity	Prevalence
I	Severe	Chronic non-spherocytic hemolytic anemia in the presence of normal erythrocyte function	Uncommon; occurs across populations
II	Severe	<10%	Uncommon, more common in Asian, African and Mediterranean populations
III	Moderate	10–60%	10% of black males in US
IV	Mild to none	60–150%	Rare
V	None	>150%	Rare

stippling and polychromasia, with evidence of intravascular hemolysis. Supravital staining reveals presence of **Heinz bodies**. Heinz bodies are aggregates of denatured, precipitated hemoglobin within red blood cells. Hemoglobin protein globin chains are denatured through oxidative damage by reactive oxygen species. Oxidation of reactive sulfhydryl (S-H) groups creates disulfide bonds that change the conformation of the globin protein chains, resulting in precipitation of the hemoglobin molecule.

The final diagnosis is made by demonstration of reduced enzyme activity in the red cell of affected children. Affected persons demonstrate an activity <10%. The reduced enzyme activity is better demonstrated sometime after the acute hemolytic episode, is over because immediately after the hemolytic episode, the younger RBCs are predominant which have higher enzyme levels.

Treatment   **G6PD Deficiency-Induced Hemolysis**

Treatment includes blood transfusion and supportive care during an attack of hemolysis. It is best to prevent exposure to drugs which may precipitate acute hemolysis in susceptible persons.

PYRUVATE KINASE (PK) DEFICIENCY

This is an autosomal recessive disorder due to (i) deficiency of pyruvate kinase enzyme in the red cell; or (ii) its reduced activity. Clinical deficiency may present in (a) neonatal period with severe anemia and hyperbilirubinemia or (b) in childhood with anemia, jaundice, and splenomegaly.

Neonatal jaundice may warrant an exchange transfusion. Occasional packed red cell transfusion is required for severe anemia and aplastic crisis. Splenectomy may reduce hemolysis in some patients but is not curative.

METHEMOGLOBINEMIA

Iron is present in ferrous state in normal hemoglobin. Methemoglobin refers to an abnormal hemoglobin where iron is present in ferric form. Methemoglobin cannot release oxygen to the tissues because of very high affinity for oxygen. In normal children, it accounts for less than 1% of the total hemoglobin, because of presence of the enzyme NADH cytochrome reductase, which converts any methemoglobin formed in the blood to normal oxyhemoglobin.

Pathophysiology

Methemoglobinemia refers to the state of excess accumulation of methemoglobin. Signs and symptoms of hypoxia appear because methemoglobin is unable to release oxygen to the tissues. Cyanosis appears when methemoglobin exceeds 15% of the total hemoglobin. There may be associated dizziness, tachycardia, dyspnea, and altered sensorium. Death may occur.

Clinical Features

A child with definite central cyanosis, mild dyspnea, and without a murmur/heart failure should be suspected of having methemoglobinemia. Majority of cases are due to agents that increase the auto-oxidation of hemoglobin in the red cell. Rarely some children may have congenital metabolic defects.

Case Study | Methemoglobinemia

A 2-year-old boy was brought by the mother with history of swallowing moth balls (naphthalene) following which he developed vomiting, fever, and red-color staining of his diapers. Investigations revealed hemoglobin of 5 g/dL, hematocrit of 15%, LDH of 500 IU/L (reference range, 0 to 100 IU/L). His peripheral smear revealed polychromasia and occasional bite cells.

What is your diagnosis?
The boy seems to have developed methemoglobinemia due to moth ball ingestion. It is a life-threatening condition characterized by the inability of hemoglobin to carry oxygen because the ferrous part of the heme molecule is oxidized to a ferric state. Acquired methemoglobinemia is due to medications or chemicals that cause the rate of methemoglobin formation to exceed its rate of reduction. Naphthalene is an oxidizing drug and results in G6PD deficiency. In this case the baby has developed severe intravascular lysis as evidenced by the LDH value and the extremely low hemoglobin. Presence of bite cells in the peripheral smear suggests the formation of Heinz bodies and their subsequent removal by the spleen.

What are the clinical features of moth ball intoxication?
Signs and symptoms of acquired methemoglobinemia usually occur within 20 to 30 minutes of drug administration. At methemoglobin levels greater than 0.15 g/dL, cyanosis is apparent. Weakness, headache, and dizziness occur at methemoglobin levels of 0.30 to 0.40 g/dL; at levels greater than 0.45 g/dL, dyspnea, acidosis, cardiac arrhythmias, heart failure, seizures, and coma ensue; death occurs at levels greater than 0.70 g/dL.

How will you diagnose the condition?
The diagnosis of methemoglobinemia is based on clinical assessment when respiratory status does not explain the cyanosis that a patient has and is refractory to oxygen therapy. Arterial blood is chocolate brown, and the blood gas analysis indicates a PaO$_2$ that is inappropriately high or normal. Pulse oximeter readings are normal. The definitive diagnostic test is multiple wave length co-oximetry.

How will you treat the condition?
Remove the inciting agent and provide supportive care. Specific antidote is intravenous methylene blue in a dose of 1 to 2 mg/kg of a 1% solution administered over 5 minutes. However, doses of methylene blue should not exceed 7 mg/kg because of its oxidizing properties at high doses.

Commonly used drugs that can cause methemoglobinemia include sulfonamides, primaquine, nitrates and nitrites. Substances used in chemical factories such as nitrobenzene and aniline, explosive plants, and household chemicals such as marking ink, naphthalene balls, shoe polish (containing nitrobenzene), colored crayons, perfumes, etc. may cause methemoglobinemia.

Management

The color of the blood becomes brown. Diagnosis is confirmed by co-oximetry test. PaO$_2$ concentrations are usually normal despite cyanosis. Methylene blue is administered intravenously in acute poisoning. Withdrawal of the incriminating agent is sufficient in chronic slow poisoning.

PAROXYSMAL NOCTURNAL HEMOGLOBINURIA

A rare hemolytic anemia, paroxysmal nocturnal hemoglobinuria (PNH) is characterized by increased susceptibility of the red cells to complement lysis resulting in intravascular hemolysis. PNH occurs due to an X-linked somatic mutation in the hematopoietic stem cells designated as phosphatidylinositol glycan class A (PIGA) which leads to loss of glycosylphosphatidylinositol (GPI)-anchored proteins present in all cell lines including RBCs. Classically, RBCs are destroyed while patients sleep because of their increased sensitivity to complement lysis, and upon arising the patient notices hemoglobinuria. Diagnosis of PNH can be done by flow cytometry. Sugar water test and the Ham test, have also been used.

RBC Enzyme Defects

1. Glucose-6-phosphate dehydrogenase (G6PD) deficiency is the most common RBC enzyme defect, inherited as an X-linked recessive disorder, almost exclusively affecting males.
2. Clinical manifestations of G6PD deficiency include neonatal jaundice and acute hemolytic anemia arising from oxidative stress on RBCs induced by some medications, an infection, or ingestion of fava beans.
3. Following drugs can precipitate hemolysis in G6PD deficient individuals: Chloroquine, primaquine, nitrofurantoin, dapsone, chloramphenicol, vitamin K, acetylsalicylic acid, nalidixic acid, methylene blue, rasburicase, sulphamethoxazole, and sulphasalazine.
4. Blood tests can detect G6PD deficiency by measuring the G6PD enzyme activity.
5. Treatment of hemolysis in G6PD deficient individuals includes blood transfusion and supportive care during an attack of hemolysis.

Kaplan M, Hammerman C. The need for neonatal glucose-6-phosphate dehydrogenase screening: a global perspective. *J Perinatol.* 2009;29 Suppl 1:S46–52.

Nair H. Neonatal screening program for G6PD deficiency in India: need and feasibility. *Indian Pediatr.* 2009;46:1045–9.

Tripathy V, Reddy BM. Present status of understanding on the G6PD deficiency and natural selection. *J Postgrad Med.* 2007;53:193–202.

8.12 AUTOIMMUNE HEMOLYTIC ANEMIA

Autoimmune hemolytic anemia (AIHA) is an uncommon group of disorders characterized by destruction of red blood cells by autoantibodies which may occur suddenly, or it may develop gradually. It can occur at any age and has a predilection for female sex. While, in most cases no cause can be ascertained, it may sometimes be associated with disorders like systemic lupus erythematosus (SLE), Crohn disease, rheumatic illnesses, and lymphoproliferative disorders. Rarely it may follow the use of certain drugs, such as penicillin, or certain viral infections. It is of two types:

- *Warm antibody hemolytic anemia* The autoantibodies (usually IgG type) attach to and destroy red blood cells at temperatures equal to or in excess of normal body temperature. The hemolysis is extravascular.
- *Cold antibody hemolytic anemia* The autoantibodies (usually IgM type) become most active and attack red blood cells only at temperatures well below normal body temperature. The hemolysis is mostly intravascular.
  - *Paroxysmal cold hemoglobinuria* (Donath-Landsteiner syndrome) It is a rare type of cold antibody hemolytic anemia. Destruction of red blood cells results from exposure to cold, even if the cold exposure is limited to a small area of the body, such as when the person drinks cold water or washes hands in cold water. An antibody binds to red blood cells at low temperatures and causes destruction of red blood cells within arteries and veins after warming. It occurs most often after a viral illness or in otherwise healthy people, although it occurs in some people with syphilis.
  - *Cold agglutinin syndrome* It is a type of cold antibody hemolytic anemia, seen more frequently in older age group and characterized by C3 mediated hemolysis. IgM antibodies bind to RBCs in cold conditions and cause agglutination followed by complement activation and intravascular hemolysis.

CLINICAL FEATURES

If the hemolysis is mild or gradual, patients are asymptomatic. Pallor, weakness, and jaundice occur if the hemolysis is more severe or rapid. When destruction persists for a few months or longer, the spleen may enlarge. People with paroxysmal cold hemoglobinuria may have severe pain in the back and legs, headache, vomiting, and diarrhea. The urine may be dark brown.

DIAGNOSIS

The hemoglobin is around 4–7 g/dL with normal red cell indices. Spherocytes are seen in peripheral smear especially in warm autoimmune hemolytic anemia. Pancytopenia may also be seen. Coombs test can aid the diagnosis. Direct antiglobulin test (DAT) or direct Coombs test detects increased amounts of autoantibodies attached to red blood cells while the indirect antiglobulin or indirect Coombs test can detect their presence in serum. DAT is positive in 95% of warm AIHA. Presence of IgM in serum suggests cold AIHA. This is accompanied by agglutination of RBCs in cold temperatures which reverses on warming. Other tests (antiphospholipid antibody, ANA, and VDRL) can be done to ascertain the specific etiology.

Treatment	**Autoimmune Hemolytic Anemia**

If symptoms are mild no treatment is needed. If red blood cell destruction is increasing, corticosteroids (such as prednisone) are the first choice for treatment. High doses are used at first, followed by a gradual reduction of the dose over many weeks or months. When people do not respond to corticosteroids or when the corticosteroid causes intolerable side effects, rituximab or immunosuppressants like cyclosporine or azathioprine can be given. Splenectomy can be offered in refractory cases. When red blood cell destruction is severe, blood transfusions are sometimes needed, but they do not treat the cause of the anemia and provide only temporary relief. The best treatment for paroxysmal cold hemoglobinuria is avoidance of exposure to cold.

Autoimmune Hemolytic Anemia

1. Autoimmune hemolytic anemia (AIHA) is characterized by destruction of red blood cells by autoantibodies.
2. It is predominantly of two types:
   - *Warm antibody hemolytic anemia:* IgG type auto-antibodies destroy red blood cells at temperatures equal to or in excess of normal body temperature resulting in extravascular hemolysis.
   - *Cold antibody hemolytic anemia:* IgM type auto-antibodies become most active and attack red blood cells only at temperatures well below normal body temperature resulting in intravascular hemolysis. It includes paroxysmal cold hemoglobinuria (most often after a viral illness and in syphilis) and cold agglutinin syndrome (complement mediated hemolysis).
3. Direct antiglobulin test (DAT) or direct Coombs test detects increased amounts of autoantibodies attached to red blood cells while the indirect antiglobulin or indirect Coombs test can detect their presence in serum.
4. Corticosteroids are useful in cases with severe hemolysis. Rituximab or immunosuppressants like cyclosporine or azathioprine can be given if patient is unresponsive to corticosteroids.

8.13 BLEEDING AND COAGULATION DISORDERS

Abnormalities in platelets, vessel wall, or clotting factors can prevent hemostasis resulting in hemorrhage. The following is a basic classification of bleeding disorders:

i. *Platelet disorders* Thrombocytopenia, platelet function defects
ii. *Coagulation disorders* Congenital or acquired
iii. *Vascular disorders* Henoch-Schönlein purpura, scurvy, and Ehlers-Danlos syndrome.

APPROACH TO DIAGNOSIS

A careful and detailed history followed by a clinical examination should enable one to identify children with a high probability of having an underlying bleeding disorder.

History

- Features of abnormal bleeding such as prolonged bleeding after minor trauma, epistaxis not relieved by fifteen minutes of pressure along the entire side of the nose, menstrual periods lasting longer than seven days with passage of clots, and ecchymotic patches inconsistent with degree of trauma, should lead to suspicion of a bleeding or coagulation disorder.
- Family history of bleeding is especially relevant for hemophilia which has X-linked inheritance.
- *Type of bleeding:* Mucosal membrane bleeding, petechiae and bruising are associated with qualitative or quantitative platelet disorders and von Willebrand disease (vWD). Spontaneous, deep muscle and joint bleeding are commonly seen with coagulation factor deficiency.
- *Time of onset of syndrome:* Acute onset over a period of days to weeks is suggestive of acquired disorders like immune thrombocytopenic purpura (ITP) or vitamin K deficiency. Bleeding following trauma in which there is a good initial hemostasis followed by persistent oozing due to failure to form a firm clot is suggestive of a factor XIII deficiency and disorders of fibrinolytic pathway.
- *General condition of the patient (sick/well appearing):* A healthy looking child with petechiae or ecchymotic patches without significant anemia is most probably a case of ITP. A sick patient is likely to suffer from aplastic anemia, or malignant disorder, or liver disease, or DIC.

Physical Examination

The following clinical features need to be checked for: presence of petechiae, mucosal bleeds, hematoma, joint mobility and swelling, retinal bleeding, hematuria, jaundice and presence of anemia, hepatomegaly, splenomegaly, and lymphadenopathy. **Table 8.9** depicts differences between coagulation factor deficiencies and platelet or vessel wall abnormalities.

- Presence of significant anemia along with thrombocytopenia and lymphadenopathy or hepatosplenomegaly suggests underlying leukemia, or lymphoma.
- Anemia and thrombocytopenia without any other significant finding is suggestive of aplastic anemia or immune-mediated pathology (Evans syndrome).
- Patients with platelet or vessel abnormality usually have spontaneous and superficial bleeds like petechiae, ecchymosis, hematomas, epistaxis, etc.
- Children with coagulation factor deficiencies do not develop petechiae but may have superficial bleeds like ecchymotic patches or subcutaneous hematoma and they characteristically manifest with deep bleeding into the muscle or joints.

Table 8.9 Clinical Features to Distinguish Bleeding and Coagulation Disorders		
Clinical sign/symptom	*Platelet/vascular abnormality*	*Coagulation factor deficiency*
Ecchymosis	Small and superficial	Large and deep
Petechiae	Frequent	Never
Mucosal hemorrhage	Frequent	Uncommon in hemophilia and acquired defects
Muscle/joint or internal bleeding following trauma/surgery	Uncommon Immediate. Stops with pressure	Frequent hemorrhage Delayed (1–2 days later). Does not stop with pressure

• Patient with abnormal collagen matrix and vessel wall may have loose joints and lax skin associated with easy bruising.

Laboratory Evaluation

1. *Platelet count* A healthy child has a platelet count of 150–400 × 10⁹/L. Accurate results are obtained by electronic counts but an experienced pathologist can also comment on the adequacy of platelets on a peripheral smear. A normal peripheral smear shows platelets in clumps. Thrombocytopenia is defined as a reduction in number of platelet (<1,50,000/mm³). Defect in platelet function is known as thrombasthenia.

   Thrombocytopenia due to decreased platelet production is associated with a decrease in mean platelet volume and decreased number of megakaryocytes in the bone marrow. Presence of coexisting abnormalities in leukocytes and erythrocytes indicates involvement of the bone marrow aspirate. Presence of coexisting abnormalities in leukocytopenia in conjunction with abnormalities in coagulation, suggests consumptive coagulopathy including DIC.

2. *Peripheral smear examination* This is important to evaluate rule out to the involvement of other cell lines especially in cases of leukemia, and aplastic anemia.

3. *Bleeding time* It is the time required for the cessation of bleeding from a puncture site. The normal range is 4–7 minutes. The bleeding time is prolonged if the circulating platelets are reduced in number as in idiopathic thrombocytopenic purpura (ITP) or if there is a functional intrinsic platelet defect leading to platelet deficiency even if the number is normal, eg, Glanzmann thrombasthenia.

4. *Prothrombin time (PT)* This indicates the integrity of the extrinsic and common pathway of coagulation (Fig. 8.19). The normal value is 12 sec, but it should always be assessed in relation to a control done from a normal person simultaneously. Prothrombin time is prolonged in deficiency of factors II, V, VII and X **(Table 8.10)**.

5. *Activated partial thromboplastin time* (APTT) This demonstrates the intrinsic and common pathways of

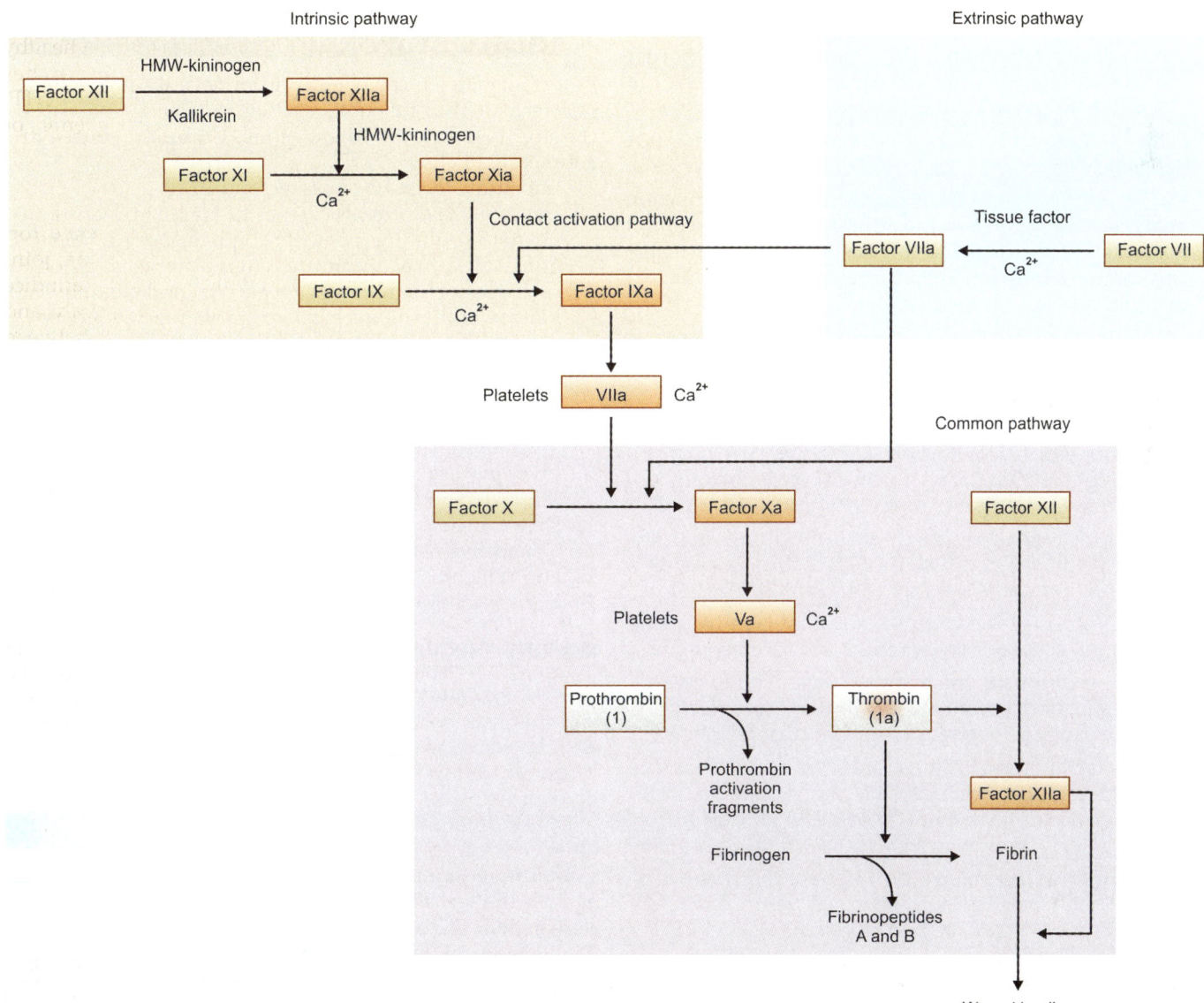

Fig. 8.19 Coagulation cascade

Table 8.10 Approach to a Child with Bleeding Disorder

GC	BT	PT	APTT	P/C	Probable diagnosis
Well	N	N	↑	N	Hemophilia A or B
Well	N	↑	N	N	Factor VII deficiency
Well	N	↑	↑	N	Vitamin K deficiency
Sick	↑	↑	↑	↓	DIC, liver disease
Well	↑	N	N	↓	ITP
Sick	↑	N	N	↓	Aplastic anemia, leukemia
Well	↑	N	N	N	Qualitative platelet defects

GC: General condition, BT: Bleeding time; PT: Prothrombin time; APTT: Activated partial thromboplastin time; P/C: Platelet count

coagulation. The normal values are 25–40 seconds but should be compared with a control value. APTT is prolonged in deficiency of factors V, VIII, IX, X, XI, XII.

- An increase in PT with normal APTT indicates deficiency of factor VII.
- A normal PT with increased APTT indicates factor VIII, IX, XII deficiency.
- Both PT and APTT are deranged in generalized disorders like vitamin K deficiency and liver disorder or disseminated intravascular coagulation (DIC) in which both pathways are affected.

6. *Factor assays* can be done to diagnose isolated factor deficiencies.

7. *Platelet function* can be analyzed using a platelet function analyzer which can test the adhesion and aggregation properties of platelets. But this is not routinely available and can be helpful in patients in whom platelet function disorder is being suspected.

Bleeding and Coagulation Disorders

1. Thrombocytopenia is defined as a reduction in number of platelet (<1,50,000/mm³). Defect in platelet function leading to bleeding is known as thrombasthenia.

2. Superficial and mucosal bleeding are usually associated with qualitative or quantitative platelet disorders and von Willebrand disease (vWD).

3. Spontaneous, deep muscle and joint bleeding are commonly seen with coagulation factor deficiency.

4. Presence of significant anemia along with thrombocytopenia and lymphadenopathy or hepatosplenomegaly suggests underlying leukemia, or lymphoma.

5. Prothrombin time (PT) indicates the integrity of the extrinsic and common pathway of coagulation and is prolonged in deficiency of factors II, V, VII, and X.

6. Activated partial thromboplastin time (APTT) demonstrates the intrinsic and common pathways of coagulation and is prolonged in deficiency of factors V, VIII (hemophilia A), IX (hemophilia B), X, XI, and XII.

7. Both PT and APTT are deranged in generalized disorders like vitamin K deficiency and liver disorder or disseminated intravascular coagulation (DIC).

Lusher JM. Clinical and laboratory approach to the patient with bleeding. In: Nathan DG, Orkin SH, Ginsburg D, Look AT. *Nathan and Oski's Hematology of Infancy and Childhood,* 6th edition. Philadelphia: Saunders; 2003.p 1515–1526.

Scott JP, Raffini LJ, Montgomery RR. Hemostasis. In: Kliegman RM, Stanton BF, St. Geme JW III, Schor NF, Behrman RE. *Nelson Textbook of Pediatrics, 19th edition.* Philadelphia: Saunders, Elsevier; 2011.p.1693–9.

8.14 PLATELET DISORDERS

Defects of platelets can be either in terms of absolute number or in terms of their function, resulting in defective hemostasis causing bleeding manifestations. Common causes are enumerated below:

1. Idiopathic thrombocytopenic purpura
2. *Drug-induced thrombocytopenia:* Heparin, valproate, phenytoin, quinine, penicillin, cephalosporins, NSAIDs, gold salts, procainamide, chemotherapy, digoxin, rifampicin, ethambutol, vancomycin, and clindamycin.
3. Marrow infiltration, eg, leukemia, storage disorders
4. Aplastic anemia
5. Hypersplenism
6. *Infections* Parvovirus, rubella, mumps, varicella, hepatitis C, EBV, malaria, HIV, and septicemia.
7. Megaloblastic anemia
8. Liver disease
9. Massive blood transfusion
10. Disseminated intravascular coagulation
11. Connective tissue disorders, eg, SLE
12. von Willebrand disease
13. Hemolytic uremic syndrome

IMMUNE THROMBOCYTOPENIC PURPURA (ITP)

This is the commonest cause of thrombocytopenia in children and characterized by isolated destruction of platelets due to antiplatelet antibodies (usually IgG) produced by the body. These antibodies are directed against platelet-surface glycoproteins.

The autoimmune phenomenon is usually seen 2–4 weeks after viral infection. Because of the similarity between the viral antigen and the platelets, the antibodies produced against the virus binds with the platelets and cause their destruction. The antibody-platelet complex attaches to the Fc receptors on the macrophages in the reticuloendothelial system especially the spleen and the platelets are destroyed. There is a compensatory increase in the number of immature megakaryocytes in the bone marrow.

Clinical Features

ITP may be acute, persistent, chronic, or recurrent.
- *Acute (or Newly diagnosed) ITP* refers to all new cases at diagnosis up to 3-month duration.
- *Persistent ITP* refers to ITP between 3 and 12 months from diagnosis
- *Chronic ITP* refers to thrombocytopenia persisting longer than 12 months.
- *Recurrent ITP* refers to return of thrombocytopenia after at least 3 months of remission, sustained without treatment.

Acute ITP is the usual presentation in children, while chronic ITP occurs mainly in adults. ITP may be labeled as primary in the absence of an underlying disorder or secondary ITP where a specific etiology has been identified like SLE. Peak prevalence of ITP in children occurs in the age group 2–4 years. Spontaneous remission occurs in more than 80% of cases in children but is uncommon in adults.

Acute ITP

The incidence is equal in both boys and girls. There is sudden and spontaneous onset of mucocutaneous bleeds including petechiae, gum bleed, or epistaxis. History of antecedent viral infection like measles or rubella may be present in some patients. Skin is only site of bleeding in majority of patients. Petechiae are usually pinpoint to pinhead sized skin bleeds which are macular and not blanchable (Fig. 8.20). They are numerous and may be present over any part of the body. Epistaxis and gum bleeds are less common. Some children may have hematuria, menorrhagia and melena. Intracranial bleed is rare and may be fatal.

The child is otherwise well without significant anemia. There is remarkable absence of any physical sign apart from the skin bleeds. Usually, there is no anemia or splenomegaly. Anemia, if present is proportional to the severity of bleeding. Spleen may be just palpable in less than 10% of patients. There is no hepatomegaly or significant lymphadenopathy. Presence of anemia out of proportion to the severity of blood loss, significant splenomegaly, hepatosplenomegaly, or significant lymphadenopathy should arouse the suspicion of an alternate diagnosis such as leukemia.

The disease is usually self-limiting and majority of the patients are asymptomatic within 6 months of onset of symptoms. Treatment seems to have a little effect on the course or duration of the disease.

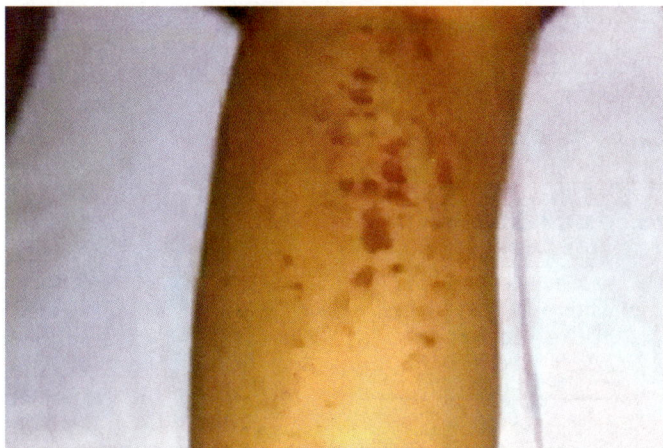

Fig. 8.20 A child with ITP showing skin bleeds

Diagnosis

Thrombocytopenia is universal with counts being <20,000/mm^3 in many children. The RBCs and leukocytes are normal. Hemoglobin may decrease in cases of severe bleeding. The bone marrow examination shows normal erythroid and myeloid series with normal or increased number of megakaryocytes, which are morphologically normal. Bone marrow examination is not warranted in a typical case of ITP (a well-looking child with sudden appearance of petechiae all over the body, isolated thrombocytopenia and no other physical finding). Bone marrow should be examined to rule out the suspicion of leukemia, or aplastic anemia, or when planning to start steroids in ITP. Other tests like Coombs test, antinuclear antibody tests, serology for hepatitis B and C and HIV, antiphospholipid antibody, and thyroid function tests may be considered.

Treatment	Acute ITP

Majority of the children do not require any treatment. Proper counseling of the parents about the self-limiting and benign nature of the disease is of utmost importance. Any kind of therapy is not beneficial in mild to moderate symptoms. 70–80% of children with acute ITP improve spontaneously. About 55–75% of these patients recover within 4 weeks and 90% improve within 4–6 months.

Therapeutic intervention has only shown to probably rapidly increase the platelet counts to a relatively safe level. The time to remission and severity remains unaffected by treatment. Treatment may be offered in circumstances where follow up is difficult or child stays in a remote location.

Decision to intervene or start pharmacotherapy should be based on the clinical picture of the child rather than the platelet count alone. Isolated skin bleed do not warrant any definitive treatment. Treatment is indicated (i) when the platelet count <10,000 mm^3 irrespective of bleeding, (ii) presence of significant mucosal or internal bleeding; or suspected intracranial bleed, irrespective of the platelet count. Remember that you need to treat the patient and not his platelet count.

First line therapy includes corticosteroids, anti-D, and intravenous immunoglobulin (IVIG).

1. Corticosteroids

Corticosteroids raise the platelet count to a safe level by several mechanisms: (i) inhibition of phagocytosis and antibody synthesis, (ii) improved platelet production, (iii) increased endothelial stability. Prednisolone is given in a dose of 2mg/kg/day for 3–4 weeks. Alternately, prednisolone in a dose of 4mg/kg/day for 4 days followed by gradual tapering to complete the total duration of treatment of 2–3 weeks has been also tried. Intravenous or oral methylprednisolone has also been used. Usually, the initial response takes 8–10 days.

2. IVIG (intravenous immunoglobulin)

IVIG raises the platelet count rapidly in 90–95% of children within 1–2 days. The rise is faster than that with steroids. It helps by decreasing the phagocytosis of antibody coated platelets in spleen by binding to the Fc receptors. It is given in a single dose of 0.8 g/kg. The therapy is expensive. Side effects include flu-like symptoms, and rarely anaphylaxis (more so in IgA deficient patients), or aseptic meningitis.

3. Anti-D globulin

This is effective only in Rh-positive individuals in a dose of 50–70 g/kg intravenously. It is as effective as IVIG and much cheaper. The anti-D antibody binds to the Rh-positive RBCs and this complex goes and binds to the Fc receptors and blocks them. This prevents Fc receptor mediated destruction of the platelets. This phenomenon may also cause mild hemolytic anemia in the individual.

4. Splenectomy

Splenectomy is reserved for children >4 years of age with life-threatening bleeding not responding all other modalities, severe ITP, or chronic ITP.

5. Platelet transfusion

Platelet transfusion has no role in most patients. Whatever new platelets are transfused, they are rapidly destroyed by circulating autoantibodies. It may be rarely be indicated in patients with severe life-threatening bleed to immediately raise the platelet count and tide over of the crisis for a very short duration of time.

6. Supportive

Restriction of physical activity, avoidance of contact sports, use of helmets and knee/elbow caps while playing are advisable to prevent trauma which can precipitate bleeding. Use of antiplatelet drugs like aspirin and non-steroidal anti-inflammatory drugs should be avoided.

Chronic ITP

About 15–20% of the children with acute ITP continue to have symptoms beyond 12 months and are labeled as chronic ITP. These children have a more insidious onset of symptoms. Chronic ITP is common in children above 10 years of age. Girls are affected 2–3 times more often than boys. Other causes of thrombocytopenia like SLE, HIV and von Willebrand disease must be ruled out.

These children are managed by medical therapy (IVIG, steroids, anti-D) as and when required depending upon the bleeding manifestations. Children not going into remission and having repeated significant bleeding manifestation for more than 1–2 years may benefit from splenectomy.

Refractory ITP

A patient with ITP who has failed to respond to first line therapy as well as splenectomy and continues to experience clinically significant bleeding. Some other drugs like azathioprine, rituximab, cyclosporine A, mycophenolate mofetil, and danazol can also be tried in such cases. Latest modalities include ramiplostim, eltrombopag, and recombinant thrombopoietin and thrombopoietin receptor agonists.

Platelet Disorders

1. Immune thrombocytopenic purpura (ITP) is commonest cause of thrombocytopenia in children and is characterized by isolated destruction of platelets due to antiplatelet antibodies.
2. ITP may be acute (thrombocytopenia up to 3 months duration), persistent (3–12 months duration), chronic (>12 months duration), or recurrent.
3. A child with ITP appears otherwise well without significant anemia and has usually superficial bleeding.
4. Bone marrow should be examined to rule out the suspicion of leukemia or aplastic anemia or when planning to start steroids in ITP.
5. Spontaneous remission occurs in more than 80% of cases of ITP in children. Treatment is indicated (*i*) when the platelet count <10,000 mm^3 irrespective of bleeding, (*ii*) presence of significant mucosal or internal bleeding; or suspected intracranial bleed, irrespective of the platelet count. First line therapy includes corticosteroids, anti-D, and intravenous immuno-globulin (IVIG).
6. Platelet transfusion has no role in most patients.

Blanchette V, Bolton-Maggs P. Childhood immune thrombocytopenic purpura: diagnosis and management. Hematol Oncol Clin North Am. 2010;24:249–73.

Breakey VR, Blanchette VS. Childhood immune thrombocytopenia: a changing therapeutic landscape. Semin Thromb Hemost 2011;37:745–55.

Bredlau AL, Semple JW, Segel GB. Management of immune thrombocytopenic purpura in children: potential role of novel agents. Paediatr Drugs. 2011;13:213–23.

Cooper N, Bussel JB. The long-term impact of rituximab for childhood immune thrombocytopenia. Curr Rheumatol Rep. 2010;12:94–100.

Grainger JD, Rees JL, Reeves M, et al. Changing trends in UK management of childhood ITP. Arch Dis Child. 2012;97:8–11.

CONGENITAL QUALITATIVE DEFECTS

Sometimes the platelet count is normal but the child continues to bleed. The defect herein may lie in the platelet function or the clotting cascade (Fig. 8.21).

- *Glanzmann thrombasthenia* is an autosomal recessive disorder with normal platelet count in which platelets

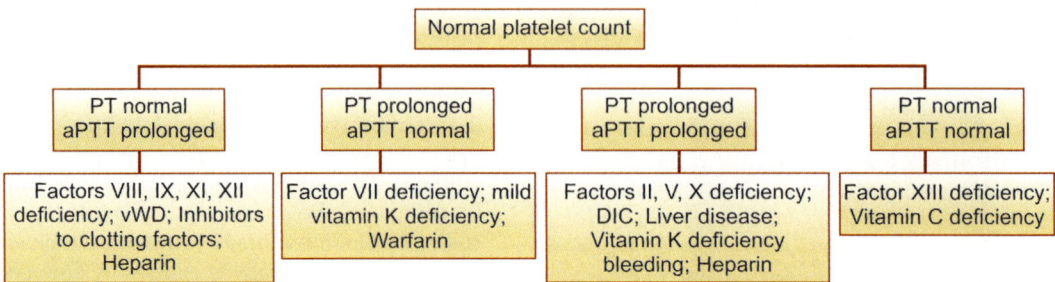

Fig. 8.21 Algorithm for initial bleeding workup of patient with normal platelet count. aPTT: Activated partial thromboplastin time; PT: Prothrombin time, TT: Thrombin time

contain defective or low levels of glycoprotein IIb/IIIa. Therefore, no fibrinogen bridging of platelets to other platelets can occur leading to prolonged bleeding time.

- *Bernard-Soulier syndrome* is also an autosomal recessive disorder associated with thrombocytopenia. The receptor for von Willebrand factor, ie, glycoprotein Ib on platelet surface is lacking. These patients have mild symptoms of easy bruisability or epistaxis, menorrhagia, etc. These patients have low platelet counts and large (giant) platelets. Platelet transfusion is required in the case of significant bleeding.

- *Wiscott-Aldrich syndrome* is an X-linked recessive disorder characterized by eczema, immunodeficiency and platelet function defect along with thrombocytopenia.

- *von Willebrand disease* is characterized by a platelet function defect along with deficiency of von Willebrand factor leading to factor VIII deficiency in the plasma.

8.15 CONGENITAL COAGULATION DISORDERS

HEMOPHILIA

Hemophilia is characterized by prolonged bleeding especially in a male child, often with a family history, with a normal prothrombin time, and prolonged partial thromboplastin time. Coagulation defect is (i) either due to deficiency of factor VIII (hemophilia A); (ii) deficiency of factor IX (hemophilia B), or (iii) deficiency of factor XI (hemophilia C). Hemophilia A and B are inherited as X-linked recessive disorders; affecting only the males, and females are carrier. Hemophilia C is inherited in an autosomal recessive manner.

Prevalence

Hemophilia A occurs more commonly, ie, 1 in 10,000 male births, than hemophilia B which has an incidence of 1 in 40,000 male births. Approximately 1 woman in 5,000 is a carrier for hemophilia A, and 1 in 20,000 is a carrier of hemophilia B.

Severity

Individuals with less than 1% active factor are classified as having severe hemophilia, those with 1–5% active factor have moderate hemophilia, and those with mild hemophilia have between 5 and 40% of normal levels of active clotting factor.

Clinical Manifestations

Hemophilia A and B cannot be differentiated clinically. Mild deficiency may go unnoticed till adolescence or adulthood, there is no spontaneous bleed. Moderate deficiency usually presents as severe bleeding following trauma or surgery; spontaneous bleed is occasional. The diagnosis is only made when these children have heavy bleeding following a surgery, dental procedure, or accident. Children with severe disease have spontaneous bleeding in the joints and muscles.

- The symptoms can present right from the neonatal period. Circumcision is the commonest event leading to excessive bleeding in the neonatal period. Some neonates may present with large cephalhematoma following a difficult delivery.

- In most children, manifestations start appearing in the latter half of the infancy when the child starts crawling or walking, and are prone to falls and injuries. These children bleed profusely for days, following minor cuts and injuries. There is no other significant finding apart from the ecchymotic patches.

- Formation of an intramuscular hematoma following an intramuscular injection may be the first symptom of hemophilia.

- Hemarthrosis bleeding into joints is the most characteristic feature of severe hemophilia (Fig. 8.22). Knee joint is the most common joint to be involved, followed by elbow and ankle joints. There is progressively increasing swelling of the joints after a trivial trauma. Repeated bleeding into the same joint (target joint) leads to destruction of the joint and bones leading to physical disability and restriction in joint movements. The swelling is initially painful but the pain disappears in 3–4 days and swelling may take months to subside. In patients with severe recurrent bleeding there can be formation of contractures. Isolated hemarthrosis may be confused with rheumatic, idiopathic or septic arthritis.

- Intracranial bleed can be fatal and are not uncommon in severe hemophilia.

Investigations

Complete blood count (CBC) is usually normal in hemophiliacs. However, the activated partial thromboplastin time (aPTT) is prolonged. aPTT may be prolonged due to deficiency of factors VIII, IX, XI, or XII. Therefore, mixing studies need to be done to identify the deficient clotting factor. If mixing with normal plasma corrects the aPTT, it suggests an underlying factor deficiency, but if it remains prolonged, it could be due to presence of inhibitors of clotting cascade such as lupus or any acquired inhibitor. Prothrombin time (PT) will be normal among people with hemophilia A and B. Diagnosis is usually established by bioassay of the factor VIII or IX.

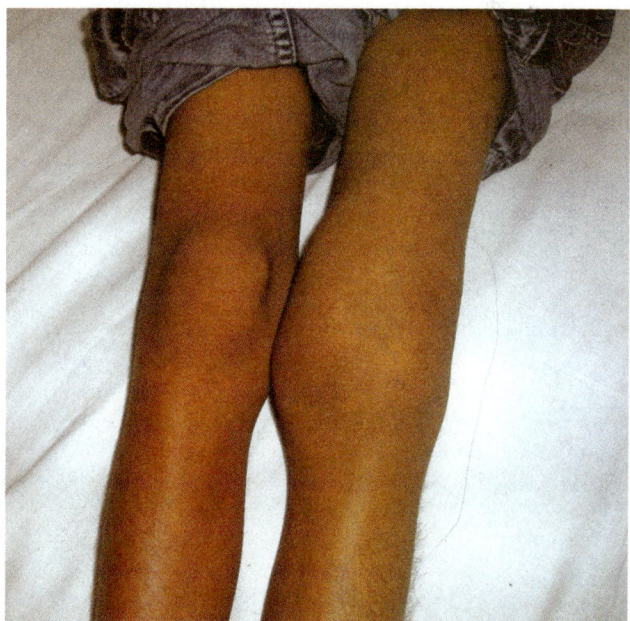

Fig. 8.22 Left knee hemarthrosis in a child with hemophilia A

Diagnosis

Laboratory investigations reveal a normal platelet count, normal PT and prolonged aPTT. Diagnosis is confirmed by assays of factors VIII and IX. The goal of treatment is to prevent life-threatening bleeding and avoid chronic damage to joints.

Treatment	**Hemophilia**

Trauma and injury should be avoided especially in infants and toddlers. Injury can be avoided by use of elbow and kneepads; using furniture with rounded instead of sharp margins; avoidance of contact sports; and use of helmet while cycling. Parents should be counseled about the disease and first aid required for bleeding.

Control bleeding

Bleeding can be controlled by replacement of the deficient factor, using their concentrates derived from plasma or recombinant technique; or appropriate blood products (plasma, cryoprecipitate, whole blood) **(Table 8.11)**.

- *Local measures* RICE (Rest, ice, compression, elevation), topical hemostatics, and splinting.
- *Non-specific measures* Tranexamic acid, epsilon-amino-caproic acid (EACA), or desmopressin can be used for minor mucocutaneous bleeding in children with mild hemophilia A. Desmopressin 0.3 mg/kg diluted in 50 mL of normal saline is infused intravenously in hemophilia A patients as it causes

release of factor VIII from stores. It can also be given subcutaneously or intranasally.
- Levels of factor VIII should be raised to at least 30% in hemarthrosis or muscle bleed. It should be raised to 100% for a life threatening intracranial bleed.
- One unit of the specific Factor concentrate per kg body weight increases the plasma concentration of Factor VIII by 2%, and Factor IX by 1%. Cost of the factor concentrates and development of antibodies against these recombinant factors because of repeated administration are the limiting factors.

Storing concentrates

Factor concentrates can be stored in a refrigerator for quite long periods (up to 6 months). However, they should not be frozen. Factor VIII is available in vials of 250, 500, and 1000 IU. Factor IX is available in vials of 300 and 600 IU.

Blood products

If factor concentrates are not available, it is possible to use fresh frozen plasma (FFP) (for hemophilia A and B), cryoprecipitate (for hemophilia A), whole blood, or prothrombin complex concentrates (for hemophilia B) as an alternative life-saving option. However, their administration entails a high risk for acquiring infections like HIV, hepatitis B and C, and CMV.
- A bag of cryoprecipitate made from one unit of FFP (200–250 mL) may contain 70–80 units of FVIII in a volume of 30–40 mL.
- One bag of FFP contains 200 IU of factor VIII and IX.

Table 8.11 Factor Replacement Therapy for Bleeding Episodes in Hemophilia (for resource-poor countries)

Type of bleed	Hemophilia A		Hemophilia B	
	Desired level (IU/dL)	Duration (days)	Desired level (IU/dL)	Duration (days)
Hemarthrosis*	10–20	1–2	10–20	1–2
Superficial muscle bleed (without compromise)	10–20	2–3	10–20	2–3
Iliopsoas bleed or deep muscle bleed (with compromise)*·				
• Initial	20–40		15–30	
• Maintenance	10–20	3–5 (or longer)	10–20	3–5 (or longer)
CNS bleed				
Initial	50–80	1–3	50–80	1–3
Maintenance	50–30	4–7	50–30	4–7
	20–40	8–14	20–40	8–14
Renal	20–40	3–5	20–40	3–5
Deep laceration	20–40	5–7	20–40	5–7
Major surgery				
Preoperative	60–80		60–80	
Postoperative	30–40	1–3	30–40	1–3
	20–30	4–7	20–30	4–7
	10–20	8–14	10–20	8–14
Minor surgery				
Preoperative	40–80		40–80	
Postoperative	20–50	1–5	20–50	1–5
Gastrointestinal bleeding				
Initial	30–50	1–3	30–50	1–3
Maintenance	10–20	4–7	10–20	4–7
Renal	20–40	3–5	15–30	3–5

*Prednisolone may be added for 1–3 days as adjunctive treatment

8

Treatment of specific hemorrhages

In case of large internal hemorrhage, hemoglobin should be checked and corrected while other measures are being planned. Ensure hemodynamic stability while factor replacement therapy is initiated. The dose of the factor used and the duration of therapy to treat the bleeding episode varies according to the nature and site of bleeding. Administer the appropriate dose of factor concentrate to raise the patient's factor level suitably as shown in **Table 8.11**.

The use of viral inactivated, plasma-derived, or recombinant concentrates are recommended for treating bleeding episodes in hemophiliacs.

In the absence of an inhibitor, each unit of FVIII per kilogram of body weight infused intravenously will raise the plasma FVIII level approximately 2 IU/dL. The half-life of FVIII is approximately 8–12 hours. The dose is calculated by multiplying the patient's weight in kilograms by the desired rise in factor level in IU/dL, multiplied by 0.5.

In absence of an inhibitor, each unit of FIX per kilogram of body weight infused intravenously will raise the plasma FIX level approximately 1 IU/dL. The half-life is approximately 18–24 hours. To calculate dosage, multiply the patient's weight in kilograms by the desired rise in factor level in IU/dL.

Factor concentrates should be infused by slow IV injection at a rate not to exceed 100 units per minute in young children.

Prophylactic therapy

Early prophylactic use of clotting factors with severe hemophilia is gaining acceptance to prevent pain and morbidity associated with bleeding disorders. Regular administration of factor concentrates can aid in maintaining the factor levels above 5%. The indications for prophylactic therapy are recurrent hemarthrosis and an episode of intracranial bleed. NSAIDs should be avoided in hemophiliacs.

CARRIER STATUS AND PRENATAL TESTING

Since hemophilia has X-linked inheritance (Fig. 8.23), men with the genetic mutation will have hemophilia, therefore a male who does not have the condition cannot be a carrier of the disease. A woman who has a son with known hemophilia is termed an obligate carrier, and no testing is needed to establish that she is a carrier of hemophilia. Women whose carrier status is unknown can be evaluated either by testing for the clotting factors or by methods to characterize the mutation in the DNA. The DNA screening methods are generally the most reliable. A hemophilia gene test can be done during pregnancy by chorionic villus sampling (CVS) test. A simple factor assay can also help ascertain carrier status. A woman who is a hemophilia carrier is likely to have low levels of factor VIII or IX. Estimation of factor VIII-C: F VIII Ag is useful; ratio <0.6 is suggestive of carrier state in Hemophilia A.

DEVELOPMENT OF ANTIBODIES (ACQUIRED HEMOPHILIA)

About 5–10% of patients with hemophilia develop antibodies against factor VIII/IX. It should be suspected whenever patients fail to respond to adequate replacement therapy. Inhibitors can be estimated by Bethesda Assay. Treatment of acquired hemophilia may be done with high doses of

Case Study   Hemophilia

A 4-year-old boy was brought by his mother to the emergency department with complaints of sudden onset weakness in both lower limbs following trivial trauma. There was no associated fever, rash, headache, vomiting, seizures or recent vaccination. The mother gave a history of easy bruisability and repeated hemarthrosis noticed since infancy in her son. His younger brother also had similar complaints of repeated skin bleeds, though his older sister was normal. Laboratory investigation revealed: Hemoglobin: 10.4 g/dL, TLC: 4600, platelet count: 2.13 lac/mm³, with an essentially normal peripheral smear, PT= 12s (C=14s), PTTK= 84s (C=32s) and a normal bleeding time. CECT (spine) revealed an extradural collection suggestive of a hematoma, extending from D7 to D11.

What is the probable diagnosis?
The child is probably suffering from Hemophilia, as his partial thromboplastin time is deranged suggesting a defect in the intrinsic pathway (factors XII, XI, IX, or VIII deficiency). Hemophilia A is due to the deficiency of clotting factor VIII, Hemophilia B is due to the deficiency of factor IX and Hemophilia C is due to the deficiency of factor XI. Hemophilia has an X-linked recessive inheritance.

How will you confirm the diagnosis?
Specific factor assays viz, factor VIII and factor IX should be done to confirm this condition. Mixing studies should be done to rule out the presence of inhibitor of factor VIII or factor IX in the plasma.

What is the specific treatment of this disorder?
Specific therapy i.e., replacement therapy in the form of fresh frozen plasma (containing factor VIII and factor IX) or cryoprecipitate (containing factor VIII, von Willebrand factor and fibrinogen) can be given for managing bleeding seen in patients of severe hemophilia. One unit of factor VIII raises the factor VIII level by 2% (t1/2 of factor VIII 8–12 hours) while one unit of factor IX raises the factor IX level by 1% (t1/2 of factor IX 18–24 hours). However, there is a risk of blood transfusion associated infections like HIV, hepatitis B and C, cytomegalovirus). To circumvent this problem, factor VIII and IX concentrates (plasma derived or recombinant) are preferred. However, for mild or moderate hemophilia, antifibrinolytic drugs like epsilon-aminocaproic acid (EACA) or tranexamic acid can be given. Desmopressin (intranasal or intravenous) can be given in mild or moderate hemophilia A.

factors VIII and IX, porcine factor VIII, activated prothrombin complex, activated factor VII, use of immunosuppressive agents and recombinant factor VIII or IX.

VON WILLEBRAND DISEASE (vWD)

Von Willebrand disease is an autosomal dominant disorder and occurs due to deficiency of von Willebrand factor (vWF). vWF is present in platelets, endothelial cella and in plasma along with F VIII. Children with vWD present with mucosal bleeding and symptoms akin to hemophilia A. Laboratory investigations reveal prolonged bleeding time with decreased F VIII levels. Ristocetin aggregation test is decreased unlike patients with hemophilia A who have a normal ristocetin induced aggregation. Management is similar to hemophilia.

8

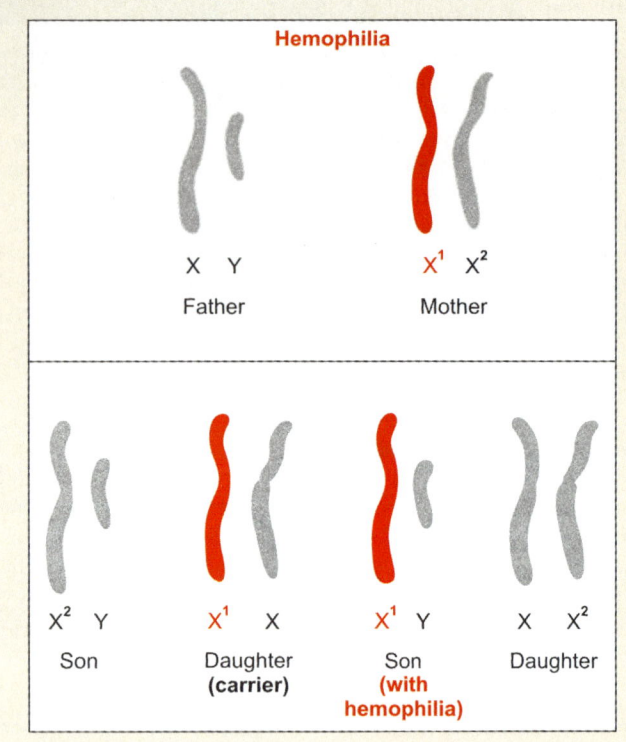

Fig. 8.23 Inheritance pattern in hemophilia

Congenital Coagulation Disorders

1. Hemophilia A and B are X-linked recessive disorders characterized by prolonged bleeding especially in a male child, often with a family history, with a normal prothrombin time, and prolonged partial thromboplastin time.
2. Diagnosis of hemophilia is confirmed by assays of factor VIII and IX.
3. Bleeding into joints is the most characteristic feature of severe hemophilia.
4. Bleeding can be controlled by replacement of the deficient factor, using their concentrates derived from plasma or recombinant technique; or appropriate blood products (plasma, cryoprecipitate, whole blood). The use of viral-inactivated, plasma-derived, or recombinant concentrates are recommended for treating bleeding episodes in hemophiliacs. One unit of the specific Factor concentrate per kg body weight increases the plasma concentration of Factor VIII by 2%, and Factor IX by 1%.
5. Local measures such as RICE (Rest, ice, compression, elevation), topical hemostatics, and splinting are important in management of acute bleeds.
6. *Non-specific measures* Tranexamic acid, epsilon-aminocaproic acid (EACA), or desmopressin can be used for minor mucocutaneous bleeding.
7. Early prophylactic use of clotting factors with severe hemophilia to maintain the factor levels above 5% is gaining acceptance as a way to prevent pain and morbidity associated with bleeding disorders.

Coppola A, Di Capna M, DiMinno MN, et al. Treatment of hemophilia: a review of current advances and ongoing issues. J *Blood Med.* 2010;1:183–195.

Iorio A, Marchesini E, Marcucci M, et al. Clotting factor concentrates given to prevent bleeding and bleeding-related complications in people with hemophilia A or B. *Cochrane Database Syst Rev.* 2011;9:CD003429.

Iorio A, Halimeh S, Holzhauer S, et al. Rate of inhibitor development in previously untreated hemophilia A patients treated with plasma-derived or recombinant factor VIII concentrates: a systematic review. *J Thromb Haemost.* 2010;8:1256–65.

Kulkarni R, Soucie JM. Pediatric hemophilia: a review. *Semin Thromb Hemost.* 2011;37: 737–744.

8.16 ACQUIRED COAGULATION DISORDERS

These are usually systemic diseases, which affect all the coagulation factors. Deficiency of coagulation factors occur either because of their decreased production (chronic liver disorders, vitamin K deficiency) or increased consumption (disseminated intravascular coagulation). Chronic liver disease is discussed in chapter on gastroenterology. Vitamin K deficiency and disseminated intravascular coagulation (DIC) are briefly described here.

VITAMIN K DEFICIENCY BLEEDING (VKDB)

Vitamin K is a fat-soluble vitamin needed for synthesis of Factors II, VII, IX and X. It is mainly derived from green leafy vegetables and some is synthesized by the colonic bacterial flora. Deficiency in neonatal period manifests as hemorrhagic disease in newborns and infants.

HEMORRHAGIC DISEASE OF INFANCY (HDN)

Vitamin K is not transported across the placenta. A state of vitamin K deficiency is seen in a newborn because of lack of body stores, hepatic immaturity, paucity of colonic bacteria, or certain maternal medications like anticoagulants or anticonvulsants. Vitamin K deficiency can also result from impaired absorption due to lack of bile salts and, prolonged use of antibiotics (impaired synthesis due to destruction of colonic flora).

Breastmilk being a poor source of vitamin K, children on exclusive breastfeeding in whom complimentary feeding is not started at appropriate time can develop vitamin K deficiency and manifest with bleeding in the latter half of infancy.

The disease is categorized into three types based on the time of appearance of symptoms:

1. *Early HDN* The newborn presents with bleeding within first 24 hours of birth. This is usually seen in newborns whose mothers have been treated with phenytoin, primidone, phenobarbital, or anticoagulants.
2. *Classical HDN* This is typically seen in newborns who have not been supplemented with prophylactic vitamin K at birth. The bleeding starts 2–7 days after birth. There can be ecchymotic patches or gastrointestinal bleeds but the neonate otherwise appears well and has no abnormal physical findings.
3. *Late HDN* This occurs at 4–12 weeks of life. High risk factors include prolonged use of broad spectrum antibiotics or presence of chronic liver disease or malabsorption.

Both PT and aPTT are prolonged and platelet count is normal. Vitamin K administration is sufficient in mild bleeding but in moderate to severe bleeding transfusion of fresh frozen plasma is also required. All newborns should be supplemented with parenteral vitamin K (1 mg) at birth as a prophylaxis to prevent its deficiency.

DISSEMINATED INTRAVASCULAR COAGULATION (DIC)

DIC is a consumption coagulopathy characterized by diffuse intravascular clotting which consumes the coagulation factors and the platelets resulting in their deficiency.

Causes

1. *Malignancy* Acute myeloid leukemia (mainly promyelo-cytic), neuroblastoma, histiocytosis X, rhabdomyosarcoma
2. *Infections* Gram-negative septicemia, *Neisseria meningitides, Staphylococcus aureus, Streptococcus pneumoniae,* malaria, rickettsial diseases, aspergillosis.
3. *Obstetric causes* Abruptio placentae, pre-eclampsia, amniotic fluid embolism.
4. *Massive tissue injury* Burns, trauma, extensive surgery
5. *Venoms/toxins* Snake bites, insect bites
6. *Neonatal causes* Birth asphyxia, septicemia, severe Rh incompatibility, hypothermia, respiratory distress syndrome, necrotizing enterocolitis, congenital infections (herpes, cytomegalovirus)
7. *Miscellaneous* Heat stroke, diabetic acidosis, acute pancreatitis.

Clinical Features

Bleeding can be superficial or deep; and can be life threatening. Tissue damage occurs because of ischemia caused by intravascular thrombus formation. Vital organs like kidneys, brain and liver are affected. Thromboembolic phenomena can lead to hematuria, oliguria, abdominal pain, ileus, vomiting, and respiratory distress.

Laboratory Diagnosis

Diagnosis of DIC is based on clinical features in addition to laboratory tests which would be characterized by: low platelet count; low levels of fibrinogen, factors II, V, X, VIII

and XIII (prolonged PT, aPTT and TT); low levels of antithrombin III and protein C; increased fibrin degradation products (FDPs) and microangiopathic hemolytic anemia.

Treatment	DIC

This is a potentially fatal condition, which should be aggressively managed by treating the precipitating condition. Transfusion of fresh frozen plasma, platelet concentrates, and packed red cells will help control bleeding and treat associated anemia. Hydrocortisone may be used in presence of purpura fulminans or meningococcemia. Heparin therapy has a role in reducing complications due to thromboembolic phenomenon. Heparin acts by activating the thrombin system and inhibition of proteolytic enzymes and factors such as thrombin, IXa and Xa. In certain conditions like severe malaria or severe Rh hemolytic disease, exchange transfusion can be useful.

Table 8.12 shows the laboratory findings which may enable us to differentiate a bleeding episode due to the

Case Study	Bleeding Disorder

A 10-year-old boy with chronic tonsillitis presented with excessive bruising. His coagulation results were as follows:
PT 18.5 seconds (Reference range, 10.8 to 13.5)
aPTT 48.1 seconds (Reference range, 28.5 to 35.5)
Platelets 325,000 (Reference range, 150,000 to 400,000)
Bleeding 5 minutes (Reference, 8 minutes)
Peripheral blood smear is unremarkable with adequate platelets.

Which coagulation tests are abnormal? How will you manage this child?

Two parameters, the PT and aPTT are elevated, and the child shows a history of recent bruising. Probably, the common pathway of the coagulation cascade is affected, specifically factors I, II, V, and X. Since this child has had a history of chronic tonsillitis, he may have been receiving prolonged antibiotics. Antibiotics may deplete the normal gut flora, a source of vitamin K synthesis. Vitamin K is the essential cofactor for the gamma carboxylation of these factors II, VII, IX, and X. Therefore, antibiotics could lead yo deranged coagulation. Administering oral/parenteral vitamin K can correct this defect.

Table 8.12 Laboratory Findings in Bleeding due to Coagulation or Platelet Disorders					
Condition	Prothrombin time	Partial thromboplastin time	Bleeding time	Platelet count
von Willebrand disease	Unaffected	Prolonged	Prolonged	Unaffected
Vitamin K deficiency or warfarin	Prolonged	Normal or mildly prolonged	Unaffected	Unaffected
Thrombocytopenia	Unaffected	Unaffected	Prolonged	Decreased
Liver failure	Prolonged	Prolonged	Prolonged	Decreased
Hemophilia	Unaffected	Prolonged	Unaffected	Unaffected
Glanzmann thrombasthenia	Unaffected	Unaffected	Prolonged	Unaffected
Factor X deficiency	Prolonged	Prolonged	Unaffected	Unaffected
Factor V deficiency	Prolonged	Prolonged	Unaffected	Unaffected
Disseminated intravascular coagulation	Prolonged	Prolonged	Prolonged	Decreased
Congenital afibrinogenemia	Prolonged	Prolonged	Prolonged	Unaffected
Bernard-Soulier syndrome	Unaffected	Unaffected	Prolonged	Decreased, or unaffected
Aspirin	Unaffected	Unaffected	Prolonged	Unaffected

various coagulation defects and platelet defects, described previously.

Acquired Coagulation Disorders

1. Hemorrhagic disease of infancy (HDN) is a state of vitamin K deficiency which may occur because of lack of body stores at birth, hepatic immaturity, paucity of colonic bacteria, or certain maternal medications like anticoagulants or anticonvulsants. All newborns should be supplemented with parenteral vitamin K (1 mg) at birth as a prophylaxis to prevent its deficiency.

2. Disseminated intravascular coagulation (DIC) is characterized by diffuse intravascular clotting and is characterized by low platelet count; low levels of fibrinogen, factors II, V, X, VIII and XIII (prolonged PT, aPTT and TT); low levels of antithrombin III and protein C; increased fibrin degradation products (FDPs) and microangiopathic hemolytic anemia.

Brousson MA, Klein MC. Controversies surrounding the administration of vitamin K to newborns: a review. *CMAJ.* 1996;154:307–15.

Franchini M, Manzato F, Salvagno GL, Lippi G. Potential role of recombinant activated factor VII for the treatment of severe bleeding associated with disseminated intravascular coagulation: a systematic review. *Blood Coagul Fibrinolysis.* 2007;18:589–93.

Shearer MJ. Vitamin K deficiency bleeding disorder (VKBD) in early infancy. *Blood Rev.* 2009;23:49–59.

Van Winckel M, DeBruyne R, Van De Velde S. Vitamin K, an update for the pediatrician. *Eur J Pediatr.*2009;168:127–134.

8.17 BLOOD AND BLOOD PRODUCT TRANSFUSION IN CHILDREN

Blood transfusion can be a lifesaving procedure, but it has risks, including infectious and noninfectious complications. A blood transfusion is usually given through an intravenous (IV) catheter, or rarely through an umbilical catheter (in neonates) or via an intraosseous line (in shock when IV access is not possible).

BLOOD GROUPS

There are four major blood groups in human, determined by the presence or absence of two antigens—A and B—on the surface of *RBCs*.

Group A Presence of A antigen on RBCs and B antibody in the *plasma*.

Group B Presence of B antigen on *RBCs* and A antibody in the *plasma*.

Group AB Has both A and B antigens on RBCs but neither A nor B antibody in the plasma.

Group O Has neither A nor B antigens on RBCs but both A and B antibody are in the plasma.

In addition to the A and B antigens, there is a third antigen called the Rh factor, which can be either present (Rh+) or absent (Rh–).

Recipients must be transfused with ABO group-specific or ABO group-compatible RBCs. Rh-positive recipients may receive either Rh-positive or Rh-negative RBCs, but Rh-negative recipients should receive Rh-negative RBCs (except when these units are in short supply and the situation is lifesaving). Transfusion of Rh-positive RBC should be avoided for Rh-negative women of child-bearing age. ABO incompatibility of RBCs can lead to complement-mediated acute hemolytic reaction, particularly in the setting of PRBC transfusion. Additionally, ABO incompatibility can cause hemolysis in hematopoietic and solid organ transplantation (graft vs host disease), and hemolytic disease of the newborn. It is important to prevent ABO incompatibility. **Table 8.13** shows compatible blood types for transfusion.

Table 8.13 Compatible Blood Types	
Recipient	*Donor*
A	A, O
B	B, O
AB	AB, A, B, O
O	O

Universal red cell donor has O negative blood type. Universal plasma donor has Type AB blood type.

DERIVING BLOOD COMPONENTS AND PLASMA DERIVATIVES

The various blood components include: red cells, platelets, fresh frozen plasma and cryoprecipitate. The plasma derivatives used for transfusion include albumin, coagulation factors and immunoglobulins.

Voluntary fit donor for blood collection is selected as per the standard criteria laid down by drug controlling authorities and National AIDS Control Organization. The Whole blood is collected as 350 ml or 450 ml in bags with CPDA-1 (citrate-phosphate-dextrose with adenine) or additive solution. Apheresis is a procedure where required single or more than one component is collected, and the rest of blood components are returned to the donor.

BLOOD COMPONENTS

After blood collection, components should be separated within 5–8 hours. Different blood components have different relative density, sediment rate and size and they can be separated by centrifugation of one unit of whole blood. In increasing order, the specific gravity of blood components is plasma, platelets, leukocytes (buffy Coat [BC]) and packed red blood cells (PRBCs). Preparing only PRBC and fresh frozen plasma (FFP) is by single-step heavy spin centrifugation (5000 G for 10–15 min). However, preparing platelet concentrates (PLTCs), PRBC concentrates, and FFP is by two step centrifugation. The two main procedures of preparing PLTC are either by platelet-rich plasma (PRP) method or BC method.

INDICATIONS FOR TRANSFUSION OF DIFFERENT BLOOD PRODUCTS

Before undertaking a blood transfusion, ensure that you are using the right blood (ABO and Rh matched), right patient [match the patient identity on the Identity (ID) band and blood pack] and right indication. Transfusion should only be used when the benefits outweigh the risks and there are no appropriate alternatives.

Indications for blood component therapy are listed in **Table 8.14.**

BLOOD PRODUCTS IN SPECIAL SITUATIONS

1. *Leukodepleted products (RBCs and platelets)* Removal of leukocytes from various blood products has been shown to minimize febrile non-hemolytic transfusion reactions, HLA alloimmunization, platelet refractoriness in multitransfused patients and prevention of transmission of leukotropic viruses. Leukodepletion involves removal of leukocytes with the help of certain specific filters or leucacytapheresis devices (apheresis machines). Leukofilteration of blood components can be done either at the time of collection and processing, postprocessing (within the blood bank), or by the side of the patient (post-storage). Leukocyte content in a blood component unit should be less than 5×10^6/unit after leukoreduction and leukoreduced RDPs should have $<8.3 \times 10^5$ WBC/unit.

Indications:
- Prevention of transmission of leukotropic viruses like CMV and EBV
- Prevention of nonhemolytic febrile transfusion reactions
- Prevention or delay of WBC alloimmunization and platelet refractoriness in selected patients requiring repeated transfusions over an extended time period.

2. *Irradiated* components can be used to prevent graft-versus-host disease due to the action of viable donor T-lymphocytes that can proliferate in a host with an impaired immune defence.

Indications
- Neonates and infants < 6 months of age
- All pediatric malignancies
- Intrauterine or neonatal exchange transfusions
- Myelosuppressive therapy (chemotherapy or irradiation)
- Patients undergoing, or candidates for, marrow or peripheral blood progenitor cell transplant
- Congenital immunodeficiency syndromes, include suspected DiGeorge syndrome
- Patients receiving anti-thymocyte globulin or purine analog therapy.

3. *Washed red blood cells or platelets* RBCs and platelets are prepared using 0.8% sodium chloride which helps to reduce plasma proteins, potassium, free hemoglobin and antibodies.

Indications
- History of anaphylactic or severe, unexplained reaction to blood components.
- Extracorporeal membrane oxygenation (ECMO) or cardiopulmonary bypass patients if fresh red blood cells are unavailable
- Paroxysmal nocturnal hemoglobinuria
- Intrauterine transfusion (fetal transfusion)

Table 8.14 Indications for Blood Component Therapy		
Blood/Blood component	*Indication*	*Dosing**
Reconstituted fresh whole blood (<7 days old) in neonates	Exchange transfusion in neonates (for neonatal jaundice, severe malaria and septicemia in neonates	Single volume exchange transfusion: 80 mL/kg body weight; double volume exchange transfusion: 160 mL/kg body weight
Packed RBC (PRBC) transfusion	Premature infant • Stable, growing, Hb <7 g/dL • Respiratory distress syndrome: Not warranting oxygen therapy, Hb < 10 g/dL; with oxygen requirement, Hb < 12 g/dL • Mildly symptomatic anemia (e.g., apnea, tachycardia, poor wt. gain), Hb <10 g/dL • Severely symptomatic (e.g., worsening apnea, hypotension, acidosis, heart disease), Hb < 12 g/dL. Term infant < 4 months of age • Symptomatic anemia (e.g., apnea, tachycardia, poor wt. gain), Hb < 7 g/dL • Perioperative anemia, Hb < 10 g/dL • Hypoxia or on ECMO, Hb < 12 g/dL • Cyanotic heart disease, Hb < 13 g/dL • Acute blood loss >10% blood volume, not responsive to other forms of therapy > 4 months of age • Acute blood loss >15% of blood volume, or anticipation thereof, or hypovolemia not responsive to other forms of therapy • Postoperatively with signs of anemia (e.g., apnea) Hb < 10 g/dL	10–15 mL/kg of PRBCs are transfused at 5 mL/kg/h and the transfusion should be completed within 4 hours. RBC compatibility testing must be performed before RBC transfusion.

Contd...

8

	Table 8.14 Indications for Blood Component Therapy *(Contd...)*	
Blood/Blood component	*Indication*	*Dosing**
	• Severe cardiopulmonary disease, Hb < 12 g/dL • Patients receiving chemotherapy or irradiation, or patients with chronic anemia not responsive to medical therapy, Hb < 7 g/dL (symptomatic patients may be transfused at a higher hemoglobin level) • Chronic hemolytic anemias like thalassemia, complications of SCD, Hb <9 g/dL	
Fresh Frozen Plasma	• INR > 1.5–2 times the mean normal value in a non-bleeding patient • Warfarin overdose with major bleeding • Support during DIC • Bleeding patient with liver disease • During or within 24 hours of ECMO • For correction of vitamin K deficiency in bleeding patient • Protein C, protein S, anti-thrombin III deficiencies, or other single-factor • Deficiency where no product is available and patient is bleeding • Bleeding secondary to vitamin K deficiency	The dose of 12–15 mL/kg should be administered at a rate of 10–20 mL/kg/h. Once thawed, FFP should be used within 24 hours.
Cryoprecipitate (concentrated Factor VIII:C, von Willebrand factor, fibrinogen, Factor XIII and fibronectin)	• Acute DIC: Bleeding and fibrinogen < 100 mg/dL) • Hypofibrinogenemia: thrombolytic therapy • Dysfibrinogenemia • Hemophilia A with active bleeding or invasive procedure planned, unresponsive to DDAVP and/or factor concentrates • Fibrin glue production	Fibrinogen replacement: 1 unit of cryo per 5 kg patient weight will increase fibrinogen by about 100 mg/dL.Dosing in hemophilia A depends upon the factor VIII level/type of bleedingvon Willebrand Factor replacement: 1 unit per 10 kg patient weight will usually be enough to control bleeding. Cryoprecipitate of the same ABO group must be given; Rh matching is not needed.
Platelet transfusion	Platelet thresholds in neonates: • Stable neonate: <20,000/µL • Unstable or sick neonate: <30,000–50,000/µL • Active bleeding or invasive procedure: < 50,000/µL Platelet transfusion thresholds in older children • Non-infected, clinically stable: <10,000/µL • Critically ill patients: <100,000/µL • Patients with induction therapy for leukemia, requiring lumbar puncture or insertion of a central venous line: <20,000–40,000/µL • Bleeding child with platelet function defects Platelet transfusions are not usually indicated in patients with rapid platelet destruction associated with ITP unless a life-threatening bleeding episode is probable, heparin-induced thrombocytopenia (HIT) and thrombotic thrombocytopenic purpura (TTP). Platelets should be ABO-compatible to reduce the risk of hemolysis caused by donor plasma.	1 unit RDP for every 10 kg increases platelet count by approximately 50 × 10^9/L (50,000/cu mm). 0.2 unit/kg of RDP will raise the platelet count to 50 × 10^9/L (50,000/cu mm.)
Granulocyte transfusion	• Bacterial sepsis in an infant < 2 weeks of age with neutrophil count < 3 × 10^9/L. • Bacterial sepsis or disseminated fungal infection that is unresponsive to antibiotics in a patient > 2 weeks of age with neutrophil count < 0.5 × 10^9/L and whose neutrophil count is expected to recover. • Infection that is unresponsive to antibiotics and the presence of a qualitative neutrophil defect, regardless of neutrophil count.	

* The dose of blood components for infants and children should always be carefully calculated and prescribed in mL (compared to 'units'as in adults) to avoid volume overload.

- For patients with hyperkalemia with poor renal function (until hyperkalemia resolves)
- Ig A deficient individuals.

4. *Platelet transfusion (RDP and SDP)* Random donor platelets (RDP) are prepared from donated blood within 4 to 6 hrs of collection by centrifugation. Each RDP contains approximately 5.5×10^{10} platelets. Single Donor Platelets (SDP) are prepared by platelet aphaeresis machine. One unit of SDP is equivalent to 5 to 10 units of RDP. Platelets are stored at 22°C on an agitator and must not be frozen. Their life span is 3–4 days. For indications see **Table 8.14**.

5. *Albumin transfusion* Human albumin is a physiological plasma-expander and has specific indications as it is costly and has limited availability. Preparations of 5%, 20%, and 25% are available for use. Albumin infusion is generally well tolerated, but we must watch for immediate hypersensitivity reactions (fever, rigors, nausea, vomiting, urticaria, hypotension, increased salivation, and effects on respiration and heart rate).

Indications:

- *Paracentesis:* 5 g of albumin per liter of ascetic fluid removal
- Therapeutic plasmapheresis
- Refractory ascites in cirrhotic patients with serum albumin <2g/dL
- Nephrotic syndrome with serum albumin <2 g/dL or hypovolemia or pulmonary edema
- Extensive burns (>30%)

ADVERSE REACTIONS TO BLOOD TRANSFUSION

All patients receiving blood transfusion must be monitored during the transfusion because of the possible life-threatening nature of acute transfusion reactions. Any adverse reaction to the transfusion of blood or blood components should be reported to Blood Bank. Reactions may be categorized into reactions that present in proximity to the transfusion and those that present later. Acute transfusion reactions (ATRs) present within 24 hours of transfusion and vary in severity from mild febrile or allergic reactions to life-threatening events.

- *Febrile non-hemolytic transfusion reactions* These are usually mild, characterized by fever, shivering, muscle pain and nausea. Use of leukodepleted blood components can minimize (FNHTR). These can occur up to 2 hours after completion of the transfusion and are more common in multi-transfused patients receiving red cells. Mild FNHTRs (pyrexia >38°C, but <2°C rise from baseline) can often be managed simply by slowing (or temporarily stopping) the transfusion and use of antipyretic drugs like paracetamol. In the case of moderate FNHTRs (pyrexia >2°C above baseline or >39°C or rigors and/or myalgia), the transfusion should be stopped. If the symptoms worsen, or do not quickly resolve, consider the possibility of a hemolytic or bacterial reaction. Patients with recurrent FNHTRs can be pre-medicated with oral paracetamol given at least one hour before the reaction is anticipated. Patients who continue to react should have a trial of washed blood components.

ACUTE TRANSFUSION REACTIONS

- *Febrile reactions* One in eight patients receiving a transfusion may develop fever with or without chills. These are usually rise of 1°C temperature from baseline and warrant symptomatic therapy. These are mediated by cytokines released in response to antibodies reacting to leukocyte antigens. Watch the vitals carefully to distinguish from bacterial sepsis.

- *Allergic transfusion reactions* These may range from mild urticaria to severe reactions manifesting with laryngeal edema and bronchospasm or anaphylaxis. Symptoms often improve if the transfusion is slowed and an antihistamine (e.g. chlorpheniramine) is administered orally or intravenously.

- *Acute hemolytic reaction* The commonest cause is clerical errors like mislabeled pretransfusion specimen, ABO incompatibility, etc. It may manifest with fever, chills, constricting pain in the chest, tachycardia, hypotension, and hemoglobinemia with subsequent hemoglobinuria and hyperbilirubinemia. Rarely, patient may develop uncontrollable bleeding due to disseminated intravascular coagulation.

- *Delayed hemolytic reactions* These can occur 4–8 days after blood transfusion, but may develop up to one month later. Delayed hemolytic reactions occur in patients who have developed antibodies from previous transfusion or pregnancy but, at the time of pretransfusion testing, the antibody in question is too weak to be detected by standard procedures. It may go undetected. It manifests as falling hematocrit with or without hemoglobinuria and jaundice. A positive direct antiglobulin (Coombs) test (DAT) is suggestive.

- *Transfusion-associated circulatory overload (TACO)* Typical features include acute respiratory distress, tachycardia, raised blood pressure and evidence of positive fluid balance. The treatment of TACO involves stopping the transfusion and administering oxygen and diuretics.

- *Transfusion-related acute lung injury (TRALI)* Classical TRALI is caused by antibodies in the donor blood reacting with the patient's neutrophils, monocytes or pulmonary endothelium and these subsequently sequester in the recipient's lungs. Most cases present within acute onset (within 2–6 hours) severe breathlessness and cough with frothy pink expectoration (non-cardiogenic pulmonary edema). It is often associated with hypotension, fever and rigors and transient peripheral blood neutropenia or monocytopenia. Chest X-ray shows bilateral nodular shadows in the lung fields with normal cardiac size. Treatment is supportive, with high-concentration oxygen therapy and ventilatory support if required. Steroid therapy is not effective. TRALI is often confused with acute heart failure due to circulatory overload. However, diuretics should not be given in a patient with TRALI.

Management of Acute Transfusion Reaction (ATR)

You must stop the transfusion and maintain venous access with physiological saline and check vital signs; start resuscitation if necessary. Match the identification details of the patient, their ID band and the compatibility label of the component match. Examine the remaining blood in the bag for clumps or discoloration. If the presumed ATR is severe or life-threatening the transfusion must be discontinued and immediate medical review arranged. Depending upon the patient's condition, treatment may include crystalloids (for shock), diuretics (for acute hemolysis and volume overload), antipyretics, antihistaminic, antibiotics, and oxygen/ventilator support. You should return the remaining blood to the blood bank to allow prompt investigation. Also, initiate the Transfusion Reaction Report Form which must be notified to the blood bank. You may collect peripheral blood sample from the patient and a fresh urine specimen (look for hemoglobinuria) which may be sent for laboratory tests.

DELAYED TRANSFUSION REACTIONS

- *Bacterial contamination* These can range from mild pyrexial reactions to septic shock. Diagnosis is established by blood culture of both the blood component and the recipient.
- *Transfusion-transmitted infection* Conventional screening tests are based on the detection of viral antibodies in donor blood (exception: Hepatitis B). However, there is a small risk of infectious products may enter the donor if a donation was made during the window period (before a detectable antibody response). These window periods have been much reduced by the addition of antigen testing and nucleic acid testing (NAT).
- *Post-transfusion purpura (PTP)* Thrombocytopenia develops typically 7–48 days after transfusion. The typical patient is negative for a common platelet antigen (HPA-1a) and may have been sensitized earlier by receiving HPA-1a positive blood. PTP is caused by re-stimulation of platelet-specific alloantibodies in the patient that also damage their own (antigen-negative) platelets. This severe, and potentially fatal, complication has become rare since the introduction of leukodepleted blood components.
- *Graft-vs-Host disease (GVHD)* Viable T-lymphocytes in blood components are transfused and these engraft and react against the recipient's tissues because the recipient is unable to reject the donor lymphocytes because of immunodeficiency. It presents with cytopenia, fever, rash and deranged liver function, 3–4 weeks after transfusion in bone marrow transplant and solid organ transplant

Blood Transfusion

1. Apheresis is a procedure where required single or more than one component is collected, and the rest of blood components are returned to the donor.
2. Different blood components have different relative density, sediment rate and size and they can be separated by centrifugation of one unit of whole blood.
3. 10–15 mL/kg of packed red blood cells are transfused at 5 mL/kg/h.
4. Irradiated components can be used to prevent graft-versus-host disease due to the action of viable donor T-lymphocytes that can proliferate in a host with an impaired immune defense.
5. Washed Red Blood Cells or platelets can be used in patients with a history of anaphylactic or severe, unexplained reaction to blood components, despite premedication with antihistaminics.
6. Random Donor platelets (RDP) contain approximately 5.5×10^{10} platelets. One Single Donor Platelets (SDP) is equivalent to 5 to 10 units of RDP.
7. Recipients must be transfused with ABO group-specific or ABO group-compatible RBCs. Rh-positive recipients may receive either Rh-positive or Rh-negative RBCs, but Rh-negative recipients should receive Rh-negative RBCs (except when these units are in short supply and the situation is life saving).

recipients. Transfusion of irradiated blood and blood components can prevent this.

Fasano R, Luban NL. Blood component therapy. *Pediatr Clin North Am.* 2008;55(2):421–45.

Liumbruno G, Bennardello F, Lattanzio A, Piccoli P, as Italian Society of Transfusion Medicine and Immunohaematology (SIMTI) Working Party G. Recommendations for the use of albumin and immunoglobulins. *Blood Transfusion.* 2009;7(3):216–234.

Simmons DP, Savage WJ. Hemolysis from ABO Incompatibility. *Hematol Oncol Clin North Am.* 2015;29(3):429–43.

Sharma RR, Marwaha N. Leukoreduced blood components: Advantages and strategies for its implementation in developing countries. *Asian Journal of Transfusion Science.* 2010;4(1):3–8.

Gastrointestinal and Hepatobiliary Disorders

9.1 ANATOMY AND PHYSIOLOGY OF DIGESTION

Digestion of Carbohydrates

Carbohydrates in food comprise mainly of disaccharides (lactose, sucrose) and starch. Starch molecules (amylose and amylopectin) require preliminary intraluminal digestion by salivary and pancreatic amylases. These amylases convert starch into maltose, maltotriose, and dextrin residues but no glucose.

Ingested disaccharides are not absorbed as such unless these are hydrolyzed into constituent monosaccharides. The hydrolysis of the disaccharidases is performed by following enzymes present in the brush border:

- *Sucrase-isomaltase* of the proximal intestine causes hydrolysis of sucrose, isomaltose and most (75%) of the maltose.
- *Maltase-Glucoamylase* predominantly in the ileum causes hydrolysis of remaining (25%) maltose (through its N-terminal domain) and also breaks glucose from glucose (through its c-terminal domain) in dextrins.
- *Lactase* in the proximal intestine breaks lactose into glucose and galactose.

Thus, the disaccharides are ultimately broken down into glucose, galactose, and fructose. Entry of glucose and galactose into the enterocytes through the brush border membrane occurs via Na^+, K^+ATPase dependent carrier ($SGTL_1$) whereas entry of fructose occurs through another carrier (GLUTS) which is not sodium dependent.

Clinical Implications

Carbohydrate malabsorption manifests as diarrhea (because of fermentation of undigested monosaccharides and disaccharides by colonic bacteria) and malnutrition. Although pancreatic amylase deficiency (as in pancreatic insufficiency) also affects carbohydrate (starch) absorption, symptoms related to carbohydrate malabsorption are not prominent as starch is a poorer substrate for colonic bacteria than are monosaccharides.

Congenital (eg, sucrase-isomaltase deficiency) or acquired defects of intestinal digestion and absorption of disaccharides lead to fermentative diarrhea characterized by watery stools whose volume is roughly proportional to the amount of ingested carbohydrates. The stools are acidic (pH 4.0 to 5.5) and usually contain unabsorbed reducing sugars or disaccharides. The child also has abdominal distension. In these conditions, excluding the malabsorbed carbohydrate from the diet stops diarrhea in a few hours; and it is triggered again in a short period of time, if the malabsorbed carbohydrate is reintroduced in the diet. Persistent diarrhea due to lactose intolerance is one of the best examples.

Protein Digestion

Stomach Digestion of proteins starts in the lumen of the stomach, where gastric acid denatures them and activates pepsinogens I and II into the corresponding pepsins. Most of the proteins are lysed into small peptides or free amino acids by pancreatic enzymes.

Intestine Enterokinase, a glycoprotein present in the brush border membrane of enterocytes in the proximal small intestine converts trypsinogen (secreted by pancreas) into trypsin, which, activates the other zymogens into active proteases. Trypsin splits bonds at the amino end of basic amino acids (lysine and arginine); chymotrypsin splits those involving aromatic amino acids (phenylalanine, tyrosine, tryptophan); and elastase splits those involving uncharged small amino acids (such as alanine, glycine, and serine). Amino acids at the carboxy end are released from peptides by exopeptidases (carboxypeptidase A and B).

In contrast to carbohydrates, peptides enter enterocytes after preliminary digestion by brush border peptidases into amino acids. Di- or tripeptides enter the enterocytes as such, which are then split inside the cell by cytoplasmic peptidases. In fact, small peptides represent the main physiologic route of entry of amino acids in the enterocytes. Cell peptidases have their highest activities in the ileum and are able to hydrolyze almost all peptide bonds. The released amino acids are absorbed through the following systems:

i. Neutral amino acids enter the enterocytes mainly through the Na^+ dependent system whose defect results in Hartnup's disease.

ii. Proline and hydroxyproline mainly use the Na^+, Cl^- dependent imino-carrier to enter the enterocyte.

iii. Bicarboxylic acids enter through a specific Na^+ dependent, electroneutral XAG system whose defect is responsible for dicarboxylic aminoaciduria.

Clinical Implications

Protein absorption is not affected by gastrectomy as gastric acid and pepsins do not play a critical role in protein digestion. However, absence of pancreatic protease activities (as in pancreatic exocrine insufficiency) leads to fecal losses of nitrogen resulting in failure to thrive and edema. The stools are often whitish, greasy, loose (but not watery) and foul smelling because of associated fat malabsorption and resultant steatorrhea. Atrophy of the intestinal mucosa, such as those seen in celiac disease, do not usually lead to symptoms that can easily be assigned to protein or peptide maldigestion or absorption. Anorexia (and consequently, decreased protein intake) and associated protein-losing enteropathy are likely to be the more significant factors resulting in hypoproteinemia associated with celiac disease.

Fat Digestion

Fats, being insoluble in water, are absorbed through either bile salt micelles in the gut lumen or chylomicrons in the absorbing cell and circulation to reach their site of metabolic use.

Lipase originating from the gastric fundus hydrolyzes medium-chain triglycerides (MCT) and long-chain triglycerides (LCT). Free fatty acids released as a result facilitates emulsification of lipid droplets. Gastric lipase activity plays a particularly important role in neonates whose pancreatic lipase activity is low.

In the duodenum, *pancreatic lipase* acts at the oil/water interface, adsorbed to the lipid droplets. Bile salts both increase the interface by emulsifying the ingested lipid droplets, thus favoring lipase activity, and, on the contrary, by forming a film between oil and lipase, inhibit its action. Pancreatic lipase in combination with other lipolytic enzymes secreted by pancreas (carboxylesterase hydrolase, phospholipase A_2) solubilizes all forms of lipids and fat-soluble vitamins.

Primary bile acids (cholic and chenodeoxycholic acids) are synthesized in the liver from cholesterol; they are transformed by colonic bacteria into secondary acids (deoxycholic and lithocholic acids) which allow a much better micellar solubilization of the products of lipolysis. Bile acids are efficiently reabsorbed in the distal ileum.

Clinical Implications

As mechanism of fat absorption is complex involving several carriers and enzymes, causes of fat malabsorption and resultant steatorrhea are much more numerous than those of carbohydrate and protein malabsorption. Fat malabsorption may result from lipase deficiency (eg, pancreatic insufficiency); abnormal bile salt synthesis (eg, Byler disease), excretion (eg, biliary atresia), deconjugation (eg, bacterial overgrowth syndrome or tropical enteropathy), reabsorption (eg, inflammatory bowel disease); decreased absorptive surface (eg, celiac disease, short gut), defect in chylomicron formation/excretion (eg, abetalipoproteinemia), or obstruction of intestinal lymphatics (eg, intestinal lymphangiectasia).

Most frequently, fat malabsorption is secondary to intestinal mucosal atrophy as in celiac disease, and absorption of other nutrients is also affected. However, steatorrhea is usually far less severe in intestinal mucosal disorders than in exocrine pancreatic insufficiency. The moderate steatorrhea observed in conditions with subtotal villous atrophy is usually not sufficient to make the stools grossly greasy. In fact, the stool characteristic in these situations result more from the severity of associated carbohydrate fermentation.

In contrast to the long chain fatty acids, medium chain fatty acids (*coconut oil is rich in medium chain triglycerides*) are not bound by fatty acid-binding proteins, and they are not re-esterified before their uptake directly into the portal system. Thus, in certain disorders of fat absorption, the administration of medium chain triglycerides (coconut oil) provide an alternate source of energy.

> **Revision Point**
>
> **Aantomy and Physiology of Digestion**
>
> 1. Dietary carbohydrates comprise monosaccharides, disaccharides (lactose, sucrose) and starch. Starch molecules require salivary and pancreatic amylases. Disaccharides are hydrolyzed into monosaccharides (glucose, galactose, and fructose) by intestinal brush border enzymes (lactase, sucrose-isomaltase, maltase-glucoamylase).
> 2. Proteins are initially digested in the stomach by gastric acid and pepsinogens. Further, proteins are lysed into small peptides or free amino acids by pancreatic enzymes. Pancreatic trypsin however need to be activated by enterokinase, an intestinal enzyme.
> 3. Lipase originating from the gastric fundus hydrolyzes medium-chain triglycerides (MCT) and long-chain triglycerides (LCT). In the duodenum, pancreatic lipase and other lipolytic enzymes dissolve all forms of lipids and fat-soluble vitamins. Bile salts aid this process. Fats are absorbed through either bile salt micelles in the gut lumen or chylomicrons,

9.2 ACUTE DIARRHEA AND DEHYDRATION

Diarrheal diseases are one of the leading causes of childhood morbidity and mortality in developing countries in children under 5 years of age. The two main dangers of diarrhea are malnutrition and death. Dehydration is the primary cause of death in acute diarrhea.

Definitions

Diarrhea

Increase in frequency and change in consistency of stools, ie, passage of liquid or watery stools more than three times a day. Recent change in consistency of stools (as per mother's interpretation) is more important than frequency.

Dysentery

Loose stools along with passage of visible blood, abdominal cramps, and fever is defined as dysentery. Gross blood in the stools is the most reliable sign. It does not include blood streaks on surface of formed stool, blood detected only by microscopic examination, or biochemical tests and passage of digested blood (melena) in stools.

Persistent Diarrhea (PD)

A diarrheal episode lasting for more than 2 weeks. Persistent diarrhea carries a much higher risk for mortality and leads to malnutrition and malabsorption of nutrients.

What is NOT Diarrhea

- Frequent (8–10) semi-loose or pasty stools per day in an exclusively breastfed infant is not diarrhea.

- Frequent passage of formed stools in an older child is not diarrhea.
- Passage of motions immediately following a meal is often due to gastrocolic reflex and should not be taken as a sign of 'upset stomach' or diarrhea.
- Passage of frequent loose stools on 3rd, 4th days of life (*transitional stools*) is normal and should not be considered as diarrhea.

Etiology

Rotaviruses are the most common cause of acute diarrhea in children younger than 2 years. In India, rotavirus accounts for 5–10% of total diarrheal episodes in children. However, the rotavirus is isolated more frequently (25–40%) in children hospitalized with dehydrating diarrhea.

Shigella and enterotoxigenic *E. coli* are the most common bacterial pathogens causing diarrhea in under-5 children. Other common bacterial agents causing diarrhea include other forms of diarrheagenic *E. coli* such as enteroinvasive *E. coli* (EIEC), enterohemorrhagic *E. coli* (EHEC), localized adherent *E. coli* (LA-EC), diffusely adherent *E. coli* (DA-EC), aggregative adherent *E. coli* (Agg-EC), *Campylobacter,* and *Salmonella.*

In endemic areas, possibility of cholera (caused by *Vibrio cholerae*) should always be considered.

Cryptosporidium is increasingly being recognized as a cause of acute and persistent diarrhea in children, and is now considered as one of the four most common causes of moderate-to-severe diarrhea in under-five children.

Dysentery is most commonly caused by *Shigella.* EIEC and EHEC can also cause dysentery. *Entamoeba histolytica* is an uncommon cause of dysentery in children responsible for less than 5% of cases.

In addition, systemic infections like pneumonia, meningitis, and urinary tract infections can also cause diarrhea in children.

Epidemiology

Mode of Transmission

The spread occurs mostly by fecal-oral route (either with contaminated food or water). Hands contaminated with fecal matter may also spread infection directly. Flies may also spread the organisms.

Environmental Factors

Diarrheal illnesses are more common in summers and rainy season. Inadequate water supply, lack of sanitary facilities, poor personal and domestic hygiene, improper food preparation and storage, poor weaning practices, early stopping of breastfeeding, and practice of bottle feeding contribute to diarrhea.

Malnutrition

Diarrhea is more common in malnourished children. On the other hand, diarrhea leads to decreased absorption and increased loss of nutrients, decreased appetite and improper feeding during episode, all contributing to malnutrition. A vicious cycle of malnutrition–diarrhea–malnutrition is thus established (Fig. 9.1). Malnourished children have more chances to develop persistent diarrhea and are at 15–20 times higher risk for diarrhea related mortality. Diarrhea in malnourished children is more likely to be associated with a systemic infection like septicemia or meningitis.

Assessing a Child with Diarrhea

A careful history taking is required to decide whether the reported episode is actually diarrhea and to differentiate between acute, persistent, and recurrent diarrhea. The nature of stools passed is important to have an idea of possible etiology. For example, rice watery stools are passed in cholera and bloody stools are a feature of dysentery.

It is also important to ask for symptoms indicative of any systemic infection like high grade fever, cough, respiratory distress and convulsions. Examination should include the following:

- *State of dehydration* Any child reporting with diarrhea must be assessed for presence of dehydration. Simple clinical signs are very useful to classify the state of dehydration as *no* dehydration, *some* dehydration or *severe* dehydration **(Table 9.1)**.
- *State of nutrition* As discussed earlier, the state of nutrition has important bearing on the outcome of diarrhea. Therefore, the nutritional status of the child should be assessed by anthropometry.
- *Signs of systemic infections* Look for the presence of any systemic infection, especially in young infants and malnourished children. The following features could be useful to provide a clue for the presence of systemic infection in a child suffering from diarrhea:
  - i. Fever preceding the onset of diarrhea;
  - ii. Fever persisting for >72 hours after the onset of diarrhea;
  - iii. General condition of the child is poorer than his state of dehydration permits; and
  - iv. Presence of specific findings such as crepitations, bulging fontanel, etc.

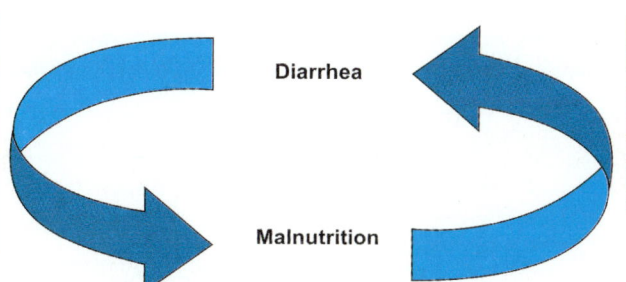

- Loss of nutrients due to poor absorption
- Increased catabolism due to infection
- Poor appetite during diarrheal episodes
- Voluntary restriction of intake due to ignorance of parents/doctors

Diarrhea

Malnutrition

- Reduced acute phase immune response
- Low secretory IgA; hence impaired mucosal immunity
- Intestinal mucosal atrophy leading to poor absorption
- Similar predisposing factors

Fig. 9.1 Diarrhea–malnutrition cycle

Table 9.1 Assessment of Dehydration

Look and feel	Signs	Dehydration	Treatment plan
• General Condition – Lethargic or unconscious* – Restless and irritable • Look for sunken eyes** • Offer the child fluid – Not able to drink or drinking poorly – Drinking eagerly (thirsty)	• **Two of the following signs** – Lethargic or unconscious – Sunken eyes – Not able to drink or drinking poorly – Skin pinch goes back very slowly	SEVERE	PLAN C
• Skin pinch on abdomen*** – Goes back slowly – Goes back very slowly	**Two of the following signs** – Restless, irritable – Sunken eyes – Drinks eagerly, thirsty – Skin pinch goes back slowly	SOME	PLAN B
	Not enough signs to classify as some or severe dehydration	NO	PLAN A

Being lethargic and sleepy are not the same. A lethargic child is not simply asleep: The child's mental state is dull and the child cannot be fully awakened; the child may appear to be drifting into unconsciousness.

**In some infants and children, the eyes normally appear somewhat sunken. It is helpful to ask the mother if the child's eyes are normal or more sunken than usual.*

***The skin pinch is less useful in infants or children with marasmus (severe malnutrition) or kwashiorkor (severe malnutrition with edema) and in obese children.*

Investigations

There is not much role of investigations in the management of acute diarrhea. Stool microscopy is not required in most of the cases. It may be useful when there is a history of mucus in stools (to confirm for bacterial diarrhea by finding of pus cells) or if the child does not respond to therapy in dysentery (to find out amebiasis as a cause of dysentery, which requires a different class of antimicrobials). Serum electrolytes should be estimated when the child has altered sensorium, seizures, abdominal distension, or marked irritability.

Treatment	**Acute Diarrhea**

Oral Rehydration Therapy (ORT)

ORT is the mainstay of management of diarrhea. It includes:
1. WHO (reduced osmolarity) oral rehydration salt (ORS) solution **(Table 9.2)**
2. Home-made sugar-salt solution
3. Food based fluids (rice water + salt, *lassi* + salt)
4. Culturally acceptable home fluids (coconut water, lemon water, plain water, *dal* water, soups)

Administration of glucose water without salt, aerated beverages and tea does not constitute ORT.

Physiological basis of ORS

In diarrhea, body water, sodium, and potassium are lost in the stools, causing dehydration and electrolyte deficit. Oral administration of glucose electrolyte solution helps to replace this deficit, provide ongoing maintenance, and also replaces the ongoing losses of fluid and electrolytes in diarrheal stools. Water, sodium and potassium in the ORS solution correct the corresponding losses; bicarbonate corrects the acidosis, while glucose facilitates sodium absorption simultaneously providing some nutrition in form of calories. The glucose linked enhanced sodium absorption in the small intestine remains largely intact during acute diarrhea.

The ORS previously recommended by WHO had an osmolarity of 311 mmol/L. Though it was effective in rehydration, the need for improved composition was felt as it did not decrease the stool output in diarrhea. Following extensive research, a new reduced osmolarity ORS was approved by international health agencies which is now the standard recommended ORS for all ages **(Table 9.2)**.

Reduced osmolarity ORS

Reduced osmolarity ORS has many additional advantages. Apart from preventing and treating dehydration, it reduces stool output by 20%, decreases incidence of vomiting by 30%, and also

Table 9.2 Composition of Reduced Osmolarity WHO ORS

Salt	By weight	Electrolyte	By osmolarity
Sodium chloride	2.6 grams	Sodium	75 mmol/L
Potassium chloride	1.5 grams	Potassium	20 mmol/L
Trisodium citrate	2.9 grams	Citrate	10 mmol/L
Glucose	13.5 grams	Glucose	75 mmol/L
		Chloride (from NaCl and KCl)	65 mmol/L
Water	To 1 liter	Total	245 mmol/L

reduces the need for supplemental intravenous fluids. Reduced osmolarity ORS works equally well for dehydration following diarrhea, dysentery, or cholera but there is a risk of asymptomatic hyponatremia in cholera. Reduced osmolarity ORS should be the first choice for correction of dehydration in all diarrheal illnesses.

A. Fluid management

1. *Treatment Plan A for prevention of dehydration*
Children without any signs of dehydration also require fluids to prevent dehydration. In such children, feeding should be continued and ORT should be given in form of home available fluids, sugar-salt solution and food-based solutions. ORS should be given to replenish the fluids lost in stools. The amount of ORS required is as follows:

<2 years	50–100 mL for every loose stool
2–10 years	100–200 mL for every loose stool
>10 years	As much as wanted by the child

Mother should be trained to prepare and give ORS at home and she should be asked to report appearance of danger signs (repeated vomiting, eating or drinking poorly, blood in stools, convulsions, lethargic or unconscious).

2. *Treatment Plan B (for some dehydration)*
All children showing signs of some dehydration should be treated at health care facility. These children require increased fluids for (*i*) correction of dehydration; (*ii*) replacement of ongoing losses; and (*iii*) maintenance.

Administer 75 mL/kg ORS in the first 4 hours. If the child wants more ORS than the calculated amount, give more. ORS should be given by a teaspoon in children <2 years of age and by frequent sips from a cup in case of older children. If the child vomits, wait for few minutes and give ORS more slowly. Feeding should be continued. Mother should be instructed to give ORT at home after discharge and asked to return to the health facility, if she notices any danger signs.

3. *Treatment Plan C (for severe dehydration)*
Severe dehydration should be corrected by intravenous fluids. If intravenous access cannot be obtained, a nasogastric tube should be placed and fluids given through that.

Ringer lactate and normal saline are the two most commonly used intravenous fluids for correction of dehydration. The total amount of fluid to be given is 100 mL/kg divided as follows:
<1 year old: 30 mL/kg in first hour and 70 mL/kg in next 5 hours
>1 year old: 30 mL/kg in first 30 min and rest in next 2.5 hours
ORS and feeding should be started as soon as the child can drink without difficulty. The child should be frequently monitored for signs of dehydration and the following danger signs:

Danger Signs in Diarrhea
1. Repeated vomiting
2. Eating or drinking poorly
3. Blood in stools
4. Convulsions
5. Lethargy/unconsciousness

B. Zinc for diarrhea
Zinc is important for various immune mechanisms in the body and modulates the host response to infection. Metaanalyses of randomized trials have demonstrated that zinc supplements given during an episode of acute diarrhea reduce the duration and severity of the episode and if given for 14 days, also lowers the incidence of diarrhea in the next 3 months.

WHO, UNICEF, and IAP therefore recommend daily 20 mg zinc supplement for 14 days for children with acute diarrhea, and 10 mg per day for infants under six months of age, to curtail the severity of the episode and prevent further occurrences in the ensuing 3 months. Zinc (zinc sulfate, gluconate or acetate) can be given either in form of syrup containing 20 mg of elemental zinc per 5 mL, or dispersible tablets of zinc sulfate, zinc gluconate, or zinc acetate containing 10 mg/ 20 mg of elemental zinc.

C. Antimicrobial therapy
As discussed earlier, most of the diarrheal episodes in children are self-limiting and antibiotics are not indicated. Indications for administration of antimicrobials include (*i*) dysentery (blood in stools), (*ii*) diarrhea due to *Vibrio cholerae*, *Cryptosporidium*, *Giardia*, or *E. histolytica*, (*iii*) associated systemic infections (pneumonia, septicemia, meningitis, etc.), and (*iv*) diarrhea in a severely malnourished child.

Treatment of dysentery
Ciprofloxacin is now the first line drug recommended by WHO for treatment of dysentery because of emergence of resistance to the commonly used drugs, ie, trimethoprim sulpha-methoxazole and nalidixic acid in a majority of isolates of *Shigella* from the developing countries. Cefixime is used as second line drug if there is no clinical response after 2 days of therapy with ciprofloxacin.

The risk of complications of dysentery are more in infants (especially non breastfed), severely malnourished children, those with dehydration, and if there is a recent history of measles. Such children should be hospitalized and given intravenous antibiotics. Figure 9.2 provides the recommended algorithm for treatment of dysentery.

Treatment of cholera
Though the mainstay of management of cholera is effective fluid therapy, appropriate antibiotics diminish the duration of diarrhea, reduce the volume of rehydration fluids needed, and shorten the duration of *V. cholerae* excretion.

The recommended antibiotic of choice for cholera is single dose doxycycline (6–8 mg/kg). Oral erythromycin (50 mg/kg/d in four divided doses) for three days is another alternative. Single dose ciprofloxacin or azithromycin are also clinically effective, and can be used if there is resistance to doxycycline or no clinical response. No chemoprophylaxis is needed for contacts.

D. Other drugs
Antimotility agents like loperamide are contraindicated for childhood diarrhea as these increase the risk of ileus. The role of probiotics and antisecretory agents such as racecadotril is also unclear and these are not recommended for routine use in childhood diarrhea.

E. Diet in diarrhea
Nutritional management is a very important aspect in management of diarrhea.
1. *Do not stop feeding* Most nutrients are well absorbed during diarrhea. This is an erroneous belief that rest to the bowel promotes early recovery.
2. *Give more food* A considerable quantity of nutrients is lost in the diarrheal stools. The dietary intake should be increased

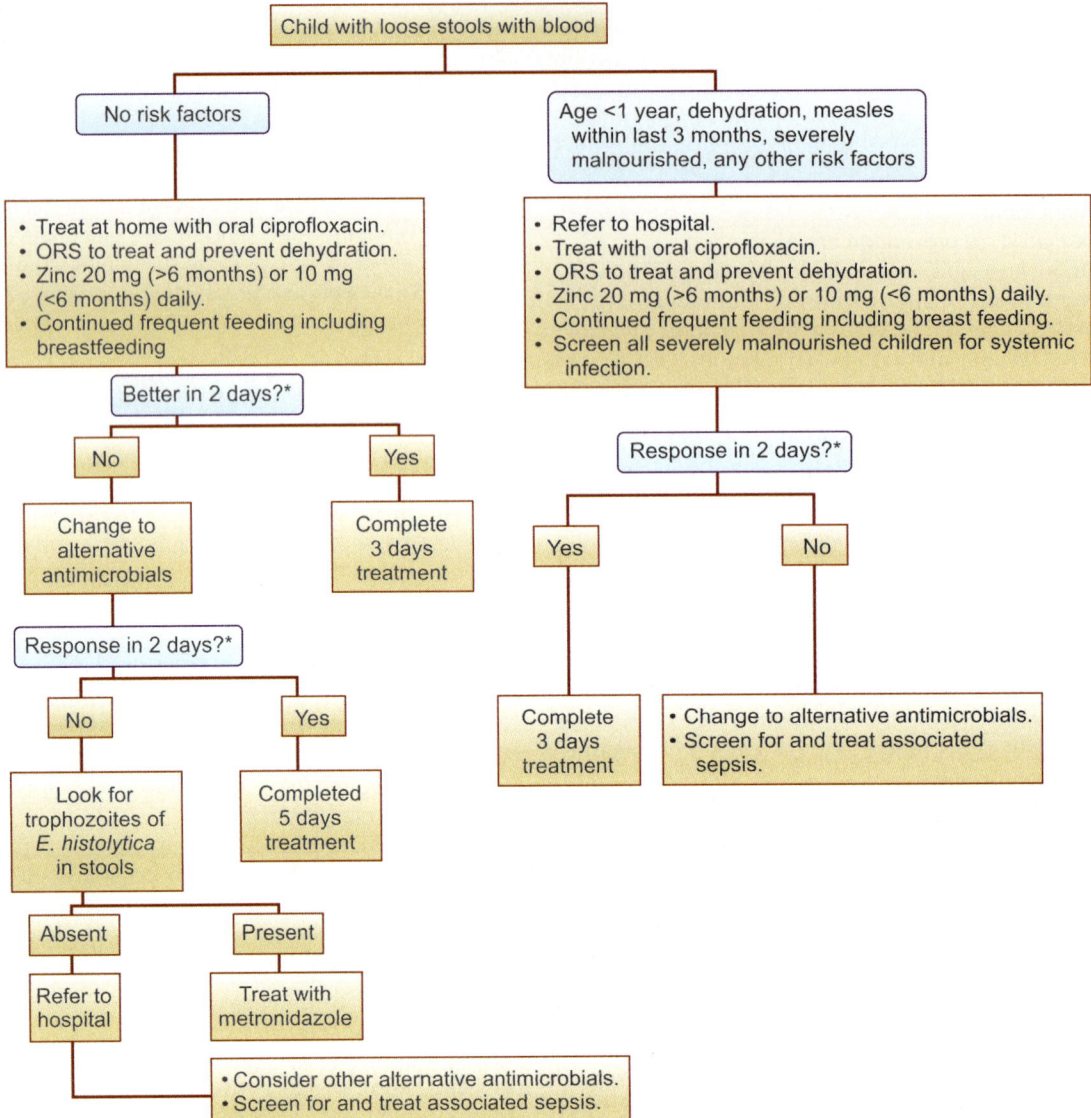

Fig. 9.2 WHO algorithm for treatment of dysentery

* Disappearance of fever, less blood in stools, improved appetite, decreased abdominal pain, return to normal activity indicate good response.

to compensate for losses and to promote rapid nutritional recovery.

3. *Continue breastfeeding* during an attack of diarrhea. Breastmilk contains viable phagocytes and other protective substances, such as secretory IgA and specific IgM, which protect against diarrhea.

4. *Do not stop milk* Transient lactose intolerance lasting for 3 to 5 days may occur during acute diarrhea. This is self-limiting and does not require dilution of milk or stopping it altogether.

5. *Give easily digestible and nutritionally balanced diet* The diet should contain adequate amount of concentrated foods, so that enough nutrients are absorbed from a small quantity of food. Milled cereals are preferred to whole cereals. A well-cooked gruel of rice and lentil (*khichri*) is usually well tolerated. Mashed bananas are also good. The diet should be iso-osmolar. These foods should be started within 4 to 6 hours of starting the treatment.

6. Soft drinks and fruit juices with high sugar content should be avoided during diarrhea.

7. Food should be given in smaller quantities at shorter intervals.

8. Contrary to the popular belief, most children tolerate small quantities of fats and oils, which are rich sources of energy, and the diarrhea does not worsen.

Prevention of Diarrhea

Diarrhea can be prevented to a large extent by improving poor dietary habits and hygiene, as follows.

Diet

1. Exclusive breastfeeding should be given for first 6 months.

2. Complementary feeding with energy-rich food mixtures containing adequate amounts of nutrients such as balanced amounts of proteins, fats, iron and vitamins

should be introduced soon after 6 months of age while continuing breastfeeding (till at least 2 years of age).

Hygiene

1. Wash hands before preparation or administration of food.
2. Protect food from contamination during preparation, storage or at the time of administration.
3. Mothers should be guided to use clean containers, avoiding exposure of food to dust, flies or cockroaches.
4. Water given to the child or used for preparing feeds should be clean and potable, preferably boiled during epidemics.
5. Vegetables and fruit should be washed and peeled before these are fed to the child.

Case Study | **Acute Diarrhea**

A 30-month-old girl, resident of a slum cluster presents to you with 3 days history of watery diarrhea and vomiting. There is no history of fever or any other complaints. There is history of similar illness in many children of neighborhood. On examination, the child looks irritable, weighs 10.0 kg and is thirsty. Her height is 86 cm. Vitals are normal and systemic examination is non-contributory.

Q1. Assess and classify dehydration in this child.

The child has an acute onset diarrhea. The occurrence of similar illness in neighborhood suggests an infectious etiology through a common source such as contaminated water. The assessment required in this child would include assessment for dehydration, nutritional status, and presence of any other co-existing illness.

Assess hydration

Assessment for dehydration should include evaluation of four signs; (*i*) general condition, (*ii*) skin pinch, (*iii*) intake of fluids or thirst and (*iv*) presence of sunken eyes. This child is irritable and thirsty suggesting two signs of 'some' dehydration. Other examination should include examination for sunken eyes and skin pinch. Presence of both 'skin pinch going back very slow' and sunken eyes will upgrade the dehydration to 'severe' as two of the criteria of severe dehydration would be satisfied. If sunken eyes are not present, or the skin pinch goes back slowly but not very slowly, hydration status would still be 'some dehydration' as two defining criteria for severe dehydration would not be satisfied. Even if both the signs are absent, ie, skin pinch does not go back slowly and no sunken eyes; the hydration status would be classified as 'some dehydration' as two defining criteria for this are already met. For further discussion, let us assume that the child did not meet the criteria for having severe dehydration and is classified as having 'some dehydration'.

Q2. Plan fluid and nutritional therapy for this child.

Assess nutrition

Next step is to evaluate the nutritional status. The expected (50th percentile) weight for height of 86 cm for a girl is 11.6 kg as per WHO growth standards. Thus, this child's weight-for-height is lying between −1 Z-score (10.7 kg) and −2 Z-score (9.8 kg), classifying her as NOT having malnutrition.

Classifying nutritional status is important for management as severely malnourished children require a different approach to fluid therapy (*see* Chapter 3) and also antibiotics might be needed assuming infection. However, this child is not having severe malnutrition. The child's history does not suggest any other co-existing infection as it is a short duration diarrhea and there is no fever or any other signs suggesting infection. Investigations are unlikely to be contributory in the management of this child. A stool hanging drop examination and culture may be needed if cholera is prevalent in the area and program guidelines need reporting for this illness.

Plan fluid

Thus 'this child is classified as having '*Acute watery diarrhea with some dehydration*', the fluid therapy for this child would be 'Plan B', ie, oral correction of dehydration with ORS.

The ORS packet should be dissolved in one liter of clean water and kept covered. The child needs 750 mL (75 mL/kg) of this solution in next 4 hours. The child should be given sips of ORS from a glass or a spoon. Do not give too much ORS at one time as it might induce vomiting. Even if the child vomits, ORS should be continued and it should be given more slowly. Preferably, the rehydration should be completed in the health facility itself checking the amount taken by child and state of her hydration hourly. Breastfeeding can be continued during this period if the child is breastfed and sips of plain water are also allowed.

After correction of dehydration, normal feeding is to be resumed and mother instructed to give her energy-rich foods in small amounts frequently. Mother should be trained in mixing and preparing ORS and should be counseled to give the child ORS and other home-available fluids at home till diarrhea continues. It should be emphasized to complete 14 days of zinc administration.

Apart from rehydration and zinc therapy, nutritional counseling is to be done to improve the dietary intake once the child gets well, in order to prevent onset of malnutrition. Also, counsel the mother about steps to prevent future diarrheal episodes.

Drug therapy

You also need to decide about any other treatment needed in this child besides correction of dehydration and nutritional status. Antimicrobial treatment is not indicated in this child as there is no dysentery, child is not severely malnourished and there is no sign of any other infection. Zinc (in form of oral tablets or suspension) should be given in dose of 20 mg per day to be continued for 14 days to reduce the severity of diarrheal episode and also to prevent future episodes. The child may be sent back from health facility after correction of dehydration and training of mother in giving ORS and medications. Mother should be instructed to bring back the child in case of danger signs such as convulsions, lethargy, not taking anything orally or vomiting everything.

Environment

1. Proper sewage disposal.
2. Good water supply.
3. Proper excreta/toilet facilities.

Vaccine

Effective vaccines against rotavirus are now available. The schedule needs to be preferably completed before 6 months. Rotavirus vaccines will not prevent diarrhea because of other causes; emphasis of prevention should be on handwashing and general hygiene measures.

Revision Point

Acute Diarrhea and Dehydration

1. Acute watery diarrhea is a self-limiting disorder and can be successfully managed with ORT, zinc supplementation and continued feeding. It subsides within 5–7 days in a large majority of cases.
2. Acute diarrhea is most frequently caused by rotavirus and *E.coli.*
3. Dehydration is the primary cause of death in acute diarrhea. Children are classified as having No, Some, or Severe dehydration.
4. Children with No dehydration can be managed at home with oral fluids; those with Some dehydration need oral rehydration therapy with WHO's reduced osmolarity ORS (75 mL/kg in 4 h); and those with Severe dehydration need intravenous fluids (Ringer lactate or normal saline 100 mL/kg)
5. Antibiotics have no role in acute watery diarrhea except in dysentery, cholera, and children with severe malnutrition or co-existing systemic infections.
6. Bloody diarrhea is referred to as dysentery. Shigella is the most common causative organism. Ciprofloxacin is the drug of choice; non-responders are given cefixime. Serious hospitalized patients are treated with ceftriaxone.
7. All children with diarrhea or dysentery should be given zinc supplementation for 14 days.

Bhatnagar S, Lodha R, Choudhury P, et al. Indian Academy of Pediatrics. IAP Guidelines 2006 on management of acute diarrhea. *Indian Pediatr.* 2007;44:380–9.

Dabas A, Shah D, Bhatnagar S, Lodha R. Epidemiology of *Cryptosporidium* in pediatric diarrheal illnesses. Indian Pediatr. 2017;54:299–309.

Hahn S, Kim S, Garner P. Reduced osmolarity oral rehydration solution for treating dehydration caused by acute diarrhoea in children. *Cochrane Database Syst Rev.* 2002;1:CD002847.

Kotloff KL, Nataro JP, Blackwelder WC, Nasrin D, Farag TH, Panchalingam S, et al. Burden and aetiology of diarrhoeal disease in infants and young children in developing countries (the Global Enteric Multicenter Study, GEMS): a prospective, case-control study. *Lancet.* 2013;382:209–22.

Lazzerini M, Wanzira H. Oral zinc for treating diarrhoea in children. *Cochrane Database Syst Rev.* 2016;12:CD005436.

Liu J, Platts-Mills JA, Juma J, Kabir F, Nkeze J, Okoi C, et al. Use of quantitative molecular diagnostic methods to identify causes of diarrhoea in children: a reanalysis of the GEMS case-control study. *Lancet.* 2016;388:1291–301.

Musekiwa A, Volmink J. Oral rehydration salt solution for treating cholera: <270 mOsm/L solutions vs >310 mOsm/L solutions. *Cochrane Database Syst Rev.* 2011;12:CD003754.

National Rotavirus Surveillance Network., Kumar CP, Venkatasubramanian S, Kang G, Arora R, Mehendale S. Profile and trends of rotavirus gastroenteritis in under 5 children in India, 2012–2014. Preliminary report of the Indian National Rotavirus Surveillance Network. *Indian Pediatr.* 2016;53:619–22.

World Health Organization. The treatment of diarrhoea: A manual for physicians and other senior health workers. Geneva: *WHO;* 2011.

9.3 PERSISTENT DIARRHEA

Diarrhea starting as an acute episode and lasting for more than 14 days is labeled as persistent diarrhea. Stools are often watery and may lead to dehydration. Persistent diarrhea is more common in children below the age of 2 years and in malnourished children.

Persistent diarrhea needs to be differentiated from *chronic diarrhea* which occurs due to an underlying pathology such as celiac disease, tropical sprue, and congenital and metabolic diseases. Chronic diarrhea is more insidious in onset continuing for months, stools are not watery and do not usually lead to dehydration (see Section 9.4).

Pathophysiology

Diarrhea starts as an acute episode due to infection with a microorganism. Most often, the illness subsides in a period of about 5–7 days. However, sometimes the diarrhea continues because of:

i. Persistent infection because of poor nutritional status or impaired immunological defenses;
ii. Presence of systemic infection such as urinary tract infection, pneumonia or protracted septicemia; or
iii. Malabsorption, particularly of carbohydrates and fats due to loss of intestinal brush border, and associated enzymatic dysfunction.

Nutritional losses further contribute to malnutrition and a vicious cycle is set up. Thus, the child is not able to recover from diarrhea. Infrequently, protein intolerance may also develop. Faulty feeding practices and overuse of antibiotics compound the problem.

Clinical Features

Growth faltering, worsening of malnutrition, and *death* are the major consequences of persistent diarrhea. Despite passage of frequent loose stools, the hydration usually remains good. Dehydration may develop if purge rate is high or when oral intake is inadequate because of associated systemic infection. Continued diarrhea may worsen the pre-existing malnutrition, predispose to systemic infections and may result in death.

Investigations

Send stool specimen for microscopic examination (especially for pus cells, RBCs, and trophozoites or cysts of *E. histolytica, Cryptosporidium,* or *Giardia*) and culture. Obtain stool pH to determine lactose intolerance (suggested by the stool pH of <5.5 on two separate occasions). Screen for other systemic infections, especially urinary tract infections.

Treatment	Persistent Diarrhea

Children with persistent diarrhea should be admitted if they are less than 4 months of age, are dehydrated or having severe malnutrition or a systemic infection. Assess the child for dehydration as described in the Section on acute diarrhea and manage as per Plan A, B or C. The mainstay of management is dietary therapy.

Dietary therapy

1. *Breastfeeding* Encourage exclusive breastfeeding in infants less than 6 months of age. Continue breastfeeding in older infants and children up to 2 years of age.
2. *Diet A: Reduced lactose diet* Initially, put the child on a reduced lactose diet. Limit the quantity of top milk to 50 mL/kg/day; it need not be stopped altogether or diluted with water. The feeds may be given in the form of a milk rice gruel, milk *sooji* gruel, rice with curds or *dalia*. Offer 6–7 feeds per day. The total caloric intake should be 150 kcal/kg/d. If oral intake is not satisfactory, feed through a nasogastric tube. About 60% children will improve on this diet alone.
3. *Diet B: Lactose free diet* If the child does not respond to Diet A, they are shifted to a lactose free diet. This does not contain any milk. Milk protein is replaced by chicken or egg. Cereals are allowed. A typical diet providing 90 kcal and 2.5 g of protein per 100 g of portion can be prepared by mixing egg white (½ egg), puffed rice powder (3 tsp), glucose (1½ tsp), oil (1½ tsp) and water (120 ml).
4. *Diet C Monosaccharide-based diet* 10% children with persistent diarrhea may not respond either to Diet A or B. These children are given a monosaccharide-based diet that is free of cereals and is largely based on egg/chicken. Besides it contains oil, glucose and water. No milk is allowed.
5. *Vitamins and minerals* Provide vitamin A (2 lac units to those >8 kg and 1 lac units to those weighing less than 8 kg) as a single dose. Start daily zinc supplementation (10–20 mg/day). Give all other vitamins and minerals in twice the recommended daily allowance. Introduce iron only when diarrhea stops.
6. *Monitoring* Record weight, stool frequency and signs of dehydration daily.
7. *Antimicrobials* Start them as indicated by presence of blood in stools, associated systemic infection or as per reports of urine and stool microscopy and culture. All severely malnourished children would also require treatment with antibiotics.

Revision Point

Persistent Diarrhea

1. Diarrhea starting as an acute episode and lasting for more than 14 days is labeled as persistent diarrhea.
2. Persistent diarrhea needs to be differentiated from *chronic diarrhea* which usually occurs due to an underlying pathology such as celiac disease, tropical sprue, and congenital and metabolic diseases.
3. *Growth faltering, worsening of malnutrition* and *death are* the major consequences of persistent diarrhea.
4. Children with persistent diarrhea should be hospitalized if they are less than 4 months of age, are dehydrated or having severe malnutrition or a systemic infection.
5. The mainstay of management is dietary therapy. Three diets are primarily used: Diet A: Reduced lactose diet; Diet B: Lactose-free diet; and Diet C: Monosaccharide-based diet.

Prognosis

Though only about 5–10% of episodes of diarrhea in under-five children last for more than 14 days, persistent diarrhea is responsible for one-third to one-half of diarrhea related mortality. The case fatality rate of persistent diarrhea is about 20 times higher than that of acute diarrhea; the prognosis being poorer in severely malnourished children, and in those with persistent dysentery.

Abba K, Sinfield R, Hart CA, Garner P. Pathogens associated with persistent diarrhea in children in low and middle income countries: systematic review. *BMC Infect Dis*. 2009;9:88.

Ahmed ER, Moinuddin MD, Molla M, et al. Persistent Diarrhea Research Group. Childhood diarrheal deaths in seven low- and middle-income countries. *Bull World Health Organ*. 2014;92:664–71.

Bernaola Aponte G, Bada Mancilla CA, Carreazo NY, Rojas Galarza RA. Probiotics for treating persistent diarrhea in children. *Cochrane Database Syst Rev*. 2013;8:CD007401.

Bhan MK, Bhandari N, Bhatnagar S, Bahl R. Epidemiology and management of persistent diarrhoea in children of developing countries. *Indian J Med Res*. 1996;104:103–14.

Bhutta ZA, Molla AM, Issani Z, Badruddin S, Hendricks K, Snyder JD. Dietary management of persistent diarrhea: comparison of a traditional rice-lentil based diet with soy formula. *Pediatrics*. 1991;88:1010–9.

Grimwood K, Forbes DA. Acute and persistent diarrhea. *Pediatr Clin North Am*. 2009;56:1343–61.

9.4 MALABSORPTION SYNDROMES AND CHRONIC DIARRHEA

Malabsorption syndromes are characterized by chronic diarrhea, abdominal distension, and failure to thrive.

Chronic diarrhea is the direct consequence of malabsorption, which results in malnutrition and failure to thrive. Chronic diarrhea here refers to primarily conditions associated with "abnormal stools" which continues or recurs over several months.

Etiology

Chronic diarrhea can be categorized into one or more of the 3 major pathophysiologic etiologies; ie (*i*) impaired intraluminal digestion, (*ii*) intestinal malabsorption, and (*iii*) fermentation.

- *Chronic diarrhea due to impaired intraluminal digestion* is seen in conditions such as cystic fibrosis, deficiencies of other pancreatic enzymes, lipase deficiency, and bile duct atresia. Stools are loose and pasty, obviously greasy with undigested fat oozing like oil when it is passed in a pot. The oil may float on the surface of the water in the toilet with an offensive cheesy smell.
- *Chronic diarrhea due to intestinal malabsorption* occurs because of mucosal changes in the intestinal wall. The most important of these changes is the villous atrophy. This occurs in celiac disease, cow milk protein allergy (CMPA), giardiasis, immunodeficiency and malnutrition. Stools are loose or liquid, often with an acidic smell, and rarely greasy. These children have modest steatorrhea, abnormal d-xylose test, and abnormal intestinal histology. Intestinal biopsy is necessary.
- *Chronic diarrhea due to fermentation* is seen in congenital deficiencies of certain mucosal enzymes digesting mono-/disaccharides. Diarrhea due to fermentation is liquid, acidic (pH less than 5.5) and often passed with flatus, and

its volume is variable, roughly proportionate to the amount of malabsorbed carbohydrate that has been ingested.

Diagnosis

A child suspected to have chronic diarrhea and malabsorption should have the following investigations:

i. Repeated stool examination especially for Giardia;

ii. Fecal fat excretion studies for evidence of fat malabsorption;

iii. D-xylose test (blood levels and urinary excretion) and hydrogen breath tests for carbohydrate malabsorption;

iv. Estimation of fecal α_1-antitrypsin levels and fecal elastase levels;

v. Intestinal biopsy; and

vi. Specific tests, eg, sweat chloride for cystic fibrosis, exocrine pancreatic function tests; and serology for celiac disease and HIV.

CELIAC DISEASE

Celiac disease is a T-lymphocyte mediated small intestinal enteropathy induced by gluten (a protein found in wheat, barley, oats, rye, and triticale) in genetically predisposed individuals. Gluten triggers an autoimmune reaction causing inflammation and damage to the small intestinal mucosa.

Also known as *gluten enteropathy*, it is a lifelong disorder which may present either in childhood or in adults with malabsorption, recurrent diarrhea, short stature, and non-responding anemia. Removal of gluten from the diet leads to full clinical remission and restoration of the small intestinal mucosa to normal.

Clinical Presentation

Celiac disease is known for its variable clinical presentation:

In a *typical* case, the common features include: Chronic diarrhea, abdominal distension, muscle wasting, failure to thrive, anemia, vomiting, anorexia and irritability. Onset occurs after introduction of wheat in the diet, but there might be a long latent period between introduction of wheat and the onset of symptoms. The child may pass foul greasy and bulky stools or has recurrent episodes of diarrhea. The appetite decreases and weight gain stops.

In *atypical* cases, diarrhea is not present but anemia and short stature are prominent findings. The diagnosis in these children is usually delayed beyond 5 years of age.

There is a high degree of association of celiac disease with other autoimmune disorders such as type-1 diabetes mellitus and autoimmune thyroiditis; and screening tests are warranted for these disorders in children with celiac disease.

Diagnosis

The perception of celiac disease has changed from an uncommon gastrointestinal disease to a common multiorgan disease strongly dependent on the haplotypes human leukocyte antigen (HLA)-DQ2 and HLA-DQ8.

Detection of circulating antibodies to gliadin, recticulin, endomysium, and/or tissue transglutaminase, suggests the diagnosis. IgA antiendomyseal antibody (EMA), IgA

Case Study | **Celiac Disease**

A 5-year-old boy belonging to a middle-income group North Indian family has been coming to the pediatric outpatient clinic for last one year with non-specific abdominal pain, poor appetite and inadequate weight gain. On one such visit, his records were examined in detail.

He was noted to have microcytic hypochromic anemia on several occasions and thus received iron containing medications every time for varying periods. He had history of several episodes of diarrhea subsiding on its own or on receiving medications. His examination revealed pallor and a slightly protuberant abdomen. On asking, mother reported that the child often develops abdominal fullness after meals. The child's weight was 12 kg and height was 91 cm. Other systemic examination was non-contributory.

A diagnosis of short stature and anemia was made and celiac disease was suspected to be a cause of the child's problems.

Q1. What made clinician think of celiac disease?

In this child, presence of short stature and refractory anemia along with GI symptoms such as recurrent diarrhea and protuberant abdomen made the clinician suspect celiac disease.

The mode of presentation of celiac disease may be quite variable. Though many children with celiac disease have a history of diarrhea, it may not always be typical greasy, bulky and foul smelling stools. Associated short stature (child's height is 83% of expected for age signifying severe stunting but weight for height is 92% signifying no wasting) suggests some chronic disease. Also, presence of anemia despite receiving hematinics several times suggest ongoing nutritional problem.

Any child whose rate of growth is slow, accompanied by recurrent or refractory iron deficiency anemia, irrespective of presence of GI symptoms, should be investigated for presence of celiac disease.

Q2. Discuss the investigations required to confirm or refute the diagnosis.

Diagnosis of celiac disease requires demonstration of IgA antiendomysial antibodies or IgA tissue-transglutaminase (TTG) antibodies along with demonstration of mucosal changes (like total or subtotal villous atrophy) in intestinal biopsy.

Serology is useful as initial test and both antiendomysial antibodies and tissue transglutaminase antibodies have comparable sensitivity and specificity. However, these should not be relied on for final diagnosis for the purpose of instituting therapy because false negative as well as false positive tests are known to occur. Small intestinal endoscopy and biopsy while the child is still eating a gluten containing diet is a must for establishing the diagnosis. Other investigations such as thyroid function tests and blood glucose should be done to exlcude other autoimmune disorders, once CD is confirmed.

---

antigliadin antibody, and IgA tissue transglutaminase (tTG) antibodies characteristically occur in children with untreated celiac disease. Estimation of IgA-tTG antibodies is the most frequently used serological test for screening of celiac disease in children.

The diagnosis of celiac disease is based upon the demonstration of an abnormal small intestinal mucosa with features characteristic of celiac disease (villous atrophy, crypt elongation, increased intra-epithelial lymphocytes) in a biopsy specimen from small intestine (duodenum). Although duodenal biopsy is must for confirmation of diagnosis of celiac disease, and should be done in all cases before starting gluten-free diet, it can be avoided in few patients in which IgA-tTG levels are raised more than 10 times the upper limit of normal, along with positive anti-endomysial antibody (done by sampling on a separate occasion) and compatible HLA phenotype (DQ2 or DQ8).

Finally, it is crucial to demonstrate a clinical response to the withdrawal of gluten from the child's diet, in terms of relief of symptoms and significant weight gain.

Treatment — Celiac Disease

Stop all gluten containing foods. Gluten is a collective term used to describe the elastic protein component of the cereal grains: wheat, rye, barley, oats, and triticale. A strict gluten free diet is the cornerstone of management of celiac disease. A gluten-free diet should not contain any detectable source of gluten in it. To manage this, it requires a lot of care in terms of avoiding unintentional consumption of gluten and cross contamination with foods containing gluten.

Wheat contains the greatest amount of gluten and therefore *chapattis*, breads, cakes, biscuits, breakfast cereals, etc. are the most significant source of gluten in Indian diet. The starch derived from these cereal grains may also contain small amount of gluten, and should therefore be avoided. These starches are used as thickeners, binders, fillers, stabilizers in many types of foods.

In celiac disease, rice and maize are the main cereals to be eaten and act as wheat substitutes. *Chapattis* and breads can be made out of mixture of other flours like gram flour (*besan*), soya flour, maize flour or dried water chestnut (*singhara*) flour. It is best to make these flours at home as commercially available unlabelled flours or flours made in local mills are likely to be contaminated with wheat flour made in the same grinding

I What is Permitted in Celiac Disease?

- Rice, rice flour, South Indian foods like *Dosas, Vadas,* and *Uttapams* (except *Rawa/ Sooji* preparations like *Rawa Iddli, Rawa Dosa, Upma*, etc.)
- Maize, maize flour, corn, bajra, millets, ragi
- Pulses, and flour made out of them (*besan*, soya flour, *moong dal* flour)
- Fresh fruits, fruit juices, salads
- Vegetables and tubers (eg, potato)
- Meat, fish, poultry, eggs, cheese and milk
- Nuts (not coated/roasted)

II What is to be Avoided?

- Wheat, wheat flour and its preparations (eg, *chapattis*, breads, *dalia* porridge)
- Sooji or semolina, noodles, pastas
- Biscuits, cakes, chocolates, ice creams (unless labeled gluten free)
- Most breakfast cereals and commercial snacks
- Foods/drinks/sauces containing thickeners, stabilizers, malt
- Soya sauce/ black bean sauce

machine. Commercially available gluten-free flours are acceptable and convenient, but expensive.

A list of common foods which are allowed or forbidden in a child with celiac disease is given below. The clinical response to gluten withdrawal is dramatic. Diarrhea stops and the growth velocity improves rapidly. A lifelong strict gluten free diet is mandatory.

Revision Point

Malabsorption Syndromes and Chronic Diarrhea

1. *Malabsorption syndromes* are characterized by chronic diarrhea, abdominal distension, and failure to thrive.
2. Chronic diarrhea can be caused by (*i*) impaired intraluminal digestion, (*ii*) intestinal malabsorption or (*iii*) fermentation.
3. Celiac disease also known as *gluten enteropathy* is induced by gluten (a protein found in wheat). It is a lifelong disorder.
4. Onset of celiac disease occurs after introduction of wheat in the diet, but there might be a long latent period between introduction of wheat and the onset of symptoms.
5. Presentations of celiac disease include diarrhea, short stature, and non-responding anemia.
6. Detection of circulating antibodies to gliadin, reticulin, endomysium, and/or tissue transglutaminase, suggests the diagnosis of celiac disease. Intestinal biopsy is diagnostic.
7. Removal of gluten from the diet leads to full clinical remission of celiac disease.

Downey L, Houten R, Murch S, Longson D. Guideline Development Group. Recognition, assessment, and management of coeliac disease: summary of updated NICE guidance. *BMJ.* 2015;351:h4513

Fric P, Gabrovska D, Nevoral J. Celiac disease, gluten-free diet, and oats. *Nutr Rev.* 2011;69:107–15.

Husby S, Koletzko S, Korponay-Szabó IR, Mearin ML, Phillips A, Shamir R, et al. ESPGHAN Working Group on Coeliac Disease Diagnosis; ESPGHAN Gastroenterology Committee; European Society for Pediatric Gastroenterology, Hepatology, and Nutrition.. European Society for Pediatric Gastroenterology, Hepatology, and Nutrition guidelines for the diagnosis of coeliac disease. *J Pediatr Gastroenterol Nutr.* 2012;54:136–60.

Lau MS, Sanders DS. Optimizing the diagnosis of celiac disease. *Curr Opin Gastroenterol.* 2017;33:173–80.

Newnham ED. Coeliac disease in the 21st century: paradigm shifts in the modern age. *J Gastroenterol Hepatol.* 2017;32 Suppl 1:82–5.

9.5 APPROACH TO A CHILD WITH VOMITING

Vomiting is a common symptom of many disease states. It is caused by the violent contraction of the gastrointestinal smooth muscles. Bile or blood in the vomitus always indicates evaluation for the cause. Bilious vomiting indicates obstruction or dysmotility distal to the second part of duodenum; and blood indicates GI bleed.

Etiology

The differential diagnosis of the child with vomiting varies with the age of the child. Congenital anatomic, genetic, and

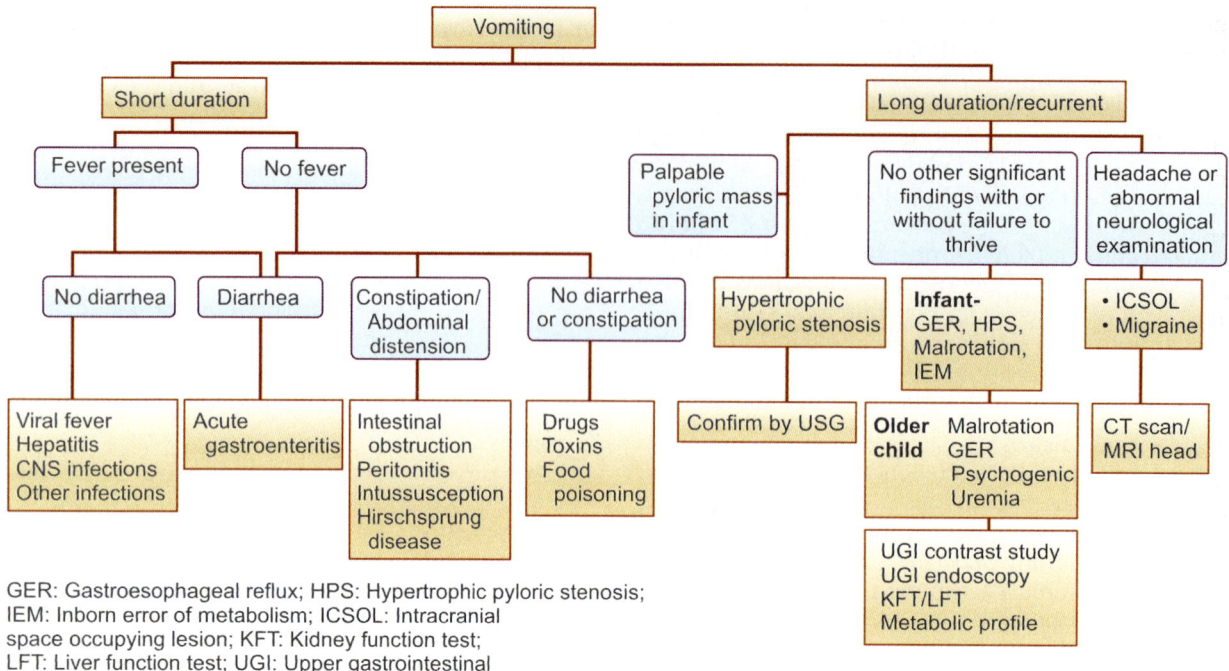

GER: Gastroesophageal reflux; HPS: Hypertrophic pyloric stenosis;
IEM: Inborn error of metabolism; ICSOL: Intracranial
space occupying lesion; KFT: Kidney function test;
LFT: Liver function test; UGI: Upper gastrointestinal

Fig. 9.3 Clinical and diagnostic approach to a child with vomiting

Table 9.3 Causes of Vomiting in Children	
Anatomical/Structural defects of GIT	*CNS causes*
Hypertrophic pyloric stenosis	CNS infections
Malrotation	Intracranial space occupying lesions
Volvulus	Benign intracranial hypertension
Intussusception	Hydrocephalus
Intestinal obstruction	Extradural/subdural/intracranial bleed
Hirschsprung disease	
Gastroesophageal reflux	
GI motility and functional disorders	*Toxic and metabolic causes*
	Food poisoning
Infections and Inflammations	Other poisonings
Acute gastroenteritis	Uremia
Pyelonephritis	Diabetic ketoacidosis
Hepatitis	Inborn errors of metabolism
Pancreatitis	Drug toxicities
Cholecystitis	*Others*
Peritonitis	Milk protein intolerance
Typhoid fever	Psychogenic

metabolic disorders are more commonly seen in the infancy. Peptic, infectious, and psychogenic causes are more prominent with increasing age **(Table 9.3)**.

Investigations

A child with prolonged or repetitive vomiting should have the following investigations: Complete blood count, serum electrolytes, blood urea nitrogen, and urinalysis. Specific indications from history and physical examination may help in obtaining other tests such as upper gastrointestinal imaging, abdominal ultrasound, CT scan or MRI of the head,

tests of liver function, serum amylase, toxicology screen, serum ammonia and urinary organic acids. Figure 9.3 outlines the clinical and investigative approach to the diagnosis in a child with vomiting.

- *Upper gastrointestinal contrast series* should be performed to diagnose or exclude hypertrophic pyloric stenosis, esophageal webs, gastroesophageal reflux, and malrotation in a young child having prolonged or repetitive vomiting associated with failure to thrive.
- *Ultrasound* is a sensitive tool to diagnose hypertrophic pyloric stenosis, in children having a palpable pyloric mass.
- *Endoscopic examination* of the esophagus, stomach, and duodenum is sometimes helpful if peptic disease or anatomic abnormality is suspected.
- *Manometric evaluation* of the esophagus, stomach, and duodenum is occasionally helpful in defining primary or secondary motor abnormalities causing emesis.

Irwin S, Barmherzig R, Gelfand A. Recurrent gastrointestinal disturbance: Abdominal migraine and cyclic vomiting syndrome. *Curr Neurol Neurosci Rep.* 2017;17:21.

Kleinman, RE, Goulet, O, Mieli-Vergani, G, Sanderson, et al. (Eds). Walker's Pediatric Gastrointestinal Disease. 6th ed. USA: People's Medical Publishing House; 2015.

9.6 GASTROESOPHAGEAL REFLUX (GER)

Gastroesophageal reflux (GER) refers to the spontaneous effortless movement of gastric contents proximally into the esophagus. When the reflux is high enough to be visualized, it is called regurgitation. GER is extremely common during infancy.

When the reflux or regurgitation results in complications (eg, failure to thrive, swallowing difficulties, apnea, pneumonia, reactive airway disease) or contributes to tissue damage or inflammation (eg, esophagitis), it is called *gastroesophageal reflux disease* (GERD).

Pathophysiology

Episodes of transient relaxation of lower esophageal sphincter allowing gastric contents to reflux into the esophagus, is considered to be the predominant mode of GER in infants and older children. Possible explanations for inappropriate relaxation of the lower esophageal sphincter may be related to the central nervous system or a developmentally exaggerated enteric reflex. Children with severe GER may also have delayed gastric emptying.

Clinical Features

Though mostly asymptomatic, severity of the symptoms of GER varies from an occasional burp to persistent emesis. GER in infancy causing no or minimal symptoms is most often physiologic and symptoms if any, resolve within 6 to 12 months. When GER results in growth failure, respiratory disease, apnea, or esophagitis, it is termed as gastroesophageal reflux disease (GERD).

The gastrointestinal symptoms of GER include vomiting, heartburn and gastrointestinal blood loss. This may result in nutritional problems such as failure to thrive and anemia. Esophagitis caused by the reflux of gastric acid results in heartburn, irritability and abnormal posturing (Sandifer-Sutcliffe syndrome). Child may start avoiding food and in severe cases, dysphagia might develop because of esophageal stricture.

In the respiratory system, GER has been suggested as an etiologic determinant of apnea, sudden infant death syndrome, asthma and recurrent pneumonia in children. However, the cause and effect relationship between GER and respiratory disease remains difficult to prove especially in infants as GER is otherwise also very common in this age group.

Diagnosis

- *24-hour esophageal pH monitoring* with a pH probe is the most sensitive and specific investigation for diagnosis of GER. Radionuclide studies with technetium 99m (99 mTc) are also useful and carry the advantage of being noninvasive and low in radiation.
- *Upper GI endoscopy* with esophageal biopsy is also needed in children having symptoms of esophagitis. The presence of intraepithelial eosinophils along with other inflammatory cells in the distal esophageal mucosa suggests the diagnosis of esophagitis secondary to GERD.
- *Contrast radiographic studies of the esophagus* have low sensitivity in diagnosing GER but may be needed when other structural abnormalities form a differential diagnosis in a child presenting with vomiting.

Treatment

A. *General Measures*
- Head and upper portion of chest should be elevated. Prone and left lateral positions reduce GER, and can be adopted post-prandially if the child is awake. However, during sleep, American Academy of Pediatrics recommends supine position in all infants to reduce risk of sudden infant death syndrome.
- Small frequent feeds reduce the amount of food in the stomach available for reflux.
- Thickening of feeds might benefit some infants and children with GER.

B. *Medications*
- **H2 antagonists** (eg ranitidine 6–8 mg/kg/day in BID or TID doses) or proton pump inhibitors (PPIs) (eg, omeprazole 2.0–2.5 mg/kg/d or lansoprazole 1.4 mg/kg/d) reduce gastric acid secretion and thus reduce associated esophagitis. However, PPIs should not be used empirically in infants, as most infants do not need medication, and PPIs may be associated with increased risk of gastrointestinal and respiratory infections. In older children, empirical *acid suppressive* therapy can be used if symptoms are typical of GERD.
- *Prokinetic agents* such as metoclopramide and domperidone (0.2–0.4 mg/kg/dose three times a day) increase pressure at the lower esophageal sphincter and hasten gastric emptying, and thus are effective in reducing GER. The safety of these drugs is however questionable.

C. *Operative procedures* to tighten the lower esophageal sphincter
- Nissen's fundoplication prevents the reflux of gastric contents proximally and may be required rarely in severe cases not responding to medical management.

Revision Point

Gastroesophageal Reflux (GER)

1. Gastroesophageal reflux (GER) refers to the spontaneous effortless movement of gastric contents proximally into the esophagus.
2. Gastroesophageal reflux disease (GERD) refers to symptomatic GER. Common symptoms include growth failure, respiratory disease, apnea, or esophagitis.
3. Diagnostic tools include 24 hour esophageal pH monitoring, upper GI endoscopy, and contrast radiographic studies of the esophagus.
4. H2 antagonists (ranitidine) or proton pump inhibitors (omeprazole or lansoprazole) are useful in management.

Benninga MA, Faure C, Hyman PE, St James Roberts I, Schechter NL, Nurko S. Childhood Functional Gastrointestinal Disorders: Neonate/Toddler. *Gastroenterology*. 2016;150:1443-55.

Cohen S, Bueno de Mesquita M, Mimouni FB. Adverse effects reported in the use of gastroesophageal reflux disease treatments in children: a 10 years literature review. *Br J Clin Pharmacol*. 2015;80:200–8.

Poddar U. Diagnosis and management of gastroesophageal reflux disease (GERD): an Indian perspective. *Indian Pediatr*. 2013;50:119–26.

Puntis JW. Gastro-oesophageal reflux in young babies: who should be treated? *Arch Dis Child*. 2015;100:989–93.

Tighe M, Afzal NA, Bevan A, Hayen A, Munro A, Beattie RM. Pharmacological treatment of children with gastro-oesophageal reflux. *Cochrane Database Syst Rev*. 2014;11:CD008550.

Van den plas Y, Rudolph CD, Di Lorenzo C, et al. Pediatric gastroesophageal reflux clinical practice guidelines: joint recommendations of the North American Society for Pediatric Gastroenterology, Hepatology, and Nutrition (NASPGHAN) and the European Society for Pediatric Gastroenterology, Hepatology, and Nutrition (ESPGHAN). *J Pediatr Gastroenterol Nutr*. 2009; 49:499.

9.7 ABDOMINAL PAIN

Abdominal pain is a very common symptom in pediatric age group. There are mainly three mechanisms by which abdominal pain is perceived. All three types of pain may be modified by a child's level of tolerance. Psychogenic and environmental factors augment or inhibit the perception of pain to varying degrees in different individuals.

Anatomical Correlates of Abdominal Pain

1. *Autonomic sensory pathways from the abdominal viscera*
   Visceral pain tends to be experienced in the dermatome from which the affected organ receives innervations. It is a dull aching sensation generally perceived in one of three regions: The periumbilical, epigastric, or suprapubic midline area.
   • Painful stimuli originating in the liver, pancreas, biliary tree, stomach, or upper bowel are felt in the *epigastrium.*
   • Pain from the distal small bowel, cecum, appendix, or proximal colon is felt at the *umbilicus.*
   • Pain from the distal large bowel, urinary tract, or pelvic organs is usually *suprapubic.*
   An example of the visceral pain is the initial pain of appendicitis which is usually felt in the periumbilical area.

2. *Somatic sensory pathways from the parietal peritoneum, abdominal wall, or retroperitoneal skeletal muscles*
   Somatic pain is usually well localized and intense (often sharp) in character. An intra-abdominal process will manifest somatic pain if an inflammatory process affecting a viscus touches a somatic organ (ie, the anterior parietal peritoneum or abdominal wall). An example of somatic pain is the localized pain of acute appendicitis in the right iliac fossa due to the inflammation affecting the nearby peritoneum.

3. *Referred pain*
   Referred pain may occur from extra-abdominal sites which share central projections with sensory pathways from the abdominal wall (referred pain). The classic example of referred abdominal pain is the shared central projections of the parietal pleura of the lung and the abdominal wall, such that abdominal pain may be the initial presentation of pneumonia.

Acute Abdominal Pain

Acute abdominal pain, or "acute abdomen," refers to abdominal pain of recent onset that triggers an urgent need for prompt diagnosis and active treatment. Although most children with acute abdominal pain have self-limiting conditions, the pain may herald a serious medical or surgical emergency. Therefore, a major challenge is to make a timely *diagnosis of the acute surgical abdomen.* Figure 9.4 outlines the clinical approach for delineating the etiology of acute abdominal pain in a child.

Chronic Abdominal Pain

This refers to long-lasting constant or intermittent abdominal pain in children, which persists for greater than 3 months duration, and affects normal activity. Chronic abdominal pain can be *organic* (disease-related) or *functional.*

Functional abdominal pain disorders, which include irritable bowel syndrome (chronic abdominal pain along with alteration in bowel movements), functional dyspepsia (pain or discomfort in upper abdomen), abdominal migraine (pain associated with nausea, anorexia, vomiting or pallor), and functional abdominal pain—not otherwise specified, are the most common causes of recurrent abdominal pain in children.

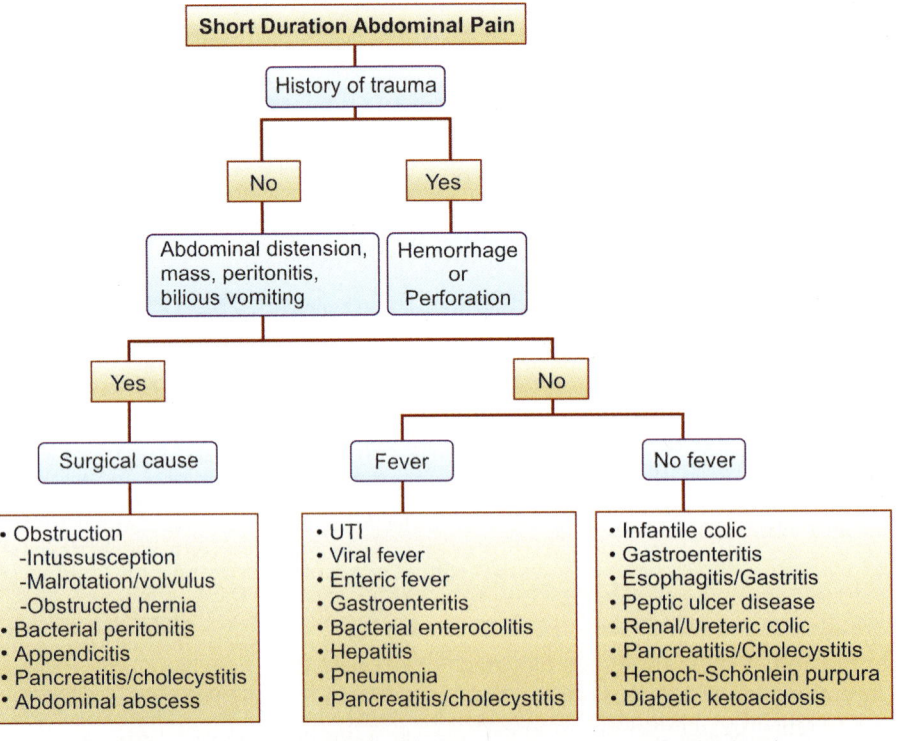

Fig. 9.4 Clinical approach to a child with acute abdominal pain

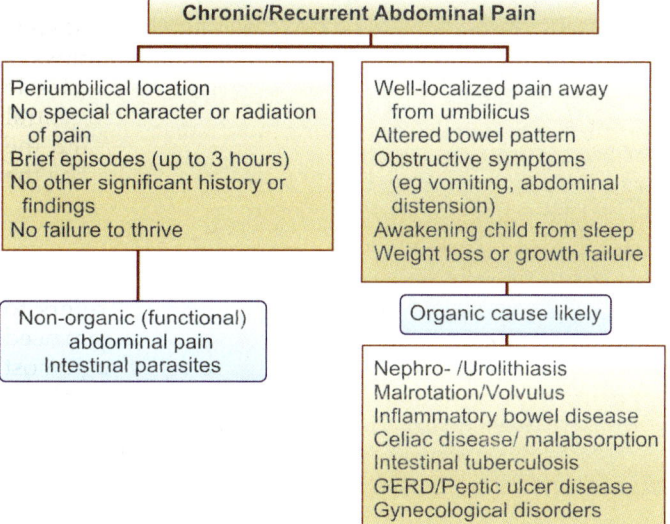

Fig. 9.5 Clinical approach to a child with chronic/recurrent abdominal pain

Other differential diagnoses of recurrent abdominal pain include a heterogeneous group of anatomic, infectious, non-infectious, inflammatory, and biochemical disorders. Approach to etiological diagnosis of a child with chronic abdominal pain is summarized in Fig. 9.5.

American Academy of Pediatrics Subcommittee on Chronic Abdominal Pain, North American Society for Pediatric Gastroenterology Hepatology, and Nutrition. Chronic abdominal pain in children. *Pediatrics.* 2005;115:e370.

Gomez-Suarez R. Difficulties in the diagnosis and management of functional or recurrent abdominal pain in children. *Pediatr Ann.* 2016;45:e388-93.

Hyams JS, Di Lorenzo C, Saps M, Shulman RJ, Staiano A, van Tilburg M. Childhood Functional Gastrointestinal Disorders: Child/Adolescent. *Gastroenterology.* 2016;150:1456–68.

Quek SH. Recurrent abdominal pain in children: a clinical approach. *Singapore Med J.* 2015;56:125–8.

9.8 CONSTIPATION

Passage of hard stools with difficulty is termed as constipation. Constipation can present as (*i*) difficulty in passing stools, (*ii*) painful or bloody stools due to fissure in ano, (*iii*) palpable abdominal masses due to fecal impaction, or (*iv*) soiling of clothes due to insensitivity to the rectal distension.

Constipation can be severe, persistent, or recurrent.

Etiology

Most children with constipation have no obvious cause (primary or functional constipation); Hirschsprung disease, hypothyroidism, and anal stenosis are important secondary causes.

Constipation is also more common in children who suffer from chronic neurological disorders including cerebral palsy, degenerative, and neuromuscular disorders.

Assessing a Child with Constipation

The chief complaints and their duration should be noted. A note should be made of the nature of toilet training, medications and compliance, and the diet and fluid intake. Any psychosocial factors or problems in schooling should be evaluated. Obtain history suggestive of neurological disorders (convulsions, mental retardation, tone abnormalities).

History of delayed passage of meconium, onset of constipation in first few months, episodes of severe unexplained diarrhea, and marked abdominal distension suggest possibility of Hirschsprung disease. Coarse facies, hoarseness of voice, umbilical hernia, and developmental delay suggest hypothyroidism. Look for any abdominal distension/masses or fissures. Per rectal examination can be useful to confirm impaction, and suggest or exclude Hirschsprung disease and anal stenosis. Neurological evaluation should include examination of spine and perineum, ankle jerk, etc.

Investigations are usually unnecessary unless there is some clue towards secondary constipation. X-ray of spine is required if examination suggests tone/tendon reflex abnormalities in lower limb or if neurogenic bladder is also present. T3, T4, TSH needs to be done if clinical features suggest hypothyroidism. Rectal biopsy is indicated for suspected Hirschsprung disease.

Treatment	Constipation

The explanation of the condition is most important, and takes time. It cannot be rushed, and must be directed both at parents and child. Go through the mechanism with parents and child using pictures and diagrams. Emphasize that withholding a stool or soiling is not deliberate. It takes a long time to get into this state and may take a long time to resolve.

- The bowel needs to be emptied. A clear-out may be more difficult to manage than the previous state of incomplete bowel emptying, eg, cramps, urgency, or perhaps more soiling. Parents and child need to be warned of this.
- When the bowel is completely cleared, it then needs to be kept empty with maintenance treatment or it will very quickly fill back.

It is desirable that a clear-out is achieved before maintenance treatment can be started. A clear-out is done using laxatives like senna, picosulphate or osmotic laxatives like polyethylene glycol (PEG). Colonic lavage might be done in hospitalized children. All children needing bowel clear-out will need maintenance treatment, usually long-term. This should not be suddenly stopped. Misinformation about long-term laxatives causing "lazy" bowels or physical dependence should be addressed. The medications used for maintenance in chronic constipation include lactulose, liquid paraffin, milk of magnesia and PEG. PEG (0.5 to 1.0 g/kg/day) has a distinct advantage over other medications in being more effective over long-term with minimal adverse effects.

The most common explanation for "intractable constipation" is the prescription of inadequate therapy or non-adherence to the prescribed regimen. A period of supervised treatment may therefore be necessary. The child should be monitored closely to determine the particular nature of the problem in their case. This is done using (*a*) history and stool charts; and (*b*) abdominal and rectal examination to ascertain that there are no masses or distension. If unsuccessful, try a different option, and consider the psychological and behavioral aspects. Involve a psychologist if appropriate.

Children must have a clear toilet training regime. They need to know that this is essential, and that they may not initially feel a recognizable desire to defecate. Children with severe constipation usually have diminished or absent rectal sensation due to chronic rectal distension and are therefore unaware of the need to defecate. A supervised visit to sit on the toilet and try to go twice per day is reasonable. A reward system such as a star chart can be helpful in some children, but must be very simple.

Colombo JM, Wassom MC, Rosen JM. Constipation and encopresis in childhood. *Pediatr Rev.* 2015;36:392–401.

Gordon M, MacDonald JK, Parker CE, Akobeng AK, Thomas AG. Osmotic and stimulant laxatives for the management of childhood constipation. *Cochrane Database Syst Rev.* 2016;8:CD009118.

Hyams JS, Di Lorenzo C, Saps M, Shulman RJ, Staiano A, van Tilburg M. Childhood Functional Gastrointestinal Disorders: Child/ Adolescent. *Gastroenterology.* 2016;150:1456–68.

Poddar U. Approach to constipation in children. *Indian Pediatr.* 2016;53:319–27.

9.9 INFLAMMATORY BOWEL DISEASE (IBD)

Ulcerative colitis and Crohn disease are idiopathic chronic conditions affecting the gastrointestinal system that are generically grouped under the term inflammatory bowel disease (IBD).

Epidemiology

Inflammatory bowel diseases are the major causes of chronic intestinal inflammation in children beyond the first year of life in developed countries. In developing countries, the diagnosis of IBD should be considered in children having recurrent or unusually prolonged dysentery like illness.

The most common age of onset of IBD is during adolescence and young adulthood. The etiological factors implicated for IBD are genetic, environmental (urban residence, psychological stress) and immunological (increased antigen uptake, defective antigen processing, abnormal vascular function and abnormalities in the production of intermediators like interleukins and eicosanoids).

Clinical Features

A. Ulcerative Colitis

The cardinal symptoms of ulcerative colitis are diarrhea, rectal bleeding, and abdominal pain. The presentation is varied depending upon the extent and severity of mucosal inflammation:

- *Mild illness* presents with insidious onset of diarrhea, later associated with passage of blood in stools (hematochezia), but usually without systemic signs of fever, weight loss, or hypoalbuminemia.
- *Severe illness* Signs of systemic illness appear later that include diarrhea, cramps, urgency, malaise, fever, anorexia, weight loss, anemia, and hypoalbuminemia. Abdominal tenderness and distension is usually present in severe forms.
- *Extra-intestinal features* About one-fourth of children develop extra-intestinal features which may occur before GI manifestation, during GI symptoms, or even after the

Table 9.4 Extra-intestinal Manifestations of Ulcerative Colitis and Crohn Disease

Musculoskeletal	*Blood*
• Arthritis including ankylosing spondylitis • Enthesopathy	• Iron deficiency anemia • Autoimmune hemolytic anemia • ITP
Skin	
• Pyoderma gangrenosum • Erythema nodosum	*Pancreas* • Pancreatitis
Eye	*Cardiorespiratory*
• Episcleritis • Uveitis	• Pericarditis • Pneumonitis
Hepatobiliary	*Growth and development*
• Sclerosing cholangitis • Autoimmune hepatitis • Cholelithiasis	• Delayed growth • Delayed puberty

surgical removal of the diseased bowel. The principal extra-intestinal manifestations of ulcerative colitis are listed in **Table 9.4**.

- *Complications* The complications of ulcerative colitis include toxic megacolon, colonic perforation, sepsis, and massive hemorrhage. Individuals with long-standing disease are at markedly increased risk of carcinoma.

B. Crohn Disease

Abdominal pain is the most common symptom of Crohn disease. This is often associated with diarrhea, poor appetite and weight loss. Abdominal pain is periumbilical but may localize to the right lower quadrant or diffusely to the lower abdomen. Diarrhea is usually not bloody, unless disease involves the right colon or there is perianal fissure.

Perinatal fistulae, large tags or recurrent perianal abscesses in any child warrant investigation to exclude Crohn disease. Extra-intestinal manifestations similar to those seen in ulcerative colitis might occur. The complications include malnutrition, narrowing of the bowel lumen from inflammation or stricture, fistulae, and intra-abdominal abscesses.

Table 9.5 outlines the differences between Crohn disease and ulcerative colitis.

Diagnosis

Laboratory Tests

No single test can confidently confirm the suspicion of IBD. The diagnosis is made on basis of clinical presentation, and substantiated by radiological and histological investigations.

- Peripheral blood counts reveal leucocytosis, microcytic anemia, and thrombocytosis. The ESR and C-reactive protein are increased and there is hypoalbuminemia. Children with significant mucosal inflammation may have normal laboratory test results.
- Stool culture should be performed to rule out infection.
- Perinuclear antineutrophil cytoplasmic antibodies (PANCAs) are seen in 60–80% of children with ulcerative colitis compared to 10–27% of those with Crohn disease.
- *Anti-saccharomyces cerevisiae* (ASCA) antibodies are commonly found in individuals with Crohn disease, but are rarely seen in ulcerative colitis.

Table 9.5 Differences between Ulcerative Colitis and Crohn Disease

	Ulcerative colitis	*Crohn disease*
Site of involvement	Rectum and colon	Entire length of gastrointestinal system (from mouth to rectum)
Pattern of involvement	Diffuse and continuous, extending proximally from rectum	Patchy (segmental)
Blood in stools	Common	Uncommon
Extra-intestinal manifestations	More common	Less common
Oral ulcers	Rare	Common
Perianal tags, abscesses, fistulas	Rare	Common
Circulating antibodies	Perinuclear antineutrophil cytoplasmic antibodies (PANCAs)	Anti-Saccharomyces cerevisiae (ASCA) antibodies
Biopsy findings	Mucosal inflammation, crypt abscesses and pseudopolyposis	Non-caseating granulomas and transmural inflammation

Radiological Studies

Radiological studies are not very helpful in ulcerative colitis except for diagnosis of complications. In Crohn disease, upper GI contrast examination with small bowel follow through may show ulcerations, thickened and nodular folds, or narrowing of the lumen of the bowel (string sign of Kantoor).

Endoscopy

Flexible sigmoidoscopy or colonoscopic inspection of colon and ileum, in conjunction with mucosal biopsies provides the most sensitive and specific evaluation of intestinal inflammation. In ulcerative colitis, the involvement is diffuse and continuous starting from rectum and extending proximally. In Crohn disease, findings on colonoscopy include patchy nonspecific inflammation, aphthous ulcers, linear ulcers, modulatory strictures, cobblestone appearance, and skip. As Crohn disease may often involve distal portions of small intenstine without involving colon, video capsule endoscopies may be required to demonstrate the lesion.

Intestinal Biopsy

Non-caseating granulomas and transmural inflammation are characteristic histological features of Crohn disease; whereas mucosal inflammation, crypt abscesses, and pseudopolyposis are typical of ulcerative colitis.

Treatment   Inflammatory Bowel Disease

Goals of therapy for IBD are (*i*) induction of remission with control of symptoms; (*ii*) prevention of relapse; (*iii*) avoidance of complications; and (*iv*) provision of the optimal quality of life.

A. Medical management

- Commonly used drugs are oral aminosalicylates (sulfa-salazine, mesalamine), oral corticosteroids, 6-mercaptopurine (6-MP), and azathioprine.
- Topical aminosalicylates and topical corticosteroids are used to treat distal colitis associated with ulcerative colitis.
- Antibiotics are used in presence of complications and for fistulous and perianal disease in Crohn disease.
- Intravenous corticosteroids and newer drugs like infliximab (a chimeric monoclonal antibody to tumor necrosis factor-α) are used to treat fulminant and refractory disease.

B. Surgical treatment

Surgical treatment might be needed for intractable disease or in presence of complications such as perforation and strictures. Provision of adequate nutrients is essential for optimal healing. Enteral nutrition is preferred to parenteral nutrition.

Inflammatory Bowel Disease (IBD)

1. Ulcerative colitis and Crohn disease are the two most common inflammatory bowel diseases (IBD).
2. The most common age of onset is during adolescence and young adulthood.
3. The cardinal symptoms of ulcerative colitis are diarrhea, rectal bleeding, and abdominal pain. Abdominal pain is the most common symptom of Crohn disease.
4. Perinuclear antineutrophil cytoplasmic antibodies (P-ANCAs) are more common in ulcerative colitis while anti-Saccharomyces cerevisiae antibodies (ASCA) are commonly found in Crohn disease.
5. Flexible sigmoidoscopy or colonoscopy and mucosal biopsies are diagnostic.
6. Commonly used drugs are oral aminosalicylates (sulfasalazine, mesalamine), oral corticosteroids, 6-mercaptopurine (6-MP), and azathioprine.
7. *Surgical treatment* might be needed for complications or intractable disease.

Fell JM, Muhammed R, Spray C, Crook K, Russell RK; BSPGHAN IBD working group. Management of ulcerative colitis. *Arch Dis Child.* 2016;101:469–74.

Griffiths AM, Buller HB. Inflammatory bowel disease. *In*: Walker WA, Durie PR, Hamilton JR, *et al.* editors. *Pediatric Gastrointestinal Disease: Pathophysiology, Diagnosis, and Management.* 3rd edition. Ontario: BC Decker; 2000. p. 613–64.

IBD Working Group of the European Society for Paediatric Gastroenterology, Hepatology and Nutrition. Inflammatory bowel disease in children and adolescents: recommendations for diagnosis—the Porto criteria. *J Pediatr Gastroenterol Nutr.* 2005; 41:1.

Kammermeier J, Morris MA, Garrick V, Furman M, Rodrigues A, Russell RK; BSPGHAN IBD Working Group. Management of Crohn disease. *Arch Dis Child.* 2016;101:475–80.

North American Society for Pediatric Gastroenterology, Hepatology, and Nutrition, Colitis Foundation of America, Bousvaros

A, *et al*. Differentiating ulcerative colitis from Crohn disease in children and young adults: report of a working group. *J Pediatr Gastroenterol Nutr*. 2007; 44:653.

Rosen MJ, Dhawan A, Saeed SA. Inflammatory bowel disease in children and adolescents. *JAMA Pediatr*. 2015;169:1053–60.

9.10 APPROACH TO HEPATOSPLENOMEGALY

1. Hepatosplenomegaly with Fever and Anemia

- *Enteric fever* History of high fever for 1–3 weeks, toxic look, mild and soft enlargement of spleen.
- *Malaria* Short or recurrent history of fever, history of chills and rigors, firm and tender enlargement of spleen.
- *Leishmaniasis* Firm and massive spleen enlargement, residence in endemic area.
- *Leukemia* Bleeding spots, lymphadenopathy, sternal tenderness.
- *Lymphoma* Lymphadenopathy.

2. Hepatosplenomegaly with Anemia, no Fever

- *Hemolytic anemia* History of blood transfusions, hemolytic facies, predominant enlargement of spleen.
- *Chronic liver disease* Firm and irregular enlargement of liver, nodular surface of liver. Presence of splenomegaly and ascites indicates associated portal hypertension. Jaundice may be present in decompensated disease.
- *Intrauterine infections* Low birth weight, onset in infancy, microcephaly or hydrocephalus, mental retardation.
- *Lysosomal storage disorders* Gaucher disease, Niemann-Pick disease.

3. Hepatosplenomegaly with Jaundice

- *Acute hepatitis* Presence of low grade fever, jaundice, anorexia, clay-colored stools. Tender hepatomegaly. Mild enlargement of spleen.
- *Decompensated chronic liver disease* Firm and irregular enlargement of liver, nodular surface of liver, ascites.
- *Hemolytic anemia* History of blood transfusions, hemolytic facies, predominant enlargement of spleen, jaundice mild without dark-colored urine.
- *Neonatal and infantile cholestasis syndromes* Seen in infants.

9.11 APPROACH TO A CHILD WITH JAUNDICE

Jaundice is yellow discoloration of the sclera, skin, and mucous membranes and occurs due to rise in serum levels of bilirubin (hyperbilirubinemia).

- Clinically apparent jaundice in neonates occurs when the bilirubin rises to more than 5 mg/dL.
- Older children and adults become icteric when the serum concentration of bilirubin reaches 2–3 mg/dL.
- Jaundice is better appreciated by examining the child in daylight rather than under artificial lighting.

Bilirubin in Body

Measurement of the total serum bilirubin concentration allows quantification of jaundice. Bilirubin occurs in plasma in four forms:

1. Unconjugated bilirubin tightly bound to albumin;
2. Free bilirubin (the form responsible for kernicterus, because it can cross cell membranes);
3. Conjugated bilirubin (the only fraction to appear in urine); and
4. Delta (δ) fraction which is conjugated bilirubin that is covalently bound to albumin. This form can represent a major proportion of serum bilirubin in children who have had conjugated hyperbilirubinemia for a time. The δ fraction permits conjugated bilirubin to persist in the circulation and delays resolution of jaundice.

Unconjugated Hyperbilirubinemia

Indirect reacting bilirubin indicates increased production of bilirubin, hemolysis, reduced hepatic removal, or altered metabolism of bilirubin. Causes are enumerated below:

I. *Increased production*

   i. Hemolysis: Rh incompatibility, ABO incompatibility, minor blood group incompatibilities, hereditary spherocytosis, G6PD deficiency, sickle cell anemia, thalassemia, sepsis, drugs.

  ii. Enclosed hematoma, eg, cephalhematoma

 iii. Polycythemia

II. *Decreased bilirubin uptake*

   i. Breast milk jaundice

  ii. Hypothyroidism

 iii. Hypoxia

III. *Decreased conjugation*

   i. Physiological neonatal jaundice

  ii. Crigler-Najjar syndrome, Types I and II

 iii. Gilbert disease

IV. *Increased enterohepatic circulation*

Pyloric stenosis, duodenal atresia, intestinal obstruction, Hirschsprung disease.

Conjugated Bilirubinemia

Conjugated bilirubinemia (defined as >20% of total bilirubin level) reflects decreased excretion by damaged hepatic parenchymal cells or disease of biliary tract, which may be due to sepsis, endocrine or metabolic disease, inflammation of the liver, or obstruction in the hepatobiliary tree **(Table 9.6)**.

The terms direct and indirect bilirubin (measured by traditional diazo methods of bilirubin estimation) are used equivalently with conjugated and unconjugated bilirubin, respectively. However, this is not quantitatively correct, because the direct fraction includes both conjugated bilirubin and δ bilirubin. Newer methods of bilirubin measurement such as Ektachem slide method allow more accurate measurement of conjugated, unconjugated, and delta-bilirubin levels separately.

Evaluation of a child with jaundice involves an appropriate and accurate history, a carefully performed physical examination, and skillful interpretation of signs and symptoms. Further evaluation is aided by judicious selection of diagnostic tests.

9.12 ACUTE HEPATITIS

Acute hepatitis is a clinical syndrome characterized by abrupt onset of jaundice associated with conjugated hyper-

Table 9.6 Causes of Conjugated Hyperbilirubinemia
Infections
• Acute viral hepatitis
• Chronic viral hepatitis
• Septicemia
• Typhoid fever
• Kala-azar
• Leptospirosis
• Brucellosis
• Cholangitis
• Infectious mononucleosis
• Disseminated tuberculosis
Autoimmune
• Autoimmune hepatitis
• Systemic lupus erythematosus
• Sclerosing cholangitis
Infiltrative Disorders
• Lymphoma
• Leukemia
• Histiocytosis
• Hepatic metastasis
Metabolic and Storage Disorders
• Lipid storage disorders (Gaucher and Niemann-Pick disease)
• Wilson disease
• α_1-Antitrypsin deficiency
• Cystic fibrosis
• Mitochondrial disorders
Toxic
• Hepatotoxic and cholestatic drugs (eg, INH, valproate)
• Snake envenomation
Extrahepatic Diseases
• Sclerosing cholangitis
• Bile duct obstruction due to stones, worms
• Mass (neoplasia, lymph nodes)
Miscellaneous
• Indian childhood cirrhosis
• Ischemic hepatopathy (associated with shock and hypoperfusion)
• Parenteral nutrition
Neonatal and Infantile Cholestasis Syndromes (*see Table 9.8*)

bilirubinemia and elevation of hepatic enzymes. Although acute hepatitis may occur alone or as a part of systemic disease, the most common cause in children is infection—usually by one of the five hepatotropic viruses (hepatitis A to E).

Etiology

Hepatitis A Virus (HAV)

HAV infections occur most often in developing countries with almost all children demonstrating evidence of past infection by the age of adolescence. The risk of infection is more in contacts of infected persons, child-care centers and travelers to endemic areas. Transmission of HAV is almost always by person-to-person contact. Spread is predominantly by the fecal-oral route (through contaminated food or water) and maternal-neonatal transmission is not recognized.

Hepatitis A virus causes only acute hepatitis syndrome and does not lead to chronicity or cirrhosis. Most infections in children younger than 5 years of age are asymptomatic or have mild, nonspecific manifestations; the illness is much more likely to be symptomatic in older children and adults.

Hepatitis B Virus (HBV)

The major route of transmission in children is from mother-to-child (perinatal transmission). Other important modes include blood products, unsafe injections, sexual contact, institutional care, and contact with carriers. No risk factors are identified in about 40% of cases.

Hepatitis B infection may present as asymptomatic infection, acute hepatitis syndrome, or chronic hepatitis. The risk of chronicity is related inversely to age; the older the age of acquisition, the lower the risk of chronic disease. Chronic carrier stage of hepatitis B predisposes to hepatocellular carcinoma. Infection during pregnancy does not influence the maternal or fetal outcome adversely.

Hepatitis C Virus (HCV)

The risk factors for transmission are exposure to contaminated blood products, sexual contact and unsafe injections. Perinatal transmission is uncommon.

Most acute infections are clinically silent, less than 25% of children become icteric. Clinically apparent acute infections are mild and progression to fulminant hepatitis is exceedingly rare. HCV is the most likely hepatotropic virus to cause chronic infection with about 85% of cases becoming chronic.

Hepatitis D Virus (HDV)

HDV cannot produce infection without HBV as a helper virus. HDV can cause an infection at the same time as the initial HBV infection (co-infection), or can infect a person who is already infected with HBV (superinfection). The routes of transmission are same as that for HBV.

Acute hepatitis is common with co-infection and is usually much more severe than for HBV alone. In superinfection, acute illness is rare and chronic hepatitis is common. However, the risk of fulminant hepatitis is highest in superinfection.

Hepatitis E Virus (HEV)

Hepatitis E virus infection occurs through fecal-oral route usually contracted through contaminated water. It occurs in outbreaks or as sporadic cases in endemic areas. The highest attack rate of overt disease occurs in adolescents and adults. HEV infection is associated with a very high mortality rate among infected pregnant women.

Drugs

Most drug-induced liver disease is cytotoxic. Some drug-induced liver disease, however, is predominantly cholestatic. Acute hepatotoxic injuries develop over a relatively short time and cause a lesion without any features of chronicity.

The most common drugs associated with hepatotoxicity in children are isoniazid, valproate, paracetamol, azathioprine, and halothane.

Autoimmune Hepatitis

Though mostly associated with chronic liver disease, 25–30% of children with autoimmune hepatitis, particularly children, the illness may mimic acute viral hepatitis. Acute liver disease may also be associated with other immune-mediated disorders like SLE, inflammatory bowel disease, and celiac disease.

Metabolic Diseases

Wilson disease may present as acute self-limited hepatitis or as fulminant hepatic failure. α_1-antitrypsin deficiency may also rarely presents as acute hepatitis.

Other Infections

Diseases like typhoid fever, kala-azar, leptospirosis, scrub typhus, and brucellosis can also cause acute hepatitis like state. Though asymptomatic elevation of hepatic enzymes is most frequently seen, frank jaundice is sometimes present.

Clinical Features

Acute viral hepatitis is ordinarily an acute self-limited illness. The incubation period is about 4 weeks for HAV and 4 months for HBV. In infants and young children, the infection may be entirely asymptomatic or manifest by a nonspecific gastroenteritis-like syndrome with no icterus.

In older children and in adults, there may be a prodromal period of several days in which fever, headache, and malaise predominate, followed by the onset of jaundice, abdominal pain, nausea, mild vomiting, and anorexia. Pruritus may accompany the jaundice. Over the next several days, as the jaundice peaks, the systemic symptoms wane. In hepatitis B infection, a serum sickness like state consisting of arthralgia or arthritis, urticaria or angioedema, and a maculopapular rash might occur. The arthritis is migratory and symmetric and subsides when jaundice begins.

On examination, marked jaundice is present with a mildly enlarged, tender liver. Occasionally, splenomegaly is noted. Mild to moderate ascites may be present in some cases especially with HAV infection. Jaundice and other symptoms usually resolve by 2 to 4 weeks after onset. In some cases, the disease progressively worsens to hepatic failure manifesting as encephalopathy and coagulopathy. Progression to fulminant hepatic failure is not seen with HCV and extremely rare with HEV except in pregnant women.

Complications

Acute Liver Failure

Currently accepted definition of acute liver failure is presence of coagulopathy (defined as INR >1.5 in presence of encephalopathy or INR >2 in absence of encephalopathy) not corrected by vitamin K administration within 8 weeks of onset of biochemical abnormalities in acute hepatitis. There is severe hepatic dysfunction affecting liver's synthetic, detoxification, and metabolic function. HAV, HBV, HDV superinfection, Wilson disease, autoimmune hepatitis, drugs (eg, paracetamol) and toxins (eg, poisonous mushrooms) are common causes of acute liver failure.

Others

Chronic hepatitis HCV, HBV, HDV superinfection, autoimmune hepatitis.

Cirrhosis and portal hypertension HCV, HBV, HDV superinfection, Wilson disease, autoimmune hepatitis.

Hepatocellular carcinoma HBV, HCV

Diagnosis

Evidence of Jaundice and Hepatic Dysfunction

Acute hepatitis is suspected clinically in any child with a short history of jaundice associated with other non-specific symptoms such as anorexia, vomiting, fever and abdominal pain. The serum bilirubin may only be mildly elevated especially in younger children or it becomes very high. The conjugated fraction is typically raised to more than 20% of total levels. Serum aminotransferase (ALT and AST) values usually peak around the time that jaundice occurs; values are often 20–100 times the upper limit of normal. Prolongation of prothrombin time (PT) indicates the need for hospitalization.

Evaluation of Cause

A detailed history is taken regarding exposure to persons having similar disease, history of travel to endemic areas, or similar cases in neighborhood for possible fecal-oral mode of transmission. Details of any blood transfusions, sexual contact/abuse, and unsafe injections are to be noted. A record of the medications recently used should be made for possible drug induced liver damage. Family history of jaundice or neurological illness should be asked for possibility of Wilson disease presenting as acute hepatitis.

Wilson disease and autoimmune hepatitis need to be considered if tests for the viral antibodies are negative. Salmonellosis, leptospirosis, scrub typhus, and brucellosis also need to be considered as a cause of acute hepatitis like illness, especially if fever is persistent.

The diagnosis of viral etiology is usually made serologically. Presence of following markers is required for diagnosis of acute infection with the respective viruses

Acute hepatitis A: IgM anti-HAV positivity

Acute hepatitis B: IgM anti-HBc along with HBsAg positivity

Acute hepatitis C: Detection of HCV RNA in serum by either PCR or branched DNA amplification technique (anti-HCV, the most commonly available serological test for HCV may become positive only after 2 months of acute infection and thus not useful in diagnosing acute hepatitis because of HCV)

HDV co-infection: IgM anti-HDV positivity along with HBsAg positivity

Acute hepatitis E: IgM anti-HEV positivity

Treatment	**Acute Hepatitis**

Treatment for acute hepatitis is purely supportive, and most children recover fully.

- Adequate rest should be ensured till the acute symptoms start resolving.
- Further liver insult should be prevented by avoiding hepatotoxic drugs.
- Adequate fluid intake should be ensured to avoid dehydration due to vomiting.
- Good nutritious diet, rich in carbohydrates and with adequate proteins is to be given. Fat restriction may be advised in initial stages to minimize vomiting but is not essential if nausea and vomiting is not marked.
- Antiviral therapy is not beneficial and is not indicated in any form of acute viral hepatitis.
- Wilson disease and AIH if presenting as acute fulminant hepatitis carry grave prognosis and usually require liver transplantation.

Treatment of acute liver failure

Acute liver failure should be managed in intensive care setting, preferably in a center having facilities for liver transplantation. The prognosis with conservative management is generally poor with survival rates not exceeding 50%.

Poor prognostic factors are: INR >5, rapid decrease in liver size without clinical improvement, Wilson disease and deeper stages of encephalopathy.

Conservative management of acute liver failure involves following:

i. *Fluid and electrolyte balance* Intravenous fluids containing glucose to prevent and correct hypoglycemia and dehydration. Strict input/output charting should be done.

ii. *Correction of coagulopathy and bleeding* by transfusion of fresh frozen plasma, platelet concentrates and blood.

iii. *Cerebral edema* should be managed by administration of mannitol. Endotracheal intubation and hyper-ventilation may be required in children having coma.

iv. *Administration of H_2 blockers* (ranitidine 1–2 mg/kg/dose 8–12 hourly) to prevent gastric bleeding.

v. *Oral lactulose* (5–40 mL) every 2–4 hourly initially till diarrhea, then titrate the dose so that the child passes 2–4 semi-loose acidic stools per day. This results in reduction of ammonia production by gut bacteria, by reducing their load.

vi. *Broad spectrum antibiotics* (eg, cefotaxime and cloxacillin) should be given to all cases as co-existent bacterial infection is present in almost 50% of cases. Oral administration of non-absorbable antibiotics such as neomycin also helps to clear the gut of bacteria thus decreasing ammonia production.

vii. *Renal care* Associated renal failure is managed by dialysis and a careful fluid administration titrated to the urine output.

viii. *Diet* In children taking orally or during recovery, protein intake should be restricted.

D'Agostino D, Diaz S, Sanchez MC, Boldrini G. Management and prognosis of acute liver failure in children. *Curr Gastroenterol Rep*. 2012;14:262–9.

Newland CD. Acute liver failure. *Pediatr Ann*. 2016 Dec 1;45(12):e433–8.

Pediatric Gastroenterology Chapter of Indian Academy of Pediatrics. Bhatia V, Bavdekar A, Yachha SK; Indian Academy of

Revision Point

Acute Hepatitis

1. Acute hepatitis is characterized by jaundice, conjugated hyperbilirubinemia, and raised liver enzymes.
2. Viral hepatitis caused by five hepatotropic viruses (hepatitis A to E) is the most common cause.
3. Hepatitis A, E are spread by feco-oral route while hepatitis B, C, D have parenteral transmission. Hepatitis B is also transmitted from mother to the newborn (vertical transmission)
4. Hepatitis A, E infections are acute; while hepatitis B, C, may become chronic.
5. Drugs, autoimmune hepatitis, and metabolic diseases (Wilson disease) are other common causes of hepatitis in children.
6. Acute viral hepatitis is an acute self-limited illness. Treatment is supportive. Acute liver failure is the most dreaded complication.

Pediatrics.. Management of acute liver failure in infants and children: consensus statement of the pediatric Gastroenterology Chapter, Indian Academy of Pediatrics. *Indian Pediatr*. 2013;50:477–82.

Wang Q, Yang F, Miao Q, Krawitt EL, Gershwin ME, Ma X. The clinical phenotypes of autoimmune hepatitis: A comprehensive review. *J Autoimmun*. 201666:98–107.

9.13 CHRONIC LIVER DISEASE

Chronic liver disease is long-term liver damage resulting from continuing inflammatory, infiltrative, metabolic, congestive, or obstructive process with a potential to lead to irreversible change in the structure of the liver and the complications of cirrhosis.

Cirrhosis refers to diffuse involvement of liver with evidence of fibrosis and regenerative nodules.

Etiology

Hepatotropic viruses including hepatitis B, C and D viruses can cause chronic liver disease and cirrhosis because of persistent hepatic inflammation. The risk of developing chronic HBV infection, defined as being positive for HBsAg for more than 6 months or being negative for IgM anti-HBc and positive for HBsAg, is related inversely to age; the older the age of acquisition, the lower the risk of chronic disease. Almost 90% children acquiring the hepatitis B infection perinatally become chronic carriers.

Other than viruses, chronic liver disease is caused by metabolic disorders such as Wilson disease, α_1-antitrypsin deficiency, hemochromatosis, and inborn errors of metabolism. Autoimmune hepatitis (Type I, II and III) is also important cause of chronic liver disease in older children.

Despite extensive investigations, a significant proportion of children having chronic liver disease are found to be having no obvious cause and are labeled as having idiopathic or cryptogenic chronic liver disease.

Clinical Presentation

1. Acute Hepatitis-like Presentation

- Chronic liver disease should be suspected whenever an episode of acute hepatitis-like illness continues for a prolonged period (usually 3 months) or when there is a relapse of apparent acute hepatitis.

- However, this cut-off period of 3 months is not strict and chronic liver disease may be suspected earlier than 3 months if there is a history suggestive of chronic liver disease or if examination or investigations suggest otherwise **(Table 9.7)**.
- Continuing abnormality of liver function after an apparent acute hepatitis also suggests chronic liver disease.
- Some children with an apparent acute hepatitis but clinical examination or investigations suggest chronic liver disease.

2. Chronic/insidious Presentation or Presentation with Complications

- Most children will present with bleeding varices, ascites, or hypersplenism—known complications of previously undiagnosed portal hypertension.
- Some children present with non-specific symptoms such as failure to thrive with or without prolonged/recurrent episodes of jaundice.
- Examination findings of firm/hard liver, firm splenomegaly, or ascites in any child with non-specific symptoms

Table 9.7 Features Suggesting Chronicity of Liver Disease

I *History*
- Relapsing disease
- Clinical or biochemical features of hepatitis persisting >12 weeks
- History of neonatal/infantile cholestasis
- Past history of acute hepatitis
- Family history of chronic liver disease
- History of some etiological disorder, eg, known HBsAg or anti-HCV positivity, Wilson disease, autoimmune disease or cystic fibrosis

II *Examination*
- Small liver
- Enlarged left lobe of liver
- Hard/irregular liver
- Firm splenomegaly
- Moderate to massive ascites
- Edema
- Growth failure/muscle wasting

III *Cutaneous Features*
- Portosystemic shunts
- Spider angiomas
- Facial telangiectasia
- Palmar erythema

IV *Investigations*
- Low serum albumin
- Raised PT despite vitamin K therapy
- High serum gammaglobulins
- Ultrasound
  - Nodular/heterogeneous liver parenchyma
  - Impaired portal vein flow velocity
  - Flat venous forms in hepatic veins
  - Increased hepatic artery pulsatility

should alert the clinician towards possibility of chronic liver disease.

- Jaundice is not an essential feature for diagnosis of chronic liver disease and would be present only in decompensated or cholestatic disease.

3. Asymptomatic Elevation of Liver Enzymes

Occasionally, the condition is discovered in children with no current or past evidence of liver disease, when liver function tests are performed as part of a routine medical examination or for complaints unrelated to the liver. Findings of raised liver enzymes, prolonged prothrombin time, or low serum albumin suggest possibility of chronic liver disease.

Associated Problems

Cholestasis

Cholestasis refers to impairment of bile flow. Involvement of liver in a chronic disease process often leads to some amount of cholestasis. This manifests as jaundice, pruritus, and acholic stools. Malnutrition and vitamin deficiencies also may occur because of malabsorption related to cholestasis.

Portal Hypertension

Involvement of the portal system in the fibrosis process leads to obstruction of portal flow leading to portal hypertension. Spleen invariably enlarges in portal hypertension and hypersplenism may occur resulting in pancytopenia. Variceal bleeding and ascites are other features of portal hypertension.

Hepatocellular Impairment

The hepatocellular function usually remains intact in chronic liver disease except in later stages when decompensation occurs. Features suggesting decompensation in CLD are: (*i*) jaundice; (*ii*) edema; (*iii*) coagulopathy not responding to vitamin K; (*iv*) pedal edema; low serum albumin; (*v*) massive ascites; and (*vi*) encephalopathy.

Nutritional Problems

Malnutrition and failure to thrive are usually seen in chronic liver disease because of cholestasis, anorexia leading to low caloric intake, and presence of chronic disease state.

Investigations

The aims of investigating a child suspected to be having chronic liver disease are (*i*) to document evidence of hepatic dysfunction and to evaluate the extent of damage; (*ii*) to detect or rule out associated complications; and (*iii*) to establish an etiological diagnosis.

A. Assessment of Hepatic Dysfunction

- *Serum bilirubin (direct and indirect)* Presence of conjugated hyperbilirubinemia usually suggests decompensation. Presence of unconjugated hyperbilirubinemia suggests co-existing hemolysis (eg, Wilson disease, autoimmune hemolytic anemia in autoimmune hepatitis).
- *Enzymes* Alanine aminotransferase (ALT, SGPT) typically shows a mild rise (2–5-fold increase) as against 20–100-fold

rise usually seen with acute viral hepatitis. Other enzymes like alkaline phosphatase and γ-glutamyl transpeptidase (GGT) may also be raised.

- *Serum albumin* is low because of impairment of synthetic function of liver and also due to malnutrition.
- *Prothrombin time* is raised because of impairment of synthesis of coagulation factors by liver or because of cholestasis associated vitamin K deficiency. In the later case, the correction of PT occurs following vitamin K administration whereas in the former, PT does not normalize after vitamin K therapy.
- *Liver biopsy* A percutaneous liver biopsy should be done in all children with chronic liver disease to (*i*) define severity of morphological changes and for evidence of chronic active hepatitis; and to (*ii*) establish the etiological diagnosis, eg, α₁-antitrypsin deficiency, infiltrative disorders. Biochemical and genetic analysis on liver tissue can also be done for diagnosis of some disorders such as Wilson disease and some inborn errors of metabolism.

Prothrombin time and platelet count must be done before liver biopsy and biopsy should be deferred if international normalized ratio (INR) >1.3 or platelet count is less than $70 \times 10^9/L$. In these situations, if the cause is identified and treatable (such as Wilson disease, hepatitis B, or autoimmune hepatitis), start specific therapy and reattempt liver biopsy when there is no coagulopathy. Otherwise, liver biopsy may be done under cover of transfusions (fresh frozen plasma, platelets and whole blood) if there is a dire need.

B. Detection of Complications of Chronic Liver Disease

- Full blood count, serum urea and electrolytes: To detect associated abnormalities: Anemia, pancytopenia, infection, and electrolyte disturbances.
- Upper GI endoscopy for evidence of varices.
- Hepatic and portal venous studies by ultrasound Doppler to detect portal hypertension.
- Ascitic fluid analysis is required in suspected spontaneous bacterial peritonitis.

C. For Etiological Diagnosis

- *Viral markers* HBsAg, HBeAg, anti-HBe, HBV DNA; anti-HCV, HCV PCR.
- *Markers for autoimmune hepatitis* Presence of raised levels of immunoglobulin G (IgG) suggests diagnosis of autoimmune hepatitis. Antinuclear antibodies (ANA) and/or anti-smooth muscle antibodies (anti-SMA) are present in Type I autoimmune hepatitis. Antibodies to liver-kidney microsomal antigen-1 (anti-LKM-1) are present in Type II autoimmune hepatitis where ANA and anti-SMA would be absent. If these three antibodies are absent but diagnosis of autoimmune hepatitis is strongly suspected, antibodies to soluble liver antigen (anti-SLA) should be detected which are raised in the rare Type III variety of autoimmune hepatitis.
- *Markers for Wilson disease* Slit-lamp examination for Kayser-Fleischer ring should be done in all suspected cases but a negative test does not rule out Wilson disease. Serum ceruloplasmin and 24-hour urinary copper excretion studies should be done. Copper content in liver biopsy should be estimated for definitive diagnosis.

- *Imaging* Ultrasound and Doppler studies can detect choledochal cyst, Budd-Chiari syndrome, and extrahepatic portal hypertension.
- $α_1$-*Antitrypsin* phenotype for diagnosis of $α_1$-antitrypsin $α_1$-deficiency. This diagnosis is also suggested if there are PAS positive, diastase resistant granules on microscopic examination of liver biopsy specimen.
- *Sweat chloride test* for cystic fibrosis.
- *Others* Fasting blood sugar, lactate and screening for inborn errors of metabolism.

Differential Diagnosis

Extrahepatic Portal Hypertension

This diagnosis should be strongly considered in a child having portal hypertension and splenomegaly. The liver is not enlarged; liver functions are normal with a normal liver biopsy. The child is well preserved, and there is no evidence of cholestasis.

Constrictive Pericarditis

Constrictive pericarditis can cause firm enlargement of liver and massive ascites and thus can mimic chronic liver disease. In constrictive pericarditis, jugular venous pressure would be elevated and associated cardiac complaints such as chest pain and discomfort might be present. ECG, chest X-ray and cardiac catheterization can help in ruling out constrictive pericarditis.

Infiltrative Disorders

Lymphoma, histiocytosis and leukemia can mimic chronic liver disease clinically. Infective disorders like kala-azar and chronic malaria can also cause a chronic liver disease like presentation. The enlargement of liver in these cases is usually regular with a smooth surface. Aspiration of bone marrow/lymph nodes can detect evidence of infiltration (lymphoma, leukemia, etc.) or infection (kala-azar, chronic malaria).

Treatment	Chronic Liver Disease

Symptomatic therapy

- *Diuretics* Spironolactone and furosemide are used if ascites is massive and causing distress to the child.
- *Stop bleeding* Coagulopathy should be corrected by giving vitamin K 5 mg intravenously and by transfusions of fresh frozen plasma if decompensation is present. Variceal bleeding is to be managed by sclerotherapy and giving transfusions.
- *Cholestasis* The choleretic agent ursodeoxycholic acid may be particularly useful in children with predominant biliary features such as itching and cholestasis.
- *Nutrition* Adequate nutritional intake should be ensured by making food calorie dense. Fat-soluble vitamins are required in 5–10 time the recommended doses.
- *Psychological support* should be given to the child and family while the child is being worked up and also if there is progression to irreversible cirrhosis.

Specific therapy

Specific therapy can be offered in viral hepatitis due to HBV or HCV, autoimmune hepatitis and Wilson disease. Corticosteroid therapy, with or without low doses of azathioprine, improves

Case Study	Acute Liver Failure

A 10-year-old girl weighing 25 kg suffering from jaundice for last 15 days is brought to the hospital with complaints of repeated vomiting and agitated behavior since last night. On examination, deep icterus is present and there are large ecchymotic patches over buttocks. She appears confused and deep tendon reflexes are exaggerated.

Q1. What investigations need to be done in this child?

Tests for hepatocellular dysfunction: The first step would be to confirm whether this jaundice is hepatocellular or hemolytic. Children with cerebral malaria can have CNS involvement in presence of hemolytic jaundice, which will be indirect type. Presence of direct hyperbilirubinemia (direct bilirubin > 20% of total) and elevated liver enzymes suggest hepatocellular involvement. Liver enzymes especially ALT will be raised manifold (20–50 times) if it is acute hepatitis due to hepatotropic viruses. Prothrombin test must be done in all cases. PT raised beyond 15 seconds (INR >1.5) will suggest acute liver failure as there is clinical evidence of encephalopathy. If PT is deranged, test should be repeated after giving vitamin K (5 mg intravenously) injection. PT >60s (INR >5) will suggest a grave prognosis, and the child should be referred to a center having facility for liver transplantation in that case.

Investigations for likely cause: IgM HAV, IgM HEV and HBsAg should be done to rule out acute hepatitis due to hepatitis A, hepatitis E, and hepatitis B, respectively. If HBsAg is positive, IgM HBcAg should be done to confirm presence of acute hepatitis B as Australia antigen positivity alone could be incidental. If these viral markers are negative, investigations for Wilson disease (serum ceruloplasmin, 24 hour urinary copper, and slit-lamp examination for Kayser-Fleischer ring) and autoimmune hepatitis (total immunoglobulins, antinuclear antibody, anti-smooth muscle antibody, anti-liver-kidney-muscle I antibody) should be done, as these disorders can occasionally present as acute hepatitis. History of drug or toxin ingestion should be recorded. If fever is a prominent symptom, tests for malaria (peripheral smear for malaria parasite, malaria antigen test), typhoid fever (blood culture, serum widal), scrub typhus (Weil-Felix test, immunofluorescence), and leptospirosis (leptospiral antibodies, immunofluorescence) should also be undertaken.

Investigations for other complications: Blood sugar should be done to rule out hypoglycemia. Platelet count should be done as child has ecchymotic patches. Kidney function tests (serum urea and creatinine) should be done to find any evidence of hepatorenal syndrome. Serum electrolytes should be done to diagnose any electrolyte disturbances (eg, hyponatremia, hypokalemia). Blood culture and urine culture should be taken to guide therapy for any co-existent infection.

Q2. Outline the management protocol.

1. Shift the child to intensive care unit after explaining the nature of disease, its severity, and its likely course to the parents. Explain possible need of blood product transfusion, and possible need of hepatic transplantation (if available) or referral to a higher center.
2. Administer IV fluids (N/4 10% dextrose) and prevent/treat hypoglycemia or any electrolyte disturbance.
3. Put a nasogastric tube for early diagnosis of any upper gastrointestinal bleeding, and also for giving lactulose and oral medications in case the child is not accepting orally.
4. Lactulose 10–20 mL 2 hourly. Increase dose if required till the child starts passing clear liquid stools. Reduce frequency of administration to 6–8 hourly thereafter.
5. Start broad spectrum antibiotics (cefotaxime + gentamicin) to treat any co-existent infections.
6. Administer ranitidine 25 mg IV 8 hourly.
7. Send sample for cross matching. Administer FFP if gastric contents are hemorrhagic or if there is bleeding from any site.
8. Monitor input/output, vital parameters and CNS status. Intubate and hyperventilate if child slips into coma.

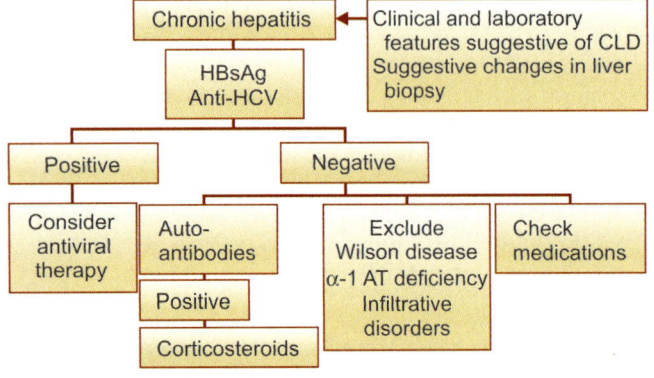

Fig. 9.6 Algorithmic approach towards management of chronic liver disease

the clinical, biochemical, and histologic features in most children with autoimmune hepatitis and prolongs survival in most children with severe disease.

A diagnostic and therapeutic approach in a child with chronic liver disease is presented in Fig. 9.6.

Roberts EA, Schilsky ML, American Association for Study of Liver Diseases (AASLD). Diagnosis and treatment of Wilson disease: an update. *Hepatology*. 2008; 47:2089.

Roberts EA, Schilsky ML, Division of Gastroenterology and Nutrition, Hospital for Sick Children, Toronto, Ontario, Canada. A practice guideline on Wilson disease. *Hepatology*. 2003; 37:1475.

Revision Point

Chronic Liver Disease

1. Chronic liver disease is long-term liver damage that may lead to *cirrhosis.*
2. It should be suspected whenever an episode of acute hepatitis like illness continues for a more than 3 months.
3. Common causes include hepatitis B, C and D virus infections, Wilson disease, autoimmune hepatitis, and other metabolic disorders.
4. Most children will present with prolonged/recurrent jaundice, bleeding varices, ascites, or hypersplenism. Jaundice is not an essential feature for diagnosis of chronic liver disease.
5. Investigations include liver function tests, prothrombin time, liver biopsy, viral marker studies, antibodies for autoimmune hepatitis, and markers of Wilson disease.
6. Treatment is symptomatic. Specific therapy can be offered in viral hepatitis due to HBV or HCV, autoimmune hepatitis, and Wilson disease.

9.14 NEONATAL AND INFANTILE CHOLESTASIS

Neonatal cholestasis is defined as prolonged elevation of conjugated bilirubin in serum, beyond the first 14 days of life. However, the onset of problem can be anytime during the infancy depending on the clinical condition causing cholestasis.

Etiology

Cholestasis in a newborn or infant may be due to a variety of abnormalities giving rise either to (*a*) mechanical obstruction of bile flow; or to (*b*) functional impairment of hepatic excretory function and bile secretion. The causes of neonatal and infantile cholestasis can be broadly categorized into intrahepatic and extrahepatic, listed in **Table 9.8.**

Pathogenesis

Cholestasis, defined physiologically as a reduction in canalicular bile flow, is caused by intrahepatic or extrahepatic obstruction. The two most likely pathogenetic mechanisms for neonatal cholestasis are (*i*) virus-induced liver injury; and (*ii*) metabolic liver disease. Autoimmune mechanisms may also be responsible for some of the forms of neonatal liver injury. Overall, the mechanisms are not well documented.

If the process predominantly involves hepatocytes or intrahepatic bile ducts, it results in intrahepatic obstruction and if the process predominantly involves extrahepatic bile ducts, it results in extrahepatic biliary obstruction.

There are areas of overlap—children with extrahepatic biliary atresia may have some degree of intrahepatic injury and in later stages intrahepatic diseases have complete obstruction simulating extrahepatic biliary atresia. Children with "idiopathic" neonatal hepatitis may in the future be determined to have a primary metabolic or viral disease. Sepsis also causes cholestasis, presumably mediated by endotoxins produced by Gram-negative bacteria.

Clinical Features

The major clinical consequences of cholestasis are related to retention of bile acids, which are dependent on bile flow for

Table 9.8 Causes of Neonatal and Infantile Cholestasis
I. Intrahepatic Disorders
A. *Cholestasis associated with Infections*
– Sepsis with possible endotoxemia* (Gram-negative sepsis or UTI)
– Syphilis*
– Toxoplasmosis
– Perinatal viral infections (CMV*, rubella, herpes simplex, HBV, HCV)
B. *Metabolic and Endocrine Disorders*
– Galactosemia
– Tyrosinemia
– α_1-antitrypsin deficiency
– Niemann-Pick disease
– Gaucher disease
– Glycogen storage disease, Type IV
– Zellweger syndrome (cerebrohepatorenal syndrome)
– Cystic fibrosis
– Neonatal hemochromatosis
– Hypothyroidism
C. *Anatomic and Structural Defects*
– Intrahepatic bile duct paucity* (Alagille syndrome)
– Persistent familial intrahepatic cholestasis (PFIC)
– Benign recurrent intrahepatic cholestasis
– Hereditary cholestasis with lymphedema (Aagenaes disease)
– Caroli disease
D. *Toxic*
– Parenteral nutrition related
– Drugs
E. *Idiopathic Neonatal Hepatitis**
II. Extrahepatic Disorders
– Extrahepatic biliary atresia*
– Choledochal cyst
– Bile duct stricture
– Mass (neoplasia, stone)

* Relatively common causes

excretion. The clinical manifestations and their pathogenesis are summarized in Fig. 9.7.

Neonatal cholestasis often presents as persistence of jaundice in the neonatal period beyond the limit for physiological jaundice (14 days). This is accompanied with passage of dark-colored urine and there might be passage of pale or clay-colored stools. Hepatomegaly is often present. Spleen may also be enlarged because of the primary disorder itself or because of portal hypertension in later stages.

The majority (about two-thirds) of infants with prolonged cholestasis can be categorized into one of the two diagnostic category of either biliary atresia or idiopathic neonatal hepatitis. It may be difficult to clearly differentiate infants with biliary atresia, who require surgical correction, from those with intrahepatic disease (neonatal hepatitis) and patent bile ducts. No single biochemical test or imaging procedure is entirely satisfactory. Diagnostic schemas incorporate clinical, historical, biochemical, and radiologic features. **Table 9.9** enumerates the differences between these two major causes of neonatal and infantile cholestasis.

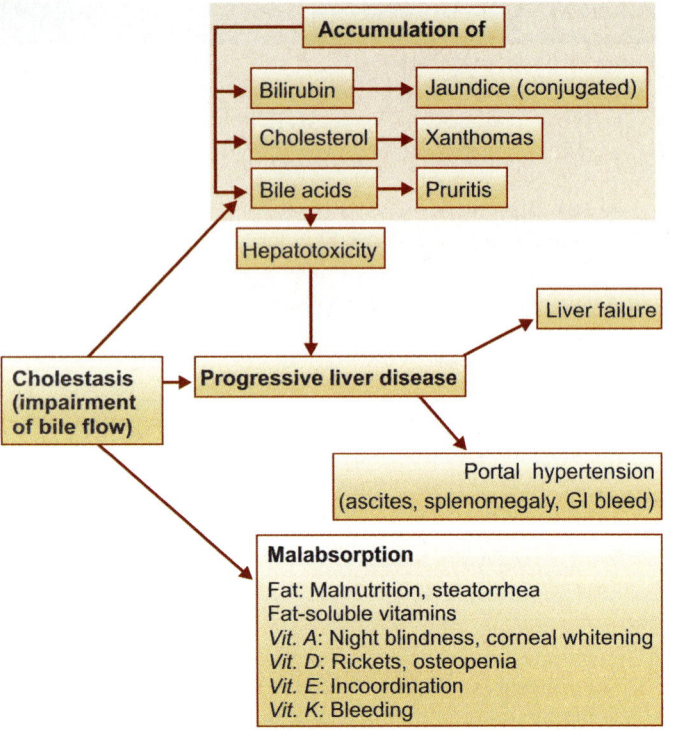

Fig. 9.7 Clinical manifestations of neonatal and infantile cholestasis

Diagnostic Evaluation of an Infant with Cholestasis

Conjugated hyperbilirubinemia in the newborn period always requires prompt evaluation and a stepwise cost-effective approach.

A. Confirmation of Conjugated Hyperbilirubinemia

Conjugated and unconjugated levels of serum bilirubin should be obtained in any child if hyperbilirubinemia persists for a prolonged period (>14 days). Unconjugated hyperbilirubinemia mostly is due to a benign cause such as breastmilk jaundice but presence of a conjugated (direct-acting) fraction of more than 2 mg/dL or more than 20% of the total bilirubin suggests cholestasis and need for further work-up. If the facilities for further work-up and treatment are not available, the infant should be referred early to a center having such facilities.

B. Determine Severity of Disease

Tests of (*i*) hepatocellular and biliary disease (ALT, AST, alkaline phosphatase, GGT); and (*ii*) hepatic function (serum albumin, prothrombin time, blood glucose, ammonia).

C. Differentiate Extrahepatic Biliary Obstruction from Intrahepatic Disorders (Table 9.9)

(*i*) Ultrasonography; (*ii*) hepatobiliary scintigraphy; and (*iii*) liver biopsy.

D. Exclude Treatable Disorders

Bacterial cultures (blood, urine), VDRL test, ultrasonography to rule out choledochal cyst; and T4 and TSH (to rule out hypothyroidism).

E. Findout other Specific Disorders

α_1-Antitrypsin phenotype, metabolic screen (urine-reducing substances, serum ammonia, serum/urine tyrosine), and sweat chloride/mutation analysis for cystic fibrosis.

Treatment	Neonatal Cholestasis

A. Supportive treatment
- *Nutritional supplementation* Nutritional care is an important part of management of cholestasis. Fats should be given in the diet in the form of medium chain triglycerides (MCT) as they do not require bile salts for absorption. Coconut oil is a good source of MCT.

Table 9.9 Differences between Idiopathic Neonatal Hepatitis and Extrahepatic Biliary Atresia

	Neonatal hepatitis	*Extrahepatic biliary atresia*
Birth weight	Low birth weight/ IUGR	Normal birth weight
Jaundice	Variable, waxing/waning	Progressively worsening
Stools	Pigmented or intermittently acholic	Persistently acholic
Failure to thrive	Early	Late
Splenomegaly	Early	Late when portal hypertension occurs
Familial cases	May be seen	Not seen
Associated malformations	Uncommon	Cardiovascular malformations, situs inversus, polysplenia, malrotation may be associated
Duodenal intubation	Bile stained flow seen	No bile staining of fluid
Ultrasonography	No specific anomaly	Absent or contracted gall bladder, triangular cord sign
Hepatic scintigraphy	Delayed uptake and delayed excretion	Normal uptake with no excretion
Liver biopsy	Diffuse hepatocellular involvement with distortion of lobular architecture, marked infiltration with inflammatory cells, and focal hepatocellular necrosis Bile ductules show a little alteration	Proliferation of bile ductules with presence of bile plugs, portal or perilobular edema and fibrosis. Basic hepatic lobular architecture intact

9

- *Vitamins* Supplementation with fat-soluble and water-soluble vitamins (vitamin A 5,000–15,000 IU daily or 50,000 IU weekly; Vitamin D 2,500–5,000 IU daily or 30,000 IU weekly; Vitamin E 50–400 IU/day; Vitamin K 2.5–5 mg twice a week; water-soluble vitamins twice the recommended daily allowance) is required to prevent or treat deficiency states.
- *Ursodeoxycholic acid* (UDCA) in the dose of 15–20 mg/kg/day is effective in relieving pruritis associated with cholestasis.
- *Diuretics* like spironolactone may be used if ascites is troublesome.

B. Specific treatment

Congenital syphilis Treat with crystalline penicillin for 10–14 days.

Extrahepatic biliary atresia All children suspected of having biliary atresia should undergo exploratory laparotomy and direct cholangiography to determine the presence and site of obstruction.

- If the cholangiogram indicates that the biliary tree is patent but of diminished caliber, cholestasis is not due to biliary tract obliteration but because of intrahepatic disease. In these cases, transection of or further dissection into the porta hepatis should be avoided.
- For children in whom EHBA is confirmed, the hepato-portoenterostomy procedure of Kasai can be carried out. The success rate for this surgery is much higher (90%) if performed before 8 weeks of life. Therefore, it is very important to refer the suspected cases early to a suitable center.

Galactosemia Lactose free formula feeding.

Choledochal cyst or other obstructive lesions Surgical removal.

If no treatable cause is found or if the disease has already progressed to irreversible cirrhotic stage, liver transplantation may be the only alternative.

Bhatia V, Bavdekar A, Matthai J, Waikar Y, Sibal A. Management of neonatal cholestasis: consensus statement of the Pediatric Gastroenterology Chapter of Indian Academy of Pediatrics. *Indian Pediatr*. 2014 Mar;51(3):203–10.

Fischler B, Lamireau T. Cholestasis in the newborn and infant. *Clin Res Hepatol Gastroenterol*. 2014;38:263–7.

Gottesman LE, Del Vecchio MT, Aronoff SC. Etiologies of conjugated hyperbilirubinemia in infancy: a systematic review of 1692 subjects. *BMC Pediatr*. 2015;15:192.

9.15 ASCITES

Collection of serous fluid within the peritoneal cavity is termed ascites. Excessive fluid in the peritoneum could be a part of generalized edema (anasarca) or it may be the sole or predominant site of fluid accumulation.

Etiology

In children, hepatic, renal, and cardiac diseases are the most common causes of ascites. Common causes are listed below:

I. Ascites with no edema or ascites out of proportion to peripheral edema
  i. *Hepatic causes*: Cirrhosis, congenital hepatic fibrosis, portal vein obstruction, Budd-Chiari syndrome
  ii. Constrictive pericarditis
  iii. Urinary ascites (perforation or leakage from urinary tract)
  iv. Chylous ascites
  v. Peritoneal tuberculosis
  vi. Acute pancreatitis
  vii. Intra-abdominal malignancies: Lymphoma, neuro-blastoma

II. Ascites with generalized edema
  i. *Renal causes*: Nephrotic syndrome, acute glomerulo-nephritis, renal failure
  ii. *Cardiac causes*: Congestive heart failure, constrictive pericarditis
  iii. *Polyserositis*: Systemic lupus erythematosus, dengue fever, sepsis
  iv. Severe malabsorption

Clinical Features

The clinical hallmark of ascites is abdominal distention, but this may also be caused by other conditions, including gaseous distension, fecal retention, abdominal masses, and obesity. History of generalized and progressively increasing abdominal distension usually suggests ascites. The physical signs suggesting ascites are fullness of flanks, fluid thrill, shifting dullness, and umbilical herniation. Small amount of fluid may be detectable only by ultrasonography.

Evaluation of Cause

The causes of ascites differ according to whether it is a part of generalized edema or it is the predominant or sole manifestation. When the ascites is disproportionately more in relation to edema, hepatic, peritoneal, or intra-abdominal causes are more likely.

Age

Ascites in a neonate usually suggests urinary ascites or chylous ascites as a cause. In the later neonatal period and infancy, cholestatic syndromes are important causes of ascites.

Clinical Evaluation

Findings suggestive of an underlying liver disorder (jaundice, firm hepatomegaly, shrunken liver, cutaneous stigmata) indicate chronic liver disease (with or without portal hypertension) as a cause of ascites. History of contact with tuberculosis and associated pulmonary findings suggest tuberculosis as the cause of ascites. Presence of significant lymph nodes suggests tuberculosis or lymphoma as possible diagnosis.

Ascitic Fluid Analysis

Exudative ascites is seen with tuberculosis, malignancies, and infections whereas transudative ascites is seen with chronic liver disease and when ascites is a part of generalized edema (anasarca). To differentiate transudate from exudates, the preferred method is determination of serum-ascitic albumin gradient (SAAG: Serum albumin concentration–ascitic fluid albumin concentration). Ascites is transudative when a child's SAAG level is greater than or equal to 1.1 g/dL, and exudative when levels are less than 1.1 g/dL. However, these cut-offs are not absolute and there is usually a considerable degree of overlap between the causes of exudative and transudative ascites.

Ascitic fluid should also be sent for cytologic examination, gram stain and cultures especially if infection is suspected. Lymphocytic pleocytosis is seen with tuberculosis and a predominant polymorphic response is obtained in bacterial peritonitis. Hemorrhagic ascites is seen with pancreatitis, malignancies and rarely in tuberculosis. Milky fluid is obtained in chylous ascites.

Imaging and Biochemistry

Ultrasound examination estimates quantity of fluid and is also helpful to diagnose the etiology. Intra-abdominal lymph nodes are enlarged in tuberculosis and lymphoma. Coarsening of hepatic echotexture suggests chronic liver disease. Portal venous Doppler studies may suggest presence of portal hypertension. CT scan of the abdomen may be required to assess intra-abdominal malignancies or cysts.

Liver function tests and *UGI endoscopy* are required to assess presence of CLD and portal hypertension.

Chest X-ray and *Mantoux test* are done for assessment of tuberculosis as a cause of ascites.

Treatment	Ascites
1. Low salt diet	
2. Diuretics like spironolactone and furosemide	
3. Intravenous albumin (0.5–1 mg/kg/day) in refractory cases	
4. Repeated large volume paracentesis with volume expansion to minimize risks of hypovolemia.	
5. Treatment of the cause:	
• Antitubercular therapy ± steroids for peritoneal tuberculosis	
• Antibiotics if spontaneous bacterial peritonitis is present	
• Treatment of cause of chronic liver disease (eg, interferons for HBV, HCV; steroids for AIH)	
• Portal hypertension is controlled by medications (eg, propranolol) or surgical methods (eg, portosystemic shunting)	
• Liver transplantation may be the only alternative if hepatic decompensation, cirrhosis and portal hypertension are present.	

9.16 UPPER GASTROINTESTINAL BLEEDING

Upper gastrointestinal (GI) bleeding in children usually manifests as *hematemesis* (fresh blood in vomitus), *melanemesis* (altered blood leading to brownish 'coffee ground' vomitus), or *melena* (black, tarry stools).

The minimum quantity of blood required to produce melena is 50–100 mL. Melena may persist for 3–5 days after acute GI bleed and cannot be used as an indicator of ongoing bleeding. Melena may be seen very rarely in lower GI bleeding if bleeding is very slow or if the child is constipated. Sometimes, massive GI bleed may present as *hematochezia* (passage of unaltered blood in stools) due to rapid transit of blood through the gut.

Etiology

Table 9.10 enumerates the age-specific causes of upper GI bleeding in children.
- Hematemesis on first or second day of life in a well-appearing child is most commonly due to swallowed maternal blood.
- On 3rd to 7th days, bleeding in a well child is usually due to vitamin K deficiency bleeding (VKDB).
- In a sick-appearing neonate, upper GI bleeding is usually the result of stress bleed or DIC.
- In infants, GERD may cause small amount of UGI bleed.
- Streaks of blood in vomitus following forceful vomiting are usually due to Mallory-Weiss tear.
- Variceal bleeding is the most common cause of severe upper GI bleeding in children. The varices are secondary to either cirrhotic portal hypertension or more commonly as a result of extrahepatic portal hypertension.

Evaluation of a Child with Upper GI Bleeding

A prioritized diagnostic and therapeutic approach to the child with suspected gastrointestinal blood loss is critical to avoid a delay in diagnosis. Important clues to the diagnosis are obtained with a careful history, physical examination, and knowledge of the potential causes of upper GI bleeding in infants and children.

History and Examination

- Treatment with drugs like aspirin or other NSAIDs suggests drug-induced gastritis or ulcer as a cause.
- History of umbilical sepsis or catheterization in neonatal period is suggestive of extrahepatic portal hypertension due to portal/splenic vein thrombosis.
- History of recurrent pain abdomen, regurgitation, and retrosternal burning is suggestive of GERD or peptic ulcer.
- Presence of jaundice, firm hepatomegaly, shrunken liver, or cutaneous stigmata (palmar erythema, spider nevi, gynecomastia) is suggestive of variceal bleed due to cirrhosis.
- Presence of splenomegaly suggests portal hypertension as a cause. However, spleen may regress after massive hematemesis to reappear again only after child is stabilized with volume resuscitation and transfusions.

Table 9.10 Etiology of Upper Gastrointestinal Bleeding in Children		
Newborn	*Infant*	*Child/Adolescent*
Swallowed maternal blood	Stress gastritis	Esophageal/Gastric varices
Hemorrhagic disease of newborn	Gastroesophageal reflux disease (GERD)	Acid peptic disease
Stress gastritis or ulcer	Mallory-Weiss tear	Mallory-Weiss tear
Vascular anomaly	Vascular anomaly	Caustic ingestion
Coagulopathy	GI duplication	Vasculitis (Henoch-Schönlein purpura)
Milk protein sensitivity	Esophageal/gastric varices	Crohn disease
Malrotation	Bowel obstruction and webs	Bowel obstruction

Note: In order of frequency of occurrence and/or importance

Investigations

- Send the blood sample immediately for grouping and cross matching. A complete blood count, electrolytes and LFT should be done.
- *Upper GI endoscopy* is the preferred method to evaluate the upper GI tract for a source of bleeding. Any child with significant upper GI bleed should be stabilized by volume resuscitation, transfusions and medical therapy and thereafter referred to an endoscopist experienced with children. Endoscopy is performed under intravenous sedation or general anesthesia. Upper GI endoscopy is best avoided if the child is clinically unstable, such as in shock or profound anemia and every effort should be made to stabilize the child first by conservative management.
- *Abdominal ultrasound* is useful in assessment of chronic liver disease and portal hypertension. Doppler flow studies can identify portal blood flow dynamics.

Treatment — Variceal Bleeding

A. Initial assessment and stabilization

Any child who presents with hematemesis or malena should be considered a potential emergency. The initial goal in the treatment of any child with upper gastrointestinal bleeding is to provide hemodynamic stability including oxygen delivery, fluid and blood resuscitation, and correction of coagulopathy, and metabolic or electrolyte abnormality. Presence of significant tachycardia suggests that the child has lost about 20% of blood volume whereas presence of shock indicates about 40% blood loss.

- Make a quick assessment of child's vitals including heart rate, blood pressure and oxygen saturation.
- Establish a venous line and draw blood samples for counts, grouping and cross matching.
- Start crystalloid infusion with Ringer's lactate or normal saline till blood transfusion can be given.
- Give oxygen if shock or hypoxemia is present.
- Pass a Ryle's tube and give gastric lavage with normal saline and then maintain continuous drainage to assess amount of continuing blood loss.
- Monitor vitals including pulse rate, blood pressure, respiration and oxygen saturation. Urine output and fluid intake/output should be measured if shock is present.

B. Pharmacological treatment

- *Octreotide* This is synthetic analogue of somatostatin and can be given as a bolus or by infusion. This is the drug of choice. A loading dose of 1 µg/kg is given as an intravenous infusion over 30 min followed by 0.5–1 µg/kg/hour.
- *Vasopressin* It acts by causing splanchnic vasoconstriction, thus decreasing the blood supply to the portal vein and the varices. It is used in dose of 0.33 units/kg in 20 minutes, followed by intravenous infusion of 0.33 units/kg/hour.
- *Somatostatin* It also acts by causing splanchnic vaso-constriction but has a very short half-life. In adults, it is given in the dose of 250 µg, IV bolus, followed by continuous infusion of 250 µg/hour.
- *Antacids* H_2 blockers (ranitidine) and proton pump inhibitors (omeprazole, pantoprazole) decrease gastric acid secretion and thus prevents clot lysis by inhibiting activation of pepsinogen.

Case Study — Upper Gastrointestinal Bleeding

A 7-year-old boy weighing 20 kg presents with bouts of hematemesis and passage of black tarry stools for last 6 hours. He has weak peripheral pulses, severe pallor, and marked tachycardia. He had reported to outpatient department about a week back with vague abdominal pain and discomfort where the doctors detected a spleen enlargement of 5 cm without any other abnormality. His blood tests, including liver function tests were found to be normal at that time, and he was advised to continue follow-up for investigations.

Q1. Identify the likely cause of bleeding.

This boy has massive hematemesis resulting in circulatory failure. The most likely cause is portal hypertension as massive hematemesis in children is almost always due to variceal bleeding. Another pointer towards portal hypertension in this child is detection of splenomegaly on a previous outpatient visit. Remember that spleen regresses during episode of massive bleeding, and may be absent on examination at this time. The cause of portal hypertension is likely to be extrahepatic (pre-hepatic) as his clinical examination and liver function tests were normal.

Q2. Outline the emergency treatment required to control bleeding.

1. Establish an intravenous line.
2. Send blood sample for cross matching, and arrange whole blood. Transfuse blood as early as possible. This child will need two units of blood immediately as he would have lost about 40% of his blood volume. Meanwhile, administer crystalloids (eg, Ringer lactate, normal saline) and colloids (eg, dextran) to restore intravascular volume.
3. Administer oxygen as there would be hypoxia due to severe anemia and circulatory collapse.
4. Put a nasogastric tube to estimate the ongoing bleed.
5. Give octreotide 20 µg as IV infusion over 30 minutes. Start octreotide infusion 10–20 µg/hour through infusion pump. (*Referring the child for endoscopy at this stage would be dangerous as child is in circulatory failure*).
6. Administer ranitidine 20 mg intravenously 8–12 hourly to take care of any associated portal gastropathy.
7. Monitor vital parameters and record amount of ongoing bleed. Titrate the blood transfusions as per the estimated loss, and vital parameters of the child.
8. Once the child is stabilized, he should be referred for endoscopy to directly visualize the varices.
9. Endoscopic variceal banding or endoscopic sclerotherapy should be done preferably in that sitting itself.
10. Child should be well sedated/anesthetized before the procedure.

C. Endoscopic treatment

Endoscopic sclerotherapy and endoscopic variceal ligation are effective for controlling esophageal variceal bleeding. The commonly used sclerosants are ethanolamine oleate and alcohol. Variceal ligation is more safe than sclerotherapy but requires special equipment and expertise.

D. Mechanical methods

Sengstaken-Blakemore Tube stops bleeding mechanically by balloons that compress esophageal and gastric varices (mechanical tamponade). It is very effective in controlling hemorrhage but is associated with high incidence of re-bleeding once the tube is removed.

E. Surgical methods

Emergency surgical methods like portosystemic shunting, esophageal transaction and liver transplantation are associated with high morbidity and mortality and should be reserved for the most refractory cases.

Arora NK, Ganguly S, Mathur P, Ahuja A, Patwari A. Upper gastrointestinal bleeding: etiology and management. *Indian J Pediatr.* 2002;69:155–69.

Fox VL. Gastrointestinal bleeding in infancy and childhood. *Gastroenterol Clin North Am.* 2000; 29:37.

Gøtzsche PC, Hróbjartsson A. Somatostatin analogues for acute bleeding oesophageal varices. *Cochrane Database Syst Rev.* 2008;3: CD000193.

Revision Point

Upper Gastrointestinal Bleeding

1. Upper gastrointestinal (GI) bleeding in children usually manifests as hematemesis (fresh blood in vomitus) or melena (black, tarry stools).
2. Esopahgeal or gastric varices (secondary to portal hypertension) are the most important causes of severe upper GI bleeding.
3. Presence of splenomegaly suggests portal hypertension as a cause.
4. Upper GI endoscopy is done to find the source of bleeding.
5. The initial goal in the treatment of any child with upper gastrointestinal bleeding is to provide hemodynamic stability, including oxygen, fluid, and blood transfusion.
6. Octreotide is the drug of choice for stopping the bleed. Other alternatives include vasopressin and somatostatin.
7. Endoscopic sclerotherapy and endoscopic variceal ligation are effective for controlling esophageal variceal bleeding.

9.17 COMMON SURGICAL PROBLEMS

Infants and children having various gastrointestinal and hepatobiliary complaints such as vomiting, constipation, abdominal distension, and jaundice occasionally have a condition requiring surgical management. However, these children often present to physician or pediatrician and it is important to recognize the subgroup of children requiring surgery.

It is sometimes difficult to clearly distinguish medical causes from those requiring surgery but a high index of suspicion should be kept. In doubtful or borderline cases, conservative management should be continued till more clear symptoms/signs of surgical cause are manifested. The following clinical symptoms/signs in gastrointestinal manifestations suggest need for surgical consultation or management.

When to Suspect a Surgical Problem

- Presence of palpable abdominal mass in an infant having recurrent/persistent vomiting→*Hypertrophic pyloric stenosis.*
- Recurrent abdominal distension and vomiting in an infant or young child presenting with constipation→ *Hirschsprung disease.*
- Gaseous abdominal distension along with vomiting and absolute constipation→*Intestinal obstruction.*
- Bilious vomiting or bilious gastric aspirates in any child→ *Intestinal obstruction; atresias.*
- Abdominal pain with vomiting and small amount of mucoid/bloody stools in an infant→*Intussusception.*
- Multiple air-fluid levels in straight X-ray abdomen of a child having abdominal distension→*Intestinal obstruction.*
- Persistent acholic stools in neonatal cholestasis→ *Extrahepatic biliary atresia.*
- Passage of fresh blood in non-diarrheal stools→*Rectal polyp, hemorrhoids, Meckel diverticulum.*

HYPERTROPHIC PYLORIC STENOSIS

Idiopathic hypertrophic pyloric stenosis (IHPS) is the most common surgical cause of vomiting in infants. It is more common in males.

Clinical Features

Non-bilious vomiting is the initial symptom of pyloric stenosis. The vomiting may or may not be projectile initially but is usually progressive, occurring immediately after feeding. Vomiting may follow each feed, or it may be intermittent. The vomiting usually starts at about one month of age but may develop as early as the 1st week of life and as late as the 5th month. After vomiting, the infant is hungry and wants to feed again. As vomiting continues, a progressive loss of fluid, hydrogen ion, and chloride leads to hypochloremic metabolic alkalosis. If not recognized early, it leads to chronic malnutrition and dehydration.

A palpable pyloric mass may be located in the mid-epigastrium. The mass is easier to palpate just after an episode of vomiting. After feeding, there may be a visible gastric peristaltic wave that progresses across the abdomen.

Differential diagnosis of this condition includes any condition which presents with recurrent or persistent non-bilious vomiting in infancy.

Investigations

Ultrasound examination confirms the diagnosis in the majority of cases, allowing an earlier diagnosis in infants with suspected disease but no pyloric mass on physical examination. Barium studies demonstrate an elongated pyloric channel, a bulge of the pyloric muscle into the antrum (shoulder sign), and parallel streaks of barium seen in the narrowed channel, producing a "double tract sign".

Treatment | **Hypertrophic Pyloric Stenosis**

The preoperative treatment is directed toward correcting the fluid, acid–base, and electrolyte losses. Intravenous fluid therapy is begun with N/2 in 5% dextrose or dextrose normal saline (DNS), with the addition of potassium chloride in concentrations of 40 mEq/L. Fluid therapy should be continued until the infant is rehydrated and alkalosis has been corrected. After rehydration is complete, the infant is referred for surgery. The surgical procedure of choice is the Ramstedt pyloromyotomy.

INTUSSUSCEPTION

Intussusception is the invagination of a part of the intestine into itself. It is the most common abdominal emergency in early childhood and the second most common cause of intestinal obstruction, after pyloric stenosis.

Pathophysiology

The most common type of intussusception is ileocolic, but some are ileoileocolic, jejunojejunal, jejunoileal, or colocolic. Most of the cases occur in infancy. Intussusceptions cause compression of the intramural and mesenteric veins, leading to edema and hemorrhage in the bowel wall ultimately leading to ischemia and infarction.

Diagnosis

The typical child is a previously healthy infant who develops severe abdominal pain manifesting with pallor and drawing up of the legs. The attacks are separated by periods of apathy and are followed by vomiting and the passage of "currant jelly" stool. The child may develop a sausage-shaped abdominal mass, usually in the right upper quadrant or mid-epigastrium. Many children do not develop typical manifestations of severe abdominal pain, blood or mucus in stools or a palpable abdominal mass. The differential diagnosis includes gastroenteritis and other forms of obstruction, including malrotation with volvulus.

Management

Intussusception is important to recognize early as delay in diagnosis may lead to fatal complications. When the diagnosis of intussusception is suspected, the first step is to stop oral feeds, start intravenous fluids and decompress the stomach with a nasogastric tube. Plain radiographs and ultrasonography are useful screening tests for intus-susception. A contrast (air or radiopaque) enema under fluoroscopy is an alternative diagnostic test, which can also be used to achieve reduction of the intussusception.

Non-operative reduction is attempted by giving hydrostatic pressure through a barium column or by air pressure. If peritonitis or pneumoperitoneum is present or if perforation occurs following attempts at non-operative reduction, laparotomy is required.

HIRSCHSPRUNG DISEASE

Hirschsprung disease, or congenital aganglionic megacolon is a gut motility disorder caused by abnormal innervation of the bowel. Hirschsprung disease is the most common cause of lower intestinal obstruction in neonates. In older children, it presents as intractable constipation.

Pathophysiology

The aganglionic segment begins in the internal anal sphincter and extends proximally to involve a variable length of gut. The Hirschsprung lesion is limited to the rectum and sigmoid in 75% of cases and in about 8% it affects the entire colon. Increased prevalence of Hirschsprung disease is seen with Down syndrome and many other congenital syndromes and malformations.

Dheeraj Shah

Clinical Features

Most of the infants have history of delayed passage of meconium (beyond 24 hours). Commonly this symptom gets unnoticed and child may be normal for a variable period thereafter. In the typical presentation, the infant has increasing difficulty with the passage of stools, starting in the first few weeks of life associated with a gaseous abdominal distension. The stools, when passed, may consist of small pellets, may be ribbon-like, or may have a fluid consistency.

Rectal examination demonstrates empty rectum with a normal anal tone and is usually followed by an explosive discharge of foul-smelling feces and gas. Intermittent attacks of intestinal obstruction from retained feces may be associated with pain and fever. Inadequate nutrient intake and insufficient weight gain may occur.

Differential Diagnosis

Hirschsprung disease must be differentiated from meconium plug syndrome, meconium ileus, hypothyroidism and intestinal atresia. In older children, it is to be distinguished from functional constipation.

Diagnosis

Absence of gas in the pelvis on plain radiograph of the abdomen with the infant in the prone position suggests Hirschsprung disease and a need for further studies. Radiological evidence of an intestinal cutoff sign (gaseous distension with abrupt cutoff at the level of the pelvic brim) may be seen. A single-contrast barium enema is the standard method for localizing the transition zone between the contracted aganglionic segment and the dilated hyper-trophied colon proximal to the aganglionic segment.

Rectal manometry and rectal suction biopsy are most reliable diagnostic tests for confirmation of Hirschsprung disease. The biopsy specimen can be stained for acetylcholinesterase, which may facilitate interpretation. Children with aganglionosis demonstrate a large number of hypertrophied nerve bundles that stain positively for acetylcholinesterase with an absence of ganglion cells.

Treatment	Hirschsprung Disease

Medical therapy
The role of medical intervention is to stabilize the child by restoring fluid and electrolyte balance, especially if enterocolitis is present, and to perform adequate evacuation of the colon with warm saline enemas through a rectal tube. Broad-spectrum antibiotics should be used in children with suspected enterocolitis.

Surgical therapy
Surgical intervention would be required in most cases. The options include a temporary colostomy followed by a definitive surgery later or a definitive surgical procedure as soon as the diagnosis is established. The prognosis of surgically treated Hirschsprung disease is generally satisfactory; the great majority of children achieve fecal continence. Postoperative problems include recurrent enterocolitis, stricture, prolapse, perianal abscesses, and fecal soiling.

Respiratory Disorders

10.1 ANATOMY AND PHYSIOLOGY OF RESPIRATION

An understanding of the anatomy and physiology of the respiratory system is fundamental to the comprehension of pathophysiology and management of respiratory diseases. The respiratory system consists of the chest wall, the airways, the lungs, and the pleura.

The Chest Wall

The chest wall consists of the bony cage (consisting of the obliquely oriented ribs, the sternum anteriorly and the vertebral column posteriorly), the intercostal muscles and the dome shaped diaphragm. Inspiration results in an expansion in volume of the thoracic cavity in three planes—vertical (flattening of dome of diaphragm as it contracts); transverse (bucket handle action of obliquely placed ribs); and anteroposterior (raising the sternal ends of the ribs). On the contrary, quiet expiration is usually a passive process. Forced expiration, however, predominantly follows an active contraction of the abdominal wall muscles.

Chest wall of the infant is slightly different from the older child or adult:
- Ribs are oriented much more horizontally and the diaphragm is flatter and less domed—unable to duplicate the bucket handle movement.
- Rib cage is softer and more compliant.
- Functional residual capacity is higher than expected.
- Limited ability to maintain adequate ventilation in lung disease, resulting in greater retraction of the soft chest wall.

All the above handicaps result in greater retraction of the soft chest wall in an underlying disorder of respiratory system in infants.

Airways

The *upper respiratory tract* includes the nose, pharynx, and larynx. The *lower respiratory tract* consists of the trachea, bronchial tree, and lungs.

The larynx or glottis is the passage for air between the pharynx above and the trachea below. It extends from the fourth to the sixth cervical vertebral levels. The trachea commences in the neck below the larynx and ends in the thorax at the level of sternal angle (lower border of fourth thoracic vertebra) by dividing into right and left principal (main) bronchi. The right principal bronchus is wider, shorter and more vertical than the left. Each principal bronchus divides into lobar (secondary) bronchi, each of which gives rise to segmental (tertiary) bronchioles, which again divide into respiratory bronchioles that terminate in the alveoli.

Lungs and the Pleura

The lungs and the pleura lie on either side of the mediastinum in the thoracic cavity. Each pleura has two layers—parietal layer that lines the thoracic wall, and the visceral layer covering the surface of the lungs. The two layers are continuous with each other and enclose within themselves a potential space called pleural cavity, which contains a small amount of tissue fluid called pleural fluid.

The lungs are soft and spongy organs which are conical in shape. Each lung has a blunt apex, a concave base, a convex costal surface, and a concave mediastinal surface. The hilum of the lung receives the bronchi, blood vessels, and the nerves. The right lung is slightly larger than the left and is divided by the oblique (major) and horizontal (minor) fissures into three lobes—the upper, middle, and lower lobes. The left lung is divided by a similar oblique fissure into two lobes—the upper and the lower lobes. Each lung contains anatomical, functional, and surgical units called broncho-pulmonary segments. These segments are pyramidal in shape with apex towards the lung root and are supplied by individual segmental bronchus, artery, lymph vessels, and nerves. The main bronchopulmonary segments are as follows:

	Right Lung (10 Segments)	*Left Lung (10 Segments)*
Superior lobe	Apical, posterior, and anterior	Apical, posterior, anterior, superior lingular, inferior lingular
Middle lobe	Lateral, medial	—
Inferior lobe	Superior basal (apical), medial basal, anterior basal, lateral basal, posterior basal	Superior basal (apical), medial basal, anterior basal, lateral basal, posterior basal

Pulmonary Mechanics and Work of Breathing

The movement of air in and out of the lungs requires a sufficient pressure gradient between alveoli and atmosphere during inspiration and expiration. The pressure in the space between the lungs and chest wall (*intrapleural pressure*) is subatmospheric. During inspiration, the intrathoracic volume increases due to contraction of inspiratory muscles (mainly diaphragm); and the intrapleural pressure becomes more negative which draws air into the lungs. At the end of inspiration, due to the recoil of lung and chest wall, the pressure in the airway increases and forces air out of the lungs.

The presence of surfactant in the alveoli prevents them from collapsing completely at the end of expiration. It serves to maintain the stability of pulmonary tissue by reducing the surface tension of fluids that coat the lung. Surfactant is composed of lipoprotein secreted by the alveolar cells of the lung. The major constituents of surfactant are dipalmitoyl phosphatidylcholine (lecithin), phosphatidyl glycerol, apoproteins, surfactant proteins (SP-A, SP-B, SP-C, and SP-D), and cholesterol. With advancing gestational age, increasing amounts of phospholipids are synthesized and stored in type II alveolar cells.

Pulmonary Gas Exchange

The main function of the respiratory system is to remove carbon dioxide from and add oxygen to the systemic venous blood. Gas exchange occurs by the process of diffusion and equilibration of alveolar gas with pulmonary capillary blood. This diffusion depends on the alveolar capillary barrier and amount of available time for equilibration.

In health, the equilibration of alveolar gas and pulmonary capillary blood is complete for both oxygen and carbon dioxide. In diseases in which alveolar capillary barrier is abnormally increased (*alveolar interstitial diseases*) and/or when the time available for equilibration is decreased (increased blood flow velocity), diffusion is incomplete. Because of its greater solubility in liquid medium, carbon dioxide is 20 times more diffusible than oxygen.

Therefore, diseases with diffusion defects are characterized by marked alveolar-arterial oxygen (A-a) O_2 gradients and hypoxemia. Significant elevation of CO_2 does not occur as a result of a diffusion defect unless there is coexistent hypoventilation. The total blood oxygen content is composed of the dissolved oxygen and the oxygen bound to hemoglobin. Oxygen delivery to the tissues is a product of oxygen content and cardiac output.

Lung Volumes and Capacities

- *Tidal volume* (V_T) The amount of air that is moved in and out of the lungs during each breath (6–7 mL/kg body weight at rest).
- *Inspiratory capacity* (IC) The amount of air inspired by maximum inspiratory effort after tidal expiration.
- *Expiratory reserve volume* (ERV) The amount of air exhaled by maximum expiratory effort after tidal expiration.
- *Residual volume* (RV) The volume of gas remaining in the lungs after maximum expiration.
- *Vital capacity* (VC) The amount of air moved in and out of the lungs with maximum inspiration and expiration. Forced vital capacity refers to the vital capacity with the patient exhaling with maximum speed and effort.
- *Functional residual capacity* (FRC) The amount of air left in the lungs after tidal expiration.
- *Total lung capacity* (TLC) is the volume of gas occupying the lungs after maximum inhalation.

Lung Function Tests or Spirometry

Lung functions can be measured by spirometry that consists of blowing of air with a maximal expiratory effort both in terms of force of exhalation and duration of exhalation.

- The child is asked to blow out into the spirometer as rapidly as possible till the lungs are fully emptied out.
- The spirometer measures FEV_1 (forced expiratory volume in first second) and FVC (forced vital capacity) among various other parameters.
- FEV_1 is the most widely used parameter to measure the mechanical properties of the lungs. In a normal person, the FEV_1 is about 75% to 85% of the FVC. FEV_1 is reduced in obstructive and restrictive disorders. The FEV_1/FVC ratio helps in differentiating between obstructive, restrictive, and mixed disorders.
- *Obstructive diseases* FEV_1 is reduced disproportionately to the FVC, reducing the FEV_1/FVC ratio below the lower limit of normal and indicates airflow limitation.
- *Restrictive disorders* FEV_1, FVC, and total lung capacity are all reduced, and the FEV_1/FVC ratio is normal or even elevated. Thus the absolute value of these two parameters and their ratio gives a good idea about the respiratory physiology of the disease. A child can have obstructive (asthma), restrictive (eg, pneumonia, interstitial lung diseases), or a mixed disorder (atelectobronchiectasis).

Regulation of Respiration

Respiration is delicately controlled by a complex interaction between controller mechanism (which receives inputs from sensors and sends commands to effectors), sensors, and effectors.

Controller Mechanism

1. *Voluntary control of respiration* is exerted by cerebral motor cortex and limbic forebrain structure. The control system uses information from sensory neurons such as pain, touch, temperature, smell, vision, and emotions; and sends impulses directly to the respiratory muscles through corticobulbar and corticospinal tracts. This form of control protects from aspiration and inhalation of noxious gases. Patients with CNS injury and toxic or metabolic encephalopathies may lose voluntary control of respiration.
2. *Automatic control of respiration* is mediated by a group of neurons called pre-Botzinger complex (preBotC) located in the medullary region of the brainstem. PreBotC is responsible for maintaining respiratory rhythmicity and various patterns of respiration, and has receptors for neurotransmitters like substance P, and acetylcholine, etc.
   - *Apneustic center* is a group of neurons located in the lower pons and stimulates preBotC, resulting in prolonged inspiratory gasps (*apneuses*) interrupted by transient expiratory efforts.
   - *Pneumotaxic center* is another group of neurons in the upper pons, involved in inhibiting the activity of preBotC.

The apneustic and pneumotaxic centers fine-tune the rhythmic respiratory activity generated by preBotC neurons.

10

Sensors

Depending on the type of stimulus required to stimulate them, sensors are termed chemoreceptors and mechano-receptors. Chemoreceptors, in turn, can be central or peripheral.

1. *Central chemoreceptors* These are located in the posterior hypothalamus, cerebellum, locus ceruleus, raphe, and multiple nuclei within the brainstem. Central chemo-receptors sense a change in the chemical composition of the extracellular fluid of the brain and respond to the changes in the H^+ concentration; an increase in H^+ concentration stimulates ventilatory response of the controller, and *vice versa*.

2. *Peripheral chemoreceptors* These are located in carotid bodies just above the bifurcation of the common carotid arteries, and aortic bodies above and below the aortic arch. In contrast to central chemoreceptors, peripheral chemoreceptors respond to changes in partial pressures of oxygen and carbon dioxide.

Mechano-receptors or Lung Receptors

1. *Stretch receptors* (located within the airway smooth muscle): These are stimulated by lung inflation, and the impulse is conducted via the vagus nerve. The main effect of these receptors is to decrease the respiratory rate by inhibition of inspiratory muscle activity and an increase in exhalation time (Hering-Breuer inflation reflex).

2. *Irritant receptors* (in between the epithelial cells in the airway mucous membrane): These are stimulated by particulate matter, noxious gases, and chemical fumes in the inspired gas, and also by cold air. Stimulation of irritant receptors results in bronchoconstriction and hyperpnea *via* the vagus nerve.

3. *J receptors* (juxta-capillary, in the alveolar walls close to the pulmonary capillaries): The pulmonary capillary engorgement and interstitial and alveolar wall edema provide stimuli for activation of the J receptors, resulting in shallow and rapid respirations and dyspnea as is seen in left heart failure, ARDS, and interstitial diseases.

4. *Muscle receptors* (the diaphragm and the intercostals): Distortion of the diaphragm and the intercostals inhibits inspiratory activity when large negative intrathoracic pressure is required to move air, such as in airway obstruction.

5. *Arterial baroreceptors:* These are located in aortic arch and carotid sinuses; and are activated by changes in arterial blood pressure. A decrease in blood pressure results in hyperventilation and an increased blood pressure causes hypoventilation.

6. *Pain and temperature receptors* (especially pronounced in the neonates and young infants): A painful stimulus causes breath holding followed by hyperventilation. Increased skin temperature causes hyperventilation, and hypothermia results in hypoventilation.

Effectors

The important effectors of respiration are the diaphragm, intercostals, and abdominal muscles. Accessory effectors are sternocleidomastoids and paraspinal muscles that contribute in times of need. The effectors can be seriously impaired in malnutrition, spinal injury, and neuromuscular disease.

Gaultier C, Amiel J, Dauger S, *et al*. Genetics and early disturbances of breathing control. *Pediatr Res*. 2004;55:729–33.

Gaultier C. Abnormalities of the chemical control of breathing: Clinical correlates in infants and children. *Pediatr Pulmonol*. 2001;23:114–7.

Gozal D. New concepts in abnormalities of respiratory control in children. *Curr Opin Pediatr*. 2004;16:305–8.

Nogués MA, Benarroch E. Abnormalities of respiratory control and the respiratory motor unit. *Neurologist*. 2008;14:273–88.

Parmigiani S, Solari E, Bevilacqua G. Current concepts on the pulmonary surfactant in infants. *J Matern Fetal Neonatal Med*. 2005;18:369–80.

Ranu H, Wilde M, Madden B. Pulmonary function tests. *Ulster Med J*. 2011;80:84–90.

Swaminathan S. Pulmonary function testing in office practice. *Indian J Pediatr*. 1999;66:905–14.

Revision Point   **Anatomy and Physiology of Respiration**

1. Human respiration is materialized by both external (breathing and ventilation) and internal/cellular respiration.
2. The right lung has three lobes and two fissures and the left has two lobes and one fissure. Each lung has 10 bronchopulmonary segments. Muscles of respiration are the intercostal muscles and diaphragm.
3. Gas exchange occurs on a large surface area when gas moves in and out of the alveolus and blood flows through the pulmonary capillary vessels.
4. Oxygen is primarily carried in the blood bound to hemoglobin and a small amount is dissolved in the plasma.
5. The primary processes contributing to hypoxemia (abnormally low arterial blood oxygen) are hypo-ventilation, diffusion impairment, shunt, ventilation/perfusion mismatch and low venous PO_2.

10.2 COUGH

Cough is a reflex action of deep inspiration followed by forced, rapid expiration, usually to protect and clear the airway of secretions, foreign material, or irritants.

Etiology

Cough can be caused by a multiplicity of diseases located in a variety of anatomical sites. The most common cause of an acute cough in children is an acute viral URI which normally subsides in 7–14 days. If cough persists for longer than this, other possible causes must be considered systematically **(Table 10.1)**.

Typology

For clinical purposes, cough in children is categorized as acute (<2 weeks), subacute (2–4 weeks), and chronic (>4 weeks). Most of the acute and subacute cases of cough (due to upper respiratory infection) resolve in 2–3 weeks. Based on the underlying disorder, chronic cough can be subdivided as *specific* cough and *nonspecific* cough (no identifiable etiology). The classifications can, however, be overlapping.

Table 10.1 Causes of Cough in Children
I. Infectious causes
• *Viral upper respiratory infection*: Respiratory syncytial virus, adenovirus, parainfluenzae virus, influenza virus, and rhinovirus
• *Sinusitis*: Streptococci, Moraxella, and *H. influenzae*
• Pneumonia and lower respiratory tract infections: *Streptococcus pneumoniae*, *H. influenzae*, Gram-negative bacilli, *Staphylococcus aureus*, *Chlamydia*, *Mycoplasma*, and viral pneumonia
• Bronchiolitis
• Bronchiectasis or lung abscess
• Whooping cough like syndrome: Pertussis, parapertussis, respiratory syncytial virus, adenovirus, influenza
II. Congenital anomalies
• Compression/abnormality of airway
• Tracheoesophageal fistula
• Tracheobronchomalacia
• Aberrant mediastinal vessels
• Bronchopulmonary-foregut malformation
III. Allergic
• Rhinitis: Allergic or vasomotor
• Asthma
IV. Others
• Immunodeficiency syndromes
• Foreign body aspiration or ingestion
• Cystic fibrosis
• Immotile cilia syndrome
• Psychogenic or habitual

- *Acute cough* Acute viral infection of the upper respiratory tract is the most common cause, especially during the winter months. Pneumonia, aspiration, and congestive heart failure are the other common causes of cough of short duration and recent onset. Figure 10.1 presents an algorithm for suspecting the various causes for cough.

- *Recurrent cough* Recurrent respiratory tract infections need investigations for an underlying heart disease or developmental disorder of lung parenchyma or airways. In early childhood, as many as 6–8 upper respiratory tract infections may occur annually in a child. Viral infections can also trigger recurrent episodes of asthma. Other causes for recurrent cough include postnasal drip, aspiration syndromes, and immunodeficiency disorders.

- *Persistent cough* Any child with cough lasting beyond 2–3 weeks requires a detailed systematic evaluation to rule out tuberculosis, bronchial asthma, congenital anomalies of airway, foreign body, and cystic fibrosis.

Clues from History

- Onset of cough is *sudden* or *hyperacute* in foreign body aspiration and in most acute bacterial infections; *subacute* in whooping cough; and *gradual* in tuberculosis.
- Aggravation with exercise, or early morning, or nocturnal cough points towards asthma.
- Cough aggravated during or after feeding indicates aspiration.
- Cough worsening in the recumbent posture suggests gastroesophageal reflux.

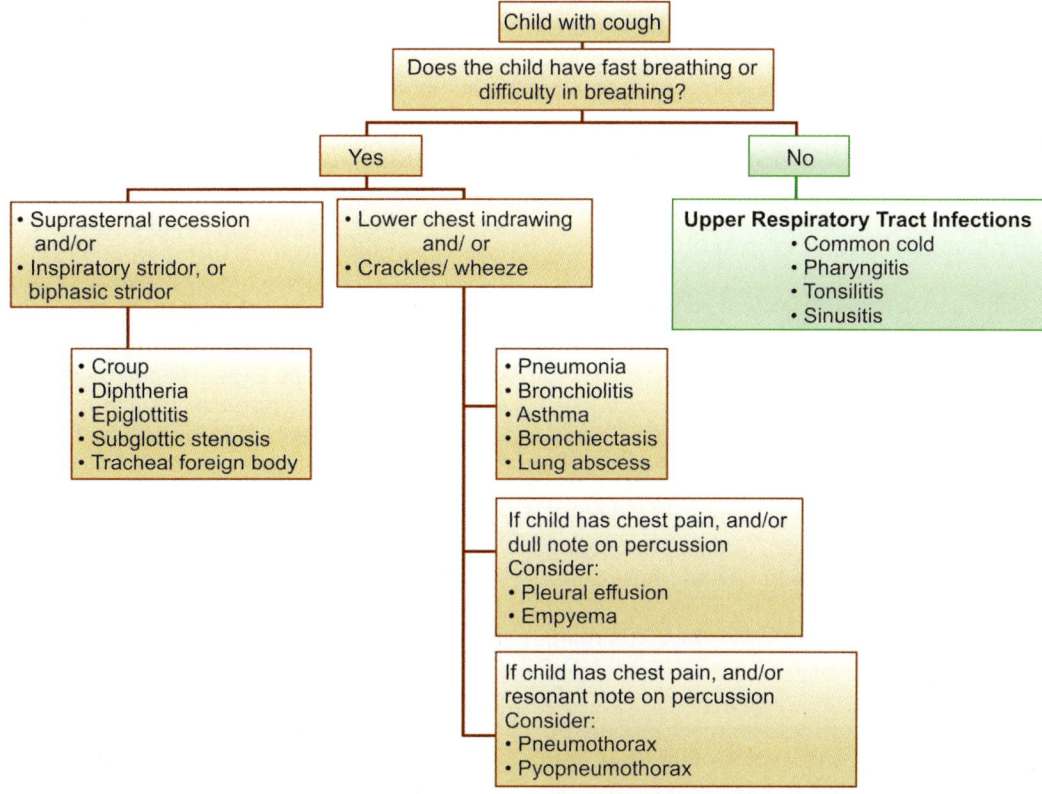

Fig. 10.1 Approach to a child with cough

10

- Cough worsening on cold exposure suggests hyperactive airways.
- Use of medications in the past, and their response especially to bronchodilators can determine asthma as a cause of cough.
- *Seasonal variations* Spring or seasonal changes may trigger asthma and allergic causes of cough.
- A dry hacking cough is suggestive of tracheal irritation.
- Overcrowding, malnutrition, parental smoking, family or personal history of atopy are important points to be elicited.

Character of cough Paroxysms of cough with a whoop are suggestive of pertussis or other whooping cough syndromes. Stridor is suggestive of upper tracheal, subglottic, or laryngeal involvement. High pitched wheezing is suggestive of small airway disease like asthma. Classical cough types suggesting underlying etiology are as follows:

Characteristic cough type	Probable etiology
Barking	Acute laryngotracheobronchitis, tracheomalacia, habit cough
Honking	Psychogenic
Whooping	Pertussis
Staccato	Atypical (Chlamydia) pneumonia

Sputum Cough in children is seldom associated with bringing up of sputum. This is particularly true for younger children as they do not generate enough pressure to bring up secretion. Sputum production, the type of sputum and its timing should be noted. Purulent sputum suggests bronchiectasis. In some children there may be hemoptysis (coughing up blood) that suggests tuberculosis, bronchiectasis, pulmonary hydatidosis or pulmonary hemosiderosis. Sputum production in asthma is minimal, clear, and mucoid.

Physical Examination

General Physical Examination

- A healthy child with chronic cough may have asthma while wasting may be associated with tuberculosis, bronchiectasis, and immunodeficiency.
- Peripheral lymphadenopathy with or without matted lymph nodes may be associated finding with tuberculosis.
- Clubbing is usually associated with prolonged suppurative respiratory disease.

Upper Respiratory Examination

- Nasal blockage with thick purulent nasal secretions and mouth breathing suggests adenoidal hypertrophy and sinusitis.
- Mucopurulent secretions on the posterior pharyngeal wall associated with cobblestone appearance of the pharyngeal mucosa are considered suggestive of chronic post-nasal drip.
- Examination of the ears to rule out otitis media is essential.

Chest Examination

Any chest deformity, overinflation, or asymmetry should be noted. Shift of the mediastinum by palpation of the apex beat and trachea should be noted. The chest asymmetry should be correlated with difference in the chest movement/

expansion as the loss of chest movement marks the affected side. A stony dull percussion note suggests pleural effusion. Rhonchi, wheeze, and prolonged expiratory phase suggests asthma. Coarse crackles are suggestive of bronchiectasis. Unequal breath sounds should raise the suspicion of foreign body aspiration.

Investigations

- *Blood* Leucocytosis suggests infection, a raised ESR may be indicative of chronic infective/inflammatory conditions, and eosinophilia is indicative of allergic disorders. A lymphocytic leukemoid reaction is characteristic of pertussis.
- *Chest X-ray* is required in all cases of chronic cough and additionally lateral and other views may be needed in some patients. In a suspected case of foreign body aspiration, obtain both expiratory and inspiratory films.
- *Barium swallow* Non-ionic contrast studies of the upper gastrointestinal tract may demonstrate gastroesophageal reflux, or extrinsic pressure from a mediastinal mass.
- *Computed tomography* of the thorax can be used for suspected mediastinal masses, and obstruction of airways. High-resolution CT can be used to evaluate diseases of the lung parenchyma, especially in bronchiectasis, interstitial lung disease, and cystic fibrosis.
- *Pulmonary function tests* may be helpful in older children especially in cases of asthma, other obstructive or restrictive airway disease.
- *Bronchoscopy* may be helpful in detection and removal of a foreign body, identifying a lesion in the major airways, or investigating persistent segmental or lobar collapse.

Treatment	Cough

The etiology of cough should guide its treatment. The treatment of specific etiologies of cough has been discussed in subsequent sections. Systematic reviews have shown that frequently used over-the-counter drugs (eg, diphenhydramine, cromones, antihistamines, and anticholinergics) have little efficacy and many adverse effects when used in the treatment of nonspecific chronic cough. Antimicrobials are sometimes used for chronic wet cough (eg, uncomplicated sinusitis), however studies have shown that the benefit is only marginal as compared to placebo. Addressing the environmental triggers (pollutants, tobacco smoke, etc.) that can exacerbate cough, plays an important role in treatment of chronic, nonremitting cough. Parents should be informed about the approximate time-length of resolution of cough, to reduce their anxiety.

Revision Point

Cough

1. Infections and allergic causes account for majority of cases of cough.
2. Generally, acute cough is largely due to infections.
3. Recurrent cough is due to environmental causes or allergic etiology.
4. Persistent cough may be evaluated for anatomical abnormality in airways.

Chang AB, Berkowitz RG. Cough in the pediatric population. *Otolaryngol Clin North Am.* 2010;43:181–98.

Chung KF. Pathophysiology and therapy of chronic cough. *Minerva Med.* 2005;96:29–40.

Kelley LK, Allen PJ. Managing acute cough in children: evidence-based guidelines. *Pediatr Nurs.* 2007;33:515–24.

Landau LI. Acute and chronic cough. *Paediatr Respir Rev.* 2006;7:S64–7.

Mc Garvey LP, Elder J. Future directions in treating cough. *Otolaryngol Clin North Am.* 2010;43:199–211.

Mc Garvey LP. Does idiopathic cough exist? *Lung.* 2008;186:S78–81.

Ramanuja S, Kelkar PS. The approach to pediatric cough. *Ann Allergy Asthma Immunol.* 2010;105:3–8.

Shields MD, Bush A, Everard ML, *et al.* British Thoracic Society Cough Guideline Group. BTS guidelines: Recommendations for the assessment and management of cough in children. *Thorax.* 2008;63:iii1–iii15.

Weldon DR. Differential diagnosis of chronic cough. *Allergy Asthma Proc.* 2005;26:345–51.

Woodcock A, Young EC, Smith JA. New insights in cough. *Br Med Bull.* 2010;96:61–73.

10.3 ACUTE PHARYNGITIS

Pharyngitis is an inflammation of the mucous membranes and underlying structures of the throat, characterized by fever, sore throat, and pharyngeal exudates. It is caused by several different groups of micro-organisms; while nasopharyngitis is mostly viral, tonsillopharyngitis is mostly bacterial. *Tonsillitis* refers to inflammation of the pharyngeal tonsils.

Etiology

Many viral and bacterial agents are capable of producing pharyngitis, either as a separate entity or as part of a generalized illness **(Table 10.2)**.

Viral Causes

Respiratory viruses, such as rhinovirus (60%), influenza, parainfluenza, coronavirus, adenovirus frequently cause acute pharyngitis in children. Ebstein-Barr virus sometimes causes pharyngitis as part of infectious mononucleosis (characterized in addition by rash, mild splenomegaly, generalized lymphadenopathy). Coxsackievirus causes herpangina ie, pharyngitis associated with ulcers in oral cavity.

Bacterial

Group A beta-hemolytic streptococci (GAS) are the most common bacterial cause of acute pharyngitis accounting for 15–30% of cases of acute pharyngitis in children. The streptococcal pharyngitis by itself is a self-limiting, short lived illness but is a formidable problem due to the risk of non-suppurative complications like rheumatic fever.

Other causative bacteria for acute pharyngitis include *Haemophilus influenzae,* and *Streptococcus pyogenes.* Diphtheria is still seen in areas where immunization coverage is inadequate. Groups C and G beta-hemolytic streptococci can cause pharyngitis with clinical features similar to those seen with group A. Groups C and G outbreaks are common in older children and related to ingestion of contaminated food products.

Epidemiology

Most cases of acute pharyngitis occur during the colder months, when the respiratory viruses are prevalent. Spread amongst family members is frequent, with children being the reservoir of infection. Group A streptococci are common etiological agents in the age group 5–15 years.

Clinical Manifestations
Streptococcal Pharyngitis

Acute group A streptococcal pharyngitis has certain clinical characteristics and epidemiological patterns. Onset is acute with high grade fever and sore throat. There is difficulty and pain in swallowing. Fever may be accompanied by headache,

Pathogen	Clinical syndrome
Bacteria	
Group A streptococcus	Pharyngotonsillitis, scarlet fever
Group C and group G Streptococcus	Pharyngotonsillitis
Neisseria gonorrhoeae	Tonsillopharyngitis
Corynebacterium diphtheriae	Diphtheria
Mixed anaerobes	Vincent angina
Fusobacterium necrophorum	Lemierre syndrome, peritonsillar abscess
Viral	
Adenovirus	Pharyngoconjunctival fever
Herpes simplex viruses 1 and 2	Gingivostomatitis
Coxsackievirus	Herpangina
Rhinovirus, Coronavirus	Common cold
Influenza A and B	Influenza
Parainfluenza	Cold, croup
Epstein-Barr virus	Infectious mononucleosis
Cytomegalovirus	CMV mononucleosis
HIV 1 and 2	Primary acute HIV infection

Table 10.2 Causative Organisms for Acute Upper Respiratory Tract Infections

10

nausea, vomiting, abdominal pain, and sometimes, a rash. Examination of the throat reveals inflammation of the pharynx and tonsils. Tonsils are red and enlarged, often covered by patchy white exudates or pus points. Pharyngeal congestion or ulcers may be observed. Examination of neck often reveals tender cervical lymphadenopathy. The child looks toxic and sick. However, none of these findings is specific for group A streptococcal (GAS) pharyngitis. Many patients may exhibit milder signs and symptoms. An attempt should be made to differentiate viral pharyngitis from the streptococcal disease so that the antibiotics are used rationally.

The absence of fever or the presence of diarrhea, characteristic exanthema/enanthem, and similar illness in the household suggests a viral etiology rather than group A streptococcal pharyngitis. The degree of fever or erythema is a poor clinical feature to differentiate between the two etiologies. The absence of pharyngeal exudates and tender lymphadenopathy are good pointers in favor of a viral etiology.

Viral Pharyngitis

Pharyngitis caused by adenovirus is also associated with fever, erythema of the pharynx, enlarged tonsils with exudates, and enlarged cervical lymph nodes. It can be associated with conjunctivitis–pharyngoconjunctival fever, with pharyngitis lasting up to 7 days, the conjunctivitis persisting for 14 days and both resolving spontaneously.

Enteroviruses (coxsackievirus, echovirus) can cause outbreaks of pharyngitis in summer. The pharynx may be erythematous, but tonsillar exudates and cervical adenopathy are unusual. Herpangina is caused by coxsackievirus or echovirus and is characterized by fever and painful, discrete, gray-white papulovesicular lesions on an erythematous base in the posterior oropharynx. These lesions become ulcerative and usually resolve within 7 days.

Pharyngeal Diphtheria

Pharyngeal diphtheria is characterized by a greyish brown pseudomembrane that may be limited to one or both tonsils or may extend widely to involve the nares, uvula, soft palate, pharynx, larynx, and tracheobronchial tree. Soft tissue edema and prominent cervical and submental lymphadenopathy may create a bull-neck appearance.

Diagnosis

1. Throat Culture

Culture of a specimen obtained by throat swab is required for the microbiologic confirmation of Group A streptococcal pharyngitis. If taken appropriately, a single throat swab has a sensitivity of 90–95% in detecting Group A streptococci.

Obtain the throat swab specimen by vigorous swabbing of both tonsils and posterior pharynx. Avoid touching the tongue or oropharynx to avoid contamination. Even with appropriately collected specimens, false-negative results may be obtained if patient receives antibiotics prior to specimen collection.

Culture of the diphtheria bacilli from the swab obtained from the larynx or the pharynx is necessary for confirmation of pharyngeal diphtheria.

2. Rapid Antigen Detection Tests (RADTs)

RADTs have been developed for the identification of Group A streptococci directly from throat swabs, as throat swab cultures are time consuming with delays in diagnosis. This rapid identification and treatment can reduce the spread of Group A streptococci and speed up clinical improvement. Currently available RADTs have specificity of 95% or greater as compared to cultures; the sensitivity varies between 80 and 90%. Enzyme immunoassays are better than latex agglutination tests.

Streptococcal antibody tests like anti-streptolysin O (ASO) and antideoxyribonuclease B (anti-DNase B) have no role in the diagnosis or treatment of acute streptococcal pharyngitis as these reflect past and not present immunologic events. It takes several weeks for them to become positive.

Treatment	Acute Pharyngitis

Specific Treatment

Antimicrobial therapy is indicated for documented streptococcal infection, either by throat culture or RADT. Early initiation of antimicrobial therapy results in shortening of the clinical course of illness. The goals of pharmacotherapy are to reduce the morbidity and to prevent complications. A 10-day treatment with penicillin is the preferred option. Amoxicillin is a widely used alternative. Therapeutic options are detailed below:

1. *Oral penicillin V* Children: 250 mg twice or thrice daily for 10 days.
2. *Oral amoxicillin* 30–40 mg/kg/day for 10 days.
3. *Intramuscular single dose benzathine penicillin G* 1.2 mU (patients >27 kg); 0.6 mU (patients <27 kg).
4. *Oral erythromycin* 40–50 mg/kg/day for 10 days.
5. *Oral azithromycin* 12 mg/kg/day once a day for 5 days.
6. *Oral cephalexin* 50 mg/kg/day for 10 days.

Pharyngeal diphtheria requires oral or parenteral penicillin for 14 days along with administration of antitoxin. Three negative cultures at 24-hour intervals should be obtained before the patient is declared free of the organism. Bedrest for 2–3 weeks is recommended for all patients to reduce the risk of cardiac complications.

Treatment for viral pharyngitis is mainly supportive.

Supportive Management

Warm fluids or gargling may have a soothing effect on the throat. Antipyretics (paracetamol 15 mg/kg/dose) and analgesics are used for relief of pain or pyrexia. First generation anti-histaminics; ie, chlorpheniramine, and promethazine may relieve rhinorrhea by 25–30% due to anticholinergic action. Routine use of cough suppressants (dextromethorphan, codeine) and expectorants (guaifensin, ammonium citrate, and ambroxol, etc) is of no value and may be harmful.

Complications

Group A streptococci can be associated with suppurative and non-suppurative complications. Suppurative complications include peritonsillar abscess, retropharyngeal abscess, cervical lymphadenitis, sinusitis, otitis media, and mastoiditis.

Acute rheumatic fever, acute poststreptococcal glomerulonephritis, and poststreptococcal reactive arthritis are recognized non-suppurative sequelae of Group A streptococcal pharyngitis. These can be prevented by effective treatment of streptococcal pharyngitis as described above. Treatment started as late as by the 9th day of illness can prevent these complications.

Recurrent Streptococcal Pharyngotonsillitis

Recurrence of tonsillitis requires the management of each episode as an acute episode. Tonsillectomy is indicated only under the following circumstances:

1. More than 7 episodes of tonsillitis in last 1 year (*true bacterial tonsillitis and not mere sore throat or URI*) OR 5 or more episodes per year over a 2-year period.
2. Enlarged tonsils that create significant upper airway obstruction.
3. An abscess in the tonsils.

Following tonsillectomy, the incidence of pharyngitis is reduced significantly for 1–2 years.

Pharyngitis

1. Self-limiting viral infections are the most common cause of upper respiratory infections. Group A Streptococcus (GAS) is the most common bacterial cause of acute pharyngitis.
2. Clinical distinction between viral and bacterial etiology of pharyngitis is difficult.
3. Throat swab culture and rapid diagnostic tests are recommended if there is clinical suspicion of GAS pharyngitis.
4. Penicillin (for 10 days) is the first line treatment of GAS pharyngitis.
5. Antibiotics given within 9 days of onset of symptoms can prevent acute rheumatic fever

Altamimi S, Khalil A, Khalaiwi KA, *et al.* Short versus standard duration antibiotic therapy for acute streptococcal pharyngitis in children. *Cochrane Database Syst Rev.* 2009;1:CD004872.

Baltimore RS. Re-evaluation of antibiotic treatment of streptococcal pharyngitis. *Curr Opin Pediatr.* 2010;22:77–82.

Gereige R, Cunill-De Sautu B. Throat infections. *Pediatr Rev.* 2011;32:459–68.

Merrill B, Kelsberg G, Jankowski TA, Danis P. Clinical inquiries. What is the most effective diagnostic evaluation of streptococcal pharyngitis? *J Fam Pract.* 2004;53:734,737–8,740.

Munir N, Clarke R. Indications for tonsillectomy: the evidence base and current UK practice. *Br J Hosp Med (Lond).* 2009;70:344–7.

Shah R, Bansal A, Singhi SC. Approach to a child with sore throat. *Indian J Pediatr.* 2011;78:1268–72.

Shulman ST, Bisno AL, Clegg HW, et al. Clinical Practice Guideline for the Diagnosis and Management of Group A Streptococcal Pharyngitis: 2012 Update by the Infectious Diseases Society of America. *Clinical Infectious Diseases* 2012;55(10):e86–102.

Van Driel ML, De Sutter AI, Keber N, *et al.* Different antibiotic treatments for group A streptococcal pharyngitis. *Cochrane Database Syst Rev.* 2010;10:CD004406

Wessels MR. Clinical practice. Streptococcal pharyngitis. *N Engl J Med.* 2011; 364:648–55.

10.4 STRIDOR AND CROUP

Stridor is a loud, harsh, medium-pitched, musical sound produced by turbulent airflow through a partially obstructed airway. It is a symptom, and not a diagnosis or disease. Stridor is primarily inspiratory, but can also be biphasic.

Inspiratory stridor suggests an extrathoracic lesion (eg, laryngeal, nasal, pharyngeal) while *biphasic stridor* suggests a subglottic or glottic anomaly or a severe obstruction of the extra-thoracic airway.

Pathophysiology

Gases produce pressure equally in all directions; however, when a gas moves in a linear direction, it produces pressure in the forward vector and decreases the lateral pressure. When air passes through a narrowed flexible airway in a child, the lateral pressure that holds the airway open can drop precipitously (*venturi principle*) and cause the tube to collapse. A similar process obstructs airflow and produces stridor in cases with upper airway obstruction.

Causes of Acute Stridor

1. *Laryngotracheobronchitis (croup)* This is a viral infection of the larynx and subglottic region and is the most common cause of acute stridor in children, especially in children aged 6 months to 2 years (*see* details later).
2. *Epiglottitis* This is a medical emergency occurring most commonly in children aged 2–7 years, due to fulminant inflammation of the supraglottic structures: Epiglottis, arytenoids, aryepiglottic folds, and uvula, due to infection by *Haemophilus influenzae type B*. It is not that common in India. Clinically, the child appears toxic. The disease is characterized by an abrupt onset of high-grade fever, sore throat, dysphagia, respiratory distress, and drooling of saliva. Mother complains of noisy breathing during inspiration. The patient assumes a characteristic posture with chin thrust forward and tripod position of the upper limbs with wrists flexed, with a characteristic low-pitched stridor. The disease can be life-threatening.
3. *Diphtheria* It is commonly seen in partially or completely unimmunized children. Throat examination reveals a thick pharyngeal membrane spreading to the adjacent larynx. This results in airway obstruction. The child appears sick and toxic out of proportion to the degree of fever. The child may have swelling with edema of the neck (bull neck) due to local toxin release. The child may have inspiratory stridor or biphasic stridor depending upon the degree of obstruction. Urgent airway management may be required.
4. *Bacterial tracheitis* It is relatively uncommon and mainly affects children younger than 3 years. It is a secondary infection (most commonly due to *Staphylococcus aureus*) following a viral process (commonly croup or influenza) and is characterized by severe airway obstruction, high fever, toxicity, and subglottic narrowing. Associated barking cough is a characteristic feature.
5. *Foreign body* Aspiration of foreign body should be suspected in children with history of coughing and choking preceding the onset of stridor. Commonly aspirated foreign bodies are food items like nuts and seeds, coins, beads, whistle, etc.
6. *Retropharyngeal abscess* It is a complication of bacterial pharyngitis observed in children younger than 6 years. The child presents with abrupt onset of high fever, difficulty in swallowing, refusal to feed, sore throat, hyperextension of the neck, stridor, and respiratory distress.
7. *Allergic reaction* (ie, anaphylaxis) It occurs within 30 minutes of an adverse exposure. Hoarseness and inspiratory stridor may be accompanied by allergic

10

symptoms (eg, dysphagia, nasal congestion, itching eyes, sneezing, and wheezing).

Causes of Chronic Stridor

1. *Laryngomalacia* This is the most common cause of inspiratory stridor in the early infancy and accounts for up to 75% of all cases of stridor in young infants. Stridor is typically exacerbated by activity, crying, or feeding. Placing the patient in a prone position with the head up improves the stridor; while in supine position the stridor worsens. Stridor due to laryngomalacia is usually benign, self-limiting, and improves as the child reaches age of 1 year. If significant obstruction or failure to thrive is present, surgical correction (supraglottoplasty) may be considered.

2. *Congenital subglottic stenosis* It can present with inspiratory or biphasic stridor. Symptoms can be evident at any time during the first few years of life and can cause recurrent episodes of stridor. Congenital subglottic stenosis occurs due to incomplete canalization of the subglottis and cricoid rings leading to narrowing of the subglottic lumen. Acquired stenosis is most commonly caused by prolonged intubation or due to a neglected foreign body.

3. *Vocal cord paralysis* It can be congenital or secondary to trauma at birth or during cardiac or intrathoracic surgery. The left vocal cord is more commonly affected as the left recurrent laryngeal nerve may get damaged secondary to ligation of patent ductus arteriosus.
   - Children with *unilateral paralysis* present with a weak cry or hoarseness. Stridor may improve when lying with the affected side down.
   - *Bilateral vocal cord paralysis* is a more serious entity. Children usually present with aphonia and a high-pitched biphasic stridor that may progress to severe respiratory distress. It is usually associated with CNS abnormalities, such as Arnold-Chiari malformation or increased intracranial pressure, aggressive traction during delivery, hydrocephalus, and hypoxia.

4. *Laryngeal webs* These are caused by an incomplete recanalization of the laryngeal lumen during embryogenesis. Most (75%) are in the glottic area. Infants with laryngeal webs have a weak cry and biphasic stridor.

5. *Congenital laryngeal cysts* These are a less frequent cause of stridor. They are usually found in the supraglottic region in the epiglottic folds. Patients may present with stridor, hoarse voice, or aphonia, or cysts may cause obstruction of airway lumen if they are very large.

VIRAL CROUP (LARYNGOTRACHEOBRONCHITIS)

Croup is a heterogeneous group of acute and infectious processes in children (between 6 months and 6 years of age) that manifest most commonly with characteristic inspiratory stridor, barking cough, hoarse voice, and varying degrees of respiratory distress. The word 'Croup' is derived from Anglo-Saxon word 'Kropan' which means 'crying aloud'.

Viral croup is the most common cause of upper airway obstruction in children 6 months to 6 years of age with peak incidence at the age of 12–24 months. It is usually a mild and self-limiting illness, but it occasionally may progress to severe obstructive illness requiring hospitalization and emergency care.

Etiology

Parainfluenza type 1 (50%), parainfluenza types 2 and 3, respiratory syncytial virus (RSV), influenza A and B, and rhinovirus account for the majority of cases. Approximately 15% of patients have a strong family history of croup.

Clinical Presentation

The illness usually starts like a common cold with symptoms of rhinorrhea, cough, sore throat, and fever. Features of upper airway obstruction, ie, inspiratory stridor, hoarseness, and barking cough develop over next 2–3 days. In most cases, symptoms usually resolve within a week. A few children develop symptoms of severe airway obstruction characterized by intercostal recession, tachypnea, irritability, lethargy, and cyanosis; and need hospitalization. These symptoms usually occur due to inflammation of larynx, trachea and bronchus (hence the term 'laryngotracheobronchitis'). However, it is specifically the subglottic inflammation and resultant swelling that compromises the airway and results in stridor and difficult breathing.

It is imperative to rule out other entities like acute epiglottitis, bacterial tracheitis, foreign body, spasmodic cough, and laryngeal diphtheria because the management would differ in each case.

Assessment of the Severity

- *General appearance* Agitation, restlessness, head nodding, hypotonia, and lethargy are the signs of hypoxia due to severe airway obstruction.
- *Degree of respiratory distress* Stridor at rest, intercostal or subcostal indrawing, tachypnea, and pulses paradoxus indicate moderate to severe obstruction.
- *Stridor* The loudness of stridor is not a good indicator of severity of obstruction. However, presence of biphasic stridor indicates fixed obstruction (like foreign body, subglottic stenosis, or hemangioma).
- *Cyanosis or extreme pallor* Either of the two indicates severe obstruction.
- *Oxygen saturation* Falling saturation is a late and unreliable sign to assess the degree of respiratory distress and not a good substitute for clinical assessment.

Investigations

The diagnosis of viral croup is essentially based on the history and clinical examination. Investigations are necessary when the diagnosis is not clear. X-ray of chest and soft tissue neck can help rule out a foreign body. Typical 'steeple sign' which refers to steeple like narrow subglottic area on plain neck X-ray (Fig. 10.2) is present in less than 50% of children with croup.

Treatment	Viral Croup

Treatment depends upon the severity of croup and includes humidified oxygen, oral or parenteral steroids, and inhaled adrenaline.

1. *Humidified air* It has been widely advocated in the past without any scientific validation, but it still can be used as home remedy in children with mild croup.

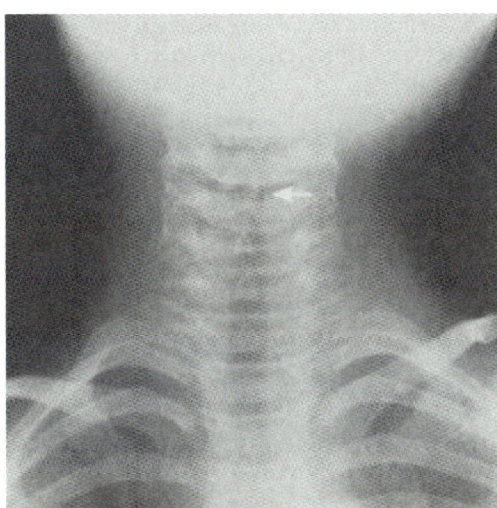

Fig. 10.2 Classical 'Steeple' sign seen in plain X-ray neck

2. *Oxygen therapy* Oxygen is the most important treatment for a child with moderate or severe croup who has considerable upper-airway obstruction or SpO_2 <92%.
3. *Oral or inhaled steroids* Steroids can improve the symptoms of croup within 6–8 hours after starting the treatment. They also result in shorter duration of hospital stay, lesser need of endotracheal intubation, and decreased need for adrenaline nebulization. Oral corticosteroids are preferred as they are inexpensive, easy to administer, readily available, and produce measurable improvements within hours. The recommended doses of dexamethasone are 0.15–0.3 mg/kg (oral or IM) and doses of prednisolone (suspension or tablets) are 1–2 mg/kg. Nebulized budesonide (2 mg) has been shown to be equally efficacious. This can be repeated 12 hourly for up to 48 hours. The choice of route is based upon the availability and the child condition.
4. *Nebulized adrenaline* It is indicated in children with moderate to severe croup with stridor at rest and marked intercostal or subcostal indrawing. Administer 1:1000 dilution solution of nebulized adrenaline 0.5 mL/kg of body weight to maximum of 5 mL. It has a rapid onset of action on bronchial and tracheal epithelial vascular permeability, thereby decreasing airway edema, which, in turn, increases the airway radius and improves airflow, with improvement in croup severity score within 30 minutes. However, it has a temporary action on the airway obstruction and only gives time to basic pathology to resolve. If stridor persists, the dose can be repeated after 2–4 hours.
5. *Antimicrobials* These have no role in treatment of viral croup, even to prevent secondary bacterial infection.
6. *Discharge* Child can be sent home when there is no stridor at rest. Parents need to be educated for monitoring of worsening of symptoms.

Charles J, Britt H, Fahridin S. Croup. *Aust Fam Physician.* 2010;39:269.

Development Group. Evidence based guideline for the management of croup. *Aust Fam Physician.* 2008;37:14–20.

Fitzgerald DA, Kilham HA. Croup: assessment and evidence-based management. *Med J Aust.* 2003;179:372–7.

Fitzgerald DA. The assessment and management of croup. *Paediatr Respir Rev.* 2006;7:73–81.

Mazza D, Wilkinson F, Turner T, Harris C. Health for Kids Guideline. Croup-assessment and management. *Aust Fam Physician.* 2010;39:280–2.

Sobol SE, Zapata S. Epiglottitis and croup. *Otolaryngol Clin North Am.* 2008;41:551–66.

Stroud RH, Friedman NR. An update on inflammatory disorders of the pediatric airway: epiglottitis, croup, and tracheitis. *Am J Otolaryngol.* 2001;22:268–75.

Syed I, Tassone P, Sebire P, Bleach N. Acute management of croup in children. *Br J Hosp Med.* 2009;70:M4–6.

10.5 APPROACH TO A CHILD WITH FAST BREATHING

Fast breathing or tachypnea is a condition where the rate of breathing is more than the normal upper limit for that age group. Worrisome fast breathing which signifies a significant underlying lung problem has been defined by the WHO as follows:

Age group	Respiratory rate cut-off
Young infant (<2 months)	>60/minute
Infant (2 mo–1 yr)	>50/minute
Children (1–5 yr)	>40/minute
School children (>5 yr)	>30/minute

It is important that the respiratory rate is counted for full 60 seconds when the child is calm and quite; otherwise there is a risk of both under and over reading of rapid breathing. Increased work of breathing is witnessed as head bobbing, sweating over forehead, lower chest indrawing and mentation changes like initially irritability and later on altered sensorium or drowsiness. Fast breathing coupled with labored or increased work of breathing or cyanosis is termed as *respiratory distress* or *dyspnea* **(Box 10.1)**.

Pathogenesis

Fast breathing occurs after the activation of sensory systems involved in respiration. The central chemoreceptors (located in medulla) and peripheral chemoreceptors (carotid and aortic bodies) are responsible for detection of changes in oxygen and carbon dioxide concentration. An increase in carbon dioxide stimulates central receptors and results in an increase in ventilation. Hypoxia stimulates respiration

10

Box 10.1 Signs of Respiratory Distress in Children

1. Tachypnea (cut off for respiratory rate)
   Age 0–2 months: >60/min
   Age 2–12 months: >50/min
   Age 1–5 Years:> 40/min
2. Dyspnea
3. Retractions (suprasternal, intercostal, or subcostal)
4. Grunting
5. Nasal flaring
6. Apnea
7. Altered mental status
8. Pulse oximetry measurement <90% on room air

through its effects on the peripheral receptors, which may cause breathlessness in patients who have underlying lung disease.

Upper airway mechanoreceptors and pulmonary vagal receptors are important in shaping the pattern of breathing. The afferent impulses from these receptors project to the CNS and are processed there. Based on the response to afferent information, the CNS sends an efferent impulse *via* the phrenic nerve to the diaphragm and the other respiratory muscles to increase respiration.

Etiology

Fast breathing may be physiological, eg, after running or exercise, or it may occur due to underlying disease process which may be respiratory or non-respiratory. Common causes of tachypnea are listed below:

I. Upper respiratory tract involvement
   - Croup
   - Retropharyngeal abscess
   - Foreign body aspiration
   - Diphtheria
   - Laryngospasm

II. Lower respiratory tract involvement
   - Pneumonia,
   - Bronchiolitis
   - Asthma
   - Pleural effusion or empyema and hemothorax
   - Pneumothorax
   - Atelectasis
   - Hypersensitivity pneumonitis

III. Non-respiratory causes
   - Congestive heart failure due to heart disease or severe anemia
   - CNS infections and cerebral edema
   - Metabolic acidosis as in renal failure, diabetic ketoacidosis, renal tubular acidosis, etc.
   - Psychogenic hyperventilation, anxiety, panic attacks

Clinical Features

A child with respiratory distress may have tachypnea with cyanosis, nasal flaring, grunting, wheezing, chest wall retractions, or stridor. It is important to characterize tachypnea or dyspnea in terms of onset, frequency, intensity, duration, triggers (exposures), provoking activities (ambulation, eating, changing position), associated respiratory symptoms, and strategies or actions (medications, positions) that provide relief.

There are very varied causes of respiratory distress in a child. History and clinical examination usually provides enough clues to shortlist a few probable causes for further investigation.

- Fever, cough and rapid breathing with or without lower chest indrawing are the commonest presentation of lower respiratory tract infections like pneumonia, bronchiolitis and virus induced wheeze in young children.
- *Nocturnal cough and dyspnea* may be indicative of asthma, CHF or gastroesophageal reflux disease.
- Dyspnea occurring mainly after exercise indicates congestive heart failure or exercise induced asthma.
- *Episodic dyspnea* may be caused by asthma or less often by heart failure (eg, in congenital heart diseases) whereas persistent or progressive dyspnea suggests chronic conditions like interstitial lung disease, persistent congestive heart failure, or pulmonary hypertension.
- The symptoms of fever, sore throat, and acute respiratory distress with stridor may suggest epiglottitis.
- Pleuritic chest pain associated with rapid but shallow breathing could be caused by pleuritis, pneumonia, pneumothorax, or pulmonary embolism,
- Any history of dysphagia or recurrent vomiting with intermittent wheezing may indicate gastroesophageal reflux with aspiration.

Physical Examination

The general appearance and vital signs can be used to determine the severity of dyspnea by observing respiratory effort, use of accessory muscles, mental status, and ability to speak. An examination of the neck, thorax, lungs, heart, and extremities is always needed.

- The neck area might reveal a shift of the trachea, jugular venous distention, suprasternal recessions, an enlarged thyroid gland, or an adenopathy.
- Stridor is indicative of upper airway obstruction.
- Inspection of thorax might show an increased anteroposterior diameter or chest wall deformity.
- Palpation might reveal subcutaneous emphysema.
- Dullness on percussion is indicative of consolidation or effusion. Absent breath sounds may be consistent with pneumothorax or pleural effusion.
- Wheezing indicates turbulent airflow, which can be caused by asthma or left ventricular failure.
- Crepitations are suggestive of pneumonia or pulmonary edema.
- Rapid or irregular pulse may indicate dysrhythmia. An S_3 gallop suggests a left ventricular dysfunction in congestive heart failure.
- A loud P_2 is characteristic of pulmonary hypertension or cor pulmonale.
- Extremities should be checked for cyanosis or clubbing to rule out a congenital cyanotic heart disease, or a chronic lung disease.

Management

A general approach to diagnosis and management of fast breathing in a child is summarized in Fig. 10.3. The basic investigations needed for these children include X-ray chest, ECG, blood gas, serum electrolytes, hemoglobin, and blood

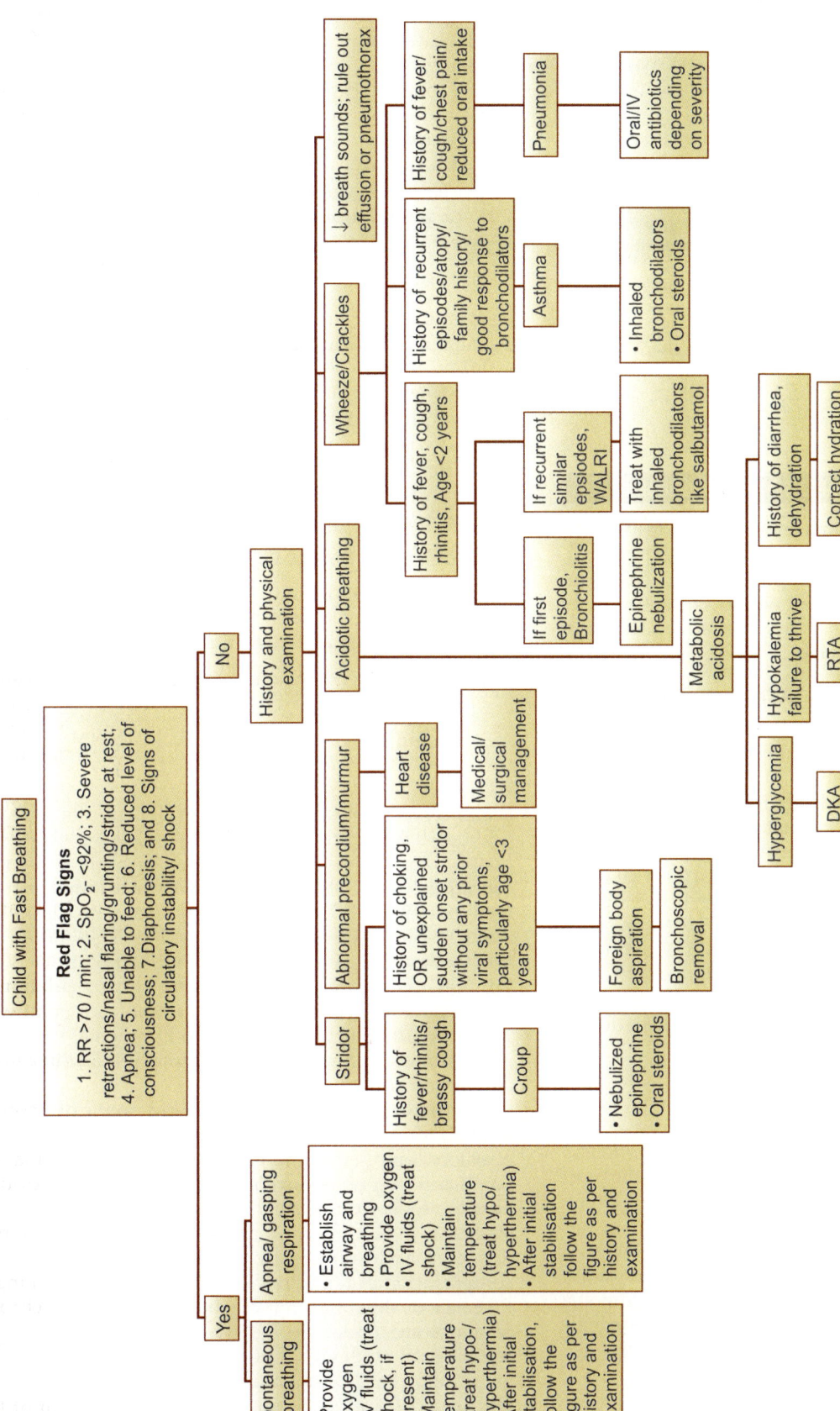

Fig. 10.3 Approach to a child with fast breathing

counts. Specific situations may necessitate laryngoscopy, bronchoscopy, pulmonary function tests, and a complete biochemical evaluation.

The treatment of a child presenting with fast breathing or respiratory distress includes maintaining the temperature, airway, breathing, and circulation; followed by administering the definitive treatment based on history and physical examination.

> Gove S. Integrated management of childhood illness by outpatient healthworkers: technical basis and overview. The WHO Working Group on Guidelines for Integrated Management of the Sick Child. *Bull World Health Organ*.1997; 1:7–24.
> Grant GB, Campbell H, Dowell SF, *et al*. World Health Organization Recommendations for treatment of childhood non-severe pneumonia. *Lancet Infect Dis*. 2009;9:185–96.
> Kercsmar CM. Current trends in neonatal and pediatric respiratory care: conference summary. *Respir Care*. 2003;48:459–64.
> Sigillito RJ, De Blieux PM. Evaluation and initial management of the patient in respiratory distress. *Emerg Med Clin North Am*. 2003;21:239–58.

10.6 COMMUNITY ACQUIRED PNEUMONIA

Community acquired pneumonia refers to an acute infection of the lung parenchyma in a previously healthy child, typically acquired outside of hospital setting. The child should not have been hospitalized within 14 days prior to the onset of symptoms or has been hospitalized less than 4 days prior to onset of symptoms.

Acute Respiratory Infections (ARI) and Pneumonia

Acute respiratory infections (ARI) in children less than 5 years old are the leading cause of childhood morbidity and mortality in the world. More than 95% of all episodes of clinical pneumonia in young children worldwide occur in developing countries. Recent estimates from India suggest that in children under 5 years of age, ARI constitutes 24% of the childhood burden of disease and 14% of deaths. Community based studies from different parts of the country have reported the annual incidence of ARI as 2.5–6.4 episodes per child per year. About 0.23–12.5% of children with ARI are estimated to have lower respiratory tract infection (LRTI). Mortality estimates suggest that 2.3 million children less than 5 years of age die every year in India and 20% of these deaths are due to ARI.

Etiology

Age is a good predictor of the likely pathogen of pneumonia and can help narrow the list of etiological agents. The etiology can be viral or bacterial. *Streptococcus pneumoniae* is the most common etiological agent causing pneumonia at all ages. Gram-negative agents are common under 2 months of age, while *Haemophilus influenzae* is most common between 2 months and 2 years of age. *Staphylococcus aureus*, *Mycoplasma*, and *Chlamydia*, are the other important causes of pneumonia in under-five children. **Table 10.3** outlines the probable agents at various age groups in order of common prevalence.

Clinical Features

Children with suspected pneumonia present with non-specific triad of fever, cough, (may or may not be productive), and fast breathing. Severe cases have associated dyspnea or

Table 10.3 Causative Organisms for Pneumonia	
0–2 months of age	• Gram-negative organisms • *Streptococcus pyogenes* • *Chlamydia* • Viruses
2 mo–5 yrs of age	• *Streptococcus pneumoniae* • *H. influenzae* • *Streptococcus pyogenes* • Viruses
>5 yrs of age	• *Mycoplasma pneumoniae* • *Streptococcus pneumoniae* • *Staphylococcus aureus* • Viruses • *Mycoplasma pneumoniae* • *Streptococcus pyogenes* • *H. influenzae*

difficult breathing. Constitutional symptoms such as chest pain, malaise, lethargy, abdominal pain, headache, nausea, and vomiting may predominate.

Fast Breathing for Diagnosis of Pneumonia

- Clinically defined pneumonia is based on signs and symptoms of lower respiratory tract dysfunction. WHO defines *pneumonia* as a condition presenting with cough and fast breathing. Presence of lower chest indrawing indicates '*severe pneumonia*'. However, it must be remembered that other clinical syndromes like bronchiolitis, croup, asthma also present similarly. In a hospital setting, these conditions need to be excluded clinically (*see* relevant sections).
- Rapid respiration (as defined by WHO cut-offs stated in *Section* 10.5) identifies children who have a very high probability of having pneumonia and are therefore candidates for antibiotic therapy. While a simple sign as tachypnea is useful to identify most cases with significant lower respiratory tract involvement, a clinician should use this tool merely as the beginning point and utilize other clinical skills including auscultation to recognize pneumonia with a fair degree of certainty.
- The presence of grunt, crackles, and bronchial breathing is suggestive of pneumonia but except crackles, these signs are seen uncommonly.
- Often there may be presence of signs suggesting other complications of pneumonia like para-pneumonic effusions, empyema, and pneumothorax.
- Small children often have refusal to feed and some may also have gastrointestinal signs such as vomiting and diarrhea.
- Referred abdominal pain can occur with lower lobe consolidation or if pleurisy develops.
- Presence of skin boils; rapid progression or deterioration of symptoms; presence of empyema or pneumothorax, or radiological evidence of pneumatocele strongly suggest Staphylococcal pneumonia.
- Clinical differentiation between viral and bacterial pneumonia is difficult. However, the presence of preceding viral catarrh, wheezing, and non-toxic look suggests a viral pathology.

- Asthma is suspected if there is history of recurrent (3 or more) episodes; presence of predominant wheeze and hyperinflation; presence of family or personal history of atopy; and a good response to bronchodilator.
- Bronchiolitis should be considered if the child is between 2 months–2 years of age, and has presented with a wheezy illness for the time, preceded by symptoms of viral upper respiratory tract. X-ray will reveal hyperinflation.
- Consider a diagnosis of croup, if there is associated stridor.

Assessing Severity of Pneumonia

Based on the various clinical parameters one could assess and classify the severity. WHO criteria for assessment of severity are simple and useful at all levels of care. It suggests that in children with cough, cases with tachypnea alone are considered as *pneumonia* and given domiciliary treatment, where as those with chest indrawing, and retractions are treated as *severe pneumonia* in the hospital. Children with severe indrawing, refusal to feed or altered sensorium; or signs of imminent respiratory failure like cyanosis, irritability, or erratic breathing are considered to have *very severe pneumonia*. Another criteria for assessment of severity of illness is given in **Box 10.2**.

Indications for Hospitalization

Hypoxemia is a good indicator of the severity of pneumonia, and if facility exists, pulse oximetry should be performed on every child deemed ill enough to be admitted. Oxygen saturation of <92% or presence of cyanosis, respiratory rate >70 min, and inability to feed are indications to admit the child and treat with oxygen and parenteral antibiotics. Further, all children below the age of 3 months with pneumonia should also be hospitalized.

The child should be transferred to intensive care unit if there is a failure to maintain SaO_2 >92% in 60% oxygen, or is having peripheral circulatory failure, or having gasping respiration or apnea.

Complicated pneumonia Common complications of community acquired pneumonia are listed in **Table 10.4**.

Investigations

Radiological shadows are taken as gold standard for diagnosing pneumonia. However, there is marked inter and intra-individual differences in interpretation of skiagrams.

Table 10.4 Complications of Community Acquired Pneumonia

A. Pulmonary
1. Pleural effusion or empyema
2. Pneumothorax
3. Lung abscess
4. Bronchopleural fistula
5. Necrotizing pneumonia
6. Acute respiratory failure

B. Metastatic
1. Meningitis
2. Central nervous system abscess
3. Pericarditis
4. Endocarditis
5. Osteomyelitis
6. Septic arthritis

C. Systemic
1. Systemic inflammatory response syndrome or sepsis
2. Hemolytic uremic syndrome

Therefore, skiagram of the chest is not indicated routinely. Indications of getting an X-ray chest are:
- Severe or very severe pneumonia;
- Diagnosis of child under 5 years of age with fever of 39°C of unknown origin;
- Suspected complications such as a pleural effusion or pneumothorax;
- Children with atypical features; and
- Children deteriorating or not responding after 48 hours of treatment.

Diffuse interstitial infiltrates on chest skiagram suggests viral infection, whereas homogeneous opacity with air bronchogram suggests consolidation due to bacterial cause. Necrotising pneumonia as in staphylococcal infection may show evidence of breakdown in the form of thin cavities (pneumatoceles). The chest skiagram usually clears within 3–4 weeks and radiological clearance usually lags behind clinical recovery.

Microbiological tests are of no use routinely. Acute phase reactants like TLC, DLC, CRP are not diagnostic but may be useful to monitor the response to treatment. A negative test may be more useful in excluding the diagnosis as compared to confirmation on the basis of a positive test. A high white blood cell count with neutrophilia suggests bacterial

Box 10.2 Criteria for Assessment of Severity of Illness in Community Acquired Pneumonia (Modified from IDSA Guidelines for CAP 2011)

Major criteria	*Minor criteria*
1. Need for Mechanical ventilation/NIPPV	1. Tachypnea/Apnea
2. Fluid refractory shock	2. Increased work of breathing (eg, retractions, nasal flaring, grunting)
3. Severe hypoxemia (FiO_2 > that feasible in general ward)	3. Multilobar infiltrates
	4. Altered mental status
	5. Hypotension
	6. Presence of effusion
	7. Comorbid conditions (eg, immunodeficiency)
	8. Unexplained metabolic acidosis

Children having > 1 major or > 2 minor criteria are considered having severe disease and should be admitted in an intensive care unit with continuous cardiorespiratory monitoring.

pneumonia. Blood culture may be positive in 10–15% of cases with acute bacterial pneumonia. These tests provide helpful clues but by themselves do not definitely distinguish between viral and bacterial pneumonia.

| Treatment | **Pneumonia** |

Supportive Therapy

- *Oxygen* Requirement of oxygen is guided by pulse oxymetry and clinical signs of hypoxia. Rapid breathing and chest retractions are good correlates of hypoxia. Higher the hypoxia, faster is the breathing and severe the retractions except in the pre-terminal phase when the effort can go down due to exhaustion. Importantly, severely malnourished children may not be able to increase their respiratory rate as much as others even in the presence of significant disease.
- *IV Fluids* Parenteral fluids are administered if the patient is dehydrated, has tachypnea severe enough to make the child unable to drink, or has impending respiratory failure.
- *Fever management* High grade fever increases oxygen requirement. Fever is controlled by paracetamol and sponging.
- *Bronchodilators* These are indicated in presence of wheeze and help to decrease the work of breathing.
- *Chest physiotherapy* It helps in preventing atelectasis.

Antibiotic Therapy

Empiric antibiotic therapy is based on knowing the most likely pathogen in each community. Selection of antibiotic is also dictated by the age of the child, and epidemiological factors, and sometimes the results of the chest radiography.

Domiciliary treatment
Oral amoxicillin for 5–7 days is given to children with pneumonia who are being treated at home. Second line therapy (oral co-amoxiclav or chloramphenicol for 5–7 days) is advised if no improvement occurs in 48 hours. In children below 2 years, one can also use a combination of oral ampicillin and chloramphenicol. Oral azithromycin is another alternative second line drug for older children.

Hospital management
Children with severe pneumonia and those less than 3 months of age are always treated in hospital with injectable ampicillin. Second line therapy consists of injectable co-amoxiclav or third generation cephalosporins, eg, cefotaxime or ceftriaxone. An aminoglycoside may be added for those below 3 months of age, or for those having 'very severe pneumonia'.

Co-amoxiclav or else a combination of one of the 3rd generation cephalosporin with cloxacillin is preferred in children in suspected or proven staphylococcal pneumonia. Most children treated for mild disease shall need treatment for 5–7 days while those on second line therapy need prolonged antibiotics for 7–10 days. The uncomplicated staphylococcal disease is treated for 2 weeks while those having empyema or pneumothorax are treated for 4–6 weeks. The patient is initially treated with parenteral antibiotics and put on oral formulations as soon as the fever and tachypnea starts settling down and child is able to take orally.

Response to Therapy

Clinical response consists of absence of fever, and improvement in breathing. The end of treatment X-ray is not needed in every case except when the response is delayed or incomplete, or there are associated complications. In case the child does not show significant improvement (improvement in breathing rate and signs of distress) even after 48 hours, the child should be investigated for any complication. Second line therapy may then be started. Children with staphylococcal disease, however, respond more slowly and may show significant improvement only after 96 hours of therapy.

LOBAR PNEUMONIA

Lobar pneumonia in children is usually caused by *Streptococcus pneumoniae*. The disease presents with acute onset high grade fever with cough and rapid breathing. It may be associated with chest pain over the involved side.

On examination, the child has tachypnea and lower chest indrawing. There may also be other signs of respiratory distress including nasal flaring, intercostal and subcostal retractions, and inability to feed. Severely hypoxic children can have air hunger, irritability, drowsiness, or cyanosis.

The trachea is usually central but may be shifted to the side of lobar pneumonia, only if there is an underlying or associated collapse. Chest examination reveals no chest asymmetry, decreased chest movements on the involved side, and normal to decreased breath sounds on the ipsilateral side. On percussion, there is impaired note. Vocal fremitus and resonance is increased over the involved area. Breath sounds may be *bronchial* in character. There may not be any adventitious sounds initially and crackles appear once the resolution starts. Lobar pneumonia is sometimes complicated by a parapneumonic effusion. Total leukocyte count is high with neutrophilic predominance. X-ray chest shows a homogeneous lung opacity in a lobar configuration; which causes a loss of cardiac or diaphragmatic silhouette if middle or lower lobe, respectively are involved. An air bronchogram may be seen as the air in the solidified opaque lung marks out the airways.

- Presence of pneumatoceles (thin walled cavities) on chest radiograph suggests staphylococcal pneumonia.
- *Mycoplasma* can also give rise to a lobar pneumonia with acute symptoms though more often it presents as an *atypical pneumonia* where the signs are far more than the symptoms.

As pneumococcus is the commonest bacteria responsible for lobar consolidation, the specific treatment of choice is penicillin given for 7–10 days. Management of fever, hydration, and oxygen supplementation are other important supportive therapies needed.

BRONCHOPNEUMONIA

Bronchopneumonia is primarily a disease of young children. Most common bacterial organisms causing broncho-pneumonia include *Streptococcus* sp, *Haemophilus influenzae*, and *Staphylococcus aureus*.

It presents as acute onset fever with cough and fast breathing. In severe cases the child may also have respiratory distress with or without cyanosis. On examination, the child has rapid breathing, nasal flaring, and lower chest indrawing. Signs of hypoxia in form of irritability or drowsiness, inability to feed due to respiratory distress, altered sensorium, cyanosis, and diaphoresis may appear depending upon the severity of the disease. Chest examination may reveal bilateral diffuse crackles with or without wheezing. Wheezing is more often seen with viral pneumonia as compared to bacterial disease.

Chest X-ray reveals patchy homogeneous or inhomogeneous alveolar opacities scattered all over a segment or a lobe or more than one lobe of one or both lungs. Apart from the supportive therapy described above, these children are treated with systemic antibiotics. First line agents are ampicillin and gentamicin. Amoxiclavulinic acid or ceftriaxone should be used as second line agents.

GRAM-NEGATIVE PNEUMONIA

Young infants (less than 3 months old) and children with underlying severe malnutrition usually develop pneumonia due to Gram-negative organisms. *Klebsiella pneumoniae*, *Pseudomonas* sp., and *E.coli* are the most important agents. The clinical presentation is very similar to the Gram-positive organisms. Third generation cephalosporins are the agent of choice for treatment. Aminoglycosides may be added in severe cases.

VIRAL PNEUMONIA

Pneumonia due to influenza viruses, parainfluenza virus, respiratory syncytial virus, and paramyxoviruses clinically mimic bacterial pneumonias, except that these children do not appear toxic. There often is also presence of eye congestion, rhinitis, and diarrhea. The degree of hypoxia can be as severe as with bacterial pneumonia. Wheezing is seen more often with viral pneumonia.

Interstitial pneumonia is the typical finding on chest X-ray; it shows as a lacy reticular pattern of increased bronchovesicular markings over the lung fields; this may be associated with interstitial thickening. The blood counts and acute phase reactants like C-reactive protein are usually normal in such cases. The treatment is largely supportive. The antibiotics are used only if the clinical distinction from bacterial pneumonia is difficult. However, at a community level where no facilities are available to differentiate, WHO and national policy are to treat all children as bacterial pneumonia.

PERSISTENT AND RECURRENT PNEUMONIA

Definitions

• *Persistent* or *non-resolving pneumonia* is defined as the persistence of symptoms and documentation of non-resolving radiographic abnormalities in a child with lower respiratory tract infections for more than 1 month despite a course of adequate antibiotic therapy.

• *Recurrent pneumonia* is defined as at least 2 distinct episodes of radiologically established pneumonia within the same year or 3 or more such episodes over any time period. For the diagnosis of recurrent pneumonia, there must be documented complete resolution of clinical and radiological findings between acute episodes.

• Distinguishing between recurrent and persistent pneumonia may be difficult at times.

Case Study | **Pneumonia**

A 5-year-old boy weighing 18 kg reported with history of high grade fever and cough for 1 week. He also complained of pain over the right side of chest for 2 days. His appetite had decreased over the last one week. On examination, his temperature and hydration were normal. Pulse rate was 90/min and respiratory rate was 42/min. He had lower chest indrawing and nasal flaring. Auscultation of chest revealed crackles over both the lung fields.

Justify the provisional clinical diagnosis.

In view of rapid breathing with lower chest indrawing in a case of fever with cough, the most probable clinical diagnosis is acute lower respiratory infection, ie, pneumonia. The presence of crackles on chest auscultation further supports the diagnosis. Pneumonia is severe because of presence of lower chest indrawing.

List the relevant investigations you would ask for.

Pulse oximetry and complete blood counts shall be needed. As the patient has severe disease, a chest radiograph should also be obtained.

Outline the principles of management of this child.

This child has no rhinorrhea or viral prodrome (suggestive of viral disease) and also because the bacterial pneumonias are common in our country, the specific therapy will be oral or injectable penicillin, ampicillin or amoxicillin. Paracetamol needs to be administered and oxygen saturation should be monitored. Antibiotics should be given for at least 7 days.

Evaluation of Recurrent or Persistent Pneumonia

It is important to establish whether the pneumonia is *unilobar* or *multilobar*. Common causes of unilobar persistent pneumonia include a foreign body, bronchial tumor, congenital malformations, tuberculosis, or Hodgkin disease. Unilateral localized disease is more likely due to local problems like intra- or extra-luminal obstruction while diffuse or multilobar disease is more often due to systemic disorders of immunity (**Table 10.5**). Further work-up is guided by the clinical clues and distribution of pneumonia. *Severe, Persistent, Unusual, Recurrent* pneumonia (*SPUR mnemonic*) should prompt investigation for immune deficiency states.

Bhutta ZA. Dealing with childhood pneumonia in developing countries: how can we make a difference? *Arch Dis Child.* 2007;92:286–8.

Bradley JS, Byington CL, Shah SS, *et al*. Pediatric Infectious Diseases Society and the Infectious Diseases Society of America. The management of community-acquired pneumonia in infants and children older than 3 months of age: clinical practice guidelines by the Pediatric Infectious Diseases Society and the Infectious Diseases Society of America. *Clin Infect Dis.* 2011;53:e25–76.

Carbonara S, Monno L, Longo B, Angarano G. Community-acquired pneumonia. *Curr Opin Pulm Med.* 2009;15:261–73.

Chisti MJ, Tebruegge M, La Vincente S, *et al*. Pneumonia in severely malnourished children in developing countries—mortality risk, aetiology and validity of WHO clinical signs: a systematic review. *Trop Med Int Health.* 2009;14:1173–89.

Durbin WJ, Stille C. Pneumonia. *Pediatr Rev.* 2008;29:147–58;159–60.

India Clinical Epidemiology Network (India CLEN) Task Force on Pneumonia. Rational use of antibiotics for pneumonia. *Indian Pediatr.* 2010;47:11–8.

Mathew JL, Patwari AK, Gupta P, *et al*. Acute respiratory infection and pneumonia in India: a systematic review of literature for advocacy and action: UNICEF-PHFI series on newborn and child health, India. *Indian Pediatr.* 2011;48:191–218.

10

Table 10.5 Common Causes of Persistent and Recurrent Pneumonia

I. Unilobar Pneumonia

1. Intraluminal obstruction
   - Foreign body
   - Endobronchial granulation, eg, tuberculosis
   - Bronchial tumor – Hemangioma, adenoma, carcinoid, etc.
2. Extra-luminal compression
   - Lymphadenopathy: Infectious (tuberculosis), or non-infectious (Hodgkin disease, sarcoidosis)
   - Vascular rings and slings
   - Esophageal foreign body
3. Structural abnormalities
   - *Congenital anomalies:* Congenital cystic adenomatoid malformation, congenital lobar emphysema, broncho-genic cyst, pulmonary sequestration
   - Bronchiectasis

II. Multilobar Pneumonia

1. Aspiration syndromes
   - *Impaired swallowing:* CNS or neuromuscular disorders, anatomic abnormalities like cleft palate, laryngeal cleft, etc.
   - *Regurgitation:* Tracheoesophageal fistula (TEF), or gastro-esophageal reflux (GER)
2. Infections
   - Drug resistant organisms or unusual organisms
   - Fungal pneumonia
   - *Pneumocystis jiroveci* pneumonia
   - Hydatidosis
3. Asthma
4. Allergic bronchopulmonary aspergillosis
5. Structural abnormalities
   - Tracheobronchomegaly
   - Cartilage deficiency/ incomplete cartilage
   - Segmental bronchomalacia
6. Congenital heart disease
   - Left to right shunt eg, ventricular septal defect, atrial septal defect, patent ductus arteriosus
7. Defense mechanism aberrations
   - Cystic fibrosis
   - Primary ciliary dyskinesia
8. Immunodeficiency disorders
   - *Primary*: Antibody deficiency, cell-mediated immuno deficiency, complement deficiency, phagocytic defect
   - *Secondary*: HIV, iatrogenic (steroids, immunosuppressive drugs, post-radiotherapy, etc.), malignancy (leukemia and lymphoma, etc.)
9. Others
   - Interstitial or diffuse lung disease
   - Pulmonary hemosiderosis
   - Hypersensitivity pneumonitis
   - Alpha-1 antitrypsin deficiency
   - Pulmonary alveolar proteinosis
   - Bronchopulmonary dysplasia

Pneumonia

1. Pneumonia may be classified as *simple* (broncho-pneumonia, lobar pneumonia) or *complicated* (effusions, empyema, abscesses, cavities, pneumo-thorax, etc.).
2. Viruses are frequent pathogens in children younger than 2 years.
3. Among the bacterial causes of pneumonia in young children, *Haemophilus influenzae* (below 2 years) and *Streptococcus pneumoniae* (after 5 years of age) are the most common.
4. Malnutrition, low birth weight, and lack of exclusive breastfeeding, predispose to pneumonia.
5. Children with pneumonia usually present with fever, tachypnea, productive cough, and chest pain.
6. Chest X-rays are not routinely necessary in patients being treated on OPD basis with a strong clinical suspicion of pneumonia.
7. Amoxicillin is the first line antibiotic in a dose of 50 mg/kg/day, given in two or three divided doses.
8. Children with severe or very severe pneumonia (as per WHO definitions) should be hospitalized for parenteral antibiotics and also offered supportive therapy.
9. Persistent or nonresolving pneumonia is defined as the persistence of symptoms and radiographic abnormalities in a child with lower respiratory tract infections for more than a month despite a course of adequate antibiotic therapy.
10. Recurrent pneumonia is defined as at least two distinct episodes of radiologically established pneumonia within the same year or 3 or more such episodes over any time period.

Thomson A, Harris M. Community-acquired pneumonia in children: what's new? *Thorax.* 2011;66:927–8.

Woods CR. Acute bacterial pneumonia in childhood in the current era. *Pediatr Ann.* 2008;37:694–702.

10.7 PARAPNEUMONIC EFFUSIONS AND EMPYEMA

Pleural effusions occurring in association with pneumonia are called *parapneumonic effusions*. Most pleural effusions associated with pneumonia resolve without any specific therapy directed towards the effusion. About 10% will require drainage or other specific intervention. These effusions are called complicated parapneumonic effusions; and they may develop into *empyema* (presence of frank pus in the pleura), if inadequately treated.

Etiology

Staphylococcus aureus, Streptococcus pneumoniae, H. influenzae, Streptococcus pyogenes, E. coli, Klebsiella, and *Pseudomonas* are the most commonly implicated organisms. Anaerobes and mixed infections are also reported.

S. pneumoniae is the commonest organism causing empyema in developed countries. *H.influenzae* pneumonia with empyema was common earlier but its incidence has decreased following immunization. In India, *Staphylococcus aureus* is the commonest organism at all ages, followed by *S.pneumoniae*. Frank tubercular empyema occurs rarely in about 2% cases of tubercular pleurisy. Group A Streptococcus is less commonly implicated but it can produce large pleural effusions that progress rapidly to produce empyema.

Pathophysiology

There are three stages in formation of empyema thoracis, ie, exudative, fibrinopurulent, and organising stage, as classified by American Thoracic Society.

1. *Exudative phase (Stage I)* Initial infection of the pleura with pathogenic organisms causes edema of the connective tissue layers within pleural membranes leading to exudation of proteinaceous fluid in the pleural cavity. The pH, glucose, and LDH levels in pleural fluid are normal. The deepest layers of the pleura are relatively impervious to infection so that the infection tends to localise in the pleural cavity itself. This stage is characterized by thin pleural fluid with relatively low cell count. The visceral pleura underlying the lung remain mobile. Most cases at this stage do well with antibiotic therapy alone. This stage lasts for 24–72 hours.

2. *Fibrinopurulent (Stage II)* If the infection stays unabated, the inflammation continues with formation of fibrin layers on the epithelial surface in the pleural cavity, particularly the parietal pleura. In the fibropurulent stage (stage II) the pleural fluid becomes thicker, turbid, proteinaceous, and cellular. The pH and glucose values decrease and LDH levels increase. This stage usually lasts for 7–10 days. Chest drainage is very important intervention for such children along with antibiotic therapy.

3. *Organisational stage (Stage III)* Finally, the thickened fibrinous layer gets organized and vascularized. There is growth of fibroblasts into the exudates on both the surfaces of pleura, resulting in a fibrinous layer. This may begin within 2 weeks but usually takes 4–6 weeks to develop a thick ring over the lung. This late stage usually is marked by flattened hemithorax with crowding of the overlying ribs and scoliosis. These children would often need surgical decortication.

Clinical Presentation

Most children present with a febrile illness of varying duration, associated with chills, chest pain, cough, and dyspnea. The pain typically gets worse on deep inspiration or cough.

On examination, the child has rapid breathing with signs of distress. Trachea and the rest of mediastinum is shifted (pushed) to the opposite side. The affected side of chest shows decreased movements with dull percussion note. The breath sounds are diminished over the involved area. Vocal resonance and vocal fremitus are also decreased. Pleural rub, a leathery rubbing sound, may be heard in the early stages. In chronic cases, the shoulder may be drooping on the affected side with a contracted rib cage due to pleural fibrosis.

Empyema usually occurs as a complication of pneumonia, therefore, a high index of suspicion should be kept in children with pneumonia who do not show significant response to antibiotics; or those who have a recent history of measles; or, those with co-existing staphylococcal infection elsewhere in body; and in infants who often have non-specific findings like lethargy, poor feeding, irritability, groaning, and rapid breathing.

Investigations

Chest Radiography

The pleural effusion is best detected by radiograph of the chest. Small amounts may be detected on a lateral decubitus film. X-ray of chest commonly shows a linear opacity along the lung and chest wall. The costophrenic angle is blunted. In massive effusion, the whole hemithorax may be opaque with shift of the mediastinum to opposite side. It is not possible to differentiate between empyema and a parapneumonic effusion on plain chest radiography.

Ultrasonography is useful in diagnosing effusion, which is seen as hyperechoic collection between lung and chest wall. It is particularly useful in detecting loculated effusion as it gives better information about the size, site, and echogenicity of fluid. Transudates are usually anechoic while exudates are echoic. Ultrasonography is useful in differentiating pneumonia from fluid collection in children with an opacified lung field on chest radiograph. It is also a good modality to differentiate effusion from pleural thickening, when the pleural tap is dry.

CT of chest is useful if diagnosis is still not certain or if surgical intervention is planned for a non-resolving empyema or due to a persistent bronchopleural fistula.

Pleural Fluid

Pleural fluid should be sampled in every case to find its nature and to determine the cause. Pleural fluid should be analysed for pH, glucose, protein and lactic dehydrogenase (LDH). Microscopic examination is essential to see the cells in pleural fluid. Polymorphonuclear predominance suggests an empyema, while lymphocytic predominance suggests tuberculosis. However, these differences are not diagnostic of either. Pleural fluid should also be sent for Gram stain, culture and sensitivity for pyogenic organisms.

The effusion should be categorized as either a *transudate* (pleural fluid protein <3 g/dL, low LDH, low sugar, few cells) or *exudate* (pleural fluid protein >3 g/dL, cell count >5000 per cubic mm, pleural serum LDH ratio >0.6, and a pleural pH of less than 7.3). Exudative fluid tends to gel or form a cobweb on standing. A straw colored exudate in a child with long history of symptoms is usually due to tuberculosis, the acute pyogenic cases usually have thin or thick pus.

Complicated parapneumonic effusion is characterized by pH <7.1, glucose <40 mg/dL, proteins >3 g/dL, and LDH >1000 IU/L. This distinction is important because complicated effusions (empyema) are best managed by drainage.

Complications of Empyema

Pyopneumothorax Pneumothorax associated with complicated parapneumonic effusion or pyothorax often results from the rupture of a peripheral pulmonary microabscess in the pleural cavity. Large air escape may cause tension pneumothorax, with significant respiratory distress.

As this type of pneumothorax is intercurrent with pleural infection, the treatment is the same as that for complicated

10

parapneumonic effusion at the acute stage, requiring drainage by a large-bore chest tube. The total drainage of the pleural material, with complete expansion of the lung, is usually enough to close the leakage area of the pulmonary parenchyma.

Bronchopleural fistula This is a sinus tract between the bronchus and the pleural space that may result as a complication of pleuropulmonary infections and can develop at any point of time during the course of illness. Acute respiratory distress due to tension pneumothorax may occur if a large fistula develops. The diagnosis must be suspected when there is a constant release of air in under water seal through the chest tube; or there is a new or increasing air-fluid level on chest radiographs, if patient has no chest tube in place.

Medical management includes dependent drainage and reduction of the pleural space, antibiotics, and nutritional supplementation. Surgical closure of the fistula is attempted when the medical management fails.

Treatment	Empyema

The two important decisions to be made under these circumstances are (a) choosing appropriate antibiotics, and (b) whether intervention, if any, is required for draining the effusion.

- *If the pleural fluid aspirate is frank pus,* the preferred therapy is injectable cloxacillin with ceftriaxone; or co-amoxiclav alone. Vancomycin may be used instead of cloxacillin in non-responders suspected to have methicillin resistant staphylococcal infection.
- These children need pleural drainage and a *chest tube drain with under water seal* should be instituted without delay.
- The chest tube under water seal should be placed in the most dependent part or the largest loculation.
- More than one tube insertions may be required if there are multiple significant loculations.
- The bag should be emptied out regularly so that the pressure gradient added by the drained pus does not impair further drainage from the pleural space. In addition, this help in assessing the average daily drainage.
- The tube is usually removed when the daily drainage becomes thinner, is less than 30 mL per day for 2–3 days, and there is no air leak on spontaneous breathing or coughing.
- A chest skiagram is done prior to removal of the tube to confirm that underlying lung has expanded.
- While one should switch to oral antibiotics (where feasible) once the toxemia and fever starts settling and the tube drain comes out (usually about 10–14 days), but the therapy should continue for a total duration of 4–6 weeks.
- *Intrapleural fibrinolytics* Streptokinase, urokinase, and alteplase can be used to facilitate drainage in thick loculated empyema.
- *Supportive treatment* It includes oxygen (if SpO_2 <92%), fluid therapy (if dehydrated or unable to drink), analgesics (for pain at chest tube site), and antipyretics (for fever).

The clinical response to therapy should be assessed with parameters such as decrease in fever, normalization of laboratory parameters such as total leukocyte count, C-reactive protein, decrease in drain volume, clearing in chest X-ray, and improvement in general well-being of patient.

Surgical Management

Surgery is indicated in cases with failure of medical therapy (persisting sepsis and large pleural collection), chronic empyema, and persistent bronchopleural fistula. Surgical modalities in use include: (*i*) Video-assisted thoracoscopic surgery (VATS); and (*ii*) open thoracotomy.

Video assisted thoracoscopic surgery (VATS) It is a minimally invasive procedure, which allows washing fibrin out of the pleural cavity and placing a well-located chest tube under direct visualization. If performed at an early stage, it reduces the need for other surgical procedures.

It is especially recommended for complicated parapneumonic effusion at the fibrinopurulent stage, since it allows breaking down the adhesions and removing fibrin and the infected material, with the release of all pulmonary surfaces, including the diaphragmatic ones, allowing complete reexpansion of lung. It has been shown in studies that it significantly reduces the need for pulmonary resection, duration of chest drainage and the hospital stay.

Thoracotomy The pleural drainage of the empyema can be carried out by thoracotomy, which is useful for the drainage of the pleural fluid, breakdown of adhesions and removal of fibrin and, when necessary, resection of the necrotic lung tissue, or bronchopleural fistula. This surgical procedure was called decortication in the past. Thoracotomy was recommended for effusions at the fibrinopurulent or organizational stages, which could be performed by classical posterolateral incision, or by mini-thoracotomy. Due to complications such as deformity of the chest wall, significant blood loss and higher probability of resection of the pulmonary parenchyma and of the bronchopleural fistula, or postoperative pneumonia, the procedure is currently performed only in cases of complicated effusion at the organizational stage.

Pleurostomy It has been used in children with complicated effusion at the organizational stage, with a poor health state, for whom anesthesia or a large surgery is of high risk. This procedure should only be used after confirming that the lung is adhered and encased, with no risk of collapse after the pleural cavity is opened. This opening allows the drainage of secretions, washing of the pleural cavity and gradual pulmonary re-expansion. Another advantage of this method is the possibility of earlier discharge from hospital. Nevertheless, it is important that the pleural opening be located on the lowermost part of the fluid cavity, in order to avoid the accumulation of intrathoracic secretion below the pleurostomy level.

Becker A, Amantéa SL, Fraga JC, Zanella MI. Impact of antibiotic therapy on laboratory analysis of parapneumonic pleural fluid in children. *J Pediatr Surg.* 2011;46:452–7.

Hawkins JA, Scaife ES, Hillman ND, Feola GP. Current treatment of pediatric empyema. *Semin Thorac Cardiovasc Surg.* 2004;16:196–200.

Hilliard TN, Henderson AJ, Langton Hewer SC. Management of parapneumonic effusion and empyema. *Arch Dis Child.* 2003;88:915–7.

Krenke K, Peradzyñska J, Lange J, *et al.* Local treatment of empyema in children: a systematic review of randomized controlled trials. *Acta Paediatr.* 2010;99:1449–53.

Narayan Prasad A. Intrapleural fibrinolytic therapy in a neonate. *Indian J Pediatr.* 2011;78:1154–6.

Nyambat B, Kilgore PE, Yong DE, *et al.* Survey of childhood empyema in Asia: implications for detecting the unmeasured burden of culture-negative bacterial disease. *BMC Infect Dis.* 200811;8:90.

Padman R, King KA, Iqbal S, Wolfson PJ. Parapneumonic effusion and empyema in children: retrospective review of the duPont experience. *Clin Pediatr.* 2007;46:518–22.

| Case Study | Empyema Thoracis |

A 3-year-old girl weighing 12 kg presented to the hospital emergency with history of fever, cough, vomiting and decreased appetite for 15 days. She had received some oral drugs for 10 days but her symptoms continued to persist. She had developed difficulty in breathing and left sided chest pain for the last 2 days. She is taking rapid but short breaths. She prefers to lie on the left side. Her pain increases on coughing.

Outline the differential diagnoses based on history. Justify your approach.

The symptoms of fever, cough and chest pain indicate respiratory illness, which has been progressive (chest pain and breathing difficulty for two days) and of a long duration with significant severity (decreased oral acceptance and breathing difficulty), therefore, the most probable diagnosis would be *severe pneumonia*. Difficulty in breathing and chest pain on left side indicate either synpneumonic effusion or pneumothorax on left side. Tuberculosis should also be kept as a differential diagnosis, since it may also present with similar features in highly endemic areas.

On examination, she was lethargic, had a temperature of 39° C, pulse rate of 120/min and the blood pressure was 96/50 mm Hg. The respiratory rate was 58/min and spO$_2$ was 85%. Child had nasal flaring, with significant chest indrawing. Trachea was shifted to right. The left side of the chest appeared bulging when inspected from the foot end of the patient lying supine. The chest movements were decreased on the left side and it was stony dull to percussion. Auscultation revealed decreased breath sounds with decreased vocal resonance on left side. The heart sounds were better heard on the right side of the chest suggesting a shift of the mediastinum.

What is the most probable diagnosis? Justify.

The shifting of mediastinum to right side, increased left hemithoracic volume (bulge) with decreased chest movements, suggest that the lesion is on the left side. On percussion, the left side was stony dull and auscultation revealed ipsilateral decrease in breath sounds. All these findings suggest a left sided pleural effusion. Looking at the poor general condition of the patient and features of severe respiratory distress (tachypnea, chest indrawing, hypoxia and lethargy) there is a high likelihood of pyogenic infection.

List the investigations required to confirm the diagnosis, in order of priority.

1. Chest skiagram in erect posture.
2. Pleural tap and fluid examination: Gross and microscopic examination. Gram staining, bacteriological culture; and biochemical examination.
3. Complete hemogram including differential leukocyte count.
4. Blood culture.

Describe the initial management of this child.

This child has significant respiratory distress and hypoxemia. She should be admitted and immediately put on oxygen supplementation to maintain SpO$_2$ above 92%. She will need supportive therapy in form of antipyretics like paracetamol and maintenance intravenous fluids. Further specific treatment shall be guided by the pleural fluid examination.

On pleural tapping, frank thick pus was aspirated and sent for microbiological testing.

Outline the specific therapeutic plan for this child.

This child has empyema. The pus in the pleural cavity should be drained with an intercostal thoracostomy tube using an under water drainage. She should be given injectable antibiotics covering for staphylococcal infection, eg, a combination of cloxacillin/amoxyclavulinic acid with an aminoglycoside (gentamicin or amikacin). Antibiotic therapy shall need to be given for 4–6 weeks, of which initial 10–14 days therapy should be intravenous. Chest tube can be removed when the drainage is less than 20–30 mL per day for two consecutive days and there is no suggestion of a bronchopleural fistula. A nutritious diet with high protein is given.

Revision Point

Empyema

1. Empyema is mostly a complication of bacterial pneumonia.
2. *Staphylococcus aureus* is the most common causative pathogen.
3. Very young children may present with predominantly abdominal signs and symptoms.
4. Ultrasonography is a better modality than CT scan to differentiate free from loculated fluid.
5. Thoracocentesis is ultimately required for differentiation of uninfected parapneumonic effusion from empyema.
6. Initial therapy consists of IV cloxacillin and gentamicin. Total duration of treatment is 4–6 weeks.
7. Intercostal drainage with a chest tube is the mainstay of therapy

Schneider CR, Gauderer MW, Blackhurst D, *et al.* Video-assisted thoracoscopic surgery as a primary intervention in pediatric-parapneumonic effusion and empyema. *Am Surg.* 2010;76:957–61.

Soares P, Barreira J, Pissarra S, *et al.* Pediatric parapneumonic pleural effusions: experience in a university central hospital. *Rev Port Pneumol.* 2009;15:241–59.

Utine GE, Ozcelik U, Yalcin E, *et al.* Childhood parapneumonic effusions: biochemical and inflammatory markers. *Chest.* 2005; 128:1436–41.

10.8 APPROACH TO A CHILD WITH WHEEZE

Wheeze is a musical high-pitched sound resulting from oscillations in narrowed airways. Wheezing is heard mostly during expiration as a result of critical airway obstruction.
- *Polyphonic wheezing* It refers to musical sounds of varied pitch, due to widespread but variable narrowing of the airways as seen in bronchiolitis, bronchitis, and bronchial asthma.

10

- *Monophonic wheezing* It refers to a single-pitch sound produced during expiration, due to localized obstruction of the larger airways, as in foreign body or extraluminal compression of the airway, eg, due to enlarged lymph node or vascular rings, etc.

Pathophysiology

Wheeze is produced by oscillation of the airway walls when their lumen is severely compromised. Younger children (under 5 years of age) are more prone to wheezing due to several causes. As the resistance to airflow through a tube is inversely related to the fourth power of the tube's radius, smaller children can have wheeze with even a marginal narrowing of their airways. The higher compliance of the chest wall in younger children results in collapse of the intrathoracic airways due to the inward pressure produced in expiration. The airway compliance in younger children is further increased by the different tones of smooth muscle and cartilage rings of the trachea.

Risk Factors associated with Early or Preschool Wheezing

These include influences of certain genes (*ORMDL3* and *GSDMB* genes on chromosome 17q21), prenatal environment (uncontrolled maternal asthma or maternal smoking); and postnatal environment (rapid weight gain in early infancy, exposure to tobacco smoke or traffic-related particles, endotoxins, paracetamol, day care attendance and older siblings). Having older siblings or attending day care increases the chances of respiratory viral infections (Respiratory syncytial virus and human Rhinovirus being the most common viruses), thus increasing the risk of preschool wheezing.

Etiology

Most wheezing in infants is caused by infection (generally bronchiolitis), but many other entities can manifest with wheezing, as listed below:

1. Infection
   - *Viral* Respiratory syncytial virus (RSV), parainfluenza virus, influenza virus, rhinovirus C, and human metapneumovirus
   - *Bacterial* *Streptococcus pneumoniae*, *Chlamydia trachomatis*, *Mycoplasma*, tuberculosis
2. Asthma
3. Anatomic abnormalities
   - *Central airway abnormalities*: Laryngomalacia, tracheomalacia, bronchomalacia
   - *Extrinsic airway anomalies* resulting in airway compression: Mediastinal lymphadenopathy from tuberculosis or tumor, vascular ring or sling, mediastinal mass or tumor, duplication cyst, and esophageal foreign body
4. *Mucociliary clearance disorders* Cystic fibrosis, primary ciliary dyskinesias, bronchiectasis
5. *Aspiration syndromes* Gastroesophageal reflux disease (GERD)
6. *Others* Congenital heart disease with left-to-right shunt (increased pulmonary edema), foreign body.

Phenotypes of Wheezers

The most common phenotype seen in children is *"episodic viral wheeze"* where viral respiratory infection results in wheezing and respiratory distress, but there are no interval symptoms. The other phenotype is labeled as *multi-trigger wheeze* (preschool asthma). Children with this phenotype have clinical behavior similar to asthma and they have exacerbations in response to multiple triggers (viral infections, cold air, crying, exercise). They also have interval symptoms and commonly have family history of atopy.

Clinical Assessment of a Child with Wheeze

- *Triggers* Viral infections of the respiratory tract are the most common predisposing factors leading to airway obstruction and wheeze. This phenomenon of wheeze associated respiratory infection is not uniquely associated with viral infections; and can also be seen with bacterial infections of lower respiratory tract. All these disorders are collectively termed as wheeze associated lower respiratory tract infections (WALRI). Other triggers include running, laughing, crying, cold weather, fumes, and dust, *etc*. (usually seen in asthma).
- *Type of cough* A spasmodic cough which is more at night or in early morning, is characteristic of wheezy disorders. In a few cases, isolated spasmodic cough may be the only indication of a wheezy disorder (cough variant asthma).
- *Age of onset* and *duration of wheezing* Onset of wheezing in infancy indicates bronchiolitis, WALRI, GERD, or congenital heart disease. While children with severe and persistent asthma can present early, yet any child with infantile onset should be diligently assessed for asthma mimickers like congenital airway malformations, vascular ring, GERD, and cystic fibrosis. Asthma is, however, the most frequent cause of recurrent wheezing in children after five years of age.
- *Associated symptoms* Vomiting/regurgitation of feeds suggests GERD. History of atopy, eczema, or rhinitis should alert to possibility of asthma.
- *Birth history* Need for prolonged ventilation or oxygen therapy in neonatal period can predispose to chronic lung disease of infancy which can present with tachypnea with crackles and wheeze.
- *Past history* Recurrent respiratory tract infections, malabsorption, failure to thrive suggest immuno-deficiency or mucociliary disorders including cystic fibrosis or α-1 antitrypsin deficiency.
- *Family history* Ask for history suggestive of asthma, cystic fibrosis, tuberculosis in siblings, parents, and grandparents.
- *Social history* Parental smoking habits, overcrowding at home, presence of pets, moulds, cockroaches should be enquired for.
- *Physical examination* Record vitals, oxygen saturation (SpO$_2$), signs of respiratory distress including character of wheeze, pulsus paradoxus, and timing and presence of stridor. Look for signs of atopy: Dermatitis, sneezing, hives, boggy turbinates, *etc*.
- *Presence of atypical features* like clubbing, recurrent multisystemic infections, chronic diarrhea, failure to thrive, feeding difficulties, recurrent or persistent radiological shadows, localized monophonic wheeze, *etc*. should alert to a possibility of non-asthmatic wheezing.

Differential Diagnosis

In the first 2 years of life, wheezing is mostly caused by acute viral respiratory infections such as bronchiolitis and WALRI. After first 2 years of age, wheezing is often due to asthma particularly if the child has a definite history of afebrile episodes. Sometimes children with pneumonia present with wheeze. It is important to consider pneumonia as an alternative diagnosis, particularly in the first 2 years of life. The differential diagnoses of the common causes of wheezing and their salient features are detailed below:

1. Asthma

- History of recurrent wheeze, some unrelated to coughs and colds
- Family or personal history of asthma/eczema/hay fever
- Hyperinflation of the chest and prolonged expiration
- Reduced air entry (if very severe airway obstruction)
- Good response to bronchodilators

2. Bronchiolitis

- First episode of wheeze in a child aged <2 years
- Wheeze episode at time of seasonal bronchiolitis
- Hyperinflation of the chest and prolonged expiration
- Reduced air entry (if very severe, airway obstruction)
- Poor/no response to bronchodilators

3. Wheeze associated with Lower Respiratory Cough or Cold

- Wheeze always related to coughs and colds
- No family or personal history of asthma/eczema/hay fever
- Prolonged expiration
- Good response to bronchodilators

4. Foreign Body

- History of sudden onset of choking or wheezing
- Wheeze may be unilateral
- Air trapping with hyper-resonance and mediastinal shift
- Signs of lung collapse: Reduced air entry and impaired percussion note
- No response to bronchodilators

5. Pneumonia

- Fever
- Cough with fast breathing
- Lower chest wall indrawing
- Crackles or bronchial breathing on auscultation

Investigations

- *Chest X-ray* A posteroanterior view might reveal infiltrates in a child having severe respiratory distress. Hyperinflation is common in bronchiolitis, asthma, and viral pneumonia. Signs of chronic diseases and airway compression may be found in asthma mimickers. In a child with repeated wheeze, there is no need for a chest radiograph with every episode. Radiographs are preferred only in the initial assessment for diagnosis or when the clinical evidence is contradictory.
- *Response to bronchodilator* A trial of bronchodilator may be diagnostic as well as therapeutic because it can reverse conditions such as WALRI and asthma but will not affect a fixed obstruction. Bronchodilators potentially can worsen a case of wheezing caused by tracheal or bronchial malacia.
- *Sweat chloride test* to evaluate for cystic fibrosis.
- *Bronchoscopy* Diagnostic and therapeutic for foreign body.
- *Radionuclide studies* (GI scintiscan) or 24-hour esophageal pH monitoring for gastroesophageal reflux disease.
- *Upper gastrointestinal contrast X-rays* to look for extrinsic airway compression as seen with a vascular ring.

Management

Treatment depends on the underlying etiology, however, the first and foremost priority is establishing airway and breathing and maintaining oxygenation. Presence of severe respiratory distress warrants hospitalization.

Chung KF, Bolser D, Davenport P, et al. Semantics and types of cough. *Pulm Pharmacol Ther.* 2009;22:139–42.

de Benedictis FM, Bush A. Infantile wheeze: rethinking dogma. *Arch Dis Child.* 2016 Oct 4.[Epub ahead of print]

Ducharme FM, Tse SM, Chauhan B. Diagnosis, management, and prognosis of preschool wheeze. *Lancet.* 2014;383:1593–604.

Eigen H. Differential diagnosis and treatment of wheezing and asthma in young children. *Clin Pediatr.* 2008;47:735–43.

Granell R, Henderson AJ, Timpson N, et al. Examination of the relationship between variation at 17q21 and childhood wheeze phenotypes. *J Allergy Clin Immunol.* 2013; 131: 685–94.

Lasso-Pirot A, Delgado-Villalta S, Spanier AJ. Early childhood wheezers: identifying asthma in later life. *J Asthma Allergy.* 2015;8:63–73.

Scott M, Kurukulaaratchy RJ, Arshad SH. Definitions are important and not all wheeze is asthma. *Thorax.* 2011;66:633; 633–4.

Shah D, Gupta P. Pertinent issues in diagnosis and management of wheezing in under-five children at community level. *Indian Pediatr.* 2010;47:56–60.

Tenero L, Piazza M, Piacentini G. Recurrent wheezing in children. *Transl Pediatr.* 2016;5:31–6.

Weiss LN. The diagnosis of wheezing in children. *Am Fam Physician.* 2008;77:1109–14.

Wing A. "Why does he wheeze?": wheezing and asthma in young children. *J Fam Health Care.* 2006;16:87–9.

10.9 BRONCHIOLITIS

Bronchiolitis is a self-limiting condition caused by respiratory syncytial virus (RSV) infection, in children between 2 months and 2 years of age. The disease preceded by cough, cold and rhinitis, is characterized by presence of fever, rapid breathing with signs of airway obstruction, wheezing, and hyperinflation of lungs.

Etiology

Respiratory syncitial virus (RSV) is the most common underlying viral infection. Other viruses, eg, influenza, parainfluenza, adenovirus, coronaviruses, and rhinoviruses have also been implicated in children with bronchiolitis.

Epidemiology

RSV infection is severe in boys, particularly those between 2 and 5 months of age. Poverty, crowding, urban environment, exposure to cigarette/ tobacco smoke, prematurity, chronic lung disease like bronchopulmonary dysplasia, and cystic fibrosis, and underlying heart disease predispose to severe disease. Most cases occur in winters.

10

RSV infection spreads more often due to large droplets than the small particle aerosol. The virus can remain in large droplets for several hours contaminating fomites like table tops, nebulizing chambers, towels and tap hands, etc. Hence, handborne infection control measures are relevant to nosocomial and intrafamilial spread just as with rhinovirus.

Pathogenesis

The incubation period is about 4 days and the virus is excreted for variable periods (0–3 weeks). The inflammation typically involves smaller bronchi and respiratory bronchioles causing necrosis and destruction of ciliary epithelium. There is inflammatory infiltration of the peribronchiolar tissue. Edema and congestion of submucosa occur with increased mucus production.

Clinical Presentation

The initial symptoms are of an upper respiratory tract viral infection, such as fever, nasal obstruction, rhinorrhea, and an irritating cough. Within next 4–6 days, the child develops respiratory distress, increased cough, and sometimes an audible wheeze. Sicker infants report with poor feeding and lethargy. Most infants with bronchiolitis present with significant tachypnea, mild-to-moderate hypoxia, and visible signs of respiratory distress, such as nasal flaring and retractions.

On examination, chest is often overexpanded. The liver and spleen are palpable as they get pushed down by overinflated lungs. There typically is an audible or auscultable wheeze, crackles or rhonchi, and poor air movement. The disease has a waxing and waning course which can make the family very anxious. Based on the ability to feed, the respiratory effort, and oxygen saturation, the disease is classified as mild, moderate, or severe.

I. Mild Bronchiolitis

- Normal ability to feed
- Little or no respiratory distress
- Oxygen saturation 95% or more
- Fever >38.5° C, in ~50% of infants

II. Moderate Bronchiolitis

- Can appear short of breath during feeding
- Moderate respiratory distress, with some chest wall retractions, nasal flaring
- Usually hypoxemic, corrected to SaO_2 >95% by oxygen supplementation

III. Severe Bronchiolitis

- May be lethargic, or unable to feed
- Severe distress, with marked chest wall retractions, nasal flaring, and grunting
- May have increasingly frequent or prolonged apneic episodes
- Have hypoxemia, which usually may not be corrected by supplemental oxygen.

Diagnosis

Diagnosis is essentially clinical and should be suspected in child between 2 month and 2 years of age, who for the first time presents with an episode that starts with upper respiratory tract infection and later develops findings consistent with bronchiolitis, including wheezing, and respiratory distress with lower chest retraction. Investigations contribute little. Chest X-ray is indicated only if moderate (or worse) respiratory difficulty is present, or in case of a diagnostic uncertainty. The radiographic findings of bronchiolitis include hyperinflation and patchy infiltrates that are typically migratory. X-ray finding are attributable to postobstructive atelectasis and peribronchial cuffing.

Differential Diagnosis

Congenital anomalies, such as vascular ring, congenital heart disease, gastroesophageal reflux, aspiration pneumonia or foreign body aspiration can mimic the symptoms of bronchiolitis. Airway malacia (tracheomalacia and/or bronchomalacia) can be difficult to differentiate from bronchiolitis.

Treatment	Bronchiolitis

Most mild cases need only symptomatic supportive therapy in form of continued feeding, antipyretics, nasal clearance, and occasionally local decongestants. In moderate to severe cases, where oxygen saturation is less than 92% or there is a combination of clinically significant respiratory distress, a respiratory rate above 60 per minute, and difficulty in feeding—oxygenation is the mainstay of treatment.

1. *Humidified oxygen*
Oxygen should be administered by a nasopharyngeal cannula or mask kept little away from the face, if the infant does not tolerate the conventional masks, hoods, or prongs. As far as possible, one should opt to use the least distressful and non-threatening manner of giving oxygen. Persistent hypoxemia with or without severe distress, despite high oxygen flow, requires immediate assessment for ventilator assistance.

2. *Supportive therapy*
Place the child in sitting posture or against the shoulder of the mother with head and chest elevated at 30° with neck extended. Oral and nasal secretions should be frequently suctioned.

3. *Fluid therapy*
Oral feeding is encouraged. Intravenous fluid (maintenance therapy) should be administered in children who cannot feed or have moderate-to-severe respiratory distress, marked tachypnea (>60/min), or apnea. Regular maintenance IV fluids are administered.

4. *Drugs*
- The role of bronchodilators in acute bronchiolitis is controversial. Since mucosal edema is an important component of airway obstruction in bronchiolitis, a combined α-adrenergic and β-adrenergic agonist, such as epinephrine may be useful.
- Response to bronchodilators is erratic and unpredictable. A child unresponsive to supportive management and adrenaline nebulization may be given a trial of inhaled salbutamol. Further continuation depends on response to the initial

dosages. Unlike asthma, the lack of response should not prompt more aggressive bronchodilator therapy. Recently, nebulized (3%) hypertonic saline has been shown to have some benefit.

- Irritability is often due to hypoxia and improves with oxygen. Sedatives should not to be used, as they can result in respiratory depression.
- ICU management will be needed if there is progression to severe respiratory distress or any significant apneic episodes or persistent desaturation despite oxygen.
- There is no role of RSV immunoglobulin during acute episodes.
- RSV is the most common cause of bronchiolitis but specific antiviral therapy (ribavirin) of symptomatic infants has been of limited value. It has been used for infants with congenital heart disease or chronic lung disease without any convincing evidence of benefit.
- Antibiotics and steroids are not indicated.

Discharge

An infant is considered ready for discharge if there is no need of supplemental oxygen for at least 10 hours, there is minimal or no chest recession, normal feeding has been resumed, and the child is active.

Prognosis

Case fatality rate is less than 1 percent. Death occurs due to respiratory failure or apnea. The symptoms usually persist for a median of 12 days. The incidence of subsequent wheezing is higher in children who have had bronchiolitis.

Prevention

- Pooled hyperimmune RSV specific intravenous gammaglobulin (RSV IgG) and palivizumab (a monoclonal antibody, given IM) lowers the severity and incidence of acute bronchiolitis in children with history of prematurity; and those with concomitant chronic lung disease, or congenital heart defect.
- Palivizumab is a humanized monoclonal antibody-produced by recombinant DNA technology—used in the prevention of respiratory syncytial virus (RSV) infections. It is recommended for infants that are high-risk because of prematurity or other medical problems such as

Revision Point

Bronchiolitis

1. Bronchiolitis is a clinical syndrome in children less than 2 years of age characterized by fever, cough, cold, tachypnea and/or wheezing.
2. Bronchiolitis is primarily caused by respiratory syncytial virus.
3. Risk factors for severe disease and/or complications include gestational age less than 37 weeks, age less than 12 weeks, chronic pulmonary disease, congenital and anatomic defects of the airways, congenital heart disease, immunodeficiency and neurologic disease.
4. Bronchiolitis is diagnosed clinically. Chest radiographs and laboratory tests are not routinely indicated.
5. Management is supportive. Bronchodilators may work in some patients.

significant lung or congenital heart disease. It reduces the risk of hospitalization due to RSV infection by about half. Palivizumab is used only for prevention, not for treatment, and once initiated for a given RSV season (usually November–March), it needs to be continued for the full duration of that season. It is an expensive treatment, given as once a month intramuscular (IM) injection.

Dawson-Caswell M, Muncie HL Jr. Respiratory syncytial virus infection in children. *Am Fam Physician*. 2011;83:141–6.

Fitzgerald DA. Preventing RSV bronchiolitis in vulnerable infants: the role of palivizumab. *Paediatr Respir Rev*. 2009;10:143–7.

Fitzgerald DA. Viral bronchiolitis for the clinician. *J Paediatr Child Health*. 2011;47:160–6.

Gadomski AM, Brower M. Bronchodilators for bronchiolitis. *Cochrane Database Syst Rev*. 2010;12:CD001266.

Hartling L, Bialy LM, Vandermeer B. Epinephrine for bronchiolitis. *Cochrane Database Syst Rev*. 2011;6:CD003123.

Hartling L, Fernandes RM, Bialy L, *et al*. Steroids and bronchodilators for acute bronchiolitis in the first two years of life: systematic review and meta-analysis. *BMJ*. 2011;342:d1714.

Schuh S. Update on management of bronchiolitis. *Curr Opin Pediatr*. 2011;23:110/4.

Turner T, Wilkinson F, Harris C, Mazza D; Health for Kids Guideline Development Group. Evidence based guideline for the management of bronchiolitis. *Aust Fam Physician*. 2008;37:6–13.

Zhang L, Mendoza-Sassi RA, Wainwright C, Klassen TP. Nebulized hypertonic saline solution for acute bronchiolitis in infants. *Cochrane Database Syst Rev*. 2008;4:CD006458.

10.10 BRONCHIAL ASTHMA

Asthma is a chronic inflammatory condition of the airways associated with variable airflow obstruction that is often reversible. It is characterized by recurrent episodes of wheezing, cough, and difficulty in breathing, which respond to treatment with bronchodilators and anti-inflammatory drugs. Any child with more than 3 episodes of wheezing is likely to have asthma particularly in the presence of personal or family history of atopy.

Etiology

Although the etiopathogenesis of asthma is not clear, it may be postulated that it results from early environmental exposures in a genetically predisposed individual. Respiratory exposures include inhaled allergens, respiratory viral infections, and chemical and biologic air pollutants such as environmental tobacco smoke.

In the predisposed host, immune responses to these common exposures can be a stimulus for prolonged, pathogenic inflammation and aberrant repair of injured airway tissues, making the airways hyperresponsive. These pathogenic processes in the growing lung during early life adversely affect growth and differentiation of airways, leading to alteration of airways at mature ages. Once asthma has developed, ongoing exposures appear to worsen it, and increase the risk of severe exacerbations.

Clinical symptoms of asthma may be produced following viral infections or exposure to allergens. Infection or an allergen causes narrowing of the airways by three mechanisms:

  i. Contraction of the smooth muscles surrounding the airways in the lung (bronchospasm);
 ii. Swelling of the mucosal lining of the airways; and
iii. Increased secretions in the lumen of the airways.

10

Genetic predisposition is an important factor for asthma. Therefore, a family history of asthma should be taken in every child who presents with wheezing. The airways become narrow in response to moulds, dustmite, etc. and pollutants (dust, smoke, etc.) Apart from allergens, wheezing can get precipitated in response to viral infections, exercise and certain drugs.

The common triggers for inducing asthma are physical exertion and hyperventilation (laughing), cold or dry air, airway irritants (eg, smoke) and viral infections (eg, RSV, rhinovirus, adenovirus).

The risk factors for persistent childhood asthma are as follows:
- Parental asthma
- Allergy (allergic rhinitis, atopic dermatitis, food allergy)
- Wheezing apart from colds
- Bronchiolitis or pneumonia requiring treatment
- Male gender
- Low birth weight
- Environmental tobacco exposure

Clinical Manifestations

The classical triad of cough, wheeze, and breathlessness need not be present in all children with asthma. The most common symptoms of asthma are intermittent dry cough and expiratory wheezing. There may be associated shortness of breath and chest tightness or pain. The symptoms are aggravated at night or early morning, and with physical activity such as running. The parents often give a history of symptomatic improvement with bronchodilator treatment.

Physical examination reveals prolonged expiration or wheezing with or without signs of respiratory distress. Crackles may be heard due to presence of mucus and inflammatory exudate. Presence of crackles therefore does not always constitute a proof of pneumonia or superadded infection and, thus does not by itself justify antibiotic therapy. Children with bacterial infections have toxic look and may have spiking fever with chills. In severe exacerbations, the greater extent of airways obstruction causes labored breathing and respiratory distress. In extreme conditions, airflow may be so limited that wheezing may not be heard (referred to as silent chest).

However, an asthmatic child may present without abnormal signs, emphasizing the importance of the medical history in diagnosing asthma. Deeper breaths can sometimes elicit otherwise undetectable wheezing. In clinic, quick resolution (within 10 min) or convincing improvement in symptoms and signs of asthma with administration of a short-acting inhaled β-agonist is supportive of the diagnosis of asthma.

Differential Diagnosis

The common conditions masquerading as asthma include: allergic rhinosinusitis; laryngotracheobronchomalacia; vocal cord dysfunction; foreign body aspiration; and gastro-esophageal reflux disease.

Investigations

1. *Hemogram* Eosinophilia may be found in 5–10% cases.
2. *X-ray chest* It is done in the initial visit to rule out other conditions that can mimic as asthma.

3. *Spirometry* It helps in demonstration of the degree of reversible airflow obstruction
4. *Peak expiratory flow rate (PEFR)* It has a limited role in the diagnosis of asthma but can be used in the follow up to assess the response to long term management.
5. *Serum IgE, RAST, skin allergy testing* These tests help in diagnosis of atopy and not asthma. There role is limited because of the cumbersome nature of the tests and costs involved.
6. *Fractional exhaled nitric oxide (FeNO)* It is used as a marker of airway inflammation and has been used for evaluation of difficult asthma.

Treatment	Acute Asthmatic Episode

The first step in treating acute asthmatic episode is to assess the severity of the episode. The types of drug used, and their doses are largely governed by the severity of the attack.

Red Flag Signs
Step 1 is to look for presence of Red Flag signs (**Box 10.3**). If 'Red flag' signs are absent, grade the severity of exacerbation using pulmonary score as given in **Table 10.6.**

Box 10.3 Red Flag Signs of Asthma
1. Altered sensorium (drowsy or very agitated)
2. Bradycardia
3. Poor pulse volume
4. Cyanosis
5. Excessive use of accessory muscles or a state of exhaustion
6. Vocalization limited to 1–2 words
7. Silent chest on auscultation
8. SpO$_2$ on room air <92%

A. Mild Attack
Mainstay of drug therapy includes rapidly acting bronchodilators and steroids (Fig. 10.4).

Alert child with no cyanosis and no signs of severe respiratory distress The acute episode is managed by administration of inhaled salbutamol either by nebulization or by metered dose inhaler (MDI) with spacer. Nebulized salbutamol is given as 2.5 mg per dose and 3 such doses are given at 20 min intervals. Alternatively, 4–5 puffs of salbutamol metered dose inhaler can be given instead of a nebulized dose in the same fashion (one puff doses, 3–4 min apart). The child should be reassessed after 1 hour for resolution of respiratory distress and rhonchi on auscultation of chest.

- *If the respiratory distress has resolved completely*, and there are occasional or no rhonchi on auscultation, this is considered as a *good response* and the child should be kept under observation for the next 4 hours to see that the response is sustained. If the child continues to stay well and does not have fast breathing, he can be discharged on inhaled or oral salbutamol.
- *If the response is partial or poor* ie, tachypnea has improved partially; rhonchi have decreased, child is stable and able to take orally; oral steroids (prednisone 1 mg/kg/d in 2–3 divided doses) are started and the child is kept under observation for the next 4 hours to see that there is no deterioration. Such a child can then be sent home on oral steroids and oral/inhaled salbutamol.

Score	Respiratory rate/min Age <6yrs	Respiratory rate/min Age >6yrs	Wheezing *	Accessory muscle usage
0	<30	<20	None	No apparent activity
1	31–45	21–35	Terminal expiration with stethoscope	Questionable increase
2	46–60	36–50	Entire expiration with stethoscope	Increase apparent
3	>60	>50	During inspiration and expiration without stethoscope	Maximum activity

Table 10.6 Pulmonary Score for Grading Severity of an Episode of Asthma

Add Score   0–3: **Mild**; 4–6: **Moderate**; >6: **Severe**

* If wheezing absent (due to minimal air flow), score = 3.

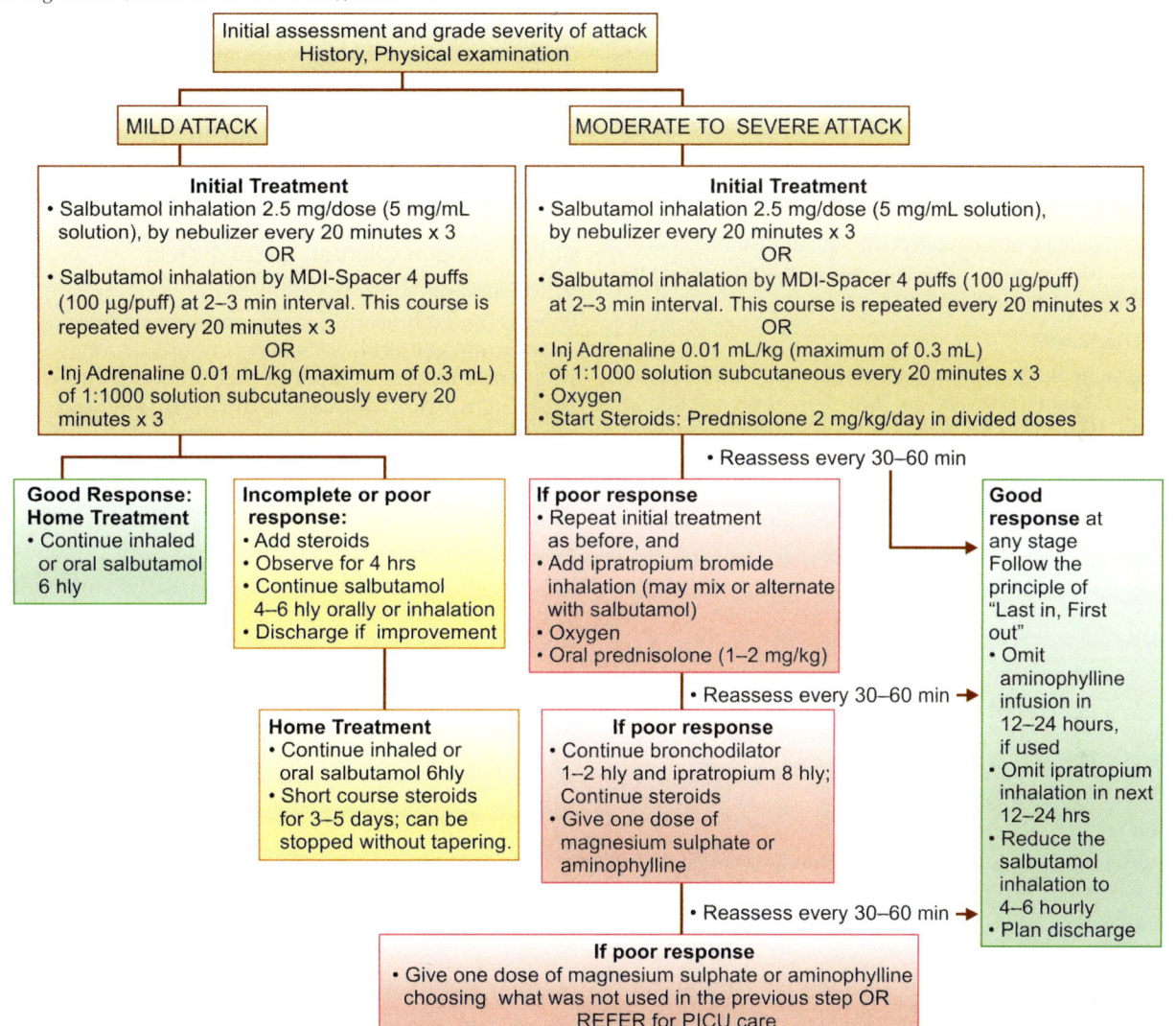

Fig. 10.4 Management algorithm for treating acute asthma in a hospital

- *Children with poor response or deterioration* are treated as moderate to severe attack.

B. Moderate to Severe Attack

These children should be hospitalized and administered oxygen in a non-threatening manner. The initial salbutamol inhalation should be given as for a mild attack. Alternatively, adrenaline is administered 0.01 mL/kg 1:1000 solution subcutaneously every 20 min up to three times. Initial dose of steroids (oral prednisolone 1–2 mg/kg) should be given promptly, if not started

so far. Nebulized ipratropium bromide is added (given as 3 nebulized doses at 20 min interval in the first hour and then continued every 8 hours for next 24–48 hours depending on the severity and response to therapy. The child is continuously monitored for sensorium, respiratory rate, oxygenation, and chest findings. The child is reassessed after 30–60 minutes.

- *Good response* If the child starts improving or is stable, salbutamol inhalations are continued at 1, 2, or 4 hourly intervals depending upon the time for which the response to initial treatment is sustained. Ipratropium bromide should subsequently be continued only at 8 hourly intervals. Once the good response is seen, ipratropium inhalation is stopped and then gradually the interval between salbutamol inhalations is increased till it is every 6 hours or so.

- *Partial response* Inhaled salbutamol is continued as before for another hour and continued at 1 or 2 hourly intervals depending upon the time for which the response to initial treatment is sustained. Systemic steroids are also continued.

- *Sustained poor or no response* Intravenous infusion of magnesium sulfate (50 mg/kg in 30 mL saline over 20–30 min) or aminophylline (0.8 mg/kg/hr infusion) can be added. If the non-response continues, an ICU transfer should be considered and intravenous terbutaline drip may be started.

Subsequently, medications are decreased once the patient starts showing a good and sustained response. The drug added last is removed first ("last in, first out" principle). Aminophylline infusion is usually stopped in 24 hours followed by withdrawal of ipratropium inhalation in next 24 hours. Then gradually decrease frequency of salbutamol inhalation to 4–6 hourly.

Daily maintenance fluids appropriate for age are given in those very distressed or vomiting. Breastfeeding and oral fluids intake should be encouraged in those able to take orally.

When to Discharge?

The child can be discharged when he/she is able to take orally, does not need oxygen therapy, and is on 4–6 hourly salbutamol inhalations. The recorded PEFR should be >75% of the predicted. The parents should be given a self-management plan about therapy and prevention of environmental triggers.

C. Treatment of a Child with Acute Life Threatening Asthma

Features of life threatening asthma include (*i*) cyanosis, silent chest, or feeble respiratory effort; (*ii*) fatigue or exhaustion; (*iii*) agitation or reduced level of consciousness; and (*iv*) peak expiratory flow rate (PEFR) <30% of predicted value; and (*v*) oxygen saturation of <90%. These children require urgent care and management, as detailed below:

- Start oxygen and maintenance intravenous fluids.
- Injection adrenaline is administered subcutaneously.
- Simultaneously initiate combined therapy with inhaled salbutamol and ipratropium.
- Start systemic steroids (Inj hydrocortisone 5–10 mg/kg) also simultaneously.
- Consider magnesium sulfate administration (50 mg/kg) as IV infusion over 30 minutes.
- Plan and arrange transfer to an intensive care unit for mechanical ventilation if there is no significant response in the first hour. Continue treatment as a severe attack till transfer occurs to a facility with intensive care capacities.
- *ICU care* Children needing ventilator support should be given gentle ventilation using low tidal volumes (7 mL/kg) and prolonged expiration (I:E - 1:2 to 1:3). The aim is to maintain normoxemia; some degree of hypercapnia is acceptable.

Follow-up Care

Asthma is a chronic and recurrent condition. A long-term treatment plan should be made based on the frequency and severity of symptoms. This may include intermittent or regular treatment with bronchodilators, regular treatment

with inhaled steroids or short course of oral steroids depending upon the severity. Most children have episodic wheeze with no intercurrent symptoms. Such patients do not need any treatment in between the episodes. The children with more than weekly day time symptoms or more than twice weekly night time symptoms have persistent disease and need long term treatment. It is important to enquire about symptoms like cough on running, laughing, night time or early morning coughing; as in between exacerbations the symptoms like breathlessness may not be seen or appreciated in many cases.

Long-term Management of Asthma

Children with persistent symptoms need long term therapy. Inhaled corticosteroids (ICS) form the mainstay of long-term therapy. While the benefits of inhaled corticosteroids far outweigh the side effects (ie, growth suppression); in severe cases, their risk benefit in under five children with wheezing is less favorable.

A. Wheezing in Children under 5 Years

While asthma is the commonest diagnosis in children over 5 years of age presenting with recurrent wheezing, it is not so common in young wheezers (under 5 years) where it may frequently be due to causes other than asthma. The current understanding divides the under five wheezers (albeit artificially) into two main asthma phenotypes *viz.* Episodic viral wheezers and Multi-trigger wheezers. This excludes atypical wheezers which are asthma mimickers and not asthma phenotypes.

Episodic viral wheeze It is most common in preschool children. Wheezing occurs in discrete episodes, the child being well in between episodes. These children are usually born with smaller airways and it predisposes them to wheeze with viral respiratory infections (further narrowing of airways occurs due to inflammation and edema). As these children grow older their airways grow in size and the frequency and severity of disease progressively decrease. Use of long term therapy of any kind (ICS or leukotriene antagonists) provides limited benefit in preventing or modifying long term outcome.

Multi-trigger wheeze Wheezing may be seen in some children on exposure to cold air, crying, laughter, exercise, etc. Such cases are considered closer to asthma phenotype of the older children and adults. It should be strongly suspected particularly if there is a family history of asthma/atopy.

Atypical wheezers usually have failure to thrive and may have features like clubbing, history of choking and regurgitation or serious bacterial infections, and may have underlying conditions such as gastroesophageal reflux disease, foreign body, immunodeficiency and cystic fibrosis that mimic asthma.

Diagnosis of asthma is more likely in young children who have recurrent wheezing in the presence of any of the identifiable risk factors for development of persistent asthma as indicated by (*i*) atopic dermatitis; (*ii*) family history of asthma; (*iii*) physician diagnosed allergic rhinitis; (*iv*) greater than 4% peripheral blood eosinophilia; or (*v*) wheezing episodes apart from episode of common cold.

Treatment	**Long-term Management of Wheezing in an Under 5 Child**

In children under 5 years if the frequency and severity of symptoms is significant (as described for persistent asthma in older children), daily long-term therapy with controllers should be started. Usually the therapy is withdrawn after 8 weeks and reintroduced if only the persistent symptoms recur.

- Leukotriene antagonists (eg, montelukast) are the less effective option used in this setting. Being an oral drug it is easier to give than ICS but is not as effective as ICS. Montelukast may be used to treat severe and frequent episodic wheezers but it is of limited efficacy.
- The clinical benefits of inhaled corticosteroids for episodic wheeze are not very clear as some studies have shown that it does not reduce the severity or frequency of attacks unlike the multi-trigger wheeze.
- The details of managing wheezing in under 5 child is detailed in Fig. 10.5. This includes management of both acute episode and thereafter.

Treatment	**Long-term Management of Asthma in Older Child**

Long-term management of asthma should be aimed at: (*i*) Freedom from symptoms; (*ii*) normal daily activities; and (*iii*) normal growth. To achieve these goals, the strategies should be: (*a*) Education to enhance patient's and family's knowledge and skills for self-management; (*b*) Appropriate selection of medications to address patient's needs; (*c*) Identification and management of precipitating factors/triggers and co-morbid conditions that may worsen asthma; and (*d*) Periodic assessment and monitoring of disease activity.

1. Patient Education

The parents of the child who needs long-term treatment should be explained that asthma is a chronic disease with intermittent exacerbations and that the drugs can only control and not cure asthma. However, they should be reassured that most children outgrow their symptoms. The doctor should emphasize the need for compliance with long-term controller therapy and maintaining a diary of symptoms. Parents should be told about dealing with asthma-triggers and home management of an acute attack.

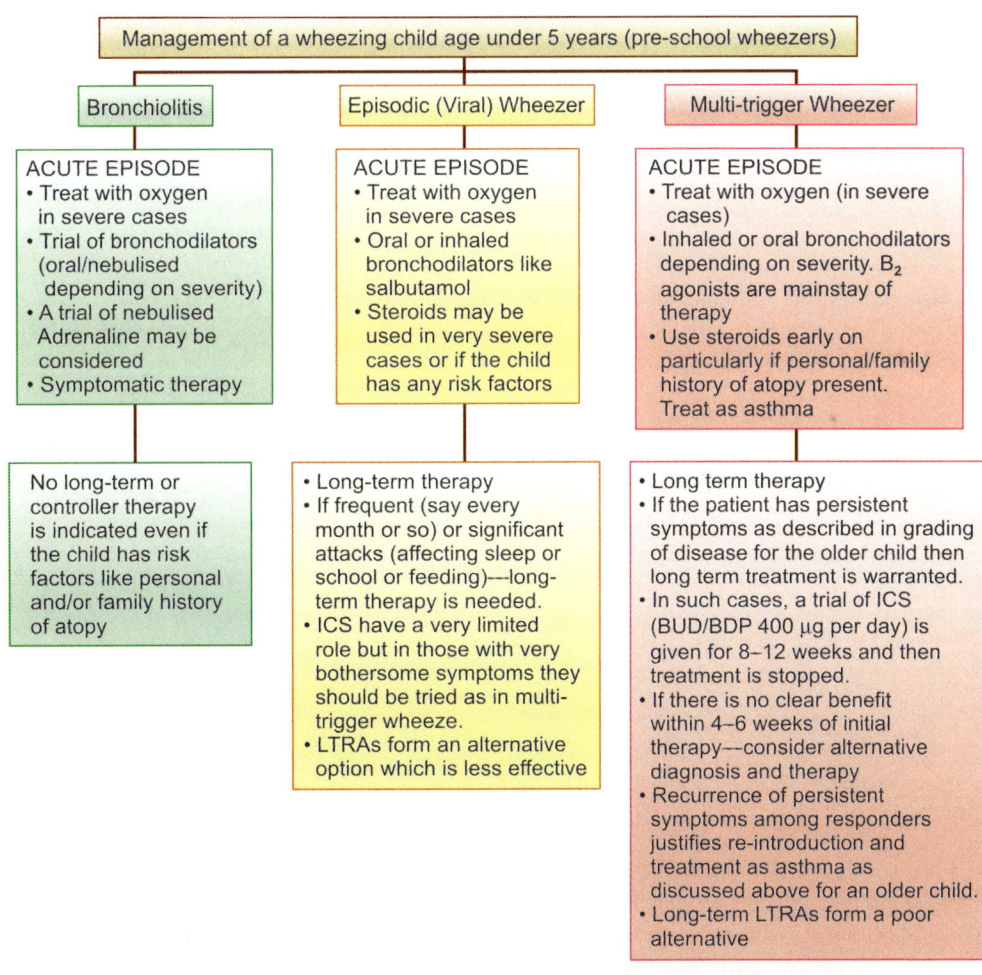

Fig. 10.5 Management of a wheezing child age under 5 years

2. Drugs

Inhaled corticosteroids These are the most effective controller drugs. Beclomethasone dipropionate, budesonide, and fluticasone propionate are commonly used and have comparable efficacy and adverse effect profile in equivalent doses. Low dose refers to usage of beclomethasone or budesonide at <200 µg /day, medium dose at 200–400 µg/day, and high dose at >400 µg/day. Metered dose inhaler with volume holding chamber (spacer) should be used preferably for effective airway deposition in children.

Long acting β2 agonists (LABA) Salmeterol and formoterol are the most commonly used long acting β2 agonists and act synergistically with inhaled corticosteroids. They are not recommended for use alone as controller therapy.

Leukotriene receptor antagonists (LTRA) Montelukast is the most commonly used drug in this category. It is used as add-on drug with inhaled corticosteroids in treatment of asthma (preferred in children <5 years).

3. Drug Delivery Devices

Inhaled drugs are preferred over oral drugs because of the following advantages: Smaller doses, quicker action, and safer profile.

Metered dose inhaler (MDI) with spacer It is suitable for all age groups and for all the controller regimes. Spacer or volume holding chambers eliminate the need for coordination of actuation and inhalation while using an MDI. Use of spacer also limits the deposition of inhaled steroid in the oropharynx, thereby decreasing the occurrence of local side effects of inhaled steroids (ie, thrush and dysphonia). In children less than 4 years face mask may be added to spacer.

Dry powder inhaler (DPI) DPI can be used in children above 6 years, as they can generate inspiratory flow of 30–60 L/min which is required for optimal drug delivery using DPI. However, it cannot be used during acute attacks as the patient may not be able to generate sufficient flows. Moreover, the oropharyngeal drug deposition is also more as compared to MDI with spacer.

Nebulizer Oxygen driven nebulizers are used in hospitalized patients with acute severe episodes. These are not recommended for home use as MDI and DPI ensure adequate drug delivery and are relatively cheaper and more convenient for daily controller therapy.

4. Selection of Medications

Selection of medications for long term control of asthma is based on assessment of severity and grading of disease.

Assessment of severity The assessment of severity in patients and level of control (in patients on long-term therapy) is assessed in two domains: (a) Impairment due to disease; and (b) risk factors for poor asthma control (**Table 10.7**).

Grading of disease severity Initial therapy is guided by the current symptom severity and subsequently constantly adjusted as per level of control achieved. Asthma severity is graded after patient has been on controller treatment for several months. The grading of severity is done by step of therapy at which control is achieved (**Table 10.8**).

Since the diagnosis of asthma is most commonly made in children above 5 years, the treatment discussed here is applicable for this age group only. The drug therapy should be based on the grading of asthma (**Table 10.9**). The appropriate regime should be started and titrated upwards or downwards according to the achievement of control.

Children with persistent asthma as signified by day time symptoms which are more frequent than twice weekly in the past 1–2 months and night time symptoms at least once a week or frequent are considered to have persistent disease and need long-term controller medication for asthma. The preferred medication for those needing long-term therapy is detailed in **Table 10.9**.

5. Manage Precipitating Factors and Co-morbidities Triggers

- *Allergens* dust mite antigen, moulds and spores, cockroach antigen, pollens, animal dander, etc.
- *Irritants* Smoke, mosquito repellent mats, sprays, weather changes, cold baths, etc.

Table 10.7 Classification of Level of Control of Childhood Asthma	
A. *Impairment* Characteristics (in past 4 weeks) 1. Daytime symptoms > 2 times/week 2. Any limitations of activity 3. Any nocturnal awakening due to asthma 4. Need for rescue/"reliever" treatment>2 times/ week	**Level of Control** **Controlled :** None of these **Partly controlled :** 1–2 of these **Uncontrolled :** 3 or more features
B. *Risk factors for poor asthma control* Assess these factors at diagnosis and periodically *Modifiable* 1. Uncontrolled asthma symptoms 2. Inadequate ICS (not prescribed, poor adherence, incorrect technique) 3. Low FEV1 4. Co-morbidities: Obesity, rhinosinusitis, confirmed food allergy 5. Exposures: Smoking, allergen exposures if sensitized 6. Sputum or blood eosinophilia *Non modifiable* I. Ever intubated or ICU admissions II. >1 severe exacerbations in the last 12 months	

Ref: Asthma by Consensus, 3rd ed.

Table 10.8 Grading of Severity of Asthma based on Control Achieved at Different Steps

Control achieved at step	Grading of asthma
Step 1	Intermittent asthma
Step 2	Mild asthma
Step 3	Moderate asthma
Step 4 or above	Severe asthma

Ref: Asthma by Consensus, 3rd ed.

Step of treatment	Preferred controller choice	Other controller option	Reliever
Step 1	No controllers	As needed SABA	
Step 2	Low dose ICS	I. LTRA II. Slow release theophylline	
Step 3	<12 yr: Medium dose ICS >12yr: Low dose ICS with LABA	1. Low dose ICS + LTRA 2. Medium dose ICS	As needed SABA
Step 4	Medium dose ICS with LABA	• Medium dose ICS + LTRA • High dose ICS	
Step 5	Low dose oral steroids	1. Anti-IgE	

- All patients must be given Asthma Education: Knowledge about disease and written asthma action plan, allergen prevention and plan for regular review.
- At each visit re-assess the child for diagnosis, symptom control/risk factors, lung function and inhaler technique
- Re-adjust treatment including medications, device demonstration and trigger avoidance
- Review response for symptoms, exacerbations, lung function and adverse effects of drugs

Ref: Asthma by Consensus, 3rd ed.

Table 10.9 Long-term Drug Therapy for Asthma in Children Aged 5 Years or More

	Intermittent	Mild Persistent	Moderate Persistent	Severe Persistent
Day time symptoms	Twice or less per week, usually once-a-month episode	More than twice per week, more than once-a-month episodes	Daily	Throughout the day
Night time awakenings	Twice or less per month	3–4 time per month	Once or more per week (not daily)	7 nights/week
Activity limitation	None	Minor	Some	Extreme
FEV$_1$ % predicted	>80%, normal between attacks	≥ 80%	60–80%	<60%
Management • First choice	No long term daily medication needed	Low dose ICS	Low dose ICS +LABA/LTRA/ theophylline OR medium dose ICS	Medium to high dose ICS + LABA/LTRA
• Other option		LTRA/cromolyn/ nedocromil/ theophylline	Medium/high dose ICS + LTRA/ theophylline	Systemic steroid (oral)

Note: At every grade of severity, the acute attacks should be treated with reliever drug including short-acting β2 agonists. Appropriate environmental and trigger control should be part of the management strategy.
SABA: Short acting beta-agonist; ICS; inhaled corticosteroids; LTRA: leukoriene receptor (eg, monteleukast); LABA: long acting beta-agonist

- *Precipitants* Viral infections, drugs (aspirin, other NSAIDS), diet (food additives like monosodium glutamate)
  The appropriate actions are avoidance of exposure (to allergens, irritants) as well as timely initiation of inhaled bronchodilator therapy.

Co-morbid Conditions
- *Allergic rhinosinusitis* Inadequate control of allergic rhinosinusitis may contribute towards poor control of asthma.

Montelukast may be effective in such cases. Intranasal steroid sprays can also be tried along with second generation antihistaminics.
- *Gastroesophageal reflux disease (GERD)* GERD is suspected in younger children with poor asthma control. Antireflux treatment should be given in proven cases.

6. Periodic Assessment and Monitoring of Disease Activity
The child should be kept under regular follow up. Based on the

Case Study | A Child with Recurrent Wheeze

A 7-year-old boy weighing 29 kg presented to the hospital emergency department with history of coryza for last 2 days and cough for 1 day. The cough was dry and each bout of coughing was followed by vomiting. The child did not have adequate night sleep because of cough. He was also having breathing difficulty for past few hours. There was a past history of several such episodes for last 5 years, often afebrile, which could be managed with oral drugs and nebulization at home, but for last 1 year he had been having this problem nearly every month. He had also received nebulization on couple of emergency visits. In between these episodes the child used to be relatively better but develops short bouts of cough after running or climbing stairs. The father had history of a similar illness during his childhood.

On examination, he was responding to questions but had difficulty in breathing. His respiratory rate was 32/ min and SpO$_2$ was 94% in room air. His temperature and hydration were normal and pulse rate was 100/ min. He had mild lower chest retractions. Auscultation of chest revealed polyphonic wheeze in both lung fields. The rest of the systemic examination was normal.

What is the most likely diagnosis? Justify your answer.

Mild to Moderate persistent bronchial asthma is the most probable diagnosis. The points favoring diagnosis of asthma are: (*i*) repeated episodes of cough and breathing difficulty requiring nebulization; (*ii*) exercise induced symptoms; (*iii*) mostly afebrile episodes; positive family history; (*iv*) and polyphonic wheeze on auscultation of chest.

Disease severity has been assessed as mild to moderate persistent because he is symptomatic in between the episodes. It is not severe because the child does not have daily or frequent night symptoms.

List the relevant investigations needed to confirm your diagnosis.

Usually no further investigation is needed as asthma is a clinical diagnosis. A good clinical response to bronchodilators is reliable clinical indicator of the diagnosis in such a patient.

Describe the initial management of this condition.

This patient should be managed with inhaled short acting β2 agonist like salbutamol, given by nebulization (3 doses: 0, 20 and 40 min). In case the response is not sustained he may be admitted and given frequent repeat doses of the drug and oral steroid (tab prednisone) is added. Further therapy is guided by the response to treatment and the severity of the episode.

Outline the long term management of this condition? What follow up advice will you give to the parents?

The long term management includes following:

- Educating the parents about the child's problem and its probable consequences on his health.
- Finding out any triggers or precipitants or any co-morbid condition leading to persistence of symptoms, making the parents aware of such conditions.
- Selection of low to medium dose inhaled corticosteroid say budesonide 100 µg 2 puffs twice a day, to be given to the patient by metered dose inhaler with spacer.
- Checking compliance and technique of drug administration as well as growth monitoring on every follow up visit.
- Stepping up or down on treatment depending upon the response.

control, if a child has complete or near complete absence of symptoms for 6–8 weeks, the therapy is stepped down on 4–8 weekly intervals, decreasing the drugs by about 25% on each visit. It is possible to withdraw the drugs completely in a proportion of children with persistent asthma amongst children.

In those who have inadequate control, the treatment may need stepping up, provided the inhalation technique is fair.

Untreated or poorly controlled asthma can result in failure to thrive. Therefore, growth velocity should be monitored in children on daily controller regimes. These children also need periodic eye examination to look for posterior subcapsular cataract.

Peak expiratory flow (PEF) monitoring offers a quantitative measure of impairment of airway function, establishes the individual patient's personal best and evaluates responses to change in controller therapy. It can be used in children >5 years with moderate to severe persistent asthma.

Spirometry is helpful to document normalization of lung function in a child of asthma who has been initiated on controller regime. It is also useful in assessing the response to bronchodilator.

Remission A child with asthma is said to be in remission if he neither had symptoms of airflow obstruction nor taken therapy for the past 12 months. Such a patient should be advised to avoid triggers and is followed up every 3–6 months for a period of 1–2 years.

7. Dealing with Poor Asthma Control

In case of poor response to controller treatment, the following steps are needed:

- Rule out alternative diagnosis.
- Ascertain adherence of patient/parents with prescribed regime.
- Check the technique of use of drug delivery device.
- Eliminate triggers.
- Check concurrent medical condition.
- Consider short course oral steroid.
- Step up controller regime after objective monitoring.
- Specialist referral in cases not responding to above measures.

Revision Point

Bronchial Asthma

1. Bronchial asthma is most likely diagnosis in children with recurrent wheezing.
2. Childhood asthma most often starts before school age and is increasing in prevalence across the world.
3. All that wheezes is not asthma. Likewise, isolated cough without wheeze or chronic wet cough needs evaluation.
4. Spirometry is an integral component of asthma management.
5. Inhaled corticosteroids are the mainstay in the treatment of childhood asthma.
6. Strict adherence to an asthma action plan reduces exacerbations, morbidity and mortality

American Thoracic Society/European Respiratory Society Task Force on Asthma Control and Exacerbations. An official American Thoracic Society/European Respiratory Society statement: asthma control and exacerbations: standardizing endpoints for clinical asthma trials and clinical practice. *Am J Respir Crit Care Med.* 2009;180:59–99.

Asthma Guidelines Working Group of the Canadian Network for Asthma Care. Summary of recommendations from the Canadian Asthma Consensus guidelines, 2003. *CMAJ*. 2005;173:S3–11.

British Thoracic Society Scottish Intercollegiate Guidelines Network. British Guideline on the Management of Asthma. *Thorax*. 2008;63:iv1–121.

Global Allergy and Asthma European Network; Grading of Recommendations Assessment, Development and Evaluation Working Group. Allergic Rhinitis and its Impact on Asthma (ARIA) guidelines: 2010 revision. *J Allergy Clin Immunol*. 2010;126:466–76.

Inhalation devices. *CMAJ*. 2005;173:S39–45.

Pedersen SE, Hurd SS, Lemanske RF Jr, *et al*. Global Initiative for Asthma.Global strategy for the diagnosis and management of asthma in children 5 years and younger. *Pediatr Pulmonol*. 2011;46:1–17.

Roddick LG, Clements B, Wales S, Henry RL; Children's Hospitals Australasia. Guidelines for weaning of bronchodilator therapy. *J Paediatr Child Health*. 2005;41:696–7.

10.11 TUBERCULOSIS

Tuberculosis is a chronic illness caused by *Mycobacterium tuberculosis*, starting from a primary focus in lung, lymph node, or intestine. Children contract the disease from infectious cases, commonly adults in the family.

Tuberculosis can affect any organ or system of the body. Common manifestations in children include tubercular lymphadenitis (presenting with swelling in neck or axillae) or pulmonary tuberculosis (presenting with prolonged fever, cough, and weight loss). Severe forms are common in young infants and malnourished children; these include miliary tuberculosis and tubercular meningitis that carry a very high risk of mortality, and sequelae in survivors.

Nearly 3.4 million children in India have the disease while 94 million are at the risk of infection. The overall prevalence of infection in the 0–14 years age group is estimated between 8.6 and 10%.

Peculiarities

Tuberculosis is a formidable enemy due to (*a*) slowly dividing stubborn causative organism which has a sturdy wall impervious to antibiotics; (*b*) need for prolonged therapy (at least six months); (*c*) problems related to its definitive diagnosis; (*d*) availability of limited (though at present quite effective) drugs for treatment; and (*e*) misuse of the available drugs by the providers, resulting in emergence of drug-resistant strains.

Etiopathogenesis

Tuberculosis is caused by an acid fast bacillus—*Mycobacterium tuberculosis*. Few cases may be due to *Mycobacterium bovis*. Pulmonary tuberculosis is an airborne infection. When any infective case of tuberculosis coughs, large numbers of live bacilli are coughed into the air where they remain suspended for a variable period depending on the size of the droplet and airflow conditions. Pulmonary infection occurs when small aerosolized particles containing few live but virulent tubercle bacilli are inhaled from a contagious source. The infection leads to formation of a *tubercle* or *granuloma* which may develop central caseous necrosis and liquefaction and can heal by fibrosis and calcification. The liquefaction is usually associated with the development of clinical disease. Expulsion of caseous liquefied material from an airway leads to cavity formation.

Tubercle bacilli are usually inhibited in solid, caseous and nonliquefied lesion due to acidic pH, low oxygen tension, and fatty acids. Thus solid lesions in all organs have small bacillary population $\sim 10^2-10^5$ organisms. However, the high oxygen tension in the walls of the cavity promotes active replication resulting in 10^7-10^9 organisms. The bacilli replicate poorly in fibrous and calcified lesions. The bacilli can survive for years in solid caseum and may remain insensitive to chemotherapy in this dormant state.

In general, lung and kidney lesions have higher bacillary load than other lesions. The primary type of tubercular lesion in children usually has fewer bacilli than the progressive primary and reactivation type disease of the periadolescent age group. The lesions of pulmonary tuberculosis may vary within same region of a lung from resolution, calcification, and liquefaction to fibrosis.

Pathogenesis

The portal of entry for *Mycobacterium tuberculosis* is lung in >98% cases, where after multiplication, most of the bacilli are killed and the remaining survive within alveolar macrophages which carry them through lymphatic vessels to the regional lymph nodes. The primary complex (*Ghon complex*) of tuberculosis includes local infection at the portal of entry and the regional lymph nodes that drain the area (the hilar or paratracheal lymph nodes).

- The parenchymal portion of the primary complex often heals completely by fibrosis or calcification after undergoing caseous necrosis and encapsulation. Occasionally, this portion continues to enlarge, resulting in focal pneumonitis and pleuritis. If caseation is intense, the center of the lesion liquefies and empties into the associated bronchus, leaving a residual cavity.

- The foci of infection in the regional lymph nodes develop some fibrosis and encapsulation, but viable *M. tuberculosis* can persist for decades within these foci. The hilar and paratracheal lymph nodes can compress regional bronchus and extrinsic compression of the bronchus can result in atelectasis or hyperinflation of distal alveoli depending on whether the obstruction of bronchus is complete or partial, respectively. Inflamed caseous nodes can erode through bronchial wall, causing endobronchial tuberculosis or a fistula tract.

- From the primary complex the tubercle bacilli are often carried through the blood and lymphatic vessels to most of the organs like liver, spleen, brain, kidneys, and bones.

- *Disseminated tuberculosis* results if the number of circulating bacilli is large and the host's cellular immune response is inadequate such as in HIV infected persons. It refers to concurrent involvement of two non-contiguous organs or involvement of blood or bone marrow by tuberculosis process.

- *Miliary tuberculosis* results from massive hematogenous spread of the bacilli resulting in multiple, tiny, discrete foci of 1–2 mm size, uniformly distributed in the lungs or other viscera. It is characterized by snow-storm appearance in the chest X-ray.

- Development of disease in other organs appears to follow the *Wallgren's time table of tuberculosis*. Disseminated and meningeal tuberculosis are early manifestations, often occurring within 2–6 months of acquisition. Significant

10

lymph node or endobronchial tuberculosis usually appears within 3–9 months. TB pleuritis usually occurs in 3–9 months, bone and joint disease in 1–3 years and renal disease in 5–25 years following the primary infection.

- Extrapulmonary manifestations develop in 25–35% of children with tuberculosis, compared with about 10% of immunocompetent adults with tuberculosis.

Reactivation tuberculosis most commonly occurs in lungs (upper lobes), 1 year after the primary infection. It is caused by endogenous regrowth of bacilli persisting in partially encapsulated lesions. It is rare in children but is common among adolescents and young adults.

Reinfection also can occur in persons with advanced HIV or AIDS. In immunocompetent persons the response to the initial infection with *M. tuberculosis* usually provides partial protection against reinfection when a new exposure occurs, however, this is not so in high burden communities.

Natural History

Exposure The child comes into contact with a source—usually an adult—who has contagious pulmonary disease. All exposed children are not infected.

Tubercular infection Those infected develop hypersensitivity to tubercular proteins and can be identified by a positive tuberculin (Mantoux) test, usually after three months of getting infected. There are no signs and symptoms of the disease.

Tubercular disease The disease is characterized by appearance of symptoms and signs. Radiological lesions appear in pulmonary involvement. The nature of radiographic abnormalities and clinical manifestations depend on host reaction.

Not all patients pass through all the stages. The likelihood of developing disease is maximal in the period just after infection. Approximately 5% of individuals develop pulmonary tuberculous disease within 5 years of the initial infection, whereas nearly 90% may never develop the disease.

- Children below 6 years of age have the highest rates of acquisition of tubercular disease and also have the most severe disease.
- Certain childhood diseases like measles, whooping cough, severe malnutrition act as predisposing factors for flaring up a latent tubercular infection into the disease.

Clinical Manifestations

History

Fever and cough of more than 2 weeks of duration associated with weight loss or failure to thrive, or enlarged glands in the neck lasting for more than 2 weeks, without associated sore throat, are the most common clinical presentations of pulmonary tuberculosis, and tubercular lymphadenitis, respectively. Clinical suspicion should be stronger if there is a history of contact with an adult patient of tuberculosis, whether within or outside family.

Children with primary pulmonary tuberculosis, unlike adults, may often be asymptomatic or may have non-specific symptoms including night fever and chills, fatigue, malaise, anorexia, and weight loss.

Examination

Physical examination may reveal one or more of the following: malnutrition, lymphadenopathy (non-tender, matted, that sometimes become fluctuant or develop cold abscess and/or sinuses), chest signs, hepatomegaly, splenomegaly, meningeal signs, altered sensorium, neurological deficit, pleural effusion, or ascites.

Coarse crepitations can be heard over bronchiectatic areas. Bronchial breathing may be heard over large consolidations, collapsed segments or cavities. The pulmonary disease may often be without significant chest findings even in presence of pneumonia. Absence of physical findings despite large lesions seen on radiograph is quite suggestive of tuberculosis.

A tuberculous pleural effusion is usually characterized by acute onset fever with sharp localized chest pain, particularly during inspiration. On examination there is tachypnea or respiratory distress; shift of mediastinum to opposite side with moderate to large effusions; dullness to percussion on the involved side; and decreased breath sounds and vocal resonance on the involved site.

Extrapulmonary disease including peripheral lymphadenopathy, skeletal system, central nervous system, gastrointestinal tract, genitourinary system, eyes, ears, heart and skin is less common than the pulmonary disease. However, children are more likely to develop extrapulmonary disease than immunocompetent adults. Peripheral lymphadenitis is the commonest form of extrapulmonary disease seen.

Diagnosis

The diagnosis of tuberculosis in children is extremely challenging due to difficulties in demonstrating acid fast bacilli, which is the gold standard. In addition, the clinical symptoms and signs of tubercular disease are non-specific and common symptoms of cough, fever, failure to gain weight can lead to both over and under diagnosis. Definitions used for diagnosis of tuberculosis are summarized in **Box 10.4**.

1. Mycobacterial Detection and Isolation

Demonstration of acid fast bacilli on stain or detection of *Mycobacterium tuberculosis* in culture should be attempted in

Box 10.4 Definitions for Diagnosis of Tuberculosis
Presumptive TB
It refers to a patient who presents with symptoms or signs suggestive of TB (previously known as a "TB suspect").
Bacteriologically confirmed TB case
It refers to a patient in whom a biological specimen is positive by smear microscopy, culture or WHO approved rapid diagnostic such as Xpert MTB/RIF
Clinically diagnosed TB case
A patient who does not fulfil the criteria for bacteriological confirmation but has been diagnosed with active TB by a clinician or other medical practitioner who has decided to give the patient a full course of TB treatment. This definition includes cases diagnosed on the basis of X-ray abnormalities or suggestive histology and extra-pulmonary cases without laboratory confirmation. A significant proportion of cases in children belong to this category.

all children suspected to have tuberculosis. Body specimens including gastric washings, sputum, pleural fluid, bronchoalveolar lavage, cerebrospinal fluid, peritoneal fluid, abscess, and biopsy material are used. Sputum, gastric aspirates/lavage and fluid aspirates from the involved lymph nodes are the most useful specimens for best yield of *M. tuberculosis*. Pleural fluid, ascitic fluid, and cerebrospinal fluid are mostly smear negative because of a very low bacillary load at these sites.

Specimens to be Used

Sputum Unless endobronchial tuberculosis is present, children <6 years of age usually do not have a cough deep enough to produce sputum for analysis. However, where feasible, sputum analysis is best accomplished in the morning. WHO recommends to obtain a minimum of two samples on separate days. Sputum collection is possible in older children with extensive and cavitatory disease, particularly if the patient has a wet cough.

Gastric aspirate Early morning gastric aspirate is a preferred specimen for most young children with suspected TB for detecting AFB or isolating *M.tuberculosis*. The child is kept fasting for about 6 hours (at night) and an appropriate size intragastric tube is passed in the morning. Initially the aspirate is drawn from the stomach and then a further washing with 15–30 mL saline is taken. The contents so recovered are then immediately transferred to the laboratory. This specimen can also be collected as an ambulatory procedure after 4–6 hours fasting.

Induced sputum Induction of sputum by 3% nebulized hypertonic saline can be tried in other children (after the age of 4 months). The patient is pretreated with nebulized bronchodilators prior to induction. Following saline nebulisation, chest physiotherapy is done to loosen up the secretions and the samples are collected from the throat or nasopharynx.

Bronchoalveolar lavage Bronchoscopy and lavage is often needed when evaluating a persistent pneumonia. TB remains an important cause of persistent pneumonia in our country.

Direct Smear

The body secretions or aspirates are drawn into smears over a clean slide and stained with Ziehl-Neelsen stain for detecting acid fast bacilli (AFB). Use of fluorescent dyes like auromine-O, etc. can improve the sensitivity of this test. Use of fluorescence microscopes with LED bulbs and auramine-rhodamine staining instead of conventional staining and microscopic examination can also make the detection of mycobacteria faster.

Culture Techniques

Culture of specimens containing tubercle bacilli is a much more sensitive method of detecting *mycobacteria* than are direct smears. The solid media traditionally used is an egg based Lowenstein-Jensen medium. The growth of mycobacteria takes 6–8 weeks for colonies to appear.

There are some automated systems such as *Mycobacterium growth indicator tube (MGIT 960), BACTEC 460, MB/BacT* which detect the growth of mycobacteria much earlier than conventional culture media (LJ or Middlebrook medium). The average time for growth detection is 11–13 days by automated systems as compared to 6–8 weeks for conventional techniques.

2. Tuberculin Skin Test (Mantoux test)

The Mantoux test (most common method of tuberculin skin test) consists of intradermal injection of 0.1 mL solution containing 1 tuberculin unit (TU) of purified protein derivative with RT-23, into the volar surface of the forearm, using a short-bevel 25-gauge needle. The area of induration around the site of injection is measured 48–72 hours later at its largest transverse diameter.

- *Induration of 10 mm or more is considered as positive*. If the child fails to show up for reading, it is acceptable to read the result for up to 1 week after testing if the result is positive. Any child who reports late and has a result at 4–7 days which would be classified as negative should be re-tested on the other arm.

- *Erythema without induration should be considered as a negative reaction*. However, erythema of more than 10 mm in the absence of induration mandates re-testing. This phenomenon could occur if the test injection was inadvertently made too deeply. No child should be tested more than twice in 1 month if the injection has been administered subcutaneously.

- A positive tuberculin skin test is a useful diagnostic test for detecting infection. However, a *negative tuberculin skin reaction may not necessarily exclude the diagnosis* of tuberculosis. False negative tuberculin skin tests may occur with severe systemic tuberculosis, anergy, immuno-deficiency, immunosuppression, malnutrition, infections such as measles, as also, improper dilutions, bacterial contamination, or exposure of PPD to heat or light.

Often the laboratories use higher strengths like 5TU or 10TU. These are likely to give higher reactions and probably more false positives. Using standard preparations are essential for the correct interpretation of this simple but useful test. The poor availability of standard preparations are a real problem. Currently, testing with 1 or 2 TU Tuberculin RT23 and using a 10 mm cut off is considered acceptable by most experts.

3. Roentgenographic Examination

Chest X-ray is an important diagnostic tool for evaluating pulmonary tuberculosis despite the fact that there is no radiological appearance specific to tuberculosis. Initial studies include AP and lateral views. Lateral decubitus views help to determine if an effusion is freely moving or loculated. Fluoroscopy of the main airways helps differentiate the presence of hilar adenopathy (which remains immobile throughout respiration) from prominent pulmonary vasculature.

There is no routine role for the CT scan or MRI in the evaluation of the symptomatic tuberculosis infected child with a normal chest radiograph.

Typical radiological shadows seen in tuberculosis are infiltrations in lung parenchyma, hilar or paratracheal lymphadenopathy, consolidation with or without collapse, miliary shadows, and pleural effusion.

10

4. Tissue Diagnosis

Aspiration cytology Fine needle aspiration of cytological fluid from the lymph node swellings and other involved areas in the solid or solidified tissues can be used for either cytopathology or demonstrating AFB.

Histopathological diagnosis Tissue biopsy of pleura, lymph node, liver and transbronchial biopsy may show the presence of caseating granulomas if and when these organs are involved.

Body fluid cytology Exudative (protein >3 g/dL) lymphocytic fluid aspirates from the pleura or peritoneal or pericardial sacs is suggestive of tuberculosis. AFB staining of the aspirates may occasionally be positive for tuberculous bacteria.

5. Antigen-based Test

Interferon gamma release assays (IGRAs)—Elispot and Quantiferon Gold are newer tests using ESAT-6 and CFP-10 protein antigen. These antigen based tests are used to identify Interferon-γ production in the infected individuals on antigen challenge *in vitro*. They cannot differentiate between the infected and diseased individuals. However, unlike tuberculin they do not produce false positive result due to BCG vaccination.

6. Molecular Diagnosis

Polymerase chain reaction It is a promising tool for rapid diagnoses of tuberculosis but has the problems of cost, technique, contamination, and false positivity. With the existing experience, WHO does not recommend the use of PCR for regular workup of tubercular suspects. Several studies have shown a poor reproducibility and high false positivity in clinical specimens.

There are two new genotypic methods known as *Transcription mediated amplification (TMA)* and *nucleic acid amplification (NAA)*. Both these techniques use chemical, rather than biological amplification to produce nucleic acid, so that within a few hours these tests distinguish between *M.tuberculosis* complex and nontubercular mycobacteria in an AFB positive specimen. These tests are highly sensitive (96%) and specific (100%) for *M.tuberculosis* on specimens that are smear positive for AFB. However, there are occasional false-negative or false positive results being reported, which are either due to the presence of dead bacilli or due to contamination.

GeneXpert is a cartridge based heminested real time PCR based point of care test which can provide results in a couple of hours. It not only identifies *the organism* but can also simultaneously identify rifampin resistance. WHO recommends it as the initial diagnostic test in individuals suspected of MDR-TB or TB-HIV co-infection.

7. Discarded Tests

BCG test This test is no longer recommended for diagnosis of tuberculosis. Reasons are threefold. The BCG test utilizes a very high load of several antigen and is prone to a risk of high false positivity. The preparation being live makes it impossible to estimate the real strength of antigen used. Its validity in countries like India where routine BCG vaccination is undertaken is further suspect.

Immunodiagnosis WHO has called for abandoning the ELISA tests for serodiagnosis of tuberculosis because of their inadequate sensitivity, specificity or reproducibility under various clinical conditions. Government of India has since banned the usage of these tests in the country.

Most of the newer techniques are costly, technically difficult and have till date an unacceptable sensitivity and specificity. For these reasons, the triad of (*i*) positive tuberculin skin test; (*ii*) an abnormal chest radiograph; and (*iii*) history of exposure to an adult with probable or definite tuberculosis, remains the most commonly employed method for diagnosing tuberculosis in children. Often a non-response of symptoms, particularly with persistence of the radiological shadows to potent antibiotics, is used as an additional ground for suspecting tuberculosis.

Figure 10.6 depicts a diagnostic algorithm for identifying children with pulmonary tuberculosis, as recommended by Revised National Tuberculosis Control Program, in 2015.

Treatment	Childhood Tuberculosis

The therapy for tuberculosis is based on the bacillary load, level of drug resistance and the bacillary sub-populations. In general, combination chemotherapy is used to kill the large number of the actively multiplying organisms.

Combination of three or four drugs like rifampin (R), isoniazid (H), pyrazinamide (Z), and ethambutol (E) are effective against most prevalent strains except for the multidrug resistance cases. In countries where the initial INH resistance is more than 5%, (like India) or HIV burden is high (like Africa) only four drug initial regimes are recommended. The RNTCP in India has, therefore, now done away with the 3 drug regime referred to as category III treatment.

Now, the initial *intensive phase* of 2 months is with 4 drugs (RHZE) and is followed by 4 months of *continuation phase* using 2 drugs (rifampin and INH). The drug dosage for various drugs and drug regimens for different sets of patients are given in **Tables 10.10 and 10.11.**

The following recommendations are made pertaining to treatment categories and regimens:

- *New case* A patient who is recently diagnosed and has never received anti-TB drugs or received for less than 4 weeks duration.
- In children with tubercular meningitis on Category I treatment, the four drugs used during the intensive phase can either be HRZE or HRZS. The patients where AFB can not be demonstrated but are considered to have relapsed/ failed on treatment must be investigated thoroughly for alternative diagnosis or co-morbid conditions with similar symptoms before embarking on category II treatment.
- Routinely no other adjunct treatment is required in most cases. Steroids are indicated in patients with CNS tuberculosis, severely ill miliary cases, pericardial and pleural tamponade, and genitourinary tuberculosis.
- Under Revised National Tuberculosis Control Program, these drugs are given under direct observation (DOT) on thrice weekly basis whereas for unsupervised treatment the same combination and duration of drug is used on a daily basis. The intermittent treatment is acceptable as it provides drugs under direct supervision thus decreasing the chances for incomplete or inadequate treatment.
- Drug dosages for intermittent therapy are higher than daily dosage.

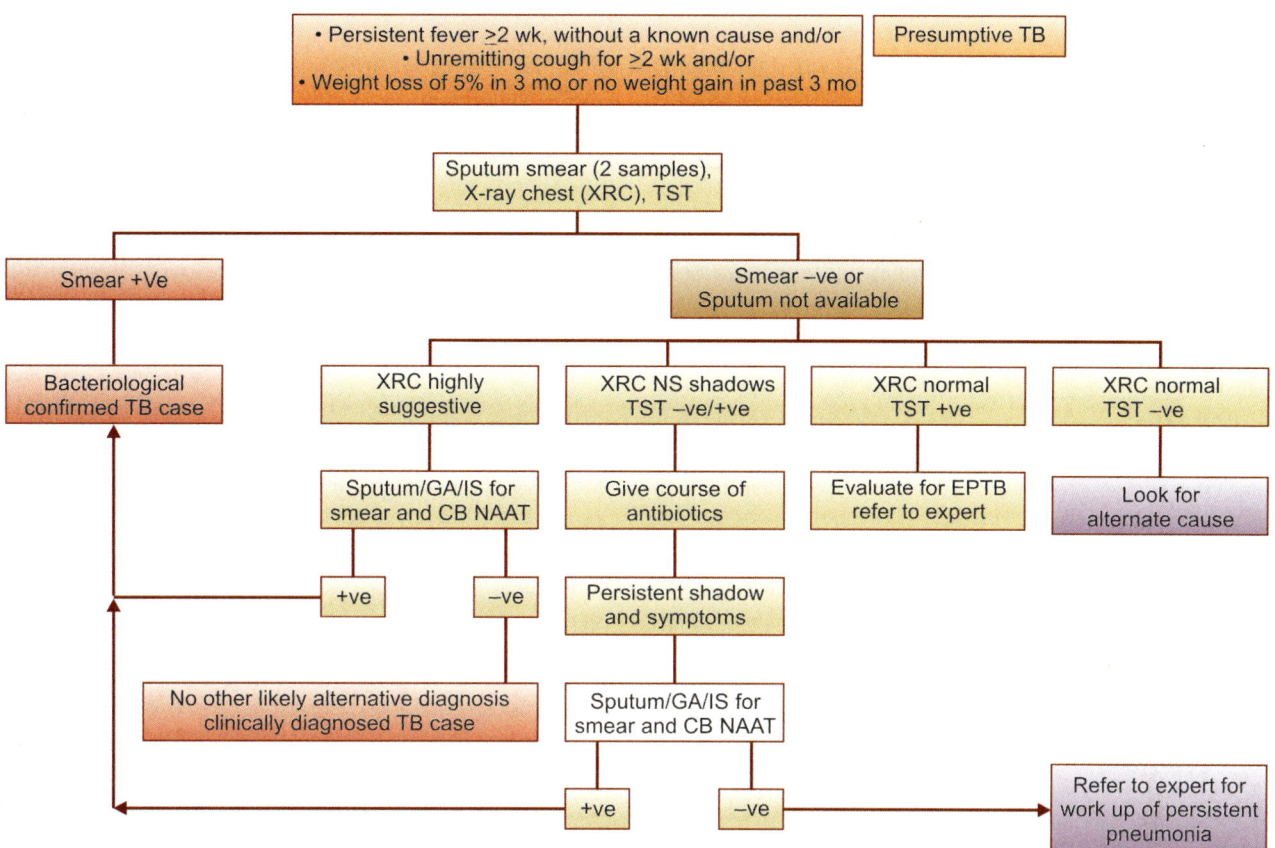

Fig. 10.6 Diagnostic algorithm for the diagnosis of pulmonary tuberculosis in children (RNTCP 2015)

Table 10.10 Anti-tuberculous Drugs and their Dosages		
Drug (symbol)	*Daily dosages*	*Major side effects*
Streptomycin (S)	15–20 mg/kg/day	Tinnitus
Rifampin (R)	10–15 mg/kg/day	Hepatotoxicity, gastritis, flu like illness
Isoniazid (H)	10 mg/kg/day	Peripheral neuropathy, hepatoxicity
Pyrazinamide (Z)	30–35 mg/kg/day	Arthralgia, hepatotoxicity
Ethambutol (E)	20 mg/kg/day	Oculotoxicity

Table 10.11 Treatment Categories and Regimens for Childhood TB, as per RNTCP				
	RNTCP 2012		*RNTCP 2015*	
Treatment category	*Type of patients*	*Treatment regimens*	*Type of patients*	*Treatment regimens*
New case	• Smear +ve/–ve (PTB) • EPTB	$2H_3R_3Z_3E_3 + 4 H_3R_3$	• Bacteriologically confirmed TB • Clinically diagnosed TB • Extrapulmonary TB	$2HRZE^{\#} + 4HRE^{@}$
Previously treated case	• Relapse, failure or Defaulter	$2H_3R_3Z_3E_3 +$ $1H_3R_3Z_3E_3 + 5H_3R_3E_3$	• Bacteriologically confirmed recurrent • Microbiological positive failure/defaulter • Other*	$2HRZES + 1HRZE+$ $5HRE$

\# If there is poor or no clinical response after completion of 8 weeks of intensive phase it can be extended by one more month.

@ In TB Meningitis, spinal TB, miliary/disseminated TB and osteoarticular TB the recommended duration of continuation phase is seven months, making the total duration of therapy as 9 months (2 IP+7CP). The duration of continuation therapy may be further extended by 3 more months (making the total duration to be 12 months); as per the discretion of the treating physician or in cases of delayed response

*Others include Patients with either Sputum smear negative or EPTB and now having recurrenceCompared to 2012 guidelines, RNTCP in 2015 recommends three drugs (HRE) in continuation phase of new patients. Further 2015 guidelines recommend daily treatment regimen. It is planned to implement these changes in a district-wise phased manner throughout the country, so presently the RNTCP regimen being used in a particular district should be followed. Patients receiving non-DOTS ATT should be advised daily ATT.INH = Isoniazid, R = Rifampicin, Z = Pyrazinamide, E = Ethambutol, S = Streptomycin. PTB = Pulmonary TB, EPTB = Extrapulmonary TB.

Monitoring of treatment

Check for compliance and adherence to prescribed treatment along with response to treatment. The child should be monitored for side effects including gastric intolerance, drug induced hepatitis, ocular or peripheral neurotoxicity, and arthritis. As most side effects are usually mild, antitubercular therapy does not need to be stopped and symptomatic therapy alone may suffice in most cases. The most frequent side effects are pain abdomen, nausea and vomiting due to gastritis which respond well to antacids and H_2 blockers like ranitidine.

Hepatic toxicity

Antitubercular drugs are hepatic enzyme inducers, and can cause asymptomatic biochemical derangement without increase in bilirubin level. This derangement may be tolerated till the enzymes are elevated to 5 times the normal range. However, if the patient has symptoms suggestive of hepatotoxicity, particularly development of icterus on ATT, it is prudent to stop hepatotoxic drugs irrespective of the enzyme levels. The drugs are withheld till the serum bilirubin becomes normal and the enzymes also start touching the normal range. In most cases the regular four drugs treatment can be restarted after the liver

---

Case Study | **Prolonged Cough and Fever**

An 18-month-old boy weighing 6 kg was brought with history of cough and fever for 20 days. He had received multiple courses of antibiotics over last two weeks but the symptoms did not improve. He had not been accepting feeds well and developed difficulty in breathing for 2 days. There is no history of repeated similar complaints or infections of the other systems (eg. diarrhea, ear discharge, deep abscesses) in the past. Mother of this child was receiving some treatment for cough and hemoptysis from a DOTS center for the past 2 months. There was no BCG scar present over the left deltoid.

On examination, the child looked severely malnourished, temperature was 37°C, pulse rate 110/min, and the respiratory rate was 48/min. There was significant pallor. The cervical lymph nodes were enlarged; size of largest node being 2 × 2 cm. He had lower chest indrawing and had a SpO_2 of 88%. The chest was normal on percussion; auscultation revealed few crepitations in both lung fields. Liver was enlarged 4 cm below the costal margin and was firm in consistency. Spleen was also palpable 2 cm below the left costal margin. The child was lethargic but was responding to parents' commands. The meningeal signs were negative, cranial nerves and motor and sensory examinations were normal. No other abnormality was seen.

What is the most probable diagnosis?

The history of cough and fever indicate pulmonary involvement. The pointers towards tuberculosis are:
• Long duration of illness (cough and fever for >2 weeks)
• No response to antibiotics
• Contact with a case of tuberculosis (mother likely on ATT)
• Severe malnutrition (predisposes to tuberculosis)
• Not received BCG

Provisional diagnosis: Severe pneumonia with hepatosplenomegaly with anemia with severe malnutrition; Disseminated tuberculosis.

List the investigation you will need to confirm this diagnosis.

The investigations required are chest X-ray, collection of gastric washings for 2 consecutive days after an overnight or 4–6 hours fasting to stain for AFB and culture for mycobacteria, tuberculin skin test (Mantoux test), ultrasonography of the abdomen, CSF examination (for evidence of meningeal spread of tuberculosis as the patient is lethargic), complete blood count with peripheral smear, fine needle aspirate from involved lymph nodes (for cytology, AFB staining), liver biopsy, and HIV serology. Routine culture for TB should be sent only if the facilities are available but effort must be made for TB culture whenever drug resistance is suspected (MDR contact or a retreatment case)

His chest X-ray showed small nodules evenly distributed in bilateral lung fields like a snow storm. Ultrasonography of the abdomen revealed multiple granulomas in the liver and the spleen, while an examination of the CSF was normal. He was seronegative for HIV antibodies.

Outline the plan of management to treat this child.

This baby will be treated with a 4 drug regime containing rifampin, INH, pyrazinamide, and ethambutol, preferably given as an observed treatment. This 4 drug intensive phase lasts for 2–3 months depending upon the response. Since she has miliary disease with suggestion of alveolocapillary block (she is hypoxic), she should in addition receive oral steroids in form of prednisone therapy for initial 4–6 weeks. The responsive patients are then put on 2 drug (rifampin and INH) continuation phase for a total of 7 months. The total duration of therapy is 9–10 months.

As the child has severe acute malnutrition, he should be screened and treated for hypoglycemia, hypothermia, infections, electrolyte imbalances, dehydration and micronutrient deficiencies. His anemia and vitamin A deficiency should be treated and deworming should be done. Feeding is to be started slowly and cautiously aiming 100 kcal/kg/d of energy and 1–1.5 g/kg/d of protein intake in the stabilization phase (first 7 days) and it is increased to 150–220 kcal/kg/d and 4–6 g/kg/d in the transition phase (2–6 weeks). The daily weight gain should be monitored, the desired one being >10 g/kg/d. The patient should be provided sensory stimulation and emotional support. The child is fit for discharge when he attains 90% weight for length, and parents should be advised regular follow up and immunization at discharge.

enzymes have fallen and bilirubin has reverted back to normal. Most pediatricians prefer to re-introduce drugs sequentially every 3–4 days, though some may add all together. In case the patient is seriously ill, then a combination of non-hepatotoxic drugs like streptomycin, ethambutol, and flouroquinolones may be used in the interim period.

Other reactions

Arthralgia due to pyrazinamide is easily managed with non-steroidal anti-inflammatory drugs. If the uric acid levels are very high and associated with gout like symptoms, allopurinol may be added. Severe skin reactions and oculotoxicity also require a review of therapy and exclusion of the offending drug. Pyridoxine is useful for isoniazid induced paraesthesias. Most children however, tolerate the treatment very well.

DRUG RESISTANT TUBERCULOSIS

Drug resistance in *mycobacteria* is defined as decrease in sensitivity to commonly used anti-mycobacterial drugs. This is an important reason for failure of primary first line drugs. It is primarily a microbiological diagnosis. Various types of drug resistance are described below:

- *Multidrug-resistant tuberculosis* (MDR TB) It is caused by strains of *Mycobacterium tuberculosis* that are resistant to at least isoniazid (INH) and rifampicin (RMP) with or without resistance to other first line drugs.
- *Polyresistance* Strains of *Mycobacterium tuberculosis* that are resistant to combination of drugs other than both isoniazid and rifampicin are called polyresistant.
- *Extensively resistant tuberculosis* (XDR TB). Infection by multidrug resistance (MDR) strains of Mycobacterium with additional resistance to any fluoroquinolone and one of the three second line injectable drugs amikacin, kanamycin or capreomycin, is labelled as XDR-TB.
- *Pan-drug or totally drug resistant tuberculosis* (TDR-TB) is caused by strains of mycobacteria resistant to all known antitubercular drugs.

Treatment	Drug Resistant Tuberculosis

Polydrug resistance tuberculosis can usually be managed by a five drug combination of first line drugs, as in category 2 drugs of RNTCP. However, the management of MDR and XDR TB is

Revision Point	Tuberculosis

1. Tuberculosis is a chronic illness caused by *Mycobacterium tuberculosis*, starting from a primary focus in lung, lymphnode, or intestine.
2. Children contract the disease from infectious cases, commonly adults in the family.
3. CB-NAAT (cartridge based nucleic acid amplification test) is a rapid and reliable detection tool for diagnosis of TB.
4. RNTCP now recommends three drugs (HRE) in continuation phase of new patients. Further 2015 guidelines recommend daily treatment regimen.
5. All new cases are treated for 6 months with 2HRZE + 4 HRE. TB Meningitis, spinal TB, miliary/disseminated TB and osteoarticular TB are treated for at least 9 months (2HRZE + 7 HRE).

difficult as the drugs available are few, do not have pediatric formulations, expensive, toxic and less effective. Such cases should only be managed at specialized centers.

Bhargava A, Jain Y. The Revised National Tuberculosis Control Programme in India: time for revision of treatment regimens and rapid upscaling of DOTS-plus initiative. *Natl Med J India*. 2008;21:187–91.

Chugh S. Paediatric Bhargava A, Jain Y. The Revised National Tuberculosis Control Programme in India: time for revision of treatment regimens and tuberculosis and DOTS strategy under RNTCP. *J Indian Med Assoc*. 2008;106:799–802.

IAP Working Group. Consensus statement of IAP Working Group: status report on diagnosis of childhood tuberculosis. *Indian Pediatr*. 2004;41:146-55.

Lodha R, Menon PR, Kabra SK. Concerns on the dosing of anti-tubercular drugs for children in RNTCP. *Indian Pediatr*. 2008;45:852–4.

WHO guidelines for the programmatic management of drug-resistant tuberculosis: 2011 update. *Eur Respir J*. 2011;38:516–28.

Working Group on Tuberculosis, Indian Academy of Pediatrics (IAP). Consensus statement on childhood tuberculosis. *Indian Pediatr*. 2010;47:41–55.

10.12 BRONCHIECTASIS

Bronchiectasis is defined as an abnormal, permanent dilatation of one or more branches of the tracheobronchial tree, clinically recognized as a suppurative lung disease, with affected children presenting with chronic wet cough with significant expectoration, clubbing, and coarse crepitations in the chest.

Etiology

The most common underlying etiology in our set-up is post-infectious, often due to tuberculosis. Bronchiectasis can occur secondary to congenital or acquired disorders affecting the lung parenchyma, listed in **Table 10.12.**

Clinical Features

Children with bronchiectasis usually have chronic wet cough with intermittent febrile exacerbations. They bring up significant amount of foul smelling sputum and occasionally may also have hemoptysis. Dyspnea may be seen in severe long standing illness.

On examination, they usually have digital clubbing and in severe cases may also have cyanosis. Respiratory examination reveals localized or generalized coarse crackles with or without rhonchi. They may show other symptoms depending upon the etiology, eg, malabsorption and failure to thrive is

Table 10.12 Etiology of Bronchiectasis	
Congenital	*Acquired*
1. *Gross structural defects*: Tracheomalacia, bronchomalacia, pulmonary sequestration	1. *Infections*: Tuberculosis, pneumonia, measles
2. *Ultrastructural defects*: Primary ciliary dyskinesia	2. *Obstruction*: Foreign body, enlarged lymph node
3. *Metabolic defects*: Cystic fibrosis, alpha-1 antitrypsin deficiency	3. *Immune disorders*: Allergic bronchopulmonary aspergillosis, autoimmune disease
4. *Immunodeficiency*: Hypogammaglobulinemia	

10

seen in children with underlying cystic fibrosis while chronic or recurrent sinusitis may be seen in children with immunodeficiency or ciliary dyskinesia (*Kartagener Syndrome*).

Diagnosis

On plain radiograph of chest, bronchiectasis appears as ring like densities, or rail track like dilated bronchi. Post-infective cases may show areas of atelectasis. CT chest is diagnostic with a typical signet ring appearance of the dilated bronchi. Further investigations are indicated for the underlying cause like tests for tuberculosis and fungal infections, serum immunoglobulin levels, and sweat chloride test for cystic fibrosis.

Chang AB, Redding GJ, Everard ML. Chronic wet cough: Protracted, chronic suppurative lung disease and bronchiectasis. *Pediatr Pulmonol.* 2008;43:519–31.

Jordan TS, Spencer EM, Davies P. Tuberculosis, bronchiectasis and chronic air flow obstruction. *Respirology.* 2010;15:623–8.

Redding GJ. Bronchiectasis in children. *Pediatr Clin North Am.* 2009;56:157–71.

Treatment	Bronchiectasis

- Airway clearance techniques and chest physiotherapy form the mainstay of medical therapy.
- This may be assisted by use of mucolytic agents like N-acetyl cysteine, or bromhexine.
- Chronic cachexia can be prevented by proper supportive care in form of supplemented nutrition and by maintaining adequate hydration.
- The role of antibiotics is limited to acute exacerbations as indicated by appearance of fever, change in the nature of sputum from mucoid (white) to purulent (yellow- greenish yellow). The choice of antibiotics depends on the isolate from sputum/bronchoalveolar lavage.
- Surgical resection is possible in those with localized disease and the indications are: recurrent severe infections, bleeding from localized bronchiectasis, and severe failure to thrive.

Cardiovascular Disorders

11.1 NORMAL CARDIAC ANATOMY

Unoxygenated blood from systemic circulation (systemic venous return) enters the right atrium via the superior vena cava and inferior vena cava (Fig. 11.1). Right atrium also receives blood from coronary sinus. Right atrium opens into right ventricle via tricuspid valve. Tricuspid valve apparatus attaches both to the ventricular septum and to the right ventricle free wall and is more apically attached than the mitral valve.

Right ventricle is coarsely trabeculated, smoothening towards the outflow tract. The pulmonary valve connects right ventricle to the main pulmonary artery. Pulmonary valve is supported by the subpulmonary infundibulum, and sits higher than aortic valve. Normal pulmonary valve is tricuspid and sits left and anterior to the aortic valve. Main pulmonary artery bifurcates into right and left pulmonary arteries, which connect to respective lungs.

Right pulmonary artery has a straighter course, crosses posterior to ascending aorta and below the right bronchus (ep-arterial right bronchus) to join right lung hilum while left pulmonary artery crosses over the left bronchus (left bronchus–hyp-arterial) before joining left hilum.

Pulmonary blood flow returns to left atrium via four pulmonary veins, two from each lung, and join posterior wall of left atrium. Left atrial appendage is crescent shaped. Left atrium is connected to left ventricle via mitral valve, which is bileaflet, and does not have septal attachment of chordae. The left ventricle is smoothly trabeculated and outflows into the aorta via aortic valve. Aortic valve is tricuspid and sits posterior and right of the pulmonary valve. Right coronary artery arises from right aortic sinus and left coronary artery from left aortic sinus.

Both atria are separated by interatrial septum while both ventricles are separated by interventricular septum. Normal pressure range in all cardiac chambers at birth and in childhood is shown in Fig. 11.2.

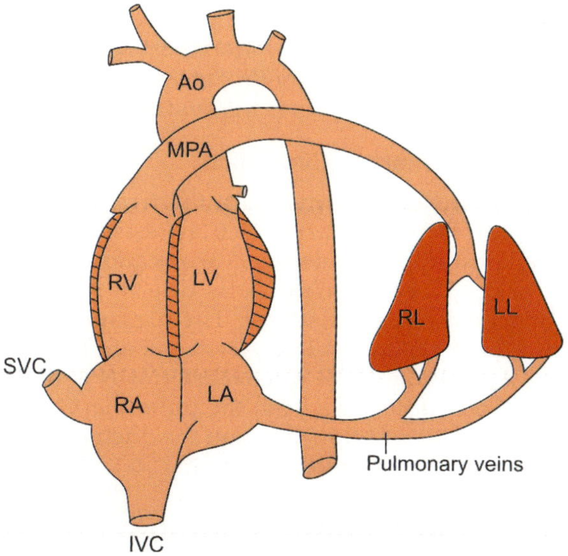

11.2 FETAL CIRCULATION

The heart assumes its normal four-chambered shape by the end of 6 weeks of intrauterine life. After that, changes consist mainly in the growth of the heart as a whole. However, significant differences exist between the fetal circulation and postnatal circulation. Unique aspect of the fetal cardio-vascular circulation is its interface with placenta.

Fig. 11.1 Line diagram depicts course of circulation after birth. Desaturated blood, ie, systemic venous return (via SVC and IVC) enters right atrium, through tricuspid valve to right ventricle and then to pulmonary arteries. Oxygenated blood, ie, pulmonary venous return (4 pulmonary veins) comes to left atrium and through mitral valve enters left ventricle and then aorta

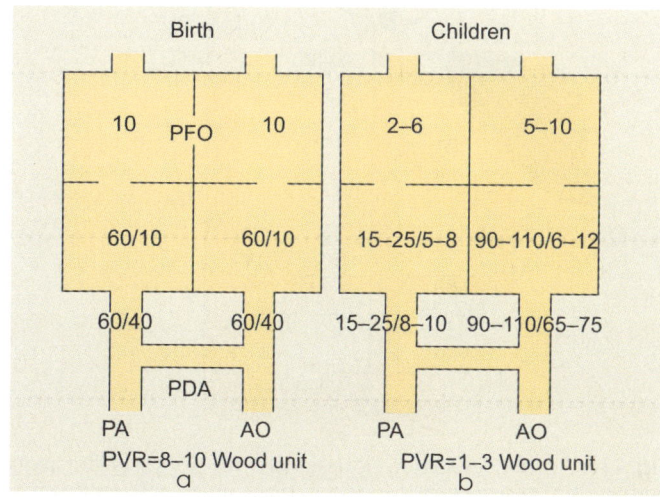

Fig. 11.2 Pressures in cardiac chambers (in mmHg): (a) At birth; and (b) in children. PFO: Patent foramen ovale; PDA: patent ductus arteriosus; PVR: pulmonary vascular resistance

Oxygenated blood enters the fetal circulation via placental transfer. Umbilical vein carries oxygenated blood, which enters the fetus at the umbilicus and course through liver to join the portal vein. The ductus venosus provides a low resistance bypass between the portal vein and the inferior vena cava so most of the umbilical venous blood shunts through the ductus venosus to the inferior vena cava. Eustachian valve directs inferior vena cava blood across the foramen ovale to the left atrium. The inferior vena cava blood comprises the streams of hepatic veins, umbilical veins, and that reaching the inferior vena cava directly from lower extremities and kidneys. Deoxygenated blood from upper extremity returns via superior vena cava to right atrium and is preferentially directed to the right ventricle. The right ventricle pumps this blood into pulmonary arteries, and across the patent ductus arteriosus into the descending aorta. Due to this streaming of blood in the fetal heart, coronary and carotid arteries get most oxygenated blood while lower body gets perfused with less oxygenated blood. Oxygen saturation and partial pressure in different chambers during fetal life is given in Fig. 11.3.

During fetal life, as lungs are relatively high resistance unit, only a small amount of blood from right ventricle flows through the pulmonary arteries and veins. Thus, little of the right ventricular output reaches the left ventricle through the lungs; the rest goes through the ductus arteriosus into the descending aorta. The two ventricles are, therefore, acting together in parallel. The left ventricle supplies the head and upper extremities while the right ventricle supplies the trunk, viscera, and the lower extremities.

The fetal cardiac output is approximately 450 mL/kg/minute, the ratio between right ventricular and left ventricular output being approximately 1.3:1. In postnatal life, the two ventricles are connected in series and therefore, the outputs of right and left ventricles are approximately identical.

Circulatory Adjustments at Birth

Circulatory adjustments occur immediately following birth, and continue to occur for a variable period of time following birth. This change is brought about because of a shift of the main organ responsible for gas exchange from placenta (in fetus) to lungs (in neonate). A summary of these changes is given below:

1. Loss of Low-resistance Placental Circulation

Clamping of the umbilical cord results in loss of low resistance placental circulation. This causes a sudden increase in systemic vascular resistance, aortic blood pressure, and the left ventricular systolic pressure. The left ventricular diastolic pressure also rises, causing increase in left atrial pressure.

2. Closure of Ductus Venosus

Ductus venosus closes because of a sudden reduction of flow, secondary to cessation of placental circulation. The exact pathophysiology is not known. Flow through the ductus venosus disappears by the 7th day of postnatal life.

3. Closure of Foramen Ovale

The loss of placental flow results in a decrease in the volume of blood returning to the right atrium. The right atrial pressure decreases. The left atrial pressure becomes higher as described in 1 above, and exceeds the right atrial pressure. As a result, septum primum comes closer to septum secundum to close the flow across foramen ovale (functional closure). This occurs by 3rd month of life. Anatomical closure of the foramen ovale occurs over a period of months to years.

4. Increased Pulmonary Circulation

Sudden expansion of lungs with the first few breaths causes a fall in pulmonary vascular resistance and an increased flow into the pulmonary trunk and arteries. The pulmonary artery pressure falls due to lowering of pulmonary vascular resistance. The pressure relations between the aorta and pulmonary trunk are reversed so that the flow through the ductus arteriosus is reversed. Instead of blood flowing from the pulmonary artery to aorta, the direction of flow through the ductus arteriosus is from the aorta to pulmonary trunk.

5. Closure of Ductus Arteriosus

During fetal life, patency of ductus arteriosus is maintained by the combined relaxant effect of low oxygen tension and endogenously produced prostaglandins. In full term neonate, oxygen is the most important factor controlling ductus closure. When PaO_2 of the blood passing through the ductus increases to 50 mmHg, the ductal wall constricts. This

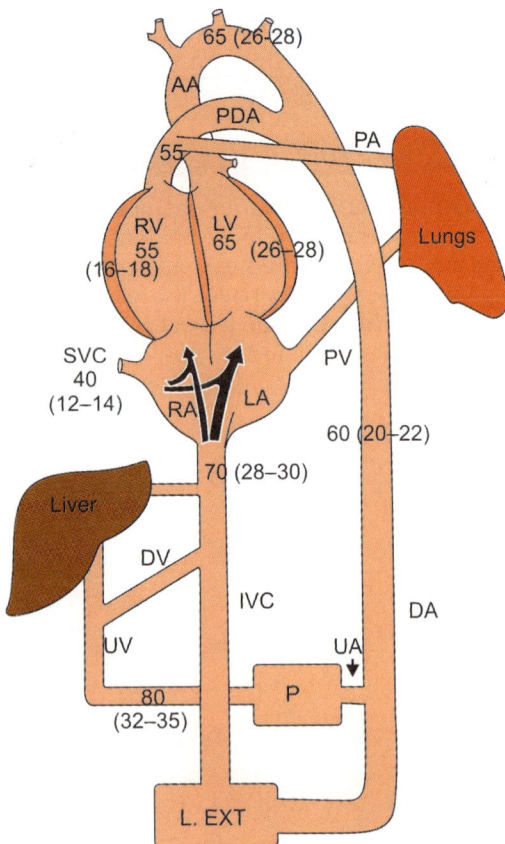

Fig. 11.3 Fetal circulation. Figures indicate oxygen saturation with partial pressure of oxygen in parentheses. P: placenta; UV: umbilical vein; UA: umbilical artery; DV: ductus venosus; PV: pulmonary vein; DA: descending aorta; IVC: inferior vena cava; SVC: superior vena cava; PA: pulmonary artery

effect of oxygen may be direct or mediated by its effects on prostaglandin synthesis.

In full term neonates the ductus arteriosus closes within 10 to 21 days. This results in the establishment of the postnatal circulation, which is in series. The ductus arteriosus of preterm baby is less responsive to oxygen. Some functional patency and flow can be demonstrated through the ductus arteriosus for a few days after birth.

Appearance of Murmur in Neonates with Heart Defects

Immediately after birth, the pulmonary pressure and resistance is equal or only slightly lower than the systemic pressure and resistance (Fig. 11.2a). Therefore, even if there is a communication between the two sides, eg, atrial or ventricular septal defect or patent ductus arteriosus, there is very little flow from left to the right side. Thus an atrial or ventricular septal defect, or a PDA does not manifest at birth or in first few days after birth.

The pulmonary vascular resistance falls fairly rapidly to reach normal adult levels by two to three weeks in normal babies. This results in markedly lower pulmonary pressure as compared to systemic pressure (Fig. 11.2b). The fall in pulmonary vascular resistance and pressure is however slower in the presence of a ventricular septal defect or patent ductus arteriosus and the pulmonary vascular resistance reaches adult values around 6 to 10 weeks. The ventricular septal defect or patent ductus arteriosus murmurs tend to appear by the middle or the end of the first week of life. They gradually increase in intensity as the pressure and resistance in the pulmonary circuit fall. The maximum shunt becomes apparent only by 6 to 10 weeks or more, when the pulmonary vascular resistance may have reached its nadir.

In atrial septal defect, the right ventricular hypertrophy, present at birth, prevents a left to right shunt. This right ventricular hypertrophy takes at least 6 months to regress. The shunt of atrial septal defect therefore does not manifest till at least 6 months of life.

A. Dependent Shunt

The clinical manifestations of atrial, ventricular or aorto-pulmonary communication show rapid changes in the first few weeks or months of life, because of their dependency on the fall of pulmonary vascular resistance. These shunts therefore are also known as 'dependent' shunts.

B. Obligatory Shunt

On the other hand, the murmur of obstructive lesions and valvular leaks are audible immediately after birth. Obstructive lesions (aortic or pulmonary stenosis) and valvular leaks (mitral, aortic, pulmonary, or tricuspid regurgitation) would be operative from birth. Some other defects such as left ventricular to right atrial shunt, arteriovenous fistula are also functional from birth as the flow through these defects is not dependent on the fall of pulmonary vascular resistance and these are called 'obligatory' shunts.

Friedman AH, Fahey JT. The transition from fetal to neonatal circulation: normal responses and implications for infants with heart disease. *Semin Perinatol*. 1993;17:106–21.

Revision Point

Fetal Circulation

1. Fetal circulation is a circulation in parallel while neonatal/adult circulation is in series.
2. Circulatory adjustments at birth are brought about because of a shift from placental dependence for gas exchange in the fetus to pulmonary gas exchange in the neonate.
3. Changes from fetal to neonatal circulation include loss of placental circulation with clamping of the umbilical cord; increase in systemic vascular resistance; closure of ductus venosus, foramen ovale, and ductus arteriosus; fall in pulmonary vascular resistance; and an increased flow into the pulmonary trunk and arteries.

Rudolph AM. Congenital cardiovascular malformations and the fetal circulation. *Arch Dis Child Fetal Neonatal Ed*. 2010;95:F132–6.
Sansoucie DA, Cavaliere TA. Transition from fetal to extrauterine circulation. *Neonatal Netw*. 1997;16:5–12.

11.3 DIAGNOSIS OF HEART DISEASE

1. NADA'S CRITERIA

In any child with heart murmur the decision should be made whether it is organic or is it the so-called functional murmur. Assessment of child for the presence of heart disease is facilitated by Nada's criteria, which are categorized as *Major* and *Minor*.

Major criteria	Minor criteria
1. Systolic murmur grade III or more	1. Systolic murmur less than grade III in intensity
2. Diastolic murmur	2. Abnormal second sound
3. Cyanosis	3. Abnormal ECG
4. Congestive heart failure	4. Abnormal chest X-ray
	5. Abnormal blood pressure

Presence of 1 Major or 2 Minor criteria suggests the presence of a heart disease

Cyanosis

Cyanosis is of two types: Central and peripheral. Central cyanosis is present in fingers, toes, and mucous membranes of the mouth and tongue. Presence of central cyanosis implies low systemic arterial oxygen saturation. Peripheral cyanosis is due to peripheral vasoconstriction.

Central cyanosis can occur because of (*i*) inadequate pulmonary blood flow (pulmonary stenosis, right to left shunt); or (*ii*) inadequate oxygenation of pulmonary blood flow (lung pathology). Pulmonary hypoxia also results in *polycythemia* and *clubbing of* fingers and toes. Third cause of central cyanosis is methemoglobinemia, which occurs due to excessive production of methemoglobin following exposure to oxidant drugs, chemicals, or toxins. Methemoglobin cannot bind oxygen, resulting in functional anemia and failure of delivery of oxygen to tissues. However, clubbing does not occur in methemoglobinemia.

Central cyanosis thus indicates presence of heart disease if methemoglobinemia and lung disease can be ruled out.

11

Abnormal Blood Pressure

It is important to use the right size of cuff to obtain correct readings. Compare with the normal range for age as shown below. The blood pressure cuff should cover at least two-thirds of the length of the arm and most of the circumference. If the cuff is small, it would give erroneously high reading. Appropriate cuff size for different ages is: infant—2.5 cm; 1 month to 1 year—5 cm; 1 to 8 years—9 cm; older children—12.5 cm. Normal blood pressure values (mm Hg) follow:

Age	Systolic	Diastolic
1 to 3 months	75±5	50±5
4 to 12 months	84±5	65±5
1 to 8 years	95±5	65±5
9 to 14 years	105±5	65±5

In a child suspected to be having heart disease, blood pressure is taken in all the four limbs. Different size cuff should be used to measure arm and leg blood pressure. Hypertension with upper limb blood pressure more than in the legs suggests coarctation of aorta. High blood pressure with wide difference between the systolic and diastolic readings suggests aortic run-off. Severe aortic stenosis would result in narrow pulse pressure.

Congestive Cardiac Failure

Presence of congestive cardiac failure usually indicates the presence of underlying heart disease. Newborn infants can develop congestive cardiac failure from non-cardiac causes; eg, hypoxia, sepsis, hypoglycemia, hypocalcemia, polycythemia, and anemia. Signs and symptoms of congestive heart failure are discussed in detail later in this chapter.

2. HEART SOUNDS

The first heart sound is produced by closure of atrio-ventricular valves (mitral and tricuspid) at the onset of systole and normally a single component is audible. Second heart sound is produced due to closure of semilunar valves (aortic and pulmonary) at the end of systole; aortic component occurring before the pulmonary component. Correct evaluation of second heart sound is very crucial in the precise evaluation of heart defects.

Normal second heart sound denotes (i) normal intensity of both components, ie, aortic closure sound (A_2) and pulmonary closure sound (P_2); and (ii) normal split and variation with respiration.

During expiration, both the components are superimposed on each other and only a single second sound is heard. During inspiration, the aortic component can be heard before the pulmonary component, producing a split sound (Fig. 11.4).

Abnormal Second Sound

Abnormalities of the second sound always indicate presence of heart disease. It has been included as a minor criterion only because interpretation of auscultation of second sound is prone to subjective variation.

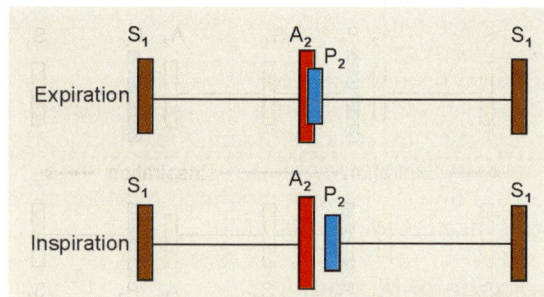

Fig. 11.4 Line diagram showing normal splitting second heart sound (S_2) with respiration ie, single second heart sound during expiration and splitting into A_2 and P_2 component during inspiration

Abnormalities of the Aortic Component (A_2) of the Second Sound

Intensity

A_2 may be accentuated or diminished in intensity. A_2 is *accentuated* in conditions where the aortic valve closes against a higher pressure in the left ventricle, as in systemic hypertension, and aortic regurgitation. A_2 is *diminished* in intensity or may be inaudible when the movement of aortic valve is compromised as in fibrosis or calcification, or when the aortic valve is absent.

Timing

A_2 can occur early or late in timing. A_2 is *delayed* when the left ventricular outflow time is increased resulting in late closure of aortic valve as in aortic stenosis, aortic regurgitation, left ventricular failure, and large patent ductus arteriosus. Another cause of delayed A_2 is left bundle branch block.

A_2 occurs *early* in conditions where the left ventricle empties earlier than usual. This may occur because of alternative exits for left ventricular outflow as in mitral regurgitation (backflow to left atrium) or ventricular septal defect (shunting of left ventricle flow to right ventricle).

Abnormalities of the Pulmonary Component (P_2) of the Second Sound

Intensity

P_2 is *accentuated* in intensity when the pulmonary valve closes against a higher pressure as in pulmonary arterial hypertension from any cause. P_2 is soft in pulmonary stenosis; but only when there is right ventricular dysfunction, or there is a right to left atrial shunt leading to decreased pulmonary blood flow. P_2 is absent when the pulmonary valve is absent or atretic.

Timing

P_2 is *delayed* in conditions that result in delayed emptying of right ventricle because of outflow obstruction (pulmonary stenosis), increased volume (atrial septal defect and total anomalous pulmonary venous drainage); or right bundle branch block.

Abnormalities in Splitting of the Second Sound (S_2)

- Normally, S_2 is single in expiration and split in inspiration with the louder A_2 preceding the P_2 (Fig. 11.4).

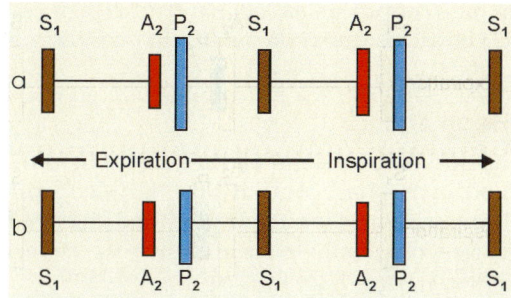

Fig. 11.5 Second heart sound is (a) wide and variably split in ventricular septal defect; and (b) wide and fixed split in atrial septal defect with large left to right shunt

- *Wide splitting of the second sound is defined* as splitting during expiration due to an early A_2 or late P_2 that results in an A_2–P_2 interval of 0.3 sec or more during expiration.
- *Wide and variable split* refers to a split >0.3 sec during expiration that increases further during inspiration (Fig. 11.5a). It is observed in pulmonary stenosis, mitral regurgitation, and ventricular septal defect with large left to right shunt. In pulmonary stenosis it is due to a delay in P_2 whereas in mitral regurgitation and ventricular septal defect it is due to an early A_2.
- *Wide and fixed split* When A_2–P_2 interval is more than 0.3 sec, but remains unchanged during expiration or inspiration (Fig. 11.5b). This is characteristic of atrial septal defect, right bundle branch block, and total anomalous pulmonary venous connection.
- *Narrow or absent split* This can occur in conditions where A_2 is delayed. A farther delay will result in paradoxically split S_2. Pardoxical split in second sound can be diagnosed when the split is more during expiration, than in inspiration. This is characteristic of critical aortic stenosis, large PDA, and severe aortic regurgitation.
- *Single S_2* A single second sound is either A_2 or P_2 or a combination (overlap) of both. The decision whether it is A_2 or P_2 or a combination of both A_2 and P_2 depends on the overall clinical picture. Truncus arteriosus, pulmonary atresia, and aortic atresia have a single S_2.

3. MURMURS

Systolic Murmurs

Systolic murmur can be *ejection systolic* or *pansystolic*. A pansystolic murmur is always abnormal irrespective of its intensity. The causes of pansystolic murmur are (*a*) ventricular septal defect, (*b*) mitral regurgitation, and (*c*) tricuspid regurgitation.

An ejection systolic murmur on the other hand may be due to an organic cause or it may be "functional" murmur. An ejection systolic murmur associated with a thrill is always organic. Systolic murmurs less than grade III do not exclude heart disease, *per se*.

- *Pansystolic murmur* A murmur starting with the first heart sound (partially masking it) and ending with the second heart sound without change in character is a pansystolic murmur (Fig. 11.6a). They are usually soft and blowing if due to AV valve regurgitation, and harsh if due to VSD.
- *Ejection systolic murmur* Murmur audible during the phase of ejection, ie, after the first heart sound and ending with

or before the second heart sound is called ejection systolic murmur (Fig. 11.6b). The ejection murmurs are crescendo and decrescendo; the peak may be in the middle of systole or later giving a diamond shape to the murmur. The ejection murmur could be pulmonary or aortic being produced at the respective valves either due to obstruction to the flow or increased flow across the normal valve. A murmur starting with the first heart sound and ending before mid systole is early systolic murmur and a murmur starting late in systole ending with the second heart sound is late systolic murmur.

Diastolic Murmurs

Presence of a diastolic murmur is almost diagnostic of a heart disease. Rarely one can hear a diastolic murmur which is not pathological is flow murmur (across tricuspid or mitral valve) in condition of high cardiac output as severe anemia or aortic regurgitation. Diastolic murmur in both these conditions disappears after correcting the underlying cause.

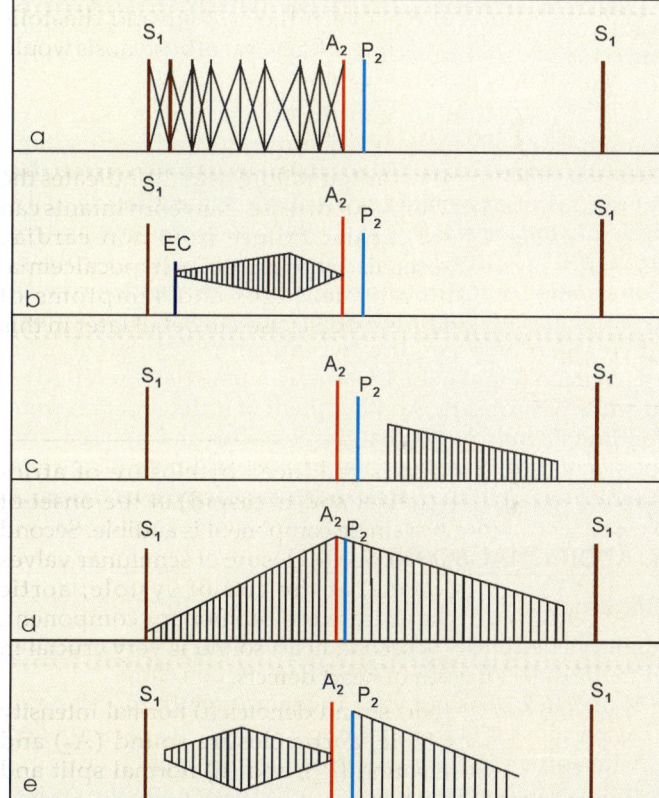

Fig. 11.6 Line diagram representing various types of murmurs: (a) Pansystolic murmur starts with first heart sound (masking first heart sound) and ends with aortic component of second heart sound with same intensity; (b) Ejection systolic murmur starts after first heart sound with a gap, increases in insensity, peaks in later part of systole and then intensity decreases; (c) Delayed diastolic murmur starting with a gap from second heart sound and extending into diastole to variable duration, ends before first heart sound; (d) Continuous murmur in a child with restrictive PDA, starts in systole, peaks in later part of systole and continue into diastole convering second heart sound with same character; (e) Systolic and early diatolic murmur in a patient with aortic stenosis and aortic regurgitation

- *Delayed diastolic murmurs* These are low pitched rumbling in character heard after the second heart sound (Fig. 11.6c). They are audible either in tricuspid or mitral area and are due either to obstruction or increased flow across the respective valves. The diastolic murmur heard in the late diastolic phase and ending with the first heart sound is late diastolic or presystolic murmur, this corresponds to atrial systole.
- *Early diastolic murmurs* are heard with the aortic or pulmonic component of the second heart sound. They indicate regurgitation of the respective valves.

Continuous Murmurs

A continuous murmur begins in systole and continues without interruption or change in character through the second heart sound (Fig. 11.6d). It may occupy whole or part of diastole. Causes of continuous murmur include: (*i*) patent ductus arteriosus; (*ii*) coronary arterio-venous fistula; (*iii*) ruptured sinus of Valsalva fistulae into the right side; (*iv*) restrictive aortico-pulmonary septal defect; (*v*) systemic arteriovenous fistula over the chest; (*vi*) bronchial collateral murmurs; (*vii*) pulmonary arteriovenous fistula; (*viii*) peripheral pulmonic stenosis; (*xi*) venous hum; and (*x*) small atrial septal defect associated with severe mitral stenosis.

The impression of continuous murmur due to a combination of a pansystolic murmur and regurgitant diastolic murmur occurs most commonly in ventricular septal defect associated with aortic regurgitation. This difficulty may also occur in combinations of mitral and/or tricuspid regurgitation with aortic regurgitation. Combination of aortic stenosis and aortic regurgitation never gives an auscultatory impression of a continuous murmur since a gap between the two murmurs can always be appreciated (Fig. 11.6e). These murmurs are also referred as **to and fro murmurs**. Another point of differentiation from continuous murmur is that the character and frequency of the systolic and diastolic components are different in to and fro murmurs, but they are similar in a continuous murmur.

4. ADDITIONAL SOUNDS

Clicks

High-pitched clicky sounds heard after the first heart sound with the onset of ejection are called ejection clicks.
- If the click does not vary in intensity with the phase of respiration, it is constant ejection click and is associated with aortic valve stenosis or aortic dilatation.
- If the click becomes louder during expiration the click is called *inconstant* and is associated with pulmonary valvular stenosis.
- Some clicks are audible in the middle of systole and are called *mid systolic clicks*. These could be due to mitral valve or tricuspid valve prolapse, and atrial or ventricular septal aneurysm.

Third Heart Sound

Low pitched sound heard after the second heart sound in early diastolic phase of cardiac cycle is called third heart sound. It could be from right side or left side of the heart. It indicates rapid filling of the respective ventricle, which could

be due to high output states, failing ventricles or restrictive filling of ventricles (most of the filling occurring in early diastolic phase).

Fourth Heart Sound

The sound audible at the end of diastole just before the first heart sound, in the phase of atrial filling is called fourth heart sound. The sound may be either right sided or left sided and indicates non-compliant ventricle of the respective side.

5. CHEST X-RAY

Chest X-ray provides information on visceral situs, cardiac size, position and configuration, pulmonary vasculature, pulmonary arterial and venous hypertension, and pulmonary pathology.

What is a Good X-ray Chest?

A. Proper Centering without Any Rotation

If the centering is correct both clavicles should be at the same level. The shadow of the spine should not be rotated. In this position, the right border of the cardiac silhoutte is made up by superior vena cava, right atrium, and inferior vena cava; while the left border is made up of aortic knuckle, main pulmonary artery, left atrial appendage if enlarged, and the left ventricle (Fig. 11.7).

B. Correct Exposure

The space between 2nd and 3rd vertebra should be visible if the penetration is adequate. If the whole spine is clearly seen, the chest X-ray is over penetrated and then the vasculature will be underestimated. On the contrary, if the spine is not at all seen the chest X-ray is under penetrated, and this will lead to overestimation of vasculature changes.

C. Proper Inspiratory Film

A proper inspiratory film should have diaphragm at the level of 9th intercostal space. If the film is taken when the inspiration is not complete the level of the diaphragm will be higher and the cardiac size will be wrongly overestimated.

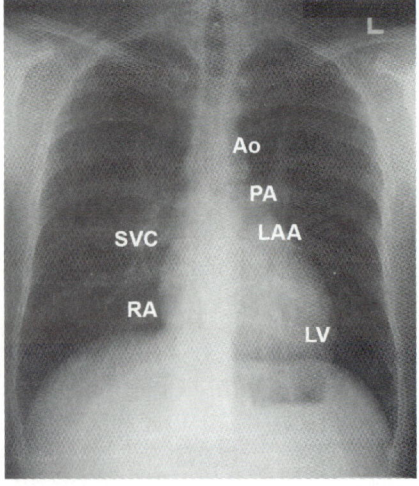

Fig. 11.7 Normal cardiac silhoutte. SVC: superior vena cava; RA: right atrium; Ao: aortic knuckle; PA: pulmonary artery; LAA: left atrial appendage; LV; left ventricle

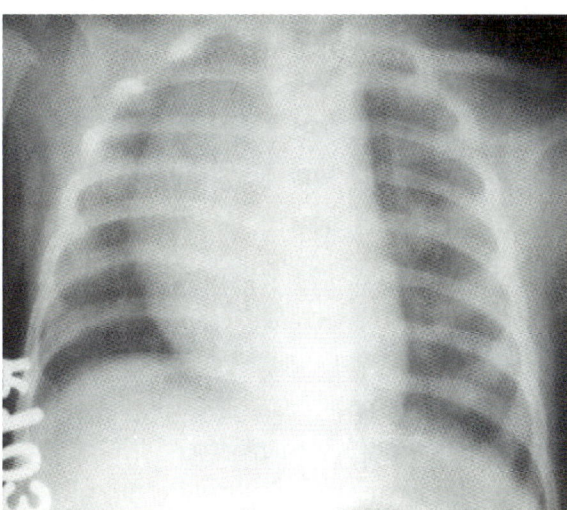

Fig. 11.8 Chest X-ray frontal view of an infant referred as dextrocardia. X-ray showed thymic shadow on right cardiac border giving the impression of dextrocardia. Cardiac size is normal with normal pulmonary vascularity

D. Alterations in Cardiac Position

One should always remember to look for extraneous causes to explain the altered cardiac position like hiatus hernia, pneumothorax or hyperinflation, shifting the heart to opposite side. Collapse or hypoplasia of lung causes shift to the same side. Thymic shadow should be looked for before commenting on abnormal cardiac position, cardiomegaly, or wide mediastinum (Fig. 11.8).

Diagnosis of Situs

In normal situs (situs solitus) the gas bubble in stomach is seen on left side and the liver shadow is seen on the right side (Fig. 11.9a). The right dome of the diaphragm being higher than the left dome. If the stomach gas bubble is seen on the right side and the liver shadow with the higher diaphragm is seen on the left side it will indicate that one is dealing with situs inversus (Fig. 11.9b). A midline liver indicates asplenia or polysplenia associated with complex heart disease (Fig. 11.9c).

Bronchial division can also give a clue to the situs. The left main bronchus is longer and has a more acute angle with trachea as compared to the right main bronchus. If the right and left bronchi are lateralized normally it indicates normal situs and if vice versa ie inversely lateralized it will indicate situs inversus. If they are identical it indicates as asplenia or polysplenia.

Heart Size

For the assessment of heart size, cardiothoracic (CT) ratio is calculated. The cardiac dimension is measured from middle of the spine to maximum cardiac shadow on right and left side. The thoracic dimension is the widest internal thoracic dimension (Fig. 11.10). Cardiothoracic ratio of more than 60% in neonates, 55% in infants and 50% in children is taken as cardiac enlargement. While calculating this ratio it is necessary that the chest X-ray is obtained during inspiration and is well-centered. Expiratory film causes false increase in cardiothoracic ratio.

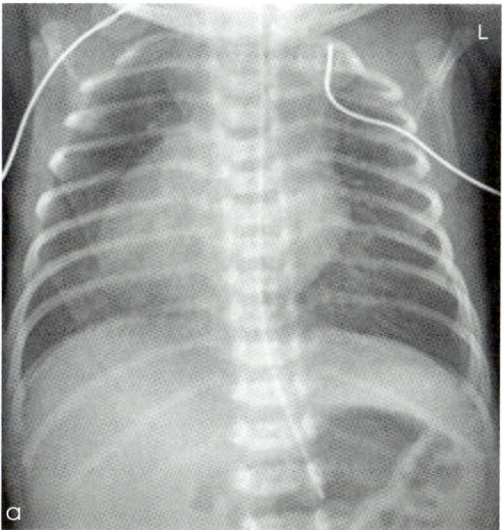

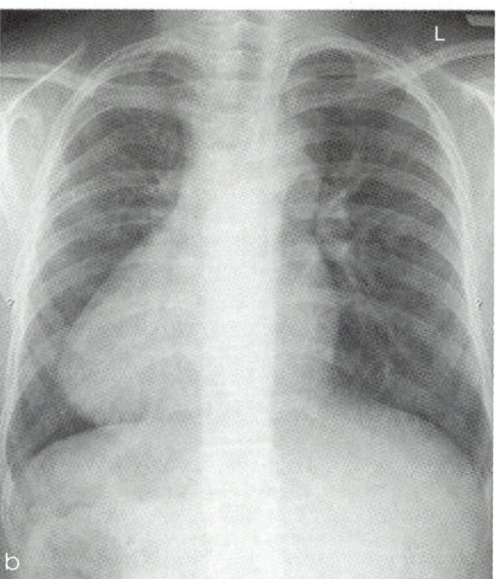

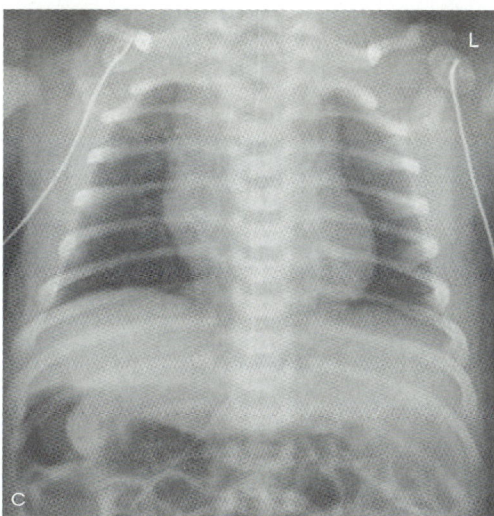

Fig. 11.9 a–c Chest X-rays frontal view with dextrocardia; (a) Situs solitus (gastric bubble on left) with dextrocardia; (b) Situs inversus (gastric bubble on right) with dextrocardia; and (c) Isomerism (midline transverse liver) with mesocardia

11

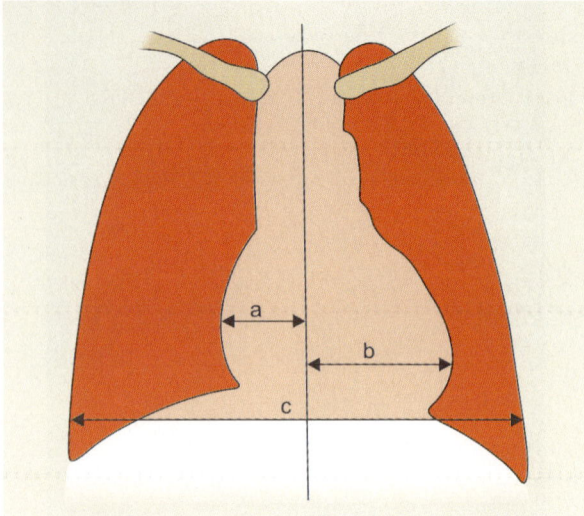

Fig. 11.10 Cardiothoracic ratio: (a +b)/c

Cardiac Configuration

- Left ventricular enlargement results in shifting of the apex of the heart downwards and outwards, evidenced by an obtuse cardiophrenic angle (Fig. 11.11a).
- Right ventricular enlargement is indicated by lifting up of the apex, resulting in an acute cardiophrenic angle (Fig. 11.11b). As right ventricle is an anterior structure, RV enlargement is best characterized in a lateral view film, as

obliteration of retrosternal space between pericardium and sternum.
- Enlargement of the right atrium is indicated by an enlarged contour of the right heart border (which is formed by the right atrium) occupying more than 2½ intercostal spaces.
- Enlargement of left atrium is best judged by seeing the carinal angle. Normally it is less than 70°. A carinal angle >90° is specific for left atrial enlargement.
- Lateral enlargement is evidenced by double contour of right heart border. Straightening of left heart border due to dilated left atrial appendage is an indirect evidence of LA enlargement.

Vascularity of Lungs

Increased Pulmonary Vascularity

The main pulmonary artery is prominent with normally related great vessels. The hilar pulmonary arteries are also prominent and the pulmonary arteries can be traced till the lateral third of the lung fields. Additionally more than four end-on vessels are seen in each lung field (the end on vessel being more than twice the size of accompanying bronchus)

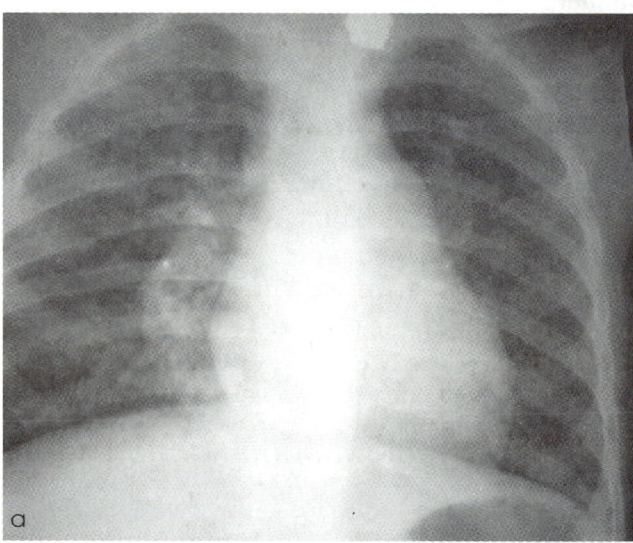

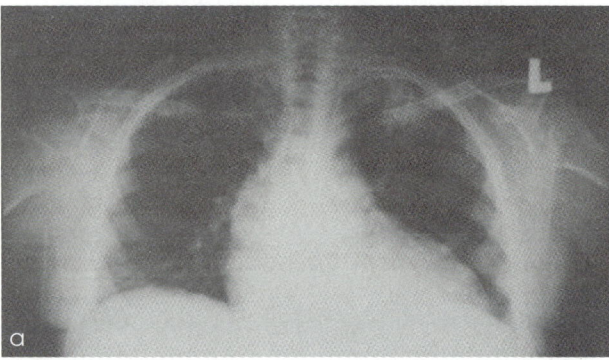

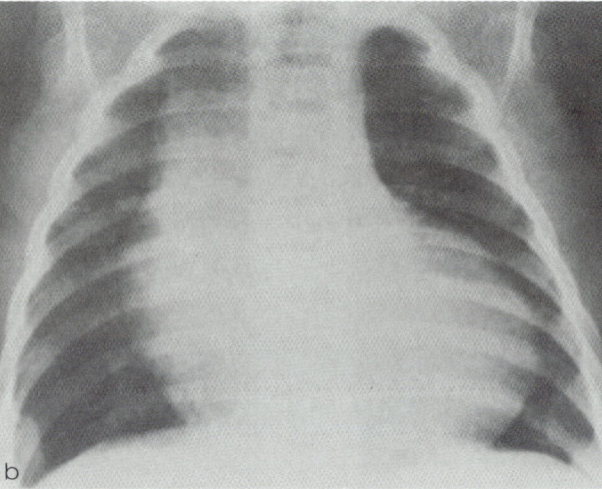

Fig. 11.11 Cardiomegaly with (a) left ventricular apex; and (b) right ventricular apex

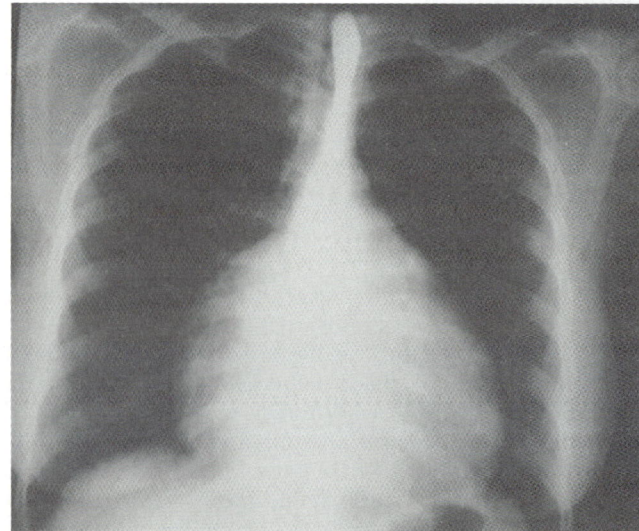

Fig. 11.12 Pulmonary vasculature; (a) plethora and (b) oligemia

(Fig. 11.12a). Three or more end-on vessels on one side, or five or more on both lung fields combined, indicate increased vascularity.

Decreased Pulmonary Vascularity

The main pulmonary artery is not prominent and hilar branches appear small. The peripheral pulmonary vessels are thinned out (stringy vasculature). The overall lung fields appear dark (Fig 11.12b).

Pulmonary Arterial Hypertension (PAH)

The main pulmonary artery dilates. Right pulmonary artery diameter of more than trachea indicates significant PAH. If the PAH is severe, with prominent hilar vessels there is sudden tapering of the vessels called pruning. Pruning means that more than a 50% reduction in vessel diameter at any branching level. It is generally clearly seen at the junction of medial and middle third of lung fields.

Pulmonary Venous Hypertension (PVH)

In the initial stages with mild elevation of pulmonary venous pressures the upper lobe vessels dilate with constriction and blurring of the lower zone vessels. With further increase in pulmonary venous pressures the interstitial lung water increases leading to increased lymphatic drainage resulting in cuffing of fluid around bronchi, background haze, Kerley's lines, septal and interstitial edema. Very severe elevation of pulmonary venous pressures results in collection of edema fluid towards the hilum resulting in "Bat's wing" appearance.

6. ELECTROCARDIOGRAPHY

ECG is primarily used to detect abnormalities of cardiac conduction, arrhythmias, and chamber (atrial or ventricular) hypertrophy. Major abnormalities and their causes are listed below:

P Wave

Absent P wave Sinoatrial block, atrial fibrillation

Tall P wave (> 3 mm) Right atrial enlargement

Prolonged P wave duration (wide and often notched) Left atrial enlargement

PR Interval

Short PR interval delta wave-WPW syndrome, Pompe's disease

Prolonged PR interval Atrial septal defect, Ebstein's anomaly, toxicity of digitalis or quinidine, hyperkalemia, profound hypoxia, myocarditis (rheumatic, viral, diphtheria)

Variable PR interval Mobitz type I second degree atrioventricular block

Mean Frontal Plane QRS Axis

Normal At birth: around 120°; By age of 1 year: between +60° and +90°; Adults: +30° to +60°. Transition from +120° to between +30° and +60° may occur somewhat early or late but presence of QRS axis beyond +120° after the age of 6 months is possibly abnormal, and beyond the age of 1 year it should always be considered abnormal and is suggestive of right ventricular hypertrophy.

If the value for the mean vector of QRS complex falls outside the range of normal values for age, then there is deviation of QRS. The commonest cause of right axis deviation in children is right ventricular hypertrophy. The most common causes of left axis deviation in childhood are related to abnormal intraventricular conduction associated with atrioventricular septal defect, or tricuspid atresia. Concentric left ventricular hypertrophy generally does not cause left axis deviation.

QRS Amplitude

Low voltage QRS complex is defined as QRS amplitude less than 5 mm in all limb leads and less than 10 mm in all precordial leads (Fig. 11.13). It is a nonspecific finding that may be seen in myocarditis, pericardial effusion, myxedema, and generalized edema.

Normal newborn ECG may show low voltage QRS complexes due to vernix caseosa fat being a poor conductor.

Ventricular hypertrophy The right ventricle forces are directed anteriorly (height of R wave in V1) and to the right (depth of S wave in lead V6). Conversely the posterior forces generated by left ventricle are reflected by depth of S wave in V1 while the leftward forces are reflected by the height of the R wave in V6.

QT Interval

Prolonged QTc interval QTc should not exceed 0.44 sec, except in infants <6 months, QTc up to 0.49 sec may be normal. Causes of prolonged QTc include hypocalcemia, long QT syndrome, and anti-arrhythmic drugs: quinidine, procainamide, and amiodarone.

Short QT interval Hypercalcemia, digitalis effect.

Atrial Enlargement

Criteria for atrial enlargement will not be valid with ectopic atrial rhythm.

Right atrial enlargement Tall, peaked P wave in lead II (>3 mm), or biphasic or tall P wave in V1.

Left atrial enlargement Broad notched P wave (P wave > 0.10 sec in children, >0.08 sec in infants) in lead II, or deep, slurred biphasic P wave in V1.

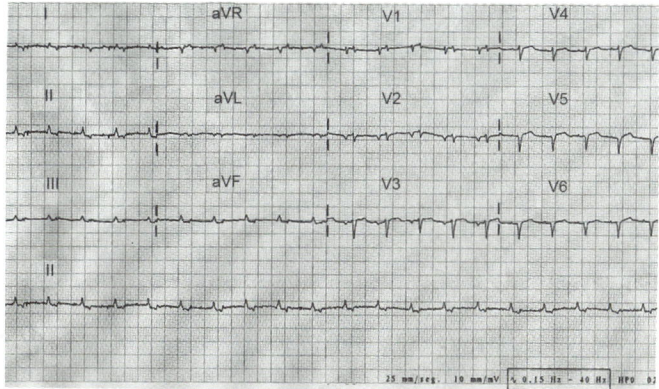

Fig. 11.13 ECG from 12-year-old girl with thiamine deficiency presented with severe ventricular dysfunction, pericardial and pleural effusion and ascites. ECG showing sinus tachycardia (HR-124/minute) and generalized low votage QRS complexes

Ventricular Hypertrophy

Criteria for an ECG determination of ventricular hyper-trophy are based on whether QRS voltages in specific leads exceed normal values. Right ventricle is anterior, superior and to the right, so that the increased forces are to right, anterior and superior suggest right ventricular hypertrophy (RVH). Left ventricle is to left, posterior, and inferior and increased forces directed to the left, inferior and posterior suggest left ventricular hypertrophy (LVH). Leads V1 and V2 may be used to judge anteroposterior forces, while leads V5 and V6 to judge left-right forces and lead aVF to judge inferior-superior forces.

Left Ventricular Hypertrophy

- *R wave* greater than 98th percentile for age in V6, S wave greater than 98th percentile for age in V1
- *Tall R wave in aVF* This may also be present in RVH, in the absence of RVH this criteria is helpful in supporting a diagnosis of LVH
- *T wave abnormality* A left ventricular strain pattern consists of inverted T wave in inferior leads (II, III, aVF) and left precordial leads (V5, V6), or a wide QRS-T angle (>100°)
- *Deep Q wave in V5, V6* more in favor of volume overloaded left ventricle. Deep Q waves are not seen in severe left ventricular hypertrophy.

Right Ventricular Hypertrophy

- R wave greater than 98th percentile for age in V1
- S wave greater than 98th percentile in V6
- R/S ratio in V1 abnormally high; and in V6 abnormally low

7. ECHOCARDIOGRAPHY

Echocardiography, in addition to defining cardiac anatomy, also provides hemodynamic details of the lesion, assessment of pulmonary artery pressure, ventricular function, and valvular physiology. It is also useful in following up a child with heart disease, during difficult cardiac surgery, in immediate postoperative period, and also during catheter intervention as balloon atrial septostomy, device closure, and pericardiocentesis, etc.

- *Two-dimensional echocardiography* provides a realtime image of cardiac structures with the use of several standard views and has replaced cardiac angiography for the preoperative diagnosis of many of the heart defects.
- *M-mode echocardiography* is used mostly for the measurements of cardiac chambers, wall thickness and cardiac function. It also provides information about motion of valves and interventricular septum.
- *Doppler echocardiography* is used to assess the flow velocities across various valves and communications.
- *Three-dimensional echocardiography* has been used for measurements of volume and ejection fraction of unusual ventricular geometries; visualization of device placement; and simulation of intraoperative preoperative anatomy.

Frank JE, Jacobe KM. Evaluation and management of heart murmurs in children. *Am Fam Physician*. 2011;84:793–800.

Somerville J, Grech V. The chest X-ray in congenital heart disease. *Paediatr Cardiol*. 2011;11–13: in four parts.

Surawicz B, Childers R, Deal BJ; American Heart Association Electrocardiography and Arrhythmias Committee. AHA/ACCF/HRS recommendations for the standardization and interpretation of the Electrocardiogram. *Circulation*. 2009;119:e235–40.

11.4 CONGENITAL HEART DISEASE

The incidence of congenital heart disease (CHD) is 8/1000 live births, excluding patent ductus arteriosus in preterm, bicuspid aortic valve and mitral valve prolapse. The incidence is higher in stillborns, abortuses, and premature babies. **Table 11.1** shows relative frequency of congenital heart defects.

Table 11.1 Prevalence of Congenital Heart Defects	
Lesion	Relative prevalence (%)
Ventricular septal defect (VSD)	16–50
Atrial septal defect (ASD)	8–10
Patent ductus arteriosus (PDA)	6–8
Tetralogy of Fallot (TOF)	3.36–9.7
Complete transposition of great vessels (d-TGA)	5–7
Pulmonary stenosis (PS)	5.8–11.6
Valvular aortic stenosis (AS)	3.7–7.6
Atrio-ventricular septal defect (AVSD)	4
Hypoplastic left heart syndrome (HLHS)	3.4
Peripheral pulmonary stenosis (PPS)	2–3
Tricuspid atresia	1.2
Total anomalous pulmonary venous connection (TAPVC)	0.8–1.5
Ebstein anomaly	0.38–1

Age at Presentation

Most of the congenital heart defects are well tolerated during the intrauterine life. This is due to the parallel circulation in fetus in contrast to circulation in series after birth. Lesions that can cause problems during fetal life include atrioventricular valve regurgitation (mitral/tricuspid regurgitation); aortic valve regurgitation; restriction of foramen ovale; restriction of ductus arteriosus; and cardiomyopathies.

Transposition, hypoplastic left heart syndrome, Fallot tetralogy, and coarctation of aorta are the most common lesions presenting within first two weeks after birth.

Etiology

Most cases of congenital heart disease have multifactorial etiology and result from a combination of genetic and environmental stimulus. In some there is definite association with chromosome abnormalities, including trisomy of chromosome 21, 18 and 13, Turner syndrome and micro-deletions of chromosome 22q11. Almost 90% of children with trisomy 18 have heart disease. In trisomy 21, 50% of children have heart disease—commonest being atrioventricular septal defect in 40%.

Known teratogens, such as maternal insulin-dependent diabetes, rubella, and drug exposure, can be implicated in others. CHD may be associated with specific dysmorphic features suggesting a syndrome, which may show monogenic inheritance (eg, William, Marfan, Noonan, etc.). However, in the majority of cases of isolated CHD, no single

Table 11.2 Common Syndromes Associated with Heart Defects		
Syndrome	*Heart defect*	*Chromosomal defect*
Goldenhar syndrome	Tetralogy of Fallot	22q11
Congenital rubella syndrome	PDA	20p12 (*Jagged1* gene)
Holt-Oram syndrome	ASD, VSD	12q2
Turner syndrome	Coarctation of aorta	5q35
Trisomy 21	Endocardial cushion defect	21q22
Noonan syndrome	Pulmonary stenosis	12q24
Ellis-van Crevald syndrome	Single atrium	4p16
Williams syndrome	Supravalvular aortic stenosis	7q11(*elastin* gene)
Marfan syndrome	Mitral valve prolapse	15q21(*fibrillin* gene)

underlying cause can be identified. A list of some syndrome associated with heart defects is provided in **Table 11.2.**

Classification

Group I: *Acyanotic heart disease*
- *Left to right shunts* (volume overload) Ventricular septal defect (VSD), atrial septal defect (ASD), patent ductus arteriosus (PDA), aortopulmonary window
- *Obstructive lesions* Aortic stenosis, coarctation of aorta, pulmonary stenosis (PS)

Group II: *Cyanotic heart disease*
- *Decreased pulmonary blood flow* Fallot tetralogy (TOF), tricuspid atresia with PS, single ventricle with PS, double outlet right ventricle with PS, TGA with VSD with PS.
- *Increased pulmonary blood flow* d-Transposition of great arteries (dTGA), truncus arteriosus, total anomalous pulmonary venous connection (TAPVC), single ventricle without PS.

Clinical Features

A heart disease is likely to be congenital in origin in presence of one or more of the following:
1. Presentation in neonatal period or infancy
2. Presence of central cyanosis
3. Presence of parasternal murmur
4. Associated extracardiac anomalies: Specially of ear, kidneys, and skeleton

Presentations of congenital heart disease according to the type of defect are detailed below.

A. Left-to-Right Shunts

The three common left-to-right shunts are VSD, ASD, and PDA. Their presentation is quite similar, yet the age at onset of symptoms varies. VSD and PDA may present in infancy while ASD presents in later childhood. Children with left to right shunts are characterized by absence of cyanosis. They are prone to have frequent chest infections and land up in congestive heart failure. Examination reveals a precordial bulge, and hyperkinetic precordium. Chest X-ray will demonstrate cardiomegaly and plethoric lung fields.

B. Obstructive Lesions

These lesions are also acyanotic. There is no history of frequent chest infections. Precordial bulge is absent and the apex beat is forcible or heaving due to concentric hypertrophy of the respective ventricle without cardiac enlargement. There is no cardiomegaly on chest X-ray and pulmonary vasculature is normal.

Obstructive lesions can be right sided (pulmonary stenosis) or left sided (aortic stenosis or coarctation of aorta). ECG can help in differentiating between a right or left sided obstruction; and also helpful in indicating the severity of the obstruction.

C. Right-to-Left Shunts

Right-to-left shunts are characterized by presence of cyanosis, clubbing, and polycythemia. These children can be categorized into two groups: (*i*) Those with decreased pulmonary blood flow; and (*ii*) those with increased pulmonary blood flow. Children with increased pulmonary blood flow are mildly cyanotic; those with normal or diminished pulmonary blood flow are moderately to severely cyanotic.

Right-to-left shunt with decreased pulmonary blood flow is seen in tetralogy of Fallot and is due to pulmonary stenosis (and other conditions with similar physiology, ie, good mixing at ventricular level and PS). These children may have a typical history of hypercyanotic spell and squatting episodes. There is no CHF, no cardiomegaly, a quiet precordium, and no chest infections. Chest X-ray shows oligemic lung fields.

Increased pulmonary blood flow with cyanosis is seen in d-transposition of great arteries (TGA), secondary to reversed origin of great vessels; TAPVC, and truncus arteriosus. These children do not have hypercyanotic spells but are characterized by presence of CHF, recurrent chest infections, and cardiomegaly. On chest X-ray, pulmonary vascularity is increased and pulmonary arteries are dilated, along with cardiomegaly.

Risk of Recurrence

- Incidence of congenital heart disease in general population is 0.6–0.8%.
- Incidence in second pregnancy after a child with heart disease is 2–6%.
- Risk further increases if previous two children have the heart disease.
- Recurrence risk with left sided obstructive lesions is higher than other heart defects.

- The recurrence rate of CHD in offspring of either parent with a heart disease is variable, ranging from 3–5%. A higher recurrence risk when the mother rather than the father is affected has raised the possibility of mitochondrial inheritance in some cases.
- Diseases with a single gene disorder and/or chromosomal abnormalities are associated with a high recurrence rate. In Marfan, Noonan, and Holt-Oram syndromes, there is a 50% risk of recurrence in offspring.
- Risk is also higher if 1st degree relatives have a congenital heart disease.

In the above situations, fetal echocardiography is recommended at 16–18 weeks of gestation. However, a negative study cannot guarantee the absence of congenital heart disease.

Congenital Heart Disease

1. Acyanotic heart diseases consists of left-to-right shunts and obstructive lesions. Left-to-right shunts include VSD, ASD, and PDA. All of them have increased pulmonary blood flow, cardiomegaly, CHF, and repeated chest infections.
2. Common obstructive congenital heart diseases are coarctation of aorta, pulmonary stenosis, and aortic stenosis. Severe pulmonary stenosis, however may present with cyanosis.
3. Cyanotic children are classified into (a) those with decreased pulmonary blood flow (↓PBF), eg, tetralogy of Fallot; and (b) those with increased pulmonary blood flow (↑PBF), eg, TGA, TAPVC.

Humayun KN, Atiq M. Clinical profile and outcome of cyanotic congenital heart disease in neonates. *J Coll Physicians Surg Pak.* 2008;18:290–3.

Qu JZ. Congenital heart diseases with right-to-left shunts. *Int Anesthesiol Clin.* 2004;42:59–72.

Rao PS. Diagnosis and management of cyanotic congenital heart disease: part I. *Indian J Pediatr.* 2009;76:57–70.

Saxena A. National consensus meeting on "Management of Congenital Heart Diseases in India" held on 26th august 2007 at the All India Institute of Medical Sciences, New Delhi, India, supported by The Cardiological Society of India. Indian Heart J. 2007;59:515–21.

Syamasundar Rao P. Diagnosis and management of cyanotic congenital heart disease: part II. *Indian J Pediatr.* 2009;76:297–308.

Waldman JD, Wernly JA. Cyanotic congenital heart disease with decreased pulmonary blood flow in children. *Pediatr Clin North Am.* 1999;46:385–404.

LEFT-TO-RIGHT SHUNTS

11.5 VENTRICULAR SEPTAL DEFECT

Ventricular septal defect (VSD) refers to an abnormal communication between the two ventricles present since birth. Time of clinical manifestation depends on the size and location of defect. Ventricular septal defects are classified into 4 types:

1. *Perimembranous ventricular septal defects* These are the commonest type of ventricular septal defects, located in the membranous part of the interventricular septum. Some of the perimembranous ventricular septal defects have a tendency for spontaneous reduction in size or at times to get closed by attachment of the septal leaflet of the tricuspid valve to the defect. Less commonly, aortic valve cusp gets prolapsed into the defect, causing restriction of the defect but at the risk of distortion of aortic valve leading to development of aortic regurgitation.

2. *Doubly committed* or *Subpulmonary ventricular septal defects* These defects involve the infundibular septum and so are committed to both aortic and pulmonary outflows. As the right coronary cusp of the aortic valve remains unsupported, chances of developing aortic regurgitation are higher than in perimembranous septal defects.

3. *Trabecular defect* These defects can be single or multiple and may occur in isolation or in association with defects in other locations. These types of defects have the highest tendency towards spontaneous reduction of size and closure.

4. *Inlet ventricular septal defects* These defects occur in inlet part of the ventricular septum. There may be loss of normal offsetting of the atrioventricular valves. Inlet VSDs never close naturally.

Size of Defect

Anatomically, ventricular septal defects are classified as *large* if the defect is larger than two-thirds of the aortic orifice diameter, *moderate* if the size of the defect is less than two-third but larger than one-third of the aortic orifice diameter; and *small* if its size is less than one-third of the aortic orifice diameter. Depending on the pressure gradient between the two ventricles, ventricular septal defects are classified as:

- *Restrictive (small)* Gradient between two ventricles 64 mmHg and above.
- *Moderately restrictive* Gradient between two ventricles between 25 and 64 mm Hg.
- *Non-restrictive (large)* No significant pressure gradient between the two ventricles (<25 mm Hg).

Hemodynamics

Because of communication, a pressure gradient between the two ventricles, and the different vascular resistances in the systemic and pulmonary circuits; shunting of oxygenated blood occurs from left ventricle to right ventricle.

Large Non-restrictive Defect

Due to a large defect, the pressure between the two ventricles equalizes very early in systole. Thus shunting of blood from left to right ventricle produces a short systolic murmur. Pressure increases in the right ventricle due to additional flow coming from the left ventricle. Due to transmission of increased right ventricular flow and pressure to pulmonary artery, P_2 becomes loud and its closure is delayed. On the other hand, aortic valve closes early due to faster emptying of left ventricle. This result in a widely split second heart sound that remains variable with respiration. Increased flow across the pulmonary valve also results in an ejection systolic murmur at the pulmonary area. Large pulmonary flow translates into a larger pulmonary venous return into left atrium and subsequently increased flow across the mitral valve, passing through the normal mitral valve, the large volume of blood (pulmonary blood flow: Systemic blood flow ratio more than 2:1) results in a delayed diastolic murmur at the apex. If the degree of shunt is more than 1.5:1 but less than 2:1, then only a third heart sound (left

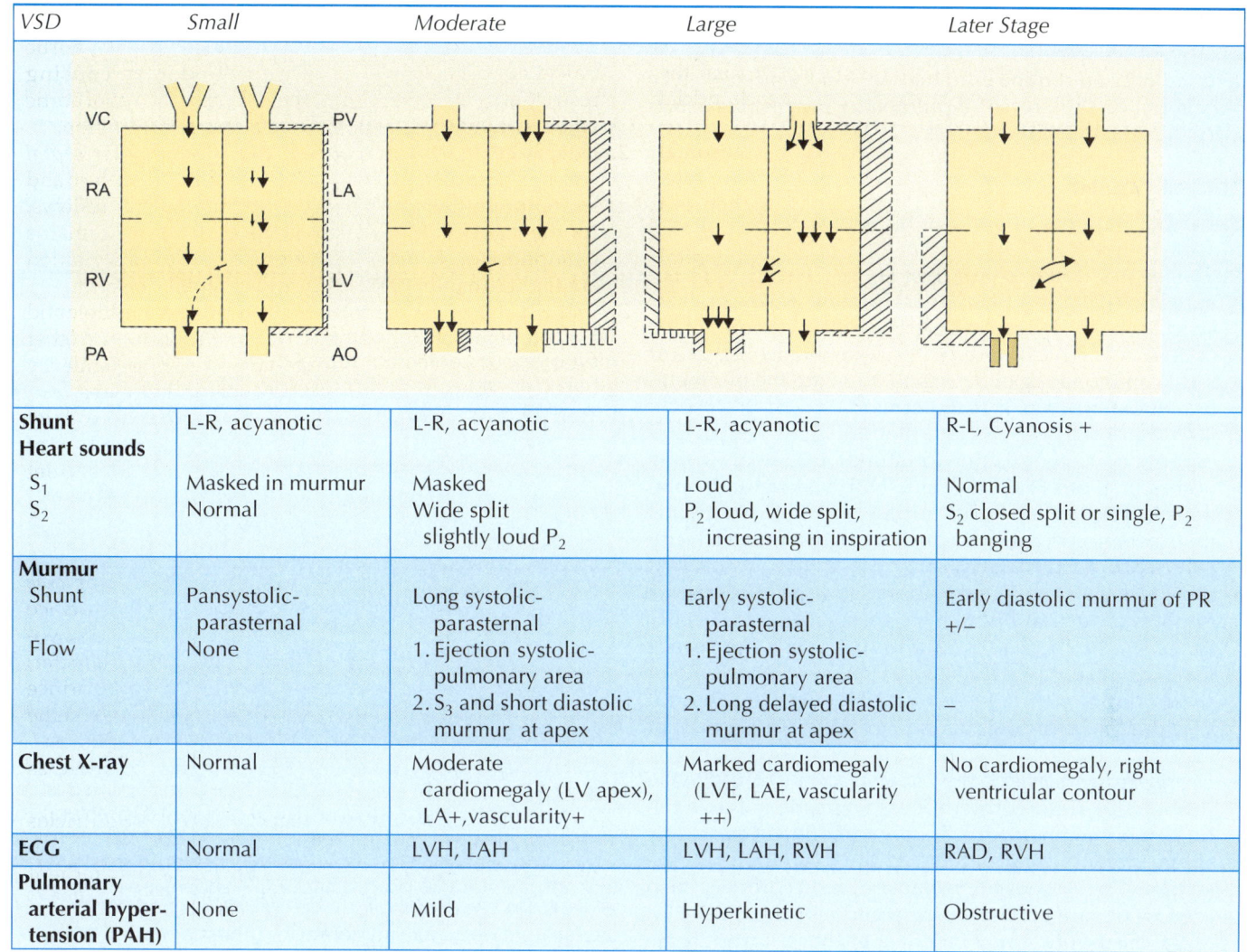

VSD	Small	Moderate	Large	Later Stage
Shunt **Heart sounds**	L-R, acyanotic	L-R, acyanotic	L-R, acyanotic	R-L, Cyanosis +

S_1
S_2
	Masked in murmur
	Normal
		Masked
		Wide split
		   slightly loud P_2
			Loud
			P_2 loud, wide split,
			   increasing in inspiration
				Normal
				S_2 closed split or single, P_2
				   banging

Murmur
Shunt
 	
Flow
	Pansystolic-
	   parasternal
	None
		Long systolic-
		   parasternal
		1. Ejection systolic-
		   pulmonary area
		2. S_3 and short diastolic
		   murmur at apex
			Early systolic-
			   parasternal
			1. Ejection systolic-
			   pulmonary area
			2. Long delayed diastolic
			   murmur at apex
				Early diastolic murmur of PR
				+/–
				
				–

Chest X-ray	Normal	Moderate
		   cardiomegaly (LV apex),
		   LA+,vascularity+
			Marked cardiomegaly
			   (LVE, LAE, vascularity
			   ++)
				No cardiomegaly, right
				   ventricular contour

ECG	Normal	LVH, LAH	LVH, LAH, RVH	RAD, RVH
Pulmonary **arterial hyper-** **tension (PAH)**	None	Mild	Hyperkinetic	Obstructive

Fig. 11.14 Hemodynamics of ventricular septal defect

ventricular S_3) will be audible. In lesser degree of shunts, there is no diastolic sound at apex (Fig. 11.14).

Restrictive (small) Defects

The left ventricle starts contracting before the right ventricle, the flow of blood from left to right ventricle starts very early in systole and a high pressure gradient will be maintained between the two ventricles throughout the systole. The murmur thus starts early partially masking the first sound, and continuing through the systole. This is heard as a pansystolic murmur parasternally, best over 3rd–4th left intercostal space.

Clinical Presentation

Large/Non-restrictive Ventricular Septal Defect

The pressures in both ventricles are equal soon after birth but with fall in pulmonary vascular resistance (PVR), which occurs by 6–10 weeks of age, left to right shunt increases and the child becomes symptomatic having features of congestive cardiac failure. Features of a large shunt such as fast breathing, feed intolerance, failure to gain weight, excessive sweating, and recurrent chest infections appear.

Examination shows failure to thrive, hyperkinetic precordium, cardiomegaly, tachycardia, tachypnea, systolic murmur at left 4th intercostal space, wide and variable second heart sound with loud pulmonary component, ejection systolic murmur at left upper sternal border, and delayed diastolic murmur at apex.

Large left to right shunts are usually associated with pulmonary arterial hypertension (PAH), characterized by loud P_2 and ejection systolic murmur at pulmonary area; caused by increased blood flow through the pulmonary bed. This is known as the *hyperkinetic* variety of PAH. With passage of time, sustained increased pulmonary blood flow leads to irreversible changes in pulmonary vascular bed. Pulmonary vascular changes result in increased resistance to pulmonary blood flow. This chain of events suggests the onset of *obstructive pulmonary arterial hypertension*. Ultimately, pulmonary vascular resistance exceeds the systemic vascular resistance. The flow across the shunt now operates from right ventricle to left ventricle. This is known as 'reversal of shunt.' Clinically, there is a forcible parasternal heave, S_2 becomes single, P_2 is very loud, and mitral murmur disappears. Cyanosis appears due to right to left shunt across the VSD (*Eisenmenger syndrome*).

11

Restrictive (small/moderate) Ventricular Septal Defect

Small ventricular septal defects are asymptomatic and are detected only on routine examination. Moderate size left to right shunt can be present if pulmonary flow is more than twice the systemic flow (Qp/Qs > 2:1).

Natural Course

Untreated patients of ventricular septal defects have a variable course:

1. *Spontaneous closure or reduction in size* Overall, approximately 60–70% of VSDs either decrease in size or close spontaneously. Muscular defects are the commonest type of defects to close or reduce in size spontaneously. Next most common type of defects to do so are the perimembranous ventricular septal defects.

2. *Pulmonary stenosis* Development of right ventricular outflow tract stenosis due to infundibular hypertrophy occurs in about 9% of patients with ventricular septal defects. Right ventricular outflow tract obstruction is more common in patients who have right aortic arch with ventricular septal defects.

3. *Development of pulmonary vascular obstructive disease* Reports show that pulmonary vascular disease occurs in 12.4% of long term survivors with moderate ventricular septal defects, while it occurs in *majority* of the patients with *non-restrictive* ventricular septal defects, sometimes occurring as early as two years of age.

4. *Development of aortic valve prolapse and aortic regurgitation* Prolapse of right coronary cusp of aortic valve is ten times more common with doubly committed ventricular septal defects than defects of the perimembranous septum. The reasons for prolapse of right coronary cusp are loss of support for the cusp and also the distortion of the cusp due to suction effect of the jet through the septal defect.

5. *Bacterial endocarditis* The incidence of infective endocarditis has been estimated as 0.9% per year. The risk is small, therefore, restrictive ventricular septal defects with normal pulmonary artery pressure and normal left ventricular dimensions, without pulmonary stenosis or aortic valve prolapse, are not considered as an indication for surgery.

Diagnosis

Electrocardiography

- *Small ventricular septal defect* Normal ECG
- *Moderate shunts* Left ventricular hypertrophy and left atrial overload pattern
- *Large shunts with hyperkinetic pulmonary artery hypertension* Biventricular hypertrophy (Fig. 11.15).
- *Large shunt with severe obstructive pulmonary vascular disease* Severe right ventricular hypertrophy
- *Follow-up*
  a. If the ECG normalizes it indicates that VSD is becoming smaller.
  b. If it shows progressive increase in RVH, it suggests that the child is either developing PAH or PS (Fig. 11.16). Both these developments require prompt workup for surgical consideration.

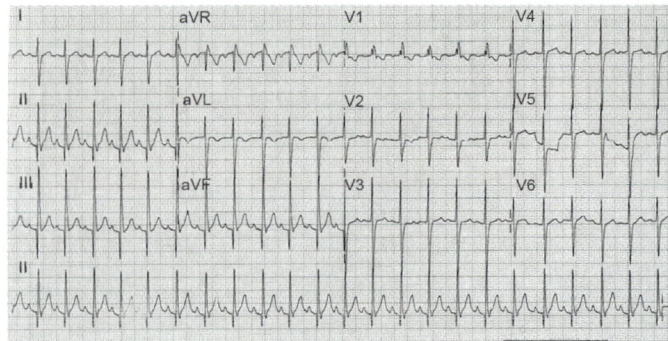

Fig. 11.15 ECG from 6 months old child with nonrestrictive perimembranous ventricular septal defect showing normal 'P' wave axis, sinus tachycardia (HR-150/minute), right axis deviation (QRS+160°), biventricular hypertrophy (chest leads in ½ voltage)

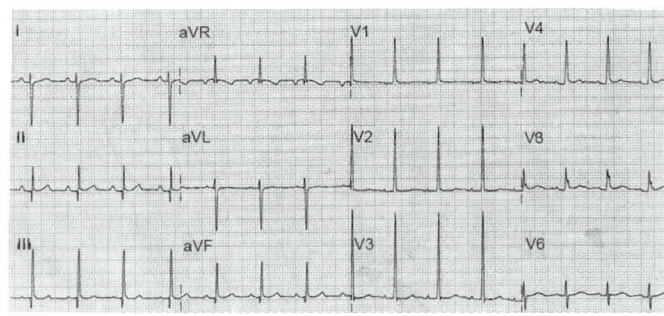

Fig. 11.16 ECG from a 6 years old child with small muscular VSD, severe pulmonary stenosis (RVOT gradient-110 mmHg). To start with, this child had nonrestrictive muscular VSD and mild pulmonary stenosis. On follow-up, VSD became smaller and pulmonary stenosis progressed. ECG showed normal sinus rhythm (HR-75/minute), right axis deviation (QRS + 140°), and severe right ventricular hypertrophy (chest leads in ½ voltage)

  c. If there is progressive increase in LVH a careful evaluation for aortic regurgitation is required.

Chest X-ray

The magnitude of changes depends upon the degree of shunt. With small shunt, chest X-ray will be normal. Moderate shunts produce left ventricular type of cardiomegaly. Presence of left atrial enlargement and pulmonary plethora indicates increased pulmonary blood flow and a large left to right shunt (Fig. 11.17).

Echocardiography

Echocardiography shows the site of defect, number of defects, assessment of pulmonary artery pressure, left atrial and left ventricular dimensions, associated pulmonary stenosis, condition of aortic valve, coarctation of aorta, etc.

Cardiac Catheterization

With availability of echocardiography, cardiac catheterization is rarely done for VSD. Indications for cardiac catheterization include the following:
- Large VSD with severe PAH if there is an issue of operability-to assess pulmonary vascular resistance and pulmonary vasculature reactivity with vasodilators.

Case Study | **Ventricular Septal Defect**

A 4-month-old girl was brought to emergency department with complaints of fast breathing, poor feeding, fever and cough since three days. She was born at term gestation with birth weight of 2.8 kg. She was doing well till 2 months of age, when mother noticed feeding problems in form of suck-rest-suck cycle and sweating over forehead while feeding. Mother was also concerned about her poor growth.

On examination, the child looked thin and weighed 3 kg. She was febrile and had tachypnea (RR 65/min with sub-costal and intercostals retractions) and tachycardia (HR 170/min). Pulse volume was low and all the peripheral pulses were felt. Blood pressure was 66/48 mm Hg in right arm. SpO_2 was 98% in all four limbs. Neck veins were dilated. Precordial examination revealed hyperdynamic left ventricular apex outside the mid-clavicular line in 6th intercostal space. First heart sound was normal; P_2 component of second heart sound was loud; S_3 gallop was heard at apex. Grade 3/6, pansystolic murmur was heard in left lower parasternal region with radiation to entire precordium. Short mid diastolic murmur was heard at apex. Liver was felt 4 cm below right costal margin. Respiratory system examination revealed crepitations in bilateral infraclavicular and axillary areas.

Q. What is the most likely diagnosis?

This child has acyanotic congenital heart disease. According to Nadas criteria, presence of CHF and systolic murmur grade 3 (both major criteria), abnormal S_2, abnormal chest X-ray, abnormal ECG (all minor criteria), indicate a cardiac condition. She has feeding problems and has presented with CHF (evidenced by suck-rest-suck cycles, tachypnea, tachycardia, weak pulses, cardiomegaly, prominent neck veins and hepatomegaly) and lower respiratory tract infection. There was no cyanosis. This favors left to right shunt physiology. Size of the shunt is large as suggested by presence of CHF, S3 gallop, and mid-diastolic murmur at apex. Presence of pan-systolic murmur indicates a ventricular septal defect.

Q. Describe the findings in X-ray and ECG of this child, shown below.

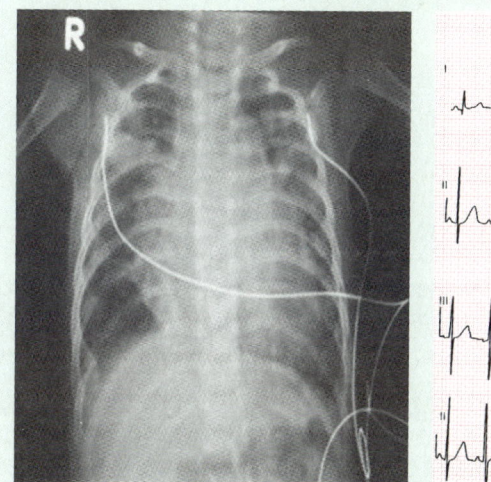
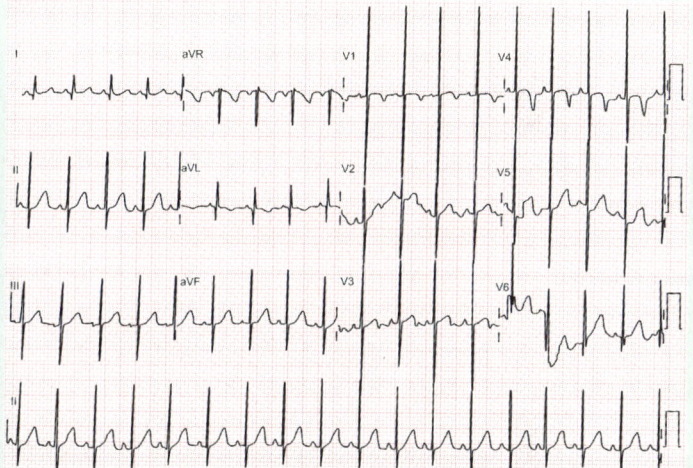

Chest X-ray shows cardiomegaly with cardio-thoracic ratio 0.7. The apical contour is left ventricular type. There is increased pulmonary blood flow. Areas of consolidation are visible in both lung fields. ECG characteristically shows large equidiphasic QRS complexes in mid-precordial chest leads indicating biventricular enlargement due to large VSD. This is called **Katz-Wachtel phenomenon.**

Q. How will you manage child?

Acute management involves treatment of respiratory infection and control of CHF. Oxygen should be started to relieve respiratory distress. I/V fluids and antibiotics need to be started. Inj furosemide and oral spironolactone will be required. Calorie dense feeds are to be given initially by NG tube till oral intake improves. Iron supplementation for treatment or prevention of anemia has to be initiated after control of infection. Echocardiography will confirm the diagnosis. Surgery involving patch closure of VSD is indicated soon after the chest infection is controlled. In the interim period diuretics should be continued.

Q. Is there no role of digitalis/enalapril?

Role of digoxin in patients with heart failure due to left to right shunts is not well defined. It is not used in current pediatric cardiology practice. Angiotensin converting enzyme inhibitors (enalapril) reduce the systemic vascular resistance (blood pressure) hence help in reducing afterload of failing left ventricle. This helps in improving the cardiac output and also reduces the shunt fraction. Hence enalapril can be added as a third line agent if combination of furosemide and spirolactone does not control the symptoms of heart failure. Remember, definite treatment is surgery.

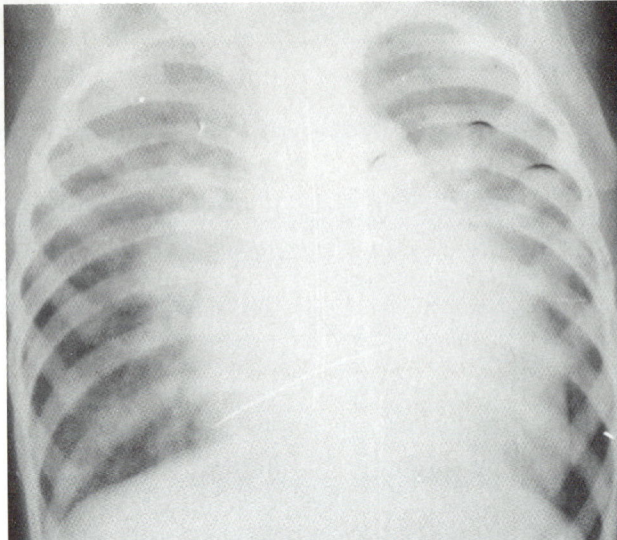

Fig. 11.17 X-ray chest from a patient with large ventricular septal defect; at the age of 5 months showing cardiomegaly (LV type apex) with enlargement of MPA segment. Pulmonary vasculature is markedly increased. The aortic shadow is not prominent

• Small VSD but clinical findings not correlating with echocardiography
• Multiple VSDs
• Device closure of VSD

Treatment	**Ventricular Septal Defect**

Medical management

The medical treatment consists of control of congestive cardiac failure. This includes administration of digoxin, diuretic, ACE inhibitors, and control of anemia and infections. Digoxin is indicated only for ventricular dysfnction. Adequate high caloric diet is essential to sustain growth in face of increased demands. Follow up is needed for development of pulmonary stenosis, pulmonary arterial hypertension, or aortic regurgitation.

Surgical management

Early surgical treatment (before 6 months) is indicated in large defects and if CHF is not controlled by medical management. Association of aortic regurgitation is also indication for surgery, irrespective of the size of defect.

• *Operative treatment* consists of closure of the ventricular septal defect with the use of a dacron or pericardial patch. It is being done for more than 4 decades with very good results and less than 1% risk.
• *Percutaneous device closure* (Fig. 11.18) is indicated in children weighing more than 10 kg with muscular VSD, or residual VSD after surgery, with good results.

Aguilar NE, Eugenio Lopez J. Ventricular septal defects. *Bol Asoc Med P R*. 2009;101:23–9.

Danford DA, Martin AB, Fletcher SE, et al. Children with heart murmurs: can ventricular septal defect be diagnosed reliably without an echocardiogram? *J Am Coll Cardiol*. 1997;30:243–6.

Shrivatsava S, Saxena A, Iyer K, *et al.* Pediatric Cardiac Society of India recommendations for timing of surgery/catheter intervention in left-to-right shunts. *Indian Heart J*. 2006;58:169–71.

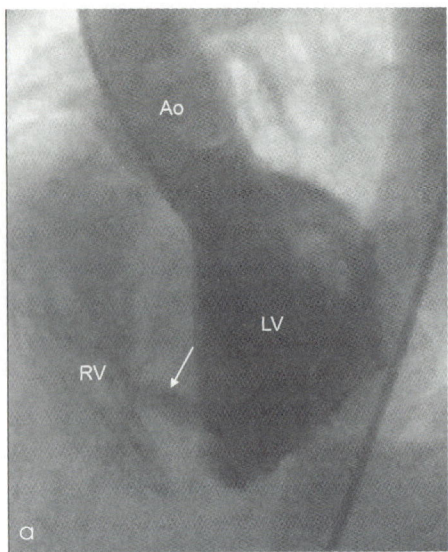

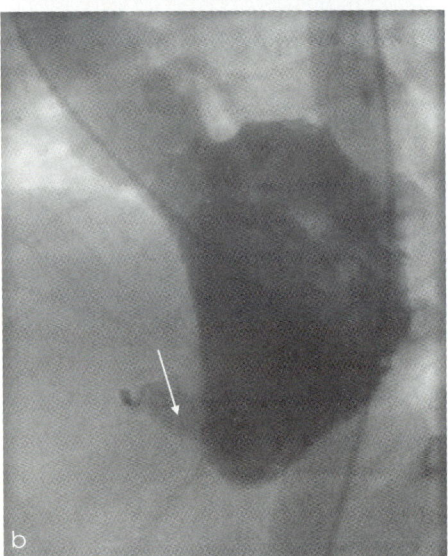

Fig. 11.18 Left ventricular angiography in long axial oblique view: (a) Angiogram showing muscular VSD (arrow) filling right ventricle; (b) LV angiogram after device closure of muscular VSD showing device in situ (arrow), no residual flow

Revision Point

Ventricular Septal Defect (VSD)

1. VSD is an acyanotic heart disease with left to right shunt.
2. Moderate to large sized VSD present after 6 weeks of age, with feeding difficulties, suck-rest-suck cycle, and repeated respiratory infections.
2. Clinical examination reveals a pansystolic murmur in left parasternal region, along with a wide split P2 varying with respiration.
3. Small VSD is asymptomatic and may close spontaneously. Moderate to large VSD will require closure.

Working Group on Management of Congenital Heart Diseases in India. Consensus on timing of intervention for common congenital heart disease. *Indian Pediatr*.2008;45:117–26.

11.6 PATENT DUCTUS ARTERIOSUS

In adult circulation, blood flows from right ventricle to lungs *via* pulmonary artery for oxygenation. Since the fetus does not use the lungs (oxygenation is provided through the mother's placenta), flow from the right ventricle needs an outlet. The ductus arteriosus is a normal fetal structure between pulmonary artery and aorta, allowing the right ventricular outflow to bypass the pulmonary circulation. It shunts the left pulmonary artery flow to the aorta just beyond the origin of the left subclavian artery. Exposure to the high levels of oxygen at birth causes the ductus to close within 24 hours. Persistence of this fetal structure beyond 10 days of life in a term baby is considered abnormal.

Epidemiology

Patent ductus arteriosus represents 5–10% of all congenital heart diseases, excluding those in premature infants. It occurs in approximately 8 of 1000 live births. Females are 2–3 times more likely than males to have patent ductus arteriosus.

Hemodynamics

Patent ductus arteriosus results in a left to right shunt from the aorta to the pulmonary artery (contrary to right-to-left shunt that operates in fetal life). *The flow from aorta to pulmonary artery occurs both during systole and diastole, as a pressure gradient is present throughout the cardiac cycle between the two great arteries.* This leads to overloading of the pulmonary circulation.

1. The flow of blood from aorta to pulmonary artery results in a continuous murmur, which starts in systole after the first sound, reaches a peak at the second sound, and continues in diastole without change in character. Murmur may diminish in intensity and is audible during only a part of the diastole.
2. Shunt results in increased flow to the pulmonary circulation.
3. Left atrium receives a large volume of blood from overloaded pulmonary circulation. Transfer of this volume to left ventricle across a normal mitral valve results in a mitral diastolic murmur (preceded by S_3) along with a loud S_1. Intensity of this murmur is directly proportional to the size of left-to-right shunt across the ductus.
4. The large volume of blood in the left ventricle causes a prolongation of the left ventricular systole and an increase in the size of the left ventricle to accommodate the extra volume. The prolonged left ventricular systole results in *delayed closure of the aortic* valve and a late A_2. With large left-to-right shunts the S_2 *may be paradoxically split* (Fig. 11.19).
5. The large left ventricular volume ejected into the aorta results in *dilatation of the ascending aorta and arch of aorta.* A dilated ascending aorta results in an *aortic ejection click.*
6. Greater volume burden is placed on the left side of the heart, causing both left atrial and left ventricular enlargement.

Clinical Picture

Children with large patent ductus arteriosus present with congestive cardiac failure at around 6–10 weeks of age. Mild to moderate defects present after infancy with frequent chest infections, effort intolerance, and palpitation. Large defects may be associated with pulmonary arterial hypertension.

*   Pulse is high volume and bounding in character. Pulse pressure is wide due to continuous leak of systemic flow from aorta to pulmonary artery.

	Small PDA	Large PDA
Hemodynamics of PDA	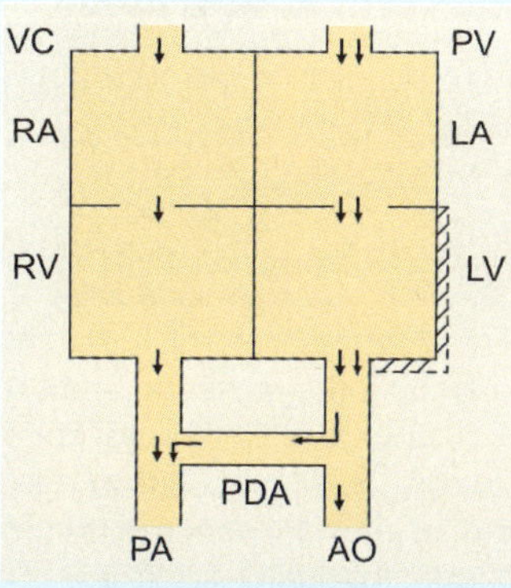	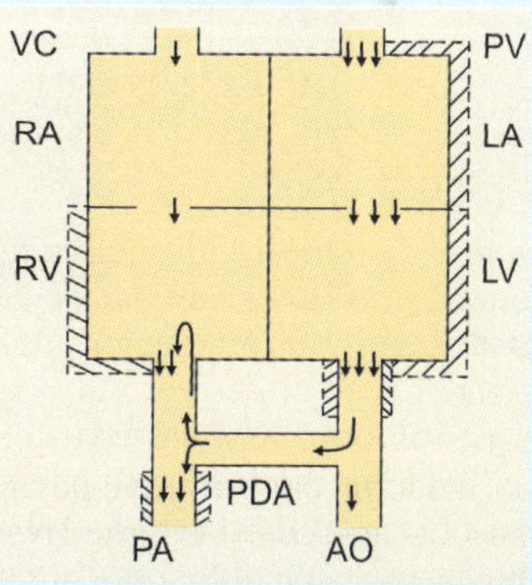
Characteristic	L-R, acyanotic	L-R, acyanotic, increased pulmonary flow
Heart sounds S_1 S_2	May be masked in murmur Masked in murmur	Loud P_2 loud, paradoxically split
Murmur Shunt Flow	Continuous Nil	Ejection systolic at pulmonary area Delayed diastolic at apex with S_3
Chest X-ray	Normal	Cardiomegaly (LA, LV, Aorta, MPA)
ECG	Normal	LVH, LAH

Fig. 11.19 Hemodynamics of patent ductus arteriosus

- Inspection of the precordium reveals prominent carotid pulsations, and a hyperkinetic precordium. Apex is shifted down and out due to left ventricular overload.
- Palpation may reveal a thrill at the second left interspace. P_2 component of second sound may be palpable in large size shunts.

Heart Sounds

The first sound is accentuated. The second heart sound is split normally, or single, or pardoxically split, depending on the size of the shunt. A large shunt causes paradoxical split due to marked delay in emptying of left ventricle (thus causing delayed A_2, after P_2).

Murmurs

Continuous murmur is a hallmark of PDA. It indicates presence of difference in pressure between the aorta and pulmonary artery during both systole and diastole. The murmur starts after the first sound, overlaps the second sound and continues into diastole without any change in the character. Therefore, it may be difficult to assess the second sound, being masked by continuous murmur. The continuous murmur is best heard below the left clavicle.

Ejection systolic murmur PDA with significant shunts result in markedly increased pulmonary flow and subsequent pulmonary artery hypertension. Thus pressure gradient

---

Case Study | Patent Ductus Arteriosus

An 8-month-old boy was brought to out-patient department with complaints of poor growth. He was born at term gestation with birth weight of 2.4 kg. He was well in the neonatal period. He developed feeding problems in form of suck-rest-suck cycle and prolonged feeding time in second month of life. During third and fifth month of age he was hospitalized with complaints of fever, reduced oral acceptance, cough, and fast breathing. On examination child looked thin and weighed 4.8 kg. He was afebrile and had tachypnea and tachycardia. Heart rate was 140/min, respiratory rate was 50/min and sub-costal retractions were present. Pulses were bounding in character and all the peripheral pulses were easily felt. Blood pressure was 90/40 mm Hg in right arm. SpO_2 was 98% in all four limbs. There was no cyanosis. Precordial examination revealed hyperdynamic left ventricular apex outside the mid-clavicular line in 6th intercostal space. First heart sound was normal; P_2 component of second heart sound was loud; S_3 gallop was heard at apex. A continuous murmur without thrill was heard in left infraclavicular region. A short mid-diastolic murmur was heard at apex. Liver was felt 2 cm below right costal margin. Other systemic examination was normal. Chest X- ray of the patient is shown here.

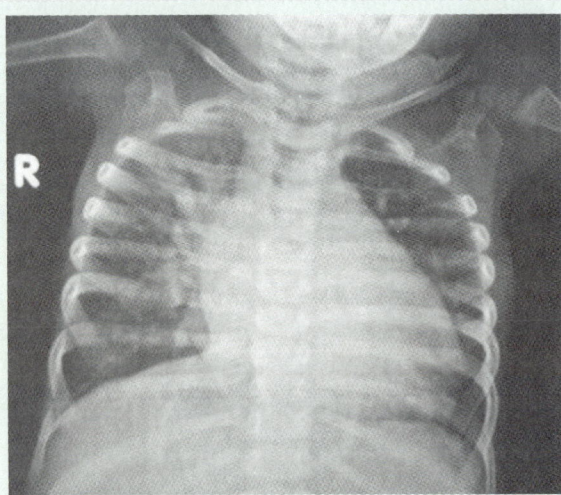

Q1. What is the likely diagnosis?

This boy has acyanotic congenital heart disease. According to Nadas criteria, presence of murmur (1 major criteria), abnormal S_2, abnormal blood pressure, abnormal chest X-ray (3 minor criteria), diagnosis of CHD is justified. He has feeding problems and two episodes of lower respiratory tract infections requiring hospitalization. This favors left to right shunt physiology. Size of shunt is large as suggested by presence of S_3 gallop and mid-diastolic murmur at apex. Presence of continuous murmur at left infra-clavicular area along with bounding pulses and wide pulse pressure indicates patent ductus arteriosus. The child also has failure to thrive.

Q2. What does the X-ray depict?

Chest X-ray shows cardiomegaly (cardiothoracic ratio 0.65). The apical contour is left ventricular type. The structures forming left heart border are prominent and merging with each other. Aortic knuckle and pulmonary artery shadow are prominent with a shadow occupying the space between them, this is ductal shadow. Left atrial dilation is depicted by prominent LA appendage. Pulmonary vascular markings are present till the outer 1/3 of lung fields and there are multiple dilated end-on vessels visible. This indicates increased pulmonary blood flow.

Q3. How will you confirm the diagnosis and treat?

Echocardiography will confirm the diagnosis. Treatment is closure of PDA. Diuretics, commonly furosemide is started to control symptoms. Iron supplementation for treating anemia should be started. Depending on size of PDA, either transcatheter device closure is planned or surgical PDA ligation is carried out.

between aorta and pulmonary circulation diminishes during diastole, causing disappearance of the diastolic component of the continuous murmur. Presence of ejection systolic murmur instead of a continuous murmur thus indicates a larger size shunt. In these cases, evaluation of S$_2$ is possible because of its distance from the murmur.

Apical diastolic murmur Large shunts also result in a delayed diastolic murmur at apex due to increased flow through mitral valve along with a third heart sound.

Obstructive Pulmonary Arterial Hypertension

This results in reversal of shunt (Eisenmenger syndrome) across the PDA and the flow murmurs disappear. Second heart sound remains normally split with very loud pulmonary component. These patients are considered inoperable. Right-to-left shunt through the PDA causes differential cyanosis with cyanosis in toes but not in fingers.

Investigations

Electrocardiography Left ventricular dominance or hypertrophy is the most common finding. Associated aortic stenosis or coarctation of aorta should be suspected if the ECG shows LVH out of proportion to the degree of the shunt or if the ECG shows ischemic changes in the left precordial leads.

Hyperkinetic pulmonary arterial hypertension (PAH) results in biventricular hypertrophy while obstructive PAH manifests with severe right ventricular hpertrophy.

Chest X-ray There is cardiomegaly with a left ventricular apex. Left atrium is also enlarged depending on the degree of shunt. Lung fields are plethoric. Aorta is prominent.

Echocardiography Echocardiography can define PDA size, direction of shunt, pressure gradient across PDA to assess pulmonary artery pressure, evidence of volume overload and, any associated heart defect.

Cardiac catheterization and angiography are useful in adolescents and adults to assess anatomy and pulmonary vascular resistance.

Differential Diagnosis

Continuous murmur can also be produced by (*i*) AV fistula, (*ii*) bronchial collaterals, (*iii*) venous hum, (*iv*) small aorto-pulmonary septal defect, (*v*) atrial septal defect with mitral stenosis, and (*vi*) VSD with aortic regurgitation.

Treatment — Patent Ductus Arteriosus

PDA in Preterm Baby
Medical therapy Intervene if baby is in heart failure. Indomethacin, a prostaglandin synthetase inhibitor is administered orally (0.1 mg/kg/dose, 12 hourly for three doses) to close the ductus. Indomethacin is contraindicated if the neonate is having renal or hepatic insufficiency or bleeding tendency. Ibuprofen can also be used as an alternative therapy (10 mg/kg 1st dose followed by 5 mg/kg/dose 2 doses at 12-hrly intervals orally).

Surgical ligation If above drugs fail or are contraindicated.

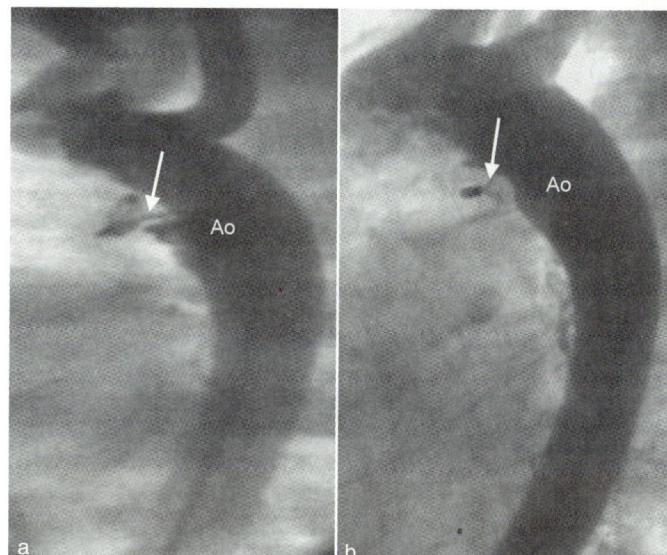

Fig. 11.20a and b Descending aortogram: Post coil closure of PDA showing (a) coil in situ (arrow), (b) device in situ (arrow), no residual flow

PDA in Term/older Child
Initial treatment is directed at control of congestive heart failure. Small PDA in full term baby may close up to 3 months of age. Large ductus would require surgical closure at appropriate time.
- *Large/moderate* PDA, with congestive heart failure, pulmonary arterial hypertension: early closure by 3–6 months.
- *Moderate* PDA, no congestive heart failure: 6 months–1 year; if failure to thrive, closure can be accomplished earlier.
- *Small* PDA: at 12–18 months.
- *Silent* PDA diagnosed only on echocardiography without any auscultatory findings: Closure not recommended.

Mode of closure can be individualized. Options available include device closure, coil occlusion (Fig. 11.20), or surgical ligation. While surgical ligation is preferred in children <6 months of age, or those with very large PDA; device or coils are preferred in older children.

Revision Point

Patent Ductus Arteriosus (PDA)

1. Patent ductus arteriosus (PDA) refers to a communication between the proximal descending thoracic aorta and the main pulmonary artery. It is essential in fetal life, and closes within the first few hours to days in all neonates after birth.
2. Persistent patency of the ductus arteriosus (DA) leads to a wide range of hemodynamically significant problems.
3. Continuous murmur peaking around the second sound is characteristic of PDA. Second sound may be paradoxically split.
4. Most preterm ducts are managed by conservative medical therapy.
5. Spontaneous closure of PDA in term babies is rare. PDA usually always need to be closed. Definitive treatment involves transcatheter closure or surgical closure.

11

Capozzi G, Santoro G. Patent ductus arteriosus: patho-physiology, hemodynamic effects and clinical complications. *J Matern Fetal Neonatal Med*. 2011;24Suppl 1:15–6.

Giliberti P, De Leonibus C, Giordano L, Giliberti P. The physiopatho-logy of the patent ductus arteriosus. *J Matern Fetal Neonatal Med*. 2009;22 Suppl 3:6–9.

Mercanti I, Boubred F, Simeoni U. Therapeutic closure of the ductus arteriosus: benefits and limitations. *J Matern Fetal Neonatal Med*. 2009;22 Suppl 3:14–20.

Ohlsson A, Walia R, Shah S. Ibuprofen for the treatment of patent ductus arteriosus in preterm and/or low birth weight infants. *Cochrane Database Syst Rev*. 2008 Jan 23;(1):CD003481.

11.7 ATRIAL SEPTAL DEFECT

Atrial septal defect (ASD) is an abnormal communication between the two atria and is classified into five types:

1. *Ostium secundum atrial septal defect* It is the commonest type of atrial septal defect, comprising two-thirds of all atrial septal defects. This type of defect occurs in the central part of the atrial septum and involves whole or part of the flap of foramen ovale.

2. *Sinus venosus, superior vena cava (SVC) type atrial septal defect* The defect lies in the posterosuperior portion of the atrial septum. The anatomical components of this defect are overriding and straddling of the superior vena cava, and anomalous drainage of right pulmonary veins to right atrium.

3. *Sinus venosus, inferior vena cava (IVC) type atrial septal defect* This type of defect occupies the posteroinferior part of the atrial septum and is associated with straddling and overriding of inferior vena cava, and may be associated with anomalous drainage of right lower pulmonary vein to right atrium.

4. *Coronary sinus type ASD* The coronary sinus is unroofed, the left superior vena cava drains directly into the left atrium and opening of the coronary sinus into the right atrium acts as the site for atrial shunting.

5. *Ostium primum ASD* The defect occupies the lower most part of the atrial septum. It is a part of atrioventricular septal defect and frequently associated with deformities of the mitral or tricuspid valves or a small VSD.

Hemodynamics

The hemodynamics of the atrial septal defect is characterized by overloading of right atrium, right ventricle, and pulmonary artery. With normal pulmonary artery pressure, the shunt at atrial level is dominantly left to right (during systole) with small phasic right to left shunting during diastole. However, the atrial shunt remains silent as the pressure gradient between the two atria is not enough to cause turbulent flow.

Right atrium enlarges to accommodate extra blood coming from the interatrial left to right shunting. Increased flow from right atrium to right ventricle across a normal tricuspid valve results in a diastolic murmur at the left lower sternal border. Right ventricle also enlarges to accommodate increased volume coming to it. Volume overload of the right ventricle results in an increased pressure and flow across the pulmonary valve to the pulmonary artery and lungs. An ejection systolic

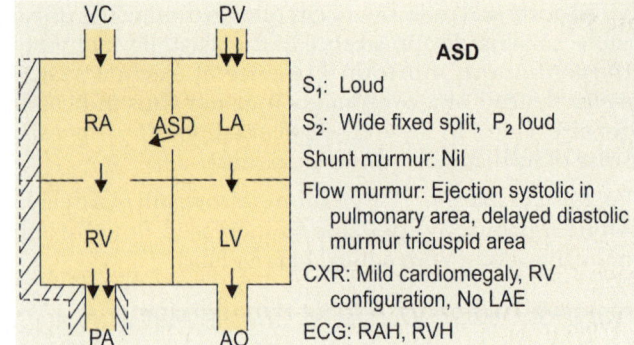

Fig. 11.21 Hemodynamics of atrial septal defect

murmur is thus produced by increased flow across a normal pulmonary valve. Pulmonary valve closure is delayed due to increased time taken for emptying of right ventricle. P_2 is thus delayed. On the left side, A_2 occurs early because of siphoning of the systemic flow through interatrial shunt and a relatively lesser volume of oxygenated blood flowing to left ventricle and subsequently aorta. This results in wide spilt second heart sound. The split however does not increase in inspiration as right atrium is already overloaded and cannot accommodate extravenous return during inspiration. With phasic variations in respiration, the quantum of left-to-right shunt across the atrial septal defect changes but there is no net increase in right sided flow with inspiration. The split of second sound is thus wide and fixed (Fig. 11.21).

Clinical Features

Most patients with atrial septal defects usually remain asymptomatic with murmur detected on routine evaluation. Some of them present with exertional dyspnea, palpitation, or poor weight gain. In a rare subset, the patients with atrial septal defect develop congestive heart failure; in some series 5–10% of cases of isolated ASDs can develop CHF in infancy. ASD usually presents in adolescent and adulthood with exercise intolerance, rhythm abnormalities, or features of pulmonary hypertension.

Inspection of precordium may reveal a parasternal impulse. Palpation may reveal mild cardiomegaly and a systolic thrill in less than 10% patients. First heart sound is loud due to loud tricuspid components and second is widely split and does not vary during respiration. P_2 is accentuated. An ejection systolic murmur at second left intercostal space and a delayed diastolic murmur at tricuspid area is audible.

Around 10–15% of patients with large atrial septal defects develop pulmonary arterial hypertension usually by the 3rd or 4th decades of life, more so in female patients. With the development of pulmonary arterial hypertension, (i) cardiomegaly persists; (ii) flow murmurs across the right ventricular outflow and tricuspid valve disappear; (iii) second heart sound remains wide and either fixed or variable split; P_2 becomes louder and (iv) murmurs of tricuspid regurgitation and pulmonary regurgitation may appear.

Associated mitral valve disease has been demonstrated in 20–30% of patients. Presence of pansystolic murmur of mitral regurgitation in a patient with atrial septal defect may point to cleft mitral valve, mitral valve prolapse, or rheumatic mitral valve disease.

Case Study | Atrial Septal Defect

An 8-year-old boy was brought to outpatient department for complaints of not gaining weight as compared to peers. He was a term born neonate with birth weight of 2.9 kg. He did well in his neonatal and infantile period. Presently he is studying in 4th standard and fared well academically. There were no school absences for sick-leaves.

On observation he was active and cheerful with normal intellect. Weight was 15 kg and height was 125 cm. General physical examination was normal. Pulse rate was 86/min, it was regular in rhythm, normal volume and all peripheral pulses were felt. Saturation was 99% in all four limbs. CVS examination revealed left precordial bulge. Diffuse pulsations were seen and felt at left middle and lower parasternal area. Epigastric pulsations were felt. S1 was normal. S2 was wide split without any change during respiration. Grade 3/6 ejection systolic murmur was heard in pulmonary area. Other systemic examination was normal.

Q. What is the characteristic finding in this child that can lead to diagnosis?

Wide and fixed splitting of second heart sound is the auscultatory hallmark of Atrial Septal Defect. The left-to-right shunt happens between left atrium and right atrium. Blood from right atrium is received by right ventricle which becomes volume overloaded. Already volume overloaded RV cannot further increase its capacity of receiving more blood during inspiration, hence S2 is wide and fixed split. These children usually present after 5 year of age with failure to gain weight, respiratory infection, or congestive heart failure.

Q. What is the cause of murmur?

Left to right shunt in ASD happens between LA and RA both of which are low pressure chambers. Hence there is no murmur at the level of shunt. The extra volume of blood received by RA traverses the tricuspid and pulmonary valves to reach lungs. Flow through tricuspid valve produces a diastolic murmur, which is difficult to appreciate. Flow through pulmonary valve produces ejection systolic murmur that is heard at pulmonary area.

Q. X-ray of this child is given below. Describe the findings.

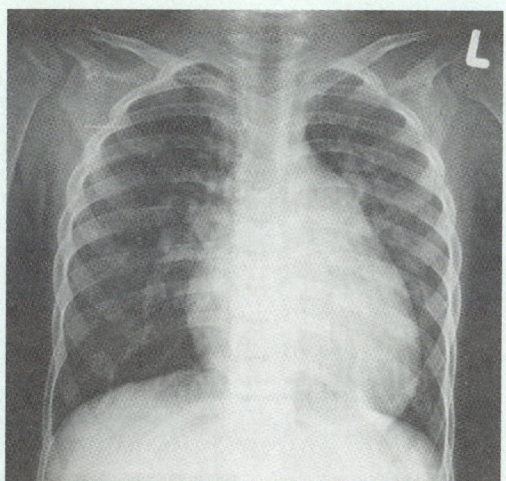

Chest radiograph shows cardiomegaly with CT ratio 0.6. Right atrium is dilated as it occupies more than three intercostal spaces. Cardiac apex is RV type as it forms acute angle with diaphragm. MPA (main pulmonary artery) segment is dilated and pulmonary vascularity is increased.

Q. How will you manage the patient?

Definitive diagnosis is made by echocardiogram which shows the location and size of defect. Ostium primum and sinus venosus ASDs need surgical patch closure. Ostium secundum ASD can be closed percutaneously using ASD device provided the rims of the defect are adequate to hold the device.

Diagnosis

Electrocardiography ECG features in ostium secundum defect include right axis deviation, varying grades of right atrial and right ventricular hypertrophy, and RBBB pattern. Left axis deviation (−30° to −60°) suggests an ostium primum ASD (Fig. 11.22).

Left axis deviation of more than −60° suggests a complete atrioventricular canal defect. SVC type of sinus venosus ASD may cause abnormal P axis.

Presence of significant right ventricular hypertrophy suggests associated pulmonary arterial hypertension or pulmonary stenosis. On the other hand, if the ECG shows additional left ventricular hypertrophy, one should carefully evaluate for mitral regurgitation which could be caused by an associated mitral valve prolapse, rheumatic mitral valve disease, or cleft mitral leaflet.

Chest X-ray X-ray is normal with small left to right shunt. With larger shunt, there will be cardiomegaly, right atrium and right ventricle enlargement, prominent pulmonary artery, and increased pulmonary vascularity (Fig. 11.23).

11

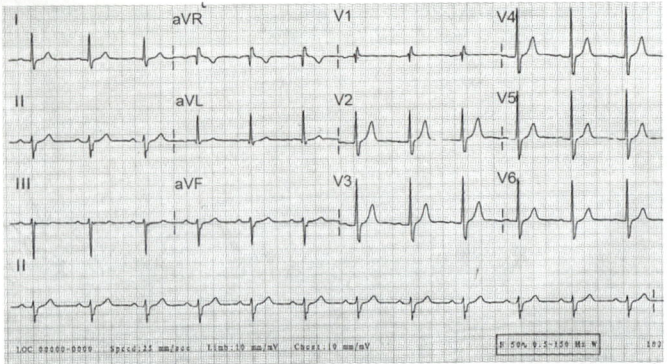

Fig. 11.22 ECG from a 16 years old adolescent with ostium primum ASD, cleft mitral valve, and moderate mitral regurgitation. ECG shows sinus rhythm, normal 'P' wave axis, PR interval (0.20 sec), and QRS axis in left upper quadrant (minus 45°), incomplete RBBB

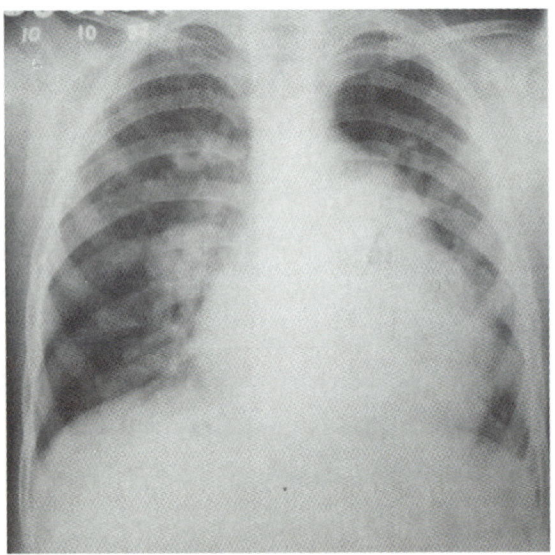

Fig. 11.23 X-ray chest PA view from a child with atrial septal defect with large left-to-right shunt. The X-ray chest shows moderate cardiomegaly, right atrial enlargement and dilated MPA. Also notice prominent hilar PA with evidence of increased pulmonary blood flow indicative of large shunt at atrial level

Echocardiography Echocardiography is helpful in complete evaluation of ASD–the type and size of ASD, degree of shunt, pulmonary arterial pressures, and associated defects.

Treatment	**Atrial Septal Defect**

Elective closure of ostium secundum ASD in patients with right ventricular overload is advised by age of 2–4 years. Indications for surgery at an earlier age include persistent CHF or evidence of pulmonary arterial hypertension. For fossa ovalis ASD, there are two treatment options:

- *Percutaneous device closure* This modality can be offered only in fossa ovalis ASD with adequate rims in children above 10 kg and size of ASD being not very large for the patient.
- *Surgery* Surgery is the only treatment option for large fossa ovalis ASD or with deficient rims, sinus venosus ASD, and ostium primum ASD. It is a well-established mode of closure with minimal risk (<1%).

Prophylaxis for infective endocarditis is not advised as bacterial endocarditis is rare in patients of isolated ostium secundum atrial septal defect, unless there is associated mitral valve disease.

Revision Point

Atrial Septal Defect (ASD)

1. Most atrial septal defects are secundum ASD (75%) and occur in central part of atrial septum in fossa ovalis; 20% are primum ASD (20%) and occur in the region of the endocardial cushion.
2. The classical hallmark of ASD is wide fixed splitting of the second heart sound. CHF occurs only in later childhood.
3. Most children are asymptomatic. 25% of patients with ASD die by 30 years, 50% by 37 years, 75% by 50 years and 90% by 60 years. Most adults develop heart failure.
4. Enlarged right atrial size leads to atrial arrhythmias especially AF. Half of patients aged 40 years have paroxysmal or permanent atrial fibrillation.
5. Secundum ASD can be managed with nonsurgical transcatheter repair. Open heart surgical correction is required for primum defects.

Butera G, Biondi-Zoccai G, Sangiorgi G, *et al*. Percutaneous versus surgical closure of secundum atrial septal defects: a systematic review and meta-analysis of currently available clinical evidence. *EuroIntervention*. 2011;7:377–85.

Johri AM, Rojas CA, El-Sherief A, *et al*. Imaging of atrial septal defects: echocardiography and CT correlation. *Heart*. 2011;97:1441–53.

Peters F, Khandheria BK, Sussman M, Essop MR. Ostium secundum atrial septal defect and partial anomalous pulmonary venous connection. *Eur Heart J Cardiovasc Imaging*. 2012 Feb 28. [Epub ahead of print]

Ueda H, Yanagi S, Nakamura H, *et al*. Device closure of atrial septal defect. *Circ J*. 2012 Feb 16. [Epub ahead of print]

RIGHT-TO-LEFT SHUNTS

11.8 TETRALOGY OF FALLOT

Tetralogy of Fallot is one of the commonest cyanotic congenital heart diseases, comprising up to 3.5 to 9.0% of total patients with congenital heart disease. It has following anomalies:

1. Pulmonary stenosis
2. Ventricular septal defect (large and malaligned)
3. Overriding of aorta over the septal defect
4. Right ventricular hypertrophy

Hemodynamics

The most characteristic and hallmark feature of this entity is the sub-pulmonary stenosis resulting in right ventricular outflow obstruction (Fig. 11.24). Pulmonary stenosis causes concentric right ventricular hypertrophy. The right ventricle effectively decompresses into the left ventricle through a large ventricular septal defect and, therefore, there is no cardiomegaly. For the same reason, congestive heart failure

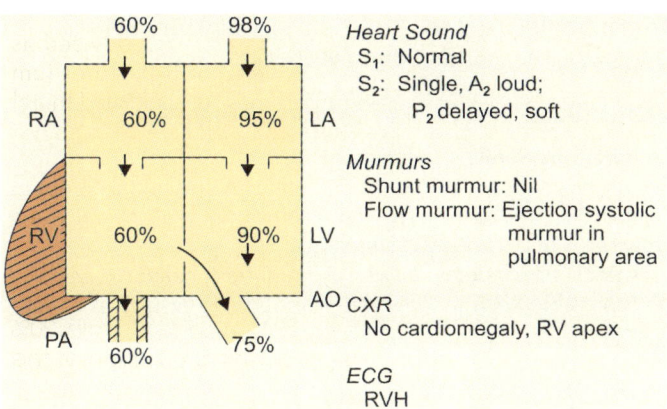

Fig. 11.24 Hemodynamics of tetralogy of Fallot. There is VSD and severe PS. Right-to-left shunt is at the level of VSD leading to systemic arterial desaturation. Values shown are oxygen saturation (%) in different cardiac chambers

does not occur. The child develops congestive heart failure only if there is anemia, infective endocarditis, hypertension, or myocarditis. There is no shunt murmur at the level of the ventricular septal defect, as right and left ventricular pressures are identical.

Flow from right ventricle into pulmonary artery across the stenosed right ventricular out flow produces an ejection systolic murmur. With increasing severity of obstruction, the flow to the pulmonary artery decreases with concomitant decrease in the duration and intensity of the murmur and increase in the degree of cyanosis. Thus the severity of pulmonary stenosis is directly proportional to the degree of cyanosis and inversely proportional to the loudness of the pulmonary ejection murmur in tetralogy of Fallot. Right ventricular outflow obstruction also results in delayed soft P_2 which is usually inaudible.

Clinical Features

Child can present at any time after birth depending on the severity of the pulmonary stenosis. Symptomatology includes central cyanosis, exertional dyspnea, and effort intolerance. During infancy and early childhood, cyanotic/anoxic spells may be the main presenting feature.

Cyanotic spells These spells usually occur after waking up from sleep or after exertion, feeding, excessive crying, or defecation. Spells are defined as deepening of cyanosis associated with tachypnea, tachycardia, and followed by lethargy or at times unconsciousness or convulsions. Sometimes minor spells occur in the form of unprovoked, inconsolable cry followed by sleep.

Squatting Children with tetralogy of Fallot usually present with a history of getting relief with assuming a squatting (knee-chest) posture following exertional dyspnea. Squatting helps to abort spell by many mechanisms. There is compression of abdominal aorta and kinking of femoral arteries which leads to increased systemic vascular resistance and thus improves blood flow through stenosed pulmonary valve. There is compression of femoral veins, which causes decrease in venous return of hypoxic blood from lower limbs. This leads to reduction in tachypnea, which is an important part of vicious cycle culminating in a cyanotic spell.

Physical examination reveals following findings:
- Cyanosis with clubbing, absence of CHF and normal sized heart. In some children, infundibular stenosis is less severe so that cyanosis never develops (*pink tetralogy*).
- Mild parasternal lift.
- Systolic thrill in 2nd, 3rd left intercostal spaces in 30% of cases.
- Normal first heart sound, single second sound (only A_2 is heard; P_2 is inaudible due to decreased pulmonary blood flow).
- An ejection systolic murmur in pulmonary area that ends before the second heart sound.
- Occasionally a constant ejection click may be present (due to dilated aorta).
- An inconstant ejection click may be present rarely if pulmonary stenosis is predominantly at the valvular level.

Features of congestive cardiac failure are absent in tetralogy of Fallot as right ventricle is decompressed into the left ventricle through a large ventricular septal defect. Only few conditions can result in cardiac failure in tetralogy of Fallot: (*i*) anemia; (*ii*) infection; (*iii*) aortic regurgitation due to dilated aortic root or secondary to infective endocarditis; (*iv*) pulmonary regurgitation in association with 'absent pulmonary valve syndrome'; or (*v*) functionally restrictive (small) ventricular septal defect which occurs in less than 5% of patients with tetralogy of Fallot. As the right ventricle is not effectively decompressed via the septal defect, the chances of right ventricular failure increase with increasing severity of the pulmonary stenosis.

An early diastolic murmur in a child with a diagnosis of tetralogy of Fallot may be attributed to aortic or pulmonary regurgitation.

TOF Physiology

Certain cardiac lesions have same pathophysiology as of tetralogy of Fallot; ie, restriction to the pulmonary blood flow and good intracardiac mixing. Children with these lesions have presentation similar to TOF and are grouped as TOF physiology. These conditions are as follows:
1. Double outlet right ventricle (DORV) with pulmonary stenosis.
2. Complete or corrected transposition of great vessels with VSD and pulmonary stenosis.
3. Tricuspid artesia with pulmonary stenosis
4. Single ventricle with pulmonary stenosis.
5. Atrioventricular septal defect with pulmonary stenosis.

Diagnosis

ECG There is right axis deviation and right ventricular hypertrophy. P waves may be peaked, and tall in 30% cases. Extreme right axis deviation suggests DORV with PS; or TGA with VSD-PS (Fig. 11.25).

Chest X-ray Cardiac size is normal and lung vascularity is decreased. Aortic knuckle is prominent and there is absence of main pulmonary artery (pulmonary bay). The apex is upturned because of right ventricular hypertrophy and with absence of main pulmonary artery segment may give an appearance of '*Boot shaped heart*' (Fig. 11.26). In tetralogy, 30% of the cases may have right aortic arch.

11

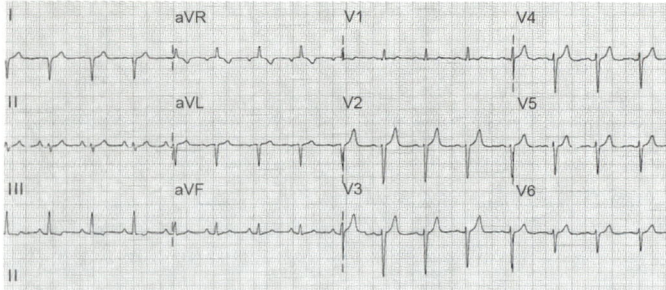

Fig. 11.25 ECG from an 8 years old child with tetralogy of Fallot showing sinus rhythm, normal 'P' wave axis, right axis deviation, right ventricular hypertrophy (chest leads in ½ voltage), early transition from 'R' in V1 to rS in V2

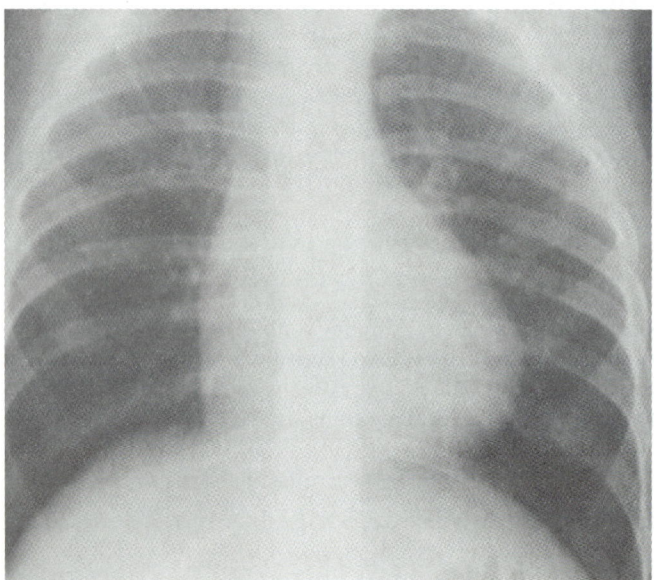

Fig 11.26 X-ray chest in tetralogy of Fallot showing normal heart size, RV type apex, and presence of pulmonary bay and diminished pulmonary vascular markings. Right aortic arch is also seen

Echocardiography is essential to document ventricular septal defect with aortic override, pulmonary outflow obstruction, and right ventricular hypertrophy. Cardiac catheterization and angiography are required only when echocardiographic evaluation is not satisfactory, or for better delineation of collateral vessels and coronary arteries.

Course and Complications

The pulmonary stenosis increases in severity with age with resultant increase in cyanosis and exercise intolerance, considerably limiting the child's activities. Severity and frequency of cyanotic spells increases and may even prove fatal. Anemia, by decreasing the oxygen carrying capacity further precipitates cyanotic spells and also increases the chances for heart failure, and as the microcytic red blood cells are more prone for sludging, there are higher chances for cerebrovascular accidents.

Neurological complications may occur in patients with tetralogy of Fallot as a result of (*i*) anoxic infarction during anoxic spells or due to anemia; (*ii*) paradoxical embolism as there is a right to left shunt; (*iii*) higher chances for venous

thrombosis due to sluggish circulation because of polycythemia; and (*iv*) brain abscess.

Treatment	**Tetralogy of Fallot**

A. Cyanotic Spells

While managing a cyanotic spell, care should be taken not to agitate the child further. This is possible by doing all the following measures in a least invasive manner.

1. *Check and maintain airway* Administer inhaled oxygen.
2. If possible keep in *knee-chest position*, or at least with legs flexed.
3. *Inject morphine* 0.1 mg/kg body weight. If needed, infusion of 10–60 µg/kg/h can be given.
4. *Correct metabolic acidosis* by giving 1 mL/kg of 7.5% sodium bicarbonate 1:1 dilution, slow intravenous.
5. *Correct anemia* and hypovolemia.
6. *Administer β blocker* Heart rate and blood pressure must be carefully monitored while giving beta blockers. Beta blockers act by several mechanisms:
   - Decrease heart rate thus reducing myocardial oxygen consumption;
   - Relieve infundibular spasm, allows more blood to lungs;
   - Beta blockers also cause overactivity of alpha receptors leading to increase in systemic vascular resistance. Subsequently right to left shunt across the VSD decreases and pulmonary blood flow increases;
   - Shift oxygen dissociation curve to right, relieving more oxygen at tissue level; and
   - Reset respiratory centre by reducing hyperapnea reflex.
   - Injection metoprolol is the agent of choice given 0.1 mg/kg over 5 minutes. Repeat every 5 minutes for a maximum of 3 doses. It can also be given in 1–5 µg/kg/minute infusion. This is to be followed by oral metoprolol 0.25–0.5 mg/kg/dose, 6 hourly. The traditional alternative is IV propranalol, 0.1 mg/kg IV (during spell). This is followed by oral propanolol (2–4 mg/kg/day 6–8 hourly) for long term use.
7. *Vasopressors* Injection methoxamine (0.1 to 0.2 mg/kg/dose) IV/IM.
8. Persistent spells may need general anesthesia, or mechanical ventilation.

After managing the spell, a complete diagnosis should be made by doing a systematic EchoDoppler evaluation. Precipitating factors should be looked into. If after treatment of precipitating factors the spells subside, surgical intervention can be appropriately planned. If the spells are not controlled, palliation with shunt surgery (modified Blalock Taussig, ie, connection between the subclavian artery and pulmonary artery on either side) or balloon dilation of the right ventricular outflow tract should be contemplated urgently if patient is not suitable for total correction.

B. Surgery

Palliative treatment consists of creating a communication between systemic and pulmonary circulation, to increase the pulmonary blood flow. Blalock-Taussig shunt creates an anastomosis between the subclavian and right or left pulmonary artery with interposition of graft.

Definitive treatment This consists of closure of VSD, and resection of infundibular stenosis, resulting in total correction. *Ideal management plan* for a patient with tetralogy of Fallot is as follows:

Case Study | **Tetralogy of Fallot**

A 1-year-old girl was brought to emergency room with complaints of excessive cry followed by unconsciousness since last 10 minutes. She had such episodes almost thrice in last 3 months. She had cyanosis and had grade II pan-digital clubbing. There was conjunctival suffusion. She was diagnosed to have congenital heart disease at 4 months of age when evaluated for cyanosis. Saturation was 75% in all four limbs. After stabilization, examination revealed RV type of diffuse apex. S_1 was normal, S_2 was single. A grade 3/ 6 ejection systolic murmur was heard at left upper para-sternal border. Her weight and length were normal for age. Her chest X-ray is shown below.

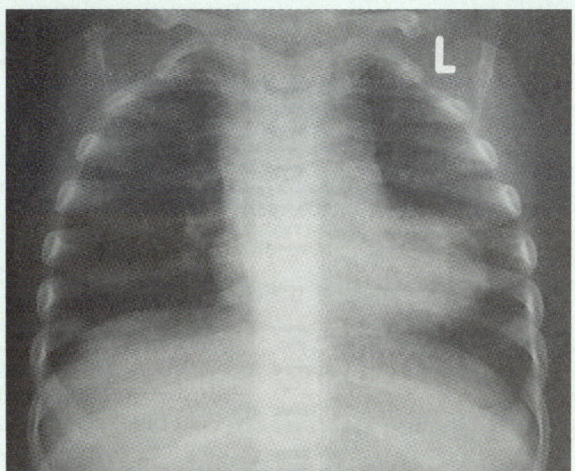

Q 1. What is the diagnosis?

The child was brought in a cyanotic spell. This indicates a congenital cyanotic heart disease with decreased pulmonary blood flow. Differential diagnoses will include TOF or TOF variants like DORV/VSD/PS, tricuspid atresia, single ventricle PS, or TGA/VSD/PS. Ejection systolic murmur in pulmonary area occurs due to blood flowing through stenotic pulmonary valve. Chest X–ray shows boot-shaped heart because right ventricle forms the apex and pulmonary bay is concave due to small pulmonary artery. There is pulmonary oligemia as seen by absence of vascular markings beyond medial third of lung fields.

Q 2. What is a cyanotic spell?

A cyanotic spell is characterized by episodic deepening of cyanosis associated with hyperpnea due to sudden decline in pulmonary blood flow, leading to limpness, syncope, seizure, stroke, or death. An infant may present with excessive cry.

Q 3. How will you manage this child, now?

- Keep the child in knee-chest position, preferably on mother's shoulder.
- Administer oxygen by hood/face-mask.
- Inject Morphine 0.1 mg/kg subcutaneously or intramuscular to calm the child and reduce hyperpnea.
- Secure an I/V line and inject fluid bolus 10 mL/kg normal saline.
- Inject sodium bicarbonate 1 mEq/kg to correct acidosis.
- Inject propranolol 0.1 mg/kg to reduce heart rate and counter infundibular contraction.

Most children come out of spell at this stage, but if it does not improve, further treatment includes phenylephrine, ketamine, or general anesthesia with intubation. Emergency Blalock-Taussig shunt may be required in resistant cases.

- *Stable, minimally cyanosed* Total correction around 6–9 months of age or earlier according to the institution policy.
- *Significant cyanosis (SaO$_2$ <70%) or history of spells despite therapy* Age < 3 months: Systemic to pulmonary artery shunt. Age >3 months: Shunt or correction depending on anatomy and surgical centre's experience. Children having undergone palliation in infancy should be evaluated one year later electively for total correction.
- Children with additional large aortopulmonary collaterals need percutaneous coil closure of these collaterals before total correction.

Bailliard F, Anderson RH. Tetralogy of Fallot. *Orphanet J Rare Dis*.2009;4:2.

Duro RP, Moura C, Leite-Moreira A. Anatomophysiologic basis of tetralogy of Fallot and its clinical implications. *Rev Port Cardiol*. 2010;29:591–630.

Fox D, Devendra GP, Hart SA, Krasuski RA. When 'blue babies' grow up: What you need to know about tetralogy of Fallot. *Cleve Clin J Med*. 2010;77:821–8.

Sharkey AM, Sharma A. Tetralogy of Fallot: anatomic variants and their impact on surgical management. *Semin Cardiothorac Vasc Anesth*. 2012;24. [Epub ahead of print]

Tubbs RS, Gianaris N, Shoja MM, *et al*. "The heart is simply a muscle" and first description of the tetralogy of "Fallot". Early contributions to cardiac anatomy and pathology by bishop and anatomist Niels Stensen (1638-1686). *Int J Cardiol*. 2012;154:312–5.

Ueda H, Yanagi S, Nakamura H, *et al*. Device closure of atrial septal defect. *Circ J*. 2012 Feb 16. [Epub ahead of print]

van Roekens CN, Zuckerberg AL. Emergency management of hypercyanotic crises in tetralogy of Fallot. *Ann Emerg Med*. 1995;25:256–8.

Zhao K, Wang H, Han H, *et al*. Staged procedures versus primary repair for tetralogy of fallot and small left ventricle. *Heart Surg Forum*. 2012;15:E37–9.

11.9 TRANSPOSITION OF GREAT ARTERIES

When the aorta arises from the right ventricle and the pulmonary artery arises from the left ventricle, the malformation is known as '*complete transposition of great arteries*' (d-TGA). It is a condition with *ventriculoarterial discordance* and atrioventricular concordance. The defect clinically presents with both cyanosis and congestive heart failure in infancy. Transposition of great arteries (d-TGA) accounts for 5 to 7% of all congenital cardiac malformations, with male predilection. Increased prevalence is noted in infants of diabetic mothers, and with prenatal exposure to sex hormone therapy.

Physiologically corrected transposition of great arteries (l-TGA) is characterized by atrioventricular as well as ventriculo-arterial discordance. Left atrium is connected to morphological right ventricle, which is then connected to aorta. Right atrium flow, on the other side opens up into pulmonary artery through the morphologic left ventricle. As the route of blood flow is corrected physiologically, hemodynamics and clinical presentation in corrected transposition of great arteries are determined by other associated cardiac defects (VSD, PS, Ebstein anomaly, complete heart block) which are present in up to 98% of these children.

Hemodynamics of Complete Transposition

The right atrium receives systemic venous blood (deoxygenated) and empties into the right ventricle, from which the aorta arises. On left side, the left atrium after receiving pulmonary venous (oxygenated) blood empties into left ventricle from which the pulmonary artery arises. This arrangement is compatible with life only if there is a mixing between the two circulations through a shunt, which can be at the level of atria, ventricle, or great arteries. Clinical variants are described below.

1. Complete Transposition of Great Arteries with Intact Ventricular Septum (Fig. 11.27)

The mixing between the systemic and pulmonary circulation occurs through a patent foramen ovale, atrial septal defect, or patent ductus arteriosus. Patent foramen ovale, being too small, does not ensure adequate mixing of the two circulations. Consequently, these babies present within the first week of life with fast breathing, severe hypoxia, and cyanosis. Another site of mixing could be through a patent ductus arteriosus. Mixing occurs at high pressure, so the baby will present early with signs of cardiac failure. Rarely, bronchopulmonary collaterals can also be a site for mixing.

Physical examination reveals severe cyanosis, features of congestive cardiac failure, normal first heart sound, single second heart sound (as pulmonary arteries are posterior to aorta so pulmonary component is not audible), and S_3 gallop. Murmurs are not significant; a short ejection systolic murmur in parasternal area is the most common.

2. Complete Transposition of Great Arteries with Ventricular Septal Defect

A. *Without Pulmonary Stenosis* (TGA+VSD without PS)

Presence of large ventricular septal defect results in mixing between the two circuits. As the pulmonary vascular

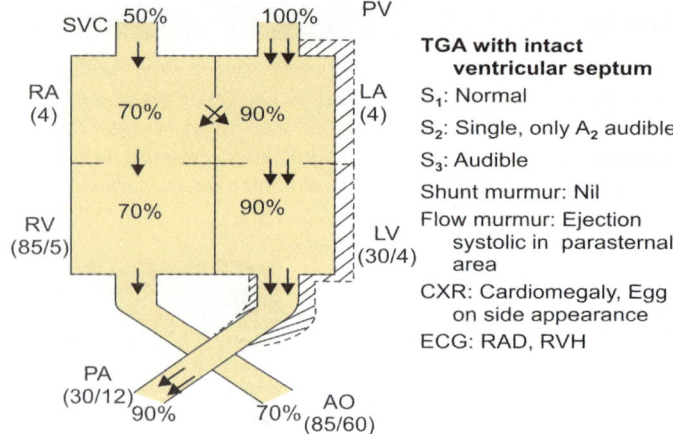

Fig. 11.27 Hemodynamics in an infant of complete transposition of great vessels with large ASD. There is bidirectional shunt at the level of ASD. Values given are oxygen saturation (%) in different cardiac chambers

resistance falls after birth, due to presence of a large ventricular septal defect, the pulmonary blood flow increases markedly. With increase in pulmonary blood flow there is greater pulmonary venous return, resulting in a rise in the left atrial pressure if atrial communication is restrictive. Therefore such babies become symptomatic in the first ten to fifteen days of life with features of a large shunt, congestive cardiac failure, and pulmonary venous congestion. Marked cyanosis may not be a feature in these children. In presence of a large atrial septal defect, which is *not* usually the case, the child presents at the age of four to six weeks with features of congestive failure and mild cyanosis that increases on crying.

On examination there may be mild cyanosis, cardiomegaly, signs of congestive cardiac failure, normal first heart sound, and single or normally split second heart sound with a loud pulmonary component. S_3 gallop may be present. One may hear an ejection systolic murmur grade 2/6 in the left parasternal area and a delayed diastolic murmur at the mitral area.

B. *With Pulmonary Stenosis* (TGA+VSD with PS)

These children present with marked cyanosis from birth without any congestive cardiac failure and are grouped under *tetralogy of Fallot physiology*. The differentiating feature is marked cyanosis since birth with mild cardiomegaly as both circulations in the complete transposition are overloaded.

The first heart sound is heard normally, while the second heart sound is single, and there may be an ejection systolic murmur grade 2–3/6 at the left upper parasternal border.

Natural History

Untreated patients of d-transposition of great arteries have very high mortality: 30% die within the first week of life; 50% within the first month of life; 70% within 6 months, and 90% succumb within the first year of life.

Development of pulmonary vascular obstructive disease occurs early in d-transposition, more commonly with ventricular septal defect or associated large patent ductus arteriosus. Children with patent ductus arteriosus who have

Case Study | Transposition of Great Arteries

A 4-month-old infant was brought to emergency room with complaints of bluish discoloration of lips and nails since birth. His birth weight was 4.0 kg. There was history of gestational diabetes in mother which was controlled on insulin. Baby was sick looking. The mother also complained of feeding difficulties, recurrent episodes of fever with cough and suck-rest-suck cycles. There was tachycardia (HR 160/min), tachypnea (RR 70/min) with deep central cyanosis. Pulses were felt in all four limbs. SpO_2 was 65% in all four limbs. Diffuse left parasternal pulsations and epigastric pulsations were felt. S_1 was normal. S_2 was loud and single. There was a ejection systolic murmur over left parasternal border. Respiratory system examination revealed bilateral basal crepitations.

Q. What is the clinical diagnosis?

The child was born as large for gestational age to a mother with gestational diabetes mellitus. He has presented with features of increased pulmonary blood flow (evidence of respiratory infections + CHF), and right ventricular dominance. This presentation indicates presence of transposition of great arteries (TGA). Presence of murmur indicates a shunt, most probably a VSD. The diagnosis is TGA with VSD.

Q. How will you manage the patient?

We will confirm the diagnosis by echocardiography. Medications for control of heart failure are started. Iron supplementation is initiated. Patient is taken for surgery as soon as possible. Definitive treatment is arterial switch operation (ASO) with VSD patch closure.

Eisenmenger physiology show differential cyanosis. Cyanosis is less in the lower limbs than the upper limbs, since blood of higher oxygen saturation from pulmonary artery is shunted to descending aorta.

Diagnosis

Electrocardiography reveals right axis deviation with right ventricular hypertrophy. Patients with d-TGA with VSD show biventricular hypertrophy. *Chest X-ray* shows mild to moderate cardiomegaly. The great vessels are transposed giving the configuration of 'egg on side' due to narrowing of pedicle. There is associated pulmonary plethora (Fig. 11.28). *Echocardiography* is required to reveal the detailed anatomy.

Treatment | Transposition of Great Arteries (TGA)

The first step is to control the congestive heart failure. It is important to maintain hydration, temperature, and electrolyte and sugar levels. In neonates, it may help to keep the ductus open by infusion of prostaglandins. However, this is only a short term measure. Rashkind Balloon atrial septostomy should be attempted as soon as possible if the saturations are low and the interatrial communication is small.

Jatene arterial switch This procedure should be performed within the first 4 weeks of life. The pulmonary artery is shifted to RV above the aortic valve; and the aorta and coronary arteries are shifted to LV above the pulmonary valve. If the age at presentation is more than 8 weeks, assess left ventricle by

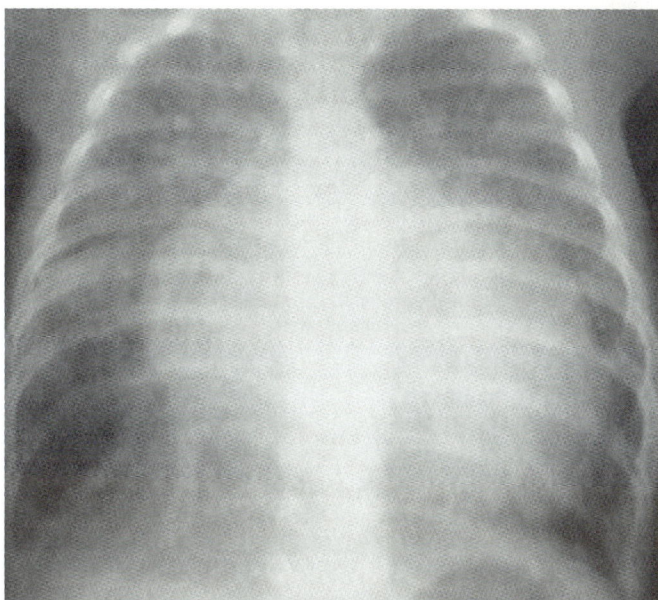

Fig. 11.28 Characteristic 'Egg on side' appearance in complete transposition of great arteries with large VSD. Note presence of cardiomegaly with narrow pedicle and increased pulmonary vascular markings. Right side of egg is formed by dilated right atrium and left side of egg is formed by dilated right ventricle. There is narrow pedicle because aorta and pulmonary artery are placed anterior and posterior to each other. Also there is thymic hypoplasia which reduces the width of superior mediastinum.

echocardiography carefully before recommending the arterial switch operation.

- *If the left ventricle is regressed* Senning's/Mustard atrial switch at 3–6 months or a rapid two-stage arterial switch where the left ventricle is prepared by pulmonary artery banding and BT shunt followed by arterial switch.

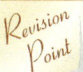

Revision Point | Transposition of Great Arteries (TGA)

1. When the aorta arises from the right ventricle and the pulmonary artery arises from the left ventricle, the malformation is known as 'complete transposition of great arteries' (d-TGA). TGA is the most common cardiac cause for neonatal cyanosis.

2. This arrangement is compatible with life only if there is a mixing between the two circulations through a shunt, which can be at the level of atria (ASD), ventricle (VSD), or great arteries (PDA).

3. TGA with a shunt presents in early infancy with severe cyanosis, features of congestive cardiac failure, normal first heart sound, single second heart sound, a short ejection systolic parasternal murmur, and S3 gallop.

4. Egg-on-side cardiac silhouette on chest X-ray is diagnostic of TGA.

5. Arterial switch operation, done in the first few weeks of life is the benchmark of present day care in TGA. In good centers this surgery carries less than 5% mortality.

6. Balloon atrial septostomy (BAS) is performed, if arterial switch operation is not being done immediately.

11

- If a ventricular septal defect is there, it can also be closed at the same time.
- For corrected transposition, the surgical options vary with the associated lesions.

Graham TP Jr, Markham L, Parra DA, Bichell D. Congenitally corrected transposition of the great arteries: an update. *Curr Treat Options Cardiovasc Med.* 2007;9:407–13.

Hazekamp M, Portela F, Bartelings M. The optimal procedure for the great arteries and left ventricular outflow tract obstruction. An anatomical study. *Eur J Cardiothorac Surg.* 2007;31:879–87.

Hornung TS, Calder L. Congenitally corrected transposition of the great arteries. *Heart.* 2010;96:1154–61.

Martins P, Castela E. Transposition of the great arteries. *Orphanet J Rare Dis.* 2008;3:27.

Prifti E, Crucean A, Bonacchi M, *et al.* Early and long term outcome of the arterial switch operation for transposition of the great arteries: predictors and functional evaluation. *Eur J Cardiothorac Surg.* 2002;22:864–73.

Squarcia U, Macchi C. Transposition of the great arteries. *Curr Opin Pediatr.* 2011;23:518–22.

Warnes CA. Transposition of the great arteries. *Circulation.* 2006;114:2699–709.

11.10 TOTAL ANOMALOUS PULMONARY VENOUS CONNECTION

Total anomalous pulmonary venous connection (TAPVC) is defined as the anomalous drainage of all the pulmonary veins in to the right atrium, instead of left atrium. This results in a mixture of all the oxygenated blood coming from the lungs, with the systemic venous return (deoxygenated blood) in the right atrium. Presence of interatrial communication is necessary to sustain life, and therefore an atrial septal defect or patent foramen ovale is considered a part of the complex.

Maternal exposure to lead paint and pesticides has been found to be associated with higher incidence of total anomalous pulmonary venous connection in offsprings.

Classification

Total anomalous pulmonary venous connection is classified by Darling, *et al.* according to the site of drainage:

1. *Type I: Supracardiac variety* Pulmonary veins drain into innominate vein, superior vena cava or, azygos vein. This is the most common type of defect, seen in 40 to 50% of all TAPVC.
2. *Type II: Cardiac variety* Pulmonary veins drain directly into the right atrium or via coronary sinus; 20 to 30% of cases.
3. *Type III: Infradiaphragmatic* Pulmonary veins drain into the portal system, hepatic vein, or IVC (13 to 24%).
4. *Type IV: Mixed* (5 to 10%).

Hemodynamics

Right atrium receives unoxygenated blood from both vena cavae and also oxygenated blood coming from pulmonary veins. This mixed blood flows to the left atrium (Figs 11.29 and 11.30) through a interatrial communication (foramen ovale or ASD). Due to complete mixing of systemic and pulmonary venous blood in right atrium, saturation in all four cardiac chambers and both the great vessels is equal around 85%. But in few cases, blood streaming effects

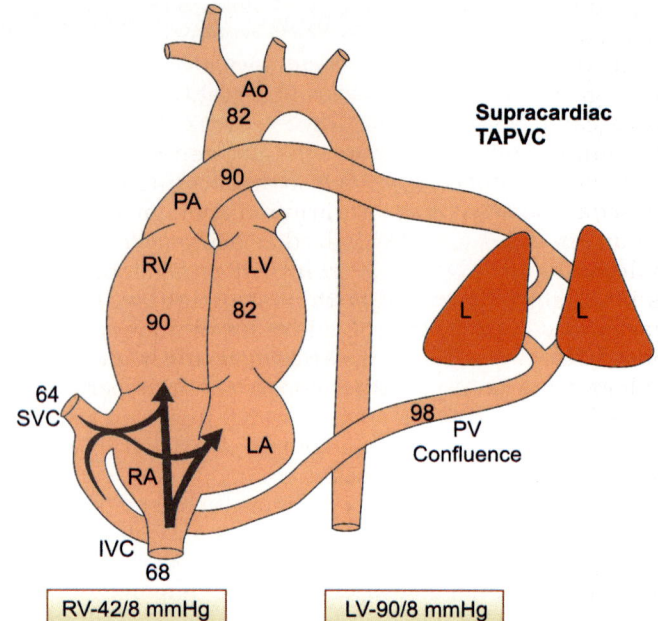

Fig. 11.29 Hemodynamics in total anonalous pulmonary venous connection to superior vena cava (supracardiac variety). Values given are oxygen saturation (%). RV pressures are moderately elevated as compared to LV pressure

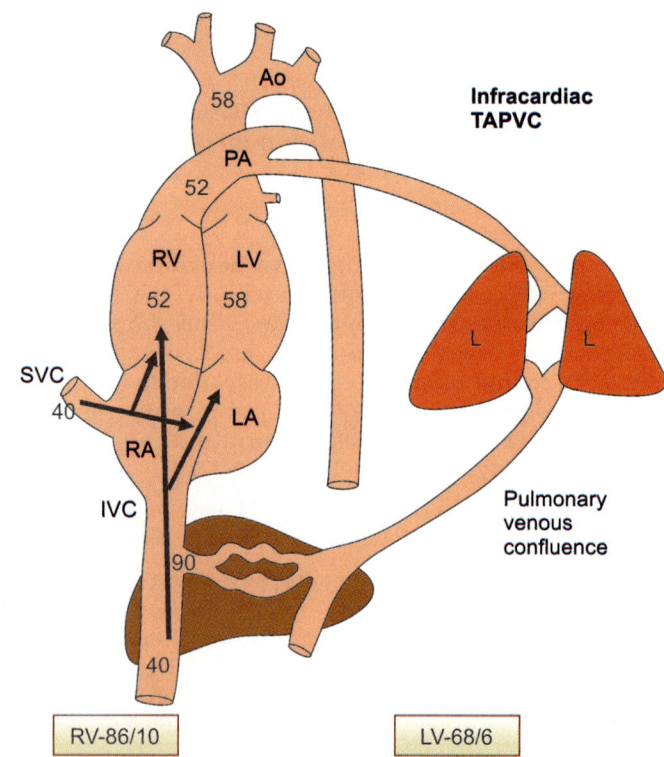

Fig. 11.30 Hemodynamics in a neonate with total anonalous pulmonary venous connection to portal system cava and through inferior vena cava (infracardiac). Values given are oxygen saturation (%). RV systolic pressure is severly elevated as compared to LV pressure and there is severe systemic arterial desaturation

caused by embryological flow dynamics lead to variable saturations.

Blood coming from the superior vena cava tends to flow into right ventricle and pulmonary circulation; while inferior vena caval blood tends to flow across the interatrial communication. Therefore, the oxygen saturation of pulmonary artery is higher than in the aorta in supracardiac defect; and lower than in aorta in infradiaphragmatic defects.

Further, TAPVC is categorized as being *with* or *without* pulmonary venous obstruction. Infradiaphragmatic TAPVC is invariably associated with obstruction, while other varieties can exist with or without pulmonary venous obstruction. Obstructive variants result in decreased pulmonary blood flow and pulmonary arterial hypertension. Non-obstructive TAPVC presents with features of congestive cardiac failure due to increased pulmonary blood flow. Non-obstructive presentation is more common.

Clinical Features

Non-obstructive Total Anomalous Pulmonary Venous Connection

These children are usually asymptomatic at birth. Signs of congestive heart failure appear in two-thirds of them by 3–6 months of age and the remaining one-third become symptomatic by one year.

Cyanosis may be so mild as to be clinically unapparent, except in the presence of cardiac failure and in the patients who survive long enough to develop pulmonary arterial hypertension.

Besides features of cardiac failure, patient may have cardiomegaly, hyperkinetic precordium, normal or accentuated first heart sound, wide and fixed second heart sound with loud pulmonary component, ejection systolic murmur grade 2 to 4/6, and delayed diastolic tricuspid flow murmur.

Obstructed Total Anomalous Pulmonary Venous Connection

These patients present in the neonatal period with respiratory distress and marked cyanosis. Examination reveals normal heart size with a parasternal heave, normal first heart sound, normally split second heart sound with a loud pulmonary component, and no significant murmur.

Investigations

ECG shows right atrial enlargement, right axis deviation, and evidence of right ventricular overload.

Chest X-ray shows cardiomegaly, right ventricular configuration, and increased pulmonary blood flow in non-obstructed TAPVC. In total anomalous pulmonary venous connection to the innominate vein, dilatation of the vertical vein on left side, and the dilated innominate vein and superior vena cava on the right side results in the characteristic '*figure of 8*' or '*Snowman*' *appearance* (Fig. 11.31). The upper circle of '8' is formed by the dilated venous channels on both sides while the lower circle is formed by the cardiac shadow itself (after one year of age).

In total anomalous pulmonary venous connection to the superior vena cava, the thoracic roentgenogram shows dilated superior vena cava along with cardiomegaly (Fig. 11.32).

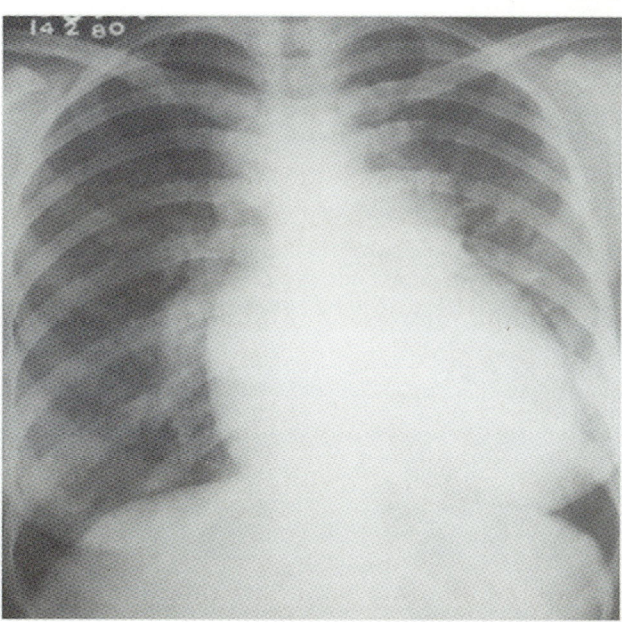

Fig. 11.31 Characteristic 'Snowman appearance' or 'figure of 8' in patient with supracardiac TAPVC draining into left innominate vein through vertical vein. Upper part of figure of 8 is formed by ascending vertical vein, dilated innominate vein and dilated SVC and the lower part of figure '8' by the cardiac shadow. The pulmonary vasculature is increased

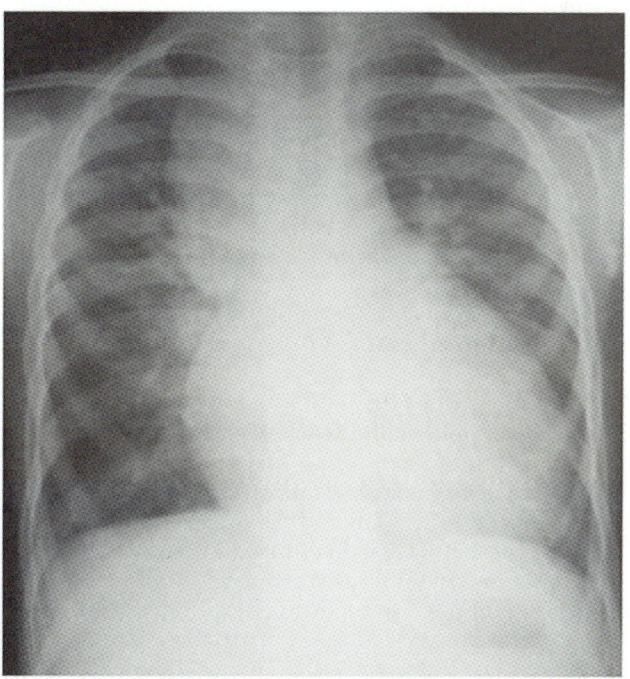

Fig. 11.32 Another patient with supracardiac TAPVC to right SVC. Note the prominent right SVC shadow along with presence of cardiomegaly, RA enlargement and increased pulmonary vasculature

In children with obstructed total anomalous pulmonary venous connection, the characteristic finding is white lung, ie, ground glass appearance of bilateral lung fields as a result of pulmonary edema, with a normal sized heart.

Echocardiography is helpful to demonstrate the site of anomalous connection, presence or absence of obstruction, and associated pulmonary hypertension. Cardiac catheterization and angiography are useful in doubtful cases or for assessment of the pulmonary vascular resistance and its reactivity.

Treatment	Total Anomalous Pulmonary Venous Connection

Medical management consists of control of congestive cardiac failure, treatment of chest infections, and supportive measures. The treatment is surgical and should be under-taken at earliest.

Kanter KR. Surgical repair of total anomalous pulmonary venous connection. *Semin Thorac Cardiovasc Surg Pediatr Card Surg Annu*. 2006:40–4.

Lee ML, Wu MH, Wang JK, Lue HC. Echocardiographic assessment of total anomalous pulmonary venous connections in pediatric patients. *J Formos Med Assoc*. 2001;100:729–35.

Snellen HA, van Ingen HC, Hoefsmit EC. Patterns of anomalous pulmonary venous drainage. *Circulation*. 1968;38:45–63.

Stein P. Total anomalous pulmonary venous connection. *AORN J*. 2007;85:509–20.

Yap SH, Anania N, Alboliras ET, Lilien LD. Reversed differential cyanosis in the newborn: a clinical finding in the supracardiac total anomalous pulmonary venous connection. *Pediatr Cardiol*. 2009;30:359–62.

11.11 PARTIAL ANOMALOUS PULMONARY VENOUS CONNECTION

When one or more, but not all, pulmonary veins connect to the systemic venous system then it is defined as partial anomalous pulmonary venous connection. Usually the left sided pulmonary veins connect to derivatives of the left cardinal system (coronary sinus, left superior vena cava, left innominate vein) and the right-sided pulmonary veins connect to the derivatives of the right cardinal system (right superior vena cava, inferior vena cava). The commonest site of anomalous drainage is the innominate vein. Atrial septal defects are a usual association except in partial anomalous pulmonary venous connection to the inferior vena cava, where the atrial septum is usually intact.

Hemodynamics

The basic physiological disturbance in partial anomalous pulmonary venous connection is similar to an atrial septal defect, which is increased pulmonary blood flow as a consequence of recirculation of oxygenated blood through the lungs. The factors that determine the hemodynamic state are: Number of anomalously connected pulmonary veins; site of anomalous connection; compliance of receiving chamber; and presence and size of atrial septal defect.

- When a single pulmonary vein connects anomalously, the anomalously draining blood flow is about 33% of the total pulmonary blood flow so that the lesion is rarely recognized clinically.
- When pulmonary veins of one lung connect anomalously, it results in anomalous drainage of about 66% of the total pulmonary blood flow. This is due to greater compliance of the right atrium, which is the receiving chamber.

Clinical Features

Depending on the number of anomalously connected veins, symptoms secondary to increased pulmonary blood flow

appear. Pulmonary arterial hypertension is not a common occurrence with partial anomalous pulmonary venous connection except with partial anomalous connection of right sided pulmonary veins to the inferior vena cava (Scimitar syndrome), with intact interatrial septum.

On examination, children are usually acyanotic. Cardiac evaluation reveals normal first heart sound, wide and fixed split second heart sound (if there is associated atrial septal defect, which is usually the case) and an ejection systolic murmur at the left upper sternal border due to increased pulmonary blood flow across the right ventricular outflow tract. One also finds a delayed diastolic murmur at the left lower sternal border due to increased blood flow across a normal tricuspid valve. With an intact interatrial septum the second heart sound will be wide but variably split. Congestive heart failure and pulmonary arterial hypertension are rare.

Investigations

ECG findings are comparable to uncomplicated atrial septal defect. Chest X-ray reflects the increased pulmonary blood flow and right ventricular dilatation. In Scimitar syndrome, associated hypoplasia of the right lung, dextroposition, lung sequestration, and right lung parenchymal abnormalities should also be looked for. Echocardiography demonstrates the anomalous number of pulmonary veins, site of anomalous connection, presence or absence of pulmonary arterial hypertension, and associated defects.

Treatment	Partial Anomalous Pulmonary Venous Connection

Children with single pulmonary vein connecting anomalously do not need surgical intervention. Surgery is indicated, if two or more pulmonary veins connect anomalously, resulting in pulmonary overcirculation or respiratory insufficiency. Surgical modalities include re-routing of pulmonary veins to the left atrium and closure of atrial septal defect, if present.

Abbasi K, Abbasi A, Tazik M, *et al*. Anomalous right-sided pulmonary venous connection to the superior vena cava. *Monaldi Arch Chest Dis*.2009;72:37–9.

El Bardissi AW, Dearani JA, Suri RM, Danielson GK. Left-sided partial anomalous pulmonary venous connections. *Ann Thorac Surg*. 2008;85:1007–14.

Peters F, Khandheria BK, Sussman M, Essop MR. Ostium secundum atrial septal defect and partial anomalous pulmonary venous connection. *Eur Heart J Cardiovasc Imaging*. 2012 Feb 28. [Epub ahead of print].

11.12 TRICUSPID ATRESIA

Triscuspid atresia is a rare congenital cyanotic heart disease accounting for 1–3% of all children with congenital heart diseases. There is complete absence of tricuspid valve with no direct communication between right atrium and right ventricle. This is invariably associated with some degree of right ventricular hypoplasia. Great vessels origin can be concordant or discordant.

Hemodynamics (Fig. 11.33)

As there is no outlet from the right atrium to the right ventricle; the entire systemic venous return enters the left

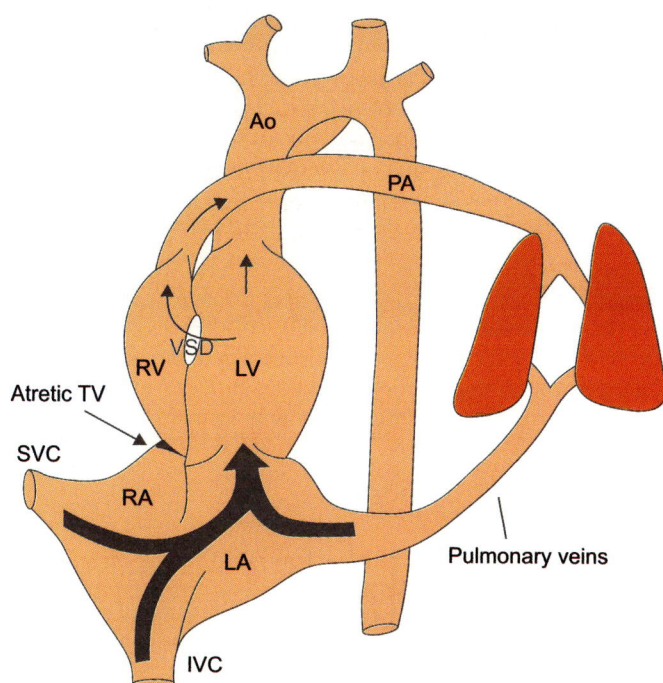

Fig. 11.33 Line diagram showing course of circulation in a child with tricuspid atresia, small VSD, concordant ventriculo-arterial connection and pulmonary stenosis

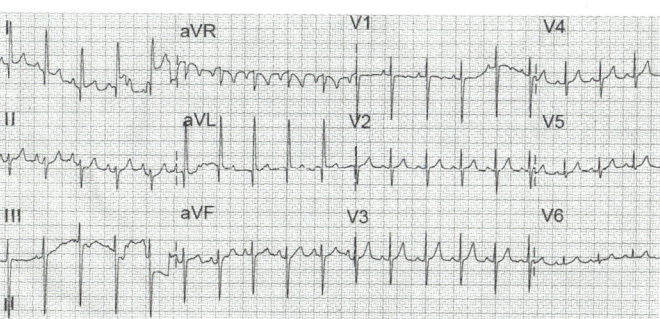

Fig. 11.34 ECG from a 5-months-old infant with tricuspid atresia, VSD, severe PS. ECG shows sinus rhythm, tall P waves, normal 'P' wave axis, left axis deviation (frontal QRS axis of minus 45°, counterclock wise loop), absence of RV forces in chest leads, left ventricular hypertrophy (chest leads in ½ voltage)

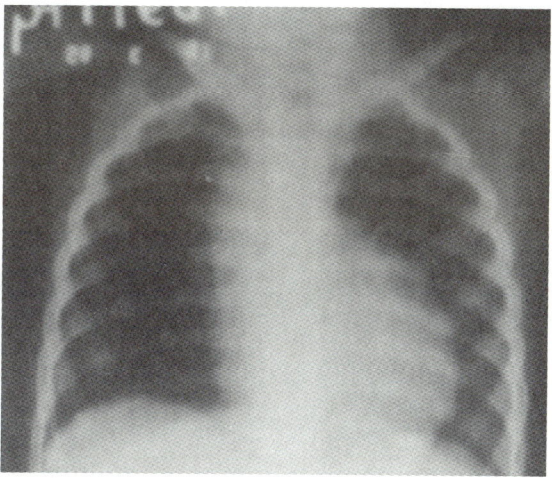

Fig. 11.35 X-ray chest in a child with tricuspid atresia showing normal heart size, LV type apex, prominent right atrial border merging with SVC shadow, absent MPA segment with decreased pulmonary vasculature

side of the heart via the foramen ovale or an associated atrial septal defect. Systemic venous blood mixes with pulmonary venous return in left atrium and enters left ventricle. Left ventricular blood usually flows into the right ventricle via a VSD and also directly to aorta. Pulmonary blood flow (and thus the degree of cyanosis) depends on the size of the VSD and the presence and severity of pulmonary stenosis. Intact ventricular septum leads to condition of pulmonary atresia and baby presents in neonatal period with severe cyanosis as the ductus starts constricting.

Clinical Features

Cyanosis is usually evident at birth, the extent depending on the degree of limitation to pulmonary blood flow. There may be an increased left ventricular impulse, in contrast to the majority of other causes of cyanotic heart disease. Second heart sound is single and there is a pansystolic murmur on the left sternal border. Clinical presentation in older children is identical to Fallot tetralogy.

Diagnosis

Left axis deviation, right atrial overload, and left ventricular hypertrophy are characteristic ECG features of tricuspid atresia (Fig. 11.34). Lung fields are oligemic. Right atrium and superior vena cava are prominent on chest X-ray (Fig. 11.35). Echocardiography reveals atretic right AV valve, stretched PFO or ASD, usually normal mitral valve, VSD, and ventriculo-arterial connections. Cardiac catheterization may be needed in some patients to assess pulmonary artery pressure.

Treatment	**Tricuspid Atresia**

Surgical management consists of pulmonary artery banding at 8–10 weeks in patients with increased pulmonary blood flow.

Blalock Tuussig shunt is advisable in patients with decreased pulmonary blood flow, if saturation falls below 70%. These palliative procedures should be followed by a Glenn shunt at 6–8 months and later Fontan completion after 2–3 years.

Revision Point

Tricuspid Atresia

1. Tricuspid atresia (TA) is defined as congenital absence or agenesis of the tricuspid valve. It is the third most common cyanotic congenital heart defect.
2. Nearly 50% of children with TA present with cyanosis on their first day of life and 80% become symptomatic by the end of one month. A subgroup (those with TGA) may present with CHF.
3. Left axis deviation in ECG in a cyanotic infant is characteristic and virtually diagnostic of tricuspid atresia.
4. Fontan procedure, a "corrective" surgery is performed in patients older than 2 years. Early presenting infants need a effective palliation (Blalock Taussig Shunt) before reaching the age of surgery.

Case Study | Tricuspid Atresia

A 5-month-old infant was brought with complaints of progressively deepening cyanosis since last two months. He was a term born neonate with 2.5 kg birth weight. The neonatal period was uneventful. There was no history of feeding difficulty or cyanotic spells. His weight and length were normal for age. Examination revealed central cyanosis, grade II pan-digital clubbing, and conjunctival suffusion. Oxygen saturation (SPO$_2$) was 75% in all four limbs. Examination revealed LV (left ventricular) type of apex in 4th left intercostal space in mid-clavicular line. There was no epigastric impulse. S$_1$ was normal, S$_2$ was single. There was grade 3/6 ejection systolic murmur at left upper and mid para-sternal region. There were no findings suggestive of CHF or a respiratory infection.

Q. What is the clinical diagnosis?

The child is having a congenital cyanotic heart disease. Presence of progressively deepening cyanosis and absence of symptoms of increased pulmonary blood flow (No CHF, No respiratory infections) points towards tetralogy of Fallot (TOF) or its variants (eg, DORV with VSD with PS, tricuspid atresia, single ventricle with PS, or TGA with VSD with PS). Apex is localized to one intercostal space and LV type. Also there is absence of epigastric impulse, indicating that left ventricle is the dominant chamber. This effectively rules out all conditions listed above except tricuspid atresia. Cyanotic heart disease with left ventricular dominance is almost diagnostic of tricuspid atresia.

Q. ECG of this child is shown below. Describe the findings?

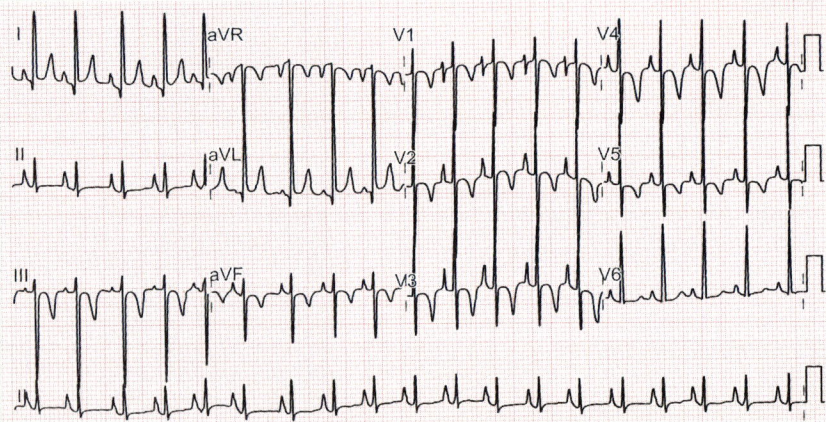

ECG shows tall peaked P waves in lead II. These are called *Himalayan* P waves. Their presence indicates huge right atrial enlargement. QRS axis is -30 degree. For a five-month infant, this is left axis deviation. Looking at chest leads there are deep S waves in right sided leads, *ie,* V1, V2, V3; and monophasic R in left sided leads V6. This indicates left ventricle dominance and left ventricle hypertrophy. In a patient diagnosed to have TOF physiology, presence of LAD and LVH are characteristic of tricuspid atresia.

Q. How will you manage this child?

Echocardiogram is done to confirm the diagnosis. Iron supplementation is started. Right ventricle being hypoplastic, only palliative surgery can be done. It involves direct connection of systemic veins (SVC and IVC) to pulmonary arteries bypassing the atretic tricuspid value and hypoplastic right ventricle.

Sittiwangkul R, Azakie A, Van Arsdell GS, *et al*. Outcomes of tricuspid atresia in the Fontan era. *Ann Thorac Surg*. 2004;77:889–94.

11.13 TRUNCUS ARTERIOSUS

Truncus arteriosus refers to a common trunk arising from heart giving rise to aorta, pulmonary arteries, and coronary arteries. The truncal valve is committed to both ventricles. There is associated large conotruncal outlet ventricular septal defect.

Clinical Features

Both ventricles are at systemic pressure and eject blood into the truncus. After birth, as pulmonary vascular resistance falls by 2–4 weeks of life, pulmonary blood flow increases enormously and infant presents with features of congestive cardiac failure. Because of large pulmonary blood flow, cyanosis may not be evident clinically. Examination reveals tachypnea, tachycardia, wide pulse pressure, and bounding pulses. This is accompanied by cardiomegaly, hyperkinetic precordium, single loud S$_2$, and ejection systolic murmur. S$_3$ and delayed diastolic murmur is heard at the apex due to increased flow across mitral valve.

If left unoperated, pulmonary vascular resistance increases and pulmonary blood flow falls. This leads to appearance of cyanosis along with clinical improvement in CHF.

Investigation

ECG shows right, left, or biventricular hypertrophy. Chest X-ray reveals cardiomegaly with increased pulmonary blood flow, absence of main pulmonary artery segment shadow, and dilated ascending aorta. Aortic arch is right sided in 26–50% of cases. Echocardiography demonstrates large VSD, overriding common truncus, morphology of truncal valve, origin of pulmonary arteries from truncus (common origin or separate origin or absent of one branch pulmonary artery), presence of arch anomalies, and dilated ventricles.

Treatment — Truncus Arteriosus

Stabilize with decongestive medications. If CHF is controlled, surgery can be deferred till 6–8 weeks of age. If CHF remains uncontrolled despite therapy, surgery is indicated immediately. Surgical treatment consists of total repair using right ventricle to pulmonary artery conduit. Pulmonary artery banding is done if total repair not possible.

Revision Point

Truncus Arteriosus

1. Truncus arteriosus refers to a common trunk arising from heart giving rise to aorta, pulmonary arteries, and coronary arteries.
2. CHF develops by 2–4 weeks of life, with wide pulse pressure, and bounding pulses. This is accompanied by cardiomegaly, hyperkinetic precordium, single loud S_2, and ejection systolic murmur.
3. Surgical treatment consists of total repair using right ventricle to pulmonary artery conduit.

Elzein C, Ilbawi M, Kumar S, Ruiz C. Severe trunkal valve stenosis: diagnosis and management. *J Card Surg*. 2005;20:589–93.

Restivo A, Piacentini G, Placidi S, *et al*. Cardiac outflow tract: a review of some embryogenetic aspects of the conotrunkal region of the heart. *Anat Rec A Discov Mol Cell Evol Biol*. 2006;288:936–43.

11.14 ANOMALOUS ORIGIN OF LEFT CORONARY ARTERY FROM PULMONARY ARTERY (ALCAPA)

Anomalous origin of left coronary artery from pulmonary artery (ALCAPA) leads to myocardium being supplied by desaturated blood under low pressure, causing myocardial ischemia. This may translate into myocardial infarction of the (*i*) anterolateral free wall of left ventricle, and (*ii*) papillary muscle of the mitral valve, which leads to mitral regurgitation.

Hemodynamics

ALCAPA does not manifest in fetal life due to almost equal pressures and equal oxygen saturation in pulmonary artery and aorta. This results in normal myocardial perfusion and no potential stimulus exists for collateral development. After birth, oxygen content of pulmonary artery falls, and thus anomalous coronary artery originating from it, also starts getting desaturated blood supply. Myocardial damage ensues and collateral flow develops.

Clinical Presentation

Usual presentation is by the age of 1–2 months (subsequent to falling pulmonary artery pressure). The child may occasionally present in neonatal period with features of CHF (tachycardia, tachypnea, excessive sweating) but rarely the presentation may be delayed to late childhood or even adult. Combination of left ventricular dysfunction and mitral regurgitation leads to congestive cardiac failure (tachypnea, tachycardia, feeding difficulty) and excessive cry due to chest pain, which is easily mistaken for infantile colic.

Examination reveals cardiomegaly, congestive hepatomegaly, gallop rhythm, and pansystolic murmur of mitral regurgitation. Rarely a continuous murmur may be heard in 2nd left interspace due to retrograde flow from left coronary artery to pulmonary artery, via collaterals.

Diagnosis

Characteristic ECG pattern may demonstrate anterolateral myocardial infarction with deep Q waves in 1, aVL and V4–V6 with ST segment elevation and T wave inversion (Fig. 11.36). As the child grows older, and if he survives (80–90% die within the first year if untreated), ST and T wave changes may disappear and Q waves diminish in size. ECG features of LVH and LAD are common especially in older patients. Some patients may not show typical infarct pattern but only show ST-T changes and/or left ventricular hypertrophy.

Chest X-ray shows cardiomegaly and features of pulmonary venous hypertension.

Two-dimensional *echocardiography* shows left ventricle dilatation with dysfunction, sclerosis of anterior papillary muscle of mitral valve, dilated right coronary artery, and origin of left coronary artery from pulmonary artery.

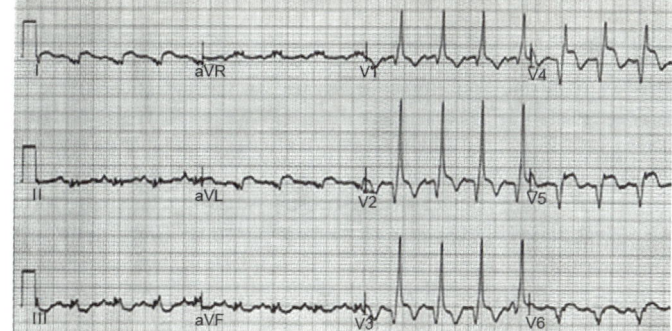

Fig. 11.36 ECG from 3 months old child with anomalous origin of left coronary artery from pulmonary artery with severe LV dysfunction. ECG shows deep Q wave in lead I, aVL, all chest leads V1–V6, presence of sign of myocardial ischemia (ST-T wave changes in all the chest leads), (Chest leads in ½ voltage)

Treatment — ALCAPA

Surgery (reimplantation of left coronary to aorta) at the time of diagnosis is the only treatment option. Medical stabilization consists of decongestive medication.

Birk E, Stamler A, Katz J, *et al*. Anomalous origin of the left coronary artery from the pulmonary artery: diagnosis and postoperative follow up. *Isr Med Assoc J*.2000;2:111–4.

Brotherton H, Philip RK. Anomalous left coronary artery from pulmonary artery (ALCAPA) in infants: a 5 years review in a defined birth cohort. *Eur J Pediatr*.2008;167:43–6.

Farouk A, Zahka K, Siwik E, *et al*. Anomalous origin of the left coronary artery from the right pulmonary artery. *J Card Surg*.2009;24:49–54.

Leong SW, Borges AJ, Henry J, Butany J. Anomalous left coronary artery from the pulmonary artery: case report and review of the literature. *Int J Cardiol*.2009;133:132–4.

Peña E, Nguyen ET, Merchant N, Dennie G.ALCAPA syndrome:not just a pediatric disease. *Radiographics*.2009;29:553–65.

Walsh MA, Duff D, Oslizlok P, *et al*. A review of 15-year experience with anomalous origin of the left coronary artery. *Ir J Med Sci*.2008; 177:127–30.

11.15 EBSTEIN ANOMALY OF THE TRICUSPID VALVE

Ebstein anomaly consists of downward apical displacement of septal and posterior leaflet of tricuspid valve into the right ventricle. The right ventricle is thus divided into two parts by the abnormal tricuspid valve: a thin-walled *"atrialized"* portion is continuous with the cavity of the right atrium; smaller *functioning portion* consists of normal ventricular myocardium. The right atrium is grossly dilated.

Hemodynamics

Tricuspid valve is usually regurgitant; the degree of regurgitation being extremely variable. The effective output from the right side of the heart is decreased because of the poorly functioning small right ventricle and tricuspid valve regurgitation. Sometimes right ventricular function is so compromised that it is unable to generate enough force to open the pulmonary valve in systole, producing "functional" pulmonary atresia. The increased volume of right atrial blood shunts through the foramen ovale to the left atrium, producing cyanosis.

Clinical Features

The severity of symptoms and the degree of cyanosis is highly variable and depends on the degree of displacement of the tricuspid valve, severity of tricuspid regurgitation, presence and size of atrial communication, and the severity of right ventricular outflow tract obstruction. In many patients, cyanosis is mild and the patient may present in adolescence with fatigue or palpitations. On palpation, the precordium is quiet. Multiple heart sounds are typical of Ebstein anomaly that includes split S_1, split S_2 and systolic sound produced by the sail like anterior tricuspid leaflet, S_3, and S_4. A soft pansystolic murmur is audible over most of the precordium resulting from tricuspid regurgitation. A scratchy diastolic murmur may also be heard at the left sternal border. This murmur is superficial and may mimic a pericardial friction rub.

Newborn infants with severe forms of Ebstein anomaly present with marked cyanosis, and massive cardiomegaly. Death may occur as a result of cardiac failure and hypoxemia, if the neonate is not treated appropriately.

Diagnosis

ECG shows tall peaked 'P' waves, prolonged PR interval, low voltage QRS complex in right sided leads and wide QRS complex (right bundle branch block) (Fig. 11.37). Delta wave as a feature of Wolff-Parkinson-White syndrome may be present; patients may have episodes of supraventricular tachycardia. There is no right ventricular hypertrophy.

Chest X-ray Heart size varies from normal to massive cardiomegaly due to enlargement of the right atrium and ventricle (Fig. 11.38). The pulmonary vasculature can be normal or decreased.

Echocardiography shows the degree of displacement of the tricuspid valve leaflets, a dilated right atrium, right ventricular outflow tract obstruction, and atrial communi-

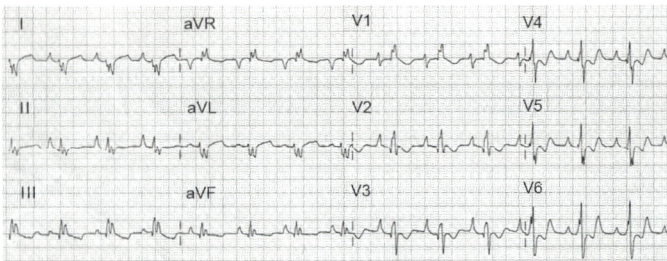

Fig. 11.37 ECG from 14 years old child with Ebstein anomaly of tricuspid valve. ECG shows sinus rhythm (HR-100/minute), PR interval 0.20 sec, tall 'P' wave (Himalayan 'P' wave-RA enlargement), low voltage wide QRS complex, frontal QRS axis of + 100°

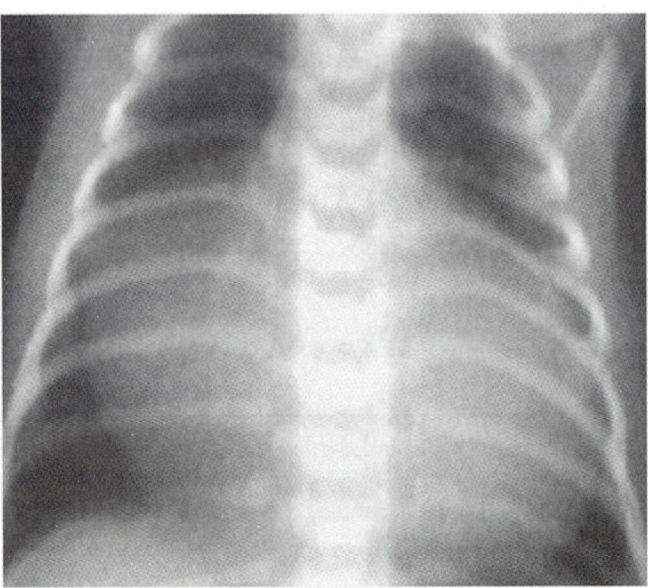

Fig. 11.38 X-ray chest findings in patients with Ebstein anomaly of tricuspid valve showing marked cardiomegaly with absent MPA shadow, gross RA enlargement with diminished pulmonary vascular markings

cation if present. Pulsed and color Doppler examination demonstrates the degree of tricuspid regurgitation.

Treatment	Ebstein Anomaly

Newborn with severe cyanosis If severe hypoxemia is persisting, maintaining ductal patency with PGE1 may be necessary. Rarely, a Blalock Taussig shunt may be required. If severe cyanosis is not there, conservative management in the newborn is recommended; with fall of pulmonary vascular resistance, the baby would tend to stabilize.

Older children Surgical intervention is advised for all symptomatic patients with cyanosis, CHF, or cardiomegaly. Recurrent arrhythmias may need radiofrequency ablation. Surgical management depends upon severity of Ebstein anomaly and functional right ventricle. The options are:
a. Tricuspid valve repair for good right ventricle cavity;
b. Tricuspid valve repair + Glenn shunt (directing SVC blood to RPA) for small right ventricle cavity; and
c. Fontan pathway (directing SVC → RPA; IVC → LPA) for severe variety with non-functioning right ventricle.

Bove EL, Hirsch JC, Ohye RG, Devaney EJ. How I manage neonatal Ebstein's anomaly. *Semin Thorac Cardiovasc Surg Pediatr Card Surg Annu.* 2009;63–5.

Cherry C, DeBord S, Moustapha-Nadler N. Ebstein's anomaly: a complex congenital heart defect. *AORN J.* 2009;89:1098–110.

Paranon S, Acar P. Ebstein's anomaly of the tricuspid valve: from fetus to adult: congenital heart disease.*Heart.* 2008;94:237–43.

11.16 EISENMENGER SYNDROME

Eisenmenger syndrome is characterized by severe, non-reactive, pulmonary vascular obstructive disease resulting in a right to left shunt at the atrial, ventricular or pulmonary arterial level. The condition develops secondary to long standing pulmonary arterial hypertension associated with left to right shunt lesions (VSD, PDA, AP window and less commonly ASD).

These children present with cyanosis, clubbing, fatigue, effort intolerance, dyspnea, history of chest infections in childhood, parasternal impulse, palpable P_2, and pulmonary ejection click. Differential cyanosis (where the fingers remain pink and the toes show cyanosis and clubbing) is diagnostic of pulmonary artery hypertension with patent ductus arteriosus. There is no significant flow murmur. Pulmonary regurgitation murmur may be audible. In patients with ASD, murmur of tricuspid regurgitation may be audible.

ECG reveals right axis deviation and right ventricular hypertrophy. Chest *X*-ray show prominent pulmonary artery at hilum and oligemic lung fields.

Treatment　　Eisenmenger Syndrome

Heart lung transplant is the only surgical treatment for these patients. Medical treatment consists of treating congestive heart failure and supportive management. Children should be advised to maintain adequate hydration, iron supplementation, and avoid going to high altitude. Children with severe polycythemia (hematocrit more than 60%) get symptomatic relief after phlebotomy. Intermittent use of oxygen may help.

Beghetti M, Tissot C. Pulmonary arterial hypertension in congenital heart diseases. *Semin Respir Crit Care Med.* 2009;30:421–8.

Berman EB, Barst RJ. Eisenmenger's syndrome: current management. *Prog Cardiovasc Dis.* 2002;45:129–38.

Moons P, Canobbio MM, Budts W. Eisenmenger syndrome: A clinical review. *Eur J Cardiovasc Nurs.* 2009;8:237–45.

OBSTRUCTIVE LESIONS

These lesions are acyanotic. There is no history of frequent chest infections. Precordium is not bulging and the apex beat is forcible or heaving. Obstructive lesion may be right-sided (pulmonic stenosis) or left-sided (aortic stenosis, coarctation of aorta). Heart size is usually normal and the lungs are normally vascularized.

11.17 AORTIC STENOSIS

Left ventricular outflow obstruction can occur at three levels: at the valve (valvular); above the valve (supravalvar); or below the valve (subvalvar).

• *Valvar aortic stenosis* Valvar aortic stenosis occurs in 3–6% of patients with congenital cardiovascular malformations,

with male predominance (4:1). Stenosis results from a unicuspid or a bicuspid aortic valve. Unicuspid aortic valve becomes symptomatic early in life. Bicuspid aortic valve resulting in significant obstruction mostly presents in later age; only 10% present in infancy.

• *Supravalvar stenosis* occurs due to obstruction at the aortic root, superior to the aortic valve.

• *Subvalvar aortic stenosis* This variety is categorized as *(i) membranous*: membrane located below the aortic annulus; *(ii) fibromuscular*: fibromuscular tissue extending from the septal wall of the left ventricle to the anterior leaflet of the mitral valve; or *(iii) hypertrophic*: obstruction occurs due to hypertrophy of left ventricle outflow tract.

Hemodynamics

The essential hemodynamic abnormality produced by the obstruction to left ventricular outflow consists of a pressure gradient between the left ventricle and aorta during systole. Obstruction of the aortic valve results in build-up of systolic pressure in the left ventricle. This causes concentric hypertrophy of the left ventricle. Ejection of left ventricular flow into aorta is prolonged because of outflow obstruction. This results in delayed closure of the aortic valve and a delayed A_2. Turbulent flow across the obstruction results in an ejection systolic murmur best heard over aortic area or suprasternal notch. This murmur starts after the first sound, reaches a crescendo in mid or late systole (depending on the severity of aortic stenosis) and ends with a decrescendo before or with the aortic component of the second sound (diamond shaped murmur). The most characteristic feature of the aortic stenosis is a thrill in the neck, suprasternal notch, and at the aortic area. Peripheral pulses are of low amplitude and prolonged duration with severe obstruction.

Clinical Features

Children with mild to moderate aortic stenosis are asymptomatic. Severe aortic stenosis presents with easy fatiguablity, exertional dyspnea, chest pain, or syncope. Critical aortic stenosis can present in the neonatal period with feeding difficulty and circulatory collapse. Pulse and blood pressure are normal with mild aortic stenosis. Pulse is low volume and pulse pressure is narrow in severe aortic stenosis.

Apical impulse is forceful or heaving in severe aortic stenosis. Systolic thrill is felt in suprasternal notch. Presence of systolic thrill in the second right intercostal space indicates moderately severe aortic stenosis. First heart sound is normal. The first sound is followed by an ejection click in valvular aortic stenosis, but is absent in supra and subvalvular stenosis, which precedes the start of the murmur. The aortic ejection click is well heard at the apex, and along the left sternal border. A delayed A_2 results in a narrow split. With *moderate* aortic stenosis, A_2 overlaps P_2 resulting in a single sound. *Severe* aortic stenosis is characterized by a paradoxical split (A_2 occurring after P_2). Presence of 4th heart sound also indicates a severe stenosis. Aortic stenosis is characterized by a diamond shaped ejection systolic murmur; severe the stenosis, closer is the peak of the murmur to the second sound. Aortic regurgitation murmur is usually audible in subvalvular aortic stenosis.

11

Supravalvar aortic stenosis may be associated with characteristic 'Elfine facies' of *William syndrome*. Other characteristics of this syndrome include mental retardation, dental abnormalities, strabismus, and idiopathic hypercalcemia caused by hypervitaminosis D. The defect occurs due to a gap in the chromosome 7 that results in a deletion of the elastin gene. Only 20% of children with supravalvular aortic stenosis have characteristic features of William's syndrome; another 20% have familial type of supravalvular aortic stenosis but do not have William's syndrome. Remaining children with supravalvular aortic stenosis are sporadic. A loud A_2 and prominent left arm pulses are good pointers to supravalvular variety.

Diagnosis

ECG Left ventricular hypertrophy and or ST and T-wave changes on the left sided leads in the electrocardiogram favor severe aortic stenosis (Fig. 11.39). However, one can have normal ECG even with severe aortic stenosis. ECG does not help in identifying the site of aortic stenosis.

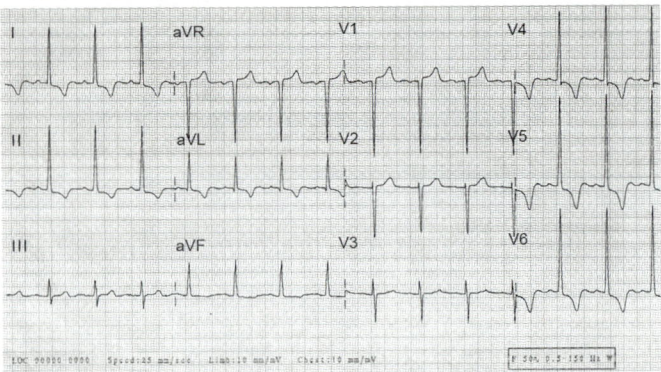

Fig .11.39 ECG from a child with critical aortic stenosis. ECG shows sinus rhythm, normal 'P' wave axis, QRS axis +40°, LVH, inverted 'T'wave in V4, V5, V6

Chest X-ray Chest X-ray shows post-stenotic dilatation of the ascending aorta in valvar aortic stenosis (Fig. 11.40). This is characteristically absent in supravalvar and subvalvar aortic

---

Case Study	Congenital Aortic Stenosis

An 11-year-old girl was brought to emergency department with left sided chest pain. It was a squeezing type of sub-sternal chest discomfort that was sudden in onset when she was playing. It got relieved after resting for a while. It was the first episode of such kind. She had a normal neonatal and infantile life. Her school performance was average. There was a past history of a syncopal attack, 6 months back which resolved spontaneously. No medical attention was sought at that time.

On examination her vitals were stable. Blood pressure was 96/76 mm Hg in right arm. Pulse was low volume, slow rising and delayed peaking and all peripheral pulses were felt. There was a systolic thrill in the suprasternal notch. Carotid thrill was also present. The apex was heaving and palpable in left 5th intercostal space in mid clavicular line. S_1 was normal. S_2 was normal in intensity with narrow split A_2-P_2. A constant click was heard at apex and right upper sternal border, just after S_1. Grade 3/6, harsh, late peaking ejection systolic murmur was heard at right upper sternal border. Other systemic examination was normal.

Q. What is the clinical diagnosis?

Precordial pain, syncopal attack, low volume pulse, thrill in the suprasternal notch and carotids, and grade 3/6 systolic murmur in the aortic area, are almost diagnostic of aortic stenosis. The character of the pulse described above is characteristically *pulsus parvus et tardus* which is also present in aortic stenosis. Presence of click indicates valvar AS with bicuspid aortic valve.

Q. ECG of this child is shown below. Describe the findings.

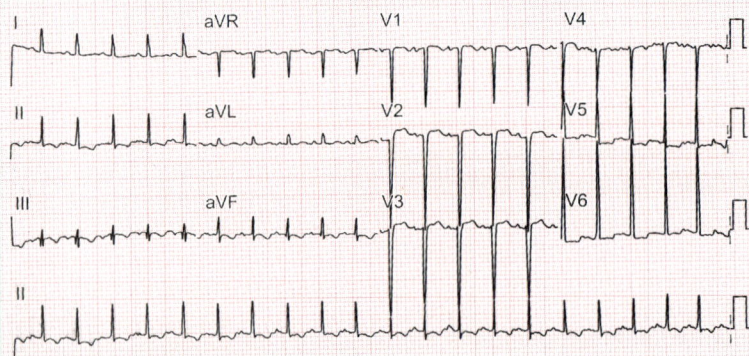

P wave in V1 is biphasic and the terminal part is negative, indicating LA enlargement. QRS axis is +30 degree. V1 has deep monophasic S wave and V6 has tall monophasic R wave. This indicates LVH. T waves in left precordial leads are negative indicating LV strain pattern. ECG is compatible with our clinical diagnosis of severe aortic stenosis.

Q. How will you manage the patient?

As the child is symptomatic with exertional angina, activity limitation will be advised. The diagnosis will be confirmed by echocardiography. If there is pure valvar AS without any regurgitation, percutaneous balloon dilation of aortic valve can relieve stenosis. Aortic regurgitation is a potential complication of balloon valvuloplasty.

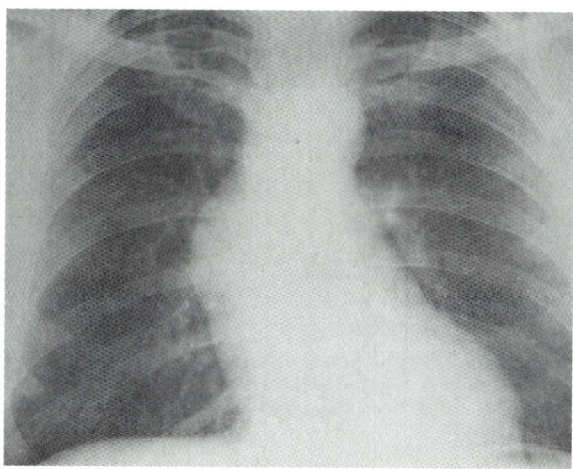

Fig. 11.40 Characteristic X-ray findings in a child with valvular aortic stenosis with preserved left ventricular function. Note the presence of normal heart size with dilated ascending aorta suggestive of the diagnosis

stenosis. Cardiomegaly indicates severe aortic stenosis with left ventricular failure.

Echocardiography Doppler echocardiography can quantitate the gradient across the aortic valve very accurately. It also documents the site of stenosis, severity of stenosis, ventricular function, and associated defects.

Treatment — Congenital Aortic Stenosis

Aortic stenosis is a progressive lesion which can cause sudden death. These children therefore need to be monitored periodically for increasing severity of symptoms, blood pressure, pulse pressure, second heart sound, and ECG changes. Doppler echocardiography should be done at regular intervals to monitor the gradient.

- *Valvar aortic stenosis* Balloon aortic valvotomy is the preferred tool for non-operative relief of aortic stenosis, both in infants and older children. Balloon dilatation is indicated if the mean pressure gradient across the aortic valve is more than 40 mmHg, or there is evidence of left ventricular dysfunction.
- *Aortic valve replacement* It is required in children with thick, fibrosed, or calcified valve; narrow aortic root; or significant aortic regurgitation. Operated children will require life-long anticoagulants.

Congenital Aortic Stenosis

1. Aortic Stenosis refers to a fixed left ventricular outflow tract obstructive lesion at the level of aortic valve (valvar AS), above (supravalvar AS) or below (subvalvar AS).
2. Aortic stenosis can present in neonatal period, remain asymptomatic, or present anytime in childhood.
3. In older children, exertional dyspnea, angina pectoris, and syncope are the characteristic features in moderate to severe stenosis. A thrill in the suprasternal notch with weak pulses is almost diagnostic.
4. Balloon valvuloplasty is the treatment of choice with excellent outcome.

- *Ross procedure*, ie, replacement of diseased aortic valve with patient's pulmonary valve and using homograft in place of pulmonary valve is another option for the pediatric age group. As homograft is in pulmonary position, rate of degeneration is slower and pulmonary regurgitation is tolerated well. These patients do not need anticoagulants.

Carabello BA. Aortic stenosis: from pressure overload to heart failure. *Heart Fail Clin.* 2006;2:435–42.

Horstkotte D, Loogen F. The natural history of aortic valve stenosis. *Eur Heart J.* 1988;9S:57–64.

O'Rourke RA. Aortic valve stenosis: a common clinical entity. *Curr Probl Cardiol.* 1998;23:434–71.

Resnekov L. Aortic valve stenosis. Management in children and adults. *Postgrad Med.* 1993;93:107–10, 113–4, 117–22.

Singh GK. Aortic stenosis. *Indian J Pediatr.* 2002;69:351–8.

Suys B, De Groote K, Decaluwe W, *et al.* Congenital left heart outflow abnormalities in the newborn. *Acta Cardiol.* 2006;61:210–1.

Syamasundar Rao P. Diagnosis and management of acyanotic heart disease: part I - obstructive lesions. *Indian J Pediatr.* 2005;72:496–502.

11.18 COARCTATION OF AORTA

Coarctation of aorta is a congenital narrowing of aorta. The most common site is located just distal to the origin of left subclavian artery. The indentation in aorta spares the medial wall. Associated defects are common and include bicuspid aortic valve (60–80%), ventricular septal defects (40%), associated valvar and subvalvar aortic stenosis, and atrio-ventricular valve abnormalities.

Hemodynamics

The narrowing of the aorta obstructs the systemic blood flow through the constricted segment of the aorta; thus increasing left ventricular pressure and workload. Collateral vessels develop, between the branches of the subclavian and intercostal arteries, bypassing the coarct segment of the aorta and supplying circulation to the lower extremities. Coarctation also results in systemic hypertension, the exact pathophysiology of which is not known.

Clinical Features

The clinical presentation of coarctation of aorta generally follows one of the three patterns: (*a*) an infant with congestive cardiac failure; (*b*) a child or adolescent with arterial hypertension; or (*c*) a child with a heart murmur.

When coarctation presents in infancy, it often presents as a catastrophic event. After birth as ductus closes, baby presents with congestive cardiac failure and shock. Multiorgan failure, particularly renal failure and necotizing enterocolitis, and subsequent death occur rapidly unless appropriate management is urgently provided.

Severe lesions present in infancy with poor feeding, growth failure, tachypnea, edema, acidosis, and congestive heart failure. A child or adolescent usually presents with intermittent claudication, pain and weakness of legs, and exertional dyspnea. Femoral pulses are weak and delayed as compared to brachial arterial pulses. Carotid pulse is prominent. Arterial pulsations can be felt in the suprasternal notch. Blood pressure measurement reveals hypertension. Characteristically, the blood pressure in upper extremities is more than that in the lower limbs, exactly opposite to what one would expect in a normal child. Degree of hypertension correlates with the severity of coarctation.

The heart size is normal with a left ventricular forcible or heaving apex. A systolic thrill may be palpable in the suprasternal notch. S_1 is loud and followed by a ejection click. S_2 is normally split with a loud A_2. Auscultation reveals a non-specific ejection murmur along the left sternal border which may also be heard over the back in the interscapular region. Collateral circulations in the chest wall may produce faint continuous murmurs and palpable collaterals over back.

Diagnosis

ECG shows left ventricular hypertrophy. In newborn period and infancy, the ECG may show right ventricular hypertrophy. Associated ST and T wave changes on left sided leads indicate associated aortic stenosis or endocardial fibroelastosis.

Thoracic roentgenogram shows a normal sized heart. Ascending aorta and the aortic knuckle are prominent. Aortic segments proximal and distal to the site of coarctation are dilated resulting in a typical '3' sign (Fig. 11.41a). Barium swallow shows the characteristic 'E' sign and confirms the site of coarctation (Fig. 11.41b). The characteristic notching of the lower borders of the ribs (3 to 8) (Fig. 11.41c) tends to appear only after the age of 4–5 years. Rib notching will be unilateral if origin of subclavian artery is stenosed or it arises distal to the site of coarctation.

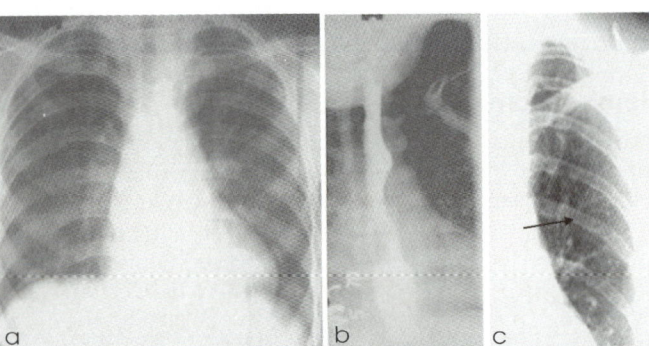

Fig. 11.41 Characteristic radiologic findings in patient with coarctation of aorta: (a) X-ray chest showing characteristic '3' sign (arrow at the site of coarctation); (b) barium swallow showing 'E or reversed 3' sign; (c) findings of rib notching (arrow) in presence of long standing coarctation of aorta

Echocardiography and *Doppler studies* can determine the site and severity of obstruction.

Treatment	**Coarctation of Aorta**

Medical management consists of control of congestive heart failure and systemic hypertension. Definitive treatment consists of surgical repair for infants < 6 months of age; balloon dilatation or surgery for children > 6 months of age (Fig. 11.42); and balloon dilatation with stent deployment in children >10 years of age.

Timing of Intervention

1. With left ventricular dysfunction/congestive heart failure or severe upper limb hypertension (for age)—*Immediate intervention.*

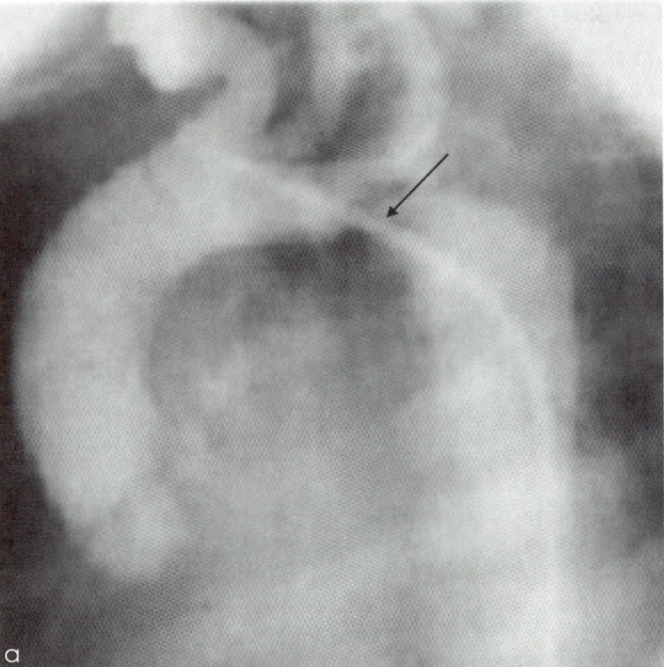

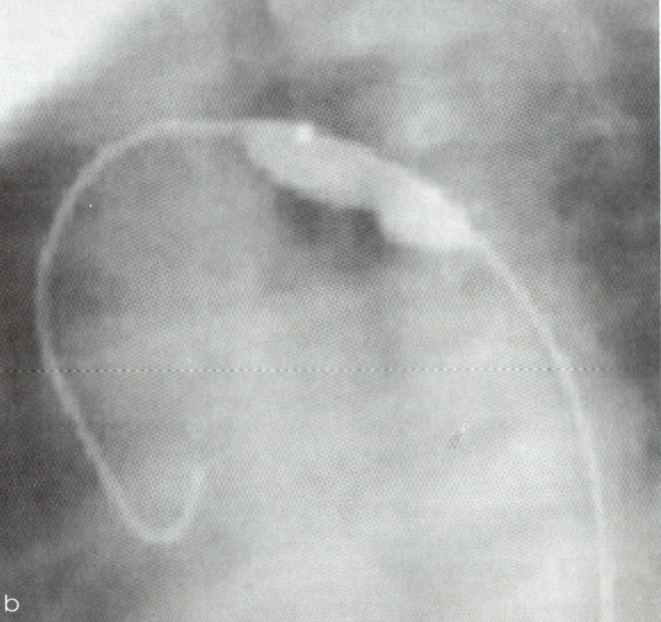

Fig. 11.42 (a) Aortogram from a patient with severe juxtaductal coarctation of aorta (arrow); (b) percutaneous baloon dilatation of coarctation of aorta is being done under fluoroscopic guidance

2. Normal left ventricular function, no congestive heart failure and mild upper limb hypertension—*Intervention beyond 3–6 months of age.*

3. No hypertension, no heart failure, normal ventricular function—*Intervention at 1–2 years of age.*

Systemic hypertension can persist following relief of obstruction if the obstruction is relieved late and re-coarctation of aorta can also occur. Re-coarctation is amenable to treatment by balloon angioplasty.

Abbruzzese PA, Aidala E. Aortic coarctation: an overview. *J Cardiovasc Med.* 2007;8:123–8.

Hager A. Hypertension in aortic coarctation. *Minerva Cardioangiol.* 2009;57:733–42.

Kanter KR. Management of infants with coarctation and ventricular septal defect. *Semin Thorac Cardiovasc Surg.* 2007;19:264–8.

Kenny D, Hijazi ZM. Coarctation of the aorta: from fetal life to adulthood. *Cardiol J.* 2011;18:487–95.

Tomar M, Radhakrishanan S. Coarctation of aorta—intervention from neonates to adult life. In*dian Heart J.* 2008;60(4 Suppl D):D22–33.

Case Study	Coarctation of Aorta

A 15-year-old adolescent boy was detected to have high blood pressure during a school health camp. He was growing well and participated in all activities without any symptom. There was no family history of hypertension. On examination, pulses in bilateral radial and brachial arteries were well felt. However, the femoral pulses and dorsalis pedis were feeble. Four limb blood pressures are mentioned below. JVP was normal. Apex was felt in fourth left intercostal space in mid-clavicular line. Heart sounds were normal and there were no precordial murmurs. A continuous murmur was however heard over back at interscapular area, bilaterally.

Right arm: 170/90 mmHg
Right leg : 110 systolic
Left arm : 170/90 mmHg
Left leg : 110 systolic

Q. What is the diagnosis?

Patient is suffering from coarctation of aorta. The presence of upper limb hypertension with feeble lower limb pulses and radio-femoral delay leads to the diagnosis. Due to the presence of obstruction between arch of aorta and descending aorta there is systolic blood pressure difference between arm and leg. Upper limb blood pressure is higher and pulse volume is good compared to the lower limbs. Very severe coarctation limits blood flow to descending aorta. Blood supply to lower part of body is maintained by collateral blood vessels arising from branches of subclavian arteries. Intercostal arteries have major role in collateral circulation, which dilate and produce notching at the lower border of ribs seen on chest X-ray. These collateral vessels produce continuous murmur which is heard at back.

Q. What is the importance of four limb blood pressure recording?

The diagnosis of coarctation can be easily missed if pulses are not examined in all four limbs. While evaluating a patient with hypertension, it is crucial to take blood pressure measurement with appropriate size cuff in both upper limbs and at least one lower limb. Different size cuff should be used for arm and leg blood pressure recording.

Coarctation of Aorta

1. Coarctation of aorta indicates a narrowing along the course of the aorta at some point.
2. There is no cyanosis. Neonates and infants can present with CHF, cardiovascular collapse, renal failure and acidosis. Children and adolescents may present with hypertension, or an incidental murmur.
3. Arterial pulses below the coarctation are diminished in amplitude and delayed in timing compared with the proximal pulses (radiofemoral delay).
4. Systolic blood pressure is elevated proximal to the coarctation, and a systolic pressure gradient is present between the arm and leg (difference more than 20 mm Hg).
5. Investigations reveal rib-notching (chest X-ray), E-shaped indentation on barium esophagogram, and LAD and LVH on ECG.

11.19 PULMONARY STENOSIS WITH INTACT VENTRICULAR SEPTUM

Congenital obstruction of right ventricular outflow is most commonly due to valvar pulmonary stenosis, but it may be subvalvular or supravalvular and can involve the main and branch pulmonary arteries in some cases. Pulmonary stenosis with or without other associated lesions occurs in 25 to 30% of all patients with congenital heart defects.

Associated syndromes with right ventricular outflow obstruction are congenital rubella, Noonan syndrome, William syndrome, LEOPARD syndrome; associated systemic diseases are gout and neurofibromatosis.

Isolated pulmonary valve stenosis is found in 80–90% of all patients with right ventricular outflow obstruction, 8–10% of patients have associated other congenital heart disease. Pulmonary valve can be tricuspid (commonest), quadricuspid, bicuspid or dysplastic. Dysplastic pulmonary valve is more commonly found with Noonan syndrome.

Hemodynamics (Fig. 11.43)

Pulmonary stenosis results in an increase in the right ventricular systolic pressure to maintain flow across right

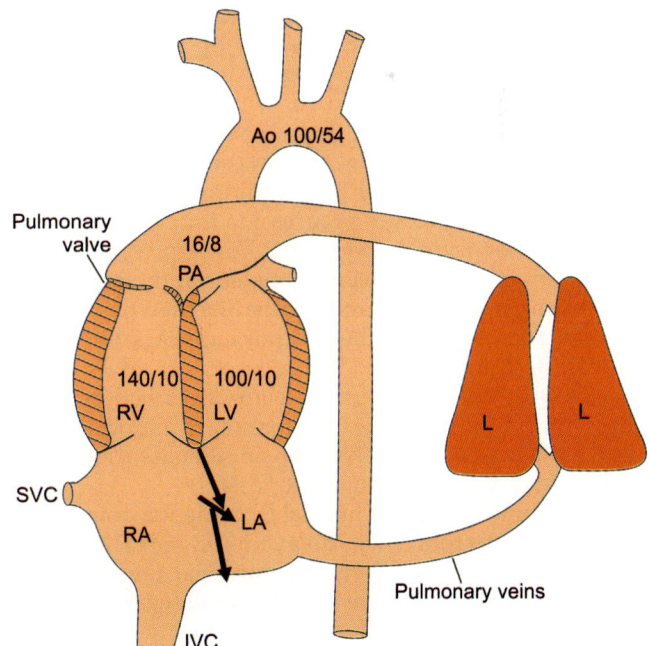

Fig. 11.43 Line diagram showing severe pulmonary stenosis with intact ventricular septum. Pulmonary valve is thickened and domed with pressure gradient of 124 mmHg and suprasystemic RV pressure. There is right to left shunt across PFO. L-lung. Values shown are pressures in mmHg in different cardiac chambers

ventricular outflow tract. This causes concentric right ventricular hypertrophy. Because of the obstruction, right ventricle ejection phase prolongs and causes delayed pulmonary closure of valve. P_2 therefore is delayed resulting in a wide variable split second sound. In valvar pulmonary stenosis a pulmonary ejection click (inconstant) is audible just after the first heart sound. The click is better heard during expiration but disappears or becomes softer during inspiration. Severity of pulmonary stenosis is inversely proportional to the distance between S_1 and click. This click is produced by sudden opening and excursion of the valve leaflets before the systolic ejection starts. Intensity of click depends on the degree of excursion of the leaflets. During inspiration, there is increased systemic venous return to RV, this increased RV volume pushes the pulmonary valve leaflets to a partially opened position even before the systole could start. Hence effective systolic excursion of leaflets is reduced during inspiration leading to reduced click intensity in this phase of respiration.

This click is followed by the murmur. Flow across the narrow right ventricle outflow causes ejection systolic murmur best heard at upper left parasternal area. Duration of murmur increases with the increasing severity of pulmonary stenosis. Severe pulmonary stenosis, ultimately results in right ventricle failure and tricuspid regurgitation. With development of right ventricular failure, peripheral cyanosis also appears due to decreased peripheral perfusion. If there is interatrial communication, more commonly patent foramen ovale, central cyanosis appears as a result of right to left shunt across the atrial communication.

Clinical Features

The symptoms with obstructive lesions of the right ventricular outflow tract obstruction are of early fatigability and exercise intolerance. Children with *mild stenosis* are asymptomatic but may rarely progress to moderate or severe stenosis with development of symptoms. Chances of progression are common during the growing period. Children with *moderate stenosis* are also usually asymptomatic except for some complaints of exercise intolerance. As chances of progression to *severe obstruction* are there, they require regular follow up. With severe obstruction, exercise intolerance appears and there may be syncope, palpitation and rarely angina like chest pain. If there is a patent foramen ovale, then cyanosis appears due to right to left atrial shunt.

Facies with pulmonary stenosis are described as 'moon facies', round face with hypertelorism. Examination may reveal evidence of Turner, Noonan or other associated non-cardiac issues with pulmonary stenosis.

Examination will reveal normal S_1, wide variable split S_2 with ejection systolic click, delayed and soft P_2, ejection systolic murmur, S_3 with right ventricular failure, and S_4 with critical stenosis. Severe lesions may have cyanosis.

Assessment of Severity

- *Symptomatic patients*—more severe stenosis
- *Cyanosis*—more severe stenosis
- *Evidence of heart failure*—critical stenosis
- *The closer the ejection click to first heart sound*—more severe the stenosis

- *The wider the splitting of second heart sound (delayed P_2)*—more severe the stenosis
- *The longer the murmur*—more severe the stenosis
- *Later the peaking of murmur*—severe the stenosis.

Diagnosis

ECG Moderate and severe cases demonstrate right axis deviation, right atrial enlargement, and right ventricular hypertrophy (Fig. 11.44). Children with Noonan syndrome can have left axis deviation despite presence of severe pulmonary stenosis. This is due to intraventricular conduction abnormalities.

Chest X-ray shows normal size heart, prominent main and left pulmonary artery with normal vasculature (Fig. 11.45). In valvar pulmonary stenosis, the pulmonary arteries (mostly main and left pulmonary arteries) show post-stenotic dilatation. Cardiomegaly and thinned out pulmonary vasculature appears with critical pulmonary stenosis and

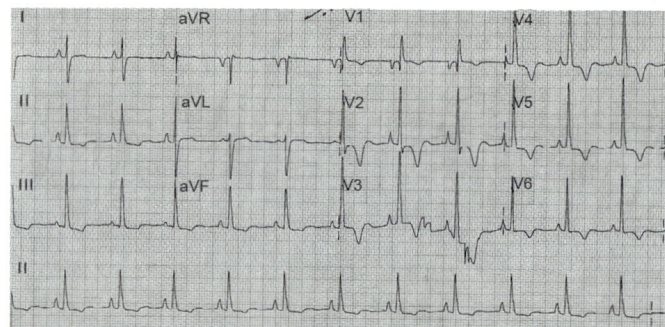

Fig. 11.44 ECG from 12 years old child with severe valvar pulmonary stenosis (suprasystemic RV pressure) with intact interventricular septum. ECG shows normal sinus rhythm, normal 'P' wave axis, RA enlargment (tall 'P' wave), right axis deviation (frontal QRS axis +100°), severe RVH, presence of RV strain pattern (q wave in lead V1, T wave inversion in V1–V6), absence of transition

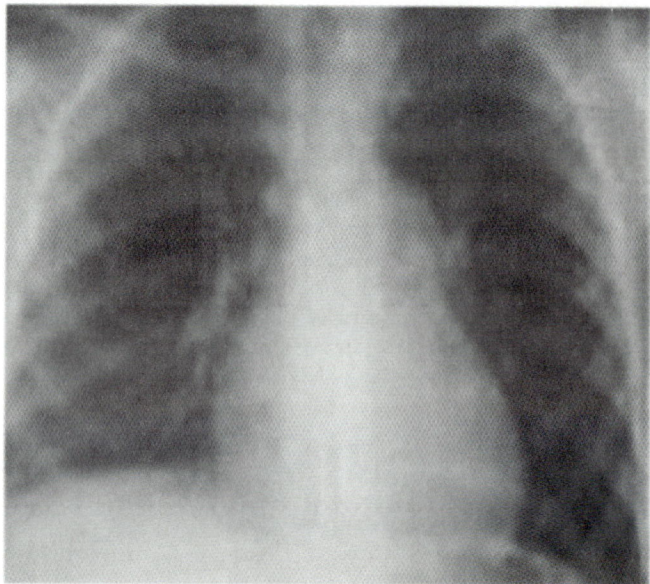

Fig. 11.45 X-ray chest of patient with valvular pulmonary stenosis (PS). Notice normal heart size with dilated MPA and LPA and normal pulmonary vascular markings

right ventricular dysfunction or with associated significant tricuspid regurgitation.

Echocardiography can diagnose the site of stenosis, severity of stenosis, ventricular function, associated defects; and also define the need for intervention.

Treatment	**Pulmonary Stenosis**

Balloon pulmonary dilatation is indicated if the peak systolic gradient is >60 mmHg with domed pulmonary valve. Surgical treatment is indicated if the pulmonary valve is dysplastic or there is subvalvular, supravalvular, or branch pulmonary artery obstruction.

Pulmonary Stenosis

1. Pulmonary stenosis can be valvar, subvalvar, or peripheral (involving the pulmonary artery).
2. Majority of children with PS are diagnosed due to incidental detection of a murmur. Those with long standing moderate to severe stenosis present with exertional dyspnea and fatigue.
3. Moderate and severe degree of stenosis is associated with right ventricular hypertrophy (RVH).
4. Balloon pulmonary valvuloplasty is the treatment of choice for moderate and severe PS.

Almeda FQ, Kavinsky CJ, Pophal SG, Klein LW. Pulmonic valvular stenosis in adults: diagnosis and treatment. *Catheter Cardiovasc Interv.* 2003;60:546–57.

Franch RH. Recognition and management of valvular pulmonic stenosis. *Heart Dis Stroke.* 1994;3:365–70.

Odenwald T, Taylor AM. Pulmonary valve interventions. *Expert Rev Cardiovasc Ther.* 2011;9:1445–57.

Sommer RJ, Rhodes JF, Parness IA. Physiology of critical pulmonary valve obstruction in the neonate. *Catheter Cardiovasc Interv.* 2000;50:473–9.

11.20 ACUTE RHEUMATIC FEVER

Acute rheumatic fever occurs in 5–15 years age group and is more common in children from poor socio-economic background.

Etiology

This is most likely an immunological response resulting in damage to the heart by antibodies. These antibodies are produced in response to a primary infection of the throat by group A beta hemolytic streptococci. A history of preceding sore throat may be present. However, more than 50% children with rheumatic fever do not have a definite history of sore throat.

Following untreated streptococcal sore throat, there is a latent period that may last from 10 days to several weeks. During this period, antibodies form to the streptococcal antigen. These antibodies have the capacity to react with human connective tissue specially the cardiac muscle. This antigen antibody reaction results in rheumatic fever.

Although the inciting bacterial agent is well known, susceptibility factors remain unclear. The location of the streptococcal infection seems to play an important role. The clinical syndrome typically follows a streptococcal pharyngitis, but streptococcal cellulitis has never been implicated. Genetics may contribute, as evidenced by an increase in family incidence. No significant association with class I human leukocyte antigens (HLA) has been found, but an increase in class II HLA antigens DR2 and DR4 has been found in black and white patients, respectively. Evidence suggests that elevated immune-complex levels in blood samples from patients with acute rheumatic fever are associated with HLA-B5.

Incidence

The incidence of an acute rheumatic fever episode following streptococcal pharyngitis is 0.5–3%. The peak age is 5–15 years. Most major outbreaks occur under conditions of poverty and overcrowding where access to antibiotics is limited. Rheumatic heart disease accounted for 25–50% of all cardiac admissions in India. Regions of major public health concern include the Middle East, the Indian subcontinent, and some areas of Africa and South America. As many as 20 million new cases occur each year. The introduction of antibiotics has been associated with a rapid worldwide decline in the incidence of acute rhuematic fever.

No general clear-cut sex predilection has been reported, but its manifestations seem to be sex variable. For example, certain clinical manifestations (ie, chorea and tight mitral stenosis) are predominant in females, while males are more likely to develop aortic regurgitation.

Clinical Features

The earliest and most common presentation is of fever and migratory joint pains, following streptococcal sore throat. Large joints such as knees, ankles, elbows, or shoulders are typically affected. Another subset of children may present with fever, tachypnea, tachycardia and palpitation, suggestive of heart involvement. Carditis (with progressive congestive heart failure, a new murmur, or pericarditis) may be the presenting sign of unrecognized past episodes and is the most lethal manifestation. Sydenham chorea is the least common presentation that manifests with gradual onset of abnormal choreoathetoid movements. Acute attacks usually resolve within 12 weeks.

Guidelines for the clinical diagnosis of acute rheumatic fever originally suggested by Dr. T. Duckett Jones, were subsequently revised by the American Heart Association in 1965 and updated in 1992. The latest revision of Jones criteria has been published in 2015.

The disease is diagnosed based on the presence of major, minor, and essential criteria, as follows:

A. Major Criteria

1. Carditis
2. Polyarthritis
3. Subcutaneous nodules
4. Chorea
5. Erythema marginatum

B. Minor Criteria

1. *Clinical*

- Fever
- Arthralgia
- Previous rheumatic fever or rheumatic heart disease

2. Laboratory

- *Acute phase reactants* Leucocytosis, elevated sedimentation rate and C reactive protein.
- Prolonged PR interval in the electrocardiogram

C. Essential Criteria

Evidence for Recent Streptococcal Infection

- Increased antistreptolysin "O" titer
- Positive throat culture
- Recent scarlet fever

'2 Major' or '1 Major and 2 Minor' criteria are required in the presence of 'Essential criteria' to diagnose acute rheumatic fever.

2015 Modifications to Jones Criteria

- According to revised Jones criteria (2015), population has been divided into low risk and moderate/high risk categories on the basis of incidence of ARF in school aged children (>2/lac/year) and prevalence of RHD in population (>1/1000).
- To increase the sensitivity of diagnostic criteria, monoarthritis and polyarthralgia have been included as major criteria and monoarthralgia as minor criteria for moderate/high risk population.
- Subclinical carditis diagnosed by echocardiography as pathological mitral regurgitation and aortic regurgitation, in the absence of clinical carditis, has been included as major criteria in new revised Jones criteria.

Carditis

Carditis occurs in 50–70% of all children with acute rheumatic fever. It can occur as the first manifestation of rheumatic fever in a previously healthy child or can recur in a child who already has an established rheumatic heart disease. It involves all the 3 layers of the heart, ie, pericardium, myocardium and endocardium (*pancarditis*).

- *Pericarditis* is suggested by presence of chest pain and a pericardiac friction rub on auscultation. The pericardial effusion is never massive and therefore lacks signs of tamponade or passive venous congestion.
- *Myocarditis* presents with tachycardia, cardiomegaly, and congestive failure. In the past, much attention was paid to Carey Coomb's murmur, a delayed diastolic murmur best heard at the apex. It was supposed to be a marker of inflammation of the mitral valve papillary muscle complex and due to associated mitral regurgitation. However, we realize now that myocarditis occurs due to interstitial tissue involvement and not due to myocyte damage.
- *Endocarditis* Endocardial involvement is indicated by valvular murmurs. There may be appearance of new murmur, or change in the character or intensity of pre-existing murmurs. Mitral, aortic, and tricuspid valves are involved, in that order of frequency. Pulmonary valve is very rarely involved. Endocarditis of the involved valves results in acute regurgitant lesion of the respective valve. Mitral regurgitation is present in 95% children with carditis; of these, one-fourth also have associated aortic regurgitation. Isolated aortic regurgitation occurs in only 5% children. Tricuspid regurgitation does not occur in isolation, though it may be associated with aortic or mitral regurgitation in 10–30% children.

Arthritis

Arthritis usually involves multiple large joints, particularly the knees, ankles, elbows, and wrists. Hips and smaller joints of hands and feet are rarely involved. Typically, a series of painful joints is followed by another series of painful joints. Involved joints become swollen, red, hot and painful. Migratory polyarthritis is usually associated with a febrile illness. There is no residual damage to the joints, after the arthritis subsides.

Western literature reports joint involvement in 80% of affected children; corresponding data from India indicate arthritis or arthralgia in only 30 to 50% children with acute rheumatic fever.

Subcutaneous Nodules

Subcutaneous nodules appear on bony prominence like elbows, shins, occiput, and spine and are non-tender. Nodules of rheumatic fever are better seen than palpated. They measure between a few mm to a cm. Lesions appear late, 6–8 weeks after onset of acute rheumatic fever. They occur in about 5 to 20% of cases of rheumatic fever in India. Children who have subcutaneous nodules almost always have carditis. Nodules usually last from a few days to weeks; persistence up to one year has been reported.

Chorea

Sydenham chorea or chorea minor (referred to as Saint Vitus Dance) is a disease characterized by rapid, uncoordinated, non-repetitive, involuntary jerking movements affecting primarily the face, fingers, feet and hands. The child is clumsy and drops things because of a poor grip. Hand writing is badly affected. Movements disappear during sleep. Diagnosis can be confirmed by physical examination, as tests detailed in **Table 11.3**. It is reported to occur in 20–30% of patients with acute rheumatic fever. The disease is usually latent, occurring up to 6 months after the acute infection, but may occasionally be the presenting symptom of rheumatic fever. Sydenham chorea is more common in females than males.

Table 11.3 Physical Signs of Sydenham Chorea

Procedure	Result
1. Ask the child to lift the arms and stretch the hands above the head	Forearms tend to pronate
2. Ask the child to stretch the arms and hands forwards towards you	Wrist is flexed and fingers are hyperextended
3. Ask the child to grip your fingers tightly	Unable to do so. There is alternate relaxation and tightening of the grip (milk maid grip)
4. Ask the child to protrude out the tongue	Unable to maintain tongue outside the mouth. It keeps going in and out (darting)

Erythema Marginatum

Erythema marginatum rash is reddish, macular and non-itching, serpiginous, predominantly observed on trunk. It is very rarely observed in Indian children.

Essential Criteria

Demonstration of anti-streptococcal antibodies is preferred over antigens, as the essential criteria for evidence of recent streptococcal infection, because of several reasons. Firstly, Group A streptococcal antigen detection tests are specific but not very sensitive. In contrast, antistreptococcal antibodies usually reach a peak titer (in Todd units) at the time of onset of rheumatic fever and are more useful. Moreover, specific antibodies to streptococcal antigens also indicate true infection rather than mere carriage of the organism. However, children without acute rheumatic fever may have an isolated positive antistreptolysin O (ASO) titer. This may also be found in children with certain related diseases such as rheumatoid arthritis and Takayasu arteritis. Therefore, rising ASO titers should be combined with a careful clinical evaluation and the discovery of other antistreptococcal antibodies to support the diagnosis of acute rheumatic fever.

Antistreptococcal antibodies include ASO, anti-deoxyribonuclease B (anti-DNAse B), antistreptokinase, and antihyaluronidase. These antibodies target extracellular products produced by streptococci. Although age, geographic location, and season affect the titers, an elevated titer of at least one of these antibodies indicates streptococcal infection in 95% of patients. ASO is found in 80–85% of children with acute rheumatic fever. For comparison, the sensitivity of ASO titer (adults with >240 Todd U and children with >320 Todd U) is 80%. The sensitivity increases if multiple antibody titers or paired sera are tested.

The sensitivity of throat culture as evidence of recent streptococcal infection is only 25–40%.

Course of the Disease

The cardiac involvement may result in a permanent damage to the valves. This causes a long lasting heart lesion (aortic or mitral regurgitation, mitral stenosis, tricuspid regurgitation), that is classically referred to as "Rheumatic Heart Disease".

A child who develops rheumatic heart disease is prone to have recurrent episodes of acute rheumatic fever, if the streptococcal focus is not eradicated. Fresh bout of rheumatic fever on a pre-existing rheumatic heart disease may result in further damage to the already diseased valves or involvement of other valves, which were hitherto normal.

Treatment	**Acute Rheumatic Fever**

A. Restriction of Activity

All patients should be restricted to bed rest and monitored closely for carditis. When carditis has been documented, a 4 weeks period of bedrest is recommended. Immobilization may have to be continued for longer time especially in the presence of congestive failure. As soon as the signs of acute inflammation subside, patients should resume active ambulation as tolerated.

B. Diet

Restrict salt intake only if features of congestive heart failure are present, otherwise give normal nutritious diet rich in iron to prevent anemia.

C. Penicillin

One of the primary goals of treating acute rheumatic fever is to eradicate streptococci from the pharynx. Penicillin is the drug of choice in persons who are not at risk of allergic reaction. A single parenteral injection of benzathine benzyl penicillin (1.2 mega units) or 10 days course of oral Penicillin-V or injectable procaine penicillin (4 lac units IM, twice a day) is considered adequate therapy. Oral cephalosporins, rather than erythromycin, are recommended as an alternative in children who are allergic to penicillin. However, be cautious of the 20% cross-reactivity of the cephalosporins with penicillin.

By promptly treating streptococcal pharyngitis in susceptible hosts, repetitive exposure to pathologically reactive antigens can be avoided. However, management of the current infection will probably not affect the course of the current attack and does not alter the course, frequency, or severity of cardiac involvement.

D. Suppressive Therapy

Aspirin and steroids are used to suppress activity in acute rheumatic fever. These agents need to be given for the entire duration of rheumatic activity which is approximately 12 weeks in 80% of the patients. Aspirin is the preferred drug to treat isolated arthritis, while steroids are preferred for treatment of carditis. Consensus Guidelines on Pediatric Acute Rheumatic Fever and Rheumatic Heart Disease Working Group Cardiology Chapter of Indian Academy of Pediatrics has advocated the following regimes for treating acute rheumatic fever in children).

Arthritis ± Mild Carditis (aspirin preferred)

Regime I Aspirin is started in a dose of 100 mg/kg/day for 2–3 weeks. Once symptoms start resolving, taper dosages to 60–70 mg/kg/day, for next 9 weeks. For older children 50 mg/kg/day.

Regime II Aspirin 50 to 60 mg//kg /day for 12 weeks. Children who do not tolerate aspirin should be treated with naproxen 10–20 mg/kg/day. Switch over to steroids, if there is no response to aspirin in four days.

Moderate to Severe Carditis (steroids preferred)

Regime I Start prednisolone (2 mg/kg/d, maximum 80 mg/day) till ESR normalizes-usually 2 weeks. Taper over next 2–4 weeks, reduce dose by 2.5–5 mg every 3rd day. Start aspirin 50–75 mg/kg/d simultaneously, to complete total 12 weeks of therapy.

Regime II Prednisolone same doses × 3–4 weeks, taper slowly to cover total period of 10–12 weeks.

Non-responders should be given a trial of intravenous methyl prednisolone (30 mg/kg/day for 3 days), if there is no response to oral steroid therapy. Steroids are a more potent suppressive agent as compared to aspirin. However, there is no proof that the use of steroids results in less cardiac damage as compared to aspirin. It is known that steroids act faster and are superior—at least in the initial phases.

E. Management of Chorea

Chorea is a late manifestation of rheumatic fever and by the time a patient presents with chorea, the sedimentation rate as well as the ASO may be normal. The patient as well as the parents should be reassured and told about the self-limiting course of the disease. Protracted Sydenham chorea has responded to haloperidol. Complete physical and mental rest is essential because the manifestations of chorea may be exaggerated by emotional trauma. Recently, glucocorticoids have been used for treating chorea considering this as a sign of acute rheumatic fever. Because chorea disappears with sleep, adequate sedation should be provided. Chorea requires long-term penicillin prophylaxis, even if there are no other manifestations of rheumatic fever. Long-term studies have shown that over a follow up for 10 years, 10% may develop mitral stenosis; and after 20 years follow-up, 20% may develop mitral stenosis.

11

Prevention of Rheumatic Fever

For rheumatic polyarthritis, prophylaxis should be continued for 5 years after the last episode or till 18 years of age, whichever is later. Prophylaxis needs to be given till at least the age of 35 years in patients with rheumatic heart disease. Ideally, this should continue lifelong. The principles of treatment include the following:

- The risk of rheumatic fever recurrence is greatest during the first 3–5 years following the attack.
- Prophylaxis must continue indefinitely in children with established heart disease or in those frequently exposed to streptococci.
- Treatment for an indefinite period is required among patients with frequent exposure to streptococci or for those who are difficult to monitor.
- Drug regimes for prophylaxis of rheumatic fever are given in **Table 11.4.**

The decision to withdraw the antibacterial drugs should be individualized after carefully assessing the risk of repetitive exposures.

Diagnosis of Rheumatic Fever (in established RHD)

For the diagnosis of activity, one has to go back to the Jones criteria.

- Presence of cardiac involvement cannot be used as a major criterion since it may be the result of a previous attack of rheumatic fever.
- Presence of a pericardial friction rub is evidence of active carditis.
- If the patient has well documented cardiac findings then the appearance of a new murmur or a significant increase in a pre-existing murmur is very suggestive for active rheumatic fever.
- History of arthralgia or arthritis within a period of less than 12 weeks is suggestive of active rheumatic fever specially if associated with elevated sedimentation rate, C reactive protein and antistreptolysin 'O' titer.
- Elevated antistreptolysin 'O' titer goes in favor of active rheumatic fever. If initial titer is low then a rising titer in repeat sample indicates rheumatic activity.

RHEUMATIC HEART DISEASE

The sequels of rheumatic fever consist of mitral, aortic and tricuspid valve disease and very rarely pulmonary valve involvement. Other manifestations are atrial arrhythmias, thromboemoblism, and cardiac hemolytic anemia. Post-inflammatory scarring is presumed to be responsible for delayed sequel. Postrheumatic scarring is more prevalent in girls, with male-to-female ratio of approximately 0.4:1.

Chronic valvular deformities occurring as a result of rheumatic carditis may cause congestive heart failure. In pediatric age group, the mitral valve involvement manifests predominantly as mitral regurgitation and much less commonly as mitral stenosis while aortic valve involvement presents exclusively with regurgitation. Tricuspid valve involvement usually results in regurgitation but rarely stenosis can occur. Rheumatic aortic stenosis has never been described in children.

Acute Rheumatic Fever

1. Acute rheumatic fever is an inflammatory autoimmune disorder that affects several organs of the body characterized by arthritis, carditis, chorea, rheumatic nodules, erythema marginatum and fever caused by Group A beta hemolytic streptococci.
2. Peak incidence is seen between ages 5 and 15 years.
3. Diagnosis is based on revised Jones criteria 2015 and confirmation of streptococcal infection.
4. Carditis is the leading cause of valvular involvement. Mitral and aortic valves are mostly involved.
5. Acute rheumatic fever is treated with aspirin and/or steroids depending on the presence of carditis.
6. Primary prevention consists of appropriate treatment of all episodes of streptococcal sore throat.
7. Children with residual heart disease require lifelong prophylaxis with penicillin.

American Heart Association. Revision of the Jones Criteria for the Diagnosis of Acute Rheumatic Fever in the Era of Doppler Echocardiography: A Scientific Statement From the American Heart Association. *Circulation.* 2015;131:1806–1818.

Drug	Dose	Sore throat treatment (duration)	Secondary Prophylaxis (interval)
Benzathine Penicillin G	1.2 million unit (>27 kg) (deep IM inj) after sensitivity test 0.6 million unit (<27 kg) (after sensitivity test) contraindication: penicillin allergy	Single dose Single dose	Every 21 day Every 15 days
Penicillin-V (oral)	Children: 250 mg qid Adult: 500 mg tid contraindication: penicillin allergy	10 days 10 days	Twice a day Twice a day
Azithromycin (oral)	12.5 mg/kg/day once daily	5 days	Not recommended
Cephalexin (oral)	15–20 mg/kg/dose bid	10 days	Not recommended
Erythromycin (oral)	20 mg/kg/dose max 500 mg	Not recommended	Twice a day

Table 11.4 IAP Drug Regime for Rheumatic Fever Prophylaxis*

* *Consensus Guidelines on Pediatric Acute Rheumatic Fever and Rheumatic Heart Disease Working Group on Pediatric Acute Rheumatic Fever and Cardiology Chapter of Indian Academy of Pediatrics 2008.*

Case Study | Acute Rheumatic Fever

A 13-year-old boy was brought to out-patient department with breathlessness for two days. He was an active school going student who was faring well in his studies. About 10 days back, he had high grade fever with sore throat followed by pain in right ankle. This later involved the left knee, elbow, and right knee over next 3–4 days. This was not associated with swelling over the joints. The pain subsided after taking treatment from local practitioner. Since last 2 days the boy started having, breathlessness and mild abdominal distension. He was 4th in birth order and lived in a joint family under overcrowded conditions.

On examination he was thin built and sick looking. He was afebrile but has tachycardia (HR 120/min) and tachypnea (RR = 40/min). Pulse was normal volume and all peripheral pulses were felt. The child had pedal edema and JVP was raised. Apical impulse was hyperdynamic and felt in 6th intercostal space just outside the mid clavicular line. S_1 and S_2 were normal. S_3 gallop and pericardial rub were present. Grade 3/6 pansystolic murmur was heard at apex. Respiratory system examination was normal. Liver span was 11 cm.

Q. What is the clinical diagnosis? Justify.

Suspected diagnosis is acute rheumatic fever. The present case fulfils 1 major (carditis) and 2 minor (polyarthralgia and fever) criteria for diagnosis of ARF. Carditis is supported by presence of pericardial rub (indicating pericarditis) pedal edema, S_3 gallop, tachypnea, tachycardia, raised JVP (due to myocarditis) and a regurgitant (systolic) murmur of mitral valve (due to endocarditis). Throat swab culture and anti-streptococcal antibody titers should be done to document supportive evidence of antecedent Group A beta hemolytic streptococcal infection.

Q. How will you manage this child?

A. *Immediate management*

We will advise bedrest, prop-up the child, administer oxygen by face mask, and administer IV fluids (2/3 of normal maintenance). These supportive measures will have to be accompanied with administration of intravenous diuretics to reduce afterload.

The child will need to be started on steroids (prednisolone 2 mg/kg/d) in 2–3 divided doses for 3 weeks, after which they can be tapered. Aspirin will have to be started once we start tapering steroids (60–80 mg/kg/day) and continued for 9 weeks. Thus, total of 12 weeks of anti-inflammatory therapy is needed.

B. *Eradication of streptococci*
- One dose of I/M Benzathine penicillin 12 lac IU after sensitivity testing
- Alternatively oral or I/V penicillin can be administered for 10 days

C. *Secondary prophylaxis*
- 12 lac IU benzathine penicillin administered I/M every 3 weekly
- He should be under regular follow up to evaluate residual valvar lesion and thus decide for duration of prophylaxis.

De Rosa G, Pardeo M, Stabile A, Rigante D. Rheumatic heart disease in children: from clinical assessment to therapeutical management. *Eur Rev Med Pharmacol Sci.* 2006;10:107–10.

Gordon N. Sydenham's chorea, and its complications affecting the nervous system. *Brain Dev.* 2009;31:11–4.

Jackson SJ, Steer AC, Campbell H. Systematic Review: Estimation of global burden of non-suppurative sequelae of upper respiratory tract infection: rheumatic fever and post-streptococcal glomerulonephritis. *Trop Med Int Health.* 2011;16:2–11.

Lee JL, Naguwa SM, Cheema GS, Gershwin ME. Acute rheumatic fever and its consequences: a persistent threat to developing nations in the 21st century. *Autoimmun Rev.* 2009;9:117–23.

Lennon D, Kerdemelidis M, Arroll B. Meta-analysis of trials of streptococcal throat treatment programs to prevent rheumatic fever. *Pediatr Infect Dis J.* 2009;28:e259–64.

Mayosi BM. Protocols for antibiotic use in primary and secondary prevention of rheumatic fever. *S Afr Med J.* 2006;96:240.

Saxena A. Diagnosis of rheumatic fever: current status of Jones Criteria and role of echocardiography. *Indian J Pediatr.* 2000;67:S_1 1–4.

Saxena A. Diagnosis of rheumatic fever: current status of Jones Criteria and role of echocardiography. *Indian J Pediatr.* 2000;67:283–6.

Sethi S, Kaushik K, Mohandas K, *et al.* Anti-streptolysin O titers in normal healthy children of 5–15 years. *Indian Pediatr.* 2003;40:1068–71.

Sharma M, Sharma D. Subcutaneous nodules. *Indian Pediatr.* 2000;37:556.

Singh S. Aspirin in acute rheumatic fever. *Indian Pediatr.* 1998;35:1159–60.

Soudarssanane MB, Karthigeyan M, Mahalakshmy T, *et al.* Rheumatic fever and rheumatic heart disease: primary prevention is the cost effective option. *Indian J Pediatr.* 2007;74:567–70.

Working Group on Pediatric Acute Rheumatic Fever and Cardiology Chapter of Indian Academy of Pediatrics. Consensus guidelines on pediatric acute rheumatic fever and rheumatic heart disease. *Indian Pediatr.* 2008;45:565–73.

VALVULAR HEART DISEASES

11.21 MITRAL REGURGITATION

Mitral regurgitation, is the abnormal leaking of blood from the left ventricle through the mitral valve into the left atrium, when the left ventricle contracts, ie, there is regurgitation of blood back into the left atrium.

Pathophysiology

Mitral regurgitation is the most frequent sequel of rheumatic fever. In acute stage, mitral regurgitation is due to active carditis leading to ventricular dilatation, mitral valvulitis, or rarely rupture of chordae. In chronic rheumatic mitral valve disease, the underlying lesion is retractile fibrosis of the valvular apparatus, causing loss of leaflet coaptation. The secondary dilatation of the mitral annulus tends to further decrease the contact between leaflets. This leads to mitral regurgitation. In addition, there is often some degree of mitral stenosis due to fusion of commissures.

Hemodynamics

Hemodynamics of the mitral regurgitation are different in (*a*) the acute phase, (*b*) the chronic compensated phase, and (*c*) the chronic decompensated phase. These are described below.

Acute Phase

Acute mitral regurgitation occurs during acute rheumatic carditis, as a part and parcel of rheumatic endocarditis. This can occur on a normal (hitherto undiseased) or a previously damaged valve. Usually, it occurs secondary to inflammation of the mitral leaflets resulting in non cooptation of leaflets. There is a sudden volume overload of both the left atrium and the left ventricle due to regurgitant stream. In the acute setting, the stroke volume of the left ventricle is increased - this results is dilation of left ventricle and the ventricular contractions are more forceful. Acute increase in left atrial pressure due to significant mitral regurgitation is transmitted to pulmonary circulation through the increased back-pressure via pulmonary veins, because the left atrium does not get adequate time to expand in acute regurgitation. Clinically, this manifests as pulmonary venous hypertension. Subsequently, there may be fall in forward stroke volume and low cardiac output, manifesting as left ventricular failure.

Compensated Phase

If the mitral regurgitation develops slowly or if not intervened in acute phase, the individual will enter the chronic compensated phase of the disease. In this phase, the left ventricle dilates and develops eccentric hypertrophy in order to better manage the larger than normal stroke volume. The stroke volume and ejection fraction is increased. Thus features of left ventricular failure are absent. Volume overload of the left atrium causes its enlargement. Therefore, the left atrial pressure increases in systole (due to regurgitant bloodstream) and drops in diastole (due to increased capacity to hold blood). The net result is that mean left atrial pressure stays near normal. Thus, there is no pulmonary venous hypertension and no congestion in the lungs. This stage is not associated with pulmonary arterial hypertension unless there is associated stenosis of the mitral valve.

Decompensated Phase

Patient with chronic severe mitral regurgitation will eventually develop left ventricular dysfunction. In this phase, the ventricular myocardium is no longer able to contract adequately to compensate for the volume overload of mitral regurgitation, and the stroke volume of the left ventricle will decrease. The decreased stroke volume causes a decreased forward cardiac output and an increase in the end-diastolic volume, increased filling pressures of the left ventricle and increased pulmonary venous congestion. The individual develops symptoms of congestive heart failure. Patient in compensated stage can also deteriorate secondary to development of arrhythmia (commonly atrial fibrillation), anemia or infection. The left ventricle further dilates during this phase. This causes a dilatation of the mitral valve annulus, which may worsen the degree of mitral regurgitation.

The decreased forward output is not adequate during phases of exertion, thus the usual presentation is *easy fatigability*, which is the most common symptom of mitral regurgitation. The other common symptom is palpitation due to enlarged left ventricle and compensatory tachycardia.

Symptoms

The symptoms associated with mitral regurgitation are dependent on which phase of the disease process the individual is in.

Acute mitral regurgitation will have the signs and symptoms of decompensated congestive heart failure, ie, easy fatigability, shortness of breath, pulmonary edema, orthopnea, and paroxysmal nocturnal dyspnea. Cardiovascular collapse with shock (cardiogenic shock) may be seen in individuals with acute mitral regurgitation due to papillary muscle rupture or rupture of a chordae. This usually occurs in setting of bacterial endocarditis and is rare in uncomplicated acute rheumatic fever.

Chronic compensated mitral regurgitation may be asymptomatic, with a normal exercise tolerance and no evidence of heart failure. Chronic uncompensated mitral regurgitation will present with exertional dyspnea, palpitations, and congestive failure. These individuals may be sensitive to small shifts in their intravascular volume status, and are prone to develop volume overload (congestive heart failure).

Physical Examination

The pulse in mitral regurgitation has a good volume. Pulse pressure is relatively wide with a rapid upstroke, often called as a small water hammer pulse. Features of congestive failure include pedal edema, tachycardia, and hepatomegaly. Cardiomegaly may be absent in acute rheumatic mitral regurgitation, developing in a hitherto normal heart. In chronic mitral regurgitation, cardiac apex is forcible and displaced down and out indicating a left ventricular enlargement. Precordium is hyperkinetic.

Cardiovascular findings depend on the severity and duration of mitral regurgitation. With moderate to severe mitral regurgitation, there will be cardiomegaly with hyperdynamic cardiac impulse. The mitral component of the first heart sound is usually soft and may be masked by the pansystolic murmur best heard at the apex, and radiating to the back. This may be associated with a systolic thrill. The loudness of the murmur does not correlate well with the severity of regurgitation. Pulmonary arterial hypertension is characterized by a loud pulmonary component of the second heart sound. A third heart sound and delayed diastolic murmur suggests a severe mitral regurgitation. Presence of pulmonary arterial hypertension suggests acute or chronic uncompensated mitral regurgitation.

Diagnosis

Electrocardiogram Features of left atrial enlargement and left ventricular hypertrophy suggest a long standing and severe mitral regurgitation. There may be associated atrial flutter or fibrillation in chronic mitral regurgitation.

Chest X-ray There is cardiomegaly with a left ventricular configuration. Cardiomegaly is proportionate to the severity of mitral regurgitation. Elevation of left bronchus suggests left atrial enlargement. Acute rheumatic mitral regurgitation with left ventricular dysfunction will have features of pulmonary venous hypertension on chest X-ray.

Echocardiogram Two-dimension echocardiography shows valvular pathology (annular dilatation, non-coaptation, ruptured or elongated chordae, cusp perforation), dilated left atrium, and left ventricular function. Color flow mapping can quantitate mitral regurgitation non-invasively. Doppler interrogation of tricuspid regurgitation jet (if present) is used to assess pulmonary arterial systolic pressure.

Differential Diagnosis

All those conditions that manifest with a pansystolic murmur (tricuspid regurgitation, VSD) should be considered in the differential diagnosis of mitral regurgitation. While murmur of tricuspid regurgitation increases in inspiration—that of mitral regurgitation becomes louder in expiration. Murmur of VSD is characteristic because of its non-radiating nature with maximum loudness over parasternal area.

Etiology of acquired mitral regurgitation includes bacterial endocarditis, dilated cardiomyopathy, hypertrophic cardiomyopathy, ischemia, trauma, and left atrial myxoma. Congenital defects of the mitral valve are seen in Marfan syndrome and Type I mucopolysaccharidosis. Left ventricular fibroelastosis and anomalous origin of left coronary artery from pulmonary artery are the other two important differential diagnoses of mitral regurgitation.

Treatment — Mitral Regurgitation

The treatment of mitral regurgitation depends on the acuteness of the disease and whether there are associated signs of hemodynamic compromise.

Medical management

In acute severe mitral regurgitation and decompensated mitral regurgitation, the patient needs propped up nursing, oxygen administration, intravenous diuretics, digitalis, after load reducing agents and treatment of concurrent illness. In acute mitral regurgitation secondary to rupture of a papillary muscle or chordae tendinae, the treatment of choice is urgent mitral valve repair/replacement. Individuals with chronic mitral regurgitation can be treated with vasodilators to decrease afterload. In the chronic state, the most commonly used agents are ACE inhibitors.

Surgical therapy

Indications of surgery for chronic mitral regurgitation include significant left ventricular dilatation, any evidence of left ventricular dysfunction (LVEF <60%), and development of pulmonary arterial hypertension. There are two surgical options for the treatment of mitral regurgitation—mitral valve replacement and mitral valve repair. In the double orifice technique for mitral valve repair, the opening of the mitral valve is sewn closed in the middle, leaving the two ends still able to open. This ensures that the mitral valve closes when the left ventricle pumps blood, yet allows the mitral valve to open at the two ends to fill the left ventricle with blood before it pumps. The same idea can be used with a minimally-invasive catheter technique which installs a clip to hold the middle of the mitral valve closed (not practiced in India).

De Rosa G, Pardeo M, Stabile A, Rigante D. Rheumatic heart disease in children: from clinical assessment to therapeutical management. *Eur Rev Med Pharmacol Sci*. 2006;10:107–10.

Veasy LG, Tani LY. A new look at acute rheumatic mitral regurgitation. *Cardiol Young*. 2005;15:568–77.

Walsh WF. Medical management of chronic rheumatic heart disease. *Heart Lung Circ*. 2010;19:289–94.

11.22 MITRAL STENOSIS

Mitral stenosis is characterized by the narrowing of the orifice of the mitral valve of the heart. It occurs in 25% of patients with chronic rheumatic heart disease and in association with mitral insufficiency in another 40%. Progressive fibrosis (ie, thickening and calcification of the valve) takes place over time, resulting in enlargement of the left atrium and formation of mural thrombi in that chamber.

The stenotic valve is funnel-shaped, with a "fish mouth" resemblance.

On auscultation, S_1 is initially accentuated but becomes reduced as the leaflets further thicken and calcify. P_2 becomes loud as pulmonary arterial hypertension develops. S_2 is followed by opening snap (OS) heard at apex. The closer the OS to A_2, more severe is the mitral stenosis. Diastolic murmur with presystolic accentuation is heard at apex.

Pathophysiology

The initial insult of rheumatic carditis involves the mitral leaflets, causing tiny translucent nodules along the line of closure of the leaflets. At this point, even though there is no significant obstruction of the mitral valve, one may hear a diastolic rumble (the *Carey Coombs murmur*) or a blowing systolic murmur at the apex. Usually it takes more than a decade from the onset of rheumatic carditis until significant symptomatic obstruction of the mitral valve occurs. This results from thickening, fibrosis, and possible calcification of the valve cusps. But in India we see severe mitral stenosis even in pediatric age group suggesting a more fulminant course and recurrent attacks. Same is seen in other third world nations. Boys are affected twice as common as girls up to 12 years of age.

When mitral stenosis is symptomatic, the anatomic features consist of thickened mitral cusps with or without calcific deposits, fusion of the valve commissures, and shortening and fusion of the chordae tendinae. The posterior leaflet of the mitral valve tends to become immobile and plastered to left ventricular posterior wall.

Hemodynamics

Normally the mitral valve opens during left ventricular diastole, to allow blood to flow from the left atrium to the left ventricle, resulting in equalization of pressures in the left atrium and the left ventricle during ventricular diastole. The result is that the left ventricle gets filled with blood during early ventricular diastole, with only a small portion of extra blood contributed by contraction of the left atrium (the "atrial kick") during late ventricular diastole.

When the mitral valve orifice is reduced to less than 50% of normal, the valve causes an impediment to the flow of blood into the left ventricle, creating a pressure gradient across the mitral valve. As the gradient across the mitral valve increases, the amount of time necessary to fill the left ventricle with blood increases. Eventually, the left ventricle requires the atrial kick to fill with blood. As the heart rate increases, the amount of time that the ventricle is in diastole and can fill up with blood (called the diastolic filling period) decreases. When the heart rate goes above a certain point, the diastolic filling period is insufficient to fill the ventricle with blood and pressure builds up in the left atrium, leading to pulmonary venous hypertension and congestion.

With increase in severity of mitral stenosis, increased left atrial pressure is transmitted to the pulmonary vasculature and causes pulmonary hypertension. Severe elevations of pulmonary capillary pressures cause an imbalance between the hydrostatic pressure and the oncotic pressure, leading to extravasation of fluid from the vascular tree and pooling of fluid in the lungs (*pulmonary edema*). Significant mitral stenosis with tricuspid regurgitation also results in diminished cardiac output, manifesting as small volume pulse.

Pulmonary Arterial Hypertension

As mitral valve obstruction increases, left atrial, pulmonary venous, and wedge pressures increase. An increase in wedge pressure causes an obligatory increase in the pulmonary artery mean pressure if blood is to flow across the pulmonary bed. Most patients with mitral stenosis have passive pulmonary hypertension; however, in some patients, pulmonary artery pressure rises out of proportion to the increase in wedge pressure. Under this circumstance, the gradient across the pulmonary bed may be even greater than the obstruction across the narrowed mitral valve. Such patients have *'reactive pulmonary hypertension'* due to associated pulmonary vasculature spasm. Obstructive pulmonary vascular disease is very rare in mitral stenosis.

Functional Tricuspid Regurgitation

Pulmonary arterial hypertension results in increased pressure in the right ventricle, as the right ventricle tries to maintain the pulmonary flow with high pulmonary pressure. The right ventricle hypertrophies. Increased pressure in right ventricle may result in backward flow of blood in systole to right atrium through a normal tricuspid valve, manifesting as *functional tricuspid regurgitation*. Mitral stenosis and pulmonary arterial hypertension may or may not be necessarily followed by tricuspid regurgitation; however, it is associated with right ventricular hypertrophy. This may also cause the right ventricle to enlarge. In absence of tricuspid regurgitation, the right ventricular hypertrophy is concentric and does not result in cardiomegaly. In some patients, the tricuspid valve is organically involved by the rheumatic process.

Arrhythmia

The constant pressure overload of the left atrium will cause the left atrium to increase in size. As the left atrium increases in size, it becomes more prone to develop arrhythmia, most commonly atrial fibrillation. When atrial fibrillation develops, the atrial kick is lost (since it is due to the normal atrial contraction) and the patient becomes more symptomatic.

In individuals with severe mitral stenosis, the left ventricular filling is dependent on the atrial kick. The loss of the atrial kick due to atrial fibrillation can cause a precipitous decrease in cardiac output and sudden congestive heart failure.

Symptoms

Patients with mild mitral stenosis may be asymptomatic. With increasing severity of stenosis, patient presents with effort intolerance and dyspnea. With critical lesion, the patients present with orthopnea, paroxysmal nocturnal dyspnea and even overt pulmonary edema. Other important symptoms consist of cough, hemoptysis, atypical angina, and congestive cardiac failure. Symptoms may be precipitated by tachycardia, atrial fibrillation, anemia or rheumatic reactivation. Congestive failure is usually associated with moderate or severe pulmonary arterial hypertension.

Dyspnea, orthopnea, and *paroxysmal nocturnal dyspnea* are the usual features of pulmonary venous hypertension. As pulmonary venous pressure increases, fluid is driven out of the pulmonary capillaries. This transudate decreases the compliance of the lungs and increases the work of breathing. The resultant symptom is dyspnea. With exercise this process is accelerated. The supine position increases pulmonary venous pressure, leading to the symptoms of orthopnea and paroxysmal nocturnal dyspnea.

Hemoptysis results from a significant increase in pulmonary venous pressure following development of bronchial varices, and it may be one of the first sign of mitral stenosis. Such hemoptysis can be massive, requiring emergency intervention (balloon valvotomy/surgery). Profuse hemoptysis of this type is an indication for urgent mitral valve intervention. The other potential causes of hemoptysis in patients with mitral stenosis are blood-streaked sputum associated with attacks of dyspnea, in association with attacks of bronchitis, accompanying acute pulmonary edema or due to pulmonary embolism.

Palpitations With increasing severity of mitral stenosis, left atrium dilates and chances of arrhythmia increases leading to complaints of palpitation.

Right sided failure In critical mitral stenosis with development of severe pulmonary arterial hypertension, there will be dilatation and hypertrophy of right ventricle and tricuspid annulus. Dilated tricuspid annulus causes appearance of tricuspid regurgitation which will be of high velocity (PAH secondary to severe pulmonary venous hypertension). These patients present with features of right ventricular failure.

Physical Examination

Pulse is low volume in severe mitral stenosis. There is dyspnea and features of right ventricular failure as elevation of jugular venous pressure, ascites, hepatomegaly and pedal edema. Precordium reveals a normal sized heart with a tapping apex, parasternal heave and diastolic thrill at the apex. P_2 is palpable and there are epigastric pulsations. Pulsations may also be observed in the pulmonary area.

1. *First heart sound is loud* and may be palpable (*tapping apex beat*) because of increased force in closing the mitral valve. It may be the most prominent sign.
2. *Loud P_2* If pulmonary hypertension secondary to mitral stenosis is severe, the P_2 (pulmonic) component of the second heart sound (S_2) will become loud.
3. An *opening snap* which is a high pitched additional sound is heard after the A_2 (aortic) component of the second heart sound (S_2), which correlates to the forceful opening of the mitral valve. The mitral valve opens when the pressure in the left atrium is greater than the pressure in the left ventricle. In individuals with mitral stenosis, the pressure in the left atrium correlates with the severity of the mitral stenosis. As the severity of the mitral stenosis increases, the pressure in the left atrium increases, and the mitral valve opens earlier in ventricular diastole reducing the interval between A_2 and opening snap.
4. A *mid-diastolic rumbling murmur* with presystolic accentuation will be heard after the opening snap. The

murmur is best heard at the apical region with bell of stethoscope. Its duration increases with worsening of stenosis. A diastolic thrill might be present when palpating at the apical region of the precordium.

5. A *pansystolic murmur of tricuspid regurgitation* may also be audible at the left sternal border, this murmur increases with inspiration.

Investigations

Electrocardiogram shows 'P' mitrale, right axis deviation, and right ventricular hypertrophy.

Chest X-ray Heart size is normal and there are features of left atrial enlargement, and pulmonary venous and arterial hypertension.

Echocardiography shows rheumatic involvement of mitral valve leaflets which are thickened with short and fused chordae and subvalvular apparatus, dilated left atrium and right ventricle, and reduced mitral valve area. Doppler interrogation of mitral inflow can quantify the severity of stenosis by pressure gradient across mitral valve while tricuspid regurgitation jet peak velocity is used for assessment of pulmonary arterial hypertension. The transmitral gradient as measured by Doppler echocardiography is the gold standard in the evaluation of the severity of mitral stenosis. The mitral valve area can be calculated in 2D echocardigram and also by Doppler velocity across the mitral valve.

Treatment — Mitral Stenosis

Mild stenosis
Intervention is not indicated in asymptomatic patients with mild mitral stenosis but 6 monthly follow up (clinical and echocardiography) is required along with rheumatic and bacterial endocarditis prophylaxis.

Moderate and severe mitral stenosis
These children need to be digitalized and given diuretics; and prepared for mitral valvuloplasty–either percutaneously by balloon or surgical intervention that can be done as closed or open procedure. If the mitral valve is severely fibrosed or calcified, surgical mitral valve replacement is needed. The disadvantage of mitral valve replacement is lifelong anticoagulant to prevent thrombosis of prosthetic valve.

To determine which patients would benefit from percutaneous balloon mitral valvuloplasty, a scoring system has been developed. Scoring is based on 4 echocardiographic criteria: Leaflet mobility, leaflet thickening, subvalvar thickening, and calcification. Individuals with a score of >8 tend to have suboptimal results. Superb results with valvotomy are seen in individuals with a crisp opening snap, score <8, and no calcium in the commissures. If mitral valve is pliable, non-calcified, and mitral regurgitation is not significant; percutaneous transmitral commissurotomy provides good results. Balloon valvotomy can relieve commissural fusion but cannot accomplish much for subvalvar fusion and shortening of the chordae tendinae. The more the subvalvar pathology in an individual patient, the less satisfactory the final result is likely to be.

Although the immediate results of percutaneous mitral balloon dilatation are often quite gratifying, the procedure does not provide permanent relief from mitral stenosis. Regular follow-up is mandatory, to detect restenosis. Long-term follow up data from patients undergoing percutaneous mitral balloon dilatation indicates that up to 70–75% individuals can be free of restenosis 10 years following the procedure. The number decreases to about 40% after 15 years of mitral balloon dilatation.

American College of Cardiology/American Heart Association Task Force on Practice Guidelines. ACC/AHA 2006 guidelines for the management of patients with valvular heart disease: a report of the American College of Cardiology/American Heart Association Task Force on Practice Guidelines (writing committee to revise the 1998 Guidelines for the Management of Patients With Valvular Heart Disease): developed in collaboration with the Society of Cardiovascular Anesthesiologists: endorsed by the Society for Cardiovascular Angiography and Interventions and the Society of Thoracic Surgeons. *Circulation*. 2006;114:84–231.

Glancy DL. Mitral stenosis: I. Anatomical, physiological, and clinical considerations. *J La State Med Soc*. 2003;155:91–5, quiz 96, 119.

Jamieson WR, Cartier PC, Allard M, *et al.* Surgical management of valvular heart disease 2004. *Can J Cardiol*. 2004;20:7E–120E.

Regitz-Zagrosek V, Seeland U, Geibel-Zehender A, Gohlke-Bärwolf C, Kruck I, Schaefer C. Cardiovascular diseases in pregnancy. *Dtsch Arztebl Int*. 2011;108:267–73.

Subramaniam V, Herle A, Mohammed N, Thahir M. Ortner's syndrome: case series and literature review. *Braz J Otorhinolaryngol*. 2011;77:559–62.

11.23 AORTIC REGURGITATION

Rheumatic involvement of the aortic valve results is distortion and retraction of the aortic cusps, leading to aortic regurgitation. Aortic valve involvement in rheumatic heart disease usually occurs in combination with mitral valve involvement. Clinically pure aortic regurgitation, without associated mitral valve disease is rare and occurs in 5 to 8% patients. The mitral valve is pathologically involved in all cases.

Hemodynamics

Chronic Severe Aortic Regurgitation

In *chronic severe aortic regurgitation*, the volume of blood that regurgitates into the left ventricle during diastole increases slowly with time. To accommodate this regurgitant volume, the left ventricle slowly dilates, its walls undergoing minimal thickening, and its compliance increases. This pattern of increased chamber radius with minimal increase in ventricular wall thickness is known as eccentric hypertrophy. It allows the affected ventricle to operate at a larger end-diastolic volume with little or no rise in end-diastolic pressure. As long as systolic function is preserved, such ventricles are capable of ejecting an abnormally large total stroke volume (normal stroke volume plus regurgitant stroke volume). In this manner, systemic perfusion is maintained, left ventricular ejection fraction is preserved, left ventricular diastolic pressure remains low, and symptoms of heart failure do not develop. In effect, the ventricle is operating at a much greater end-diastolic volume with a normal end-diastolic pressure (ie, its compliance has increased). Ejection of the large total stroke volume results in a widened arterial pulse pressure. The size of the ventricle is directly related to the quantum of regurgitation blood.

Acute Aortic Regurgitation

Acute aortic regurgitation is very rare with acute rheumatic fever and mostly occurs after acute perforation or destruction as in bacterial endocarditis. The clinical presentation and hemodynamic is in sharp contrast to the situation just described in patients with chronic aortic regurgitation. In these individuals, eccentric hypertrophy is not present and ventricular compliance is normal and remains so despite the sudden regurgitant volume overload. This over load is poorly tolerated because the left ventricle is now "overfilled" and operating on the steep or non-compliant portion of its diastolic pressure—volume relationship. If the volume of acute aortic regurgitation is large, end-diastolic left ventricular pressure is markedly increased, even approaching aortic diastolic pressure. The normal left ventricle, neither hypertrophied nor dilated, cannot acutely increase its total left ventricular stroke volume sufficiently to maintain forward stroke volume in this setting. There is a resultant precipitous rise in left ventricular end-diastolic pressure without a change in forward cardiac output. Because left ventricular stroke volume is not markedly increased, arterial pulse pressure remains unchanged, and the bounding arterial pulses of chronic aortic regurgitation are absent. Regurgitation of aortic blood into the relatively non-compliant left ventricle has several consequences. The marked rise in left ventricular diastolic pressure can lead to increase in left atrial and pulmonary capillary pressures of sufficient magnitude to produce pulmonary edema.

Clinical Features

Children with chronic compensated aortic regurgitation, in absence of complications usually are asymptomatic. Symptoms usually consist of palpitation, prominent precordial pulsations, and chest pain. Features of congestive cardiac failure appear with progressive severity of aortic regurgitation.

The large stroke volume and forceful left ventricular contractions results in *palpitations*, which is the most common symptom of aortic regurgitation. Peripheral vasodilatation results in excessive sweating and heat intolerance. In severe aortic regurgitation with failing left ventricle, dyspnea on effort can progress to orthopnea and to overt signs of pulmonary edema. Signs of aortic regurgitation are as follows:

1. *The pulse pressure is wide* The wider the pulse pressure, the more severe the aortic leak. Pulse is collapsing; good volume and typically known as *water-hammer pulse*.
2. Increased stroke volume and wide pulse pressure results in peripheral signs of AR. These can be clinically identified as (*i*) prominent carotid pulsations (*Corrigan sign*); (*ii*) visible arterial pulsations over the extremity vessels (*dancing peripheral arteries*); and (*iii*) visible pulsations of the abdominal aorta. Arteriolar pulsations may be seen over the nail bed (*Quincke sign*), uvula, lips, ear lobes, and in the eye grounds.
3. *De Musset sign* Nodding of head occurs with each systole due to sudden filling of the carotid vessels in severe aortic regurgitation.
4. *Hill' sign* There is also exaggeration of the systolic pressure difference between the brachial and femoral arteries. Normally the systolic pressure in the brachial artery (upper limb) is less than that in the femoral artery; the difference being less than 20 mm Hg. In aortic regurgitation, this pressure difference is exaggerated.

Systolic pressure difference between 20 and 40 mm Hg suggests mild aortic regurgitation, 40–60 mm Hg suggests moderate aortic regurgitation; and a difference of more than 60 mm Hg indicates severe aortic regurgitation.

5. *Femoral bruit* Apply pressure over the proximal end of femoral artery by putting the chest piece of stethoscope over it, to partially occlude the femoral artery. A systolic murmur is heard. And if the pressure is applied distally, a diastolic murmur is heard. This combination of systolic and diastolic murmur is known as *Duroziez sign*.
6. If the stethoscope is placed over the femoral artery without occluding the vessel, *pistol shot sounds* are heard in moderate to severe aortic regurgitation.
7. Inspection and palpation of the precordium will reveal a *hyperkinetic apex*. The apex is shifted down and out because of left ventricular enlargement. With large leaks, the whole *precordium is pulsatile*. Pulsations are also visible in the neck. A diastolic thrill may be palpated at the upper parasternal border.
8. S_1 is soft, S_2 may be heard because of a loud A_2 or it may be masked by the regurgitant diastolic murmur.
9. The characteristic murmur of aortic regurgitation is a hollow, high pitched blowing, decrescendo *diastolic murmur*, best heard along the left sternal border. The murmur typically radiates to the apex. It is best heard with the diaphragm of stethoscope with the patient sitting and leaning forward.
10. With moderate to severe aortic regurgitation an additional ejection systolic murmur may be heard at the second right interspace. This murmur radiates to the neck and may be associated with a systolic thrill. The systolic murmur is the result of a functional aortic stenosis because of passage of large stroke volume, across the regurgitant valve. It can be differentiated from organic AS due to presence of a wide pulse pressure and associated diastolic murmur.

Acute Severe AR

Children with acute onset aortic regurgitation present with dyspnea on exertion, orthopnea, dry minimal productive cough aggravated by recumbence, paroxysmal nocturnal dyspnea and dyspnea at rest while lying down supine. Symptoms reflecting the reduction in cardiac output are more subtle and are often over-shadowed by those due to pulmonary congestion. Symptoms of low cardiac output include fatigue on exertion, apathy, agitation, and/or deterioration in intellectual function reflecting impaired cerebral perfusion. Heart failure is almost invariably present in acute aortic regurgitation. Heart failure is usually progressive, severe, and eventually fatal in the absence of effective therapy.

Severe acute aortic insufficiency may elevate left ventricular diastolic pressure to such a degree that the latter exceeds left atrial pressure and actually causes premature closure of the mitral valve. Finally, the often present compensatory tachycardia shortens diastole. Premature mitral valve closure results in absence or marked softening of the first heart sound. Blood entering the left ventricle from the left atrium flows through these relatively coapted mitral leaflets often giving rise to a low-pitched mid-to-late-diastolic (Austin-Flint) rumbling murmur.

Physical Examination

In acute severe aortic regurgitation, forward ventricular stroke output is reduced. The pulse pressure is not appreciably widened, systolic blood pressure is normal or only slightly elevated, and diastolic arterial pressure is usually slightly elevated. Tachycardia is the rule. The precordium is relatively quite as compared to the laterally displaced, heaving, apical impulse reflecting left ventricular volume overload and eccentric hypertrophy of chronic compensated AR.

The second heart sound is also soft and may be absent if one or more aortic valve leaflets have been damaged to the point of little or no diastolic coaptation. An ejection-type murmur of variable intensity is often heard localized to the base. The diastolic murmur characteristic of chronic severe aortic regurgitation (high-pitched, decrescendo, and lasting throughout most of diastole) is usually absent. Instead one hears a nondescript short early diastolic murmur of mixed frequencies in patients with acute severe aortic regurgitation. The murmur is often soft. An Austin-Flint (mid-diastolic rumble) murmur is often present in acute severe aortic regurgitation. A third sound is also frequently present. A fourth heart sound is usually absent. Rising pulmonary pressures lead to an increase in right ventricular afterload with resultant right ventricular failure. Therefore, jugular venous distension with a prominent *a* wave may be present. In contradistinction to chronic severe aortic regurgitation, prominent neck pulsations in acute aortic regurgitation are venous in origin rather that arterial (bounding carotid arteries secondary to wide pulse pressure). Pulse alternans is often present in patients with acute aortic regurgitation.

Differentiating features between an acute and chronic AR are provided in **Table 11.5**.

Investigations

Electrocardiogram ECG may be normal in mild regurgitation. ECG of chronic severe aortic regurgitation shows evidence of left ventricular hypertrophy and LV volume overload (prominent q wave and tall T wave). In acute aortic regurgitation, ECG shows tachycardia and non-specific ST-T wave changes.

Chest X-ray It shows cardiomegaly of left ventricular type and dilated ascending aorta (aortic root). In acute aortic regurgitation there will be features of pulmonary venous hypertension, and mild or no cardiomegaly; aortic root is normal.

Echocardiography Two-dimensional echocardiography shows dilated left ventricle, thickened aortic valve and mitral valve, dilated ascending aorta and flutter of anterior mitral leaflet. Color flow mapping is used to look for presence of aortic regurgitation and quantify the leak.

Differential Diagnosis

Aortic regurgitation should be differentiated from conditions associated with a wide pulse pressure that include patent ductus arteriosus, mitral regurgitation, ventricular septal defect with AR, AV fistula, rupture of sinus of Valsalva, anemia, hyperpyrexia, and thyrotoxicosis.

Rheumatic aortic regurgitation also needs to be differentiated from other causes of diastolic murmur such as pulmonary regurgitation and congenital aortic valve disease (bicuspid aortic valve, diseases of ascending aorta, Hurler syndrome, and Marfan syndrome).

Table 11.5 Clinical Manifestations of Severe Aortic Regurgitation: Acute and Chronic		
Clinical findings	*Acute AR*	*Chronic AR*
Congestive cardiac failure	Present, early and sudden	Late and insidious
Arterial pulse		
Tachycardia	Present	Normal or increased heart rate
Rate of rise	Not increased	Increased
Systolic pressure	Normal to decreased	Increased
Diastolic pressure	Normal to decreased	Decreased
Pulse pressure-volume	Near normal	Increased
Peripheral signs of AR	Absent	Present
Left ventricular impulse	Near normal, not hyperdynamic	Laterally displaced, hyperdynamic
Auscultation		
First heart sound	Soft	Normal
Second heart sound		
Aortic component	Soft	Normal or decreased
Pulmonary component	Normal or increased	Normal
3rd heart sound	Common	Common with failure
4th heart sound	Common	Absent
AR murmur	Short, medium pitched	Long, high pitched
Austin flint murmur	Mid diastolic	Presystolic, mid diastolic or both
Chest X-ray	Features of pulmonary venous hypertension Aortic root and arch: normal, may have mild cardiomegaly	Usually normal lungs, dilated aortic root, cardiomegaly
Electrocardiogram	Tachycardia, non-specific ST-T wave changes	LVH (left ventricular hypertrophy)

11

Case Study | **Rheumatic Heart Disease**

A 13-year-old boy was brought to outpatient department with complaints of palpitation and increased precordial activity for 1 year. He was a healthy adolescent otherwise. There had been no complaints of any significant illness requiring medical attention in the past (specifically sore throat or joint pain). On examination his vital parameters were within normal limits. Respiratory rate was 30/min. Pulse rate was 90/min with normal rhythm. It was a high volume, bounding pulse with water hammer character. All the peripheral pulses were very well felt. Blood pressure was 110/60 mmHg in arms and 150/60 mmHg in legs. JVP was normal.

On precordial examination, hyperdynamic apical impulse was felt in left 6th intercostal space in anterior axillary line. S_1 was soft in intensity, S_2 was normal. S_3 gallop was heard at apex. There was no S_4. At apex, grade 3/6 high frequency, pansystolic murmur was heard with radiation to axilla. There was grade 3/6 mixed frequency, early diastolic murmur at right second and left third intercostal space at parasternal border. Other systemic examination was normal.

Q. What is the diagnosis? Justify.

Patient is suspected to have mitral regurgitation (MR) and aortic regurgitation (AR). Supportive findings are water hammer pulse, wide pulse pressure, Hill sign, cardiomegaly, hyperdynamic apex, soft S_1, and murmurs of AR and MR. There is no history of rheumatic fever in past; but only 30–50% of patients give such history. In view of high prevalence region, it should be considered rheumatic in etiology and confirmed by echocardiogram.

Q. What maneuvers can enhance the AR murmur?

Sitting and leaning forward position with breath held in expiration and fisting of both hands.

Q. How will you manage this child?

Benzathine Penicillin 12 lac IU should be administered I/M every 3 weekly. ACE inhibitors are first line medications as they reduce the peripheral resistance and reduce regurgitation. Definitive treatment is surgery. Mitral and aortic valve repair should be aimed. If repair is not possible, valve replacement is suggested. Prosthetic valves are at high risk of dysfunction due to thrombosis, hence anticoagulants are required to maintain INR 2–2.5.

Treatment | **Aortic Regurgitation**

Symptomatic chronic aortic regurgitation should be treated surgically by aortic valve replacement. Till surgery, congestive heart failure needs to be controlled by angiotensin converting enzyme (ACE) inhibitors and frusemide. Surgery in rheumatic AR should be contemplated only when the symptoms persist despite adequate treatment of associated anemia, rheumatic activity, and medical management of congestive heart failure, respiratory infections, and endocarditis.

In acute severe aortic regurgitation, patient needs general supportive measures, pharmacological management, and surgical intervention. General supportive measures include nursing in propped up position and high flow oxygen. If in pulmonary edema, patient may need ventilation. At the same time, patient should be started on intravenous frusemide, and intravenous vasodilator (nitroprusside). If acute aortic regurgitation is secondary to infective endocarditis and cannot be stabilized by medical management, family needs to be counseled about high risk of emergency surgery and chances of recurrence of infection.

Revision Point

Aortic Regurgitation

1. Aortic regurgitation in RHD is associated with mitral valve disease (regurgitation or stenosis) in approximately 40% cases. Clinically isolated AR without associated clinical mitral valve disease is rare.
2. Palpitation is the earliest symptom in patient of AR. Examination reveals signs of peripheral runoff including a wide pulse pressure, and a high pitched diastolic murmur. Left ventricular failure is common.
3. Symptomatic chronic aortic regurgitation should be treated surgically by aortic valve replacement. Till surgery, congestive heart failure needs to be controlled by angiotensin converting enzyme (ACE) inhibitors and frusemide.

11.24 TRICUSPID REGURGITATION

Tricuspid regurgitation is documented in 25–50% children with rheumatic heart diseases. This includes children with mitral stenosis who may develop an organic or functional tricuspid regurgitation. It rarely occurs alone. Tricuspid regurgitation associated with pure mitral regurgitation is almost always organic in nature.

Hemodynamics

Tricuspid regurgitation results in a backward leak of blood from right ventricle to right atrium during systole. Volume overload of the right atrium causes right atrial enlargement. Right ventricle also suffers from volume overload because of increased flow from right atrium, it also gets enlarged. Besides volume overload, right atrium and right ventricle pressures also increase. Systolic backflow from right atrium into systemic venous circulation results in prominent jugular venous pulse, and hepatic pulsations.

Clinical Features

- There are no specific symptoms of tricuspid regurgitation. The lesion however contributes to fatigue due to decreased systemic output.
- Peripheral features of tricuspid regurgitation include raised jugular venous pressure, prominent "v" waves in jugular venous pulse with rapid y descent, a hepatojugular reflux, and a pulsatile liver. If the y descent is not rapid, associated tricuspid stenosis should be suspected.
- Cardiac examination reveals a loud P_2 due to pulmonary arterial hypertension and a pansystolic murmur best heard in tricuspid area (left lower sternal border) increasing on inspiration. The murmur needs to be differentiated from pansystolic murmur of MR. Tricuspid valve murmur increases on inspiration while mitral murmur increases during expiration. Moreover, the pansystolic murmur of

tricuspid regurgitation does not radiate to the axilla or back. Severe TR is also characterized by S_3 or a delayed diastolic murmur (due to functional tricuspid stenosis).

Treatment	Tricuspid Regurgitation

Congestive heart failure needs to be managed with decongestive measures (digoxin, frusemide, propped up position, bed rest) along with management of mitral valve disease and rheumatic activity.

Bland EF, Jones TD. Rheumatic fever and rheumatic heart disease. *Circulation* 1951;4:836

Pisacane C, Pacileo G, Santoro G, *et al.* New insights in the pathophysiology of mitral and aortic regurgitation in pediatric age: role of angiotensin-converting enzyme inhibitor therapy. *Ital Heart J.* 2001;2:100–6.

Steer AC, Carapetis JR. Prevention and treatment of rheumatic heart disease in the developing world. Nat *Rev Cardiol.* 2009;6:689–98.

Walsh WF. Medical management of chronic rheumatic heart disease. *Heart Lung Circ.* 2010;19:289–94.

11.25 CONGESTIVE HEART FAILURE

Congestive heart failure (CHF) refers to a clinical state of systemic and pulmonary congestion resulting from inability of the heart to maintain effective circulation. The defect may lie in (*i*) pumping of blood from heart into the systemic circulation (systolic failure); or (*ii*) receiving the blood from peripheral circulation into the heart (diastolic failure).

Systolic failure is more common than diastolic failure. The latter is characteristically seen is constrictive pericarditis, hypertrophic cardiomyopathy, and restrictive heart disease.

Pathophysiology

Heart failure may result from (*a*) an excessive volume overload (left to right shunt, regurgitation); (*b*) pressure overload on normal myocardium (left or right sided outflow obstruction), or (*c*) ventricular dysfunction (anomalous origin of left coronary artery from pulmonary artery, electrolyte imbalance, myocarditis, cardiomyopathy). Arrhythmias, pericardial diseases and combination of various factors can also result in CHF.

The resultant decrease in cardiac output triggers physiological responses aimed at restoring perfusion of the vital organs, ie, (*i*) renal retention of fluid; (*ii*) renin-angiotensin mediated vasoconstriction; and (*iii*) sympathetic overactivity.

- Excessive fluid retention increases the cardiac output by increasing the end diastolic volume (preload), but also results in symptoms of pulmonary and systemic congestion. Clinically this manifests as edema, and pulmonary edema.
- Vasoconstriction (increase in afterload) tends to maintain flow to vital organs, but it is disproportionately elevated in patients with CHF and increases myocardial work. This causes cardiomegaly, hepatomegaly, raised jugular venous pressure, and poor peripheral perfusion.
- Similarly, sympathetic over-activity results in increased contractility, peripheral vasoconstriction, which also increases myocardial requirements. Clinically, this manifests in marked tachycardia and S_3 gallop.

An understanding of the interplay of the four principal determinants of cardiac output—preload, afterload, contractility, and heart rate is essential in optimizing the therapy of congestive heart failure.

Etiology

CHF during Fetal Life

Restricted foramen ovale and restricted ductus arteriosus during fetal life, fetal heart block or tachyarrhythmias, severe tricuspid regurgitation, myocardial dysfunction, and twin to twin transfusion can initiate CHF in fetal life that may present at birth.

CHF on First Day of Life

Myocardial dysfunction secondary to asphyxia, hypoglycemia, hypocalcemia, or sepsis is usually responsible for congestive heart failure on the first day of life, rather than a structural heart defect. Significant tricuspid regurgitation secondary to hypoxia induced papillary muscle dysfunction or Ebstein anomaly of the tricuspid valve; atrioventricular septal defect with AV regurgitation; and cerebral arteriovenous fistula can also result in congestive failure. CHF with Ebstein anomaly/tricuspid regurgitation improves as the pulmonary artery pressure falls over the next few days.

CHF in First Week of Life

CHF in the first week of life is often precipitated by the closure of the ductus arteriosus leading to catastrophic deterioration in the seemingly healthy neonate. These disorders **(Table 11.6)** can be life threatening yet they are potentially curable, implying a need for early diagnosis and management. Important tips follow:

- Peripheral pulses and oxygen saturation (by a pulse oximeter) should be checked in both the upper and lower extremities. A lower saturation in the lower limbs means right to left ductal shunting and occurs due to severe pulmonary hypertension. Lower pressure in lower limbs occurs with coarctation of aorta.
- An atrial or ventricular septal defect does not lead to failure in the early neonatal period. Therefore, we should look for additional cause (eg, aortic stenosis, coarctation of aorta, AV regurgitation, multiple sites of shunt, transposition or obstructed TAPVC).

Table 11.6 Causes of CHF in First Week of Life

I. *Structural heart defects*
- *Critical left sided obstructive lesions*: Aortic stenosis; coarctation of aorta, hypoplastic left heart syndrome
- *Critical right sided obstructive lesion*: Pulmonary stenosis with intact ventricular septum
- *Regurgitant lesions of valves*: Ebstein anomaly, AV septal defect, mitral regurgitation, aortic regurgitation
- Obstructed total anomalous pulmonary venous connection
- d-Transposition of great vessels

II. *Myocardial dysfunction:* Sepsis, electrolyte imbalance, asphyxia, hypocalcemia, glycogen storage disease, endocrine disorders

III. *Arrhythmias:* Tachyarrhythmias, congenital heart block

- Premature infants have a poor myocardial reserve and there is precipitous fall in pulmonary vascular resistance, and a shunt lesion as patent ductus arteriosus (PDA) may result in CHF in the first week in them.
- Metabolic disorders as glycogen storage disorder, adrenal insufficiency due to enzyme deficiencies, or neonatal thyrotoxicosis could also present with CHF in the first few days of life.

CHF Beyond First Week of Life

Structural Heart Defects

Shunt lesions manifest with CHF during this period, and the most common cause of CHF is a ventricular septal defect that presents around 6–8 weeks of age. This is because the volume of the left to right shunt increases as the pulmonary resistance falls. Although a murmur of VSD is apparent by one week, the full-blown picture of CHF occurs around 6–8 weeks. CHF can appear in the first week of life if there are multiple sites of shunt, or associated obstructive or regurgitant lesions. Other left to right shunts as PDA, and aortopulmonary window present similarly. Single ventricle, transposition of great vessels with VSD, truncus arteriosus presents with mild cyanosis and CHF. The fall in pulmonary vascular resistance is delayed in presence of hypoxic lung disease and at high altitude this could somewhat alter the time course accordingly.

Left coronary artery arising from the pulmonary artery (ALCAPA), a rare disease presenting in this age group merits separate mention, since it is curable and often missed. As the pulmonary artery pressure decreases in the neonatal period, these babies suffer from episodes of excessive crying with sweating (angina equivalent) and myocardial infarction. The electrocardiogram may show pathologic 'q' wave or left ventricular hypertrophy with or without ST-T changes. These infants are often misdiagnosed as having "dilated cardiomyopathy" due to associated myocardial dysfunction.

Others

1. *Arrhythmias:* Tachyarrhythmias, complete heart block
2. *Metabolic and endocrinal causes:* Hypocalcemia, glycogen storage disease, hyperthyroidism

Causes of CHF in Older Children

1. Rheumatic fever and rheumatic heart disease
2. Congenital heart disease complicated by anemia, infection, endocarditis, or development of other valvular lesions like aortic regurgitation
3. Hypertension
4. Myocarditis and primary myocardial disease

Clinical Manifestations

The clinical picture of CHF results from a combination of "relatively low output" and compensatory responses to increase it.

Diagnosis of CHF in small children and infants is difficult and needs a high index of suspicion. The most common symptom is feeding difficulty. Mother complains that the baby does not suck the breast continuously for a longer period. He sucks for some time and then stops feeding. After some time, he is again ready for sucking. This occurs because the baby gets breathless after sucking at the breast as the process involves effort. This situation is similar to 'effort intolerance' in older children. Due to poor feeding, the child fails to gain weight. The child may also have excessive sweating especially on forehead associated with feeding. On examination, these children are also found to have tachycardia, gallop rhythm, hepatomegaly and cardiomegaly.

Congestive heart failure in older children is characterized by tachypnea, tachycardia, gallop rhythm, pedal edema, decreased urinary output, raised jugular venous pressure, poor peripheral pulses, hepatomegaly, cardiomegaly, and basal crepitations **(Table 11.7)**.

Treatment	Congestive Heart Failure

The treatment of CHF includes general supportive measures, management of the precipitating events, control of the congested state, and identification and treatment of the cause.

A. General measures

Position and nursing Nursing the infant with head end elevated, judicious use of sedation and temporarily denying oral intake to avoid aspiration in the distressed infant, are useful practices.

Nutrition Infants with CHF require high caloric feeds (120–150 kcal/kg/day). Nasogastric feeding may be required. Salt intake need to be minimized in older children.

Oxygen Role of oxygen should be cautiously considered as oxygen may sometimes worsen the CHF in patients with left to right shunts due to its pulmonary vasodilating and systemic vasoconstrictor effects. Similarly, it may constrict PDA in

Table 11.7 Manifestations of Congestive Heart Failure		
Neonate	*Infant*	*Older Child*
1. Persistent tachycardia (>160/minute)	1. Poor weight gain	1. Tachycardia
2. Tachypnea (>60/minute)	2. Feeding difficulty	2. Tachypnea
3. Hepatomegaly (>3 cm)	3. Tachycardia	3. Gallop rhythm
4. Feeding difficulty	4. Tachypnea with grunting and	4. Pedal edema
5. Poor peripheral perfusion	intercostal retraction	5. Raised JVP
6. Presence of S3	5. Hepatomegaly	6. Hepatomegaly
7. Cardiomegaly on chest X-ray	6. Excessive sweating	7. Cardiomegaly
	7. Poor peripheral perfusion	8. Chest crepitations
	8. Presence of S3, gallop rhythm	

neonates and may be detrimental to patients with ductus arteriosus dependent lesions. However, in patients with pulmonary edema and hypoxia, raising alveolar PO_2 by oxygen supplementation is required and regularly used.

B. Treatment of the precipitating events

Almost always, the worsening in clinical state of a patient with CHF can be traced to a precipitating event. These factors include infection, anemia, electrolyte imbalances, arrhythmia, rheumatic activity, infective endocarditis, pulmonary embolism, drug interactions, drug toxicity, or non-compliance and other system disturbances. Treatment of underlying precipitating event leads to considerable improvement.

C. Treatment of congested state

Conventional medical management of congestive heart failure includes 3 main approaches:

1. Reducing the pulmonary or systemic congestion
   Diuretics: Frusemide, chlorthiazide, aldactone, etc
2. Increasing myocardial contractility
   Inotropes: Digoxin, other inotropes, and other measures
3. Reducing the disproportionately elevated afterload
   Vasodilators: ACE inhibitors, etc.

Diuretics

Diuretics afford quick relief in pulmonary and systemic congestion. Frusemide (1 mg/kg) is the agent of choice. For chronic use, 1–4 mg/kg of frusemide or 20–40 mg/kg of chlorothiazide in divided dosage are used. It is important to monitor body weight, blood urea, serum electrolytes (at least twice weekly initially).

Hypokalemia is one of the major concern in children on frusemide therapy. However, potassium supplementation is usually not required with <2 mg/kg of frusemide or equivalent doses of other diuretics. A daily supplementation of 1–1.5 mEq/kg of potassium may be required if there is significant hypokalemia. Secondary hyperaldosteronism does occur in infants with CHF and addition of spironolactone 1 mg/kg single dose conserves potassium.

Metabolic alkalosis, hypomagnesemia and hyponatremia are the other problems. Infants tolerate hyponatremia much better than adults. The treatment for hyponatremia is rarely required even when serum sodium is as low as 120 mEq/L. Reducing the dose of diuretics, restriction of free water intake, and liberalizing salt for a short period would restore the serum sodium except in patients with a very low cardiac output.

In refractory failure, a combination of diuretics having different sites of action should be tried and intravenous rather oral preparation should be used. Dopamine in a renal vasodilating dose (2–5 mg/kg/min) may be useful as a diuretic although scientific data is limited.

Digoxin

Despite some controversy regarding the use of digoxin in patients with left to right shunt, it remains the mainstay of treatment of CHF in infants and children. Rapid digitalization (over 24 hours) should be resorted to in babies with severe CHF. A total dose of 30–40 micrograms/kg body weight orally (intravenous doses—75% of the oral dose) would digitalize term infants and children. For most other circumstances, starting with an oral maintenance dose (8–10 micrograms/kg/day in two divided doses) with no loading dose is adequate. Prolongation of PR interval can be an early feature of digitalis toxicity.

It is the physician's responsibility to ensure that the patient receives the correct dosages, simply because the mistakes in this regard can prove fatal. Nausea and vomiting are commonest signs of toxicity but severe toxicity may be present without these. If the child regurgitates a dose, it may be prudent to give the next dose 12 hours later. Bradycardia and blocks are commoner in children than ectopy during toxicity. The individual tolerance varies, but the safety margin is not high. Digoxin should be avoided in patients with myocarditis.

Vasodilators

Vasodilators include arteriolar dilators (hydralazine), venodilators (nitroglycerine, nitrates), and combined arteriovenodilators (ACE inhibitors, angiotensin receptor blockers, calcium channel blockers). The last group of drugs is used most frequently.

Angiotensin converting enzyme inhibitors

These drugs mainly act by reducing the afterload. However, they may also decrease the preload and increase plasma potassium level. These therefore can be combined well with a diuretic; and in this case potassium supplements are not needed. ACE inhibitors are especially useful in the presence of hypertension, mitral or aortic regurgitation. In children with left to right shunts, ACE inhibitors have been found useful in patients with large shunts or in those with an elevated systemic vascular resistance. These drugs should not be used in patients with stenotic lesions.

ACE inhibitors can lead to severe hypotension in volume-depleted patients hence diuretics may have to be reduced initially. A test dose (one fourth of the usual dose) should be given first, as some patients react with exaggerated hypotension to the initial dose. Patients with pre-existing renal failure (serum creatinine >1.5 mg/dL) should not receive ACE inhibitors. ACE inhibitors precipitate renal failure in bilateral renal arterial stenosis. Dry cough may occur in some cases, angioedema rarely occurs. Optimal dosages are variable. Enalapril in an oral dose from 0.1 to 0.5 mg/kg/day has been used in children. Captopril is used in a dosage of 0.2–2 mg/kg/dose 8 hourly.

Angiotensin receptor blockers

Losartan, candesartan, irbesartan, and valsartan have been extensively used in adults. Data in children are limited. In an open-label study conducted to characterize the pharmaco-kinetics and antihypertensive response to irbesartan in children, it was well tolerated and may be a treatment option for pediatric hypertensive patients. However, there is no report of its use in CHF in the pediatric age group.

Nitroglycerin Intravenous nitroglycerin is safe and very effective therapy for pulmonary edema. It is predominantly a venodilator and also a weak arteriolar dilator. The blood pressure needs to be monitored frequently. The addition of an ionotrope such as dobutamine may be required if the child develops hypotension (systolic BP <90 mmHg). With careful noninvasive monitoring, nitroglycerin may be administered with a micro drip set, although the use of an infusion pump is preferable. Dosages are titrated from 0.5 to 1.0 micro-grams/kg/min.

Sodium nitroprusside

A potent arterial dilator, sodium nitroprusside requires careful monitoring of intra-arterial pressure. It is rapid acting and severe hypotension may occur within minutes. Careful titration is required. The dosage ranges from 0.5 to 1 micrograms/kg/min. The infusion fluid needs to be protected from sunlight. Renal failure enhances its toxicity.

11

It is most useful for treatment of acute left ventricular failure in presence of hypertension and for acute mitral or aortic regurgitation in postoperative patients.

Nifedipine This calcium channel blocker causes peripheral vasodilation and is useful in patients with coarctation of aorta or pulmonary arterial hypertension. The advantages are a rapid onset of action, safety and sublingual administration. It can be used in infants also in a dose of 0.1–0.3 mg/kg/dose sublingual 6 hourly.

Hydralazine It is an infrequently used vasodilator for the treatment of CHF now. Chronic use results in tachyphylaxis. The dosage is 1–7 mg/kg/day in divided doses.

Inotropes

Inotropes other than digoxin are used for short-term support of circulation or to tide over the crisis. Their long-term use is not associated with improved long-term survival. Dopamine is currently the most widely used inotrope for acute support in pediatric practice. It has the advantages of peripheral vasoconstriction and raising blood pressure at moderate to high doses (6–10 micrograms/kg/min). At higher doses (20 micrograms/kg/ min), intense vasoconstriction raises blood pressure but it is counterproductive as it increases myocardial work. Dopamine also increases pulmonary vascular resistance and causes tachycardia. Both these factors may be detrimental to some patients (eg, mitral stenosis). For hypotension in the preterm neonate, dopamine is particularly effective at low dosage.

Dobutamine is a synthetic sympathomimetic agent and causes increase in contractility with relatively less tachycardia or rise in blood pressure. It is compatible with dopamine in the same infusion and often a combination of dopamine and dobutamine is used to provide inotropic support. The individual variations are wide and dosages of 5–20 micrograms/kg/min are generally used.

Epinephrine, norepinephrine and isoprenaline are potent, naturally occurring sympathomimetics used during post-operative low output only. Isoprenaline, a beta stimulant is a pulmonary and systemic vasodilator and causes tachycardia. Rarely, nor-epinephrine has been found effective in septic shock unresponsive to other treatment.

Phosphodiesterase inhibitors (Milrinone)

This phosphodiesterase inhibitor inotropic agent, used in refractory failure, also has pulmonary vasodilating properties. Dose is 0.3–0.7 micrograms/kg/min in children, mainly in postoperative or refractory failure. Thrombocytopenia and hepatic dysfunction limit its use. It should not be mixed in dextrose containing solutions or with frusemide.

Miscellaneous

Beta blockers Paradoxically, some patients with dilated cardiomyopathy may respond to beta-blockers. The rationale relates to downgrading of beta receptors due to chronic catacholamine stimulation. The therapy is best undertaken in hospital as careful monitoring is required. Carvedilol, a nonselective beta blocker with alpha-1 blocking and anti-oxidative properties has proven to be beneficial in a majority of adult patients with congestive heart failure. Although the experience from adult patients may be extrapolated to older children, symptomatic infants remain a subset for whom dosage, safety and efficacy need to be established in larger studies. It has been recently reported that carvedilol is well tolerated in infants with dilated cardiomyopathy and there is significant improvement in their functional status. Optimal timing of starting therapy, dosage and long-term effects need to be investigated with multi-institutional trials. A recent multi-center study has suggested carvedilol as an adjunct to standard therapy for pediatric heart failure. It improves symptoms and left ventricular function. Side effects are common but well tolerated. Further prospective studies are required to determine the effect of carvedilol on survival and to clearly define its role in pediatric heart failure therapy.

L Carnitine Metabolic cardiomyopathy associated with carnitine deficiency responds to replacement with L-carnitine in a dosage of 50 to 100 mg/kg/day in divided doses. Its role in other cardiomyopathies is not proved.

Prostaglandins E1 As described earlier, neonates with duct dependent lesions as transposition of great arteries, coarctation of aorta, aortic stenosis in failure or hypoplastic left heart syndrome etc. improve remarkably with PGE1 infusion. The therapy is initiated at 0.05 micrograms/kg/min if an adequate response is seen; the dose may be reduced subsequently. Apnea may occur during the infusion and ventilatory support should be available. Irritability, seizures, hypotension and hyperpyrexia are rare.

Other options

Extracorporeal membrane oxygenation (ECMO) was initially developed for respiratory failure. Its use, however, has evolved into an excellent method of preoperative and postoperative support in the treatment of infants and children with acquired and congenital heart disease. Along with ECMO, the left ventricular assist device (LVAD) and the intra-aortic balloon pump (IABP) have also found a place in the management of children with heart failure. There is a 74% survival rate and the long-term outcome has been excellent in most cases.

A combination of external implantable pulsatile and continuous-flow external mechanical support now can be used to bridge pediatric patients with end stage cardiomyopathy to orthotopic heart transplantation. Such a combination has been found to complement each other to significantly extend the lives of a wide range of pediatric patients with severe cardio-myopathies and myocarditis.

Biventricular pacing Biventricular pacing therapy is an innovative therapy for improving cardiac output in adult patients with severe heart failure. However, recently this technique had been used in a six month young infant with tetralogy of Fallot and atresia of the left pulmonary artery in whom biventricular stimulation led to improved left ventricular function and successful weaning from extracorporeal circulation.

Cardiac transplantation Pediatric heart transplantation has become an accepted method of treatment for certain pediatric heart diseases in western countries. Pediatric heart transplantation can provide good intermediate term survival for selected pediatric patients. Cardiac transplantation has since become a standard therapeutic option for certain disorders in which poor cardiac output without other surgical options exists in the face of maximized medical therapy. The most common disorder requiring transplantation is dilated cardiomyopathy, other forms of cardiomyopathy (ie, restrictive cardiomyopathy, arrhythmogenic right ventricular dysplasia/cardiomyopathy, and hypertrophic cardiomyopathy with poor ventricular function), and hypoplastic left heart.

Treatment of the Cause

It is extremely important, particularly for infants with persistent CHF in the first few months of life to arrive at an accurate early diagnosis for the cause of CHF and planning definitive measures.

Survival is determined by early correction of treatable cause as infection, electrolyte imbalance, arrhythmias, structural heart defects as shunt lesions, complete transposition of great vessels, anomalous origin of left coronary artery from pulmonary artery and critical left or right-sided obstructive lesions. Timely intervention is crucial and the results of catheter and surgical intervention are excellent for structural defects.

Revision Point

Congestive Heart Failure (CHF)

1. CHF may occur due to ventricular systolic dysfunction, diastolic dysfunction, or abnormal ventriculoarterial coupling. There are associated with an exaggerated, inappropriate, or abnormal afterload on a normal myocardium.
2. An underlying structural heart disease must be carefully looked for in children with heart failure.
3. Diagnosis of heart failure in children is largely clinical. The cause can be usually confirmed on echocardiography.
4. Conventional drug therapy includes digoxin, frusemide, spironolactone, and inotropes. Adjunctive therapy includes ACE inhibitors (captopril/enalapril) and beta-blockers (carvedilol).

Bautista-Hernandez V, Sanchez-Andres A, Portela F, Fynn-Thompson F. Current pharmacologic management of pediatric heart failure in congenital heart disease. *Curr Vasc Pharmacol*. 2011;9:619–28.

Chaturvedi V, Saxena A. Heart failure in children: clinical aspect and clinical evaluation, diagnostic testing, and initial medical management. *Eur J Pediatr*. 2010;169:269–79.

Chaturvedi V, Saxena A. Heart failure in children: clinical aspect and management.management. *Indian J Pediatr*. 2009;76:195–205.

Frobel AK, Hulpke-Wette M, Schmidt KG, Läer S. Beta-blockers for congestive heart failure in children. *Cochrane Database Syst Rev*. 2009;1:CD007037.

Hoffman TM. Newer inotropes in pediatric heart failure. *J Cardiovasc Pharmacol*. 2011;58:121–5.

Hsu DT, Canter CE. Dilated cardiomyopathy and heart failure in children. *Heart Fail Clin*. 2010;6:415–32.

Hsu DT, Pearson GD. Heart failure in children: part II: diagnosis, treatment, and future directions. *Circ Heart Fail*. 2009;2:490–8.

Jefferies JL, Hoffman TM, Nelson DP. Heart failure treatment in the intensive care unit in children. *Heart Fail Clin*. 2010;6:531–58.

Kantor PF, Mertens LL. Clinical practice: heart failure in children. Part II: current maintenance therapy and new therapeutic approaches. *Eur J Pediatr*. 2010;169:403–10.

Kantor PF, Mertens LL. Clinical practice: heart failure in children. Part I: Kaufman BD, Shaddy RE, Shirali GS, Tanel R, Towbin JA. Assessment and management of the failing heart in children. *Cardiol Young*. 2008;18:63–71.

Madriago E, Silberbach M. Heart failure in infants and children. *Pediatr Rev*. 2010;31:4–12.

Margossian R. Contemporary management of pediatric heart failure. *Expert Rev Cardiovasc Ther*. 2008 ;6:187–97.

O'Connor MJ, Rosenthal DN, Shaddy RE. Outpatient management of pediatric heart failure. *Heart Fail Clin*. 2010;6:515–29.

Penny DJ, Vick GW 3rd. Novel therapies in childhood heart failure: today and tomorrow. *Heart Fail Clin*.2010;6:591–621.

11.26 INFECTIVE ENDOCARDITIS

Infective endocarditis is a microbial infection of the endocardial surface of the heart. It should be considered in any child presenting with (*a*) prolonged fever and (*b*) one of the following: congenital or rheumatic heart disease, post-operative cardiac surgery, indwelling lines, pathological murmur, and embolic phenomenon.

Pathogenesis

An underlying structural heart disease, or iatrogenic manipulation of heart (surgery, central catheter) may result in denudation of endocardial epithelium; this exposed raw area serves as a nidus for platelet and fibrin deposition. This initial insult is known as non-bacterial thrombotic endocarditis, that on exposure to bacteremia, subsequently manifests as infective endocarditis.

Etiology

The most common agent is *Streptococcus viridans*, followed closely by *Staphylococcus aureus*, and enterocococci (*S. bovis, S. faecalis*)

Uncommon organisms causing infective endocarditis include: *Streptococcus pneumoniae, Haemophilus influenzae, Staphylococcus epidermidis, Coxiella burnetii, Neisseria gonorrhoeae, Brucella, Chlamydia psittaci, Chlamydia trachomatis, Chlamydia pneumoniae, Pasteurella multocida, Campylobacter fetus*, and HACEK (*Hemophilus parainfluenzae, H. aphrophilus, H. paraphrophilus, Actinobacillus, Cardiobacterium, Eikenella*, and *Kingella*) group of organisms.

Fungal endocarditis should be suspected in sick neonates, immunosuppressed, and those on prolonged antibiotic or steroid therapy. *Aspergillus* and *Candida* are the common etiological agents.

Culture negative endocarditis contributes to approximately 10% of all cases.

Clinical Manifestations

There is a history of preceding dental, urinary, intravenous, or cardiac procedure in a child with underlying congenital or rheumatic heart disease. Typically, the child will have prolonged low grade fever, fatigue, chest pain, arthralgia, myalgia, bodyache, dyspnea, malaise, night sweats, weight loss, or neurological manifestations (stroke, seizures, headache).

Examination reveals elevated temperature (90%), murmur (100%), tachycardia, and tachypnea. Embolic phenomena can present as Roth spots in eye, hemiparesis (CNS), hematuria (kidney), petechiae, splinter nail bed hemorrhages, Osler nodes in skin, septic pulmonary embolism, and distant infection as arthritis, meningitis, or splenic abscess. Other important clinical findings include clubbing, Janeway lesions, and splenomegaly.

Diagnosis

Essential investigations include 3 blood cultures taken from 3 different sites over a period of 3 hours, ESR, hemoglobin, C-reactive protein, urine microscopy, chest X-ray, ECG; and echocardiography for evidence of valve vegetations, prosthetic valve dysfunction or leak, or myocardial abscess.

11

Duke Criteria for the Diagnosis of Bacterial Endocarditis

A. Major Criteria

1. *Positive Blood Culture*

    i. Typical microorganism for infective endocarditis from two separate blood cultures *Streptococci viridans*, *Streptococci bovis*, HACEK group, *Staphylococcus aureus* or community acquired enterococci in the absence of a primary focus, Or

    ii. Persistently positive blood culture, defined as recovery of a microorganism consistent with infective endocarditis from at least 3 blood cultures drawn more than 12 hours apart, or all of three or a majority of four or more separate blood cultures, with first and last drawn at least 1 hour apart; Or

    iii. Single positive blood culture for *Coxiella burnetii* or antiphase 1 IgG antibody titer >1:800.

2. *Evidence of Endocardial Involvement*

    i. Positive echocardiogram: Oscillating intracardiac mass, on valve or supporting structures, myocardial abscess, or new partial dehiscence of prosthetic valve or patch.

    ii. New valvular regurgitation.

B. Minor Criteria

1. *Predisposition*: Predisposing heart condition or intravenous drug use.

2. Fever >38.0°C (100.4°F)

3. *Vascular phenomena*: Major arterial emboli, septic pulmonary infarcts, mycotic aneurysm, intracranial hemorrhage, conjunctival hemorrhages, Janeway lesions.

4. *Immunological phenomena*: Glomerulonephritis, Osler nodes, Roth's spots, rheumatoid factor.

5. *Microbiological evidence*: Positive blood culture but not meeting major criterion.

Definitive infective endocarditis
A. *Pathological criteria*
Microorganism: demonstrated by culture or histology in a vegetation or in an intracardiac abscess or pathological lesions: vegetation or intracardiac abscess present, confirmed by histology showing active carditis
B. *Clinical criteria*
Two major or one major and three minor or five minor
Possible endocarditis
One major and one minor or three minor criteria

Treatment **Infective Endocarditis**

Antibiotics are the mainstay of management, aimed at eradication of the micro-organism in vegetations. Decongestive medication (digitalis, salt restriction, and diuretic therapy) and avoidance of physical exertion is required when patient is in congestive cardiac failure. The child should be started on empirical antibiotic therapy on a strong suspicion, that can be changed depending upon clinical response and the reports of blood cultures **(Table 11.8)**. Surgical intervention is indicated for:

a. Severe aortic or mitral valve regurgitation with intractable heart failure, not stabilizing on medical treatment;

b. Dehiscence of an intracardiac patch, rupture of aortic sinus or rarely, a mycotic aneurysm requires an emergency operation; and

c. Other surgical indications include failure to sterilize the blood despite adequate antibiotic levels, a myocardial abscess, recurrent emboli, and failure of medical management.

Removal of vegetations and in some instances, valve replacement may be lifesaving, and sustained antibiotic administration will most often prevent reinfection.

Fungal endocarditis is difficult to manage and has a poor prognosis regardless of treatment. The drugs of choice are amphotericin B and 5-fluorocytosine. Surgery to excise infected tissue is occasionally attempted, usually with limited success.

Endocarditis Prophylaxis

Prophylactic antibiotics should be given as a single dose 30–60 minute before dental procedures, tonsillectomy, or adenoidectomy in all children having a congenital heart disease, prosthetic cardiac valves, or previous infective endocarditis. Ampicillin, cephalexin, clindamycin, or azithromycin can be used.

Infective Endocarditis

1. The diagnosis of infective endocarditis (IE) is based on clinical findings (prolonged fever and splenomegaly in a child with an underlying heart disease or having immune compromised status), positive blood cultures, laboratory results, and an echocardiogram. The modified Duke criterion is the most commonly used diagnostic criteria for IE.

2. Common blood culture isolates in IE include *Staphylococcus aureus*, *Streptococcus viridians*, enterococci, and coagulase-negative staphylococci.

3. The principles of management include prolonged antimicrobial therapy, monitoring for complications, and timely surgical intervention if needed.

American Heart Association. Infective Endocarditis in Childhood: 2015 Update: A Scientific Statement From the American Heart Association. *Circulation.* September 2015.

Akpunonu BE, Bittar S, Phinney RC, Taleb M. Infective endocarditis and the new AHA guideline. *Geriatrics*. 2008;63:12–9.

Hoyer A, Silberbach M. Infective endocarditis. *Pediatr Rev.* 2005;26:394–400.

Kohli V. Infective endocarditis. *Indian J Pediatr*. 2002;69:333–9.

Nishimura RA, Carabello BA, Faxon DP, et al. ACC/AHA 2008 guideline update on valvular heart disease: focused update on infective endocarditis: a report of the American College of Cardiology/American Heart Association Task Force on Practice Guidelines endorsed by the Society of Cardiovascular Anesthesiologists, Society for Cardiovascular Angiography and Interventions, and Society of Thoracic Surgeons. *Catheter Cardiovasc Interv.* 2008;72:E1–12.

Milazzo AS Jr, Li JS. Bacterial endocarditis in infants and children. *Pediatr Infect Dis J.* 2001;20:799–801.

	Table 11.8 Treatment of Infective Endocarditis		
Etiologic agent	*Drug*	*Route*	*Duration of therapy (wk)*
Streptococcus viridans, S. bovis (minimal inhibitory concentration [MIC] <0.1 mg/mL)	Penicillin G *or* Penicillin G plus gentamicin	IV IV IV	4–6 2–4 2
S. viridans, S. bovis (MIC >0.1 mg/mL)	Penicillin G plus gentamicin	IV IV	4–6 2

S. viridans or enterococci (*S. bovis* or *S. faecalis*) (MIC >0.5 mg/mL)	Penicillin G *or*
	    ampicillin plus
	    gentamicin
		IV
		IV
		IV
			4–6
			4–6
			4–6

S. viridans, S. bovis (penicillin allergy)	Vancomycin plus gentamicin if resistant	IV IV	4–6 4–6
Staphylococcus aureus	Nafcillin *or* oxacillin plus optional gentamicin	IV IV	6–8 2

S. aureus (methicillin resistant) (penicillin allergy)	Vancomycin plus
	    optional trimetho-
	    prim–sulfamethoxazole
		IV
		IV,
		PO
			6–8
			4–8

S. aureus (with prosthetic device, methicillin–sensitive)	Nafcillin/oxacillin plus
	    gentamicin plus rifampin
	    IV/PO
		IV
		IV
		at least 6
			At least 6
			2

S. aureus (with prosthetic device, methicillin–resistant)	Vancomycin
	    plus gentamicin
	    plus rifampin
		IV
		IV
		IV/PO
			At least 6
			2
			at least 6

S. epidermidis	Vancomycin plus optional rifampin	IV IV/PO	6–8 6–8
Haemophilus species	Ampicillin plus optional gentamicin	 IV	4–6 2–4

HACEK group	Ceftriaxone or
	    ampicillin—Sulbactum or
	    ciprofloxacin
		IV	4
			4
			4

Culture negative
Native valve
	1. Ampicillin –Sulbactum
	        plus gentamicin
	2. Vancomycin plus
	        gentamicin plus
	        ciprofloxacin
		IV
		
		IV
			4–6
			4–6
			4–6
			4–6
			4–6

Prosthetic valve (early-less than or equal to 1 year)	Vancomycin plus
	    gentamicin plus
	    cefipime plus
	    rifampin
		IV
		IV/IM
		IV
		IV/PO
			6
			2
			6
			6

Drug doses:

Inj aqueous Crystalline penicillin 200,000–300,000 U/kg/24 hr every 4–6 hourly, not to exceed 20 million U/24 h;
Inj gentamicin 3 mg/kg, 3 divided doses IV /IM; Inj ceftriaxone 100 mg/kg /24 hr IV/IM once daily;
Inj vancomicin 40 mg/kg/day in 2–3 divided doses IV; Inj nafcilin/Oxacillin –200 mg/kg/day in 4–6 equally divided doses IV;
Inj ampicillin sodium 300 mg/kg/day in 4–6 equally divided doses IV; rifampicin –20 mg/kg/day 3 divided doses IV/Oral
Inj ampicillin-sulbactum 300 mg/kg/day 4–6 equally divided doses IV; Inj ciprofoxacin-20–30 mg/kg/day IV/oral 2 divided doses

11.27 CARDIOMYOPATHY

Cardiomyopathy refers to a myocardial disease without any structural deformity of the heart. It can be *primary* (unknown etiology) or *secondary* to a systemic disease. WHO classifies cardiomyopathies in 3 basic types of functional impairment on the basis of predominant pathological features:

1. *Dilated cardiomyopathy* This is the most common form, characterized by ventricular dilatation, impaired systolic function, and often symptoms of congestive cardiac failure.
2. *Hypertrophic cardiomyopathy* This is recognized by disproportionate left ventricular hypertrophy, asymmetrical or symmetrical involvement of the

11

interventricular septum, with preserved systolic function until late in the course of disease. Hypertrophic cardiomyopathy may occur (*a*) without flow obstruction, or (*b*) with obstruction. Obstructive type is also known as idiopathic hypertrophic subaortic stenosis (IHSS).

3. *Restrictive cardiomyopathy* The least common form, marked by impaired diastolic filling.

DILATED CARDIOMYOPATHY

Cardiomegaly and congestive heart failure are the most common presentations. CHF is secondary to impaired systolic function of one or both ventricles. Abnormalities of diastolic dysfunction are also recognized. Children with dilated cardiomyopathy usually present in the first two years of life with about half in the first year. Both sexes are similarly affected.

Etiology

Most cases remain idiopathic but, in few cases it is possible to establish a cause and effect relationship: these conditions are recognized as 'specific cardiomyopathies' such as metabolic cardiomyopathies. In 'idiopathic group', factors as genetic origin, altered immune response, and viral infection (coxsackie B virus and adenovirus) have been implicated.

Clinical Manifestations

The clinical presentation of a child with dilated cardiomyopathy is usually related to heart failure and depends on the age and acute or chronic nature of the disease. Decreased exercise tolerance, breathlessness on exertion or feeding difficulty is common.

- Infants may present with fever, severe heart failure, respiratory distress, distant heart sounds, weak pulses, and tachycardia out of proportion to the fever, mitral insufficiency caused by dilatation of the valve annulus, a gallop rhythm, acidosis, and shock. Some may present with insidious onset of CHF.
- Older children may have a history of nocturnal cough and orthopnea. Intercurrent infections, frequently of upper respiratory tract, increase myocardial demands and worsen the symptoms.
- In some children, presentation can be related to arrhythmias.
- Physical examination reveals a child with tachycardia, tachypnea, and hepatomegaly.
- Occasionally presentation may be with pain abdomen due to acute liver distension.
- Peripheral pulses are weak, and there is cardiomegaly. Third heart sound is common; murmur of mitral and tricuspid insufficiency may be present.

Diagnosis

Chest roentgenogram demonstrates cardiomegaly and features of pulmonary edema. ECG reveals sinus tachycardia; reduced QRS complex voltage, and ST segment and T wave abnormalities. Arrhythmias may be the first clinical manifestation; presence of fever and a large heart strongly suggest acute myocarditis. Arrhythmias of atrial or ventricular origin can occur.

Echocardiography demonstrates dilated left ventricle, ventricular dysfunction, mitral valve regurgitation, normal coronary arteries, and no structural heart defects.

Myocarditis can be confirmed by *endomyocardial biopsy* though not routinely recommended. This is performed during cardiac catheterization and can also detect other causes of cardiomyopathy as carnitine deficiency, storage disease, and mitochondrial defects.

Treatment	Dilated Cardiomyopathy

1. Treat congestive heart failure. Supportive measures include complete rest, fluid restriction, and nursing in propped up position. Decongestive medication consists of digoxin (2/3rd of required dose orally, used with caution as patients with myocarditis may be more susceptible to the digitatis toxicity), frusemide (intravenous or oral depending upon clinical condition) and ACE inhibitors. Dobutamine, dopamine or milrinone may be helpful if child is in very low output stage.
2. Arrhythmias if present should be treated.
3. For infants and children having cardiogenic shock, extra-corporeal membrane oxygenation (ECMO) may be indicated.
4. In larger adolescents, implantation of a left ventricular assist device has been performed, usually as bridge to cardiac transplantation, which is the treatment of choice in patients with refractory heart failure.
5. Trials are currently under way evaluating the efficacy of intravenous gamma globulin, which is given in dose of 2 g/kg in slow infusion over 20–24 hours.
6. The role of corticosteroids for treatment of acute viral myocarditis is still controversial.

Hsu DT, Canter CE. Dilated cardiomyopathy and heart failure in children. *Heart Fail Clin.* 2010;6:415–32.
Silva JN, Canter CE. Current management of pediatric dilated cardiomyopathy. *Curr Opin Cardiol.* 2010;25:80–7.

HYPERTROPHIC CARDIOMYOPATHY

This condition is also known as idiopathic hypertrophic subaortic stenosis or asymmetric left ventricular septal hypertrophy (with or without left ventricle outflow tract obstruction). Rarely there can be symmetrical hypertrophy and involvement of both ventricles. Ventricular hypertrophy and diastolic dysfunction are the characteristic finding.

Pathophysiology

The mitral valve is displaced anteriorly by hypertrophy of papillary muscles, and the left ventricular cavity is distorted by the massive generalized hypertrophy. Systolic anterior motion of the mitral valve and hypertrophied interventricular septum may cause substantial obstruction.

The hypertrophied fibrosed stiff muscles have a decreased distensibility so the dominant pathophysiological abnormality is impaired relaxation. This abnormality of diastolic dysfunction can result in elevation of the left ventricular end diastolic pressure, with resulting pulmonary congestion and dyspnea. This is the most common symptom in hypertrophic cardiomyopathy in infancy and childhood. Similar elevation of RA pressure occurs when right ventricle is affected. Varying degrees of mitral or tricuspid regurgitation are common.

Etiology

In most cases, the condition is inherited as an autosomal dominant disorder, with incomplete penetrance. Affected individuals are heterozygous. Five separate genes (on chromosome 1, 7, 11, 14, and 15) are currently known to produce hypertrophic cardiomyopathy. However, some cases are sporadic and non-genetic.

Clinical Features

Children often lack symptoms. Not infrequently, the disease is detected because of the presence of a murmur, often thought to be innocent or an arrhythmia. There is no correlation between the severity of the disease and the symptoms.

Weakness, fatigue, dyspnea on effort, palpitations, angina pectoris, dizziness, and syncope may occur. There is risk of sudden death even in asymptomatic children. The pulse is brisk because of the early systolic ejection of blood from the ventricle. There is a prominent left ventricular lift and double apical impulse. Heart sounds are normal and 4th heart sound may be heard. Obstructive variety is characterized by a blowing pansystolic murmur best heard at apex due to accompanying mitral regurgitation and ejection systolic murmur over lower left sternal border.

Diagnosis

ECG shows left ventricular hypertrophy with or without ST segment depression and T wave inversion. Signs of the Wolf-Parkinson-White syndrome and other intraventricular conduction defects may be present. Chest X-ray may show mild to moderate cardiomegaly with prominence of the left ventricle. The echocardiogram shows asymmetric left ventricular hypertrophy predominantly affecting the interventricular septum; and systolic anterior motion of the mitral valve. Doppler studies demonstrate the presence of a left ventricular outflow tract gradient and mitral regurgitation.

Treatment	Hypertrophic Cardiomyopathy

There is no standardized therapy. Beta blockers and calcium channel blockers are useful in obstructive variety. The patients are prone to develop ventricular arrhythmias. The prognosis of hypertrophic cardiomyopathy is unpredictable, especially in the asymptomatic patient, who may remain stable for years. Some children may progress to chronic congestive heart failure, and others are at risk for sudden death caused by arrhythmia.

- Competitive sports and strenuous physical activity should be discouraged.
- Digitalis is contraindicated.
- Aggressive diuresis and the infusion of isoproterenol or other inotropic agents should also be avoided.
- β-adrenergic blocking agents (propranolol) in high dose (5–18 mg/kg) and calcium channel blocking agents (verapamil) have been used with some success in decreasing the degree of outflow obstruction.
- Surgical ventricular septal myotomy, resection of the left ventricular outflow tract, or mitral valve replacement may be needed, if the left ventricular outflow obstruction is severe.

Semsarian C; CSANZ Cardiac Genetics Diseases Council Writing Group. Guidelines for the diagnosis and management of hypertrophic cardiomyopathy. *Heart Lung Circ*.2011;20:688–90.

RESTRICTIVE CARDIOMYOPATHY

Poor ventricular compliance leading to abnormal diastolic dysfunction is the major abnormality. Systolic function is also impaired in later stages. Endocardial fibroelastosis and endomyocardial fibrosis are the two common variants in children.

Clinical manifestations closely simulate those of constrictive pericarditis. In its full blown form, restrictive cardiomyopathy results in dyspnea, edema, ascites, hepatomegaly, increased venous pressures, and pulmonary congestion. The heart is mildly or moderately enlarged without a significant murmur. Sometimes, mitral or tricuspid regurgitant murmur can be heard. Heart sounds are distant.

The electrocardiogram shows low voltage and nonspecific ST-T wave changes.

Roentgenographic examination shows mild to moderate cardiomegaly. Differential diagnosis from constrictive pericarditis is critical, as the latter is a treatable entity while former is a slowly progressive disease with poor long-term outcome.

The prognosis for restrictive cardiomyopathy is generally poor. Treatment is directed towards relief of edema with diuretics and decongestants. Cardiac transplantation is the last management option.

Cardiomyopathies

1. Cardiomyopathies refer to diseases of cardiac muscles which can be *acute* or *chronic*.
2. Myocarditis is an acute inflammatory disease of the myocardium and the most common known cause of dilated cardiomyopathy in children.
3. WHO classifies cardiomyopathies in 3 basic types: *dilated, hypertrophic*, and *restrictive*.
4. Dilated cardiomyopathy is characterized by the ventricular dilation and systolic dysfunction resulting into congestive heart failure.
5. Hypertrophic cardiomyopathy, a genetically inherited disease, is associated with disproportionate left ventricular hypertrophy, asymmetrical involvement of the interventricular septum, with preserved systolic function until late in the course of disease.
6. Restrictive cardiomyopathy is a rare cardiomyopathy marked by impaired diastolic filling; and has poor prognosis.
7. Treatment includes management of heart failure symptoms and prevention of arrhythmia, thromboembolic complications, and sudden death.
8. Heart transplantation is the therapy of choice for end-stage cardiomyopathies refractory to medical therapy.

Georgakopoulos D, Tolis V. Hypertrophic cardiomyopathy in children, teenagers and young adults. *Hellenic J Cardiol*.2007;48:228–33.

Maron BJ. Hypertrophic cardiomyopathy in childhood.. *Pediatr Clin North Am*.2004;51:1305–46.

Shaddy RE. Cardiomyopathies in adolescents: dilated, hypertrophic, and restrictive. *Adolesc Med*. 2001;12:35–45.

Talwar KK, Poddar P. Beta blockers in cardiomyopathy: status report 2010. *Indian Heart J*. 2010;62:123–5.

| Case Study | Hypertrophic Obstructive Cardiomyopathy |

A 14-yr-old adolescent was brought to outpatient with complaints of gradual onset exertional dyspnea for 1 year. He was otherwise asymptomatic. There was no past history of any illness or acute event. There was a family history of sudden death in a cousin aged 20 years. On examination, vitals were stable. Pulse was brisk volume. Blood pressure was 110/70 mmHg in right arm. JVP was normal. Precordial examination revealed heaving apex with double impulse in left 5th intercostal space in mid-clavicular line. S1 was loud. S2 was narrow split. S4 was heard at apex. Grade 3/6 harsh, ejection systolic murmur was heard at left 3rd and 4th intercostal space at sternal border. Upon dynamic auscultation, murmur intensity and duration increased upon standing, inspiration, and exercise. Other system examination was normal.

Q. What is the diagnosis? Explain the basis of dynamic auscultation.

Patient has hypertrophic obstructive cardiomyopathy. Symptoms, family history, and clinical findings, all point towards the diagnosis. Obstruction to LV outflow occurs due to abnormal hypertrophy of subaortic interventricular septum (IVS). Whenever there is reduction in preload or afterload to left ventricle, the ventricular cavity volume decreases. This leads to the hypertrophied IVS coming closer to anterior mitral leaflet enhancing outflow obstruction and increasing the length and intensity of murmur. Similar physiology happens during enhanced contractile state of ventricle. Reverse happens with increased preload and afterload; and reduction in contractile state.

Q. What is the mechanism of sudden death in HOCM?

The hypertrophied myocardium on histopathology shows disorganized array of myocytes arranged obliquely or perpendicular to each other, rather than normal parallel arrangement. This impairs transmission of normal electrical impulses and predisposes to abnormal depolarization and repolarization; serving as nidus for ventricular tachyarrhythmias leading to sudden cardiac death.

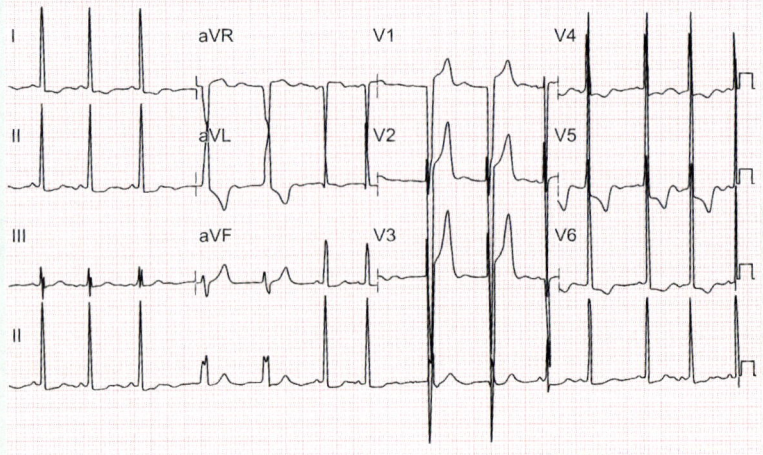

Q. What does ECG depict?

ECG shows very tall R wave in left precordial leads measuring 45 mm in V6 and very deep S wave in right precordial leads. Note that the ECG is half standardized. This shows severe LVH. T wave inversion in left precordial leads indicates strain pattern. Two ventricular premature beats are seen in rhythm strip.

Q. How will you manage?

Sports participation is restricted. Medical management with high dose beta blockers or calcium channel blockers will be initiated. In the light of family history of sudden death patient is at risk of sudden cardiac death, hence primary prevention with ICD (Implantable cardioverter-defibrillator) will be done. After echocardiogram evaluation, if the obstruction is severe, surgical septal myectomy is indicated.

Towbin JA. Hypertrophic cardiomyopathy. *Pacing Clin Electrophysiol.* 2009;32:S23–31.

Wong ML, Tay JS, Wong JC, Chan KY. Cardiomyopathy in paediatrics. *J Singapore Paediatr Soc.* 1991;33:40–4.

11.28 PERICARDITIS

Pericardial inflammation results in an accumulation of fluid in the pericardial space. The fluid may be serous, fibrinous, purulent, or hemorrhagic depending on the cause of the pericarditis.

In a healthy child, there is normally 10–15 mL of fluid in the pericardial space. For every small increment of fluid, the pericardial pressure rises slowly; once a critical level is reached, there is a rapid rise in pressure, culminating in severe cardiac compression and features of *cardiac tamponade*. Inhibition of ventricular filling during diastole, elevated systemic venous and pulmonary venous pressures and shock occur.

Etiology

1. Infectious
   - *Viral*: coxsackievirus B, Epstein-Barr virus, influenza virus, adenovirus;
   - *Bacterial*: *Streptococcus, Pneumococcus, Staphylococcus, Meningococcus, Mycoplasma,* tularemia; *H. influenzae*

- Tuberculosis
- *Fungal*: Histoplasmosis, actinomycosis
- *Parasitic*: Toxoplasmosis, echinococcus
2. *Connective tissue diseases:* Rheumatoid arthritis, rheumatic fever, SLE, systemic sclerosis, sarcoidosis
3. *Metabolic:* Uremia, hypothyroidism
4. *Nutritional:* Thiamine deficiency
5. *Hematoncology:* Bleeding diathesis, malignancy (primary, metastatic), radiotherapy–induced
6. *Others:* Trauma, postcardiac surgery, aortic dissection, and idiopathic

ACUTE PERICARDITIS

Purulent pericarditis is most often associated with bacterial infections such as pneumonia, epiglottitis, meningitis, or osteomyelitis. Usually there are signs and symptoms of the primary infection. Once the purulent process is established, the course is fulminant, terminated by acute cardiac tamponade and death. The most common organisms implicated in purulent pericarditis are *Staphylococcus aureus*, *Haemophilus influenzae* type b, and *Neisseria meningitidis*. Tuberculous pericarditis rarely occurs in children. Extensive treatment with antituberculous chemotherapy with steroid is required.

Clinical Manifestations

The first symptom of pericardial disease is often precordial pain. The major complaint is a sharp, stabbing sensation over the precordium; the pain may be exaggerated by lying supine and relieved by sitting, especially leaning forward. Because there is no sensory innervation of the pericardium, the pain is probably referred pain from diaphragmatic and pleural irritation. Cough, dyspnea, abdominal pain, vomiting, and fever may also occur. The presence of symptoms or signs associated with other organs depends on the cause of the pericarditis.

- The presence of a pericardial friction rub is helpful but is a variable sign in acute pericarditis, apparent when the effusion is small.
- When the effusion is larger, muffled heart sounds may be the only auscultatory finding.
- Narrow pulses, tachycardia, neck vein distention, and a pulsus paradoxus suggest significant fluid accumulation and cardiac tamponade. Normally there is slight decrease in systolic arterial pressure during inspiration. With cardiac tamponade, this normal phenomenon is exaggerated due to decreased filling of the left side of the heart with the inspiratory phase of respiration. This is known as *pulsus paradoxus*. Pulsus paradoxus may also be seen in patients with chronic obstructive pulmonary disease due to a marked increase in intrathoracic pressure.

Investigations

ECG reveals tachycardia, low voltage QRS complexes in limb leads (damping effect of pericardial fluid), and ST segment elevation (due to pressure on the myocardium by fluid or exudate which produces a current of injury), and generalized T-wave inversion (as a consequence of associated myocardial inflammation).

Chest X-ray Large pericardial effusion causes an enlarged cardiac shadow with the usual "water-bottle" configuration. In most instances, the lung fields are clear. With constrictive pericardial disease, the heart is relatively small and calcification may be present.

Echocardiogram is done for diagnosis of pericardial effusion and to evaluate its size, progression; and hemodynamic effects.

Treatment	Acute Pericarditis

Pericardiocentesis (diagnostic or therapeutic) or open pericardial drainage is required along with appropriate intravenous antibiotics.

CONSTRICTIVE PERICARDITIS

Constriction process usually takes months or years after the initial episode of pericarditis, but occasionally it may be an acute, rapidly progressive process particularly after purulent pericarditis. Tuberculosis is the most common cause of constrictive pericarditis in India.

Hemodynamics

Thickened pericardium forms a rigid cage around the heart, primarily restricting the diastolic filling. The rigid pericardium leads to separation of intracardiac and intrathoracic pressures and elevation and almost equalization of filling pressures of both ventricles. Myocardium is involved in later stages.

Clinical Manifestations

Signs and symptoms occur secondary to (*i*) restrictive diastolic dysfunction and elevated filling pressure; and (*ii*) decreased cardiac output. Raised jugular venous pressure, ascites, dyspnea, and hepatomegaly are characteristic findings.

- Child usually presents with easy fatigability, and breathlessness.
- Hepatomegaly and ascites are usually out of proportion to the other signs and symptoms. Liver is typically pulsatile on bimanual palpation.
- Neck veins are prominent and demonstrate inspiratory filling (*kussmaul's sign*).
- Pulse is low volume and pulse pressure is narrow. Pulsus paradoxus may be present.
- Precordium is quiet with a normal sized heart.
- Heart sounds are muffled and there may be a pericardial friction rub or an early S_3.

Investigations

Chest X-ray reveals a small heart, prominence of superior vena cava and right atrium, shaggy cardiac borders, patchy atelectasis, pleural effusion, and rarely calcification of the pericardium. ECG shows low voltage complexes, tachycardia, and nonspecific ST-T wave changes.

Echocardiography Typically demonstrates thickened pericardium, and normal systolic function of both ventricles. Cardiac catheterization is the gold standard for the hemodynamic assessment and diagnosis of constrictive pericarditis.

11

Case Study | **Constrictive Pericarditis**

A 17-year-old adolescent boy was brought to out-patient department with progressively increasing breathing difficulty and abdominal distension for last six months. He started having swelling over feet 6 months back which gradually progressed and involved abdomen also. Breathlessness used to occur on exertion (exertional dyspnea) initially which progressed to resting dyspnea. Examination revealed tachycardia, pedal edema, icterus, and markedly distended neck veins. Abdominal examination revealed large ascites (with fluid thrill) and hepatomegaly. Despite anasarca, patient looked cachexic. Apical impulse was feebly felt in left 5th intercostal space in mid clavicular line. S_1 and S_2 were distantly heard. Pericardial knock was heard at apex. There were no significant murmurs. Air entry was reduced and there was dullness to percussion in both the basal lung fields.

Q. What is the clinical diagnosis?

Patient is suffering from a chronic disease has presented with signs of right heart failure (edema, ascites, hepatomegaly, pleural effusion), left heart failure (dyspnea, orthopnea), distant heart sounds, and pericardial knock. This points towards diagnosis of constrictive pericarditis. Any child presenting with marked ascites and prominent neck veins should alert to this possibility.

Q. How will you confirm the diagnosis?

CT/MRI chest will confirm the diagnosis. Pericardial thickening and enhancement can be seen. Chest X-ray may demonstrate a small-sized heart and pericardial calcification. ECG will show low voltages in limb leads. Echocardiogram will show exaggerated respiratory variation in ventricular filling.

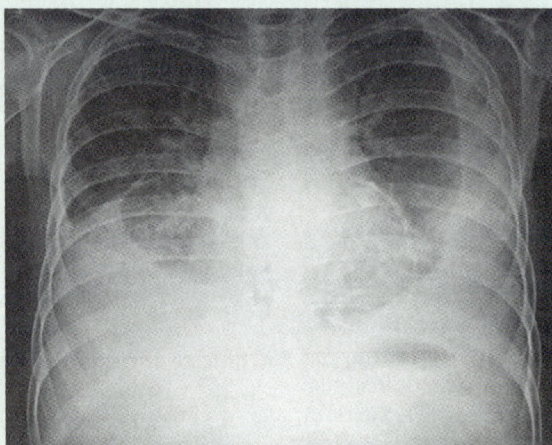

Q. What does the X-ray depict?

Bilateral cardiophrenic angles are blunt indicating peural effusion. Features of pulmonary venous congestion are present in lung fields in form of kerley lines and interlobar fissure edema. Pericardium shows linear radio-opaque shadow around left cardiac silhouette. This is pericardial calcification.

Q. How will you manage this child?

Diuretics are administered and salt restriction is started. Empirical ATT with steroids is initiated as tuberculosis is a common cause of constrictive pericarditis. Early surgery, after intensive phase of ATT, is performed which involves extensive pericardial excision.

Treatment | **Constrictive Pericarditis**

Decongestive medications include digoxin, diuretics and fluid restriction. Attempts should be made to rule out any tuberculous focus. If there is evidence of tuberculosis, appropriate therapy should be given. Radical pericardiectomy with decortication of the pericardium over a wide area of the heart including the systemic and pulmonary veins is the only effective treatment for constrictive pericarditis. In most patients, surgical intervention elicits a rapid response characterized by increased cardiac output and prompt diuresis. The long-term prognosis is usually excellent.

Demmler GJ. Infectious pericarditis in children. *Pediatr Infect Dis J.* 2006;25:165–6.

Durani Y, Giordano K, Goudie BW. Myocarditis and pericarditis in children. *Pediatr Clin North Am.* 2010;57:1281–303.

Pericarditis

1. Viral pericarditis is the most common cause of acute pericarditis in children. Other less common causes are trauma, myocarditis, systemic lupus erythematosus (SLE) and purulent pericarditis.
2. Bacterial pericarditis usually occurs due to staphylo-coccal and *Haemophilus* infections. Appropriate antibiotics with urgent drainage of pericardial space are the standard of care. Some children would require surgical pericardiectomy.
3. Tubercular pericarditis is an important cause of constrictive pericarditis in India.
4. Noninfectious causes of pericardial involvement include systemic lupus erythematosus, rheumatic fever, systemic onset juvenile idiopathic arthritis, uremia and hypothyroidism.

11.29 CARDIAC ARRHYTHMIAS

ELECTRICAL CONDUCTION IN HEART

Cardiac conduction system consists of the following components:
1. SA node (sinoatrial node)
2. AV node (atrioventricular node)
3. Bundle of His with right and left bundle branches
4. Purkinje fibres

SA node is known as pacemaker of heart and is located in right atrium. Electrical activity arises in pacemaker cells of SA node, travels through the wall of atria and internodal fibres and reaches AV node. SA nodal activation causes contraction of atria. From AV node, impulse travels along *bundle of His* lying in the interventricular septum and goes to right and left ventricle through right and left bundle branches. Ultimately the electrical impulse spreads diffusely to the myocardium through Purkinje fibers (Fig. 11.46). Normal range of resting heart rate is given in **Table 11.9.**

Table 11.9 Normal Range of Heart Rates According to Age	
Birth–1 week	90–160/min
1 week–1 year	100–170/min
1–2 years	80–150/min
3–7 years	70–135/min
7–10 years	65–130/min
11–15 years	60–120/min

Electrical activity is followed by mechanical events in the myocardium. When electrical impulse reaches AV node, there is a period of delay (0.12 second) before the impulse is transmitted to ventricles. Hence there is a time gap between atrial contraction and ventricular contraction.

Normal Electrocardiogram (ECG)

Normal ECG has five waves in following sequence P, Q, R, S, and T wave (Fig. 11.47). P wave depicts atrial depolarization. Next three waves occur together forming QRS complex, which depicts ventricular depolarization. T wave depicts ventricular repolarization. Atrial repolarization merges with the QRS complex, hence is not seen as a distinct wave (Fig. 11.48).

Definition and Classification

Cardiac arrhythmias are disturbances in (*a*) origin or (*b*) propagation of electrical activity through the cardiac conduction tissue. Because mechanical events follow electrical events in heart, cardiac arrhythmias can result in abnormal cardiac function. Arrhythmias can be associated with fast heart rate, normal heart rate, or low heart rate. Depending upon heart rate, arrhythmias are classified as either *tachyarrhythmia* (fast heart rate) or *bradyarrhythmias* (slow heart rate) (**Table 11.10**). Symptoms occurring due to arrhythmias are listed in **Box 11.1**.

TACHYARRHYTHMIAS

1. Sinus Tachycardia

Rhythm originating in SA node with heart rate inappropriately high for the age is defined as sinus tachycardia. It has gradual onset and termination as compared to SVT which has abrupt onset and termination. It occurs due to high sympathetic tone or withdrawal of

Table 11.10 Classification of Cardiac Arrhythmia
A. *Tachyarrhythmia*
1. Sinus tachycardia
2. Supraventricular tachycardia
• Atrial tachycardia
• Atrioventricular re-entry tachycardia (AVRT)
• Atrioventricular nodal re-entry tachycardia (AVNRT)
• Permanent Junctional reciprocating tachycardia (PJRT)
• Junctional ectopic tachycardia (JET)
3. Ventricular tachycardia
B. *Bradyarrhythmia*
1. Sinus bradycardia
2. Heart block
• First degree heart block
• Second degree heart block
• Third degree heart block/complete heart block
3. Bundle branch block

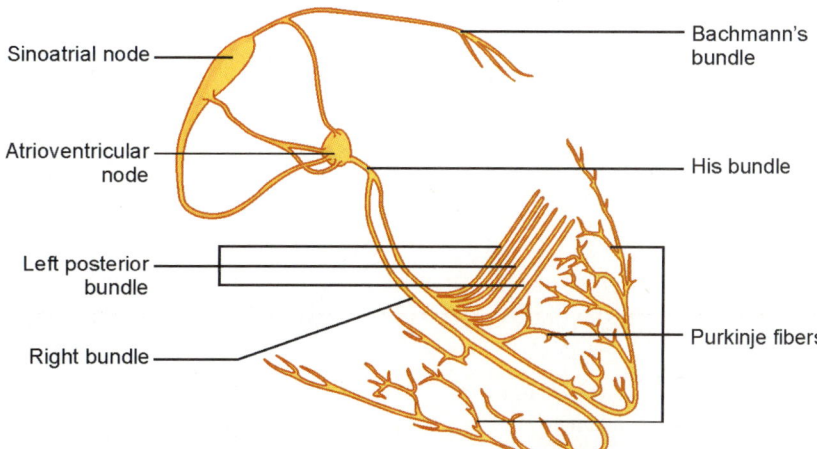

Fig. 11.46 Cardiac conduction system

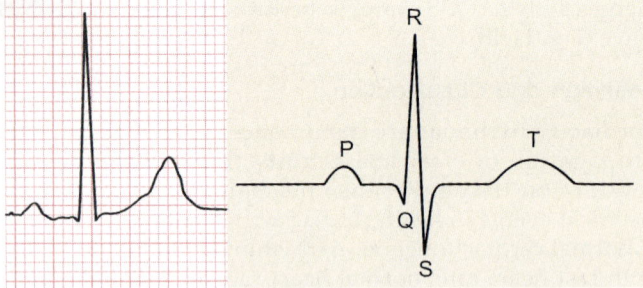

Fig. 11.47 Depicting waveforms in ECG

Box 11.1 Symptoms due to Arrhythmia

1. Asymptomatic
2. Palpitation
3. Missed beat sensation
4. Syncope
5. Prominent neck pulsations
6. Sudden cardiac death
7. Tachypnea, tachycardia, respiratory distress, heart failure (in neonates and infants)
8. Tachycardiomyopathy

---

parasympathetic tone. It can occur due to fever, anemia, hypotension, shock, anxiety, thyrotoxicosis, and drugs like atropine and caffeine. Treatment involves managing the underlying cause.

2. Supraventricular Tachycardia

Supraventricular tachycardia (SVT) is the commonest arrhythmia in pediatric age group. It is a broad term for all the arrhythmias originating above the bifurcation of bundle of His. It includes atrial tachycardia, AVRT, AVNRT, JET, WPW syndrome, and PJRT. These are described here individually.

Atrial Tachycardia

The electrical impulse originates from a focus in atria other than the SA node. Impulse travels to ventricles through AV node as it does normally. It is an automatic tachycardia that occurs when an ectopic focus in atrium becomes more excitable than the SA node. It can be either (i) unifocal, (ii) multifocal, or iii) intra-atrial re-entrant tachycardia (IART or atrial flutter).

Heart rate is around 250–350/min. ECG shows P waves followed by QRS complex of normal morphology. P wave morphology is different from sinus P wave. Ventricles have 1:1 response to atrial activity. But at higher rates 2:1 or 3:1 response can occur due to refractoriness of AV node at higher rates. If prolonged, atrial tachycardia can cause tachycardia-cardiomyopathy. Treatment involves reduction of ventricular rate by beta-blockers, or calcium channel blockers. Class IA, IC and III antiarrhythmic agents are used for long-term suppression. In refractory cases, radio-frequency ablation (RFA) of ectopic atrial focus is recommended.

Atrio-ventricular Re-entry Tachycardia (AVRT)

Normally the electrical conduction between atria and ventricles occurs through AV node only, because the rest of atrio-ventricular junction is electrically insulated. Sometimes *accessory* pathways exist between atria and ventricles. These are abnormal conduction pathways which have different refractory period and conduction velocity compared to AV node. Pathways which have slower velocity of conduction have short refractory period and those which have faster velocity of conduction have longer refractory period. Accessory pathways can conduct impulse from atria to ventricle or from ventricle to atria. Mechanism of AVRT involves a self propagating electrical circuit with impulse re-entry into atria and ventricles involving AV node and accessory pathway as shown in Fig. 11.49.

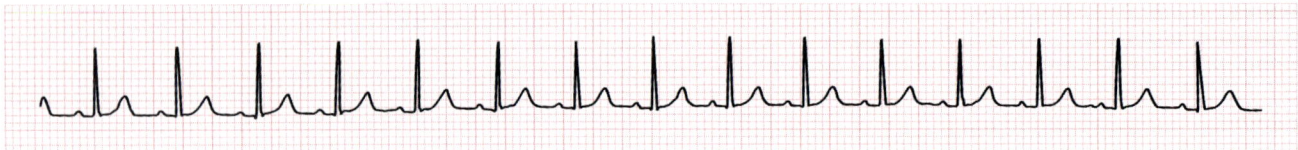

Fig. 11.48 ECG of a 3-year-old child showing normal sinus rhythm

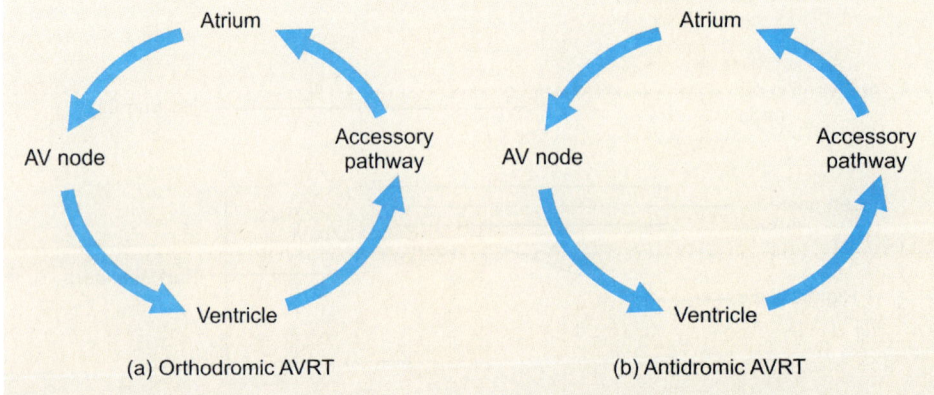

Fig. 11.49 Depicting the mechanism of accessory pathway mediated supraventricular tachycardia

If the impulse travels from atria to ventricles through AV node and goes retrogradely from ventricle to atria through accessory pathway, it is called *Orthodromic AVRT* (ORT); if it is in opposite direction it is called *Antidromic AVRT* (ART). Heart rate varies between 200–300/min. ECG in ORT has narrow QRS complex, as the ventricular activation is happening normally through AV node. Wide QRS complex occurs in ART because ventricular activation is happening by the impulse conducted through accessory pathway. In individuals who have accessory pathways, a premature atrial contraction may find the AV node refractory and hence the impulse may get transmitted to ventricle through the accessory pathway and the returning impulse may find AV node excitable (but the accessory pathway is refractory at this time) and hence get conducted to atria retrogradely through AV node. This vicious cycle continues and establishes re-entrant tachycardia.

Infants present with poor feeding, irritability, or shock. Older children present with anxiety and palpitations. Before starting management, 12 lead ECG should be taken. Figure 11.50 shows ECG strip of patient with SVT, showing fast heart rate and narrow QRS complexes. Causative factors like fever or excessive crying should be addressed first. If the vitals of child are stable vagal maneuvers are tried. If tachycardia does not get terminated he should be given adenosine injection.

Method of giving adenosine is very important. As it gets rapidly lysed in blood, it has to be injected rapidly followed by saline flush so that it reaches heart quickly without its effect being lost peripherally. Cannula for injection should be placed as proximally on limbs as possible. Side effects include severe bronchospasm or sudden cardiac arrest. One should anticipate the problems and be prepared to handle them. If vitals are unstable immediate synchronized cardioversion is done.

For preventing recurrence, oral beta-blockers are given. As children grow, the accessory pathways get obliterated and hence treatment can be stopped after three months if there is no recurrence. In older children, radiofrequency ablation of accessory pathway is done if medical management fails or if the frequency of episodes is more.

Atrioventricular Nodal Re-entry Tachycardia (AVNRT)

AVNRT is similar to AVRT except that the re-entry happens within the AV node. Some fibers in AV node have different refractory period and conduction velocity compared to others which establishes AVNRT. It is uncommon in children as compared to adults.

Junctional Ectopic Tachycardia

It is an automatic tachycardia with impulse originating within or immediately adjacent to AV node. Impulse then travels to both atria and ventricles from this focus. It commonly occurs in post-operative cases and treatment involves sedating the patient, correcting fever, and treating electrolyte disturbance. Amiodarone is used in unresponsive cases.

3. Ventricular Tachycardia

Abnormal electrical focus is located in ventricles which gives rise to ventricular tachycardia. It is called sustained if it lasts more than 30 seconds. QRS complexes are wide in morphology and QRS axis is different from baseline axis. *Torsades de pointes* is a type of VT in which QRS morphology keeps on changing. Etiology includes postoperative state in which ventriculotomy was done, myocarditis, metabolic disturbance including dyselectrolytemia, Brugada syndrome, and drug toxicity (digoxin).

If children with VT present in hemodynamically compromised state, DC cardioversion is done. In stable children lignocaine may be used. Electrolyte disturbance is corrected. Magnesium loading is drug of choice for *torsades*. In refractory cases amiodarone is used. Beta blockers are administered for long-term suppression. If a focus is identified, radiofrequency ablation is done. ICD implantation is done for myocarditis.

BRADYARRHYTHMIAS

1. Sinus Bradycardia

Rhythm originating in SA node with heart rate inappropriately low for the age, is defined as sinus bradycardia. It can occur during sleep, trained athletes, hypothyroidism, or medications like beta blocker, calcium channel blocker. It is generally asymptomatic and is diagnosed incidentally. Treatment is required in an occasional patient with reduced cardiac output or arrhythmia resulting from slow heart rate. Atropine administered subcutaneous or intramuscular increases the heart rate. If patient has recurrent symptomatic episodes in form of syncope, pacemaker implantation may be required.

2. AV Block

Heart block is simply defined as condition in which the atrial electrical impulse is conducted with delay or not conducted at all to the ventricles when AV node is not physiologically refractory. Block can occur at AV node, His bundle or bundle branches. Heart blocks generally lead to low heart rates.

First Degree Heart Block

First degree heart block has greater than normal delay in transmission of electrical activity from atria to ventricles. All P waves are conducted to the ventricles. There is atrio-

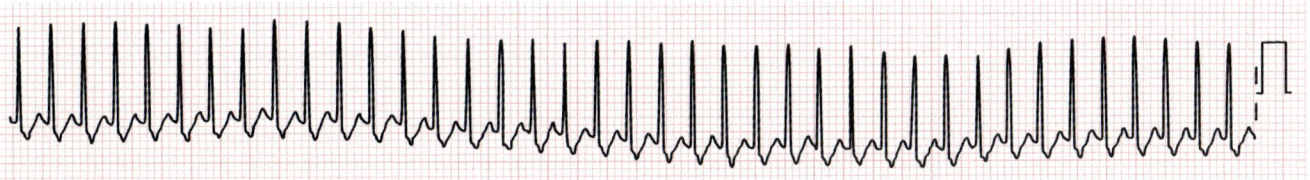

Fig. 11.50 ECG of an infant with SVT (supraventricular tachycardia), requiring adenosine

11

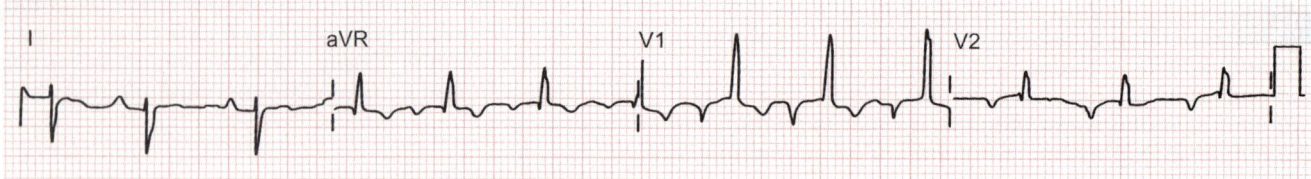

Fig. 11.51 ECG strip showing prolonged PR interval

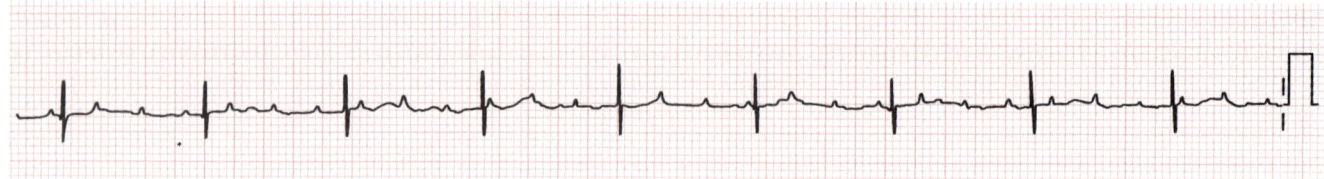

Fig. 11.52 ECG of a neonate with complete heart block

ventricular synchrony with 1:1 A-V conduction. It manifests as prolonged PR interval in ECG (Fig. 11.51). It can occur due to congenital heart disease like Ebstein anomaly, endocardial cushion defect; acute rheumatic fever; myocarditis; or due to drug toxicity like digoxin. It is generally asymptomatic condition and treatment is not required unless drug toxicity is suspected.

Second Degree Heart Block

In *second degree heart block*, few P waves are not conducted and few are conducted to ventricles. In *Mobitz type I* heart block (*Wenckebach phenomenon*) there occurs progressively increasing PR interval such that one P is not followed by QRS, and this cycle repeats. It occurs in myocarditis, cardiomyopathy, and in postsurgical patients. It generally does not progress. Underlying cause should be treated. Unlike Mobitz type I which has variable conduction block, Mobitz type II has fixed conduction block. In Mobitz type II heart block there is 2:1 or 3:1 block, *ie*, each QRS complex occurs after 2 or 3 P waves. It may progress to third degree heart block. Sometimes pacemaker implantation is required.

Third Degree Heart Block

Third degree heart block is also called complete heart block. There is complete dissociation between the atria and ventricles with no impulse being conducted from atria to ventricles. Both the atria and ventricles contract independent of each other. Atrial pacemaker may be located anywhere in atria, ie, SA node or any ectopic atrial focus. Ventricular pacemaker may be located at His bundle or more distally in bundle branches.

ECG shows constant P-P interval and constant R-R interval. But there is no synchronicity between occurrence of P waves and QRS complexes (Fig. 11.52).

- *Congenital* complete heart block may occur due to maternal autoimmune conditions (SLE, Sjogren syndrome). It has narrow QRS morphology as the block occurs above the level of bundle of His.
- *Acquired* complete heart block can occur after cardiac surgery, diphtheria, cardiomyopathy, myocarditis, prosthetic valves compressing on conduction tissue. It has wide QRS morphology as the block occurs more distally below the bundle of His.

Children may be asymptomatic if the ventricular rate is sufficient for maintaining cardiac output. If patient is symptomatic due to heart block (low ventricular rate, dizziness, syncopal attacks, low cardiac output, ventricular dysfunction, heart failure), pacemaker implantation has to be done.

3. Bundle Branch Block

It is due to blocked conduction at right or left bundle branches. In RBBB (right bundle branch block) activation of right ventricle occurs after that of left ventricle. There is RSR´ pattern in V1 with prolonged QRS duration. It can occur in postoperative state after right ventriculotomy or myocarditis. In LBBB (left bundle branch block) activation of left ventricle occurs after that of right ventricle. There is wide slurred R or RSR´ in V5-6. LBBB is always pathological and occurs postoperative, in hypertrophic cardiomyopathy, and in myocarditis.

Table 11.11 summarizes the diagnostic criteria and treatment for common types of arrhythmias.

Brugada J, Blom N, Sarquella-Brugada G, et al; European Heart Rhythm Association.; Association for European Paediatric and Congenital Cardiology. Pharmacological and non-pharmacological therapy for arrhythmias in the pediatric population: EHRA and AEPC-Arrhythmia Working Group joint consensus statement. *Europace*. 2013;15(9):1337-82.

Srinivasan C. Diagnosis and acute management of tachy-arrhythmias in children. *Indian J Pediatr*. 2015;82(12):1157–63.

Rhythm disorder	Diagnostic characteristic	Treatment
Table 11.11 Diagnostic Criteria and Treatment for Common Types of Arrhythmias		
Tachyarrhythmias		
1. Sinus tachycardia	• P:QRS 1:1 • Each P wave is followed by QRS complex • Normal P and QRS axis • Normal P and QRS morphology	• Treat underlying cause
2. Atrial tachycardia	• P:QRS 1:1 or 2:1 or 3:1 • Each P wave is followed by QRS complex; but may be blocked sometimes • Abnormal P axis and morphology • Normal QRS axis and morphology	• Beta blockers and calcium channel blockers for rate control • Class IA, IC, III drugs for long term use • Radiofrequency ablation (RFA) for refractory cases
3. AVRT/AVNRT	• P:QRS 1:1 • P wave may occur on the QRS complex or just after it • P morphology and axis is abnormal • QRS axis and morphology is normal	• Vagal maneuvers (ice pack application, Valsalva) • Adenosine 0.1 mg/kg rapid bolus. Can be repeated up to three times • Beta blockers to prevent recurrence • RFA, if high frequency or poor medical control in older patient
4. Ventricular tachycardia	• P:QRS ≤ 1:1 • Wide QRS complex • Abnormal QRS axis	• Lignocaine • Correct electrolytes • Inj Magnesium for Torsades • Amiodarone for refractory cases* • RFA if a focus is identified • ICD
Bradyarrhythmias		
1. Sinus bradycardia	• P:QRS 1:1 • Each P wave is followed by QRS complex • Normal P and QRS axis, morphology	• Not required in asymptomatic • Atropine to increase heart rate acutely • Pacemaker in symptomatic
2. First degree heart block	• P:QRS 1:1 • Each P wave is followed by QRS complex • Prolonged PR interval • Normal P and QRS axis, morphology	Not required
3. Second degree heart block *Mobitz type I (Wenckebach phenomenon)*	• P:QRS = 1:1 • Prolongation of PR interval with each successive beat, until there is a non-conducted P wave, the cycle repeats • Normal P and QRS axis • Normal P and QRS morphology	Not required
Mobitz type II	• P:QRS 2:1 or 3:1 • QRS complex occurs after 2 or 3 P waves • Normal P and QRS axis • Normal P and QRS morphology	Pacemaker implantation, as it has high chance of progression to third degree heart block
4. Third degree heart block	• Constant P-P and R-R interval • No relation between P and QRS • Normal P axis and morphology	Pacemaker implantation
Congenital *Acquired*	Normal QRS axis and morphology QRS duration is wide	
5. Bundle branch block	• P:QRS 1:1 • Each P wave is followed by QRS complex • Normal P axis and morphology	
RBBB LBBB	RSR′ pattern in V1-2 Broad slurred R or RSR′ pattern in V5–6	Not required Pacemaker or CRT if ventricular dysfunction

*If a patient with tachyarrhythmia presents in hemodynamically unstable state, cardioversion is done

Savitri Srivastava, Munesh Tomar, Updated and Revised by Sakshi Sachdeva and Piyush Gupta.

11

Disorders of Kidneys and Urinary Tract

12.1 ANATOMY AND PHYSIOLOGY OF KIDNEY

Kidneys maintain the volume and composition of body fluid by filtration of the blood and selective reabsorption or secretion of filtered solutes. They are located behind the peritoneum, on the posterior wall of the abdomen on each side of the vertebral column, at the level of 9–12th ribs. The left kidney is placed slightly higher in the abdomen than the right, due to the presence of the liver on right side.

The kidneys receive their blood supplies directly from the aorta via the renal arteries; blood from kidneys is returned to the inferior vena cava *via* the renal veins.

Urine excreted from the kidneys passes down the fibromuscular *ureters* and collects in the *bladder*. The bladder muscle (the *detrusor muscle*) is capable of distending to accept urine up to 700–1000 mL without high pressure damage to the renal system. When urine is passed, the *urethral sphincter* at the base of the bladder relaxes, the detrusor contracts and urine is voided *via* the *urethra***.**

ANATOMY

The kidney has a pale outer region, the *cortex* and a darker inner region, the *medulla*. The medulla is divided into 8–18 conical regions, called the *renal pyramids*.The base of each pyramid starts at the corticomedullary border and the apex ends in the *renal papilla* which merges to form the *renal pelvis* and then onto form the ureter. In humans, the renal pelvis is divided into two or three spaces, ie, the *major calyces*, which in turn divide into further *minor calyces*. The walls of the calyces, pelvis, and ureters are lined with smooth muscle that can contract to force urine towards the bladder by peristalsis (Fig. 12.1).

The cortex and the medulla are made up of nephrons, which are the functional units of the kidney. Each kidney contains about 1.3 million of nephrons (Fig. 12.2). Nephrons are responsible for ultrafiltration of the blood and reabsorption or excretion of products in the subsequent filtrate. Each nephron is made up of a filtering unit, the glomerulus, proximal convoluted tubule, loop of Henle and distal convoluted tubule. About 125 mL of filtrate is formed by the kidneys every minute as blood is filtered through the glomerulus. This filtration is uncontrolled.

The *proximal convoluted tubules* control absorption of glucose, sodium, water and other in this region.

The *loop of Henle* is responsible for concentration and dilution of urine by utilizing a counter-current multiplying

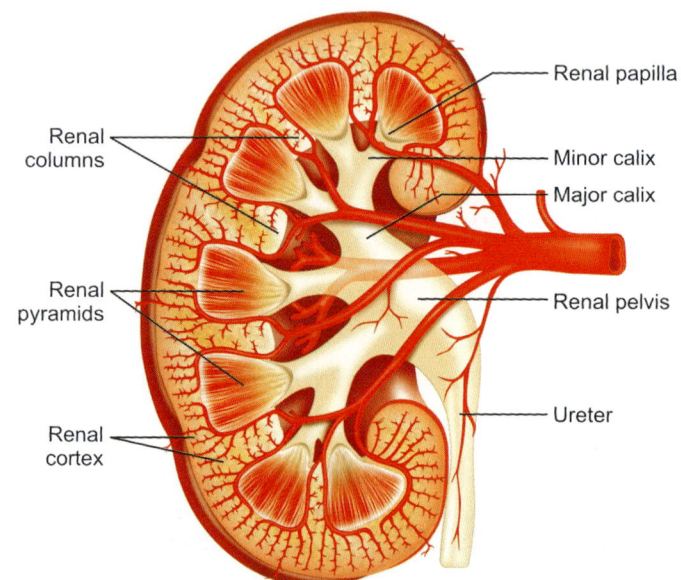

Fig. 12.1 Gross anatomy of the kidney

mechanism. It is water-impermeable but can pump sodium out, which in turn affects the osmolarity of the surrounding tissues and will affect the subsequent movement of water in or out of the water-permeable collecting duct.

The *distal convoluted tubule* is responsible for absorbing water back into the body; 99% of the water is normally reabsorbed, leaving highly concentrated urine to flow into the collecting duct and then into the renal pelvis.

Juxtaglomerular Apparatus

The *juxtaglomerular complex* consists of macula densa cells, which are special distal tubular epithelial cells, which detect chloride concentration and modified smooth muscle cells, juxtaglomerular cells, in the walls of the afferent and efferent arterioles. These cells produce renin.

Renin is an enzyme which converts the plasma protein angiotensinogen to angiotensin I. Angiotensin converting enzyme (ACE) which is formed in small quantities in the lungs, proximal tubule and other tissues, converts angiotensin I to angiotensin II, which causes vasoconstriction and an increase in blood pressure. Angiotensin II also stimulates the adrenal gland to produce aldosterone and causes water and sodium retention which together increase blood volume.

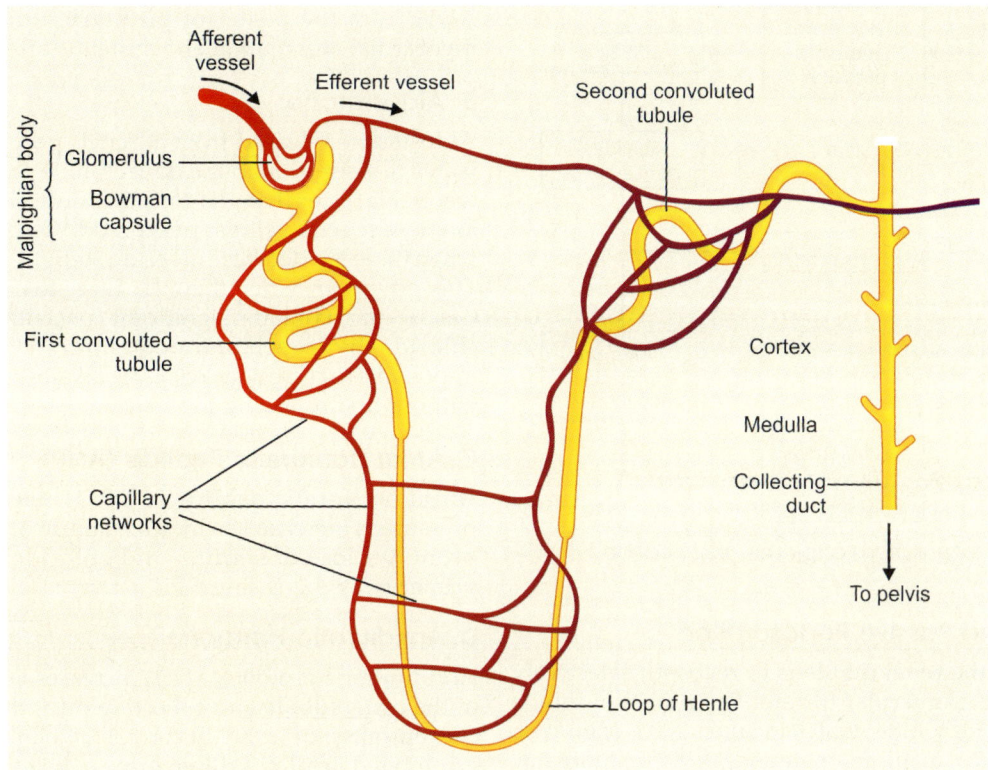

Fig. 12.2 Structure of the nephron

FUNCTIONS OF THE KIDNEY

- Regulation of the water and electrolyte content of the body.
- Retention of substances vital to the body such as protein and glucose.
- Maintenance of acid–base balance.
- Excretion of waste products, water-soluble toxic substances and drugs.
- Endocrine functions.

REGULATION OF THE WATER AND ELECTROLYTE

Renal blood supply is normally about 20% of the cardiac output. Approximately 99% of the blood flow goes to the cortex and 1% to the medulla. The cortex is the outer part of the kidney containing most of the nephrons. The medulla is the inner part of the kidney and contains the specialized nephrons in the juxtamedullary region, immediately next to the medulla. These nephrons have a greater concentrating ability.

The kidney is unique as it has two capillary beds arranged in series, the glomerular capillaries which are under high pressure for filtering and the peritubular capillaries which are situated around the tubule and are at low pressure (Fig. 12.3). This permits large volumes of fluid to be filtered and reabsorbed. Urine is formed as a result of a three-phase process: (*i*) Simple filtration; (*ii*) selective reabsorption; and (*iii*) passive reabsorption.

A. Filtration

Filtration takes place through the semipermeable walls of the glomerular capillaries, which are almost impermeable

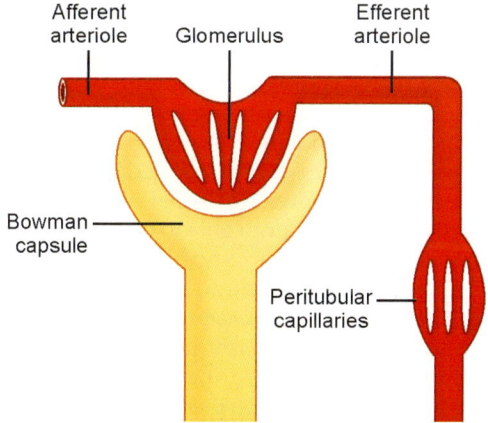

Fig. 12.3 Glomerular capillaries which are under high pressure for filtering and the peritubular capillaries

to proteins and large molecules. Glomerular filtrate is thus virtually free of protein and has no cellular elements. About 20% of renal plasma flow is filtered each minute (125 mL/min). This is called the glomerular filtration rate (GFR). The driving hydrostatic pressure is controlled by the afferent and efferent arterioles and provided by arterial pressure. This process is called *autoregulation*.

When there is a decrease in GFR, renin is released from the juxtaglomerular apparatus, which stimulates angiotensin II production causing constriction of the efferent arteriole (Fig. 12.4). Both these act to increase the hydrostatic pressure in the glomerular capillary bed and return GFR to normal.

12

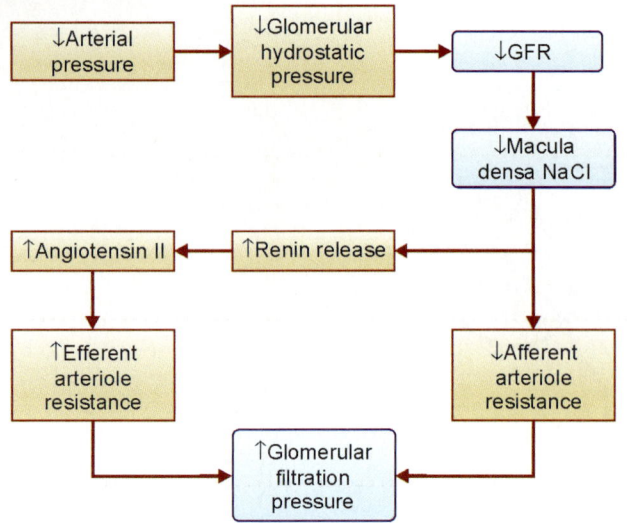

Fig. 12.4 Regulations of glomerular filtration

B. Selective and Passive Reabsorption

The function of the renal tubule is to reabsorb selectively about 99% of the glomerular filtrate. The proximal tubule reabsorbs 60% of all solutes, which includes 100% of glucose and amino acids, 90% of bicarbonate and 80–90% of inorganic phosphate and water. Reabsorption is by either active or passive transport.

Active transport requires energy to move solute against a concentration gradient. It is the main determinant of oxygen consumption by the kidney. Passive transport occurs down an electrochemical, pressure or concentration gradient. Most of the solute reabsorption is active with water being freely permeable and therefore moving by osmosis.

The final concentration of urine depends upon the amount of antidiuretic hormone (ADH) secreted by the posterior lobe of the pituitary. In presence of ADH, the distal tubule and collecting duct become permeable to water. As the collecting duct passes through the medulla with a high solute concentration in the interstitium, the water moves out of the lumen of the duct and concentrated urine is formed. In the absence of ADH, the tubule is minimally permeable to water; also large quantity of dilute urine is formed.

There is a close link between the hypothalamus of the brain and the posterior pituitary. There are cells within the hypothalamus, osmoreceptors, which are sensitive to changes in osmotic pressure of the blood. If there is low water intake, there is a rise in osmotic pressure of the blood and *vice versa*. Nerve impulses from the hypothalamus stimulate the posterior pituitary to produce ADH, when the osmotic pressure of the blood rises. As a result, water loss in the kidney is reduced and water gets reabsorbed in the collecting duct.

KIDNEY AND THE HORMONES

A. Renin

Renin increases the production of angiotensin II which is released when there is a fall in intravascular volume, eg, hemorrhage and dehydration. Angiotensin II leads to constriction of the efferent arteriole to maintain GFR, release of aldosterone from the adrenal cortex, increased release of

ADH from the posterior pituitary, thirst and inotropic myocardial stimulation and systemic arterial constriction.

B. Aldosterone

Aldosterone released from adrenals promotes sodium and water reabsorption in the distal tubule and collecting duct, where Na^+ is exchanged for potassium (K^+) and hydrogen ions by a specific cellular pump. Aldosterone is also released when there is a decrease in serum sodium ion concentration. This can occur, when there are large losses of gastric juice. Gastric juice contains significant concentrations of sodium, chloride, hydrogen and potassium ions. Therefore, it is impossible to correct the resulting alkalosis and hypokalemia without first replacing the sodium.

C. Atrial Natriuretic Peptide (ANP)

Atrial natriuretic peptide (ANP) is released when atrial pressure is increased as in heart failure or fluid overload. It promotes loss of sodium and chloride ions and water, primarily by increasing GFR.

D. Antidiuretic Hormone

Antidiuretic hormone (ADH) increases water permeability of the distal tubule and collecting duct, thus increasing the concentration of urine. In contrast, when secretion of ADH is inhibited, it allows dilute urine to be formed. This occurs mainly when plasma sodium concentration falls leading to stimulation of osmoreceptors. The hormones interact when blood loss or dehydration occurs to maintain intravascular volume.

E. Vitamin D

Other substances produced by the kidney are 1,25-dihydroxy-vitamin D (the most active form of vitamin D) which promotes calcium absorption from the gut and erythropoietin which stimulates *red cell production*.

F. Erythropoietin

It is produced by kidney and helps in erythropoiesis and maintains hemoglobin level in presence of other hematopoietic factors.

MEASUREMENT OF RENAL FUNCTION

A simple means of estimating renal function is to measure pH, blood urea nitrogen, creatinine and basic electrolytes (including sodium, potassium, chloride, and bicarbonate). Other tests and ratios involved in estimating renal functions are mentioned in **Table 12.1**.

Glomerular Filtration Rate

The glomerular filtration rate (GFR) is calculated by product of urine concentration of a substance (mg/dL) and urine flow rate (mL/min), divided by plasma concentration of substance (mg/dL). It is corrected to body surface of 1.73 m². The value is 40 mL/min/1.73 m² in term newborns and increases thereafter to adult values (100–120 mL/min/1.73 m²) by 2 years of life.

The level of plasma creatinine reflects muscle mass and its serum concentration is used to calculate GFR. The revised Schwartz formula for GFR is: 0.413 × height (cm)/serum

Table 12.1 Measurements of Renal Functions

Measurement	Calculation	Details
Renal plasma flow	$RPF = \dfrac{\text{effective RPF}}{\text{extraction ratio}}$	Volume of blood plasma delivered to the kidney per unit time. Para-aminohippuric acid (PAH) is a renal analysis tool used to provide an estimate
Renal blood flow	$RBF = \dfrac{RPF}{1 - HCT}$ (Hct is hematocrit)	Volume of blood delivered to the kidney per unit time. In humans, the kidneys together receive roughly 20% of cardiac output, amounting to 1 L/min in a 70 kg adult male
Glomerular filtration rate	$GFR = K_f \left([P_C - P_i] - \sigma[\pi_C - \pi_i] \right)$	Volume of fluid filtered from the renal glomerular capillaries into the Bowman's capsule per unit time. Estimated using inulin. Usually a creatinine clearance test is performed but other markers, such as the plant polysaccharide inulin or radiolabelled EDTA, may be used as well
Filtration fraction	$FF = \dfrac{GFR}{RPF}$	Measures efficiency of reabsorption
Anion gap	$AG = [Na^+] - ([Cl^-] + [HCO_3^-])$	Cations minus anions. Excludes K^+ (usually), Ca^{2+}, $H_2PO_4^-$. Aids in the differential diagnosis of metabolic acidosis
Clearance (other than water)	$C = \dfrac{UV}{P}$ where U = concentration, V = urine volume/time, U*V = urinary excretion, and P = plasma concentration	Rate of removal
Free water clearance	$C = V - C_{osm}$ or $V - \dfrac{U_{osm}}{P_{osm}} V_{CH_2O}$	The volume of blood plasma that is cleared of solute-free water per unit time
Net acid excretion	$NEA = V \left(U_{NH_4} + U_{TA} - U_{HCO_3} \right)$	Net amount of acid excreted in the urine per unit time

creatinine (mg/dL). It is useful when muscle mass is normal and renal function is stable and GFR is in the range of 15–75 mL/ 1.73 m^2/min.

ACID–BASE FUNCTION

The pH in the body is kept under tight control as almost all enzyme activities in the body are dependent on the pH. The lungs and kidneys work together to produce a normal extracellular fluid and arterial pH of 7.35–7.45. Carbon dioxide (CO_2), when dissolved in the blood is an acid and is excreted by the lungs. The buffer, sodium bicarbonate is filtered by the glomerulus and then reabsorbed in the proximal tubule. The sodium is absorbed by a sodium/ hydrogen ion pump (Na^+/H^+) exchanging Na^+ for H^+ on the luminal proximal border of the tubular cell. A sodium/ potassium pump (Na^+/K^+) forces Na^+ through the cell from tubular fluid in exchange for potassium. The H^+, released as the tubular secretion of acid (above), forms carbonic acid with the bicarbonate (HCO_3^-).

$$H^+ + HCO_3^- <=> H_2CO_3 <=> H_2O + CO_2$$

Carbonic anhydrase, found in the proximal tubular cells, catalyses the reaction to carbon dioxide (CO_2) and water (H_2O). The CO_2 diffuses into the cell where it again forms carbonic acid in the presence of carbonic anhydrase. The carbonic acid ionises to H^+ and HCO_3^-. The H^+ is then pumped out of the cell back to the lumen of the tubule by the Na^+/H^+ pump and the sodium is returned to the plasma by the Na^+/K^+ pump. Water is absorbed passively. Other buffers include inorganic phosphate (HPO_4^-), urate and creatinine ions, which are excreted in urine as acid when combined with H^+ ions secreted in the distal nephron.

Ammonia is produced enzymatically from glutamine and other amino acids and is secreted in the tubules. Ammonia (NH_3) combines with secreted H^+ ions to form a non-diffusible ammonium ion (NH_4^+) which is excreted in the urine. Ammonia production is increased in severe metabolic acidosis up to 700 mmol/day.

EXCRETION OF WASTE PRODUCTS

The filtration of waste products occurs as blood flows through the glomerulus. Some substances not required by the body and some foreign materials (eg, drugs) may not be cleared by filtration through the glomerulus. Such substances are cleared by secretion into the tubule and excreted from the body in the urine.

12

Anatomy and Physiology of Kidney

1. Glomerular filtration rate gradually increases after birth and reaches adult level by 2 years of age.
2. Major functions of kidneys are to maintain fluid and electrolyte balance, acid–base homeostasis, and removal of nitrogenous waste products from the body.
3. Erythropoietin is produced by kidney and second hydroxylation of vitamin D also takes place in the kidney producing 1,25-dihydroxycholecalciferol.
4. Revised Schwartz formula (0.413 × height (cm)/serum creatinine (mg/dL) is useful for calculation of glomerular filtration rate in children with chronic kidney disease.

12.2 URINARY TRACT INFECTIONS

Urinary tract infection (UTI) is common in infancy and childhood and may be the first sign of an underlying urinary tract abnormality. Failing to identify and treat UTI may cause progressive renal damage, resulting in scarring in around 10–40% of children. Renal damage can have grave consequences like poor renal growth, impaired glomerular function, hypertension, and end stage renal disease.

DEFINITION

Urinary tract infection is identified by growth of a significant number (usually, $>10^5$ in a clean catch mid-stream sample) of organisms of a single species in the urine, in the presence of symptoms. To establish the diagnosis of UTI, clinicians should require urinalysis demonstrating both *pyuria* and the presence of a *positive urine culture*.

PREVALENCE

In the first year of life, UTI is more common in boys (3.7%) than in girls (2%). Later, the incidence changes, with UTI becoming more common in prepubertal girls (3%) compared to prepubertal boys (1%). The rate of UTI for uncircumcised boys is 4 to 20 times higher than that for circumcised boys.

CLASSIFICATION

A. Classification according to Site

- *Cystitis (infection of the lower urinary tract)* Cystitis refer to inflammation of the urinary bladder mucosa, usually associated with symptoms like dysuria, stranguria, frequency, urgency, incontinence, hematuria, and suprapubic pain. These symptoms are rarely observed in newborns and infants.
- *Pyelonephritis (infection of the upper urinary tract)* This is a diffuse infection of the renal pelvis and parenchyma. The child usually presents with symptoms including fever ≥39°C, loin pain and systemic toxicity. Infants and young children may have nonspecific signs such as poor appetite, lethargy, irritability, vomiting, or diarrhea.

B. Classification according to Episode

- *First episode of UTI*
- *Recurrent UTI* Second and all subsequent episodes of UTI

C. Classification according to Symptoms

- *Asymptomatic bacteriuria* This refers to significant bacteriuria in the absence of symptoms of UTI and absence of leucocytes in urine. It indicates colonization of the bladder by non-virulent bacteria that are incapable of activating a symptomatic response. *The key to distinguishing true UTI from asymptomatic bacteriuria is the presence of pyuria.* Asymptomatic bacteriuria is a benign condition, which does not cause renal injury and should not be treated. Eradication of these organisms is often followed by symptomatic infection with more virulent strains.
- *Symptomatic UTI* When UTI is associated with specific voiding symptoms, suprapubic pain, or non-specific symptoms like fever, vomiting, and poor appetite without any obvious focus of infection.

D. Classification according to Complicating Factors

- *Simple UTI* UTI with low grade fever, dysuria, frequency, urgency without features of complicated UTI.
- *Complicated UTI* Presence of fever >39°C, systemic toxicity, persistent vomiting, dehydration, renal angle tenderness, and raised creatinine.

In view of the risk of renal parenchymal damage associated with delayed treatment, UTI in children, for all practical purposes, is considered to involve the upper tract and should be treated promptly. The distinction between simple and complicated UTI is necessary because it has implications for therapy.

ETIOLOGY

Escherichia coli is the most common cause of community acquired urinary tract infections (80% cases). Other common organisms causing UTI include Gram-negative organisms like *Klebsiella*, *Proteus*, *Enterococcus*, *Citrobacter*, *Salmonella* and Gram-positive organisms like *Staphylococcus aureus*, *Streptococcus faecalis*, and *Enterococcus*. Infection with *Candida* may be seen in immunocompromised children or neonates in intensive care settings, receiving prolonged antibiotic therapy.

PATHOGENESIS

Urinary tract infection is usually an ascending infection from urethra to bladder and the kidneys. Therefore, the fecal flora predominates. In newborn infants however, the spread may be hematogenous.

PREDISPOSING FACTORS

- *Sex* Boys younger than 1 year of age are vulnerable. *After infancy*, girls tend to have a higher incidence of UTI. They have a shorter urethra that puts them at higher risk of retrograde infection. Uncircumcised boys also carry a higher risk of UTI if the prepuce is not retracted and cleaned regularly.
- *Urethral instrumentation* Catheterization of urethra, if done in a non-sterile technique or if kept for prolonged periods (as in intensive care settings) predisposes to UTI. However, in those children who require prolonged catheterization, it is recommended not to routinely change catheters, unless there is obstruction or any other significant reason. Routine

change of urinary catheters result in micro-traumas which predispose to UTI.

- *Obstructive uropathy* Congenital anomalies leading to obstruction to outflow of urine cause urinary stasis within the urinary tract that serves as a good medium for bacterial multiplication and subsequent UTI.
- *Bladder bowel dysfunction (BBD)* Infrequent voiding which may be functional or secondary to underlying defects of bladder also leads to urinary stasis and subsequent UTI. Constipation is a common predisposing cause of UTI in children.
- *Vesicourethral reflux* This is the most significant risk-factor predisposing to upper UTI. It is discussed in detail later.

CLINICAL FEATURES

Neonates Newborns with pyelonephritis or urosepsis usually present with nonspecific symptoms like failure to thrive, jaundice, vomiting, hyperexcitability, lethargy, or hypothermia.

Infants Young children, especially those less than 2 years of age may present with fever without a focus, or fever with excessive cry, diarrhea, or vomiting.

Older children They present with lower urinary tract symptoms including dysuria, stranguria, frequency, urgency, incontinence, or suprapubic pain. Fever, systemic toxicity, flank pain or renal angle tenderness suggest an upper urinary tract involvement. Recent onset of enuresis or foul-smelling/turbid urine should also alert to the possibility of UTI.

PHYSICAL EXAMINATION

A complete physical examination is required to exclude any other source of fever. When UTI is suspected, one should search for signs of constipation, palpable or painful kidneys, palpable bladder, stigmata of spina bifida or sacral agenesis. The genitalia should be examined for phimosis, labial adhesion, post-circumcision meatal stenosis, abnormal urogenital confluence, cloacal malformations, vulvitis, or epididymoorchitis.

DIAGNOSIS

A. Urine Sampling

Urine sample must be collected before any antimicrobial agent is given. Care must be taken to adhere to the right technique of obtaining urine for urinalysis or culture, as this affects the rate of contamination and influences the interpretation of the results.

Newborns, infants, and non-toilet-trained children **Suprapubic aspiration** is the most sensitive method for obtaining an uncontaminated urine sample. Ultrasound guidance may be used to demonstrate the presence of urine in the bladder. **Bladder catheterization** may be an alternative to suprapubic aspiration, although the rates of contamination are higher. A plastic bag attached to the genitalia has a high rate of contamination, and should therefore be discouraged.

Toilet-trained children In toilet-trained children, a **clean voided midstream urine sample** has a good rate of accuracy.

The genitalia should be cleaned beforehand to reduce the contamination rate.

B. Urinalysis

1. Urine Microscopy

The specimen must be fresh (within 1 hour after voiding maintained at room temperature or < 4 hours after voiding with refrigeration) to ensure sensitivity and specificity of the urinalysis.

- *Significant pyuria* is defined as >10 leukocytes per mm^3 in a fresh uncentrifuged sample, or >5 leukocytes per high power field in a centrifuged sample.
- Pyuria may also occur in conditions such as fever, glomerulonephritis, renal stones or presence of foreign body in the urinary tract. *Pyuria in the absence of significant bacteriuria is not sufficient to diagnose UTI*.

2. Rapid Dipstick-based Tests

The dipstick tests that have commonly been used include the biochemical analyses of leukocyte esterase and nitrite. They indicate the presence of leukocyte esterase (as a surrogate marker for pyuria) and urinary nitrite (which is converted from dietary nitrates in the presence of most gram-negative enteric bacteria in the urine).

Urine nitrite test The conversion of dietary nitrates to nitrites by bacteria requires approximately 4 hours in the bladder. Hence, this test is not a sensitive marker for children, particularly infants, who empty their bladders frequently. Negative nitrite test results do not rule out UTI. Moreover, not all urinary pathogens reduce nitrate to nitrite. The test is helpful when the result is positive because it is highly specific.

Leukocyte esterase test The reported sensitivity of this test in various studies is around 83% while its specificity is much lower at around 72%, which reflects the non-specificity of pyuria. False-positive results are seen in conditions other than UTI where pyuria may occur, like fever resulting from any condition, after vigorous exercise, glomerulonephritis, renal stones, etc.

C. Urine Culture

The diagnosis of UTI is made on the basis of quantitative urine culture results in addition to evidence of pyuria. Urine specimens should be processed promptly. If this is not possible, then it should be refrigerated at 4°C for up to 12–24 hours, to prevent the growth of organisms that can occur in urine at room temperature. Also, specimens that require transportation to another site for processing, should be transported on ice.

Urine culture results are considered positive or negative on the basis of the method of collection and the number of colony forming units (CFUs) that grow on the culture medium (**Table 12.2**). The cut off for significant colony counts differs with different methods of urine collection because the same organism which colonizes the distal urethra and periurethral region may cause UTI. Thus, a low colony count may be present in a specimen obtained through voiding or catheterization when bacteria are actually not present in bladder urine.

Table 12.2 Colony Count Criteria for the Diagnosis of UTI

Method of collection of urine	Colony count
Suprapubic aspiration	Any number of organism
Urethral catheterization	>50,000 CFU*/mL
Mid-stream, clean catch	>10^5 CFU*/mL

*CFU—colony forming unit; *Source*: Guidelines of the Indian Society of Pediatric Nephrology

Treatment — Urinary Tract Infection

A. Treatment of UTI

Children less than 3 months of age and those with complicated UTI should be hospitalized and treated with parenteral antibiotics. Treatment should be promptly started, after collecting urine sample for investigations.

Children above 3 months of age with simple UTI should be treated with oral antibiotics. There is no need for parenteral antibiotics in simple UTI

Antimicrobials for Treatment of UTI

The choice of antibiotic should be guided by local antimicrobial sensitivity patterns and may be adjusted later according to sensitivity testing results. A third generation cephalosporin (cefotaxime or ceftriaxone) is preferred. A list of antibiotics along with their dosages and schedule is provided in **Table 12.3**.

Duration of Treatment

The duration of therapy is 10–14 days for infants and children with complicated UTI and 7–10 days for uncomplicated UTI.

In those receiving parenteral therapy, once the child shows clinical improvement with resolution of fever and toxicity (usually within 24 to 48 hours), the route of administration of antimicrobials can be changed to oral to complete the course of therapy.

With successful treatment, urine usually becomes sterile after 24 hours and leukocyturia normally disappears within 3–4 days.

Indications of Repeat Urine Culture

A repeat urine culture is not necessary, unless there is persistence of fever and toxicity despite 72 hours of adequate antibiotic therapy. In patients with prolonged fever and lack of clinical improvement, treatment resistant uropathogens or the presence

Table 12.3 Antibiotics for Treatment of Urinary Tract Infection in Children

Antibiotic	Dose (mg/kg/day)
Parenteral	
Ceftriaxone	75–100 (2 divided doses)
Cefotaxime	100–150 (2–3 divided doses)
Amikacin	10–15 (single daily dose)
Gentamicin	5–6 (single daily dose)
Ampicillin	100 (in 3 divided doses)
Oral medications	
Cefixime	8–10 (in 2 divided doses)
Co-amoxyclav	Amoxycillin 30–40 (in 3 divided doses)
Ciprofloxacin	15–20 (in 2 divided doses)
Ofloxacin	15–20 (in 2 divided doses)
Cephalexin	50–70 (in 2–3 divided doses)
Cotrimoxazole	6–10 (of trimethoprim) (2 divided doses)

of congenital uropathy or urinary tract obstruction should be considered. In such cases, immediate ultrasound examination is necessary.

Supportive Therapy

- Maintenance of adequate hydration by encouraging a liberal fluid intake which also helps to alleviate dysuria.
- Antipyretics are used to relieve fever.
- Alkalinization of urine is not necessary.

B. Evaluation After the First UTI

In India, the diagnosis of UTI is often missed or delayed as underlying congenital urogenital anomalies remain undetected due to absence of routine antenatal ultrasound in pregnant women. Hence, it is recommended that all children with the first UTI should undergo radiological evaluation to rule out underlying congenital abnormalities or renal parenchymal damage (**Table 12.4**).

- *Infants <1 year* All infants with UTI should be screened by ultrasonography, followed by micturating cystourethrography (MCU) and DMSA (dimercaptosuccinic acid) scintigraphy.
- *Older children (1–5 years old)* These children should undergo ultrasonography and DMSA scan. Significant reflux and scars or urinary tract anomalies are likely to be obvious on ultrasonography or scintigraphy. MCU should be done only in those children having abnormalities on either of the above investigations.
- *Children older than 5 years* They require to be evaluated by ultrasonography alone. Further investigations (DMSA and MCU) are necessary only if this is abnormal.
- In children with recurrent UTI all three investigations (USG, MCU and DMSA) should be done.

Urinary Tract Ultrasonography

An ultrasonogram provides information on kidney size, number, location, presence of hydronephrosis, dilatation of ureters, urinary bladder anomalies and post-void residual urine. Ultrasonography should be done soon after the diagnosis of UTI.

Renal Scintigraphy

DMSA scintigraphy is a sensitive technique for detecting renal parenchymal infection and cortical scarring. Patients having hydronephrosis without any evidence of VUR should be evaluated by diuretic renography using 99mTc-labeled diethylenetriamine penta-acetic acid (DTPA) or mercaptoacetylglycine (MAG-3). These techniques assess the renal function and give an idea about obstructive/non-obstructive drainage. DMSA scan should be carried out 2–3 months after the diagnosis and treatment of UTI.

Micturating Cystourethrogram (MCU)

MCU detects vesicoureteric reflux (VUR) and provides anatomical details regarding the bladder and the urethra. MCU should be done 2–3 weeks after UTI.

Indications

- All children below 1year of age with their first attack of UTI.
- All children between 1 and 5 years if ultrasound and/or DMSA scan are abnormal and in children above 5 years, if ultrasound is abnormal.

Precautions

MCU should be done under cover of prophylactic antibiotics, in order to prevent infection following catheterization.

- Amoxicillin is administered orally in a dose of 50 mg/kg, 1 hour before the procedure and 25 mg/kg 6 hours later.
- Gentamicin (2–3 mg/kg) may be given 30 minutes before the MCU by intramuscular route.

Table 12.4 Radiological Investigations After First Episode of Urinary Tract Infection			
Age group	Radiological investigations which are mandatory	Timing of investigations post-UTI	Additional radiological investigations
<1 year	i. Ultrasonography of kidneys, ureters and bladder ii. Micturating cystourethrography iii. DMSA scan	Just after UTI 2–3 weeks after UTI 2–3 months after UTI	None
1–5 years	i. Ultrasonography of kidneys, ureters and bladder ii. DMSA scan	Just after UTI 2–3 months after UTI	If either USG or DMSA is abnormal, MCU should be done
>5 years	i. Ultrasonography of kidneys, ureters and bladder	Just after UTI	If USG is abnormal, both MCU and DMSA should be done

Table 12.5 Antimicrobials for Prophylaxis of Urinary Tract Infection		
Drug	Dosage (mg/kg/d)	Remarks
Cotrimoxazole	2 (trimethoprim) + 10 (sulphamethoxazole) bedtime dose	Avoid in infants <3 months of age and G6PD as single deficiency
Nitrofurantoin	1–2 as single daily dose	Gastrointestinal upset. Avoid in infants <3 months of age, G6PD deficiency and renal insufficiency
Cephalexin	10 as single daily dose	Drug of choice in first 3–6 months of life

C. Prevention of Recurrent Urinary Tract Infection

Parents should encourage their children to have adequate fluid intake and regular voiding with complete emptying of bladder each time. Constipation should be avoided. Parents should be instructed to seek prompt medical evaluation (ideally within 48 hours) in case of future febrile illnesses, to ensure that recurrent infections can be detected and treated promptly.

Bowel Bladder Dysfunction

Children often have a voiding disorder, characterized by abnormal patterns of micturition without any neuronal or congenital anatomical abnormalities. These children have associated constipation. Such a functional voiding disorder along with constipation is known as bowel bladder dysfunction (BBD). Recurrent UTI is common in such children.

D. Prophylaxis for Urinary Tract Infection

Antibiotic prophylaxis (long-term, low dose) is recommended to prevent recurrent febrile UTI episodes in following situations:
  i. UTI below 1 year of age, while awaiting imaging studies,
  ii. Children with vesicoureteral reflux (VUR)
  iii. Children with frequent febrile UTI (3 or more episodes in an year).

The commonly used drugs for prophylaxis include cotrimoxazole, nitrofurantoin and cefalexin, usually as a single bedtime dose, which is one-fourth of regular dose (**Table 12.5**).

Antibiotic prophylaxis is not required in patients with urinary tract obstruction (e.g., posterior urethral valves), urolithiasis, and neurogenic bladder, and in patients on clean intermittent catheterization. In case of breakthrough UTI, change of the medication being used for prophylaxis is usually not necessary. Also, there is no role for antibiotic cycling for prophylaxis.

Follow-up Children on antibiotic prophylaxis are kept on close follow-up for occurrence of breakthrough UTI. An MCU is repeated after 12–18 months to evaluate for resolution of reflux. A DMSA scan is repeated, in patients having breakthrough UTI, to detect fresh renal scarring.

E. Vesicoureteric Reflux

Vesicoureteral reflux refers to backward flow of urine from the bladder into ureters. If urine is infected, it facilitates the movement of bacteria from the bladder to upper urinary tract and cause renal parenchymal infection. VUR is found in 30–50% children and 40–50% infants presenting with UTI. Its severity is graded using the International Study Classification from Grade I to V.

Conventional therapy for VUR has been antibiotic prophylaxis and surgical intervention. However, systematic reviews have concluded that the outcomes following surgical repair *versus* prophylaxis were similar in terms of the number of breakthrough UTI and risk of renal scarring. A recent multicentric, randomized, placebo-controlled trial showed that antimicrobial prophylaxis given to children with vesicoureteral reflux after the first or second urinary tract infection resulted in a substantially reduced risk of recurrence of UTI, but did not reduce the risk of future renal scarring.

The schedule of antibiotic prophylaxis as recommended by ISPN is shown in **Table 12.6**. In children with Grade III–V VUR, repeat imaging should be done after 18–36 months. In such children radionuclide cystogram, with lower radiation exposure is preferred for follow-up evaluation.

Table 12.6 Recommended Duration of Antibiotic Prophylaxis for Vesicoureteric Reflux (VUR)
Grade I and II
• Antibiotic prophylaxis till the age of 1 year.
• If breakthrough febrile UTI occurs, antibiotics to be re-started
Grade III, IV, V
• Antibiotic prophylaxis to continue till 5 years of age.
• If breakthrough febrile UTI occurs, surgery is to be considered.
• Prophylaxis is to be continued after 5 years of age if bowel bladder dysfunction is present

12

Case Study | Urinary Tract Infection

A 20-month-old boy was brought with fever for 4 days, associated with vomiting and poor feeding. The child was sick looking with temperature of 39°C. No other abnormal findings were observed.

In such a child without any focus for fever, if you suspect urinary tract infection, what additional points will you ask in history?

If we suspect UTI, we should enquire about the infant's urinary stream—whether he has a poor stream, whether urine stream is interrupted, whether he appears to have difficulty and seems to apply undue pressure while micturition, whether urine flows in drops, instead of a good projectile stream. These features would be suggestive of bladder outlet obstruction like posterior urethral valve (the most common congenital cause of obstructive uropathy in boys), which is known to cause urinary retention, secondary vesicoureteric reflux, and pyelonephritis.

Further, we should enquire about constipation. We should also enquire about any weakness in lower limbs since birth, any history of lumbosacral spine surgery which would suggest neurogenic bladder. Additionally, any document of antenatal ultrasound should be asked for, to look for any congenital urogenital anomaly.

How will you collect urine sample from this child? What investigations will you ask for and how will you send the samples? How will you confirm the diagnosis of UTI?

As the child is 20 months old, he is not expected to be toilet-trained. So collecting a mid-stream, clean-catch specimen is not possible. Urine should be collected by catheterization.

Two samples of urine should be collected and sent for microscopy and culture. The urine samples must be sent fresh for urinalysis and should be plated for culture within 2 hours. If delay is inevitable, the samples should be refrigerated and can be kept up to 12–24 hours.

Urinary tract infection will be confirmed if both the following are present:
i. Urine microscopy showing leukocytes >5/high power field in a centrifuged sample
ii. Urine culture showing growth of a single organism with >50,000 CFU/mL (colony forming unit)

What further investigations should be done in this child after confirmation of UTI? When should these investigations be done?

As per Indian Society of Pediatric Nephrology (ISPN) guidelines, this child, belonging to the age group 1–5 years needs to be evaluated by ultrasonography of kidneys and urinary tract, as well as a DMSA scan. The ultrasonography should be done soon after the urinary tract infection. DMSA scan should be done at least after 3 months. If either of the above investigations reveals some abnormalities, the child should also undergo a micturating cystourethrogram.

Hoberman A, Chesney RW. RIVUR Trial Investigators. Antimicrobial prophylaxis for children with vesicoureteral reflux. *N Engl J Med*. 2014;371:1072–3.

Indian Society of Pediatric Nephrology, Vijayakumar M, Kanitkar M, Nammalwar BR, Bagga A. Revised statement on management of urinary tract infections. *Indian Pediatr*. 2011;48:709–17.

Revision Point

Urinary Tract Infections

1. The diagnosis of urinary tract infection is made only when both significant pyuria (>5 white cells/hpf) and significant bacteriuria (>10^5 CFU/mL of a single organism, in a mid-stream clean-catch specimen of urine) are present.
2. In toilet-trained children, urine must be collected as a mid-stream clean-catch specimen for analysis. In children who are not toilet-trained, either a catheterized sample or a sample by suprapubic aspiration must be taken. Urine should never be collected from urobags for analysis.
3. For management purposes, UTI must be classified as *simple* or *complicated*, depending upon the presence or absence of fever, loin pain and toxicity.
4. If indicated, a micturating cystourethrogram should be done after 2–3 weeks and DMSA should be done 2–3 months following the episode of UTI.
5. Prophylaxis for UTI is required in i) infants <1 year of age awaiting all investigations, ii) presence of vesico-ureteral reflux, iii) recurrent UTI.

Mori R, Lakhanpaul M, Verrier-Jones K. Diagnosis and management of urinary tract infection in children: summary of NICE guidance. *BMJ*. 2007;335:395–7.

Stein R, Dogan HS, Hoebeke P, Koèvara R, *et al*. European Association of Urology; European Society for Pediatric Urology. Urinary tract infections in children: EAU/ESPU guidelines. *Eur Urol*. 2015;67:546–58.

Subcommittee on Urinary Tract Infection, Steering Committee on Quality Improvement and Management, Roberts KB. Urinary tract infection: clinical practice guideline for the diagnosis and management of initial UTI in febrile infants and children 2 to 24 months. *Pediatrics*. 2011;128:595–610.

12.3 HEMATURIA

DEFINITION AND ETIOLOGY

Hematuria refers to the presence of more than 5 red blood cells (RBCs) per µL in fresh uncentrifuged urine specimen or >5 per high power field in centrifuged specimen. Hematuria may be *gross* (visible to the naked eye) or *microscopic* (detected only on urine microscopy).

The incidence of gross hematuria has been reported as 0.13% and the majority has an easily recognizable and an apparent cause. Asymptomatic isolated microscopic hematuria occurs in 0.41 to 4% of school-aged children.

The causes of hematuria in children and newborn are given in **Tables 12.7 and 12.8**, and vary from benign (eg, urinary tract infection) to a serious one (malignancy).

PATHOPHYSIOLOGY

RBCs can originate from any point along the urinary tract but the most common site of bleeding is from the glomeruli. Thus, hematuria is usually classified as *glomerular* and *non-glomerular*.

Glomerular hematuria In glomerular disorders, RBCs cross the endothelial-epithelial barrier of the glomeruli and enter the capillary lumen through the discontinuities in the capillary wall, which leads to dysmorphism of the RBCs.

Table 12.7 Causes of Hematuria in Children	
Glomerular causes	*Non-glomerular causes*
Primary 1. Post-streptococcal glomerulonephritis (most common) 2. IgA nephropathy 3. Benign familial hematuria 4. Rapidly progressive glomerulonephritis 5. Membranoproliferative glomerulonephritis 6. Focal segmental glomerulosclerosis 7. Alport syndrome 8. Acute interstitial nephritis **Systemic** 1. Hemolytic uremic syndrome (HUS) 2. Henoch-Schönlein purpura (HSP) 3. Goodpasture syndrome 4. Systemic lupus erythematosus (SLE) 5. Polyarteritis nodosa 6. Thrombotic thrombocytopenic purpura 7. Systemic infections (malaria, leptospirosis, infective endocarditis, snake bite envenomation, DIC)	1. Urinary tract infection (most common) 2. Nephrolithiasis (most common) 3. Viral hemorrhagic cystitis 4. Hypercalciuria 5. Trauma 6. Tumors (Wilms tumor, rhabdoid tumors) 7. Tuberculosis 8. Strenuous exercise 9. *Vascular*: Renal artery/vein thrombosis, A-V malformations 10. *Anatomic abnormalities:* Ureteropelvic junction obstruction, posterior urethral valves, urethral diverticula/prolapse, autosomal dominant polycystic kidney disease, multicystic dysplastic kidney 11. Coagulopathies 12. *Hemoglobinopathies* Sickle cell disease 13. *Drugs* NSAID, cyclophosphamide, anticoagulants 14. Menstruation

Table 12.8 Causes of Hematuria in Newborn
1. Renal artery/vein thrombosis
2. Autosomal recessive polycystic kidney disease
3. Urinary tract infection
4. Obstructive uropathy
5. Coagulopathies
6. Trauma
7. Bladder catherization

During this passage, the morphology of RBC is modified (*dysmorphic RBCs*) by its intrinsic deformability, intra-glomerular capillary pressure, size of the gaps, thickness of the glomerular basement membrane, variation in urine pH, and osmotic pressure, and effects of the renal tubular enzymes.

Glomerular bleeding is usually smoky brown or coca cola colored due to hematin formation from hemoglobin in an acidic environment (Fig. 12.5). RBC cast develop when RBCs are entangled in the glomerular protein matrix.

Non-glomerular hematuria It is caused by direct injury to the tubulointerstitium by infections, stones, or ischemic necrosis of the papilla. Nonglomerular bleeding is usually bright red or pink in color (Fig. 12.6). The shape of RBCs remain normal (isomorphic RBC). RBC casts are absent.

Distinguishing features of glomerular versus non-glomerular hematuria are listed in **Table 12.9**.

EVALUATION OF A CHILD WITH HEMATURIA

Step 1

History and Physical Examination

Eliciting a good history helps us to narrow down the various etiologies of hematuria. The history should include the color of urine (smoky brown color or bright red color), onset, duration, frequency (recurrent: IgA nephropathy, Alport syndrome, thin glomerular basement membrane disease),

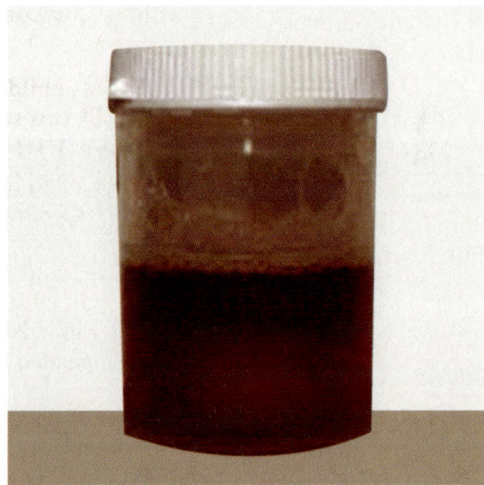

Fig. 12.5 Cola-colored urine in post-streptococcal glomerulo-nephritis

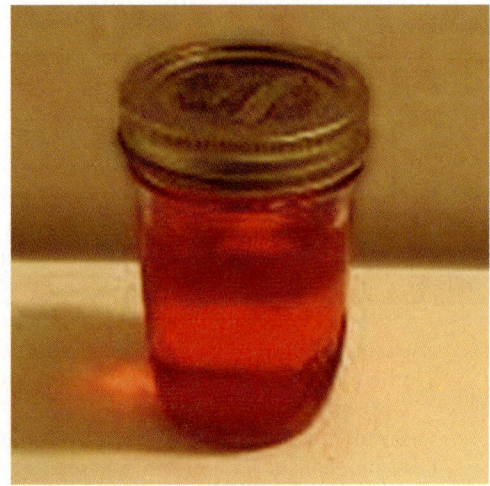

Fig. 12.6 Hematuria in a boy with vesical calculus

12

Table 12.9 Distinguishing Features of Glomerular from Non-glomerular Hematuria

Features	Glomerular hematuria	Non-glomerular hematuria
Color	Smoky brown or coca cola color	Bright red/pink color
Proteinuria	2+ or more	Less than 2+
Dysmorphic RBCs	More than 20%	Less than 15%
RBC cast	Present	Absent
Blood clots	Absent	May be present

with or without pain, timing of hematuria (hematuria at the onset of micturition suggests urethral bleeding, continuous hematuria throughout micturition suggests bleeding from ureter/kidneys), and terminal hematuria (at the end of urination) suggests bleeding from bladder. History should also differentiate true hematuria from other causes of red urine. Some of the causes of pseudohematuria are listed in **Box 12.1**.

Also elicit history of any recent trauma, strenuous exercise, headache, visual disturbances, seizures, and features of heart failure.

- History of sore throat or impetigo 2–4 weeks prior to the onset of hematuria favors post-streptococcal glomerulo-nephritis.
- History of fever, dysuria, flank pain that may radiate down to the groin favors urinary tract infection or nephro-lithiasis.

The physical examination should include measurement of blood pressure, assessment for edema and recent weight gain, abdomen examination for tenderness/masses, skin examination for rash/purpura/eczema, and examination of genitalia.

Step 2

Urine Analysis

Urine dipstick A positive test indicates presence of RBCs, hemoglobin, or myoglobin in urine. The reagent strip utilizes the pseudoperoxidase activity of hemoglobin or myoglobin to catalyse the reaction between hydrogen peroxide and the chromogen tetramethyl benzidine to produce an oxidized chromogen which has a ***green-blue color.*** It is important to briefly dip the strip in the urine, tap off excess urine and read the strip at the recommended time interval (usually 1 minute). The test can detect as small as 150 µg/L of hemoglobin in urine. Urine dipsticks have a sensitivity of 100% and specificity of 99%.

Microscopy A 10 mL of freshly voided urine, preferably passed in the morning, collected by mid-stream clean-catch method should be subjected for microscopic examination as

RBCs are better preserved in fresh concentrated and acidic urine. This urine is centrifuged at 3600 revolutions per minute for 5 minutes and the presence of more than 5 RBCs per high-power field (under 40X suggests microscopic hematuria). Identification of dysmorphic RBCs require light microscopy that can be confirmed by staining with Wright's stain or phase contrast microscopy. RBC morphology should be examined at least in 10 high power fields and the presence of more than 20% dysmorphic RBC is suggestive of glomerular hematuria (Fig. 12.7).

Step 3

Additional Investigations

Further evaluation is guided by the history, physical examination and initial urine analysis findings. Some of the investigations ordered are urine culture (UTI), Urine calcium-creatinine ratio (hypercalciuria), urine spot protein/creatine ratio or 24-hour urine protein excretion (glomerular hematuria), blood urea/serum ceratinine (renal failure), serum C3 (post-streptococcal glomerulonephritis), ASO titre (post streptococcal glomerulonephritis), antinuclear antibodies (SLE), USG abdomen and pelvis with Doppler (UTI, urolithiasis, tumors, anatomic abnormalities), CT

Case Study	**Hematuria**

A 10-year-old boy is brought to the outpatient department for passing red-colored urine. His mom says that it is scary and the family is very anxious.

What should be the first step?
Confirm presence of hematuria by urine microscopic examination.

Urine analysis reveals cola-colored urine and microscopy shows plenty of RBCs with 30% dysmorphic of RBCs.

What is your impression?
The findings are suggestive of glomerular hematuria.

How will you further proceed with this case?
The age of presentation and urine microscopy favors the possibility of post-streptococcal glomerulonephritis (PSGN). History of sore throat or skin lesions 2–4 weeks preceding the onset of this illness adds to the diagnosis of PSGN. Also one should enquire about history of reduced urine output/headache/visual disturbances/seizures/breathlessness to rule out complications of PSGN if any. Clinical examination should include assessment for pedal edema, measurement of blood pressure and performing a thorough systemic examination. Further investigations should include ASO titer and serum C3 levels.

Box 12.1	**Causes of Pseudohematuria (Red Urine NOT due to RBCs in Urine)**	
1. *Drugs*	Chloroquine, phenazopyridine, rifampicin, deferoxamine, nitrofurantoin, iron-sorbitol, phenolphthalein	
2. *Food*	Beetroot, black berries, food coloring	
3. *Metabolites*	Porphyrins, methemoglobinuria, bile pigments, homogentisic acid, urates, tyrosine, melanin	
4. *Others*	Hemoglobinuria, myoglobinuria	

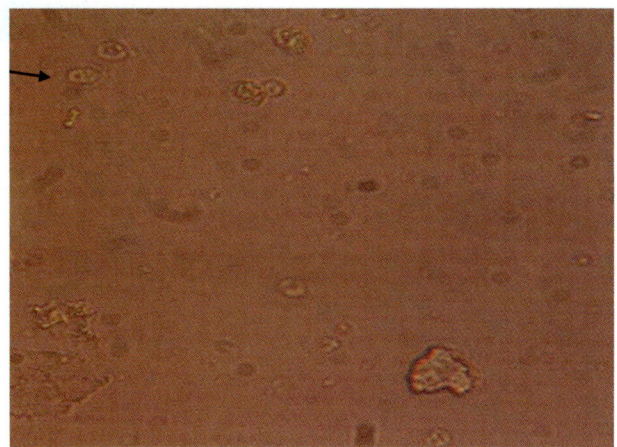

Fig. 12.7 Dysmorphic RBCs seen in urine microscopy

abdomen (renal masses or vascular malformations), complete hemogram with peripheral smear (sickle cell disease, HUS, HSP), coagulation profile (PT, aPTT) for coagulopathies, and renal biopsy.

The indications of renal biopsy in children with hematuria are listed in **Box 12.2**. An algorithmic approach to evaluation of hematuria is given in Fig. 12.8.

Box 12.2 Indications for Renal Biopsy in Children with Hematuria
1. Significant proteinuria
2. Abnormal renal function tests
3. Recurrent persistent hematuria
4. Serologic abnormalities (abnormal complement, ANA, or dsDNA levels)
5. Recurrent gross hematuria
6. A family history of end-stage renal disease

Treatment	Hematuria

Treatment of hematuria depends on the underlying etiology. Supportive treatment includes restriction of physical activity, plenty of fluid intake, alkalinization of urine (to prevent acute tubular, necrosis), and blood transfusion (in presence of severe anemia).

Pade KH, Liu DR. An evidence-based approach to the management of hematuria in children in the emergency department. *Pediatr Emerg Med Pract*. 2014;11:1–13.

Pan CG, Avner ED. Clinical evaluation of the child with hematuria. *In:* Kliegman RM, Stanton BF, St.Geme JW, Schor NF, Behrman RE,

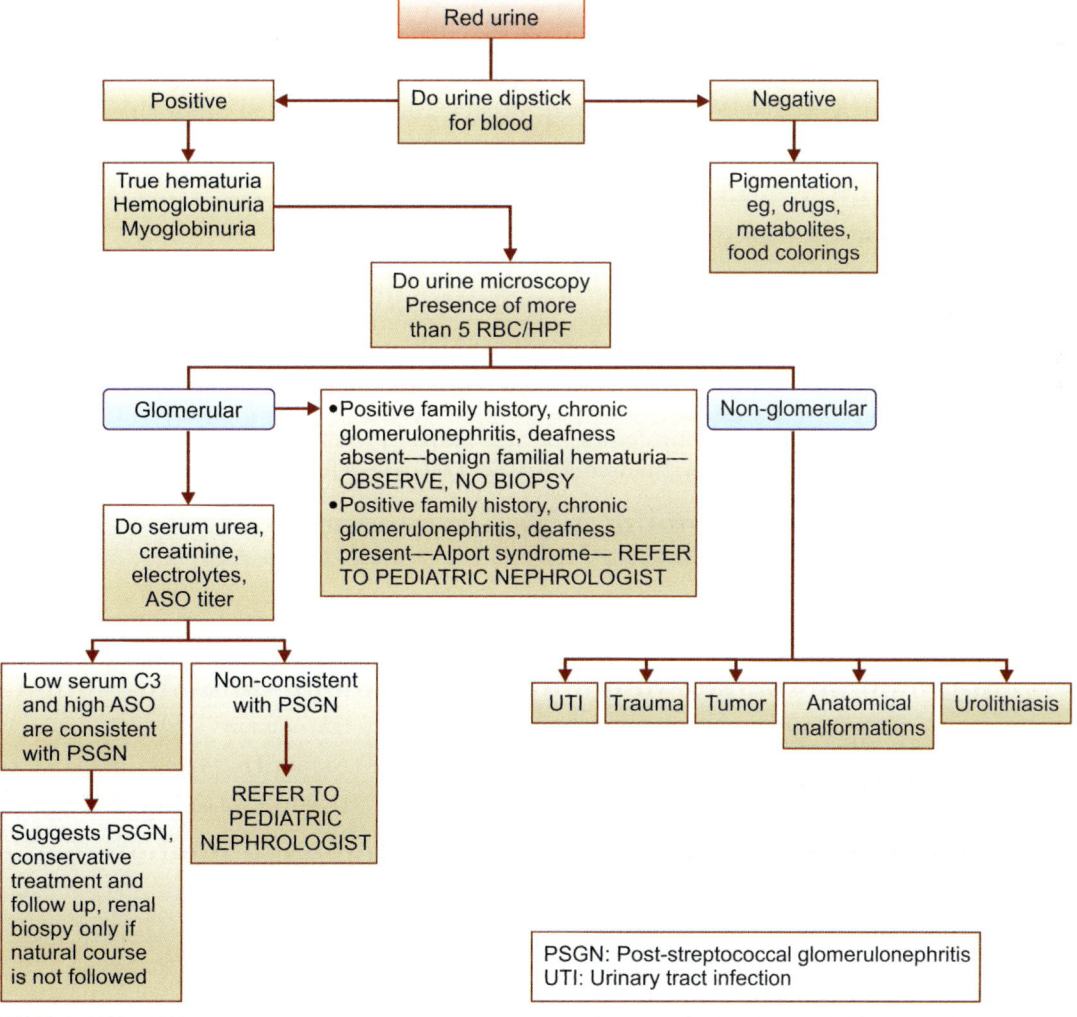

Fig. 12.8 Algorithmic approach to a child with red urine/hematuria

Hematuria

1. Hematuria is defined as presence of >5 RBC/HPF in a centrifuged urine sample. It needs to be differentiated from other common causes of red urine such as hemoglobinuria, myoglobinuria, and drug intake (eg, rifampicin).
2. The most common screening test for hematuria is urine dipstick which is confirmed by urine microscopy.
3. Glomerular causes should be differentiated from Non-glomerular causes of hematuria on the basis of dysmorphic RBCs and RBCs casts.
4. Glomerulonephritis, urinary tract infection, and renal stones are the most common causes.
5. Management of hematuria depends upon the underlying etiology.

editors. *Nelson Textbook of Pediatrics*. 20th ed. Philadelphia: Elsevier; 2016.p.2494–6.

Phadke KD, Vijayakumar M, Sharma J, Iyengar A; Indian Pediatric Nephrology Group. Consensus statement on evaluation of hematuria. *Indian Pediatr*. 2006;43:965–73.

Vijayakumar M, Nammalwar BR. Diagnostic approach to a child with hematuria. *Indian Pediatr*. 1998; 35:525–32.

12.4 GLOMERULONEPHRITIS

Glomerulonephritis refers to a group of diseases characterized by inflammation and proliferation of cells within the glomerulus. The inflammatory changes may be triggered by immunological mechanism following insult with an infectious agent or sometimes by non-immune mediated injury.

Glomerulonephritis may manifest clinically as (*a*) *acute nephritic syndrome* (most common), (*b*) asymptomatic hematuria and/or proteinuria, (*c*) nephrotic syndrome, or (*d*) rapidly progressive glomerulonephritis (RPGN).

- *Acute nephritic syndrome* is defined as acute onset of hematuria (gross or microscopic) and proteinuria in the presence of edema, hypertension, and oliguria.
- *Nephrotic syndrome* is characterized by heavy proteinuria leading to hypoalbuminemia, edema, and hyperlipidemia.

Table 12.10 compares salient features differentiating acute nephritic and nephrotic syndrome.

ETIOLOGY

The most common cause of acute nephritic syndrome is post-infectious glomerulonephritis that occurs following a Group A beta-hemolytic streptococcus (GABHS) infection. Chronic glomerulonephritis caused by systemic lupus erythematosus nephritis and membranoproliferative glomerulonephritis may present as acute nephritic syndrome. Other conditions presenting with acute nephritic syndrome are listed in **Table 12.11**.

ACUTE POST-INFECTIOUS GLOMERULONEPHRITIS

Acute post-streptococcal glomerulonephritis (PSGN) continues to be the most common cause of acute nephritis in children globally and it primarily occurs in developing countries. The annual incidence ranges from 9.5 to 28.5 per 100,000 individuals in underdeveloped nations. Acute glomerulonephritis follows pharyngeal or skin infection with GABHS (Group A beta-hemolytic streptococci) in over 90% of the cases hence the term 'acute post-streptococcal glomerulonephritis' is often used synonymously with AGN.

Besides GABHS, acute post-infectious glomerulo-nephritis (PIGN) may result from various other infective agents (**Box 12.3**). Acute glomerulonephritis may also evolve after infection at other sites such as pneumonia, meningitis, sepsis or deep-seated abscess and chronic bacterial infections (ventriculo-peritoneal shunts, subacute bacterial endocarditis).

ACUTE POST-STREPTOCOCCAL GLOMERULONEPHRITIS

Post-streptococcal glomerulonephritis is an immune-mediated glomerular injury that occurs 1–4 weeks after GABHS (*Streptococcus pyogenes*) infection. Longer latent period of 2–4 weeks is seen after skin infections as compared to 1–2 weeks seen after throat infection.

Table 12.10 Differences between Nephritic and Nephrotic Syndrome		
	Nephritic syndrome	*Nephrotic syndrome*
Onset	Acute	Insidious
Edema	Minimal, turgid, usually periorbital, sometimes generalized	Massive, pitting, generalized often involves scrotal region
Hypertension	Present in more than two-thirds patients	Uncommon
Urine output	Decreased	Normal/Decreased
Circulatory volume	Hypervolemia	Hypovolemia
Hematuria	50–70% gross, microscopic in all cases	20 % have microscopic hematuria
Proteinuria	1+ or 2+ on dipstick spot Up/Uc 0.2 to 2	>2+ on dipstick spot Up/Uc >2
Serum cholesterol	Normal	Increased
Serum albumin	Normal/ minimal decrease	Low
Glomerular filtration rate	Decreased	Normal

Spot Up/Uc—spot urinary protein creatinine ratio

Table 12.11 Conditions Presenting as Acute Nephritic Syndrome

| 1. Acute post-infectious glomerulonephritis |
| 2. Membranoproliferative glomerulonephritis |
| 3. IgA nephropathy |
| 4. Henoch-Schönlein purpura nephritis |
| 5. Systemic lupus erythematosus nephritis |
| 6. Vasculitis |
| 7. Goodpastrue syndrome (anti-GBM disease) |
| 8. Hemolytic uremic syndrome |

Box 12.3 Infectious Agents Associated with Acute Post-infectious Glomerulonephritis

1. *Bacterial* Streptococcus Group A, C, G, *Streptococcus viridans, Staphylococcus (aureus, albus)*, Pneumococcus, *Neisseria meningitidis, Mycobacteria, Salmonella typhi, Klebsiella pneumoniae*, and *Escherichia coli.*
2. *Viral* coxsackievirus, echovirus, cytomegalovirus, Epstein-Barr virus, hepatitis B, C, HIV, rubella, measles, varicella, influenza, adenovirus, and mumps.
3. *Fungal Coccidioides immitis.*
4. *Protozoal Plasmodium malariae, Plasmodium falciparum, Schistosoma mansoni, Toxoplasma gondii,* and filariasis.

Epidemiology

PSGN is still the most common glomerulopathy in developing countries. It occurs after throat or skin infection by certain nephritogenic strains.

- M serotypes 2, 47, 49, 55, 57, and 60 are associated with nephritis following skin infections and types 1, 2, 3, 4, 12, 25, and 45 following upper respiratory infection.
- In tropical countries like India with hot and humid climate it is seen after pyoderma in summer while in temperate climate it occurs in winter months post-streptococcal pharyngitis.

Pathogenesis and Pathophysiology

Deposition of immune complexes (antigen–antibody complexes) in glomerular tufts is the key pathogenic event. Several mechanisms have been proposed for the event:

1. Formation of immune complexes in circulation and deposition in glomeruli.
2. Implantation of nephritogenic antigen in glomeruli and formation of immune complexes *in situ.*
3. *Molecular mimicry* Antibodies form against streptococcal antigens and bind to normal glomerular antigens due to cross reactivity among them.
4. Activation of complement pathway directly by implanted antigen in glomeruli.

Due to certain M serotypes being non-nephritogenic, recent studies have refuted M proteins as "the nephritogenic antigen" in pathogenesis of PSGN. Investigators have proposed nephritis-associated plasmin receptor (NaPlr), streptococcal pyrogenic exotoxin B (SPEB), and its zymogen precursor as nephritogenic. Formation of immune complexes by above mechanisms induces cascade of events, ie, complement pathway activation, production of cytokines, infiltration of leukocytes, and cellular proliferation in glomerular mesangium and endocapillary.

The inflammatory reaction in glomerular tufts decreases the glomerular filtration rate (GFR). The reduction in GFR causes decreased reabsorption of solutes and water in the proximal tubules hence causing sodium and water retention. This results in expansion of extracellular volume, edema, and hypertension. The serum albumin levels are normal or slightly reduced hence do not play role in hemodynamics. The increased ECF volume appropriately suppresses renin-angiotensin-aldosterone axis. The C3 levels are low due to alternate complement pathway activation. C4 levels when low denote classic complement pathway activation also.

Clinical Features

PSGN most frequently affects children from 3 to 12 years of age but may affect any age group. Males are twice more commonly affected than females. The onset of disease is usually 1–2 weeks after an antecedent pharyngitis and 3–4 weeks after pyoderma. The clinical manifestations depend on severity of kidney involvement.

Mild cases may present with microscopic hematuria with some proteinuria with or without hypertension. A typical patient of PSGN presents with sudden onset of gross hematuria, edema, oliguria, hypertension, and mild azotemia. Active or healed skin lesions might be seen over the extremities. Prodromal symptoms such as malaise, low-grade fever, lethargy, anorexia, and headache may be present.

Gross hematuria is present in 30–70% of patients while microscopic hematuria is a universal finding. Urine is smoky or cola colored. Gross hematuria may be present for a few hours in a day and usually subsides in 1–2 weeks. Microscopic hematuria may last for an year. A few patients may have relapses of gross hematuria after vigorous exercise or viral illness later.

Edema is present in majority of patients and often noticed in morning as mild periorbital puffiness. It results due to retention of salt and water. Unrestricted fluid and salt intake may cause edema in peripheries, sometimes causing pleural effusion, and ascites.

Oliguria is often present. Anuria is infrequent and when persistent, requires close monitoring for rapidly progressive glomerulonephritis.

Hypertension is mild and present in 70% of patients. It manifests as headache, blurred vision, seizures, and sometimes altered sensorium. It is transient and resolves after onset of diuresis and recovery of renal function. Severe hypertension requiring multiple antihypertensives and persisting beyond 4 weeks suggests rapidly progressive glomerulonephritis (RPGN) or chronic glomerulopathy.

Course of Disease and Complications

The acute phase usually lasts for 4–6 weeks (Fig. 12.9). Gross hematuria resolves in 1–2 weeks. Azotemia, edema, and hypertension resolve once diuresis ensues. However, microscopic hematuria may persist for 1–2 years.

Patients may present with one or more complications of acute glomerulonephritis.

1. *Acute pulmonary edema* Salt and water retention causes expansion of extracellular fluid volume resulting in

circulatory congestion which is the most common complication. Severe hypertension and hypervolemia may lead to pulmonary edema.

2. *Hypertensive encephalopathy* 10% of cases of PSGN may present with altered sensorium due to sudden increase in blood pressure which impairs cerebral autoregulation resulting in cerebral edema.

3. *Acute kidney injury* Most cases would have modest derangement of renal functions. However, 1% patients of PSGN may develop oligoanuria, severe hypertension, anemia, rapidly increasing BUN, and creatinine. Hyperkalemia, hyperphosphatemia, metabolic acidosis, and uremia refractory to medical treatment would require dialysis.

4. *Nephrotic syndrome* 2% of cases may present with edema, gross hematuria, hypertension, and massive proteinuria.

Laboratory Evaluation

Examination of *urine specimen* reveals 1+/2+ proteinuria, dysmorphic RBCs, and RBC casts in most cases. Nephrotic range proteinuria, WBCs, and WBC casts may be found infrequently.

Hemogram may reveal mild anemia which is dilutional due to expansion of ECF volume. Thrombocytopenia is rare, and when present suggests other etiology such as systemic lupus erythematosus and hemolytic uremic syndrome.

Tests for *renal function* often show modest rise in blood urea, creatinine and potassium. Worsening of renal functions suggested by rapid increase in blood urea and creatinine suggest RPGN and requires prompt evaluation and management.

Tests for *complement studies* show low CH 50 (total complement activity) and low C3 levels (alternate complement pathway activation). C4 levels may decrease in few cases which denotes classic complement pathway activation. 15% of PSGN patients may demonstrate normal complement levels.

Chest X-ray is indicated when the patient has respiratory distress.

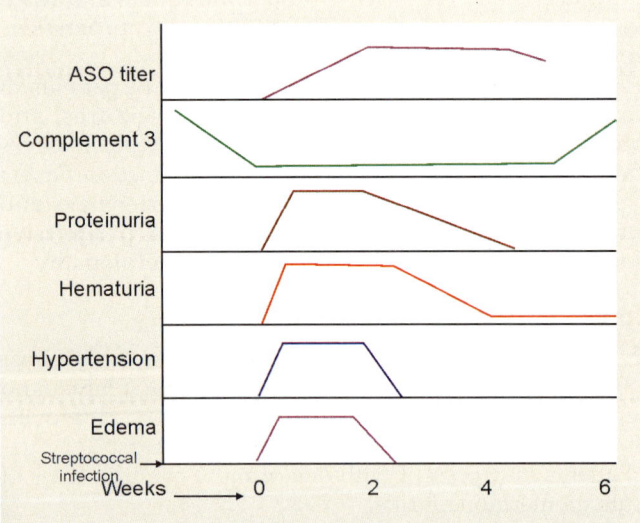

Fig. 12.9 Clinical course of post-streptococcal glomerulonephritis

Tests for Evidence of Streptococcal Infection

1. *Culture from throat and skin* depending upon site of infection
2. *Anti-streptolysin-O titer (ASO, normal levels <200 U/L)* ASO levels increase in nephritis associated with pharyngitis. Titers done early may be normal hence serial titers are more relevant. Mean time of significant titers is 3 weeks and continue to rise till 4 weeks. The sensitivity of ASO titers is 60–97% and specificity is 80% as reported in various studies.
3. *Anti-deoxyribonuclease-B and anti-hyaluronidase antibodies* They increase in nephritis associated with pyoderma. When two antibodies are tested, sensitivity increases from 60 to 80%.
4. *Streptozyme test* A slide hemagglutination test that detects antibodies to deoxyribonuclease-B, nicotinamide adenine dinuclease (NADase), streptolysin-O, hyaluronidase and streptokinase.

Renal Biopsy

Renal biopsy is not required for diagnosis of PSGN but is done when indicated to rule out other conditions. Indications of renal biopsy are (1) rapidly progressive disease; (2) Gross hematuria, hypertension and/or deranged renal functions persisting for more than 2 weeks; (3) Normal complement levels; (4) Evidence of systemic disease; and (5) Persistent low C3 for more than 12 weeks.

Light microscopy shows diffuse hypercellularity of endothelial and mesangial cells and infiltration of the glomerular tuft with polymorphonuclear cells. Immuno-fluorescence microscopy shows granular deposits of IgG and C3 in capillary loop and mesangium.

Differential Diagnosis

A child presenting with acute nephritic syndrome with low C3 and evidence of recent streptococcal infection is most likely a case of PSGN. However, some other conditions can present with similar picture of acute nephritic syndrome.

1. *IgA nephropathy* Children present with gross hematuria within 24–48 hours of upper respiratory tract infection. It is also called 'synpharyngitic hematuria'. Recurrent episodes are common. Urinalysis is often found normal at presentation since it is transient. Complement levels are normal.
2. *Membranoproliferative glomerulonephritis* Mean age of presentation is 10 years. It is a chronic glomerulonephritis. Sometimes may present as acute exacerbation of chronic glomerulonephritis after an episode of upper respiratory tract infection. Proteinuria is often massive. Renal functions may be deranged at presentation. It is sometimes diagnosed when renal biopsy is done for persistent low C3 levels in a child diagnosed as PIGN.
3. *Systemic lupus erythematosus* SLE is more common in adolescent females. It is a chronic glomerulonephritis but may present with acute nephritic syndrome with nephrotic range proteinuria. Other systemic features (fever, rash, arthritis, anemia, thrombocytopenia, CNS involvement) may be present. C3 and C4 levels are low. ANA, double-stranded DNA antibodies are present. Renal biopsy establishes the diagnosis.
4. *Henoch-Schönlein purpura* It presents after a viral prodrome with fever, palpable purpuric rash (lower limbs),

abdominal pain, joint pain and swelling. Involvement of gastrointestinal system and joints may be several days to weeks after rash. Renal involvement is found in 50% of the cases, usually presents as hematuria, gross or microscopic. Proteinuria, hypertension, acute renal failure, and nephrotic syndrome may be present. Complement levels are normal. It is a clinical diagnosis as laboratory findings are nonspecific.

Approach to diagnosis of a child with acute nephritic syndrome is depicted in Fig. 12.10.

| Treatment | **Post-streptococcal Glomerulonephritis** |

Treatment of patient with acute PSGN is supportive until the resolution of symptoms occurs. Eradication of triggering agent by administration of antibiotics after onset of symptoms does not ameliorate the severity of nephritis.

1. Bedrest and limitation of activity is advised.
2. *Fluid and sodium restriction* Low salt diet and restriction of fluids remains the mainstay of management in mild cases.
3. *Diet* Potassium restricted diet if hyperkalemia is present. Protein restriction is required if azotemia is present.
4. *Edema* Fluid and sodium restriction along with loop diuretics decrease edema.
5. *Hypertension* Furosemide (1–2 mg/kg/day in 2–3 divided doses) is the drug of choice for control of hypertension in AGN and it also decreases hyperkalemia. Higher doses may be given for pulmonary edema. Oral nifedipine 0.25–0.5 mg/kg every 4–6 hours is given if BP is not controlled with diuretics. In patients with hypertensive emergency intravenous labetalol or nitroprusside infusion is given for 24 to 48 hours.
6. *Hyperkalemia* Potassium is restricted in diet. Sodium polystyrene sulfonate resin in dose of 0.5–1 g/kg/per dose every 4–6 hourly can be given orally. If still uncontrolled other measures as glucose insulin infusion and nebulization with salbutamol, may help.
7. *Dialysis* This is done in patients with refractory hyperkalemia, acidosis, uremia, hypertension and fluid overload.
8. *Antibiotics* These are indicated in children with active streptococcal pharyngitis or pyoderma or when throat culture is positive. Single dose of benzathine penicillin 0.6 million units or oral penicillin V 125 mg, every 6 hours for 7–10 days, are adequate treatment. Erythromycin or azithromycin is the treatment of choice in children allergic to penicillin. The antibiotic therapy limits the spread of nephritogenic streptococci to susceptible contacts but does not alter the course of AGN.

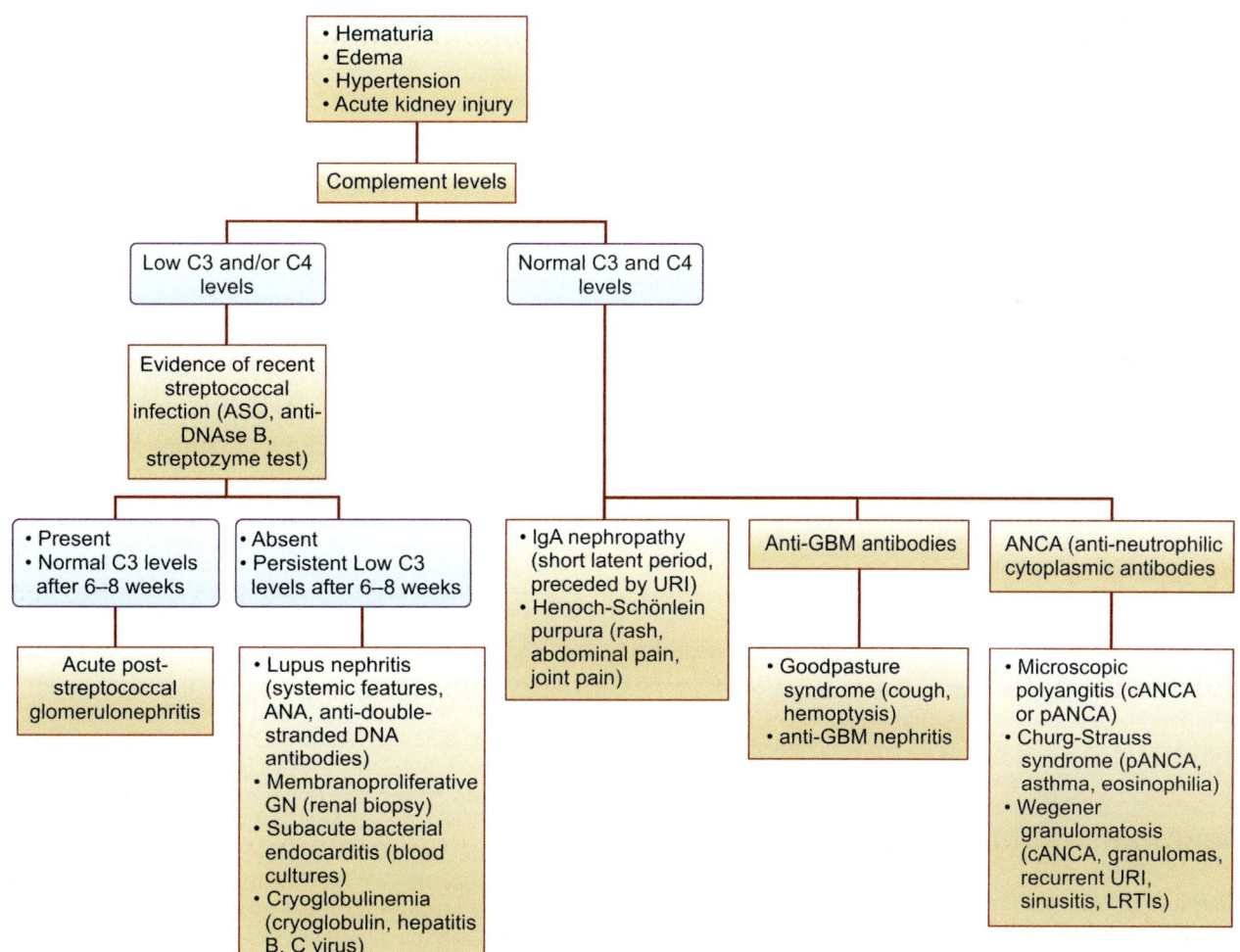

Fig. 12.10 Approach to a case of acute nephritic syndrome

12

| Case Study | Acute Nephritic Syndrome |

A 7-year-old boy presented with puffiness around eyes more in early morning and headache for 4 days. He was passing cola-colored urine. The day before he passed urine only twice and that too in small volumes.

What is your working hypothesis, based on the history?

The child has presented with edema, hematuria (to be confirmed by urine examination), oliguria, and hypertension (to be confirmed by BP measurement). The symptoms point towards a possible diagnosis of acute glomerulonephritis.

What other leading questions need to be asked?

- *Symptoms of systemic disorders* Fever, rash, joint pains (systemic lupus erythematosus, Henoch-Schönlein purpura), abdominal pain (Henoch-Schönlein purpura), cough, hemoptysis (Goodpasture syndrome)
- *Complications of the disease* Seizures, altered sensorium (hypertensive encephalopathy), rapid breathing, difficulty in breathing (pulmonary edema).
- *Past history* History of antecedent sore throat or cutaneous infection (streptococcal infection). Latent period between sore throat and onset of symptoms since shorter period of 2–4 days is suggestive of IgA nephropathy.

The child had chickenpox 1 month back; later, a few lesions developed purulent discharge. He was prescribed oral antibiotics for a week by his pediatrician but they discontinued after 3 days. On examination, he was tachypneic with respiratory rate of 32/min, PR 98/min, BP 164/100 mmHg and JVP was raised. He had periorbital puffiness and pedal edema. He had hyperpigmented spots all over body. Chest examination revealed bilateral basal crepitations. Liver was palpable 4 cm below right subcostal margin. Heart sounds and neurological examination were normal.

What is the probable diagnosis now? Outline the investigation to be done to confirm the diagnosis?

The child presented with gross hematuria, edema, oliguria, and hypertension (acute nephritic syndrome) 1 month after superadded bacterial infection of varicella, the probable diagnosis is acute post-streptococcal glomerulonephritis.

The relevant investigations are urine routine microscopy, blood urea, serum creatinine, serum electrolytes, serum albumin, cholesterol, chest X-ray, ECG, C3 level, ASO titer, and anti-DNAse B.

Urine examination revealed urine protein 2+, full field RBCs, 30% dysmorphic, a few WBCs. Other investigations revealed blood urea 65 mg/dL, serum creatinine 1.2 mg/dL, sodium 138 mEq/L, potassium 5 mEq/L, serum albumin 3.4 mg/dL, cholesterol 180 mg/dL, C3 34 mg /dL, ASO titer 300 U/L, anti DNAse B 2000 U/mL. Chest X-ray revealed bilateral fluffy infiltrates and ECG was normal.

Interpret above findings in view of clinical diagnosis.

The child has hematuria of glomerular origin (RBCs, RBC casts, dysmorphic RBCs), azotemia (raised urea and creatinine), low C3, and evidence of past streptococcal infection (elevated ASO and DNAse B). All these favor the diagnosis of post-streptococcal glomerulonephritis. Chest X-ray findings suggest associated pulmonary edema.

Outline your priorities in immediate management of this child.

We need to take care of pulmonary edema and hypertension. Intravenous furosemide 1–2 mg/kg needs to be urgently administered.

Prevention

Adequate treatment of streptococcal infection with a 10-day course of antibiotic therapy prevents the transmission of nephritogenic strains during epidemics and also protects against glomerulonephritis. Hence, it is important to diagnose streptococcal pharyngitis which is suggested by temperature >38°C, tonsillar exudate, soft palate petechiae, and anterior cervical lymphadenopathy.

Prognosis

Majority of children of PSGN recover completely without any sequelae. Recurrences are extremely rare. 1% of cases may develop rapid progressive course which has guarded prognosis. Management of complications adequately decreases mortality. There is scant long-term data of AGN due to other infections (non-streptococcal) but in general have favorable outcome. Progression to chronic glomerulonephritis occurs in less than 2% of cases which may slowly progress to end-stage renal disease.

Revision Point

Acute Glomerulonephritis

1. Most common cause of acute nephritic syndrome is post-infectious glomerulonephritis that occurs following a Group A beta-hemolytic streptococcus (GABHS) infection.
2. PSGN is characterized by sudden onset of gross hematuria, edema, oliguria, hypertension, and mild azotemia.
3. Clinical presentation of acute nephritic syndrome along with low complements and evidence of recent streptococcal infection establishes the diagnosis.
4. The acute phase usually lasts for 4–6 weeks.
5. Salt and fluid restriction along with loop diuretics remain mainstay of management.
6. Prognosis is good and recurrences are extremely rare.

Eison TM, Ault BH, Jones DP, Chesney RW, Wyatt RJ. Post-streptococcal acute glomerulonephritis in children: clinical features and pathogenesis. *Pediatr Nephrol.* 2011;26:165–180.

Gunasekaran K, Krishnamurthy S, Mahadevan S, *et al.* Clinical characteristics and Outcome of post-infectious glomerulonephritis in children in Southern India: A prospective study. *Indian J Pediatr.* 2015;82:896–903.

Kambham N. Postinfectious Glomerulonephritis. *Adv Anat Pathol.* 2012;19:338–47.

Stratta P, Musetti C, Barreca A, Mazzucco G. New trends of an old disease: the acute post-infectious glomerulonephritis at the beginning of the new millennium. *J Nephrol.* 2014;27:229–39.

RAPIDLY PROGRESSIVE GLOMERULONEPHRITIS

Rapidly progressive glomerulonephritis (RPGN) is characterized by acute nephritic syndrome with rapid deterioration in renal function (>50% decrease in GFR) within days to weeks and histopathological evidence of crescents affecting >50% of glomeruli. Rapidly progressive glomerulonephritis and crescentic glomerulonephritis term is often used synonymously. RPGN is caused by varied renal disorders. Certain conditions may have similar presentation of RPGN but are without crescents as in hemolytic uremic syndrome.

Pathogenesis

Crescents are formed by infiltration of inflammatory cells and proliferation of parietal and visceral epithelial cells in Bowman space. Severe glomerular injury is caused by immune complexes (systemic infections) and antibodies to glomerular and cellular antigenic components (ANCA, anti-GBM, ANA, double-stranded DNA antibodies).

Classification

Crescentic glomerulonephritis is categorized as:

1. *Immune complex mediated glomerulonephritis* It is most common cause of RPGN in children accounting for 50–75% of causes in most series. This group include diseases that result in granular deposits of immunoglobulins and/or complements along capillary wall and mesangium in immunofluorescence microscopy. Primary glomerulonephritis as Ig A nephropathy, post-infectious glomerulonephritis and systemic diseases like systemic lupus erythematosus are diseases which lead to immune complex mediated glomerulonephritis.

2. *Pauci-immune glomerulonephritis* 15–40% cases are caused by pauci-immune glomerulonephritis. Small vessel vasculitis as in microscopic polyangiitis, Wegener's granulomatosis and renal limited vasculitis cause extensive crescent formation and necrotizing glomerulonephritis without or minimal deposition of immune complexes. 80% of cases have ANCA (anti neutrophilic cytoplasmic antibodies) in blood.

3. *Anti-glomerular basement antibody-mediated glomerulonephritis* It causes RPGN in 12–15% of cases. It is most severe form of RPGN. Immunofluorescence shows linear deposits of immunoglobulin G with or without C3 along capillary walls.

Clinical Features

Most common presentation is of acute nephritic syndrome with rapid derangement of renal functions often complicated by hypertensive emergency and acute pulmonary edema. Investigations and clinical features of different categories of RPGN are listed in **Table 12.12**.

Table 12.12 Causes, Clinical Features, and Diagnosis of Rapidly Progressive Glomerulonephritis			
	Causes	*Other clinical features*	*Specific investigations*
Immune complex mediated *Low serum complement C3*	Post-infectious glomerulonephritis	H/o antecedent streptococcal infection, evidence of septic foci	↑ ASO, ↑ anti-DNAse B, renal biopsy—diffuse proliferative GN with IgG and C3 deposits in mesangium and along capillary walls
	Membranoproliferative glomerulonephritis	Acute nephritic syndrome post-viral prodrome, anemia	Low C3 ± low C4, renal biopsy—mesangial proliferation and thickening of the peripheral GBM with C3 and IgG deposits
	Systemic lupus erythematosus	Fever, malaise, joint pain, anemia, seizures	Low C3, low C4, ANA, anti-dsDNA, renal biopsy—diffuse proliferation with sub endothelial deposits and full house (deposits of all Ig class) in IF
Normal complement	IgA nephropathy	H/o recurrent episodes of gross hematuria after URI	↑Serum IgA, renal biopsy—mesangial hypercellularity with mesangial IgA deposits
	Henoch-Schönlein purpura	Fever, joint pain, abdominal pain, palpable purpura	Essential clinical diagnosis Renal biopsy s/o mesangial hyper-cellularity with mesangial IgA deposits
Pauci-immune Systemic vasculitis	Microscopic polyangiitis	Vasculitic rash over lower limbs	pANCA +,extra-renal non-granulomatous lesions, renal biopsy—necrotizing crescentic glomerulonephritis
	Wegener granulomatosis	Cough, sinusitis, subglottic stenosis, nasal deformity	cANCA (70–90%) extra-renal granulomatous lesions, renal biopsy—focal necrotizing crescentic glomerulonephritis
	Churg-Strauss syndrome	Recurrent wheezing episodes	Eosinophilia, renal biopsy—necrotizing crescentic glomerulonephritis
No systemic vasculitis	Renal limited vasculitis	No extrarenal features	Renal biopsy—necrotizing crescentic glomerulonephritis
Anti-glomerular basement antibody mediated	Goodpasture syndrome Anti-GBM nephritis	Hemoptysis, pulmonary hemorrhage	Presence of anti-GBM antibodies, Renal biopsy—crescentic glomerulonephritis with linear IgG deposition along the glomerular capillaries in IF

Treatment   Rapidly Progressive Glomerulonephritis

Management of a child with RPGN includes supportive management of fluids, electrolytes, hypertension, nutrition, and specific therapy. High dose steroids and cytotoxic therapy constitute the mainstay of specific management. Intravenous pulse methylprednisolone is given in a dose of 15–20 mg/kg for 3 to 6 days followed by oral prednisolone 1.5–2 mg/kg/day for 4 weeks. Steroids are then tapered over 3 months and then continued on alternate days for 6 months to one year. Alternatively, Intravenous pulse cyclophosphamide in a dose of 500–750 mg/m^2 every 3–4 weeks for 6 pulses is given along with steroids or oral cyclophosphamide in a dose of 2–2.5 mg/kg/day for 12 weeks.

Maintenance immunosuppression is with azathioprine, alternate day prednisolone, or mycophenolate.

Plasmapheresis may be required in patients who do not respond to pulse steroid therapy, in anti-GBM nephritis, and in ANCA associated RPGN.

Prognosis

Outcome of RPGN has improved in last few years. 60–70% of patients have recovery of renal function. Resolution of renal parameters depends on underlying disease, histopathology, proportion of crescents, extent of tubulo-interstitial scarring and fibrosis. Post-streptococcal crescentic GN has better prognosis than lupus, MPGN, pauci-immune or anti-GBM associated RPGN.

12.5 PROTEINURIA

Proteinuria is classified *as transient* or *persistent*. While the former is usually benign, the latter indicates the presence of an underlying renal disorder and is recognized as a marker and mediator of progressive renal insufficiency, as well as a risk factor for cardiovascular disease. Therapeutic measures to control persistent proteinuria are therefore, considered an integral part of renoprotective strategies.

DEFINITIONS

1. On a 24-hour urinary sample, *proteinuria* is defined as more than 100 mg/m^2/day (or >4 mg/m^2/hour). Proteinuria of more than 1 g/m^2/day is known as *nephrotic range proteinuria*.
2. On a spot urine sample, proteinuria is defined as urinary protein/creatinine ratio (U Pr/Cr) of $\geq$0.5 mg/mg in infants, and $\geq$0.2 mg/mg in children. Nephrotic range proteinuria is defined as urinary protein/creatinine ratio (U Pr/Cr) of >2 mg/mg on a spot urine sample.
3. Persistent proteinuria, defined as proteinuria of $\geq$1+ by dipstick on multiple occasions, is abnormal and needs to be investigated further. Nephrotic range proteinuria is manifested by 3+ or 4+ proteinuria on dipstick testing.
4. Albuminuria is defined as urine albumin/creatinine ratio >30 mg/g.

EPIDEMIOLOGY

The prevalence of transient proteinuria in a single urine specimen due to exercise, fever or infection, in children and adolescents is relatively common and has been reported in different studies to be between 5% and 15%. However, persistent proteinuria on repeated testing is much less common (less than 0.5%) in child population. The prevalence of nephrotic syndrome in childhood is low; approximately 2 to 3 cases per 100,000 children.

MECHANISMS OF PROTEIN HANDLING BY THE KIDNEYS

The glomerular barrier is a complex membrane with selective permeability. It prevents the passage of macromolecules such as albumin (molecular weight 65 kD). In addition to the size barrier, the glomerular capillary wall also contains negative charges because of the presence of heparan sulfate proteoglycans. These negative charges repel albumin, which is negatively charged. The proximal tubules also absorb most of the low molecular weight (LMW) proteins, such as insulin or β_2-microglobulin, which are filtered across glomeruli.

Consequently, healthy children excrete minute amounts of proteins, ie, less than 100 mg/m^2/day or <4 mg/m^2/hour. Out of these, albumin comprises less than 30%, and Tamm-Horsfall protein (a glycoprotein secreted by the ascending limb of loop of Henle) comprises 50% of the total. The rest is comprised of small quantities of plasma proteins filtered by glomeruli, eg, immunoglobulins, transferrin, and β_2-microglobulin. This modest amount of physiological proteinuria is not usually detected on routine dipstick testing.

In children with renal disorders, excessive urinary protein losses may be caused by either increased glomerular permeability (*glomerular proteinuria*) or decreased reabsorption of LMW proteins (*tubular proteinuria*). In the absence of nephrotic syndrome, glomerular proteinuria may be the only sign of renal damage in many patients with early chronic kidney disease (CKD).

How does Persistent Proteinuria Cause Renal Injury?

A number of mechanisms have been mentioned by which proteinuria may induce renal insufficiency:

1. Injury may occur after the release of lysosomal enzymes into the cytoplasm of protein-reabsorbing tubules.
2. Iron that is filtered into the tubular fluid bound to transferrin may be directly cytotoxic or may have indirect effects as a consequence of iron-catalyzed synthesis of reactive oxygen metabolites.
3. Renal tubules may be obstructed by proteinaceous casts.
4. Activation of the alternative complement cascade by proximal tubules may be harmful.
5. Ischemic tubular injury may follow the release of vasoconstricting molecules.
6. Release of fibrosis-promoting factors from renal cells activated/injured by proteinuria may result in interstitial fibrosis.
7. Filtration of cytokines or chemokines may provoke cell proliferation, inflammatory cell infiltration, and activation of infiltrating cells.
8. Filtration of novel antigens may function as antigen-presenting cells and initiate a cellular immune response.
9. Filtration of lipoproteins and absorption by proximal tubules may activate inflammatory pathways causing cell injury.

Estimation of Proteinuria

1. Dipstick Method

A frequently used screening method for detection of proteinuria is urinary dipstick, which primarily detects albumin, leaving LMW proteins undetected. A color reaction between urinary albumin and tetrabromophenol blue produces various green hues based on the concentration of albumin in the sample, which is graded as follows: Trace (15 mg/dL); 1+ (30 mg/dL); 2+ (100 mg/dL); 3+ (300 mg/dL); and 4 + (2000 mg/dL).

Because it is the concentration of urine protein that is measured, false-negative results may occur with very dilute urine. Conversely, false-positive results may occur with very alkaline or concentrated urine specimens in the presence of contaminating antiseptics, such as chlorhexidine and benzalkonium chloride, or after the administration of radiographic contrast, eg, after intravenous pyelogram (IVP). **Box 12.4** summarizes the causes of false-positive or false-negative dipstick results.

An alternative method is to measure urinary protein in patients with suspected proteinuria by dipstick using protein precipitation with sulfosalicylic acid. This technique provides a more quantitative estimate of all the urinary proteins including LMW proteins.

2. Heat Coagulation Test

In a test tube, take 2 mL of urine sample. The test tube is then inclined and the surface is heated on a flame. The formation of a coagulum indicates the presence of albumin.

3. Urinary Protein/Creatinine Ratio

In contrast to adults, since an accurately timed or 24-hour urine collection may not be feasible or possible in children, the urinary protein/creatinine ratio (U Pr/Cr) of an untimed (spot) urine specimen (preferably first morning sample) is commonly used for estimation of protein excretion in children. This U Pr/Cr ratio has been shown to correlate with the 24-hour urine protein excretion, especially since an early morning spot testing rules out confounding factors such as postural proteinuria. A value of >0.2 is abnormal in children older than 2 years.

Etiology

Proteinuria in children can be etiologically classified as *transient, orthostatic, overflow,* or *persistent* proteinuria.

Box 12.4 Causes of False-positive or False-negative Dipstick Results
A. False-positive results
1. Concentrated urine
2. Alkaline urine
3. Contamination by antiseptics (eg, chlorhexidine, benzalkonium) and antibiotics (eg, penicillins)
4. Administration of radiographic contrast
5. Gross hematuria
6. Contamination by vaginal secretions
B. False-negative results
1. Diluted urine
2. Acidic urine
3. Microalbuminuria/low molecular weight proteinuria

1. Transient or Functional Proteinuria

At least 30–50% of children with proteinuria may have transient, non-recurring proteinuria. Transient proteinuria is known to occur with fever, strenuous exercise, emotional stress, exposure to extreme cold, epinephrine administration, abdominal surgery or congestive heart failure and after seizures. It resolves spontaneously after the cessation of the precipitating factor, and an exhaustive diagnostic work-up is usually not recommended.

2. Orthostatic (Postural) Proteinuria

Orthostatic proteinuria accounts for up to 60% of all cases of asymptomatic proteinuria reported in children, with an even higher incidence in adolescents. Variations in the quantity of daily protein excretion have been observed. If all laboratory tests (such as blood urea, serum creatinine, serum albumin, serum cholesterol) and clinical findings (such as blood pressure, growth) are normal except for persistently elevated protein excretion, the possibility of orthostatic proteinuria should be investigated, particularly if the child is older than 6 years of age. This is best done by using the **orthostatic test**.

The child is instructed to urinate just before going to bed at night and to discard the urine. He or she must remain supine all night and urinate the next morning immediately after arising. This urine sample is kept separate and labeled "supine" or "recumbent." Additional urine samples are then collected and pooled during the next 12 to 16 hours, while the patient maintains normal daily activity. The final sample should preferably be collected in the evening, just before the patient goes to bed; this pooled sample should be labeled "active" urine. The duration of collection time for the latter sample can be shortened to 12 hours or less. In patients with orthostatic proteinuria, the supine sample will be free of protein, but the active sample will contain protein. Children with orthostatic proteinuria usually have U Pr/Cr less than 1.0. Yearly follow-up is recommended for children diagnosed with this condition.

3. Overflow Proteinuria

Overflow proteinuria occurs when the plasma concentration of certain small proteins exceeds the capacity of the tubules to reabsorb the filtered protein. Examples include the presence of immunoglobulin light chains in the urine in multiple myeloma, hemoglobinuria in intravascular hemolysis, myoglobulinuria in rhabdomyolysis, and amylasuria in acute pancreatitis.

4. Persistent Proteinuria

The finding of at least two positive urine tests showing proteinuria, out of three specimens would suggest persistent proteinuria and warrants a work-up. Persistent proteinuria can be secondary to glomerular or tubular etiologies.

Glomerular proteinuria

Nephrotic syndrome and acute post-streptococcal glomerulonephritis are the main causes of glomerular proteinuria in children.
- In nephrotic syndrome patients have heavy or "nephrotic range" proteinuria, defined as a protein excretion greater than $1 \text{ g}/\text{m}^2/\text{day}$ (or a U Pr/Cr greater than 2.0).

12

- Proteinuria in acute post-infectious glomerulonephritis (most commonly post-streptococcal) is usually 1+ or 2+, is accompanied by hematuria, and generally has a good outcome without long-term sequelae.
- Other important causes of proteinuria include focal segmental glomerulosclerosis, membranous nephropathy (which may occur due to hepatitis B), Henoch-Schönlein purpura nephritis, lupus nephritis, and membrano-proliferative glomerulonephritis. Human immunodeficiency virus (HIV) infection has emerged as an important cause of proteinuria and nephrotic syndrome in both adults and children.

Other congenital and acquired renal tract or urinary tract anomalies such as hydronephrosis, polycystic kidney disease, reflux nephropathy, and renal dysplasia may also manifest with proteinuria.

Tubulointerstitial Nephropathies

Proteinuria, with or without hematuria, occurs in patients with tubulointerstitial diseases of diverse etiologies. When the glomerular filtration rate is normal, the proteinuria is usually of tubular origin. As the glomerular filtration rate decreases as a result of significant nephron loss, hemodynamic mechanisms contribute to glomerular proteinuria.

In general, the proteinuria of tubulointerstitial disease is mild (less than 1.0 g per 24 hours). Characteristically, tubular proteinuria is predominantly composed of LMW proteins. Some tubular diseases that can manifest as isolated LMW proteinuria during childhood include Dent disease, Lowe syndrome, and Fabry disease.

Approach to Evaluation of Proteinuria

The initial evaluation of proteinuria should comprise a complete history, including a family history of renal disease, recent upper respiratory infections, gross hematuria, changes in weight, and changes in urine output. The physical examination should include measurements of height, weight, and blood pressure, identification of edema, ascites and pallor, and palpation of the kidneys in newborn infants. A urinalysis should be performed, and blood obtained for determination of electrolyte, blood urea nitrogen, creatinine, serum albumin levels, as well as a complete blood cell count and C3 complement. A quantitative assessment of urinary protein excretion should be made, using a spot urine sample for the U Pr/Cr ratio.

Treatment	Proteinuria

Management depends on the underlying etiology of proteinuria. Nephrotic syndrome in children should be managed as per guidelines of the Indian Pediatric Nephrology Group. Post-infectious glomerulonephritis is usually self-limited, and a renal biopsy is not indicated, except in atypical circumstances such as rapidly rising creatinine levels, persistent hypertension, absence of hypocomplementemia at diagnosis or persistent nephrotic range proteinuria. Other etiologies such as polycystic kidneys may be detectable by renal ultrasonography. Orthostatic proteinuria usually has a benign course, and extensive work up is not required apart from annual follow up.

Restrictions on the child's lifestyle and physical activity are not necessary. Avoiding excessive salt intake is desirable; routine protein intake in the diet should be allowed. In some patients with a glomerular disease resulting in heavy proteinuria unresponsive to corticosteroids or cytotoxic agents, therapy with an angiotensin converting enzyme (ACE) inhibitor can bring about a significant reduction of proteinuria. ACE inhibitors and angiotensin-receptor blockers have an established antiproteinuric effect that appears to be unrelated to their other diverse effects, including control of hypertension. The mechanism of the antiproteinuric effect is that selective vasodilatation of the efferent arteriole lowers the filtration pressure and, hence, the amount of albumin in the ultrafiltrate; as well as anti-TGF-β activity (since TGF-β is a fibrogenic cytokine).

Prognosis

Long-term follow-up studies have documented the benign nature of orthostatic proteinuria, although rare cases of glomerulosclerosis have been identified later in life in patients who were initially found to have proteinuria with an orthostatic component. Transient proteinuria, which is most often associated with fever, stress, dehydration, or exercise, is not considered to be indicative of underlying renal disease.

Case Study	Post-streptococcal Glomerulonephritis

A 6-year-old boy is referred to the pediatric outpatient department with complaints of puffiness of the face, accompanied by 2+ proteinuria (done at another hospital), and oliguria. There is no history of cola-colored urine. However, there is history of pyoderma over the legs 3 weeks ago, which are now healed. BP is recorded to be 128/90 mmHg (>95th centile for height, age and sex).

What is the most likely cause of proteinuria in this child?
Post-streptococcal glomerulonephritis (PSGN) is the most likely diagnosis, since there is a history of pyoderma 3 weeks ago, following which sub-nephrotic range proteinuria, oliguria, and hypertension have been documented.

What other investigations are needed to confirm the diagnosis?
Microscopic hematuria is required to confirm the diagnosis. Hence, a urinalysis is required to be done. Blood urea, serum creatinine, anti-streptolysin-O (ASO) and C3 levels should be performed in all cases of suspected PSGN.

Urinalysis demonstrated RBC casts with 20 RBC per HPF. Blood urea was 30 mg/dL and serum creatinine was 0.4 mg/dL. Serum C3 levels were very low. ASO was 400 units/L.

What is the role of immunosuppressive therapy as an anti-proteinuric measure in this case?
The investigations confirm PSGN. Most cases of PSGN are benign and self-limiting. They however, require appropriate management in the form of control of hypertension, no added salt in diet, fluid intake and urine output measurement, fluid regulation, furosemide for edema, and penicillin V for streptococcal infection eradication. Immunosuppressants (methylpredni-solone, etc.) should not be prescribed, except in the rare cases of PSGN complicated by rapidly progressive glomerulonephritis, which manifest with rapidly rising creatinine levels and severe acute kidney injury.

Persistent Proteinuria as An Indicator of Renal Disease and its Progression

On basis of population-based studies in adults with chronic kidney disease (CKD), persistent proteinuria is considered both a maker of renal disease as well as its progression. It reflects the severity of underlying renal damage. In children, proteinuria has been significantly correlated with a decline in glomerular filtration rate, both in glomerular and tubular disorders. Current strategies to prevent CKD progression, a concept known as *renoprotection*, aim at controlling blood pressure and reducing urinary protein excretion.

Persistent Proteinuria as a Risk Factor for Cardiovascular Disease

Obesity is considered an independent risk factor for CKD, hypertension, and cardiovascular disease in children and adults. Obesity-related glomerulopathy, presenting as proteinuria and progressive renal dysfunction, is increasing even in children. Severe persistent proteinuria may be a long-term risk factor for atherosclerosis in children. As the severity of proteinuria increases, it is associated with a variety of metabolic disturbances that contribute to cardiovascular disease, eg, hypercholesterolemia, hypertriglyceridemia, and hypercoagulability. Leakage of proteinuria into the urine reflects generalized endothelial damage and capillary injury. In some patients, factors such as hypertension, renal insufficiency, and steroid therapy may also contribute to the risk for cardiovascular disease.

Fig. 12.11 depicts the algorithm for diagnostic evaluation of children with proteinuria.

Revision Point

Proteinuria

1. Persistent proteinuria indicates the presence of an underlying renal disorder and is recognized as a marker and mediator of progressive renal insufficiency, as well a risk factor for cardiovascular disease.
2. Therapeutic measures to control persistent proteinuria are considered an integral part of renoprotective strategies.
3. Glomerular proteinuria is more severe than tubular proteinuria.

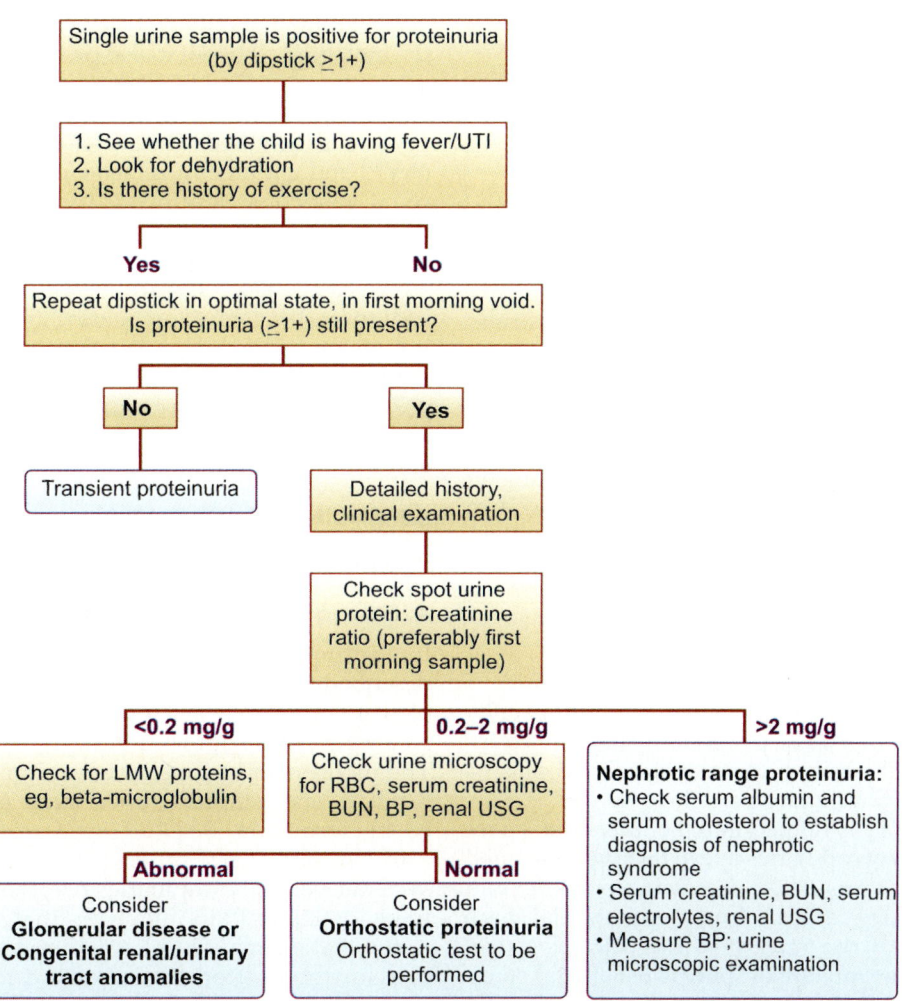

Fig. 12.11 Algorithm for diagnostic evaluation of children with proteinuria

12

Abitbol CL, Chandar J, Onder AM, Nwobi O, Montané B, Zilleruelo G. Profiling proteinuria in pediatric patients. *Pediatr Nephrol.* 2006;21:995–1002.

Haraldsson B, Nyström J, Deen WM. Properties of the glomerular barrier and mechanisms of proteinuria. *Physiol Rev.* 2008;88:451–87.

Hogg RJ, Portman RJ, Milliner D, Lemley KV, Eddy A, Ingelfinger J. Evaluation and management of proteinuria and nephrotic syndrome in children: recommendations from a pediatric nephrology panel established at the National Kidney Foundation conference on proteinuria, albuminuria, risk, assessment, detection, and elimination (PARADE). *Pediatrics.* 2000;105:1242–9.

Houser MT, Jahn MF, Kobayashi A, Walburn J. Assessment of urinary protein excretion in the adolescent: effect of body position and exercise. *J Pediatr.* 1986;109:556–61.

Indian Pediatric Nephrology Group, Indian Academy of Pediatrics, Bagga A, Ali U, Banerjee S, Kanitkar M, Phadke KD, Senguttuvan P, Sethi S, Shah M. Management of steroid sensitive nephrotic syndrome: revised guidelines. *Indian Pediatr.* 2008;45:203–14.

Litwin M, Grenda R, Sladowska J, Antoniewicz J. Add-on therapy with angiotensin II receptor 1 blocker in children with chronic kidney disease already treated with angiotensin-converting enzyme inhibitors. *Pediatr Nephrol.* 2006;21:1716–22.

Rademacher ER, Sinaiko AR. Albuminuria in children. *Curr Opin Nephrol Hypertens.* 2009; 18:246–51.

Wühl E, Schaefer F. Therapeutic strategies to slow chronic kidney disease progression. *Pediatr Nephrol.* 2008;23:705–16.

12.6 EDEMA

Edema is characterized by an increase in interstitial fluid volume and tissue swelling that can either be localized or generalized. Severe generalized edema is known as anasarca. More localized interstitial fluid collections include ascites (peritoneal cavity) and pleural effusions (pleural cavities).

PATHOGENESIS

The extracellular fluid consists of plasma (in capillaries) and interstitial volume (in interstitial space). The movement of fluid between these spaces is determined by the balance of hydrostatic and oncotic pressures in these compartments, and the permeability of the capillary wall that separates them. This is summarized in the following equation:

Net filtration = K_f (change in hydrostatic pressure) − σ (change in oncotic pressure)

$$J_v = K_f(P_c - P_i) - \sigma(\pi_c - \pi_i)$$

K_f = the ultrafiltration coefficient accounting for capillary wall permeability and surface area
σ = reflection co-efficient
P_c = capillary hydrostatic pressure
P_i = interstitial hydrostatic pressure
π_c = capillary oncotic pressure
π_i = interstitial oncotic pressure
σ = reflection co-efficient

For edema to be detected, the interstitial volume is usually expanded by several liters. The physical forces that govern the exchange of fluid between the interstitial and plasma spaces are known as Starling forces.

At equilibrium, fluid is filtered into the interstitial space at the arterial portion of capillaries due to relatively elevated capillary hydrostatic pressure. At the venous portion, fluid tends to go back into the capillary from the interstitial space as a consequence of the increased oncotic pressure. Remaining fluid in the interstitial space is usually taken up by lymphatics. Edema formation results from a derangement of one or more of Starling forces across a capillary bed that

promotes net fluid movement from the plasma to the interstitial space. This can involve one or more of the following mechanisms:

i. Increase in capillary hydrostatic pressure (congestive heart failure);
ii. Decrease in capillary oncotic pressure (hypoalbuminemic state);
iii. Increase in the permeability of the capillary (drug, viral or bacterial infection and allergic angiedema); and
iv. Obstruction of lymphatic flow (malignancy with obstruction).

Role of Kidneys

Edema in congestive heart failure is due to stimulation of sodium retention by the kidneys. Fall in cardiac output is associated with a decrease in effective arterial blood volume. As a consequence, the kidneys attempt to correct this deficit in arterial blood volume by activating sympathetic nervous system and renin-angiotensin system. Renin acts on angiotensin to release angiotensin I, which is broken down to angiotensin II. Angiotensin II has generalized vasoconstrictor properties and causes constriction of efferent renal arterioles. This increases sodium reabsorption from proximal tubule independently. It also stimulates production of aldosterone by zona glomerulosa, which in turn enhances sodium reabsorption by collecting tubule. In heart failure, not only aldosterone secretion is elevated but the biologic half life of it also prolonged.

In acute glomerulonephritis, renal failure and nephrotic syndrome, the arterial blood volume as well as the interstitial volume is increased. The secretion of arginine vasopressin (AVP) and endothelin is also elevated that contributes to renal vasoconstriction, sodium retention, and edema. Arterial distension and/or sodium load also stimulate release into circulation of atrial natriuretic peptide (ANP), which causes arteriolar and venous dilatation, excretion of sodium and water by augmenting glomerular filtration rate, inhibiting sodium reabsorption in proximal tubule and inhibiting release of renin and aldosterone.

Regardless of whether sodium retention is the primary or secondary event, the kidneys play an important role in generalized edema.

EDEMA IN DISEASE STATES

Physiology is described in **Table 12.13**.

A. Edema of Cardiac Diseases

In addition to activation of renin-angiotensin system as described above, the defective systolic emptying of chambers of heart and impairment of ventricular relaxation promotes an accumulation of blood in heart and venous circulation. The increase in venous blood volume causes increase in capillary and lymphatic hydrostatic pressure and leads to edema formation.

In *impairment of right ventricular function*, pressures in systemic veins and capillaries rise, thereby augmenting the transudation of fluid into interstitial space and enhancing peripheral edema. The elevated systemic venous pressure is also transmitted to thoracic duct with consequent reduction of lymph drainage with further increase in accumulation of fluid.

Table 12.13 Physiological Mechanisms and Diagnosis of Diseases Causing Edema

Clinical condition	Mechanism of edema	Clinical findings	Investigations
Nephrotic syndrome	↑Cytokine, ↑aldosterone, ↓ oncotic pressure	Anasarca, frothy urine, dependent edema	Spot urine protein/creatinine >2 mg/mg, or 24-hour urinary protein >40 mg/m²/hr, serum albumin and cholesterol
Acute kidney injury	↑intravascular volume	Oliguria, hypertension, orthopnea, dependent edema	Serum urea, creatinine, serum electrolytes, urinalysis, ABG analysis, chest X-ray, ultrasound
Congestive heart failure	↓ cardiac output, ↑renin, ↑angiotensin, ↑aldosterone	Orthopnea, paroxysmal nocturnal dyspnea, dependent edema, raised JVP, bilateral basal crepts, tender hepatomegaly	Chest X-ray, ECG, echocardiogram
Cirrhosis	Portal hypertension, ↑aldosterone, ↑prostaglandin, ↓oncotic pressure	Hematemesis, malena, varices, caput medusae, ascites, dependent edema, palmar erythema, spider angiomata	Ultrasound scan of the liver, liver biopsy, serum albumin, prothrombin time and INR
Kwashiorkor	↓Oncotic pressure	Weight between 60 and 80th percentile, dependent edema, pshychomotor changes, dermatoses, hypopigmented hairs	Serum albumin
Idiopathic edema	↑Renin, ↑angiotensin or ↑aldosterone	Dependent edema	Serum albumin
Inflammation	Cytokine mediated	Redness, heat, swelling, pain	Acute phase reactants, blood culture
Deep venous thrombosis	Venous obstruction, lymphatic obstruction	Phlegmasia cerulea dolens, Homan's sign, lymphadenopathy	Doppler flow study of superficial and deep veins, lymphogram

In *left sided dysfunction*, there is increase in pulmonary venous and capillary pressure leading to pulmonary edema.

B. Nephrotic Syndrome and Other Hypoalbuminic States

There is decreased oncotic pressure due to massive protein losses into urine. This facilitates shift of water into interstitial compartment and leads to hypovolemia and activation of renin-angiotensin system.

C. Cirrhosis Edema

This is characterized by obstruction to hepatic venous outflow, expansion of splanchnic blood volume and increased hepatic lymph formation. Intrahepatic hypertension also acts a potent stimulus for renal sodium retention and systemic vasodilation and reduction of effective arterial blood volume as well. The secondary hypoalbuminemia due to reduced hepatic synthesis also reduces plasma oncotic pressure and blood volume, which in turn activate renin-angiotensin system, renal sympathetic nerves and sodium retention.

Serum aldosterone is elevated by liver failure due to defective metabolism of this hormone. Initially fluid accumulates in peritoneal cavity but later on peripheral edema and generalized edema may appear.

Treatment — Edema

Treatment should always focus on correcting the underlying cause of the edema.

Localized edema Local edema caused by infection, hypothyroidism, or an autoimmune reaction, should be treated with antibiotics, thyroid replacement, and steroids, respectively. *Generalized edema* Restrict salt and water intake. Diuretics are usually recommended for generalized edema of unknown etiology. If the edema is the result of decreased cardiac function, inotropic agents such as digoxin or dobutamine may be useful in addition with afterload reduction with angiotensin converting enzyme (ACE) inhibitors or angiotensin receptor blockers. In nephrotic syndrome, furosemide and/or spironolactone, prednisolone or other immunosuppressives are the therapeutic modality. Similarly, if edema seems to be caused by glomerulosclerosis or hyperfiltration, angiotensin converting enzyme inhibitors may be beneficial. In cases of acute kidney injury, dialysis may be required for volume removal. Nutritional support is required for patients of kwashiorkor.

Diuretics should not be used for prolonged period. Since it also stimulates the production of aldosterone, it may aggravate cyclical edema of adolescents. In fact, the metabolic alkalosis that arises from the inhibition of chloride reabsorption may actually result in a worsening of the edema because of a decrease in oncotic pressure. This may be a contributing factor in the production of the idiopathic edema associated with the use of diuretics.

Albumin infusions (20% salt poor albumin, 0.5–1g/kg over 30–60 min and furosemide 1–2 mg/kg, IV) are helpful in transient management of patients. Ascites reinfusion, in which ascitic fluid is transferred back into the vascular space either by removal and subsequent reinfusion through a peripheral vein or by continuous reinfusion with a peritoneal-atrial, or LeVeen shunt can be useful in treatment of children with cirrhosis. Head out immersion treatment can increase extravascular hydrostatic pressure, thereby shift fluid into intravascular compartment but the effect lasts only as long as the body is immersed under water, so it is not a practical solution. Support stockings and limb elevation provide the same effect.

Revision Point

Edema

1. Edema in renal diseases starts from periorbital region. Degree of edema is more in nephrotic syndrome than acute glomerulonephritis.
2. Main etiology of edema in nephrotic syndrome is decreased plasma oncotic pressure due to hypoalbuminemia and aggravated by activation of renin-angiotensin system.
3. Measures to reduce edema include salt restriction, diuretic therapy (furosemide and/or spironolactone), and infusion of salt poor albumin (20%) in presence of features of hypovolemia.

Elwell RJ, Spencer AP, Eisele G. Combined furosemide and human albumin treatment for diuretic-resistant edema. *Ann Pharmacother.* 2003;37:695–700.

Hwang SJ, Tsai JH, Lai YH, Chen JH. Plasma atrial natriuretic peptide and natriuretic responses to water immersion in patients with nephrotic syndrome. *Nephron.* 1991;58:330–338.

Teoh CW, Robinson LA, Noone D. Perspectives on edema in childhood nephrotic syndrome. *Am J Physiol Renal Physiol.* 2015 Oct 1;309(7):F575–82.

van de Walle JG, Donckerwolcke RA. Pathogenesis of edema formation in the nephrotic syndrome. *Pediatr Nephrol.* 2001;16: 283–293.

12.7 NEPHROTIC SYNDROME

DEFINITION

Nephrotic syndrome is a common renal disorder in children characterized by generalized edema in association with a biochemical triad comprising of massive proteinuria (>40 mg/m^2/h), hypoalbuminemia (serum albumin <2.5 g/dL) and hypercholesterolemia (serum cholesterol >200 mg/dL). The disease is known to be associated with recurrent remissions and relapses.

In most (90%) children with idiopathic nephrotic syndrome, the disease is sensitive to therapy with oral corticosteroids, and is termed **Steroid Sensitive Nephrotic Syndrome (SSNS)**. The prognosis in these cases is favorable. Approximately 10% children with nephrotic syndrome, who do not respond to therapy with corticosteroids (at the end of 4 weeks of therapy), are classified as **Steroid Resistant Nephrotic Syndrome (SRNS)**, and have an adverse outcome.

PREVALENCE

An estimate on the annual incidence of nephrotic syndrome is 2–7 per 100,000 and it is found to be more among South Asians. In India, the incidence is about 9–10/lac population.

ETIOLOGY

It is *primary (idiopathic)* in 95% cases. *Secondary causes* can be identified in less than 5% cases. Nephrotic syndrome occurs due to alterations of permselectivity at the glomerular capillary wall associated with podocytopathy, resulting in inability of the kidney to restrict the urinary loss of protein.

Primary Nephrotic Syndrome

Primary (idiopathic) nephrotic syndrome is histopathologically dominated by **minimal change disease (MCD)** (approximately 80% of cases). An overwhelming majority of these cases are typical cases of steroid sensitive nephrotic syndrome and do not require a kidney biopsy. Hence, the true incidence of MCD may be even higher.

Other histopathological variants in primary (idiopathic) nephrotic syndrome include *focal segmental glomerulosclerosis (FSGS)* and *mesangioproliferative glomerulonephritis (MesPGN)*. Rare histopathological entities include *membranous nephropathy* and *membranoproliferative glomerulonephritis* (MPGN). These histopathological variants often manifest with steroid resistant nephrotic syndrome or atypical clinical features such as gross hematuria, uremia, and persistent hypertension; necessitating a renal biopsy, which establishes the histopathological diagnosis.

Secondary Nephrotic Syndrome

It occurs in systemic lupus erythematosus, Henoch-Schönlein purpura, sickle cell disease, malaria, Hodgkin disease, intrauterine infections, amyloidosis, and infections like HIV, Parvovirus B19, and hepatitis B and C virus infections. It can also follow administration of NSAIDs, penicillamine, gold, toxins, and allergens. Suspicion of a secondary etiology requires confirmation with a renal biopsy.

PATHOGENESIS

The precise pathogenesis of childhood nephrotic syndrome still remains an enigma. Infections such as viral upper respiratory infections trigger a Th2 cytokine bias, increasing the levels of IL-4, IL-10, and IL-13. It is postulated that these interleukins may bind to receptors located on podocytes, causing effacement of their foot processes. This leads to disruption of the glomerular filtration barrier resulting in massive albuminuria, thereby leading to hypoalbuminemia. Hypoalbuminemia reduces the plasma oncotic pressure, leading to fluid shift from the intravascular to the interstitial compartment. Fluid shift manifests in the form of periorbital edema, anasarca, pleural effusion, ascites, pedal edema or anasarca. The liver synthesizes lipoproteins to compensate for the loss of LDL receptors (LDL-r which are proteins) in the urine, and resulting in hypercholesterolemia.

Evidence for an immunological basis for the disease was historically noted by the observation of the disease going into remission after exposure to measles (which suppresses the cell-mediated immunity), and precipitating by bee or wasp sting. This led to the introduction of steroids, which now have an established place in the management of the disease.

Evidence for a genetic basis for childhood nephrotic syndrome also exists in the form of familial clustering of the disease (even in steroid sensitive patients), in a few cases. Genetic mutations in genes such as *NPHS2, WT1, NPHS1, ACTN4*, and *LAMB2* are reported in congenital nephrotic syndrome (age of onset less than 3 months) as well as infantile nephrotic syndrome. Genetic studies in pediatric nephrotic syndrome are currently recommended for familial steroid resistant nephrotic syndrome, congenital nephrotic syndrome, and initial steroid resistance (first episode of nephrotic syndrome being steroid resistant).

CLINICAL FEATURES

Age of Onset

The median age of onset of MCNS is 4 years (range 2 to 6 years). Onset before 1 year of age or more than 15 years of age is a predictor of non-Minimum Change Disease and requires renal biopsy to establish the histopathological variant.

Presenting Features

The classical presenting feature is that of a viral upper respiratory tract infection in association with periorbital edema followed by edema all over the body (anasarca). This might include pedal edema, ascites, pleural effusion, scrotal/penile/vulval edema. Edema can also occur over the sacral area (dependent body parts) in children who are bed-ridden. The edema is pitting in nature, and is often accompanied by oliguria.

Children with initial episode of nephrotic syndrome tend to present with more edema than those with relapses. This is because the parents recognize proteinuria early at home (often even before the onset of significant edema) in cases of relapse, which leads to early presentation to the hospital.

Although mild transient hypertension is quite common (due to activation of the renin-angiotensin-aldosterone axis, consequent upon fluid shift from the intravascular to the interstitial compartment), it is important to note that persistent or severe hypertension is an atypical finding and points towards a non-Minimal Change Disease. Similarly, even though transient microscopic hematuria is quite common, gross (macroscopic) hematuria is unusual.

Complications as Presenting Features

Other presenting clinical features in children with nephrotic syndrome that could be related to the development of complications include the following:
a. *Serious infections* such as spontaneous bacterial peritonitis (fever, abdominal pain, guarding or rigidity over the abdomen, mucoid diarrhea, sick looking child), pneumonia (fever, dyspnea, cough, lung crepitations), cellulitis (fever with inflamed limb), or rarely urinary tract infections, etc. Spontaneous bacterial peritonitis is the most common severe infection, caused by *Streptococcus pneumoniae*.
b. *Thromboembolic complications* arising from cerebral venous thrombosis, deep vein thrombosis or renal vein thrombosis (because of hypercoagulable state due to loss of antithrombin III in urine, protein C deficiency compounded by volume depletion, sepsis and diuretic use).
c. *Hypovolemic shock.*

Clues to Secondary Etiology

Although primary idiopathic nephrotic syndrome is most common, one should always look out for any features suggestive of secondary etiology of nephrotic syndrome such as malar rash (lupus), palpable purpura (Henoch-Schönlein purpura), hepatosplenomegaly or arthritis (lupus), gross hematuria or cola colored urine (IgA nephropathy, lupus, membranoproliferative glomerulonephritis).

Features of Steroid Toxicity

Children with long-standing disease and/or those on prolonged steroid therapy may present with short stature, poor height gain, posterior subcapsular cataract, glaucoma, abdominal striae, moon face, hypertension, epigastric pain, fractures, etc.

INVESTIGATIONS

It is essential to demonstrate the biochemical triad comprising of (a) massive proteinuria, (b) hypoalbuminemia (serum albumin <2.5 g/dL) and (c) hypercholesterolemia (serum cholesterol >200 mg/dL).

Proteinuria

Massive proteinuria is defined as urine albumin 3+ or 4+ in an early morning urine specimen, either by urine dipstick, or by 20% sulphosalicylic acid test, or by heat coagulation test. Another useful test is the spot urine albumin:creatinine ratio performed on an early morning urine specimen (a value more than 2 indicates nephrotic range proteinuria). Other methods of demonstrating nephrotic range proteinuria include estimating urine protein in 24-hour urine sample ($>1\,g/m^2/24$ hour or $>40\,mg/m^2/$hour). However, collection of 24-hour urine samples in children is often cumbersome and difficult. Hence, a spot urine albumin: creatinine ratio on an early morning sample is considered a very useful test.

Plasma Proteins

Total serum protein is reduced and albumin level is <2.5 g/dL. Serum IgG and IgA are reduced and IgM levels can be elevated. Complement C3 level is normal.

Hyperlipidemia

There are increased serum levels of cholesterol, triglycerides, low density (LDL) and very low density lipoproteins (VLDL). Levels of high density lipoprotein (HDL) may be low, normal or elevated. The hyperlipidemia is due to increased synthesis of lipoproteins in response to hypoalbuminemia and decreased lipoprotein lipase activity.

Other Investigations during the Initial Episode

a. *Blood urea, serum creatinine:* These are usually normal in MCD nephrotic syndrome.
b. *Serum sodium, potassium:* Hyponatremia may be noticed due to hemodilution. Hypokalemia may be noticeable during diuresis.
c. *C3:* Indicated in children with gross hematuria only.
d. Mantoux test and chest radiographs if clinically indicated to rule out TB.
e. HBsAg and antinuclear bodies if clinical examination suggests features of hepatitis or lupus, respectively.

Routinely performing blood and urine cultures in the absence of clinical indications is not advised. Similarly, abdominal paracentesis for ascites in children with nephrotic syndrome should not be done as a routine. This procedure should be reserved for clinical suspicion of peritonitis (*diagnostic tap*) or therapeutic management of severe ascites leading to breathing difficulty (*therapeutic tap*).

Renal Biopsy

Most children with nephrotic syndrome do not require renal biopsy. Indications for renal biopsy are listed in **Box 12.5**.

Box 12.5 Indications of Renal Biopsy in Nephrotic Syndrome
A. **At onset of nephrotic syndrome:** 　1. Age <1 year 　2. Gross hematuria, persistent microscopic hematuria, low C3 levels 　3. Sustained hypertension 　4. Renal failure not attributable to hypovolemia 　5. Suspected secondary cause, eg, lupus, IgA nephropathy, etc. B. **After initial treatment:** 　6. Proteinuria persisting despite 4 weeks of daily prednisolone at 2 mg/kg/day 　7. Before starting treatment with cyclosporine A or tacrolimus

Differential Diagnosis

Differential diagnoses include other renal causes of anasarca such as acute nephritic syndrome and acute kidney injury. Acute nephritic syndrome (most commonly due to post-streptococcal glomerulonephritis) presents with gross or microscopic hematuria (often with cola-colored urine) in association with sub-nephrotic range proteinuria (urine protein:creatinine ratio 0.2–2); often accompanied by hypertension, oliguria or edema (lesser edema than nephrotic syndrome).

Other causes of anasarca such as acute liver failure, constrictive pericarditis, protein losing enteropathy, congestive heart failure should be ruled out by appropriate history, examination, and investigations.

Treatment	**Nephrotic Syndrome**

1. Salt Restriction and Diet

Children with nephrotic syndrome should be advised 'no added salt' during periods of edema (eg, relapses) to prevent edema from increasing. Salt should not be added to salads and fruits, and high salt foods such as pickles, snack items should be avoided during edema. No more than 30% of diet should be derived from fat; and saturated fat should be restricted in the diet in view of hypercholesterolemia. A balanced diet, adequate in proteins (1.5–2 g/day) is recommended. In children with persistent proteinuria, 2–2.5 g/kg/day protein is recommended.

2. Diuretics

Diuretics are not routinely advised in children with nephrotic syndrome to decrease edema. Their use can be accompanied by hazards such as reduction in intravascular volume (that is already often low in nephrotic syndrome) as well as thrombotic complications. Diuretics are advised only in cases with massive ascites leading to respiratory distress; or persistent weight gain

to the extent of more than 10%. In these situations alone, oral frusemide (1–3 mg/kg daily), spironolactone (2–4 mg/kg/day), hydrochlorthiazide (1–2 mg/kg/day) or metolazone (0.1–0.3 mg/kg/day) can be administered.

In refractory edema or refractory ascites (refractory to diuretics and steroid therapy), intravenous 20% human albumin infusion (1 g/kg) is recommended; and this can be accompanied by a careful aseptic abdominal paracentesis for massive refractory ascites. Albumin infusions are also administered for management of hypovolemic shock.

3. Control of Hypertension and Dyslipidemia

Hypertension, if present, can be treated with furosemide (1–2 mg/kg/day), enalapril (0.2–0.5 mg/kg/day) or amlodipine (0.1–0.6 mg/kg/day).

Statins are not recommended for management of steroid sensitive nephrotic syndrome. In steroid resistant nephrotic syndrome, they may be administered in the presence of persistent dyslipidemia for more than 3–6 months (despite dietary control/exercise).

4. Identify and Treat Infections

Urinary tract infections, tuberculosis, and peritonitis need to be identified and treated aggressively before starting steroid therapy. Children with nephrotic syndrome are more prone to develop infections due to low serum IgG levels, defective cell-mediated immunity and defective opsonization of capsulated antigens due to loss of complements in urine. Spontaneous bacterial peritonitis is the most common severe infection, caused by *Streptococcus pneumoniae* and *E.coli*. These children present with tense and tender ascites. Aspiration of the ascitic fluid will reveal pus cells or polymorphs. Spontaneous bacterial peritonitis should be treated with penicillin G and aminoglycosides or third generation cephalosporins (cefotaxime or ceftriaxone).

5. Specific Therapy

Prednisolone is the mainstay of management in nephrotic syndrome. The duration of administration of prednisolone for the initial episode is different from duration of treatment of relapse. Serious infections (if any) such as peritonitis, pneumonia and cellulitis, should be managed with appropriate antibiotics (eg, intravenous ceftriaxone for 10–14 days in spontaneous bacterial peritonitis) before starting steroids.

Terms used in Childhood Nephrotic Syndrome
For the management of children with nephrotic syndrome; it is essential to know some terminologies (**Table 12.14**).

A. *Management of initial episode*
The first episode of steroid sensitive nephrotic syndrome is treated with oral prednisolone at a dose of 2 mg/kg/day (maximum 60 mg) in single or divided doses for 6 weeks, followed by 1.5 mg/kg (maximum 40 mg) as a single morning dose on alternate days for the next 6 weeks (total duration 12 weeks). Prednisolone is abruptly discontinued thereafter.

Pneumococcal vaccine (to prevent spontaneous bacterial peritonitis and pneumonia) and varicella vaccine are advised 4–6 weeks after stopping steroids. Live vaccines should never be administered while on steroids.

Remission is usually achieved in majority of children with MCNS after 10–14 days of starting prednisolone. *Those who do not go into remission despite treatment with prednisolone at a dose of 2 mg/kg (60 mg/m^2/day) for 4 weeks are categorized as steroid resistant nephrotic syndrome (SRNS),* and require renal biopsy for further management.

Table 12.14 Terminologies used in the Management of Childhood Nephrotic Syndrome

Remission	Urine albumin nil or trace for 3 consecutive days
Relapse	Urine albumin 3+ or 4+ for 3 consecutive days, having been in remission previously
Infrequently relapsing nephrotic syndrome	Less than 2 relapses in six months of initial response, or less than 4 relapses in any twelve months
Frequently relapsing nephrotic syndrome	2 or more relapses within six months of initial response, or 4 or more relapses in any twelve months
Steroid dependent nephrotic syndrome	2 consecutive relapses when on alternate day steroids or within 14 days of discontinuation of steroids
Steroid resistant nephrotic syndrome	Absence of remission despite therapy with 4 weeks of daily prednisolone in a dose of 2 mg/kg per day

B. *Management of relapse*

The disease recurs in the majority; more than 75% relapse subsequently and almost half show frequent relapses or steroid dependence.

Infrequently relapsing nephrotic syndrome

Each relapse should be treated with prednisolone 2 mg/kg/day daily (maximum 60 mg) in two divided doses till remission (urine albumin nil/trace for 3 consecutive days) followed by 1.5 mg/kg on alternate days (maximum 40 mg) as single dose in the morning for 4 weeks. Hence, the usual duration of treatment of a relapse is 5–6 weeks. Prednisolone is abruptly discontinued thereafter.

Parents should be taught to perform and grade urine albumin with dipstick and maintain a diary at home. In an event of 3+ or 4+ albumin for 3 consecutive days, they should be asked to contact the hospital for initiation of treatment of a relapse. This is important to detect the relapse before the appearance of significant edema.

C. *Frequently relapsing and steroid dependent nephrotic syndrome*

Frequent relapses are more common in children (*i*) who are less than 3 years of age at onset of disease, (*ii*) who take more than 2 weeks to achieve remission; and those (*iii*) who relapse within 6 months of initial treatment.

If the definition of frequently relapsing or steroid dependent nephrotic syndrome is satisfied (as in **Table 12.15**), then, after treatment of the relapse (for 5–6 weeks, as mentioned in the preceding section), the prednisolone is not discontinued, but tapered by 0.25 mg/kg every 4 weeks and brought down to less than 0.5 mg/kg on every alternate day, so that remission is maintained. This minimum dosage of prednisolone on every alternate day is administered to maintain remission for a period 9 to 18 months, along with calcium carbonate and vitamin D supplements to prevent osteoporosis.

If, on the contrary, the prednisolone threshold, to maintain remission, is higher than 0.5 mg/kg or if features of corticosteroid toxicity are seen, additional use of the following immuno-modulators is suggested, that would act as steroid-sparing agents:

1. **Levamisole** 2–2.5 mg/kg on alternate days orally for a period of 24 months with prednisolone. The main side effect of levamisole is leukopenia; flu-like symptoms, hepatotoxicity, are rare. The leukocyte count should be monitored every 3–4 monthly.
2. **Cyclophosphamide** 2–2.5 mg/kg daily for 12 weeks orally (cumulative dosage should not exceed 168 mg/kg) with alternate day prednisolone. Leukopenia and gonadal toxicity are the chief adverse effects. The leukocyte count should be monitored every 2 weekly during this 12-week period of administration of the drug.
3. **Mycophenolate mofetil** 800–1200 mg/m^2/day orally daily for 24 months along with alternate day tapering doses of prednisolone. The principal side effects include gastro-intestinal discomfort, diarrhea and leukopenia. The leukocyte count should be monitored every 3–4 monthly.
4. **Cyclosporin** 4–5 mg/kg/day orally daily for 24 months along with alternate day tapering doses of prednisolone. It is often possible to discontinue prednisolone after about 6–9 months. Adverse effects include hypertension, gum hypertrophy, hirsutism, acne and nephrotoxicity; hypercholesterolemia may occur. Estimation of serum creatinine is required every 3 months and a lipid profile annually.
5. **Tacrolimus** Tacrolimus is administered at a dose of 0.1–0.2 mg/kg daily orally for 24 months. Adverse effects include hyperglycemia, diarrhea and neurotoxicity (which may manifest as headache, seizures). Estimation of serum creatinine and blood glucose is required every 3 months.

STEROID RESISTANT NEPHROTIC SYNDROME

These cases should be referred to a pediatric nephrologist. Renal biopsy is mandatory for initiating appropriate therapy. If the renal biopsy shows FSGS, MesPGN or MCD, treatment with calcineurin inhibitors (cyclosporin or tacrolimus) for 2 years or intravenous cyclophosphamide (monthly pulses for 6 pulses) is initiated. ACE inhibitors (enalapril), alternate day tapering doses of prednisolone and calcium/vitamin D supplements are administered additionally. Rituximab (anti-CD20 monoclonal antibody) can be given (375 mg/m^2 weekly infusions for 4 weeks) in case of non-response to calcineurin inhibitors. Further management of steroid resistant nephrotic syndrome is beyond the scope of this chapter.

MONITORING ADVERSE EFFECTS OF STEROIDS

A close monitoring of growth velocity (height gain/year) and blood pressure, and evaluation for features of steroid toxicity is essential. These include Cushingoid features and ophthalmological complications (posterior subcapsular cataract and glaucoma). Annual ophthalmological screening of children receiving long-term steroids for these complications is recommended. Calcium and vitamin D supplements should be prescribed for children receiving long-term steroids to prevent osteoporosis.

Steroids should never be prescribed on an empty stomach, to prevent peptic ulcers. Usually, proton pump inhibitors or H2 blockers are not required when steroids are administered after food. However, for children experiencing epigastric symptoms even after taking steroids after food, proton pump inhibitors or H2 blockers should be prescribed.

Eddy AA, Symons JM. Nephrotic syndrome in childhood. *Lancet Lond Engl.* 2003;362:629–39.

Habashy D, Hodson E, Craig J. Interventions for idiopathic steroid-resistant nephrotic syndrome in children. *Cochrane Database Syst Rev.* 2004;CD003594.

Hahn D, Hodson EM, Willis NS, Craig JC. Corticosteroid therapy for nephrotic syndrome in children. *Cochrane Database Syst Rev.* 2015;CD001533.

Indian Pediatric Nephrology Group, Indian Academy of Pediatrics, Bagga A, Ali U, Banerjee S, Kanitkar M, Phadke KD, *et al.* Management of steroid sensitive nephrotic syndrome: revised guidelines. *Indian Pediatr.* 2008;45:203–14.

Case Study	Nephrotic Syndrome

A 4-year-old girl presents with periorbital and pedal edema for 5 days accompanied by abdominal distension along with mildly decreased urine output. There is no past history of similar edema episodes. There is no history of fever, cough, respiratory distress, jaundice, dyspnea, palpitations, joint pain, abdominal pain, limb swelling, or red colored urine.

List the probable diagnoses in this patient based on history and justify.

In view of history of generalized edema and oliguria, possibilities of nephrotic syndrome, post-streptococcal glomerulonephritis, and acute kidney injury should be considered.

The blood pressure is 98/62 mm Hg. There is no palpable purpura, malar rash, cola-colored urine, jaundice, arthritis, or hepatosplenomegaly. The child has urine albumin 4+ by sulphosalicylic acid test, and urine protein:creatinine ratio on an early morning specimen is 3.4. There are no RBC on urinalysis. Serum albumin is 1.8 mg/dL and serum cholesterol is 442 mg/dL. Blood urea is 24 mg/dL and serum creatinine is 0.5 mg/dL.

Mention the most likely diagnosis and justify the same.

The investigations point towards nephrotic syndrome, most probably of Minimum Change Disease (MCD) etiology. The biochemical triad comprising of massive proteinuria, hypoalbuminemia (serum albumin <2.5 g/dL) and hyper-cholesterolemia (serum cholesterol >200 mg/dL) is present in this case, satisfying the definition of nephrotic syndrome.

Will you perform a renal biopsy to confirm the diagnosis?

Renal biopsy should not be performed since there are no atypical features, and the age of onset is between 1 and 15 years of age. Blood urea and serum creatinine are usually normal in Minimum Change Disease (MCD), the most common variant of childhood nephrotic syndrome.

LONG-TERM OUTCOME

The long-term outcome of steroid sensitive nephrotic syndrome is excellent, with studies reporting that between two-thirds to 80% of these children outgrow the disease by puberty. There is a tendency to fewer relapses per year after the first decade of life in majority of cases.

On the contrary, the long-term prognosis of steroid resistant nephrotic syndrome is usually poor, with 50% of cases progressing to chronic renal failure at the end of 10 years.

The most important prognostic factor is steroid responsiveness, and not the histopathological variant.

Nephrotic Syndrome

1. Nephrotic syndrome is a common renal disorder in children characterized by repeated relapses and remissions.
2. It is characterized by a triad of biochemical triad comprising of (*a*) massive proteinuria, (*b*) hypo-albuminemia (serum albumin <2.5 g/dL) and (*c*) hypercholesterolemia (serum cholesterol >200 mg/dL).
3. Most cases respond to steroids and have an excellent long-term prognosis.
4. Renal biopsy is not usually required. Steroid resistant nephrotic syndrome, however, always requires a renal biopsy.

Indian Society of Pediatric Nephrology, Gulati A, Bagga A, Gulati S, Mehta KP, Vijayakumar M. Management of steroid resistant nephrotic syndrome. *Indian Pediatr.* 2009;46:35–47.

12.8 HEMOLYTIC UREMIC SYNDROME

Hemolytic uremic syndrome (HUS) is characterized by a triad of Coombs' negative microangiopathic hemolytic anemia, thrombocytopenia, and acute kidney injury (AKI). It is the most common cause of AKI in children below 3 years of age.

CLASSIFICATION

According to seasonal variation it was earlier described as epidemic form (affects younger children mainly during summer, preceded by diarrhea) and sporadic form (older children, occurs throughout year, no diarrheal prodromal illness). Presently, it is classified into 3 variants, ie., D+, D–, and with co-existing disease/condition.

- D+ (diarrhea associated): *Typical HUS* caused by Shiga toxin producing *E. coli* (STEC)
- D– (not associated with diarrhea prodrome): *Atypical HUS.* It can occur in hereditary conditions (mutations in complement factor H (CFH), complement factor I, membrane co-factor protein), autoimmune (anti-CFH antibodies, dysregulation of alternate complement pathway), cobalamin C defects, and diacylglycerol kinase E mutation.
- *Co-existing disease/condition* Secondary HUS may follow bone marrow or solid organ transplantation, or associated with cancer chemotherapy, autoimmune disorders (systemic lupus erythematosus, antiphospholipid syndrome, scleroderma), drug-induced (cyclosporine A, tacrolimus, sirolimus, clopidogrel), and HIV infection.

ETIOPATHOGENESIS

About 75% cases of D+ HUS are caused by Shiga toxin producing *E.coli.* Most important serotype is 0157 with or without flagella type H7. However, in Indian subcontinent or Africa, *Shigella dysenteriae* type 1 is the major cause. *Streptococcus pneumoniae* and influenza A (H1N1) can also lead to HUS.

The pathology of HUS is broadly described as *thrombotic microangiopathy* (TMA) in which mixed platelet-fibrin thrombi occur in capillaries, arterioles, and sometimes arteries in the absence of vascular inflammation and fibrin deposition. Toxin-induced endothelial injury, cell retraction, or detachment expose procoagulant material in the subendothelial matrix and cause local thrombosis. Red cells and platelets get injured while traversing these damaged vessels. Though microvascular injury occurs mainly in kidneys, other organs specially brain may be affected.

Three sub-types of microangiopathy are recognized, depending upon renal tissue involved:
 i. Glomerular TMA (D+ HUS);
 ii. Arterial TMA (D–HUS); and
iii. Cortical necrosis with TMA, following bacillary dysentery in India and Bangladesh.

CLINICAL MANIFESTATIONS

A. Typical HUS (D+)

A prodromal phase of acute dysentery with abdominal pain and vomiting precedes by 1–15 days. The onset of illness is sudden causing acute kidney injury (AKI); about 50% of patients are anuric. If urine output is there, hematuria and proteinuria are consistent features. Hypertension and hypervolemia are also present at the time of presentation.

Systemic manifestations include severe hemorrhagic colitis (10–20%), central nervous system involvement (20%), hepatitis (40%), and acute pancreatitis (20%). The nervous system involvement leads to focal or generalized seizure, stupor, coma, hemiparesis, cortical blindness, and brain stem involvement. Myocarditis, cardiogenic shock, and pulmonary edema are the other manifestations.

B. Atypical HUS (D–)

There is no preceding dysentery. These cases represent only 10% of HUS in children. Renal failure has a remitting and relapsing course. Decline in renal function leads to end-stage renal disease in most patients over a period of months to years. Neurological symptoms can also occur.

INVESTIGATIONS

Peripheral smear reveals evidence of red cell fragmentation as schistocytes, burr cells, and helmet cells. Coombs test is negative and there is reticulocytosis and thrombocytopenia. Coagulation tests are normal. Plasma urea and creatinine are increased. Urine microscopy may reveal microscopic hematuria and proteinuria. Stool/rectal swab culture is done for detection of STEC. Assay of C3, C4, anti-CFH antibodies and screening for mutations in CFH, CFI membrane co-factor protein by direct sequencing or next generation sequencing can also be performed in cases of atypical HUS. High plasma levels of homocysteine and methylmalonic acid can be detected in cobalamin C defect associated HUS.

Treatment	Hemolytic Uremic Syndrome

Treatment is supportive with management of AKI, anemia, hypertension, and correction of fluid and electrolyte disturbances. Acute kidney injury is present in 95% of STEC-HUS and 85% of atypical HUS and dialysis is required in 50–60% of cases. Early peritoneal dialysis or hemodialysis is the most effective way of preventing complications and should be

instituted as soon as patients with HUS become oligoanuric. Use of antibiotics in enterocolitis has been associated with an increased risk of HUS and it should be avoided.

Supportive therapy is effective in STEC-HUS, while plasma exchange/transfusion in addition to anti-C5 antibody (eculizumab) has been found to be beneficial in recovery of renal function in atypical HUS and reduction in mortality.

Case Study	Hemolytic Uremic Syndrome

A 2-year-old girl presented in emergency with passage of decreased urine output for 24 hours. There was a history of frequent passage of stool mixed with blood 10 days back, and now developed decreased urine output and swelling over the body.

What physical findings you will look for in this patient?
I will look for puffiness of face, pedal edema, acidotic breathing, and evidence of skin and mucous membrane bleeding, and will record blood pressure for evidence of hypertension.

What is most likely diagnosis?
The most likely diagnosis in this patient is hemolytic uremic syndrome (HUS) as she had history of dysentery followed by oliguria, edema, and bleeding but other causes of AKI should be excluded.

Mention relevant investigations to confirm diagnosis.
Hemoglobin for degree of anemia, complete blood count, peripheral blood smear examination for thrombocytopenia, and features of hemolysis such as fragmented RBCs, schistocytes, burr cells, and reticulocytosis. Renal function tests (serum urea, creatinine, sodium, potassium) must be done to assess the severity of acute kidney injury. Also get C3, C4, and assay of anti-CFH antibody.

Outline management of this patient.
The child should have restricted fluid intake (400 mL/m²/day) and institution of early peritoneal or hemodialysis. If dialysis facility is not available, then plasma transfusion/plasma exchange is advised for dilution and removal of toxins. Hypertension should be treated with calcium channel blocker and/or beta blocker. Meticulous recording of urine output, renal function tests, and blood pressure should be done in the follow up.

OUTCOME

Early mortality of HUS in children is less than 3%, and largely due to acute cerebral edema and hindbrain herniation. 20–30% of survivors experience adverse renal outcome and include proteinuria, hypertension, and renal impairment. An adverse outcome is more likely in D-HUS and if the patient required more than 14 days of dialysis during the acute stage HUS. The best predictive feature of long-term renal outcome is the duration of anuria. Risks of chronic renal insufficiency are very high in case of cortical necrosis or when >50% of glomeruli show microangiopathy.

Carter S, Hewitt I, Kausman J. Long-term remission with eculizumab in atypical haemolytic uraemic syndrome. *Nephrology* (Carlton). 2017 Feb;22 Suppl 1:7–10.
Fakhouri F, Zuber J, Frémeaux-Bacchi V, Loirat C. Haemolytic uraemic syndrome. *Lancet*. 2017 Feb 25.
Jokiranta TS. HUS and atypical HUS. *Blood*. 2017 May 25;129(21): 2847–2856.

Hemolytic Uremic Syndrome

1. Hemolytic uremic syndrome (HUS) consists of a triad of microangiopathic hemolytic anemia, thrombocytopenia, and acute kidney injury.
2. Typical HUS follows dysentery and caused by Shiga toxin producing *E.coli*; Atypical HUS occurs mostly because of genetic mutations of complement system.
3. Peripheral smear reveals evidence of red cell fragmentation as schistocytes, burr cells, and helmet cells. Coombs' test is negative and there is reticulocytosis and thrombocytopenia.
4. Treatment is mainly supportive. Dialysis is required in 50–60% cases of HUS.
5. Early mortality of HUS in children is <3%. Adverse renal outcome occurs in 20–30% of survivors.

Loirat C, Fakhouri F, Ariceta G, *et al.* An international consensus approach to the management of atypical haemolytic uremic syndrome in children. *Pediatr Nephrol.* 2016;31:15–39.

Zhang K, Lu Y, Harley KT, Tran MH. Atypical hemolytic uremic syndrome: a brief review. *Hematol Rep.* 2017 Jun 1;9(2):7053.

12.9 ACUTE KIDNEY INJURY

Acute kidney injury (AKI) is a clinical condition characterized by rapid decline in glomerular filtration rate leading to oliguria/anuria, retention of nitrogenous waste products (urea, creatinine), and electrolyte and acid–base disturbances.

Oliguria is defined as urine output <0.5 mL/kg/hour in neonates, <1 mL/kg/hour in infants; and < 500 mL/m²/day in older children. Although the kidneys perform multiple roles (eg, metabolic, endocrine, fluid and electrolyte balance), but the GFR is accepted as the index of functioning renal mass, which is calculated by the following formula:

$$\text{GFR (mL/min/1.73m}^2) = K \times \frac{\text{Height (cm)}}{\text{Cr (mg/dL)}}$$

K = 0.33 for LBW infant <1 year, 0.45 for AGA infants <1 year, 0.55 for children and adolescent females, and 0.70 for adolescent males.

CLASSIFICATION

AKI is classified using the criteria of **R**isk, **I**njury, **F**ailure, **L**oss, and **E**nd-stage renal failure (**RIFLE**). The adult RIFLE criteria is based on changes in serum creatinine from baseline, an abrupt decrease in urine output, and the length of renal replacement required at later stages. A modified pediatric RIFLE (pRIFLE) criteria has been used for child patients in the intensive care unit setting (**Table 12.15**).

ETIOLOGY

I. In Neonates

(*i*) septicemia; (*ii*) birth asphyxia; (*iii*) obstructive uropathy; (*iv*) renal vein thrombosis; (*v*) multicystic dysplastic kidney.

II. In Older Children

The AKI may be classified into *Pre-renal azotemia* caused by acute renal hypoperfusion with intact renal parenchyma; *Renal azotemia* caused by acute diseases of renal parenchyma of tubular damage due to ischemic insult or toxins; and *Post-renal azotemia* because of obstructive uropathy. The different causes of AKI are presented in **Table 12.16**.

PATHOPHYSIOLOGY

Regardless of the cause of renal failure, reduction in renal blood flow represents a common pathologic pathway for decrease in GFR. The decreased renal blood flow eventually leads to ischemia and cell death. This initial ischemic insult triggers production of oxygen free radicals and enzymes that continue to cause cell injury even after restoration of blood flow. The tubular cell damage results in disruption of tight junctions between cells, allowing back leak of glomerular filtrate and further decrease in GFR. In addition, dying cells slough off into tubules forming obstructing casts, which further decrease GFR and lead to oliguria.

CLINICAL FEATURES

A child with AKI presents with oliguria or anuria associated with facial puffiness, pedal edema, and acidotic breathing. There may be associated hematuria, hypertension, convulsions, and encephalopathy. There may be a history of preceding events like gastroenteritis, viral exanthems, boils and drugs intake like penicillin, sulphonamides, vancomycin, amphotericin B, or aminoglycosides.

LABORATORY INVESTIGATIONS

A. Renal Functions

Urea and electrolytes Blood urea and serum creatinine are increased. Serum sodium is either normal or decreased, and potassium is increased or low (HUS). Serum calcium level

Table 12.15 Pediatric-modified RIFLE (pRIFLE) Criteria		
	Estimated CCl	*Urine output*
Risk	eCCl decrease by 25%	<0.5 mL/kg/h for 8 h
Injury	eCCl decrease by 50%	<0.5 mL/kg/h for 16 h
Failure	eCCl decrease by 75% or eCCl<35 mL/min/1.73 m²	<0.3 mL/kg/h for 24 h or Anuric for 12 h
Loss	Persistent failure >4 weeks	
End stage	End-stage renal disease (persistent failure >3 months)	

(eCCl estimated creatinine clearance, calculated using the Schwartz formula)

Table 12.16 Etiology of Acute Kidney Injury		
Pre-renal	*Renal*	*Post-renal*
1. Hypovolemia • Hemorrhage • GI losses • Hypoproteinemia • Burns • Renal or adrenal diseases with salt wasting 2. Hypotension • Septicemia • DIC • Hypothermia • Hemorrhage • Heart failure 3. Hypoxia • Pneumonia • Respiratory distress syndrome	1. Glomerulonephritis • Poststreptococcal • SLE • MPGN • RPGN • Anaphylactoid purpura 2. Acute tubular necrosis • Heavy metals/drugs • Chemicals • Hemoglobin/ myoglobin • Shock • Ischemia 3. Hemolytic uremic syndrome 4. Renal vein thrombosis 5. Acute interstitial nephritis (drugs/ infection) 6. Developmental • Cystic disease • Hypoplasia/dysplasia 7. Hereditary nephritis	1. Obstructive uropathy • Ureteropelvic junction obstruction • Ureterocele • Posterior urethral valve • Tumor 2. Vesicoureteric reflux 3. Acquired • Stones • Blood clots

is normal or reduced and phosphate is increased. Arterial blood gas analysis shows features of metabolic acidosis (decreased pH and low bicarbonate).

Relation of serum creatinine with GFR
- Creatinine 1.0 mg/dL—normal GFR
- Creatinine 2.0 mg/dL—50% reduction in GFR
- Creatinine 4.0 mg/dL—70–80% reduction in GFR
- Creatinine 8.0 mg/dL—90–95% reduction in GFR

Renal failure indices These help in differentiating functional oliguria from intrinsic renal failure. Common indices are urinary sodium, osmolality, functional excretion of urea and sodium, and ratios of blood urea creatinine, and urine *vs.* plasma osmolality. Expected values are listed in **Table 12.17**.

Urine examination It should be done for proteinuria, hematuria, pus cells, eosinophils, red cell casts or granular casts. Urine culture should also be done to rule out associated urinary tract infection.

B. Other Investigations

Hematological parameters Hemoglobin may be low due to severe hemolysis, dilutional anemia, and precipitation of pre-existing nutritional anemia. Total leucocyte counts are either normal or increased as in HUS (mostly neutrophils), or allergic interstitial nephritis (eosinophilia). Peripheral blood smear may show features of hemolysis in HUS, malaria and G6PD deficiency. Absolute platelet count is decreased in acute kidney injury secondary to HUS, lupus nephritis, and disseminated intravascular coagulation.

Imaging Chest X-ray is done to rule out cardiomegaly and pulmonary edema.

Table 12.17 Renal Failure Indices		
Index	*Functional oliguria*	*Intrinsic renal failure*
Urinary sodium (mEq/L)	<20 (<30)	>40 (>60)
Urinary osmolality (mOsm/kg)	>500 (>400)	<300 (<350)
Blood urea creatinine ratio	>20:1	<20:1
Urine plasma osmolaity ratio	>1.5(>2)	<0.8–1.2 (<1.1)
FENa (%)	<1*(<3)	>1(>10)
Fractional excretion of urea *	<35%	>35%

*This is more sensitive and specific than FENa in differentiating between pre-renal and renal cause of ARF especially when diuretics have been administered.

$$\text{Fractional excretion of Na}^+ (\text{FENa}) = \frac{\text{Urine Na}^+ \times \text{Serum creatinine}}{\text{Urine creatinine} \times \text{Serum sodium}} \times 100$$

Exceptions (intrinsic renal failure with FENa <1%) are urinary tract obstruction, acute glomerulonephritis, hepatorenal syndrome, and radiologic contrast induced acute tubular necrosis.

*Pre-renal ARF with FENa >1% (patients on diuretics, pre-existing chronic renal failure and patient with bicarbonaturia)

ECG It is done to detect hyperkalemia. Look for tall tented T wave, widening of QRS complex, ST segment depression, prolongation of PR interval, absent P wave, and complete heart block.

USG abdomen Renal ultrasonography is required to rule out hydronephrosis, hydroureter, loss of corticomedullary differentiation, stones, clots, and tumors.

Color Dopper flow is indicated for suspected renal vein thrombosis and renal arterial stenosis/thrombosis.

Renal biopsy Indicated for children in whom pre-renal and post-renal AKI has been excluded and cause of intrinsic AKI is unclear, eg, vasculitis, glomerulonephritis, and interstitial nephritis.

BIOMARKERS OF AKI

The rise in serum creatinine in AKI is a late phenomenon and it occurs when 50% of the renal function is already lost. Certain urinary biomarkers such as neutrophil associated gelatinase lipocalin A (NGAL), kidney injury molecule-1, N-acetyl-beta-D–glucosaminidase activity, interleukin-18, and plasma cystatin C have been found to be helpful to detect early AKI. Of these, NGAL is considered better and has modest sensitivity and specificity for early diagnosis of AKI following cardiac surgery, sepsis, and contrast induced nephropathy.

Treatment — Acute Kidney Injury

Recovery from AKI is mainly dependent upon restoration of renal blood flow. In pre-renal involvement, correction of dehydration and restoration of renal blood flow is usually sufficient. With intrinsic renal conditions, removal of toxins and initiation of therapy for glomerular disease results in normalization of renal function. Relief of urinary obstruction in post-renal cause results in prompt normalization of blood flow to renal tissue.

A. Pre-renal AKI

Immediate correction of dehydration is achieved by intravenous administration of 20 mL/kg of normal saline or Ringer lactate over 20 minutes. Repeat the same dose if dehydration persists. After volume resuscitation, hypovolemic patients usually void within 2 hours.

Consider diuretic therapy (furosemide 2–4 mg/kg IV), if the child does not pass urine, as a single dose. Failure to pass urine following diuretic treatment requires evaluation for intrinsic or post renal causes of AKI.

B. Treatment of Intrinsic (renal) AKI

Patients with normal intravascular volume should be given 5% or 10% dextrose, 400 mL/m^2/24 h (insensible loss) plus amount of fluid lost in urine/stool/blood (mililitre for mililiter) by N/2 saline. Children with marked hypervolemia may require further restriction of fluid. Further, composition of fluid can be changed according to electrolyte report. Fluid intake, urine/stool output, weight and serum biochemistry need to be monitored on daily basis. **Table12.18** summarizes a problem based management approach in a child with AKI.

Table 12.18 Management of Complications of Acute Kidney Injury		
Problem	*Treatment*	*Remarks*
Fluid overload	Fluid restriction: 400 mL/m^2/day of 5% dextrose for insensible losses; N/2 saline for urine output (replace mL by mL), single dose of furosemide in oliguric patients	Monitor other losses and replace as appropriate
Pulmonary edema	(i) Oxygen; (ii) dopamine 5–10 µg/kg per minute, (iii) furosemide (one dose only) 2–4 mg/kg IV	Monitor by CVP line; peritoneal dialysis with hypertonic glucose/hemodialysis
Hypertension	*Symptomatic:* (i) Nitroprusside 0.5–8 µg/kg per minute infusion or labetalol infusion 0.25–3 mg/kg/hr; (ii) furosemide (one dose only) 2–4 mg/kg IV; (iii) nifedipine 0.25 mg/kg orally *Asymptomatic:* Salt restriction, furosemide treatment	Watch for fluid overload and hypernatremia; consider dialysis
Hyperkalemia	*Acute emergency*: Calcium gluconate (10%), 0.5–1 mL/kg over 5–10 minutes *Less urgent*: (i) Salbutamol 5–10 mg nebulization (ii) Sodium bicarbonate (7.5%), 1–2 mEq/kg over 15–20 minutes (iii) Glucose (50%) 0.5–1 g/kg with 0.1–02 units/kg insulin (iv) Calcium resonium 1g/kg/day	Stabilizes cell membranes; prevents arrhythmia Shifts potassium into cells Shifts potassium into cells Shifts potassium into cells Given orally or rectally
Hyponatremia	(i) Fluid restriction; (ii) if sensorial alteration or seizures, 3% saline 6–12 mL/kg; 30–90 min or; (iii) mEq of Na required = 0.6 × wt (kg) × 125–observed Na	Hyponatremia mostly due to fluid excess; 12 mL/kg of 3% saline raises sodium by 10 mEq/L
Anemia	(i) Packed red blood cells 3–5 mL/kg; (ii) Consider exchange transfusion	Monitor blood pressure
High serum phosphate	(i) Phosphate binders (calcium carbonate, acetate); (ii) Dietary phosphate restriction	Avoid aluminum-containing agents
Metabolic acidosis	NaHCO$_3$ (7.5%) mEq = 0.3 × wt (kg) × 12 – observed HCO$_3$	If intractable, consider dialysis

Dialysis

Clinical indications Deteriorating neurological status, intractable seizures, congestive heart failure, pulmonary edema, hypertension, features of volume overload, bleeding diathesis due to uremic platelet dysfunction, and anuria >24 hours.

Biochemical indications Blood urea >200 mg/dL, rate of rise of blood urea >20 mg/dL/day, hyperkalemia >6 mEq/L, refractory hyperphosphatemia, and persistent metabolic acidosis.

Peritoneal dialysis does not require vascular access and sophisticated equipment, so it is preferred dialytic procedure in younger children.Older patients can be put on continuous *veno-venous* hemofiltration (CVVH) or intermittent hemodialysis depending upon the facility and expertise available.

Supportive care

Nutritional support Requirements are as follows: Energy 20–30 kcal/kg/d; carbohydrate 3–5 g/kg/d; fat 0.8–1 g/kg/d; protein intake of 0.8–1.0 g/kg/d in non-catabolic AKI patients without need for dialysis; 1.0–1.5 g/kg/d in patients with AKI on renal replacement therapy; and 1.7 g/kg/d in patients on continuous renal replacement therapy and hypercatabolic patients. Protein should be of high biological value. Vitamin and micronutrients should be supplemented.

Treat anemia with fresh blood transfusion (if Hb <7g/dL), as old blood contains increased amount of potassium. Use antibiotics to treat the infection. Doses of the antibiotics are modified as per **Table 12.19.**

Antimicrobials needing dose reduction in acute kidney injury Antibiotics which do not require dose modifications at all are azithromycin, cefaclor, cloxacillin, chloramphenicol, and linezolid. Antibiotics which can be given at normal dose safely up to a fall of GFR of 40 mL/min/1.73 m^2 include ceftriaxone, cefotaxime, cefixime, ciprofloxacillin, cefuroxime axetil, ampicillin, amoxicillin, trimethoprim, clarithromycin, erythromycin, clindamycin, and metronidazole.

Case Study | **Acute Kidney Injury**

A 4-year-old boy presented with history of high grade fever, frequent loose stools, and vomiting for 2 days, followed by decreased urine output, mild periorbital puffiness, and fast breathing. There is no history of dysentery, sore throat, skin lesions, headache, red urine, seizures.

On physical examination, child was well nourished and had puffiness of face with pedal edema. There was no evidence of skin or mucosal bleeding. His pulse was 92/ min, regular, fair volume, RR 22/min, BP 160/90 mmHg, and JVP was not raised. He had acidotic breathing. Microscopic examination of urine showed only hyaline casts.

Mention the most likely diagnosis. Justify.

Presence of edema and oliguria, preceded by infective diarrhea, points towards a possibility of acute kidney injury. Since there is no dehydration, AKI is unlikely to be pre-renal in origin. Probable etiology is acute tubular necrosis.

Enumerate relevant investigations to confirm your diagnosis in order of priority.

The relevant investigations in order of priority are: (*i*) peripheral blood smear to look for evidence of hemolysis and thrombocytopenia (to rule out HUS); (*ii*) serum urea and creatinine to classify AKI as per pRIFLE criteria, (*iii*) ABG analysis for evidence of metabolic acidosis, anion gap, and hyperkalemia; (*iv*) C3 and C4 levels to reveal type of glomerulonephritis (low C3 in PIGN, and MPGN and both C3 and C4 low in SLE nephritis); and (*v*) serum electrolytes for evidence of hyperkalemia and treatment as per severity of hyperkalemia.

List important complications in this child.

Expect hyperkalemia, cardiac arrhythmias, metabolic acidosis, hypertensive encephalopathy, and left ventricular failure.

Table 12.19 Dose Modification of Antibiotics According to Glomerular Filtration Rate (GFR)

Drug	GFR : 40	GFR : 10	Anuric
Paracetamol	Normal dose	50%,↑ interval	50%, ↑ interval
Amikacin	40% od	20% od	10% od
Gentamicin	60% bid	10% od	5% od
Ceftriaxone	Normal dose	80% od	50% od
Ceftazidime	50% bid	15% od	10% od
Vancomycin	30% od	5% od	15 mg/kg, followed by 1.9 mg/kg/day
Ciprofloxacillin	Normal dose	50% od	33% od
Amoxicillin	Normal dose	30% bid	15% od
Amoxicillin + clavulinic acid	Normal dose	25% bid	15% od
Phenobarbitone	80%	30%	25%
Phenytoin	Normal dose	Normal dose	Normal dose
Ranitidine	Normal dose	50% bid	50% bid
Steroids	Normal dose	Normal dose	Normal dose

od: Once a day; bid: two times a day

12

Outcome

Acute kidney injury consists of 3 phases: Oliguric phase, diuretic phase, and post-diuretic recovery phase. *Oliguric phase* lasts for about 5–10 days, followed by *diuretic phase* leading to increase in urine output (2–3 liters/day) and it is due to inability of damaged tubules to concentrate urine which results in loss of excess fluid. In *recovery phase*, general condition improves and there is normalization of renal function.

Outcome of the AKI depends upon the nature of underlying disease process and stage of AKI. It carries a mortality of 20–50%. The risk of mortality is 2.5 times higher in risk, 5.4 times in injury and 10.1 times in failure stage of AKI. Recovery of AKI due to pre-renal causes like HUS, acute tubular necrosis, and interstitial nephritis is good.

Poor prognostic features include anuria >72 hours, cortical necrosis, AKI in infancy, sepsis, shock, and fluid overload. Medical management may be necessary for prolonged period of time to treat sequel of AKI including CKD, hypertension, renal tubular acidosis, etc.

Acute Kidney Injury

1. AKI is classified using the **RIFLE** (**R**isk, **I**njury, **F**ailure, **L**oss, and **E**nd-stage renal failure) criteria.
2. The common causes of AKI in newborns are sepsis and birth asphyxia, while acute tubular necrosis following severe dehydration due to acute gastroenteritis is the leading cause in children.
3. The most useful biomarker for early detection of AKI is neutrophil gelatinase-associated lipocalin A (NGAL).
4. Hyperkalemia in AKI is a serious biochemical abnormality and can be treated with salbutamol nebulization, intravenous calcium gluconate administration, glucose-insulin infusion, and dialysis.
5. Recovery of renal function is good in acute tubular necrosis, while it is poor in cortical necrosis.

Benoit SW, Devarajan P. Acute kidney injury: emerging pharmacotherapies in current clinical trials. *Pediatr Nephrol.* 2017 Jun 10.

Burdmann EA, Chakravarthi R. Peritoneal dialysis in acute kidney injury: lessons learned and applied. *Semin Dial.* 2011;24:149–56.

Ciccia E, Devarajan P. Pediatric acute kidney injury: prevalence, impact and management challenges. *Int J Nephrol Renovasc Dis.* 2017 Mar 29;10:77–84.

Daschner M. Drug dosage in children with reduced renal function. *Pediatric Nephrol.* 2005;20:1675–86.

Elella RA, Habib E, Mokrusova P, et al. Incidence and outcome of acute kidney injury by the pRIFLE criteria for children receiving extracorporeal membrane oxygenation after heart surgery. *Ann Saudi Med.* 2017 May-Jun;37(3):201–206.

Filho LT, Grande AJ, Colonetti T, Della ÉSP, da Rosa MI. Accuracy of neutrophil gelatinase-associated lipocalin for acute kidney injury diagnosis in children: systematic review and meta-analysis. *Pediatr Nephrol.* 2017 Jun 14.

Goldstein SL. Acute kidney injury in children: prevention, treatment and rehabilitation. *Contrib Nephrol.* 2011;174:163–72.

KDIGO Clinical Practice Guideline for Acute Kidney Injury: Evaluation and general management of patients with and at risk for AKI. Kidney Int Supplements http://www.kidney-international.org; 2012.

Mohrer D, Langhan M. Acute kidney injury in pediatric patients: diagnosis and management in the emergency department. *Pediatr Emerg Med Pract.* 2017 May;14(5):1–24. Epub 2017 May 2.

Uchino S, Bellomo R, Goldsmith D, et al. An assessment of the RIFLE criteria for acute renal failure in hospitalized patients. *Crit Care Med* 2006; 34: 1913–1917.

12.10 CHRONIC KIDNEY DISEASE

Chronic kidney disease (CKD) It is defined as abnormalities of kidney structure or function, present for >3 months, with or without decreased GFR; OR any patient who has GFR <60 mL/min/1.73 m^2 lasting for at least 3 months with or without kidney damage (structure or function).

End-stage renal disease (ESRD) This is characterized by decline of renal function to a degree when life cannot be sustained without replacement of renal function either in form of dialysis or transplantation.

ETIOLOGY

Congenital anomalies are the most common cause of CKD in children below 5 years. Glomerulonephritis is responsible for most cases of CKD in older children.

1. *Congenital anomalies of kidney and urinary tract (60% cases)* Hypoplasia, dysplasia ± reflux nephropathy, obstructive nephropathy.
2. Focal segmental glomerulosclerosis (5–10%)
3. *Glomerulonephritis* (5–10%) Lupus nephritis, Henoch-Schonlein purpura, IgA nephropathy, membrano-proliferative glomerulonephritis.
4. *Hereditary* Familial juvenile nephronophthisis, Alport syndrome, autosomal recessive polycystic kidney disease, familial nephrotic syndrome.
5. *Metabolic* Cystinosis, oxalosis
6. *Vascular* Renal vein thrombosis
7. *Renal cortical necrosis* Hemolytic uremic syndrome (atypical)
8. *Other* Prune-belly syndrome, bilateral Wilms tumor.

STAGES OF CHRONIC KIDNEY DISEASE

National Kidney Foundation Disease Outcome Quality Initiative (KFDOQI)

Stage	GFR (mL/min/1.73m^2)	Description
1	>90	Kidney damage with normal or increased GFR
2	60–89	Kidney damage with mild decrease in GFR
3	30–59	Moderate decrease in GFR
4	15–29	Severe decrease in GFR
5	<15 (or on dialysis)	Kidney failure

Systemic hypertension, acidosis, and proteinuria are the most important independent risk factors for progression of CKD. Other factors are underlying renal disease, polymorphic genetic variation, hyperphosphatemia, dyslipidemia, and insulin resistance.

CLINICAL PRESENTATION

The onset is usually insidious. The clinical manifestations are usually nonspecific and include fatigue, anorexia, headache, lethargy, vomiting, polyuria, polydipsia, and growth failure. On physical examination, majority of patients are anemic and have high blood pressure. In children with

Table 12.20 Clinical Manifestations of Chronic Kidney Disease

Renal	Edema, hematuria, proteinuria, hypertension
Metabolic	Hypocalcemia, metabolic acidosis, hypekalemia/hypokalemia, hyperphosphatemia, hyperglycemia, and hyperlipidemia
Hematological	Anemia, bleeding tendency
Cardiovascular	Congestive heart failure, hypertension, pericarditis
Gastrointestinal	Anorexia, vomiting, GERD, gastroduodenal ulcer
Neurological	Fatigue, poor concentration, headache, drowsiness, loss of memory, slurred speech, muscle weakness and cramps, psychosis, ataxia, tremors, asterixis, seizures, coma, mental retardation, peripheral neuropathy (motor, sensory or autonomic), and encephalopathy.
Dermatological	Pruritus, dermatitis
Reproductive	Delayed sexual development
Musculoskeletal	Muscle weakness, growth retardation, renal osteodystrophy
Miscellaneous	Failure to thrive, polyuria, dehydration

congenital renal abnormalities, growth retardation, and osteodystrophy are present. In any child having severe unexplained anemia, growth retardation, hypertension and acidotic breathing, CKD is most likely diagnosis. Other clinical manifestations are mentioned in **Table 12.20**.

Anemia in CKD

Anemia is common in children with CKD and manifests in stage 3 and 4 or when GFR falls to 25–35 mL/min/1.73 m². The causes of anemia include erythropoietin deficiency, iron deficiency, blood loss (phlebotomy, hemodialysis, gastrointestinal), hemolysis, malnutrition, B_{12} or folate deficiency, bone marrow suppression, chronic or acute inflammation, carnitine deficiency, and associated systemic diseases such as SLE, or malignancy. The etiology of iron deficiency in CKD include blood losses, poor dietary intake, poor absorption and depletion of iron store during recombinant human erythropoietin therapy (rHuEPO). Clinical manifestations include fatigue, depression, decreased quality of life, decreased exercise tolerance, impaired cognitive function, and loss of appetite.

Renal Osteodystrophy

Renal osteodystrophy occurs usually late in children with CKD and is characterized by osteopenia, osteoporosis/ rickets, osteosclerosis, and osteitis fibrosa cystica. *Osteitis fibrosa cystica* is characterized by increased osteoclast and osteoblast activity and excessive woven bone, high bone turnover, increased quantity of unmineralized bone matrix (osteoid).

The clinical manifestations include muscle weakness, bony pain, fractures with minor trauma, and valgus and varus deformities of long bones. Slipped femoral epiphysis, bowing of lower extremities, soft tissue calcification, rachitic rosary and Harrison sulcus may be present. Pathophysiology of osteodystrophy is depicted in Fig. 12.12.

Short stature is the sequelae of childhood CKD (30–60% of children with ESRD may grow up to become stunted adults). The causes include protein and calorie malnutrition, fluid and electrolyte disturbances, renal osteodystrophy, end organ hyporesponsiveness to growth hormone, and anemia. Growth failure is severe in children who develop renal

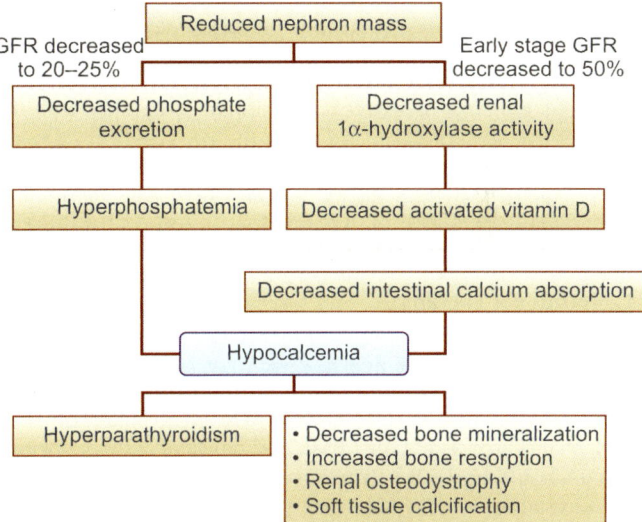

Fig. 12.12 Pathophysiology of renal osteodystrophy

insufficiency in the first 2 years of life as children normally attain one-third of their final adult height during this period.

INVESTIGATIONS

Renal Functions

The first and most important step in evaluation is calculation of GFR of the patient as detailed in chapter of AKI. Initial evaluation includes complete blood count, serum creatinine, urea, electrolytes, calcium, phosphorus, alkaline phosphatase, iPTH, total protein/albumin, uric acid, cholesterol, triglycerides, serum iron, TIBC, percentage saturation of transferrin, serum ferritin, reticulocyte count, and arterial blood gases. Urine analysis should look for hematuria, proteinuria, casts, and specific gravity.

Imaging

X-rays of wrist, long bones, chest, and spine should be done every 6 months in children with CKD.

Early radiographic findings are features of osteopenia (thinning of cortices and trabeculae gives ground glass appearance), salt and pepper skull, epiphyseal thickening and fraying of metaphysis but no cupping, late epiphyseal ossification, and slipped epiphysis.

Late radiological features are secondary to hyperparathyroidism and include subperiosteal cortical resorption of distal phalanx, end of clavicle, ischium, pubis, sacroiliac joints, metaphyseal–diaphyseal junction of long bones, lucent metaphyseal bands, bowing of long bones, rugger jersey spine, brown tumor of ribs and jaw.

USG of KUB should also be done for kidney size, hydronephrosis, calculi, cystic and solid lesions of kidney.

Others

Decreased serum calcium, increased phosphate, increased alkaline phosphatase, normal PTH level, and increased iPTH level are usual findings in children with renal osteodystrophy.

Renal biopsy can be undertaken to demonstrate the glomerular pathology.

Treatment	Chronic Kidney Disease

The aim of treatment is to replace absent/diminished renal functions which progressively deteriorate in parallel with the progressive loss of GFR and slow the progression of renal dysfunction. Hyperkalemia is usually not observed until GFR decreases to less than 10 mL/min/1.73m². Management of hyperkalemia, acidosis, and hypertension should be done as already described in **Table 12.18**.

1. Nutritional Therapy
Poor nutritional status in children with CKD is due to anorexia, altered taste, frequent illnesses, and dietary restriction. Dietary changes are required when GFR is less 25 ml/min/1.73m².

Usually children with CKD should have energy intake of 100% of RDA required as per age, BMI, and physical activity. Protein intake should be 100–140% RDA in stage 3 CKD, 100–120% RDA in stage 4 and 5 CKD, and 100% + allowance for dialysis loss in stage 5. Vitamins and trace elements are to taken 100% RDA. About 50% of energy should be from carbohydrate, 35–40% from fat, and rest proteins. The recommended allowance of protein is 2.2 g/kg/day in children less than 6 months and 0.9–1.9 g/kg/day for older one. Patients who are on hemodialysis should be given additional protein of 0.4 g/kg/day, whereas those on peritoneal dialysis; additional 0.7–0.8 g/kg/d for losses because of larger surface area of peritoneum. Proteins of high biological values like eggs, milk, meat, fish are recommended.

Fat-rich diet should be given but "heart healthy fats" (corn oils, safflower, soy, olive, peanut oils) should be consumed. Omega-3 fatty acids have beneficial effect on cardiovascular status in patients of CKD. Therapeutic dose is 3–8 g/d in the form of fish oil supplements.

Weight, height, head circumference, and mid-arm circumference should be measured every 3–6 months to look for nutritional status and detect growth retardation in children.

Hypertensive children of more than 2 years old should consume less than 1.5 g/day of salt. Recommended intake of phosphate in CKD is 600–800 mg/day, when phosphate binders are started. Low phosphate containing foods are animal flesh proteins; while eggs, dairy products, legumes have higher phosphate protein ratio. Calcium supplements if given with meals bind phosphate but empty stomach increases calcium absorption.

2. Hypertension
Antihypertensive therapy is prescribed to target BP less than 50th centile as for age, gender and height. ACE inhibitors are preferred due to its antiproteinuric effect. They should be avoided if GFR <30 mL/1.73m²/min/, may cause fall in GFR and can also lead to hyperkalemia.

3. Treat Anemia
The management of anemia includes recombinant human erythropoietin (rHuEPO) and iron therapy. rHuEPO is started when hemoglobin falls below 10 g/dL. It may be given subcutaneously (half-life 14–25 h) and intravenously (half-life 5.6–7.5 h).

The initial dose for subcutaneous rHuEPO receiving peritoneal dialysis is 100 units/kg/week in 2 divided doses and may be increased to 150 units/kg/week in severe anemia. Dose for intravenous administration is 150 units/kg/week in 3 divided doses and may be increased to 200–300 units/kg/week in severe anemia in children less than 5 years old. The goal is to increase Hb by 1–2 g/dL per month.

Another preparation such as Darbepoetin alfa (0.45µg/kg) can be given once in a week and long acting Mircera once per month. Dose relationship of rHuEPO of 2000 units is equivalent to 10 µg of Darbepoetin alfa and 30 microgram of Mircera. Complications of recombinant erythropoietin therapy include iron deficiency, hypertension, seizures, and pure red cell aplasia.

Oral iron and folic acid should be given along with erythropoietin. The dose of iron is 3–6 mg/kg/day in children not on hemodialysis. Iron therapy should be stopped in children with transferrin saturation more than 50% and serum ferritin more than 500 ng/mL.

4. Correct Acidosis
Children with CKD should receive sodium bicarbonate 2–3 mEq/kg/day to target serum bicarbonate levels at 20–22 mEq/L.

5. Manage Growth Failure
Gradual loss of standard height must be expected in children and adolescents on long-term dialysis. General measure of treatment is adequate calorie and protein intake, dialysis and hormonal replacement therapy. There is variable response for starting to catch up growth after renal transplantation and depend on impairment of renal function and glucocorticoid dosage.

Hormonal treatment includes calcitriol and growth hormone. The administration of GH markedly increases systemic (mainly hepatic) and local IGF-1 production (in growth cartilage) in children with CKD who remain <3rd centile for height or growth velocity <2 SD despite optimal medical support.

The dose of recombinant human growth hormone (rHuGH) is 0.05 mg/kg/d, subcutaneously with periodic adjustment of dose to achieve normal height velocity. Daily dosing is more effective than three times administration per week. The response of growth hormone depends on residual renal function, target height, initial target height deficit, duration of treatment and age at start of treatment (younger age more response). The adverse effects of rHuGH are pseudotumor cerebri, hyperinsulinemia, increased risk of atherosclerosis, and accelerated progression of renal failure by increasing GFR.

6. Management of Renal Osteodystrophy
The dietary management includes limitation of foods such as milk, cheese, nut, chocolate, and organ meat. Low phosphorus

formula milk (Similac PM 60/40) and fresh or frozen breastmilk pretreated with sevelamer are recommended for infants with renal osteodystrophy. Though phosphate is easily dialyzable but efficacy of removing phosphate is limited because of concomitant intake of calcitriol (0.25–0.50 microgram or 5–10 ng/kg/day) and phosphate binders, which result in 50% absorption. National Kidney Foundation Disease Outcome Quality Initiative (KFDOQI) recommended target ranges for serum PTH and Ca × P product as mentioned below.

Stages of CKD	II	III	IV	V
PTH level (pg/mL)	35–70	35–70	70–110	200–300
Ca × P product	age ≤12 years: <65 mg²/dL²; age ≥12 years: <55 mg²/dL²			

Initial treatment restricts dietary phosphorus intake when phosphate or parathyroid hormone levels begin to rise. Serum phosphorus levels should be maintained between 2.7 and 4.6 mg/dL in patients with stages 3 and 4 CKD, and between 3.5 and 5.5 mg/dL in individuals with stage 5 CKD.

Calcium-based binders Calcium acetate, carbonate, and phosphate have limited phosphate binding capacity and prolonged administration leads to hypercalcemia. Hence, it should be given with meals. Calcium acetate binds more phosphate; improved phosphate control and has decreased incidence of hypercalcemia. Calcium carbonate has fewer gastrointestinal side effects.

Sevelamer hydrochloride It is a hydrogel of polyallylamine and efficient phosphate binders. It is resistant to digestive degradation and hypercalcemia occurs less frequently. It also acts as bile acid sequestrant and decreases total cholesterol and LDL cholesterol.

Vitamin D therapy It is indicated in vitamin D level below the established range for child's age or in child with PTH level above target for that stage. Both vitamin D_2 (25-hydroxy) or vitamin D_3(1,25 dihydroxy) can be given. In a patient with severe vitamin D deficiency (25-OH-vitamin D <5 ng/mL), vitamin D_3 is given 60000 IU/week for 4 weeks, followed by 60000 IU every other week for 3 months. Moderate deficiency (25-OHD 5–15 ng/mL) can be treated with 60,000 IU every other week for 3 months. Mild vitamin D deficiency (25-OHD 16–30 ng/mL), should be treated with 60000 IU every 4 weeks for 3 months. However, if secondary hyperparathyroidism persists despite vitamin D_2 therapy, calcitriol (5–10 ng/kg/day) is also recommended.

7. Renal Replacement Therapy
The initiation of dialysis should be considered when GFR is less than 15 mL/1.73m²/min. Peritoneal dialysis is indicated in all patients less than 2 years. In children above 5 years, hemodialysis/hemodiafiltration is performed. Differences between the two are summarized in **Table 12.21**. Hemodiafiltration is preferred over hemodialysis as the latter removes both small (urea, creatinine, phosphate) and large (β₂ microglobulin, cytokines) molecules and results in better appetite and growth.

Renal transplantation is the ultimate goal as it provides most normal lifestyle and possibility for rehabilitation for the child and family.

Table 12.21 Peritoneal Dialysis vs Hemodialysis	
Peritoneal dialysis	*Hemodialysis/ hemodiafiltration*
Daily sessions are required	Usually three per week required
Less restrictive diet	More restriction on fluid and dietary intake
Can be done at home and technically easier	Hospital setting required
Complications	*Complications*
Malfunction of catheter, infection of exit site, peritonitis, negative body image	Thrombosis, stenosis of access, and catheter sepsis

8. Immunization
All children with CKD should receive standard immunization according to schedule. Live vaccines to be withheld in CKD related to children with glomerulonephritis on immunosuppressive medications. All children should receive MMR, varicella, and pneumococcal vaccines before renal transplantation. They should also receive yearly Influenza vaccine.

PROGNOSIS

Early diagnosis (antenatal screening), treatment of etiology, reduction of proteinuria, control of blood pressure, correction of anemia, acidosis, maintenance of calcium, phosphorus and iPTH in normal range and modification of drug doses based on GFR are some of the factors that may retard the progression of CKD and improve the prognosis.

Chronic Kidney Disease

1. CAKUT is the most common cause of CKD in children below 5 years while chronic glomerulonephritis is the main etiology above 5 years of age.
2. Hypertension, proteinuria, and acidosis are the independent risk factors for progression of CKD.
3. Anemia, growth retardation, hypertension, azotemia, and features of renal osteodystrophy are diagnostic features of CKD.
4. Medical management includes correction of anemia, control of proteinuria, hypertension, acidosis, hyperphosphatemia, and vitamin D and calcium carbonate supplementation.
5. Dialytic therapy (peritoneal/hemodialysis) and renal transplantation has improved survival in these children.

Copelovitch L, Warady BA, Furth SL. Insights from the chronic kidney disease in children (CKiD) study. *Clin J Am Soc Nephrol.* 2011;6:2047–53.

Geary DF, Hodson EM, Craig JC. Interventions for bone disease in children with chronic kidney disease. *Cochrane System Rev.* 2010:CD008327.

Greenberg JH, Kakajiwala A, Parikh CR, Furth S. Emerging biomarkers of chronic kidney disease in children. *Pediatr Nephrol.* 2017 Jun 17.

Hanudel MR, Salusky IB. Treatment of pediatric chronic kidney disease-mineral and bone disorder. *Curr Osteoporos Rep.* 2017 Jun; 15(3):198–206

Hogg RJ, Furth S, Lemley KV *et al.* National Kidney Foundation's Kidney Disease Outcomes Quality Initiative clinical practice guidelines for chronic kidney disease in children and adolescents: evaluation, classification, and stratification. *Pediatrics.* 2003;111: 1416–21.

Ketteler M, Block GA, Evenepoel P, et al. Executive summary of the 2017 KDIGO Chronic Kidney Disease-Mineral and Bone Disorder (CKD-MBD) Guideline Update: what's changed and why it matters. *Kidney Int.* 2017 Jul;92(1):26–36.

Poustie VJ, Smyth RL, Watling RM. Oral protein calorie supplementation for children with chronic disease. *Cochrane System Rev.* 2010: CD001914.

Roderick PJ, Willis NS, Blakeley S, Jones C.Correction of chronic metabolic acidosis for chronic kidney disease patients. *Cochrane System Rev.* 2010;3:CD001890.

Waller S. Parathyroid hormone and growth in chronic kidney disease. *Pediatr Nephrol.* 2011;26:195–204.

12.11 HYPERTENSION

Hypertension is a relatively uncommon finding in children as compared to adults, yet the numbers identified seems to be increasing. The causes for increase in blood pressure are attributed to obesity, change in dietary habits, decreased physical activity, and increasing stress. Overall, 1–5% children suffer from this condition.

FACTORS AFFECTING BLOOD PRESSURE

- Blood pressure (BP) is considerably lower in childhood and increases steadily as the growth and maturation occurs.
- There is a direct association between weight and BP and this is evident as early as five years of age. Height or stature is independently related to BP at all ages.
- The BP is slightly higher in boys as compared to girls in the first decade of life and this difference widens after onset of puberty. Therefore the norms of BP in the pediatric age group are specific for age, gender, and height.
- Children with a family history of hypertension tend to have higher blood pressure.
- Low birth weight has been identified as a risk factor for hypertension.

PRIMARY *VS* SECONDARY HYPERTENSION

Hypertension is classified as *primary* (essential) or *secondary* to a renal, cardiovascular, or endocrine disorder. Most children with sustained, severe, or symptomatic hypertension have an underlying etiology, and are at risk for acute and chronic complications. There is an emerging consensus that primary or essential hypertension is a multifactorial disorder resulting from an interaction of various genetic and environmental factors and tracks into adulthood.

Definitions

According to the 4th Report from National High Blood Pressure Education Program, hypertension in children is defined as systolic or diastolic blood pressure exceeding the 95th percentile for age, gender, and height, on at least three separate occasions, 1–3 weeks apart.

- *Pre-hypertension* is defined as systolic or diastolic blood pressure between 90th and 95th percentile. Adolescents having blood pressure >120/80 mmHg, but below the 95th percentile are also included in this category.
- *Hypertension* is further classified as stages 1 and 2.
- *Stage 1 hypertension* is defined as systolic or diastolic blood pressure values exceeding the 95th percentile and up to 5 mm above the 99th percentile. *Stage 2 hypertension* is systolic or diastolic blood pressure values 5 mm or more above the 99th percentile. Stage 1 hypertension needs a reconfirmation over a 2–3 weeks period however those with stage 2 hypertension should be managed on an urgent basis.

The recordings of high BP should always be repeated on at least 3 occasions, weeks apart (hypertensive emergency being an exception). Also the recording should be repeated at the same visit after 5–10 minutes of rest. The subsequent readings tend to normalize in borderline cases due to accommodation of the child to the measurement procedure. It is important to recognize *white coat hypertension*, which is a transient rise of blood pressure in response to medical environment or the observer recording the BP. Repeated readings in a quiet or home environment especially with an ambulatory measuring device help in excluding white coat hypertension.

Measurement of Blood Pressure

Standard mercury based sphygmomanometer is not used any more due to the environmental toxicity of mercury. Digital and aneroid manometers are more frequently used nowadays.

An appropriate sized cuff should be used for the measurement. It is recommended that the bladder width of the cuff should be at least 40% of the mid-arm circumference and it should cover 80–100% of the arm circumference. Use of a small-sized cuff may lead to overestimation of the BP. An approximate size of various BP cuffs to be used at different ages is given in **Table 12.22**. The BP tables are based on auscultatory measurements hence the preferred method of measurement is auscultation with an aneroid device. The tables of normative blood pressure data are provided in the report of the 4th Task Force and should be referred to.

Children over the age of 3 years who are seen in medical care settings should have their BP measured at least once during every health care episode. Children under age of 3 should have their BP measured in special circumstances that include history of prematurity, nursery stay, congenital heart disease, genitourinary structural lesions, urinary tract infections, or having received drugs known to cause hypertension (steroids, phenylepherine, etc.).

Table 12.22 Appropriate Cuff Sizes for BP Measurement		
Age	*Cuff width (cm)*	*Cuff length (cm)*
Newborn	4	8
Infant	6	12
Child	9	18
Adolescent	10	24
Adult	13–16	30–38
Thigh cuff	20	42

Etiology

Hypertension in children is usually secondary and related to an identifiable and treatable cause. Almost 70–90% cases are due to renal parenchymal and renovascular causes. However, the distribution of causes varies with age. In infancy, coarctation of aorta and renal vessel thrombosis constitute a major group, while renal causes prevail beyond first year of life. Hypertension can occur due to the use of certain drugs (steroids), while central nervous system lesions and endocrine disorders (pheochromocytoma, Cushing syndrome, hyperthyroidism) are relatively uncommon causes.

Essential hypertension is being recognized more frequently in children beyond 10 years of age (especially in obese).

Transient causes of raised BP like acute glomerulonephritis, drug therapy, raised intracranial tension should always be ruled out before starting a detailed evaluation.

Some causes of persistent hypertension are given in **Table 12.23**.

Evaluation of Hypertension

History and Examination

- *Symptoms* Irritability, excessive crying, failure to gain weight, poor feeding, low-grade fever are the only symptoms in children younger than 2–3 years. In older children presence of abdominal pain, hematuria, swelling, nocturia may suggest *renal parenchymal disease.*
- A recent or recurrent history of edema, hematuria and hypertension suggests *renal glomerular disorders.*
- Presence of anemia, short stature and poor growth are pointers towards *chronic kidney disease* (CKD).
- History of palpitations, headache, sweating and weight loss is present with *neuroendocrine tumors* (pheochromocytoma).

Table 12.23 Causes of Sustained Hypertension in Children

I. Renal parenchymal diseases
  i. Chronic glomerulonephritis
  ii. Reflux nephropathy
  iii. Obstructive uropathy
  iv. Polycystic kidney disease, renal dysplasia

II. Renovascular hypertension
  i. Idiopathic aortoarteritis (Takayasu disease)
  ii. Renal artery stenosis
  iii. Renal artery/vein thrombosis

III. Cardiovascular disease
  i. Coarctation of aorta

IV. Endocrine disorders
  i. Pheochromocytoma
  ii. Cushing syndrome
  iii. Congenital adrenal hyperplasia
  iv. Primary hyperaldosteronism

V. Tumors
  i. Wilms tumor
  ii. Neuroblastoma

VI. Essential hypertension

Adapted from: Bagga, *et al.* Indian Pediatrics 2007;44:103–21.

- Hypertension associated with muscle cramps and weakness occurs in conditions of *primary mineralocorticoid excess.*
- Onset around adolescence occurs in some varieties of congenital adrenal hyperplasia (11β-hydroxysteroid dehydrogenase and 11β-hydroxylase enzyme deficiencies).
- Joint pains, rashes, and swelling occur in connective tissue disorders especially systemic lupus erythematosus and vasculitis.
- Presence of *fundal changes* and cardiac chamber hypertrophy (target organ damage) are indicative of longstanding disease.
- A *positive family history* is present in essential hypertension, polycystic kidney disease, neurofibromatosis, and glucocorticoid remediable hypertension.

Investigations

A diagnostic evaluation workup is outlined in **Table 12.24**. Phase I investigations are recommended for all hypertensive children while Phase II investigations should be done selectively depending upon the clinical clues and results of initial evaluation. Long-standing hypertension can cause changes in kidney that may manifest as CKD. Investigations like the fasting blood sugar levels and the lipid profile should be done for the obese patients.

The commonest causes are renal parenchymal and renovascular hence initial investigations should be aimed at ruling out conditions like acute post-streptococcal glomerulonephritis, renal artery stenosis, chronic glomerulonephritis.

Table 12.24 Evaluation for a Hypertensive Child

Investigations

Phase I evaluation (essential)
1. Complete blood counts
2. Blood urea, and serum creatinine, sodium, potassium, calcium, uric acid, cholesterol
3. Urine routine microscopy
4. Chest X-ray, ECG. Echocardiography for coarctation
5. Fundus examination for hypertensive changes
6. Renal ultrasound

Phase II (depending upon initial evaluation)
1. Doppler ultrasound of kidneys for renal artery stenosis
2. Diethylenetriamine penta-acetic acid (DTPA) scan
3. Dimercaptosuccinic acid (DMSA) scan for renal scarring
4. Micturating cystourethrogram (MCUG) to rule out reflux
5. Urinary catecholamines for pheochromocytoma
6. MRI abdomen/Metaiodobenzylguanidine (MIBG) scan for pheochromocytoma
7. ASLO, C3 for acute glomerulonephritis
8. ANA, dsDNA for lupus nephritis
9. p-ANCA and c-ANCA for vasculitis
10. Renal biopsy in persistent proteinuria, hematuria
11. Renal angiography for renal artery stenosis
12. T3, T4, TSH for hyperthyroidism
13. Plasma cortisol, ACTH for steroid/catecholamine mediated hypertension
14. Plasma renin activity, plasma aldosterone for mineralocorticoid disorders

- *Ultrasonography* Structural abnormalities of the kidneys can be identified with a good renal ultrasound. In a child with hematuria, proteinuria, and hypertension elevated ASLO titers with low C3 are diagnostic of post-streptococcal glomerulonephritis.
- *Ultrasound Doppler* This can be used for screening of renal artery stenosis, though its sensitivity is low.
- *MR angiography* of abdominal aorta and renal vessels can easily identify renal artery stenosis in almost all cases.
- *Echocardiography* An ECHO can identify left ventricular hypertrophy that may occur due to long-standing hypertension (target organ damage) or coarctation of aorta.

ESSENTIAL HYPERTENSION

Primary or essential hypertension was considered to be a rather uncommon cause of pediatric hypertension till a few years back. Its pathophysiology though not well understood appears to be multifactorial. Genetic predisposition, environmental factors, lifestyle and fetal factors appear to influence blood pressures. Obesity and stress among school going children is emerging as an important cause of borderline or raised recordings in older and adolescent children. Obesity is primarily a lifestyle disease and seems to be catching on children worldwide, thanks to the ever-increasing modern household gadgets and lack of physical activity. Obesity acquired during childhood, to some extent tracks into adult life. The BMI of a hypertensive child should be calculated and tables referred for the centiles. The values of more than 95th centile are diagnostic of obesity. Before labeling a young child with essential hypertension, reasonable efforts should be made to rule out secondary causes.

Treatment	**Hypertension**

A. Principles of Therapy

- The goal of treatment for hypertensive children is directed at reducing the BP to below 95th centile. In patients with concurrent diseases the BP should be lowered below 90th centile. The KDIGO 2012 guidelines for management of chronic kidney disease recommend that in children with CKD the BP should be lowered to 50th centile.
- Patients with severe hypertension (BP >99th centile) or with target organ damage should be started on antihypertensives immediately and all efforts should be made to identify an underlying cause.
- Patients with BP between 90 and 95th centile or >95th centile without target organ damage should be managed with non-therapeutic measures initially for 3–6 months and if these measures are ineffective, antihypertensives should be considered.
- Patients with stage 2 hypertension are at risk for hypertensive crises, which are classified as *emergencies* or *urgencies,* based on the respective presence or absence of end organ damage (eg, hypertensive encephalopathy, intracerebral bleeding, acute left ventricular failure, and renal failure). These complications are related to the rate of rise and duration of hypertension, rather than absolute blood pressure values. In such situations the BP should be reduced in a controlled manner.

B. Non-pharmacological Methods

1. Dietary changes

Salt restriction (max 1 g/d for 4–8 yr and 1.5 g/d for older children) is recommended for all hypertensive patients. A 'no added salt diet' is often sufficient to achieve this. Intake of food products high in sodium (processed and canned foods, fast foods) should be avoided. Increased potassium intake, through vegetables and fruits, is associated with modest reduction of systolic and diastolic blood pressure in adults with essential hypertension. An increased intake of fresh vegetables and fruits, whole grains and non-fat dairy products is recommended. These foods are low in sodium and saturated fat and rich in minerals (potassium, calcium, magnesium) and fiber. The family should be motivated to change food habits in general.

2. Lifestyle changes

Weight reduction is recommended for those with obesity (BMI >95th centile for that age and gender). Regular physical activity and exercise of 30–60 minutes/day for at least 4 days per week is recommended for all hypertensive children.

C. Drug Therapy

Step 1

- *Angiotensinogen convertase enzyme (ACE) inhibitors* These drugs (enalapril, lisinopril, ramipril) should be considered as the first line drugs in patients with renal parenchymal diseases like chronic glomerulonephritides, lupus and CKD (stages 1–3). Besides reducing BP, this class of drug also has a role in modifying the progression of renal disease. Enalapril can be given in doses of 0.2–0.6 mg/kg/day. However, ACE inhibitors should be avoided till a renovascular cause has been sufficiently ruled out.
- *Diuretics* Frusemide (2–6 mg/kg/day) and thiazides (hydrochlorothiazide in doses of 2–3 mg/kg/day) can be used for patients with renal conditions associated with fluid retention like nephrotic syndrome, acute glomerulonephritis, and chronic kidney disease.
- Patients with transient hypertension like post-streptococcal glomerulonephritis can be managed with diuretics like frusemide (2–6 mg/kg/day) alone.

Step 2

If the hypertension is not controlled on ACE inhibitors and diuretics, *calcium channel blockers* like amlodipine (0.1–0.5 mg/kg/day) or *beta blockers* like atenolol (1–2 mg/kg/day) can be added. Nifedipine, because of its short duration of action should not be used for management of chronic hypertension. It can be used for control of BP in hypertensive urgency without target organ damage. Since it is given sublingual in emergency situations, it should not be used in patients with hypertensive encephalopathy as it may cause an unpredictable fall in BP.

Step 3

If the hypertension is not controlled on maximum doses of these drugs consider *peripheral α-receptor blocker* like prazosin (30–150 µg/kg/dose in 6–8 hrly doses) or *central adrenergic agonist* like clonidine (15–30 µg/kg/day in 6–8 hrly doses). Rarely minoxidil can also be added at doses of 0.1–0.2 mg/kg/day.

Hypertensive Emergency

Hypertensive emergency can be managed with IV sodium nitroprusside infusion at doses of 0.5–5 µg/kg/min for the first 48–72 hours and further control can be done with the above-mentioned drugs. The aim should be to reduce BP gradually,

Drug class	Dose, route	Comments
Table 12.25 Antihypertensives for Hypertensive Emergencies		
Most useful Esmolol (β-blocker)	100–500 µg/kg per min IV infusion	Very short-acting; constant infusion preferred. May cause profound bradycardia
Labetalol (α- and β-blocker)	Bolus: 0.2–1.0 mg/kg per dose up to 40 mg/dose infusion; 0.25–3.0 mg/kg per hr, IV bolus or infusion	Asthma and overt heart failure are relative contraindications
Nicardipine (calcium channel blocker)	1–3 µg/kg per min, IV infusion	May cause reflex tachycardia
Sodium nitroprusside (vasodilator)	0.5–10 µg/kg per min, IV infusion	Monitor cyanide levels with prolonged use (>72 hr) or in renal failure
Hydralazine (vasodilator)	0.2–0.6 mg/kg per dose, IV, IM	Should be given every 4 hr when given IV bolus

Other drugs that can be used: IV fenoldopam, oral clonidine, isradipine, minoxidil though these drugs are used rarely

Case Study | Hypertension

A 4-year-old boy, being evaluated for short stature and anemia, was found to be hypertensive. His weight was 8 kg and height 88 cm.

What history would you elicit from this child to identify the cause of hypertension?
This case scenario points to a chronic kidney disease. I would like to ask for any symptoms of difficulty in passing urine or dribbling to rule out urinary obstruction like posterior urethral valves, neurogenic bladder; and also ask the history of repeated episodes of fever, pyuria, urinary hesitancy, or frequency for recurrent UTI. History of painful hematuria should be elicited to identify renal stone disease.

What initial investigations would you like to do to identify the cause?
A urinalysis for proteinuria and pyuria should be done. Blood urea, creatinine, Na, K, Ca, P, alkaline phosphatase, and venous blood gas would help in identifying the severity of renal disease. A hemogram should be done to identify the type of anemia. An ultrasound of the KUB region identifies structural abnormalities of the kidney.

How will you identify target organ damage?
A fundus examination would help in identifying constriction in retinal vessels. Any retinal bleeds due to hypertensive emergency can be identified. An ECHO should be done to detect left ventricular hypertrophy due to long-standing hypertension.

Ultrasonography shows bilateral hydronephrosis and a distended bladder with thickened walls. The child has a serum creatinine of 4 mg/dL. What further investigations should be planned?
The child has structural abnormality of the renal tract. Since the bladder is abnormal, a micturating cystourethrogram (MCUG) should be done to rule out posterior urethral valves or a neurogenic bladder.

What is the diagnosis? Which antihypertensive should be used in this child?
The child has a chronic kidney disease (CKD). The child has a calculated eGFR of 12.1 mL/min/1.73m² by Schwartz formula which categorizes him as CKD stage 4. Since the GFR is low the safe antihypertensive would be a calcium channel blocker like amlodipine in doses of 0.5 mg/kg/day as two divided doses. If the BP is not controlled on this drug then a β-blocker like atenolol can be added. Diuretic like frusemide can be added if there is a decrease in urine output or edema. Diuretic should also be added if the ECHO shows features of left ventricular hypertrophy. ACE inhibitors like enalapril, ramipril, and receptor blockers like losartan, ibesartan should be avoided below a GFR of 30 mL/min/1.73m². Their use at low GFR is associated with significant hyperkalemia.

one third of the planned reduction over first 6 hours, next third over 12–36 hours and the last third over 36–72 hours. Rapid reduction of BP can worsen perfusion to critical organs like heart and brain. Other drugs that can be used in an emergency situation are listed in **Table 12.25**.

Bagga A, Jain R, Vijaykumar M, Kanitkar M, Ali U. Evaluation and management of hypertension. *Indian Pediatr.* 2007;44:103–121.

Flynn JT, Alderman MH. Characteristics of children with primary hypertension seen at a referral center. *Pediatr Nephrol.* 2005; 20: 961–966.

Munter P, He J, Cutler JA, Wildman RP, Whelton BK. Trends in blood pressure among children and adolescents. *JAMA.* 2004;291: 2107–13.

Hypertension

1. Hypertension in children is defined as systolic or diastolic BP more than 95th centile for that age, gender, and height measured on 3 separate occasions 1–3 weeks apart.
2. Renal parenchymal and renovascular diseases are the commonest causes of hypertension in children.
3. An appropriate sized BP cuff should be used for measurement of BP in children.
4. ACE inhibitors and ARBs are the preferred anti-hypertensives except in situations where the renal functions are moderately deranged.

National Heart, Lung and Blood Institute Joint National Committee on Prevention, Detection, Evaluation and Treatment of High Blood Pressure. The Seventh Report of the Joint National Committee on prevention, detection, evaluation and treatment of high blood pressure: The JNC 7 report. *JAMA*. 2003;289:2560–72.

National High Blood Pressure Education Program Working Group. The Fourth report on the diagnosis, evaluation and treatment of high blood pressure in children and adolescents. *Pediatrics*. 2004;114 (suppl):555–76.

Pickering TG. Principles and techniques of blood pressure measurement. *Cardiol Clin*. 2002;20:207–23.

Vaughan CJ, Delanty N. Hypertensive emergencies. *Lancet*. 2000;356:411–7.

12.12 RENAL TUBULAR ACIDOSIS

Renal tubular acidosis (RTA) is defined as a chronic disorder characterized by hyperchloremic metabolic acidosis due to inability of the renal tubules to retain HCO_3^- or to secrete H^+ in the presence of normal or minimally impaired glomerular filtration rate.

In children, most cases of RTA are primary disorders due to specific genetic abnormalities in the transporters or enzymes involved in the processes of HCO_3^- reabsorption, HCO_3^- regeneration, and H^+ secretion. These clinically manifest in infancy or early childhood. RTA secondary to drugs, toxins or due to systemic diseases are more common in adults.

RENAL ACID–BASE HOMEOSTASIS

The renal proximal tubule plays a pivotal role in maintaining the systemic acid–base balance by reabsorbing approximately 80% of filtered bicarbonate (HCO_3^-) and 65% of filtered Na^+ from the glomerulus along with water. Luminal Na^+/H^+ exchanger and the basolateral Na^+–HCO_3^- co-transporter are responsible for this process which is mostly dependent on Na^+.

The distal tubules are metabolically active and mainly responsible in sodium, potassium, and divalent cation homeostasis leading to adjustments in urine concentration and pH. Dietary protein metabolism leads to formation of "non-volatile acids", buffering of which results in Na^+ salts of the acids which are excreted by the kidneys principally with NH_4^+. The process of excretion of NH_4^+ culminates in regeneration of HCO_3^- in the blood, which was consumed in buffering the non-volatile acids.

Titratable acid refers to the process whereby secreted hydrogen ion (H^+) is eliminated with urinary buffers that determine the urinary pH in the distal tubule.

TYPES OF RTA

Four types of RTA can be characterized based on clinical and molecular criteria. Those with autosomal recessive pattern of transmission may be the first in the family to manifest the disease if the parents are carriers.

1. Type 1: Distal RTA

Distal RTA was the first RTA to be identified and hence names as 'classical RTA' or 'type 1'. Majority of primary distal type 1 RTA are due to an autosomal recessive defect in H^+ ATPase. It results due to decreased distal H^+ ion secretion leading to failure to lower pH maximally and excrete acid as ammonium, which ultimately leads to development of hyperchloremic metabolic acidosis, hypokalemia, early development of nephrocalcinosis and sometimes sensory deafness. Some patients with obstructive uropathy have inability to acidify urine along with impaired K^+ secretion and develop hyperkalemic distal type 1 RTA.

2. Type 2: Proximal RTA

In proximal type 2 RTA there is impaired HCO_3^- ion absorption in the proximal tubule resulting in urinary HCO_3^- ion wastage. Isolated form of proximal RTA is extremely rare and more commonly it is associated with generalized dysfunction of the proximal tubule as part of Fanconi syndrome (ie, cystinosis). Low molecular weight proteinuria, hyperaminoaciduria, glucosuria, hypophosphatemia with relative hyperphosphaturia, and hypouricemia with relative hyperuricosuria are all features of proximal tubular dysfunction.

3. Type 3 RTA

Type 3 RTA has features of both, type 1 and type 2 RTA. In Middle East and North America, type 3 RTA is associated with osteopetrosis, cerebral calcifications, and intellectual disability due to loss of function mutation in the gene coding carbonic anhydrase II.

4. Type 4 RTA

Type 4 RTA is mostly due to acquired causes such as obstructive uropathy, hypoaldosteronism, and drugs causing aldosterone resistance, eg, amiloride. It is caused mainly by impaired ammoniagenesis resulting from sustained hyperkalemia produced by either aldosterone deficiency or resistance. In patients with obstructive uropathy (aldosterone resistance) it is often associated with decreased glomerular filtration rate.

CLINICAL PRESENTATION

Most children with RTA present early in infancy or childhood with history of vomiting, polyuria, polydipsia and liking for salty food. Delay in diagnosis is common due to non-specific symptoms and leads to failure to thrive, short stature, rickets and bony deformities. Children with distal type 1 RTA have hypercalciuria, nephrocalcinosis, and nephrolithiasis. Children with proximal type 2 RTA usually present as Fanconi syndrome which may be secondary to any systemic diseases (cystinosis, galactosemia, fructose intolerance, tyrosinemia, Wilson disease, Lowe syndrome). Long-standing obstructive urological symptoms are seen in RTA due to obstructive nephropathy.

DIAGNOSIS

1. Plasma Anion Gap

Metabolic acidosis is characterized by low plasma HCO_3^- (<22 mEq/L) and low blood PCO_2 (<40 mmHg) and is further classified according to plasma or serum anion gap. Anion gap is calculated as $(Na^+ + K^+) - (Cl^- + HCO_3^-)$, and depicts the difference between unmeasured anions and cations and is affected by changes in plasma concentrations of albumin, phosphate, and divalent ions. Increased anion gap metabolic acidosis is a consequence of retention of anions other than Cl^- as seen in diabetic ketoacidosis, advanced chronic kidney disease, lactic acidosis, toxins and inborn errors of metabolism. Normal AG metabolic acidosis is termed as 'hyperchloremic', because the drop in HCO_3^- ion is matched by an equivalent rise in Cl^- ion levels and is seen in diarrhea (gastrointestinal loss of HCO_3^-) and RTA (decreased renal reabsorption of HCO_3^-, and/or decreased urinary NH_4^+ excretion). *All types of RTA are characterized by normal anion gap metabolic acidosis (12±4 mEq/L).*

2. Urinary ammonium and Urinary Anion Gap

Urinary NH_4^+ and pH should be evaluated in the same sample when the child is acidotic. The normal renal response to metabolic acidosis includes lowering of urine pH and increased production and urinary elimination of NH_4^+. Measurement of urinary NH_4^+ is cumbersome, hence not done by most laboratories. Urinary anion gap ($Na^+ + K^+ - Cl^-$) is considered an indirect index of urinary excretion of NH_4^+ in presence of hyperchloremic metabolic acidosis. Raised levels of urinary NH_4^+ have corresponding high levels of Cl^- and hence the urinary anion gap becomes negative, implying a preserved mechanism of urinary acidification. *Inappropriately low urinary NH_4^+ has low urinary Cl^-, and lead to positive urinary anion gap as seen in distal type 1 RTA ($Na^+ + K^+ > Cl^-$).*

3. Bicarbonate Load Test

Calculation of fractional excretion (FE) of HCO_3^- when the plasma HCO_3^- is normal and urine to blood (U-B) pCO_2 difference when an alkaline urine pH is achieved, helps in characterization of RTA. This is done by bicarbonate loading, an easy to perform test.

Oral HCO_3^- is administered at a dose of 4 mEq/kg for 2–3 days to achieve plasma HCO_3^- level of > 22 mEq/L and urine pH of >7.5. However, in some patients this dose is not sufficient to normalize plasma due to huge urinary bicarbonate loss as occurs in type 2 proximal RTA. Intravenous infusion of 3.75% sodium bicarbonate at a rate of 0.3 to 0.8 mL/min can be used in such cases, which cause an increment of 2–3 mEq/L/hr in the plasma HCO_3^- level. FE HCO_3^- is calculated by the formula given below, the normal values are <5%.

$$FEHCO_3 \ (\%) = \frac{\text{urine } HCO_3^- \times \text{plasma creatinine}}{\text{plasma } HCO_3^- \times \text{urine creatinine}} \times 100$$

Urine pCO_2 levels in the setting when the urinary pH is higher than the blood pH, is a sensitive index of distal tubular H^+ secretion. H^+ combines with HCO_3^- in the tubular lumen to form H_2O and CO_2. High CO_2 generated in lumen gets trapped in the renal medulla and finally leads to high urine pCO_2. When the urine pH is above 7.7 and urine HCO_3^- above 80 mEq/L, the U-B pCO_2 gradient is more than 20 mmHg. Interpretation of bicarbonate load test is described in **Table 12.26**.

4. Tubular Phosphate Excretion

The fractional excretion (FE) of phosphate determined on a timed (6-hr, 12-hr, 24-hr) urine specimen, is useful for detecting phosphate wasting, which provides supportive evidence for presence of type 2 proximal RTA, as in Fanconi syndrome. Tubular reabsorption of phosphate (TRP) can be calculated as $100 - FEPO_4^-$; normally 88–95% phosphate is reabsorbed.

$$\text{FE phosphate} = \frac{\text{urine phosphate} \times \text{plasma creatinine}}{\text{plasma phosphate} \times \text{urine creatinine}} \times 100$$

5. Frusemide + Fludrocortisone Test

Simultaneous oral administration of furosemide (2 mg/kg) and fludrocortisone (0.02 mg/kg) to healthy subjects decreases the urine pH to <5.3 and increases urinary NH_4^+ levels up to $85 \pm 23 \ \mu Eq/min$. Patients with type 1 distal RTA

Table 12.26 Differential Diagnosis of RTA According to the Biochemical findings in Presence of Metabolic Acidosis				
	Normal	*Type 1 RTA*	*Type 2 RTA*	*Type 4 RTA*
Serum chloride	98–102 mEq/L	High	High	High
Serum anion gap	12±4 mEq/L	Normal	Normal	Normal
Serum potassium	3.5–4.5 mEq/L	Low/normal	Low	High
Urine ammonium	57 ± 4.3 µEq/L (1–16 months) 80.0±3.7 µEq/L (7–12 year)	Low	Normal	Low
Urine anion gap	Negative	Positive	Negative	Positive
FEHCO₃⁻	<5%	<5%	>10–15%	5–10%
Urine pCO₂ (mmHg)	>60–70	Low	Normal	Normal
U-B pCO₂ (mmHg)	>20–30	<20	>20	>20
Urine pH	<5.3–5.5	>5.5	<5.5	<5.5
Urine spot Ca/Cr	<0.2	High	Normal	Normal
FEPO₄⁻	5–12%	Normal	>15%	Normal

FEHCO₃⁻: Fractional excretion of HCO₃⁻; U-B: Urine-Blood
Ca/Cr: Calcium/Creatinine; FEPO₄⁻: Fractional excretion of PO₄⁻

Case Study — Renal Tubular Acidosis

A 4-year-old boy presented with complaints of not growing well, and a 1-day history of irritability and vomiting. His length was <3rd centile, weight was <5th percentile and weight/height was <-3SD. Blood pressure was 88/60 mmHg. He was alert and calm, with normal skin turgor. Systemic examination was normal. Serum HCO_3^- was 16 mEq/L and pCO_2 was 30 mmHg (suggestive of metabolic acidosis). He had history of previous admission for similar complaints in past numerous times.

What are the relevant questions to be asked in history?

History of polyuria, polydipsia, and diarrhea should be obtained. To evaluate for the cause of growth retardation, detailed dietary and psychosocial history is essential. Specific history for salt cravings, muscle weakness, fatigue, and muscle cramps should be elicited.

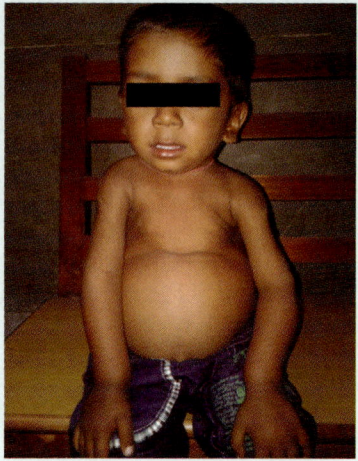

How will you further investigate this child?

The first step in the evaluation is the calculation of plasma anion gap. Hyperchloremic metabolic acidosis (normal anion gap) is the usual finding in all the cases of RTA. Further, urine anion gap (indicative of the urinary NH_4^+) will be calculated.

Laboratory values on admission were: Blood pH, 7.30; serum sodium, 138 mEq/L; potassium, 2.8 mEq/L; chloride, 113 mEq/L; bicarbonate, 16 mEq/L; urea, 33 mg/dL; and creatinine, 0.2 mg/dL. Urinalysis showed: pH, 7; no glucosuria or albuminuria. Urinary electrolytes were indicative of impaired NH_4^+ excretion (urine anion gap = +70), suggestive of distal RTA. $FEHCO_3^-$ was 4% and U-B pCO_2 was 15 mmHg. Diagnostic evaluation for sepsis was negative.

What do the investigations show?

The reports are indicative of normal anion gap metabolic acidosis with normal kidney function tests with an impaired urinary acidification. A positive anion gap was indicative of distal type 1 RTA in this case. For further characterization of the RTA, serum potassium levels and bicarbonate loading test needs to be done.

What further investigations would you like to do?

Ultrasonography of the kidneys to look for nephrocalcinosis, urinary calcium-to-creatinine ratio, urinary citrate levels, and evaluation of hearing are needed.

Ultrasound showed diffuse nephrocalcinosis bilaterally. The urinary calcium-to-creatinine ratio was 0.73 mg (normal <0.2). The urinary citrate was 80 mg/g creatinine (normal, 180 mg/g creatinine). Evaluation for sensorineural hearing abnormality was negative.

What is your impression now?

The alkaline urine pH consistently above 5.5 in the presence of metabolic acidosis and the presence of nephrocalcinosis suggest the diagnosis of renal tubular acidosis (RTA).

How will you treat this child?

The mainstay of treatment of distal RTA is long-term administration of alkali to balance the net acid production. Alkali supplementation as polycitra (1mEq of K^+, 1 mEq of Na^+ and 2mEq of HCO_3^- per mL) will be provided to maintain a normal serum concentration of >22 mEq/L. Normalization of serum HCO_3^- and growth are good indicators for treatment.

---

fail to acidify the urinary pH <5.3 and there is minimal increase in NH_4^+ excretion over the basal values.

Figure 12.13 summarizes the practical protocol of evaluating a suspected case with RTA.

Treatment — Renal Tubular Acidosis

Long-term supplementation of alkali corrects the biochemical abnormalities, improves growth, prevents renal stones and skeletal abnormalities due to RTA. A combination of sodium and potassium citrate is recommended at a dose of 3–4 mEq/kg/day of alkali, titrated to plasma HCO_3^- levels (>22 mEq/L) in children with type 1 distal RTA. Citrate salts correct the hypocituria and prevents nephrolithiasis. Children require lifelong treatment and have excellent prognosis if diagnosis is made early and adequate amounts of alkali is continuously administered. Additional potassium supplementation is required in majority of the patients.

Due to massive bicarbonate wasting in type 2 proximal RTA, the dose of alkali required is high, approximately 5–15 mEq/kg/day in children. Addition of hydrochlorothiazide (2 mg/kg/day) decreases the extracellular volume which causes enhanced HCO_3^- reabsorption; this however also has a side-effect of increased urinary potassium wastage. For the same reason, treatment with potassium citrate is recommended. Polycitra contains 1mEq of K^+, 1 mEq of Na^+ and 2 mEq of HCO_3^- per mL. Children with Fanconi syndrome require additional supplements like phosphate (50–100 mg/kg/day) for treatment of rickets.

Santos F, Ordóñez FA, Claramunt-Taberner D, Gil-Peña H. Clinical and laboratory approaches in the diagnosis of renal tubular acidosis. *Pediatr Nephrol.* 2015;30:2099–107.

Santos F, Gil-Peña H, Alvarez-Alvarez S. Renal tubular acidosis. *Curr Opin Pediatr.* 2017 Apr;29(2):206–210.

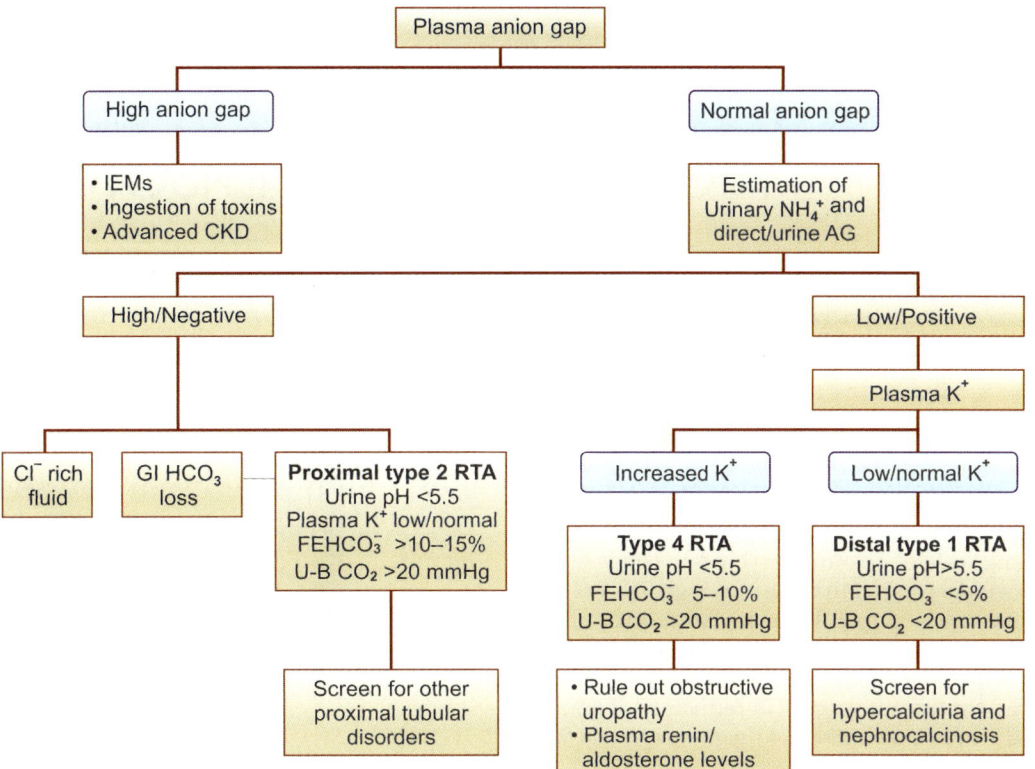

Fig. 12.13 Summarizes the practical protocol of evaluating a suspected case with RTA

Renal Tubular Acidosis

1. Renal tubular acidosis (RTA) is defined as a chronic disorder characterized by hyperchloremic metabolic acidosis (with a normal anion gap) due to inability of the renal tubules to retain HCO_3^- or to secrete H^+ in the presence of normal or minimally impaired glomerular filtration rate.
2. Four types of RTA can be characterized based on clinical and molecular criteria. Distal RTA (Type 1) is the classical variant.
3. Most children with RTA present early in infancy or childhood with history of vomiting, polyuria, polydipsia, liking for salty food OR with non-specific symptoms such as failure to thrive, short stature, rickets, and bony deformities.
4. Early appropriate alkali therapy results in favorable outcome in most of the cases.

OP Mishra and Rajniti Prasad (Anatomy and Physiology, Edema, HUS, AKI, CKD); Sriram Krishnamurthy (Nephrotic Syndrome, Proteinuria); Kirtisudha Mishra (UTI); Kanika Kapoor (Glomerulonephritis); R Ganesh (Hematuria); Mukta Mantan (Hypertension); and Abhijeet Saha (RTA)

Neurological Disorders

13.1 NEURAL TUBE DEFECTS (SPINAL DYSRAPHISM)

Neural tube defects are also known as spina bifida. They may be hidden, ie, without being apparent (*spina bifida occulta*) or present as meningocele or meningomyelocele (*spina bifida manifesta*). The incidence in North India is as high 3.9–9/1000 live births. Spina bifida is usually associated with other problems such as paraplegia, bladder and bowel dysfunction, hydrocephalus, and infection. The last decade has demonstrated significant success in reduction of neural tube defects by a simple intervention, ie, *periconceptional folic acid supplementation* to the mother.

Various types of neural tube defects (NTD)/spina bifida are depicted in Fig. 13.1.

Classification

Neural tube defects are categorized as *primary* (95%) and *secondary* (5%).

- *Primary defects* occur early at 17–28 days of gestation, due to failure of closure of neural tube. These include occipital or frontal anencephaly, encephalocele and meningomyelocele.
- *Secondary defects* occur after the neural tube has closed, due to defect in the mesoderm. These include meningocele, lipomeningocele, and dorsal dermal sinus.

Meningocele and Meningomyelocele

Meningocele This is a hernial protrusion of a sac-like cyst from the vertebral column. It contains meninges, and is filled with spinal fluid. It does not contain any neural elements. 80% are located on lumbosacral spine.

Meningomyelocele This is also a hernial protrusion from the vertebral column. However, it also contains a portion of spinal cord with its nerves, besides CSF and meninges. It is the most common neural tube defect, and associated with hydrocephalus in 90% cases. Arnold- Chiari malformation Type II and agenesis of corpus callosum are the other associated defects. Arnold-Chiari malformation Type II is characterized by myelomeningocele and a small posterior fossa with descent of brainstem and cerebellar tonsils.

Etiology

Primary neural tube defects have multi-factorial inheritance. Maternal risk factors include exposure to drugs (anticonvulsants: Valproate and carbamazepine; oral contraceptive

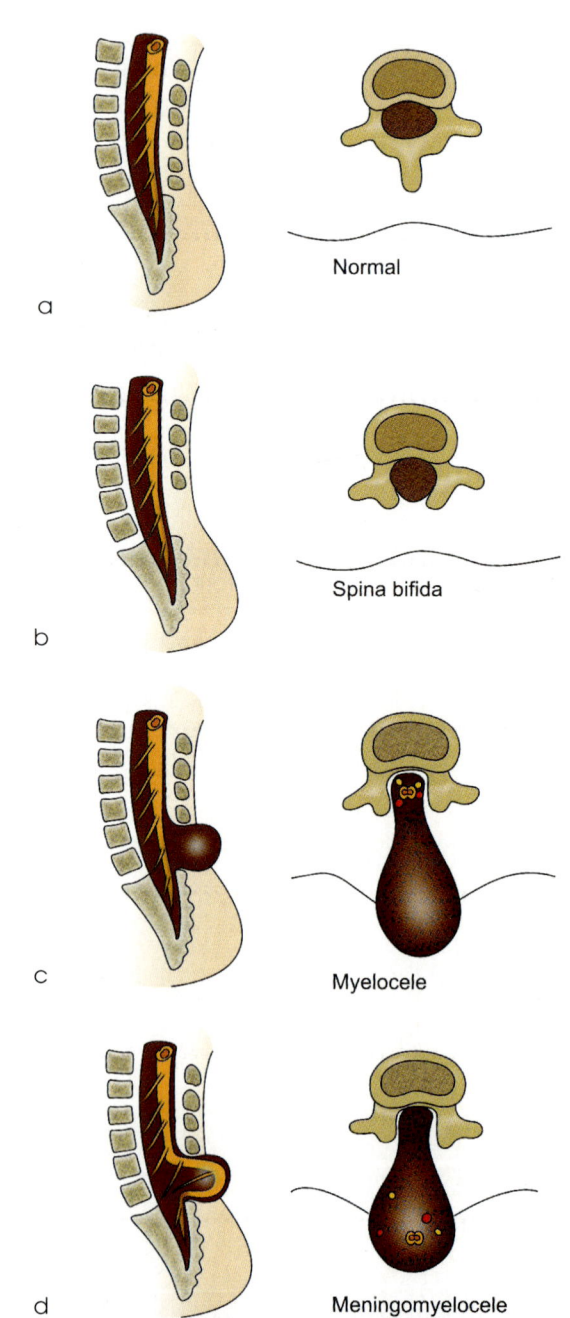

Fig. 13.1 Types of neural tube defects: (a) Normal, (b) spina bifida, (c) myelocele, and (d) meningomyelocele

drugs, trimethoprim, and antimetabolites), alcohol, or radiation; insulin dependent diabetes mellitus (IDDM), and folate deficiency. Chromosomal abnormalities including trisomy 13 and 18 have been associated with neural tube defects. High doses of exogenous estrogens and clomiphene also seem to have some indirect association with neural tube defects.

Recurrence risk for isolated neural tube defects is 2–4% after having 1 child affected with NTD. With two affected siblings, the risk is approximately 10%.

Clinical Evaluation of a Child with Neural Tube Defect

Obtain history of intake of anti-epileptic drugs, teratogens, and whether detected in antenatal ultrasounds. Ask for any history of affected siblings in the past. Also ask for lower limb movements, urine stream, and bladder and bowel incontinence.

- *Examine the back* for meningocele (Fig. 13.2a), tuft of hair (Fig. 13.2b), and open defects.
- Evaluate the anal reflex in all children suspected to have NTD.
- Evaluate for hydrocephalus: Measure head circumference, look for split sutures, examine fontanels.
- Perform local examination for nature of lesion, leaking/infected, rostral level to aid neurological assessment.
- Neurological examination of lower limbs for sensory and motor deficits.
- *Evaluate bladder function:* About 90% have bladder dysfunction in terms of urinary retention, flaccid or spastic bladder, or detrusor sphincter dyssynergia.

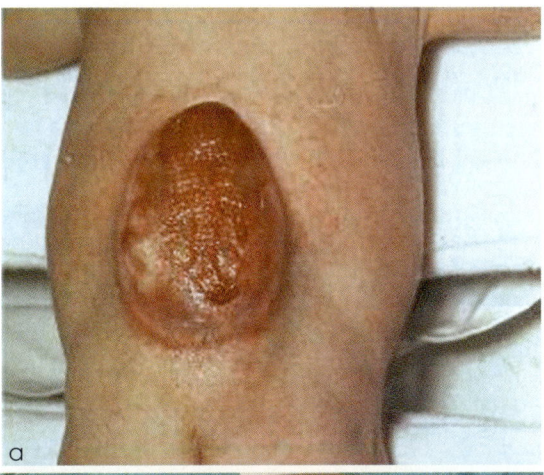

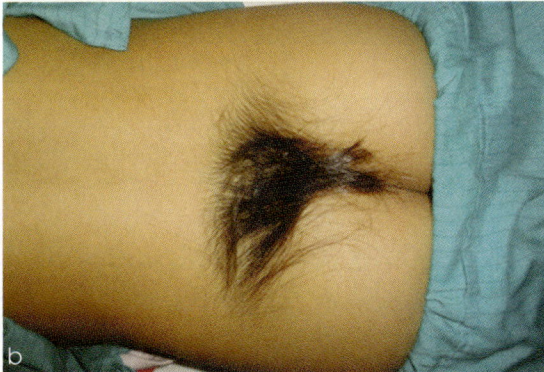

Fig. 13.2 (a) Meningomyelocele; (b) tuft of hair over the lumbosacral spine. The child had underlying tethered cord

- *Investigations* include neuroimaging, ultrasound of kidney, X-ray of chest and spine, and culture from lesion, if leaking. Neuroimaging involves MRI of brain and spine in all children to evaluate the extent of lesion, and for associated abnormalities such as hydrocephalus and Arnold-Chiari malformation.

Complications and Prognosis

Delay in intervention may result in worsening of neurologic deficit, infection (local or ventriculitis), and progressive hydrocephalus.

Late complications include hydrocephalus (80–90%), urinary tract problems (UTI, VUR), fecal incontinence or constipation, developmental dysplasia of hip, congenital talipes equinovarus, sexual dysfunction (erection and ejaculation), intellectual deterioration, epilepsy (10–30%), ocular problems (30%), shunt infection (25%), and psychosocial problems.

Long-term multidisciplinary approach for management is required. Of all cases, 2% die during initial hospitalization and 15% succumb by 10 years of age.

Treatment	Neural Tube Defect

Keep the child nil per orally (NPO) and maintain temperature. Cover the lesion by sterile saline moist dressings. Nurse the baby prone or lateral. Rule out other cardiac, pulmonary, genitourinary, and gastrointestinal malformations.

1. Surgery

Early closure of the defect prevents neurological deterioration. Open lesions draining CSF should be closed within 24 hours and closed lesions within 48 hours of birth. If the lesion is infected, administer parenteral and/or intrathecal antibiotics. This is to be followed by surgery.

Lorber's criteria Surgery is not done if there is (*i*) severe paraplegia at or above L3 level; (*ii*) kyphosis or scoliosis; (*iii*) gross hydrocephalus; (*iv*) associated gross congenital anomalies; (*v*) intracerebral birth injuries; or (*vi*) pre-existing ventriculitis. These children are given supportive therapy only. About 5–10% still survive.

2. Supportive Management

A. *Prevent Infection*
- Position infant to prevent urinary/fecal contamination
- Clean the defect carefully with sterile saline, apply sterile dressings.
- Avoid urethral contamination with stool.
- Ensure good perineal hygiene.
- Administer antibiotics for an open defect.
- Ensure adequate fluid intake.

B. *Prevent Trauma related to Delicate Spinal Lesion*
- Careful handling of infant.
- Place in prone/side-lying position.
- Apply protective devices around sac.
- Modify routine nursing activities (feeding, comforting).

C. *Prevent Skin Disintegration due to Continual Dribbling of Urine and Feces*
- Keep perianal area clean and dry.
- Diapering is contraindicated until the defect has been repaired and healing is advanced or epithelialization has taken place.
- Change diapers as soon as soiled, if diapered.

D. *Prevent Increased Intracranial Pressure (ICP)*
- Measure head circumference daily.
- Observe for signs of increased intracranial pressure.

E. *Prevent or Minimize Lower Extremity Deformity*
- Carry out passive range of motion exercises.
- Carry out muscle stretching when indicated.
- Maintain hips in slight to moderate abduction and feet in neutral position.

3. Family Support
Parents are encouraged to become involved in care of the child.
- They need to learn how to continue the care at home that has been initiated in the hospital—positioning, feeding, skin care, and range of motion exercises when appropriate.
- Parents are taught clean intermittent catheterization technique when advised.
- The family needs to know the symptoms of anticipated complications and how to reach assistance when needed.
- In cases where the defect has not been repaired, parents are taught to care of the lesion.
- As the child grows and develops, it is important that the parents encourage and stimulate the infant to accomplish age-appropriate developmental tasks within the limits imposed by the disabilities.

Prevention

Two major interventional strategies have been accepted for prevention of neural tube defects: (*i*) Antenatal screening with subsequent termination of affected pregnancies; and (*ii*) folic acid supplementation. Role of folic acid in primary and secondary prevention of neural tube defects is the most important discovery in the recent past.

- *Primary prevention* includes folate supplementation (400 μg per day) to all prospective mothers beginning at least 1 month prior to attempting conception and continuing till at least 3 months after conception or preferably throughout pregnancy.
- A mother with a previous child with neural tube defects should be advised 4 mg per day of folate supplementation in the periconceptional period. **Folate supplementation reduces recurrence risk by 70%.** Additionally, prenatal diagnosis should be offered.
- Counseling of family with a previous child with NTD is essential. The risk of recurrence is 4% with 1 affected child, 10% with 2 affected children and 25% with 3 affected children.

Revision Point

Neural Tube Defects
1. Neural tube defects usually occur at 17–28 days of gestation due to failure of closure of neural tube.
2. Periconceptional folic acid supplementation is a successful strategy for prevention of neural tube defects.
3. Hydrocephalus and spastic bladder with vesico-ureteric reflux are common complications/comorbidities; hence it is important to assess these children with brain neuroimaging and ultrasound for kidney-ureter-bladder.

- Food fortification with folic acid is another practical public health base approach.
- *Secondary prevention* includes prenatal screening and selective termination of affected fetuses. The condition can be diagnosed by ultrasonography (pickup rate 100%), elevated maternal blood α-fetoprotein level at 16–18 weeks (accuracy 60–70%), or elevated amniotic fluid α-fetoprotein and acetylcholinesterase levels (accuracy 97%).

Blencowe H, Cousens S, Modell B, *et al.* Folic acid to reduce neonatal mortality from neural tube disorders. *Int J Epidemiol.* 2010;39 Suppl 1:i110–21.

Bulas D. Fetal evaluation of spine dysraphism. *Pediatr Radiol.* 2010;40:1029–37.

Liptak GS, Dosa NP. Myelomeningocele. *Pediatr Rev.* 2010;31:443–50.

Sandler AD. Children with spina bifida: key clinical issues. *Pediatr Clin North Am.* 2010;57:879–92.

13.2 HYDROCEPHALUS

Hydrocephalus is characterized by (*i*) dilatation of the cerebral ventricles; and (*ii*) increased cerebrospinal fluid (CSF) pressure.

CSF is predominantly (80–90%) formed by the choroid plexus of the lateral, third and fourth ventricles by an active transport process across the endothelium of capillaries in the villous process of the choroid plexus. The arachnoid villi are the primary site of CSF absorption. Hydrocephalus results if there is an increase in the production and/or decrease in the absorption of CSF.

Etiology

Causes of hydrocephalus are detailed in **Table 13.1**. Hydrocephalus may be *congenital* or *acquired*.
- Aqueductal stenosis is the most common cause (10%) of congenital hydrocephalus. Other causes of congenital hydrocephalus include congenital infections and other structural malformations.
- Infections, intraventricular hemorrhage and malignancies are responsible for acquired hydrocephalus in 20%, 10% and 20% cases respectively.
- About 10–15% cases are idiopathic, ie, without an apparent cause.

Classification

Hydrocephalus can be classified as *communicating* and *non-communicating* types depending on the site of obstruction.

Table 13.1 Etiology of Hydrocephalus	
Communicating hydrocephalus	*Non-communicating hydrocephalus*
Meningitis: Tubercular, pneumococcal	Aqueductal stenosis
Leukemia	*Malformations:* Chiari, Dandy-Walker
Sub-arachnoid hemorrhage Intrauterine Infection Achondroplasia	*Mass lesions:* Abscess, hematoma, posterior fossa tumors, vein of Galen malformation
Metabolic: Mucopolysaccharidosis, Gaucher disease	Klippel-Feil syndrome

- *Communicating hydrocephalus* is the commonest cause of hydrocephalus in children. The ventricular system is patent and the site of block is in the basal subarachnoid cisterns, subarachnoid sulci or at the arachnoid villi. Meningitis is the most common cause of communicating hydrocephalus.
- *Non-communicating hydrocephalus* There is blockage of CSF pathway at or proximal to the outlet foramina of the fourth ventricle. The cause is usually congenital.

Clinical Features

These depend on age at onset, duration, and severity.

Early onset (0–2 Years)

50% of children may be asymptomatic. Vomiting, drowsiness, failure to thrive, shrill cry, and delayed motor milestones are common symptoms.
- There is progressive increase in head circumference.
- Head shape is abnormal and overshadows face (Fig. 13.3).
- There is frontal bossing and triangular facies.
- The skin of scalp is shiny and tense with dilated veins and sparse hair.
- The anterior fontanel is open, large and non-pulsatile.
- Open squamo-parietal suture beyond the first month is an early sign of hydrocephalus.
- Ocular signs such as 6th nerve palsy, sunset sign (Fig. 13.3), ptosis and nystagmus may be present. Papilledema is rare at this age.
- Spasticity of lower limbs due to compression of periventricular white matter may develop.
- Pseudobulbar palsy may be present and results in regurgitation, dysphonia, and stridor.

Late onset (2–10 years)

Papilledema, headache, and vomiting are usual presenting features.
- Increasing head size is present in only 60% children.
- *McEwen's sign* (crack pot resonance on percussion of the skull) can be elicited.
- Pyramidal signs may be seen in 40%, psychomotor retardation and gait anomaly in 30%, and epilepsy in 20% children.

Arrested hydrocephalus

A large proportion of both congenital and acquired hydrocephalus may undergo spontaneous arrest and may not require active surgical intervention. The clinician needs to follow-up a patient to distinguish arrested from progressive hydrocephalus.

Diagnosis

The purpose of neuroimaging is to assess the severity and etiology of the disease. Ultrasonography is especially helpful for screening neonates. In the older population, a computed tomography (CT) or magnetic resonance imaging (MRI) with or without contrast will assess the degree of ventriculomegaly (Fig. 13.4) and the possible etiology.

Treatment	Hydrocephalus

The goals of therapy for hydrocephalus include the following:
1. Decreasing intracranial pressure (ICP) to safe level; and
2. Maximizing the potential for neurological development by preserving brain parenchymal thickness.

The integrity of CSF pathways must be preserved to prevent ventricular coaptation and give chance in the future for life without shunt dependency.

Medical therapy

Mild ventriculomegaly or gross hydrocephalus in delayed presenters (more than 6 months of age) may benefit from medical treatment. However, the institution of medical therapy requires careful follow-up to assess the ventriculomegaly, mental and cognitive development and fundus changes.

Osmotic therapy is useful for transient reduction in CSF pressures while definitive therapy is being instituted. Hypertonic saline (3% NaCl) is indicated as first choice agent. Mannitol 20% is the drug of choice in a normotensive child. Carbonic anhydrase inhibitors like acetazolamide in doses of 50–100 mg/kg/day can reduce CSF production. Frusemide also decreases CSF production. Dehydration, altered acid-base balance, and dyselectrolytemia are potential complications associated with the use of these drugs especially in the neonatal period.

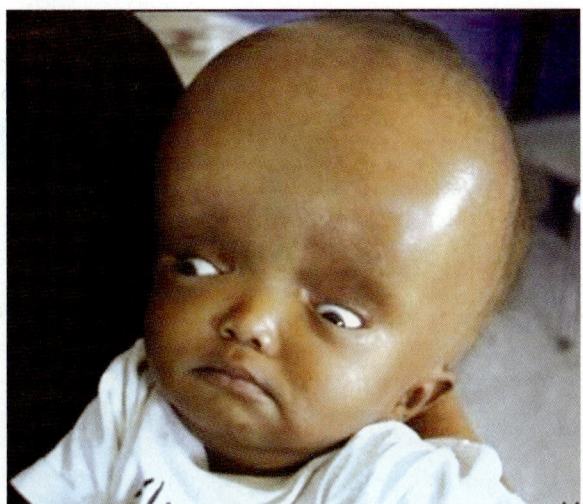

Fig. 13.3 A child with hydrocephalus and sunset sign.

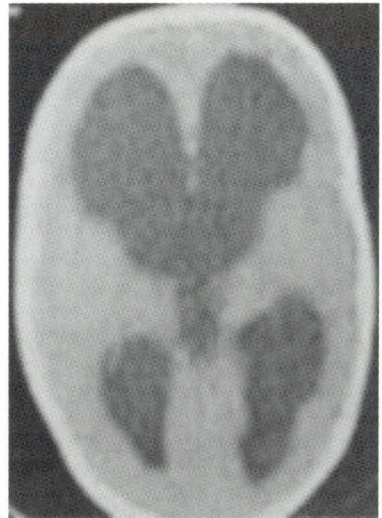

Fig. 13.4 CT scan showing ventricular dilatation

Surgical treatment

The conventional modality of surgical treatment is ventriculoperitoneal shunting. The indications for shunt surgery are as follows:

- Cortical mantle <2 cm on initial imaging in infant <6 months of age at presentation;
- Evidence of thinning of cortical mantle, features of raised ICP like papilledema and delayed milestones despite adequate medical therapy on follow-up; and
- Evidence of papilledema or periventricular ooze (on CT scan) on initial or subsequent assessment.

Patients who present late with gross hydrocephalus (>6 months old, mantle <1 cm, optic atrophy) may be offerred shunt surgery based on treating team's discretion. The candidates deemed fit for shunt surgery are counseled and explained regarding the need for follow-up and the possibility of multiple revisions.

Sites of CSF shunting include ventriculoperitoneal (VP) shunts, ventriculoatrial shunts and ventriculopleural shunts. Ventriculoperitoneal (VP) shunt is the most popular and accepted shunt (Fig. 13.5). In this, a shunt (tube) is placed between the enlarged ventricle that drains out CSF into the peritoneal cavity. Complications of shunt surgery include malfunction, shunt infection, over drainage (slit ventricle syndrome), wound infection, abdominal hernia, peritonitis, and shunt migration, etc. **(Table 13.2)**.

Endoscopic third ventriculostomy (ETV) The procedure involves creating an outlet in floor of third ventricle so that CSF can escape into extracerebral subarachnoid space and be absorbed into superior sagittal sinus. Well accepted indications of ETV include: aqueductal stenosis; arachnoid cyst and associated hydrocephalus; neoplastic etiology, eg, tectal plate tumors; and intraventricular neurocysticercosis. Complications of ETV include bleeding and neurological deficits.

POST-MENINGITIC HYDROCEPHALUS

Meningitis of pyogenic, tubercular, and non-bacterial origin are the most common cause of acquired hydrocephalus in

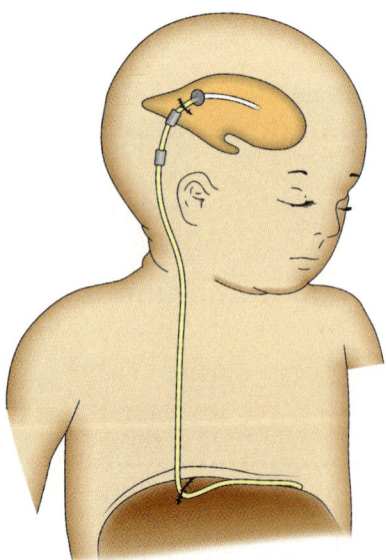

13 **Fig. 13.5** Ventriculoperitoneal shunt, catheter threaded beneath skin

Table 13.2 Complications of Ventriculoperitoneal (VP) Shunts	
Common to all types	*Unique to VP shunts*
1. Malfunction: Obstruction, disconnection, migration	1. Inguinal hernia
2. Infection	2. Ascites
3. Overdrainage	3. Cyst formation
4. Seizures	4. Intestinal volvulus
5. Pneumocephalus	5. Bowel perforation
6. Isolated ventricle syndrome	6. Intra-peritoneal spread of infection/malignancy

India. The incidence of hydrocephalus after meningitis ranges between 1 and 5%. There is obliteration of the subarachnoid space leading to decreased CSF absorption and communicating hydrocephalus.

- Children with mild ventriculomegaly and no features of raised intracranial pressure are treated with acetazolamide and osmotic decongestants.
- In the absence of active infection and low CSF cell/protein, patients with features of raised intracranial pressure (papilledema, rigidity, periventricular ooze) are advised shunt surgery.
- In children with high CSF cell/protein content, external ventricular drainage is instituted to decrease intracranial pressure.

Revision Point

Hydrocephalus

1. Hydrocephalus is characterized by accumulation of excessive amount of cerebrospinal fluid in the cerebral ventricles and/or subarachnoid spaces, resulting in ventricular dilation and increased intracranial pressure (ICP).
2. Presentation of hydrocephalus depends upon the timing of onset relative to closure of cranial sutures, the duration and rate of rise in ICP.
3. Children with suspected hydrocephalus should undergo neuroimaging and a detailed physical examination, including fundoscopy to evaluate for papilledema.
4. Surgical treatment of hydrocephalus consists of CSF shunt insertion or endoscopic third ventriculostomy.

Dinçer A, Özek MM. Radiologic evaluation of pediatric hydrocephalus. *Childs Nerv Syst.* 2011;27:1543–62.

Kandasamy J, Jenkinson MD, Mallucci CL. Contemporary management and recent advances in paediatric hydrocephalus. BMJ. 2011;343:d4191.

Prusseit J, Simon M, von der Brelie C, *et al.* Epidemiology, prevention and management of ventriculoperitoneal shunt infections in children. *Pediatr Neurosurg.* 2009;45:325–36.

13.3 SEIZURES AND EPILEPSY

Seizure is defined as a paroxysmal involuntary disturbance of brain function that may manifest as an impairment or loss of consciousness, abnormal motor activity, behavioral abnormality, sensory disturbances or autonomic dysfunction. Seizures affect 4–7% of children.

Seizures occurring during the course of an acute illness are termed as *provoked seizures*. Febrile seizures are the most important cause of provoked seizures and affect 3–5% of all children.

Epilepsy is defined as two or more unprovoked seizures occuring more than 24 hours apart. The prevalence of epilepsy (4–9/1000 population) is higher in developing countries due to high incidence of neurocysticercosis, CNS infections, birth asphyxia, and consanguinity related metabolic diseases.

Seizure *versus* Non-seizure

Most important initial step is to distinguish seizure from a non-seizure event. Disorders mimicking seizures include jitteriness; benign neonatal sleep myoclonus (in neonates); breath holding spells and shuddering attacks in infants; and syncopal attacks, night terror, pseudoseizures in childhood and adolescence. Up to 20 to 25% of patients referred to Neurology Clinics, as epileptics do not have epileptic seizures.

A sequenced account of the event, precipitating factors, reproducibility, and the gain expected out of the event are helpful in establishing the diagnosis. The timing of the event, injury, specific distribution and pattern of abnormal movements, post-event deficits, and loss of consciousness, points towards a true seizure. Observation of the child during an episode, electroencephalography (EEG), and sometimes a video EEG, may be helpful.

Provoked *versus* Un-provoked Seizures

As mentioned above, provoked or *acute symptomatic seizures* are seizures during the course of acute illnesses. Common causes of provoked seizures are: (*a*) Febrile seizures; (*b*) metabolic events: Blood sugar <36 mg/dL, serum calcium <5 mg/dL, serum magnesium <0.8 mg/dL, serum sodium <115 mg/dL; (*c*) acute CNS infections: Meningitis, encephalitis; (*d*) drug intoxication; hypoxia; (*e*) stroke; and (*f*) head trauma.

- Seizures are considered acute symptomatic if they occur within 7 days of cerebrovascular disease, trauma, CNS infections or anoxia.
- For acute symptomatic seizures due to metabolic illnesses, the blood sample upon which classification is based is operationally defined as within 24 hours of the seizure.

Etiology

Recurrent seizures are thought to accrue from a genetic predisposition and underlying neuropathologic changes. The attributed causes for epilepsy in children include malformations, infections, neoplasms, toxic/metabolic/asphyxial injury, and trauma of the central nervous system.

Classification of Epilepsy

ILAE (International League Against Epilepsy) has classified epilepsy as generalized, focal, and unknown (**Table 13.3**).
- *Generalized epilepsy* Epilepsy is considered generalized if the seizures after starting at a point rapidly engage bilaterally distributed networks and may manifest with motor or non-motor seizures.

Table 13.3 Classification of Seizures	
Generalized onset seizures	
Motor	*Non-motor (absence)*
• Tonic-clonic	• Typical
• Clonic	• Atypical
• Myoclonic	• Myoclonic
• Myoclonic-tonic-clonic	• Eyelid myoclonia
• Myoclonic-atonic	
• Atonic	
• Epileptic spasms	
Focal onset seizures	
Motor onset	*Non-motor onset*
• Aware	• Aware
• Impaired awareness	• Impaired awareness
• Unknown awareness	• Unknown awareness
• Automatisms	• Autonomic
• Atonic	• Behavioral arrest
• Clonic	• Cognitive
• Epileptic spasms	• Emotional
• Hyperkinetic	• Sensory
• Myoclonic	• Focal to bilateral tonic-clonic
• Tonic	
• Focal to bilateral tonic-clonic	
Unknown onset seizures	
Motor	*Non-motor*
• Tonic-clonic	Behavior arrest
• Epileptic spasms	
Unclassified seizures	

- *Focal epilepsy* The term focal has replaced partial to describe epilepsy associated with seizures that are inferred from clinical or EEG data to originate in networks limited to one hemisphere.
- *Generalized and focal epilepsy* This term should be used for epilepsies that have both generalized and focal seizures. This category includes several epilepsy syndromes (such as Dravet syndrome or Lennox-Gastaut syndrome), but may also be relevant for epilepsies associated with diffuse or focal structural, genetic, or metabolic etiologies.
- *Unknown if generalized or focal epilepsy* This term is used for epilepsies with seizures in which it cannot be clearly determined whether onset is focal or generalized. A key example is epileptic spasms, which may appear generalized despite being caused by a focal lesion. The term unknown should also be used in an individual who presents with a generalized tonic-clonic seizure and normal examination but whose EEG and neuroimaging is either non-informative or unavailable.

Clinical Features

Generalized Seizures

Generalized seizures are further classified into **motor** and **non-motor seizures**.

A. *Motor Seizures*

The motor seizures include tonic-clonic, tonic, clonic, myoclonic, and atonic seizures in addition to epileptic spasms.
- The term *tonic* refers to continuous stiffening of the extremities.

13

- *Clonic* refers to the rhythmic alternating contraction and relaxation of muscles.
- A *tonic-clonic* seizure is the one that starts with continuous stiffening and is then followed by a clonic phase of rhythmic jerks.
- *Myoclonus* is defined as sudden shock like contraction of muscles and may manifest as sudden jerk involving limbs, trunk, or head.
- *Atonic* (akinetic) seizures are drop attacks. They are so brief that consciousness has been regained by the time the child strikes the floor.

B. *Non-motor Seizures*

The non-motor seizures are the absence seizures. Typical absence seizures can be subtle or distinct, and they always recur during the course of several hours or days. Absence seizures typically begin in young school-aged children. They consist of brief (3–30 seconds) staring spells, accompanied by a cessation of activity. They are classically precipitated by hyperventilation.

Focal Seizures

Focal seizures have also been classified into focal seizures with motor onset and focal seizures with non-motor onset. Of note, the terms simple partial, complex partial, and secondarily generalized have been eliminated, since they were difficult to define pragmatically and were often used incorrectly. The term "focal to bilateral tonic-clonic" is used to describe a seizure that begins focally but then spreads to engage bilateral networks.

Diagnostic Evaluation

The aim should be to answer the following key questions while evaluating a child with seizures:
- Is it a seizure?
- First event or recurrent seizures?
- Febrile or afebrile (if afebrile, any other prvocative factor)?
- Is it focal or generalized or other?
- Is it symptomatic or idiopathic?
- Are there comorbidities?
- Is it syndromic?

Investigations

More than 80% of epilepsy in the community can be managed without any investigations.
- *Electroencephalography (EEG)* is not required routinely. It is useful to differentiate seizures from non-seizures, classify seizures types and localize epileptogenic foci in intractable epilepsy. Provocation procedures like sleeping deprivation, hyperventilation and photic stimulation should be used.
- *Hyperventilation to provoke absence seizures if suspected*. This is an important, simple and quick diagnostic test. To perform an adequate hyperventilation test, the patient is asked to breathe in and out deeply for up to 3 minutes. At the completion of hyperventilation, the patient is asked to count to 30, this is most revealing as the stream of speech and content is interrupted by an absence seizure.
- *Neuroimaging* It should be considered in every child with epilepsy, and first episode of unprovoked seizure.

Neuroimaging can be avoided if the diagnosis of febrile seizures is certain.CECT is the first investigation. This is important because in developing countries, neuro-cysticercosis is an important cause of epilepsy. It is also required to rule out other intracranial space occupying lesions in children with features of raised intracranial pressure along with focal deficits. MRI is preferred to look for migration defects and structural brain lesions.

Treatment	Seizures

Figure 13.6 provides an algorithm for antiepileptic management in childhood epilepsy. A detailed description follows:

Management Issues in First Seizure
- *Provoked seizure*—Acute symptomatic treatment only.
- *Generalized tonic clonic*—Withhold long-term antiepileptic drugs (AEDs) unless mentally retarded, neurological deficit, inflammatory granuloma, first episode is status epilepticus, or early medical help is inaccessible.
- *Focal*—Evaluate and treat.
- *Absence*—Treat.
- *Myoclonus*—Evaluate and treat.

Choice of Antiepileptic Drugs
It depends upon the seizure type, age and gender of the patient, epileptic syndrome diagnosis if possible, premorbid conditions, cost of therapy and safety profile. The efficacy of the four first line antiepileptic drugs (phenytoin, phenobarbital, carbamazepine and valproate) in the management of common epileptic disorders including generalized tonic clonic and focal seizures is nearly similar. In view of lower cost, ease of administration and fewer side effects, phenytoin is the usual drug of choice. The rational choice of antiepileptic drugs in various seizure types is as follows:
- *Generalized tonic clonic* Phenytoin, sodium valproate.
- *Focal* Carbamazepine, phenytoin.
- *Absence* Sodium valproate, ethosuximide, lamotrigine.
- *Myoclonus* Sodium valproate, benzodiazepines.
- *Infantile spasms* ACTH, sodium valproate, benzodiazepines.
- *Mixed* Sodium valproate.
  The overview of first line AEDs are detailed in **Table 13.4.**

Rational Antiepileptic Therapy
- Single first line drug for seizure type is used.
- If seizures are persistent, the dosage is increased to maximum tolerated clinically.
- If the seizures are still persistent, replace the first drug by a different first line drug.
- If seizures are still persistent use two first line drugs.
- If still uncontrolled, add newer antiepileptic drugs many of which are available for seizure control (eg, lamotrigine).

Discontinuing Antiepileptic T herapy
There is a need to discontinue antiepileptic drugs since most children with epilepsy achieve remission. Moreover, prolonged use of any drug is not bereft of its side-effects. Usually, antiepileptic drug is given for 2 years, after the last seizure was documented.

Relapse The risk of relapse is 30%. Certain patients have a high risk of relapse and in these patients discontinuing AED is not advisable. These patients include: Seizure onset during infancy, juvenile myoclonic epilepsy, intractable seizures, seizures due to previous serious CNS insults (head trauma, structural malformations and migration defects), and severe neuro-developmental retardation.

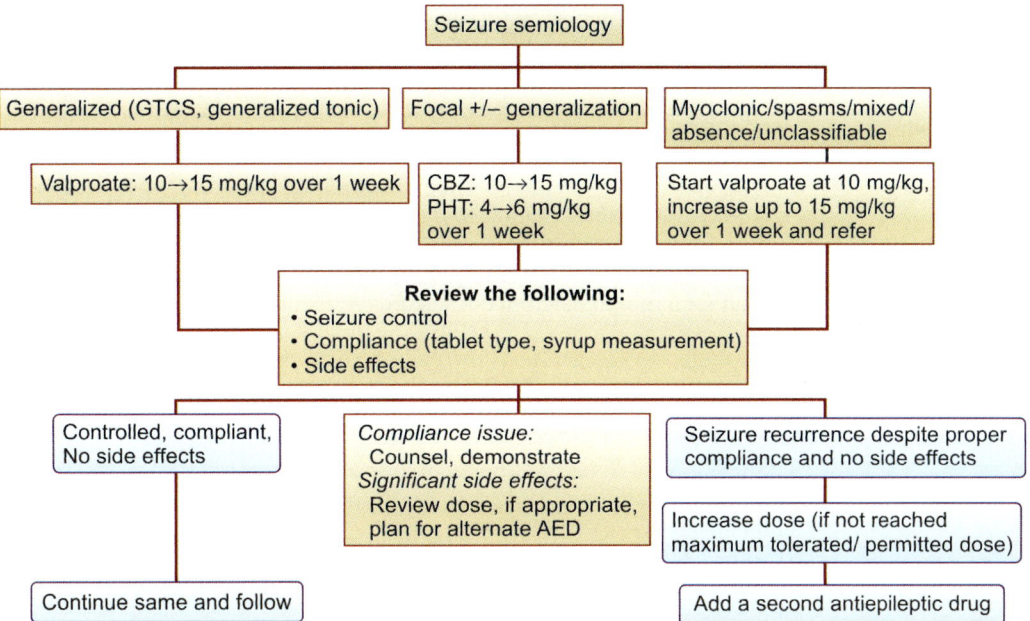

Fig. 13.6 Algorithm for anti-epileptic management in childhood epilepsy. CBZ: Carbamazepine; PHT: Phenytoin

Table 13.4 First Line Antiepileptic Drugs		
Drug	*Dose (mg/ kg/ d)*	*Side effects*
Phenobarbitone*	3–5	Drowsiness, hyperkinesia (mid-childhood), drug dependence
Phenytoin	3–8	Gingival hyperplasia, hirsutism, dermatitis, blood dyscrasias, ataxia, Stevens-Johnson syndrome, liver damage, nystagmus, lymphadenopathy, interferes with calcium metabolism, encephalopathy
Carbamazepine	10–30	GI disturbances, hepatitis, skin rash, diplopia, ataxia, bone marrow depression, sedation, urinary retention, nausea, Stevens-Johnson syndrome
Sodium valproate	10–60	Idiosyncratic reaction, fatal hepatic necrosis, nausea, vomiting, sedation, weight gain, hair loss, hyperammonemia

*Particulary useful in neonates

Increasing duration of antiepileptic drug therapy beyond 2 years of seizure free period does not decrease the risk of subsequent relapse. Acute symptomatic epilepsy due to inflammatory granulomas may allow earlier tapering.

Prescription Tips for Antiepileptic Medications
- Preferably use one brand only. Some brands have different strength formulation, so substitution may be lead to drug toxicity; eg, Suspension Dilantin (phenytoin) has a strength of 125 mg/5 mL in contrast to Syrup Eptoin (phenytoin) having 30 mg/5 mL. Also, the pharmacokinetics of different brands of same drug differs.
- Always prescribe syrups in mL, never as teaspoonful.
- Do not use bottle caps, spoons for measuring syrups, always use syringe.
- Shake syrup/suspension bottle before use.

STATUS EPILEPTICUS

Operational Definition of Status Epilepticus
1. Continuous seizure activity for ≥5 min.
2. ≥2 seizures without interictal recovery of consciousness to baseline.
3. Brought seizuring to emergency room.

Status epilepticus is a medical emergency consisting of persistent (lasting for more than 5 minutes) or recurring seizures. It may be further classified into early status epilepticus (5–30 minutes) and established status epilepticus (30–120 minutes). Longer the seizure more is the neuronal damage and it becomes difficult to control. Management of status epilepticus is detailed in **Table 13.5**.

- *Refractory status epilepticus* may be defined as persistent seizures beyond 120 minutes despite therapy with benzodiazepines, phenytoin, phenobarbitone or valproate and warranting general anesthesia. Treatment options for refractory status include midazolam infusion, phenobarbitone coma, thiopentone, ketamine, magnesium, steroids, and ketogenic diet.
- *Super-refractory status epilepticus* continues or recurs 24 hours or more after the onset of anesthetic therapy and this includes recurrence on reduction or withdrawal of anesthesia.

13

Status epilepticus	Time frame	Drugs	Supportive therapy	EEG
Incipient	<5 min	• *IV access not available*: Intranasal midazolam (0.2 mg/kg) OR buccal midazolam (0.2 mg/kg) OR IM midazolam (0.2 mg/kg/d) OR rectal diazepam (0.2–0.5 mg/kg) • *IV access available:* IV lorazepam (0.1 mg/kg; max 5 mg) over 1 min OR IV midazolam (0.1 mg/kg) over 1 min OR IV diazepam (0.2 mg/kg; max 10 mg) Wait for 5 min to determine if seizure terminates	Airway, Breathing, Hemodynamics, Temperature, Euglycemia, Maintain Eucalcemia. Search for and treatment of the underlying cause	Continuous EEG Monitoring
Early	5–30 min	• Repeat BZD • Phenytoin (20 mg/kg IV) at 1 mg/kg/min (max 50 mg/min)		
		CONSULT PEDIATRIC NEUROLOGY SERVICES		
Established	30–120 min	*If seizures persist 10 min after phenytoin infusion:* Valproate (20 mg/kg IV) at 5 mg/kg/min (contraindicated in cases of suspected metabolic disorders, severe thrombocytopenia and hepatic dysfunction) OR Levetiracetam (20 mg/kg IV) at 5 mg/kg/min (preferred in cases of hepatic dysfunction and metabolic disorders) OR Phenobarbitone (20 mg/kg IV) at 2 mg/kg/min (monitor for hypotension/respiratory depression) If seizures persist 5 min after infusion of any of the above drugs, consider use of the other drug		
		SHIFT TO PICU		
Refractory	>120 min	• *If seizure continues beyond 2 hours*, then initiate *coma* with IV midazolam 0.2 mg/kg bolus (max 10 mg) over 2 min followed by infusion at 1 microgram/kg/min. • If seizures persist 5 min after initial midazolam bolus, then administer additional midazolam bolus of 0.2 mg/kg bolus. Continue infusion. • *If clinical seizures persist after another 5 min*, then administer another midazolam bolus of 0.2 mg/kg, and increase infusion to 0.2 mg/kg/hr. Repeat as needed. • *If seizures persist at maximum midazolam* (generally 2 mg/kg/hr) or midazolam infusion is not tolerated, consider transition to thiopentone. Thiopentone 5 mg/kg IV over 20 seconds followed by 3–5 mg/kg/hr infusion (monitor hemodynamics). • Continue pharmacologic coma for 24 hours after last seizure with EEG goal of burst-suppression. • Continue initial medications in maintenance doses. • Ensure an additional anticonvulsant is administered to provide coverage during weaning (eg, topiramate). • Reduce midazolam (by 0.05 mg/kg/hr) or thiopentone every 3 hours with frequent EEG review. If no clinical or electrographic seizures then wean until off. • Continue EEG for at least 24 hours after end of infusion to evaluate for recurrent electrographic seizures.		
Super-refractory	≥24 hours after onset of coma	Consider: • Ketamine: 1 mg/kg IV followed by 1–5 mg/kg/hr infusion • Magnesium: 50 mg/kg IV over 30 min • Pyridoxine: 30 mg/kg IV • Methylprednisolone pulse If no resolution within 2 days of pulse: • Intravenous immunoglobulin (IVIG) 0.4 g/kg/d × 5 days • 4:1 ketogenic diet		

Table 13.5 Suggested Protocol for Management of Status Epilepticus

INTRACTABLE EPILEPSY

A task force of the International League against Epilepsy proposed that drug-resistance be defined as the failure of adequate trials of two tolerated, appropriately chosen and administered anti-seizure drugs (whether as monotherapy or in combination) to achieve seizure freedom. They also recommended replacing the term "intractable" with "drug-resistant" epilepsy. The risk of seizure relapse in these individuals remains high, usually greater than 70%. Treatment options for intractable epilepsy include epilepsy surgery, ketogenic diet, and vagal nerve stimulation.

Seizures and Epilepsy

1. Seizure is a paroxysmal event representing clinical expression of abnormal, excessive, synchronous discharges of neurons residing primarily in the cerebral cortex.
2. An individual is considered to have epilepsy if he/she has at least two unprovoked seizures occurring more than 24 hours apart.
3. Epilepsy is classified into generalized, focal, and unknown based on unilateral/ bilateral involvement.
4. Choice of antiepileptics depends on seizure type, age and gender of patient and epileptic syndrome.
5. Withdrawal of antiepileptic drug therapy should be considered in most children after two years without seizures.

Berg AT, Berkovic SF, Brodie MJ, *et al.* Revised terminology and concepts for organization of seizures and epilepsies: report of the ILAE Commission on Classification and Terminology, 2005–2009. *Epilepsia.* 2010;51:676–85.

Fisher RS, Cross JH, French JA, et al. Operational classification of seizure types by the International League Against Epilepsy: Position paper of the ILAE Commission for Classification and Terminology. *Epilepsia.* 2017;58(4):522–530.

Owens J. Medical management of refractory status epilepticus. *Semin Pediatr Neurol.* 2010;17:176–81.

Shorvon S, Ferlisi M. The treatment of super-refractory status epilepticus: a critical review of available therapies and a clinical treatment protocol. *Brain.* 2011;134:2802–18.

Vendrame M, Zarowski M, Alexopoulos AV, *et al.* Localization of pediatric seizure semiology. *Clin Neurophysiol.* 2011;122:1924–8.

13.4 FEBRILE SEIZURES

Febrile seizures are the most common seizure disorder in childhood. Approximately 2–4% of all children below 5 years may experience febrile seizures.

Definition

A febrile seizure refers to a seizure in infancy or childhood, usually occurring between 6 months and 5 years of age, associated with fever but without evidence of intracranial infection or defined cause. Seizures with fever in children who have suffered a previous non-febrile seizure are excluded from this definition. Febrile seizures are not considered a form of epilepsy, which is characterized by recurrent non-febrile seizures.

The median age of occurrence is 18–22 months. The infections commonly encountered in children with febrile seizures include infections of the middle ear, upper respiratory tract, urinary tract, and gastrointestinal system. *Generally accepted criteria for febrile seizures include:*

- Convulsion associated with an elevated temperature >38°C;
- Age of the child between 6 and 60 months;
- Absence of central nervous system infection or inflammation;
- Absence of acute systemic metabolic abnormality that may produce convulsions; and
- No history of previous afebrile seizures.

Febrile seizures are further divided into simple and complex febrile seizures.

Simple febrile seizures These constitute up to 85% of febrile seizures. They are generalized seizures, lasting less than 15 minutes, not recurring within 24 hours, and with no post-ictal neurological abnormalities.

Complex febrile seizures These are focal, prolonged or recurrent within 24 hours or associated with postictal neurological abnormalities including todd paresis. They constitute around 15% of febrile seizures.

Febrile status This is a febrile seizure with duration of 30 minutes or more, either one long lasting or a series of shorter seizures without regaining consciousness interictally.

Factors Predisposing to Febrile Seizures

There is significant genetic susceptibility to febrile seizures. The risk of another child having febrile seizures is 1 in 5 with one affected sibling; and 1 in 3 if both parents and a previous child have had febrile seizures.

Predictors of a first febrile seizure These include a high degree of fever at initial presentation, family history of febrile seizures, and delayed neonatal discharge >28 days.

Recurrence Risk and Prognosis

The average recurrence rate after a first febrile seizure is 30–40% but this is dependent on complex interplay between genetic and environmental factors. Of these, 75% of recurrences would occur within 1 year of first episode.

Risk factors for recurrent febrile seizures These include: Age <18 months at onset, family history of febrile seizures, shorter duration of fever prior to the onset of seizure, and low peak of temperature at the time of the seizure.

Risk of epilepsy The overall risk of subsequent epilepsy after febrile seizures is 2–2.5%. The risk factors are: Complex febrile seizures (each complex feature of febrile seizures is an independent predictor of later afebrile seizures), pre-existing neurological or developmental abnormality, and a family history of epilepsy.

Evaluation

History aims to rule out possible CNS infections, determine cause of fever, describe seizures semiology, ascertain family risk factors, and determine neurodevelopment of the child. Clinical examination includes observation of postictal phase, to look for CNS infections like meningitis, and to look for signs of raised intracranial pressure.

13

Investigations are oriented towards finding the cause of fever and to rule out meningitis. Serum electrolytes, blood glucose, calcium, magnesium and blood counts are not routinely needed.

Lumbar puncture (LP) LP is indicated in a child with fever and seizure whenever a doubt of meningitis exists, because of (*i*) abnormal neurological examination, especially meningeal signs; (*ii*) focal seizure with suspicious physical findings (rash or petechiae, cyanosis, hypotension, grunt, etc.); and (*iii*) ongoing seizure activity at the time of arrival in the hospital.

- Lumbar puncture should be strongly considered in infants younger than 12 months, presenting first time with seizure, because the clinical signs and symptoms associated with meningitis may be minimal or absent in this age group.
- In a child between 12 and 18 months of age, an LP should be considered, because clinical signs and symptoms of meningitis may be subtle.
- In a child older than 18 months, a lumbar puncture is recommended only if intracranial infection is suspected.
- In infants and children who have had febrile seizures and have received prior antibiotic treatment, clinicians should be aware that treatment can mask the signs and symptoms of meningitis. As such, a lumbar puncture should be strongly considered.

EEG and *neuroimaging* These investigations need not be performed in the routine evaluation of a neurologically healthy child with a first simple febrile seizure.

Case Study | **Febrile Seizure**

A 2-year-old girl was brought with the history of fever, cough and cold for 1 day, and 1 episode of generalized tonic-clonic seizure. The parents noted the temperature after the seizure: It was 102°F.

What other information would you like from the history?
The following information should be asked from the parents:
1. Duration of seizure?
2. Did she have only one seizure during this episode, or more?
3. Does she have any features suggestive of meningitis? Is she lethargic, irritable? Does she have vomiting, head banging?
4. Has she had any seizures in the past?
5. Is she developmentally normal?
6. Is there any family history of febrile seizures or epilepsy?

The parents say this was the only seizure during this febrile illness, and it lasted 2 minutes. She has been active and playful after the seizure. She has not had any seizures in the past. She is developmentally normal. There is no family history of febrile seizures or epilepsy.

What would you like to see in the examination?
First assess the vitals, airway, breathing, and circulation. Look for features of meningitis such as irritability, lethargy, bulging fontanel, neck rigidity, and Kernig sign.

On examination, the girl was febrile, but alert and conscious. The vitals were stable. She had no features of meningeal irritation. She had cough and cold, but no fast breathing or chest indrawing. The chest was clear on auscultation.

What is the likely diagnosis?
The likely diagnosis is upper respiratory tract infection with simple febrile seizure, as this was a seizure occurring with fever in a previously normal child, without any evidence of central nervous system infection and the seizure was brief (<15 min), generalized, and single.

What investigations will you perform?
No investigations are needed in this scenario. No neuroimaging or EEG is indicated for simple febrile seizure. As the child is 2 years old, and has clinically no features suggestive of meningitis, lumbar puncture is not indicated.

How will you treat this child?
The parents should first be explained the benign nature of simple febrile seizures, and their anxiety should be allayed. Long-term anti-epileptic treatment is not indicated. The parents should be explained that the child may have seizures during fever in the future, but is likely to be free of seizures after 5 years of age. They should be advised to give 6 hourly paracetamol (15 mg/kg/dose) for 48–72 hours when the child has fever.

The most important thing is to explain to the parents what to do if the child has a seizure again. They should not panic. They should lay the child in a safe place, and loosen all the tight clothing. They should wipe off any secretions from the mouth and nose. After the seizure is over, they should turn over the child to her side, and lay her in the recovery position. Explain that most seizures stop within 5 minutes. If the seizure lasts longer than 5 min, they should give abortive treatment with any of the following: Intranasal/buccal midazolam, or rectal diazepam. If the seizure does not stop 5 minutes after this treatment, they should repeat the dose, and bring the child to the hospital.

If they stay in a remote place, with no immediate access to medical facilities, intermittent clobazam prophylaxis may be considered (1 mg/kg/day in 2 divided doses) for 48–72 hours during the febrile episode. However, the risk of sedation and ataxia with this treatment must be explained.

Treatment	**Fetrile Seizure**

During the Seizure

Any child with a febrile seizure needs to be managed as for any other acute seizure. The decision to admit should be individualized but admission is usually not necessary. Children, especially those with a first febrile seizure, should be hospitalized if any of the following are present: (*i*) Lethargy beyond postictal state; (*ii*) unstable clinical status; (*iii*) age <18 months; (*iv*) complex features; (*v*) uncertain home situation; or (*vi*) unclear follow up. Any child with the slightest suspicion of meningitis should be admitted and investigated.

Long-term Management

The primary goal of long-term management of febrile seizure is to prevent recurrences. Treatment options include: (*a*) Intermittent prophylaxis; and (*b*) Prolonged daily prophylaxis.

Antipyretics are not effective in preventing recurrent febrile seizures, but are useful in making the child more comfortable. Tepid water sponging is advised if temperature remains high, despite drug therapy.

Intermittent prophylaxis

Diazepam administered intermittently either rectally or orally at the onset of fever has been shown to be effective in preventing recurrence of febrile seizures. It may be prescribed in complex febrile seizures and also in simple febrile seizures, if the parents are extremely anxious or if the health facility is far from place of residence.

Diazepam is generally given in a dose of 0.3 to 0.5 mg/kg (max 10 mg) orally or rectally and repeated every 8–12 hours for 3 days, if temperature is 38°C or more.

Intermittent clobazam (1 mg/kg/day for 3 days) given orally has also been found to be useful in preventing febrile seizure recurrences. This therapy does not decrease the incidence of later epilepsy in children with febrile seizures.

Abortive treatment

This must be explained to all parents. Buccal or intranasal midazolam, or rectal diazepam may be used. All the parents must be taught home management of seizures including recovery position.

Continuous prophylaxis

Indications for continuous prophylaxis include recurrent complex seizures with failed intermittent prophylaxis, abnormal neurodevelopment and positive family history of epilepsy. Sodium valproate is preferred to phenobarbitone. Neither of them is effective in reducing the risk of epilepsy in children with febrile seizure.

Febrile Seizure

1. Simple febrile seizures are characterized by seizures associated with febrile episode, that last less than 15 minutes, have no focal features, and occur once in a 24-hour period. These are mainly generalized tonic-clonic seizures.
2. Complex febrile seizures are characterized by episodes that do not fulfill pre-mentioned criteria.
3. LP should be strongly considered in infants younger than 12 months to rule out meningitis.
4. Intermittent benzodiazepine prophylaxis may be given if the parents are extremely anxious or if the health facility is far from place of residence.

Mohebbi MR, Holden KR, Butler IJ. FIRST: a practical approach to the causes and management of febrile seizures. *J Child Neurol.* 2008;23:1484–8.

Nordli DR, Moshé SL, Shinnar S. The role of EEG in febrile status epilepticus (FSE). *Brain Dev.* 2010;32:37–41.

13.5 COMA

The word "coma" is derived from the Greek word "Coma" meaning deep sleep. It is a state of decreased consciousness from which the child cannot be aroused by ordinary verbal, sensory or physical stimuli. Consciousness is maintained by the interaction of the reticular activating system with the cerebral hemispheres. Thus, coma results from lesions involving the reticular formation of the brainstem, the hypothalamus, and connections with the cerebral hemispheres.

Definition

Alterations in the state of consciousness in infants and children include delirium, stupor, and coma.

- *Delirium* is marked by confusion, disorientation, irrationality, and perhaps excitability.
- *Lethargy* is characterized by drowsiness and a lack of interest in the environment.
- *Obtundation* is an increase in the depth of the lethargy.
- *Stupor*, a state of unconsciousness from which the child may be aroused momentarily, often precedes coma.
- *Coma* This is a state of unarousable unresponsiveness, and is the most profound degree to which arousal and consciousness are impaired.

Etiology

The common causes of coma are detailed in **Table 13.6**. In clinical practice, coma is often associated with CNS infections, and encephalopathy secondary to systemic infections, intoxication, dyselectrolytemia, hepatitis, uremia, ketoacidosis, and poisoning.

Glasgow Coma Scale

This scale is useful for evaluating progress of children with disturbed consciousness. The Glasgow Coma Scale is scored between 3 and 15, 3 being the worst, and 15 the best. It is composed of three parameters: Best eye response (E), best verbal response (V), and best motor response (M). A score of 13 or higher correlates with mild brain injury; a score of 9 to 12 correlates with moderate injury; and a score of 8 or less represents severe brain injury (**Table 13.7**).

Approach to Diagnosis of Coma

The airway, breathing and circulatory status should be immediately attended. If respiratory depression or circulatory collapse is present, the therapeutic measures include intravenous line, intubation, assisted ventilation and normalization of blood pressure. A proper detailed history of events preceding coma, background illnesses, exposure to drugs and toxins provides useful information.

Table 13.6 Etiologic Classification of Coma

I. Central Nervous System Disturbances
1. Trauma
2. Disturbances in circulation (hemorrhage, cerebral vascular occlusions)
3. Acute infantile hemiplegia
4. Central nervous system infections (cerebral abscess, meningitis—bacterial, tubercular, encephalitis, subdural empyema, cerebral malaria, enteric/shigella encephalopathy, sepsis)
5. Hypertensive encephalopathy
6. CSF shunt obstruction
7. Increased intracranial pressure (mass lesions in brain, demyelinating disorders of CNS)
8. Post-convulsion coma

II. Metabolic Disorders
1. *Metabolic acidosis:* Diabetic ketoacidosis, organic acidemias
2. Ammonia encephalopathy: Disorders of the urea cycle, Reye syndrome, hepatic coma, valproic acid
3. Leigh syndrome
4. Hypoglycemia
5. Renal insufficiency
6. Hypoxemia
7. Tetany
8. Acute hyponatremia, hypernatremia, hypomagnesemia, hypermagnesemia, hypocalcemia, hypercalcemia
9. Heat stroke, heat exhaustion
10. Hypothermia and septic shock

III. Drugs, Poisons
1. Sedatives, barbiturates, phenothiazines
2. Narcotics
3. Lead poisoning
4. Salicylate poisoning
5. Kerosene poisoning
6. Organic phosphate (parathion) poisoning

History in Comatose Child

1. *Events leading to onset* Sudden onset coma in an otherwise normal and awake child suggests convulsions or intracranial hemorrhage. A preceding history of sleepiness or unsteadiness suggests ingestion of drug or toxin. A history of fever or recent illness suggests an acute infectious etiology (sepsis, meningitis, encephalitis), but other disorders in which encephalopathy is usually preceded by a febrile illness must be considered. These include acute disseminated encephalomyelitis (ADEM), Reye syndrome, mitochondrial encephalopathy, and other inborn errors of metabolism.
2. Drug or toxin exposure.
3. History of trauma.
4. Personal or family history of seizure disorder.
5. Personal or family history of migraine.
6. History of dog bite.
7. Recent immunizations.
8. History of recurrent episodes of encephalopathy are characteristic of some inborn errors of metabolism (urea cycle defects, organic acidemias and fatty acid oxidation defects), but may also be present in migraine, epilepsy, substance abuse, and Munchausen syndrome by proxy.

9. *Other concurrent systemic illness,* eg, jaundice (hepatic failure), pneumonia (hypoxic encephalopathy), diarrhea (dyselectrolytemia), dysentery (Shigella encephalopathy).
10. *Past medical illness* Children with diabetes mellitus may have altered sensorium because of hypoglycemia or ketoacidosis; children with congenital heart disease are more susceptible to brain abscess or infarction; children with renal failure may develop uremic encephalopathy; and children with liver disease may develop hepatic encephalopathy.

Examination of Comatose Child

Temperature

Presence of fever suggests an infective process, eg, sepsis, pneumonia, meningitis, encephalitis, or a brain abscess; but may also indicate abnormality of hypothalamic temperature regulatory mechanisms. Hyperthermia may also be a result of heat stroke.

Heart Rate

Tachycardia may be a result of fever, hypovolemic or septic shock, heart failure or arrhythmias. Bradycardia may result from raised intracranial pressure or as a result of myocardial injury (due to myocarditis, hypoxia, sepsis, or toxins).

Respiration

Tachypnea with other features of respiratory distress signifying increased work of breathing is an indicator of lung pathology, eg, pneumonia, pneumothorax, empyema, or asthma.

- *Quiet tachypnea* is indicative of acidosis which may be present in diabetic ketoacidosis, uremia, or some poisonings (eg, ethylene glycol).
- *Cheyne-Stokes respiration,* in which periods of hyperpnea alternate with periods of apnea is usually caused by bilateral hemispheric or diencephalic injuries, but can result from bilateral damage anywhere along the descending pathway between the forebrain and upper pons. Other causes include metabolic disorders such as uremia and diffuse anoxia.
- A sustained, rapid, deep breathing, called *central neurogenic hyperventilation* occurs in lesions ventral to the aqueduct or the fourth ventricle.
- *Apneustic breathing,* characterized by a long inspiratory pause, is seen with lesions of the lateral tegmentum of the lower half of the pons.
- *Ataxic breathing,* haphazard breaths and pauses without a predictable pattern, follows damage of the dorsomedial medulla.
- *Ondine's curse* which refers to loss of automatic breathing during sleep, occurs with lower brainstem dysfunction.

Odor of Breath

The odor of exhaled breath can be helpful in diagnosis in some conditions, eg, diabetic ketoacidosis (fruity odor), hepatic coma (fetor hepaticus), uremia (musty), and alcohol intoxication.

Blood Pressure

Hypertension may be the cause of alteration in sensorium in hypertensive encephalopathy or may be a compensatory

Table 13.7 Pediatric Modification of Glasgow Coma Scale (GCS)

Glasgow Coma Score	Pediatric modification	
Eye opening		
>1 year	**0–1 year**	
4 Spontaneously	4 Spontaneously	
3 To verbal command	3 To shout	
2 To pain	2 To pain	
1 No response	1 No response	
Best motor response		
>1 year	**0–1 year**	
6 Obeys	6 Spontaneous	
5 Localizes pain	5 Localizes pain	
4 Flexion withdrawal	4 Flexion withdrawal	
3 Flexion abnormal (decorticate)	3 Flexion abnormal (decorticate)	
2 Extension (decerebrate)	2 Extension (decerebrate)	
1 No response	1 No response	
Best verbal response		
>5 years	**0–2 years**	**2–5 years**
5 Oriented and converses	5 Cries appropriately, smiles, coos	5 Appropriate words and phrases
4 Disoriented and converses	4 Cries	4 Inappropriate words
3 Inappropriate words	3 Inappropriate crying/screaming	3 Cries/screams
2 Incomprehensible sounds	2 Grunts	2 Grunts
1 No response	1 No response	1 No response

Score is the sum of the individual scores from eye opening, best verbal response, and best motor response, using age-specific criteria.

mechanism to maintain cerebral perfusion in children with increased intracranial pressure or stroke.

Skin and Mucous Membranes

Cyanosis suggests poor oxygenation, pallor suggests anemia or shock, and jaundice is indicative of liver dysfunction. Rashes may be seen in infective conditions like meningococcemia or rickettsial diseases. The presence of neurocutaneous stigmata suggests seizures as a cause of encephalopathy.

Neurological Examination

The head and scalp should be examined for evidence of head trauma, eg, cephalhematoma, lacerations, ecchymosis. Presence of hemorrhage overlying mastoid (Battle's sign) or around eyes (raccoon eyes), CSF rhinorrhea, or otorrhea is suggestive of basilar skull fracture.

The important variables in locating the site of abnormality are state of consciousness, pattern of breathing (discussed above), pupillary size and reactivity and motor responses.
- Lethargy (difficulty in maintaining the aroused state) is usually caused by mild depression of hemispheric function.
- Stupor (responsive only to pain) and coma (unresponsive to pain) are caused by extensive disturbance of hemispheric function or involvement of the diencephalon and upper brainstem.
- The presence of oculocephalic (doll's eye), oculovestibular, and corneal reflexes are indicative of intact brainstem function. The trunk, limb, position, spontaneous movements, and response to stimulation must be observed to look for any focal deficits (suggestive of post-ictal Todd's palsy or structural abnormality).
- Decerebrate rigidity is ominous and suggests brainstem dysfunction.

Ocular Examination

Pupils Pupillary size, shape, symmetry and response to light provide valuable clues to brainstem and third nerve dysfunction. The pupillary light reflex is very resistant to metabolic dysfunction. Abnormalities especially when unilateral indicate structural lesions of the midbrain or oculomotor nerve. Exceptions include topical administration of mydriatics or use of atropine during cardiopulmonary resuscitation. Drugs and toxins which may rarely cause unreactive pupils include barbiturates, succinylcholine, lidocaine, phenothiazines methanol, and aminoglycoside antibiotics. Hypothermia and acute anoxia may also cause unreactive pupils, which, if persistent for several minutes after the insult, carry a poor prognosis. Hypothalamic damage causes unilateral pupillary constriction and Horner syndrome. Midbrain lesions cause mid-position fixed pupils and pontine lesions cause small but reactive pupils.

Fundus Fundus examination must be performed to look for papilledema and retinal hemorrhages. Signs of meningeal irritation may be present in meningitis, encephalitis and subarachnoid hemorrhage.

Systemic Examination

Chest examination is helpful to detect underlying pneumonia or empyema. Cardiovascular examination may suggest congenital or rheumatic heart disease, both of which predispose the patient to endocarditis and subsequent intracranial abscess dissemination. Abdominal examination is important to detect hepatosplenomegaly which may be present in many infective conditions and liver disease.

Laboratory Tests for Children with Coma

1. *Blood examination* Complete blood cell count; In febrile coma, malarial parasite should be carefully examined for; Evaluation of clotting mechanism; Examination of blood smear for sickling; Blood glucose; Blood ammonia, blood lactate, hepatic enzymes, blood urea, serum creatinine, serum bicarbonate, chloride, sodium and serum calcium; Blood cultures.
2. *Urinalysis* Microscopic; chemical for albumin, acetone, glycosuria, salicylates. Glycosuria may be present in patients who have meningitis or other CNS disease.
3. *Examination of the CSF* is an important diagnostic procedure in patients with coma of unknown etiology. Possible contraindications to lumbar puncture include increased intracranial pressure and shock.
4. *Neuroimaging* CT of the head is the diagnostic procedure of choice if a head injury is suspected or confirmed. MRI is especially helpful in detecting hemorrhage, including traumatic hematomas, cerebral ischemia, or edema.
5. If the possibility of *poisoning* exists, gastric lavage may be indicated for diagnostic as well as therapeutic reasons.
6. In patients thought to have encephalitis, *virologic and serological investigations* are carried out if possible.
7. *EEG* is indicated for children with unexplained stupor or coma.

Treatment	Coma

Initial Stabilization in the Emergency Room
Check airway patency, intubate if Glasgow Coma Score <8, or there is pooling of secretions; check breathing, give 100% oxygen, use bag and mask/tube if breathing efforts are unsatisfactory; check circulation, give intravenous normal saline or Ringer lactate 20 mL per kg to maintain blood pressure and peripheral perfusion; give inotropic support/antihypertensives as required; seizure control with diazepam/midazolam; raised ICP/impending herniation-head elevation 15°–30°, hyperventilation, mannitol; metabolic support, 2 mL per kg of 25% glucose IV, consider specific antidotes in case of known poisoning.

General Measures and Monitoring
Monitor vital signs and neurological parameters to detect any life-threatening events like raised ICP or herniation syndrome. Maintain patency of airways and provide oxygenation, optimal fluid intake and output management. Correction of acid–base and electrolyte disturbances. Temperature control is important. Urinary catheterization is often required to guide fluid therapy and prevent stasis. Adequate nutrition should be maintained by nasogastric feeding in children with prolonged coma.

Specific Management
Depending upon the cause of coma, specific therapy is life-saving. Examples include:
1. *Antidotes* Naloxone should be used in case of suspected opiate poisoning. Flumazenil is useful for benzodiazepine overdose.
2. *Antibiotics* for underlying infections
3. *Antiviral drugs* Acyclovir for herpes encephalitis
4. *Antimalarials* for cerebral malaria
5. *Neurosurgical intervention* in traumatic brain injury and hydrocephalus
6. *Steroids* in Acute disseminated encephalomyelitis

The clinical course of each child should be monitored closely and documented on a daily basis. Particular attention should be paid to changing level of consciousness, fever, seizures, autonomic nervous system dysfunction, increased intracranial pressure, and speech and motor disturbances. Nosocomial infection in these children is an important complication, which must be looked for and treated.

Prognosis

The prognosis of coma mainly depends upon its etiology, duration and depth. Recovery is best in children with coma due to primary epilepsy, whereas anoxia has the worst outcome. These children should be followed up for early identification of developmental disabilities, learning and behavior problems, as well as other neurological sequelae such as motor, visual or hearing deficit and seizure disorder.

REYE SYNDROME

Reye syndrome is a systemic disorder of mitochondrial function presenting with anicteric hepatic encephalopathy, hypoglycemia, and raised intracranial pressure. The disorder occurs during or after a viral infection. The occurrence is higher following salicylate use for symptomatic relief.

Characteristic Features

Reye syndrome is a biphasic illness. A viral prodrome with infection of the upper respiratory or gastrointestinal tract or varicella is followed 5–7 days later by abrupt onset of encephalopathy heralded as profuse, effortless vomiting. Raised intracranial tension from brain swelling is implicated as the cause of neurological injury and death. A number of metabolic disorders can present with a Reye syndrome like presentation **(Table 13.8)**. 'Classic' Reye syndrome is a diagnosis of exclusion. Investigations reveal hypoglycemia, hyperammonemia, and increased concentration of hepatic enzymes. Liver biopsy demonstrates microvescicular steatosis.

Table 13.8 Metabolic Disorders Resembling Reye Syndrome	
1.	Urea cycle defects
2.	Organic acidurias
3.	Defects in fatty acid oxidative metabolism
4.	Fructosemia
5.	Systemic carnitine deficiency
6.	Hepatic carnitine palmitoyl transferase deficiency

Treatment and Prognosis

Management requires precise diagnostic evaluation to exclude metabolic disorders resembling Reye syndrome. Affected children must be admitted in an intensive care unit. Treatment is mainly supportive; measures to decrease intracranial pressure, appropriate therapy for hypoglycemia and coagulopathy.

Prognosis depends on the duration of disordered cerebral function during the acute stage of illness. In mild disease, the recovery is rapid and complete, but patients with severe disease may die or develop neurodevelopmental sequel.

Coma

Revision Point

1. Trauma, infections, metabolic derangements, and intoxications are the most common etiologies of coma in children.
2. Glasgow Coma Scale is useful for evaluating progress of children with disturbed consciousness.
3. Neurologic examination in coma patients includes assessment of arousal, cranial nerve examination including fundoscopy, and motor examination. In addition, systemic examination including abdominal examination and animal/snake bite should be assessed.

Kirkham FJ, Newton CR, Whitehouse W. Paediatric coma scales. *Dev Med Child Neurol.* 2008;50:267–74.

Michelson DJ, Ashwal S. Evaluation of coma and brain death. *Semin Pediatr Neurol.* 2004;11:105–18.

Shemie SD, Pollack MM, Morioka M, *et al.* Diagnosis of brain death in children. *Lancet Neurol.* 2007;6:87–92.

CNS INFECTIONS

13.6 PYOGENIC MENINGITIS

Meningitis is the inflammation of the leptomeninges with variable involvement of the encephalon. Acute meningitis is usually bacterial or viral. Acute viral meningitis is usually a mild and self-limiting illness while bacterial meningitis is a serious illness that is fatal if untreated.

Etiological Agents

Haemophilus influenzae, *Streptococcus pneumoniae*, and *Neisseria meningitidis* are the most common agents causing meningitis in children. Uncommon agents include Gram-negative bacteria: *E coli*, *Pseudomonas*, *Proteus* (in hospital acquired infections, immunocompromised children and neonates), *Staphylococcus aureus,* and *S. epidermidis* (in patients with ventriculoperitoneal shunt, neurosurgical procedures, head trauma) and Group A Streptococcus.

Haemophilus influenzae meningitis usually occurs between the age of 1 month to 2 years. Age-related etiology of acute bacterial meningitis is depicted as follows:

Age	Common bacterial pathogens
<1 month	*E. coli, Streptococcus agalactiae, Listeria monocytogenes, Klebsiella* sp.
1–23 months	*Streptococcus pneumoniae, N. meningitidis, H. influenzae, S. agalactiae, E. coli*
>2 years	*N. meningitidis, S. pneumoniae*

Clinical Features

Fever, headache, and neck stiffness of short duration (less than 7 days) constitute the classical symptom triad of meningitis. However, acute meningitis should be suspected in any sick child with high grade fever and presence of any of the following: Nausea, vomiting, irritability, excessive crying and anorexia; head banging in a younger child; headache/photophobia in older children; and altered sensorium. Seizures may be present in 20–30% of children at presentation.

Examination reveals presence of meningeal signs, ie, neck rigidity, Kernig sign, and Brudzinski sign. Focal CNS deficits such as hemiparesis, visual loss and features of raised intracranial pressure such as bulging anterior fontanelle in infants, papilledema, bradycardia, hypertension, and brisk deep tendon reflexes may be present. Petechial hemorrhage or rash indicate meningococcal or arboviral infection. Other extra CNS manifestations include arthralgia, disseminated intravascular coagulation, shock, and presence of a septic focus elsewhere, eg, pneumonia.

Differential diagnoses include other causes of meningism: Subarachnoid hemorrhage, tonsillopharyngitis, apical pneumonias, typhoid, pyelonephritis, and bacillary dysentery.

Investigations

Lumbar puncture Examination of cerebrospinal fluid (CSF) is the most important investigation for a patient suspected to have meningitis. CSF picture in meningitis caused by different etiological agents is detailed in **Table 13.9.**

Following therapy, CSF Gram stain and culture becomes negative within 24–48 hours and glucose normalizes within 72 hours. Increase in cells and proteins may persist for days following therapy. Repeat CSF analysis may be indicated in partially treated cases, poor clinical response to therapy, Gram-negative meningitis, and shunt infections.

Table 13.9 CSF Picture in Meningitis Caused by Different Etiological Agents				
Parameter *(normal)*		*Pyogenic*	*Viral*	*Tubercular fungal*
Gross appearance (clear)	Turbid	Clear to turbid	Clear, cobweb coagulum forms on standing	Turbid
Sugar (≥2/3rd of blood sugar)	<40 mg/ dL	Normal	<50 mg/dL	30–40 mg/dL
Protein (<40 mg/dL)	100–500 mg/dL	Normal or slight increase	Up to 300 may be increased >500 mg/dL	100 (20–500) mg/dL
Total cells (<10/cumm)	Up to several thousand	Up to 100/mm³	25–100 (rarely >500)/mm³	Up to 50/mm³
Predominant cell type (no neutrophils)	Neutrophils	Lymphocytes	Lymphocytes	Lymphocytes

13

Other tests include Gram staining on a centrifuged specimen of CSF and culture/sensitivity of CSF. Counter immunoelectrophoresis, latex agglutination, and enzyme linked immunosorbent assay (ELISA) of CSF are particularly useful in eliciting the etiology in a case of partially treated meningitis, where culture of CSF may not grow any organism.

Other investigations include complete blood counts, blood culture, buffy coat Gram stain for intracellular organisms in leucocytes, petechial scrapings microscopy and culture for meningococcus and chest X-ray. CT scan is not routinely performed. It is indicated only when complications are suspected.

Treatment — Pyogenic Meningitis

A. Antibiotic Therapy

Empiric antibiotics are initiated based on the likely pathogen, age, drug susceptibility patterns and underlying health status **(Table 13.10)**. Therapy should be modified once the offending organism is isolated and its antibacterial susceptibility is determined.

- In most of the children, therapy is initiated with cefotaxime or ceftriaxone.
- Ampicillin is added in infants younger than 3 months.
- Addition of vancomycin to the initial regimen is suggested in areas where penicillin-resistant pneumococcal infections have been documented.
- Immunocompromised children require additional cover for possible Gram-negative bacilli and *Pseudomonas*.
- Children with ventriculoperitoneal shunts or those having undergone neurosurgical procedures are treated with a combination of antistaphylococcal antibiotics with a third-generation cephalosporin (vancomycin plus ceftriaxone).
- Empirical and targeted therapy, duration of therapy and doses used are shown in **Table 13.11**.

Table 13.10 Empiric Antibiotic Therapy in Meningitis

Age	Common bacterial pathogens
<1 months	E. coli, Streptococcus agalactiae, Listeria monocytogenes, Klebsiella sp.
1–23 month	Streptococcus pneumoniae, Neisseria meningitidis, Haemophilus influenzae, S. agalactiae, E. coli
> 2yrs	N. meningitidis, S.pneumoniae
CSF leak	S. pneumoniae, H. influenzae b, hemolytic streptococci.
Penetrating trauma	S. aureus, Coagulase negative staphylococci, Gram-negative bacilli
CSF Shunt	Coagulase negative staphylococci, S. aureus, Gram-negative bacilli, Propionibacterium acnes.

B. Role of Steroids

The pathogenesis and outcome of acute bacterial meningitis is a consequence of both the micro-organism and the host response to the infection. It is expected that anti-inflammatory agents may be effective to reduce the mortality and morbidity. Steroids have been suggested for use as they can; (*i*) decrease meningeal inflammation and brain edema; (*ii*) modulate production of cytokines; and (*iii*) decrease the incidence of hearing loss or other neurological complications. Concerns with use of steroids include the potential to reduce penetrance of antimicrobials into cerebrospinal fluid, masking of antimicrobial failure by preventing secondary fever, and potential adverse effects such as gastrointestinal bleeding.

Dexamethasone has been shown to be of clear benefit in adults but the same cannot be said about its use in children. Significant benefit of adjunctive dexamethasone (0.15 mg/kg/dose every

Table 13.11 Antibiotic Therapy for Meningitis

Microorganism/Susceptibility	First line therapy	Duration
Streptococcus pneumoniae		
Penicillin susceptible	Penicillin G/Ampicillin	
Penicillin resistant	Ceftriaxone/Cefotaxime	10–14 d
Cephalosporin resistant	Ceftriaxone + Vancomycin ± Rifampin	
Neisseria meningitidis	Penicillin G/Ceftriaxone	7 d
Haemophilus influenzae	Ceftriaxone/Cefotaxime	7–10 d
Staphylococcus aureus		
Methicillin susceptible	Cloxacillin	
Methicillin resistant	Vancomycin ± Rifampin	28 d
Staphylococcus epidermidis	Vancomycin ± Rifampin	
E. coli and other Enterobacteriaceae	Ceftriaxone	14–21 d
Pseudomonas	Ceftazidime/Cefepime ± Aminoglycoside	14–21 d
Enterococcus		
Ampicillin susceptible	Ampicillin + Gentamicin	
Ampicillin resistant	Vancomycin + Gentamicin	14–28 d
Vancomycin resistant	Linezolid	

Ampicillin: 200 mg/kg/d, q4h; *Amikacin*: 15 mg/kg/d, q12–24; *Cefotaxime*: 200 mg/kg/d, q6h; *Ceftriaxone*: 100 mg/kg/d, q12h; *Ceftazidime*: 150 mg/kg/d, q8h; *Gentamicin*: 7.5 mg/kg/d, q8h; *Meropenem*: 120 mg/kg/d, q8h; *Cloxacillin*: 100–200 mg/kg/d, q6h; *Penicillin G*: 400,000 U/kg/d, q4h; *Vancomycin*: 60 mg/kg/d, q6h; *Rifampicin*: 10 mg/kg/d.

6 hours for 2 days) particularly in prevention of hearing loss in *H. Influenzae* b meningitis and pneumococcal meningitis has been seen. When used, dexamethasone should be given in dose of 0.15 mg/kg/dose 6 hourly for 2 days, starting with or shortly before the first dose of antimicrobial therapy. There is no role of steroids after the antibiotics have already been initiated. Also, steroids are not indicated in neonatal meningitis.

C. Supportive Measures

Feeding
Initially, the child should not be fed orally, to reduce the chance of vomiting and aspiration. Feeding can be initiated 24–48 hours later once the child is stable and acute problems have resolved.

Fluid management
Hyponatremia can worsen the course and outcome of meningitis. Syndrome of inappropriate antidiuretic hormone secretion (SIADH) is thought to be the underlying cause in most such children. As a consequence fluid restriction (two-thirds of maintenance) was widely advocated and used. However, in India, there is high likelihood of dehydration in children secondary to fever, vomiting, poor oral intake, late presentation, hot environment and other factors. Hence, it would be prudent to restrict fluid only in those patients in whom hyponatremia is clearly due to SIADH or those with increased intracranial pressure. A recent Cochrane review also supports maintaining intravenous fluids rather than restricting them in the first 48 hours, in settings with high mortality rates, and where patients present late.

Isotonic fluids should be used to prevent hyponatremia and cerebral edema. Vasopressors, such as dopamine, dobutamine and adrenaline may be used to support blood pressure and perfusion as per the clinical situation.

Seizures
Seizures should be treated aggressively. Phenytoin is the preferred drug in this setting, because it does not depress the respiratory centers, and it may also benefit the patient by inhibiting the secretion of ADH.

Monitoring
Careful monitoring of heart rate, blood pressure, capillary refill, respiration and temperature should be done. Monitor for signs of raised intracranial pressure. During hospital stay repeated evaluations should be aimed at identification of SIADH, seizure activity, focal deficits, and development of subdural effusions. Body weight, serum electrolytes, urine volume, and specific gravity should be determined at admission and observed closely (12 hourly) for the first 24–36 hours in the hospital and daily till clinical stabilization.

Complications
Acute complications are common with bacterial meningitis. These include raised intracranial pressure, cranial nerve palsies, vasculitis/infarction, subdural empyema, brain abscess, hydrocephalus, shock, disseminated intravascular coagulopathy, seizures, and syndrome of inappropriate ADH secretion (SIADH). Neurological sequelae are common in survivors of meningitis, and include hearing loss, cognitive impairment, epilepsy, and developmental delay.

Prevention
Immunoprophylaxis Haemophilus (Hib) vaccine is effective in reducing the burden of severe hemophilus disease in children <2 years of age. Meningococcal vaccine is given only during epidemics.

Chemoprophylaxis (for household contacts): For *H. influenzae*, rifampicin 20 mg/kg/day (max 600 mg) single dose for 4 days and for meningococcus, rifampicin 20 mg/kg/day (max 600 mg) in 2 divided doses for 2 days or single dose ciprofloxacin 500 mg.

NEONATAL MENINGITIS

Neonatal meningitis is a serious disease with high morbidity and mortality. 30% of early neonatal sepsis and around 80% of late neonatal sepsis are associated with meningitis. Common etiological agents include Gram-negative bacteria like *E. coli*, *Klebsiella*, and *Staphylococcus*. Uncommon agents include *Listeria*, group B streptococcus (developed countries) and other Gram-negative bacteria (*Proteus*, *Pseudomonas*, Enterobacter, etc.)

Treatment should include agents active against all suspected pathogens, in doses sufficient to achieve bactericidal concentrations in the CSF. Empiric therapy generally includes ampicillin in addition with either an aminoglycoside or a third generation cephalosporin. This combination has been shown to be synergistic against several common Gram-positive and Gram-negative organisms. Once a pathogen has been isolated, antibiotic therapy can be tailored to the pathogen.

BRAIN ABSCESS

Brain abscess should be suspected in a child presenting with high grade fever, partial seizures, and focal neurological deficit. Conditions predisposing to brain abscess include otitis media, mastoiditis, sinusitis, congenital cyanotic heart disease, trauma to skull, pulmonary suppuration, and neurosurgical procedures (ventriculoperitoneal shunt).

Etiology

The common microorganisms causing brain abscess include *Staph aureus*, streptococci, anaerobes, and Gram-negative organisms such as *Proteus*, *Pseudomonas*, *Citrobacter*, and *Haemophilus*. Fungal etiology must be considered in immunocompromised children. Tubercular etiology must be considered in an appropriate clinical setting.

Clinical Features

Fever, headache, nausea, vomiting and other features of raised intracranial tension; focal neurological signs, ie, focal seizures, cranial nerve palsies, aphasia, ataxia, visual field defects; irritability, drowsiness, and stupor (40–50%) are the typical presentations of brain abscess.

Investigations

CECT brain or contrast enhanced MRI brain are the most useful investigations (Fig. 13.7). Lumbar puncture is not helpful and should be avoided.

13

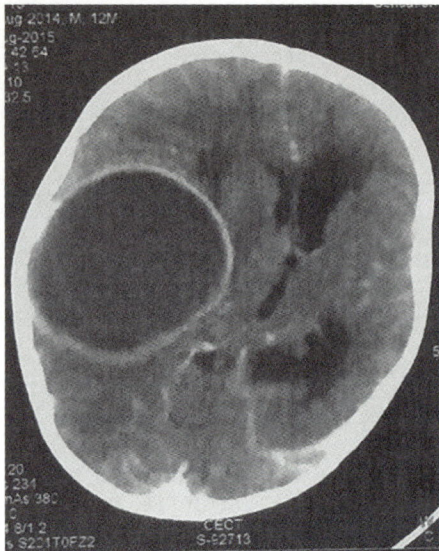

Fig. 13.7 Contrast enhanced CT scan of head showing brain abscess in right frontotemporal region with midline shift in a child with cyanotic heart disease

Treatment	**Brain Abscess**

Medical Therapy

Antibiotics should be selected keeping in mind the polymicrobial etiology and specific organisms suspected in an individual case depending upon the predisposing condition. The recommended regime consists of an intravenous third generation cephalosporin (ceftriaxone) plus metronidazole. Anti-staphylococcal antibiotics may be added if *Staphylococcus* is among the suspected etiological agents. Meropenem monotherapy may also be used. The antibiotic therapy should be given for at least 4–6 weeks duration with radiological monitoring. A follow-up CT scan should be done 1–2 weeks after the initiation of the therapy. The antibiotic duration will be guided by the radiological resolution.

Surgical Management

CT guided aspiration or surgery are indicated in large and easily accessible abscess, impending rupture of the abscess, and impending herniation. Surgery is also indicated in multiloculated abscess, lesions in posterior fossa, abscess size larger than 2.5 cm, fungal abscess, and abscess with gas.

CHRONIC MENINGITIS

Persistence of symptoms and signs of meningitis for more than 4 weeks associated with CSF pleocytosis is referred to as chronic meningitis. Etiology can be bacterial (tubercular, partially treated pyogenic meningitis), fungal (cryptococcal, *Candida*), parasitic (*Acanthamoeba*), or helminthic (cysticercosis). Non-infective causes of chronic meningitis include collagen vascular diseases (SLE, Wegner's granulomatosis, polyarteritis nodosa), and malignancies (leukemia, lymphoma).

Chronic meningitis can have an acute or insidious onset. A case of chronic meningitis with acute onset can be mistaken for partially treated meningitis. Despite the wide range of agents, an overwhelming majority of these cases in developing countries are tuberculous in etiology.

RECURRENT MENINGITIS

This is defined as ≥2 separate episodes of meningitis resulting from a different pathogen than the first episode or from the same organism but occurring more than 3 weeks after completion of therapy for the initial episode.

A child with recurrent meningitis should be investigated for skull fractures; and cranial malformations such as craniospinal dermal sinuses, dermoid cysts, occult intra-nasal encephaloceles, transethmoid meningoceles, and spinal dural defects. Thus, these children should have a CECT (thin sections) of the temporal bones and anterior skull base including the paranasal sinuses; and radionuclide cisternography.

Children with recurrent meningitis should be investigated for immunodeficiency disorders (primary or secondary to HIV infection) if a cranial anomaly is ruled out.

Revision Point

Pyogenic Meningitis

1. *Haemophilus influenzae, Streptococcus pneumoniae,* and *Neisseria meningitidis* are the most common agents causing meningitis in children.
2. Fever, headache, and neck stiffness constitute the classical symptom triad of meningitis.
3. In most children, initial therapy is third generation cephalosporin; vancomycin is added where penicillin-resistant pneumococcal infections have been documented.
4. Duration of treatment varies from 7 to 21 days.

Brouwer MC, McIntyre P, de Gans J, *et al.* Corticosteroids for acute bacterial meningitis. *Cochrane Database Syst Rev.* 2010;8; CD004405.

Dubos F, Martinot A, Gendrel D, *et al.* Clinical decision rules for evaluating meningitis in children. *Curr Opin Neurol.* 2009;22:288–93.

Karageorgopoulos DE, Valkimadi PE, Kapaskelis A, *et al.* Short versus long duration of antibiotic therapy for bacterial meningitis: a meta-analysis of randomised controlled trials in children. *Arch Dis Child.* 2009;94:607–14.

Kim KS. Acute bacterial meningitis in infants and children. *Lancet Infect Dis.* 2010;10:32–42.

Mace SE. Acute bacterial meningitis. *Emerg Med Clin North Am.* 2008;26:281–317.

Scarborough M, Thwaites GE. The diagnosis and management of acute bacterial meningitis in resource-poor settings. *Lancet Neurol.* 2008;7:637–48.

13.7 CNS TUBERCULOSIS

Neurotuberculosis is represented by different and possibly concomitant forms: Tubercular meningitis, miliary tuberculosis with tubercular meningitis, tuberculous encephalopathy, tuberculous vasculopathy, space occupying lesions (tuberculomas, tuberculous abscess), spinal tuberculosis (with or without paraplegia), tuberculous arachnoiditis (myeloradiculopathy), non-osseous spinal tuberculoma, and spinal meningitis. The most frequent manifestations are tuberculous meningitis (TBM) and tuberculoma.

Pathogenesis

Mycobacterium tuberculosis reaches the CNS by the hematogenous route secondary to disease elsewhere in the body.

13

CNS tuberculosis develops in two stages. Initially small tuberculous lesions (called Rich's foci) develop in the CNS, either during the stage of bacteremia of the primary tuberculous infection or shortly afterwards. These initial tuberculous lesions may be in the meninges, the subpial or subependymal surface of the brain or the spinal cord, and may remain dormant for years after initial infection. Later, rupture or growth of one or more of these small tuberculous lesions produces various types of CNS tuberculosis.

Pathology

Tubercular meningitis is characterized by thick, gelatinous exudates around the sylvian fissures, basal cisterns, brainstem, and cerebellum. Hydrocephalus often occurs as consequence of obstruction of the basal cisterns, outflow of the fourth ventricle, or occlusion of the cerebral aqueduct. Hydrocephalus frequently develops in children and is associated with a poor prognosis. The brain tissue immediately underlying the tuberculous exudate shows various degrees of edema, perivascular infiltration, and a microglial reaction, a process known as 'border zone reaction'. Inflammatory changes in the vessel wall may be seen, and the lumen of these vessels may be narrowed or occluded by thrombus formation. The vessels at the base of the brain are most severely affected, including the internal carotid artery, proximal middle cerebral artery, and perforating vessels of the basal ganglion. Cerebral infarctions are most common around the sylvian fissure and in the basal ganglia.

Clinical Features

In most patients with tuberculous meningitis there is a history of vague ill health lasting 2–8 weeks prior to the development of meningeal irritation. These nonspecific symptoms include malaise, anorexia, fatigue, fever, myalgias, and headache. The prodromal symptoms in infants include irritability, drowsiness, poor feeding, and abdominal pain. Eventually, the headache worsens and becomes continuous.

Usually the disease presents with a long duration of fever (>7days), irritability, seizures, altered sensorium, cranial nerve palsies, and motor deficits. Children are usually malnourished and not vaccinated with BCG. Neck stiffness may be present, deep tendon reflexes are brisk, plantars are upgoing, and ankle clonus may be present. There are features of raised intracranial tension.

Cranial nerve palsies occur in 20–30% of patients and may be the presenting manifestation of tuberculous meningitis. The sixth cranial nerve is most commonly affected. Vision loss due to optic nerve involvement may occasionally be a dominant and presenting illness. Ophthalmoscopic examination may reveal papilledema and choroid tubercles. Other features include focal neurological deficits such as hemiplegia, movement disorders (such as chorea and hemiballismus), and seizures (seen in 10–15%).

Staging

Stage 1: Alert and oriented, no focal neurological deficit. Patients have vague symptoms: anorexia, lethargy, headache, listlessness.

Stage 2: Signs of meningeal irritation, seizures, cranial nerve palsies, focal neurological deficits.
Stage 3: Coma, decerebrate posturing.

Differential Diagnosis

The differential diagnosis of tubercular meningitis includes partially treated pyogenic meningitis, viral meningo-encephalitis, brain abscesses, acute disseminated encephalo-myelitis, and other causes of chronic meningitis including primary amebic meningoencephalitis.

Diagnosis

A high index of clinical suspicion is needed to diagnose tubercular meningitis. Usually, a history of contact with an open case of tuberculosis can be obtained in one-fourth to one-fifth of the cases. Physical signs of meningeal irritation and other focal neurological deficits help in localization of the disease. Fundus examination may reveal choroid tubercles. Evidence for tuberculosis occurring elsewhere in the body should be carefully looked for (chest X-ray, abdominal ultrasound, lymph node cytology) and is one important pointer to the diagnosis. Tuberculin test may be positive, but a negative test does not exclude the diagnosis of TBM. Testing for HIV infection should always be considered in any child with CNS tuberculosis.

Lumbar Puncture

The CSF is usually under pressure (30–40 cm H_2O). It may be clear or opalescent and on standing, a pellicle or cobweb coagulum may form in the center of the tube. CSF cell count is increased to 60–400/mm^3 and early in the disease, polymorphonuclear cells predominate. Protein content of the CSF is increased above 40 mg/dL. CSF sugar content may be low or normal. It is usually reduced to about two-third of the blood sugar. However, CSF can be completely normal in 6–16% of cases of TBM with a proved diagnosis on autopsy. In about 10% cases, the CSF could be almost simulating pyogenic meningitis.

Definitive diagnosis of tubercular meningitis depends upon the detection of the tubercle bacilli in the CSF, either by smear examination of the sediment after centrifuging or teasing the cobweb or by bacterial culture, though this is not practically possible in our setting.

Neuroimaging

CT and MRI brain are useful for diagnosis and monitoring management of increased intracranial pressure. They may reveal thickening, intense contrast enhancement of meninges especially in basilar region (Fig. 13.8) and infarcts in thalamus, basal ganglion and internal capsule region. Hydrocephalus is usually of the communicating type due to blockage at the level of cisterns. Associated periventricular ooze suggests high pressure.

Other Diagnostic Tests

The positivity rate of both smears and cultures are low. CB-NAAT for *Mycobacterium tuberculosis* is available, and is the current modality for diagnosis of tubercular meningitis.

Specific antigen and antibody tests in CSF are also available. The LAM antigen and 17 KDa antigen are good candidates. These are more useful if tested early in the disease. The antibody detection tests are unable to differentiate between acute infection and past infection.

13

Serological tests are not recommended for diagnosis of tuberculosis as per the WHO policy statement. The currently available commercial serodiagnostic tests provide inconsistent and imprecise findings, because of high proportions of false-positive and false-negative results.

Treatment	**Tubercular Meningitis**

Early diagnosis and prompt treatment are more important than the drug regimen used. Clinical response to antituberculosis therapy in all forms of neurotuberculosis is excellent if the diagnosis is made early before irreversible neurological deficit is established. Chemotherapy should be started with four bactericidal antituberculosis drugs (**Table 13.12**).

The general principles of treatment are outlined below:

1. *Antitubercular treatment* The recommended regimen is 2 HRZE + 7 HRE (INH, rifampicin, pyrazinamide and ethambutol for 2 months, followed by INH, rifampicin, and ethambutol to complete minimum 9 months of therapy). This can even be extended to 12 months.

2. *Steroids* Either prednisolone (1–2 mg/kg/d) or dexamethasone (0.6 mg/kg/day in 4 divided doses) should be given concomitantly for 6–8 weeks. Steroids lowers CSF protein and globulin, modulate cytokine production and may reduce the incidence of hydrocephalus and infarction.

3. *Anti-epileptic medication* Phenytoin must be given in children with seizures, and those who undergo ventriculo-peritoneal shunt surgery.

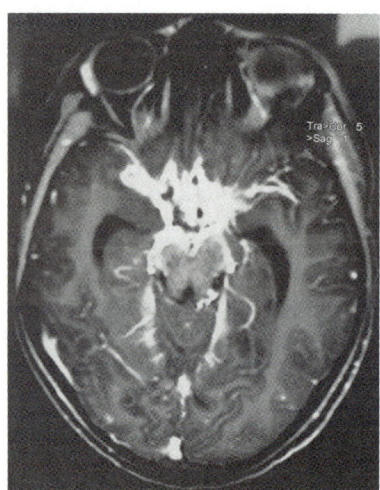

Fig. 13.8 Contrast enhanced T1W axial MRI image showing thick basilar exudates in a case of tubercular meningitis

4. *Raised intracranial pressure* In the acute stage, mannitol is given. In patients with shock, or renal failure, mannitol is contraindicated. In these patients, hypertonic saline (3%) at infusion rate of 0.1–1 mL/kg/hour is given. Later, acetazolamide may be started (30–50 mg/kg/day) in 2–3 divided doses. Acetazolamide, being a carbonic anhydrase inhibitor decreases CSF production. Detailed management of raised ICP is described elsewhere in the chapter.

5. *Surgical management* It is warranted in progressive hydrocephalus and tubercular abscess. Ventriculoperitoneal shunt is indicated in children with obstructive hydrocephalus. In patients with communicating hydrocephalus, trial of medical management is warranted in the early stages. Medical management consists of treatment with acetazolamide and glycerol. If the patient worsens despite medical management, then ventriculoperitoneal shunt must be performed. Endoscopic third ventriculostomy (ETV) is also an alternative option.

Prognosis

Prognosis of TBM depends on the stage at which disease is detected and treated. Stage I has an excellent prognosis and almost all survive without sequel. Stage II is associated with 25% mortality; of the survivors, 50% have neurological sequel. The highest mortality rates are for Stage III. Almost 50% of TBM Stage III children die, and of the rest almost everyone have sequelae. Motor disability and mental retardation are common sequelae. The motor sequel include hemiplegia and quadriplegia. Other sequelae include vision impairment, hearing impairment, epilepsy, cranial nerve palsies, hydrocephalus, hypothalamic disturbances (precocious puberty, obesity), and behavior problems such as hyperactivity and aggressive behavior.

TUBERCULOMA

Tuberculoma consists of conglomerate mass of tissue made up of small tubercles. These are intracranial space occupying lesions. They are frequently infratentorial in children. Symptoms include seizures, focal neurological deficits, ataxia, etc. and depend on site and size of the lesion. Diagnosis is made by neuroimaging. If the lesion is small, there could be a diagnostic confusion with the ring enhancing lesions of neurocysticercosis.

Size of tuberculoma is generally >20 mm in maximum dimension in contrast to cysticercous granulomas which are smaller. Tuberculomas are also more likely to cause midline shift and a thick irregular margin. They are more common in posterior fossa (Fig. 13.9). The various morphological

	IAP 2012	*WHO 2014*
Table 13.12 Regimens and Doses of Antitubercular Drugs		
Isoniazid	10 mg/kg (max = 300mg) for 6 months (8–9)	10 (7–15) mg/kg, Max = 300 mg for 6 months (9–12)
Rifampin	10–12mg/kg (max = 600 mg) for 6 months (8–9)	15 (10–20) mg/kg for 6 months (9–12)
Pyrazinamide	30–35 mg/kg (max = 2000 mg) for 2 months	35 (30–40) mg/kg for 2 months
Ethambutol	20–25 mg/kg (max =1500 mg) for 2 months OR	20 (15–25) mg/kg for 2 months OR
Streptomycin	15–20 mg/kg (max =1000 mg) for 2 months	15 (12–18) mg/kg for 2 months

In TB meningitis, the recommended duration of continuation phase is 7 months, making the total duration of therapy as 9 months (2 IP + 7CP). The duration of continuation therapy may be further extended by 3 more months (making the total duration to be 12 months); as per the discretion of the treating physician or in cases of delayed response

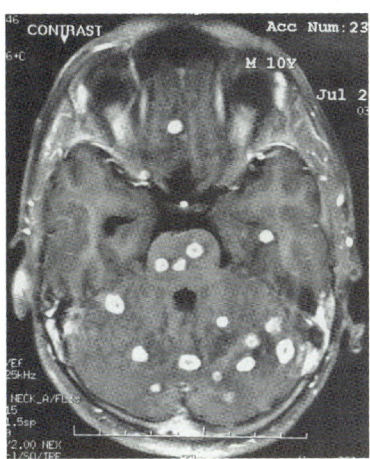

Fig. 13.9 Contrast enhanced MRI image showing multiple irregularly contrast-enhancing lesions. Likely to be tuberculomas

CNS Tuberculosis

1. Mycobacterium tuberculosis reach the CNS by the hematogenous route secondary to disease elsewhere in the body.
2. Usually the disease presents with a long duration of fever (>7 days), irritability, seizures, altered sensorium, cranial nerve palsies, and motor deficits.
3. Investigations include neuroimaging and CSF analysis. Treatment involves antitubercular therapy with steroids.

features described for tuberculoma are the disc or nodule, ring, or enplaque forms. The enplaque lesions appear as focal areas of blush. Calcification may sometimes be observed. MRI has been found to delineate the lesions better than CT scan. Newer MRI techniques like MR spectroscopy,

Case Study | Meningitis

A 6-month-old boy is brought to the casualty with complaints of fever for the last 2 days, and excessive crying and vomiting for the last 12 hours. He also had an episode of stiffening of body.

Enumerate the most likely causes.
CNS infection (meningitis, encephalitis, brain abscess) is the first possibility in view of fever, excessive, crying, vomiting, and probable seizures. Other possibilities at this stage include febrile seizure, dyselectrolytemia, and malaria.

Outline the main points you would like to examine in this child.
First assess the ABC and stabilize the vitals. Assess the sensorium is the child restless and irritable, lethargic, or comatose? Feel for a bulging anterior fontanel. Measure the head size and feel the sutures. See if any rash is present. Look for movements of the limbs are they reduced? Look for neck rigidity and kernig sign. Assess the tone, tendon reflexes, and cranial nerves. Palpate for hepatosplenomegaly.

On examination, the child was restless and irritable. He cried inconsolably. He was febrile, had a pulse rate of 140/min, respiratory rate of 48/min without any chest indrawing. The anterior fontanel was bulging. There was no rash. He had neck rigidity and a positive Kernig sign. The tone was increased in all 4 limbs, with brisk deep tendon reflexes. The chest was clear, and there was no hepatosplenomegaly. During the examination, he had a seizure, with tonic posturing of all 4 limbs, and uprolling of eyeballs lasting 1 minute.

Justify the most likely diagnosis.
The likely diagnosis is pyogenic meningitis. The child has signs of meningeal irritation and increased intracranial pressure, along with a short duration of fever.

Enlist the investigations you will perform.
The most important investigation is the lumbar puncture. This should be performed as soon as the child is stabilized. If the procedure is getting delayed for any reason, or the child is not stable, empirical antibiotics should be started immediately.

The CSF should be assessed for gross appearance, cytology, biochemistry (a simultaneous blood sugar must be assessed to see the CSF/blood sugar ratio), Gram stain, culture, and latex agglutination test.

The following blood investigations must be obtained: Complete blood count, blood culture, blood sugar, blood urea, serum creatinine, and serum electrolytes (sodium, postassium, calcium). A chest X-ray must be performed.

The CSF was grossly turbid. Cytology revealed 8,500 polymorphs/cumm. The protein was elevated (550 mg/dL), and the sugar was reduced (15 mg/dL), against a blood sugar of 87 mg/dL). Gram stain of CSF did not reveal any organism. The latex agglutination was positive for Haemophilus influenzae. The culture was sterile.

Discuss the management of this child.
Pending the CSF results, empirical antibiotic, a 3rd-generation cephalosporin–ceftriaxone or cefotaxime must be started immediately. As the child had a seizure, anti-epileptic–phenytoin must be given. Hypocalcemia, hypoglycemia, or hyponatremia should be treated if present. Mannitol should be given for 24–48 hours as the child had features of raised intracranial pressure. Maintenance IV fluids must be given. Feeds can be started after 1–2 days when the child is stabilized and symptoms of raised intracranial tension (vomiting) have subsided.

Provide a monitoring plan during the hospital stay.
Vitals must be monitored. Seizures must be watched for. The sensorium should be observed and documented on a daily basis. The head circumference must be monitored 24–48 hourly to monitor for subdural effusion/empyema. It is also important to record body weight, urine output, and blood pressure to monitor for SIADH.

Diffusion weighted imaging (DWI), magnetization transfer MR imaging (MTR) and 3D-CISS (constructive interference in steady state) may also help in differentiating between neurocysticercosis and tuberculoma.

Tuberculomas are treated with the same antitubercular regimen as tubercular meningitis. Additionally, anti-epileptics are given for 2 years of seizure free period, if the patient has seizures.

Be NA, Kim KS, Bishai WR, *et al*. Pathogenesis of central nervous system tuberculosis. *Curr Mol Med*. 2009;9:94–9.

Garg RK. Tuberculous meningitis. *Acta Neurol Scand*. 2010;122:75–90.

Rajshekhar V. Management of hydrocephalus in patients with tuberculous meningitis. *Neurol India*. 2009;57:368–74.

Rowe JS, Shah SS, Marais BJ, *et al*. Diagnosis and management of tuberculous meningitis in HIV-infected pediatric patients. *Pediatr Infect Dis J*. 2009;28:147–8.

13.8 ENCEPHALITIS

Encephalitis is an inflammatory process that affects brain tissue. *Encephalopathy* implies cerebral dysfunction due to circulating toxins, poisons, abnormal metabolites or intrinsic biochemical disorders affecting neurons but without inflammatory response.

Encephalitis is almost always accompanied by inflammation of the adjacent meninges, thus the term meningo-encephalitis. Practically, the diagnosis of encephalitis is made based on neurological manifestations, recovery of infectious agent, serologic evidence of infection and relevant epidemiological findings.

Etiology

Acute encephalitis may be (*i*) *primary*: Direct invasion and replication of the microbe leading to tissue necrosis, eg, encephalitis due to herpes simplex, arboviruses and rabies; or (*ii*) *parainfectious*: A post-infectious inflammatory response characterized by immune-mediated central nervous system damage, demyelination with preservation of neurons and their axons. Clinical manifestations in such a type of injury are variable and recovery is likely. Distinction between primary infectious and parainfectious process is however difficult. The common etiologic agents for acute encephalitis and acute meningoencephalitis are listed below:

1. *Viruses* Herpes simplex 1 and 2, varicella zoster virus, mumps virus, measles virus, Japanese B encephalitis virus, rabies virus, Ebstein-Barr virus, influenza virus, enteroviruses, adenovirus, HIV, slow virus infections, prion diseases.
2. *Bacteria* H. influenzae, N. meningitidis, S. pneumoniae, M. tuberculosis, Spirochetes: *Borrelia, Leptospira, Treponema pallidum*
3. *Fungi Cryptococcus neoformans*, coccidioidomycosis, blastomycosis, histoplasmosis, *Aspergillus, Candida*
4. *Protozoal Plasmodium falciparum, Naegleria, Acanthamoeba, Toxoplasma*
5. *Helminths Schistosoma*
6. *Others Chlamydia, Rickettsia, Mycoplasma*.

Clinical Manifestations

Common signs and symptoms include fever, sensorial alterations, ranging from irritability to deep coma, seizures and neurologic deficits. Antecedent history of viral infections, exanthem or vaccination should be enquired. Extrapyramidal symptoms may be present in Japanese encephalitis. Epidemic forms of encephalitis suggest some arboviral diseases. Mumps encephalitis can precede or be associated with parotitis.

Investigations

Children with suspected viral; encephalitis require a prompt neurodiagnostic evaluation that typically includes an electroencephalogram (EEG), a neuroimaging study [computed tomography (CT) or magnetic resonance imaging (MRI)], and a lumbar puncture, in addition to a detailed microbiological evaluation.

Lumbar Puncture

Lumbar puncture reveals mild pleocytosis (initially polymorphonuclear and later lymphocytic), slightly elevated protein, and normal sugar. Red blood cells in a non-traumatic lumbar puncture is characteristic of herpes simplex virus (HSV) encephalitis. Viral cultures, serology and PCR (if available) may be performed on the CSF. Positive identification of viral infection in the CNS helps to curtail investigations, rationalize treatment, and improve the reliability of prognosis.

CSF PCR is now considered as the primary diagnostic test for CNS infections caused by CMV, EBV, VZV, and enteroviruses. The sensitivity and specificity of CSF PCR varies with the virus being tested. CSF HSV PCR has a sensitivity of ~96% and specificity of ~99%. HSV CSF PCR may be negative during the initial illness. In such cases, whenever there is strong suspicion of HSV encephalitis, CSF HSV PCR should be repeated 3–7 days later.

EEG

The EEG typically shows diffuse slow-wave activity in encephalitis indicating diffuse cerebral dysfunction and is not of diagnostic value. Periodic lateralized epileptiform discharges (PLED) is a characteristic EEG finding in HSV and other focal encephalitis.

Neuroimaging

CT and MRI brain can help to differentiate viral encephalitis from metabolic or toxic disorders and acute disseminated encephalomyelitis. MRI appears to be significantly more sensitive. In Japanese encephalitis, CT shows non-enhancing low-density areas in the thalamus, basal ganglia, midbrain, pons and medulla. MRI shows extensive involvement of the thalamus, midbrain, cerebrum and cerebellum. The characteristic CT findings in HSV encephalitis are poorly defined with areas of low density in the anteromedial portion of the temporal lobe with contrast enhancement. MRI shows prolonged T_1 and T_2 relaxation times in the medial temporal lobe, the insular cortex, and the orbital surface of the frontal lobe, particularly the cingulate gyrus.

Treatment	Encephalitis

Specific Therapy

It is important to distinguish HSV from other viruses that cause encephalitis. This is particularly important because intravenous

13

acyclovir is the specific treatment for HSV encephalitis. Acyclovir (15–20 mg/kg/dose IV q 8 hourly) should be given for 21 days. Oral acyclovir is not effective.

Supportive Treatment

Treatment of viral meningoencephalitis caused by other viruses is only supportive. Symptomatic relief with analgesics and antipyretics is very useful. The child should be kept well hydrated with plenty of oral fluids. Intravenous fluids may be occasionally necessary. Airway protection, prevention of aspiration, prompt treatment of seizures, and lowering the raised intracranial pressure are some of the important measures.

Prognosis

10–40% of patients die during the acute stage. Many of the survivors have severe neurological sequel in the form of cognitive impairment, behavioral abnormality, focal weakness, seizures, language impairment and a variety of movement disorders especially following Japanese encephalitis. In 5–30% of children with Herpes encephalitis, the neurological evolution of the disease is characterized by acute clinical relapses in which the resurgence of cerebral viral replication or an immunoinflammatory disorder is implicated.

Prevention

CNS viral infections by measles, mumps, polio and varicella are preventable through appropriate vaccination against these viruses. Post-exposure prophylaxis and vaccination of the high risk individuals is an effective strategy against rabies. There are 3 types of JE vaccines, mouse-brain derived inactivated vaccine, cell-culture (hamster kidney cell derived) derived inactivated vaccine and cell-culture derived live attenuated JE vaccine (SA 14–14-2). Among them live attenuated vaccine is the most efficacious (>95%). Control of insect vectors and adequate personal protection reduce the incidence of arboviral infections.

 Revision Point

Encephalitis

1. Encephalitis is inflammation of the brain parenchyma and is associated with neurologic dysfunction.
2. Common signs and symptoms include fever, sensorial alterations, ranging from irritability to deep coma, seizures and neurologic deficits. Initial investigations include neuroimaging and CSF analysis.
3. Treatment of HSV encephalitis involves acyclovir; treatment of other viral meningoencephalitis is primarily supportive.

Thompson C, Kneen R, Riordan A, *et al*. Encephalitis in children. *Arch Dis Child*. 2012;97:150–61.

Steiner I. Herpes simplex virus encephalitis: new infection or reactivation? *Curr Opin Neurol*. 2011;24:268–74.

Kneen R, Michael BD, Menson E, *et al*. National guideline for the management of suspected viral encephalitis in children. *J Infect*. 2011 Nov 18.

Kumar G, Kalita J, Misra UK. Raised intracranial pressure in acute viral encephalitis. *Clin Neurol Neurosurg*. 2009;111:399–406.

Misra UK, Kalita J. Overview: Japanese encephalitis. *Prog Neurobiol*. 2010;91:108–20.

13.9 NEUROCYSTICERCOSIS

Neurocysticercosis is the most common parasitic infestation of the central nervous system in humans caused by tissue-invading larval forms of the pork tapeworm *Taenia solium* (*Cysticercus cellulosae*). In India, it contributes to 1% of all space occupying lesions and 5% of late onset epilepsies. In normal children over 3 years with unprovoked recent onset seizures, more than one-third are due to inflammatory granulomas.

Epidemiology

Man, the only natural definite host, is the most important multiplier, reservoir and disseminator of the infection to pigs, the intermediate host, which harbors the larva. Humans are unique in that they can harbor both adult and metacestode stages. Pork eating is not the only cause. Infestations of vegetables and water by cysts acquired from human excreta are the most important cause of the infestation.

Pathophysiology

The CNS involvement in cysticercosis is protean and may involve the parenchyma, meninges, subarachnoid space, ventricles and the spinal cord. The live larva presents as cystic lesion in the brain without any perifocal edema and excites very little host reaction. As the larva dies, the lesion changes from the hypodense cyst to a ring with enhancing margins. Later this ring becomes a disc with reduction of perilesional edema. The size gradually dwindles to disappear, persists, or gets calcified. The larval life may vary from few days to several years.

Clinical Features

Cysticercosis may remain symptomatic and be picked up during incidental neuroimaging. When symptomatic, seizures are the commonest symptom (90%). Seizures in NCC may be acute symptomatic or remote symptomatic. Other manifestations include raised intracranial pressure (10–15%), neurological deficits (10%), subcutaneous nodules, and ocular cysts (5–7%).

Investigations

Neuroimaging is currently the method of diagnosis. CT scan suffices in most cases. Non-contrast CT scan identifies active/live cysts as hypodense cystic lesions. Scolex may be visualized in one-third of patients as an intracystic high attenuation lesion. Contrast enhanced CT scan identifies the ring stage better (Fig. 13.10). Calcification, ventricular size, intraventricular cystic lesions, evidence of raised ICP should also be looked for. MRI is superior in identifying active cystic lesions, intraventricular lesions, smaller lesions, and posterior fossa lesions.

It is important to differentiate tuberculoma from NCC, which has already been mentioned. Chronic brain abscesses, tumors, infarcts, vascular malformations and other infestations like toxoplasmosis may produce similar imaging picture.

13

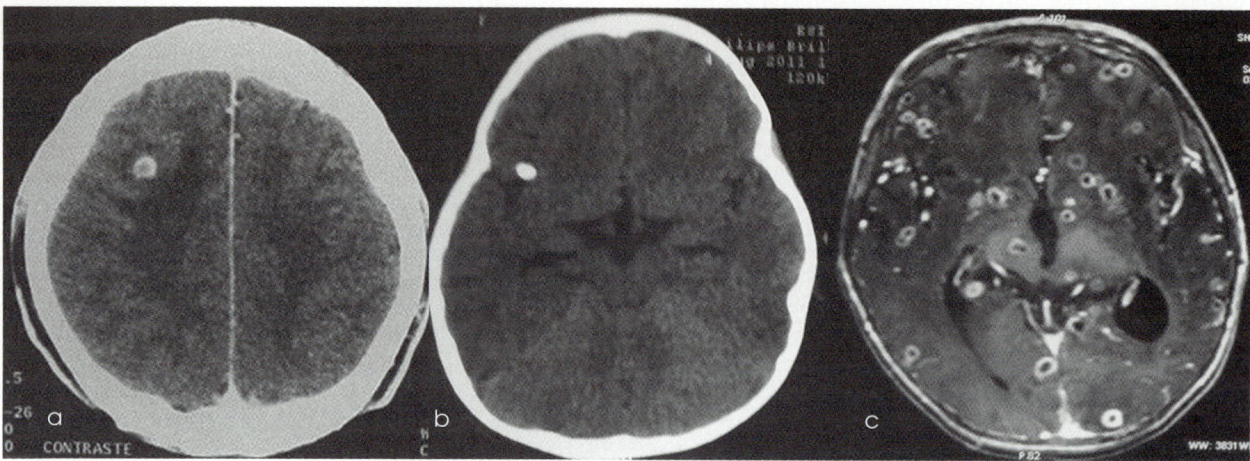

Fig. 13.10 Neurocysticercosis: Contrast enhanced CT head showing (a) ring enhancing lesion in right frontoparietal region and (b) a calcified lesion in right perisylvian region. Contrast enhanced T1W axial MRI image shows multiple ring enhancing lesions (c)

Treatment — Neurocysticercosis

Treatment consists of antiepileptic drugs to control seizures, reduce the raised intracranial pressure, and cysticidal therapy. The indications for cysticidal therapy are not definitive but debatable:

- All live cysts need treatment.
- Single enhancing lesions represent dying larva. Whether therapy promotes quicker resolution as compared to natural remission in these lesions is controversial.
- Cysticidal therapy consists of albendazole (15 mg/kg/day) for 7–28 days. Praziquantel has also been used (50 mg/kg/day) for 15 days or as a single day dose.
- Always check the fundus for intraocular cysts before cysticidal treatment.
- Cysticidal therapy is contraindicated in multicystic disease (>5 cysts), intraventricular cysts, and intraocular (intracranial) cysticercosis.
- Initiation of cysticidal therapy enhances perilesional edema and worsens symptoms. Corticosteroids (oral dexamethasone 0.6 mg/kg/day) must be given from 2 days before to 3 days after starting cysticidal therapy. In case of multiple neurocysticercosis, steroids may have to be given for longer periods.

A scheme management of neurocysticercosis is outlined in **Table 13.13** and Fig. 13.11.

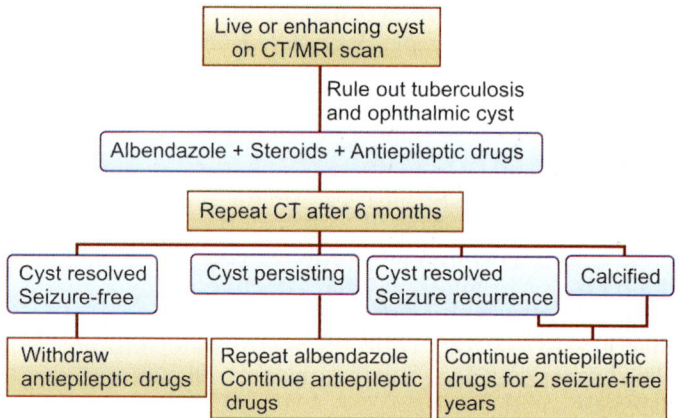

Fig. 13.11 Treatment protocol for neurocysticercosis at AIIMS, New Delhi

Abba K, Ramaratnam S, Ranganathan LN. Anthelmintics for people with neurocysticercosis. *Cochrane Database Syst Rev.* 2010;3:CD000215.

do Amaral LL, Ferreira RM, da Rocha AJ, *et al.* Neurocysticercosis: evaluation with advanced magnetic resonance techniques and atypical forms. *Top Magn Reson Imaging.* 2005;16:127–44.

Singhi P, Singhi S. Neurocysticercosis in children. *Indian J Pediatr.* 2009;76:537–45.

Table 13.13 Management of Neurocysticercosis			
Lesion	*Cysticidal therapy*	*Steroids*	*Others*
Parenchymal live or degenerating cysts			
<5	Yes	Yes	—
>5	No	Yes	—
Parenchymal calcified cyst	No	Occasionally	—
Cysticercotic encephalitis	No	Yes	Close monitoring
Ventricular cyst	No	No	Neuroendoscopic removal
Sub-arachnoid cysts	Yes	Yes	Shunt for hydrocephalus
Spinal cyst	No	No	Surgical
Ophthalmic cyst	No	No	Surgical resection

Neurocysticercosis

1. Cysticercosis is caused by the larval stage (meta-cestode) of the pork tapeworm *Taenia solium.*
2. Parenchymal cysts are associated with seizures and headache, while extraparenchymal cysts are associated with symptoms of elevated intracranial pressure.
3. Neuroimaging is currently the method of diagnosis and CT scan suffices in most cases.
4. Treatment consists of antiepileptic drugs to control seizures, reduce the raised intracranial pressure, and cysticidal therapy.

13.10 ACUTE DISSEMINATED ENCEPHALOMYELITIS (ADEM)

Acute disseminated encephalomyelitis (ADEM) is an acute inflammatory demyelinating disorder of the CNS characterized by new onset focal or multifocal neurological signs and symptoms (including encephalopathy) along with neuroimaging evidence of multifocal demyelinating lesions. ADEM frequently follows a viral illness or antecedent event such as immunization. ADEM typically follows a *monophasic* course although *polyphasic* and *recurrent* forms are also known.

Etiology

Although many viral agents associated with ADEM also cause acute viral encephalitis, ADEM usually occurs much later after the onset of infection and differs clinically by virtue of greater white matter involvement with respective neurologic symptoms. Neuropathologic examination of ADEM consistently discloses widespread perivenular inflammation and myelin disruption.

Clinical Features

Onset is acute; sometimes explosive and subacute.

- *Neurological signs and symptoms* Aphasia, seizures, bilateral optic neuritis, visual field defects, motor and sensory deficits, ataxia, dysmetria and movement disorders occur as isolated features or in various combinations.
- *Systemic symptoms* Fever, malaise, headache occur prior to the onset of neurological problems, beginning 4–42 days following the antecedent event.
- *Behavioral and mental status changes* Irritability, emotional lability, depressed level of consciousness ranging from lethargy to coma is common.
- Meningismus and seizures may also occur.
- The differential diagnosis includes encephalitis, Lyme disease, vasculitis, and neoplasms.

Investigations

CSF findings are variable. CSF may or may not show a mild to moderate lymphocytic pleocytosis, elevation in protein content and detectable levels of myelin basic protein. The presence of oligoclonal bands is variable. CSF studies are most valuable for excluding other illnesses.

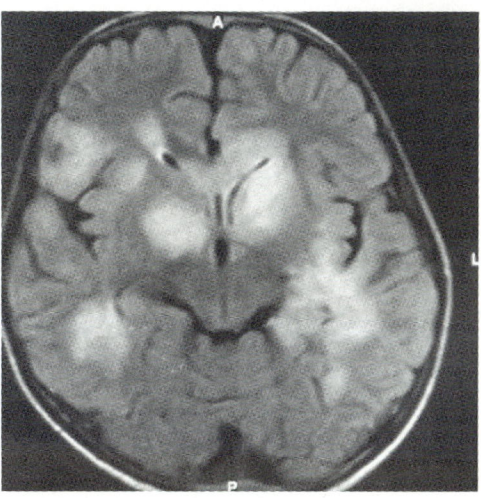

Fig. 13.12 Bilateral multiple patchy white matter and deep gray matter T2W hyperintensities highly suggestive of acute disseminated encephalomyelitis (ADEM)

MRI is the neuroimaging study of choice. Hyperintense lesions seen on T2-weighted images are often diffuse and highly variable in size and number (Fig. 13.12). These include few to multiple predominantly white matter lesions throughout the brain (subcortical white matter, grey-white junction, periventricular regions, corpus callosum, basal ganglia, thalamus, midbrain, brainstem, cerebellar white matter) and spinal cord. Enhancement with gadolinium is variable.

Treatment	Acute Disseminated Encephalomyelitis (ADEM)

Corticosteroids (methylprednisolone and dexamethasone) are the mainstay of treatment, targeted at the immune-mediated processes. The most common treatment regimens include a course of intravenous methylprednisolone (30 mg/kg/day) or dexamethasone (0.5–1 mg/kg/day) for 3–5 days. A slow 2–6 weeks oral prednisolone taper is advised in children with impairment of consciousness, brain stem or spinal cord involvement, and those with MRI findings of large lesions with mass effect. The dose is 1–2 mg/kg/day for 10–14 days followed by 4 weeks taper.

Children who fail to respond to methylprednisolone or who have a fulminant course, intravenous IVIG (400 mg/kg/day for 5 days) may be tried. Plasma exchange may also be beneficial is such patients.

Acute Disseminated Encephalomyelitis (ADEM)

1. ADEM is a demyelinating disease of the central nervous system that typically presents as a monophasic disorder associated with multifocal symptoms and encephalo-pathy.
2. The diagnosis of ADEM is based upon the clinical and radiologic features. The differential diagnosis of ADEM includes other inflammatory demyelinating disorders, such as multiple sclerosis and neuromyelitis optica.
3. Corticosteroids are the mainstay of treatment.

13

Prognosis

Childhood ADEM has a favorable outcome. Survival rate of 100% with complete functional recovery in 57–89% has been noted in studies. Rarely the patients may have relapses with similar symptoms as the first episode (recurrent ADEM) or new symptoms (multiphasic ADEM).

Banwell B, Bar-Or A, Giovannoni G, *et al*. Therapies for multiple sclerosis: considerations in the pediatric patient. *Nat Rev Neurol*. 2011;7:109–22.

Dale RC, Brilot F, Banwell B. Pediatric central nervous system inflammatory demyelination: acute disseminated encephalomyelitis, clinically isolated syndromes, neuromyelitis optica, and multiple sclerosis. *Curr Opin Neurol*. 2009;22:233–40.

Noorbakhsh F, Johnson RT, Emery D, *et al*. Acute disseminated encephalomyelitis: clinical and pathogenesis features. *Neurol Clin*. 2008;26:759–80.

13.11 RAISED INTRACRANIAL PRESSURE

Raised intracranial pressure (ICP) is a common neurological complication in critically ill children. It may occur secondary to (*i*) increase in brain volume, (*ii*) increased cerebral blood flow, or (*iii*) increase in cerebrospinal fluid (CSF) volume. Usual causes include head trauma, CNS infections, and intracranial space occupying lesions.

When to Suspect?

Clinical symptoms and signs depend on the nature of the primary brain insult, the extent of compartmentalization, the presence and location of a mass lesion, and the rate of increase in intracranial pressure. Raised ICP should be suspected based on the features given below:

Features in non-comatose patients	Features in comatose patients
1. Irritability	1. Abnormal posturing
2. Headache/vomiting	2. Abnormal pupillary responses
3. Confusion and decreased alertness	3. Hypertension
4. Neck retraction	4. Bradycardia
5. Tense fontanel	5. Irregular respiration
6. Papilledema	6. Papilledema

Approach to Child with Raised ICP

1. Assess and maintain airway, breathing and circulatory function.

2. Look for potentially life-threatening signs of herniation (asymmetric pupillary dilatation, tonic posturing, irregular respiration). If these signs are present then measures to decrease intracranial pressure should be rapidly instituted.

3. *Cushing's triad* (bradycardia, hypertension and irregular breathing) is a late sign of herniation.

4. After the initial stabilization, a thorough history and clinical examination is performed to determine the possible etiology and further course of management.

5. The imaging study of choice for the patient with raised intracranial pressure presenting to the emergency room is a computed tomography (CT) scan. A contrast study is helpful to identify features of infection (meningeal enhancement, brain abscess, etc.) and tumors.

6. If CT is normal, and the patient has clinical features of raised ICP, then an MRI with MR venogram must be obtained when the patient is stabilized. MRI can pick up early stroke, venous thromboses, posterior fossa tumors and demyelinating lesions which might be missed on CT.

Treatment	**Raised Intracranial Pressure**

- Airway protection and ventilation if required. Hyperventilation in case of impending herniation.
- Maintain mean arterial BP at least above the 50th centile for age to maintain cerebral perfusion pressure.
- Mild head end elevation 15–30°.
- Provide adequate sedation and analgesia. Minimize stimulation of the patient.
- Prophylactic use of IV lignocaine before any painful procedure.
- Aggressive treatment of fever; may give paracetamol 6 hourly.
- Achieve normoglycemia, normocalcemia, normocarbia, and normal hemoglobin.
- *Mannitol* 0.25–1 g/kg, then 0.25–0.5 g/kg, 2–6 hourly, up to 48 hours, intravenously.
- *Hypertonic saline*: Preferable to mannitol in the presence of hypotension, hypovolemia, and renal failure. Dose 0.1–1 mL/kg/hour, target sodium 145–155 mEq/L.
- *Glycerol* is another alternative osmotic agent for treatment of raised ICP. It is used in the oral (0.5–1 mL/kg/day, q 6 hrly) or intravenous forms.
- *Acetazolamide* (20–100 mg/kg/day, q 8 hrly, max 2 g/day) is a carbonic anhydrase inhibitor that reduces the production of CSF. It is particularly useful in children with hydrocephalus, high altitude illness and benign intracranial hypertension.
- *Steroids* Glucocorticoids are very effective in ameliorating the vasogenic edema that accompanies tumors, inflammatory conditions, infections and other disorders associated with increased permeability of blood brain barrier, including surgical manipulation. Dexamethasone is the preferred agent due to its very low mineralocorticoid activity (dose: 0.4–1.5 mg/kg/day, q 6 hrly). Steroids are not routinely indicated in individuals with traumatic brain injury.
- *Treat seizures* as seizures can further increase the ICP.
- *CSF drainage* ventricular tap in patients with hydrocephalus.
- *Surgery* should be undertaken when a lesion amenable to surgical intervention is identified as the primary cause of raised ICP. Common situations where this neurosurgical intervention

Revision Point

Raised Intracranial Pressure (ICP)

1. In children, elevated ICP is most often a complication of traumatic brain injury, tubercular meningitis, hydrocephalus, brain tumors, and intracranial infections.
2. The key clinical findings include early morning headache, projectile vomiting, abnormalities of vertical gaze, vision loss, papilledema, ataxia, altered sensorium, and motor deficits.
3. Hyperosmolar therapy involving mannitol or hypertonic saline is the usual first treatment.

is preferentially employed are acute epidural or subdural hematomas, brain abscess, or brain tumors.

• Invasive intracranial pressure monitoring may also be done, where available.

Sankhyan N, Vykunta Raju KN, Sharma S, *et al.* Management of raised intracranial pressure. *Indian J Pediatr.* 2010;77:1409–16.

Standridge SM. Idiopathic intracranial hypertension in children: a review and algorithm. *Pediatr Neurol.* 2010;43:377–90.

13.12 BRAIN TUMORS

Primary brain tumors constitute the most common solid tumor of childhood. 15–20% of all intracranial tumors occur in children under 15 years of age, with the peak occurrence between 4 and 8 years of age. Only 1–2% of all brain tumors occur in children under 2 years of age.

• *Neonates* Brain tumors are uncommon and represent congenital tumors. They are most common in the supratentorial region. Common primary brain tumors in the neonatal period are teratomas, embryonal tumors, and glioblastoma multiforme.

• *Older children* (2–10 years) Primary brain tumors are generally more benign and around 70% of these are infratentorial in location.

• *Supratentorial tumors* These tumors occur in the sellar or suprasellar region in the cerebrum, or diencephalon. Sellar and suprasellar tumors comprise approximately 20% of childhood brain tumors. Most frequent supratentorial tumors in the cerebral hemispheres are astrocytomas (50%), embryonal tumors (15%), and ependymomas (15%). In the suprasellar region, 75% of tumors are craniopharyngiomas.

• *Infratentorial tumors* include pilocytic astrocytoma, medulloblastoma, ependymoma, and brainstem glioma.

• Dysembryoplastic neuroepithelial tumors and ganglio-gliomas are considered *developmental tumors* and frequently associated with cortical dysplasia.

Clinical Features

Children present in variable manners depending upon the site, type, and rate of growth of the tumor and age of the child. Two distinct type of presentation include: (*i*) Raised intracranial pressure (posterior fossa mass); and (*ii*) Focal neurological signs and seizures (supratentorial tumors).

Supratentorial masses typically cause herniation downward, through the tentorial incisura. Infratentorial masses produce upward herniation. Transtentorial herniation classically produces pressure on the midbrain with secondary effects on eye movements and pupillary constriction (the blown pupils).

A list of common manifestations follows:

1. *General symptomatology* Altered personality—irritable, lethargic, hyperactive and forgetful and decline in academic performance.

2. *Raised intracranial pressure* Headache, vomiting, diplopia, papilledema, bulging fontanel in infants, and increasing head size.

3. *Headache* tends to occur in the morning and is relieved on standing, dull generalized and steady and may be intermittent and worsened by coughing, sneezing or during defecation. Headache is relieved by vomiting.

4. *Seizures* and *diplopia* are common symptoms of posterior fossa tumors.

5. *Nystagmus* Unilateral cerebellar tumor causes horizontal nystagmus that is exaggerated on looking to the side of lesions. Tumors located in the posterior cerebellar vermis or 4th ventricle produce nystagmus in all direction of gaze. Brainstem tumors may results in horizontal, vertical and rotatory nystagmus.

6. *Visual disturbances* Blurring is a serious symptom that indicates marked vasoconstriction and impending cerebellar herniation. Visual loss manifesting as clumsiness or developmental delay associated with roving eye signs is a feature of optic nerve glioma and compressive pituitary lesion.

7. *Abnormal movements* Ataxia associated with posterior fossa lesions; truncal ataxia is typical of tumors of cerebellar vermis. Involvement of anterior cerebellum results in marked gait disturbance that is typically broad based. Tumor of cerebellar hemispheres produces ipsilateral extremity ataxia and dysdiadochokinesis.

8. Coma and altered sensorium.

Treatment	Brain Tumors

CNS tumors in children constitute a diverse group in terms of prognosis. Surgical resection, radiation therapy, and chemotherapy are possible therapeutic options with variable response depending on the type of the tumor. Age-related factors in the vulnerability of the CNS to adjuvant therapy pose many challenging management problems.

Revision Point

Brain Tumors

1. Primary malignant central nervous system (CNS) tumors are the second most common childhood malignancies, after hematologic malignancies; and are the most common pediatric solid organ tumor.

2. Children with brain tumors may present with nonspecific signs and symptoms (eg, headache, vomiting, developmental and behavioral problems, ataxia, cranial nerve palsies, impaired vision, seizures, papilledema, macrocephaly).

3. Surgical resection, radiation therapy, and chemotherapy are possible therapeutic options with variable response depending on the type of the tumor.

Dhall G. Medulloblastoma. *J Child Neurol.* 2009;24:1418–30.

Grondin RT, Scott RM, Smith ER. Pediatric brain tumors. *Adv Pediatr.* 2009;56:249–69.

Paldino MJ, Faerber EN, Poussaint TY. Imaging tumors of the pediatric central nervous system. *Radiol Clin North Am.* 2011;49:589–616.

Sievert AJ, Fisher MJ. Pediatric low-grade gliomas. *J Child Neurol.* 2009;24:1397–408.

13.13 STROKE

Stroke is defined as the sudden occlusion or rupture of cerebral vessels resulting in focal cerebral damage and neurological deficits. Stroke in childhood is relatively rare, resulting in lack of recognition and delay in diagnosis. Stroke occurs because of *ischemia* or *hemorrhage*. Ischemic stroke is further categorized as arterial ischemic stroke (AIS) and sinovenous thrombosis (SVT).

Etiology

Etiology of stroke in children is multifactorial; multiple risk factors coexist unlike unifactorial etiology in adults. Heart disease (congenital or acquired), vascular malformations, metabolic disorders, and hematological abnormalities are the most common causes.

A. Ischemic Stroke

- *Cardiac* Congenital heart disease, endocarditis, arrhythmias, Kawasaki disease, cardiomyopathy, post-cardiac surgery.
- *Hematologic* Iron deficiency anemia, hemoglobinopathies, leukemia, lymphoma, procoagulant states.
- *Inflammatory* CNS infections and vasculitides.
- *Metabolic* Homocysteinemia, Fabry disease, mitochondrial diseases, urea cycle disorders, and lipid abnormalities.
- *Vasculopathies* Moyamoya disease, transient arteriopathy, dissections, and fibromuscular dysplasia.
- *Miscellaneous* Trauma, child abuse.

B. Hemorrhagic Stroke

- *Vascular anomalies* Arteriovenous malformations, venous angioma, cavernous malformation, aneurysm.
- *Vasculopathies* Ehlers-Danlos syndrome, pseudoxanthoma elasticum, moyamoya disease.
- *Intravascular* Hemophilia, ITP, hypertension, vasculitides, and trauma.

Evolution of Stroke

The clinical features at presentation vary with age of the patient, the type of stroke and extent of involvement. The clinical picture is partly dependent upon the primary disease responsible for the hemiparesis. *Embolism* produces a rapidly evolving clinical picture, with maximum involvement within a few minutes. *Thrombosis* is slower in development and may progress either intermittently or progressively during a period of hours or days. There may be a prodromal period of days to weeks, consisting of febrile upper respiratory infections or frontal headache contralateral to the hemiparesis.

A. Arterial Ischemic Stroke (AIS)

It is the most common clinical type of stroke accounting for nearly two-thirds of children with stroke. Anterior circulation is affected in >80% of patients and middle cerebral artery is the most common vessel involved. It typically presents with acute onset neurological deficit such as hemiparesis, with or without seizures. Aphasia is a prominent feature in older children. Infarcts in posterior circulation and large infarcts involving middle cerebral artery may present with alteration of sensorium.

- Seizures indicate *cortical involvement*.
- In patients with lesions at *internal capsule* there is dense hemiplegia (uniform involvement of lower as well as upper limb) with facial nerve palsy of upper motor neuron type on the same side as the hemiplegia.
- In *brainstem stroke*, there are cranial nerve palsies with hemiplegia on the opposite side (crossed hemiplegia).
- Focal signs may be absent in neonates or young infants, in whom lethargy and seizures may be the only manifestation of clinical stroke.

B. Cerebral Sinovenous Thrombosis (CSVT)

CSVT commonly occurs in the setting of acute illnesses, eg, sepsis or dehydration and head and neck infections. It is more common in neonates. Sinovenous thrombosis usually presents with decreased level of consciousness, headache, and focal neurologic signs such as hemiparesis, and cranial nerve palsies. Signs of raised intracranial pressure typically develop gradually over hours and days. *Hemiparesis is not a usual feature of CSVT*. Diffuse neurologic signs and symptoms such as headaches and papilledema are commonly seen. The primary neurologic manifestations of CSVT in the neonates comprise seizures and diffuse neurologic signs. Underlying risk factors, including prothrombotic states, may predispose the patient to thrombosis, while acute illnesses often act as triggering factors. The most frequently involved sites are lateral sinuses and sagittal sinus.

C. Hemorrhagic Stroke

Causes of hemorrhagic stroke include arteriovenous malformations and rarely, aneurysms, and bleeding diathesis. The hemorrhage can be parenchymal or extra-cerebral. Onset is dramatic in hemorrhagic stroke with loss of consciousness and seizures. Signs of raised intracranial pressure and mass effect are usual. Meningismus indicates subarachnoid hemorrhage.

Diagnostic Evaluation

The purpose of diagnostic evaluation includes:
  i. Confirmation of the presence of a cerebrovascular lesion;
 ii. Exclusion of other types of neurological dysfunction; and
iii. Identification of etiology of the stroke.

The presence of multiple risk factors in an individual patient necessitates detailed work up in all children, as follows:
1. *Neuroimaging* Plain CT scan. MRI if CT scan is normal. Specialized techniques include magnetic resonance angiography, diffusion weighted imaging, perfusion imaging, and digital subtraction angiography.
2. *Cardiovascular assessment* Chest X-ray, ECG, carotid Doppler studies, and echocardiography.
3. *Hematological studies* Complete blood count, platelet count, ESR, peripheral smear, tests for sickling, procoagulant work up (protein C, protien S, anti-thrombin III, lupus anti-coagulant, anti-cardiolipin antibodies, anti-β_2 GP1 antibodies, etc.), anti-nuclear antibodies.
4. *Biochemical tests* Serum cholesterol, triglycerides, lipoprotein fractions, lactate, ammonia, uric acid, and blood gas.

Case Study | Sudden Hemiparesis

A 7-year-old boy presented with complaint of sudden onset weakness of the right upper and lower limbs since the last 24 hours.

What more would you like to ask in the history?
Ask questions to (*a*) localize the lesion; and (*b*) look for the etiology.

Questions to localize the lesion:
- Ask whether the patient is left or right handed? This is important to assess the dominance.
- Were there any seizures, altered sensorium, or aphasia (lesion in cortex)?
- Is the weakness of same severity in the upper and lower limbs (lesion likely in internal capsule or below) or of different severity (lesion likely in corona radiata)?
- Are there any cranial nerve deficits—facial deviation, drooping of eyelids, squint, etc. Presence of a cranial nerve lesion contralateral to the side of the hemiplegia (crossed hemiplegia) indicates a brainstem lesion.

Questions for etiology
- Was there weakness following a seizure (post-ictal paralysis—Todd's palsy)?
- Was there any headache or vomiting (suggestive of raised intracranial pressure, or space occupying lesion)?
- Was there any preceding rash, or chickenpox (post varicella vasculopathy?)
- Was there any head/ neck trauma?
- Any recent febrile illness or immunization?
- Did the child have any similar episodes in the past?
- Does the child have any history of heart disease or cardiac surgery?
- Was the child developmentally normal?

On probing, there was no history of seizure, altered sensorium, headache, or vomiting. There was no preceding febrile illness, chickenpox, immunization, or head trauma. The child was developmentally normal and there was no history of prior episodes of similar illness. He is right handed.

On examination, the child is conscious, co-operative and oriented. His speech and memory are normal. He has a right upper motor neuron type facial palsy. The tone is reduced in the right upper and lower limbs. He has hemiplegia (power 2/5) in the right upper and lower limbs. The deep tendon reflexes are brisk on the right side, and normal on the left side. The abdominal and cremasteric reflexes are absent on the right side. The right plantar response is extensor, while the left plantar response is flexor.

Where would you localize the lesion?
The lesion is unlikely to be in the cortex as there are no seizures, altered sensorium or aphasia. As the severity of the hemiplegia is similar in the upper and lower limb (dense hemiplegia), the lesion is unlikely to be in the subcortical white matter/ corona radiata. As there is a supranuclear facial palsy on the same side as the hemiplegia, the lesion is above the brainstem. The lesion is most likely in the left internal capsule.

Apart from the neurological examination, what are the other essential features to be examined?
The following features must be seen during the examination: (*i*) Peripheral pulses, radio-femoral delay (for cardiac cause); (*ii*) blood pressure in 4 all limbs (for coarctation, vasculitis); (*iii*) carotid bruit; (*iv*) neurocutaneous markers; (*v*) dysmorphic facies (eg, Down syndrome); (*vi*) cardiac examination; and (*vii*) hepatosplenomegaly.

How will you investigate the child?
MRI with MR angiography is the investigation of choice. MRI will demonstrate the infarct, rule out other pathologies (eg, ICSOL, ADEM). MR angiography is important to look for vessel narrowing and vasculopathy. If this is not available, or will take time, a CT scan should be performed to exclude a bleed.

   If an infarct is confirmed on MRI/CT, the following investigations must be performed: (*i*) Echocardiogram; (*ii*) complete blood counts with peripheral smear; (*iii*) iron studies; (*iv*) coagulation profile; (*v*) fasting lipid profile; and (*vi*) investigations for pro-coagulant state (protein C, protein S).

   The MRI showed a small infarct in the right internal capsule. No etiology could be found despite the investigations.

How will you treat this child?
The child should be started on aspirin (3–5 mg/kg/day), which is given for a period for 2 years. Rehabilitation (physiotherapy, occupational therapy) must be started early.

Treatment — Stroke

The treatment of stroke in children is primarily directed toward stabilizing systemic factors and management of the underlying causes. Various antithrombotic and non-antithrombotic therapies are available. The use of anti-coagulant therapy appears to be increasing in ischemic stroke. The risk of recurrence or progression of cerebral thromboembolism should be balanced against the risk of treatment, particularly bleeding. If risks of anticoagulation therapy (eg, hemorrhage, hypertension, or an existing bleeding tendency) are present, initial anticoagulation may not be feasible.

1. *Heparin/low molecular weight heparin* Used for anticoagulation after stroke in children with high risk of recurrence or extension of thromboembolic stroke and minimum risk of secondary hemorrhage.
2. *Antiplatelet agents* The traditional role for aspirin in AIS is for prevention of recurrent stroke after TIA or stroke.
3. *Oral anticoagulation* Warfarin is used for the secondary prevention of stroke in congenital or acquired heart disease, severe hypercoagulable states, arterial dissection, and recurrent AIS or TIA while on aspirin.

Anticoagulants are also being used in childhood CSVT patients without significant hemorrhage complications.

Revision Point

Stroke

1. Stroke is defined as the sudden occlusion or rupture of cerebral vessels resulting in focal cerebral damage and neurological deficits.
2. The etiology is usually multifactorial.
3. The mainstay of management is aspirin for arterial ischemic stroke and heparin for venous thrombosis.

Cárdenas JF, Rho JM, Kirton A. Pediatric stroke. *Childs Nerv Syst*. 2011;27:1375–90.

Ibrahimi DM, Tamargo RJ, Ahn ES. Moyamoya disease in children. *Childs Nerv Syst*. 2010;26:1297–308.

Jordan LC, Hillis AE, Medscape. Challenges in the diagnosis and treatment of pediatric stroke. *Nat Rev Neurol*. 2011;7:199–208.

Lo WD. Childhood hemorrhagic stroke: an important but understudied problem. *J Child Neurol*. 2011;26:1174–85.

Lopez-Vicente M, Ortega-Gutierrez S, Amlie-Lefond C, *et al.* Diagnosis and management of pediatric arterial ischemic stroke. *J Stroke Cerebrovasc Dis*. 2010;19:175–83.

13.14 GUILLAIN-BARRÉ SYNDROME

Guillain-Barré syndrome (GBS) includes a spectrum of acquired, immune-mediated disorders causing dysfunction or degeneration in peripheral, spinal sensory and motor nerve roots, and sometimes, cranial nerves. The hallmark clinical picture is that of a previously well individual who develops symmetric ascending flaccid paralysis that evolves acutely or subacutely, and is associated with loss of tendon stretch reflexes.

Epidemiology

GBS is the most common paralytic illness affecting children in countries with established immunization programs. The incidence of GBS has been estimated in population-based studies to be between 0.25 and 1.5 cases per 100,000 children under 16 years of age.

Etiopathogenesis

Guillain-Barre syndrome is presumed to be an immune-mediated disorder. Antecedent events such as infections and recent immunizations have been noted in many patients. Amongst the infections, *Campylobacter jejuni* is the commonest pathogen identified. The pathogenesis is explained by molecular mimicry mechanisms. Gangliosides are important surface molecules of the nervous system. Antibodies formed against the ganglioside-like epitopes in the liposaccharide moiety of *C. jejuni* cross react with peripheral nerves causing damage. Host susceptibility also seems to be important. Cytomegalovirus is another common trigger of GBS, with a prevalence ranging from 10 to 22%. It is especially common in young girls. CMV-related GBS is characterized by a prominent involvement of the cranial and sensory nerves.

Clinical Features

Symptoms are preceded by an antecedent event in about two thirds of patients: Usually a respiratory infection or gastroenteritis.

The commonest manifestation is limb weakness, more proximal than distal. The initial phase is generally relentless and rapid. Between 50 and 75% of patients develop maximal weakness within 2 weeks and 90–98% within 4 weeks of onset. The duration of the plateau phase is usually short, ranging from several days to 4 weeks. Facial palsy is the most common cranial nerve involved (in 53%), followed by bulbar weakness, ophthalmoplegia, and tongue weakness. Respiratory muscle weakness (intercostal and/or diaphragm) may require mechanical ventilation.

Autonomic dysfunction has been reported in 12.5–25% of children with GBS. Manifestations are usually intermittent and include postural hypotension, supraventricular tachycardia, bradycardia, and fluctuating blood pressure. Urinary retention may occur. Pain is a common symptom, occurring in up to 67% of the children.

Natural History

The prognosis for children with Guillain-Barré syndrome is better than that for adults. Generally, by one year, about two-thirds have made a complete recovery. Ventilator support is needed in about 25% of the patients. The death rate varies among different series, ranging up to 13%. About 25% of deaths occur during the first week and about 50% during the first month. Cardiac arrest as a result of autonomic dysfunction is the commonest cause of death and accounts for 20–30% of deaths. Treatment with either plasmapheresis or IVIg significantly improves the outlook for recovery.

Clinical Subtypes

GBS is a clinical syndrome that includes the following pathological and electrophysiological subtypes, with independent immunopathogenesis. These subtypes can be differentiated based on the electrodiagnostic criteria.

A. Acute Inflammatory Demyelinating Polyneuropathy (AIDP)

AIDP is the most common form of GBS in Western countries and accounts for 85–90% of the patients with GBS. Electrodiagnostic and pathological studies show typical demyelination suggesting that the immune target is within the Schwann cell surface membrane or the myelin. Global areflexia or simultaneous onset of weakness in upper and lower limbs may point towards demyelinating subtype (vs axonal subtype). Nerve conduction velocity is slowed in 2 or more motor nerves, suggestive of demyelination.

B. Acute Motor Axonal Neuropathy (AMAN)

In China and Japan, a considerable number of patients develop pure motor axonal degeneration. This is often triggered by enteric infection by *Campylobacter jejuni* and is frequently associated with antiganglioside antibodies (GM1, GM1b, GD1a, or GalNAc-GD1a). Electrophysiological studies demonstrate reduction of compound muscle action potential without significant conduction slowing.

C. Acute Motor and Sensory Axonal Neuropathy (AMSAN)

The neurophysiological and pathological findings indicate axonal degeneration of both motor and sensory nerves. The disease course is typically fulminant, generally with slow and incomplete recovery. This group probably has the most severe form of immune mediated axonal damage in GBS.

D. Miller Fisher Syndrome

Miller Fisher syndrome is characterized by a unique clinical triad of ataxia, ophthalmoplegia, and areflexia. This disorder is closely associated with antibodies against the ganglioside GQ1b. The antibody recognizes epitopes expressed in the nodal regions of the ocular motor nerves.

Investigations

Cerebrospinal Fluid

A characteristic laboratory finding supporting the diagnosis of GBS is albuminocytological dissociation or a disproportionate elevation of CSF protein in the absence of significant evidence of inflammation (ie, >10 mononuclear cells/mm^3 of CSF) after the first week of symptoms of the disease. This feature is due to breakdown of the blood nerve barrier within the subarachnoid space surrounding the spinal nerve roots.

Electrophysiological Studies

Features differ according to the clinicopathological type **(Table 13.14)**.

Neuroimaging

Magnetic resonance imaging can be useful in diagnosis, especially when the electrophysiological findings are equivocal. It is a sensitive but non-specific test. Spinal nerve root enhancement with gadolinium on MRI is a non-specific feature seen in inflammatory conditions and caused by disruption of the blood-nerve barrier. Selective anterior root enhancement appears to be strongly suggestive of GBS. Moreover, MRI spine may be used to rule out myelopathy which closely mimics GBS clinically.

Table 13.14 Electrophysiological Features in Guillain-Barré Syndrome Subtypes

1. *Acute inflammatory demyelinating polyneuropathy*
   - Reduced conduction velocity
   - Conduction block or abnormal temporal dispersion
   - Prolonged distal latency
   - Absent F wave or prolonged F wave latency
2. *Acute motor axonal neuropathy*
   - Absent or reduced compound muscle action potential (CMAP) amplitude.
   - Normal motor distal latency and conduction velocity
   - Normal sensory nerve action potential (SNAP)
3. *Acute motor sensory axonal neuropathy*
   - Absent or reduced SNAP
   - Absent or reduced CMAP amplitude
   - Normal motor distal latency and conduction velocity

Differential Diagnosis

The differential diagnosis of GBS includes transverse myelitis, poliomyelitis, traumatic neuritis, viral myositis, and periodic paralysis. Transverse myelitis is characterized by the presence of early bladder and bowel involvement, sensory loss, and a sensory level. Poliomyelitis is characterized by the presence of fever, and asymmetric weakness. Traumatic neuritis is characterized by the history of intramuscular injection in the gluteal region preceding the weakness in the limb. In viral myositis, there will be pain and tenderness, but no areflexia or hypotonia. In periodic paralysis, there will be history of recurrent episodes of paralysis with recovery in between. The salient differentiating features between the major differential diagnoses are described in the following section.

Treatment Guillain-Barré Syndrome

Optimal management and treatment of GBS is critically important. Although many patients with the condition are desperately ill and paralyzed, their chances of leading a full and productive life for many years thereafter are high if they can make it through the acute stages. Treatment of GBS is subdivided into techniques for managing severely paralyzed patients requiring intensive care and ventilator support, and specific therapy to lessen the nerve damage.

Immunotherapy

Immunotherapy is the mainstay of treatment. Intravenous immunoglobulin (IVIg) 2 g/kg over 2–5 days or plasmapheresis done within 2–4 weeks of symptom onset are recommended. Plasma exchange possibly reduces the levels of circulating proinflammatory cytokines and cell adhesion molecules. IVIg acts by binding anti-idiotypic antibodies, downregulation of B-cell mediated antibody production, or complement binding. The treatment is warranted in non-ambulatory patients but their role in mildly affected GBS patients who are mobile is uncertain. Patients who have not responded to initial IVIg treatment may benefit from a second course of IVIg.

Supportive treatment
- *Watch for respiratory involvement* In the early stages, patients must be observed frequently for the possibility of incipient respiratory failure. Vital capacity must be monitored on a

13

frequent basis, often every 2 hours, and assisted respiration must be undertaken if the vital capacity falls to 15 mL/kg body weight, and before the patient becomes exhausted or hypoxic. Tracheal intubation is the preferred initial measure, but if mechanical ventilator assistance is required for more than a few days, a tracheostomy is preferable. Intubation and mechanical ventilation are required for 25–33% of these patients, and therefore respiratory support is the most important form of supportive treatment.

- *Provide hemodynamic support* Continuous monitoring of blood pressure and heart rate is important to prevent death from arrhythmia and hemodynamic instability resulting from autonomic involvement. Hypotension secondary to dysautonomia, which occurs in approximately 10% of severely affected patients, is treated by intravenous volume infusion and the use of vasopressor agents.

- *Nutritional issues* must be considered early. Repletion of nutrients should be undertaken, either through feeding tube, gastrostomy, or parentally, within 5 days for patients who cannot swallow.

- *Nursing care* Patients need to be turned at least every 2 hours. Frequent turning is necessary to avoid skin breakdown and pressure ulcers. Regular chest physiotherapy and close attention to pulmonary hygiene is essential as broncho-pneumonia is a common complication of GBS.

- *Complications* Deep vein thrombosis and pulmonary embolism are 2 further complications of GBS. Prophylactic subcutaneous heparin along with intermittent positive pressure leg boots are recommended.

- *Physical therapy* should be initiated within 1 or two hours of admission. Pain must be properly controlled with analgesics, and ameliorated by early initiation of rehabilitation techniques such as frequent passive limb movement. Passive movement is also useful to prevent contractures.

Outcome and Prognosis

Most series indicate that the prognosis for children who develop GBS is better than that for older age groups. Generally, by one year, about two-thirds have made a complete recovery. Ventilator support is needed in about a quarter of the patients. The death rate varies among different series, ranging up to 13%. About 25% of deaths occur during the first week and about 50% during the first month. Cardiac arrest as a result of autonomic dysfunction is the commonest cause of death and accounts for 20–30% of deaths.

Guillain-Barré Syndrome (GBS)

1. GBS is often triggered by an antecedent infection that evokes an immune response, which in turn results is an acute polyneuropathy.
2. Typical clinical features of GBS are ascending, progressive, symmetric muscle weakness and absent deep tendon reflexes.
3. Immunotherapy involving IVIG is the mainstay of treatment.

Hughes RA, Swan AV, van Doorn PA. Intravenous immuno-globulin for Guillain-Barré syndrome. *Cochrane Database Syst Rev.* 2010; 6:CD002063.

Hughes RA, Wijdicks EF, Benson E, Stevens JC; Multidisciplinary Consensus Group. Supportive care for patients with Guillain-Barré syndrome. *Arch Neurol.* 2005;62:1194–8.

van Doorn PA, Ruts L, Jacobs BC. Clinical features, pathogenesis, and treatment of Guillain-Barré syndrome. *Lancet Neurol.* 2008;7:939–950.

van Doorn PA. What's new in Guillain-Barré syndrome in 2007-2008? *J Peripher Nerv Syst.* 2009;14:72–4.

Winer JB. Guillain-Barré syndrome: clinical variants and their pathogenesis. *J Neuroimmunol.* 2011;231:70–2.

13.15 ACUTE FLACCID PARALYSIS

Acute flaccid paralysis (AFP) is defined as sudden onset of weakness and floppiness in any part of the body in a child <15 years of age or paralysis in a person of any age in whom polio is suspected.

Etiology

Common causes of AFP in India include poliomyelitis, Guillain-Barré syndrome (GBS), transverse myelitis, and traumatic neuritis. Their differentiating features are detailed in **Table 13.15**.

Epidemiology

In 2011, only one confirmed case of wild poliovirus (P1 type) was reported from West Bengal as compared to 741 cases in 2009 and 42 cases in 2010. No case of poliomyelitis has occurred in India after January 2011.

Experience in other parts of the world indicates that at least 1 case of non-polio AFP occurs for every 1,00,000 population children aged <15 years per year. This is referred to as the *background rate* of AFP among children. The other non-polio causes of AFP, such as Guillain-Barré syndrome (GBS), transverse myelitis, traumatic neuritis, account for this background rate, regardless of whether acute poliomyelitis exists in the community.

Surveillance for Acute Flaccid Paralysis

Surveillance is carried out for all cases of acute flaccid paralysis and not just for poliomyelitis. Therefore, all AFP cases should be reported, regardless of the final diagnosis. Because paralytic poliomyelitis is one cause of AFP, maintaining a high sensitivity of AFP reporting will ensure that all cases of paralytic poliomyelitis are detected, reported, and investigated, resulting in preventive control measures to interrupt transmission of disease. The aim of AFP surveillance is to detect poliovirus transmission and the earlier stool is collected the greater the chance that poliovirus may be detected. Additional conditions that need notification as AFP are listed in **Table 13.16**.

Collection of Stool Sample

Special effort should be made to obtain 2 stool specimens from AFP cases within 14 days of onset of paralysis. Outbreak response efforts should be started promptly without waiting for the laboratory results, which might take up to 8 weeks. All cases that are classified as "discarded," not polio, require thorough justification and should be reported with the final diagnosis. When a case of AFP is seen late in the field, stool specimens may be collected up to 60 days after onset of

Table 13.15 Differential Diagnosis of Acute Flaccid Paralysis

Feature	Poliomyelitis	Guillain-Barré syndrome	Transverse myelitis	Traumatic neuritis
Fever	Present; biphasic course ±	Prodromal illness may be present	Prodromal illness may be present	Absent
Symmetry	Asymmetric onset	Usually symmetrical	Usually symmetrical	Asymmetric
Sensations	Intact; diffuse myalgias ±	Variable	Impaired below the level of the lesion	May be impaired in the distribution of the affected nerve
Respiratory insufficiency	±	±	±	Absent
Cranial nerves	Affected in bulbar and bulbo-spinal variants	Usually affected	Absent	Absent
Radicular signs	May be present (aseptic meningitis ±)	Present	Absent	Absent
Bladder-bowel complaints	Absent	Transient due to auto-nomic dysfunction	Present	Absent
Nerve conduction studies	Motor studies may be abnormal	Abnormal	Normal	Abnormal
CSF studies	Lymphocytic Pleocytosis; normal/increased protein	Albuminocytologic dissociation	Variable	Normal
MRI spine	Usually normal	Usually normal	Classical findings	Normal

Table 13.16 Additional Inclusions in Acute Flaccid Paralysis

1. Isolated facial palsy
2. Isolated bulbar palsy
3. Unproved hypokalemia
4. Neck flop
5. Floppy baby
6. Flaccid hemiplegia
7. Post-ictal weakness (Todds paralysis)
8. Post-diphtheritic polyneuritis

paralysis. The chances of finding poliovirus in the stool after that length of time are extremely remote.

Adequate specimen can be defined as 2 specimens, at least 24 hours apart, collected within 14 days of paralysis onset; each of adequate volume (8–10 g) and arriving at a WHO accredited laboratory in good condition. Good condition means no desiccation, no leakage, adequate documentation and evidence that the reverse cold chain was maintained. Surveillance is carried out for all cases of AFP, not just for poliomyelitis.

Diagnosis of Poliomyelitis

A case is classified as polio if wild poliovirus is isolated from the stool specimen. Cases with inadequate stool specimens and having residual weakness, who have died or are lost to follow-up undergo additional investigation and are presented for review by the National Expert Review Committee (ERC). The ERC classifies the case as "compatible with polio" or "discarded as non-polio AFP."

Acute Flaccid Paralysis (AFP)

1. Common causes of AFP in India include poliomyelitis, Guillain-Barré syndrome (GBS), transverse myelitis, and traumatic neuritis.
2. For AFP surveillance, special effort should be made to obtain 2 stool specimens from AFP cases within 14 days of onset of paralysis
3. A case is classified as polio if wild poliovirus is isolated from the stool specimen.

Field Guide— Surveillance of acute flaccid paralysis. 3rd Edition. New Delhi: Ministry of Health and Family Welfare, *Government of India*. 2005.

Francis PT. Surveillance of acute flaccid paralysis in India. *The Lancet*. 2007;369:1322–3.

13.16 MOVEMENT DISORDERS

Movement disorders are neurologic disorders caused by abnormalities in the basal ganglia and characterized by the presence of abnormal involuntary movements. Movement disorders are broadly categorized as *hyperkinetic* and *hypokinetic*.

Hyperkinetic movement disorders are abnormal, repetitive, involuntary movements and include tics, stereotypies, chorea, dystonia, myoclonus, and tremor.

Hypokinetic movement disorder, are also referred to as akinetic/rigid disorders. The primary movement disorder in this category is parkinsonism, manifesting primarily in adults. Hypokinetic disorders are relatively uncommon in children.

13

Types of Movement Disorders

- *Chorea* It refers to an involuntary, quasipurposive, irregular hyperkinetic disorder in which movements or movement fragments with variable rate and direction occur unpredictably and randomly. The movements are more proximal and are jerky.
- *Athetosis* is defined as slow, writhing, continuous, involuntary movements, usually occurring distally.
- *Dystonia* is characterized by sustained muscle contractions, frequently causing twisting and repetitive movements, or abnormal postures.
- *Myoclonus* refers to quick, shock-like movements of one or more muscles. It may be epileptic or non-epileptic.
- *Parkinsonism* is a neurologic syndrome characterized by presence of two or more of the cardinal features of Parkinson's disease, including tremor at rest, bradykinesia, rigidity, and postural instability.
- *Stereotypies* are defined as involuntary, patterned, coordinated, repetitive, nonreflexive movements that occur in the same fashion with each repetition.
- *Tics* are involuntary, sudden, rapid, abrupt, repetitive, nonrhythmic, simple or complex movements or vocalizations. Tics are usually preceded by an uncomfortable feeling or urge that is relieved by carrying out the movement.
- *Tremor* refers to oscillating, rhythmic movements about a fixed point, axis, or plane that occur when antagonist muscles contract alternately. Usually this involves oscillation around a joint and produces a visible movement.

Common Causes

1. Cerebral palsy—especially the dyskinetic type
2. Post-encephalitic sequel—especially after TBM, Japanese B encephalitis
3. Autism and mental retardation—commonly associated with stereotypies
4. Wilson disease
5. Organic acidemias, Leigh syndrome—commonly associated with dystonias and choreoathetoid movements.
6. Tourette syndrome: Tics
7. Sydenham chorea

Revision Point

Movement Disorders

1. Movement disorders should be categorized into hyper- and hypo-kinetic disorders.
2. Acute ataxia is disturbance in the coordination of movement. In children, it is most commonly manifested as an unsteady gait.
3. Although many causes of acute ataxia are benign, patients with life-threatening processes must be quickly identified by history, examination, imaging, and laboratory investigations.

---

13 ### 13.17 CEREBELLAR ATAXIA

The cerebellum and its major connections are subject to a number of diseases. One of the most relevant consequences of cerebellar dysfunction is ataxia, a neurological dysfunction of motor coordination, which may affect fundamental activities such as gaze, speech, gait and balance. Ataxia can also be caused by injuries to the spinal cord (spinocerebellar tracts and posterior columns) and peripheral sensory nervous system (*sensory ataxia*).

Etiology

The etiology of cerebellar ataxias is complex and includes toxic, metabolic, immune, and genetic causes. Ataxias can be categorized by its onset and course: Most frequent presentation consists of a chronic progressive disease starting in infancy or adolescence.

Acute Ataxia

A few forms of ataxias present as acute diseases, such as drug intoxication like phenytoin, acute post-infectious cerebellitis, brain tumors with bleed, brainstem encephalitis, and neuroblastoma.

Paroxysmal Ataxia

Some forms present as acute recurrent diseases like basilar migraine, benign paroxysmal vertigo, dominant recurrent ataxia, episodic ataxia, intermittent variant of maple syrup urine disease, etc.

Chronic or Progressive Ataxia

Common causes include ataxia-telangiectasia, Friedreich ataxia, brain tumors (cerebellar astrocytoma, cerebellar hemangioblastoma, ependymoma, medulloblastoma) or congenital malformations (Chiari and Dandy-Walker malformations).

Hereditary forms represent an important subgroup of the chronic ataxic disorders and include metabolic ataxia (urea cycle disorders, pyruvate dehydrogenase deficiency, leukodystrophies and Refsum disease), autosomal recessive degenerative ataxia, progressive autosomal dominant spinocerebellar ataxias and mitochondrial disorders (myoclonic epilepsy with ragged red fibers, neuropathy ataxia and retinitis pigmentosa (NARP), and Kearns-Sayre syndrome).

Approach to Ataxia

An approach to childhood ataxias is provided in Fig. 13.13. Important work-up of a child with ataxia include following investigations:

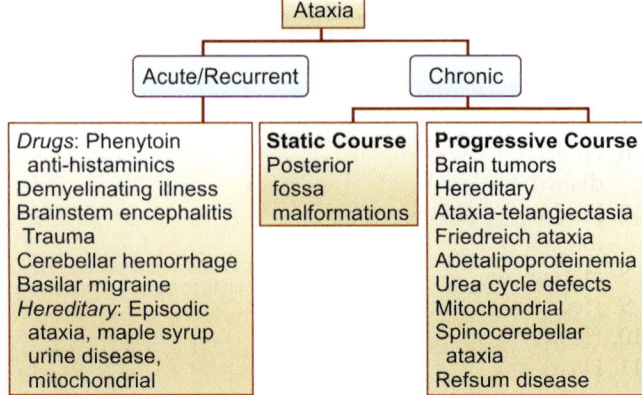

Fig. 13.13 Approach to a child with ataxia

1. MRI brain
2. Hemogram, RBC indices, peripheral smear for acanthocytes
3. Lipid profile
4. ABG, serum ammonia, lactate, sugar
5. Urinary ketones
6. TMS/GCMS
7. CSF studies
8. Serum AFP levels
9. Immunoglobulin profile
10. Vitamin E and B_{12} levels
11. Electrophysiological studies
12. Muscle/nerve biopsy
13. Enzyme/genetic studies.

Ala A, Walker AP, Ashkan K, *et al*. Wilson's disease. *Lancet*. 2007;369:397–408.

Brancati F, Dallapiccola B, Valente EM. Joubert Syndrome and related disorders. *Orphanet J Rare Dis*. 2010;8:5:20.

Delgado MR, Albright AL. Movement disorders in children: definitions, classifications, and grading systems. *J Child Neurol*. 2003;18 Suppl 1:S1–8.

Finsterer J. Ataxias with autosomal, X-chromosomal or maternal inheritance. *Can J Neurol Sci*. 2009;36:409–28.

Gilbert DL. Acute and chronic chorea in childhood. *Semin Pediatr Neurol*. 2009;16:71–6.

Müller U. The monogenic primary dystonias. *Brain*. 2009;132:2005–25.

Pandolfo M. Friedreich ataxia. *Semin Pediatr Neurol*. 2003;10:163–72.

13.18 HEADACHE

Headaches are very common during childhood and become increasingly frequent during adolescents. Headaches may be classified as primary or secondary:

a. *Primary headache* Headache itself is the illness and is not attributable to any other disorder.

b. *Secondary headache* Headache is the symptom of identifiable structural, metabolic or other abnormality. Symptoms that may suggest secondary headache include "worst ever" headache in the life, recent headache onset, increasing severity or frequency, occipital location, awakening from sleep because of headache, morning headaches with vomiting, and headache associated with straining.

International Classification of Headache Disorders (2005)

1. Migraine
2. Tension type headache
3. Cluster headache
4. Other primary headaches
5. Headache attributed to head/neck trauma
6. Headache attributed to cranial/cervical vascular disorder
7. Headache attributed to non-vascular intracranial disorder
8. Headache attributed to a substance or its withdrawal
9. Headache attributed to infection
10. Headache attributed to disorder of homeostasis
11. Headache attributed to disorder of cranium/neck/eyes/ears/nose/sinuses/teeth/mouth/other facial or cranial structures
12. Headache attributed to psychiatric disorder
13. Cranial neuralgias and central causes of facial pain
14. Others

Chronic Daily Headache

A primary headache syndrome that occurs >15 days a month and lasts for >4 hours a day. This entity includes chronic migraine, chronic tension type headache, and new daily persistent headache.

MIGRAINE

Migraine is a common, chronic, incapacitating neurovascular disorder, characterized by attacks of severe headache, autonomic nervous system dysfunction, and in some children, an aura involving neurological symptoms. It is a disorder in which neural events result in the dilation of blood vessels, which, in turn, results in pain and further nerve activation. Messenger molecules like nitric oxide and calcitonin-gene-related-peptide may be involved. The mechanism of cortical spreading depression may be involved in migraine with aura.

Clinical Features

It is the second most common cause of chronic recurrent headache in schoolchildren. Many of the children with migraine have positive family history. The migraine spectrum includes the following:

- *Common types* Migraine without aura; migraine with aura; migraine aura without headache.
- *Uncommon types* Basilar migraine; familial hemiplegic migraine; migranous infarction; migraine with prolonged aura.
- *Migraine equivalents* Cyclical vomiting, abdominal migraine, and benign paroxysmal vertigo.

Criteria for Pediatric Migraine (2013 International Classification of Headache Disorders)

1. ≥5 attacks fulfilling features 2–5 listed below
2. Headache attack lasting 1 to 72 hours.
3. Headache has at least 2 of the following four features:
   a. Unilateral location;
   b. Pulsating quality;
   c. Moderate to severe intensity; or
   d. Aggravated by or causing avoiding of routine physical activities.
4. At least 1 of the following accompanies headache:
   a. Nausea and/or vomiting; or
   b. Photophobia and phonophobia (may be inferred from their behavior).
5. Not attributed to another disorder.

Treatment	Migraine

Recommendations for the acute treatment of migraine in children and adolescents

Ibuprofen is effective; sumatriptan nasal spray is effective; acetaminophen is probably effective. There is lack of data to support or refute use of oral triptan preparations and subcutaneous sumatriptan.

13

Recommendations for preventive therapy of migraine in children and adolescents

Flunarizine is probably effective for preventive therapy; Pizotifen, nimodipine and clonidine not recommended. There is insufficient evidence regarding use of cyproheptadine, amitriptyline, divalproex sodium, topiramate, levetiracetam; and conflicting evidence for propranolol or trazodone.

Revision Point

Headache

1. Headache in children and adolescents may be due to a primary headache disorder or secondary to an underlying medical condition.
2. The evaluation of headache in children includes a thorough neurological examination, with particular emphasis on clinical features suggestive of intracranial pathology
3. Headache of migraine tends to have a throbbing or pulsatile quality, with or without aura.

Dodick DW. Pearls: headache. *Semin Neurol.* 2010;30:74–81.

Hershey AD. Current approaches to the diagnosis and management of paediatric migraine. *Lancet Neurol.* 2010;9:190–204.

Ozge A, Termine C, Antonaci F, *et al.* Overview of diagnosis and management of paediatric headache. Part I: diagnosis. *J Headache Pain.* 2011;12:13–23.

Termine C, Ozge A, Antonaci F, *et al.* Overview of diagnosis and management of paediatric headache. Part II: therapeutic management. *J Headache Pain.* 2011;12:25–34.

13.19 CEREBRAL PALSY

Cerebral palsy is a symptom complex encompassing a group of *non-progressive motor impairment syndromes* characterized by abnormalities of movement, posture, and tone, with varying accompaniments.

It usually results from an early insult of limited nature or anomalies in the early stages of brain development. Cerebral palsy is also considered as a static encephalopathy. Early identification has significant implications for the family and necessitates early intervention to achieve the maximum holistic potential of the child.

Characteristic Features

The hallmark of the condition is motor dysfunction, comprising of abnormal muscle tone (hypertonia more often than hypotonia), abnormal posture (decerebrate, decorticate, or flaccid), and disorder of movement. Deep tendon reflexes are usually brisk and plantars are upgoing.

As the child grows, the movement disorder can appear worse because every effort to move is confronted by the force of gravity. The clinical expression of the case depends on the extent and area of brain damage, growth of the child, and co-existing developmental problems. Associated problems in a child with cerebral palsy include intellectual disability (50–75%); seizures (25–35%); behavioral problems (30–50%); speech, hearing and language disorders (15–20%); ocular problems: Strabismus, refractory errors, field defects (50–70%); extrapyramidal abnormalities (10%); feeding difficulties; and malnutrition.

Etiology

1. *Prenatal* Nutritional deficiency of iodine, iron, and calories; intrauterine infections; chorioamnionitis; hypertension, diabetes; teratogens: Drugs, smoking, alcohol; cerebral malformations; and poor antenatal care.
2. *Perinatal* Prematurity/IUGR; birth asphyxia; hyperbilirubinemia; infections/meningitis; and seizures.
3. *Postnatal* CNS infections, trauma, hemorrhage, and hypoxia.

The extent to which asphyxia is responsible for cerebral palsy is debated but certainly it is not as important a cause as thought previously. Mild asphyxia is definitely not a cause of cerebral palsy. Asphyxia occurs because of a developmental malformation in the brain and may be a result and not cause of the problem. Current estimates of asphyxia as a contributor to cerebral palsy figure ≤10% in developed countries.

Classification

Spastic Cerebral Palsy

It is the most common type. There is increased muscle tone, tendency to develop deformities and contractures and poor development of postural mechanisms. Seizures often develop, as the child grows older. It can be either of hemiplegic, diplegic or quadriplegic type.

- *Quadriplegia* All limbs are affected; arms more than the legs. Only 10% learn to walk. Bowel and bladder control is absent.
- *Hemiplegia* Spastic hemiplegia accounts for around one-third of cerebral palsy cases and is usually seen in term babies.
- *Diplegia* This subtype is characteristic of preterm infants with associated intraventricular hemorrhage and periventricular leucomalacia. The entire body is affected; but lower limbs and trunk are involved much more than the upper limbs.

Other Forms of Cerebral Palsy

- *Dyskinetic* Impaired volitional activity manifested as uncontrolled and purposeless movements that disappear during sleep. The subtypes include *dystonic and choreoathetoid*.
- *Hypotonic* It is characterized by marked motor delay, decreased tone and intellectual disability.
- *Ataxic* It is a relatively uncommon form of cerebral palsy. Defective postural function and disturbed equilibrium makes sustained control against gravity difficult.
- *Mixed* A combination of spasticity and choreoathetosis is seen most commonly, athetosis with ataxia may occur.

Evaluation

The diagnosis of cerebral palsy is essentially clinical. It involves a detailed prenatal, natal and postnatal history and careful physical and neurodevelopmental examination to identify deficit type and topography, which is required for management. Associated problems such as vision and hearing impairment, seizures, feeding difficulties, etc. need to be looked for. In severe and long-standing cases the diagnosis of cerebral palsy is not difficult. *Early markers* of cerebral palsy are as follows:

1. Tone abnormalities;
2. Brisk muscle stretch reflexes;
3. Asymmetrical movements;
4. Persistence of abnormal neonatal reflexes;
5. Delayed emergence of protective/postural reflexes;
6. Early hand preference;
7. Prominent fisting; 'cortical thumb'; and
8. Toe walking.

Investigations

Laboratory tests are not necessary to confirm diagnosis. Brain imaging studies may be useful in elucidating the etiology of cerebral palsy and suggesting a prognosis. Ultrasound brain is useful to detect intraventricular hemorrhage and periventricular leucomalacia in preterm neonates. CT and MRI can help to diagnose other diseases that may be confused with cerebral palsy like slow degenerations, and migration disorders. These children need to be routinely screened for visual and auditory problems.

Treatment	Cerebral Palsy

A multidisciplinary approach is essential. A physician should have an elementary idea of all the modalities required for holistic management. This includes physiotherapy and motor training, training in activities of daily living, management of feeding difficulties, and early developmental stimulation.
- Developmental stimulation is the key to management and includes: Visual stimulation, tactile stimulation, auditory stimulation, sensory stimulation, head movement, holding head, and babbling.
- Educational problems, visual problems and communication problems need to be addressed.
- Treatment of epilepsy and drug treatment of spasticity should be instituted when indicated.
- Rehabilitate the child at his own home, and in his familiar surroundings, rather than big institution.
- Good family support is the key to success in rehabilitating a child with cerebral palsy.

Cerebral Palsy

1. Cerebral palsy is motor dysfunction, comprising of abnormal muscle tone, abnormal posture, and disorder of movement.
2. Associated comorbidities include seizures, behavioral problems, speech, hearing and language disorders, feeding difficulties, and strabismus and visual impairement.
3. Management is multidisciplinary involving developmental stimulation, management of epilepsy, spasticity and visual and communication problems.

Aisen ML, Kerkovich D, Mast J, *et al*. Rethlefsen SA. Cerebral palsy: clinical care and neurological rehabilitation. *Lancet Neurol*. 2011;10:844–52.

Heinen F, Desloovere K, Schroeder AS, *et al*. The updated European Consensus 2009 on the use of botulinum toxin for children with cerebral palsy. *Eur J Paediatr Neurol*. 2010;14:45–66.

Singhi PD. Cerebral palsy-management. *Indian J Pediatr*. 2004; 71:635–9.

Intellectual disability (formerly called mental retardation) is characterized by a triad of following: (*i*) Limitation in intellectual functioning including learning, reasoning, and problem solving, abstract thinking, and judgment. This limitation in intellectual ability typically corresponds to an intelligence quotient (IQ) that is 2 standard deviations or more below the mean; scores are typically less than 70; (*ii*) Limitations in adaptive functioning in at least one of three domains: Conceptual, social, and practical; and (*iii*) Onset before 18 years of age.

The term *intellectual disability* has now replaced *mental retardation*. This disability originates before the age of 18 years. Children less than 5 years with subnormal intelligence are now labeled as having *global developmental delay*.

Global Developmental Delay

Global developmental delay can be operationally defined as a significant delay in 2 or more developmental domains. These domains may include gross and fine motor, cognition; speech and language; and personal social or activities of daily living.
- If the delay is restricted to a single domain, then either gross motor delay or developmental language impairment can be inferred to exist.
- If there is a sufficient impairment in social interaction and communication and there is presence of restricted repetitive behavior, a diagnosis of autism spectrum disorder can be made.

Classification and Etiology

Mild	: Score 50–55 to 70
Moderate	: Score 35–40 to 50–55
Severe	: Score 20–25 to 35–40
Profound	: Score <20–25

Severe intellectual disability is linked to genetic syndromes, chromosomal abnormalities, intrauterine infections, perinatal insult, maternal drug abuse and exposure to teratogen. Mild cases are usually secondary to environmental causes.

Approach to a Child with Intellectual Disability

Developmental History

A detailed developmental history is the first step. The timing of developmental milestones in each domain should be determined. Comparing a child with other children of same age or recalling the child's developmental status at a specific personal milestone (eg, first birthday) may aid the parents to recall the milestones. One should ascertain whether the delay is global or restricted to a single domain. Probing for autistic features is essential. Current developmental attainment in all domains and functional status with regard to activities of daily living must be documented. A scholastic history and probing for a need for any supplemental educational resources is important in a school going child.

Is There Any Regression?

Next important question to answer is, 'Is there any regression? This is important to ascertain as further etiological work up and prognostication hinges on this important answer. Figure 13.14 shows the concept of regression. Moreover, the history of regression may be missed in cases of very early onset of regression, abnormally slow early development or a prolonged evolution of a slowly degenerative process. It is also necessary to exclude *pseudo-regression*. Various factors may cause an apparent regression in an otherwise static encephalopathy like increasing spasticity, new onset movement disorder, new onset seizures or deterioration in control of previously well controlled epilepsy, drug side effects or progressive hydrocephalus.

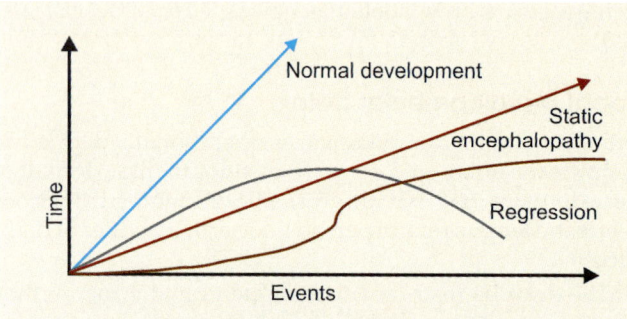

Fig. 13.14 Patterns of development

Other Pertinent History

The history of comorbidities must be elicited. These may include epilepsy, hearing or visual impairments, language problems, behavioral and sleep disturbances, feeding difficulties, drooling, gastroesophageal reflux, constipation, malnutrition, dental problems and orthopedic issues. The past medical history including presence of any chronic medical conditions, prior hospitalization, past and current medications prescribed and immunization status must be documented. The current rehabilitation status and parental access to appropriate rehabilitation services must be determined. The evaluation of the social support system is also essential. The socioeconomic status of the family, educational status of the caregiver, family size and the attitude of the family towards the child's illness should be evaluated. Elicit a detailed antenatal, perinatal and family history **(Table 13.17)**.

At the end of history, the physician should be clear regarding the presence of a static or a progressive encephalopathy, current developmental status of the child in each domain, current rehabilitation status, possible timing of the underlying cause and presence of associated comorbidities.

Physical Examination

The next step is physical examination. It starts during the initial history taking with observation of the child's spontaneous exploration of the surroundings. A child-friendly environment, ensuring physical proximity of the child with the caregiver, establishing a rapport with the child and deferring direct manipulation to the end of the examination always helps. Undressing the child always

Table 13.17 Vital Antenatal, Perinatal and Family History

Antenatal history	Perinatal history
Details of antenatal care	Timing of rupture of membranes,
Prenatal adverse events:	Maternal fever
PIH, GDM, per vaginal	Antepartum hemorrhage
bleeding, infections	Meconium staining
Maternal drugs/radiation	Timing of labor, duration,
Fetal movements	presentation
Liquor: Poly/	Mode of delivery, trial of labor
oligohydramnios	before CS
	Abnormal fetal heart rate moni-
	toring, Apgar's resuscitation
	Resuscitation details, weight and
	OFC at birth
Family history	Respiratory distress, need for
3 generation pedigree of	oxygen
child's family	Jaundice
Search for other affected	Birth injuries
family members	Any admission to NICU
Parental consanguinity	Duration of post-delivery
Geographic origin	hospital stay
Mother's prior gestational	Any evidence of neonatal
history, pregnancy losses,	encephalopathy, recurrent
early neonatal or infantile	vomiting, inadequate weight
deaths	gain

allows for a complete examination. The current somatic measurements for height and weight must be obtained. Look for abnormal head size or shape. The previous occipito-frontal circumference (OFC) should be obtained and plotted. The OFCs of the parents should be obtained in case of abnormal head size. Do not forget to measure the fontanels. Observe for any dysmorphic features. Down facies is easily recognizable but for the rest, the help of a dysmorphologist is indispensable for an accurate recognition of specific syndromes. The spine should be carefully inspected for any deformity or dysraphism. Possible stigmata of a neuro-cutaneous disorder warrant careful inspection. Eye/skin/hair abnormalities and organomegaly may provide useful clues **(Table 13.18)**. A detailed neurological examination and a formal developmental assessment completes the physical examination.

Evaluate

Once the history and physical examination are completed, sufficient information is usually obtained either to provide a diagnosis of a specific neurodevelopmental disability or to guide further laboratory investigations. In the quest for the search of etiology, one should not forget the referral of the child to specialty ancillary services which may include psychology, occupational therapy, speech therapy, play therapy, physiotherapy, audiology, ophthalmology, ENT services, dietician and social services (in appropriate settings). Such services along with pediatric neurology and developmental pediatrics are part of a *multidisciplinary team* to facilitate management of a child with global developmental delay.

A broad approach to investigate a child with global developmental delay/Intellectual disability is depicted in Fig. 13.15.

Table 13.18 Intellectual Disability: Important Clues in Physical Examination	
Microcephaly	Primary, cerebral malformations, intrauterine infections, fetal alcohol syndrome, HIV infection, Rett's syndrome, Seckel syndrome, Down syndrome, Cornelia de Lange syndrome, and Rubinstein-Taybi syndrome
Cataract	Down syndrome, galactosemia, Lowe syndrome, congenital rubella syndrome
Cherry red spot	Tay-Sachs disease, GM1 gangliosidosis, Niemann-Pick disease
Chorioretinitis	Intrauterine infections, mucopolysaccharidoses, Lowe syndrome
Dislocated lens	Homocystinuria
Retinitis pigmentosa	Laurence-Moon-Biedl syndrome, mucopolysaccharidoses
Synophrys	Cornelia de Lange syndrome
Coarse facies	Mucopolysaccharidoses, mucolipidoses, mannosidosis, fucosidosis, sialidosis
Hepatosplenomegaly	Mucopolysaccharidoses, Niemann-Pick disease, Gaucher disease, GMI gangliosidosis, glycogen storage disease
Broad thumbs and toes	Rubinstein-Taybi syndrome
Abnormal fat pad distribution	Congenital disorders of glycosylation, Cornelia de Lange syndrome
Short stature	Hypothyroidism, Seckel syndrome, Cornelia de Lange syndrome, mucopolysaccharidoses

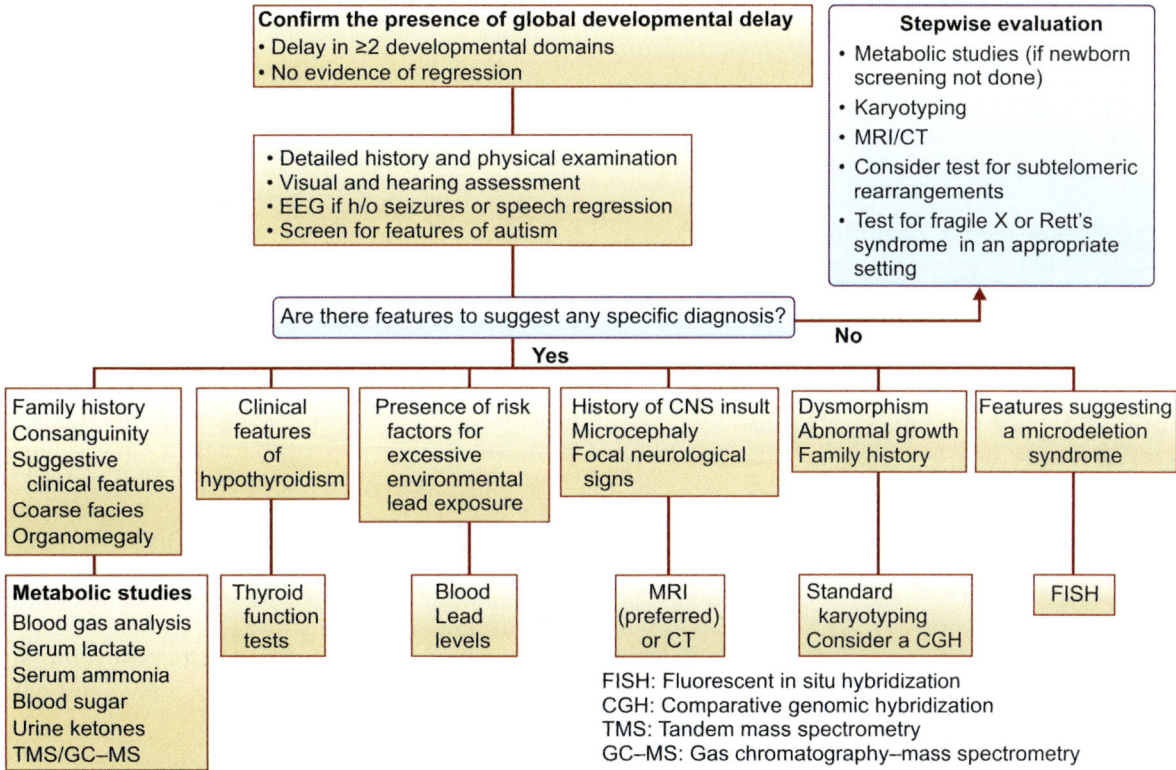

Fig. 13.15 Approach to a child with developmental delay and intellectual disability

Periventricular calcifications and lissencephaly—pachygyria in a patient with congenital CMV infection is shown in Fig. 13.16.

Risk of Recurrence

Risk of recurrence will depend on the etiology. Risk of recurrence in *de novo* chromosomal disorders is low (usually <1%). In translocation Down syndrome cases when one of the parents is a balanced translocation carrier the recurrence risk is variable. It varies from 2.5% if the father carries a 14/21 translocation to 100% if either parent carries a 21/21 translocation. In an autosomal recessive disorder risk of recurrence is 25% for the sibling. In autosomal dominant disorder the risk of recurrence for the sibling is 50% if one of the parents is affected. In X-linked recessive disorders risk of recurrence for boys is 50% whereas females usually do not manifest. Environmental causes, when identified, recurrence is unlikely unless the causative agent keeps on operating, eg, lead exposure, intrauterine exposure to teratogens.

13

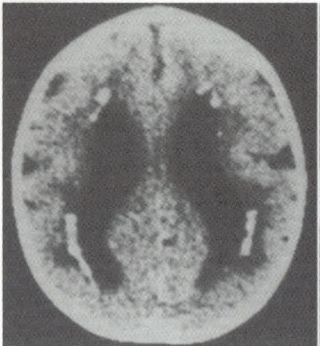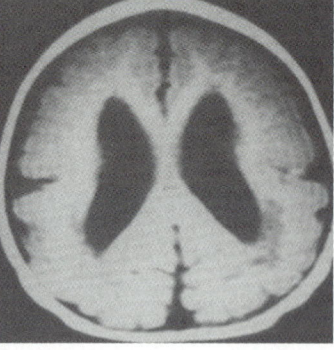

Fig. 13.16 Periventricular calcifications and lissencephaly—pachygyria in a patient with congenital CMV infection

Prevention

Strategies at primary level can go a long way to prevent GDD/ID, eg, iodine supplementation, adequate nutrition, prevention of anemia, avoidance of toxins like lead, avoid consanguinity, avoid very young and advanced age pregnancies, periconceptional folic acid, good antenatal, intranatal and perinatal care, screening for intrauterine infections and prenatal screening by maternal serum markers. Genetic counseling and prenatal diagnosis; early diagnosis and treatment where possible; and early rehabilitative interventions and support, are helpful.

Intellectual Disability

1. ID involves impairment in intellectual functioning, and adaptive functioning with onset before 18 years of age.
2. Global developmental delay can be operationally defined as a significant delay in 2 or more developmental domains.
3. It is important to rule out regression before deciding etiological workup

McDonald L, Rennie A, Tolmie J, *et al*. Investigation of global developmental delay. *Arch Dis Child*. 2006; 91:701–705.

Moeschler JB, Shevell M, American Academy of Pediatrics Committee on Genetics. Clinical genetic evaluation of the child with mental retardation or developmental delays. *Pediatrics*. 2006;117:2304–16.

Sharma A, O'Sullivan T, Baird G. Clinical evaluation of child development from birth to five years. *Psychiatry*. 2008;7:235–241.

Shevell MI. The evaluation of the child with a global developmental delay. *Semin Pediatr Neurol*. 1998;5:21–26.

Shevell M, Ashwal S, Donley D, *et al*. Practice parameter: Evaluation of the child with global developmental delay: Report of the Quality Standards Subcommittee of the American Academy of Neurology and The Practice Committee of the Child Neurology Society. *Neurology*. 2003;60;367–380.

13.21 NEURODEGENERATIVE DISEASES

Degenerative brain diseases are characterized by progressive loss of already acquired intellectual, motor, and sensory abilities following a period of normal development. This needs to be differentiated from delayed development (Fig. 13.14). These disorders can manifest at any age and may involve other body systems. Most degenerative brain disorders are inherited as autosomal recessive.

Classification

Degenerative brain disorders are classically categorized as the (*a*) diseases of gray matter; and (*b*) diseases of white matter.
- *Gray matter disorders* present with abnormalities of cognition, seizures, visual and hearing problems. They usually present early in infantile period.
- *White matter disorders* involve long tracts and classically present with loss of motor skills, spasticity, or ataxia.

This classification is too simple and usually applicable only in the early stages of the disease. The distinction becomes almost impossible in later stages as the end-stage picture of all of them is generally similar. Broad differences between gray and white matter diseases are summarized in **Table 13.19**.

Table 13.19 Symptoms of Neurodegeneration	
Gray matter disease	*White matter disease*
1. Psychomotor regression (young children)	1. Spasticity
2. Dementia (older children)	2. Babinski sign
3. Seizures	3. Ataxia
4. Extrapyramidal symptoms	4. Peripheral neuropathy
5. Visual loss	5. Optic atrophy
6. Hearing impairment	*Examples:*
Examples: Tay-Sachs disease, Niemann-Pick disease	Metachromatic leukodystrophy, adrenoleukodystrophy

Disorders Primarily Involving White Matter (Leukodystrophies)

Leukodystrophies comprise a heterogeneous group of progressive disorders that affect myelin development. A genetically determined molecular abnormality is responsible for metabolic deficits in myelin sheaths or myelinating cells, resulting in the destruction or failed development of central white matter.

Leukodystrophies are clinically characterized by predominance of motor disturbances, especially pyramidal and cerebellar features, with slow mental deterioration, and low incidence of seizures and myoclonus.

Examples of leukodystrophies are metachromatic leukodystrophy, adrenoleukodystrophy, and globoid cell leukodystrophy.

Disorders Primarily Involving Gray Matter

These disorders are clinically characterized by early cognitive decline, seizures, myoclonus, vision impairment, and late motor regression. They may be associated with visceral involvement in the form of hepatosplenomegaly. Examples include GM1 gangliosidoses and Tay-Sachs disease.

System Degeneration Involving Basal Ganglia

These disorders are characterized by dystonia, rigidity, tremors, and parkinsonian features. Examples include Wilson disease and pantothenate kinase associated neurodegeneration (PKAN).

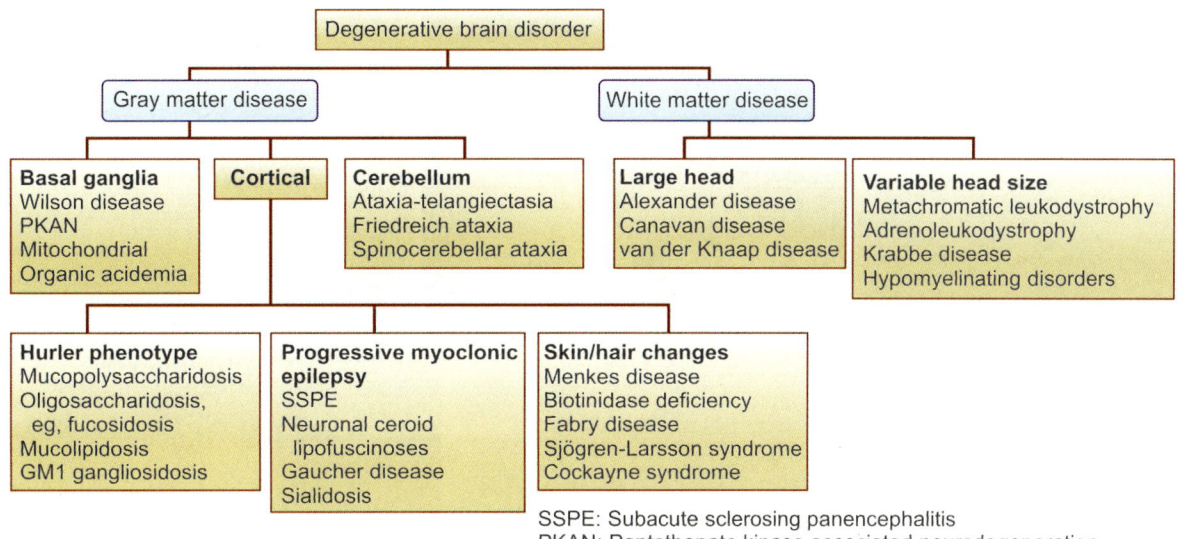

SSPE: Subacute sclerosing panencephalitis
PKAN: Pantothenate kinase associated neurodegeneration

Fig. 13.17 Approach to a child with degenerative brain disorder

Neurodegenerative Disorders

1. Neurodegenerative diseases are characterized by progressive loss of previously acquired intellectual, motor, and sensory abilities following a period of normal development.

2. Leukodystrophies comprise a heterogeneous group of progressive disorders that affect myelin development and present with early tonal abnormalities.

3. Gray matter degenerative brain diseases are characterized by early cognitive decline, seizures, myoclonus, and vision impairment.

System Degeneration Involving Cerebellum

These disorders are characterized by ataxia, incoordination, dysarthria and other cerebellar features. Examples include ataxia-telangiectasia, Friedreich ataxia and spinocerebellar ataxia.

A broad clinical approach to a child with degenerative brain disorder is shown in Fig. 13.17.

De Siqueira LF. Progressive myoclonic epilepsies: review of clinical, molecular and therapeutic aspects. *J Neurol.* 2010;257:1612–9.

Gutierrez J, Issacson RS, Koppel BS. Subacute sclerosing panencephalitis: an update. *Dev Med Child Neurol.* 2010;52:901–7.

Rosencrantz R, Schilsky M. Wilson disease: pathogenesis and clinical considerations in diagnosis and treatment. *Semin Liver Dis.* 2011;31:245–59.

Schiffmann R, van der Knaap MS. MRI-based approach to the diagnosis of white matter disorders. *Neurology.* 2009;72:750–9.

13.22 NEUROCUTANEOUS SYNDROMES

These disorders include dysplasias or neoplasm of organs derived from the embryonic ectoderm, ie, skin, central nervous system (CNS, peripheral nervous system) and eyes. Structures derived from the mesoderm (blood vessels, bone, and cartilage) and the endoderm (epithelial lining of the gastrointestinal tract) can also be affected.

NEUROFIBROMATOSIS

Neurofibromatosis (NF) is a group of heterogeneous diseases with NF-1 and NF-2 as two genetically distinct subtypes. Both are transmitted as autosomal dominant traits with almost complete penetrance. NF-1 has been mapped to chromosome 17 and there is spontaneous mutation rate of about 50%. NF-2 is an autosomal dominant disorder that has been mapped to the chromosome 22. The NF-2 usually presents at a later age than the NF-1 children.

Clinical Manifestations

Café au lait spots (Fig. 13.18a), freckling, cutaneous neurofibromas, Lisch nodules in eye, macrocephaly, learning disability, and mental retardation. Enlargement of cutaneous and subcutaneous tumors over many years can cause massive hemihypertrophy of the extremities or the face (elephantiasis neuromatosa).

Diagnosis

In children with NF-1, cranial MR demonstrates optic gliomas, gliomas of brainstem or craniocervical junction, plexiform neurofibromas, and mesodermal dysplasias. NF-2 is characterized by intracranial and intraspinal schwannomas, meningiomas, and other tumours, but not neurofibromas. The major feature of NF-2 is the presence in nearly all affected individuals of bilateral vestibular schwannomas. Cutaneous manifestations are much less frequent than in NF-1.

TUBEROUS SCLEROSIS

Tuberous sclerosis is inherited as an autosomal dominant trait, due to a possible deletion on chromosome 9; although lesions of chromosome 11 have also been implicated.

Clinical Features

Classically, tuberous sclerosis is characterized by the clinical triad of mental retardation, epilepsy, and characteristic nodular lesions on face known as adenoma

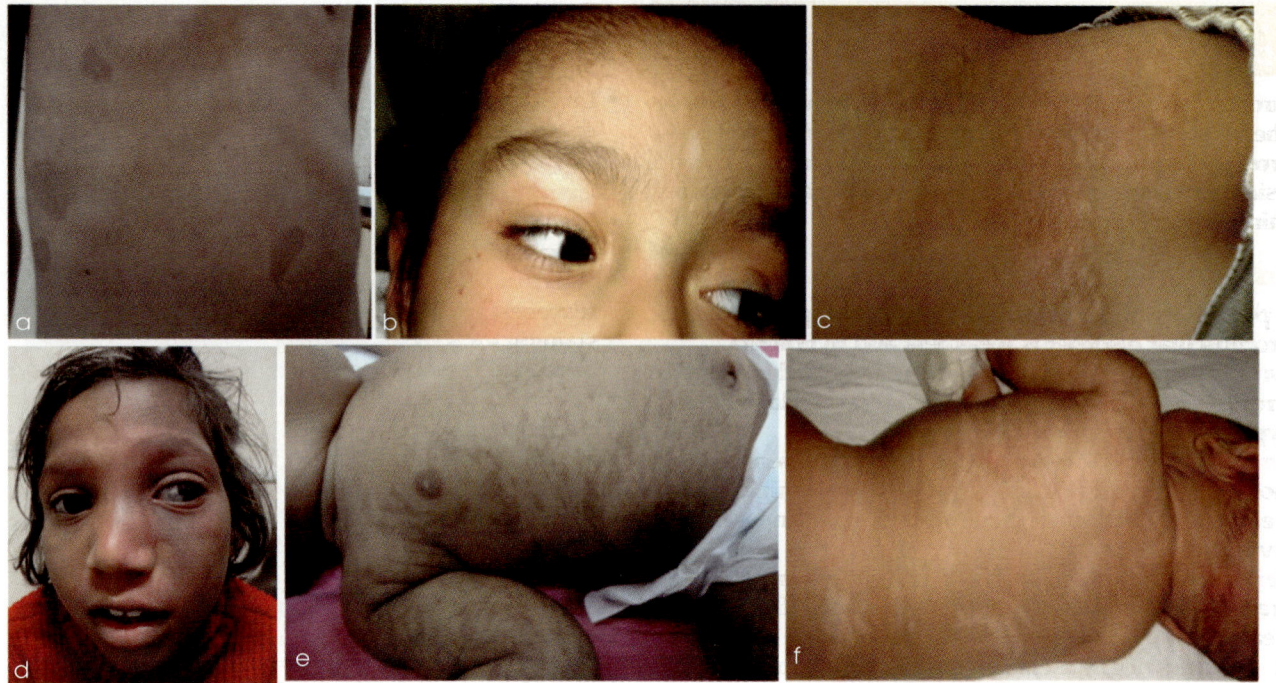

Fig. 13.18 Markers of neurocutaneous syndromes. (a) Cafe au lait macules, (b) ash-leaf macules; (c) shagreen patch; (d) port-wine stain; (e) incontinentia pigmenti, and (f) hypomelanosis of Ito

sebaceum. Other cutaneous lesions consist of ash-leaf macules (Fig. 13.18b), cafe au lait spots, shagreen patches (on back) (Fig. 13.18c), and subungual fibromas. Intracranial manifestations consist of cortical tubers, white matter abnormalities, subependymal nodules, and subependymal giant cell astrocytoma.

The peak age of presentation is between 8 to 16 years of age. These children may also present as myoclonic epilepsy. Other manifestations include retinal hamartomas, renal hamartomas, cardiac rhabdomyomas, and lymphangioleiomyomatosis.

STURGE-WEBER SYNDROME

The two essential pathognomonic features of Sturge-Weber syndrome are the (*i*) cutaneous vascular nevus (nevus flammens, port-wine nevus) usually of the upper eyelid or the supraorbital region (Fig. 13.18d) and (*ii*) the leptomeningeal angiomatosis usually overlying the ipsilateral occipital lobe.

Seizures occur in approximately 90% of the affected children. Other clinical components of this syndrome are hemiparesis, hemianopsia, and intellectual disability. Angiomatosis of the choroid of the eye may give rise to buphthalmos.

Neuroimaging demonstrates calcification of the cortex which can be seen with plain radiographs (*rail road calcification*). This is shown with CT to underlie the pial angiomatosis, however the calcification may be more extensive with the involvement of the frontal lobe or bilateral involvement. CT is superior to MR in displaying calcification, however, these calcifications are not usually visible until after 1–2 years of life.

ATAXIA-TELANGIECTASIA

The pathological features of this phakomatosis include (*i*) ocular or cutaneous telangiectasias; and (*ii*) cerebellar atrophy with predominant involvement of the anterior vermis and dentate nuclei. Atrophy of the olivary nuclei with degeneration of the posterior columns of the spinal cord may also be seen. MRI brain demonstrates marked cerebellar atrophy.

Affected children present with cerebellar ataxia, which manifests when the child starts to walk. This is followed by progressive neurological deterioration and eventually the children are wheelchair bound and exhibit oculomotor abnormalities, dysarthric speech, choreoathetosis, endocrine abnormalities, and myoclonic jerks.

Revision Point

Neurocutaneous Syndromes

1. Neurocutaneous syndromes include dysplasias or neoplasm of organs derived from the embryonic ectoderm.
2. Neurofibromatosis and tuberous sclerosis are autosomally dominant inherited disorders.
3. Sturge-Weber syndrome is characterized by facial hemangioma, leptomeningeal angiomatosis, with/without buphthalmos.

Asthagiri AR, Parry DM, Butman JA, *et al*. Neurofibromatosis type 2. *Lancet*. 2009;373:1974–86.

Comi AM. Presentation, diagnosis, pathophysiology, and treatment of the neurological features of Sturge-Weber syndrome. *Neurologist*. 2011;17:179–84.

Franz DN, Bissler JJ, McCormack FX. Tuberous sclerosis complex: neurological, renal and pulmonary manifestations. *Neuropediatrics*. 2010;41:199–208.

Reynolds RM, Browning GG, Nawroz I, *et al*. Von Recklinghausen's neurofibromatosis: neurofibromatosis type 1. *Lancet*. 2003;361:1552–4.

13.23 APPROACH TO NEUROMUSCULAR DISORDERS

Neuromuscular disorders can be due to disorder anywhere in the motor unit: Anterior horn cell, peripheral nerves, neuromuscular junction, and muscle. A careful history and physical examination helps in localization of the disorder within the motor unit.

Localization of Lesion

The predominant presenting complaint of a patient with a neuromuscular disorder is weakness and hypotonia.

- *Anterior horn cell* involvement (eg, spinal muscular atrophy) is associated with wasting, fasciculations, and hyporeflexia.
- *Peripheral nerve* involvement (eg, hereditary sensory and motor neuropathies) is associated with predominant distal weakness, distal wasting, hyporeflexia, and sensory involvement.
- *Neuromuscular junction* involvement (eg, myasthenia gravis) is associated with fatigable and fluctuating weakness.
- *Muscle disease* (eg, muscular dystrophies) is associated with proximal weakness, relatively preserved bulk and reflexes.
- A clinical approach to neuromuscular disorders is given in Fig. 13.19.

History and Examination

Mode of Inheritance

- X-linked recessive in Duchenne and Becker muscular dystrophy.
- Autosomal dominant in facioscapulohumeral dystrophy.
- Autosomal recessive in sarcoglycanopathies and congenital muscular dystrophies.

Course of Disease

- Muscular dystrophy is associated with inexorable weakness.
- Metabolic disease and ion channelopathies, eg, periodic paralysis are associated with episodic course.
- Inflammatory disorders such as dermatomyositis are associated with waxing and waning course and pain.

Involvement of Other Organs

- Cardiac disease often accompanies Duchenne muscular dystrophy and myotonic dystrophy.
- Skin rash is seen in dermatomyositis.

- Eye involvement is noted in myotonic dystrophy, congenital muscular dystrophies, and mitochondrial diseases.
- Liver involvement may be seen with mitochondrial disorders, acid maltase deficiency and carnitine deficiency.

Laboratory Evaluation

- Creatinine phosphokinase (CPK), a muscle enzyme is elevated in most muscular dystrophies.
- *Muscle biopsy* Diagnosis is made by specific morphological features, immunohistochemistry (absent or reduced staining for specific protein) and histochemistry (absent or reduced enzyme function).
- *Electrophysiological testing* Nerve conduction studies and electromyography help in localization of lesion to nerve, muscle, or neuromuscular junction; and assessment of severity and temporal course.
- *Other diagnostic tests* These include nerve biopsy, and antibody testing (eg, acetylcholine receptor antibodies in myasthenia gravis).
- *Molecular genetic testing* is now available for many neuromuscular disorders, eg, spinal muscular atrophy and Duchenne muscular dystrophy. Genetic testing is helpful not only for confirmation of diagnosis but also for prenatal diagnosis in subsequent pregnancies.

> *Revision Point*
>
> **Approach to Neuromuscular Disorder**
>
> 1. Anterior horn cell, peripheral nerve, neuromuscular junction, and muscle constitute lower motor neuron.
> 2. Muscular disorders primarily have proximal weakness.
> 3. Neurological disorders usually present with distal weakness.

Jackson CE. A clinical approach to muscle diseases. *Semin Neurol.* 2008;28:228–40.

13.24 MUSCULAR DYSTROPHIES

Muscular dystrophies include a group of *genetically determined, progressive, primary disorders of muscle.* These disorders usually present with proximal muscle weakness, waddling gait, difficulty in running, climbing stairs and getting up from floor, frequent falls, weakness of arms or face, ocular symptoms, enlargement or wasting of muscles and recurrent chest infections. Motor milestones may be achieved later than expected.

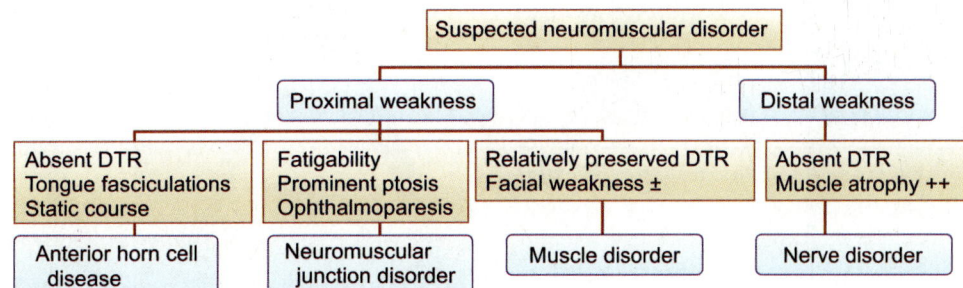

Fig. 13.19 A clinical approach to neuromuscular disorders. DTR: Deep tendon reflexes

DUCHENNE MUSCULAR DYSTROPHY

Duchenne muscular dystrophy (DMD) is the commonest muscular dystrophy. It is a severe disorder, resulting in early confinement to wheelchair by 13 years of age and often death by the age of 20 years. Becker muscular dystrophy (BMD) is a milder form of the same disease with later onset and a slower progression.

The incidence of DMD is approximately 1 in 3500 male births with a high mutation rate corresponding to one-third of the incidence. The incidence of BMD is 5.4/100,000 with a mutation rate which is about 5% of that for DMD. One-third of new cases have no previous family history.

Genetics

Duchenne and Becker muscular dystrophies display an X-linked recessive pattern of inheritance. Expression of the disease is essentially confined to males. Females are affected only if there is a loss or inactivation of the X chromosome carrying the normal allele.

DMD Gene

The gene responsible for Duchenne and Becker muscular dystrophies (the *DMD* gene) maps to the short arm of the X chromosome at band Xp21 and extends over 79 exons, and a 2.5 Mb genomic region. Approximately 60% of affected individuals have a deletion of one or more exons of the gene. Another 6% have duplication of exons, while the remaining 35% have a variety of subtle mutations, including point mutations. The mutation rate in Becker muscular dystrophy is much lower.

Dystrophin

This high molecular weight cytoskeletal protein is the primary product of the *DMD* gene. It is part of the dystrophin–glycoprotein complex, an ensemble of membrane-associated proteins that span the muscle sarcolemma, providing linkage between the intracellular cytoskeleton and the extracellular matrix. Dystrophin is expressed in skeletal muscle, smooth muscle, brain, peripheral nerves, and several other tissues. Boys with DMD have a little or no functional dystrophin; whereas in the milder disease BMD, dystrophin may be reduced in amount or altered in size.

Clinical Features

In the classical Duchenne type of muscular dystrophy, perinatal history is normal. Early development of the child is normal or slightly delayed. The median age at walking is 18 months. When the child starts walking in early part of the second year, he may appear clumsy while walking on even surface and may fall when walking or running on uneven ground. The gait is waddling with a compensatory lumbar lordosis. The toddler has difficulty in climbing up the stairs. He places his hand on the next step to lift himself up and always uses the support of the railing or the wall. The diagnosis is suspected, especially if there is a positive family history.

Hypertrophy of calf muscles may be observed by the age of 4–5 years. The child has difficulty in standing up from the recumbent position. He turns to side, lifts his trunk up by supporting his weight on his arms and then stands up as if climbing upon his body by supporting it with his hand. This is known as *Gower sign*. It indicates weakness of the pelvic girdle muscles (Fig. 13.20). The weakness of shoulder girdles is demonstrated by his inability to raise his hand above his shoulder and inability to comb his hair.

Distribution of the apparently (pseudo) hypertrophied and atrophied muscles is characteristic. The calf muscles, glutei, deltoid, serratus anterior, brachioradialis, and tongue muscles may appear large (Fig. 13.21). Sternal head of the pectoralis major and supraspinatus are atrophied. The condition shows relentless progression, with weakness and wasting that affects the proximal lower extremity muscles more profoundly. Eventually all the muscles atrophy. As the disease progresses, contractures that limit function, especially at the ankles and hips, develop. Scoliosis is common, following wheelchair dependency, which typically occurs about 12 years of age. Death in DMD most commonly results from pulmonary insufficiency and respiratory infections at about 20 years of age. Prolonged immobilization like plaster cast after a fracture hastens weakness of the muscles.

Cardiac involvement in Duchenne muscular dystrophy is common. Its onset is usually after the age of 10 years and increases in incidence with age affecting almost all patients beyond the age of 18 years. The average intelligence quotient

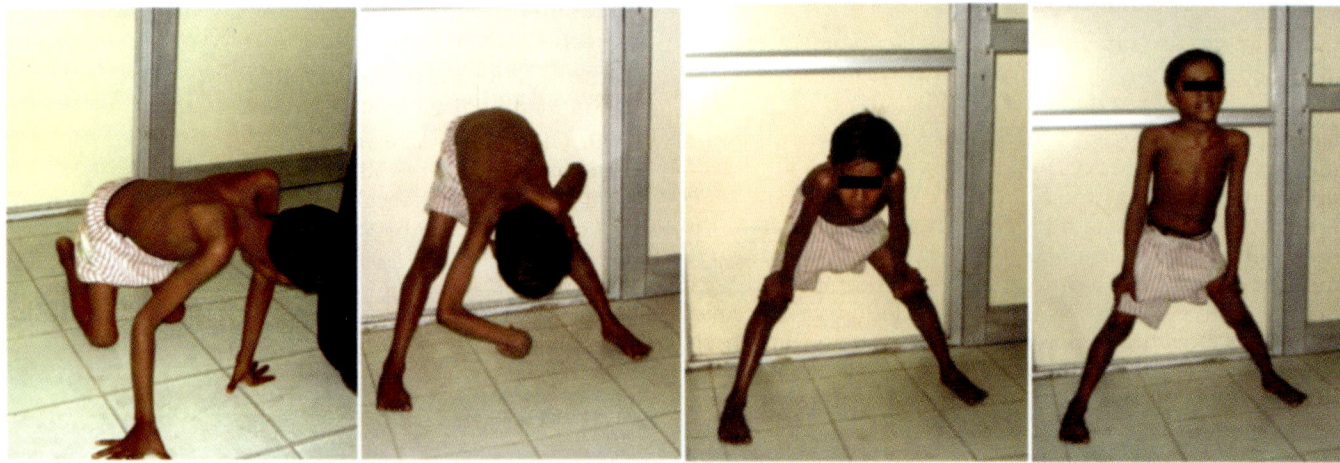

Fig. 13.20 A child with Duchenne muscular dystrophy with positive Gower sign

13

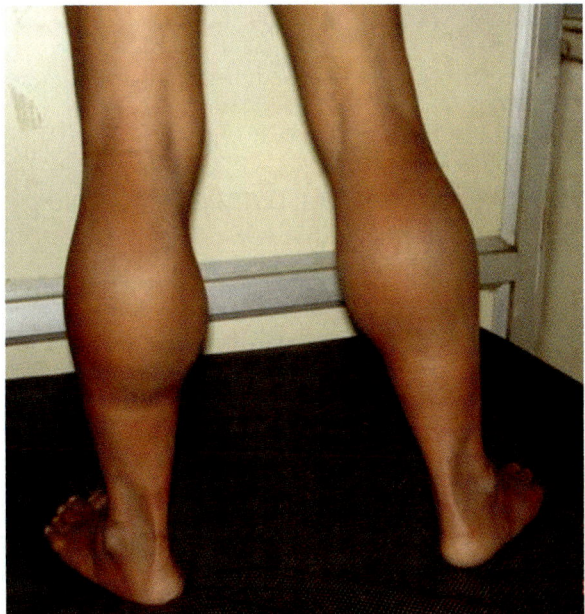

Fig. 13.21 A child with Duchenne muscular dystrophy with calf hypertrophy. Differentials include other limb-girdle muscular dystrophies, hypothyroidism, spinal muscular atrophy type III, and cysticercosis

is approximately one standard deviation below the mean. One-third of these children have an IQ below 75 which is non-progressive.

In Becker muscular dystrophy, the pattern of muscle-wasting closely resembles that seen in Duchenne. The natural history of the illness permits distinction between Duchenne and Becker muscular dystrophies. The majority of Becker patients will initially experience difficulties between the ages of 5–15 years, although an onset in the third and fourth decade, or even later, can occur. By definition, Becker patients ambulate beyond age 13 years, allowing clinical distinction from Duchenne. Becker patients have a reduced life expectancy, but the majority of patients survive at least into the fourth or fifth decade.

Diagnosis

The serum levels of the enzyme, creatine phosphokinase (CPK), are elevated in the patients especially in early stages even before the clinical manifestations become obvious. It can reach levels in the 15,000–20,000 U/L range and even higher. Levels may reduce in very advanced disease.

Histopathology of muscle fibers show diffuse changes of degeneration and regeneration, variation in size and central nuclei of the muscle fibers (more often in BMD). Ultimately, replacement of the muscle by fat and connective tissue leads to a picture of end-stage degeneration. In contrast, the muscular atrophies secondary to neurological disease show bundles of degenerated muscle fibers interspersed with bundles of normal muscle fibers. The definitive diagnosis of DMD is based on dystrophin deficiency in the muscle biopsy. Immunohistochemistry for dystrophin I, II and III reveals absent dystrophin in DMD and reduced, patchy dystrophin staining in BMD. In such cases, Western blot analysis of the protein helps to identify alteration in amount or altered molecular weight of dystrophin.

Multiplex PCR and the more sensitive *multiplex ligation-dependent probe amplification* (MLPA) are commonly employed genetic techniques for detection of mutations. In deletion negative patients linkage studies using CA repeat markers are used for carrier detection and prenatal diagnosis. A small proportion has duplications and rest have point mutations. Neither the size of the deletion nor its location bears any consistent relation to the clinical severity of the condition.

Treatment   **Duchenne Muscular Dystrophy**

There is no effective treatment. Trial with antisense oligo-nucleotide seems to hold promise.

1. *Maintain ambulation* Prolonged immobilization should be avoided as it hastens deterioration in muscle function. Ambulation is maintained by physiotherapy, exercises, daily walking and use of tricycle. Cardiomyopathy and congestive cardiac failure are managed by conventional approaches.
2. *Supportive therapy* Respiratory exercises should begin as soon as the diagnosis is made. Respiratory complications are managed by appropriate antibiotic therapy, and postural drainage. Appropriate immunizations should be done. Emotional support is given to the patient and the family. Contractures are postponed by range of motion exercises.
3. *Drug therapy* There is no cure till date. Various drugs have been tried with limited success. Steroids have some benefit. Administration of prednisolone may result in improved strength within 3–6 months of therapy, and reduce the rate of progress. The loss of ambulation may be postponed by up to 3–5 years. It is given in a dose of 0.75 mg/kg/day.
4. *Prenatal diagnosis* Prevention and counseling is of paramount importance and is often neglected by the physicians. Prenatal diagnosis is conducted if the index patient has a disease related mutation in the family or if linkage is informative. A chorionic villus sample at 11th week of gestation is taken to perform the tests. The identification of fetal sex is the first step. Further tests are necessary only for a male fetus. These include a multiplex PCR to detect a deletion or linkage studies using CA repeat markers.

EMERY-DREIFUSS MUSCULAR DYSTROPHY (EDMD)

EDMD is an X-linked disorder characterized by a specific pattern of contractures at elbow, ankle, and neck, cardio-myopathy, conduction disturbances and slowly progressive weakness in adult life. *The contractures precede the weakness.* The muscle weakness is proximal in upper limbs and predominantly distal in lower limbs.

The CPK levels are moderately elevated. There is deficiency of nuclear proteins emerin and Lamin A/C. The EDMD gene has been localized to the end of the long arm of the X chromosome at band Xq28.

LIMB-GIRDLE MUSCULAR DYSTROPHIES (LGMD)

These disorders are inherited as either autosomal dominant (LGMD 1A–E) or autosomal recessive (LGMD 2A–I) disorders. Genes involved in LGMD encode structural proteins of the sarcolemma, the sarcomere, the nuclear lamina, and enzymes such as calpain-3. *Calpainopathies* and *Sarcoglycanopathies* are the common types of LGMD.

Muscle weakness occurs in a limb-girdle distribution with sparing of the facial, extraocular and pharyngeal muscles. The degree of weakness may vary from mild to severe and the time of onset may vary from early to late onset. Calf hypertrophy is common in the recessively inherited phenotypes, and may be associated with muscle cramps and myalgia. Intelligence is normal. Cardiomyopathy is not frequent.

Serum CPK levels are elevated and tend to be higher in the recessive than dominant LGMD cases. Myopathic EMGs and muscle biopsy features of nonspecific dystrophic changes are characteristic. Immunohistochemistry and Western blot analysis are required for characterization and precise diagnosis. Treatment remains supportive.

CONGENITAL MUSCULAR DYSTROPHIES (CMD)

These children present with hypotonia and proximal muscular weakness at birth or within the first few months of life. Inheritance is autosomal recessive. Congenital muscular dystrophies are recognized as *syndromic* or *non-syndrome*.

- *Non-syndromic dystrophies* Merosin positive and negative congenital muscular dystrophies and collagen VI related disorders.
- *Syndromic variety* Fukuyama congenital muscular dystrophy, muscle-eye-brain disease, and Walker Warburg syndrome.

Pathophysiology

The connection between muscle to its extracellular matrix is disturbed due to a defect of α-dystroglycan, a major extracellular matrix receptor on muscle, or molecules of the extracelluar matrix itself, eg, merosin. As α-dystroglycan is widely expressed in muscle, brain and eye; the typical constellation resulting from these defects affect all three organs (the muscle-eye-brain spectrum).

Most affected children might eventually be able to stand with some support, but few learn to walk. Muscle weakness is usually non-progressive, but many joint contractures develop with immobility. CNS abnormalities include lissencephaly, pachygyria, pontocerebellar hypoplasia, and cerebellar cysts. Eye abnormalities include congenital myopia, glaucoma, and retinal hypoplasia.

Diagnosis

Serum creatinine kinase may be mildly to moderately elevated. Muscle biopsy shows signs of dystrophy, a marked increase in endomysial and perimysial connective tissue, and fiber size variability. Deficiency of merosin can be shown by Western blot analysis or muscle immunohistochemistry and also with chorionic villous material for prenatal diagnosis. Magnetic resonance imaging of the brain in children with merosin deficient congenital muscular dystrophy invariably shows white matter changes.

Fukuyama Congenital Muscular Dystrophy

The best characterized of the entities presenting with severe central nervous system defects, ocular abnormalities, and muscle disease is Fukuyama congenital muscular dystrophy. The condition is found predominantly in Japan, occurring

at a frequency of 7–12/100,000. Functional disability is severe. Most children never learn to walk, are bed-ridden before 10 years of age, and most die by 20 years of age. Severe mental retardation is observed in all cases. Seizures are common. It is inherited as an autosomal recessive trait.

FACIOSCAPULOHUMERAL DYSTROPHY—FSHD (LANDOUZY-DÉJÉRINE DISEASE

It is a relatively benign muscular dystrophy showing autosomal dominant inheritance. Both sexes in several generations are affected. The age of onset is around puberty. Progress of weakness is slow. Facial, shoulder girdle, and proximal arm muscles are involved. Affected children cannot close the eyes forcefully, whistle, or hold air in the oral cavity. Smiling or grimacing produces faint muscle movements. Winging and elevation of scapulae occur due to weakness of the scapular muscles. Foot drop results from weak peroneal and anterior tibial muscle. Asymmetric involvement is typical. Pelvic-girdle involvement is late and less marked. Hypertrophy does not occur. Neurological involvement occurs in form of sensorineural hearing loss. Some patients may develop exudative retinopathy. Smooth and cardiac muscles are notably spared, as is mental function. Serum creatinine kinase may be slightly elevated. Both muscle biopsy and EMG frequently show changes suggestive of a neurogenic origin, along with myopathic changes. Diagnosis relies on demonstrating the presence of contraction of the D4Z4 repeats in one copy of 4q35.

Revision Point

Muscular Dystrophy

1. Duchenne muscular dystrophy (DMD) is the commonest muscular dystrophy. It is inherited as X-linked recessive pattern.
2. In Emery-Dreifuss muscular dystrophy contractures are usually out of proportion to weakness.
3. Limb-girdle muscular dystrophies are a group of disorders with muscle weakness occurring in a limb-girdle distribution with sparing of the facial, extraocular, and pharyngeal muscles.

Bushby K, Finkel R, Birnkrant DJ, *et al*. Diagnosis and management of Duchenne muscular dystrophy, part 1: diagnosis and pharmacological and psychosocial management. *Lancet Neurol.* 2010;9:77–93.

Straub V, Bushby K. The childhood limb-girdle muscular dystrophies. *Semin Pediatr Neurol.* 2006;13:104–114.

Wattjes MP, Kley RA, Fischer D. Neuromuscular imaging in inherited muscle diseases. *Eur Radiol.* 2010;20:2447–460.

13.25 FLOPPY INFANT

Floppy infant is described as an infant with marked hypotonia of all the muscles. It is a common diagnostic problem in pediatric practice, particularly in the newborn period and early infancy. *A clinical diagnosis of hypotonia is usually suggested by bizarre and unusual postures of the infant, diminished resistance to passive movements or an excessive range of joint mobility.* These infants are usually relatively immobile. After the neonatal period, they usually present with delay in motor milestones.

Causes of Severe Hypotonia

The diagnosis of the precise etiological cause of hypotonia is difficult without detailed investigations. When assessing a floppy infant, the first decision to make is whether one is dealing with a neuromuscular problem or whether the hypotonia is symptomatic of a disorder in the central nervous system or some other system. In other words, one needs to differentiate between a weak or paralyzed infant with associated hypotonia, and a hypotonic infant without significant weakness. The distinction is usually fairly easy in practice, on the basis of whether the infant has or has not got a significant degree of weakness in association with the hypotonia. An approach to a floppy infant is given in Fig. 13.22.

The various causes of floppy infant syndrome are detailed in **Table 13.20**.

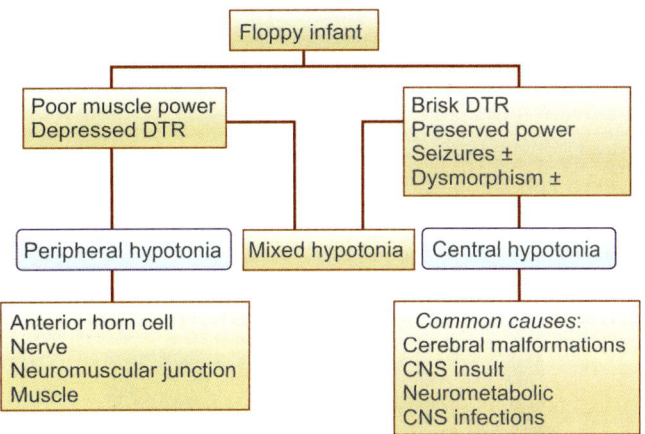

Fig. 13.22 An approach to a floppy child

Diagnosis of Floppy Infant

A normal term infant appears hypertonic by adult standards, while the preterm infant is hypotonic. The muscle tone increases as the gestational maturity proceeds. The floppy infant assumes a frog-legged position (Fig. 13.23). The muscles appear flabby. There is diminished resistance to passive movement of the limbs and the range of movement of the peripheral joints is increased. On ventral suspension, the baby assumes the position of a rag doll. When pulled up from the supine to the sitting position, the baby has a head lag.

If the hypotonia is of neuromuscular origin the main causes are likely to be spinal muscular atrophy (Werdnig-Hoffmann disease), congenital myotonic dystrophy, congenital muscular dystrophy, one of the congenital myopathies or other less frequent conditions. The degree and distribution of weakness may help to distinguish between these causes. Careful assessment should also be made of associated features which can be helpful in pointing to some of the disorders **(Table 13.21)**.

Investigations

Routine nerve conduction and electromyography (EMG) are helpful in trying to establish a neuromuscular cause, either a denervation process or a myopathy. In all cases with weakness this should be followed by a biopsy, which is the only accurate way of establishing a definitive diagnosis, since the serum enzymes as well as EMG may be completely

Table 13.20 Causes of Floppy Infant Syndrome	
Peripheral hypotonia	*Central hypotonia*

Infantile spinal muscular atrophy
Congenital muscular dystrophy
Congenital myotonic dystrophy
Neonatal congenital myasthenia
Congenital myopathies
Metabolic myopathies
• Glycogenoses (types II, III, IV, V, VII)
• Mitochondrial myopathies
• Lipid storage myopathies
• Periodic paralysis
Neuropathies
• Hereditary motor and sensory neuropathies (types I, II, III)
• Congenital hypomyelination syndrome
• Giant axonal neuropathy
• Acquired: Guillain-Barré syndrome
   Poliomyelitis
    Diphtheritic paralysis
   Arsenical neuropathy
Other neuromuscular disorders
• Infant botulism
• Spinal cord injury
• Epidural abscess
• Transverse myelitis (stage of shock)
• Polymyositis
	• Chromosomal disorders:
	  Trisomies
	  Prader-Willi syndrome
	• Cerebral malformations
	• CNS insult
	• Hypoxia
	• Intra-cranial hemorrhage
	• Neurometabolic
	  Pompe disease
	  Mitochondrial disorders
	  Lowe syndrome
	  Organic acidemia
	• CNS infections
	  Intra-uterine infections
	  Meningitis/sepsis
	• Connective tissue disorders
	  Congenital laxity of ligaments
	  Ehlers-Danlos and Marfan syndromes
	  Osteogenesis imperfecta

Table 13.21 Differential Diagnosis of the Floppy Infant based on the Associated Clinical Features

Associated signs	Suggestive disorder
Respiratory problems	Spinal muscular atrophy, congenital muscular dystrophy
Feeding difficulties	Spinal muscular atrophy, myasthenia gravis (neonatal), Prader-Willi syndrome
Ptosis/ophthalmoplegia	Mitochondrial myopathy, congenital muscular dystrophy, myasthenia gravis
Facial weakness	Congenital myotonic dystrophy, congenital muscular dystrophy
Multiple contractures/ Arthrogryposis/dislocated hips	Congenital muscular dystrophy, congenital myotonic dystrophy

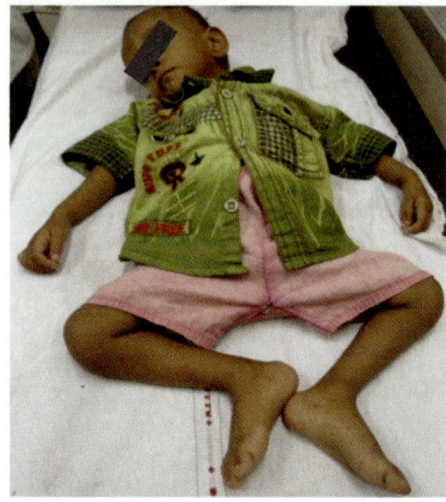

Fig. 13.23 "Frog like" posture in a floppy child

normal in some of these floppy infants with congenital myopathies, even in the presence of marked weakness.

SPINAL MUSCULAR ATROPHY

Childhood spinal muscular atrophy (SMA) is a common autosomal recessive disorder characterized by muscle weakness due to degeneration of motor neurons in the spinal cord and brain stem nuclei. It is inherited as autosomal dominant, X-linked recessive or sporadic.

The incidence is 1 in 6700 to 1 in 25000 live births and prevalence is 0.12 to 25 per 10000. Progression of the disease is due to loss of anterior horn cells, thought to be caused by apoptosis. Positional cloning strategies have revealed several gene candidates including the gene for the survival motor neuron (SMN) and the neuronal apoptosis inhibitory protein (NAIP). Both genes are duplicated on chromosome 5.

Subtypes

Spinal muscular atrophy is classified as follows:

Type I Werdnig-Hoffmann disease: Age at onset—0 to 6 months, patients never sits, death >90% by 10 years, age at onset determines age of death.

Type II Onset usually in the first year of life, unaided sitting possible, walking not achieved, survival >90% by 10 years.

Type III Walking without aids achieved, IIIa age at onset ≤ 3 years, IIIb age at onset >3 years, mild course, lifespan not markedly reduced.

Type IV Onset >30 years, variable severity, normal lifespan.

Diagnosis

The diagnosis is based on the following: Symmetrical weakness, proximal more than distal, accompanied by hypotonia and fasciculation of tongue. The trunk is commonly involved. Weakness in the legs is characteristically greater than in the arms. The child is alert. Feeding behavior and cry are poor. Deep tendon reflexes are absent. History of affected siblings in the family may be available. CPK is normal or mildly elevated. Fibrillation, positive sharp waves and fasciculation have been reported on electromyography which is a very useful diagnostic tool. Muscle biopsy shows neurogenic type of atrophy or that the muscle spindles are atrophied in groups. SMN (survival motor neuron) exon 7 is deleted in approximately 95% of SMA cases, although the figure is lower (64.3%) in our patient population. Prenatal diagnosis is possible.

Treatment	Spinal Muscular Atrophy

There is no effective therapy for SMA, and management till date consists of preventing or treating complications. Trials employing antisense oligonucleotide hold promise. Complications of severe weakness include restrictive lung disease, poor nutrition, orthopedic deformities, immobility and psychosocial problems. Possible therapeutic strategies include exon skipping, histone deacetylase inhibitors like sodium valproate and phenylbutyrate, neurotrophic agents, glutamate inhibitors, gene therapy, and cell therapy.

Floppy Infant

1. The first step while assessing floppy infant is to distinguish between floppy infant with weakness from a floppy infant without significant weakness.
2. Routine nerve conduction and electromyography are helpful in trying to establish a neuromuscular cause.
3. Spinal muscular atrophy, a common cause of floppy infant, is inherited as autosomal recessive disorder.

Bodensteiner JB. The evaluation of the hypotonic infant. *Semin Pediatr Neurol*. 2008;15:10–20.

Lunn MR, Wang CH. Spinal muscular atrophy. *Lancet*. 2008;371:2120–33.

Prasad AN, Prasad C. Genetic evaluation of the floppy infant. *Semin Fetal Neonatal Med*. 2011;16:99–108.

Wirth B, Brichta L, Hahnen E. Spinal muscular atrophy: from gene to therapy. *Semin Pediatr Neurol*. 2006;13:121–131.

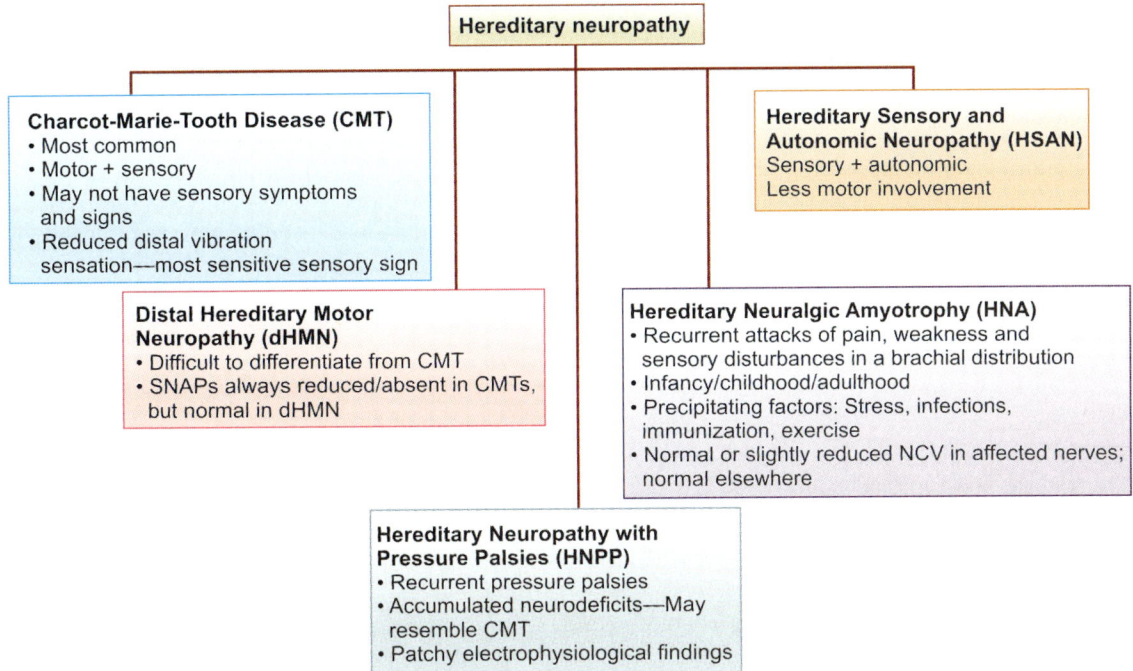

Fig. 13.24 Hereditary neuropathies in childhood. NCV: Nerve conduction velocity; CMT disease: Charcot-Marie-Tooth disease

13.26 HEREDITARY NEUROPATHIES

Hereditary peripheral neuropathies are common human genetic conditions. These clinically and genetically heterogeneous disorders produce progressive deterioration of the peripheral nerves with secondary muscle wasting and weakness in a distal distribution. The current classification of hereditary neuropathies is depicted in Fig. 13.24.

Clinical Features

A slowly progressive course, prominent sensory signs in absence of sensory symptoms, foot deformities and a family history points towards a hereditary neuropathy. Charcot-Marie-Tooth (CMT) disease is the most common hereditary neuropathy and possibly the most common peripheral neuropathy encountered in children.

The typical phenotype of a child with Charcot-Marie-Tooth disease consists of distal wasting and weakness especially of peroneal compartment ("stork-leg" like appearance) (Fig. 13.25), some distal sensory impairment, skeletal deformities, contractures and diminished or absent muscle stretch reflexes. The specific clinical features, electrophysiological characteristics, inheritance pattern and occasionally nerve biopsy features may point towards a specific hereditary neuropathy and guide the genetic testing.

The genetic screening may include testing for common subtypes like chromosome 17p (PMP) duplications and deletions, MPZ, MFN2, GJB1, and IGHMBP2. The optimal treatment remain a great challenge in the resource limited setting.

Differential Diagnosis

The common peripheral neuropathies encountered in childhood need to be entertained in the differential diagnosis.

These include demyelinating neuropathies (metachromtic leukodystrophy, adrenoleukodystrophy, diphtheria, and inflammatory polyneuropathy), predominant motor neuropathies (porphyria, lead poisoning), predominant sensory neuropathies (vitamin B_{12} and vitamin E deficiencies, vincristine induced, Friedreich ataxia); and that secondary to diabetes mellitus, and Fabry disease.

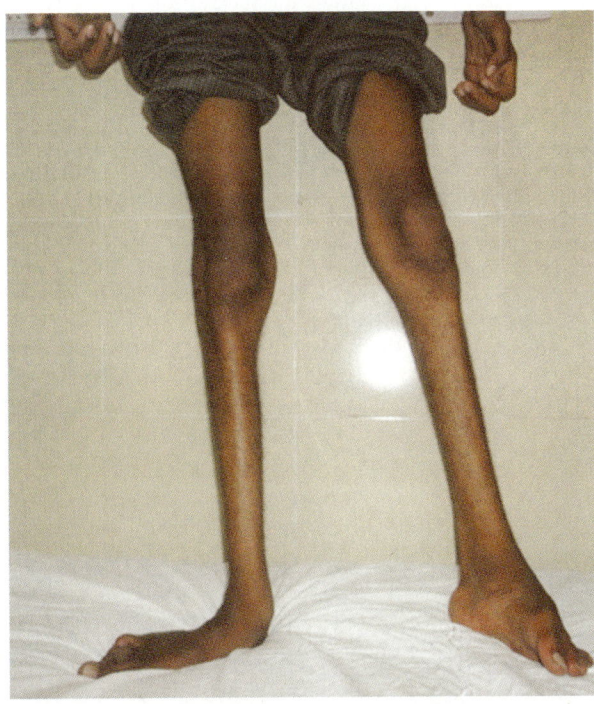

Fig. 13.25 "Stork-leg" like appearance of legs in a child with CMT1A. Also note the hand and foot deformities

13

Case Study | Limp and Loose Baby

A 3-year-old girl is brought with complaints of not being able to ever stand or walk. She had achieved neck holding at 8 months, was sitting with support at 18 months, and without support at 2 years of age. The parents also feel her to be limp and loose as compared to her sister. The birth and perinatal period were uneventful.

Q1. What other information do you want from the history?

First, we want to know whether this is an isolated motor delay or there is delay in other spheres (language, understanding, etc.) as well. We would also like to know whether there are any other associated problems—feeding difficulties, recurrent chest infections, drooping of eyelids, squint.

The parents say she is otherwise normal. She can speak sentences, is toilet trained, and can point to 3 colors. There are no other associated problems. You examine the child. She looks bright and alert. There is no facial weakness or squint. The muscle bulk is symmetrically reduced bilaterally. The tone is reduced in all 4 limbs. The antigravity movements are reduced. The power is reduced more in the proximal muscle groups as compared to the distal muscle group. The deep tendon reflexes are absent. She responds to pain and touch.

Q2. What are the other features that you should look for in the examination?

Contractures, scoliosis, tongue fasciculation

She has fasciculation of the tongue. There is no scoliosis, and there are bilateral tendo Achilles contractures.

Q3. What is the likely site of the lesion?

It is a lower motor neuron type of lesion, as it is associated with weakness, and hypotonia. Also the child is cognitively normal, making a brain cause unlikely. Amongst the lower motor neuron lesion, anterior horn cell pathology is most likely in view of proximal weakness, atrophy, fasciculations, areflexia, and normal sensation.

Q4. What is the most probable diagnosis?

Spinal muscular atrophy (type II, as the child is able to sit but unable to walk) is the most likely diagnosis. This is the most common inherited disorder of anterior horn cells.

Q5. How will you confirm the diagnosis?

Genetic testing is available for this disorder; SMN gene deletion studies by PCR should be done. This has 95% sensitivity. This may be negative in 5% of the affected children, in whom the diagnosis needs to be confirmed by electrophysiological studies (nerve conduction studies and electromyography), and muscle biopsy (which shows group atrophy, a characteristic feature of neurogenic pathology.

Q6. How will you manage this child?

Unfortunately there is no cure. The parents have to be explained the prognosis. Supportive care including physiotherapy, occupational therapy, orthosis, and immunization against common respiratory pathogens (influenza, pneumococcus) should be provided. The parents should be told about the recurrence risks (25% recurrence risk in each pregnancy, as it is an autosomal recessive disorder) need to be explained. Parents also need to be explained the need for prenatal diagnosis, which is available.

Joint Task Force of the EFNS and the PNS. European Federation of Neurological Societies/ Peripheral Nerve Society Guideline on management of chronic inflammatory demyelinating polyradiculoneuropathy. Report of a Joint Task Force of the European Federation of Neurological Societies and the Peripheral Nerve Society. *J Peripher Nerv Syst.* 2005;10:220–28.

Vavra MW, Rubin DI. The peripheral neuropathy evaluation in an office based neurology setting. *Semin Neurol.* 2011;31:102–14.

Wilmshurst JM, Ouvrier R. Hereditary peripheral neuropathies of childhood: a brief overview for clinicians. *Neuromuscul Disord.* 2011;21:763–7.

Revision Point

Hereditary Neuropathies

1. Charcot-Marie-Tooth disease is the most common hereditary neuropathy.
2. Typical phenotype of a child with Charcot-Marie-Tooth disease consists of distal wasting and weakness especially of peroneal compartment ("stork-leg" like appearance).
3. Treatment is mainly supportive.

Sheffali Gulati and Vishal Sondhi

Diabetes and Endocrine Disorders

14.1 ENDOCRINE GLANDS AND HORMONES

Endocrine glands secrete hormones, which are carried through the blood stream and produce widespread effects at distant sites. Hormones are derivatives of amino acids (eg, peptide hormones, glycoproteins, thyroxine and epinephrine) or cholesterol (eg, steroid hormones and vitamin D). The *hypothalamic-pituitary axis* is the master endocrine gland that regulates growth and water balance; and also the other endocrine glands, including thyroid, adrenal, and gonads.

Hormones and Receptors

Peptide hormones do not bind to circulating binding proteins resulting in rapid elimination and short half-life. They do not cross the plasma membrane and act on extracellular (membrane) receptors. Binding of hormones to the receptors activates a catalytic process resulting in production of a second messenger (cyclic AMP, cyclic GMP or diacyl glycerol). These second messengers act on intracellular proteins culminating in hormone effect.

Steroid and thyroid hormones bind to circulating proteins resulting in prolonged half life. They cross the cell membrane as they are lipophilic and act on intracellular receptors. The hormone-receptor complex then binds to the hormone response elements in the target gene resulting in regulation of transcription. Their effect is slower compared to the peptide hormones.

Endocrine Disorders

Hormones play an important role in the regulation of growth (eg, growth hormone (GH) and thyroxine), development (eg, thyroxine), puberty (eg, gonadotropins and sex hormones), fluid and electrolyte homeostasis (eg, vasopressin and aldosterone), blood glucose (eg, insulin, glucagon, GH, and cortisol) and serum calcium (eg, parathyroid hormone, calcitriol, and calcitonin). **Table 14.1** enlists disorders of endocrine dysfunction. They are related to abnormal production (deficiency or excess) or action (increased or decreased receptor activity) of hormones. Common disorders are discussed below.

Hormone secretion is controlled by regulatory hormones on one hand and hormone levels on the other (feedback regulation). This has significant diagnostic implications. For example, elevated pituitary hormones in a child with delayed puberty indicate primary organ defect of the gonad; while low levels suggest hypothalamic-pituitary dysfunction.

Assessment

Assessment of endocrine status involves estimation of baseline blood levels of hormones such as thyroid and parathyroid hormones. However, baseline levels of other hormones may not reflect their true assessment due to their pulsatile nature of release. This could be overcome by pooling multiple blood samples taken over time (cortisol and gonadotropins) or following stimulation tests (GH deficiency, delayed puberty, or adrenal insufficiency).

The feedback mechanism provides another basis for dynamic endocrine tests for diagnosis of hormone excess states (Cushing syndrome and GH excess).

Endocrine Glands and Hormones

1. Endocrine glands secrete hormones, which are carried through the blood stream and produce widespread effects at distant sites.
2. Hormones play an important role in the regulation of growth), development, puberty, fluid and electrolyte homeostasis, blood glucose and serum calcium.
3. Hormone secretion is controlled by feedback regulation by regulatory hormones.

14.2 GROWTH HORMONE DEFICIENCY

Growth hormone (GH), secreted by the anterior pituitary, induces production of insulin-like growth factor-1 (IGF-1) in the liver and skeletal tissue. IGF-1 acts as the final mediator of growth. The GH–IGF axis is influenced by nutritional, systemic, and endocrine disorders.

Etiology

Deficiency of GH is an important cause of short stature. It may be caused by (*i*) congenital malformations (midline defects or holoprosencephaly), (*ii*) genetic defects (mutations of GH or its receptor) , or (*iii*) acquired neurological insults (neurosurgery, trauma, radiation, and tumor).

Clinical Features

These children have normal growth at birth. Growth retardation usually becomes apparent at around one year of age. Height remains less than 3rd percentile and bone and teeth development is delayed. Midfacial crowding, doll like facies, mild obesity, and immature facial appearance are common

Hormone	Target action	Clinical syndromes	
		Deficiency	Excess
Hypothalamic-pituitary axis			
GH	Growth	Short stature	Gigantism
ACTH	Adrenal cortex	Adrenal failure	Cushing syndrome
LH, FSH	Gonads	Delayed puberty	Precocious puberty
TSH	Thyroid	Hypothyroidism	Thyrotoxicosis (rare)
Vasopressin	Fluid homeostasis	Diabetes insipidus	SIADH
Thyroid			
Thyroxine	Growth, development, temperature regulation	Hypothyroidism	Hyperthyroidism
Parathyroid			
PTH	Calcium homeostasis	Hypocalcemia	Hypercalcemia
Adrenal			
Aldosterone	Sodium homeostasis	Salt wasting crisis	Hypertension, hypokalemia
Cortisol	Glucose homeostasis	Adrenal failure	Cushing syndrome
Pancreas			
Insulin	Glucose homeostasis	Diabetes mellitus	Hypoglycemia
Gonads			
Testosterone	Male development	Delayed puberty / Genital ambiguity	Precocious puberty
Estrogen	Female development	Delayed puberty	Early puberty

Table 14.1 Important Endocrine Organs and Disorders

GH: growth hormone; ACTH: adrenocorticotropic hormone; LH: luteinizing hormone; FSH: follicle stimulating hormone; TSH: thyroid stimulating hormone; PTH: parathyroid hormone; SIADH: syndrome of inappropriate ADH secretion

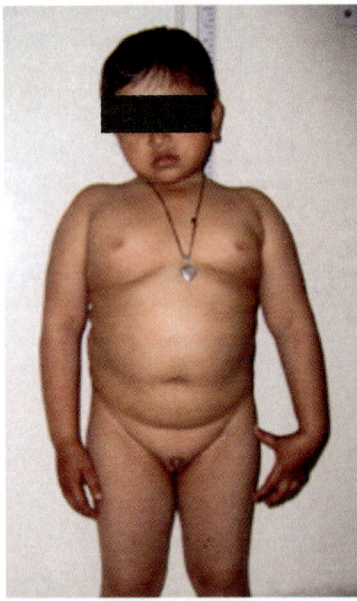

Fig. 14.1 A 9-year-old boy with growth retardation. Please note central obesity, micropenis and undescended testis. Investigations showed reduced IGF1 levels and low stimulated GH levels confirming the diagnosis of growth hormone deficiency

(Fig. 14.1). Body proportions are normal. The usual criteria for diagnosis of GHD are summarized below:
1. Height below 3rd percentile.
2. Prepubertal growth velocity less than 4 cm per year.
3. Bone age below the chronological age.
4. Peak GH levels less than 10 ng/mL during provocative stimulation tests.
5. Low IGF-1 and IGFBP-3 levels for age.
6. Resumption of growth following GH administration.

Differential Diagnosis

The most common cause of short stature is constitutional delay in growth and puberty. *Laron syndrome* or insensitivity to GH presents with severe growth retardation and elevated GH levels. *Hypothyroidism* may present with growth retardation alone in some children. *Type 1 diabetes mellitus, Turner syndrome, celiac disease, pseudohypoparathyroidism (PHP),* and *rickets* are also associated with growth retardation. Differential diagnosis of common endocrine causes of short stature is detailed in **Table 14.2**.

Nutritional causes of growth failure (malnutrition, malabsorption, celiac disease, and systemic illnesses) predominantly affect weight with secondary effect on height whereas endocrine causes predominantly affect height. Significant low weight for height age thus indicates the possibility of a nutritional cause for growth failure.

Evaluation

Evaluation for GH–IGF axis should be done preferably after all other common causes of growth retardation are excluded. Basal GH has no role in evaluating the GH–IGF axis. IGF-1 and its binding protein-3 (IGFBP-3) are used as screening tests for GH deficiency. Low levels of IGF-1 and/or IGFBP-3 should be confirmed by a GH stimulation test. This

Table 14.2 Differential Diagnosis of Short Stature

	Constitutional delay in growth and puberty	Familial short stature	Hypopituitarism (GHD)	Hypothyroidism	Turner syndrome
1. Family history	Usual	Usual	Rare	Infrequent	Rare
2. Birth weight and height	Normal	Low	Normal	Normal	Low
3. Pattern of growth	Slow from infancy	Slow from birth	Slow from a few months after birth	Slow from birth	Slow from birth
4. Epiphyseal development	Moderate, progressive retardation	Normal	Progressive retardation	Severe retardation	Variable
5. Puberty	Delayed	Normal	Delayed	Delayed	Delayed
6. GH levels	Normal	Normal	Low	Normal	Variable
7. Gonadotropin levels (after puberty)	Normal	Normal	Low except in isolated GHD	Variable	High

involves measurement of GH after physiological (exercise) or pharmacological stimulus (clonidine, glucagon, or insulin). Stimulated GH levels below 10 ng/mL are suggestive of growth hormone deficiency. This should be followed with evaluation of other pituitary hormones and brain imaging. High levels of GH suggest Laron syndrome.

Treatment	**Growth Hormone Deficiency**

GH supplementation is given as a daily night time injection (recombinant GH: 25–50 μg/kg/day) till epiphyseal closure. GH is also recommended for increasing height in children with Turner syndrome, chronic renal failure, small for gestational age infants with poor catch-up growth, Prader-Willi syndrome, and idiopathic short stature.

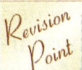

Growth Hormone Deficiency

1. Growth hormone (GH) deficiency is caused by congenital malformations, genetic defects, or acquired neurological insults.
2. It is characterized by short stature noted around 2 years of age often with a typical facies with midfacial crowding, mild obesity, and underdeveloped genitalia.
3. Clinical presentation of acute nephritic syndrome along with low complements and evidence of recent streptococcal infection establishes the diagnosis.
4. Bone age is below chronological age.
5. Diagnosis is confirmed by peak GH levels less than 10 ng/mL following a GH provocative stimulation test, and low serum IGF-1 levels.
6. GH supplementation is given as a daily nighttime injection (25–50 μg/kg/day) till epiphyseal closure for height gain.

Case Study | **Short Stature**

A12-year-old boy presented with growth retardation. His height was 131 cm and weight was 29 kg. Father's height was 173 cm and mother's height was 160 cm. There were no features of any systemic disease, chronic infections or endocrinopathies. His father had delayed onset of shaving and growth till the age of 19 years. On examination the boy was prepubertal with normal facies and body proportions.

Q1. What is the likely diagnosis?

Q2. How should he be evaluated?

Initial step of evaluation of a child with short stature is to compare height to population standards and parental height. As per growth charts, his height is below 3rd percentile and height Z score is –2.5 confirming short stature. Midparental height (mother's + father's height ÷ 2 + 6.5 cm) is 173 cm (25–50th percentile), which goes against a diagnosis of familial short stature. He has mild growth retardation, which in the presence of delayed puberty indicates the diagnosis of constitutional delay of puberty and growth. Although hypopituitarism may also present with delayed puberty and short stature; growth retardation is more severe. Screening investigations (complete blood counts, ESR, liver and renal function tests, bone age and ESR) should be done and he should be monitored for growth velocity for another year.

Screening investigations were normal. He had delayed bone age (10 years). A diagnosis of 'constitutional delay in growth and puberty (CDGP)' was made. On follow-up he had normal growth velocity (6 cm/year) but remained prepubertal till the age of 15 years (bone age 12.5 years).

Q3. What is the plan for further evaluation?

The features such as mild growth retardation, delayed bone age, paternal history of delayed puberty and normal growth velocity confirm the diagnosis of CDGP. He was given a course testosterone enanthate (50 mg intramuscularly monthly for six doses). This resulted in increase in growth velocity (10 cm/year) and improved pubertal status confirming the diagnosis. No further treatment was required.

598

Textbook of Pediatrics

Bajpai A, Menon PS. Growth hormone therapy. *Indian J Pediatr.* 2005;72:139–44.

Bajpai A, Sharma J, Menon PSN (Eds). Short Stature. *In*: Menon PSN, Bajpai A. *Practical Pediatric Endocrinology*, First edition. New Delhi: Jaypee; 2003.p.3–8.

Desai MP, Menon PSN, Bhatia V. *Pediatric Endocrine Disorders*. 3rd edition. Hyderabad: Orient Longman; 2014.79–119.

Lifshitz F, Botero D. Worrisome growth. *In*: Lifshitz F(Eds). *Pediatric Endocrinology*, 4th edition. New York: Marcel Dekker; 2003.p.1–47.

Patel L, Clayton PE. Normal and disordered growth. *In*: Brook CGD, Clayton PE, Brown RS. *Clinical Pediatric Endocrinology*, 5th edition. London: Blackwell Publishers; 2005.p.90–112.

Rosenfeld GR, Cohen P. Disorders of growth hormone/insulin like growth factor and action. *In*: Sperling MA. *Pediatric Endocrinology*, 2nd edn. Philadelphia: WB Saunders; 2002.p.211–88.

14.3 POLYURIA AND DIABETES INSIPIDUS

Polyuria is defined as urine output more than 5 mL/kg/hour or 2 L/m^2/day. At times, it may be the only manifestation of diabetes mellitus, brain tumor, or renal failure.

Physiology

Maintenance of water balance involves regulation of urine output and thirst. Hypothalamus controls thirst through osmoreceptors. Urine output is determined by solute load, hydration status, and urine concentration capacity. Fluid homeostasis involves close interaction of vasopressin, renin-angiotensin-aldosterone system, and atrial natriuretic peptide.

Antidiuretic hormone (ADH), also known as arginine vaso-pressin (AVP), secreted by the hypothalamus in response to increased plasma osmolality, acts on the collecting ducts to increase free water resorption. This results in decreased urinary output. *Renin-angiotensin-aldosterone system* is central to regulation of sodium, fluid and blood pressure. The system is activated by volume depletion and low blood pressure and results in vasoconstriction (angiotensin II effect) and salt retention (aldosterone effect).

Etiology

Polyuria may result from increased fluid intake or increased urinary losses of water:

I. **Increased Fluid Intake**
   * Iatrogenic
   * Compulsive water drinking (psychogenic polydipsia)
II. **Increased Urine Loss**
   i. *Increased solute excretion*
      * Osmotic diuresis: Diabetes mellitus, mannitol treatment
      * Salt loss: Adrenal insufficiency, diuretic, cerebral salt wasting, aldosterone resistance
   ii. *Impaired urinary concentration*
      * Diabetes insipidus: Central, peripheral
      * Renal tubular disorders: Renal tubular acidosis, Bartter syndrome.

Excessive water drinking is extremely rare and is a diagnosis of exclusion. Low urine osmolality makes it difficult to differentiate it from diabetes insipidus. Conditions with *inefficient aldosterone action* include adrenal insufficiency, isolated aldosterone deficiency, or aldosterone resistance. They present with hyponatremia, hyperkalemia, and dehydration.

DIABETES INSIPIDUS (DI)

Diabetes insipidus is caused by decreased ADH production (*central* or *neurogenic* DI) or action (*nephrogenic* DI). Urine osmolality remains low despite high plasma osmolality. Increased urine output is compensated by increased thirst. Dehydration is therefore unusual in the absence of abnor-mality in thirst mechanism. Infants are however, at a high risk of developing hypernatremic dehydration.

Central diabetes insipidus is commonly related to intracranial pathology (brain tumor, neurosurgery, trauma, or infection). *Nephrogenic diabetes insipidus* results from inherited or acquired resistance to vasopressin. Hypo-kalemia and hypercalcemia are the most common causes of nephrogenic diabetes insipidus.

I. **Central (Neurogenic) Diabetes Insipidus**
   * *Genetic defects*: Autosomal recessive, autosomal dominant, DIDMOAD syndrome
   * *Malformations*: Septo-optic dysplasia, holopros-encephaly, anencephaly
   * *Neurological insults*: Head trauma, neurosurgery, infection, brain death
   * *Infiltrative disorders*: Sarcoidosis, histiocytosis
   * *CNS tumors*: Craniopharyngioma, germinoma, pinealoma
II. **Nephrogenic (Peripheral) Diabetes Insipidus**
   * *Genetic*: X-linked vasopressin receptor mutation, autosomal recessive aquaporin mutation
   * *Acquired*: Hypokalemia, hypercalcemia, obstructive uropathy, nephrocalcinosis, exposure to drugs (lithium, demeclocycline)

Treatment	Diabetes Insipidus

* *Central diabetes insipidus* is treated by desmopressin, a vasopressin analog with prolonged duration of action. It is given intranasally (2.5–10 µg 12 hourly) or orally (50–200 µg 12 hourly). Overdose can result in hyponatremia.
* *Nephrogenic diabetes insipidus* Hydrochlorothiazide-amiloride combination (1–2 mg/kg/day) reduces urine output by decreasing delivery of free water to collecting ducts and distal tubule (site of vasopressin action). Indomethacin is added if there is no response to treatment. This should be combined with salt restriction and reduction in solute load.

APPROACH TO A CHILD WITH POLYURIA

24-hour urine output should be assessed to confirm polyuria. Subsequent work-up is guided towards identification of underlying cause.

History and Examination

Associated polyphagia and polydipsia suggest diabetes mellitus. Bony deformities or muscle weakness are indicative of renal tubular acidosis. History of head trauma, neuro-surgery, exposure to radiation, and features of focal deficits and raised intracranial tension should be evaluated. Careful search for features of histiocytosis like ear discharge, proptosis, rash, hepatosplenomegaly, lymphadenopathy, bone defects, and seborrheic dermatitis is essential. **Table 14.3** provides some useful clinical clues to the etiology of polyuria.

Table 14.3 Clues to Etiology of Polyuria	
Feature	*Diagnosis*
Midline defects	Central diabetes insipidus
Rickets	Renal tubular acidosis (RTA), renal failure
Failure to thrive	Nephrogenic diabetes insipidus, congenital adrenal hyperplasia, Bartter syndrome, RTA
Rash, seborrhea, bone defects	Histiocytosis
Hyperpigmentation	Adrenal insufficiency
Genital ambiguity	Congenital adrenal hyperplasia
Intellectual disability	CNS malformations, nephrogenic diabetes insipidus

Investigations

Initial investigations should include urine sugar and early morning specific gravity or osmolality. Blood gas, urea and serum electrolytes, calcium, and creatinine should be estimated. High plasma osmolality (>300 mOsm/kg or serum sodium >145 mmol/L) and low urine osmolality (less than 300 mOsm/kg, urine specific gravity less than 1005) are suggestive of inefficient ADH action. Patients with normal plasma osmolality and low urine osmolality (less than 700 mOsm/kg) should undergo water deprivation test. Urinary osmolality more than 700 mOsm/kg excludes diabetes insipidus. MRI of hypothalamic-pituitary region and pituitary function tests should be done in children with central diabetes insipidus. Evaluation of nephrogenic diabetes insipidus should include renal imaging and serum electrolytes. Figure 14.2 presents an algorithm for diagnosis of a child with polyuria, based on estimation of urine and plasma osmolality.

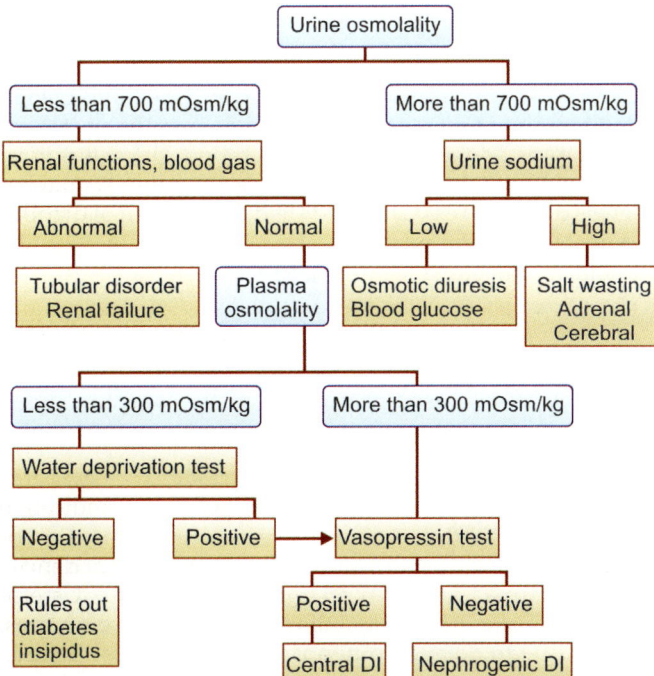

Fig. 14.2 Approach to polyuria

Water deprivation test This test is indicated in children with polyuria, low urinary osmolality and normal plasma osmolality. The aim is to increase plasma osmolality above 300 mOsm/kg (or serum sodium above 145 mmol/L) to achieve maximal renal concentration. Water deprivation is started early in the morning. The test should be stopped when urine osmolality increases above 700 mOsm/kg (or specific gravity more than 1010; excludes diabetes insipidus), plasma osmolality increases above 300 mOsm/kg (or serum sodium above 145 mmol/L; target achieved), or weight loss is more than 5% (risk of dehydration). Urine osmolality below 300 mOsm/kg with plasma osmolality above 300 mOsm/kg is diagnostic of diabetes insipidus and should be further evaluated with vasopressin.

Vasopressin response test This test is performed for differentiation of central and nephrogenic diabetes insipidus. Urine osmolality is measured one hour after vasopressin. An increase in urine osmolality by more than 50% of baseline is diagnostic of central diabetes insipidus while lower increase is suggestive of nephrogenic diabetes insipidus.

Treatment	Polyuria

Management is guided by the underlying cause. Treatment of diabetes mellitus (insulin), adrenal insufficiency (hydrocortisone), and tubular acidosis (bicarbonate) is effective in reducing urine output. Behavioral therapy is recommended for psychological polydipsia.

Revision Point

Polyuria and Diabetes Insipidus

1. Polyuria is defined as urine output more than 5 mL/kg/hour or more than 2 L/m^2/day.
2. Diabetes insipidus is caused by decreased ADH production (*central* or *neurogenic* DI) or action (*nephrogenic* DI).
3. High plasma osmolality (>300 mOsm/kg or serum sodium >145 mmol/L) and low urine osmolality (less than 300 mOsm/kg, and urine specific gravity less than 1005) are suggestive of inefficient ADH action.
4. Patients with normal plasma osmolality and low urine osmolality (less than 700 mOsm/kg) should undergo water deprivation test.
5. Urinary osmolality more than 700 mOsm/kg excludes diabetes insipidus.
6. Central diabetes insipidus is managed with desmopressin, a vasopressin analog given intranasal (2.5–10 µg 12 hourly) or orally (50–200 µg 12 hourly).

Bajpai A, Sharma J, Menon PSN. Diabetes insipidus. *In: Practical Pediatric Endocrinology*, First edition. New Delhi: Jaypee; 200.p.17–23.

Ball SG, Barber T, Baylis PH. Tests of posterior pituitary function. *J Endocrinol Invest*. 2003; 26 (7 Suppl):15–24.

Desai MP, Menon PSN, Bhatia V. *Pediatric Endocrine Disorders*. 3rd Edition. Hyderabad: Orient Longman; 2014.p.299–317.

Majzoub JA, Srivatsa A. Diabetes insipidus: clinical and basic aspects. *Pediatr Endocrinol Rev*. 2006;4 Suppl 1:60-5.

Muglia LJ. Majzoub JA. Disorders of the posterior pituitary. *In:* Sperling MA. *Pediatric Endocrinology*, 2nd edition. Philadelphia: Saunders; 2002;.p.289–322.

Ranadive SA, Rosenthal SM. Pediatric disorders of water balance. *Endocrine Clin North Am*. 2009; 38:663–72.

Rivkees SA, Dunbar N, Wilson TA, The management of central diabetes insipidus in infancy: desmopressin, low renal solute load formula, thiazide diuretics. *J Pediatr Endocrinol Metab.* 2007;20:459–69.

14.4 DIABETES MELLITUS

Diabetes mellitus is characterized by impaired insulin production and/or its action resulting in high blood glucose levels. Blood glucose higher than 126 mg/dL in the fasting state; and 200 mg/dL two hours after oral glucose challenge; and/or blood glycosylated hemoglobin (HbA1c) levels more than 6.5% are diagnostic.

Most children with type 1 diabetes have very high blood glucose levels at presentation and do not need a formal glucose tolerance test. HbA1c is also not an established parameter for diagnosis of diabetes in children.

Classification

I. **Type 1 Diabetes Mellitus** (absolute insulin deficiency due to β cell destruction)
   i. 1A (autoimmune)
   ii. 1B (non-autoimmune)

II. **Type 2 Diabetes Mellitus** (insulin resistance with relative insulin deficiency)

III. **Other Specific Types of Diabetes**
   - *Genetic disorders of β cell function*: Maturity onset diabetes of young (MODY), mitochondrial disorders
   - *Genetic disorders of insulin action*: Insulin receptor defects, lipodystrophy
   - *Exocrine pancreatic disease*: Cystic fibrosis, fibro-calculus pancreatic diabetes (FCPD), dysgenesis, hemochromatosis
   - *Genetic syndromes*: Turner, Klinefelter, Down, and Prader-Willi syndromes.
   - *Endocrinopathies*: GH excess, Cushing syndrome, hyperthyroidism
   - *Drugs:* Steroids, L-asparaginase, cyclosporine, tacrolimus, interferon, pentamidine
   - *Infections*: Congenital rubella, cytomegalovirus (CMV)

IV. Gestational Diabetes

Type 1 diabetes mellitus is the commonest type of diabetes in children. An increase in type 2 diabetes mellitus has been noted with current increase in prevalence of childhood obesity. The differentiation of type 1 from type 2 diabetes mellitus is largely clinical **(Table 14.4)**.

TYPE 1 DIABETES MELLITUS

Pathophysiology

- *Genetic factors* Most important genetic focus for type 1 diabetes lies in chromosome 6 and is linked with HLA DR3 and DR4. Genetic predisposition is present from birth.
- *Environmental factors* Implicated in the pathogenesis of type 1 diabetes include viral infections (rubella, coxsackievirus and cytomegalovirus), environmental toxins and early introduction to cow's milk. Autoimmune destruction of islet cells is the final pathway in the pathogenesis of type 1 diabetes mellitus. Antibodies

Table 14.4 Comparison of Common Forms of Childhood Diabetes Mellitus

Feature	Type 1 diabetes mellitus	Type 2 diabetes mellitus
Age at onset	Throughout childhood	Postpubertal
Presentation	Acute	Insidious
Diabetic ketoacidosis	30–40%	5–10%
Family history of diabetes	5–10%	75–90%
Obesity	Around 20%	More than 90%
Acanthosis nigricans	Absent	Usually present
Insulin requirement	Universal	Variable
Serum C–peptide levels	Low	High or normal
Insulin sensitivity	Normal	Low
Anti-islet cell antibodies	Positive in 80%	Positive in 10%
Treatment	Insulin	Diet, metformin

against islet cell and its components like insulin and glutamate dehydrogenase (GAD) are present in 70–80% children.

Natural History

In the presence of a conducive environmental setting, autoimmune process directed against islet cells is initiated. More than 80% of the pancreatic β-cell insulin synthesis and release capacity have been destroyed before the clinical features manifest.

- *Pre-diabetes phase* Evidence of autoimmunity is the only marker of disease at this stage. The amount of insulin produced is sufficient to maintain normal blood glucose levels.
- *Overt diabetes* This phase coincides with development of clinical symptoms leading to the diagnosis. With progressive destruction of β-cells, insulin secretory capacity is adequate to maintain blood glucose during physiological state but unable to regulate blood glucose levels during stress. This leads to development of diabetic symptoms in the presence of precipitating factors like infection and stress.
- *Honeymoon phase* After the initial diagnosis of diabetes and resolution of precipitating factor insulin requirements diminish. This phase lasts from 6 months to 2 years.
- *Total diabetes* This is characterized by complete β-cell destruction with no capacity for endogenous insulin synthesis or release.

Clinical Features

Children with type 1 diabetes mellitus present with polyuria, polydipsia and polyphagia. Diabetic ketoacidosis (DKA) is present in 30–40% at diagnosis. The figure is higher in India due to delayed diagnosis. Other features include recurrent infections, growth retardation, hepatomegaly and delayed puberty.

Treatment   **Diabetes Mellitus Type 1**

Goals of management include achieving good glycemic control with flexible life style and normal growth. Components of management include (*i*) insulin therapy, (*ii*) nutritional management, (*iii*) monitoring of glycemic control, (*iv*) screening for complications; and (*v*) parental/child education. This requires a multidisciplinary team approach including pediatrician/endocrinologist, diabetes educator, social worker, and nutritionist.

A. Insulin Therapy

Animal insulins have high antigenicity and complications. These have been replaced by recombinant human insulin and insulin analogs. Insulin preparations are classified as rapid, intermediate and long acting. **Table 14.5** details the characteristics of various types of insulin.

- *Rapid or short acting* Regular insulin has a delayed onset of action mandating a gap of 30–60 minutes between insulin injection and meal. Rapid acting insulin analogs (Lispro, Aspart, and Glulisine) have an immediate onset of action and can be given along with meals.
- *Intermediate acting* These preparations have been derived by chemical combination of insulin with zinc (lente) or protamine (NPH) leading to prolonged duration of action.
- *Long acting* These preparations have the advantage of prolonged duration of action requiring once daily administration. They have been developed by chemical (ultralente) or structural modification (glargine, detemir and degludec) of insulin. Long-acting insulin analogs have the advantage of stable insulin supply with no peak.

Modes of Administration
- *Syringe* Disposable plastic syringes are the commonest mode of insulin administration. They are available as 40 and 100 gradations per mL (U-40 and U-100).
- *Pen* Insulin pens have the advantage of convenience. They are not used frequently in children on mixed split regimens due to the need of two pens. They are very useful in children on basal bolus regimen.
- *Insulin pump* Insulin pumps are electronic devices connected to subcutaneous catheters. They deliver insulin at a constant rate with extra doses before meals. Their use is limited by prohibitive cost.

- *Inhaled insulin* Inhaled devices have been developed to deliver rapid acting insulin to avoid repeated injections. These devices have however been withdrawn from the market.

Dose Usual daily insulin requirement in prepubertal, pubertal and postpubertal individual is 0.6–0.8, 0.8–1.0 and 1–1.2 units per kg per day, respectively. Insulin requirement is higher in pubertal children and those in postketoacidosis phase.

Practical points Insulin should be stored at a temperature of 4–8°C. If refrigerator is not available, earthen pot or cool area of the room could be used. Insulin should never be frozen. The insulin vial should be used within three months of opening if stored in the refrigerator and one month if stored at room temperature. The site of insulin administration should be frequently rotated to avoid development of lipohypertrophy.

Administration Twice daily injection regime is the minimum beginning point for the treatment of type 1 diabetes. More intensive regimens with multiple dose insulin injections and subcutaneous insulin infusion pumps are used if required.
- *Basal-bolus regime* This involves the use of a long (ultralente, Glargine or Detemir) or intermediate acting insulin (lente or NPH) to provide basal insulin (40–50%); with a fast acting insulin given as a bolus before each meal (50–60%), usually before breakfast, lunch and dinner. This regimen provides flexibility with regard to the amount and timing of meals, and thus preferred in adolescents.
- *Mixed-split regime* This regime involves administration of a combination of intermediate (lente or NPH) and short acting insulins (regular or lispro) two times a day, before breakfast and before dinner. The regime allocates two-thirds of the daily insulin requirement to before breakfast and one-third for before dinner. The usual ratio of intermediate to short acting insulin is 2:1. This regime is indicated in children younger than 5 years of age to avoid mid-meal hypoglycemia and has the advantage of simplicity, low cost, need of less injections, and glycemic monitoring. However, it is not physiological and mandates strict diet pattern.

B. Nutritional Management

Nutritional management aims to ensure adequate growth and development with desirable glycemic control. Age appropriate healthy diet is recommended. Energy intake should be equal to the recommended dietary allowance for the age group.

		Table 14.5 Pharmacokinetic Profile of Insulin Preparations		
Preparation	*Onset*	*Peak*	*Duration*	*Indications*
Rapid acting insulin analogs Lispro Aspart	5–10 min 5–10 min	1–3 h 1–3 h	3–4 h 3–5 h	Young children on mixed–split regimen Insulin pump, bolus insulin
Short acting insulins Regular	30–60 min	2–4 h	5–8 h	DKA, mixed–split regimen
Intermediate acting insulins Lente NPH	1–2 h 1–2 h	3–10 h 2–8 h	18–24 h 16–24 h	Mixed-split regimen Mixed-split, basal–bolus regimen
Long acting insulin analogs Glargine Detemir Degludec	2–4 h 1–2 h 1–2 h	Peakless 6–12 h Peakless	20–24 h 20–24 h 48–72 h	Basal insulin Basal insulin, mixed-split regimen Basal insulin

14

Target	Less than 6 years	6 – 12 years	>12 years
Table 14.6 Suggested Levels (mg/dL) of Glycemic Control			
Blood glucose (mg/dL)			
Premeal	100–180	70–180	70–130
Bedtime	110–200	100–180	90–140
HbA1c	Less than 8%	Less than 7.5%	Less than 7.5%

Carbohydrates should provide 50–60% of total calorie intake. Total energy derived from fat should be 30–35% out of which majority of energy is derived from monounsaturated fat. Saturated and polyunsaturated fat should not account for more than 10% each of the daily caloric requirement. Rest of the calories is derived from proteins of high quality.

C. Monitoring of Glycemic Control
- *Blood glucose* Monitoring is an essential part of management of type 1 diabetes, and should be measured before all meals and at bedtime. If frequent monitoring is not possible, measurement of blood glucose at different times on different days may be performed. Glucometer is the ideal device for measurement of blood sugar.
- *Ketone monitoring* It is important in identification of diabetic ketoacidosis. Glucometers that measure blood ketone have been developed. Ketones should be tested in children with fever, blood glucose greater than 270 mg/dL and with abdominal pain and tachypnea.
- *Continuous glucose monitoring systems (CGMS)* These are inserted subcutaneously and measure interstitial glucose levels every 5–15 minutes for 5–14 days. They provide valuable information for modification of insulin doses.
- *Glycosylated hemoglobin (HbA1c)* It represents the fraction of hemoglobin that reacts to blood glucose in a non-enzymatic fashion. Its levels are indicative of blood glucose control over the previous three months. HbA1c is the best marker for glycemic control and evaluating the risk of complications. Suggested levels of glycemic control are depicted in **Table 14.6**.

Sick Day Management
A child with diabetes mellitus is prone to hypoglycemia and hyperglycemia during an acute illness. Appropriate management during illness is essential for prevention of hypoglycemia and ketoacidosis (Fig. 14.3). This involves regular monitoring of blood glucose and urine ketones. Liberal fluid intake is recommended.

Insulin should never be discontinued. Insulin dose should be increased in the presence of fever and pneumonia, conditions associated with hyperglycemia. Additional doses of regular insulin (10–20% of total daily dose) should be given in the presence of hyperglycemia and ketosis. The dose should be decreased by 10–20% in the presence of vomiting and diarrhea. Children with persistent ketosis, reduced oral intake, altered sensorium and recurrent vomiting should be brought to medical attention.

Complications
Diabetes mellitus is a serious condition associated with short and long-term complications listed below. Early identification and management of these conditions is essential for preventing severe morbidity. Major complications are listed below:
- I. *Acute* Hypoglycemia, diabetic ketoacidosis
- II. *Chronic*:
  - Vascular: Retinopathy, nephropathy, neuropathy, coronary artery disease
  - Nonvascular: Growth failure, delayed puberty, cataract, necrobiosis lipoidica diabeticorum, limited joint mobility
  - Autoimmune: Hypothyroidism, celiac disease, adrenal insufficiency

Hypoglycemia is the commonest acute complication of type 1 diabetes mellitus. Low blood sugar levels stimulate

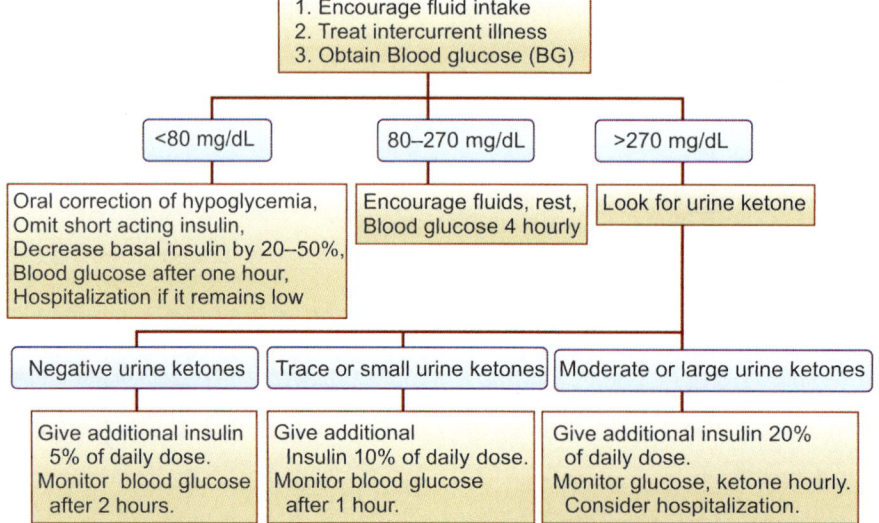

Fig. 14.3 Sick day management in type 1 diabetes mellitus

the sympathetic system leading to palpitation, sweating, tremor and anxiety. Further reduction in blood sugar levels produces neuroglucopenic symptoms—impaired mentation, headache, confusion, and convulsions. Mild and moderate hypoglycemia can be treated with oral glucose (5–15 g). Parenteral therapy with glucagon (10–20 μg/kg, maximum dose 1 mg) or dextrose (2–5 mL/kg 10% dextrose) is required for severe hypoglycemia.

Education

Diabetic education is an extremely important part of management. Initial emphasis should be on survival skills like injection technique, hypoglycemia management, and sick day guidelines. This should be followed-up with education regarding the dose adjustments, glycemic targets, and dietary advice **(Table 14.7)**.

Follow-up

Children should be reviewed two weeks after discharge and three monthly thereafter. Glycemic control should be compared to age specific targets as shown in **Table 14.5**. Follow-up should include assessment of glycemic control (child diary, logs, and HbA1c), complications of insulin therapy (lipohypertrophy and hypoglycemia), disease complications and growth. Special emphasis should be given on injection technique and glucose monitoring. In children with early morning hyperglycemia, blood glucose levels should be performed at 4 AM to differentiate between *Dawn phenomenon* (high blood glucose) from *Somogyi phenomenon* (low blood glucose) **(Table 14.8)**.

Table 14.7 Components of Diabetic Education

Category	Key points
Disease	• Lifelong disease requiring insulin treatment • Need for close follow-up • Honeymoon phase and decreased insulin requirement • Acute and long-term complications
Insulin	• Injection technique • Syringe selection according to insulin (U 100, U 40) • Insulin storage • Duration of use after opening of vial (one month in room temperature; three months in refrigerator) • Mixing of short acting and intermediate insulins • Injection site, need for rotation, lipo hyper trophy
Blood glucose monitoring	• Glucometer technique • Frequency—Before meals and bedtime
Hypoglycemia	• Identification and management; glucagon injection
Sick day guidelines	• Never stop insulin • Regular blood glucose and ketone monitoring Indications for hospitalization

Table 14.8 Comparison of Dawn and Somogyi Phenomena

Feature	Dawn phenomenon	Somogyi phenomenon
Morning blood glucose	High	High
Blood glucose at 4 am	High	Low
Pathophysiology	GH and cortisol surge	Rebound hyperglycemia
Insulin dose	Lower than required	Higher than required
Weight gain	Absent	Common
Diabetic symptoms	Common	Absent
Intervention	Increase insulin dose	Decrease insulin dose

DIABETIC KETOACIDOSIS

Diabetic ketoacidosis (DKA) is the most severe acute complication of diabetes mellitus and characterized by presence of hyperglycemia (blood glucose more than 200 mg/dL), metabolic acidosis (pH less than 7.30 and bicarbonate less than 15 mmol/L), and presence of ketones in serum and urine.

Pathophysiology

The disorder is precipitated by infection, stress, and/or trauma. It results from increased production of ketoacids (due to increased lipolysis and ketogenesis) and hyperglycemia (due to increased glycogenolysis and gluconeogenesis on one hand and decreased glucose utilization on the other). Accumulation of ketoacids produces acidosis which is responsible for Kussmaul breathing, abdominal pain, and fruity odor (acetone). Osmotic diuresis causes increased urinary losses of sodium, potassium and phosphate leading to significant deficits of these electrolytes.

Clinical Features

Most of the children present with shock and acidotic breathing, with a past history suggestive of diabetes. Altered sensorium, recurrent vomiting and abdominal pain, rapid breathing, and severe dehydration are common presenting features of diabetic ketoacidosis. A child with DKA may also present as acute abdomen, abdominal distension and tenderness.

Evaluation

Initial evaluation should include assessment of airway, breathing and circulation. The child should be assessed for presence of infection, stress, trauma, or missed insulin dose; hydration level, hemodynamic status (pulse rate, blood pressure); and level of consciousness. Initial investigation should include blood glucose, blood gas, electrolytes, and urinary or blood ketones. Hyperglycemia is associated with factitious hyponatremia with a fall in serum sodium level by 1.6 mEq/L for every 100 mg/dL increase in blood glucose. Serum sodium levels should be corrected for the levels of blood glucose by the formula given as follows.

$$Corrected\ Na = Observed\ Sodium + [(Glucose - 100)/100] \times 1.6\ mEq/L$$

Detailed evaluation for underlying infection (hemogram, chest X-ray, blood and urine cultures) should be performed.

Treatment — Diabetic Ketoacidosis

Management involves 6 steps: (*i*) correction of fluid deficit, (*ii*) metabolic acidosis, (*iii*) electrolyte disturbances, (*iv*) lowering of blood glucose, (*v*) assessment and treatment of underlying cause, and (*vi*) close monitoring for complications. Children below the age of two years, those with altered sensorium or shock and those with pH less than 7 require intensive care management.

Fluids Fluid management results in significant improvement in general condition, blood gas and glucose. Normal saline (10 mL/kg) should be infused as soon as the diagnosis of DKA is established. Repeated fluid boluses should be avoided. Subsequent fluid therapy aims at providing fluid deficit and maintenance requirement evenly over a period of at least 48 hours (total fluid 3–3.5 L/m²/day).

Insulin Insulin should be withheld during the initial hydration phase. After hydration, insulin is administered using the intravenous route at a rate of 0.1 unit/kg/hour (0.05 units/kg/h in infants). Insulin bolus is not required. Insulin should be dissolved in saline and infused intravenously using electronic infusion pumps or microinfusion sets. Insulin adheres to the surface of intravenous tubing resulting in lower rate of insulin delivery. Intravenous tubings should be flushed with insulin to saturate the binding sites. Insulin infusion should be increased in quanta of 25% to 0.2 unit/kg/h, if required.

Sodium Half normal saline is the fluid of choice in DKA. Recent studies suggest that rehydration with normal saline may also be acceptable.

Potassium Serum potassium is a poor indicator of intracellular potassium status that may be elevated due to the effect of metabolic acidosis. Correction of metabolic acidosis and administration of insulin results in migration of potassium into the intracellular compartment causing life-threatening hypokalemia. Potassium replacement (40 mEq/L) should begin only after rehydration. Potassium should be avoided in the presence of hyperkalemia (potassium more than 6 mEq/L or ECG changes of hyperkalemia) or anuria.

Dextrose Dextrose containing fluid (5%) should be added once the blood glucose falls below 270 mg/dL (10% when less than 200 mg/dL).

Acidosis correction Alkali therapy should be avoided due to risk of cerebral edema, hypokalemia and tissue hypoxia. Sodium bicarbonate should be considered only in the presence of very severe metabolic acidosis (pH <6.9) in the setting of cardiorespiratory arrest.

Box 14.1 provides a sample prescription for a 10-year-old child weighing 30 kg presenting with diabetic ketoacidosis.

Monitoring

Regular assessment of urine output, hemodynamic status and sensorium is required. Blood glucose, pH, osmolality and electrolytes should be monitored. Blood pH and ketones are the most important parameters to follow. Urine ketones have no role in monitoring of DKA as they persist for at least

Box 14.1 Management Plan for Diabetic Ketoacidosis	
A 10-year-old boy, weight 30 kg, body surface area- 1 m², Dehydration level - 10% Blood sugar-720 mg/dL, pH- 6.94, Na 140 mEq/L, K-5.5 mEq/L, presents with shock and acidotic breathing.	
Hydration phase	
Recommendation plan	Initial hydration (10 mL/kg of isotonic fluid
	Asses airway breathing and circulation
	Oxygen, catheterization, antibiotics Normal saline – 300 mL over 1 hour (repeat if required)
Dehydration correction	
Volume	Calculate maintenance and deficit to correct evenly over 48 hour Maintenance fluid for 48 hour = 1.5 L × surface area × 2 = 3 L Fluid deficit = 10% = 100 mL/kg = 3 L Total fluid required over 48 hours = 6 L
Sodium	Add 70–100 mEq/L of sodium (Use 0.45% normal saline)
Dextrose	No dextrose in fluids till blood sugar < 270 mg/dL*
Potassium	Add 40 mEq/L potassium chloride
Alkali	Not required
Plan	0.45% saline 1 L with 40 mEq/L KCl every 8 hours over 48 h
Insulin	
Recommendation	0.1 Unit/kg/hr to be started only after initial hydration.
Plan	Regular insulin 72 units in 24 mL normal saline at the rate of 1 mL/hr Flush intravenous tubing with insulin

* Add 5% dextrose when blood sugar 200–270 mg/dL and 10% dextrose when blood sugar < 200 mg/dL

48 hours even after correction. Insulin infusion rates should be lowered when the acidosis has been corrected. Transition to subcutaneous insulin should be done after correction of hyperglycemia and metabolic acidosis along with normal sensorium and adequate oral intake. Insulin infusion should be decreased in quanta of 0.01 unit/kg/h till the infusion rate of 0.05 unit/kg/h is achieved (Fig. 14.4). At this stage subcutaneous regular insulin (0.25 units/kg) should be given. Insulin infusion should be discontinued 30 minutes later.

Complications

Cerebral edema, the most serious complication of DKA, is characterized by headache, bradycardia, hypertension, change in neurological status and decreased oxygen saturation, in an otherwise improving child. Clinically apparent cerebral edema occurs in 0.7–1% cases of DKA. The condition most commonly occurs during the first 5–15 hours of therapy.

Mannitol (5 mL/kg of 20% solution) should be given immediately if any of the features of cerebral edema develop. Delay in management results in devastating consequences.

Other complications include hypoglycemia, hypokalemia and unusual infections (rhinocerebral mucormycosis).

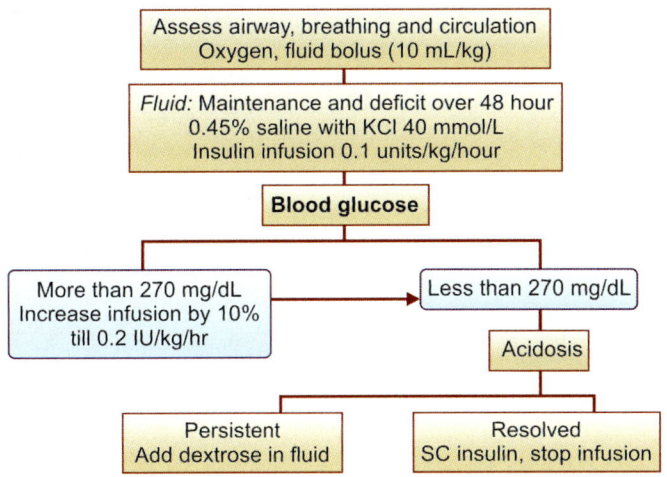

Fig. 14.4 Approach to management of DKA

CHRONIC COMPLICATIONS

Prolonged hyperglycemia is associated with long-term complications. Early identification and management of these complications is essential for reducing long-term morbidity of the diabetes. In prepubertal individuals screening for complications should be performed at the age of 11 years or after five years of disease, whichever is earlier. Evaluation for complications should be performed at two years of disease in pubertal children. Subsequent screening should be done annually. Identification of these complications should prompt tighter glycemic control and specific management **(Table 14.9)**.

TYPE 2 DIABETES MELLITUS

Previously considered to be restricted to adults, type 2 diabetes mellitus is being increasingly diagnosed in children. An increased incidence in childhood obesity appears to be related to the rise in type 2 diabetes mellitus in children. Insulin resistance, relative insulin deficiency and increased hepatic glucose production are the major pathophysiological factors in type 2 diabetes mellitus. The diagnosis is established on the basis of lack of ketosis despite no insulin therapy, presence of obesity and acanthosis nigricans and demonstration of high C-peptide and insulin levels. Treatment includes lifestyle modifications and dietary interven-

tion. Metformin (500–1000 mg 12 hourly) is the only agent approved for use in children with type 2 diabetes mellitus. Insulin treatment is required in children presenting with high blood glucose levels and/or ketoacidosis.

NEONATAL DIABETES

Onset of diabetes before the age of 6 months should prompt the possibility of neonatal diabetes. Managing neonatal diabetes is challenging as providing insulin for breastfeeding is very difficult. A significant proportion of these infants have transient diabetes that improves over a couple of months. The most common cause of persistent neonatal diabetes is potassium channel defects (in *ABCC8* and *KCNJ11* genes) that are responsive to oral sulfonylureas.

Revision Point

Diabetes Mellitus

1. Diabetes mellitus is characterized by blood glucose higher than 126 mg/dL in the fasting state; and 200 mg/dL two hours after oral glucose challenge; and/or blood glycosylated hemoglobin (HbA1c) levels more than 6.5% is diagnostic.
2. Type 1 diabetes mellitus is the commonest type in children with type 2 diabetes being increasingly diagnosed in older children.
3. Children with type 1 diabetes mellitus present with polyuria, polydipsia, and polyphagia. Diabetic keto-acidosis (DKA) is present in 30–40% at diagnosis.
4. Components of management include insulin therapy, nutritional management, monitoring of glycemic control, screening for complications, and parental/child education. This requires a multidisciplinary team approach including pediatrician/endocrinologist, diabetic educator, social worker and nutritionist.
5. Recombinant human insulin or its analogs are administered as a basal-bolus or mixed-split regime.
6. Diabetic ketoacidosis (DKA) is the most severe acute complication of type 1 diabetes and is characterized by the presence of hyperglycemia (blood glucose >200 mg/dL), metabolic acidosis (pH <7.3 and bicarbonate <15 mmol/L), and the presence of ketones in serum and urine.
7. Management of DKA includes correction of fluid deficit and electrolyte disturbances, and administration of insulin along with treatment of the underlying cause.

Table 14.9 Identification and Management of Chronic Complications of Diabetes			
Complication	*Indication*	*Procedure*	*Management*
Retinopathy Prepubertal Pubertal	Duration more than 5 year* Duration more than 2 year*	Dilated fundus	Better control, LASER
Nephropathy Prepubertal Pubertal	Duration more than 5 year* Duration more than 2 year*	Urine albumin	Better control, ACE inhibitor, control BP
Thyroid disease	At diagnosis followed by 2 yearly	TSH, thyroid antibodies	Thyroxine
Hyperlipidemia Prepubertal Pubertal	At diagnosis followed by 5 yearly Two yearly	Lipid profile	Better control, Statin

* Annually thereafter

14

Case Study | Diabetic Ketoacidosis

A 10-year-old boy presented with one-day history of diarrhea (three episodes) and vomiting (four episodes, non-projectile). On examination, he had tachycardia, cold peripheries and severe dehydration. His weight was 30 kg as against 33 kg recorded one week ago. His urine output was normal.

Q1. What are the diagnostic possibilities?

Q2. How should he be evaluated?

Gastroenteritis is the obvious cause of dehydration in the child; severe dehydration is however unlikely with this level of gastrointestinal fluid loss. Dehydration disproportionately greater than the amount of gastrointestinal loss should prompt evaluation for conditions associated with extra-intestinal fluid loss like diabetes mellitus, diabetes insipidus, and acute tubular necrosis. Dehydration due to gastrointestinal fluid loss is associated with oliguria; normal urine output in the presence of dehydration indicates renal fluid loss. Investigations should be directed towards excluding causes of renal fluid loss (blood glucose for diabetes mellitus and serum electrolytes for acute tubular necrosis and diabetes insipidus).

Urine sugar was positive (3+) with hyperglycemia (550 mg/dL, 30.6 mmol/L). Blood gases revealed severe metabolic acidosis (pH 7.01, bicarbonate 7 mmol/L, base excess −22 mmol/L).

Q3. How should he be treated?

Hyperglycemia and ketoacidosis are diagnostic of diabetic ketoacidosis (DKA). Initial management should include stabilization of airway, breathing and circulation. Oxygen should be started and normal saline bolus (10 mL/kg) should be given over one hour. Rehydration correction should be done over 48 hours. Fluid calculation should include deficit according to the level of dehydration (10%, 100 mL/kg, 3 L) and maintenance fluid (1.5 L daily, 3 L for two days). This fluid (6 L) should be should be distributed evenly over 48 hours (125 mL/hour) as half-normal saline (77 mmol/L) with potassium chloride (40 mmol/L). Insulin should be started as an intravenous infusion at a rate of 0.1 unit/kg/hour (50 unit of insulin dissolved in 50 mL normal saline, administered at 3 mL/hour). Blood glucose, blood gas and serum electrolytes should be monitored hourly.

At six hours of treatment, blood glucose was 230 mg/dL (12.8 mmol/L) with persistent metabolic acidosis (pH 7.12, bicarbonate 10 mmol/L, base excess −12 mmol/L). What is the next step?

Hyperglycemia resolves before metabolic acidosis during treatment of DKA. Reduction of insulin infusion at this point is not desirable, as this would prolong the duration of metabolic acidosis. Insulin infusion should be continued with addition of dextrose in the rehydration fluid.

Blood glucose levels remained stable after addition of dextrose in the hydration fluid. At 10 hours of treatment, clinical condition had improved with normalization of blood gas (pH 7.34, bicarbonate 20 mmol/L, base excess −4 mmol/L), sensorium and hydration status. Urine ketone were still present (3 +).

Q4. What is the plan for further management?

Improvement in clinical condition and resolution of acidosis indicate the need for transition to subcutaneous insulin. This can be done despite persistent urinary ketosis as urine ketones are unreliable marker of response to treatment in DKA. He should be advised to eat followed by subcutaneous insulin (0.25 units/kg). Insulin infusion should be discontinued thirty minutes after insulin injection.

American Association of Clinical Endocrinologists (AACE). Medical Guidelines for Clinical Practice for the Management of Diabetes Mellitus. *Endocrine Practice*. 2007;13 (supplement 1):1–68.

American Diabetes Association. Position statement: Standards of Medical Care in Diabetes—2011:. *Diabetes Care*. 2011;Suppl 1:34.

Bajpai A, Sharma J, Menon PSN. Diabetes mellitus. *In: Practical Pediatric Endocrinology*. New Delhi: Jaypee Brothers; 2003;55–7.

Daneman D. Type 1 diabetes. *Lancet*. 2006;367:847–58.

Diabetes Control and Complications Trial. The effect of long-term intensified insulin treatment on the development of microvascular complications of diabetes mellitus. *N Engl J Med*. 1993;329:304–9.

Dunger DB, Sperling MA, Acerini CL, *et al*. ESPE/LWPES consensus statement on diabetic ketoacidosis in children and adolescents. *Arch Dis Child*. 2004;89:188–94.

Glaser NS, Barnett P, McCaslin I, *et al*. Risk factors for cerebral edema in children with diabetic ketoacidosis. The Pediatric Emergency Medicine Collaborative Research Committee of the AAP. *N Eng J Med*. 2001;344:264–9.

International Society for Pediatric and Adolescent Diabetes (ISPAD). Clinical Practice Consensus Guidelines. *Pediatric Diabetes*. 2009;10 (Supplement 12):1–210.

Irani A, Menon PSN, Bhatia V. Diabetes mellitus in children and adolescents in India. Clinical Practice Guidelines 2011. Lucknow: Indian Society of Pediatric and Adolescent Endocrinology; 2011.

Menon PSN, Bajpai A. Diabetes in the developing countries. *In*: Menon RK, Sperling MA. *Pediatric Diabetes*. Boston: Kluwer Academic Publishers; 2003. p. 141–64.

Rachneil M, Perlman K, Daneman D. Insulin analogues in children and teens with type 1 diabetes: advantages and caveats. *Pediatr Clin North Am*. 2005;52:1651–75.

14.5 HYPOTHYROIDISM

Thyroid hormones are involved in the regulation of somatic and intellectual growth, intermediary metabolism and thermoregulation. There is a critical phase in the early neonatal period for the effect of thyroid hormone on mental development. This emphasizes the need for early diagnosis and appropriate management of congenital hypothyroidism.

Physiology

The thyroid gland is formed by an invagination of endoderm of the foregut in a pouch in the floor of the pharynx. The gland then migrates from foramen cecum located at the base of tongue to its position in the neck. Initial step of thyroid hormone synthesis is the transport of iodine into the thyroid cells using sodium-iodine co-transporter. Iodine is then organified to monoiodotyrosine (MIT) and diiodotyrosine (DIT). This is followed by production of thyroxine (T4) by coupling of two DIT molecules, and triiodothyronine (T3) by coupling of one DIT and one MIT molecule. *Thyroid peroxidase* (TPO), the enzyme regulating this process, is the rate-limiting enzyme in thyroid hormone synthesis. This process is controlled by thyroid stimulating hormone (TSH). TSH secretion is controlled by thyrotropin-releasing hormone (TRH) released from the hypothalamus and feedback control of T4. T3 is the active form and mostly formed in the circulation by deiodination of T4. This process is stimulated in hypothyroidism. T3 levels thus are the last to fall in hypothyroidism. TRH levels increase after birth resulting in increase in TSH, T3 and T4 levels. The levels fall rapidly by day 3 and become normal in the next few weeks. Neonatal screening for hypothyroidism should therefore be done preferably on or after day 3.

Assessment of Thyroid Function

Thyroid functions are assessed by estimation of TSH and free and total T3 and T4. TSH is the most sensitive indicator of primary hypothyroidism but has limited value in the diagnosis of central hypothyroidism. T4 levels are better indicators of thyroid status than T3 due to increased conversion of T4 to T3 during thyroid deplete state. Low free T4 (FT4) and TSH levels are suggestive of central hypothyroidism while high TSH levels indicate primary hypothyroidism. Repeated elevation in TSH with normal FT4 suggests compensated primary hypothyroidism.

Etiology

Hypothyroidism could be caused by defects in the hypothalamus, pituitary, or thyroid gland as shown below:

I. **Central**
  - *Malformations:* Septo-optic dysplasia, holoprosencephaly
  - *Genetic defects: Pit 1, PROP 1, HESX 1* mutations
  - *CNS insults:* Trauma, surgery, radiation, infection
  - *CNS tumors:* Craniopharyngioma, germinoma

II. **Primary**
  - *Dysgenesis:* Aplasia, dysplasia, ectopia of thyroid
  - *Enzyme defects:* Trapping, organification, thyroglobulin synthesis, deiodination
  - Iodine deficiency
  - *Autoimmune thyroiditis:* Hashimoto disease, polyglandular disorders
  - *Ablation of thyroid:* Surgery, radiation, infection
  - *Goitrogens:* Thiocyanates, thionamides, lithium, amiodarone
  - *Transient causes:* Transplacental passage of antibody, drugs, goitrogens

Primary Hypothyroidism

Defects in thyroid hormone synthesis, disordered development, or destruction of thyroid gland are the common causes of primary hypothyroidism.

- The syndrome of *deaf-mutism* and severe neurological handicaps is a result of prolonged iodine deficiency and is preventable by iodine supplementation. Low urine iodine concentration with residence in iodine deficient area is suggestive of the condition.

- *Thyroid dysgenesis* is the commonest cause of congenital hypothyroidism (75% of all cases). The disorder encompasses a spectrum ranging from complete to partial agenesis to ectopic thyroid. They are identified by radionuclide scan.
- *Biosynthetic defects* include disorders affecting iodine transport, peroxidation, thyroglobulin synthesis and deiodination.
- *Pendred syndrome,* a disorder of the pendrin gene, is associated with decreased intracellular transport of iodine and deafness. Smooth colloid goiter is characteristic.
- *Transient congenital hypothyroidism* may occur following transplacental passage of TSH receptor blocking antibodies, iodine exposure and treatment with drugs like amiodarone.

Autoimmune Thyroiditis

It is the commonest cause of acquired hypothyroidism. The disorder is more common in girls and presents with subtle clinical features. Goiter is often nodular and firm in contrast to soft goiter seen in dyshormonogenesis. Anti-thyroperoxidase (anti-TPO) and anti-thyroglobulin antibodies are usually present. Autoimmune thyroiditis may be associated with other autoimmune endocrinopathies such as adrenal insufficiency, type 1 diabetes and hypoparathyroidism.

Central Hypothyroidism

Central hypothyroidism is caused by defects in the hypothalamic-pituitary axis. These disorders are characterized by low TSH levels and frequently associated with other anterior pituitary hormone deficiencies. CNS malformations and genetic defects of the hypothalamic-pituitary region and isolated TSH deficiency can cause these disorders in the neonatal period. Acquired causes include head trauma, neurosurgery, radiation exposure, tumors and CNS infections.

CONGENITAL HYPOTHYROIDISM

Congenital hypothyroidism is an important preventable cause of mental retardation. Iodine deficiency, dysgenesis and defects in thyroid hormone biosynthesis are the common causes of congenital hypothyroidism. Congenital hypothyroidism may rarely be a result of hypothalamic-pituitary dysfunction, TSH receptor blocking antibodies, or intake of maternal antithyroid drugs.

Clinical Features

Features of congenital hypothyroidism are nonspecific and often difficult to identify in the neonatal period. They become more prominent with increasing age; the window period for neurological intervention has however lapsed in most of these children by this time. This emphasizes the need for neonatal screening. Clinical manifestations include hoarse cry, facial puffiness, umbilical hernia, hypotonia and lethargy. Prolonged jaundice, constipation, unexplained hypothermia and open posterior fontanels are common (Fig. 14.5).

Evaluation

Clinical Maternal thyroid disease or ingestion of antithyroid medications should be probed. Residence in iodine deficient

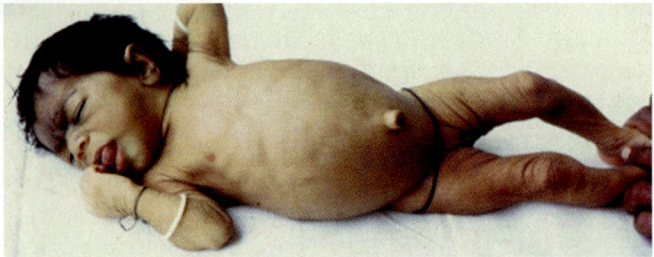

Fig. 14.5 A 3-month-old infant was brought for evaluation of abdominal distension with constipation. The infant had delayed milestones, large tongue, poor activity, dry skin, and hoarse cry. Laboratory tests confirmed hypothyroidism

area may provide a clue to the diagnosis of iodine deficiency. Goiter should prompt evaluation for transplacental passage of antithyroid drugs or disorders of thyroid hormone biosynthesis. Hypoglycemia, micropenis and midline facial defects are pointers to hypopituitarism.

Investigations Radiotracer uptake study (radioactive iodine or technetium) should be done as soon as the diagnosis is established (Fig. 14.6). Ultrasound should be done if no radiotracer uptake is identified to confirm thyroid dysgenesis. Presence of thyroid gland in this setting indicates defects in iodine transport, TSH receptor defects or transplacental passage of TSH blocking antibody. Radioactive tracer uptake by thyroid indicates the possibility of dyshormonogenesis.

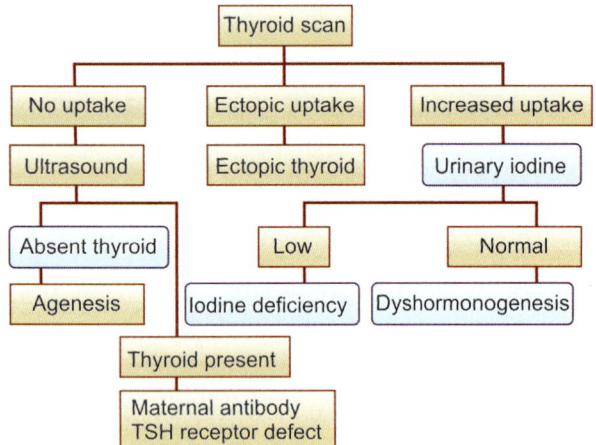

Fig. 14.6 Approach to congenital hypothyroidism

<table>
<tr><td colspan="2">Treatment   **Congenital Hypothyroidism**</td></tr>
</table>

Immediate thyroid replacement should be started. Thyroxine (T4) should be initiated at a dose of 10–15 µg/kg. T4 and TSH levels are expected to normalize over one week and one month, respectively, with this treatment. The drug should be given as tablets as liquid preparations are unreliable.

Follow-up should be done monthly during infancy, at every three months from 1–3 years and six monthly thereafter. FT4 and TSH should be measured at each visit. The dose of T4 should be adjusted to achieve FT4 levels in the upper normal range for the age.

Lifelong replacement is required in children with most forms of congenital hypothyroidism. Thyroid replacement should be stopped for a period of 1 month at the age of 3 years in children

with suspected transient congenital hypothyroidism. Treatment may be discontinued in the absence of any abnormality on investigations and normal levels of thyroid hormones. In children with central hypothyroidism, cortisol replacement should precede treatment of hypothyroidism, as thyroid replacement could precipitate adrenal insufficiency.

Outcome

Outcome is universally poor in children with congenital hypothyroidism who have been diagnosed beyond the neonatal period. Mental retardation and short stature are common. Early diagnosis and treatment before two weeks of age has resulted in normal intellectual outcomes.

Screening for Congenital Hypothyroidism

Difficulty in early identification of congenital hypothyroidism and the disastrous consequences of delayed diagnosis have led to neonatal screening for hypothyroidism. Most neonatal screening programs use dried blood sample collected at the age of 2 to 4 days. Most programs use primary TSH approach. This has the advantage of higher sensitivity compared to the T4 approach (**Table 14.10**). *Primary TSH approach* is however likely to miss children with central hypothyroidism which could be detected by T4 first approach. *T4 first approach* on the other hand has the disadvantage of missing cases with compensated hypothyroidism. Overall TSH first approach appears to be superior to T4 first approach and is becoming the most commonly practiced strategy of neonatal screening. Thyroid functions should be repeated if TSH levels are above 20 mU/L. Neonatal screening has been shown to significantly improve outcome of congenital hypothyroidism.

ACQUIRED HYPOTHYROIDISM

Acquired hypothyroidism is most commonly caused by autoimmune thyroiditis (Fig. 14.7). Rarely congenital abnormalities may manifest later in older children and at adolescence. Iodine deficiency and goitrogens are other causes of acquired primary hypothyroidism in older children. Secondary hypothyroidism due to combined hypothalamic-pituitary defects may occur as a manifestation of CNS insults or tumors.

Table 14.10 Strategies for Neonatal Thyroid Screening		
Feature	*TSH first**	*T4 first*
Investigation	TSH	T4
Cut-off for evaluation	> 20 mU/L	< 10 µg/dL
False positive	High	Low
False negative	Low	High
Detection of compensated hypothyroidism	Yes	No
Thyroid hormone resistance	Yes	No
Central hypothyroidism	No	Yes

*TSH first is the preferred strategy

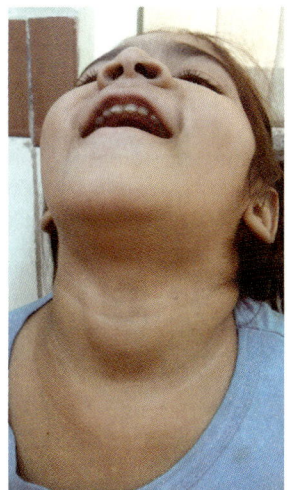

Fig. 14.7 A 10-year-old girl was brought for evaluation of progressive swelling in the neck noted for the last 3 months duration. Laboratory tests confirmed hypothyroidism. Antibodies against thyroid peroxidase were positive in high titers. Fine needle aspiration study confirmed the diagnosis of chronic lymphocytic thyroiditis (*Courtesy:* Dr Aashima Dabas)

Clinical Features

Clinical features are subtle compared to congenital hypo-thyroidism. Short stature may be the only manifestation. Cold intolerance, lethargy, constipation, delayed dentition and poor school performance may indicate the diagnosis of hypothyroidism. All children with unexplained mental retardation should be evaluated for hypothyroidism. Most children have delayed puberty; however uncontrolled longstanding the diagnosis of hypothyroidism may trigger precocious puberty. Hypothyroidism should be excluded in children with Down syndrome, Turner syndrome, celiac disease and type 1 diabetes mellitus.

Evaluation

Severe short stature and mental retardation point towards missed congenital hypothyroidism. A round uniform smooth goiter is suggestive of iodine deficiency or dyshormonogenesis; firm nodular goiter indicates auto-immune thyroiditis. Children with central hypothyroidism should be evaluated for pituitary function and MRI of the hypothalamic-pituitary region. Anti-thyroid autoantibodies such as TPO antibodies should be estimated in acquired primary hypothyroidism.

Treatment	Acquired Hypothroidism

Treatment of acquired hypothyroidism should be gradual. Thyroxine in a dose of 100 µg/m²/day is recommended. Treatment should be started at 25–50% of the dose with gradual build up every 3–4 weeks. The drug is given on an empty stomach in early morning. Feeds should be withheld for 30 minutes to avoid interference of food with the absorption of the drug. Follow-up should be done three monthly during the first two years of therapy and six monthly thereafter. The doses should be modified to maintain TSH levels in the normal range. TSH levels should be estimated during routine visit, in the presence of features of hypo- or hyperthyroidism or six weeks after modification of dose.

Case Study | **Hypothyroidism**

A 6-day-old girl was found to have high TSH levels (40 mU/L) on routine blood test at day 3 of life. Repeat thyroid profile on day 5 showed low free T4 (6 ng/mL, normal 10–22 ng/mL) and high TSH (54 mU/L, normal 0.1–5 mU/L). There were no features of hypothyroidism. There was no family history of hypothyroidism, goiter or antithyroid treatment in mother.

Q1. What is the diagnosis?

Q2. What is the plan of management?

The child has uncompensated hypothyroidism and should be started on thyroxine (10–15 µg/kg/day). Clinical features of congenital hypothyroidism are nonspecific and usually absent at diagnosis. Thyroid scan should be done before starting thyroxine to identify the underlying cause.

Q3. Thyroid scan did not show any radionuclide uptake. What is the diagnosis and plan?

Absent uptake on thyroid scan is most commonly related to thyroid agenesis but may result from transplacental passage of TSH receptor blocking antibody (TBA) or mutation of the gene for sodium-iodide transporter or TSH receptor. Identification of TBA related hypo-thyroidism is crucial due to the transient nature of the disease. Ultrasound thyroid should be done to localize thyroid gland.

Q4. Ultrasound did not show thyroid gland. What is the diagnosis now?

Absence of thyroid gland on scan and ultrasound is suggestive of thyroid dysgenesis and the need for lifelong treatment. Thyroid functions should be periodically monitored to ensure adequate supplementation.

Children with nongoitrous type of hypothyroidism need lifelong treatment. A trial of discontinuation of thyroid hormone may be considered in children with goitrous hypothyroidism after regression of the goiter. TSH levels should be repeated after a period of six weeks of discontinuation of treatment. Patients with elevated TSH levels should be restarted on thyroid hormone and would require lifelong treatment.

Hypothyroidism

1. Hypothyroidism is caused by defects in hypothalamus or pituitary (*central*) and thyroid gland (*primary*).
2. Primary hypothyroidism may be due to iodine deficiency, thyroid dysgenesis, dyshormonogenesis, or autoimmune destruction. Autoimmune thyroiditis is the most common cause of acquired hypothyroidism.
3. Clinical features of congenital hypothyroidism are nonspecific and include hoarse cry, facial puffiness, umbilical hernia, hypotonia, and lethargy.
4. Estimation of TSH and T4 levels along with ultra-sonography and/or radionuclear studies confirm the diagnosis.
5. Management include early replacement with levothyroxine with regular follow-up, clinical and hormonal evaluations.
6. Early diagnosis of congenital hypothyroidism is possible by cord blood or postnatal (at 2–4 days after birth) blood screening for TSH and/or T4.

American Academy of Pediatrics and American Thyroid Association–Newborn Screening for Congenital Hypothyroidism. Recommended Guidelines; 2006.

Bajpai A, Sharma J, Menon PSN. Hypothyroidism. *In: Practical Pediatric Endocrinology.* New Delhi: Jaypee Brothers; 2003:25–9.

Brown RS, Huang S. The thyroid and its disorders. *In:* Brooke CGD, Clayton PE, Brown RS, Savage MO (Eds.). *Clinical Pediatric Endocrinology,* 5th ed. London: Blackwell Publishers;. 2005:218–53.

Desai MP. Disorders of the thyroid gland. *In:* Desai MP, Menon PSN, Bhatia V (Eds.). *Pediatric Endocrine Disorders,* 3rd ed. Hyderabad: Orient Longman; 2014:187–219.

Fisher DA. Thyroid disorders in childhood and adolescence. *In:* Sperling MA (Ed.). *Pediatric Endocrinology,* 2nd edition. Philadelphia: Saunders; 2002:187–209.

Koch CA, Sarlis NJ. The spectrum of thyroid diseases in childhood and its evolution during transition to adulthood. Natural history, diagnosis, differential diagnosis and management. *J Endocrinol Invest.* 2001; 4.p.659.

14.6 HYPOCALCEMIA

Hypocalcemia is defined as serum total calcium lower than 8 mg/dL or ionic calcium less than 4.4 mg/dL. Estimation of serum ionic calcium is important for confirmation of hypocalcemia. Empirical formula for calculation of ionic calcium may be used if ionic estimation is not available.

$$Ionized\ Ca = Total\ serum\ Ca - 0.8 \times [Serum\ albumin\ (g/dL) - 4]$$

Calcium is needed for neurotransmission, muscular contraction, cardiac function and hormone signaling. Hypocalcemia may present as an acute emergency or as a chronic disorder.

Calcium Homeostasis

Most of the body calcium (over 95%) is stored in the bone and is in constant equilibrium with serum calcium. Parathyroid hormone (PTH), vitamin D and calcitonin are the key regulators of calcium metabolism. Calcium homeostasis involves regulation of gastrointestinal absorption, bone resorption and renal excretion.

- *Parathyroid hormone (PTH)* Hypocalcemia results in increased PTH secretion and inhibition of renal calcium excretion. PTH increases serum calcium by stimulating bone resorption (osteoclasts), calcitriol or 1,25-dihydroxy vitamin D production (proximal renal tubule) and renal calcium resorption (distal renal tubule). Thus it mobilizes calcium from bones, and decreases its excretion, to increase serum levels of calcium. PTH also increases phosphate excretion resulting in hypophosphatemia.

- *Calcitriol or 1,25-dihydroxyvitamin D* is formed by activation of vitamin D in the liver (25-hydroxylation) and kidney (1α-hydroxylation). It is the only hormone that enhances gastrointestinal absorption of calcium. 1α-hydroxylase, the rate limiting enzyme of calcitriol synthesis, is affected by serum calcium, PTH, and vitamin D levels.

- *Calcitonin,* secreted by the parafollicular cells of thyroid in response to elevated calcium levels, lowers serum calcium levels by decreasing bone resorption and increasing urinary calcium excretion.

Table 14.11 provides a summary of effects of these three hormones on calcium homeostasis in the body.

Clinical Features

Hypocalcemia in the *neonatal period* and infancy presents with subtle clinical features such as lethargy, jitteriness and poor feeding. Multifocal clonic seizures are the hallmark of neonatal hypocalcemia.

In the *postneonatal period,* the commonest presentation is with tetany (simultaneous contraction of groups of muscles). This is most readily observed in hands (adduction of thumbs along with extension of the proximal interphalangeal joints and flexion of distal interphalangeal joints) and feet (flexion and internal rotation of lower limbs) resulting in carpopedal spasm. In milder cases, latent tetany can be detected by tests of neuromuscular excitability. Tapping of facial nerve at the angle of jaw will induce contraction of facial muscles (*Chvostek sign*). Inflating of blood pressure cuff above the systolic blood pressure for more than 5 minutes may trigger spasm of the hand muscles (*Trousseau sign*).

Severe hypocalcemia may present with laryngeal spasm and cardiac failure. Prolonged QT interval (corrected QoTc more than 0.2 seconds) on ECG is suggestive of hypocalcemia.

$$QoTc = QoT / \sqrt{RR}$$

(QoT = Interval from beginning of Q wave to beginning of T wave; RR = RR interval)

Etiology

Hypocalcemia may be caused by disorders related to parathyroid glands, vitamin D deficiency, or by chelation of calcium. Major causes are listed below:

Table 14.11 Hormones Affecting Calcium Balance				
Hormone	Effect on target organ			Net effect
	Bone	Kidney	Gut	
Parathyroid hormone (PTH)	Mobilizes calcium from bones	Increases absorption of calcium	Increases absorption through calcitriol	↑Serum calcium
Calcitriol (1,25-dihydroxy vitamin D)	Stimulates PTH and mobilizes calcium from bones	Increases calcium excretion	Increases absorption	Maintains normal serum calcium
Calcitonin	Decreases calcium resorption from bones	Increases calcium excretion	–	↓Serum calcium

I. Parathyroid Related Disorders

i. *Hypoparathyroidism (decreased production)*
   - Aplasia: DiGeorge syndrome, genetic syndromes
   - Autoimmune destruction: Polyglandular auto-immune disorders I and II
   - Infiltration: Wilson disease, hemochromatosis, thalassemia
   - Transient: Hypomagnesemia, maternal hyper-parathyroidism, postsurgery

ii. *PTH resistance (pseudohypoparathyroidism) (defective action)*

II. Vitamin D Deficiency Related Disorders

- Nutritional or malabsorption
- 1α hydroxylase deficiency—Renal failure, VDDR I
- Calcitriol resistance—VDDR II
- Increased inactivation—Phenytoin, phenobarbitone

III. Chelation

Phosphate load, tumor lysis, rhabdomyolysis, top feeds

Inefficient PTH action caused by decreased production (hypoparathyroidism) or action (pseudohypoparathyroidism) is an important cause of hypocalcemia. *Phosphate levels are high* due to impaired phosphaturic action of PTH.

Hypoparathyroidism

Hypoparathyroidism may occur as part of *congenital malformations* (isolated or genetic syndromes) or acquired destruction of the parathyroid glands (autoimmune, infiltration, or surgery).

- *Autoimmune hypoparathyroidism* is the commonest type and is frequently associated with autoimmune polyendocrinopathy type 1.
- *DiGeorge syndrome*, a disorder of development of third and fourth pharyngeal arches, is caused by deletion of part of small arm of chromosome 22. It is characterized by maldevelopment of thymus (T cell immunodeficiency), parathyroid glands (hypoparathyroidism), heart (conotruncal defects), and facies (abnormal facies).
- *Hypomagnesemia* is an important cause of transient hypoparathyroidism and should be excluded in children with refractory hypocalcemia.

Pseudohypoparathyroidism

PTH resistance is caused by inactivating mutation in the gene encoding for stimulatory subunit of G protein (Gsα). This presents with clinical features of hypoparathyroidism with elevated PTH levels. Pseudohypoparathyroidism may be associated with the phenotype of Albright's hereditary osteodystrophy, ie, round facies, brachydactyly, short stature, obesity, short fourth and fifth metacarpals (brachymetacarpia), subcutaneous calcifications, and bony deformities.

Vitamin D Related Disorders

Vitamin D deficiency is the commonest cause and usually presents in infancy and puberty. Rickets may be absent. Maternal vitamin D deficiency is common resulting in reduced neonatal calcium and vitamin D stores in children. These infants develop hypocalcemia during periods of rapid bone growth (4–8 weeks of life).

Vitamin D dependent rickets (VDDR) presents with early onset severe hypocalcemia and rickets.

Increased Chelation

Increased binding of calcium to chelating agents results in reduction of ionic calcium and features of hypocalcemia. This is most commonly related to *high phosphate* levels (renal failure or release of intracellular phosphate due to hemolysis, tumor lysis or rhabdomyolysis). Increased phosphate level in cow's milk and commercial formula is an important cause of neonatal hypocalcemia. *Metabolic or respiratory alkalosis* increases albumin binding of calcium resulting in hypocalcemia.

Clinical Clues to Etiological Diagnosis

Some clinical features that may help to delineate the etiology of hypocalcemia are shown in **Table 14.12**. History of age at onset, presenting features and family history should be obtained. Neonates should be screened for prematurity, birth asphyxia, maternal hyperparathyroidism and initiation of top feeds. History suggestive of liver disease, malabsorption, malnutrition, and decreased exposure to sunlight indicates a vitamin D related cause. Congestive cardiac failure, recurrent infections and abnormal facies are suggestive of DiGeorge syndrome.

Table 14.12 Clues to Diagnosis of Hypocalcemia	
Feature	*Etiology*
Rickets	Vitamin D deficiency, renal failure, VDDR, malabsorption
Cardiac murmur	DiGeorge syndrome
Mental retardation	Pseudohypoparathyroidism, DiGeorge syndrome
Vitiligo, alopecia	Autoimmune polyendocrinopathy
Brachymetacarpia	Pseudohypoparathyroidism

Investigations

Initial investigations should include serum calcium, phosphate, alkaline phosphatase, and renal and liver function tests **(Table 14.13)**.

Since phosphate regulation is dependent on PTH, inefficient PTH action results in hyperphosphatemia with hypocalcemia. Hypocalcemia with hyperphosphatemia in the absence of phosphate load (exogenous or due to tissue lysis) and normal renal function suggests inefficient parathyroid action (Fig. 14.8).

Hypomagnesemia should be considered in children with refractory hypocalcemia and normal or low phosphate levels.

No response to vitamin D in children with rickets should prompt evaluation for renal failure, renal tubular acidosis, liver disease and malabsorption. Normal work-up for these conditions is suggestive of vitamin D dependent rickets.

Treatment	**Hypoparathyroidism**

Hypocalcemic seizure is managed by administration of 5% calcium gluconate (10 mg calcium per mL) 2 mL/kg intravenously over 5–10 minutes under cardiac monitoring. Take care to obtain blood sample for calcium before pushing in calcium,

14

Disorder	Calcium	Phosphate	ALP	25-OHD	PTH
Vitamin D deficiency	Low/Normal	Low/Normal	High	Low	High
Renal failure	Low	High	High	Normal	High
Phosphate load	Low	High	Normal	Normal	High
Hypoparathyroidism	Low	High	Normal	Normal	Low
Pseudohypoparathyroidism	Low	High	Normal	Normal	High
Hypomagnesemia	Low	Low, normal	Normal	Normal	Low

Table 14.13 Laboratory Features of Common Causes of Hypocalcemia

ALP: Alkaline phosphatase; 25-OHD: 25 hydroxyvitamin D; PTH: Parathyroid hormone

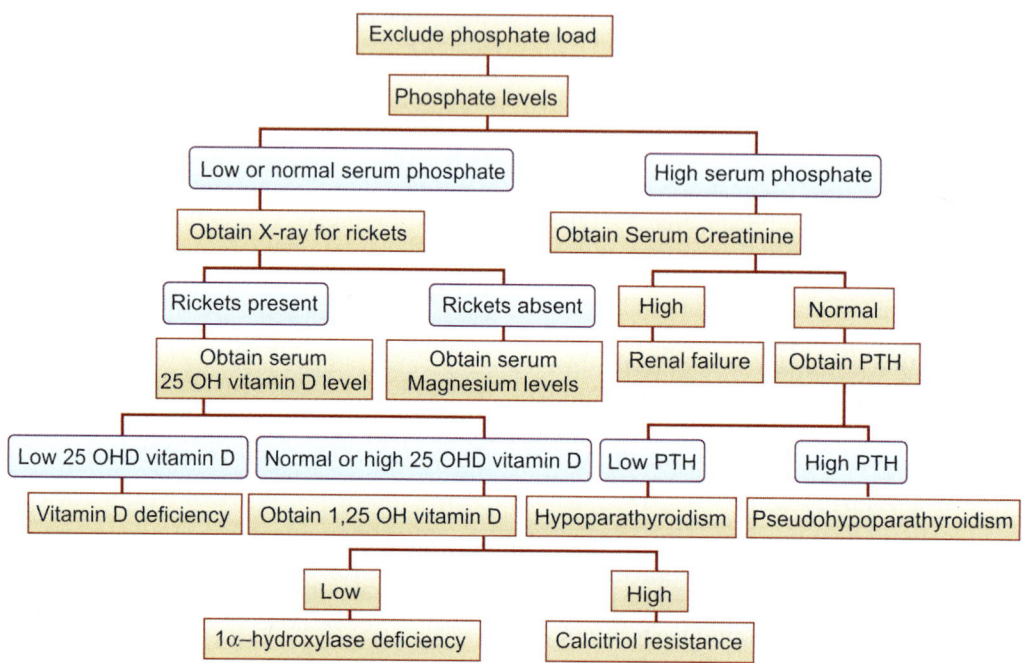

Fig. 14.8 Approach to hypocalcemia

to establish the diagnosis. Calcium gluconate 2 mL/kg should be continued every 6 hourly for at least 24 hours after the seizures are controlled (total dose 80 mg/kg/day). After 24–48 h of IV calcium, oral calcium can be started. Care should be taken to administer the drug slowly (to avoid cardiac effects) and avoid extravasation (to prevent skin necrosis).

Short course of vitamin D metabolites (calcitriol or 1α-vitamin D, 20–40 ng/kg/day in three divided doses for 2 days) should be given in vitamin D deficiency followed by high dose vitamin D (300,000–600,000 IU) to replenish vitamin D stores.

Inefficient PTH action states are treated with vitamin D metabolites (30–60 ng/kg/day) and calcium carbonate (50 mg/kg/day).

VDDR is managed with activated vitamin D and calcium phosphate. Higher doses of vitamin D are required in VDDR II.

Allgrove J. The parathyroid and disorders of calcium metabolism. *In*: Brook C, Clayton P, Brown R. *Clinical Pediatric Endocrinology*, 5th edition. Oxford: Blackwell Publishing; 2005.p.254–79.

Bajpai A, Sharma J, Kabra M, Menon PSN. Approach to a child with hypocalcemia. *Asian J Pediatr Pract*. 2001:36–42.

Revision Point

Hypocalcemia

1. Hypocalcemia is defined as serum total calcium lower than 8 mg/dL or ionic calcium less than 4.4 mg/dL.

2. Hypocalcemia in the neonatal period and infancy presents with subtle clinical features such as lethargy, jitteriness and poor feeding. Multifocal clonic seizures are the hallmark of neonatal hypocalcemia. Tetany is common in the postneonatal period.

3. Hypocalcemia may be caused by hypoparathyroidism, vitamin D deficiency, or chelation of calcium.

4. Investigations to confirm diagnosis include estimation of serum calcium, phosphate, and alkaline phosphatase along with renal and liver functions. Estimation of serum vitamin D_3, PTH, and magnesium may be necessary in a few cases.

5. Hypocalcemic seizures are managed by administration of 5% calcium gluconate 2 mL/kg IV slowly.

Diamond FB Jr, Root AW. Disorders of calcium metabolism in newborn and infant. *In*: Sperling MA. *Pediatric Endocrinology*, 2nd edition. Philadelphia: WB Saunders; 2002. 97–110.

Doyle DA and DiGeorge AM, Disorders of the parathyroid glands. *In*: Behrman RE, Klaus G, Watson A, *et al*. Prevention and treatment of renal osteodystrophy in children on chronic renal failure: European guidelines. *Pediatr Nephrol.* 2006;21:151–9.

Holick MF. Vitamin D deficiency. *N Engl J Med.* 2007;357:266–81.

Sharma J, Bajpai A, Kabra M, *et al*. Hypocalcemia: clinical, biochemical, radiological profile and follow-up in a tertiary hospital in India. *Indian Pediatr.* 2002;39:276–82.

14.7 OBESITY

Obesity implies excessive fat and not merely excess weight. Body weight is thus not a reliable criterion for defining obesity. As methods of measuring body fat are cumbersome and expensive, the following clinical parameters are used as markers of obesity.

1. *Body mass index (BMI)* BMI is the most widely used parameter to define obesity. It takes into account weight as well as the height. It is calculated by the formula:

$$BMI = weight\ (kg)\ /\ (height\ in\ m)^2$$

Children with BMI more than 85th percentile for age are considered *at-risk for obesity* while those with BMI more than 95th percentile for age are *obese*. BMI is a good indicator of body fat but may be unreliable in short muscular individuals.

2. *Weight for height* This compares the child's weight to the expected weight for his/her height. Weight for height more than 120% is diagnosed as obesity.

3. *Skin fold thickness* Skin fold thickness measured over the subscapular, triceps or biceps regions is an indicator for subcutaneous fat. Age specific percentile cut-offs should be used with values more than 85th percentile being abnormal.

4. *Waist circumference* This is a marker of abdominal adiposity, a key risk factor for metabolic and cardio-vascular effects of obesity.

Etiology

In most children obesity is caused by a combination of environmental and hereditary factors with an organic cause identified in very few cases (less than 1%). The causes of childhood obesity are listed below:

I. **Constitutional:** Environmental Factors (over 95% of all cases)

II. **Pathological**

  i. *Endocrine* Cushing syndrome, GH deficiency, hypo-thyroidism, pseudohypoparathyroidism

  ii. *Hypothalamic* Head injury, infection, brain tumor, radiation

  iii. *Drugs* Steroids, antiepileptic agents, estrogen

  iv. *Genetic syndromes* Prader-Willi syndrome, Laurence-Moon syndrome, Bardet-Biedl syndrome, Beckwith-Wiedemann syndrome, Carpenter syndrome

  v. *Monogenic disorders* Leptin deficiency/resistance, MC4 receptor gene abnormality

Differential Diagnosis

Constitutional obesity This is due to an imbalance in energy intake (increased consumption) and expenditure (decreased activity and increased inactivity). These children are *tall for their age*, a factor that differentiates them from pathological obesity. They have proportional obesity and normal development. Important environmental factors include excessive calorie intake, irregular meal pattern, frequent snacking, sedentary lifestyle, prolonged television viewing, and playing computer games. It is important to identify this subgroup of children so as to avoid unnecessary investi-gations. Advanced growth is a key pointer to this diagnosis.

Endocrine causes *Growth failure* in an obese child is an important marker of an underlying endocrine cause.

- *Cushing syndrome* is characterized by central obesity, hypertension, striae and retarded skeletal maturation.
- *Hypothyroidism* is an extremely rare cause of isolated obesity and other features are always present.
- *GH deficiency* is associated with significant short stature.
- In *pseudohypoparathyroidism,* growth retardation and hypocalcemia are dominant clinical features and obesity is a less prominent manifestation.

Genetic syndromes A variety of genetic syndromes have obesity as their major clinical feature. Many of these syndromes are associated with hypogonadism or hypotonia (Prader-Willi, Laurence-Moon, and Bardet-Biedl syndromes, **Table 14.14**).

Table 14.14 Features of Common Causes of Pathological Obesity	
Disorder	*Features*
Prader-Willi syndrome	Infantile hypotonia, hyperphagia, almond like eyes, small hand and feet, hypogonadism, behavioral abnormality
Laurence-Moon syndrome	Hypogonadism, retinitis pigmentosa, ataxia, spastic paraplegia, and peripheral neuropathy dysfunction
Bardet-Biedl syndrome	Obesity, retinitis pigmentosa, polydactyly (Fig. 14.9), renal abnormalities, intellectual disability
Beckwith-Wiedemann syndrome	Organomegaly, ear lobe creases, hemihypertrophy
Cushing syndrome	Hirsutism, central obesity, growth retardation, striae, buffalo hump, hypertension, myopathy
Hypothyroidism	Growth retardation, coarse facies, developmental delay

14

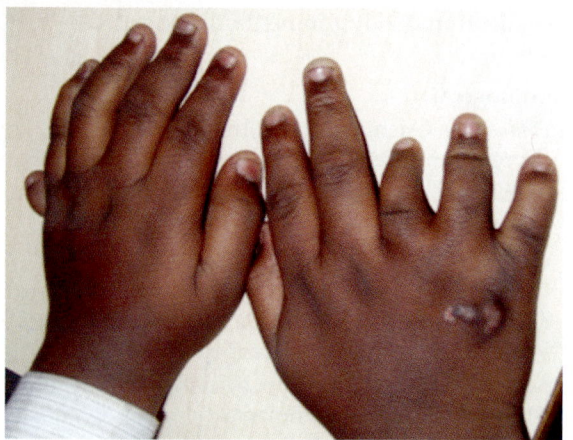

Fig. 14.9 A 14-year-old boy with obesity, polydactyly, and night blindness. Work-up was suggestive of Bardet-Biedl syndrome

Hypothalamic obesity CNS insults due to surgery, radiation, tumors and trauma results in rapidly progressive obesity. These disorders are associated with excessive appetite, signs and symptoms of CNS involvement and other hypothalamic-pituitary defects.

Monogenic obesity Monogenic obesity is seen in a very small proportion of children with obesity. They should be suspected in the presence of early onset, morbid obesity and a strong family history. *Leptin deficiency* was the first monogenic cause of obesity identified. Leptin, a polypeptide secreted by the adipocytes, induces satiety by acting on the hypothalamus. *Inefficient leptin action* (deficiency or resistance) results in uncontrolled appetite and obesity. Abnormalities in mineralocorticoid receptor (MC4) and proconvertase enzyme are also associated with obesity.

APPROACH TO AN OBESE CHILD

Initial evaluation is directed towards differentiating *constitutional* and *pathological* obesity. Normal growth, generalized pattern and lack of developmental delay or dysmorphism are suggestive of constitutional obesity; and against the need for extensive investigations **(Table 14.15)**.

Clinical Evaluation

Family history of obesity and its complications should be recorded. Detailed history of physical activity, dietary recall and periods of inactivity should be assessed. Delayed development suggests the possibility of a genetic syndrome. Features of raised intracranial tension coupled with past

Table 14.15 Comparison of Constitutional and Pathological Obesity

Feature	Constitutional obesity	Pathological obesity
Distribution	Generalized	Usually central
Growth	Accelerated	Retarded
Bone age	Advanced	Retarded
Dysmorphism	Absent	May be present

history of CNS infection, head trauma or neurosurgery indicate hypothalamic obesity. Intake of steroids and anti-epileptic drugs should be probed. Examine for specific clinical features of endocrinopathies, dysmorphic syndromes and complications (eg, hypertension and acanthosis nigricans). Special emphasis should be given to sexual maturity and ocular examination.

Investigations

Investigations for obesity are directed by the degree of obesity and associated complications (Fig. 14.10). Etiological investigations are indicated in the presence of growth failure, clinical features or developmental delay. Screening for complications is indicated if BMI is more than 95th percentile or 85–95th percentile in the presence of family history of cardiovascular complications or presence of type 2 diabetes. These should include oral glucose tolerance test, serum cholesterol, and liver function tests.

Complications

- *Cardiovascular* Hyperlipidemia, hypertension, coronary artery disease, and metabolic syndrome—a combination of insulin resistance, hypertension and hyperlipidemia.
- *Endocrine* Insulin resistance, presenting as a spectrum ranging from elevated insulin levels to impaired glucose tolerance to type 2 diabetes mellitus. A characteristic clinical feature is acanthosis nigricans, dark and rough areas on the exposed areas of skin including back of neck, axilla and thigh.
- *Respiratory* Restrictive (decreased respiratory movements due to obesity) as well as obstructive pulmonary disease (fatty deposition in the airway). The most severe respiratory complication is the obesity–hypoventilation

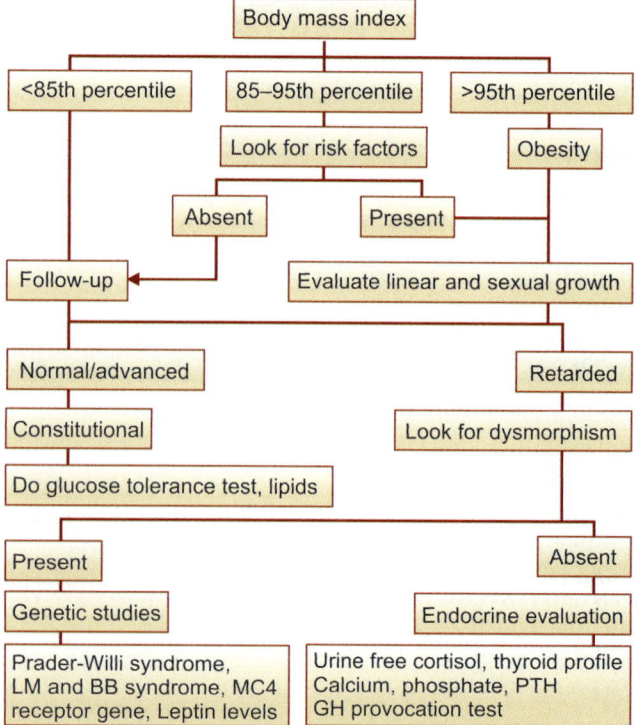

Fig. 14.10 Approach to a child with obesity

syndrome associated with hypoxia and features of cor pulmonale. In its milder form it is associated with snoring, irritability, hyperactivity and daytime somnolence.

- *Orthopedic* Slipped femoral epiphyses, flat feet, Blount's disease (tibia vara), and early onset osteoarthritis.
- *Hepatic* Insulin resistance in obesity is associated with fatty infiltration in liver. This may vary from mild infiltration with no effect to steatohepatitis to chronic liver disease. The incidence of cholelithiasis is greater in obese children.

Treatment — Childhood Obesity

Management of childhood obesity is challenging with major impetus on lifestyle measures. Specific management is available for only a few conditions. Lifestyle interventions are the cornerstones of therapy with intensive measures like drug therapy and surgery reserved for morbid cases.

Dietary measures Initial measures include mild caloric restriction and modification of dietary habits. Apart from restricting calorie intake, efforts should be directed towards improving the nutritive value of the diet. Reduction in consumption of junk foods, carbonated drinks and saturated fat along with an increase in fiber, fruits and vegetable intake are helpful in improving body composition. Regular meal consumption with fixed portion size is recommended.

Case Study | Obesity

A 10-year-old boy was referred for evaluation of obesity. There were no features of developmental delay, neurological abnormality, hyperphagia or endocrinopathies. The family history was noncontributory. His weight was 40 kg (more than 95th percentile) and height was 138 cm (97th percentile). He had generalized obesity. Examination was normal with the exception of acanthosis nigricans in the axilla.

Q1. What is the etiology?

Q2. How should he be evaluated and managed?

Initial step in the evaluation of a child with suspected obesity is to confirm the diagnosis. Body mass index (BMI) is the best clinical marker of obesity and should be compared to age specific norms. The BMI of this child (26 kg/m^2) is above the 95th percentile as per available growth standards confirming obesity. The next step is to differentiate constitutional (exogenous) obesity from pathological (endogenous) obesity. Growth (height) acceleration, absence of dysmorphism, and a normal development are indicative of constitutional obesity. In view of obesity and acanthosis nigricans he should be screened for development of complications of obesity especially hyperinsulinism (oral glucose tolerance test, liver function tests and lipid profile). Management should include lifestyle modifications (increased physical activity with reduced inactivity) and nutritional advice (mild caloric restriction, regular meals and avoidance of snacking).

Oral glucose tolerance test and lipid profile were normal. Liver function tests showed mild dysfunction. Ultrasound of abdomen showed fatty infiltration of the liver. Lifestyle interventions were effective in inducing weight loss. This was associated with resolution of hepatic dysfunction.

Lifestyle modification Increase in physical activity and reduction in sedentary lifestyle is essential. Swimming, running and playing outdoor games should be encouraged. Physical activity for at least 30–45 minutes per day should be recommended. Activities like continuous television viewing, videogames and internet surfing should be restricted.

Drugs Drug therapy is reserved for severe obesity. The only drug used in obese adolescents is *orlistat* (gastric lipase inhibitor). *Metformin* is indicated in children with insulin resistance and has the advantage of weight loss. Leptin (for those with leptin deficiency) and octreotide (for hypothalamic obesity) are indicated in specific subgroups of children.

Surgery Bariatric surgery is the last resort in treatment and indicated for morbid obesity (BMI more than 40 kg/m^2 with complications) when other measures have failed. Laparoscopic gastric banding is the procedure of choice and is directed at reducing gastric capacity. This results in reduced appetite and weight loss. Experience with bariatric surgery in children is limited but has been shown to cause significant reduction in body weight sustained for a period of one year.

Revision Point — Obesity

1. Children with body mass index (BMI) > 85th percentile for the age are considered at-risk for obesity and those with BMI >95th percentile as obese.
2. Constitutional obesity is more common in children than endocrine obesity. Presence of short stature is an important marker of an underlying cause.
3. Normal growth, generalized pattern of obesity, absence of developmental delay, and dysmorphic features suggest constitutional obesity.
4. Investigations to confirm etiology are indicated in the presence of growth failure, developmental delay, dysmorphism, and associated complications. Obese children should be screened for glucose intolerance, dyslipidemia, and liver dysfunction.
5. Management includes counseling along with appropriate education and nutritional advice, and lifestyle modifications. Drug therapy and bariatric surgery are reserved for morbid obesity.

August GP, Caprio S, Fennoy I, *et al*. Prevention and Treatment of Pediatric Obesity: An Endocrine Society Clinical Practice Guideline Based on Expert Opinion. *J Clin Endocrinol Metab*. 2008;93:4576–99.

Bajpai A, Sharma J, Menon PSN. Obesity. *In: Practical Pediatric Endocrinology*. New Delhi: Jaypee Brothers; 2003.p. 141–6.

Marwaha RK, Tandon N, Singh Y, *et al*. A study of growth parameters and prevalence of overweight and obesity in school children from Delhi. *Indian Pediatr*. 2006;43:943–52.

Reinehr T, Hinney A, de Sousa G, *et al*. Definable somatic disorders in overweight children and adolescents. *J Pediatr*. 2007;150:618–22.

14.8 PRECOCIOUS PUBERTY

Pubertal onset before the age of 8 years in girls and 9.5 years in boys is suggestive of precocious puberty. Precocious puberty is caused by premature activation of the hypothalamic-pituitary axis (*central* or *true precocious puberty*) or increased production of sex hormones independent of the hypothalamic-pituitary axis (*peripheral* or *pseudoprecocious puberty*).

14

Central precocious puberty (CPP) is now rechristened as *gonadotropin-dependent* precocious puberty. This is characterized by increased levels of LH and FSH.

Peripheral or pseudoprecocious puberty, on the other hand is *gonadotropin-independent*, and characterized by low (pre-pubertal) levels of LH and FSH.

Etiology

I. **Gonadotropin-dependent or Central Precocious Puberty (CPP)**
   • Idiopathic
   • *CNS tumors:* Hamartoma, pituitary adenoma, craniopharyngioma, glioma
   • *CNS infections:* Neurotuberculosis, meningitis
   • *CNS insults:* Head trauma, neurosurgery, cranial irradiation
   • *CNS malformations:* Arachnoid cyst, hydrocephalus, septo-optic dysplasia

II. **Gonadotropin-independent or Peripheral Precocious Puberty (GIPP)**
   Girls
   • Hypothyroidism
   • *Ovarian:* McCune-Albright syndrome, cyst, tumor, aromatase excess
   • *Adrenal:* Estrogenic adrenal adenoma
   • Exogenous exposure to estrogen
   Boys
   • *Congenital adrenal hyperplasia:* 21-hydroxylase deficiency, 11β-hydroxylase deficiency
   • *Adrenal tumor:* Adenoma, carcinoma
   • *Testicular tumor:* Seminoma, germinoma
   • Testotoxicosis
   • *hCG secreting tumor:* Germinoma, hepatoblastoma
   • *Exogenous exposure:* Testosterone cream

PRECOCIOUS PUBERTY IN GIRLS

Gonadotropin-dependent (True or Central) Precocious Puberty (CPP)

It is more common than gonadotropin-independent precocious puberty in girls. In more than 75% of girls with central precocious puberty, no underlying cause is identified. Onset after the age of six years, slow progression and lack of neurological features are suggestive of idiopathic precocious puberty.

Hypothalamic hamartoma, a neuronal migration defect, is the commonest cause of organic CPP. The disorder presents with early onset and rapid progression of puberty, seizures and uncontrolled laughter episodes (gelastic epilepsy).

Gonadotropin-independent (Peripheral or Pseudo) Precocious Puberty (GIPP)

This is rare and usually caused by *estrogenic ovarian cysts*. Fluctuating pubertal development and early vaginal bleeding (due to hyperestrogenic state) are common. In most cases the cysts are self-resolving and no treatment is required.

Early onset with recurrent ovarian cysts should raise the possibility of *McCune-Albright syndrome*, a somatic activating mutation of stimulatory G protein. The condition presents with constellation of cutaneous (multiple dark brown café au lait spots), skeletal (multiple fibrous dysplasia) and endocrine abnormalities (hyperthyroidism, rickets, GH excess).

Prolonged untreated primary hypothyroidism may induce early puberty due to action of TSH on FSH receptor. Delayed bone age and growth are characteristic. Estrogenic adrenal tumors are extremely rare.

Evaluation

Aims of evaluation include (*i*) confirmation of diagnosis; (*ii*) identification of underlying etiology; and (*iii*) determination of prognosis and treatment.

Clinical Onset, progression and extent of puberty should be recorded. Family history of precocity points towards idiopathic variant of central precocious puberty. History indicative of intracranial space occupying lesion, CNS infections, neurosurgery, radiotherapy and head trauma should be noted. Features of hypothyroidism should be looked for. *Retardation of physical growth* is indicative of hypothyroidism or concomitant deficiency of GH. Abdominal examination for adrenal or ovarian mass should be done. Features of McCune-Albright syndrome as described above should be looked for.

Investigations Initial investigations should include *bone age* and *basal gonadotropin* levels.

1. *Bone age* Advanced bone age (more than two years ahead of chronological age) is suggestive of progressive precocious puberty while normal bone age indicates slowly progressive puberty (Fig. 14.11). Retarded bone age is diagnostic of hypothyroidism.

2. *Gonadotropins* Pooled gonadotropin levels are preferred due to their pulsatile secretion. LH is a better indicator of pubertal status than FSH. LH levels in the pubertal range and LH to FSH ratio more than 1 are suggestive of onset of puberty. In equivocal cases, LH levels should be measured after GnRH injection (GnRH stimulation test).

   • Pubertal LH levels after GnRH stimulation are suggestive of central precocious puberty. These girls should have a MRI brain. Pituitary functions should be assessed if an organic cause is identified.

   • Prepubertal levels of LH following GnRH stimulation test suggest peripheral precocious puberty (gonadotropin-independent). These girls should undergo ultrasound of ovary and adrenals (for ovarian cyst and adrenal tumor) and skeletal survey (for fibrous dysplasia). Thyroid functions also should be done.

Treatment	Precocious Puberty in Girls

The aims of management are (*i*) treatment of underlying cause, (*ii*) suppression of puberty, and (*iii*) achievement of target height.

The major long-term consequence of precocious puberty is short stature. Growth is accelerated at presentation. This however occurs at the expense of disproportionate advancement in bone age resulting in premature epiphyseal fusion culminating in compromised final height. Psychosocial impact of early pubertal development and menstruation may be severe.

Central or Gonadotropin-dependent Precocious Puberty
The drugs used for pubertal suppression include medroxyprogesterone acetate (MPA), cyproterone, and GnRH analogs.

Long-acting GnRH analogs (triptorelin or leuprolide) are the commonly used agents that are effective in improving height outcome. They induce sustained stimulation and desensitization of pituitary leading to reversal of pubertal changes. Their use is

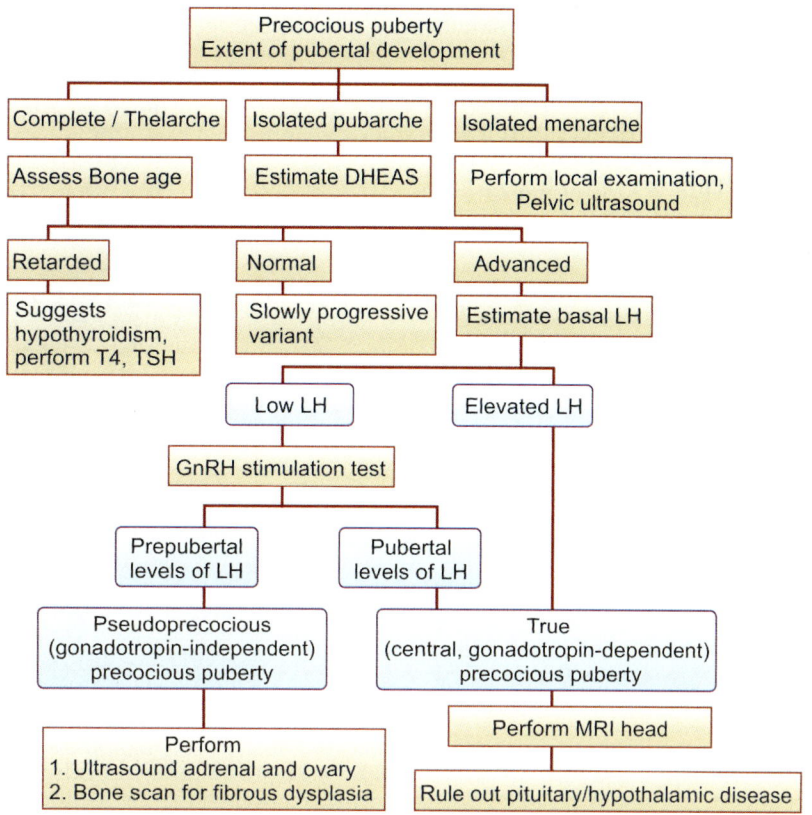

Fig. 14.11 Approach to precocious puberty in girls

however limited by high cost. GnRH analogs should be considered in girls with early onset (before 6 years of age) rapidly progressive puberty and height compromise (bone age to chronological age difference more than two years). Triptorelin or leuprolide are administered as deep intramuscular injections every 4 weeks or 12 weeks (depot preparation). The treatment is continued till the age of 11 years and bone age of 12.5 years. Following discontinuation of therapy secondary sexual characters gradually reappear. Menarche is attained around 12–18 months following discontinuation of treatment.

Medroxyprogesterone (MPA) and cyproterone are the other drugs used for pubertal suppression. MPA does not improve height outcome but may be considered in girls with intellectual disability where height is not a major concern.

Specific treatment should be initiated for girls with an organic cause (neurosurgery for brain tumor and ventriculoperitoneal shunt for hydrocephalus).

Peripheral or Gonadotropin-independent Precocious Puberty
Thyroxine replacement results in reversal of pubertal changes in hypothyroidism. Treatment for McCune-Albright syndrome is directed towards inhibiting estrogen production (aromatase inhibitors such as anastrazole or letrozole) or action (tamoxifen). Treatment of ovarian cysts is guided by size and morphological features.

INCOMPLETE VARIANTS OF PUBERTY

These disorders represent normal variants and do not require specific treatment. Their identification helps in prompt counseling and avoiding unnecessary investigations.

Isolated thelarche Isolated breast development may represent isolated thelarche or first manifestation of central precocious puberty. Normal growth, prepubertal levels of LH, age appropriate bone age and small uterine size suggest isolated thelarche. Advanced bone age, elevated LH level and increased uterine size indicate precocious puberty and need for GnRH analog therapy.

Isolated adrenarche Premature adrenarche refers to development of pubic hair and acne in the absence of breast development or menarche. Most cases occur due to physiological variation in adrenal androgen secretion. Rarely it may be secondary to excess adrenal (congenital adrenal hyperplasia due to 21-hydroxylase or 11β-hydroxylase deficiency or adrenal tumor) or ovarian (tumor or polycystic ovarian syndrome) androgen production. Girls with virilization and advanced bone age should be investigated for these disorders.

Isolated menarche Menarche in the absence of thelarche rules out central precocious puberty. Vaginal bleeding may occur early in course of estrogen excess states such as ovarian cysts, hypothyroidism and McCune-Albright syndrome. Vaginal bleeding without breast development should prompt evaluation of local causes such as infection, foreign body, sexual abuse, and tumor.

PRECOCIOUS PUBERTY IN BOYS

Precocious puberty is less common in boys compared to girls but when present is usually associated with significant organic etiology. Both gonadotropin-dependent and independent forms of precocious puberty account for similar number of cases in boys.

Gonadotropin-dependent or Central precocious puberty (CPP) Hypothalamic hamartoma, hydrocephalus and tuberculous meningitis are important causes of central precocious puberty in boys. This is characterized by increased testicular volume and elevated basal and GnRH stimulated LH.

Gonadotropin-independent precocious puberty (GIPP) This is caused by autonomous androgen production by testis and adrenals in the setting of prepubertal LH levels.

- Adrenal androgen overproduction due to *congenital adrenal hyperplasia* (21 and 11β-hydroxylase deficiency) is the commonest cause. Penile enlargement with prepubertal testicular volume is characteristic.
- *Human chorionic gonadotropin (hCG) secreting germ cell tumors* may present with precocious puberty. Testicular volume is only slightly increased as only Leydig cells are enlarged.
- *Testotoxicosis*, a disorder associated with constitutional activation of LH receptor, presents with early onset gonadotropin-independent precocious puberty.
- *Androgen secreting testicular tumor* presents with precocious puberty and unilateral testicular enlargement.

Evaluation

Clinical History should include age at onset, progression of disease, neurological features, family history of precocious puberty and androgen exposure. Detailed anthropometric and neurological examination should be performed. Pointers to CAH (hyperpigmentation and hypertension) should be identified. Estimation of testicular volume (using an orchidometer) forms an integral part of assessment of boys with precocious puberty (Fig. 14.12). Prepubertal testicular volume (less than 4 mL) is characteristic of congenital adrenal hyperplasia and adrenal tumor while unilateral enlargement is seen in testicular tumor. Pubertal testicular enlargement indicates central (gonadotropin-dependent) precocious puberty while milder enlargement is observed in hCG secreting tumor and testotoxicosis.

Investigations Initial investigations should include LH, FSH and testosterone levels and bone age (Fig. 14.13). All children with pubertal LH levels should undergo visual field examination and MRI of head including detailed pituitary evaluation. Prepubertal LH levels suggest gonadotropin-independent precocious puberty; in these cases, adrenal imaging and estimation of serum 17OHP levels should be done. The levels of hCG should be estimated if these investigations are noncontributory.

Treatment	**Precocious Puberty in Boys**

GnRH analogs are the treatment of choice and should be continued till the age of 12 years and bone age of 14.5 years is achieved. Congenital adrenal hyperplasia is treated with hydrocortisone and fludrocortisone. Surgery is the treatment of choice for adrenal and testicular tumors while radiotherapy is effective for hCG secreting tumors. Aromatase inhibitors and antiandrogens are used in the treatment of testotoxicosis. CNS pathology in treated according to the underlying condition.

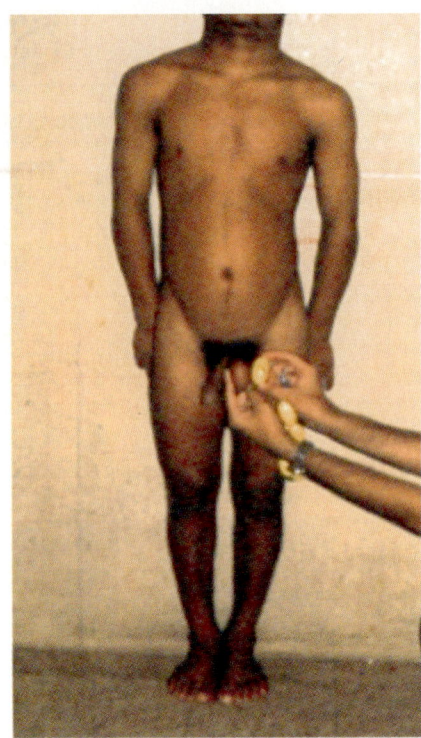

Fig. 14.12 Precocious puberty secondary to hypothalamic hamartoma. This 6-year-old boy was noticed to have progressive enlargement of penis and testes from the age of 2 years. He had hyperactivity and recurrent gelastic seizures at around the same time. MRI of brain confirmed hypothalamic hamartoma

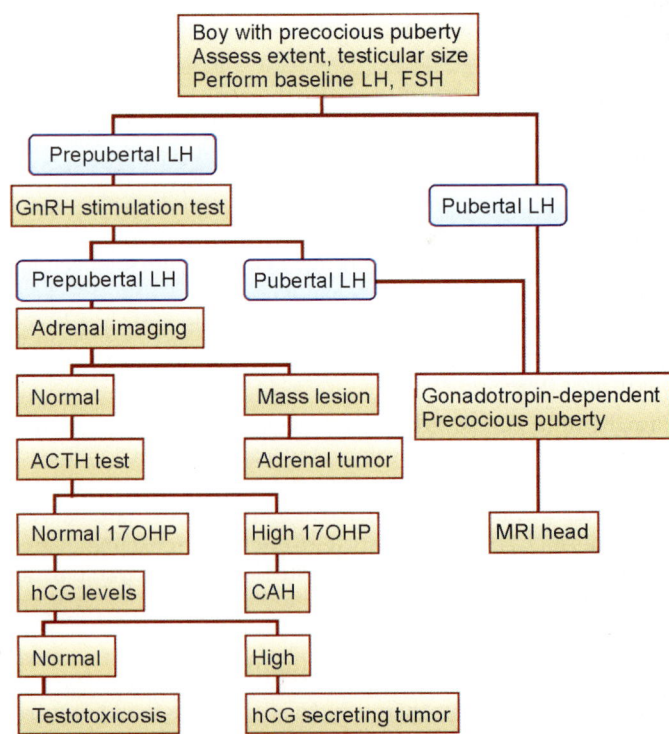

Fig. 14.13 Approach to precocious puberty in boys

Precocious Puberty

1. Pubertal onset before the age of 8 years in girls and 9.5 years in boys is suggestive of precocious puberty.
2. Precocious puberty is caused by premature activation of the hypothalamic-pituitary axis (central or true precocious puberty) (CPP) or increased production of sex hormones independent of the hypothalamic-pituitary axis (peripheral or pseudoprecocious puberty) (PPP).
3. Hypothalamic hamartoma, a neuronal migration defect, is the commonest cause of organic CPP.
4. Clinical evaluation includes sexual maturity rating using Tanner staging and assessment of bone age.
5. Pubertal levels of LH following GnRH stimulation test suggest central precocious puberty.
6. Management includes administration of depot preparations of long-acting GnRH agonist analogs.

14.9 DELAYED PUBERTY

Lack of appearance of secondary sex characters by 13 years in girls and 14 years in boys indicates delayed puberty. In a girl, absence of menarche by the age of 16 years or 5 years after pubertal onset also indicates pubertal delay.

Etiology

Delayed puberty may be caused by defects in the hypothalamic-pituitary axis, gonads, or genital tract **(Table 14.16)**. Defects in the hypothalamic-pituitary axis are associated with low gonadotropin levels (*hypogonadotropic hypogonadism*). Defects in the gonadal hormone production resulting in high gonadotropin levels result in *hypergonadotropic hypogonadism*. Detailed etiology is given in **Table 14.16**.

- *Hypergonadotropic hypogonadism in girls* is associated with defective estrogen production by ovaries and elevated gonadotropin levels. Turner syndrome, ovarian failure, and enzymatic defects in estrogen synthesis production are important causes of this condition. Patients with anatomical defects present with amenorrhea with normal breast development.
- *Hypergonadotropic hypogonadism in boys* (testicular failure) may be related to Klinefelter syndrome, partial gonadal dysgenesis, steroidogenic defects or acquired testicular injury.

Clinical Evaluation

Family history of delayed puberty provides a clue to constitutional delay in puberty. Features of chronic systemic disease should be probed. Evidence of head injury, neurosurgery and intracranial space occupying lesions suggests a defect in the hypothalamic-pituitary axis. Poor smell sensation indicates Kallmann syndrome. Girls with amenorrhea with normal secondary sexual characteristics are likely to have anatomical defects. Features of Turner syndrome (girls), Klinefelter syndrome (boys), and hypothyroidism should be looked into. Galactorrhea points towards the diagnosis of hypothyroidism or hyperprolactinemia. Features of dysmorphism and syndromes are usually evident on examination.

Table 14.16 Etiology of Delayed Puberty

I. Hypogonadotropic hypogonadism

A. *Transient*
  i. Constitutional delay
  ii. *Systemic disorders:* Chronic renal failure, liver disease, celiac disease, cystic fibrosis, RTA
  iii. *Nutritional disorders:* Malnutrition, anorexia nervosa, bulimia nervosa
  iv. *Endocrine disorders:* Hypothyroidism, hyperprolactinemia, type 1 diabetes mellitus

B. *Permanent*
Isolated hypogonadotropic hypogonadism
- Genetic—Kallmann syndrome (syndrome of defective smell, low GnRH and delayed puberty) GnRH receptor, LH, FSH, DAX1 mutations
- Dysmorphic syndromes—CHARGE, PW, LM and BB syndromes

Multiple pituitary hormone deficiency

Congenital
- Malformations—Holoprosencephaly, septo-optic dysplasia, midline defects
- Genetic disorders —PROP1, LH gene deletions
Acquired
- *Brain tumors:* Craniopharyngioma, germinoma, glioma
- *CNS insults:* Surgery, infection, radiation, trauma
- *Infiltrative disorders:* Histiocytosis, sarcoidosis, autoimmune

II. Hypergonadotropic hypogonadism

Girls
- *Ovarian failure:* Turner syndrome, gonadal dysgenesis, autoimmune
- *Steroidogenic defects:* StAR, 17α-hydroxylase, 17β-HSD, aromatase deficiency
- *Ovarian insults:* Surgery, radiation, alkylating agents, infections
Boys
- *Chromosomal abnormalities:* Klinefelter syndrome, gonadal dysgenesis
- *Steroidogenic defects:* CAH (StAR, 17α-hydroxylase, 17β-HSD), Smith-Lemli-Opitz syndrome
- *Testicular insult:* Radiotherapy, chemotherapy, trauma, torsion, infections
- *Malformations:* Vanishing testis syndrome, cryptorchidism
- *Inefficient testosterone action:* 5α-reductase deficiency, androgen insensitivity syndrome (AIS)

APPROACH TO A GIRL WITH DELAYED PUBERTY

Initial work-up is directed towards excluding systemic disorders. This should be followed by determination of serum FSH levels (Fig. 14.14). Karyotype should be done to rule out Turner syndrome if FSH levels are high. Steroidogenic defects are likely if karyotype and pelvic ultrasound are normal in this setting. In children with low/normal FSH, serum prolactin and thyroid profile should be checked to exclude reversible causes. Neuroimaging and pituitary function tests should be done if these levels are normal.

14

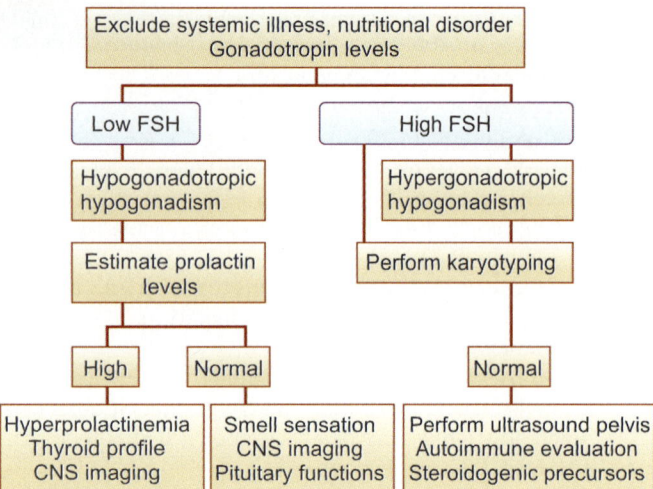

Fig. 14.14 Approach to delayed puberty in girls

APPROACH TO DELAYED PUBERTY IN BOYS

Delayed puberty is more common in boys than compared to girls and is usually related to constitutional delay. Lack of pubertal changes by the age of 14 years is suggestive of delayed puberty.

Constitutional delay is the commonest cause. Clinical features include growth retardation and delayed bone age. Family history of delayed puberty is present. Gonadotropin levels are prepubertal similar to hypogonadotropic hypogonadism.

Evaluation

Initial step includes estimation of LH, FSH and testosterone levels (Fig. 14.15). Elevated gonadotropin levels (hyper-

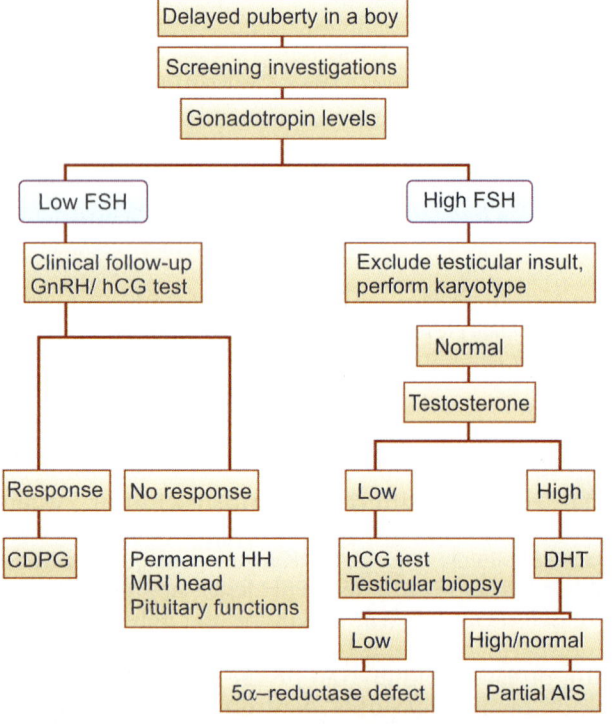

Fig. 14.15 Approach to delayed puberty in boys

gonadotropic hypogonadism) should be followed up by karyotype and evaluation for biosynthetic defects. Individuals with low LH and FSH levels may have constitutional delay of puberty or hypogonadotropic hypogonadism. They may be distinguished by hCG stimulation test or GnRH stimulation tests. These tests are nondiscriminatory in most cases and follow-up after a course of testosterone is the best management strategy. Patients with hypogonadotropic hypogonadism should undergo evaluation of hypothalamic-pituitary axis and neuroimaging.

Treatment	Delayed Puberty

All children with hypergonadotropic hypogonadism and irreversible hypogonadotropic hypogonadism need hormone replacement.

Girls Hormone replacement should be deferred till the age of 12 years to avoid deleterious effects on height. The goal of treatment is to initiate and maintain sexual characteristics and to prevent osteoporosis. Treatment should be started with low dose estrogens and gradually increased every 3 months till adult doses are reached. Progesterone (medroxyprogesterone acetate MPA 5–10 mg 12–14 days every 1–2 months) should be added after 1.5 to 2 years of initiation of treatment or once withdrawal bleeding has started.

Boys Endocrine treatment should be postponed till the age of 14 years and bone age of 14.5 years. Parenteral testosterone esters are preferred over oral preparations. Children with suspected constitutional delay of puberty are given three monthly injections of testosterone enanthate (100 mg). The course may be repeated if adequate response is not achieved. Serum testosterone levels should be estimated three months after the last dose of the drug. Normal levels indicate progression of puberty and preclude further treatment. Low testosterone levels indicate hypogonadotropic hypogonadism and the need of continued treatment.

Revision Point

Delayed Puberty

1. Lack of appearance of secondary sex characters by 13 years in girls and 14 years in boys indicate delayed puberty. In a girl, absence of menarche by the age of 16 years or 5 years after pubertal onset also indicates pubertal delay.
2. Defects in the hypothalamic-pituitary axis are associated with low gonadotropin levels (hypogonadotropic hypogonadism). Defects in the gonadal hormone production result in high gonadotropin levels (hypergonadotropic hypogonadism).
3. Clinical evaluation includes sexual maturity rating using Tanner staging and assessment of bone age.
4. Constitutional delay and chronic systemic disorders should be excluded before hormonal evaluation. Constitutional delay is the most common cause of delayed puberty in boys. Turner syndrome should be suspected in girls with elevated serum FSH levels.
5. Hormonal replacement at appropriate age helps to attain puberty with optimal height gain.

Carel J-C, Eugster EA, Rogol A, *et al*. Consensus Statement on the Use of Gonadotropin-Releasing Hormone Analogs in Children. *Pediatrics*. 2009;123:e752 –62.

Carel J-C, Leger J. Precocious Puberty. *N Engl J Med*. 2008;358:2366–77.

Klein KO. Precocious Puberty: Who Has It? Who Should Be Treated? *J Clin Endocrinol Metab*. 1999;84:2411–4.

Menon PSN. Pubertal disorders. In: Desai MP, Menon PSN, Bhatia V (Eds). Pediatric Endocrine Disorders, 3rd edition. Hyderabad: Universities Press; 2014: p. 121–178.

Rosen DS, Foster C. Delayed puberty. *Pediatr Rev*. 2001;22:309–15.

14.10 DISORDERS OF SEX DEVELOPMENT (DSD)

Disorders of sex development (DSD) are not uncommon (1 in 4000 births), and constitute a medical, social and psychological emergency. Careful clinical and laboratory evaluation is essential to identify the underlying disorder which may need emergent therapeutic intervention and decision about sex of rearing. There has been a shift from using culturally inappropriate and derogatory terms like ambiguous genitalia, intersex and hermaphroditism to more acceptable ones like disorders of sex development.

Physiology

Sex differentiation is a complex process involving a close interaction of genetic, phenotypic and psychological factors. This includes the development of gonads in accordance to the genetic signals, development of internal and external sex organs and secondary sex characters.

Gonadal differentiation Germ cells arise from the celomic epithelium of hindgut and migrate to the gonadal ridge at 4–6 weeks of gestation. There they combine with somatic cells to give rise to the bipotential gonad. Sex determining region of Y chromosome (*SRY*) is a transcriptional factor present on Y chromosome and is the most important regulator of early sexual differentiation. *SRY* acts in conjunction with other genes such as Wilms tumor gene 1 (*WT1*), *SOX* 9 and *DAX1* to induce testicular development. In the absence of *SRY* the bipotential gonad develops into ovary.

Genital differentiation Following development of testis, anti-müllerian hormone (AMH) secreted by Sertoli cells induces regression of müllerian ducts (progenitor of female reproductive tract) while testosterone produced by Leydig cells results in growth of wolffian ducts. Dihydrotestosterone (DHT), produced by action of 5α-reductase on testosterone, is responsible for male external genital development. In the absence of anti-Müllerian hormone and testosterone, müllerian ducts differentiate into fallopian tubes, uterus and the upper third of the vagina; labioscrotal swellings and

urethral folds do not fuse and give rise to labia majora and minora respectively.

Classification

These disorders were conventionally classified into four major categories of male pseudohermaphroditism, female pseudohermaphroditism, mixed gonadal dysgenesis, and true hermaphroditism. This has been now replaced by a classification based on karyotyping, and appearance of genitalia **(Table 14.17)**.

For all practical purposes, disorders of sex development may be caused by defects in gonadal differentiation (*gonadal dysgenesis*), androgen production (increased in females and reduced in males), or action (androgen insensitivity syndrome).

Etiology

I. Abnormal Gonadal Differentiation
1. SRY gene deletion
2. Mutations in genes involved in testicular differentiation (*WT1, SOX9, SF1, DAX1*)
3. 46, XY gonadal dysgenesis, 46 XX gonadal dysgenesis
4. Ovotesticular DSD (true hermaphroditism)

II. Increased Androgen Production in Females
1. Congenital adrenal hyperplasia (CAH)
2. Aromatase deficiency
3. Transplacental exposure to androgen

III. Insufficient Androgen Production or Action in Males
1. Androgen insensitivity syndrome (AIS)
2. 5α-reductase deficiency
3. Testosterone biosynthesis defects

Abnormal gonadal development Theses disorders are characterized by dysgenetic gonads with no functional tissue. Combinations of partially functional testis or ovary or ovotestis may be observed.
- *SRY gene deletion* results in 46, XY female.
- *Mutations in genes involved in the testicular differentiation* (*WT1, SOX9, SF1* and *DAX1*) also result in 46,XY gonadal dysgenesis. They are associated with renal (*WT1* mutation), skeletal (*SOX9*) or adrenal abnormalities (*DAX1*). Müllerian structures are present in contradistinction to disorders of inefficient androgen action.
- *46,XY gonadal dysgenesis* is associated with a high risk for development of gonadoblastoma.
- *46,XX gonadal dysgenesis* is usually caused by SRY translocation and presents as normal appearing male.
- *Ovotesticular DSD*, new term for true hermaphroditism, is characterized by the presence of both ovarian and testicular tissue in the same individual.

Table 14.17 Classification of Disorders of Sex Development (DSD)

Category	Previous names	Disorders
Sex chromosome DSD		45 XO Turner syndrome; 46, XX/XY gonadal dysgenesis
Ovotesticular DSD	True hermaphroditism	
46, XY DSD	Male pseudohermaphroditism	Gonadal dysgenesis, Steroidogenic defects, Androgen insensitivity syndrome, 5 α-reductase deficiency
46, XX DSD	Female pseudohermaphroditism	Androgen excess, aromatase deficiency, *SRY* insertion

* The appearance of genitalia even though normal, may be discordant to genetic karyotype

14

Increased androgen production in females These disorders are the commonest type of DSD.

- *Congenital adrenal hyperplasia (CAH)*, the commonest cause, is caused by the deficiency of steroidogenic enzymes 21-hydroxylase, 11β-hydroxylase and 3β-hydroxysteroid dehydrogenase (Please refer to section 14.11). This condition is life-threatening mandating the need for early identification and treatment (Fig. 14.16).
- *Transplacental androgen exposure* due to maternal medications or hyperandrogenism is associated with genital ambiguity in girls.
- *Aromatase deficiency*, a disease characterized by reduced conversion of testosterone to estrogen, presents with elevated androgen levels and virilization of female fetus.

Inefficient androgen production or action in males These disorders result from decreased production, activation or action of androgens.

- *Androgen insensitivity syndrome (AIS)*, an X-linked disorder of androgen action, is the commonest cause. It is characterized by resistance to androgens. The disease forms a spectrum ranging from normal female to that of male with hypospadias to infertility. Complete androgen insensitivity syndrome presents in the neonatal period as girls with inguinal masses and as primary amenorrhea in older girls. Increasing testosterone levels during puberty result in increased estrogen level and feminization. Müllerian structures are absent. High DHT levels are diagnostic.
- *5α-reductase deficiency* is associated with reduced DHT production. Increased testosterone during puberty acts on the androgen receptor leading to virilization. High testosterone and low DHT levels are diagnostic.
- *Testosterone biosynthetic defects* include deficiency of StAR, 3β-hydroxysteroid dehydrogenase, 17β-hydroxylase, and 17β-hydroxysteroid dehydrogenase enzymes.

EVALUATION OF A CHILD WITH DSD

Aims of evaluation include identification of the child requiring immediate intervention, need of further work-up and decision about the sex of rearing.

Evaluation for DSD is indicated in all infants with genital ambiguity, girls with inguinal masses (probable AIS), boys

with cryptorchidism (probable 21-hydroxylase deficiency), penoscrotal hypospadias (probable virilization disorder) and adolescent girls with amenorrhea (probable AIS).

Clinical Evaluation

Family history of DSD is helpful in diagnosis of 21-hydroxylase deficiency or AIS **(Table 14.18)**. The undescended gonads in complete AIS may be mistaken for inguinal hernia and operated. Intake of progestational drugs during first trimester and features of virilization in mother should be enquired. Failure to thrive and lethargy indicate 21-hydroxylase deficiency. Virilization during puberty is common in of 5α-reductase deficiency, while feminization indicates AIS. General examination should include assessment for facial dysmorphism and hyperpigmentation. Examination of mother and siblings for features of hyperandrogenism in the form of hirsutism, acne and change in voice should be done.

Genital Examination

The most important step is identification of gonads. Bilaterally rounded structures below the inguinal canal are most likely to be testes. The presence of gonads only on one side is suggestive of mixed gonadal dysgenesis or ovotesticular DSD. The labioscrotal region should be evaluated for the extent of fusion. The length of phallus and number of openings in the urogenital region should be recorded. Genital asymmetry indicates gonadal dysgenesis or ovotesticular DSD.

Investigations

The initial investigations should include serum electrolytes, pelvic ultrasound and karyotype. Identification of müllerian structures is crucial. Genitogram is helpful in determination of level of fusion, which is of surgical importance. Further investigations are guided by the results of clinical and laboratory evaluation. Serum 17OHP levels should be measured if müllerian structures are present. Testosterone levels should be estimated if no müllerian structures are identified. Elevated testosterone levels are suggestive of defects in androgen action while low levels indicate testosterone biosynthetic defects. These disorders can be further evaluated with hCG stimulated androgen levels. High DHT to testosterone ratio is suggestive of AIS while low levels indicate testosterone biosynthetic defects. Children with gonadal dysgenesis should undergo gonadal biopsy.

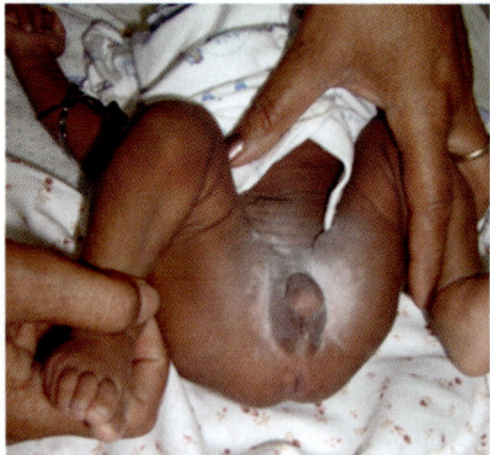

Fig. 14.16 A 14-day-old girl presented with genital ambiguity and failure to thrive. Workup was suggestive of salt wasting 21-hydroxylase deficiency

Table 14.18 Pointers to Diagnosis in DSD	
Pointer	*Likely diagnosis*
Pigmentation	Congenital adrenal hyperplasia, *SF1* defect
Genital asymmetry	Mixed gonadal dysgenesis, ovotesticular DSD
Skeletal dysplasia	*SOX* 9 defect
Polydactyly, microcephaly	Smith-Lemli-Optiz syndrome
Hypertension	CAH due to deficiency of enzyme 11- or 17-hydroxylase
Hemihypertrophy	*WT1* mutation
Renal failure	Denys-Drash syndrome

DSD: Disorders of sex development

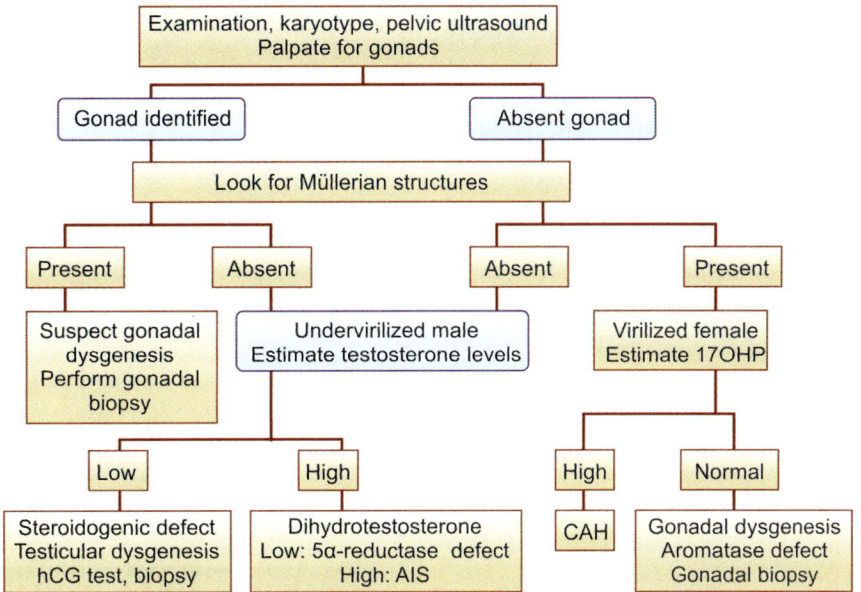

Fig. 14.17 Approach to disorders of sex development

Approach to Diagnosis

A scheme for evaluation is provided in Fig. 14.17. Müllerian structures with no palpable gonads indicate androgen excess state and need for estimation of serum 17OHP levels. Absence of Müllerian structure is suggestive of inefficient testosterone action and should be evaluated with estimation of testosterone and DHT levels. Müllerian structures with palpable gonads indicate gonadal dysgenesis or ovotesticular DSD. Absent gonads and Müllerian structures may be caused by vanishing testis syndrome or dysfunctional intra-abdominal testis. Estimation of levels of anti-Müllerian hormone (AMH) and hCG stimulation tests are helpful in differentiating these two conditions. Children with vanishing testis will have low levels of AMH and inappropriate response to hCG stimulation.

Treatment	Disorders of Sex Development

Management involves parental counseling, decision about sex of rearing, timing of surgical correction and gonadectomy. This requires a multidisciplinary team including pediatrician or pediatric endocrinologist, pediatric surgeon, geneticist, psychologist and social worker. Specific management should be initiated for conditions like 21-hydroxylase deficiency.

Parental Counseling

Birth of a child with DSD generates significant parental anxiety and stress in our society. This highlights the need for parental counseling. Most important aspect of counseling is reassurance when the child is healthy and the condition is amenable to specific treatment. Gender-specific connotation (he/she, testis, ovary) should be avoided and terms like gonads and phallus be preferably used. The process of sexual differentiation should be explained. This should be followed by explanation of child's appearance and possible diagnosis. Future implications regarding sexual and fertility prospects should be discussed. Decision about sex of rearing should be made after consultation of the management team with parents.

Decision about Sex of Rearing

Gender assignment should depend on the potential for future sexual and reproductive function, underlying abnormality, feasibility of reconstructive surgery and social acceptance and norms **(Table 14.19)**. Girls with virilization disorders have fertility potential and should be reared as females. Individuals with complete AIS should be reared as females. Decision of sex of rearing is difficult in disorders of inefficient androgen action. This should depend on genital appearance and surgical feasibility. There has been a trend of performing early surgeries before gender identity is established. Most centers perform

Table 14.19 Guidelines for Sex of Rearing in DSD		
Disorder	*Considerations*	*Gender of rearing*
CAH	Fertile female, gender appropriate	Female
Undervirilized male	Usually infertile Variable gender preference	Testosterone response Present—as male Absent—as female
Androgen insensitivity syndrome	No prospect of fertility Normal female development Risk of gonadoblastoma	Female Gonadectomy
5α-reductase defect	Virilization during puberty	Male

14

A baby, at birth, is noted to have abnormal appearing genitalia. The pregnancy was uneventful and the mother did not receive any drugs during pregnancy. There is no family history of similar illness. On examination at 24 hours of age, the child looked well, weighed 2.8 kg and was accepting breastfeeds well. Vitals were normal and systemic examination was noncontributory. Genital examination showed a small phallus with perineal hypospadias; labia were fused, and testes were palpable in the labioscrotal fold. Ultrasound of pelvis did not demonstrate ovaries.

Q1. What are the likely diagnoses?

Q2. What investigations will you perform?

The birth of an infant with abnormal appearing genitalia is a social and potential medical emergency. This necessitates rapid and organized evaluation to classify and diagnose the disorder, assign the appropriate gender, identify a possible life-threatening medical condition and initiate appropriate intervention. The diagnosis of ambiguous genitalia requires systematic history taking and physical examination including investigation of genetic studies, hormonal assays, radiological studies of internal genitalia, laparotomy and gonadal biopsy and culture of skin fibroblasts for androgen insensitivity, etc.

This child primarily has masculine features (phallus and bilateral testis) with evidence of undervirilization (small phallus and labioscrotal folds). The description fits in with a clinical diagnosis of 46,XY DSD. The underlying defect could be (*i*) inadequate production of testosterone; or (*ii*) peripheral unresponsiveness to androgen.

Investigations needed are karyotyping (to establish the genetic sex), CT or MRI (to evaluate internal genitalia, undescended gonads and adrenal anomalies), plasma steroid and testosterone levels (to detect inborn errors of testosterone biosynthesis), and gonadal biopsy later (to look for Leydig cell hypoplasia).

Revision Point

Disorders of Sex Development

1. The term Disorders of Sex Development (DSD) is used to denote a group of disorders with genital ambiguity due to abnormalities in genital development including genes, transcription factors, and/or hormones.

2. They are classified as 46,XX DSD, 46,XY DSD, sex chromosome DSD, and ovotesticular DSD.

3. The etiology of DSD includes abnormal gonadal development and differentiation, increased production or androgen in girls, and their insufficient production or action in boys.

4. Evaluation includes detailed clinical assessment, genital examination; appropriate imaging modalities; genetic and chromosomal studies; and hormonal estimations.

5. Management includes parental counseling, making decisions about sex of rearing, appropriate surgical corrections, and medical management.

6. Steroid replacement is indicated in children with congenital adrenal hyperplasia.

clitoroplasty at the age of 1 year with vaginoplasty reserved during puberty for girls with vaginal stenosis. Gonadectomy should be done in gonadal dysgenesis or ovotesticular DSD if Y cell line is present.

Ahmed, SF, Rodie M. Investigation and initial management of ambiguous genitalia. *Best Pract Res Clin Endocrinol Metab*. 2010;24:197–218.

Bajpai A, Sharma J, Menon PSN. Ambiguous genitalia. *In*: Practical Pediatric Endocrinology. New Delhi: Jaypee Brothers; 2003;97–101.

Brown J, Warne G. Practical management of the intersex infant. *J Pediatr Endocrinol Metab*. 2005: 18: 3–23.

Dreger AD, Chase C, Sousa A, *et al*. Changing the nomenclature/taxonomy for intersex: a scientific and clinical rationale. *J Pediatr Endocrinol Metab*. 2005;18:729–33.

Gupta DK, Menon PSN. Ambiguous genitalia – An Indian perspective. *Indian J Pediatr*. 1997;64:189–94.

Hughes IA, Houk C, Ahmed SF, *et al*. Consensus statement on management of intersex disorders. *Arch Dis Child*. 2006;91:554–63.

14.11 ADRENAL CORTEX DISORDERS

Physiology

Adrenal cortex produces 3 important groups of hormones involved in, fluid and electrolyte homeostasis, glucose regulation, response to stress, and sexual maturation—the glucocorticoids, mineralocorticoids, and androgens.

- *Cortisol*, the major glucocorticoid hormone has an important role in metabolism leading to increased blood glucose levels and enhanced catabolism of proteins and lipids.

- *Aldosterone*, the mineralocorticoid acts on distal renal tubules and collecting ducts to promote sodium and fluid absorption. Aldosterone deficiency causes urinary salt wasting resulting in salt wasting crisis. This results in severe hyponatremia, hyperkalemia and metabolic acidosis. Intravascular volume, serum potassium levels and renin-angiotensin system are the chief regulators of aldosterone synthesis.

- *Adrenal androgens* are involved in development of pubic and axillary hair.

- *Adrenocorticotropic hormone (ACTH)*, a polypeptide secreted by the anterior pituitary, is the principal regulator of gluco-corticoid and androgen synthesis.

The process of steroidogenesis involves conversion of cholesterol to steroid hormones in a series of enzymatic steps controlled by specific genes. The most clinically relevant step in steroidogenesis is mediated by 21-hydroxylase and essential for cortisol and aldosterone synthesis.

ADRENOCORTICAL HORMONE EXCESS

Hyperfunction of the adrenal cortex may be associated with excess production of glucocorticoids, mineralocorticoids, androgens and/or estrogen.

CUSHING SYNDROME

The most common disorder of adrenocortical hyperfunction is Cushing syndrome, characterized by generalized obesity and growth failure. It is a generic term used to describe clinical findings caused by prolonged glucocorticoid excess.

Cushing disease refers to hypercortisolism caused by an ACTH-producing pituitary tumor.

Etiology

Cushing syndrome may be caused by increased endogenous production or exogenous administration of glucocorticoids. *Glucocorticoid treatment* is the commonest cause. Increased adrenal glucocorticoid production may be related to increased ACTH levels or represent autonomous adrenal hyperfunction. Adrenal pathology is more likely in young children, while pituitary causes are more common after puberty. Etiology of Cushing syndrome is given below:

I. **ACTH-dependent**
   1. Hypothalamic lesions: Increased production of corticotropin releasing hormone (CRH)
   2. Pituitary lesions: Microadenoma, macroadenoma
   3. Ectopic lesions: Neuroblastoma, carcinoids, Wilms tumor

II. **ACTH-independent**
   1. Adrenal tumor: Carcinoma, adenoma
   2. Pigmented nodular hyperplasia
   3. McCune-Albright syndrome

III. **Exogenous**
   1. Glucocorticoid administration: Oral, parenteral, topical, inhaled ACTH.

Clinical Features

Classical features of Cushing syndrome such as central obesity, striae, moon facies and buffalo hump are rare in children. Growth failure and generalized obesity are the most common features (Fig. 14.18). Cushing syndrome should be suspected in children with obesity, growth retardation, osteoporosis, hypertension, psychosis, and hirsutism.

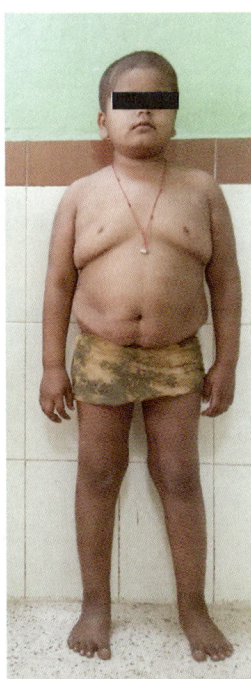

Fig. 14.18 A 10-year-old boy with Cushing syndrome. He was brought for evaluation of obesity. He had predominantly central obesity with short stature. (*Courtesy:* Dr Aashima Dabas)

ACTH-dependent Causes

Increased pituitary ACTH production is the commonest cause of endogenous Cushing syndrome. This is usually associated with increased pigmentation. Hypertension and hyperandrogenism are uncommon. Pituitary microadenoma accounts for more than 90% of all cases of childhood ACTH-dependent Cushing syndrome. Ectopic ACTH production is extremely uncommon. These children lack classical features of Cushing syndrome and present with hypertension and hypokalemic alkalosis.

ACTH-independent Causes

Autonomous adrenal production is the most common cause of Cushing syndrome in young children and may be due to adrenal adenoma, carcinoma or nodular hyperplasia.

- *Adrenal carcinoma* is likely in young children with rapid progression, hyperandrogenism, and large abdominal mass.
- *Pigmented nodular hyperplasia* is characterized by multiple, small black adrenal nodules and Cushing syndrome. Adrenal size is normal. This may occur as a part of Carney complex, a type of multiple endocrine neoplasia (MEN).
- *McCune-Albright syndrome* may also rarely present with ACTH-independent Cushing syndrome.

Evaluation

Evaluation is directed towards (*i*) confirming the diagnosis; (*ii*) identifying the underlying etiology; and (*iii*) assessing the complications.

Clinical Evaluation

Age at onset of symptoms and progression of disease should be ascertained. Adrenal carcinoma is likely with early onset and rapid progression. History of steroid intake (including inhaled and topical steroids) should be enquired. Hypertension and hyperandrogenism indicate ACTH-independent autonomous adrenal steroid production. Hyperpigmentation points towards ACTH-dependent Cushing syndrome. Features of McCune-Albright syndrome should be evaluated. Careful neurological and abdominal examination is mandatory.

Investigations

Basic investigations include estimation of ACTH and urinary free cortisol (UFC); high dose dexamethasone suppression test; and corticotropin releasing hormone (CRH) stimulation test. Diagnosis can be made using the criteria provided in **Table 14.20**. An algorithmic approach for investigating a child with Cushing syndrome is provided in Fig. 14.19.

Screening Tests

The commonly used screening tests include assessment of diurnal cortisol rhythm, overnight dexamethasone suppression test, and urine free cortisol.

- *Urine free cortisol (UFC)* is the best screening test for Cushing syndrome with levels more than 75 μg/m^2/day suggestive of Cushing syndrome.
- *Loss of diurnal rhythm* is the earliest marker of hypercortisolism. Thus, estimation of morning and evening cortisol has been used for screening of Cushing syndrome.

Table 14.20 Laboratory Findings of Common Causes of Cushing Syndrome

Disorder	UFC	HDDST	ACTH	CRH test
Adrenal lesion	High	Not suppressed	Low	Negative
Pituitary lesion				
Microadenoma	High	Suppressed	High	Positive
Macroadenoma	High	Not suppressed	High	Positive
Ectopic ACTH	High	Not suppressed	High	Negative
Exogenous	Low	Not suppressed	Low	Negative

HDDST: High dose dexamethasone suppression test; ACTH: Adrenocorticotropic hormone, CRH: Corticotropin releasing hormone; UFC: Urine free cortisol.

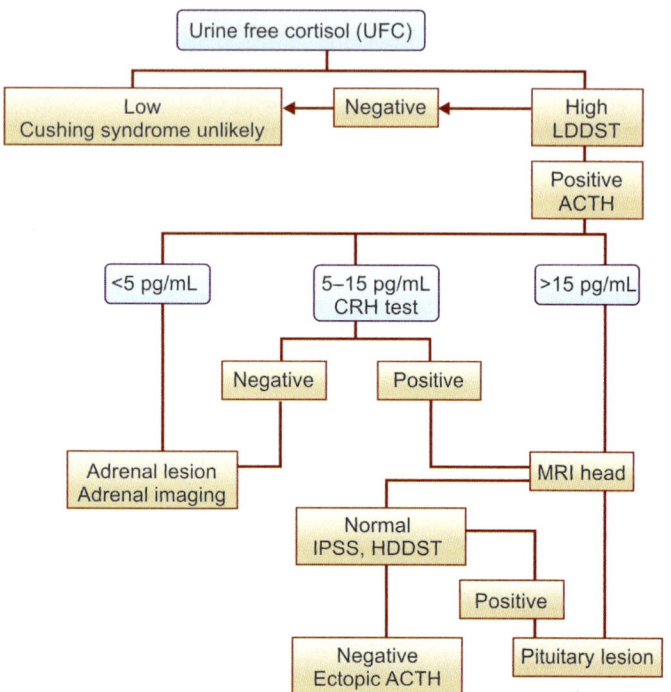

Fig. 14.19 Approach to a child with Cushing syndrome. LDDST—Low dose dexamethasone suppression test, IPSS: Inferior petrosal sinus sampling, HDDST: High dose dexamethasone suppression test, ACTH: Adrenocorticotropic hormone, CRH: Corticotropin releasing hormone. (If a reliable ACTH and/or CRH assay is not available, HDDST may be performed sequentially after LDDST, followed by the relevant imaging)

Individual variation in cortisol levels limits the diagnostic value of this test. The estimation of midnight cortisol, the time of physiological nadir of cortisol, is also a useful screening test for Cushing syndrome.

- *Overnight dexamethasone suppression test (ONDST)* involves estimation of cortisol levels after a single midnight dose of dexamethasone (0.3 mg/m²; maximum dose 1 mg). Lack of suppression of cortisol levels to less than 5 mg/dL favors the diagnosis of Cushing syndrome.

Confirmatory Tests

All children with positive screening tests need confirmation by a specific test. *Low dose dexamethasone suppression test (LDDST)* involves measurement of serum cortisol after eight doses of oral dexamethasone (5 mg/kg per dose, every six hours for two days or 1.25 mg/m²/day divided into four

doses given over two days). Serum cortisol levels greater than 5 mg/dL is diagnostic of Cushing syndrome.

Differentiation of ACTH-dependent from ACTH-independent Etiology

The most important part of evaluation is to differentiate ACTH-dependent causes from autonomous adrenal steroid production.

- *ACTH levels* These can differentiate ACTH-independent (ACTH levels <5 pg/mL) from ACTH-dependent conditions (ACTH levels >15 pg/mL). Ectopic ACTH production should be suspected in the presence of extremely high ACTH levels (>100 pg/mL).

- *High dose dexamethasone suppression test (HDDST)* It is based on the principle that high doses of dexamethasone suppress ACTH production in individuals with pituitary lesions but not in those with ectopic ACTH production. HDDST involves estimation of cortisol levels after eight doses of dexamethasone (3.75 mg/m²/day divided into four doses given over two days). Suppression of cortisol levels by greater than 50% of baseline indicates pituitary lesion, while absent or low level of suppression is suggestive of ectopic ACTH production.

ACTH-independent Presentation

Adrenal imaging should be performed to identify focal lesions. Large size, vascular invasion and loss of capsule are suggestive of adrenal carcinoma. Normal adrenal size should prompt evaluation for McCune-Albright syndrome or pigmented nodular hyperplasia.

ACTH-dependent Cushing Syndrome

MRI of the hypothalamic-pituitary region should be performed. *Inferior petrosal sinus sampling (IPSS)* should be done if neuroimaging is normal. This involves estimation of ACTH levels in the inferior petrosal sinus and peripheral blood before and after CRH stimulation. This is the best test for localization of source of ACTH production.

Treatment	**Cushing Syndrome**

Adrenal Causes

Resection of adrenal lesion is recommended in adrenal adenoma and carcinoma. Prolonged cortisol excess causes suppression of the normal contralateral adrenal. This mandates close monitoring for adrenal insufficiency in the perioperative period. Pigmented nodular hyperplasia should be treated with bilateral adrenalectomy.

Pituitary Causes

Trans-sphenoidal resection of pituitary adenoma is recommended for children with Cushing disease.

Unidentified Etiology

Treatment options include medical management or bilateral adrenalectomy. Medical management is limited by significant adverse effects. Bilateral adrenalectomy has been associated with the development of pituitary adenomas due to unmasking of pituitary lesion after removal of suppressive effect of glucocorticoids (Nelson syndrome).

Medical Treatment

Medical management of childhood Cushing syndrome with inhibitors of steroidogenesis (ketoconazole, aminoglutethimide, cyproheptadine, metyrapone, and mitotane) has been tried but is largely disappointing. Medical management may be considered in the preoperative period and in children with contraindications for surgery or relapse after surgery.

ALDOSTERONE EXCESS

Hyperaldosteronism is associated with fluid and sodium retention along with increased urinary loss of potassium. The most common clinical features of primary hyperaldosteronism are hypertension and hypokalemic alkalosis. Hypokalemia may be associated with muscle cramps and polyuria.

Etiology

Hyperaldosteronism can either be *primary*—due to increased adrenal aldosterone production or *secondary*–due to factors that activate renin–angiotensin system. Detailed etiology is listed below:

I. **Primary Hyperaldosteronism**
   - *Adrenal:* Adenoma, hyperplasia
   - Glucocorticoid remediable hyperaldosteronism (GRH)
II. **Secondary Hyperaldosteronism**
   - *Renin excess:* Renal artery stenosis, renin secreting tumor
   - *Hypovolemia:* Cardiac failure, nephrotic syndrome, liver disease
III. **Apparent Mineralocorticoid Excess**
   - Liddle syndrome, 11β-hydroxysteroid dehydrogenase deficiency, 11β-hydroxylase deficiency, and 17α-hydroxylase deficiency

Evaluation

Hypokalemic alkalosis in a child with low renin hypertension should prompt evaluation for true or apparent aldosterone excess. High aldosterone level in this setting is suggestive of primary hyperaldosteronism or glucocorticoid remediable hyperaldosteronism. The conditions may be differentiated by dexamethasone suppression test (suppression in glucocorticoid remediable hyperaldosteronism; no effect in primary hyperaldosteronism). Diagnosis of primary hyperaldosteronism should be confirmed by adrenal imaging.

Treatment	Hyperaldosteronism

Hyperaldosteronism is managed with salt restriction and antialdosterone agent, spironolactone. Physiological hydrocortisone replacement suppresses ACTH secretion in glucocorticoid remediable hyperaldosteronism resulting in resolution of hyperaldosteronism and hypertension. Surgery is the treatment of choice for adrenal adenoma.

ANDROGEN EXCESS

Increased adrenal androgen production may be related to some types of congenital adrenal hyperplasia (CAH) or adrenal tumors. Congenital adrenal hyperplasia is discussed in detail, later in this chapter.

Clinical Features

Most virilizing adrenal tumors are carcinomas. Hirsutism, premature pubarche, refractory acne, change in voice, and clitoromegaly are common presenting features in girls. The clinical features of Cushing syndrome and hypertension are common.

Diagnosis

Adrenal androgen excess should be considered in the differential diagnosis of hyperandrogenism in girls and gonadotropin-independent precocious puberty in boys. High dehydroepiandrosterone (DHEA) levels are suggestive of an adrenal source of hyperandrogenism. Dexamethasone does not suppress androgen levels in children with adrenal neoplasm unlike CAH. Hyperpigmentation should prompt evaluation for CAH with basal and ACTH-stimulated 17OHP levels. CT scan of the abdomen helps in localizing the tumor and provides information regarding the extent of tumor spread.

Treatment	Androgen Excess

Aggressive surgical treatment is recommended for adrenal carcinoma. The tumor should be excised completely without damaging its capsule. Radiotherapy or chemotherapy is usually ineffective. Steroid supplementation is effective in CAH.

ADRENAL INSUFFICIENCY

Insufficient synthesis or action of adrenal hormone can present as slowly progressive disease or acute salt wasting crisis that can be life-threatening.

Etiology

Adrenal insufficiency may be primary, secondary or due to ACTH resistance.

I. **Primary Adrenal Insufficiency**
   - Adrenal destruction: Autoimmune, hemorrhage, or infection (tuberculosis, fungi, HIV, CMV)
   - Congenital: Congenital adrenal hypoplasia, defects in steroid synthesis (21-hydroxylase. 3β-hydroxysteroid dehydrogenase, StAR deficiencies), adrenoleukodystrophy
   - Iatrogenic: Surgery, prolonged steroid treatment
II. **Secondary ACTH Deficiency**
   - Congenital: CNS malformation, genetic defects
   - Acquired: CNS insults (surgery, radiation, infection); brain tumors (glioma, craniopharyngioma)
III. **ACTH Resistance**

14

Autoimmune adrenal dysfunction is the commonest cause of primary adrenal failure (Addison disease). Infections like tuberculosis and HIV also cause primary adrenal failure. Adrenal hemorrhage in the setting of meningococcal and other bacterial infections (Waterhouse-Friderichsen syndrome) is an important cause of acute adrenal insufficiency. Congenital adrenal hypoplasia (X-linked defect in *DAX1* gene) and steroidogenic defects (StAR, 21-hydroxylase, 3β-hydroxysteroid dehydrogenase deficiencies) present with adrenal insufficiency in the neonatal period. Adreno-leukodystrophy, an X-linked peroxisomal disorder, presents with neurological features including spasticity and developmental regression and adrenal failure.

Secondary adrenal insufficiency may be caused by congenital malformations (holoprosencephaly or midline defects) genetic defects or acquired insult (neurosurgery, tumor, radiation, or infection). This is usually associated with other anterior pituitary hormone deficiencies as isolated ACTH deficiency is extremely rare. Mineralocorticoid function is preserved and salt wasting is not observed.

Prolonged steroid treatment is associated with suppression of the hypothalamic-pituitary-adrenal axis resulting in adrenal insufficiency after discontinuation of medications.

Clinical Features

- Congenital defects in steroid synthesis and congenital adrenal hypoplasia manifest in early neonatal period with polyuria, failure to thrive, recurrent vomiting, and shock.
- Acquired adrenal insufficiency presents with slowly progressive lethargy, vomiting, salt craving, fatigue, postural hypotension, fasting hypoglycemia, and episodes of shock during severe illness. Adrenal insufficiency usually manifests only after 90% of adrenal is damaged.
- Addison disease is characterized by hyperpigmentation over elbows, palmar creases, areola and genitalia. This is caused by increased production of melanocyte stimulating hormone (MSH) during the process of ACTH synthesis.

Evaluation

Investigations may reveal hyponatremia, hyperkalemia, metabolic acidosis, hemoconcentration, and hypoglycemia. This clinicobiochemical picture is characteristic of acute adrenal insufficiency and warrants immediate steroid replacement. All children suspected to have adrenal insufficiency should have urgent estimation of serum electrolytes and blood sugar.

Basal cortisol levels are low. ACTH stimulation test (cortisol estimation 60 minutes after 0.25 mg of ACTH injection IM) is the best test for adrenocortical reserve. Serum cortisol levels lower than 18 mg/dL are suggestive of adrenal insufficiency.

Next step in the evaluation of adrenal insufficiency is the estimation of ACTH levels. Elevated ACTH levels suggest primary adrenal pathology while low levels points towards pituitary defect. Further evaluation of primary adrenal insufficiency includes abdominal CT scan, estimation of antiadrenal antibodies and work-up for tuberculosis.

Treatment	**Adrenal Insufficiency**

Initial management includes correction of shock by appropriate fluids with management of hyponatremia and hyperkalemia.

Hydrocortisone should be administered immediately in a dose of 50 mg/m^2 followed by 100 mg/m^2/day. Frequent monitoring of hemodynamic parameters, urine output and serum electrolytes is required. Once the child is thermodynamically stable, hydrocortisone is tapered gradually to physiological dose (10–15 mg/m^2/day) along with the addition of fludrocortisone acetate (0.1 mg/day). Lifelong glucocorticoid and mineralocorticoid treatment is required. Glucocorticoid dose should be increased 2–3 times during minor stress (fever and mild infection) and 4–5 times in severe stress (severe infection or surgery). Patients with ACTH deficiency require lower dose of glucocorticoids (6–10 mg/m^2/day) and do not require mineralocorticoids.

CONGENITAL ADRENAL HYPERPLASIA

Congenital adrenal hyperplasia (CAH), a group of autosomal recessive defects in steroid biosynthesis, is characterized by deficiency of adrenocortical hormones on one hand and excess of steroid precursors on the other **(Table 14.21)**. CAH is the commonest adrenal disorder in childhood.

21-hydroxylase Deficiency

21-hydroxylase deficiency is the commonest form of CAH accounting for over 90% of all cases. This disorder is associated with diminished synthesis of the cortisol and aldosterone. Low cortisol levels stimulate ACTH synthesis. Elevated ACTH level in turn causes accumulation of steroid precursors and excess androgen. The disease has a spectrum of clinical features ranging from severe forms presenting in the neonatal period with salt wasting crisis, to milder types presenting with virilization alone or mild hyperandrogenism in late childhood.

Salt wasting (SW) type These children are the most severely affected and present in the neonatal period with virilization and salt wasting. The diagnosis is often missed in boys as they might lack genital ambiguity unlike girls. They usually present after the second week of life with failure to thrive, polyuria, hyperpigmentation, and shock. Early diagnosis is mandatory to prevent mortality. 21-hydroxylase deficiency should be suspected in a newborn with ambiguous genitalia, polyuria, shock, recurrent vomiting, and features of sepsis with negative septic screen. The diagnosis should be confirmed immediately by hormonal assays. If hormone studies are not available immediately, the child should be managed empirically in the lines of adrenal insufficiency.

Simple virilizing (SV) type These children synthesize enough aldosterone to prevent an adrenal crisis. They have features of androgen excess in the form of virilization in girls and peripheral precocious puberty in boys.

Non-classic (NC) type This disorder is associated with partial 21-hydroxylase deficiency. Cortisol and aldosterone levels are normal. The clinical manifestations are related to mild hyperandrogenism which presents with hirsutism, acne, and menstrual irregularities later in childhood or adolescence.

Diagnosis

The diagnosis of salt wasting type is established by the demonstration of extreme elevation of serum 17OHP levels (10000–20000 ng/dL, normal less than 90 ng/dL) in the presence of clinical and laboratory features of adrenal insufficiency. The serum 17OHP levels are elevated to a lesser

Enzyme involved	Cortisol	Aldosterone	Androgen	BP	Presentation		Diagnosis	Treatment
					Boys	Girls		
21-hydroxylase								
Salt wasting	Low	Low	High	Low	PP	Ambiguity	17OHP*	HC, FC
Simple virilizing	Low	Low, normal	High	Normal	PP	Ambiguity	17OHP*	HC, FC
Non-classic	Normal	Normal	High	Normal	Normal	Hirsutism	17OHP*	HC
11β-hydroxylase	Low	Low	High	High$	PP	Ambiguity	DOC, 11DOC	HC, SL
3β-HSD	Low	Low	Variable#	Low	Ambiguity	Ambiguity	ACTH test**	HC, FC
17-hydroxylase/ lyase	Low	Normal	Low	High$	Ambiguity	Delayed puberty	DOC, 18-OHDOC	HC, FC
StAR	Low	Low	Low	Low	Ambiguity	Delayed puberty	Low 17OHP	HC, FC

Table 14.21 Comparison of Common Types of Congenital Adrenal Hyperplasia (CAH)

HSD: Hydroxysteroid dehydrogenase; StAR: Steroidogenic acute regulatory protein; BP: Blood pressure; 17OHP: 17 hydroxyprogesterone; DOC: Deoxycorticosterone; HC: Hydrocortisone; FC: Fludrocortisone; SL: Spironolactone; PP: Precocious puberty; 11DOC: 11-deoxycorticosterone; 18OHDOC: 18-hydroxydeoxycorticosterone
* Basal and ACTH stimulated, $Due to mineralocorticoid effect of DOC, #Due to peripheral conversion of DHEA, ** Ratio of pregnenolone to progesterone, 17-hydroxypregnenolone to 17OHP and DHEA to androstenidione after ACTH stimulation.

extent in with SV and NC types. The best method of diagnosing these children is by the estimation of serum 17OHP levels before and 60 minutes after an intramuscular injection of ACTH (0.25 mg).

Treatment   Congenital Adrenal Hyperplasia

Patients with SW and SV types are treated with hydrocortisone (10–15 mg/m²/day) and a mineralocorticoid (fludrocortisone 0.1 mg/day). The dose should be increased under stressful conditions as in adrenal insufficiency. After completion of growth, synthetic glucocorticoid preparations (dexamethasone or prednisolone) can be used.

Other Variants of CAH

Enzyme deficiencies other than 21-hydroxylase deficiency account for less than 10% of cases of CAH. Patients with 11β-hydroxylase deficiency and 17α-hydroxylase deficiency present with hypertension and are managed with hydrocortisone alone **(Table 14.21)**. Deficiencies of StAR and 3β-hydroxysteroid dehydrogenase enzymes manifest as salt wasting crisis and require addition of a mineralocorticoid.

Arnaldi G, Angeli A, Atkinson AB, *et al*. Diagnosis and classification of Cushing syndrome: a consensus statement. *J Clin Endocrinol Metab*. 2003;88:5593–602.

Bajpai A, Kabra M, Menon PSN. 21-hydroxylase deficiency: clinical features, laboratory profile and pointers to diagnosis in Indian children. *Indian Pediatr*. 2004; 41:1226-32.

Boscaro M, Arnaldi G. Approach to the child with possible Cushing's Syndrome. *J Clin Endocrinol Metab*. 2009; 94: 3121–31.

Findling JW, H Raff H. Screening and diagnosis of Cushing's syndrome. *Endocrinol Metab Clin North Am.* 2005; 34: 385–402.

Migeon CJ, Lanes R. Adrenal cortex: hypo- and hyperfunction. In: Lifshitz F. *Pediatric Endocrinology*. New York: Informa Healthcare; 2007.p. 195–226.

Miller WL. The Adrenal Cortex. *In*: Brook C, Clayton P, Brown R. *Clinical Pediatric Endocrinology*, 5th edition. Oxford: Blackwell Publishing; 2005.p.293–351.

Adrenal Cortex Disorders

1. Cushing syndrome is the commonest disorder of adrenocortical hyperfunction. The clinical features include central obesity along with growth failure.
2. Diagnosis of Cushing syndrome includes detailed hormonal evaluation including estimation of plasma cortisol, urine free cortisol and ACTH along with imaging techniques. Management includes removal of adrenal or pituitary lesions.
3. Aldosterone excess is associated with fluid and sodium retention along with increased urinary loss of potassium.
4. Androgen excess is commonly due to congenital adrenal hyperplasia.
5. Adrenal insufficiency is due to primary adrenal insufficiency or ACTH deficiency and is characterized by hyperpigmentation with failure to thrive and electrolyte disturbances. It is managed by appropriate steroid replacement.
6. The most common cause of congenital adrenal hyperplasia (CAH) is 21-hydroxylase deficiency. It has a spectrum of manifestations ranging from severe forms presenting in neonatal period with salt wasting crisis with milder types presenting with virilization and mild hyperandrogenism in late childhood.
7. Patients with salt wasting and simple virilizing forms of CAH are treated with lifelong steroid replacement.

Nieman L, Biller BMK, et al. The Diagnosis of Cushing's Syndrome: An Endocrine Society Clinical Practice Guideline. *J Clin Endocrinol Metab* 2008;93:1526–40.

Pivonello R De Martino R, *et al*. Cushing syndrome. *Endocrinol Clin Metab North Am*. 2008;37:135–49.

Shulman DI, Palmert MR, Kemp SF, for the Lawson Wilkins Drug and Therapeutics Committee. Adrenal insufficiency: still a cause of morbidity and death in childhood. *Pediatrics*. 2007;119: e484–e94.

PSN Menon and Anurag Bajpai

Malignancies in Childhood

15.1 CANCER EPIDEMIOLOGY IN CHILDHOOD

Cancers are a leading cause of mortality accounting for 13% of deaths worldwide. Majority are in low-middle income countries. Though cancer is usually regarded as an adult and old age disease, it has a significant incidence in pediatric and young adolescent population. Moreover, there is a higher incidence of pediatric cancers in India in comparison to the world literature. Estimates suggest that approximately 1.5 to 5% of all cancers are contributed to by childhood cancers in our country **(Table 15.1)**. This is significantly higher than data from other countries. The reasons for this higher incidence are not clear, but may be associated with increased incidence of viral infections, which are associated with certain cancers, as well as an increased exposure to carcinogens.

World over, survival rate for childhood cancers was dismal till the 1960s, with an estimated 5-year overall survival of 28% after a diagnosis of cancer. Over the last few decades, the outcomes have been steadily improving. In the current century, the survival has improved drastically for most of the cancers, with overall outcome reaching 80% at 5 years and more than 75% at 10 years. The most impressive strides have been made in the treatment of childhood acute lymphoblastic leukemia, Hodgkin lymphoma, non-Hodgkin lymphoma and Wilms tumor, where the survival is between 80 and 100%. Similar excellent outcomes for these malignancies have not been attained in our country. There are several reasons for that including under-recognition of

pediatric cancers, late referral due to under-recognition, late diagnosis, limited pediatric oncology services, and lack of supportive care, to name a few. Though significant strides have been made in reducing childhood mortality, which has been an important MDG goal, most of effort till date has been towards improving infection related mortality. With improvements in the communicable diseases' outcome; it is essential to now place equivalent emphasis on non-communicable diseases, especially childhood cancers.

Revision Point

Cancer Epidemiology

1. Cancers account for 13% of deaths worldwide. Approximately 1.5 to 5% of children in our country may be affected by cancer.
2. Common cancers in children include leukemia, lymphoma, CNS tumors, Wilms tumor, neuroblastoma, and rhabdomyosarcoma.
3. Survival for ALL, Hodgkin lymphoma, non-Hodgkin lymphoma, and Wilms tumor is between 80 and 100%.

Ripperger T, Bielack SS, Borkhardt A, et al. Childhood cancer predisposition syndromes-A concise review and recommendations by the Cancer Predisposition Working Group of the Society for Pediatric Oncology and Hematology. *Am J Med Genet*. 2017;173:1017–37.

Schüz J, Erdmann F. Environmental Exposure and Risk of Childhood Leukemia: An Overview. *Arch Med Res*. 2016;47:607–14.

Sharma D, Singh G. Spectrum of cancer in adolescents and young adult: An epidemiological and clinicopathological evaluation. *Indian J Cancer*. 2016;53:457–9.

15.2 ACUTE LYMPHOBLASTIC LEUKEMIA

Acute leukemias of childhood are the most common childhood cancers, contributing to approximately 30–40% of all pediatric malignancies.

Acute vs chronic leukemia By definition, acute leukemia implies malignant clone expansion involving the immature marrow elements, in comparison to chronic leukemia, where there is clonal expansion of mature marrow cells. There is no specific time cut-off for definition of acute or chronic leukemia.

Epidemiology

Acute lymphoblastic leukemia (ALL) is the most common leukemia seen in pediatric age group. There is a ratio of

Table 15.1 Age-adjusted Incidence Rates (per 100,000 Population) of Childhood Cancers from India

Tumor type	Boys	Girls
Leukemia	35.7–61.3	22.3–40.2
Lymphoma	9.9–25.6	2.9–10.1
Central nervous system tumor	6.6–19.8	3.0–16.0
SNS tumor	1.5–12.6	1.8–5.3
Retinoblastoma	1.9–12.3	1.3–6.7
Renal tumor	3.1–9.5	1.8–7.0
Hepatic tumor	0.5–2.0	1.0–1.8
Bone tumor	2.8–9.0	2.3–6.2
Soft tissue sarcoma	2.8–7.2	1.6–7.6
Germ cell tumor	1.3–12.9	0.2–1.3

(*Source*: NCRP Report 2009–2011)

approximately 80 : 20 of ALL : AML cases in children. ALL has an incidence of 3–4 per 100,000 children, and has a slight male preponderance. The incidence peaks between 2 and 5 years of age.

Etiology

Majority of cases of ALL do not have any specific etiology; however predisposing features may be present in a minority. Syndromic associations include Down syndrome, Bloom syndrome, neurofibromatosis, and ataxia-telangiectasia. Other associations include immunodeficiency disorders, and radiation exposure.

Classification

A classification provided by the French-American-British (FAB) Cooperative Working Group (FAB classification) divides ALL in three morphological subtypes including FAB types L1, L2, and L3. ALL L1 is the most common subtype accounting for approximately 85–90% of ALL.

FAB (French-American-British) Classification

Based on morphology and cytochemistry of the blast cells, ALL is categorized L1, L2, L3 subtypes.
- *L1* This is the most common subtype in children. The blasts are small and homogenous with scanty cytoplasm, nil or one nucleolus, and no or minimal cytoplasmic vacuolations.
- *L2* This type is more common in adults. It is characterized by large heterogeneous blasts with indented nuclei, one or more nucleoli, abundant cytoplasm, and minimal cytoplasmic vacuolations.
- *L3* The blasts in this subtype are large and homogenous with abundant basophilic cytoplasm and prominent cytoplasmic vacuolations (Burkitt lymphoma).

This classification does not have any prognostic significance currently, as more sophisticated techniques like cytochemical staining, flow cytometry, and PCR based assays are now available to subtype the leukemia accurately. Moreover, it is not always possible to distinguish accurately between AML and ALL based on morphology alone.

Immunological Classification

Immunophenotyping is helpful in identifying the lineage of leukemia cells (T cell, mature B cell, precursor B cell) and then planning more rationale and risk adapted chemo-therapeutic regimens. In children, common precursor B-cell ALL is seen in approximately 70% cases followed by T cell ALL (15–20%). Mature B-cell ALL and pre T-cell ALL are rare in children.

Clinical Manifestations

Children with ALL typically present with a short history of a few days to months duration. Clinical features are a result of bone marrow replacement by the malignant cells, and shut down of the normal hematopoietic process.
- The majority of the children may have *fever* which is typically low grade, but occasionally can be high grade; bone pains may be present especially in the night; easy fatigability and lethargy are common systemic symptoms.
- *Bone pains* and *bony tenderness* often manifests as tiredness and refusal to walk. That occurs due to the involvement

of the long bones and periosteum by the malignancy. Arthritis may be present, and may involve several large and small joints. It may become difficult to differentiate it from a rheumatological disorder, especially juvenile idiopathic arthritis. At times, the children may be mistakenly treated for the same by steroids and methotrexate, leading to partial remission and resolution of symptoms of leukemia, before the disease resurfaces.

Presence of clinical bleeding may be there on the skin or the mucosae; rarely visceral bleeding may be present. Visceral bleeds may involve the gastrointestinal tract, the lungs, or the brain. The latter two typically occur in case of high TLC (total leukocyte count) and T-ALL subtype; and may be fatal. In the T-ALL subtype, the classical presentation is that of an older, pre-adolescent or adolescent boy, with fever, cough and mediastinal widening due to lymphadenopathy. Superior mediastinal syndrome (described later) may be present. The TLC is typically on the higher side, and hyperleukocytosis (TLC >100,000/mm^3) may be present.

Clinical examination Generalized lymphadenopathy, hepatomegaly, and/or splenomegaly are present in 50–70% of the patients. However, infrequently, there may be children with essentially normal physical examination except for mild pallor. In such cases, there may be a delay in diagnosis. Skin bleeds, arthritis, unilateral or bilateral painless testicular enlargement, retinal bleeds are other features to assess in these children. There may be petechiae, purpura, or bruises on the skin.

Laboratory features A variable degree of anemia and thrombocytopenia may be present. The TLC may be low, normal, or elevated; however, the differential leukocyte count usually has a clue as lymphocytes are typically more than expected for the age. On peripheral smear examination, there may be lymphocyte predominance, or presence of blasts.

Differential Diagnosis

Acute lymphoblastic leukemia needs to be differentiated from other disorders that also present with fever, anemia, and bleeds.
- *Infectious mononucleosis* presents with fever, lymphadeno-pathy and hepatosplenomegaly. Peripheral smear is characterized by large lymphocytes. There are no blast cells in peripheral blood.
- *Aplastic anemia* can be differentiated by characteristic absence of lymphadenopathy and hepatosplenomegaly.
- In ITP, spleen is usually not enlarged and anemia is absent, or mild—proportionate to degree of bleeds.
- *Juvenile rheumatoid arthritis* can be confused with leukemia when a child presents with joint pains, fever, hepato-splenomegaly, anemia, and lymphadenopathy. Bone marrow aspiration helps in differentiating the two conditions.
- Other malignant conditions with bone marrow involvement that have features similar to leukemia include neuroblastoma, retinoblastoma, and rhabdomyosarcoma. However, these conditions are characterized by presence of abdominal lump, ocular swelling, or a soft tissue mass, respectively.
- Differentiating ALL from *non-Hodgkin lymphoma* can be tricky at times.

15

Diagnosis

On clinical suspicion, the first investigation is a complete blood count and a peripheral smear examination. Diagnosis is confirmed by bone marrow examination which shows an increased number of leukemic blasts (normal bone marrow has less than 5% blasts; in ALL, the blasts must be more than 25%). In most of the situations, the bone marrow is nearly completely replaced by blasts. Further analysis of the blasts from the bone marrow aspiration smear allows classification and typing of the leukemia. In ALL, the cytochemistry on the bone marrow specimen will be negative for myeloperoxidase (MPO) and may be positive for periodic acid–Schiff stain (PAS).

Flow Cytometry

Flow cytometry confirms the diagnosis and helps in typing into B-ALL or T-ALL.

- The markers used for diagnosing B-ALL on flow cytometry include CD10, 19, 22, 20, 79a
- Markers for T-ALL include CD2, 3, 7
- Markers and for AML include CD13, CD33 and MPO
- Biologically, B-ALL is significantly more common than T-ALL, with 80–85% being B-ALL. T-ALL is seen typically in older children.
- Majority of the B-ALL are CD10 positive and are termed CALLA positive (CALLA stands for common acute lymphoblastic leukemia associated antigen). CD10 negativity in B-ALL is often associated with other poor prognostic markers like presence of t(4;11) or MLL gene rearrangement.
- Rarely, mixed phenotypic acute leukemia may be diagnosed on flow cytometry, when markers of either T-ALL or B-ALL may be present along with markers of AML.

A diagnostic CSF examination is required apart from a bone marrow examination to assess whether CNS disease is present or not. CNS positive status is defined as (a) presence of >5 blasts/mm^3 in the CSF examination; (b) CNS bleed; or (c) cranial nerve palsy at the time of presentation.

Risk Stratification of ALL

- Presence of high TLC beyond 50,000/mm^3; and age extremes (<1 year and >10 years) are poor risk criteria.
- Girls are usually considered to have a better outcome than boys.
- Presence of bulky disease with massive hepatosplenomegaly, large mediastinal lymphadenopathy, CNS disease or testicular involvement worsens the outcome in ALL.
- T-ALL has worse outcomes than B-ALL and these patients require upfront therapy intensification.
- Specific genetic and chromosomal aberrations confer a poor risk status. These include presence of t(9;22) or Philadelphia chromosome positivity; t(4;11) or MLL gene rearrangement; t(17;19) and intrachromosomal amplification of chromosome 21 (iAMP21).
- Presence of t(12;21) is noted in some children, and is usually associated with a good risk ALL.
- Presence of t(1;19) was traditionally considered to confer a poor risk, but with current treatment strategy, it is considered to be standard risk.
- Hypodiploidy is a poor risk factor.

Response to Therapy

It is the most important risk stratification parameter. In case of poor early response to therapy, the outcome is likely to be poorer; and therapy intensification is required. Response to therapy is assessed by clearance of blasts in the peripheral blood by day 8 of therapy and bone marrow response at the end of induction therapy by day 28 or day 35. The bone marrow should have less than 5% blasts at the end of induction. One extremely important parameter currently used worldwide for assessing response to therapy is minimal residual disease (MRD, discussed below). Presence of a low MRD implies a good response to therapy.

Concept of Minimal Residual Disease (MRD)

Minimal residual disease or MRD has become the most important risk stratification parameter in ALL over the last few years. It is now being followed universally for making important therapeutic decisions. MRD is typically assessed at the end of induction therapy for ALL by doing a flow cytometry or PCR examination from a bone marrow aspirate. This technique is used to supplement microscopic examination of bone marrow.

Overall burden of ALL equals 10^{12} cells in an average patient. Using light microscopy alone, it is possible to detect 1 malignant cell in 100 cells. This implies that once the leukemic cells decrease by two log to a value of approximately 10^{10} cells, light microscopy will not be able to detect the amount of residual disease. However, using flow cytometry/PCR based assays, it is possible to detect one malignant cell in 10$^{4-6}$ cells. Thus, this is a very sensitive technique for detecting presence of residual leukemic cells at the end of induction in B-ALL or end of consolidation in T-ALL. Presence of a high MRD at the end of induction is a poor prognostic factor, and requires intensification of therapy. On the other hand, a low MRD at the end of induction is very reassuring, and implies that the treatment is appropriate. MRD is now being used at most centers treating childhood ALL in India for risk stratification purposes.

Treatment — Acute Lymphoblastic Leukemia

ALL is highly chemosensitive, and is curable in the majority by using a combination of chemotherapeutic agents. Radiation therapy is employed infrequently, and there is no role of surgery. Chemotherapy is usually given for prolonged period of time. The treatment has 4 main parts: Remission induction or induction therapy, consolidation or intensification therapy, CNS directed therapy, and maintenance.

1. Remission Induction

It aims to decrease tumor burden and bring the bone marrow in remission. The drugs used are prednisolone, vincristine, and L-asparaginase. An anthracycline agent is added in children with high-risk leukemia. This phase typically lasts for 28–35 days, and a bone marrow assessment is done at the end to look for morphological remission as well as to assess MRD.

Often, a prephase of steroids is given (with prednisolone) for a week prior to starting other drugs, and a response in the form of reduction in peripheral blood blasts cells is assessed. A good response helps stratify the patient into good risk ALL, whereas persistence of a high number of blasts on the peripheral blood smear (taken as 1000/mm^3 in majority of the protocols) is treated as a high-risk leukemia.

2. Consolidation Therapy

Also called intensification, this phase uses different drugs than those used in induction. The aim of this phase is to further decrease the leukemic burden and to prevent development of resistance to chemotherapy. The agents used include cytarabine, cyclophosphamide, anthracyclines, etoposide, L-asparaginase, and vincristine. The intensity and duration of this phase of therapy depends on the risk stratification. In both these intensive phases, there is a significant risk of febrile neutropenia, and mortality; this should be judicially balanced against the likelihood of cure from leukemia.

3. CNS Directed Therapy

Majority of children with ALL have presence of subclinical CNS disease; approximately 5–15% may have overt CNS disease. CNS is a recognized sanctuary site; as most of the chemotherapeutic agents do not cross the blood–brain barrier. The aim of this phase is to treat the CNS seeding of leukemia, and to prevent CNS relapses. This involves intrathecal administration of chemotherapy, which typically includes methotrexate, and may involve steroids or cytarabine. This arm of treatment occurs along with induction and consolidation therapy, and continues well into maintenance.

Radiation therapy to the CNS is used rarely; and the most common indication is presence of overt CNS disease. Current treatment regimens are trying to minimize the use of radiotherapy even in this cohort as there are significant long-term side effects of CNS radiation.

4. Maintenance Therapy

This phase lasts for approximately 2 years, and aims to achieve long-term remission by clearing the remaining malignant cells. The drugs used include oral mercaptopurine and methotrexate. Some regimens use intermittent pulses of steroids and vincristine as well.

Use of imatinib in Philadelphia positive ALL starting from day 15 of induction till the end of maintenance has improved the outcome in this poor risk subset, and may prevent need for allogenic stem cell transplant in most of these patients.

A standard protocol for treatment of ALL (standard risk) is depicted in **Box 15.1**.

Box 15.1 A Common Treatment Protocol for Standard Risk ALL

Induction phase for standard risk ALL (Prephase steroids are given for 1 week in some protocols)

	Week 1	Week 2	Week 3	Week 4	Week 5
Vincristine 1.5 mg/m^2	↑	↑	↑	↑	↑
Intrathecal methotrexate	↑	↑			↑
Pegylated L-asparagine 1000 IU/m^2	↑		↑		
Dexamethasone 6 mg/m^2	▬▬▬▬▬▬▬▬▬▬▬▬▬▬▬▬				→
6-Mercaptopurine 75 mg/m^2					▬▬▬▬
Check bone marrow and MRD					↑

CNS consolidation and interim maintenance

	Week 6	Week 7	Week 8	Weeks 9–12	Weeks 13–16
Intrathecal methotrexate	↑	↑	↑	↑	↑
Vincristine 1.5 mg/m^2				↑	↑
Dexamethasone 6 mg/m^2				▬▬▬	▬▬▬
6-Mercaptopurine 75 mg/m^2 daily	▬▬▬▬▬▬▬▬▬▬▬▬▬▬▬▬▬				
Oral methotrexate 20 mg/m^2 once/week				▬▬▬▬▬▬▬▬	

Delayed intensification

	Week 17	Week 18	Week 19	Week 20	Week 21	Week 22	Week 23
Intrathecal methotrexate	↑						
Vincristine 1.5 mg/m^2	↑	↑	↑				
Doxorubicin 25 mg/m^2	↑	↑	↑				
Dexamethasone 10 mg/m^2	▬▬▬		▬▬▬				
Pegylated asparaginase 1000 IU/m^2	↑						
Cytarabine 75 mg/m^2 × 4 days					↑↑↑↑	↑↑↑↑	
Cyclophosphamide 1000 mg/m^2					↑		
6-Mercaptopurine 60 mg/m^2					▬▬▬▬▬▬▬		

Maintenance cycle. Each cycle lasts 12 weeks. There are several such cycles (8–12)

Day	1	8	15	22	29	36	43	50	57	64	71	78	84
Intrathecal methotrexate as per age	▲	▲	↑	▲	▲	▲	▲	▲	▲	▲	▲	▲	↑
Oral methotrexate 20 mg/m^2 weekly	1	8	15	22	29	36	43	50	57	64	71	78	
Cotrimoxazole (bd)	■ 1	■ 8	■ 15	■ 22	■ 29	■ 36	■ 43	■ 50	■ 57	■ 64	■ 71	■ 78	
Mercaptopurine 60 mg/m^2 (po)	▬▬▬▬▬▬▬▬▬▬▬▬▬▬▬▬▬▬▬▬▬▬▬▬▬▬▬▬▬▬▬▬▬▬▬												

5. Supportive Care

It is extremely important in ALL to prevent treatment related morbidity and mortality. For this reason, children with ALL should undergo treatment at a center which routinely treats this disease, preferably under the care of a pediatric oncologist. Presence of a departmental policy to ensure judicious transfusions, early and timely admission and initiation of antibiotics in the presence of febrile neutropenia, cotrimoxazole for *Pneumocystis jiroveci* prophylaxis are essential for a good outcome.

Relapsed ALL

Worldwide, relapsed ALL has become the 4th most common pediatric malignancy. ALL usually relapses within a period of 3 years after completion of therapy. Relapse can be medullary, with bone marrow involvement; it can be extramedullary involving CNS and testes. Whether medullary, combined or isolated extra-medullary, systemic chemotherapy is required to cure relapsed ALL.

Case Study	Acute Lymphoblastic Leukemia

A 5-year-old girl presented with low grade fever for 10 days along with lethargy. There was no obvious infective focus. Examination findings revealed moderate pallor, no lymphadenopathy, with hepatomegaly 4 cm and splenomegaly 3 cm below costal margin. A complete blood count revealed: Hb: 7 g/dL, TLC: 32,000/mm³, DLC: N20L76M3E1, Platelet count: 60,000/mm³. Evaluation for infectious etiologies including enteric fever, malaria, viral infections like EBV, and urinary tract infection was negative.

Q. What is the probable diagnosis?

Due to persistence of fever, presence of hepatosplenomegaly, thrombocytopenia, and differential counts showing presence of lymphocytosis, a possibility of acute leukemia should be considered. Presence of unexplained lymphocytosis for age in the CBC should always raise a suspicion of leukemia. At times, the peripheral smear may be normal, but the bone marrow examination would yield the diagnosis.

Peripheral smear was checked on day 5 of hospital admission, and it showed a few blast cells. Bone marrow aspirate confirmed presence of 94% blasts, which were MPO negative. On further evaluation by flow cytometry, the blasts were positive for CD10, 19, and 22; negative for CD13, 33, MPO, and CD3, 5,7. A diagnosis of CD10 positive B-ALL was considered. PCR obtained from the bone marrow studies did not have any high risk molecular abnormalities.

Q. Classify the disease and outline therapy.

She has standard risk leukemia, that should be started on 3 drugs induction with vincristine, L-asparaginase, and steroids. Simultaneous CNS prophylaxis should be started with intrathecal methotrexate. A simultaneous monitoring for tumor lysis syndrome has to be done in the initial few days of her induction therapy, and prophylactic allopurinol given. Cotrimoxazole is to be started for PCP prophylaxis. A check bone marrow examination along with evaluation of minimal residual disease is to be planned at the end of induction. Appropriate risk stratification is important to decide the therapy, and it includes tumor burden, molecular typing along with response to therapy.

Radiotherapy may be required in cases of CNS and testicular involvement at relapse. Allogenic stem cell transplant can be done in a child with high risk relapse; though the prognosis is guarded in such cases. Late relapses fare better than early relapses. Isolated extramedullary relapse has a better prognosis than bone marrow relapse.

ALL in India

Treatment of ALL in India has been showing an improving trend, with outcomes for standard risk ALL reaching 60–80% in several centers. Outcome of high risk ALL including T-ALL and Philadelphia positive ALL are still lagging, and will improve in the years to come. Currently, a multicentric trial is being conducted in major centers using a uniform risk stratification schema and chemotherapy protocol for ALL. This will help in deciding the optimal treatment specific to our population subset.

Revision Point

Acute Leukemia

1. ALL is the most common malignancy in children.
2. Diagnosis is based on bone marrow examination and flow cytometry.
3. Typically, children present with fever, pallor, bleeding manifestations, bony tenderness, lymphadenopathy, and hepatosplenomegaly.
4. High leucocyte count, age <1 year or >10 yeas, male sex, bulky disease, T-cell ALL, specific cytogenetic abnormalities and poor response to therapy are considered as poor prognostic markers.
5. Treatment consists of remission induction (with 3 drugs with or without an anthracycline agent), consolidation therapy, CNS prophylaxis, and maintenance methotrexate therapy for 2 years (with 6-MP and methotrexate).
6. Overall survival for standard risk ALL is 60–80% in India.

Athale UH, Gibson PJ, Bradley NM; POGO MRD Working Group. Minimal Residual Disease and Childhood Leukemia: Standard of Care Recommendations From the Pediatric Oncology Group of Ontario MRD Working Group. *Pediatr Blood Cancer*. 2016;63:973–82.

Burkhardt B, Mueller S, Khanam T, Perkins SL. Current status and future directions of T-lymphoblastic lymphoma in children and adolescents. *Br J Haematol*. 2016;173:545–59.

Carroll WL, Hunger SP. Therapies on the horizon for childhood acute lymphoblastic leukemia. *Curr Opin Pediatr*. 2016;28:12–8.

Ceppi F, Antillon F, Pacheco C, Sullivan CE, et al. Supportive medical care for children with acute lymphoblastic leukemia in low- and middle-income countries. *Expert Rev Hematol*. 2015;8:613–26.

Hunger SP, Mullighan CG. Acute Lymphoblastic Leukemia in Children. *N Engl J Med*. 2015;373:1541–52.

Madhusoodhan PP, Carroll WL, Bhatla T. Progress and Prospects in Pediatric Leukemia. *Curr Probl Pediatr Adolesc Health Care*. 2016;46:229–41.

Schütte P, Möricke A, Zimmermann M, et al. Preexisting conditions in pediatric *ALL* patients: Spectrum, frequency and clinical impact. *Eur J Med Genet*. 2016;59:143–51.

Seth R, Singh A. Leukemias in Children. *Indian J Pediatr*. 2015;82:817–24.

15.3 ACUTE MYELOID LEUKEMIA

Epidemiology

Acute myeloid leukemia (AML) accounts for approximately 20% of all childhood leukemias. It is a more complex disease than ALL, and is associated with poor overall survival. With the advent of excellent supportive care and availability of stem cell transplant, the outcomes of AML are gradually improving worldwide; however, they are still dismal in our country.

There is a bimodal age distribution, with one peak before 2 years of age and another at 15–20 years of age. Males and females are affected equally.

Etiology

There is no specific etiological factor for AML, however some predisposing factors are present. They include exposure to prior chemotherapy including alkylating agents or epipodophyllotoxins, syndromes including Down syndrome, Noonan syndrome, Bloom syndrome, and inherited bone marrow failure syndromes like Fanconi anemia.

Biology

Traditionally, AML is classified using the classification given by the French-American-British (FAB) Cooperative Working Group (FAB classification) which groups the disease into 8 types, from M0 to M7 **(Box 15.2)**. FAB classification of AML is based on morphology and immunostaining. With the advent of molecular diagnostics, currently the WHO classification is being followed as it has more prognostic relevance than FAB classification **(Table 15.2)**.

Box 15.2 FAB Classification of AML

M0: AML with no evidence of differentiation
M1: Myeloblastic leukemia with little maturation
M2: Myeloblastic leukemia with maturation
M3: Acute promyelocytic leukemia
M4: Acute myelomonocytic leukemia
M5: Acute monoblastic leukemia
M6: Erythroleukemia
M7: Acute megakaryoblastic leukemia

Clinical Features

The presenting symptoms of AML are due to bone marrow replacement by the malignant cells. Children often have fever, lethargy, easy fatigability, bone pains, pallor, and bleeding diathesis. Gum hypertrophy may be present. Lymphadenopathy and organomegaly may be present. Complete blood counts are often abnormal, with anemia and thrombocytopenia. Coagulopathy and DIC like picture may be seen, typically in the presence of FAB subtype M3, M4, and M5.

Presence of extramedullary mass of tumor in the form of myeloid sarcoma or chloroma is a feature of certain types of AML and is often associated with t(8;21) translocation. Chloromas may be present anywhere in the body including CNS, orbit, spine, or trunk and may cause pressure symptoms at those sites. It may cause paraparesis or proptosis if present in spine or orbit. At times, a child may present with an isolated chloroma, without features of bone marrow involvement.

Diagnosis

TLC may be low or very high, with hyperleukocytosis in a minority of patients. Diagnosis is established by bone

---

Table 15.2 WHO Classification of Acute Myeloid Leukemia 2016

A. *Acute myeloid leukemia with recurrent genetic abnormalities*
  • AML with t(8;21) (q22;q22.1); RUNX1-RUNX1T1
  • AML with inv(16) (p13.1q22) or t(16;16) (p13.1;q22); CBFB-MYH11
  • APL with PML-RARA
  • AML with t(9;11) (p21.3;q23.3); MLLT3-KMT2A
  • AML with t(6;9) (p23;q34.1); DEK-NUP214
  • AML with inv(3)(q21.3q26.2) or t(3;3) (q21.3;q26.2); GATA2, MECOM
  • AML (megakaryoblastic) with t(1;22) (p13.3;q13.3); RBM15-MKL1
  • AML with mutated NPM1
  • AML with biallelic mutations of CEBPA

B. *Acute myeloid leukemia with myelodysplasia-related changes*

C. *Therapy-related myeloid neoplasms*

D. *Acute myeloid leukemia, NOS*
  • AML with minimal differentiation
  • AML without maturation
  • AML with maturation
  • Acute myelomonocytic leukemia
  • Acute monoblastic/monocytic leukemia
  • Pure erythroid leukemia
  • Acute megakaryoblastic leukemia
  • Acute basophilic leukemia
  • Acute panmyelosis with myelofibrosis

E. *Myeloid sarcoma*

F. *Myeloid proliferations related to Down syndrome*
  • Transient abnormal myelopoiesis
  • Myeloid leukemia associated with Down syndrome

---

marrow evaluation, which will demonstrate increased leukemic blasts beyond 20%. Cytochemistry shows positive myeloperoxidase stain and Sudan Black B stains in majority of the AML. Flow cytometry is also required to subtype the leukemia accurately.

Risk Stratification

AML has a complex risk stratification system, taking several variables into account. Presence of specific cytogenetic aberrations and response to therapy are the main criteria for risk stratification. A simplified risk stratification schema is given in **Box 15.3**. Apart from the genetic abnormalities mentioned in **Box 15.3**, absence of bone marrow remission or high minimal residual disease at the end of induction signifies a high-risk AML.

Box 15.3 Risk Stratification in AML (Simplified)

Standard risk:
1. Presence of t(8;21); inversion 16; t(15;17)
2. *NPM1* mutation
3. *CEBPA* mutation

Poor risk:
1. Presence of *FLT 3-ITD* mutation
2. Monosomy 5, monosomy 7
3. Complex cytogenetic abnormalities

Treatment — Acute Myeloid Leukemia

Treatment of AML requires aggressive chemotherapy, with the aim to minimize treatment related toxicity while providing maximal chances of a cure. World over survival rates of AML have reached nearly 50%, and despite a significant increase, they still lag considerably behind ALL cure rates.

The treatment typically incorporates high doses of anthracyclines, cytarabine, and etoposide. The most common regimen used is called 3 + 7, as it uses 3 doses of daunorubicin and 7 days of cytarabine. In children, etoposide is typically added to this regimen. CNS directed therapy is in the form of intrathecal chemotherapy with methotrexate, hydrocortisone, and/or cytarabine.

In case of poor response to initial therapy, or in case of a high-risk disease, children would require allogenic stem cell transplant from a matched donor (sibling or unrelated) to achieve cure. In case of good response, further cycles of chemotherapy are continued, and they include high doses of cytarabine. Intensive supportive care is usually required for cytopenia, febrile neutropenia, neutropenic enterocolitis, and cardiac dysfunction.

Total duration of therapy is 4–6 months. There is no role of maintenance therapy in AML. Relapses can occur up to 3 years off therapy, and regular monitoring is required to assess for late effects of therapy as well as relapse. The most common late effect of therapy is related to anthracycline induced cardiac toxicity.

ACUTE PROMYELOCYTIC LEUKEMIA (APML)

This is a rare subtype of AML and treated differently. It is characterized by promyelocytes and promyeloblasts on the bone marrow examination. A characteristic finding in this subtype of leukemia is the high risk of DIC and spontaneous life-threatening bleeding which may often be the presenting complaint. The overall tumor burden is usually not high, with minimal organomegaly and low TLC, often less than $10,000/mm^3$. Aplastic anemia often constitutes a close differential, especially when children present with muco-cutaneous and/or visceral bleeds. Fever and other constitutional symptoms may be present, but are not very impressive in the majority.

Diagnosis

The diagnosis is confirmed by bone marrow examination, which shows increased number of promyelocytes as well as blasts, frequently with many *Auer rods* (termed as faggots). Granules are typically present in the malignant cells. The conclusive diagnosis is by detecting the translocation t(15;17) or PML-RARA by either FISH or PCR in the malignant cells.

Treatment — APML

Treatment of APML is by using differentiation therapy along with chemotherapy, which helps the malignant cells in maturing normally. The drug of choice is all-*trans* retinoic acid (ATRA). Another drug which can be used is arsenic trioxide. Often, either of the 2 agents is combined with chemotherapy consisting of anthracycline like daunorubicin or idarubicin along with cytarabine. Treatment of DIC requires aggressive supportive care with platelet and fresh frozen plasma infusions. Most children who survive the initial few days of induction therapy without any adverse event tend to do very well, with excellent long-term survival.

MYELOPROLIFERATIVE DISORDERS IN DOWN SYNDROME

Another specific entity is Down syndrome with AML. Children with Down syndrome are predisposed to acute leukemia, with a significantly higher risk to the tune of 10–20 times for both ALL and AML in comparison to the general population. AML is more common till about 4 years of age, after which there is a slightly higher incidence of ALL in comparison to AML.

Transient Myeloproliferative Disorder

Transient myeloproliferative disorder (TMD), also known as transient abnormal myelopoiesis, occurs commonly and almost exclusively in nearly 10% of the children with Down syndrome. It is characterized by presence of elevated TLC, hepatomegaly, and presence of circulating AML like blasts on the peripheral smear. It almost always occurs before 6 months of age, and may be present even at birth. It is difficult to differentiate from AML pathologically, however, early onset before 6 months is a big clue towards TMD.

The driving mutation is *GATA-1*, which is the same mutation causing AML in these children. It is important to make a correct diagnosis, as most cases with TMD respond spontaneously without any therapy. In a few cases having organ dysfunction, intravenous fluids, exchange transfusion, or low dose cytarabine therapy may be required. Most children do very well after recovery, however, there is an increased risk of developing AML in these children later in life.

Treatment — AML in Down Syndrome

AML in children with DS carries a very good prognosis. It is most commonly AML-M7 subtype, and responds very favorably to chemotherapy. DS children have more than normal toxicity with chemotherapy, especially cytarabine, and require modified chemotherapy regimens.

Revision Point — Acute Myeloid Leukemia (AML)

1. AML is more complex than ALL and has a poor survival
2. There are 8 subtypes (M0 to M7); flow cytometry is essential to subtype the leukemia accurately, besides a marrow examination.
3. Cytogenetic abnormalities and response to therapy determine the outcome.
4. Daunorubicin, cytarabine and etoposide are the most commonly used drugs for treatment of AML.
5. Acute promyelocytic leukemia (M3) is typically associated with high risk of DIC.
6. All-*trans* retinoic acid (ATRA) is the drug of choice for APML chemotherapy, along with anthracyclines, and cytarabine.
7. Children with Down syndrome are predisposed to develop AML or a transient myeloproliferative disorder; driven by *GATA-1* mutation.

Saida S. Evolution of myeloid leukemia in children with Down syndrome. *Int J Hematol.* 2016;103:365–72.

Taga T, Tomizawa D, Takahashi H, Adachi S. Acute myeloid leukemia in children: Current status and future directions. *Pediatr Int.* 2016;58:71–80.

Zwaan CM, Kolb EA, Reinhardt D, et al. Collaborative Efforts Driving Progress in Pediatric Acute Myeloid Leukemia. *J Clin Oncol.* 2015;33:2949–62.

15.4 CHRONIC MYELOID LEUKEMIA

Chronic myeloid leukemia (CML) accounts for approximately 1–3% of all leukemias. It was initially recognized as an entity in 1845, however, its pathophysiology became clear only by the next century when Philadelphia chromosome was discovered.

Etiopathogenesis

Exposure to ionizing radiation is considered to be a risk factor for CML. Practically all patients demonstrate chromosomal translocation t(9;22) (q34;q11) in the leukemic blast cells. This translocation is not pathognomonic of CML, as it may be rarely positive in children with ALL and AML. However, absence of this translocation makes the diagnosis of CML difficult as it is positive in >90% of the patients by routine cytogenetic testing.

Clinical Presentation

Majority of the patients present in the chronic phase of CML. Due to the *massive splenomegaly*; the primary presenting complaint is pain and dragging sensation on left side of abdomen. Occasionally, fever and systemic complaints may be present. In patients who present in the accelerated phase or blast crisis, the clinical features of leukemia (as described in the prior section) are present. High TLC may lead to features of hyperleukocytosis, which is more common in children than in adults. Approximately 90% patients are in chronic phase. In the few patients on accelerated phase, there is an increase in the spleen size, total leukocyte count, and peripheral blood examination shows increased basophilia greater than 20%. Thrombocytopenia may develop.

Diagnosis

The diagnosis is confirmed by bone marrow examination, which shows myeloid hyperplasia, with normal myeloid maturation. There are increased basophils and eosinophils, and may have some dysplasia. LAP score is low. Philadelphia chromosome or BCR-ABL transcript is detected by FISH or PCR on the bone marrow specimen.

In *accelerated phase* of CML, bone marrow examination shows presence of increased blasts between 10 and 19%; and presence of blasts at or beyond 20% is diagnostic of blasts crisis. The blast crisis may be myeloid, lymphoid, or mixed blast crisis. At times, children with ALL or rarely AML may present with Philadelphia positive disease, which needs to be differentiated from CML with blast crisis. The clinical pointers are presence of a long-standing disease, massive splenomegaly, and presence of basophilia, which are much more common in CML rather than in acute leukemias.

Treatment — Chronic Myeloid Leukemia

Historically the drugs used for treatment were busulfan, hydroxyurea, and interferon alpha. While these drugs caused improvement in symptoms in the majority, there was no improvement in the overall long-term survival. Interferon alpha therapy led to complete response in a minority of patients in comparison to the other drugs; however, had a significant side effect profile.

- Treatment of CML has been revolutionized with the discovery of tyrosine kinase inhibitor, **imatinib**. Imatinib blocks the enzyme activity of several types of tyrosine kinases, including the ones involved in CML pathogenesis. The mainstay of therapy of chronic phase CML is daily oral imatinib.
- Other second line tyrosine kinase inhibitors include dasatinib and nilotinib, and they can be tried in certain cases of imatinib failure.
- The curative treatment of allogenic stem cell transplantation is reserved for patients who have non-response or relapse on tyrosine kinase inhibitors, and is no longer considered the first line therapy. It is, however, the only curative option in case blast crisis is present.
- Monitoring of therapeutic response is done by serial and timed assessment of the number of BCR-ABL transcripts, by quantitative PCR.

JUVENILE MYELOMONOCYTIC LEUKEMIA

Juvenile myelomonocytic leukemia (JMML) is a rare neoplasm occurring solely in infancy and early childhood. It is an aggressive disease driven by overabundance of monocytic cells with organ infiltration. A less aggressive variant can occur in Noonan syndrome where spontaneous remissions are known to occur.

Clinical features Children present with fever, pallor, cough, skin rash, and may have bleeding manifestations. Typically, hepatosplenomegaly is present. It needs to be differentiated from diseases with a similar presentation, including acute leukemia, storage disorders, and infections like CMV, EBV, malaria, and kala-azar.

Diagnosis Diagnosis is made with the help of specific criteria, including presence of monocytosis on the peripheral blood film, absence of Philadelphia chromosome positivity, elevated hemoglobin F, and less than 20% blasts on the bone marrow examination.

Treatment Treatment requires stem cell transplant; however, even with SCT, the cure rates are low. Low dose chemotherapy including cytarabine and *cis*-retinoic acid are used for palliation of symptoms.

Revision Point — CML AND JMML

1. CML accounts for only 1–3% of childhood leukemia.
2. Massive splenomegaly is the hallmark of CML.
3. All patients demonstrate Philadelphia chromosome [t(9;22) (Q34;Q11)] in the blast cells.
4. CML may enter into an acute (*accelerated*) phase or develop blast crisis in 10% cases.
5. Imatinib is the drug of choice for treatment of CML.
6. JMML occurs in infancy and presents acutely with fever, bleeding, and hepatosplenomegaly. Philadelphia chromosome is negative. Cure rates are low, even with stem cell transplantation.

15

Ampatzidou M, Papadhimitriou SI, Goussetis E, *et al.* Chronic myeloid leukemia (CML) in children: classical and newer therapeutic approaches. *Pediatr Hematol Oncol.* 2012;29:389–94

Hasle H. Myelodysplastic and myeloproliferative disorders of childhood. *Hematology Am Soc Hematol Educ Program.* 2016;2016:598–604.

Hijiya N, Millot F, Suttorp M. Chronic myeloid leukemia in children: clinical findings, management, and unanswered questions. *Pediatr Clin North Am.* 2015;62:107–19.

Locatelli F, Niemeyer CM. How I treat juvenile myelomonocytic leukemia. *Blood.* 2015;125:1083–90.

Sakashita K, Matsuda K, Koike K. Diagnosis and treatment of juvenile myelomonocytic leukemia. *Pediatr Int.* 2016;58(8):681–90.

Tanizawa A. Optimal management for pediatric chronic myeloid leukemia. *Pediatr Int.* 2016;58:171–9.

15.5 HODGKIN LYMPHOMA

Lymphomas are the 3rd most common malignancy in children. They arise from the cells of lymphoid origin and typically present with enlargement of lymphoid tissue present in various parts of the body. It can be subdivided into two major subgroups: Non-Hodgkin lymphoma (NHL) and Hodgkin lymphoma (HL). Over the last several decades, chemotherapy has revolutionized the treatment of pediatric lymphomas and cure is now possible for most children suffering from lymphoma.

Hodgkin lymphoma is a success story in pediatric oncology, with one of the best cure rates amongst all oncological disorders. The current therapy includes chemotherapy and radiotherapy, and with contemporary treatment, survivals of 70 to 100% have been achieved. The current focus has now become directed towards decreasing therapy without compromising cure rates to decrease side effects of therapy including second malignant neoplasms (SMNs), cardiotoxicity, pulmonary toxicity, and infertility.

Epidemiology

Lymphomas account for approximately 10% of all pediatric malignancies. Hodgkin lymphoma contributes to about 40% of all pediatric lymphomas, occurring with a frequency of 5–7 per million. There is a characteristic age distribution with a bimodal peak. In the developing world, the first peak is early in the pre-pubertal age group. Another peak occurs in adulthood, beyond 40–50 years of age. HL is unusual in younger children below 5 years. A disproportionate sex distribution with male predominance has been reported from India. The reason for this is unknown.

Etiology

The etiology has not been clearly elucidated, however, infections like EBV and HIV are associated with an increased risk of the disease. Immunocompromised children with underlying diseases like ataxia-telangiectasia are more likely to be affected. A familial component has been detected, with siblings being at a higher risk of disease. It may be related to a possible susceptibility gene detected on chromosome 4.

Pathology

Hodgkin lymphoma can be classified into two major subtypes: (a) Classical HL and (b) nodular lymphocyte predominant HL. The various subtypes as per the WHO classification are mentioned in the **Table 15.3** and discussed

Table 15.3 WHO Classification of Hodgkin Lymphoma (Histology)

1. Classical Hodgkin lymphoma • Nodular sclerosis subtype • Mixed cellularity subtype • Lymphocyte-rich subtype • Lymphocyte-depleted subtype
2. Nodular lymphocyte predominant Hodgkin lymphoma

below. Epstein-Barr virus (EBV) infection is typically associated with mixed cellularity subtype of classic HL, and is more commonly seen in developing nations as compared to nodular sclerosis subtype of HL seen more frequently in developed countries. The cell of origin is known as **Reed-Sternberg cell**. It is a typical binucleate cell with owl's eye appearance. These malignant cells are usually few, but bulk of tumor is formed by the reactive lymphocytes and histiocytes.

Two main subtypes are described; classical HL and nodular lymphocyte predominant HL **(Table 15.3)**. Classical HL can be further divided into nodular sclerosis, mixed cellularity, and lymphocyte depleted. Their features are mentioned below.

1. *Lymphocyte predominant* This is a rare type, and is most commonly confused with benign reactive lymph node enlargement. The disease may be seen only in the paracortical regions between germinal centers. Diagnostic Reed-Sternberg (RS) cells may be sparse. Eosinophils, plasma cells, neutrophils are usually absent. This variety of Hodgkin disease is usually seen in children <10 years of age, usually localized at diagnosis (stage I/II) and carries an extremely favorable prognosis.

2. *Lymphocyte depleted* This is rare in children and usually present in advanced stage (stage III/IV) at diagnosis. Fibrosis and necrosis is commonly seen and it carries a poor prognosis. It is often associated with HIV infection.

3. *Mixed cellularity* This type is intermediate between lymphocyte predominant and lymphocyte depleted subtype in prognosis as well as proportion of neoplastic cells. There are plenty of RS cells and numerous eosinophils, plasma cells, lymphocyte, and benign histiocytes. This is the most common subtype in our country and is associated with EBV infection.

4. *Nodular sclerosis* This is the most common type of Hodgkin disease in teenagers and young adults and commonly seen in developed countries. It has a variant of RS cell called *lacunar cell*. There is thickened capsule with proliferation of collagenous bands that divide the node into nodules.

Clinical Presentation

The involved areas are typically lymph nodes, with contiguous spread to other areas. In advanced diseases, liver, spleen, bone marrow and other visceral organs may become involved. The commonest symptom is development of slowly progressive lymphadenopathy. The lymph nodes involved in HL are typically non-tender with a rubbery feel. Cervical lymph nodes are most commonly involved (75%) (Fig. 15.1) followed by mediastinal lymph nodes. Any lymph node group may be involved; however, primary involvement of infra-diaphragmatic LN is unusual.

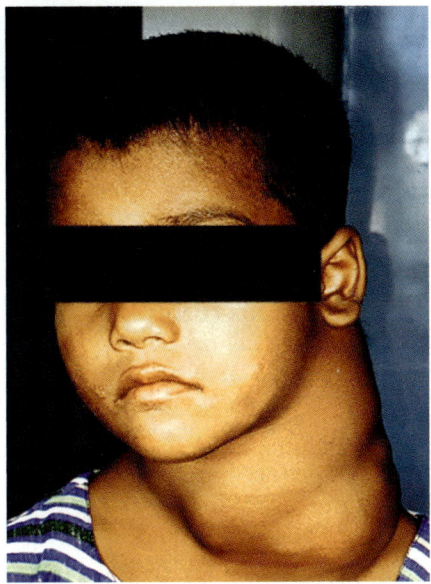

Fig. 15.1 Large cervical lymph nodes in a child with Hodgkin lymphoma

Presence of *B symptoms* is important to further stage of the disease. 'B' symptoms are present if the patient has any of the following features: Fever >100.4°F for at least 3 consecutive days, drenching night sweats, or significant weight loss (>10%) in the last 6 months. B symptoms indicate an advanced stage of disease. Presentation with advanced disease and B symptoms is common in our country, and is seen in nearly 50% patients.

Associated autoimmune phenomenon like immune thrombocytopenia and Coombs' positive hemolytic anemia may be seen infrequently, these may predate the disease or appear several years after completion of therapy.

Staging of Hodgkin lymphoma is shown in **Table 15.4**.

Investigations

Diagnosis Lymph node biopsy is mandatory for making the diagnosis. Either excision or a core needle biopsy is sufficient. Fine needle aspiration cytology (FNAC) is usually insufficient to confirm or reject the diagnosis of HL as lymph node architecture cannot be commented upon, and this

Table 15.4 Modified Ann-Arbor Staging for Hodgkin Lymphoma	
Stage	*Definition*
I	Involvement of a single lymph node region (I) or of a single extralymphatic organ/site (IE)
II	Involvement of two or more lymph node regions on same side of diaphragm (II) or localized involvement of an extra-lymphatic organ/site on same side of diaphragm (IIE)
III	Involvement of lymph node regions on both sides of the diaphragm (III), may be accompanied by involvement of spleen (IIIS) or by localized involvement of an extra-lymphatic organ or site (IIIE)
IV	Diffuse or disseminated involvement of one or more extra-lymphatic organ tissues with or without associated lymph node involvement

technique is conventionally not recommended. The background is composed of small lymphocytes, histiocytes, and eosinophils. Tumor cells stain positive for CD15 and CD30, while negative for CD45. CD20 is variably positive. However, nodular lymphocyte predominant HL (NLPHL) has a very different picture, with cells staining positive for CD45, CD20, and negative for CD15 and CD30.

Staging investigations These include chest X-ray (PA and lateral views) and an abdominal ultrasound. Chest radiograph helps in assessing presence of mediastinal enlargement. CT scan (neck to abdomen) *vs* a PET-CT is typically performed to evaluate lymph nodal groups, as well as the potential extra-nodal sites, including liver, spleen, intestine, and lung parenchyma. Either can be used to assess size and site of lesion and for comparative evaluation during restaging. However, PET scan also provides additional response to therapy, and is currently the investigation of choice.

PET may be falsely positive post recent chemotherapy (<10 days), use of colony stimulating factor, inter-current infections, and post-radiotherapy for up to 3 months. It is an expensive investigation, not widely available as of now, and requires expertise and experience to report accurately. For these multiple reasons, CT scan is frequently used rather than a PET-CT.

Evaluation of bone marrow by doing both aspirate and biopsy is recommended for advanced stage HL, typically for disease stage IIB and beyond. In coming years, it is possible that PET and MRI may become a substitute for bone marrow examination. Tumor volume estimation and ESR provide a guide to risk stratification. ESR of ≥30 mm/hour upstages a low risk patient as will presence of initial bulky tumor (tumor volume at any site of ≥200 mL).

Treatment	Hodgkin Lymphoma

Hodgkin lymphoma is an exquisitely chemosensitive and radiosensitive disease with high chances of cure after appropriate therapy. Chemotherapy alone may be curative for several patients, especially those who have low risk disease, and show a good response to initial chemotherapy cycles.

ABVD regimen used to be the benchmark of therapy; however, it is no longer considered a preferred modality for children as it has significant long-term toxicity. Some of the current treatment regimens include OEPA-COPDAC (vincristine, etoposide, prednisone, adriamycin-cyclophosphamide, vincristine, prednisone, dacarbazine),or AV-PC (adriamycin, vinblastine, prednisone, cyclophosphamide). In early stage, 3–4 cycles of chemotherapy alone may work well.

In most of the European countries, including UK, a low-risk HL would typically be treated with two cycles of OEPA chemotherapy followed by one cycle of COPDAC. The indication to add low dose involved field radiation therapy are poor early response to therapy. Bulky disease may be another reason to add radiotherapy. This strategy of intensifying treatment by adding radiotherapy is known as **response adapted therapy**, and is the benchmark of treatment of HL now. In contrast, a higher stage HL may require more intense therapy, with 4–8 cycles of multimodality, cross resistant chemotherapy. These patients also frequently require radiotherapy to achieve cure. ABVD regimen **(Table 15.5)** is typically reserved for

Table 15.5 ABVD Protocol for Treating Relapse of Hodgkin Lymphoma

Drug	Days	Doses
Doxorubicin (adriamycin)	1 and 15	25 mg/m², IV slow
Bleomycin	1 and 15	10 units/ m² IV slow
Vinblastine	1 and 15	6 mg/ m², IV slow
Dacarbazine (DTIC)	1 and 15	375 mg/ m², IV infusion over 1h

The cycles are repeated every 15 days.

children with relapsed HL in combination with ifosfamide, etoposide, and prednisolone (IEP). However, it is still a preferred first line therapy in several centers in our country due to less immediate morbidity like febrile neutropenia, and ease of administration. In addition to the chemotherapy, relapsed disease would require radiotherapy, and may require autologous stem cell transplant.

Hodgkin Lymphoma

1. Hodgkin disease is one of the highly curable malignancies.
2. Painless cervical lymph node enlargement is the most common presentation.
3. Presence of "B symptoms" (fever, night sweats, weight loss) indicates poor prognosis.
4. PET-CT is the modality of choice for initial staging and for assessment of response to therapy. CT scan can be used as an alternate.
5. Response adapted therapy is the benchmark of treatment now, which means addition of radiotherapy only in cases who have poor early response to chemotherapy.
6. Chemotherapy regimens have moved away from ABVD now to minimize long-term toxicity. OEPA-COPDAC is a preferred treatment regimen.
7. 3–4 cycles of chemotherapy alone suffice in treating low risk HL.

Giulino-Roth L, Keller FG, Hodgson DC, Kelly KM. Current approaches in the management of low risk Hodgkin lymphoma in children and adolescents. *Br J Haematol*. 2015;169:647–60.

Kelly KM. Hodgkin lymphoma in children and adolescents: improving the therapeutic index. *Blood*. 2015;126:2452–8.

Mauz-Körholz C, Metzger ML, Kelly KM, et al. Pediatric Hodgkin lymphoma. *J Clin Oncol*. 2015;33:2975–85.

Terezakis SA, Metzger ML, Hodgson DC, et al. ACR appropriateness criteria pediatric Hodgkin lymphoma. *Pediatr Blood Cancer*. 2014;61:1305–12.

15.6 NON-HODGKIN LYMPHOMA

NHL constitutes a diverse group of cancers where the malignant clone arises from the lymphoid cell. It includes all the lymphomas which are not classified as Hodgkin lymphoma. It is a heterogeneous cohort of cancers, with varying clinical presentation, diagnostic features, and therapy. NHLs are usually more frequent in males than in females, with a ratio of 2–3 : 1. Age is an important factor, and different diseases peak at different ages.

Etiopathogenesis

There are significant epidemiological variations in the incidence of childhood NHLs. The most interesting variation is in the incidence of Burkitt lymphoma (BL). There is close correlation between the incidence of HIV infection and BL, as well as EBV infection and BL. Consequently, BL is very commonly seen in equatorial Africa, where the incidence of HIV and EBV is quite high. Moreover, the characteristics of BL occurring in this area are quite different from disease which is not associated with either infection. This will be discussed in more detail in the section on BL.

Though most lymphomas are sporadic, inherited and acquired immunodeficiency syndromes are significant risk factors for development of lymphoma. These include primary immunodeficiency disorders like severe combined immunodeficiency, common variable immunodeficiency, ataxia-telangiectasia, Wiskott-Aldrich syndrome, X-linked lymphoproliferative disease, autoimmune lymphoproliferative syndrome, and acquired immunodeficiency disorders like HIV infection. The risk of developing a lymphoma is as high as 10–200 times in comparison to age matched children. Often, NHL may be the presenting complaint in some of these patients. The types of NHL as per the WHO classification are listed in **Table 15.6**.

Staging and Diagnosis

Confirmation of diagnosis is with biopsy and immunocytochemistry. Staging investigations include CT of the involved area, bone marrow aspirate and biopsy, and cerebrospinal fluid examination for malignant cytology. Other investigations required include chest radiograph, ultrasound of the abdomen, cytology from pleural or pericardial fluid if involved, serum LDH, renal function tests, and evaluation for tumor lysis syndrome. The staging system followed for NHL is St Jude staging system **(Table 15.7)**.

Table 15.6 Common Subtypes of Pediatric Non-Hodgkin Lymphoma (WHO 2016)

A. **Precursor lymphoid neoplasm**
- T-lymphoblastic lymphoma
- B-lymphoblastic lymphoma

B. **Mature B-cell neoplasm**
- Burkitt lymphoma/leukemia
- Diffuse large B-cell lymphoma
- Primary mediastinal B-cell lymphoma
- Pediatric follicular lymphoma
- Pediatric nodal marginal zone lymphoma

C. **Mature T neoplasms**
- Anaplastic large cell lymphoma
- Peripheral T-cell lymphoma

Table 15.7 St. Jude Staging System for Pediatric Non-Hodgkin Lymphoma

Stage I: Single tumor (nodal or extranodal); except mediastinum and abdomen

Stage II:
- Single tumor (extranodal) with regional node involvement
- Two or more nodal or extranodal areas on the same side of the diaphragm
- A primary gastrointestinal tract tumor (usually in the ileocecal area) with or without involvement of associated mesenteric nodes, that is completely resectable

Stage III:
- Two single tumors (nodal or extranodal) on opposite sides of the diaphragm
- Any primary intrathoracic tumor (mediastinal, pleural, or thymic)
- Extensive primary intra-abdominal disease
- Any paraspinal or epidural tumor

Stage IV: Any of the above findings with initial involvement of the central nervous system, bone marrow, or both

1. LYMPHOBLASTIC LYMPHOMA

This is the commonest subtype of NHL in children, and can be either T-lymphoblastic lymphoma or B-lymphoblastic lymphoma. It is commonest in the pre-adolescent and adolescent age group.

Clinical Presentation

They commonly present with features of superior mediastinal syndrome. They may have respiratory distress due to pleural and/or pericardial effusions. Other lymph node groups may be involved, and fever is common. Bone marrow is usually not involved, or has a blast count of <25%, if involved.

Diagnosis

A CECT of the involved area is done to assess for extent of disease. It also serves as a baseline for assessment of response to therapy. Diagnosis is confirmed by biopsy of the involved lymph nodes. Bone marrow examination and CSF for malignant cytology are done in all cases to assess for stage of disease.

Treatment	Lymphoblastic Lymphoma

It is very similar to treatment of ALL. The therapy has an initial intensive phase for a period of 6–8 months followed by a maintenance phase, with total therapy duration of 2–3 years. Initial induction phase drugs are vincristine, steroids, L-asparaginase, and dauno-doxorubicin along with intrathecal therapy with methotrexate. Other drugs used include methotrexate, cyclophosphamide, and cytarabine. Drugs used in maintenance are oral 6-mercaptopurine and methotrexate, along with intrathecal methotrexate. Radiation therapy is usually not required, except in CNS positive cases where CNS radiotherapy is given. There is usually no requirement of surgery, as the lymphoma is exquisitely chemosensitive.

Prognosis

Worldwide outcome for this disease is 80–90%. Relapsed lymphoblastic lymphoma can be treated with chemotherapy and stem cell transplant, but the outcomes are poor.

2. MATURE B-LYMPHOMA

The two main subtypes of mature B-lymphoma are Burkitt lymphoma (BL) and diffuse large B-cell lymphoma (DLBCL). BL is much more common in children than DLBCL. Together, they account for nearly 60% of childhood NHL. Both are rapidly proliferating neoplasms. Though they typically occur *de novo*; there is an increased risk in immunodeficiency disorders and certain other syndromes as mentioned above.

Burkitt Lymphoma *vs* Diffuse Large B-cell Lymphoma

Pathologically, BL has very characteristic features, with monomorphic cell population sparse deeply basophilic cytoplasm; with cytoplasmic and nuclear lipid vacuoles and tingible body macrophages scattered within, causing a 'starry sky' pattern. Immunostaining and genetic analysis along with morphology help distinguish BL from DLBCL. The typical translocation is t(8;14) in a case of BL and this is usually absent in DLBCL. Both the diseases have a very high proliferative index as demonstrated by Ki-67 positivity, with patients with BL having a near 100% Ki-67 positivity. EBV proliferation can be demonstrated in majority of the patients with endemic BL, as well as a significant number of HIV positive BL and some sporadic BL as well.

The endemic BL, which typically occurs in sub-Saharan Africa, has a characteristic presentation with rapidly progressive jaw swelling, which causes significant disfigurement. Sporadic BL, which is more common in our country, presents with extranodal disease, commonly as multiple masses in the abdomen due to enlargement of lymphoid tissue in the small intestine along with intestinal involvement, most commonly at the ileo-cecal area. This may often lead to intussusception, and the child may be operated for intestinal obstruction. Subsequently the diagnosis is established either intraoperatively or on histological examination of the resected specimen. Other common presenting symptoms are abdominal distension, GI bleeding, pain and nausea/vomiting. Head and neck area may also be involved in sporadic BL, though less commonly. DLBCL, on the other hand, involves mostly nodal areas in the neck, mediastinum, and abdomen. It may also involve the bones and present as lytic-sclerotic bony swellings. Bone marrow and CNS involvement may be present in either, and are usually asymptomatic; detected on staging investigations. Burkitt leukemia is a rare type of leukemia, where the malignant cells involve more than 25% of the bone marrow.

Treatment	Mature B-cell Lymphoma

Treatment of both the tumors consists of intensive chemotherapy. The common chemotherapeutic agents used include high dose methotrexate, cyclophosphamide, doxorubicin, vincristine, cytarabine, and prednisolone. Preventive CNS therapy includes intrathecal methotrexate, hydrocortisone, and/or cytarabine. Rituximab, which is an anti-CD20 monoclonal antibody, is being increasingly used in pediatric high-risk Burkitt lymphoma and leukemia. It is already established as a standard of care drug in adult Burkitt lymphoma. Multiple intensive cycles are given at rapid intervals. There is no role of radiotherapy. Surgery is required infrequently, and may be sometimes done upfront in situations like intussusception leading to intestinal obstruction.

Outcome

It depends on the stage of disease as well as response to therapy. Involvement of bone marrow or CNS portends poorer outcome, as does poor early response to therapy. Overall outcome of mature B-cell neoplasms in children is 80%, with outcome of >95% in early stages. Relapses occur early and are very aggressive. Despite attempts to treat relapsed disease with high dose chemotherapy and autologous stem cell transplant, the overall outcome is dismal.

Revision Point

Non-Hodgkin Lymphoma (NHL)

1. Inherited and acquired immunodeficiency syndromes are significant risk factors for development of NHL.
2. NHL can be classified as: (*a*) Precursor lymphoid neoplasm (T-cell lymphoma, B-cell lymphoma); (*b*) Mature B-cell neoplasm (Burkitt lymphoma, diffuse large B-cell lymphoma); or (*c*) Mature T-cell neoplasm (anaplastic or peripheral lymphoma).
3. T-cell lymphoma presents with features of superior mediastinal syndrome. Treatment is similar to ALL, with survival up to 80–90%.
4. Burkitt lymphoma presents as a *sporadic form* in India, with intestinal obstruction. In Africa, it typically presents with a jaw swelling (*endemic form*). Overall survival is 80% with intensive chemotherapy.

Gross TG, Biondi A. Paediatric non-Hodgkin lymphoma in low and middle income countries. *Br J Haematol*. 2016;173:651–4.

Kobos R, Terry W. Advances in therapies for non-Hodgkin lymphoma in children. *Hematology Am Soc Hematol Educ Program*. 2015;2015:522–8.

Minard-Colin V, Brugières L, Reiter A, et al. Non-Hodgkin Lymphoma in Children and Adolescents: Progress Through Effective Collaboration, Current Knowledge, and Challenges Ahead. *J Clin Oncol*. 2015;33:2963–74.

Sandlund JT, Martin MG. Non-Hodgkin lymphoma across the pediatric and adolescent and young adult age spectrum. *Hematology Am Soc Hematol Educ Program*. 2016;2016:589–97.

Sandlund JT, Perkins SL. Uncommon non-Hodgkin lymphomas of childhood: pathological diagnosis, clinical features and treatment approaches. *Br J Haematol*. 2015;169:631–46.

Sandlund JT. Non-Hodgkin lymphoma in children. *Curr Hematol Malig Rep*. 2015;10:237–43.

15.7 WILMS TUMOR

This is the most common renal tumor in younger children; however, beyond 14 years of age, renal cell carcinoma (RCC) is commoner. Bilateral disease is seen in 5–7% patients. Occasionally nephrogenic rests may be seen in the other kidney. Congenital malformations are seen in approximately 10% of children with Wilms tumor, which may be isolated or a part of a syndrome. The syndromes commonly associated with Wilms tumor are listed in **Table 15.8**. Approximately 7% children have a known syndrome with Wilms tumor. Genes associated with Wilms tumor include *WT1* on chromosome 11p13, *WTX* gene on chromosome X, and *WT2* gene at 11p15 locus.

Pathology

Typically, Wilms tumor is a triphasic tumor, consisting of elements from (i) blastema, (ii) stroma, and (iii) epithelium. High-risk histopathological features include presence of focal or diffuse anaplasia, predominance of blastemal element, or pathology like clear cell sarcoma or rhabdoid tumor of the kidney. Both latter two entities are now no longer classified as subtypes of Wilms tumor but as separate renal tumors of the childhood.

Clinical Features

The median age at diagnosis is 3 years. Most of the children present with an incidentally detected lump in the flank, felt by the mother while bathing or dressing the child. Occasionally, there may be presence of frank hematuria, though microscopic hematuria is more common. Fever, pain in the abdomen, and hypertension are other manifestations, with hypertension being present in about 25% patients. Occasionally, hypertension may be severe enough to lead to end organ damage like encephalopathy. The reason for hypertension is increased renin production. All the manifestations improve with treatment of primary disease. Wilms tumor typically involves the other kidney in about 7%. There may be local vascular invasion in 4–10% patients with involvement of the renal veins, or the inferior vena cava with rare tumor invasion up to the right atrium. The typical sites of metastasis of Wilms tumor are lungs, liver, bone, and brain, in that sequence.

Investigations and Staging

In a child with abdominal mass, an ultrasound of the abdomen is the initial investigation, and will yield information to confirm the organ of origin, cystic versus solid

Table 15.8 Syndromic Associations with Wilms Tumor			
Condition	*Locus*	*Clinical constellation*	*Risk of Wilms tumor*
WAGR syndrome	11p13, *WT1* gene	Wilms tumor, aniridia, genitourinary abnormalities, renal failure	30%
Beckwith-Wiedemann syndrome	11p15, *WT2* gene (dysregulation of imprinted gene IGF 2)	Hemihypertrophy, macroglossia, omphalocele, neonatal hypoglycemia, large for dates at birth	5%
Fraser syndrome	11p13, *WT1* gene	Pseudohermaphroditism, focal segmental glomerulosclerosis	8%
Denys-Drash syndrome	11p13, *WT1* gene	Ambiguous genitalia, diffuse mesangial sclerosis	>90%

nature of mass, extend of local spread and involvement of other organs like liver and lymph nodes. A contrast CT of the abdomen (Fig. 15.2) may have a specific **claw sign** in the involved kidney. Abdominal imaging will also confirm about the anatomy and involvement of the other kidney.

A CT scan of the chest is required to check for presence of metastasis to the lungs, and a chest radiograph is not considered adequate for this purpose any longer. There is no role of PET as an imaging modality in Wilms tumor. Staging in Wilms tumor is mentioned in **Box 15.4**.

Tissue Diagnosis

There is a divided opinion on need for tissue diagnosis in the form of core biopsy in a renal tumor. In a small tumor, a biopsy may not be done, and primary nephrectomy may be performed. On the other hand, in a large extensive tumor, or in presence of distant metastasis, it is better to confirm the diagnosis by a core biopsy enabling the administration of neoadjuvant chemotherapy. This will make surgical resection easier subsequently.

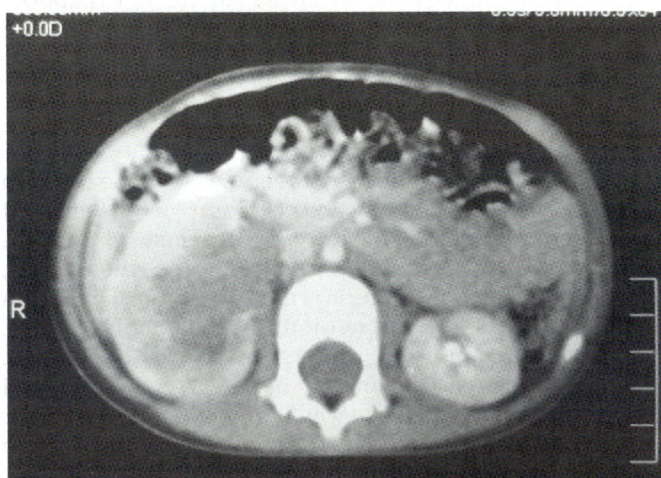

Fig. 15.2 A contrast enhanced CT of the abdomen with a large Wilms tumor replacing the entire right kidney. A normal left kidney can be seen

Box 15.4 Staging of Wilms Tumor (National Wilms Tumor Study Group)

Stage I: Tumor is limited to the kidney and is excised completely. Capsule surface intact; no tumor rupture and no residual tumor apparent beyond margins of excision.

Stage II: Tumor extends beyond the kidney but is excised completely. Regional extension of tumor, vessel infiltration, tumor biopsied or local spillage of tumor confined to the flank. No residual tumor apparent at or beyond margins of excision.

Stage III: Residual non-hematogenous tumor confined to abdomen lymph node and/or involvement of hilus, periaortic chains or beyond; diffuse peritoneal contamination by tumor spillage, peritoneal implants of tumor, tumor extends beyond surgical margins microscopically or macroscopically and tumor not completely removable because of local infiltration into vital structures.

Stage IV: Deposits beyond stage III (eg, lung, liver, bone, brain)

Stage V: Bilateral renal involvement at diagnosis.

Treatment — Wilms Tumor

Wilms tumor is a curable disease, with survival rates in the excess of 90%. Treatment is typically multimodality, with chemotherapy and surgery both required for most patients. Radiotherapy is required occasionally in the presence of certain high-risk histological features like anaplasia, stage III disease, or in the presence of metastatic disease persisting after neoadjuvant chemotherapy. Chemotherapeutic agents used typically include vincristine and actinomycin D. For higher stage disease, doxorubicin, etoposide, and platinum agents may be required.

Usually nephrectomy is performed after a few cycles of chemotherapy to enable complete and easy resection, and further chemotherapy or radiotherapy is decided on according to the extent of resection and histological features. In a small tumor, upfront nephrectomy may be done without any preoperative chemotherapy, but most children in our country present with large tumors requiring neoadjuvant chemotherapy.

Guidelines of treatment as per recommendation of International Society of Pediatric Oncology (SIOP):
1. Treatment with preoperative chemotherapy to all stage I, II and III tumors for 4 weeks.
2. Treatment with preoperative chemotherapy for 6 weeks for all stage IV tumors.
3. Surgery after 4 weeks of therapy in stage I–III tumors or after 6 weeks of therapy in stage IV tumor.
4. Staging and histology risk assessment in the post-operative specimen.
5. Radiotherapy to all patients with stage II disease with anaplasia, stage III disease and if presence of residual metastasis in stage IV disease after preoperative chemotherapy.
6. Postoperative chemotherapy with 2 drugs (vincristine and actinomycin D) to stage I–III disease, with either low or intermediate risk histology; for stage 1 disease, postoperative therapy for 4 weeks and for stage II–III disease, for 26 weeks.
7. For high-risk disease or for stage IV disease, 3–4 drugs for 26–34 weeks will be required. The drugs include etoposide, doxorubicin, carboplatin, and cyclophosphamide.

Preoperative chemotherapy for stage I, II and III Wilms tumor			
Week 1	*Week 2*	*Week 3*	*Week 4*
Vincristine Actinomycin D	Vincristine	Vincristine Actinomycin D	Vincristine

Preoperative chemotherapy for stage IV Wilms tumor			
Week 1	*Week 2*	*Week 3*	*Week 4*
Vincristine Actinomycin D Doxorubicin	Vincristine	Vincristine Actinomycin D	Vincristine
Week 5	*Week 6*		
Vincristine Actinomycin D Doxorubicin	Vincristine		

OTHER RENAL NEOPLASMS

1. *Clear cell sarcoma of the kidney (CCSK)* It used to be classified as an aggressive variant of Wilms tumor previously. However, it was realized subsequently that the cell of

origin, genetics, behavior and metastatic potential of CCSK are quite different from Wilms tumor. It is more aggressive than Wilms tumor, but is curable using multimodality therapy including chemotherapy, surgery, and radiotherapy. The staging investigations are the same, and bone scan is usually performed in addition as bone metastasis may be seen.

2. *Rhabdoid tumor of the kidney* It is now no longer classified as a subtype of Wilms tumor, but as a separate tumor. It is usually seen in the 1st year of life. This is a highly aggressive malignancy, and is at times associated with atypical teratoid-rhabdoid brain tumor. Prognosis in a metastatic disease is dismal. Even in non-metastatic disease, the outcome with multimodality therapy is relatively poor.

3. *Renal cell carcinoma* It is uncommon in young children, and its incidence increases with age. The primary modality of treatment is surgery, with poor response to chemotherapy.

Case Study | Wilms Tumor

A 2-year-old boy was brought to the OPD by his mother because she felt a mass on the right side of his abdomen while bathing him. He was otherwise well and playful. Examination revealed hypertension (BP >95th centile for age). There was a firm immobile lump in the right lumbar region, palpable bimanually. Other systemic examination was normal. Ultrasound abdomen confirmed the presence of a solid mass replacing the right kidney. A possibility of Wilms tumor was considered and diagnosis was confirmed by a fine needle aspiration of the tumor. A staging CT of the chest and abdomen showed a relatively large right renal tumor, with abdominal lymphadenopathy. The other kidney was normal. Antihypertensive was started (amlodipine) and preoperative treatment with vincristine and actinomycin was initiated, and surgery was done after 4 weeks of chemotherapy. Postoperatively, the child was staged as intermediate risk, stage 3 disease. He required radiotherapy to the abdomen in addition to further chemotherapy in view of lymph node involvement. He is currently off therapy, and well for the last 5 years.

Q. What do we learn from this case study?

1. Most children with Wilms tumor are well looking and otherwise healthy.
2. Blood pressure examination is essential in a child with a renal mass.
3. Ultrasound is the initial investigation to confirm the origin of the mass.
4. Needle aspiration or biopsy are the investigations of choice to establish the diagnosis of Wilms tumor.
5. Metastatic work up (CECT of chest and abdomen) is essential prior to initialing therapy.
6. Evaluation of the other kidney is mandatory.
7. It is preferable to give neoadjuvant chemotherapy to shrink the tumor before surgery.
8. Detailed histological evaluation of the resected specimen helps in accurate staging and further therapy decisions.
9. Wilms tumor usually has an excellent outcome.

Dome JS, Graf N, Geller JI, et al. Advances in Wilms Tumor Treatment and Biology: Progress Through International Collaboration. *J Clin Oncol.* 2015;33:2999–3007.

Godzinski J, Graf N, Audry G. Current concepts in surgery for Wilms tumor—the risk and function-adapted strategy. *Eur J Pediatr Surg.* 2014;24:457–60.

Wilms Tumor

1. Wilms tumor is the second most common renal malignancy in children.
2. Wilms tumor classically presents as a unilateral abdominal mass, it is bilateral in 5–7% cases. Other manifestations include hematuria and hypertension.
3. Radical nephrectomy is treatment of choice for unilateral diseases, preceded by chemotherapy. Radiotherapy is required in high-risk cases.
4. Overall survival is 90%.

Irtan S, Ehrlich PF, Pritchard-Jones K. Wilms tumor: "State-of-the-art" update, 2016. *Semin Pediatr Surg.* 2016;25:250–6.

Kieran K, Davidoff AM. Nephron-sparing surgery for bilateral Wilms tumor. *Pediatr Surg Int.* 2015;31:229–36.

User IR, Ekinci S, Kale G, et al. Management of bilateral Wilms tumor over three decades: The perspective of a single center. *J Pediatr Urol.* 2015;11:118.e1–6.

15.8 NEUROBLASTOMA

Etiology and Genetics

This is the commonest pediatric extra-cranial solid tumor, accounting for 8–10% of all pediatric malignancies. It has a prevalence of 1 in 7000 live births. Most cases are detected in infancy and early childhood, with ≈90% being detected by 5 years of age. The cell of origin is from the neural crest, typically from the sympathetic chain. Majority of the patients do not have any identifiable predisposing factor for the development of malignancy, however, there is a distinct but small subgroup of neuroblastoma with genetic pre-disposition and autosomal dominant inheritance. A well-known characteristic of neuroblastoma is its potential to regress spontaneously in early infancy.

Exact etiology is not known. Familial (autosomal dominant) cases account for 1–2% of all neuroblastomas. These are linked to *Phox2B* and *ALK* genes. Children with Hirschsprung disease, Beckwith-Wiedemann syndrome, and hemihypertrophy are at a higher risk of developing neuroblastoma. Most common chromosomal abnormality is the deletion of the short arm of chromosome 1. The presence of N-myc proto-oncogene amplification signifies advanced stage of tumor and poor prognosis. Loss of heterozygosity of chromosomes 1p, 11q, and/or gain of chromosome 17qq is associated with poor prognosis. Hyperdiploidy in the tumor cell is associated with a better prognosis.

Pathology

Neuroblastoma is classified as **a small blue round cell tumor**. The cells may be arranged in the form of Homer-Wright pseudorosette. The background is composed of schwannian stroma and neuropil may be seen. According to the degree of differentiation, the tumor cells may be undifferentiated neuroblastoma, ganglioneuroblastoma, or ganglioneuroma which is the most differentiated.

Spread of the tumor occurs (*i*) locally by invasion of adjacent tissues; or (*ii*) by lymphatics and hematogenously to lymph nodes and distant organs. The common sites of metastasis are lymph nodes, long bones, liver, and skin. Metastasis to lungs and brain is uncommon.

Risk Stratification Staging

There are several pathological features which denote a high-risk tumor.

- More undifferentiated tumors have a poorer outcome whereas ganglioneuroma has a better outcome.
- The genetics of a high-risk tumor include presence of *MYCN* gene amplification, chromosomal aberrations involving loss of heterozygosity of chromosome 1p and 11q or gain of chromosome 17q.
- Other features implying a high-risk neuroblastoma include a high LDH and high serum ferritin level.
- Widespread disease usually has an extremely poor outcome, except in children less than 18 months of age.
- Younger children usually have an excellent outcome, especially less than 18 months of age.
- Outcomes are good for limited stage disease.

Staging

International Neuroblastoma Staging System (INSS) is shown in **Table 15.9**. More recently, international neuroblastoma risk group consensus pre-treatment classification is being used to stage newly diagnosed neuroblastoma patients. This is a complicated staging system including age, histology, genetic risk markers including MYCN and chromosomal aberrations, as well as radiological risk grouping. Radiological risk grouping uses the terminology L1 and L2 to indicate image defined risk factors absent or present. Image defined risk factors imply unresectable tumor, or tumor close to/invading vital structures.

Table 15.9 International Neuroblastoma Staging System (INSS)

Stage 1 Localized tumor confined to areas of origin; complete gross excision, with or without microscopic residual disease; identifiable ipsilateral or contralateral lymph nodes negative microscopically.

Stage 2A Localized tumor with incomplete gross excision; identifiable ipsilateral or contralateral lymph nodes negative microscopically.

Stage 2B Localized tumor with or without complete gross excision, with positive ipsilateral lymph nodes, identifiable contralateral lymph nodes negative microscopically.

Stage 3 Unresectable unilateral tumor infiltrating across the midline, with or without regional lymph nodes involvement; or a localized unilateral tumor with contralateral regional lymph node involvement; or a midline tumor with bilateral extension by infiltration or by lymph node involvement.

Stage 4 Primary tumor disseminated to distant lymph nodes, bone, bone marrow, liver, skin and/or other organs (except as defined for stage 4S).

Stage 4S Localized primary tumor (as defined for stage 1, 2A, or 2B), with dissemination limited to skin, liver and/or bone marrow (limited to infants aged <1 year). Marrow involvement should be minimal (<10% of total nucleated cells identified as malignant by bone biopsy or by bone marrow aspirate). The results of the MIBG scan (if performed) should be negative for disease in the bone marrow.

Stage 4S is the most unusual group, comprising approximately 30% of patients with neuroblastoma. This stage occurs in infants younger than 12 months and is characterized by hepatomegaly, skin nodules, and a positive result on bone marrow biopsy. Everything else being equal, these children normally would be classified as stage 1 or 2. The 5-year survival rate of patients with 4S disease is 75%.

Clinical Features

More than 90% cases manifest before 5 years of age. The tumor can arise from any site along the sympathetic chain, though adrenals are often the primary site. Nearly two-thirds of the tumors are seen in the abdomen. Other primary sites can be there in the mediastinum, paraspinal area, and rarely the bladder. Spontaneous regression is known in neuroblastoma detected in infancy. Localized neuroblastoma is seen in nearly 40% of the patients, with the majority having disseminated disease at presentation.

Most cases originate from adrenal medulla and thus present with an abdominal lump. The most common finding on physical examination is a non-tender, firm, irregular abdominal mass that crosses the midline in contrast to Wilms tumor, which has a smooth mobile flank mass that does not cross the midline. Other findings may include hepatomegaly and blanching subcutaneous nodules (*blueberry muffin lesions*). Children with localized disease are often asymptomatic or present with abdominal lump, whereas children with disseminated neuroblastoma have constitutional symptoms. Systemic manifestations include unexplained fever, weight loss, anorexia, failure to thrive, malaise, irritability, bone pains, and changes in bowel or bladder habits.

Neuroblastoma originating from the paraspinal ganglia may invade through the neural foramina, compress the spinal cord and presents with monoplegia, paraplegia, or quadriplegia. Rarely, metastatic deposit to the retrobulbar region leads to rapidly progressive, unilateral, painless proptosis, periorbital edema, and ecchymosis of the upper lid **(Racoon sign)**. It may present with opsoclonus-myoclonus or ataxia.

Neuroblastoma originating from superior cervical ganglia or thoracic region may present with clinical manifestations of Horner syndrome or superior vena cava syndrome.

Neuroblastoma tumor cells secrete catecholamines that may cause hypertension. Vasoactive intestinal peptide (VIP) secreted by tumor cells may result in intractable secretory diarrhea **(Kerner-Morrison syndrome)**. Rarely, disseminated intravascular coagulation and tumor lysis syndrome may occur.

Metastatic Manifestations

Pepper syndrome occurs in infants with metastasis to liver. It is associated with stage 4S neuroblastoma. It has better prognosis because of spontaneous regression. Death may occur due to respiratory failure and septicemia.

Hutchinson syndrome occurs due to widespread metastasis of neuroblastoma to the bone. It usually presents with bone pains and pathologic fractures. Limping is usually the first presenting feature.

Opsoclonus-Myoclonus-Ataxia Syndrome (OMAS)

This is a well-known paraneoplastic syndrome associated with neuroblastoma. It occurs in approximately 2–4% of newly diagnosed patients of neuroblastoma and consists of rapid chaotic eye movements, myoclonus, ataxia, and developmental retardation. The pathology is thought to be immune in origin, likely due to production of anti-neural antibodies produced by the body in response to the tumor. These antibodies then cross-react with other neural tissue and lead to OMAS. Presence of OMAS is considered a good prognostic feature as it indicates body's own immune response to the cancer cells. Other infrequent paraneoplastic association of this malignancy is refractory watery diarrhea secondary to secretion of vasoactive intestinal peptide (VIP).

Diagnostic and Staging Investigations

- A biopsy of the primary site is essential to confirm the diagnosis and assess the histological risk of the tumor.
- Assessment for high-risk genetic markers is usually done on the tumor tissue for MYCN gene amplification, loss of heterozygosity of chromosome 1p and 11q, or gain of 17q.
- A CECT of the primary site is required, and typically suprarenal mass may be seen with extension across the midline, presence of calcification and vascular encasement.
- Elevation of urinary catecholamines, VMA and HVA, is seen in these tumors and assists in diagnosis.
- Bone marrow aspiration and bilateral trephine biopsy should be performed to look for metastasis. This is the commonest site for distant metastasis, and may be positive in as many as 70% patients with stage IV neuroblastoma.
- MIBG scan, which is considered the most specific and sensitive tool for assessing presence of distant bone metastasis.
- FDG or DOTATE-PET scan has an upcoming role, and may be used when MIBG scan is not available.
- Bone scan may be useful for looking at bone metastasis, but may not be required if MIBG or PET scan has been done.

Differential Diagnosis

The differential diagnosis of neuroblastoma includes polycystic disease of kidney, Wilms tumor, non-Hodgkin lymphoma, rhabdomyosarcoma, hydronephrosis, hepatoblastoma, and pheochromocytoma. In mediastinum, one should differentiate it from teratoma and duplication of esophagus; whereas in neck, lymphoma, cystic hygroma, and branchial cyst should be considered in the differential diagnosis.

Treatment	Neuroblastoma

Neuroblastoma in infancy Treatment and cure can be achieved by low dose chemotherapy or surgery alone and, at times without any therapy at all.

Low risk neuroblastoma It can be treated by surgery alone. In an incidentally detected small tumor in an infant, there may be spontaneous resolution at times, and no treatment may be required. A stage IVs tumor may require gentle chemotherapy if hepatomegaly is large enough to lead to compressive symptoms or respiratory distress.

High-risk neuroblastoma This requires multimodality therapy, despite which the cure rates are poor. Chemotherapy, surgery, autologous stem cell transplant, radiotherapy, and immunotherapy are all used to treat a child with high-risk neuroblastoma. The drugs used in chemotherapy include vincristine, carbo- and cisplatin, cyclophosphamide, etoposide, anthracyclines and others.

Some of the common regimens used are rapid COJEC and OPEC. Subsequently, surgery is performed and high dose chemotherapy along with autologous hematopoietic stem cell transplant is done.

Neuroblastoma is a radiosensitive tumor, and radiotherapy is given to the primary along with metastatic sites. Following this, oral immunotherapy in the form of *cis*-retinoic acid is given. Stage wise treatment is summarized in **Box 15.5**.

Newer modalities are being developed to improve the dismal cure rate. They include treatment with chimeric anti-GD-2 antibody (directed against neuroblastoma specific cell surface ganglioside) and radionuclide like ^{131}I labelled MIBG.

Prognosis

Age is the most significant clinical prognostic factor for neuroblastoma. Infants with neuroblastoma have a better prognosis compared with older children. The cure rate for children with stage 1, 2 and 4S is more than 90%, while of stage 3 is about 90% after surgery, chemotherapy, and radiotherapy. Children with high-risk neuroblastoma have a survival rate about 20–25%.

Aneuploidy and hyperdiploidy are associated with a favorable prognosis. The presence of N-myc amplification is associated with a poor prognosis in children older than 1 year. Other poor prognostic factors include low ratio of VMA to HVA in urine, high serum ferritin and NSE levels, and poor nutritional status.

Box 15.5 Treatment of Neuroblastoma

1. **Low risk disease:** *L2 ≤18 months, MYCN non-amplified; Stage IVs ≤12 months, MYCN non-amplified*

   a. INSS stage 1 and 2: Surgery alone.

   INSS stage 4s: Observation for older than 3 months of age. For younger children and symptomatic disease, treat as per intermediate risk

2. **Intermediate risk disease:** *L2, MYCN negative (age 18 months to 10 years) or L1, MYCN amplified (age <10 years), stage IV <12 months, MYCN non-amplified*

   This will involve at least 4–8 cycles of chemotherapy including etoposide-carboplatin and cyclophosphamide, doxorubicin, vincristine (CADO).

   Surgery is required in all cases and radiotherapy in some cases

3. **High risk:** *All others*

   Induction chemotherapy followed by surgery, autologous bone marrow/stem cell transplantation, radiotherapy and isotretinoin. Induction chemotherapy for high risk neuroblastoma comprises combination of cyclophosphamide, carboplatin, vincristine, cisplatin, and etoposide. Topotecan and doxorubicin may be required as well.

L1 and L2 stand for image defined risk factors present or absent

Neuroblastoma

1. Neuroblastoma is the most common round cell malignant tumor in children originating from the neural crest cells.
2. About 50% of primary neuroblastoma arise from the adrenal gland.
3. The disease usually presents at around 2 years of age with an abdominal lump crossing the midline.
4. Stage 4S disease occurs in infancy and characterized by hepatomegaly, skin nodules, positive bone marrow biopsy, and spontaneous remission in most cases.
5. Cure rate is more than 90%, except for high-risk neuroblastoma (survival 20–25%).

Bagatell R, Cohn SL. Genetic discoveries and treatment advances in neuroblastoma. *Curr Opin Pediatr.* 2016;28:19–25.

Mei H, Lin ZY, Tong QS. Risk stratification and therapeutics of neuroblastoma: the challenges remain. *World J Pediatr.* 2016;12:5–7.

Newman EA, Nuchtern JG. Recent biologic and genetic advances in neuroblastoma: Implications for diagnostic, risk stratification, and treatment strategies. *Semin Pediatr Surg.* 2016;25:257–64.

Pinto NR, Applebaum MA, Volchenboum SL, et al. Advances in Risk Classification and Treatment Strategies for Neuroblastoma. *J Clin Oncol.* 2015;33:3008–17.

Schulte JH, Eggert A. Neuroblastoma. *Crit Rev Oncol.* 2015;20:245–70.

Whittle SB, Smith V, Doherty E, et al. Overview and recent advances in the treatment of neuroblastoma. *Expert Rev Anticancer Ther.* 2017;17:369–86.

15.9 RHABDOMYOSARCOMA

Rhabdomyosarcoma is the commonest sarcoma in children and adolescents. It accounts for nearly 3% of the childhood cancers and 60% of all sarcomas. It belongs to the family of small blue round cell tumors. The cell of origin is mesenchymal stem cell, with myogenic differentiation.

Rhabdomyosarcoma may occur in all parts of the body except intracranially. The commonest site is head and neck followed by genitourinary system. In the head and neck area, parameningeal location is the commonest. The other sites include orbit, extremities, and retroperitoneum.

There is an increased risk of developing rhabdomyosarcoma in Li-Fraumeni syndrome, Beckwith-Wiedemann syndrome, neurofibromatosis, and Noonan syndrome.

Pathology

There are 2 main histological subtypes: Embryonal and alveolar.

- *Alveolar rhabdomyosarcoma* occurs more commonly in older children and is common in extremities and trunk. It is an aggressive tumor with a relatively poor prognosis. Majority of the cases have a translocation involving chromosome 13 which most commonly are t(1;13) or t (2;13).
- *Embryonal* rhabdomyosarcoma on the other hand is common in younger children, is less aggressive with a better outcome. It is seen more commonly in orbit, head and neck or genitourinary areas. Botyroid and spindle cell rhabdomyosarcoma are further subtypes and are considered to have a good prognosis. Embryonal variety

occurs more frequently then alveolar sub-type. Translocations are negative in embryonal rhabdomyosarcoma.

Clinical Features

The clinical symptoms depend on the location of the tumor.

- *Parameningeal tumors* Symptoms of increased intracranial pressure, compression of nearby structures, and cranial nerve palsy may be seen.
- *Limb rhabdomyosarcoma* Progressive swelling is the common symptom. Pain is not prominent, unless the swelling is very large.
- *Orbital tumors* Proptosis is the primary symptom (Fig. 15.3).
- *Genitourinary rhabdomyosarcoma* They may present with pressure symptoms, obstructive uropathy, and hydronephrosis due to bladder outflow obstruction, apart from mass symptoms.
- *Vaginal tumors* They have a specific 'bunch of grape' like appearance and are called **botyroid tumors**.

Investigations

Diagnosis is confirmed by biopsy. Usually complete excision is difficult at time of diagnosis, hence a core biopsy suffices. Morphology shows poorly differentiated small round blue malignant cells. The signs of striated muscle differentiation are often not evident. Immunohistochemistry is extremely useful in identifying the muscle-specific markers like myogenin, desmin and skeletal muscle-specific actin, which helps in differentiating the tumor from other tumors like Ewing sarcoma, lymphoma, other sarcoma, which share similar morphological features.

Further investigations include imaging of the involved area; a contrast enhanced MRI is considered the standard of care. A CT scan may be done if MRI is not available. PET scan has an upcoming role in evaluation of metastatic disease, however it is not the established standard of care. In tumors of the head and neck, CSF examination is required

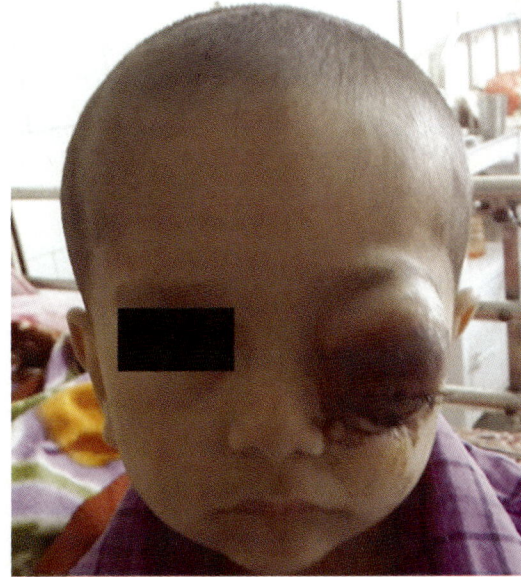

Fig. 15.3 A toddler with a large orbital rhabdomyosarcoma presenting with proptosis and loss of vision

Table 15.10 Children's Oncology Group Risk Stratification Scheme for Rhabdomyosarcoma

	Low risk	*Intermediate risk*	*High risk*
Metastasis	No	No	Yes
Histology	Embryonal	Any	Any
Stage	If group I or II—any stage If group III—stage I	If alveolar rhabdomyosarcoma: Stage 1, 2, or 3 If embryonal rhabdomyosarcoma: Stage 2 or 3	4
IRS group	I, II, or III for stage 1 I or II for stage 2 or 3	III for stage 2 or 3; I, II, or III for alveolar histology	IV

for detection of malignancy. A CT chest is required in all cases, along with a bone scan to detect spread to the lungs or the bones.

Risk Stratification

- *Age* The outcome is better for toddlers and young children, and worse for infants and young adults.
- *Invasiveness size* Tumors larger than 5 cm have a worse outcome.
- *Site of tumor* Orbit, vagina, and biliary rhabdomyosarcoma have favorable outcome.
- *Spread of diseases* Presence of distant metastases as well as local lymph node involvement are poor prognostic markers.
- *Histology* Embryonal has a better prognosis than alveolar variety.

A commonly followed risk stratification system is shown in **Table 15.10**.

Staging

Intergroup Rhabdomyosarcoma Study Committee Group System (IRS Group) staging system is commonly used for assessment of rhabdomyosarcoma **(Table 15.11)**.

Treatment	**Rhabdomyosarcoma**

Chemotherapeutic agents typically used include vincristine, cyclophosphamide, and actinomycin D. Other active agents are anthracyclines and irinotecan. Typically, neoadjuvant chemotherapy is administered followed by surgery and/or radiotherapy of the involved site. Subsequently further chemotherapy is required. The total duration of treatment extends from 6 to 12 months. In specific sites like orbit where complete resection is not possible, radiotherapy is given along with chemotherapy. Relapsed rhabdomyosarcoma may be salvaged with intensive chemotherapy, surgery and radiotherapy.

Table 15.11 Clinical Group as per the Intergroup Rhabdomyosarcoma Study Committee

Group I: Complete surgical excision, with no residual gross or microscopic disease

Group II: Microscopic residual disease
IIa: Regional disease showing microscopic margins positive
IIb: Regional disease completely resected; LN involvement positive (completely excised)
IIc: Microscopic residual disease at local site (with LN involvement present)

Group III: Gross residual disease or biopsy only

Group IV: Presence of distant metastasis

Rhabdomyosarcoma

1. Rhabdomyosarcoma is the commonest sarcoma in children and adolescents.
2. Head and neck are the most common sites of rhabdomyosarcoma. It can also occur in limbs, orbits, genitourinary system, and CNS (except intracranial).
3. Biopsy characteristically shows poorly differentiated small round blue malignant cells.
4. Treatment is with chemotherapy for 6–12 months. Surgery and radiotherapy are required. Outcome depends on the stage and risk group of the disease.

Alaggio R, Coffin CM. The evolution of pediatric soft tissue sarcoma classification in the last 50 years. *Pediatr Dev Pathol.* 2015;18:481–94.

Dasgupta R, Fuchs J, Rodeberg D. Rhabdomyosarcoma. *Semin Pediatr Surg*. 2016;25:276–83.

Shern JF, Yohe ME, Khan J. Pediatric rhabdomyosarcoma. *Crit Rev Oncog.* 2015;20:227–43.

15.10 BONE TUMORS

EWING SARCOMA

Epidemiology

Ewing sarcoma is the most common bone tumor in children, and the 2nd most common bone tumor in adolescents and young adults after osteosarcoma. It occurs in approximately 3 per million children and adolescent/young adult population.

The median age of diagnosis is between 14 and 15 years. The current WHO nomenclature is Ewing sarcoma/primitive neuroectodermal tumors and includes (*a*) classical Ewing sarcoma involving bones, chest wall tumors of ribs, and soft tissue known as Askin tumors; (*b*) soft tissue Ewing sarcoma; and (*c*) primitive neuroectodermal tumors (PNETs). All these tumors share a common genetic background and are treated on similar lines.

Clinical Features

The usual age group of presentation is adolescents, with pain at the involved site being the commonest feature. The pain is usually more at nights, and occasionally history of low grade fever may be there. Typically, there will be a history of mild trauma to which the pain is attributed, and medical attention is sought only when there is no improvement with time.

Palpable mass is the next most common symptom. Swelling, erythema, and tenderness can be noted over the local area. It is possible to mistake the tumor for an evolving abscess or osteomyelitis, leading to delay in diagnosis. This is especially pertinent in 15–20% of patients who present with constitutional symptoms including fever and weight loss. The clue is often the presence of a palpable firm to hard mass with radiology showing characteristic findings.

Pathological fracture may be seen in 10% of the patient population. Most common site of disease is the pelvic bones (25%) followed by the femur; however, any bone may be involved. Axial skeleton is involved in nearly 45% cases.

- *Chest wall Ewing sarcoma* Also known as **Askin tumor**, this usually presents with non-productive cough, pleuritic chest pain, and respiratory distress. A chest radiograph typically shows a mass in the lung with underlying rib erosion. An effusion may be present.
- Patients with *primary of the chest or pelvis* typically have minimal symptoms initially, and often present late with a large tumor mass.
- A child with a *pelvic Ewing sarcoma* may have only a limp as a presenting complaint.
- Patients with *paraspinal tumor* may present with slowly progressive paraparesis due to spinal compression.
- Metastases typically occur to the lungs, followed by bones and bone marrow. Local lymph node spread is unusual.

Investigations

The initial investigation is a radiograph of the involved site in 2 planes. This typically shows irregular bony lesions with presence of bone destruction and soft tissue mass in the diaphyseal area. Periosteal reaction can lead to an onion skin appearance of the involved site. *Codman triangle sign* (caused by detachment of periosteum) and a sunburst appearance may be seen occasionally.

CT or MRI helps in delineating the tumor in more detail. MRI helps in assessment of resectability as it provides accurate detail with respect to the neurovascular bundle, and provides a more accurate soft tissue and intramedullary delineation, whereas the CT provides an accurate extent of the bone lesion.

Work up for metastasis includes CT of the chest, and a technetium-99m whole body bone scintigraphy. There is evolving evidence for use of PET scan for evaluation of metastatic sites, but it is not an investigation of choice yet.

Confirmation of diagnosis Biopsy and histopathological examination are required for final diagnosis. It is preferable that the initial biopsy should be done by the surgeon who is going to do the final resection, so that the biopsy tract is also included in the final surgery. Histologically, ES is the prototype small round blue cell tumor, with a monomorphic cell population. The cytoplasm is scanty and nucleoli are not prominent. The cell membrane stains positive for CD99 (MIC2). The cells stain positive for periodic acid–Schiff (PAS) due to the cytoplasmic glycogen. Some of the tumors may demonstrate **Homer Wright pseudo-rossetting**.

Associated anemia is present in majority of the patients; pancytopenia may be rarely present in cases where extensive bone marrow metastasis is present. Alkaline phosphatase is not usually elevated despite bony involvement by the tumor.

Treatment	**Ewing Sarcoma**

Ewing sarcoma is a very chemosensitive and radiosensitive tumor. Multimodality therapy is usually required to achieve complete tumor control. Most of the current treatment schedules include neoadjuvant chemotherapy followed by surgery or radiotherapy of the involved site and further chemotherapy. Improvements in prosthesis and reconstructive surgery have led to increased use of limb sparing surgery with preservation of function.

The typical chemotherapy regimens include alkylating agents like ifosfamide, cyclophosphamide, anthracyclines like doxorubicin, and other agents like vincristine and etoposide. Colony stimulating factor rescue is often required for such intense chemotherapy regimens.

Prognosis

Majority of the patients (approximately 75%) have non-metastatic disease, and with current therapy, world over survival for these children is at nearly 65–70%. Larger tumor size and volume is also considered to be an adverse prognostic factor. Tumors localized to the appendicular skeleton fare better than those in the axial skeleton, possibly due to earlier diagnosis and ease of surgery.

Outcome of metastatic Ewing sarcoma, seen in 25% patients at time of diagnosis, is dismal in the best circumstances, with most patients showing initial good response to therapy followed by relapse. Patients with isolated lung metastasis fare better than patients with bone, bone marrow, or multiple metastasis.

 Revision Point

Ewing Sarcoma

1. Ewing sarcoma is a diaphyseal tumor and most commonly occurs in the pelvic bones, followed by femur, chest wall, and spine.
2. Usual age of presentation is 14–15 years with pain at the involved site.
3. Radiograph typically shows onion-skin appearance. Biopsy is diagnostic.
4. Survival in non-metastatic disease is 65–70%.

Gaspar N, Hawkins DS, Dirksen U, et al. Ewing sarcoma: current management and future approaches through collaboration. *J Clin Oncol.* 2015;33:3036–46.

OSTEOSARCOMA

Osteosarcoma is the commonest bone tumor in older children and young adults. It contributes to approximately 3% of all malignancies in children and young adults (<20 years of age). There is a bimodal age distribution, with a peak at 15 years of age, and another smaller peak at 6th to 7th decades of life.

Predisposing Factors

These including inherited cancer predisposition syndromes like Li-Fraumeni, hereditary retinoblastoma, Werner syndrome, Bloom syndrome, and Rothmund-Thompson syndrome. In older people, Paget disease of the bone and prior radiation therapy are predisposing factors. It is thought that rapid linear growing tumor in adolescence may be associated with osteosarcoma. Also, taller individuals are more at risk of developing osteosarcoma.

Clinical Features

Osteosarcoma typically occurs in long bones, with lower end of femur being the most common site. The next most common site is upper end of tibia followed by proximal fibula. The metastasis occurs typically to lung and other bones, and is seen in nearly 20% patients at presentation. Lung is the commonest site of distant metastasis. Pain and presence of a mass at the site of tumor are the commonest clinical features. Pathological fracture may be seen in a few patients at presentation. Systemic symptoms are typically absent in contrast to Ewing sarcoma.

Differences between Osteosarcoma and Ewing Sarcoma

Clinically, Ewing sarcoma is seen at all ages, and may also be seen in very young children; osteosarcoma, on the other hand, is always seen in older age group.

- Osteosarcoma almost always affects long bones, and does not occur in soft tissue alone. Ewing sarcoma can affect axial or appendicular skeleton, and extra-skeletal Ewing sarcoma may also occur in soft tissue alone.
- Osteosarcoma is predominantly a meta-epiphyseal malignancy in contrast to Ewing sarcoma which is more commonly seen in diaphysis.
- There are no familial syndromes associated with Ewing sarcoma, however osteosarcoma has a familial predisposition with Li-Fraumeni syndrome, or RB1 gene mutation.
- Onion skin appearance is typically seen in Ewing sarcoma, while sun-burst appearance is more common in osteosarcoma on the radiograph.
- Therapeutically, osteosarcoma is radioresistant whereas Ewing sarcoma is radiosensitive.

Investigations and Diagnosis

Plain radiograph of the involved site typically shows a mixed lytic-sclerotic picture. The characteristic radiological appearances include sun burst appearance, with presence of a Codman triangle secondary to periosteal new bone formation (Fig. 15.4).

Confirmation of diagnosis is by tissue biopsy. The biopsy may be open biopsy; a core needle biopsy may also suffice and is more convenient to carry out as it does not require general anesthesia. A fine needle aspiration does not yield enough tissue for an accurate diagnosis in the majority of the cases.

MRI of the involved site is required for assessing the exact extent of disease and its relation to the neurovascular bundle. It may also show up any skip metastasis in the same bone. For further staging, a CT chest and a bone scan are required to look for distant metastasis.

Enneking staging, which is based on tumor grade, tumor site, and presence or absence of metastasis is used for grading the severity.

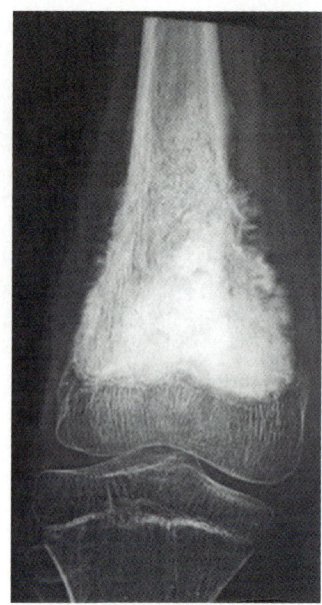

Fig. 15.4 Osteosarcoma of the lower end of femur. There is presence of lytic-sclerotic bone lesion, with Codman's triangle. The rest of the bone has osteopenia

Treatment	Osteosarcoma

Initially, the treatment for osteosarcoma was surgery only, with dismal survival rates of <20%. Once the chemosensitivity of the tumor was recognized, and chemotherapy became an integral part of therapy along with surgery, the outcome of non-metastatic osteosarcoma increased drastically to nearly 70%. The main chemotherapeutic agents active against the malignancy include methotrexate, platinum drugs, and anthracyclines. MAP (methotrexate, adriamycin and *cis*-platin) is a commonly used chemotherapeutic regimen. Radiation is ineffective.

There have been several major advances in reconstructive surgical techniques. Along with newer prosthesis, these help in preservation of limb and mobility. This has decreased the morbidity and decreased the treatment abandonment rates.

The typical treatment regimen consists of several cycles of neoadjuvant chemotherapy followed by surgery and reconstruction. Subsequently, adjuvant chemotherapy is administered. Neoadjuvant chemotherapy plays a very important role in the treatment, as it helps in shrinking the tumor and making a complete resection/limb preserving surgery feasible. Moreover, it is effective against the pulmonary and other micro-metastasis. It helps in assessing the tumor response to chemotherapy, and presence of extensive necrosis (>90%) is considered a good prognostic factor.

Revision Point

Osteosarcoma

1. Osteosarcoma typically occurs in metaphysis of long bones, presenting in adolescents.
2. Radiograph shows a sun-burst appearance. Confirmation is by tissue biopsy.
3. Osteosarcoma is radioresistant. Treatment consists of surgery and chemotherapy.

Monitoring after completion of treatment is required for several years, as late relapses are well known. Most of the relapses occur in the lung, rather than at the primary disease site. Surgical excision of metastases can be attempted. Overall outcome of relapsed disease is dismal.

Bishop MW, Janeway KA, Gorlick R. Future directions in the treatment of osteosarcoma. *Curr Opin Pediatr.* 2016;28:26–33.

Bölling T, Hardes J, Dirksen U. Management of bone tumours in paediatric oncology. *Clin Oncol (R Coll Radiol).* 2013;25:19–26.

Gorlick R, Janeway K, Lessnick S; COG Bone Tumor Committee. Children's Oncology Group's 2013 blueprint for research: bone tumors. *Pediatr Blood Cancer.* 2013;60:1009–15.

Isakoff MS, Bielack SS, Meltzer P, Gorlick R. Osteosarcoma: Current Treatment and a Collaborative Pathway to Success. *J Clin Oncol.* 2015;33:3029–35.

Kager L, Tamamyan G, Bielack S. Novel insights and therapeutic interventions for pediatric osteosarcoma. *Future Oncol.* 2017;13:357–68.

15.11 RETINOBLASTOMA

Retinoblastoma is the commonest malignant neoplasm of the eye in children. It arises from the photoreceptor elements in the fetal retinal cells. The tumor can be unilateral, bilateral (25%), or metachronous, with one eye developing the malignancy after the other. An unusual but aggressive presentation is with *trilateral retinoblastoma*, when pineal gland is involved along with both the eyes.

Genetics

The driving mutation is in retinoblastoma 1 (*RB1*) gene on chromosome 13. Majority of the patients have sporadic mutations, however, heritable *RB1* gene mutations are present in 15–25% patients.

Clinical Features

Children with bilateral tumor tend to present early, by 1 year of age. Unilateral tumors present later, typically between 2 and 5 years of age.

The earliest manifestation of retinoblastoma is *leukocoria* or white reflex in the eye. Often parents term it as a 'star shining in the eye'. It may become apparent in a photograph where instead of a red reflex, a white reflex is seen. The differential diagnosis of white reflex in the eye includes congenital cataracts, persistent hyperplastic primary vitreous, retrolental fibrodysplasia, Coats disease, *Toxocara* infection, and toxoplasmosis. These can all be ruled out by careful ophthalmologic examination.

Development of squint is the next most common symptom. Redness and pain in the eye may occur with advanced tumor and increase in intraocular pressure. Proptosis, phithisis, cervical and pre-auricular lymph node involvement are seen in more advanced, and often extraocular stage of disease.

Diagnosis

In a child with leukocoria, an indirect fundoscopic examination under anesthesia is the primary as well as the confirmatory investigation for the tumor. There is no role of tissue diagnosis by FNAC or biopsy. Moreover, there is a significant risk of extraocular spread of the tumor by doing any invasive procedure. Once the diagnosis of retinoblastoma is established, the other eye should be screened simultaneously to detect any synchronous tumor.

The most important staging investigation is imaging of the orbit and brain. A contrast MRI of the brain and orbit is the modality of choice as it helps delineate the extension of tumor along the optic nerve. Alternately, a contrast CT of the brain and orbit can be done. Apart from spread along the optic nerve, invasion of surrounding muscles, intracranial extension, meningeal enhancement, and involvement of the pineal gland needs to be assessed.

Often, a diagnostic CSF examination is done to assess spread to the meninges. This is required when the tumor has extended beyond the eye, into the orbit or the optic nerve.

Staging

The disease can be classified as *intraocular* or *extraocular*. In early stages, the disease is limited within the eye. Previously, the Reese-Ellsworth staging was used for intraocular tumors; however, it has become obsolete now. Currently, International Classification for Intraocular Retinoblastoma is followed. This classification is based entirely on indirect ophthalmoscopy examination. For disease which has spread beyond the eye and is extraocular at presentation, International Retinoblastoma Staging System is used to stage it from stages 0 through 4, with stage 0 being a conservatively (non-operatively) managed eye, and stage 4 indicating presence of distant metastasis.

Treatment	Retinoblastoma

There are 2 main aims of treatment of retinoblastoma: Saving the life of the child is the primary and most important aim; saving the vision/eye is the secondary aim. Most of the children in developed nations present with early stage intraocular disease, which is easily treatable, with salvage of the eye. In India, majority of the patients present with advanced stage extraocular disease which requires extensive therapy including enucleation and has poorer cure rates.

Retinoblastoma is sensitive to radiotherapy as well as chemotherapy.

- *Early stage disease* limited to the eye can be easily treated with focal therapy. Focal therapy typically includes laser photocoagulation, cryotherapy, thermotherapy, or local chemotherapy. Argon laser and diode laser can be used for laser photocoagulation.
- *Higher stage intraocular retinoblastoma* can be treated with primary enucleation alone. This modality can be used for group D or E disease, especially when vision is absent. Newer modalities of treatment include intra-arterial chemotherapy with melphalan and intravitreal therapy.
- *Extraocular retinoblastoma*, on the other hand, requires extensive multimodality treatment, and has poorer outcome. Typically, chemotherapy, enucleation, radiotherapy, and further chemotherapy are required.
- In case of *distant metastasis* including to brain, salvage is difficult despite multimodality therapy including autologous stem cell transplant.

Follow-up

After completion of therapy, it is important to periodically check both the eyes for tumor recurrence. Genetic testing is

15

desirable for germline mutation of retinoblastoma gene, and siblings should be screened in case it is confirmed. If genetic analysis is not feasible, siblings should be screened for retinoblastoma every 3 months till 5 years of age. Long-term problems in children with retinoblastoma with RB gene mutation are risk of secondary malignant neoplasms which include osteosarcoma, other sarcomas of bone or soft tissue, skin cancers, and pinealoblastomas.

Retinoblastoma

1. Retinoblastoma can be unilateral, bilateral, or trilateral (involving the pineal gland).
2. White reflex (leucocoria) is the earliest manifestation. Other symptoms include squint, redness, and pain is the eye.
3. Diagnosis is by ophthalmoscopic examination; tissue diagnosis is contraindicated.
4. Early intraocular disease is easily treatable with laser photocoagulation, cryotherapy, laser, or local chemotherapy. Advanced disease requires enucleation.
5. Extraocular retinoblastoma requires extensive treatment with chemotherapy, radiotherapy, and enucleation.

Chawla B, Jain A, Azad R. Conservative treatment modalities in retinoblastoma. *Indian J Ophthalmol.* 2013;61:479–85.

de Jong MC, Kors WA, de Graaf P, et al. Trilateral retinoblastoma: a systematic review and meta-analysis. *Lancet Oncol.* 2014;15:1157–67.

Kumar A, Moulik NR, Mishra RK, Kumar D. Causes, outcome and prevention of abandonment in retinoblastoma in India. *Pediatr Blood Cancer.* 2013;60:771–5.

Okimoto S, Nomura K. Clinical manifestations and treatment of retinoblastoma in Kobe children's hospital for 16 years. J Pediatr Ophthalmol Strabismus. 2014;51:222–9.

Pichi F, Lembo A, De Luca M, Hadjistilianou T, Nucci P. Bilateral retinoblastoma: clinical presentation, management and treatment. *Int Ophthalmol.* 2013;33:589–93.

Shields CL, Shields JA. New strategies in the treatment of unilateral sporadic retinoblastoma. *J Pediatr Ophthalmol Strabismus.* 2015;52:134–7.

15.12 HISTIOCYTIC DISORDERS

Histiocyte refers to cells developing from the macrophage lineage or dendritic cells lineage. Histiocytosis are a rare group of childhood hematological disorders which include Langerhans cell histiocytosis (LCH), hemophagocytic lymphohistiocytosis (HLH), Rosai-Dorfman disease (RDD), and malignant histiocytosis. These disorders share a common tendency to bones, liver, and other organs of the reticuloendothelial system. The current WHO classification of histiocytic disorders is based on the cell of origin **(Table 15.12)**.

LANGERHANS CELL HISTIOCYTOSIS

LCH is the commonest histiocytic disorder and is characterized by accumulation of Langerhans cells in various tissues of the body. However, it is overall a rare disorder, with an incidence of nearly 10% of acute leukemias.

Table 15.12 WHO Classification of Histiocytic Disorders (Revised 2016)

A. *Dendritic cell disorders*
   1. Langerhans cell histiocytosis
   2. Juvenile xanthogranuloma
   3. Solitary histiocytomas
   4. Ertheim-Chester disease

B. *Macrophage related disorders*
   1. Hemophagocytic lymphohistiocytosis
   2. Sinus histiocytosis (Rosai-Dorfman disease)
   3. Solitary histiocytoma with macrophage phenotype

C. *Malignant histiocytic disorders (partial list)*
   1. Dendritic cell or macrophage related histiocytic sarcoma
   2. Malignant histiocytic sarcoma
   3. Follicular dendritic cell sarcoma

Clinical Features

LCH is a systemic disorder presenting with variable clinical features. It may involve a single organ, or several organs. The disease commonly affects skin, bones, lymph nodes, bone marrow, CNS, liver, spleen, and lungs. Any or all organs may be affected. It is classified as either a single system disease or a multisystem disease. There are some characteristic patterns of clinical presentation. Skin rash, seborrhea, bone swellings, ear discharge, weight loss, and fever are common presenting features and are typically seen in multisystem LCH. In addition, the patient may have hepatomegaly, splenomegaly, cough with tachypnea. Bone marrow involvement is usually a part of multisystem LCH and presents with a variable degree of cytopenia. The most common symptom of CNS involvement is diabetes insipidus (DI). This happens due to pituitary involvement. However, mass lesion in the brain may also be present. Single system LCH typically involves skin or bones, though isolated lymph nodal, CNS, and lung LCH are also described.

Some of the older terminologies which are still in clinical use include **Hand-Schüller-Christian disease** which is a triad of lytic bony lesions, exophthalmos with polyuria; Letterer-Siwe disease which is a fulminant multisystem form of LCH involving the RES with hepatosplenomegaly, lymphadenopathy, skin rash, lytic bony lesions (Fig. 15.5)

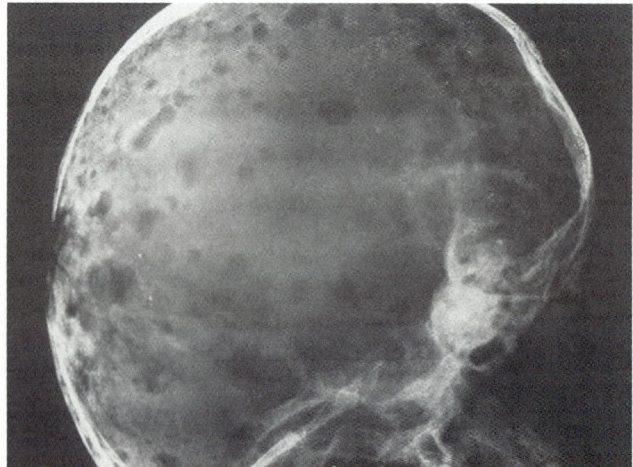

Fig. 15.5 Multiple lytic bone lesions can be seen in the skull radiograph in a child with multisystem LCH

and cytopenias; and **eosinophilic granuloma** indicating isolated lytic bony lesion.

Diagnosis

Confirmation of diagnosis is by tissue biopsy done from the most accessible tissue. Usually a core needle biopsy is sufficient. Complete excision is usually not required except in a single bone lesion where surgery with curettage will be diagnostic as well as therapeutic in most cases. The neoplastic cells are large dendritic cells which are positive for CD1a, langerin and S-100 on immunostaining. On electron microscopy, presence of **Birbeck granules** is a diagnostic feature. Further evaluation is directed by the clinical symptoms of the child. Complete blood count, liver function tests, urine osmolality and specific gravity (to assess for DI) are required in majority of the children. A skeletal survey is required to assess for bone lesions. FDG-PET is considered the most sensitive modality for detection of LCH lesions and can be used to reassess for activity after chemotherapy. For suspected brain lesions, MRI brain with pituitary cuts is required.

Risk Stratification

LCH can be classified as single system or multisystem LCH.

Single system LCH can be further classified as single lesion or multifocal disease. Presence of more than one system involvement makes it multisystem LCH. Further classification depends on presence of risk organ involvement in multisystem LCH, implying poorer prognosis and need for therapy intensification.

Multisystem disease is classified as risk organ positive (RO +) or risk organ negative (RO –) multisystem LCH. Risk organs include liver, spleen and bone marrow. Previously, lung was also considered to be a risk organ, but it is now felt that lung involvement does not lead to poor outcome, and it will be removed from the list of risk organs.

Single system LCH has an excellent prognosis, whereas multisystem LCH has guarded prognosis, especially when risk organ involvement is present.

Treatment	**Langerhans Cell Histiocytosis**

Treatment of LCH depends on the site and system involvement. A single bone lesion may be treated with curettage or with intralesional steroid injections. Multisystem LCH requires prolonged systemic chemotherapy. The most commonly agents are vinblastine, prednisolone and mercaptopurine. Other drugs that can be used to treat LCH include cytarabine, cladarabine, and indomethacin. Typically, the therapy includes an induction phase with weekly chemotherapy administration followed by maintenance phase, for a total duration of 12 months. Diabetes insipidus is usually irreversible, and requires prolonged therapy. Sclerosing cholangitis, once it sets in, may be progressive despite appropriate therapy and lead to liver transplant.

HEMOPHAGOCYTIC LYMPHOHISTIOCYTOSIS

Hemophagocytic lymphohistiocytosis (HLH), previously called class II histiocytosis, is characterized by proliferation of cells of the monocyte/macrophage lineage either in the setting of an infection or due to a genetic defect. This entity was previously subdivided into *familial erythrophagocytic lymphohistiocytosis (FEL)* which was considered to have an underlying genetic abnormality and a similar acquired syndrome known as *infection associated hemophagocytic syndrome (IAHS)*. Currently, the term HLH is used for both the conditions, and further division into primary genetic or secondary acquired is made.

- Familial HLH may occur secondary to specific genetic abnormality as well as syndromes like Chédiak-Higashi syndrome, Griscelli syndrome, and lysinuric protein intolerance.
- Infection associated HLH is commonly triggered by viruses including EBV, CMV and other viruses of the herpes family, kala-azar, tuberculosis and fungal infections.

Clinical Features

The clinical features of HLH show a high degree of overlap with sepsis and several infections; moreover, infections may co-exist with HLH (familial) or be the triggering cause of HLH (acquired). Markers like serum ferritin and bone marrow examination should be done early in a child who is suspected to have HLH. This would be indicated if there is unusual severity of an infection, lack of expected response despite appropriate therapy for an infection or if investigations for sepsis (CRP, procalcitonin, blood culture) are non-contributory in a child whose clinical behavior mimics sepsis.

HLH should be suspected in a child with an unexplained fever in the presence of cytopenia and organomegaly. Children may occasionally present with neurological symptoms secondary to CNS involvement with HLH. In children with genetic HLH, there may not always be a positive family history. A younger age at presentation favors a diagnosis of genetic HLH, however, there is considerable overlap in the ages of presentation of either type of HLH.

Diagnosis

Diagnosis of HLH is made with the help of diagnostic criteria given by the Hemophagocytic Lymphohistiocytosis Society (HLH 2004), (**Table 15.13**). There are significant therapeutic implications of genetic versus acquired nature of disease, as both the entities behave differently.

Table 15.13 Diagnostic Criteria for HLH (as per the HLH 2004 guidelines)

A. **Clinical Criteria**
  1. Fever
  2. Splenomegaly

B. **Laboratory Criteria**
  3. Cytopenias (hemoglobin <9 g/L; platelets <100 × 10⁹/L; neutrophils <1.0 × 10⁹/L)
  4. Hypertriglyceridemia or hypofibrinogenemia
  5. Hyperferritinemia (>500 µg/L)
  6. Elevated CD25 (≥2400 U/L)
  7. Low/absent natural killer function

C. **Histopathologic Criteria**   8. Hemophagocytosis in marrow, spleen, or lymph nodes with no evidence of malignancy

To make the diagnosis of HLH, at least 5 of the 8 criteria have to be met; or a genetic defect consistent with HLH should be present.

Treatment — Hemophagocytic Lymphohistiocytosis

Treatment of genetic HLH is as per the guidelines provided by HLH-2004 protocol, and include etoposide, high dose steroids (dexamethasone), cyclosporine, and intrathecal therapy with methotrexate and steroids. The definitive treatment is stem cell transplant. In case of acquired HLH, treatment of the underlying cause, which may be infection, malignancy, or rheumatological illness is important; however, therapy directed to HLH is also required, and includes high dose steroids, intravenous immunoglobulin and/or chemotherapy. Transplant is not required in this groups of patients. The outcome of secondary HLH can be excellent with appropriate therapy and supportive care.

CLASS III HISTIOCYTOSIS

These are an uncommon group of disorders which include malignant histiocytic disorders like dendritic cell or macrophage related histiocytic sarcoma, malignant histiocytic sarcoma and follicular dendritic cell sarcoma among others. These are rare and aggressive neoplastic disorders which are difficult to diagnose except for acute monocytic leukemia, and may have a guarded outcome despite chemotherapy. Most of these disorders are seen in older patients and are rare in childhood. They may occur as a primary disorder or secondary to other malignant neoplasms.

Revision Point — Histiocytic Syndromes

1. These disorders are characterized by presence of histiocytes (cells from macrophage or dendritic cell lineage).
2. They are classified as: (*a*) *Dendritic disorders*, eg Langerhans cell histiocytosis (LCH); (*b*) *Macrophage disorders*, eg, Hemophagocytic lymphohistiocytosis (HLH); and (*c*) *Malignant histiocytosis*.
3. LCH can involve single or multiple systems. Presentations include skin rash, bony swelling, fever, hepatosplenomegaly, diabetes insipidus, tachypnea and pneumonia. Presence of *Birbeck granules* is diagnostic. Prognosis is guarded in multisystem disease.
4. HLH is characterized by fever, splenomegaly, cytopenias, hyperferritinemia, hypertriglyceridemia, elevated CD25, and hemophagocytosis in marrow, spleen, or lymph nodes.
5. Prognosis for secondary HLH is excellent with chemotherapy and steroids; while genetic HLH requires stem cell transplant.

Ahuja J, Kanne JP, Meyer CA, et al. Histiocytic disorders of the chest: imaging findings. *Radiographics*. 2015;35:357–70.

Allen CE, Kelly KM, Bollard CM. Pediatric lymphomas and histiocytic disorders of childhood. *Pediatr Clin North Am*. 2015;62:139–65.

Erker C, Harker-Murray P, Talano JA. Usual and unusual manifestations of familial hemophagocytic lymphohistiocytosis and langerhans cell histiocytosis. *Pediatr Clin North Am*. 2017;64:91–109.

Ranganathan S. Histiocytic proliferations. *Semin Diagn Pathol*. 2016;33:396–409.

15.13 ONCOLOGICAL EMERGENCIES

Progressive increase in survival of pediatric cancers is noted with nearly 80% children becoming long-term survivors in the west. There is an increase in the number of patients getting treated on intensive regimens; and it is common for a pediatrician to diagnose, stabilize and refer; as well as take part in 'shared care' for a child with malignancy. With this background, it is essential to be aware of the common oncological emergencies that are encountered in day to day practice.

FEBRILE NEUTROPENIA

Definition

Febrile neutropenia is defined as a single spike of fever till 38.3°C or 38°C for more than one hour with absolute neutrophil count (ANC) <500/mm^3 or ANC <1000/mm^3 and expected to fall <500/mm^3 within the next 48 hours. Febrile neutropenia is the commonest emergency in children with cancer, and occurs most frequently after about 7–10 days of intensive chemotherapy or radiotherapy.

Pathogenesis

The leukocyte and the neutrophil count can decrease after administration of chemotherapy or radiotherapy. They may also decrease secondary to the malignancy itself, as the normal cell production decreases due to extensive bone marrow replacement by the malignant clone in patients with leukemia. If the absolute neutrophil count (ANC) falls below a certain level, there is a significantly increased risk of infections. If there is fever present as well, this condition is known as febrile neutropenia (FN).

Children at Risk

The children at risk of febrile neutropenia are characteristically the ones receiving therapy for hematological malignancy (ALL, AML, lymphoma including T-LL and Burkitt lymphoma). Other disorders at risk of febrile neutropenia include aplastic anemia, solid tumors receiving intensive chemotherapy, and post-transplant patients.

Evaluation

Obtain an extensive history and perform detailed physical examination to assess for focus of infection. Baseline investigations include a complete blood count, C-reactive protein, blood culture, assessment of kidney, and liver function tests. A routine chest radiograph is not required in the absence of symptoms. In case any central line is present, a culture should be taken from all the ports of the line.

In prolonged febrile neutropenia, further evaluation may be required including evaluation for invasive fungal infections like CT chest, galactomannan assay, and evaluation for viral infections including CMV. Typically, blood culture may be positive in 15–20% patients, and the common organisms include Gram-negative bacilli like *E.coli*, *Klebsiella* species, *Pseudomonas aeruginosa*, and Gram-positive organisms like *Staphylococcus aureus*, *S. epidermidis*, pneumococcus, and enterococcus.

Treatment — Febrile Neutropenia

Early administration of antibiotics is essential; pending even the blood counts and the culture reports. Every hospital and cancer unit has their own policy for 1st line antibiotic use in FN patients; however, the common options include 3rd generation cephalosporin drugs like cefoperazone (± sulbactam) with or without aminoglycoside, piperacillin-tazobactam with or without aminoglycoside, single agent cefepime, or carbapenem. It is essential to provide adequate cover with an anti-pseudomonal antibiotic. Typically, anti-fungal cover is initiated by day 3–5 of FN if there is no sign of recovery. The drugs that can be used are liposomal amphotericin, amphotericin B deoxycholate, and capsofungin.

Prognosis

Risk stratification of FN patients has been attempted, and low risk FN may be treated on daycare or OPD basis, rather than inpatient basis. Patients who may be considered at low risk include those whose ANC is >100/mm^3, have a low C-reactive protein, no focus of infection, and are hemodynamically stable. These patients are typically expected to recover their counts in the next 1 week or so, and are not on an intensive phase of cancer therapy. Oral antibiotic therapy may also be tried in an extremely select group of such patients.

SUPERIOR MEDIASTINAL SYNDROME

Nomenclature

Superior mediastinal syndrome implies obstruction of the structures in superior mediastinum including the superior vena cava (SVC) and the trachea. In adults, the terms superior vena cava syndrome is used separately. Children have a smaller thoracic cavity, and a mediastinal pathology causing superior vena cava syndrome generally results in superior mediastinal syndrome as well. Hence, the two terms are interchangeable in children.

Pathophysiology

Approximately one-third of the venous return to the heart is through SVC. Any mass lesion causing compression of the SVC will decrease the venous return. Most of the times, it simultaneously causes compression of trachea leading to respiratory distress. A list of possible causes along with the location is mentioned in **Table 15.14**.

Clinical Features

The patient usually presents with a history of cough, rapid breathing, and facial edema. Often, there may be complaints of snoring at night. A history of orthopnea is particularly disturbing because it denotes an advanced airway obstruction. The child in advanced stages is not able to lie down at all, and uses several pillows to prop himself up at night.

Examination would reveal facial suffusion and edema, neck vein engorgement; respiratory distress may be present. Neck nodes are usually enlarged and a careful assessment of the oral cavity is required for tonsillar enlargement. Associated pleural and pericardial effusion may be present in leukemia and lymphoma.

Sometimes an obvious chest wall bulge is present denoting an underlying mass. In advanced stages, altered sensorium may be present.

Investigations

The initial investigation is a chest radiograph. A CECT of the chest is the most useful investigation for localizing the mass and assessing the nature of mass. It will also help in planning a tissue diagnosis. At times, when the child cannot be sedated due to respiratory compromise, an ultrasound of the chest can be attempted.

An early confirmation of diagnosis is required, so that directed therapy can be started. At times, the diagnosis of leukemia may be evident from the CBC and peripheral smear examination. Often, a tissue diagnosis is required from the mass, or from any other significant lymphadenopathy. Sedation of any kind is an absolute contraindication in these children, due to the very high risk of respiratory compromise.

Treatment — Superior Vena Cava Syndrome

In case the child is too sick, and a diagnosis is taking time, empirical therapy should be initiated. Typically, the drugs used are intravenous steroids, either dexamethasone or hydrocortisone. This will help in reducing the tumor burden, decreasing the respiratory distress, and stabilizing the child. Subsequently the tissue diagnosis can be performed. At times, steroids can distort the original architecture of the tumor, and cause tumor cell necrosis, making the diagnosis difficult. At all times, the child's wellbeing takes the priority, and the treatment should be decided accordingly.

Table 15.14 Causes of Superior Mediastinal Syndrome			
Anterior mediastinum	*Middle mediastinum*	*Posterior mediastinum*	*Primary SVC involvement*
Leukemia (T-ALL*, B-ALL, AML rarely), lymphoma (T-NHL*, others), germ cell tumor, thymoma	Leukemia (T-ALL*, B-ALL, AML rarely), lymphoma (T-NHL*, others)	Neuroblastoma	Venous thrombosis after central line insertion, cardiac surgery, infections or pro-coagulant states
Tubercular lymphadeno-pathy, other infectious lymphadenopathy, thymic abscess, parathyroid adenoma	Cystic hygroma, bronchogenic cyst, infections (TB, histoplasma, fungal infection, etc.)	Neuroenteric cysts	

*Commonest causes of SMS

Supportive care

It includes anticipation and management of tumor lysis syndrome as mentioned in the section below. In leukemia and lymphoma, initial steroids significantly improve the child's condition in other malignancies like germ cell tumor and neuroblastoma, other chemotherapeutic agents are required.

Definitive therapy

It should be started as soon as feasible. Directed chemotherapy is the treatment of choice; radiotherapy may be tried in certain situations, but it carries the risk of worsening airway edema and obstruction. Treatment of superior mediastinal syndrome secondary to infections and primary venous thrombosis requires specific treatment for the primary diagnosis.

HYPERLEUKOCYTOSIS

Hyperleukocytosis is defined by presence of TLC >100,000/mm^3, in peripheral blood. The most common causes of hyperleukocytosis in children are hematological malignancies; ALL, AML, and CML. It is commonest in CML followed by AML; however, epidemiologically, it is seen most frequently in ALL as it is the commonest malignancy in children. It occurs in 8–13% of ALL cases and in 5–25% of AML cases.

Clinical Features

Hyperleukocytosis causes problem for the patient by leading to leukostasis and vascular obstruction. Leukostasis occurs secondary to the large size of leukemic blasts causing an increase in blood viscosity and vascular obstruction. There is in addition, damage to the vascular endothelium, leading to release of cytokines which aggravates the symptoms.

The symptoms commonly involve the CNS and the respiratory systems. Intracranial hemorrhage, thrombosis, and leukostasis may occur either in combination or singly. The typical manifestations are encephalopathy, features of raised intracranial pressure, and seizures.

In lungs, apart from leukostasis, pulmonary hemorrhage is a significant risk. The signs and symptoms are cough, chest indrawing, rapid breathing, and hypoxia.

Associated tumor lysis syndrome is common in children with ALL. There may be other manifestations including priapism and dactylitis.

Diagnosis

Most of the cells leading to hyperleukocytosis are leukemic blasts in ALL and AML; whereas a left shift is seen in CML, with basophilia, myelo- and metamyelocytes along with blast cells. The differential diagnosis for hyperleukocytosis includes severe infections including pertussis (which typically causes lymphocytosis with high TLC), staphylococcal sepsis, and tuberculosis. Spurious high TLC can also be seen in the presence of many nucleated RBCs which may occur in acute hemolysis, blood loss, or thalassemia. The nucleated cells get falsely counted as WBC on the coulter, and a manual check can easily rectify the error.

Treatment	**Hyperleukocytosis**

Supportive therapy

Intravenous fluids are required at a rate of 2 to 4 times normal maintenance; this helps in preventing and treating the metabolic complications as well as expanding the intravascular volume and decreasing the vascular stasis. The fluids should not contain potassium or calcium, as electrolyte imbalances like hyperkalemia may be present or develop in this situation. Support with platelet transfusions and fresh frozen plasma (in case coagulopathy is present) may be required. Packed red cells should not be transfused as they also increase the blood viscosity. In case severe anemia is present, a partial exchange transfusion or leukopharesis should be done. The other indication of these procedures is symptomatic severe hyperleukocytosis.

Definitive management

Start chemotherapy for the primary condition leading to leukocytosis. That can be done as soon as the diagnosis is established. In cases with high TLC secondary to non-malignant causes, the treatment should be appropriate antibiotics for the infection and other supportive care.

TUMOR LYSIS SYNDROME

Tumor lysis syndrome (TLS) occurs due to release of intracellular contents of cancer cells in the blood either spontaneously or soon after initiation of cancer therapy. Hyperuricemia, hyperkalemia, and hyperphosphatemia occur, followed by a secondary hypocalcemia. These together may lead to renal dysfunction, arrhythmia, encephalopathy and even death. If only the laboratory parameters are deranged, the situation is known as laboratory TLS; however, if there is evidence of organ damage (kidney, brain, heart); then the term used is clinical TLS.

The common situations which can lead to tumor lysis syndrome include tumors with a high burden and a turnover rate. These include ALL, lymphomas like Burkitt lymphoma, rarely AML, and solid tumors. The syndrome may be present prior to initiation of chemotherapy, and typically may occur till 3 to 5 days after starting chemotherapy, when there is rapid decrease in tumor burden with cancer cell lysis.

Treatment	**Tumor Lysis Syndrome**

Treatment includes aggressive intravenous hydration, use of allopurinol to prevent formation of uric acid from xanthine, and treatment of metabolic disturbances. Recombinant urate oxidase (rasburicase) helps convert uric acid to allantoin which can be excreted easily by the kidney and is the drug of choice for treating hyperuricemia due to TLS. It is recommended in patients which high risk for TLS or established TLS. Treatment of hyperkalemia and hyperphosphatemia include hydration, potassium binders, sevelemar (for hyperphosphatemia). Insulin-dextrose infusion may be required to treat severe hyperkalemia. Calcium should not be supplemented despite low records as it worsens kidney injury. It should however, be supplemented in case there is symptomatic hypocalcemia leading to tetany or arrhythmias. In case renal dysfunction has set in, hemodialysis may be required. There is currently no proven role of prophylactic urinary alkalization in the management of TLS.

Oncological Emergencies

1. *Febrile neutropenia* is characterized by fever and absolute neutrophil count <500/mm^3. It is the commonest emergency in children with cancer. Antibiotics are the mainstay of therapy (to cover Gram-negative, and *Pseudomonas* infections). Antifungals are started if there is no response in 3–5 days.

2. *Superior mediastinal syndrome* presents with cough, rapid breathing, and facial edema. It occurs due to mediastinal lymphadenopathy causing obstruction to neighboring structures including superior vena cava. Steroids followed by definitive therapy are the mainstay of therapy.

3. *Hyperleukocytosis* is defined as TLC >1,00,000/mm^3 and seen in ALL, AML, and CML. Treatment consists of IV fluids at 2–4 times maintenance and specific chemotherapy.

4. *Tumor lysis syndrome* is characterized by hyperuricemia, hyperkalemia, hyperphosphatemia, and hypocalcemia; that may lead to renal dysfunction, arrhythmia, and encephalopathy. It occurs due to release of contents of cancer cells, following start of chemotherapy. Treatment consists of aggressive IV hydration, allopurinol, rasburicase, and care of metabolic disturbances.

Burns RA, Topoz I, Reynolds SL. Tumor lysis syndrome: risk factors, diagnosis, and management. *Pediatr Emerg Care*. 2014;30:571-6; quiz 577–9.

Delebarre M, Macher E, Mazingue F, et al. Which decision rules meet methodological standards in children with febrile neutropenia? Results of a systematic review and analysis. *Pediatr Blood Cancer*. 2014;61:1786–91.

Gogia A, Sharma A, Raina V, Chopra A. Superior vena cava syndrome: Initial presentation of acute myeloid leukemia in a child. *Indian J Cancer*. 2015;52:21.

Haeusler GM, Sung L, Ammann RA, Phillips B. Management of fever and neutropenia in paediatric cancer patients: room for improvement? *Curr Opin Infect Dis*. 2015;28:532–8.

Jain R, Bansal D, Marwaha RK, Singhi S. Superior mediastinal syndrome: emergency management. *Indian J Pediatr*. 2013;80:55–9.

Jones GL, Will A, Jackson GH; British Committee for Standards in Haematology. Guidelines for the management of tumour lysis syndrome in adults and children with haematological malignancies on behalf of the British Committee for Standards in Haematology. *Br J Haematol*. 2015;169:661–71.

Knight K. Question 2: Unexpected neutropenia in a febrile, but immunocompetent, child. *Arch Dis Child*. 2015;100:1093–5.

Morgan JE, Cleminson J, Atkin K, *et al*. Systematic review of reduced therapy regimens for children with low risk febrile neutropenia. *Support Care Cancer*. 2016;24:2651–60.

Strauss PZ, Hamlin SK, Dang J. Tumor Lysis Syndrome: A unique solute disturbance. *Nurs Clin North Am*. 2017;52:309–20.

Richa Jain

Genetic and Metabolic Disorders

16.1 GENETIC BASIS OF INHERITANCE

Deoxyribonucleic acid (DNA) is the genetic material in human being and most of the organisms. DNA transmits the genetic information from parents to the offspring and a cell to the daughter cells and is a fundamental molecule of life. Segments of DNA constitute "genes" which code for various proteins which in turn govern various functions of the body. The genes are located on *chromosomes* which are formed by histone and non-histone proteins in addition to 'DNA'.

Under Human Genome Project the sequence of whole genome (constituted of 46 chromosomes) has been deciphered. It is expected that there are about 25,000 genes in human being. In addition to genetic disorders it has become clear that the genes play an important role in all medical disorders to variable extent. This is obvious because proteins produced by genes are fundamental to all biological processes. The research in the field of genetics has not only lead to a revolution in the approach to the genetic disorders, but is also likely to bring about a paradigm shift in the preventive and therapeutic aspects for common diseases, like ischemic heart disease, diabetes mellitus, autoimmune diseases, cancer, etc.

DNA

DNA is a long double-stranded molecule consisting of a series of nucleotides attached to one another. Each nucleotide consists of a deoxyribose sugar, phosphate group and a nitrogen containing base. The bases are of two types, purines (Adenine—A, Guanine—G) and pyrimidines (Thymine—T, Cytosine—C). The sugar molecules are attached to each other by phosphodiester bond connecting 5th carbon atom of a sugar (5') to 3rd carbon atom (3') of the next sugar molecule and this forms a backbone of DNA molecules. Two strands of DNA molecule are wound to form a double helix with bases pointing towards each other. The two strands of DNA run opposite to each other so that one strand run from 5' end to 3' end while the other runs from 3' end to the 5' end (Fig. 16.1). The bonds between nucleotides on opposing strands bind the two DNA strands to each other. Only complementary nucleotides pair with each other; ie, A with T, and G with C.

DNA is tightly packed in a chromosome. The total length of DNA of a cell (6 billion base pairs [bp]) in a single human cell is 1 metre. It has to be packed in a nucleus less than 10 microns. During interphase most of the DNA is uncoiled and stretched while during metaphase stage of cell division

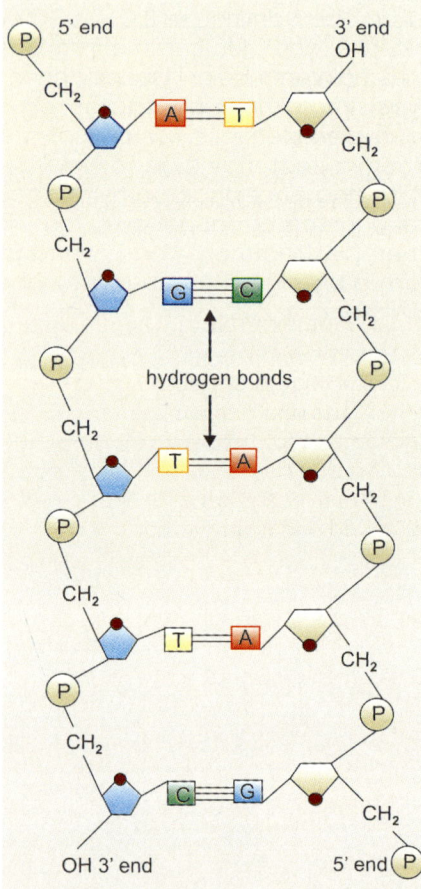

Fig. 16.1 DNA molecule. One end of a DNA strand has 5' end free and not attached to any sugar molecule and the other end has 3' end free. The other strand has an opposite orientation

the DNA gets tightly coiled onto itself and is packed to get the form of chromosomes.

Gene

A segment of DNA coding for a protein or polypeptide is called a gene. It is continuous with DNA on either side. In addition to the coding sequences, the regulatory elements like promoters and enhancers of the gene expression are also parts of the gene. These elements are near the 5' end of the gene but some may be far away from the gene and also may be on other chromosomes.

Information about regulatory elements controlling gene expression is far from complete. The sequence of nucleotides decides the sequence of amino acids in the polypeptide. A set of 3 consecutive nucleotides is called a *'codon'*. Four nucleotides generate 64 codons, which code for 20 amino acids; and 3 codons which code for 'stop signals'. Hence, more than one codon code for an amino acid. Each gene has coding sequences 'exons' intercepted with non-coding sequence 'intervening sequences' or 'introns' (Fig. 16.2).

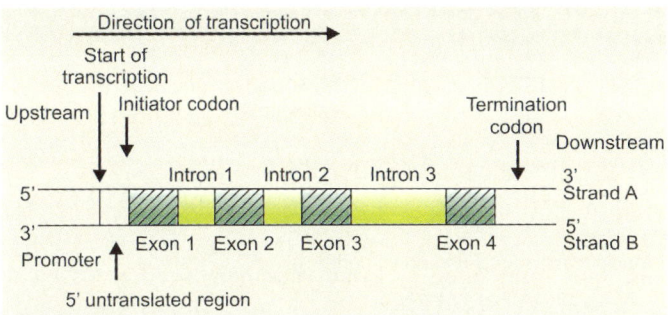

Fig. 16.2 Structure of a gene. Exons are separated by introns. The sequence of strand A represents the sequence of the gene while strand B acts as a template for RNA synthesis

Chromosomes

In human beings there are 46 chromosomes. There are 22 pairs of autosomes present in males and females. In addition, there is a pair of sex chromosomes, namely 'X' and 'Y' chromosomes. Males have one X and one Y chromosome while females have two X chromosomes and there is no Y chromosome. One set of chromosomes is inherited from one parent and one set from other. Thus, in human beings for every gene there are 2 copies; one from father and one from mother.

Mutations

The changes in the sequence of a gene in the form of substitution of a nucleotide, deletion of one or more base pairs, duplication or inversion of a segment or a gene are called *sequence variation* or *mutations*. Some mutations cause diseases, while some may be responsible for predisposition to various diseases. Some nucleotide substitutions do not change the amino acid (synonymous mutations) as an amino acid may be represented by more than one codon.

The nucleotide substitutions which do not cause diseases are present at 1 per 500 to 1000 nucleotides. These are present in all humans and known as *single nucleotide polymorphisms* or SNPs.

Alleles

The alternate forms of a gene caused due to change in the gene sequence (mutation/polymorphism) are known as *alleles*. If a person has 2 different alleles of a gene, he or she is called a *heterozygote*. If both the copies of a gene are identical, the person is a *homozygote* or *homozygous* for the allele. The persons may be homozygous for a normal (also known a 'wild') allele or a mutated allele.

Genetic Disorders

1. *Monogenic disorders* (single gene) are caused by mutation of a gene and follow Mendelian patterns of inheritance; hence they are also known as Mendelian disorders.

2. *Chromosomal disorders* are caused by gain or loss of a chromosome or a part of chromosome. Chromosomal deletion or duplication detectable under microscope contains a number of genes (5 to 10 million base pairs) and a loss or gain of even a small part of an autosome usually is associated with multiple malformations and mental retardation. Significant imbalance of genetic material in a conceptus usually leads to spontaneous abortion. The birth defects caused by smaller deletion/duplications of chromosomal segment, and which can be detected only by molecular cytogenetic techniques like microarray or fluorescent *in situ* hybridization (FISH) are known as *microdeletion/microduplication syndromes*.

3. *Multifactorial disorders* are seen more commonly amongst the relatives of a person with a disorder than among the general population but do not follow Mendelian pattern of inheritance. The increase of prevalence of such disorder amongst the relative of an affected person is explained by a model of multifactorial etiology where multiple genes and environmental factors are involved in the causation of the disease. The examples of multifactorial disorder include congenital malformations like cleft lip, Hirschsprung disease, pyloric stenosis, and many common diseases like hypertension, ischemic heart diseases, autoimmune disorders, and psychiatric illnesses.

Pedigree Drawing

Family history is an important part of clinical information, especially for genetic disorders. A pedigree is a graphical representation of data of relatives, their relationships and medical data of the individuals in the family. At least a three generations pedigree needs to be drawn (Fig. 16.3) using the standard symbols (Fig. 16.4). The person with a disorder who brings the family to notice is known as 'proband'.

The pedigree helps to decide the mode of inheritance of the disorder in the family. If the mode of disorder in concern is known, then the pedigree can be used to identify probable

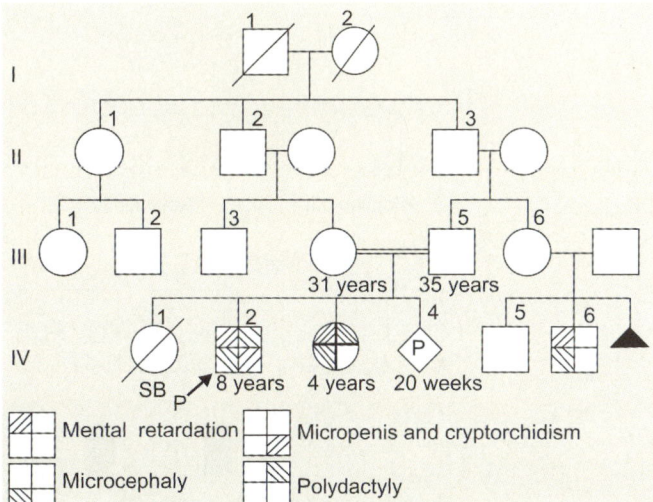

Fig. 16.3 A representative pedigree with consanguinous marriage between individuals III-4 and III-5. They have similarly affected a son and a daughter suggestive of autosomal recessive mode of inheritance. The individual IV-6 may or may not have the same disorder present in individuals IV-2 and IV-3

16

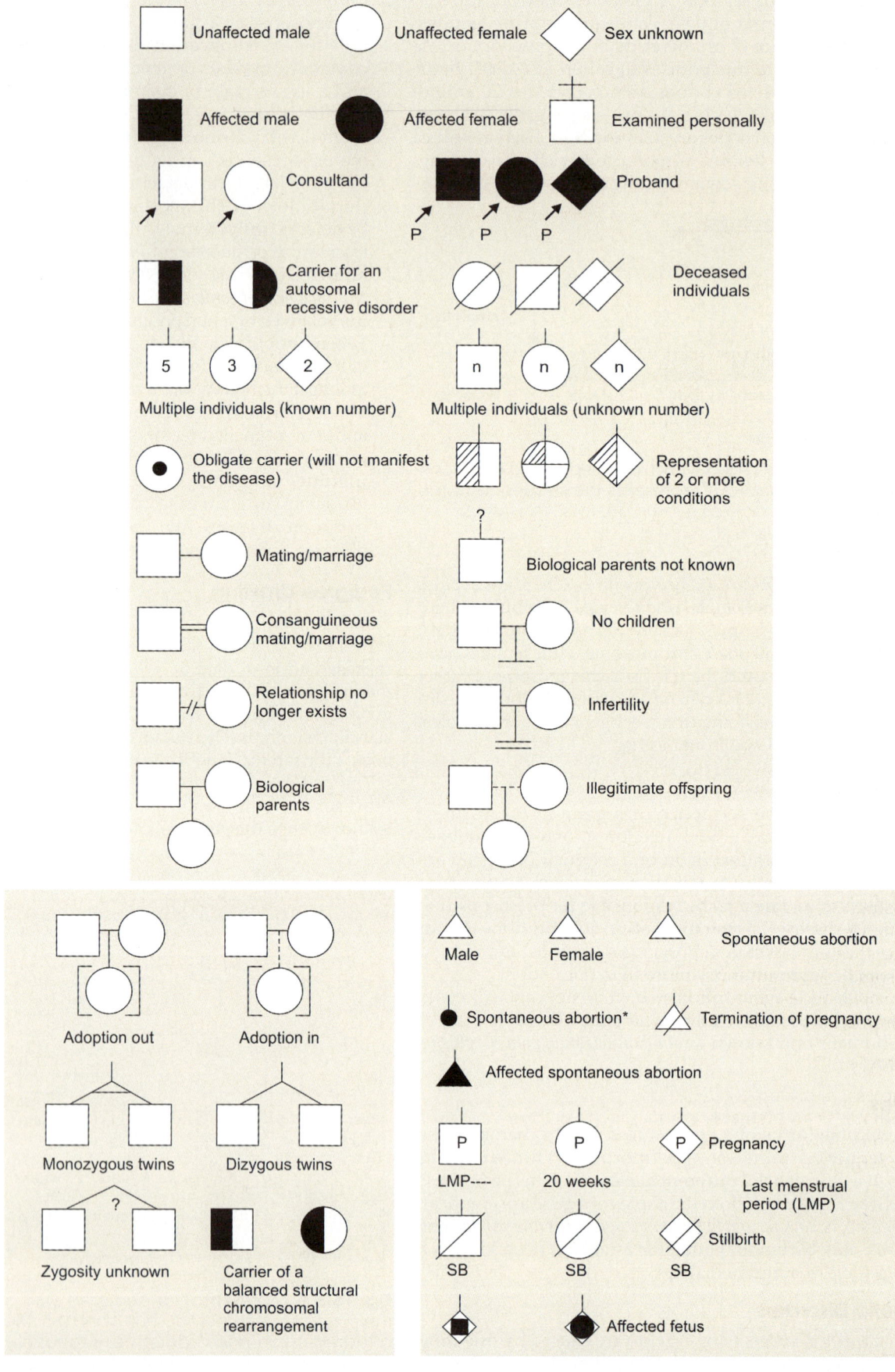

Fig. 16.4 Commonly used symbols for drawing of a pedigree; * this symbol is also used for spontaneous abortion

and obligate (definite) carriers. These carriers can be offered genetic counseling and/or genetic testing.

16.2 PATTERNS OF INHERITANCE

Mendel hypothesized 'factors' governing various traits from experiments on plants. These 'factors' are now known as genes and are primarily identified as causes of a number of disorders and traits. These disorders are known as monogenic disorders and follow Mendel's laws of inheritance and are also known as *Mendelian disorders*.

Non-Mendelian Inheritance

Many disorders do not follow Mendelian patterns of inheritance and have been known for a long time. Recent advances in molecular genetics have led to the identification of mechanism for these disorders. Non-Mendelian modes of inheritance and their common example are given below:

- *Mitochondrial* Leber hereditary optic atrophy
- *Genomic imprinting* Prader-Willi syndrome, Angelman syndrome
- *Uniparental disomy* Prader-Willi syndrome, Angelman syndrome
- *Somatic and germline mosaicism* Polyostotic fibrous dysplasia
- *Dynamic mutation* (triplet repeat disorders) Fragile X syndrome, myotonic dystrophy, Friedreich ataxia
- *Digenic/oligogenic inheritance* Hirschsprung disease, Bardet-Biedl syndrome.

16.2.1 MENDELIAN INHERITANCE

Diseases inherited in Mendelian fashion are categorized according to whether the gene is on an autosome or a sex chromosome and the trait is dominant or recessive.

1. Autosomal Dominant Inheritance

These diseases manifest even when only one copy of an autosomal gene is mutated. Thus, the disorders inherited in autosomal dominant fashion manifest in heterozygotes. Homozygotes for the dominant mutant genes may or may not be severely affected. Figure 16.5 shows a pedigree with autosomal dominant inheritance.

Examples Holt-Oram syndrome, achondroplasia, Marfan syndrome, Huntington chorea, and Waardenburg syndrome.

Characteristics

- Successive multiple generations are affected.
- Both males and females are affected in equal proportion.
- Both males and females can transmit the disease to their offspring.

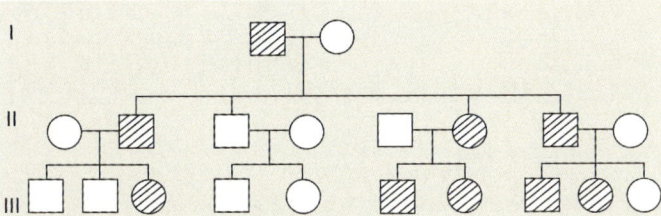

Fig. 16.5 Autosomal dominant inheritance

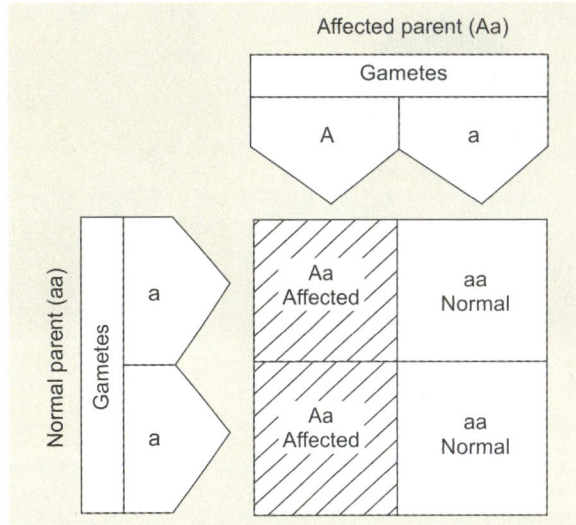

Fig. 16.6 A Punnett's square showing the possible gamete combinations for an autosomal dominant disorder in a couple with one normal spouse and one spouse with an autosomal dominant disorder

- The risk of transmission of the disease from an affected parent to the offspring is 50% (Fig. 16.6).

Penetrance and Expressivity

Reduced penetrance and variable expressivity are characteristic of autosomal dominant disorders and affect the risk of recurrence. In some autosomal dominant disorders, a person may be a carrier of a mutation but does not show manifestation. Such a phenomenon is called *incomplete penetrance*.

Variable expressivity implies variable severity of the disease, variable clinical manifestations, or variable age of onset of the disease, in different members of a family. Mother and the child shown in Fig. 16.7 have different severity of upper limb shortening and finger malformations. Variable expressivity is very common for Waardenburg syndrome. Most of the affected children may have heterochromia irides, white forelock of hair, and telecanthus (lateral displacement of inner canthi). Deafness is seen in only 50% of patients while some may have only pigmentary changes of eyes and/or hair.

Another classical example of variable severity is tuberous sclerosis. In a family of tuberous sclerosis, different individuals may have only one or two manifestations from the following: Seizure, adenoma sebaceum, hypopigmented patches on skin; while some individual may have severe form of mental retardation and/or seizure disorder with some of the above mentioned malformation.

2. Autosomal Recessive Inheritance

Autosomal recessive inheritance is due to genes located on the autosomes and the disease manifest when both the copies of the gene are mutated. The heterozygotes with one mutated copy of the gene and one normal copy of the gene are called "carriers" of the disease and do not manifest clinically (Fig. 16.8).

Examples: Thalassemia major, Friedreich ataxia, Wilson disease, spinal muscular atrophy, and ataxia-telangiectasia.

16

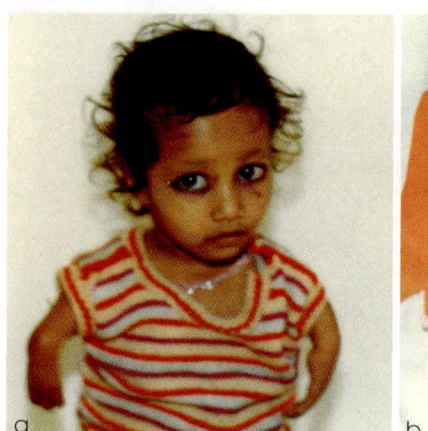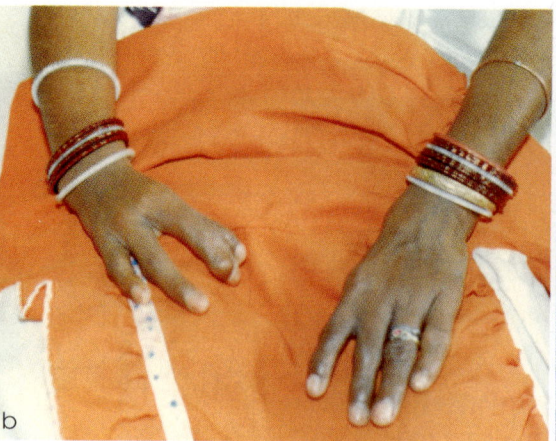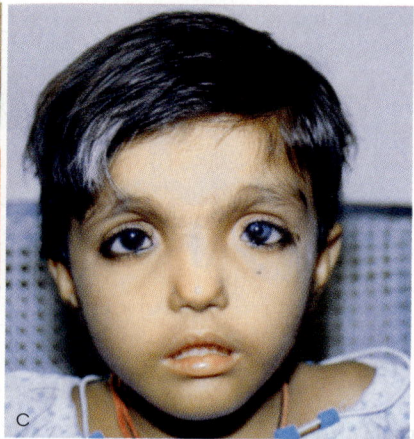

Fig. 16.7 A mother and her daughter with Holt-Oram syndrome. Expression of upper limb abnormality is more severe in the child (a) as compared to the mother (b), and Waardenburg syndrome type I—an autosomal dominant inherited syndrome of deafness (c)

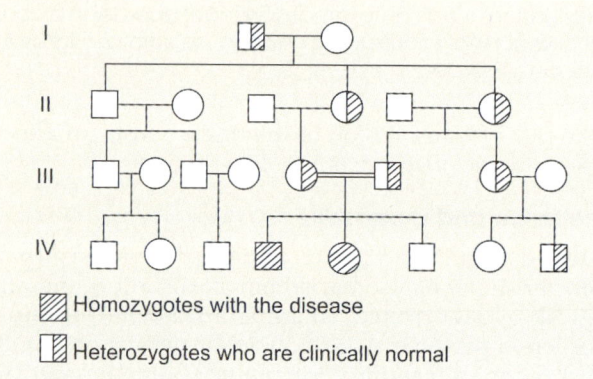

⬛ Homozygotes with the disease

▨ Heterozygotes who are clinically normal

Fig. 16.8 A pedigree showing an autosomal recessive inheritance

Characteristics

- Both males and females are affected.
- The disorder usually occurs in only one generation, mostly in a single sibship.
- Consanguinity in parents of affected child may be present especially if the disorder is rare. However, consanguinity is not essential.
- Both the parents of a person with autosomal recessive disease are not affected but are always carriers.
- The risk of recurrence of the disorder in the siblings of a child with an autosomal recessive disorder is 25% or l in 4. However, it should be noted that in a family, there can be 2, 3 or more consecutively affected children.

Sex-influenced disorders Some diseases are more common in one sex than the other. An example is gout, which is more common in males than in females. In postmenopausal women the prevalence is similar to that in males, suggesting the protective influence of hormones.

Sex-limited disorders Disorders of sex organ, though caused by autosomal genes, can occur only in the sex that has that organ; for example, familial testotoxicosis (male limited precocious puberty) occurs only in males though transmitted through females.

3. X-linked Recessive Inheritance

This is conventionally referred to as sex-linked inheritance and is due to the presence of recessive genes on the X chromosome. Males have a single X chromosome and therefore are hemizygous for most of the genes in the X chromosome. Hence, if a male has a mutated gene on the X chromosome, he will be affected. On the other hand, a female with one copy of mutated gene and the other normal copy will usually do not have manifestations of the disease.

Examples Hemophilia A, hemophilia B, Duchenne muscular dystrophy, Becker muscular dystrophy, X-linked aqueductal stenosis, mucopolysaccharidosis II (Hunter syndrome).

Characteristics

- Males are affected almost exclusively.
- All affected males are related through unaffected female (carrier) relatives.
- Male to male transmission is never observed because the X chromosome in a male is always contributed by a female.
- An affected male can pass on the disorder to his grandson through unaffected carrier daughter.
- The risk of transmitting the disease to the sons of a carrier female is 50% and the chance that her daughter will be carrier is 50% (Fig. 16.9). All daughters of an affected male will be carriers (Fig. 16.10).

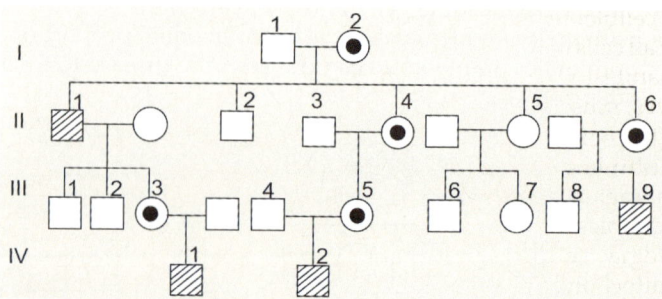

Fig. 16.9 A pedigree of an X-linked recessive disorder. Non-manifesting carrier females are denoted by a dot inside the circle

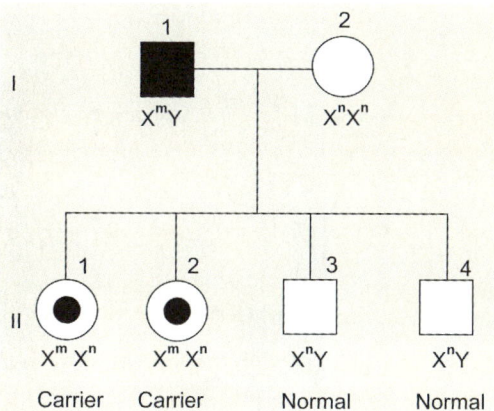

Fig. 16.10 A pedigree showing transmission of mutation of an X-linked recessive disorder from an affected father to his offspring

4. X-linked Dominant Inheritance

This is a less common form of inheritance and is caused by the presence of a *dominant disease causing allele on an* X chromosome. The pedigree of an X-linked dominant disorder superficially looks similar to that of an autosomal dominant disorder. But the number of females with the disease is more than the number of males with the disease. The disease manifestations in females are milder than in the males and there is no male to male transmission. The classical example is X-linked hypophosphatemic rickets. Some X-linked disorders are so severe in males that the affected males die *in utero* and only affected females are seen. Incontinentia pigmenti is another example of X-linked dominant disorder with lethality in males.

Fragile X mental retardation is usually labeled as *X-linked semi-dormant disorder*, as manifesting females are common.

16.2.2 NON-MENDELIAN INHERITANCE

Some genetic disorders do not seem to follow Mendel's laws of inheritance. Advances in molecular genetics have provided explanations to these non-Mendelian patterns of inheritance. These are discussed briefly:

1. Mitochondrial Inheritance

Mitochondria have thousands of copies of circular mitochondrial DNA. The mitochondrial DNA codes for ribosomal RNA, transfer RNA and some protein involved in cellular respiration. These genes are important for function of all cells of the body and hence, mitochondrial diseases can manifest with symptoms of any system of body including eyes, muscles, heart, brain, liver and endocrine glands.

Mitochondrial disorders should be suspected when multiple systems of body are involved or the patient has characteristic features of a mitochondrial disorder. Two examples are Kearns-Sayre syndrome (external ophthalmoplegia, retinitis pigmentosa, myopathy), and MELAS (mitochondrial encephalopathy, lactic acidosis, and stroke-like episodes).

Mitochondrial disorder can be transmitted only through mother as only the ovum contributes mitochondria to the

zygote. The severity and the extent of involvement vary depending on the load of mutant mitochondria in each tissue. Variability of number of mutant mitochondria in each cell and each tissue is characteristic of mitochondrial disorder. Unless the number of mutant mitochondria crosses a 'threshold'; symptoms will not appear. Similarly, the manifestations in offspring will depend on the number of mutant mitochondria transmitted to the zygote. Hence, the risk of recurrence in the offspring cannot be predicted in mitochondrial disorders.

Diagnosis of mitochondrial diseases needs testing of respiratory chain enzymes in various tissues like muscle biopsy and mutation analysis in blood and muscle biopsy specimen. Detection of mutation in prenatal sample may not be able to predict phenotype as the mutant load in sample tested may be different from that in the various organs of the body.

2. Genomic Imprinting

In Mendelian disorders, there is no difference between the function of maternally and paternally inherited copies of the gene. However, for some genes, the behaviors of paternal and maternal copies of the gene may be different. This is known as genomic imprinting. This occurs due to heritable modification of the imprinted copy of the gene.

The imprinted copy is the copy of the gene which is silenced, ie, not expressing; though the DNA sequence of the gene is normal. The important mechanism of shutting off a gene is methylation of the gene.

Methylation of a gene means that the cytosines in the CpG islands (clusters of cytosine and guanine which occur together near transcription sites of many genes) are methylated. If the maternal allele is inactive or suppressed, the gene is said to be maternally imprinted. In paternally imprinted gene, the paternal copy is silenced. The imprinting is reversible. During gametogenesis, the imprint is erased and a new one is established (Fig. 16.11).

The examples of disorders occurring due to the imprinted genes are Prader-Willi syndrome (obesity, hypogonadism,

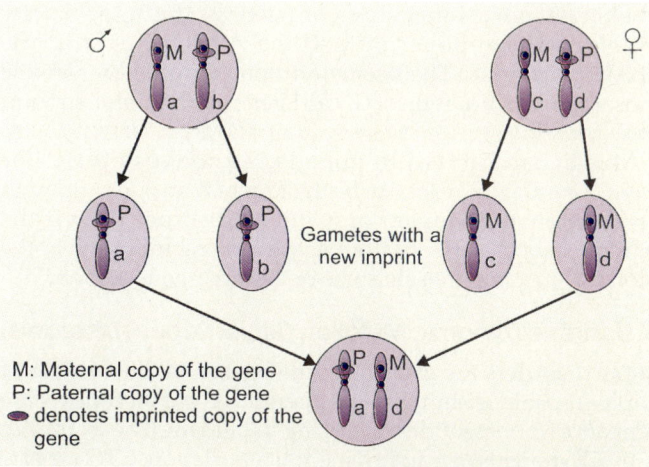

M: Maternal copy of the gene
P: Paternal copy of the gene
● denotes imprinted copy of the gene

Fig. 16.11 Establishment of new imprint during gametogenesis. Chromosome 'a', which was of maternal origin in the father, is passed on as paternal to his offspring. Similarly, chromosome 'd', which was of paternal origin in the mother, is transmitted as maternal to her offspring

and mental retardation) and Angelman syndrome (mental retardation, seizures, bursts of laughter, and ataxic gait). On chromosome 15, a small region has imprinted genes for Prader-Willi syndrome and Angelman syndrome. Prader-Willi syndrome genes are maternally imprinted and the disease occurs when paternal copy of the gene is deleted. In Angelman syndrome, the gene is paternally imprinted and hence, the disorder occurs only when the maternal copy of the gene is deleted.

3. Uniparental Disomy

The other evidence of imprinting comes from uniparental disomy. Uniparental disomy implies that both the homologous chromosomes and genes are inherited from one parent only. This can occur due to various mechanisms. Usually two events of non-disjunction are required (Fig. 16.12).

If the uniparental disomy occurs for a chromosome which has some imprinted gene, then there may be disease manifestation though there are two copies of genes with normal DNA sequence. Examples are Prader-Willi syndrome and Angelman syndrome. Paternal uniparental disomy of chromosome 15 leads to Angelman syndrome (as maternal copies of the genes are missing) and maternal uniparental disomy of 15 leads to Prader-Willi syndrome (as paternal chromosome 15 and genes on it are missing).

In uniparental disomy, both the homologous chromosomes of a parent (*uniparental heterodisomy*) may be inherited or there may be 2 copies of one chromosome of a parent (*uniparental isodisomy*). In case of uniparental isodisomy, if there is a mutated gene for a recessive disorder on that chromosome, the individual will manifest with the recessive disorder.

4. Mosaicism

Mosaicism implies presence of two types of cell lines in an individual, one with a mutation and one without the mutation. Mosaicism can be for chromosomal abnormality or a single gene mutation. Somatic mosaicism may decrease the severity of the disorder and may manifest with patchy distribution of lesions; eg, streaky pigmentary abnormalities of skin as in hypomelanosis of Ito (Fig. 16.13), or patchy involvement of bones in McCune-Albright polyostotic fibrous dysplasia. The later condition is caused by somatic mosaicism for mutation of *GNAS*1 gene for the alpha-subunit of G-protein.

Mosaicism limited to gonads is known as *germ line mosaicism*. This may lead to birth of more than one child with an autosomal dominant or X-linked disorder even if the parent is not a carrier of the disease causing mutation in the blood. Germ line mosaicism is not a rare phenomenon.

5. Unstable Dynamic Mutation (Triplet Repeat Disorders)

Some disorders are caused by an increase in the number of triplet repeats within or near a gene. The triplet repeats are repeats of 3 nucleotides occurring in tandem. The examples are CGG repeats in fragile X mental retardation, CTG repeats in myotonic dystrophy and GAA repeats in Friedreich ataxia. These repeats are usually transmitted stably from one generation to the next.

In a person with higher number of repeats, the number changes during transmission to the offspring. Increase above

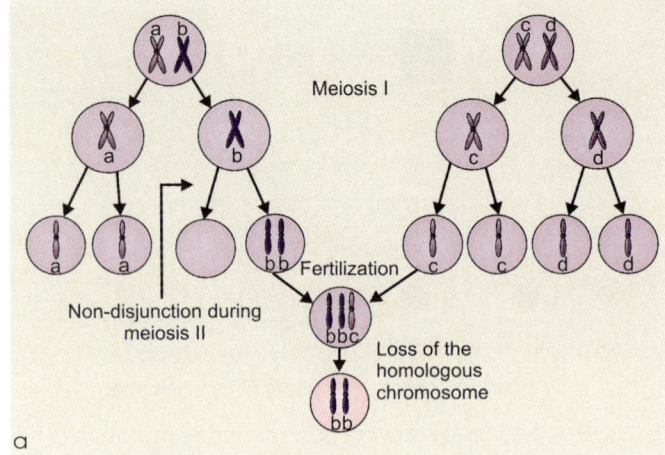

a

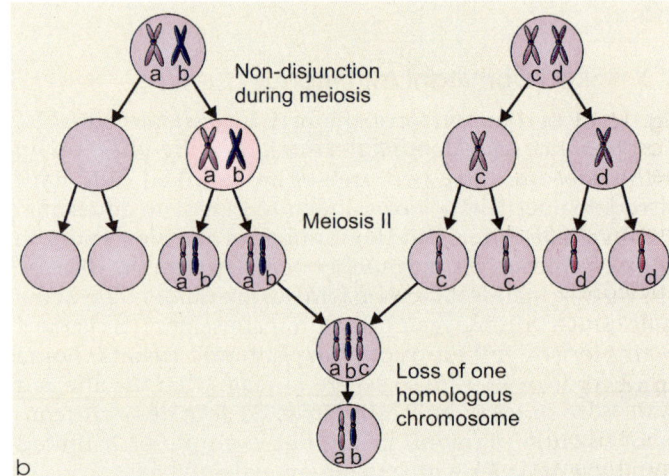

b

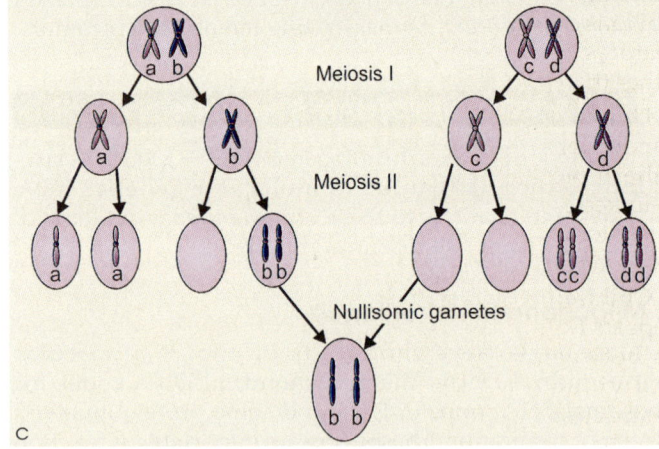

c

Fig. 16.12 Gametogenesis resulting in uniparental disomy. Two events of non-disjunction are needed for uniparental disomy. 'a' and 'b' are homologous chromosomes of a parent and 'c' and 'd' are homologous chromosomes of another parent. (a) Uniparental isodisomy, (b) uniparental heterodisomy, (c) fusion of disomic gamete of a parent with nullisomic gamete from another parent

a specific number of repeats leads to manifestations. With a higher number of repeats, there is instability and the number changes from tissue to tissue in an individual and individual to individual in a family. The increase in number of repeats over generations leads to increasing severity of

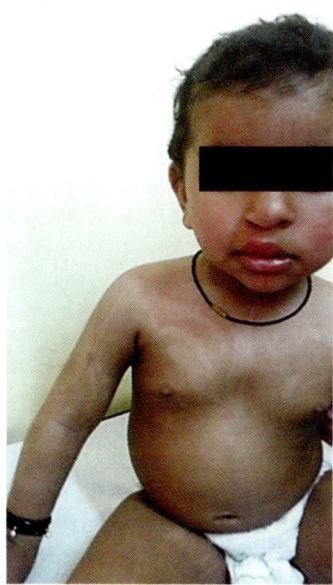

Fig. 16.13 Streak-like hypopigmentation along the lines of Blaschko. It suggests mosaicism for chromosomal or single gene mutation

manifestations and earlier age of onset, a phenomenon known as *anticipation*. Anticipation is observed in many nucleotide repeat disorders like Huntington chorea and spino-cerebellar ataxia.

FRAGILE X SYNDROME

It is the commonest cause of inherited intellectual disability and transmitted in an X-linked fashion. Fragile X syndrome accounts for 1 to 3% of cases of intellectual disability without obvious cause. Long face with prominent mandible, autistic features, and large testes in postpubertal boys are features other than intellectual disability (Fig. 16.14a).

Unlike other X-linked recessive disorder, many of the carrier females show manifestations. Thus, the mode of inheritance is described as X-linked semi-dominant or X-linked dominant with incomplete penetrance. The normal allele for the gene for fragile X syndrome—FMR1 gene has less than 50 CGG repeats (Fig. 16.14b).

Children with fragile X syndrome have more than 200 repeats (knows as full mutation). The alleles with repeats in between 50 and 200 are called *premutation alleles*. Individuals with premutation do not have mental retardation and other features of fragile X syndrome but may have ataxia and tremors in old age and females may have premature ovarian failure. The premutation allele when transmitted from mother to her offspring expands and the offspring with repeat number more than 200 have fragile X syndrome. Some females with full mutation have some features like long face, learning difficulties, or mild mental retardation. The manifestation in female depends probably on lyonization pattern, ie, the relative ratio of active X chromosomes with mutation and without mutation. A characteristic pedigree of fragile X syndrome is shown in Fig. 16.14c.

As the clinical features of fragile X syndrome are not diagnostic, testing all individuals with intellectual disability

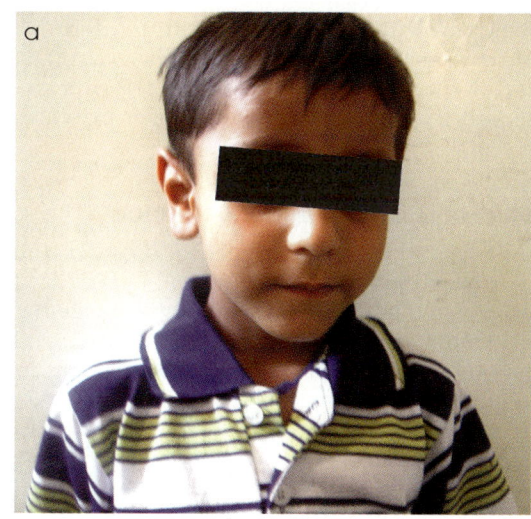

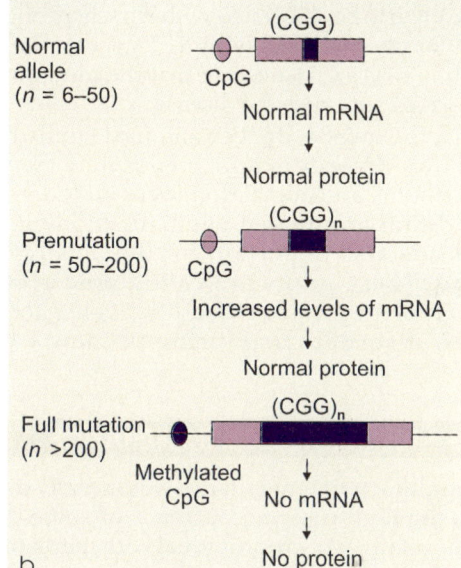

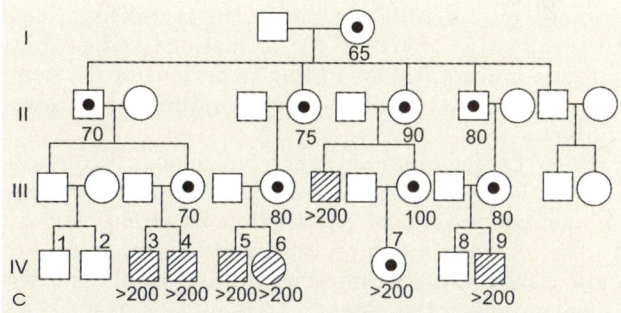

Fig. 16.14 (a) Face of a child with fragile X syndrome. The features are too subtle to be able to diagnose clinically, (b) Normal allele, premutation and full mutation alleles of FMR-1 gene showing increasing number of CGG repeats and the effect on mRNA and protein synthesis, (c) a pedigree of fragile X syndrome. The numbers of CGG repeats in carriers are shown below each individual. There is increase in the number of repeats of premutation allele over generations with subsequent conversion to mutation. Obligate carriers are shown by dot (•) inside the symbols. Affected cases are shown by shaded symbols. The number of repeats has not increased when the allele is transmitted by the father

16

and developmental delay is important to identify cases. Screening of possible female carriers in the extended family of a case of fragile X syndrome and offering prenatal diagnosis to the carriers is essential for prevention of recurrences.

6. Digenic and Oligogenic Inheritance

It has now been proved that many genetic disorders that were previously described as monogenic are, in fact, caused by mutations in two loci. Such digenic inheritance has been reported in retinitis pigmentosa and Bardet-Biedl syndrome. At least 20 genes are known for Bardet-Biedl syndrome and some pedigrees show that mutations in both copies of *BBS2* gene and in one copy of *BBS6* gene are required to manifest the disease.

Hirschsprung disease is an important example of oligogenic inheritance. Mutation in *RET* and some other genes are known to be associated with Hirschsprung disease. But not all family members with *RET* gene mutation have Hirschsprung disease, indicating that the mutation in *RET* gene alone does not cause the disease.

The variable expressivity seen amongst family members of Mendelian disorders and incomplete penetrance observed in some autosomal dominant disorders suggest that in addition to mutated gene, functioning of some other genes is also important for the development of phenotype. These genes are called **modifier genes**. Research in identification of modifier genes for various Mendelian disorders may bring up new treatment strategies.

16.2.3 MULTIFACTORIAL INHERITANCE

Model of multifactorial inheritance was initially developed to explain the high risk of recurrence of some disorders amongst the relatives of an individual with the disorder. The disorder is the combined effect of many genetic variations and environmental factors. Now many of these genetic factors are being identified in reality. This type of inheritance is seen in many congenital malformations and common disorders of adult life, including hypertension, ischemic heart disease, psychiatric diseases, and autoimmune disorders.

Factor V Leiden mutation in cerebral venous thrombosis, DR3 and DR4 alleles at HLA locus in type I diabetes mellitus, and a genetic variant of 5,10-methylenetetrahydrofolate reductase enzyme in neural tube defects, are some of the genetic risk factors identified in multifactorial disorders. Because multifactorial illnesses account for a major health burden; these are the recent thrust areas of research following completion of the human genome project.

16.3 CHROMOSOMAL DISORDERS

Cytogenetics and Karyotype

The study of chromosomes is known as *cytogenetics*. Traditional cytogenetics needs live dividing cells. The cells are cultured in tubes and the cell division is arrested by adding colchicine which is a spindle poison. The cells arrested in metaphase stage show chromosomes as discrete

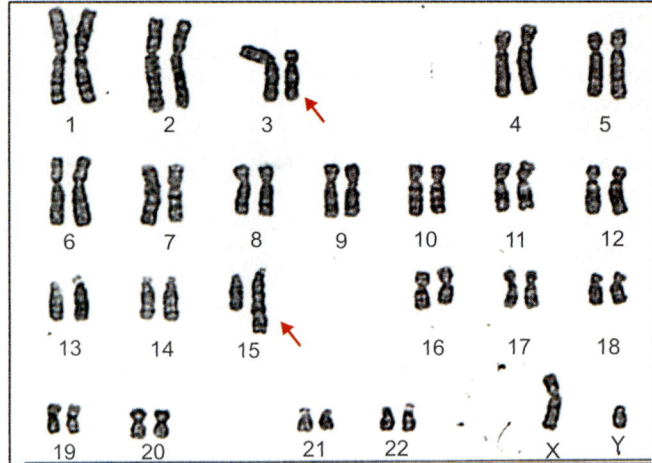

Fig. 16.15 A karyotype of a male showing 46 chromosomes with a balanced translocation between chromosomes 3 and 15. The normal chromosomes are on the left sides of the pairs and the derivatives chromosomes are shown by arrows. Note that each chromosome has different banding pattern which is used to identify chromosomes and to detect chromosomal abnormalities

bodies. During slide preparation, the chromosomes of one cell are spread in a localized area and can be counted and analyzed. A photograph of a metaphase is taken and the chromosomes are cut and arranged in pairs. Such an arrangement of chromosomes is called 'karyotype' (Fig. 16.15).

Karyotype also denotes the chromosome complement of an individual; ie, total number of chromosomes, sex chromosomes, and chromosomal abnormality, if any. The smallest chromosomal abnormality detected by traditional karyotype contains at least 5 to 10 million base pairs. Now, the analysis of whole genome by microarray based cytogenetic analysis can detect genomic imbalances as small as 10 kilobases and has found an important role in evaluation of children with mental retardation or autism.

Abnormalities of Chromosomes

Abnormalities of chromosomes can be *numerical* or *structural* and may involve autosomes or sex chromosomes. These abnormalities may present at different ages with different problems. Chromosomal abnormalities are usually unbalanced, due to gain or loss of chromosomal material. Embryo with significant chromosomal imbalance is spontaneously aborted; chromosomal anomalies account for about 50% of early spontaneous abortions. Some chromosomal imbalances of autosomes are not embryonically lethal and lead to live-born child with multiple malformations and intellectual disability. Sex chromosomal abnormalities usually lead to hypergonadotropic hypogonadism.

- *Numerical abnormalities* of chromosomes can be *aneuploidy* or *polyploidy*. Polyploidies are 69,XXX (triploidy); 92,XXYY (tetraploidy) where the total number of chromosomes is an exact multiple of haploid (23) set of chromosomes. The karyotype with number of chromosomes which is not an exact multiple of 23 is known as aneuploidy. The examples of aneuploidy are trisomy 21 (three copies of chromosomes 21), or monosomy X (only one of the sex chromosomes pair).

- *Structural abnormalities* These include *deletion* or duplication of a part of chromosome, *translocation* of a segment from one chromosome to the other (which may be balanced or unbalanced), *isochromosome* (loss of one arm of a chromosome and duplication of the other), *inversion* (of a segment in a chromosome due to two breaks and joining of the segment in an inverted manner), and *ring chromosome* (breaks in the ends of a chromosome and joining together to form a ring structure).

16.3.1 DISORDERS OF AUTOSOMES

Numerous abnormalities of chromosomes are described in liveborns, stillborns and aborted material. The three nonmosaic aneuploidies of autosomes compatible with survival are trisomy 21, trisomy 13, and trisomy 18. Syndromes of other structural abnormalities like deletions of 4p, 5p, etc. are well delineated. Use of newer techniques to study chromosomes has lead to identification of new syndromes associated with microdeletions not visible on routine chromosomal analysis (Fig. 16.16).

DOWN SYNDROME

Down syndrome is the commonest chromosomal abnormality occurring in live births. It accounts for 30% of individuals with mental handicap. The etiology of Down syndrome is an extra copy of chromosome 21 (Fig. 16.17). This may occur due to non-disjunction (trisomy)(95%), translocation (4%), or mosaicism (1%).

Translocation The extra chromosome 21 is attached to some other chromosome, commonly to 14, 21, or 22. In about 50% of such cases one of the parents may be a carrier of such balanced rearrangement (Fig. 16.18) and hence, at high risk of giving birth to offspring with trisomy 21. The risk of Down syndrome in the offspring of a female carrier of 14;21 or 21;22 translocation is 10–15%. If such balanced arrangement is seen in a male, the risk of Down syndrome in his offspring is 1 to 5%.

Clinical Features

Facial features of Down syndrome are characteristic: Flat face, hypertelorism, upslant of eyes, depressed nasal bridge, open mouth, and small ears (Fig. 16.19). Clinical diagnosis may be a little difficult in neonates and preterm babies. Other common features are listed below:

1. *Neonatal* Hypotonia, excess skin at the nape of neck.
2. *Craniofacial* Increased distance between eyes, epicanthic folds, upslant of eyes, flat face, small ears, depressed nasal bridge, flat occiput, protruding and fissured tongue.
3. *Limbs* Small hands, clinodactyly of fifth finger, simian crease, increased gap between first and second toes.
4. *Major malformations* Atrioventricular canal defects and other cardiac malformations, duodenal atresia, tracheo-esophageal fistula, and Hirschsprung disease.
5. *Other problems* Short stature, strabismus, obesity, cataract, atlantoaxial instability, risk of leukemia, and hypothyroidism.

Intellectual disability is the most important problem associated with Down syndrome. The average IQ of children

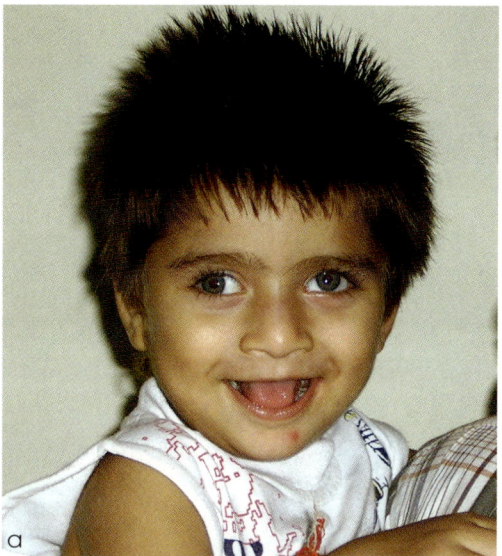

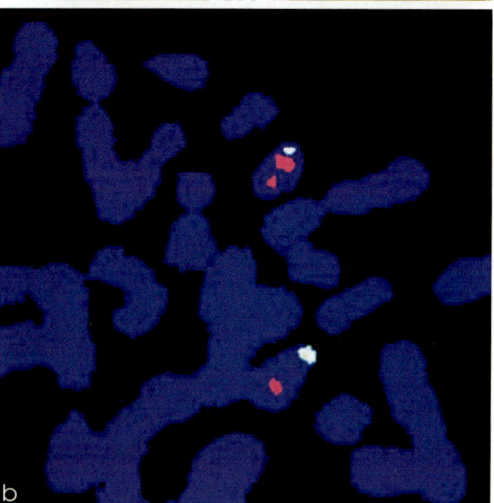

Fig. 16.16 (a) A child with Angelman syndrome. Note happy predisposition and slight prognathism, (b) Fluorescence *in situ* hybridization shows deletion of region for Angelman syndrome on one chromosome 15 (red signal near green signal for the centromere). The green signal is for centromere of chromosome 15 and the distal red signal is a control probe on chromosome 15

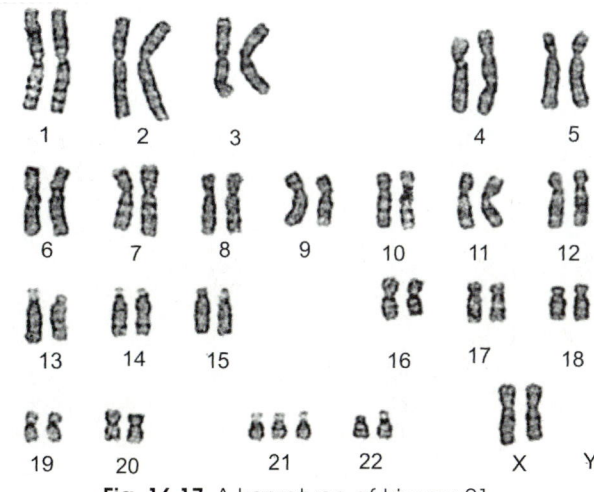

Fig. 16.17 A karyotype of trisomy 21

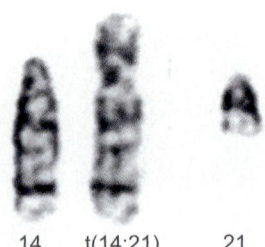

14   t(14;21)   21

Fig. 16.18 A partial karyotype showing t(14;21). The individual is a balanced carrier as she has DNA material of 2 chromosomes 21 and 2 chromosomes 14, but the number of total chromosomes is 45 as one 21 and one 14 are joined to each other

with Down syndrome is 40–60 and though late, they can talk, walk, do self-care, and lead a happy and useful life under sheltered conditions. Children with Down syndrome communicate well with the family, love the family, and can do repetitive and simple jobs with supervision.

Investigations

Examination and investigations for major malformations are the first steps, whatever may be the age of the child with Down syndrome. Chromosomal analysis (karyotyping) is essential to estimate the risk of recurrence in the family. An extra chromosome 21 (47,XX,+21 or 47,XY,+21) accounts for 95% children with Down syndrome, and the risk of recurrence of Down syndrome in the sibs of these children is 1%. Karyotypes of the parents of a case with such free trisomy 21 are not needed.

Translocation accounts for 4–5% cases of Down syndrome. In 50% of these cases one of the parents will be carrier of the translocation and hence, karyotypes of the parents need to be studied.

Management

At present, there is no curative treatment for Down syndrome but major malformations need to be surgically treated and good training can lead to better outcome. Counseling is a continued process and revisits to provide information and support are needed. The regular surveillance for hearing problem, hypothyroidism, cataract, anemia and other medical problems is necessary.

Genetic Counseling

Break the news to the family as soon as possible. Both the husband and wife should be present. The realistic information about prognosis should be given. Stress should be laid on the positive aspects like ability to lead semi-independent and fruitful life. Rare complication like risk of leukemia need not be mentioned. Explain the risk of recurrence and need for prenatal diagnosis.

Risk of Recurrence

Risk of recurrence after one child with free trisomy 21 is 1%. The risk for inherited translocation is 10–15% if the mother is carrier of balanced translocation and up to 5% if the father is the translocation carrier. Carrier of translocation between two chromosomes 21 [t(21;21)] is rare; but in such case risk of Down syndrome in the offspring is 100% irrespective of which of the parent is the carrier. Risk of recurrence in the sibling if the child has *de novo* translocation (ie, the parents' karyotypes are normal) is only 1%.

Prenatal diagnosis during the next pregnancy can be done by karyotyping of prenatal chorionic villi or amniotic fluid samples.

Prevention

A child with Down syndrome most often is born in families who do not have any family history of Down syndrome. The overall incidence of Down syndrome is 1 in 800, but it varies with the age of the mother. In a 20-year-old mother, the incidence is 1 in 1500 which gradually increases with maternal age to become 1 in 400 at 35 years and 1 in 100 at 40 years. Previously amniocentesis being invasive was offered only to women more than 35 years of age. However, most of the children with Down syndrome are born to younger mothers.

Quadruple Marker Test

Documentation of low alpha fetoprotein, low unconjugated estriol, high beta human chorionic gonadotropin, and increased inhibin in mother's blood has been used to identify women with high risk of Down syndrome in the fetus. This screening test is offered to women of all ages. Women with the risk of Down syndrome of 1 in 250 or higher identified by the screening test are offered confirmatory test by amniotic fluid karyotyping.

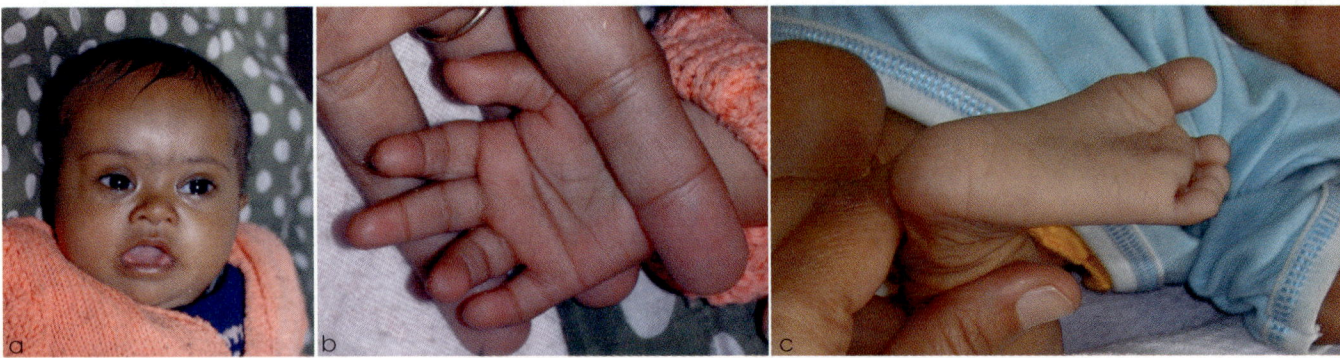

Fig. 16.19 Features of Down syndrome. (a) Flat face, upslant of eyes, hypertelorism, epicanthic folds, protruding tongue, (b) clinodactyly or hypoplastic phalanx of the little finger, and (c) sandal gap

Non-invasive Prenatal Testing (NIPT)

New technologies have made it possible to test the fetal chromosomes using free fetal DNA in mother's plasma. This test on mother's blood at 10 weeks of gestation can identify aneuploidies of chromosomes 21, 13, and 18. It can identify 99% of fetuses with trisomy 21 but confirmation by invasive test of amniocentesis or chorionic villi sampling is necessary. A small possibility of false positive and test failure makes it a screening test. At present NIPT is too costly to be routinely used as a screening test. However, as it greatly reduces the need to invasive testing; the test is of a great importance in cases of precious pregnancies.

Fetal Chromosomal Study

Complete chromosomal analysis from amniotic fluid cell by traditional cytogenetic techniques takes 10 to 15 days. Techniques based on fluorescence *in situ* hybridization (FISH) and polymerase chain reaction can test number of copies of chromosomes 21, 18, and 13 in 2 days and are used for rapid prenatal diagnosis (Fig. 16.20).

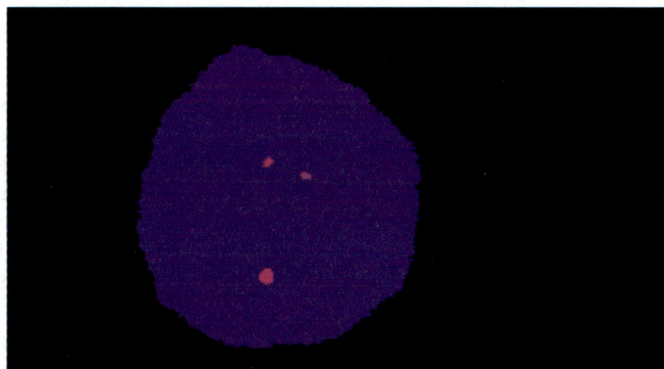

Fig. 16.20 Fluorescence *in situ* hybridization (FISH) using a probe for chromosome 21 on an interphase nucleus. Presence of 3 signals show that there are 3 copies of chromosome 21. FISH based tests are rapid and the results are available on the second day but these tests cannot look at all chromosomes like traditional karyotyping

Fetal Imaging

About 50% fetuses with Down syndrome have ultrasonographically detectable abnormalities including nuchal thickening, absent nasal bone, duodenal atresia, and congenital heart defects. Presence of these markers in fetus indicates the need of chromosomal analysis.

OTHER AUTOSOMAL ABNORMALITIES

Trisomy 18 and trisomy 13, the other trisomies seen in liveborn, usually do not survive beyond infancy. Parents need to be counseled on the same principles as that for trisomy 21.

- *Trisomy* 18 (*Edward syndrome*). It is characterized by growth retardation, characteristic clenched hands with overlapping fingers, prominent occiput, hypertonia, and cardiac anomalies (Fig. 16.21a).
- *Trisomy* 13 (*Patau syndrome*). The characteristic features include holoprosencephaly (undivided cerebrum),

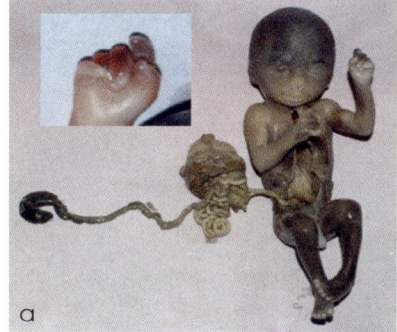
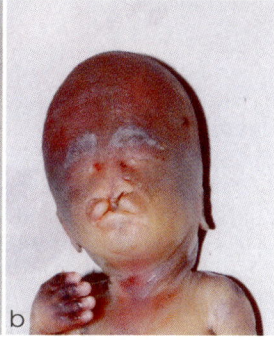

Fig. 16.21 (a) A fetus with trisomy 18. Note the typical overlapping fingers of the clenched hand. The pregnancy was terminated due to prenatal diagnosis of trisomy 18, (b) midline cleft or premaxillary agenesis seen in association with holoprosencephaly in trisomy 13

Case Study	Down Syndrome

A 33-year-old woman underwent an ultrasonography at 33 weeks of gestation because of clinical impression of polyhydramnios. The ultrasonography showed a double bubble appearance characteristic of duodenal atresia. She consulted a pediatric surgeon who told that duodenal atresia is a surgically treatable condition. Clinical geneticist told that 30% of the cases with duodenal atresia have trisomy 21. She was offered rapid prenatal diagnosis by FISH for chromosome 21 on amniotic fluid. She did not opt for prenatal tests. She delivered normally at 35 weeks of gestation and the child showed features of Down syndrome. The child was operated but died on the third day.

- **Q. What should be done immediately after birth?**
- **Q. Should the karyotype be done and what sample should be used for karyotyping?**
- **Q. When should the family be told of the diagnosis?**
- **Q. What information should be told about the prognosis?**
- **Q. When should the family given information about risk of recurrence?**

To find answers read For prenatally diagnosed cases of malformations delivery at a centre with good neonatological and surgical facilities should be planned. Immediately after delivery a quick and careful search for other malformations like tracheoesophageal fistula, anal atresia needs to be done. The karyotyping from blood of the baby should be done; preferably immediately as it is necessary to confirm diagnosis and will also helpful for estimating risk of recurrence. Before surgery, echocardiography should be done as about half of the neonates with Down syndrome have cardiac anomalies. The family needs to be given information about outcome regarding mental function. The surgery will correct duodenal atresia but the child is likely to have mild to moderate degree of intellectual disability which does not have curative treatment. Importance of karyotyping for counseling regarding next pregnancy must be mentioned and the family should be given an appointment for genetic counseling at later date.

Think it over!
  i. The parents of the family are too poor to bear the cost of the surgery for duodenal atresia.
  ii. The child is born in the family after 10 years of infertility.
  iii. The family is not very poor but the child has complex cardiac anomaly as well.

16

midline cleft lip, cardiac malformations, and polydactyly (Fig. 16.21b).

Structural chromosomal anomalies are rare but detected by karyotyping in children with malformations and developmental delay. Many malformations can now be diagnosed prenatally by ultrasonography; and about 7–10% of these fetuses have chromosomal anomalies. Chromosomal analysis needs to be done for all stillborn babies, and those with intellectual disability or developmental delay. Karyotyping of the parents of children with structural chromosomal abnormality and genetic counseling are essential to prevent recurrence.

16.3.2 SEX CHROMOSOME ABNORMALITIES

Most common anomalies of sex chromosomes are 45,X (Turner syndrome) and 47,XXY (Klinefelter syndrome). These usually present as hypergonadotropic hypogonadism in females and males, respectively. There is no significant intellectual disability.

TURNER SYNDROME (45,X)

Turner syndrome is associated with monosomy or partial monosomy of X chromosome, resulting in 45,X karyotype. Other chromosomal abnormalities associated with Turner syndrome are listed in **Table 16.1**. More than 99% of the conceptuses with 45,X karyotype are spontaneously aborted (Fig. 16.22).

Clinical Features

The characteristic features of Turner syndrome include short stature, webbed neck, cubitus valgus (wide carrying angle), wide spaced nipple, and short 4th metacarpal and metatarsal (Fig. 16.23). Some cases present as primary amenorrhea at puberty while some present as short stature in childhood. Intellectual disability is not a feature of Turner syndrome though learning deficits in specific areas may be present. Coarctation of aorta is the most frequently associated cardiovascular defect. Other notable features include horse-shoe-shaped kidney, low posterior hairline, nail hypoplasia, and multiple nevi. Turner syndrome in neonates is characterized by lymphedema of hands and feet. However, classical features are present in only 50% cases.

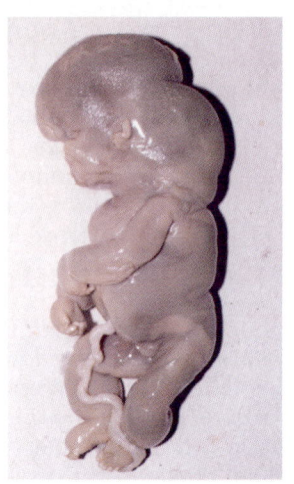
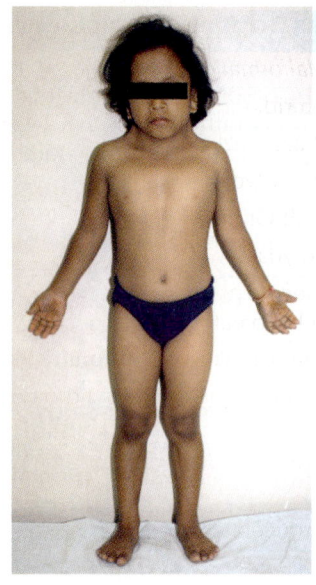

Fig. 16.22 Fetal Turner phenotype. Note a large cystic hygroma at the back of neck, and edema all over body

Fig. 16.23 A girl showing characteristic features of Turner syndrome with webbed neck and wide carrying angle

Management

Early diagnosis is useful as growth hormone therapy started from childhood results in gain of about 5–7 cm in final height. Other aspects of management include screening for cardiac and renal anomalies and surveillance for otitis media, hypertension, hypothyroidism and hormone replacement therapy for development of secondary sexual characters and establishment of menstruation. Most of the cases of Turner syndrome have infertility. Fertility may be possible by assisted reproductive techniques with donor ova.

KLINEFELTER SYNDROME (47,XXY)

Klinefelter syndrome is characterized by male hypogonadism with at least two X chromosomes and one Y chromosome (47,XXY). Other karyotypic abnormalities associated include 47,XXY/46,XY; and 47,XXXY. Rarely, structural abnormalities of X chromosome may be associated.

Majority of the patients are identified because of delayed or diminished puberty, gynecomastia, or infertility. Prepubertal boys are normal. Adults have tall stature, long legs, and female distribution of fat. Facial hair may be less. The size of the penis may be small. Small testes and oligospermia or azospermia are constant features. Intellectual disability is unusual though learning disabilities are common.

Adults have low testosterone and high gonadotropins in serum. Treatment with testosterone is useful. Surgery may be necessary for gynecomastia. Counseling and support from family is necessary to improve self-image.

Table 16.1	Chromosomal Abnormalities Associated with Turner Syndrome
45,X	Monosomy X
45,X / 46,XX	Mosaicism for 45,X and 46,XX cell lines
46,X, i(Xq)	Isochromosome of q arm of X chromosome
46,X, Xp-	Deletion of part of p arm of X chromosome
46,X, Xq-	Deletion of part of q arm of X chromosome
46,X, r(X)	Ring chromosome of X chromosome
46,XY / 45,X	Mosaicism for 45,X and 46,XY cell lines (some cases present with Turner-like features while some present with ambiguous genitalia)

16.4 CONGENITAL MALFORMATIONS

(Also *see* Section 7.17)

Malformation can be *major*, which if untreated, is associated with morbidity or mortality; or *minor*, which is usually only

Table 16.2 Genetic Defects of Monogenic Malformation Syndrome

Malformation/syndrome	Inheritance	Features	Gene
Aniridia	AD	Absence of iris	PAX6
Waardenburg syndrome	AD	Deafness, hypertelorism, heterochromia of iris, white forelock	PAX3
Synpolydactyly	AD	Polydactyly and syndactyly	HOXD13
Holt-Oram syndrome	AD	Radial ray defects, atrial septal defect	TBX5
Polydactyly	AD	Pre- or postaxial polydactyly	GLI3
Cleft lip and/or cleft palate	Multifactorial	Isolated cleft lip with or without cleft palate	IRF6
van der Woude syndrome	AD	Cleft lip, lower lip pits, hypodontia	IRF6
Popliteal pterygium syndrome	AD	Cleft lip, lower lip pits, popliteal webs (pterygia), syndactyly or absence of fingers, hypoplastic scrotum/labia	IRF6
Apert syndrome	AD	Craniosynostosis, syndactyly, aplasia of corpus callosum, cardiac defects	FGFR2
Crouzon syndrome	AD	Craniosynostosis, midface hypoplasia, proptosis	FGFR2, FGFR3

AD: Autosomal dominant; IRF6: Interferon regulatory factor-6. Mutations in one gene can give rise to different syndromes with common features.

of a cosmetic significance. 3–4% of newborns have a major malformations and 0.7% have multiple malformations. A single minor malformation is seen in 14% of neonates and 3% have two or more minor malformations.

Etiology

Chromosomal anomalies account for 5% of all congenital malformations. Single gene defects are responsible for many malformation syndromes manifesting in children and stillbirths. Isolated malformations like aqueductal stenosis, polydactyly, congenital cataract are also inherited in Mendelian fashion. Genetic defects for some malformation have been identified and this gives the information about genes involved in development **(Table 16.2)**.

Multifactorial inheritance accounts for many of the isolated malformations involving heart, central nervous system, urogenital system, lip, palate, etc. In the causation of these disorders, both genes and environmental factors play a role. Etiology of many isolated and sporadically (without family history of similar disorder) occurring malformations and malformation syndromes is still unknown.

Environmental factors like alcohol, drugs, maternal diabetes; and infections like cytomegalovirus, rubella and toxoplasmosis also account for a small number of birth defects. Drugs with definite teratogenic effects include warfarin, retinoic acid and anticonvulsants; though during pregnancy all drugs should be avoided unless necessary.

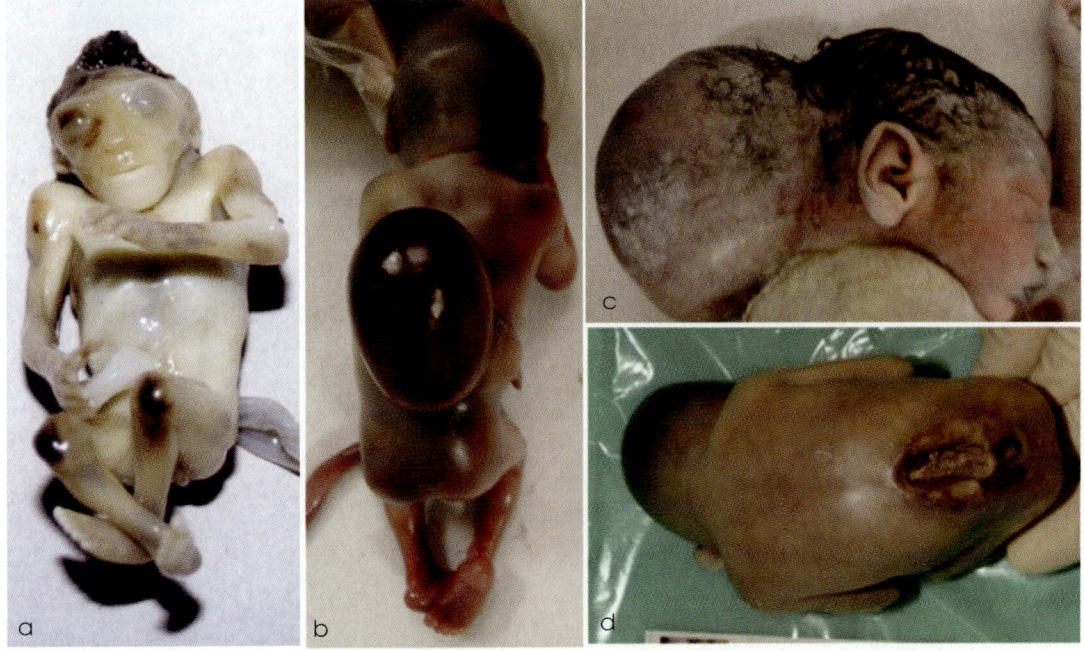

Fig. 16.24 Types of neural tube defects: (a) Anencephaly, (b) meningomyelocele, (c) encephalocele, (d) open spina bifida

Neural Tube Defects

Neural tube defects include meningomyelocele, open spina bifida, encephalocele, and anencephaly (Fig. 16.24). They need a special mention because they are the commonest congenital malformation in India occurring with the frequency of 5 per 1000 births and are preventable.

Risk of recurrence after birth of one child with neural tube defect is 5%. The risk can be reduced significantly by intake of folic acid (0.4 mg per day) by mother during peri-conceptional period. It needs to be started before planning pregnancy as by the time a woman knows that she is pregnant (first missed period) the neural tube closure is complete (day 20 after conception).

Food fortification with folic acid (0.4 mg/day) is advocated to reduce general population prevalence of neural tube defect. Prenatal screening is done by estimation of maternal serum alpha fetoprotein (elevated) and ultrasonography (to document the defect).

16.5 INBORN ERRORS OF METABOLISM

Metabolism is constituted by numerous biochemical reactions that are continuously occurring in the human body. Various enzymes catalyze these biochemical processes at the subcellular level. Defective function of an enzyme or an organelle of the cell leads to block in a metabolic pathway (Fig. 16.25). This in turn, leads to the disease manifestations.

More than 400 inborn errors of metabolism (IEM) are identified and their clinical features and biochemical defects are known. Most of them are inherited in an autosomal recessive manner while some are inherited as X-linked recessive disorders. Important groups of inborn errors of metabolism (IEM) along with some common examples are listed below:

1. *Amino acid metabolism defect* Phenylketonuria, maple syrup urine disease, alkaptonuria, tyrosinemia, urea cycle disorders like ornithine transcarbamylase deficiency
2. *Carbohydrate metabolism defect* Glycogen storage disorder (GSD) type I (von Gierke disease), GSD II (Pompe disease), galactosemia

3. *Lipid metabolism defect* Hyperlipidemias, Tay-Sachs disease, Gaucher disease, Niemann-Pick disease, metachromatic leukodystrophy
4. *Mucopolysaccharidosis (MPS) and oligosaccharidosis* Hurler syndrome (MPS I), Hunter syndrome (MPS II), Morquio syndrome, fucosidosis, mucolipidosis II
5. *Respiratory chain disorders (mitochondrial diseases)* Leigh disease, myoclonic epilepsy ragged red fibers (MERRF), Leber hereditary optic neuropathy
6. *Peroxisomal disorders* Zellweger syndrome, adreno-leukodystrophy
7. *Purine and pyrimidine metabolism defect* Lesch-Nyhan disease
8. *Mineral metabolism defect* Wilson disease, Menkes kinky hair disease, and hemochromatosis.

The above disorders usually involve multiple organ systems because either the deficient enzyme functioning is required in multiple organs (eg, MPS, respiratory chain disorders) or the deranged metabolism affects multiple organs (eg, phenylketonuria, tyrosinemia). In addition to the above mentioned disorders, there are many genetic diseases caused by deficiency of proteins; the function of which is limited to single organ system and the symptoms are limited to that particular system. Examples are hemophilia A, sickle cell disease, hypophosphatemic rickets, congenital adrenal hyperplasia, defects in thyroid hormone synthesis. These disorders are discussed in their respective chapters.

Approach to Inborn Errors of Metabolism

The signs and symptoms of inborn errors of metabolism are protean and diverse. The inborn errors of metabolism involve any system of the body and present at any age of life. The presentations can be acute, chronic or intermittent. The presentations are many times similar to the infections (septicemia, hepatitis) and non-genetic diseases (stroke). Most of the inborn errors of metabolism are rare and have prevalence of 1 per 20,000 to 1 per 40,000; even as low as 1 per 100,000 births. But though rare they must be considered in appropriate situations.

1. *Jaundice, hepatosplenomegaly* α_1-antitrypsin deficiency, galactosemia, tyrosinemia, Wilson disease, hemochromatosis
2. *Regression of milestones or developmental delay* Tay-Sachs disease, metachromatic leukodystrophy, phenyl-ketonuria, Niemann-Pick disease
3. *Acute encephalopathy, acute illness, acidosis, hypogly-cemia* Maple syrup urine diseases, urea cycle disorders, fatty acid oxidation defects, galactosemia
4. *Cardiomyopathy, with or without muscle involvement* Glycogen storage disorder II (Pompe disease), mitochon-drial disorders, carnitine transport defect
5. *Coarse facies, joint contractures, hepatosplenomegaly, ± psychomotor regression* Mucopolysaccharidosis, muco-lipidosis, fucosidosis
6. *Hepatomegaly, splenomegaly* Gaucher disease type I, Niemann-Pick disease types I and III, glycogen storage disease
7. *Congenital malformations* Zellweger syndrome, Smith-Lemli-Opitz syndrome.

An accurate diagnosis can provide appropriate treatment to the patient and the family can be provided information

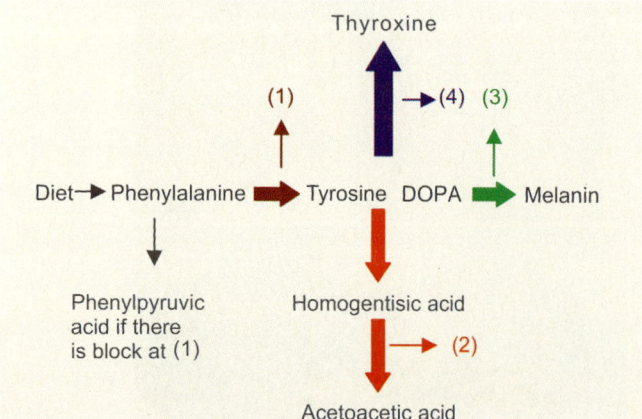

Fig 16.25 Block at (1) and (2) causes phenylketonuria and alkaptonuria respectively. The metabolites proximal to block accumulate and give rise to disease manifestations. Block at (3) and (4) gives rise to oculocutaneous albinism and hypothyroidism due to lack of end product

about risk of recurrence in the family and preventive options including prenatal diagnosis.

DEFECTS OF AMINO ACIDS

1. Phenylketonuria

Phenylketonuria is an autosomal recessive metabolic disorder caused by deficiency of phenylalanine hydroxylase thus inhibiting conversion of phenylalanine to tyrosine. Phenylalanine thus accumulates in the blood, CSF, and other tissues. High phenylalanine levels in CSF deprive brain cells of other amino acids; resulting in defective myelination and maturation. The affected and untreated children are thus severely mentally retarded and often have seizures. They may also have hyperkinesis and hypertonia.

The enzyme block also leads to deficiency of tyrosine and thus in turn melanin. Decreased melanin is responsible for fair skin complexion, blond hair, and blue iris commonly seen in children with phenylketonuria.

Excess phenylalanine gets converted to phenylpyruvic acid and other metabolites which are excreted in urine, imparting it a characteristic mushy odor. These metabolites in the urine can be detected by Guthrie test or ferric chloride test (addition of 10% $FeCl_3$ to fresh urine gives a green color).

Treatment	Phenylketonuria

Phenylalanine restricted diet Exclusion of phenylalanine from diet since the neonatal period (ie, breastmilk) is effective in preventing mental retardation. This strategy of diet modification needs diagnosis during neonatal period before the symptoms appear. This is achieved by routine screening of all neonates. The screening test is done on day 2 or 3 of life after the child has received some milk feeds (which contain phenylalanine). Neonates with high phenylalanine level in blood need further confirmatory tests before they are started on lifelong phenylalanine free diet as the phenylketonuria due to abnormalities of biopterin synthesis (a cofactor for phenylalanine metabolism) or recycling do not respond to phenylalanine restricted diet.

Drug therapy Sapropterin (tetrabiopterin (BH4) in drug form) is useful in reducing the stringency of diet control in some patients of PKU. The other new option for treatment of PKU is phenylalanine ammonia lyase (PAL) which metabolizes phenylalanine in the gut to harmless cinnamic acid and insignificant amount of ammonia.

Mother with Phenylketonuria

A high phenylalanine level during pregnancy is associated with a very high incidence of intellectual disability, microcephaly, and congenital heart defect even in the offspring who is not homozygous for phenylketonuria. Hence, strict diet control is necessary when a woman with phenylketonuria is pregnant.

2. Alkaptonuria

Deficiency of *homogentisic acid oxylase* in the liver and kidney inhibits the breakdown of homogentisic acid which is thus excreted in urine, imparting it a black color on standing. Excess homogentisic acid deposits in sclera, articular cartilages, and kidneys as a black pigment (*ochronosis*), manifesting in 3rd to 4th decades of life. Black pigment deposits can be seen in sclera, nose, and ear cartilage.

Ochronotic arthritis involves intervertebral joints, hips, and shoulder; and may cause severe spondylosis, peripheral arthropathy, tendon rupture, and bone osteoporosis. Other manifestations include aortic valve stenosis and skin pigmentation. Excess pigment in kidney manifests as renal calculi. There are no neurological manifestations. Treatment is supportive.

Nitisinone which is approved for the treatment of tyrosinemia I has been found to be successful in reducing the level of homogentisic acid in urine. However, its long-term safety and efficacy is not yet documented.

3. Homocystinuria

Homocystinuria, an autosomal recessive disorder is caused by deficiency of *cystathionine β-synthetase* enzyme in the liver. Plasma and urinary levels of homocystine are increased. Methionine and thionine also accumulate in blood. Cystine synthesis is blocked (Fig. 16.26).

Clinical features include tall stature, scoliosis, pectus excavatum, and long fingers (arachnodactyly) which are similar to Marfan syndrome. Accumulation of homocysteine causes increased stickiness of the platelets resulting in both arterial and venous vascular thrombosis, that may manifest as stroke. Lens is dislocated due to deficiency of cysteine which is essential for collagen formation. Cysteine deficiency also results in marked osteoporosis. High methionine level in the brain is responsible for intellectual disability.

Diagnosis is confirmed by demonstration of a positive urinary cyanide nitroprusside test. Treatment consists of low methionine diet and supplementation with pyridoxine.

4. Maple Syrup Urine Disease

Maple syrup urine disease is caused by accumulation of branched chain keto acids due to blockage of decarboxylation of keto acids caused by deficiency of the enzyme *keto acid decarboxylase*. This also results in elevated levels of keto acids precursors; ie, branched chain amino acids including leucine, valine, and isoleucine. These inhibit CNS myelination.

Clinical Features

Classical form presents in neonates with poor feeding, lethargy, and vomiting, associated with acidosis,

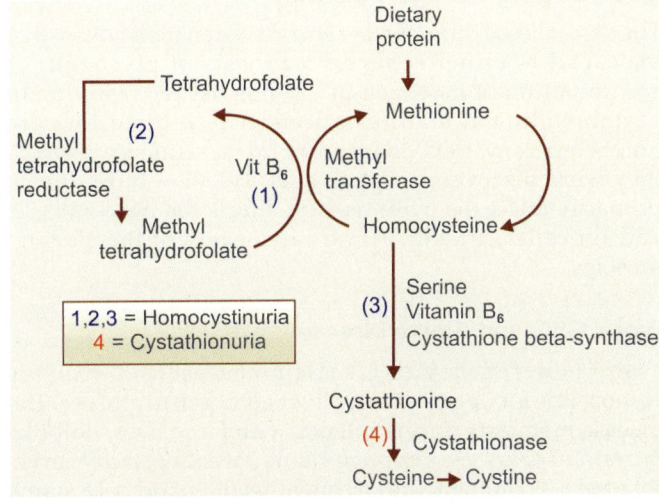

Fig. 16.26 Methionine pathway

hypoglycemia, high pitched cry, hypertonia, seizures and coma. Death may occur within a few weeks. Ketoaciduria imparts a distinct maple syrup odor to urine.

Diagnosis

Simple screening test is to add 2, 4-dinitrophenylhydrazine to urine and it gives a yellow precipitate. Ferric chloride test imparts a navy blue color to the urine. Diagnosis can be confirmed by detection of appropriate metabolites in urine by gas chromatography mass spectrometry.

Treatment	Maple Syrup Urine Disease

Treatment consists of exclusion of dietary proteins and intravenous administration of high calorie solution to prevent protein metabolism. The prognosis is poor in classical form but mild forms presenting intermittently at later age show good prognosis with special diets.

DEFECTS OF CARBOHYDRATE METABOLISM

1. Galactosemia

Deficiency of the enzyme *galactose-1-phosphate-uridyl-transferase* interferes in metabolism of galactose. Excess galactose accumulates in liver causing cirrhosis. Galactilol accumulates in eyes resulting in cataracts. Both galactose and galactilol are also excreted in urine. Disease transmission is autosomal recessive.

Clinical Features

Symptoms appear during first few weeks of life after introduction of milk feeds. The child develops lethargy, vomiting, seizures, jaundice, and septicemia. Other complications include cataract, cirrhosis of liver, and intellectual disability.

Simple treatment of avoiding milk (including breastmilk) and milk products is successful. Diagnosis by neonatal screening or on early suspicion can provide good results in this treatable disorder. Presence of reducing substance in urine is a useful screening test. Diagnosis is confirmed by the enzyme assay on blood.

2. Glycogen Storage Disorders

The defect lies at different levels of glycogen metabolism that may lead to either reduced synthesis of glycogen or accumulation of glycogen in various tissues resulting in variable clinical manifestations. These disorders are numbered from I to XIV depending on the sequence in which they were discovered. Types I, III, IV, VI, VII, IX, and X primarily affect the liver; type IIa affects the heart muscle; and types IIb, V, and VIII are disorders of the skeletal muscles.

Type I GSD: von Gierke Disease

There is deficiency of *glucose-6-phosphatase* which is responsible for degradation of liver glycogen to glucose. The disease manifests during infancy with large liver, doll-like facies, and episodes of hypoglycemia (sweating, tachycardia, seizures). Treatment with frequent feeding and corn starch feeds at night is successful.

Glycogen Storage Disease Type II (Pompe disease)

The disease involves heart muscles. An enzyme α-1,4-glucosidase is deficient. There is severe hypotonia, cardiomegaly, and hepatomegaly. Death during infancy is certain. Complete normalization of motor activities and cardiac function is possible if enzyme replacement therapy is started early or on diagnosis by newborn screening. Late onset variants manifest during late childhood or later as limb-girdle muscle weakness.

LYSOSOMAL STORAGE DISORDERS

1. Tay-Sachs Disease

This disorder is caused by deposition of sphingolipid (GM_2 ganglioside) in brain due to the deficiency of a lysosomal enzyme–*hexosaminidase A*. The child manifests by 3–6 months of age with developmental delay, hypotonia, and seizures. Presence of cherry red spot in the fundus and exaggerated startle response to noise suggests the diagnosis. Enzyme assay in serum or blood leucocytes is necessary to confirm the diagnosis. No treatment is successful. Being autosomal recessive disorder, the risk of recurrence in the siblings is 25%. The birth of similarly affected child can be prevented by prenatal diagnosis which can be done by assaying hexosaminidase A in the chorionic villi at 10 to 12 weeks of gestation or DNA based test for mutation detection.

2. Gaucher Disease

This is the commonest sphingolipidosis caused by deficiency of the enzyme *glucosylceramide β-glucosidase* (*glucocerebrosidase*). As a result, there is cerebroside deposition in the cells of reticuloendothelial system. The lipid laden cells appear large with eccentric nuclei; these can be demonstrated in the bone marrow and spleen and are known as Gaucher cells.

There are three types based on presentation.
- *Type I* (visceral involvement) presents in childhood or later with hepatosplenomegaly, bone pains, tendency to fracture, anemia and thrombocytopenia due to hypersplenism.
- *Type II* There is involvement of central nervous system in addition to hepatosplenomegaly. It presents in infants with developmental delay, spasticity, seizures and leads to early death.
- *Type III* This is a mild form presenting with hepatosplenomegaly, oculomotor involvement, with slow progression of neurological disease.

The deficient enzyme is now available as a drug and more than 1000 cases of type I Gaucher disease are being successfully treated with enzyme replacement therapy.

3. Niemann-Pick Disease

There is deficiency of sphingomyelinase resulting in accumulation of sphingomyelin in abdominal viscera and brain. Clinical presentation is similar to Gaucher disease. There is hepatosplenomegaly with or without neurological manifestations.

4. Mucopolysaccharidosis

Mucopolysaccharidosis (MPS) is a group of lysosomal storage disorders occurring due to defective degradation of mucopolysaccharides which are complex carbohydrate molecules. Six different types of mucopolysaccharidoses are known depending on clinical differences occurring due to defects in different enzymes. The children are normal at birth and signs and symptoms develop and progress as the mucopolysaccharides accumulate in various organs.

Hurler Syndrome: MPS I

MPS type I or Hurler syndrome is the most severe form. The symptoms appear by the end of first year of age in the form of corneal clouding, gibbus, joint stiffness, and coarsening of facial features (Fig. 16.27). There is hepatosplenomegaly, umbilical hernia, mental deterioration and cardiac valvular involvement. Radiographic changes in bones are characteristic. Death occurs in second decade.

The deficient enzyme is *α-L-iduronidase*. Milder forms of the disease are known as Sheie disease (MPS IS) and Hurler/ Sheie disease (MPS I S/H). Bone marrow transplantation done in early course of the disease and enzyme replacement therapy are effective.

Hunter Syndrome: MPS II

Clinical features of Hunter syndrome are similar to Hurler syndrome except corneal clouding which is absent in Hunter syndrome. Deficient enzyme is *iduronate sulfatase* and the disorder is inherited in X-linked recessive manner. Enzyme replacement therapy is available and effective if there is no neurological involvement.

Morquio Syndrome: MPS IV

Morquio syndrome is caused by the deficiency of *galactosamine-6-sulfatase* or *beta-galactosidase*. There is severe

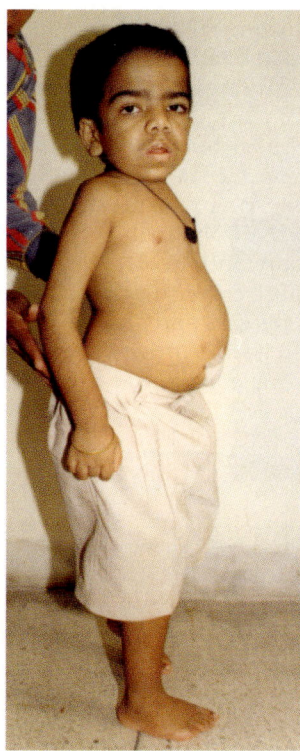

Fig. 16.27 Coarse facies, umbilical hernia, and contractures of elbow and fingers in a child with Hurler syndrome

involvement of bones leading to short stature, kyphosis, and genu valgum. Intelligence is normal.

Prenatal diagnosis of the lysosomal disorders including MPS can be made by enzyme assay on the chorionic villi or DNA based mutation detection. The enzyme deficiency needs to be confirmed in the proband before venturing on the prenatal diagnosis.

16.6 SKELETAL DYSPLASIAS

A dysplasia is an abnormal organization of cells into tissue. Usually the effects are seen in the multiple parts of the body where the tissue is present. Skeletal dysplasias usually involve all the bones to a varying degree. At present 436 genetic disorders involving bones are known and placed in 42 groups defined by molecular, biochemical, and/or radiographic criteria. Most of these conditions, are associated with one or more of 364 different genes. Achondroplasia and osteogenesis imperfecta are the commonest skeletal dysplasias. Some groups of skeletal dysplasias with representative disorders are listed below:

Group 1 (gene *FGFR3* group): Achondroplasia, thanatophoric dysplasia

Group 2 *Type II collagen group* (gene *COL2A1*): Spondyloepiphyseal dysplasia congenital, Kniest dysplasia (myopia, cleft palate), Stickler syndrome (myopia, cleft palate, mild changes of spondyloepiphyseal dysplasia, midface hypoplasia)

Group 22 *Increased bone density group*: Osteopetrosis

Group 24 *Decreased bone density group*: Osteogenesis imperfecta.

Approach to a Child with Skeletal Dysplasia

The skeletal dysplasias mainly present as disproportionate short stature; some predominantly involving spine (short trunk) (Fig. 16.28a) and some predominantly involving long bones (short limbs) (Fig. 16.28b). In the limbs there can be predominant involvement of proximal segments (*rhizomelic*), middle segments (*mesomelic*), or distal segments (*acromelic*). The skeletal dysplasias are further classified as *epiphyseal*, *metaphyseal*, and diaphyseal depending on the area involved.

The short stature may be present at birth or may become apparent in early childhood. In a child with short stature, ratio of upper segment (up to the pubic symphysis) and lower segment, arm span and measurements of different segments of the limbs are essential. Other features on clinical examination may give diagnostic clues **(Table 16.3)**.

Radiographs of all parts of the body (skeletal survey) are essential for diagnosis. Gene defects of many skeletal disorders are known and mutation detection tests are available for diagnostic purposes. Mutation detection is useful for early and definitive prenatal diagnosis.

ACHONDROPLASIA

Achondroplasia is characterized by severe short stature with predominant shortening of arms and thighs (proximal limb segments) as compared to forearm and legs; known as rhizomelic short stature (Fig. 16.28b). The disorder can be diagnosed in a neonate. The characteristic configuration

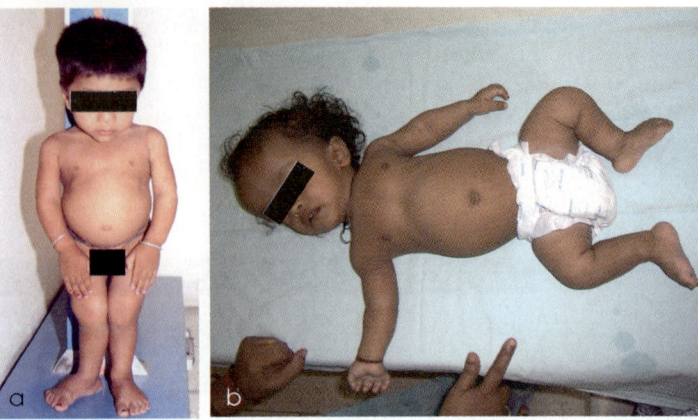
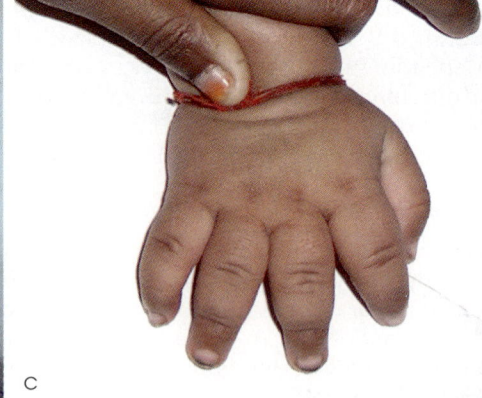

Fig. 16.28 (a) A child with spondyloepiphyseal dysplasia (predominant short trunk), (b) a child with achondroplasia (predominant rhizomelic limb shortening); (c) Typical trident hand seen in infants with achondroplasia

Table 16.3 Associated Features in Skeletal Dysplasia	
Skeletal dysplasia	*Clinical features*
Spondyloepiphyseal dysplasia congenita	Cleft palate, myopia
Osteogenesis imperfecta	Blue sclera, joint laxity, abnormalities of dentin, hearing defect, frequent fractures
Osteopetrosis severe infantile variety	Hepatosplenomegaly, anemia, optic atrophy
Cleidocranial dysplasia	Large anterior fontanel, absent or hypoplastic clavicles
Multiple epiphyseal dysplasia*	Early onset osteoarthritis of knees and hips
Diastrophic dysplasia	Club foot, cystic swelling of ear pinna
Camptomelic dysplasia	Sex reversal in XY males, bowing of bones, micrognathia
Cartilage hair dysplasia	Immunodeficiency, sparse fine hair

Body is proportionate and short stature is mild.

of hand known as trident hand is seen during infancy (Fig. 16.28c). Radiographs show short and broad long bones, narrow base of skull, square iliac bones and decreasing interpeduncular distance in lumbar vertebrae. Achondroplasia is caused by mutation in fibroblast growth factor receptor 3 (*FGFR3*) gene. A specific change (G >A transition at nucleotide 1138 of the cDNA leading to the substitution of an arginine residue for a glycine at position 380 of the mature protein) in *FGFR3* gene is responsible for 98% cases of achondroplasia. The other disorders caused by mutations in *FGFR3* gene are thanatophoric dysplasia (lethal disorder) and hypochondroplasia (causing mild short stature).

Genetic Counseling

An individual with achondroplasia is heterozygous for *FGFR 3* mutation. The other copy of the gene is normal. The risk of transmitting achondroplasia from an affected parent to the offspring is 50% and the chance that the offspring will be normal is 50%.

If both the parents have achondroplasia; the chance that the offspring will have achondroplasia is 50% and the chance that the offspring will not have achondroplasia is 25% (Fig. 16.29). Twenty five percent chances are that the child inherits achondroplasia mutation from both the parents and is homozygous for the mutated allele. Homozygosity for achondroplasia results in severely affected fetus with

marked limb shortening and narrow thorax leading to stillbirth or neonatal death.

Lethal type or homozygous achondroplasia can be detected before 20 weeks of gestation by ultrasonography. But in heterozygous achondroplasia, limb shortening and large head circumference becomes obvious only in the third trimester. Hence, for prenatal diagnosis, detection of mutation by analysis of DNA in the chorionic villi or amniotic fluid cells is the only option.

Most of the children with achondroplasia are born to clinically normal parents and are due to new mutations. In such family the chance of birth of another child with achondroplasia was considered to be negligible. But the

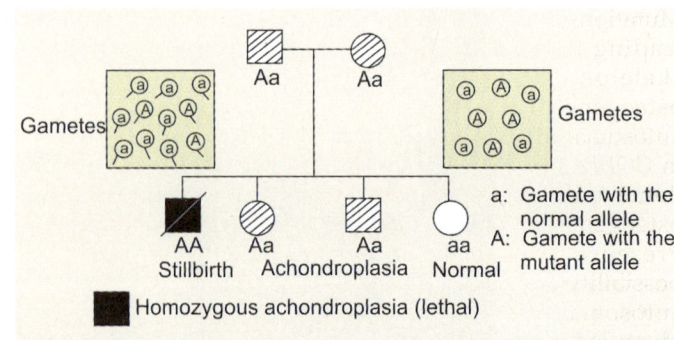

Fig. 16.29 A pedigree showing marriage of two individuals with achondroplasia

Case Study | **Inborn Error of Metabolism**

An 18-month-old girl child was brought with the complaints of regression of milestones for last 2–3 months. She was achieving her milestones normally till 11 months of age. She was standing with support and was cruising holding furniture. She was a second child born to consanguineous parents (marriage between blood relatives—cousins in the present case) and antenatal, neonatal period was uneventful.

Around 1 year of age, she stopped standing, and developed hypertonia of lower limbs. She stopped recognizing parents, and stopped speaking monosyllables. There was no history of seizures, fever, vomiting or acute illness. Examination revealed hypertonia of lower limbs, exaggerated knee jerks, and absent ankle jerks. She did not have coarsening of facial features or hepatosplenomegaly. Magnetic resonance imaging (MRI) of brain showed changes of demyelination of white matter.

Q. What are the features suggesting the possibility of inborn error of metabolism?
Q. What is the confirmatory test?
Q. What is the possible diagnosis?
Q. What is the treatment?
Q. What help can be provided to the family?

To find answers, read:

Hypertonia and scissoring of lower limbs at a glance may give an impression of cerebral palsy. But regression of milestones after a period of normal development is very strongly indicative of genetic neurodegenerative disorder. Presence of consanguinity in the family is also a strong pointer towards the possibility of an autosomal recessive disorder and most inborn errors of metabolism are inherited in autosomal recessive fashion. Absence of seizures and loss of ankle reflexes (due to involvement of peripheral nerves) is suggestive of a white matter degenerative disease. This possibility is confirmed by MRI. The age of onset of symptoms is typical for late infantile variety of metachromatic leukodystrophy. Other white matter diseases are Krabbe disease (usually presents early in the infancy), Canavan disease and Alexander disease; the later two are associated with large head.

The diagnosis of metachromatic leukodystrophy can be confirmed by assay of aryl sulphatase A in white blood cells which is deficient in metachromatic leukodystrophy. There is no treatment available and the disease progresses to vegetative state and resulting in death by 2 to 5 years.

Because the disease is inherited in autosomal recessive fashion; there is 25% risk of recurrence in the siblings of the child. Prenatal diagnosis can be provided by mutation detection or estimation of aryl sulphatase A in the chorionic villi during 10 to 12 weeks of pregnancy. DNA based mutation study can also be used for carrier detection which should be offered if there is any other consanguineous couple in the family.

The family should be given the information that there will be risk of birth of a child with the same disease in the consanguineous couples in the family and further consanguineous marriages may be avoided or tests for carrier status should be carried out in the couples in the family.

Think it over!

The family had a similarly affected child who died at 2 years of age. The child was diagnosed as cerebral palsy at 18 months of age. The physician did not think that any investigations were needed as the prognosis of the child was obviously poor. The parents were not told about the possibility of genetic etiology and risk of recurrence in the next pregnancy. As a result the family had to undergo an emotional or deal of similar illness in the next child and seeing the child deteriorate day by day resulting in death.

Whose fault?

observed risk is 1 in 400 indicating the possibility of gonadal mosaicism in some parents (Fig. 16.30).

OSTEOGENESIS IMPERFECTA

Collagen is an important component of bone tissue. Mutations in collagen genes cause defective bone formation leading to the decreased bone density throughout the skeleton. These groups of disorders are known as osteogenesis imperfecta. Types I to IV are inherited in autosomal dominant fashion and are caused by mutations in *COL1A1* or *COL1A2* genes. Other than these, one more dominantly inherited and 10 autosomal recessive types of osteogenesis imperfecta account for 10 to 20% of cases. Presence of consanguinity should point towards the possibility of recessive variety. A number of genes causing autosomal recessive osteogenesis imperfecta have been identified in last few years.

- *Type I and Type IV* osteogenesis imperfecta have variable severity with varying frequency of fractures. Height may

be normal. Defective dentin is seen in some cases of type I. Deafness is a common complication and appears at a later age. Treatment with bisphosphonates has improved the prognosis and quality of life greatly by increasing the bone density and decreasing the frequency of fractures.

- *Type* II is prenatally lethal. The affected baby is stillborn or dies during first few months. Thorax is narrow and pulmonary hypoplasia is the cause of the death. Sclera is deep blue. Inheritance is autosomal dominant or recessive. The risk of recurrence in the siblings of an affected child may be up to 25% depending on the causative gene.
- *Type III* is also a severe type of osteogenesis imperfecta. Bending of bones and recurrent fractures lead to severe deformities and physical handicap (Fig. 16.31). Sclera is blue. Type III OI is inherited as recessive or autosomal.

OSTEOPETROSIS

Osteopetrosis is a group of disorders with increased bone density (Fig. 16.32). A mild form presenting as fracture or

16

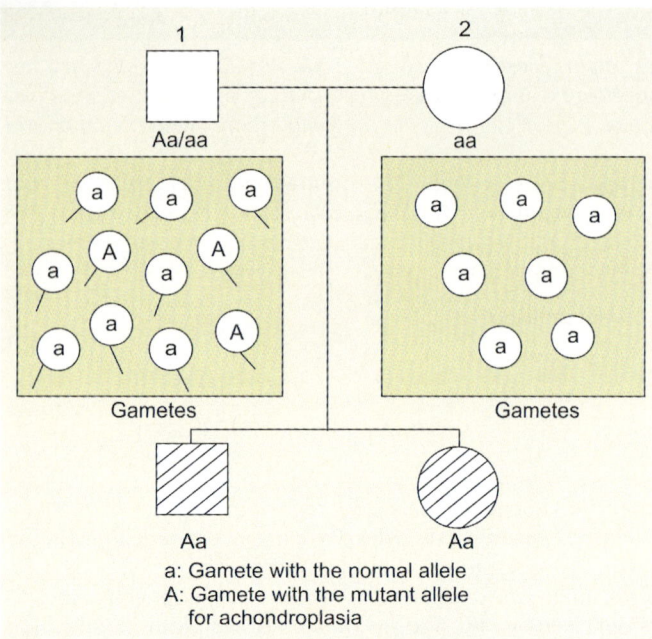

Fig. 16.30 A pedigree showing two children with achondroplasia born to the clinically normal parents suggesting the possibility of gonadal mosaicism in a parent

diagnosed incidentally in adults is inherited in autosomal dominant fashion. Severe form presenting during infancy and childhood is inherited in an autosomal recessive fashion.

Clinical Features

Infantile variety manifests with anemia, thrombocytopenia and hepatosplenomegaly due to encroachment on bone marrow. Optic atrophy and involvement of other cranial nerves occur due to narrowing of foramina at the base of the skull.

Genetic Counseling

The disorder usually occurs due to the defect in osteoclast function. Two of the causative genes are *TCIRG1* and *CLCN7*. Mutation detection helps in providing prenatal

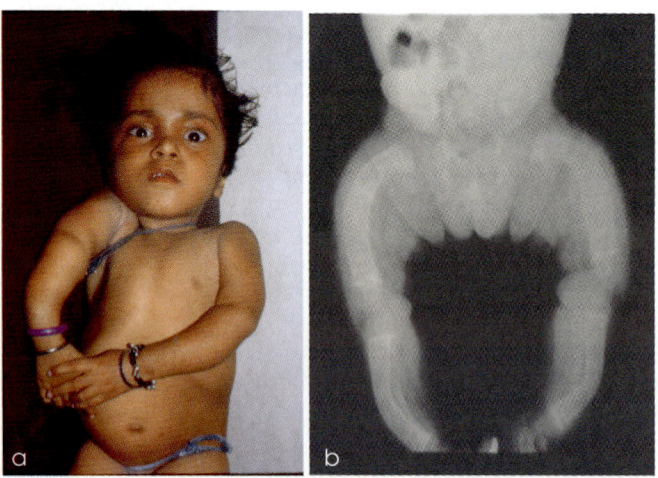

Fig. 16.31 (a) A child with severe osteogenesis imperfecta: Note bent and deformed limbs, (b) decreased bone density and bent bones with fractures

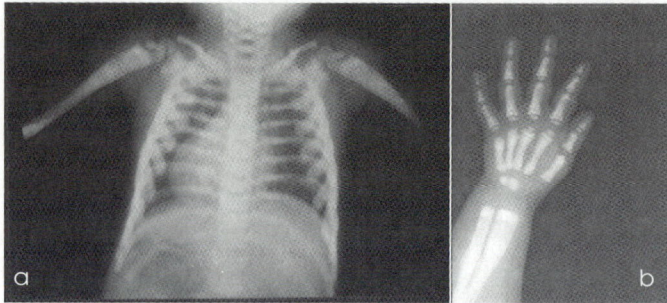

Fig. 16.32 Dense bones suggestive of osteopetrosis

diagnosis which is indicated as the disorder is severe and leads to suffering and death in childhood if untreated. The risk of recurrence in the siblings of an affected child is 25% or 1 in 4. Bone marrow transplantation is the only curative treatment. No drug treatment is effective.

LETHAL SKELETAL DYSPLASIAS

Some skeletal dysplasias are characterized by short and narrow thorax which lead to lung hypoplasia and in turn stillbirth or neonatal death. These disorders include achondrogenesis, short rib polydactyly syndromes (Fig. 16.33), thanatophoric dysplasia, Ellis-van Creveld syndrome and asphyxiating thoracic dystrophy. The diagnosis is based on radiological findings.

These conditions need to be suspected in stillborns or neonates with respiratory distress and short limbs. Whole body radiograph will give the diagnosis, so as to provide genetic counseling and prenatal diagnosis. Many of these disorders are diagnosed prenatally because of short limbs.

16.7 DNA BASED DIAGNOSIS OF MONOGENIC DISORDERS

Recent advances in ability to manipulate DNA have resulted in identification of genetic defects of more than 3000 single gene phenotypes and the numbers are ever increasing. The newer techniques to study DNA and automation of techniques have made the identification of the causative genes for monogenic disorders an easy task. DNA based diagnosis has become quick and has been increasingly used in clinical practice. The most important molecular technique is polymerase chain reaction (PCR). PCR makes multiple copies of small DNA segment/segments in a test tube on principles similar to DNA replication occurring *in vivo*.

Most of the DNA based techniques are based on various modifications of PCR and the principle of hybridization of complementary DNA strands (A with T and G with C). Accurate sequencing of DNA segments is possible. Figure 16.34 shows mutation detection in beta globin gene in patients with thalassemia. These techniques are used to identify disease causing mutation/mutations using patient's blood sample or even cell from buccal cavity mouthwash.

Whole Exome Sequencing

It is now possible to sequence the whole exome (coding regions of all genes) of an individual to identify disease

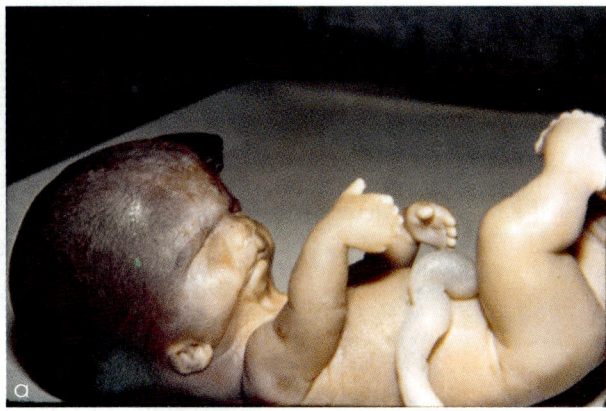

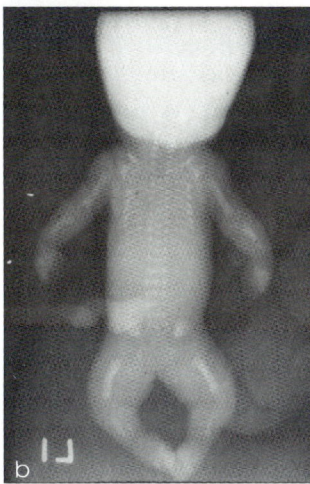

Fig. 16.33 (a) A fetus with short rib polydactyly syndrome. Note short limbs and polydactyly, (b) radiograph of a fetus with short rib polydactyly syndrome showing narrow thorax with short and horizontal ribs

causing mutations. Whole exome sequencing (WES) by high throughput sequencing methods is becoming the method of choice for disorders with heterogeneous etiologies like retinitis pigmentosa and sensorineuronal deafness, etc. or when the clinical features cannot suggest a candidate gene. WES is available in India and the cost is getting affordable to many families. The possibility of identifying the causative mutation in a patient with a monogenic disorder varies from 30 to 80% depending on the phenotype.

Allelic Heterogeneity

The mutation detection confirms the diagnosis but it should be noted that *inability to detect mutation does not rule out the disease in question.* This is because most of the diseases are known to be caused by hundreds of mutations (allelic heterogeneity—different alleles at a locus giving rise to clinically similar phenotype). Some mutations are unique to a patient or a family. So, the available tests may not be able to detect all mutations, especially in non-coding regions, promoters, etc. Now it has been observed that changes in DNA sequence far away from a gene can also affect the expression of the gene and cause a disease.

Genetic Heterogeneity

Some phenotypes are caused by more than one gene. The examples are retinitis pigmentosa, spinocerebellar ataxia, limb girdle myopathy, cardiomyopathies, and primary microcephaly. This is known as genetic heterogeneity (defects in genes at different loci giving rise to the clinically similar phenotype). Hence, mutation detection is not an easy task for many disorders.

Some of the diseases for which there is no diagnostic test other than mutation detection are spinal muscular atrophy, Huntington chorea, fragile X mental retardation,

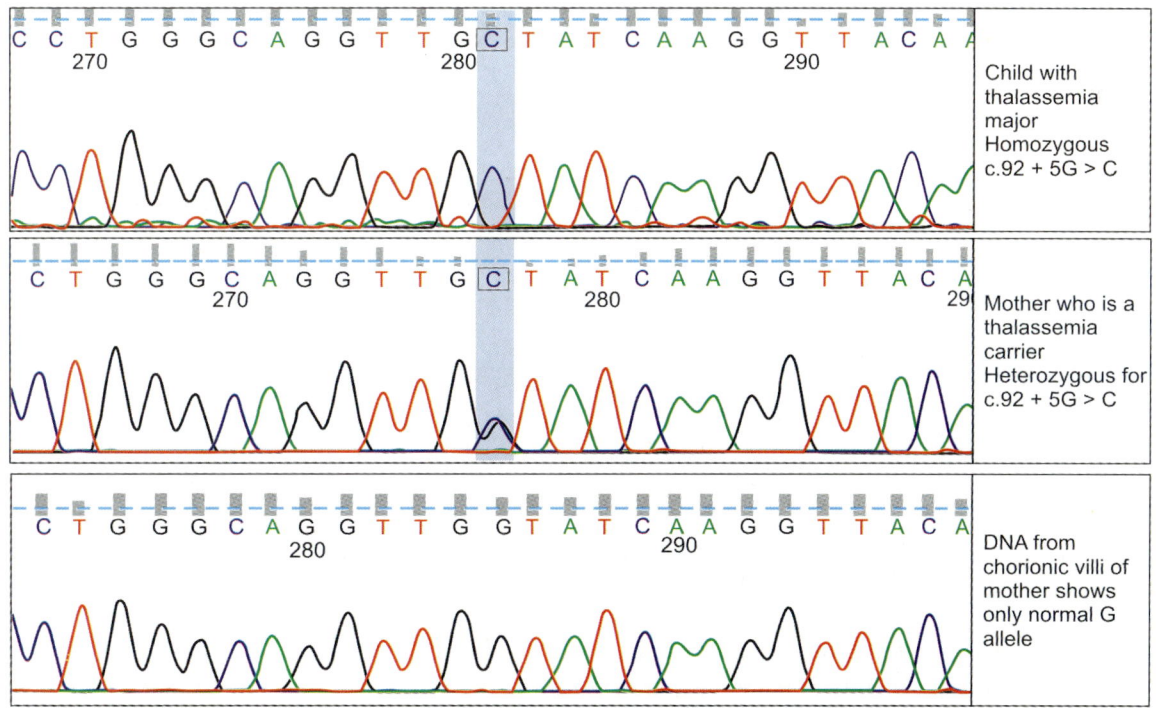

Fig. 16.34 Mutations in beta globin gene in a family with thalassemia major

spinocerebellar ataxia of various types, Charcot-Marie-Tooth disease, and hereditary spastic paraplegia.

For other diseases where diagnostic biochemical, imaging or other investigations are available, mutation detection may not be necessary for the diagnosis of the patient but is important for providing carrier detection and prenatal diagnosis.

Prenatal Diagnosis

As the DNA of all cells of the body and placenta is the same, the tests on placental biopsy (chorionic villi) or amniotic fluid cells can be used to diagnose monogenic disease involving any organ of the body. It should be noted that before prenatal diagnosis is attempted; identification of mutation in the proband or carrier parent/parents is essential.

The diseases for which prenatal diagnosis by DNA based tests are commonly available include thalassemia major, Duchenne muscular dystrophy, hemophilia A, hemophilia B, spinal muscular atrophy, fragile X mental retardation, cystic fibrosis, epidermolysis bullosa, albinism, and ichthyosis. For any monogenic disorder, availability of DNA based test should be looked for from recent literature and internet resources. Now preimplantation diagnosis by taking one cell out of blastocyst is also possible. The embryos negative for mutation can only be implanted to ensure the disease-free fetus. Feasibility of prenatal diagnosis using cell-free fetal DNA in maternal plasma has also been successfully shown and in future the invasive tests to collect fetal samples may not be necessary.

DNA based tests are now available for identifying individuals at risk of drug toxicity, diseases like diabetes mellitus, hemochromatosis, and ischemic heart disease.

16.8 TREATMENT OF GENETIC DISORDERS

Genetic disorders involve all systems of the body and have varying severity. Available treatments and outcomes vary greatly. The treatment may be as easy as avoiding some drugs in *glucose-6-phosphate dehydrogenase* (G6PD) deficiency or may be difficult as bone marrow transplantation for thalassemia major.

Successful surgical treatment of many malformations has been available for many decades and now fetal surgery for repair of defects like diaphragmatic hernia, neural tube defects is possible.

At present there is no treatment for neurodegenerative disorders, myopathies, and conditions with intellectual disability. For them the supportive treatment and rehabilitation plays an important role. Various successful strategies used for treatment of genetic disorder are discussed below.

1. *Augmentation of low level of protein* Phenobarbitone in Crigler-Najjar syndrome type II, desmopressin (DDAVP) in mild hemophilia A.
2. *Replacement of the deficient protein or enzyme* Antihemophilic factor VIII for hemophilia A, adenosine deaminase for immunodeficiency; enzyme replacement therapy for Gaucher disease, mucopolysaccharidosis I (Hurler disease), Pompe disease, and Fabry disease.

3. *Enhancement of function of a deficient protein* Biotin in biotinidase deficiency, pyridoxine in homocystinuria, high doses of vitamin D in vitamin D resistant rickets.
4. *Dietary restriction* Restriction of milk in galactosemia, phenylalanine in phenylketonuria.
5. *Drug therapy* Cholestyramine in hypercholesterolemia, penicillamine in Wilson disease.
6. *Drug avoidance* Primaquine in G6PD deficiency and phenobarbitone in acute intermittent porphyria.
7. *Treatment of phenotype* Surgical treatment of malformation, blood transfusions in thalassemia major or sickle cell disease.
8. *Organ transplantation* Kidney transplantation in polycystic kidney disease, bone marrow transplantation in thalassemia major and lysosomal storage disorders such as mucopolysaccharidosis.
9. *Organ removal* Splenectomy in hereditary spherocytosis, colectomy in familial adenomatous polyposis.

Enzyme Replacement Therapy

Enzyme replacement therapy is the recent success story and is likely to become reality for many more genetic metabolic disorders.

Gene Therapy

With knowledge of gene defects and ability to manipulate DNA (recombinant DNA technology) correction of defective gene or replacing defective gene (gene therapy) has become a reality. Gene therapy has been successful in treating monogenic immunodeficiency disorder and has shown preliminary success in thalassemia major and hemophilia B. Gene therapy has also shown promise for many more diseases including cancers, autoimmune, and infectious disorders. But still, easy permanent, and safe gene therapy appears to a distant dream. Till then, knowledge of molecular pathology of genetic disorder is likely to bring up better drug treatment for monogenic disorder and cancers. Development of ivacaftor for a specific mutation of cystic fibrosis is the proof for the same.

16.9 GENETIC COUNSELING

Familial nature of the diseases, difficult treatment, and poor outcome for many genetic disorders make genetic counseling an important part of management of patient and families with genetic disorders.

Definition

Genetic counseling is defined as 'a communicative process which deals with human problems associated with occurrence or recurrence of a genetic disorder in a family.' It helps the family to understand the diagnosis, treatment, prognosis of the disease, implications of genetic etiology in the form of risk of recurrence and ways to prevent the recurrence by way of prenatal diagnosis.

Indications

All clinical presentations suggestive of genetic disorders need to be investigated for etiology even if the disorder appears to be untreatable. Congenital malformation, stillbirths, chromosomal disorders, known monogenic disorders, intellectual disability, regression of milestones, recurrent fetal losses, and familial cancers are the indications for genetic counseling.

The Process

The person who asks for genetic counseling is called *'consultand'* and the one who provides the counseling is known as *'counselor'*. The counselor need to have knowledge of basic genetics, latest information about the disease in concern and should have good communication skills. Accurate etiological diagnosis is the first and one of the most important steps of genetic counseling. The genetic counseling should be nondirective and the decisions regarding planning of pregnancy, prenatal diagnosis and termination of pregnancy need to be taken by the family and not to be advised or forced by the counselor.

16.10 POPULATION BASED PREVENTION OF GENETIC DISORDERS

Genetic counseling offers an option of prevention of a genetic disorder in the family. But usually this is done after diagnosis of one individual with a genetic disorder in the family. Population based preventive programs aim at primary prevention of genetic disorder or birth of the first child of a genetic disorder. This can be done at different levels:

- *Food fortification* with folic acid for prevention of neural tube defects.
- *Identification of carriers* of monogenic disorders like thalassemia major, cystic fibrosis and Tay-Sachs disease by testing all couples or pregnant women and offering them genetic counseling and prenatal diagnosis.
- *Screening of all pregnancies* for common genetic disorders like Down syndrome and neural tube defects.
- *Neonatal screening* for metabolic disorders in which early diagnosis helps to provide treatment to prevent mental retardation (congenital hypothyroidism, congenital adrenal hyperplasia, biotinidase deficiency, phenylketonuria, galactosemia) or improve outcome (sickle cell disease).

Prenatal Diagnosis

Prevention of birth of a child with genetic and/or congenital disorders with poor prognosis involves termination of pregnancy when the fetus is found to be affected with a malformation or a genetic disorder. It allows an option of pregnancy and birth of child free of disorder to many couples who would otherwise refrain from planning further pregnancy for the fear of recurrence of genetic disease.

Prenatal diagnosis of congenital malformations has attained very good sensitivity and specificity due to high resolution ultrasonographic machines. Other methods of prenatal diagnosis involve obtaining fetal sample by chorionic villous sampling (10 to 12 weeks) or amniocentesis (16 weeks or later). These sampling procedures are done under ultrasound guidance and do not cause harm to the fetus. The various tests that can be done on these samples include DNA based tests for monogenic disorder, biochemical tests like enzyme assays for the diagnosis of metabolic disorders and chromosomal analysis. These tests have very minimal error rates of 1% or less.

Neonatal Screening

For adopting a screening program for a disorder, the prevalence data in the population should be available. Availability of a sensitive and simple test is another requisite for any screening program. Disorders chosen for neonatal screening include those where early intervention markedly changes the outcome.

Neonatal screening for hypothyroidism appears to be the most important and cost-effective strategy for prevention of treatable intellectual disability. The incidence of congenital hypothyroidism in India is reported to be around 1 per 2000 and treatment is easy and cheap. This stresses the need and feasibility of starting universal neonatal screening for hypothyroidism on a national level. The other disorders to be considered for newborn screening in India are congenital adrenal hyperplasia, biotinidase deficiency, galactosemia, and sickle cell disease. Screening for phenylketonuria is very rewarding but the special diets needed are very costly and implementation of neonatal screening for phenylketonuria in India may not be feasible at present.

The Future

In future, population based programs for common genetic mutations like factor V Leiden and hemochromatosis gene mutations may come up to identify individuals at risk of venous thrombosis and hemochromatosis respectively. The mutation carriers at risk of developing the disease can be provided prophylactic therapy.

Agarwal M, Joshi K, Bhatia V, et al Feasibility study of an outreach program of newborn screening in Uttar Pradesh. *Indian J Pediatr.* 2015;82:427–32.

Allanson JE, Cunniff C, Hoyme HE, *et al.* Elements of morphology: Standard terminology for the head and face. *Am J Med Genet.*2009;149A:6–28.

Battista RN, Blancquaert I, Laberge AM, et al. Genetics in health care: an overview of current and emerging models. *Public Health Genomics.* 2012;15:34–45.

Booth CH, Bobby Gaspa HB, Thrasher AT. Gene therapy for primary immunodeficiency. *Curr Opin Pediatr.* 2011; 23:659–66.

Carey JC, Cohen MMJr, Curry C, et al. Elements of morphology: Standard terminology for the lips, mouth, and oral region. *Am J Med Genet.* 2009;149A:77–92.

Cassidy SB, Allanson JE. Management of Genetic Syndromes. 3rd ed. Philadelphia: Willey Blackwell;2010

Falk MJ, Robin NH. The primary care physician's approach to congenital anomalies. *Prim Care Clin Office Pract.* 2004;31:605–19.

Fernhoff P M. Newborn screening for genetic disorders. *Pediatr Clin N Am.*2009;56: 505–13.

Frías JL, Davenport ML; Committee on Genetics and Section on Endocrinology Health supervision for children with Turner syndrome. *Pediatrics.* 2003; 111:692–702.

Gekas J, Vallée M, Castonguay L, et al. Clinical validity of karyotyping for the diagnosis of chromosomal imbalance following array comparative genomic hybridisation. *J Med Genet.*2011;48:851–5.

Ginsburg D. Genetics and genomics to the clinic: a long road ahead. *Cell.* 2011;147: 17–19.

Hendriksz CJ, Berger KI, Lampe C, et al. Health-related quality of life in mucopolysaccharidosis: looking beyond biomedical issues. *Orphanet J Rare Dis.* 2016;11(1):119.

Koene S, Smeitink J. Mitochondrial medicine. *J Inherit Metab Dis.*2001;34:247–8.

16

Srivastava A, Shaji RV. Cure for thalassemia major - from allogeneic hematopoietic stem cell transplantation to gene therapy. *Haematologica*. 2017;102(2):214–223.

Stark Z, Tan TY, Chong B, et al. A prospective evaluation of whole-exome sequencing as a first-tier molecular test in infants with suspected monogenic disorders. *Genet Med*. 2016 Nov;18(11):1090–1096.

van Karnebeek CD, Stockler S. Treatable inborn errors of metabolism causing intellectual disability: A systematic literature review. *Mol Genet Metab*.2011.

Yang CF, Yang CC, Liao HC, et al. Very Early treatment for infantile-onset pompe disease contributes to better outcomes. *J Pediatr*. 2016;169:174–80.

Case Study | Genetic Counseling for Thalassemia Major

A couple with a two-year-old child with thalassemia major has approached you for genetic counseling. The child was diagnosed as thalassemia major at 5 months of age when he presented with severe anemia (hemoglobin of 4 g/dL) and splenomegaly. The investigations showed fetal hemoglobin of 90%. The father's hemoglobin, mean corpuscular volume (MCV) and hemoglobin A_2 were 13 g/dL, 64 femtoliter (fL), and 4.5% respectively. Corresponding values for the mother were 10.5 g/dL, 56 fL and 5%, respectively.

Q. What is the risk that the next child of the couple also has thalassemia major?

Q. What can be done to avoid the recurrence of the disease in the family?

Q. What investigations are needed prior to prenatal diagnosis?

To find the answers read:

Thalassemia major is a serious disorder manifesting as severe anemia during infancy. The treatment is bone marrow transplantation or lifelong regular 2 to 3 weekly blood transfusions. Thalassemia major occurs due to homozygosity for mutated beta-globin gene. More than 300 mutations occurring in different parts of beta globin gene are known to give rise to beta-thalassemia. Each family may have any one or two of these mutations and clinical manifestations or fetal hemoglobin level does not give any clue to the mutation present in the affected child. Mostly the beta-thalassemia mutations are point mutations, ie, substitution of a base by other: eg, IVS 1–5 G to C (guanine at the 5th place of first intervening sequence is replaced by cytosine) is commonly identified mutation in India. Fifteen common mutations account for most of the cases of beta-thalassemia in India. To test for the mutation, all 3 exons of the beta globin gene need to be sequenced. The different types of mutations give rise to varying degree of decrease in beta globin synthesis. Mutation which lead to complete shutdown of synthesis of beta globins is called $\beta°$ (beta zero) mutation and causes severe type of thalassemia. The mutations which lead to decrease in synthesis of beta globin are known as beta plus (β^+).

As the disease is inherited in an autosomal recessive manner, the parents of a child with homozygous beta-thalassemia are obligate carriers. The carriers of beta-thalassemia (also known as thalassemia minor or thalassemia trait) are usually asymptomatic. They can be diagnosed by presence of microcytosis (MCV <80 fL) and hemoglobin A_2 more than 3.5%. The chance of recurrence of thalassemia major in the siblings of a child with thalassemia major is 25% or 1 in 4. Same is the case when both the spouses are detected to be heterozygous for beta-thalassemia mutations, ie, carriers of beta-thalassemia. As the disease is serious and the treatment is costly and cumbersome; prevention of birth of a child with thalassemia major is a better option. Prevention is possible by identifying couples who are carriers of beta-thalassemia and offering them prenatal diagnosis. Thalassemia carriers are detected by their blood test or because they have already given birth to a child with thalassemia major. Most of these families accept the option of prenatal diagnosis and termination of the pregnancy if the fetus is found to be affected with the disease. Prenatal diagnosis is done by testing the mutations present in the family in the DNA extracted from chorionic villi obtained between 10 and 12 weeks of gestation. Before going for prenatal diagnosis, identification of mutations in the affected child of the family or the carrier parents is essential.

Think it over!

The family asks to identify HLA type of the fetus in addition to testing for thalassemia mutations in prenatal sample. The fetus is negative for thalassemia disease but the HLA type does not match with the first child with thalassemia major and hence, the expected child cannot be donor of bone marrow for the thalassemia major child. The family thus wants to terminate the pregnancy and conceive again till they get a normal and HLA matched child who can be donor for their first child with thalassemia major. Is it ethically correct?

Case Study	Duchenne Muscular Dystrophy: Prevention of Recurrence

Prema's, 30-year-old has a 10-year-old normal daughter and a 6-year-old son with Duchenne muscular dystrophy (DMD). She is again 8 weeks pregnant. Prema has an 18-year-old brother who has similar problem and is bedridden. Prema also has a 25-year-old sister who was married 6 months ago. Her question is whether all her sons will be similarly affected.

Q. What is the chance that Prema's unborn baby has DMD?
Q. What test you will do to find out whether Prema is a carrier of DMD?
Q. Who is the proband in the family?
Q. Who should be tested for mutation detection first? Will the two affected males in the family have different mutations?
Q. What types of mutations are commonly seen in DMD?
Q. What is the earliest gestational age for prenatal diagnosis of DMD?
Q. If the mutation is not detected in the proband; can prenatal diagnosis be provided to the family?
Q. If there was no other case of DMD in the family other than Prema's son, is the prenatal diagnosis indicated?
Q. Who else in the family needs genetic counseling and carrier detection?
Q. Prema's husband asks you to test their daughter and find out whether she is a carrier of DMD or not. Should you get her tested?

To find answers read:

Duchenne muscular dystrophy (DMD) is an X-linked recessive disorder caused by a mutation in *dystrophin* gene. Onset of symptoms is usually by 3 to 5 years with difficulty in getting up from sitting posture. The muscle weakness beginning in hip girdle muscles progresses and the patient usually becomes bedridden by 12 year of age; death occurs in second decade. The pseudohypertrophy of calf muscles and raised serum creatinine phosphokinase (CPK) are diagnostic. Milder form of the disease with onset in late childhood or adolescence is called Becker muscular dystrophy. It is also caused by mutation in *dystrophin* gene and hence, is allelic to DMD.

As against the small beta globin gene, dystrophin is a very large gene of size 2 mega bases (2 million base pairs). It is on the *p* arm of the X chromosome. Most of the mutations causing DMD and BMD are deletions of varying length in the *dystrophin* gene involving different exons. These deletions lead to absent, abnormal or truncated *dystrophin* protein which leads to muscle degeneration. The detection of mutation is possible by tests on DNA of the patient. Mutation detection confirms the diagnosis but it should be noted that the available tests at present cannot detect all mutations and hence, in a clinically confirmed case the mutation may not be detected.

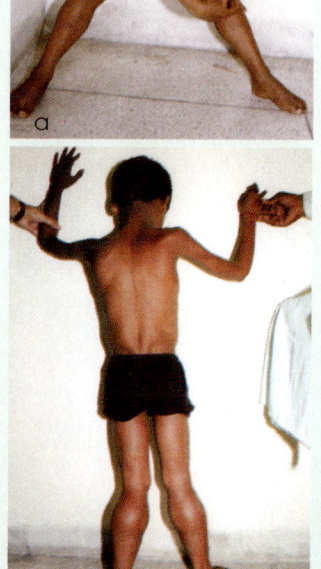

Once a mutation is detected in a child with DMD, the test for the same mutation can be used for prenatal diagnosis and detection of carriers.

If a woman has two sons with DMD or an affected son and an affected brother; then she is definitely a carrier (obligate carrier) of DMD. When a carrier woman is pregnant; the risk of the disorder is 50% if the fetus is a male and females are unlikely to be affected. So, the first step in prenatal diagnosis is to test whether the fetus is male or a female. This is done by testing for markers on Y chromosome in the DNA extracted from chorionic villi which is obtained by per abdominal sampling at 11 to 12 weeks of pregnancy. If the fetus is a male, then only further test for mutation detection is done. The family is informed whether the fetus is affected with DMD or not. According to Preconception and Prenatal Diagnostic Techniques (Prohibition of sex selection) Act, 1994

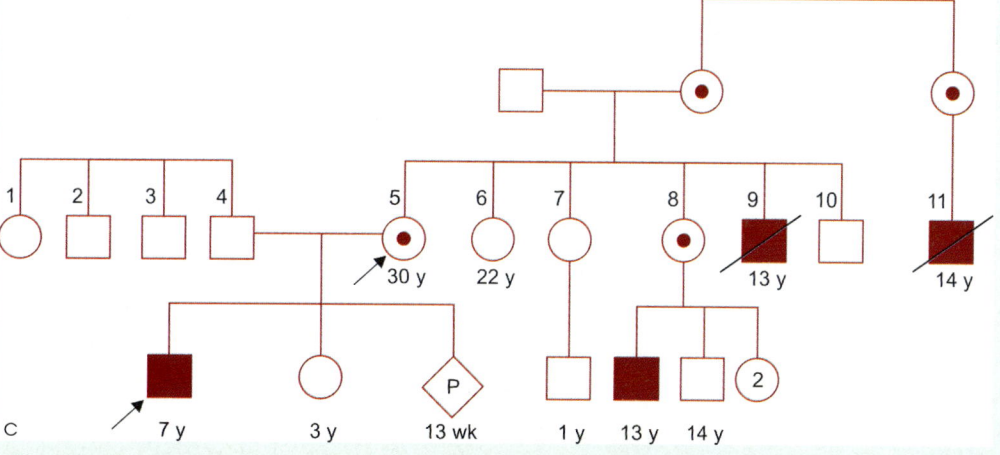

(a) A child with Duchenne muscular dystrophy. He has to take support of his thighs to get up from sitting posture, (b) prominent calf hypertrophy, (c) pedigree showing obligate carrier females (depicted with dot) who are related through males with Duchenne muscular dystrophy and will not need testing to confirm their carrier status. Individuals II-6 and II-7 will need DNA based testing using MLPA test to know their carrier status for DMD mutation

Indian law does not permit disclosure of sex of the fetus to the family. Other female relatives like sister of the proband and sister of a carrier mother can be tested by DNA based tests for identification of carriers. Carrier detection should not be done in children even if the parents insist. Only some carriers have high serum creatinine phosphokinase and hence, DNA based tests are necessary for carrier detection.

As women have two X chromosomes and carrier woman will have one normal copy of *dystrophin* gene and hence, detection of deletion in *dystrophin* gene in a carrier female is possible by multiplex ligation probe amplification (MLPA). If MLPA does not identify a mutation, sequencing of the dystrophin gene has to be done by a high throughput technique, namely next generation sequencing (NGS). This can pick up point mutations which are missed by MLPA.

If a family has only one case of DMD, the mother may or may not be carrier, If mother's blood test does not show that she is a carrier, still she should be offered prenatal diagnosis, as germ line mosaicism (ie, presence of mutation in some cells of the gonad) is reported for DMD like many other monogenic disorders including hemophilia, and achondroplasia.

Prema asks you to find out whether the baby in her womb is a carrier female. The family feels that the pregnancy should be terminated if the fetus is a carrier of DMD. Is it ethical?

Think it over!

Shubha R Phadke

Immunological and Collagen Vascular Disorders

17.1 PRIMARY IMMUNODEFICIENCY DISORDERS

Primary immunodeficiency disorders (PID) are a heterogenous group of disorders associated with defects in one or more components of immune system. Broadly, the immune system has two important components:

- *Innate immune system* It consists of barriers like skin and mucosa, cells like neutrophils and monocytes, and complement system.
- *Adaptive immune system* It consists of cell mediated immunity (T lymphocytes) and antibody mediated immunity (B lymphocytes).

Differences between innate and adaptive immunity are depicted in **Table 17.1**.

A. When to Suspect Immunodeficiency?

The usual mode of presentation of primary immunodeficiency disorders (PID) is **recurrent infections**. Most infections pertain to sinuses, respiratory tract, gastrointestinal tract, and lymph nodes.

The European Society of Immunodeficiencies (ESID) has suggested **10 warning signs** for suspecting immunodeficiency. PID should be suspected *in a child with* 2 *or more of the following* warning signs:

1. Four or more new ear infections within 1 year
2. Two or more serious sinus infections within 1 year
3. Two or more months on antibiotics with little effect
4. Two or more episodes of pneumonia within 1 year
5. Failure of an infant to gain weight or grow normally
6. Recurrent, deep skin, or organ abscesses
7. Persistent thrush in mouth or fungal infection on the skin
8. Need for intravenous antibiotics to clear infections
9. Two or more deep-seated infections including septicemia

10. Family history of PID, early deaths, or recurrent infections.

Minor infections like viral upper respiratory tract infections, recurrent bronchospasm, and recurrent urinary tract infections do not warrant investigations for PID. For recurrent meningitis, local defects (leading to exposure of meninges to external environment) should be ruled out before suspecting PID.

B. Classification of Immunodeficiency Disorders

Nearly 300 PIDs have been described till date with a prevalence of 6–10/1,00,000 population. The International Union of Immunological Societies (IUIS) has categorized the primary immunodeficiency disorders in the following 8 groups, in 2015.

1. Defects affecting cellular and humoral immunity
   Examples: Severe combined immunodeficiency disease (SCID), hyper IgM syndrome
2. Primary antibody defects
   Examples: X-linked (Bruton) agammaglobulinemia (Also known as BTK deficiency), common variable immunodeficiency (CVID), selective IgA deficiency
3. Congenital defects of phagocyte number, function, or both
   Examples: Congenital neutropenia, chronic granulomatous disease (CGD), leukocyte adhesion defect (LAD)
4. Combined immune deficiencies with associated or syndrome features
   Examples: Wiskott-Aldrich syndrome, ataxia telangiectasia, DiGeorge syndrome, hyper IgE syndrome
5. Diseases of immune dysregulation
   Examples: Familial hemophagocytic lymphohistiocytosis, autoimmune lymphoproliferative syndrome
6. Defects in Intrinsic and Innate Immunity. *Example*: Asplenia

Table 17.1 Differences between Innate and Adaptive Immunity	
Innate immunity	*Adaptive immunity*
1. Components • Barriers like skin and mucosa • Cells like neutrophils and monocytes • Complements	Components • Cell mediated immunity (T lymphocytes) • Antibody mediated immunity (B lymphocytes)
2. First line of defense	Second line of defense
3. No memory	Memory is present; hence fights recurrence of infection faster
4. No specificity (can fight against a broad range of organisms)	Consists of specific immune responses
5. Response is quick	Response slower

	Immunodeficiencies affecting cellular and humoral immunity	Primary antibody defects	Phagocytic defects
Prototype	Severe combined immuno-deficiency (SCID), Hyper IgM syndrome	X-linked agammaglobulinemia (BTK deficiency)	Congenital neutropenia, chronic granulomatous disease (CGD), leukocyte adhesion defect (LAD)
Age at presentation	Usually early after birth	After 4–6 months of age	Any time after birth
Usual infections	Bacterial, mycobacterial, viral, fungal	Usually bacterial only, occasionally with entero-viruses	Bacterial (*Staphylococcus aureus*, *Klebsiella*, *Burkholderia*) and fungal (*Aspergillus*)
Response to usual antibiotics	Slow	Usually recover	Take long duration to clear
Suggestive investigations	• Low immunoglobulins • Near absent T-lymphocytes • Lymphopenia	• Low immunoglobulins • Near absent B-lymphocytes	• Normal or high immunoglobulins • Neutropenia • Severe neutrophilia in leukocyte adhesion defect • Defective oxidative burst in Chronic granulomatous disease
Course	Die early without definitive treatment	Adult survival possible	Adult survival possible
Treatment	Hematopoietic stem cell transplantation	Periodic immunoglobulin replacement	Antibiotic and antifungal prophyl-axis, definitive therapy depends on type of defect

Table 17.2 Clinical and Investigative Profile of Common Subgroups of PID

7. Complement deficiencies
   Example: Neisserial infections seen in terminal complement deficiencies
8. Autoinflammatory disorder
   Examples: Familial Mediterranean fever, Blau syndrome
   The first three subgroups cover almost 80% of all primary immunodeficiency disorders; primary antibody deficiencies being the commonest. **Table 17.2** depicts major differences in the clinical and investigative profile of these three subgroups.

17.2 APPROACH TO SUSPECTED IMMUNODEFICIENCY

A meticulous history, targeted physical examination, and certain basic investigations can provide important clues to the type of primary immunodeficiency disorder (PID) in most instances.

A. History

History should include age at onset of infections, type of infections, organism isolated, and response to antibiotics.

1. Age at Onset

PID with *cellular or combined immune defects* and *phagocytic defects* can present with infections any time after birth whereas children with *primary antibody defects* are protected for first 4–6 months because of maternally transmitted antibodies. These antibodies gradually disappear in first few months when these children start developing infections.

Children with cellular/combined defects are usually younger at presentation. Children with severe combined immunodeficiency (SCID) usually do not survive beyond infancy because of recurrent and chronic infections with unusual organisms.

2. Type of Infections

- Children with *primary antibody defects* usually present with recurrent pneumonia, otitis media, and sinusitis in majority. Gastrointestinal infections (commonly *Giardia* and rarely *Salmonella*) account for 20% infections. Meningitis, septic arthritis, and skin infections are responsible for a small minority.
- *Phagocytic defects* usually present with suppurative infections (lymphadenitis, abscesses) and pneumonia; exception being leukocyte adhesion defect where children do not develop suppurative infections because of inability of leukocytes to reach the site of infection.
- Children with *cellular immunodeficiencies* can present with any type of infection though pneumonia and recurrent diarrhea are the commonest features.

3. Organism Isolated

- Children with *cellular PID* can develop infections due to viruses, bacteria, fungi as well as mycobacteria.
- *Primary antibody defects* present with infections due to usual organisms such as *H. influenzae*, and *Streptococcus pneumoniae*.
- *Chronic granulomatous disease* (CGD), a phagocytic defect, presents with infections due to signature organisms like *Staphylococcus aureus*, *Aspergillus*, and *Burkholderia*.
- Recurrent or systemic *Neisseria* infections with sepsis or pyogenic arthritis are associated with deficiency of C6, C7, or C5 components of complement.

4. Response to Antibiotics

Response to antibiotics is usually quick in children with primary antibody defects whereas response is usually very delayed and inadequate in phagocytic defects and cellular defects.

5. Family History

Family history of early deaths, recurrent infections, and autoimmune or collagen vascular diseases in past two generations is important. History of consanguinity may provide an important clue to an underlying autosomal recessive condition.

B. Physical Examination

- Children with primary antibody defects like BTK deficiency (X-linked agammaglobulinemia) typically have absent tonsils (Fig. 17.1), absence of palpable lymph nodes, and absence of palpable liver and spleen. Since infections here are usually bacterial and improve with usual antibiotics, some children are detected late with findings of bilateral bronchiectasis.
- Children with CGD usually present with recurrent suppurative lymphadenitis and pneumonia. They may also have generalized lymphadenopathy and hepatosplenomegaly. Hepatosplenomegaly may also be found in Chédiak-Higashi syndrome or in SCID.

Skin and Mucus Membranes

- Petechiae and ecchymosis are manifestations of Wiskott-Aldrich syndrome. Eczema is commonly associated.
- Persistent oral thrush not responding to topical antifungals may be a feature of T-cell deficiency.
- Recurrent skin abscesses are a feature of phagocytic defects. These abscesses are deeper in origin and sometimes 'cold.'
- An eczematoid rash appearing early in infancy that often involves typical and atypical sites (scalp, axilla and trunk) is characteristic of hyper IgE syndrome. Furuncle,

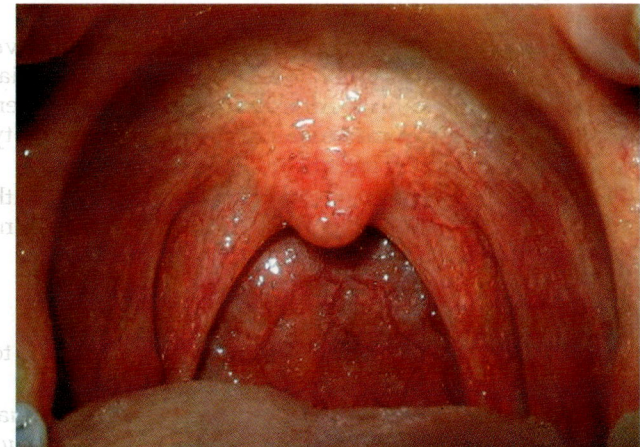

Fig. 17.1 Absent tonsils in a young child with X-linked agammaglobulinemia

carbuncle, and lung abscess are common accompaniments. Telangiectasia can be seen in ataxia telangiectasia. They usually appear by 2 years of age (rarely delayed up to 9 years).

Other Features

- Coarse facial feature may be seen in Hyper IgE syndrome.
- Dysmorphic facies may be noted in DiGeorge syndrome.
- Polyarthritis may occur in hypogammaglobulinemia and other antibody deficiencies.
- Hyperextensible joints have been described in Hyper IgE syndrome.

C. Investigations

Human Immunodeficiency virus (HIV) infection should always be ruled out before starting investigations for primary immunodeficiency disorders. Hemogram and immunoglobulin profile (IgG, IgA, IgM levels) are usually enough to pinpoint type of PID. Further work-up may require more sophisticated investigations.

Table 17.3 enlists some screening tests for immunodeficiency disorders. Abnormalities in serum immunoglobulins and their disease associations are shown in **Table 17.4**.

Table 17.3 Laboratory Evaluation for Recurrent Infections
1. *General* • Complete blood count, erythrocyte sedimentation rate • Chest X-ray (look for chronic disease and presence of thymus) • HIV serology
2. *B-cell defects* • Quantitative immunoglobulins • Isohemagglutinin titer • Antibody response to vaccine antigens (tetanus, diphtheria, *H. influenzae, S. pneumoniae*) • B cell number
3. *T lymphocyte defects* • Absolute lymphocyte count (normal result T-cell defect unlikely) • *Candida* skin test • T cell number and *in vitro* function
4. *Polymorphonuclear leukocyte defect* • Neutrophil count and morphology • Nitroblue tetrazolium reduction test • Dihydrorhodamine test
5. *Complement deficiency* • CH50 for assessment of classical pathway and AH50 for assessment of alternate pathway

Table 17.4 Abnormalities in Serum Immunoglobulin Levels	
Affected immunoglobulin	*Probable diagnosis*
Low IgG, IgA, IgM	Agammaglobulinemia
Low IgG with low IgM and/or IgA	Common variable immunodeficiency
Low IgA, IgG with normal or increased IgM	Hyper-IgM syndromes
Low IgA	Selective IgA deficiency
Low IgM	Selective IgM deficiency
Low IgG1 or G2 or G3 or G4	IgG subclass deficiency

1. Hemogram

- *Lymphocyte count less than 3000/mm³* is abnormal in first six months of life. Children with SCID usually have persistent lymphopenia after birth.
- Hemogram in primary antibody defects usually does not show significant aberrations.
- *Severe neutrophilia* (usually >50,000 per mm³) (even in absence of infection) is suggestive of leukocyte adhesion defect.
- *Neutropenia* (intermittent or persistent) may point to congenital neutropenia.
- *Persistent thrombocytopenia* in a boy with eczema and recurrent infections points towards Wiskott-Aldrich syndrome (WAS).
- Normal ESR usually rules out chronic bacterial and fungal infections.

2. Immunoglobulin Profile

Very low or undetectable IgG, IgA, and IgM levels are seen in X-linked agammaglobulinemia (BTK deficiency). Low immunoglobulins are also seen in children with SCID; however, it is difficult to interpret this investigation in first few months of life because of maternally transmitted IgG.

Children with phagocytic defects usually have higher immunoglobulin levels because of immune activation.

3. Lymphocyte Subsets

Children with SCID typically have lymphopenia and near complete absence of T lymphocytes. On the other hand, children with BTK deficiency have normal T lymphocytes and near absent B lymphocytes which explains their inability to produce immunoglobulins.

4. Tests to Assess Phagocytic Activity

- *Nitroblue tetrazolium (NBT) test* Normal neutrophils will show formation of formazan granules when mixed with NBT. This effect will be greatly enhanced if neutrophils are stimulated to enhance phagocytic activity. In contrast, neutrophils in chronic granulomatous disease (CGD) will not show formation of formazan granules even when stimulated (Fig. 17.2).
- *Dihydrorhodamine reduction (DHR) test* It depends on the principle of oxidation of DHR to rhodamine by stimulated neutrophils; this oxidative burst is defective in CGD.

5. Genetic Tests

Certain advanced tests may be needed to confirm the genetic defect associated with various PIDs. These are especially important for genetic counseling and prenatal diagnosis in next pregnancy.

17.3 PRIMARY IMMUNODEFICIENCY DISORDERS

17.3.1 IMMUNODEFICIENCIES AFFECTING CELLULAR AND HUMORAL IMMUNITY

Cell mediated immunity is needed for clearing intracellular pathogens (mycobacteria, viruses, and fungi). Cellular immune deficiency therefore predisposes to chronic mycobacterial, viral, fungal, and *Pneumocystis* infections. Oral thrush is frequent. Bacterial infections can also occur. Because these infections are not easy to treat, these children usually present with longer duration of illness. As there is no maternal transmission of cell mediated immunity, these children are predisposed to develop infections immediately after birth. Prototype condition is this category is severe combined immunodeficiency disease (SCID).

Severe Combined Immunodeficiency Disease (SCID)

SCID is a group of disorders associated with significant depletion of cell mediated immunity. Inheritance is variable being both X-linked and autosomal recessive. Usual presentation is in early infancy with severe or recurrent pneumonia, diarrhea, failure to thrive, and oral candidiasis.

Diagnosis is usually suspected because of persistent lymphopenia in a newborn or an infant. Absent thymic shadow on chest radiograph (Fig. 17.3) in a young infant may also provide a clue to this diagnosis. Near absent T-lymphocytes are diagnostic and genetic analysis is confirmatory.

These children are difficult to treat because of the profile of infections. Treatment may require broad spectrum drugs including anti-tubercular and antifungal therapy depending on the etiology. Hematopoietic stem cell transplantation is required to correct the basic defect. Gene therapy has proven to be successful in certain forms of SCID.

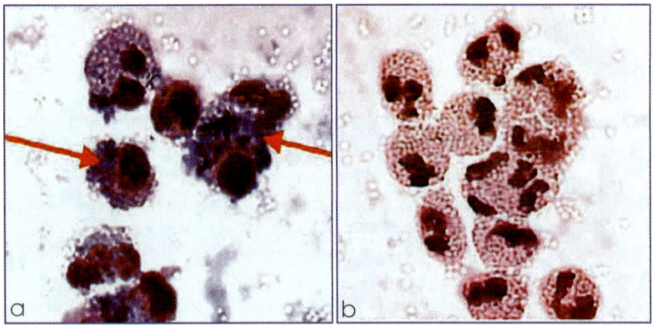

Fig. 17.2 Nitroblue tetrazolium test showing formazan granules (shown with arrows) in control (a) and no granules in a child with CGD (b)

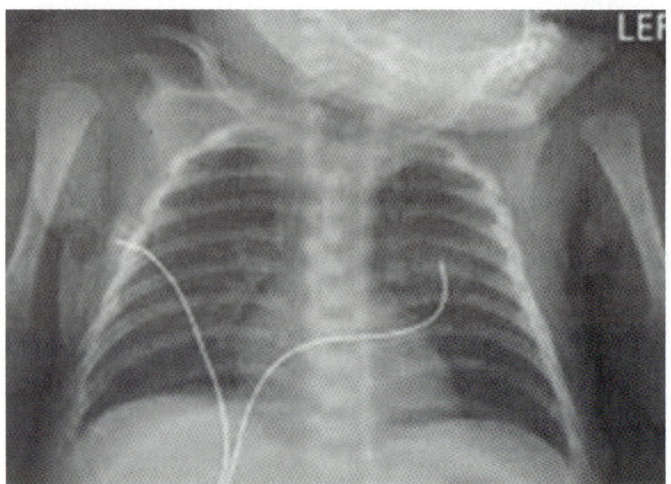

Fig. 17.3 Chest radiograph showing absent thymus and bilateral interstitial infiltrates in a child with SCID

Case Study | Severe Combined Immunodeficiency

An 8-week-old boy was hospitalized with cough and respiratory distress for last 2 weeks. Examination revealed tachypnea and mild cyanosis. There was no lymphadenopathy or hepato-splenomegaly. Chest examination was normal. BCG site showed a small papule. Investigations revealed Hb 8.9 g/dL, TLC 6400 (P92, L6, M2, E2), and platelet count 3.5×10^5 per mm^3. Blood culture was sterile and Chest X-ray showed bilateral interstitial shadows. Thymic shadow was absent in the chest radiograph (Fig. 17.3).

Are there any clues towards PID in this child?
The history and examination suggest a subacute onset severe interstitial pneumonia. This warrants investigations for underlying HIV infection. If HIV infection is ruled out, this child should be evaluated for SCID. Lymphopenia (absolute lymphocyte count of 384/mm^3) and absent thymic shadow on chest X-ray support the diagnosis of SCID.

How important is it to isolate an organism?
SCID patients can have various bacterial, mycobacterial, viral and fungal infections. Hence for appropriate management, it is important to isolate the organism. Since this child has got BCG, disseminated BCG disease is also possible in a child with SCID.

What is the likely outcome in such a child?
Hematopoietic stem cell transplantation is the mainstay of therapy and cures basic defect. Short of that, most children die during infancy.

Vaccination is contraindicated as these children do not mount an immune response and live vaccines may be harmful to them. BCG vaccine can cause disseminated BCG disease.

17.3.2 PRIMARY ANTIBODY DEFECTS

Antibody defects are the commonest PID seen world over. Antibodies are required for extracellular killing of bacteria and neutralization of toxins so antibody defects are associated with predisposition to develop bacterial infections. Most common pathogens are *Streptococcus* and Pneumococcus. Usual infections involve respiratory and gastrointestinal tracts.

Age at onset of infections is usually beyond 6 months as maternally transmitted IgG protects the newborn from infections till that time. Most infections are acute; however repeated respiratory infections can cause chronic complications like bronchiectasis. Typical prototype condition for antibody deficiency is BTK (Bruton tyrosine kinase) deficiency, also called X-linked agammaglobulinemia (XLA).

X-linked Agammaglobulinemia/BTK Deficiency

As the name suggests, this is an X-linked disease and hence manifests only in boys. Also there is near complete absence of gamma globulins (serum IgG, IgA, and IgM are very low). These boys start developing recurrent bacterial infections involving respiratory and gastrointestinal tracts usually after 6 months of age. Sinusitis and otitis media are also common. Typical clinical signs are absence of palpable lymph nodes and absence of tonsils (Fig. 17.1). Clinical examination may also show evidence of sequelae of repeated infections like bronchiectasis.

Diagnosis is confirmed by near absent levels of serum IgG, IgA, and IgM. Basic defect lies in BTK protein which is essential for development and maturation of B-lymphocytes that produce immunoglobulins. Because of BTK deficiency, these boys have very low serum immunoglobulins and near absent B lymphocytes. Genetic analysis helps in confirming the diagnosis.

Early, appropriate, and aggressive treatment of infections is important. Prevention of infections is achieved by replacement of deficient proteins, ie, immunoglobulins (IgG). IgG needs to be given periodically at an interval of 3–4 weeks. Usual dose of intravenous immunoglobulin is 400–600 mg/kg per dose. This therapy is to be given lifelong. This helps in reducing the risk of recurrent bacterial infections which are hallmark of this disease. Addition of prophylactic antibiotic (commonly cotrimoxazole) also helps in reducing the risk of infections.

Vaccination is not useful in children with XLA as they do not mount an antibody response. Ideally no vaccines should be given to these children. Oral polio virus vaccine should be avoided even in siblings because of risk of vaccine associated paralytic polio and non-clearance of vaccine virus in children with XLA.

Genetic counseling is important as this is an X-linked disease. Mothers who are carriers of mutation have 50% chance of having an affected baby boy.

Case Study | X-Linked Agammaglobulinemia

A 2-year-old boy was hospitalized with severe pneumonia. He had history of 2 previous hospitalizations for pneumonia during last 6 months that required intravenous antibiotics every time. Family history revealed death in a maternal uncle at the age of 3 years with pneumonia.

Would you think of PID in this setting?
Yes, as this child has had three severe infections requiring intravenous antibiotics.

Which group of PID is most likely in this setting?
Combined (cellular and humoral) immunodeficiency is not likely in this setting as age at onset has been late at 1.5 years and profile of infections does not suggest serious viral or fungal infections. Profile of this child fits into primary antibody deficiency.

If you are thinking of primary antibody deficiency in such a young child, would you like to examine for some specific clues to diagnosis?
Specific clues to primary antibody deficiency would be absent tonsils and absent lymph nodes. Also one should look for features of bronchiectasis as sequelae of repeated lung infections.

Name two tests which will be diagnostic of primary antibody deficiency in this child?
Near absent immunoglobulin levels and near absent B-lymphocytes would help in diagnosis of BTK deficiency. Genetic analysis would be confirmatory.

17

17.3.3 INNATE DEFECTS

Innate defects deal with defects in cells like neutrophils and complement system. Neutrophil defects can be quantitative or qualitative or both.

1. Defect in Neutrophil Number

Congenital Neutropenia

These children usually present with recurrent bacterial infections. Usual site of infection is lymph nodes and lungs. Neutropenia can be persistent or intermittent. Persistent neutropenia is easy to diagnose with all neutrophil counts being less than 1500 per cubic mm (severe neutropenia defined as neutrophil count less than 500 per cubic mm).

Intermittent neutropenia occurs cyclically and single hemogram showing normal neutrophil counts does not rule out diagnosis. Diagnosis requires multiple hemograms over duration of 6 weeks. Once diagnosed, granulocyte colony stimulating factor (G-CSF) is used to decrease risk of infections by increasing neutrophil counts.

2. Defects in Neutrophil Function

Leukocyte Adhesion Defect

The defect lies in diapedesis of neutrophils from vessels to site of infection. These children develop superficial infections without pus formation and have significant neutrophilia in circulation. Hematopoietic stem cell transplantation is curative.

Chronic Granulomatous Disease

The defect lies in oxidative burst causing impaired phagocytosis. About 70% of all CGD patients have X-linked inheritance and hence, only boys are affected. Rest of CGD cases are autosomal recessive and can occur in both sexes. These children develop infections of skin, lymph nodes, and lungs with catalase positive bacteria like *Staphylococcus aureus*, *Burkholderia cepacia*, *Serratia*, and with fungi like *Aspergillus*. Suppurative lymphadenitis (Fig. 17.4) and pneumonia are common infections seen in CGD. Hematogenous spread of infections is unusual. Hepatosplenomegaly is common.

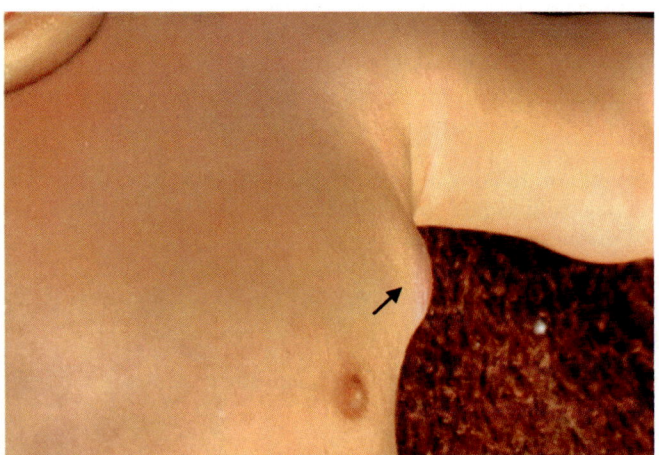

Fig. 17.4 Suppurative axillary lymphadenitis in an infant with chronic granulomatous disease

Investigations usually show polymorphonuclear leukocytosis and high immunoglobulins because of recurrent infections. Simple laboratory tests like Nitroblue tetrazolium test (NBT) and Dihydrorhodamine reduction test (DHR) help in confirming the diagnosis.

Treatment of infections is the cornerstone of management. Eradication of infections is difficult and prolonged courses of antibiotics and antifungals are needed. Once infection is adequately treated, antibiotic and antifungal prophylaxis is started for prevention of further infections. CGD is one disease where prophylaxis has been used as mainstay of management if the child remains well on the same. In case child keeps on developing infections despite prophylaxis, hematopoietic stem cell transplant is required.

Case Study	Chronic Granulomatous Disease

A 3-year-old boy presented with fever and pain abdomen for 2 weeks. He had history of recurrent episodes of suppurative lymphadenitis since early infancy. Investigations led to a diagnosis of pyogenic liver abscess for the present episode. Hemogram showed polymorphonuclear leukocytosis and thrombocytosis. Immunoglobulin profile showed elevated immunoglobulin G (IgG), immunoglobulin A (IgA) and immunoglobulin M (IgM) for age. Nitroblue tetrazolium test and Dihydrorhodamine test confirmed the diagnosis of CGD by showing reduced oxidative burst of neutrophils.

What are the clues to a phagocytic defect in this child?
Recurrent suppurative infections in the form of lymphadenitis and liver abscess suggest the possibility of phagocytic defect.

Is there a difference in clinical profile of patients with CGD from those with congenital neutropenia and leukocyte adhesion defects?
Infections in leukocyte adhesion defect are not purulent as there is a defect in transfer of neutrophils from vessels to site of infection; leading to severe neutrophilia in blood and paucity of phagocytic cells in tissues. In children with congenital neutropenia, usual infections are bacterial, and fungal infections are rare.

How will you manage this child?
Prolonged course of antibiotics will be needed for treatment of acute infection. Isolation of organism is useful in choosing appropriate antibiotics or antifungals. Once acute infection is cleared, antibiotic and antifungal prophylaxis is to be given life-long to prevent further infections. Hematopoietic stem cell transplantation will be required, if the child continues to have recurrent infections despite antibiotic and antifungal prophylaxis.

17.3.4 COMBINED IMMUNODEFICIENCIES WITH ASSOCIATED OR SYNDROMIC FEATURES

Wiskott-Aldrich Syndrome

Wiskott-Aldrich syndrome (WAS), an X-linked disorder (thus manifests only in boys) is associated with thrombocytopenia, eczema, recurrent infections (fungal, viral and due to encapsulated bacteria) and autoimmune manifestations. Autoimmunity manifests as autoimmune hemolytic anemia, arthritis, and cutaneous vasculitis.

Patients lack IgM and IgG2 subclass of immunoglobulins. Molluscum contagiosum and verrucae are also common. Persistent thrombocytopenia in any boy associated with eczema and recurrent infections should raise the possibility of this disease.

Ataxia-telangiectasia: A Defect in DNA Repair

Ataxia-telangiectasia (AT) is an autosomal recessive disease characterized by progressive cerebellar ataxia, dysarthria, oculomotor dyspraxia, oculo-cutaneous telangiectasia and immune deficiency. It is associated with chromosomal instability and increased susceptibility to malignancies, especially lymphomas and leukemias.

Immunodeficiency is both cellular and humoral. T-cell numbers are decreased. About 10% of children present with decreased serum levels of immunoglobulins IgG and IgA, and a normal or increased IgM level.

Di-George Syndrome: Thymic Defect with Additional Congenital Anomalies

Di-George syndrome is a classical T-cell defect associated with thymic hypoplasia. These children have cardiac and facial anomalies and may present with hypocalcemia due to hypoparathyroidism. Basic defect is deletion of the long arm of chromosome 22 at position q.11. Chest X-ray showing absent thymus and hypocalcemia are important clues to diagnosis.

Hyper-IgE Syndrome (Job Syndrome)

This autosomal dominant disorder presents with raised levels of IgE (>2000 IU/mL), eczematoid dermatitis at a very early age, staphylococcal skin infections, and pneumonia with pneumatocele formation. Teeth, eyes, and bony abnormalities may be associated.

Gambineri E. New frontiers in primary immunodeficiency disorders: immunology and beyond…. *Cell Mol Life Sci*. 2012;69:1–5.

Madkaikar M, Mishra A, Ghosh K. Diagnostic approach to primary immunodeficiency disorders. *Indian Pediatr*. 2013;50:579–86.

Ochs HD, Hagin D. Primary immunodeficiency disorders: general classification, new molecular insights, and practical approach to diagnosis and treatment. *Ann Allergy Asthma Immunol*. 2014;112:489–95.

Picard C, Al-Herz W, Bousfiha A, Casanova JL, Chatila T, Conley ME, et al. Primary Immunodeficiency Diseases: an Update on the Classification from the International Union of Immunological Societies Expert Committee for Primary Immunodeficiency 2015. *J Clin Immunol*. 2015;35:696–726.

Raje N, Dinakar C. Overview of immunodeficiency disorders. *Immunol Allergy Clin North Am* 2015;35:599–623.

Sobh A, Bonilla FA. Vaccination in primary immunodeficiency disorders. *J Allergy Clin Immunol Pract* 2016;4:1066–1075.

Wu EY, Ehrlich L, Handly B, Frush DP, Buckley RH. Clinical and imaging considerations in primary immunodeficiency disorders: an update. *Pediatr Radiol*. 2016;46:1630–1644:

Revision Point

Primary Immune Deficiency (PID)

1. PID are a heterogenous group of diseases with propensity to develop recurrent infections; though some patients can present with predominant autoimmunity and malignancy.
2. Clinically one should try to identify a subgroup of disorders based on age at onset and profile of infections.
3. HIV infection should always be ruled out before investigating for PID.
4. Lymphopenia points towards severe combined immunodeficiency (SCID) whereas neutropenia may point to congenital persistent or cyclic neutropenia.
5. Thrombocytopenia points to Wiskott-Aldrich syndrome.
6. Severe neutrophilia (leukemoid reaction) points to LAD whereas moderate neutrophilia can be seen in CGD.
7. Immunoglobulin profile showing panhypogammaglobulinemia points towards primary antibody deficiency (BTK deficiency) or SCID.
8. It is important to diagnose and treat infections early as recurrent infections can lead to sequelae like bronchiectasis. Isolation of organism is useful as the infections can be unusual (like in SCID, CGD) and polymicrobial.
9. Infections may require prolonged antibiotics to clear infections in children with PID.
10. Specific management for PID varies with the type. BTK deficiency children do well with immunoglobulin replacement. SCID patients need hematopoietic stem cell transplant. G-CSF (to increase neutrophil counts) is used for neutropenic disorders and life-long antibiotic and antifungal prophylaxis is used as first line management for CGD.

17.4 EVALUATION OF RHEUMATIC DISEASES

Rheumatic diseases are complex multisystemic diseases that can involve any part of the body. Some of the rheumatological conditions like juvenile idiopathic arthritis (JIA) have predominant manifestations related to joints whereas others like systemic lupus erythematosus (SLE) and vasculitis are usually multisystemic. Certain other disorders like juvenile dermatomyositis though multisystemic, have predominant manifestations involving skin and muscles.

JOINT PAIN

Joint pain is the commonest symptom of rheumatological diseases, although it can also occur in many non-rheumatological diseases. A good history and examination should be sufficient to differentiate the two.

pGALS (Paediatric gait, arms, legs and spine) examination is a good screening tool for children presenting with musculoskeletal complaints. Videos are available free at *http://www.arthritisresearchuk.org/health-professionals-and-students/video-resources/pgals.aspx*. This is a quick and easy screening examination and should be followed by a detailed examination of joints. All undergraduate and postgraduate students must incorporate this examination in their routine clinical practice.

The 3 important questions to answer, when one sees any child with joint pain, are as follows:
1. Whether the joint pain is really because of joint problem?
2. Whether there is arthritis?

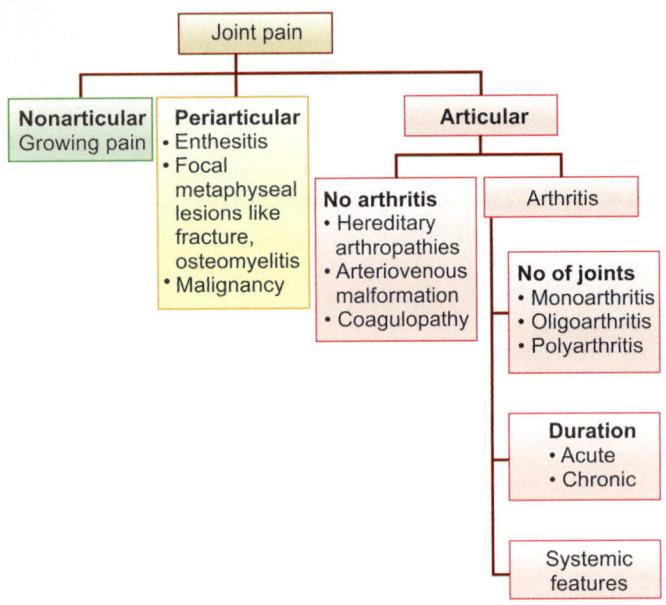

Fig. 17.5 Approach to evaluation of joint pain

Box 17.1 Red Flags in a Child with Joint Pain
- *Clinical*
  - Not able to walk or bedridden
  - Nocturnal pain
  - Bone tenderness
  - Systemic features: Pallor, bleeds, hepatosplenomegaly
- *Investigations*
  - Leukopenia or leukocytosis with lymphocytic pre-dominance
  - Thrombocytopenia (leukemia, SLE)
  - Isolated raised lactate dehydrogenase (leukemia)

3. How many joints are involved, for how long, and what are the other symptoms?
   The scheme is also depicted in Fig. 17.5.

1. Whether the so Called "Joint Pain" is Localized to Joint or is Extra-articular?

In arthritis, pain tends to be across the joint line whereas extra-articular pain is usually very pinpoint near or around the joint.

Nonarticular Pains

Typical prototype is "**growing pains**", which is a benign condition seen in children between the ages of 3–12 years. The pain is intermittent, usually bilateral and localized to shin, calves, thighs, and popliteal fossa. The child is absolutely well in between the episodes. Reassurance and symptomatic treatment usually suffice.

Periarticular Pains

Around the joints, one can have pain due to enthesitis, fractures, and osteomyelitis in the metaphyseal region.
- **Enthesitis** is defined as inflammation at the insertion of tendons or ligaments to bone. Localized pain or tenderness and/or swelling at these insertion sites is usually seen in children with enthesitis related arthritis.
- **Focal lesions like fractures or osteomyelitis in metaphyseal region** can cause pinpoint tenderness and swelling.
- *Hematological conditions* Malignancies like acute lymphoblastic leukemia can present with only "joint complaints" because of periarticular infiltration. Red flag clinical features include night pains, significant disability, pallor, bleeds, bone tenderness, and hepatosplenomegaly (**Box 17.1**).
  Less commonly, neuroblastoma can also present with diffuse bone pains. Hematological conditions like sickle cell disease and thalassemia can also present with bone pains and arthralgia.

Articular Pain

Articular involvement can occur due to arthritis or non-inflammatory causes. If there is no doubt about articular pain, one should try to answer whether there is arthritis.

2. Whether there is Arthritis?

Arthritis is defined as presence of swelling or presence of at least of two of three signs of inflammation namely redness, warmth, and diminished range of motion. Redness over the joint is hardly ever seen in inflammatory arthritis except septic arthritis. Absence of these signs of inflammation would indicate a non-inflammatory condition. Some other symptoms like early morning stiffness and gelling point to inflammatory joint pain.
- *Early morning stiffness* refers to pain and difficulty in moving the joints for about half an hour or more in the morning on waking up. *Gelling* is similar to this, but tends to happen after prolonged rest during day.
- Pain worsening during sleep points to alternative diagnosis like malignancy.
- In non-inflammatory causes, pain occurs usually when joint movement is forced beyond allowed limit due to contractures.

If there is no doubt about arthritis, one should look for number of joints involved, duration of arthritis and associated systemic features.

Non-inflammatory Articular Pain

Certain conditions like hereditary arthropathies, intra-articular arteriovenous malformation, and certain orthopedic conditions can masquerade chronic arthritis.
- *Hereditary arthropathies* usually have prominent joint contractures with or without joint swelling. Pain is usually absent except when the joints are moved beyond the allowed limit. There is usually no joint line tenderness in these patients. Family history may also give a clue.
- *Intra-articular arteriovenous malformations* can present with joint swelling, but other features of inflammation like warmth, and morning stiffness are usually absent. Superficial prominence of veins may give a clue to this diagnosis but is not always present.
- *Orthopedic conditions* like Perthes disease or avascular necrosis of the femoral head, and slipped upper femoral epiphysis can mimic hip arthritis.

3. Number of Joints Involved, Duration of Arthritis and Associated Systemic Features

Number of Joints Involved

Single joint arthritis is called *monoarthritis* whereas involvement of more than four joints with arthritis is called *polyarthritis*. Involvement of less than five joints is called oligoarthritis. Certain etiologies (septic arthritis, tubercular arthritis) involve only single joints.

Acute *versus* Chronic Arthritis

Arthritis with duration of less than 6 weeks is called *acute arthritis* whereas arthritis persisting beyond 6 weeks is called *chronic arthritis*.

Acute arthritis Acute arthritis can occur due to multiple etiologies. Short history with single joint involvement suggests a possibility of "septic arthritis". Septic arthritis should be considered as a differential for any sick looking child with acute monoarthritis. Typically, large joints are involved. Child is usually febrile and toxic. The involved joint is extremely tender, warm and swollen. In contrast, multiple joints are usually involved in rheumatic fever, and rheumatological conditions. Arthritis in rheumatic fever involves large joints and is typically migratory. A brisk response to salicylates or NSAID is diagnostic. Arthritis can also be seen in association with many rheumatological diseases like SLE, juvenile dermatomyositis, and vasculitis like HSP, Kawasaki disease.

Chronic arthritis Chronic arthritis can occur due to infectious as well as rheumatological conditions. Chronic infection like tuberculosis can present with chronic monoarthritis involving large joints. Chronic rheumatological conditions like SLE and vasculitis can present with arthritis, but usually these patients would have multisystemic involvement. JIA is the most common idiopathic cause of chronic arthritis in children, but it is important to remember that it is a diagnosis of exclusion.

Systemic Features

- Any child with arthralgia/arthritis should be examined for systemic features. Malar rash (Fig. 17.6) and oral ulcers

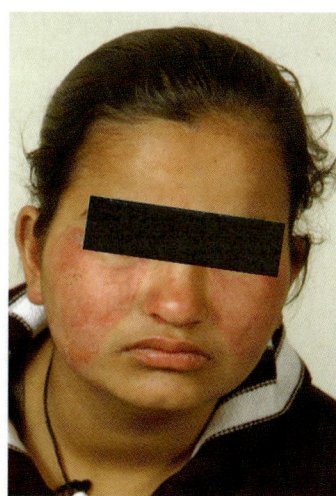

Fig. 17.6 Malar rash in a young girl with SLE

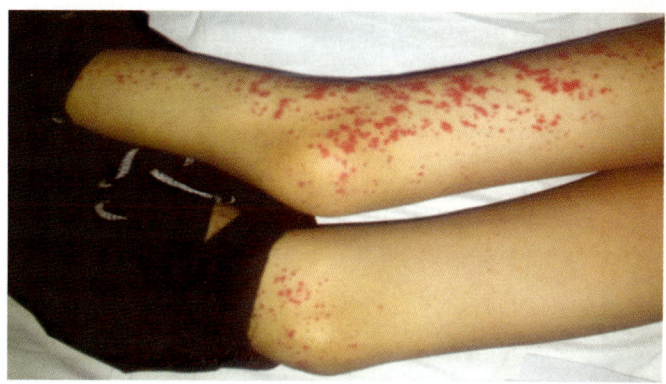

Fig. 17.7 Palpable purpuric rash in lower limbs in a child with Henoch-Schönlein purpura (HSP)

would point to systemic lupus erythematosus (SLE). High grade quotidian fever with rash appearing at the peak of fever, lymphadenopathy, and hepatosplenomegaly point to systemic arthritis. Palpable purpuric rash (Fig. 17.7) along with joint pain points towards Henoch-Schönlein purpura. Systemic examination may also give clue to diseases like HIV infection which can present with arthralgia and arthritis. Following features on clinical examination may give a clue to underlying etiology: *Skin rash* may be associated with systemic juvenile idiopathic arthritis (JIA), collagen vascular disease, vasculitis, inflammatory bowel disease, and psoriasis.

- *Gastointestinal features* (diarrhea, constipation, pain abdomen, hepatitis, and pancreatitis) are seen in inflammatory bowel diseases, collagen vascular disease, systemic vasculitis, and reactive arthritis.
- *Ocular involvement* (uveitis) is typical of oligoarticular JIA, juvenile ankylosing spondylitis, Kawasaki disease, and Behçet disease.
- *Hypertension* is associated with SLE and vasculitis.
- *Muscular involvement* with arthritis should suggest a possibility of polymyositis or dermatomyositis.
- Presence of chest pain, arrhythmia, and palpitation indicates *cardiac involvement* that occurs in association with rheumatic fever, systemic JIA, Kawasaki disease, and SLE.
- *Pulmonary involvement* as pleuritis is usually observed with SLE, systemic vaculitis, and irritable bowel disease.
- *Renal involvement* This is characteristic of SLE, and vasculitis; and manifests as hematuria or proteinuria.

Laboratory Investigations

Laboratory investigations for a child with arthritis can be categorized as (*i*) those performed on nearly all patients, and (*ii*) more specialized and selective tests that need to be individualized depending on clinical picture. All patients should have a complete blood count (CBC) with smear, ESR and C-reactive protein (acute-phase reactants) and a urinalysis. Other tests can be done depending on clinical presentation. A list of commonly advised laboratory test is provided in **Table 17.5.**

Acute Phase Reactants

Acute phase reactants are altered as a non-specific response of the body to the inflammation; these include elevation of ESR, C-reactive protein (CRP), and fibrinogen. CRP is a

Table 17.5 Laboratory Investigations in a Child with Arthritis
Hematology
• Complete blood count, ESR
• C-reactive protein
• Bleeding and coagulation profile in case suspicion of hemarthrosis
Immunology (autoantibodies)
• Rheumatoid factor
• Antinuclear antibody
• HLA B27
• ASO titers if suspicion of rheumatic fever
Biochemistry
• Renal function test
• Liver function test
• Muscle enzymes if there are features to suggest myalgia or myositis
Urinalysis
• For suspected SLE or vasculitis syndrome
Radiological
X-ray joints are usually not useful. MRI of sacroiliac joints may be required in children with SI joint involvement

reliable marker of inflammation as it rises within 24 hours of inflammation up to 10–100 times the normal value and falls rapidly on resolution of inflammation. In patients with JIA, vasculitis, and bacterial infection, the level can go up to 100–500 times.

Rheumatoid factor (RF)

Rheumatoid factor includes a group of autoantibodies to the Fc protein of IgG. Approximately 5% of healthy subjects and 75% of adults with rheumatoid arthritis have rheumatoid factor. Only 10% of children with JIA are positive for rheumatoid factor. Other conditions in which rheumatoid factor is present include subacute bacterial endocarditis, chronic active hepatitis, many viral infections, and following immunization. It may also be present in a small number of children with SLE, mixed connective tissue disease, scleroderma, and dermatomyositis.

Antinuclear Antibodies (ANA)

Antinuclear antibodies (ANA) are autoantibodies that react with various parts of the cell nuclei; it can be of IgM, IgG and IgA subclass. Parts of the nuclei that can form antigens with these antibodies include deoxyribonucleic acid (DNA), deoxyribonucleic protein, ribonucleic acid (RNA), histone, nucleoli, and non-histone unclear proteins (SML, RMP protein).

ANA is present in 98% children with SLE, 25% children with juvenile dermatomyositis, about 50% children with scleroderma, and 2–5% of healthy subjects. In juvenile idiopathic arthritis, ANA is present only in 70–80% of children with early onset oligoarthritis that typically occurs in young girls. Anti-neutrophil cytoplasmic antibody (ANCA), ie, c-ANCA—characterized by granular staining of cytoplasm—is highly specific and sensitive for the diagnosis of Wegner's granulomatosis; p-ANCA, ie, with perinuclear staining is less specific and can be present in microscopic polyarteritis nodosa, SLE, Churg-Strauss syndrome, and ingestion of certain drugs.

Anti-cardiolipin Antibodies

These antibodies are directed against negatively changed phospholipids with increased risk of arterial and venous thrombosis. These antibodies can be documented in primary antiphospholipid syndrome, SLE, and rheumatoid arthritis.

Markers of Complement Activation

The complement system is a group of proteins that react sequentially to mediate inflammation. The level of total hemolytic complement and its individual component can mirror inflammatory activity. Total serum hemolytic complement (CH50) level is low in 90% children with active lupus nephritis.

HLA Typing

Histocompatibility antigens (HLA) are controlled by genes that are localized to the sixth chromosome. Apart from recent inclusion of HLA B27 as diagnostic criteria for enthesitis related arthritis and exclusion criteria for systemic onset and polyarticular JIA, routine clinical testing is not recommended.

Others

The biochemical tests will tell us about the involvement of various organ systems. Raised ASO titer will help to reach a diagnosis of acute rheumatic fever. Immunological tests are non-specific for most of the cases of acute arthritis. Bone marrow examination is necessary to rule out a neoplastic process. Cardiac evaluation is needed to exclude carditis associated with rheumatic problems.

Synovial Fluid Examination

The synovial fluid can be categorized as normal, inflammatory, infective, or hemorrhagic; based on its color, turbidity, viscosity, cell count, glucose, total protein, Gram stain, and culture.

- A normal joint contains small amount of synovial fluid (less than 2 mL in knee joint), that is transparent, viscous, and shows good mucin clot. It contains <200 cells/mm^3, majority being lymphocytes. In septic arthritis, synovial fluid is turbid and has poor mucin clot formation; cell count is more than 100,000 with more than 80% neutrophils.
- Hemorrhagic synovial fluid is typical of a child with coagulation defect, trauma and AV malformation.
- It is difficult to identify the specific diagnosis by synovial fluid evaluation in most cases, though it can help classify arthritis in broad subdivisions.

Tissue Biopsy

Biopsy of the involved tissue can provide valuable information, but is generally avoided as it is an invasive procedure. Skin biopsy is advised for Henoch-Schönlein purpura only when some atypical features are present. Muscle biopsy is recommended only when the diagnosis is uncertain. On the other hand, renal biopsy is a must for a child with lupus nephritis for its diagnostic and prognostic value.

Berard R. Approach to the child with joint inflammation. *Pediatr Clin North Am.* 2012;59:245–62.

17.5 JUVENILE IDIOPATHIC ARTHRITIS

Juvenile idiopathic arthritis (JIA) is the commonest cause of chronic arthritis in children and is also the commonest autoimmune disease in children. It has a prevalence rate of 1 in 1000 children under the age of 16 years.

Definition

For the diagnosis of JIA, it is important that the child has ALL of the following:
1. Arthritis persisting for longer than 6 weeks (chronic arthritis)
2. Arthritis beginning before 16 years of age
3. Exclusion of other conditions associated with or mimicking arthritis

Pathogenesis

Lymphocytic inflammation of synovium makes it hyperemic and thickened and this thickened synovium (pannus) protrudes into the joint space. Pannus causes destruction of underlying articular cartilage and bones by proteolytic enzymes.

Clinical Features

Main clinical feature of JIA is persistent joint swelling in the absence of any defined cause, which begins before the age of 16 years. Other features of inflammation in joint may be:
- *Pain* Pain is common but not consistent. It is many times absent in preschool children who cannot describe their symptoms. In such children, parents may notice limp if lower limb joints are involved.
- *Stiffness* Early morning stiffness is a variable feature. Stiffness improves with movement, and is helped by a warm bath or shower.
- *Redness over joint* This is an unusual feature of JIA and is hardly ever seen.
- *Diminished range of movements* Besides joint involvement, systemic features may also be seen in JIA.
- High grade fever, transient skin rash, hepatosplenomegaly and lymphadenopathy may be seen in patients with systemic arthritis.
- Uveitis is commonly seen in patients with oligoarthritis.

Clinical Patterns of JIA

JIA is not a single disease; rather a group of heterogenous diseases. It has been classified into following categories by International League of Associations for Rheumatology (ILAR). Definition and differetiating features are summarized in **Tables 17.6** and **17.7**.
1. **Polyarthritis** (≥5 joints in first 6 months of disease)
   - Rheumatoid factor positive
   - Rheumatoid factor negative
2. **Oligoarthritis**
   - Persistent (<5 joints in the first 6 months of disease or throughout the disease course)
   - Extended (onset is oligoarticular but >4 joints affected after the first 6 months of disease)
3. **Systemic onset** (arthritis with typical rash and fever)
4. **Other categories**
   - Psoriatic arthrititis
   - Enthesitis related arthritis

Types of JIA

1. Systemic Arthritis

Systemic arthritis usually begins in early childhood with prominent extra-articular features. High grade quotidian (daily) fever is a prominent clinical feature. Typically, child is well in between two spikes of fever. Rash is erythematous, evanescent, maculopapular, and obvious only at the height of the fever. It is usually confined to the axillary region, anterior chest wall, and inside both thighs. There may be generalized lymphadenopathy and hepatosplenomegaly.

The systemic features usually resolve after a few months but may last indefinitely. The pattern of arthritis is variable, ranging from a few swollen joints to a widespread polyarthritis. This subtype is associated with a bad prognosis with severe growth delay, deforming arthritis, and complications of chronic corticosteroid use. Macrophage activation syndrome (MAS) and amyloidosis are most common complications seen in this subtype.

2. Oligoarticular JIA

Persistent oligoarthritis This subtype of JIA affects preschool girls. The knee is the most frequently affected joint, followed by the ankle and wrist. These children are at the highest risk for chronic anterior uveitis. Chronic anterior uveitis is clinically silent and insidiously progressive; it results in visual loss and blindness if not detected and treated early. Hence these children should be examined periodically for uveitis. ANA is frequently positive and predicts ocular involvement.

Extended oligoarthritis One-third of children with oligoarthritis (having <5 joint involvement in first 6 months) develop arthritis in more joints thereafter, hence this subgroup is called extended oligoarthritis. Many of these children also develop anterior uveitis. Prognosis in this subtype is similar to polyarthritis.

3. Polyarticular JIA

Polyarthritis (Rheumatoid factor (RF) negative) This subtype usually affects preschool girls who develop symmetrical arthritis of upper and lower limbs. Both large and small joints are involved. Risk of chronic anterior uveitis is less than in oligoarthritis. ANA is usually positive and RF is always negative.

Polyarthritis (Rheumatoid factor positive) This subtype is seen in older girls and behaves like rheumatoid arthritis in adults. The arthritis involves both large and small joints and can be rapidly progressive and destructive.

4. Others

Psoriatic arthritis Arthritis may predate the onset of the classic skin findings of psoriasis by many years. The articular involvement is often asymmetrical, and tends to affect both small and large joints. Extra-articular features of psoriasis can be present in first degree relatives. Asymptomatic uveitis can occur.

Enthesitis related arthritis (ERA) ERA begins after the age of 6 years and affects boys more often. Enthesitis which is described as inflammation of the point where a tendon,

17

ILAR category	Definition	Exclusion criteria
Table 17.6 ILAR Classification Criteria for JIA		
Systemic arthritis	Arthritis with or preceded by daily fever of at least 2 weeks that is documented to be daily ("quotidian") for at least 3 days and one or more of the following: • Evanescent (non-fixed) erythematous rash • Hepatomegaly and/or splenomegaly • Generalized lymphadenopathy • Serositis	a,b,c,d
Oligoarthritis	Arthritis affecting 1–4 joints during the first 6 months of disease Subcategories • *Persistent oligoarthritis*: Affecting no more than 4 joints throughout the disease course • *Extended oligoarthritis*: Affecting a total of more than 4 joints after the first 6 months of disease	a,b,c,d,e
Polyarthritis (RF negative)	Arthritis affecting 5 or more joints during the first 6 months of disease (RF negative)	a,b,c,d,e
Polyarthritis (RF positive)	Arthritis affecting 5 or more joints during the first 6 months of disease (RF positive)	a,b,c,e
Psoriatic arthritis	Arthritis and psoriasis or arthritis and at least 2 of these: Dactylitis, nail pitting or onycholysis, psoriasis in a first-degree relative	b,c,d,e
Enthesitis related arthritis	Arthritis and enthesitis or Arthritis or enthesitis with at least 2 of the following • Presence of or a history of sacroiliac joint tenderness and/or inflammatory lumbosacral pain • HLA-B27 antigen +· • Onset of arthritis in a male over 6 years of age • Acute (symptomatic) anterior uveitis • History of ankylosing spondylitis, enthesitis related arthritis, sacroiliitis with inflammatory bowel disease, Reiter syndrome, or acute anterior uveitis in a first-degree relative	a,d,e
Undifferentiated arthritis	Criteria in no category or >1 above-mentioned categories	

Exclusion criteria

a. Psoriasis or a history of psoriasis in the patient or first degree relative
b. Arthritis in an HLA-B27 positive male beginning after the 6th birthday
c. Ankylosing spondylitis, enthesitis related arthritis, sacroiliitis with inflammatory bowel disease, Reiter syndrome, or acute anterior uveitis, or a history of one of these disorders in a first-degree relative
d. Presence of IgM rheumatoid factor on at least 2 occasions at least 3 months apart
e. Presence of systemic JIA

ligament, or fascia inserts into the bone, is one of the typical clinical features. Arthritis usually involves large joints of lower limb and is usually asymmetrical. It may be a precursor illness to ankylosing spondylitis. These children are predisposed to acute recurrent symptomatic uveitis. HLA-B27 antigen may be found in 50% of patients.

Investigations

Diagnosis of JIA is clinical and no single laboratory test helps in diagnosis. Investigations in children with arthritis help in ruling out important differential diagnosis and in classifying JIA.

• ESR and CRP, if raised, are useful but up to a third of JIA patients, esp those with oligoarthritis, have normal CRP and ESR.
• Rheumatoid factor (RF) helps to classify polyarthritis.
• Antinuclear antibody (ANA) helps in determining the risk of chronic anterior uveitis.

• HLA-B27 may be positive in 50% of children with ERA.
• Coagulation studies are useful if suspecting hemarthrosis.
• Joint radiographs are hardly ever required in a typical case of JIA. However, they do help to rule out differentials like fracture, avascular necrosis, osteomyelitis, bone tumor, and skeletal dysplasia.
• Synovial fluid aspiration is usually not required; however, it is a must for any child with suspected septic arthritis.
• Synovial biopsy is hardly ever indicated for the diagnosis.

Complications of JIA

Complications can be classified as articular or extra-articular.

Articular complications These arise due to prolonged inflammation and include contractures, ankylosis, asymmetric growth, and limb length discrepancy. These complications can be reduced with early and aggressive therapy.

Table 17.7 Juvenile Idiopathic Arthritis: Classification and Subtypes

	Oligoarthritis	Polyarthritis		Systemic JIA
		Rheumatoid factor negative	*Rheumatoid factor positive*	*Systemic JIA*
Proportion of all	50–60%	30%	<10%	<10%
Joints involved (no.)	<5	≥5	≥5	Variable
Joints involved	Knees, ankles,	Asymmetric/symmetric; large/small, cervical spine	Symmetrical small and large joints	Knees, wrists, cervical spine, ankles, finger, neck, hips
Age at onset	1–5 years	2–5 years	Teenagers	Any age; commonest <5 years
Male/female ratio	4:1	3:1	9:1	1:1
Rheumatoid factor	Negative	Negative	Positive	Negative
Extra-articular features	Chronic uveitis	Chronic uveitis		Daily high fever, transient non-itchy erythematous rash, lymphadenopathy, hepato-splenomegaly, serositis
ANA	80% of those with uveitis are ANA +ve	ANA +ve in 40%	ANA +ve in 50%	
Prognosis	Resolves spontaneously Uveitis must be managed early	Generally good prognosis	Poorer prognosis with severe disability	Chronic erosive arthritis in 25%. Most have self-limiting disease
Treatment	NSAID and intra-articular steroids	NSAID and methotrexate		Biologicals: Anakinra, tocilizumab, methotrexate

Extra-articular complications These include uveitis, macrophage activation syndrome (MAS) and amyloidosis. Whereas MAS and amyloidosis are more common in systemic arthritis, uveitis is most common in oligoarthritis.

Macrophage activation syndrome This is a secondary hemophagocytic histiocytosis (HLH) occurring in children with active systemic arthritis. It is characterized by the sudden development of fever, diffuse intravascular coagulation (DIC), hepatosplenomegaly, pancytopenia, abrupt decrease in the ESR (because of low fibrinogen), very high ferritin, and elevated serum levels of liver enzymes and triglycerides. Fibrin degradation products are present and hypofibrinogenemia is induced by DIC. Bone marrow examination may show active hemophagocytosis by macrophages and histiocytes. MAS must be treated rapidly since it is associated with high mortality. The conventional approach is to administer intravenous methylprednisolone pulse therapy with or without cyclosporine.

Amyloidosis It is seen with uncontrolled systemic arthritis or polyarthritis of many years' duration and is attributed to persistent inflammation.

Chronic anterior uveitis Seen predominantly in oligoarthritis, it is often clinically silent and insidiously progressive. Presence of ANA helps in predicting the risk of uveitis. Routine follow-up for eye disease is a must in all children with JIA.

Treatment   **Juvenile Idiopathic Arthritis**

The goal of therapy is to maintain a good quality of life while preserving joint function. Early and aggressive management helps in achieving this goal. Overall management can be divided into two components:

- *Drug therapy* Nonsteroidal anti-inflammatory drugs (NSAID), glucocorticoids, disease modifying anti-rheumatic drugs (DMARDs) like methotrexate, biologic response modifiers, and miscellaneous drugs like leflunomide, sulphasalazine, thalidomide
- *Supportive management* Counseling and education about disease, physiotherapy, occupational therapy.

Pharmacotherapy

Nonsteroidal anti-inflammatory drugs (NSAID)
Treatment of children with arthritis usually begins with NSAIDs, including naproxen or ibuprofen (15–20 mg/kg per day in 2 divided doses). Anti-inflammatory effect of NSAID takes 4 to 8 weeks for full action; hence they must be continued for 4–8 weeks before their efficacy can be ascertained. Adverse effects include abdominal pain, which can be minimized by taking the NSAID with food. Mild asthma is not a contraindication to the use of NSAIDs. Naproxen has the additional risk of inducing pseudoporphyria. Majority of patients with early JIA do not respond completely to NSAIDs and need more aggressive treatment.

Glucocorticoids
Intra-articular steroid is most frequently used form of glucocorticoids in JIA. A single injection resolves signs of joint

17

inflammation in most patients for several months. Systemic steroids should be avoided if possible because of significant adverse effects. The use of oral prednisolone is limited to short-term and at low doses (5–10 mg per day) for children with severe polyarthritis or systemic arthritis (as a bridge therapy to overcome acute severe symptoms).

Methotrexate

Methotrexate is effective in approximately 70% of children with polyarthritis but much less so in systemic arthritis. It should be considered for any child whose arthritis is not well controlled with a trial of NSAIDs with or without intra-articular steroids after 4–12 weeks. It can be administered either orally or subcutaneously once a week at a dose of 10–20 mg/m^2. Effect is seen after 1–3 months. The most common adverse events are nausea, mouth ulcers, abdominal pain, elevated liver enzymes, hair loss, and bone marrow suppression. Oral folic acid supplements (1 mg/day) help to reduce side effects.

Biologic response modifiers

Tumor necrosis factor (TNF) inhibitors TNF inhibitors are more effective if administered early in the disease in combination with methotrexate and/or prednisone. Commonly used drugs are listed below:

- Etanercept (0.8 mg/kg weekly subcutaneously)
- Adalimumab, a recombinant human anti-TNF agent, at a dose of 20 or 40 mg every 2 weeks for children less than 30 kg and those weighing more than 30 kg, respectively, a dosage of 24 mg/m^2 (maximum 40 mg) every 2 weeks.

Administration of anti-TNF agents has been associated with an increased risk of tuberculosis infection. Hence, baseline screening and careful monitoring during the course of treatment are mandatory.

Abatacept This is a soluble, fully human fusion protein that comprises the extracellular portion of human CTLA4 and a fragment of the Fc region of a human IgG1. The binding between abatacept and the CD80/86 molecules prevents their interaction with the CD28 receptor and, therefore, blocks the second signal necessary for T cell activation. Abatacept is registered for use in JIA for patients older than 6 years at the dosage of 10 mg/kg intravenously every 28 days.

Tocilizumab This is an interleukin-6 (IL-6) receptor inhibitor, and used both in systemic arthritis and polyarthritis at doses of 10 mg/kg if less than 30 kg or 8 mg/kg if at least 30 kg and is given every 2–4 weeks.

Anakinra An IL-1 receptor antagonist, it has been used in systemic arthritis; however this drug is not available in India.

Supportive Therapy

Parents should be educated about the disease and its likely course. This helps in ensuring compliance. Periodic eye evaluation should be emphasized. Physiotherapy and occupational therapy help in maintaining range of movement across joint along with improving strength of periarticular muscles. An exercise program is advised to restore motion and strength of the joint. Proper nutrition, along with iron and vitamin supplements should be advised.

Surgery Need for surgery to correct contractures and limb length discrepancies have markedly reduced with advent of aggressive disease modifying agents. In children who are treated early and aggressively, one may not see any articular complications.

Prognosis

JIA is a diverse group of conditions associated with persistent arthritis. Whereas children with oligoarthritis tend to do well in terms of arthritis, children with polyarthritis and systemic arthritis may continue to have disease into adulthood.

Revision Point

Juvenile Idiopathic Arthritis

1. Diagnosis of JIA is clinical based on typical pattern characterized by persistent swelling of one or more joints (for >6 weeks), beginning before the age of 16 years, and without any clear cause being identified.
2. Differential diagnosis includes septic arthritis, neoplasia such as acute lymphoblastic leukemia, rheumatic fever, and non-accidental injury.
3. No single laboratory test is diagnostic of JIA and role of investigations lies in excluding differential diagnoses, to classify JIA and to monitor the disease.
4. Drug treatment for JIA begins with NSAIDs and intra-articular corticosteroids, with early use of methotrexate.
5. Biologic disease modifiers (etanercept, etc.) have revolutionized management of children with refractory JIA.
6. Physiotherapy and occupational therapy are important supportive therapies to prevent complications.

Blazina Š, Markelj G, Avramoviè MZ, *et al*. Management of Juvenile idiopathic arthritis: a clinical guide. *Paediatr Drugs*. 2016;18:397–412.

Cimaz R. Systemic-onset juvenile idiopathic arthritis. *Autoimmun Rev*. 2016;15:931–4.

Clarke SL, Sen ES, Ramanan AV. Juvenile idiopathic arthritis-associated uveitis. *Pediatr Rheumatol Online J*. 2016;14:27.

Giancane G, Alongi A, Ravelli A. Update on the pathogenesis and treatment of juvenile idiopathic arthritis. *Curr Opin Rheumatol*. 2017 May 22. [Epub ahead of print].

Giancane G, Consolaro A, Lanni S, *et al*. Juvenile idiopathic arthritis: diagnosis and treatment. *Rheumatol Ther*. 2016;3:187–207.

Wilson BA, Cooper M, Barber CE. Standards of care for inflammatory arthritis: A literature review. *Semin Arthritis Rheum*. 2017 Mar 6. [Epub ahead of print].

17.6 SYSTEMIC LUPUS ERYTHEMATOSUS

Systemic lupus erythematosus (SLE) is a multisystem autoimmune disease with resultant changes in skin, joints, kidneys, and other organs. It is usually described as a disease of young girls; usually above the age of 8 years.

Etiology

It is an autoimmune disorder occurring in genetically predisposed individuals, and triggered by certain factors like drugs, infection, or ultraviolet rays. The childhood SLE has a more severe course and a poor prognosis than the adult disease.

Clinical Features

Clinical features of SLE are variable and it can involve any organ system of the body. Commonly, it presents with fever, fatigue, weight loss, and anorexia. Multisystem involvement is more common though a single system may be affected at the onset. Skin, musculoskeletal, and renal systems are more commonly involved in childhood SLE. Gastrointestinal disease, liver involvement, and myocarditis are extremely rare.

Mucocutaneous Involvement

1. Malar or buttery rash (Fig. 17.6) is the most characteristic cutaneous manifestation. It is typically seen over malar eminences crossing the nasal bridge but spares the nasolabial folds.
2. Less common manifestations are discoid lupus lesions (erythematous coin shaped lesions with central hypopigmentation and peripheral hyperpigmentation and usually seen on face, ears, and scalp) and vasculitic rashes on digits, pinnae, or nares.
3. Oral cavity may show painless ulceration over hard palate.
4. Alopecia may be one of the presenting manifestations of the disease. It occurs classically in the frontal area.
5. Photosensitivity is an important characteristic of the skin lesions in SLE.

Musculoskeletal involvement Arthralgia and arthritis are very common. Arthritis however is non-erosive unlike the arthritis of JIA.

Renal involvement Renal disease is the most dreaded complication of SLE. Lupus nephritis is present in almost 75% children with SLE. It manifests as proteinuria, microscopic hematuria, hypertension, and elevated blood urea and serum creatinine. Routine urine microscopy, spot urine for protein and creatinine ratio and renal function tests are must for any child at diagnosis and periodically during follow-up. Low complement levels (C3, C4) and elevated anti-dsDNA levels are usual in children with lupus nephritis.

Neuropsychiatric involvement Neuropsychiatric involvement occurs in 20–70% of children with SLE and can involve practically any part of central or peripheral nervous system. Common manifestations include headache, seizures, altered sensorium, psychosis, stroke, transverse myelitis. Other manifestations include polyneuropathy, myelopathy, cerebellar ataxia, aseptic meningitis, and cranial nerve palsies.

Hematologic involvement Anemia, thrombocytopenia, and leukopenia are seen in 50–75% of patients. Anemia can occur due to chronic disease or autoimmune hemolysis. Coombs test may be positive. Thrombocytopenia may be the first presentation of disease presenting as spontaneous mucocutaneous bleeding or menorrhagia. Leukopenia is seen in 20–40% of cases of childhood SLE. Lymphopenia is a sensitive marker of disease activity.

Pulmonary involvement Pulmonary involvement can present as pleuritis, pneumonitis, pulmonary hemorrhage, pulmonary hypertension, and pulmonary embolism.

Cardiac involvement Symptomatic pericarditis with pericardial effusion is the most common cardiac manifestation. Myocardial and endocardial involvements are less common.

Neonatal lupus erythematosus This syndrome occurs in infants born to mothers with anti-Ro/SSA and anti-La/SSB antibodies. Mother may have SLE or another connective tissue disorder or may also be asymptomatic. In infants, it is characterized by a photosensitive skin rash and congenital heart block. Skin manifestations usually subside by 6 months of age (because of disappearance of maternally transmitted antibodies), however congenital heart block is permanent.

Investigations

Role of investigations in SLE lies in confirming the diagnosis, ruling out differential diagnosis, and assessing severity of organ involvement and associated comorbidities. For confirmation of diagnosis, one needs following investigations:

1. *Complement (C3 and C4) levels are* usually reduced in presence of active lupus nephritis.
2. *Antinuclear antibody* is positive in > 95% patients with SLE. If ANA is negative in an appropriate setting, it helps to rule out SLE; however this test has significant false positivity.
3. *Extractable nuclear antigen panel* detects different autoantibodies to subcellular structures and should be done only if ANA test is positive in high titres. This test helps in differentiating SLE from other autoimmune diseases. Anti-Smith and anti-double stranded DNA antibodies are highly specific for SLE.
   - Antibodies to ds DNA are present in 70% patients and indicate active disease and increased risk of nephritis.
   - Anti-Smith (Sm) antibodies are considered to be markers for CNS disease.
4. *Antiphospholipid antibodies* increase risk of thrombosis in children with SLE.

For assessing organ dysfunction, complete blood count, renal and liver function tests, and urine analysis are must for any child with SLE. Direct Coombs test may be needed in children with anemia. Other tests like renal biopsy, neuroimaging are done as dictated by clinical presentation.

Diagnosis

The Systemic Lupus International Collaborating Clinics (SLICC) network presented a new set of classification criteria in 2012 (SLICC-12). The classification criteria developed by SLICC are meant for research studies and clinical research, but are often used in the clinical setting for diagnosis also (**Table 17.8**).

Treatment **SLE**

Treatment of SLE is aimed at achieving good control of disease while minimizing side-effects of medications and facilitating growth and development. It is generally based on presence or absence of life or organ threatening complications.

Children with no significant life or organ threatening complications

Oral corticosteroids are started in low dose (<0.35 mg/kg/day) and then gradually tapered off. Hydroxychloroquine is used as adjunct in all patients with SLE. This drug is particularly useful in skin and joint disease and is used at a dose no more than 5–6.5 mg/kg/day. Eye screening is done at baseline and then annually to detect ocular complications associated with hydroxychloroquine. Low-dose methotrexate can be added for better control of joint and skin symptoms. Sun protection measures are must for every patient with SLE.

Table 17.8 Systemic Lupus International Collaborating Clinics (SLICC-12) Criteria for Classication of SLE (2012)

Clinical	Criteria
Acute cutaneous lupus or sub-acute cutaneous lupus	Acute cutaneous lupus: Lupus malar rash; bullous lupus; toxic epidermal necrolysis variant of SLE; maculopapular lupus rash; photosensitive lupus rash; subacute cutaneous lupus
Chronic cutaneous lupus	Classic discoid rash; localized (above the neck); generalized (above and below the neck); hypertrophic (verrucous) lupus; lupus panniculitis (profundus); mucosal lupus; lupus erythematosus tumidus; chilblains lupus; OR discoid lupus/lichen planus overlap
Nonscarring alopecia	Diffuse thinning or hair fragility with visible broken hairs (in the absence of other causes, such as alopecia areata, drugs, iron deficiency, and androgenic alopecia)
Oral ulcers or nasal ulcers	Palate, buccal, tongue, OR nasal ulcers (in the absence of other causes, such as vasculitis, Behçet's disease, infection [herpes virus], inflammatory bowel disease, reactive arthritis, and acidic foods)
Arthritis	Synovitis involving two or more joints, characterized by swelling or effusion OR tenderness in two or more joints and at least 30 minutes of morning stiffness
Serositis	Typical pleurisy for more than one day, pleural effusions, or pleural rub, OR typical pericardial pain (pain with recumbency improved by sitting forward) for more than one day, pericardial effusion, pericardial rub, or pericarditis by electrocardiography in the absence of other causes, such as infection, uremia, and Dressler syndrome
Renal	Urine protein-to-creatinine ratio (or 24-hour urine protein) representing 500 mg protein/24 hours, OR red blood cell casts
Neurologic	Seizures; psychosis; mononeuritis multiplex (in the absence of other known causes, such as primary vasculitis); myelitis; peripheral or cranial neuropathy (in the absence of other known causes, such as primary vasculitis, infection, and diabetes mellitus); OR acute confusional state (in the absence of other causes, including toxic/metabolic, uremia, drugs)
Blood	Hemolytic anemia
Leukopenia or lymphopenia	Leukopenia (<4000/mm^3 at least once) (in the absence of other known causes, such as Felty syndrome, drugs, and portal hypertension), OR lymphopenia (<1000/mm^3 at least once) (in the absence of other known causes, such as glucocorticoids, drugs, and infection)
Thrombocytopenia	Thrombocytopenia (<100,000/mm^3) at least once in the absence of other known causes, such as drugs, portal hypertension, and thrombotic thrombocytopenic purpura
Immunologic criteria	
ANA	ANA level above laboratory reference range
Anti-dsDNA	Anti-dsDNA antibody level above laboratory reference range (or >2 folds the reference range if tested by ELISA)
Anti-Sm	Presence of antibody to Sm nuclear antigen
Antiphospholipid antibody	Antiphospholipid antibody positivity as determined by any of the following: Positive test result for lupus anticoagulant; false-positive test result for rapid plasma reagin; medium- or high-titer anticardiolipin antibody level (IgA, IgG, or IgM); or positive test result for anti-beta 2-glycoprotein I (IgA, IgG, or IgM)
Complements	Low C3; low C4; OR low CH50
Direct coombs test	Direct Coombs test in the absence of hemolytic anemia

- A patient is classified as having SLE if he or she satisfies four of the clinical and immunologic criteria including at least one clinical criterion and one immunologic criterion.
- Alternatively, a patient is classified as having SLE if he or she has biopsy-proven nephritis compatible with SLE in the presence of ANAs or anti-dsDNA antibodies.

Adapted from Petri M, Orbai AM, Alarcon GS, et al. Derivation and validation of the systemic lupus international collaborating clinics classification criteria for systemic lupus erythematosus. Arthritis Rheum. 2012;64:2677–86.

For patients with life or organ-threatening complications

Aggressive treatment is used to bring disease under control rapidly and then to maintain it in that condition. The regimens include combinations of high-dose steroids, steroid sparing agents, and supportive strategies.

- *Induction of remission* Initial phase is geared to bring disease under control as early as possible and uses aggressive immunosuppression with high-dose steroids such as pulse intravenous methylprednisolone at 30 mg/kg (maximum of 1 g) for 3 consecutive days, in combination with cyclophosphamide or mycophenolate mofetil (MMF). Pulse methylprednisolone is followed by oral steroids. Whereas cyclophosphamide is used intravenously at 2–4 weekly interval during this phase, MMF is used as daily oral therapy.

- *Maintenance of induction* This can be achieved with lesser degree of immunosuppression over longer duration. Both MMF and azathioprine are used. Azathioprine should be started at 1 mg/kg/day and increased slowly to reach a maximum of 2.5 mg/kg/day. Side-effects include nausea, fatigue, alopecia, liver dysfunction, and cytopenias. MMF is usually used at a dose of 1 g/day in divided doses as maintenance treatment. Oral hydroxychloroquine at a dose of 4–5 mg/kg/day, and low-dose oral steroids are continued during the maintenance phase.

Prognosis

SLE is a disease associated with remissions and flares. Hence all patients need periodic follow-ups to identify flares and other complications like infections. All patients and parents need to be educated for strict compliance to therapy. Renal, cardiac, and hematological manifestations are the main causes of death. Five-year survival rate in India is 75%.

SLE

1. SLE is a multisystemic autoimmune disease of childhood and can involve any part of the body.
2. Mucocutaneus, renal, and musculoskeletal involvement are frequent in childhood SLE.
3. Diagnosis is based on presence of clinical manifestations in association with immunologic criteria.
4. Negative ANA helps in excluding disease. False positive ANA is frequent; hence ANA should only be prescribed in appropriate setting.
5. Management is based on severity of clinical manifestations. Minor organ involvement like mucocutaneous and musculoskeletal needs low dose steroids and hydroxychloroquine besides supportive therapy like sun protection measures. Major organ involvement in SLE requires aggressive immunosuppression to save organ and life.
6. SLE is a disease associated with remissions and flares and a life-long follow-up is mandatory.

Borgia R, Silverman E. Childhood-onset systemic lupus erythematosus: An update. *Current Opin Rheumatol*. 2015;27;483–92.

Malattia C, Martini A. Paediatric onset systemic lupus eryrhematosus. *Best Pract Res Clin Rheumatol* . 2013;27:351–62.

Silverman E, Eddy A. Systemic Lupus Erythematosus. In: Cassidy JT, Petty RE, Laxer R, Lindsley C. *Textbook of Paediatric Rheumatology*. 6th ed. Philadelphia: Elsevier Saunders. 2010:315–43.

17.7 JUVENILE DERMATOMYOSITIS

Juvenile dermatomyositis (JDM) is the most common idiopathic inflammatory myopathy of childhood. It is a chronic autoimmune disease with specific clinical features involving skin and muscles, as the name suggests. The incidence of the disease is estimated at 3.2 per 10, 00,000 children per year. The age of onset is 7 years (4–10 years). A female preponderance is seen in Western countries.

Clinical Features

Onset is usually insidious with constitutional symptoms such as fever, fatigue, anorexia, and weight loss.

Mucocutaneus Disease

Periorbital heliotrope rash (Fig. 17.8) and Gottron papules (Fig. 17.9) are pathognomonic features. The periorbital heliotrope rash is dusky, violaceous erythema of the face specially the periorbital area with accompanying edema of the eyelids. Occasionally, it may follow a butterfly distribution extended to cheeks, and forehead. *Gottron papules* are small violaceous flat-topped papules involving the extensor surfaces overlying the joints—the knuckles, dorsal wrist, elbows, and the knees.

Periungual regions become erythematous and scaly with dilated capillary loops in the nailbeds. A more macular, erythematous rash may appear on the face, neck and anterior chest (*V sign*) or on the shoulder and upper back (*shawl sign*). Subcutaneous calcifications are present in 30–70% of affected children.

Musculoskeletal

Muscle weakness is symmetric and proximal. It is usually associated with local tenderness and subcutaneus edema in severe cases. The shoulder and hip girdles are commonly

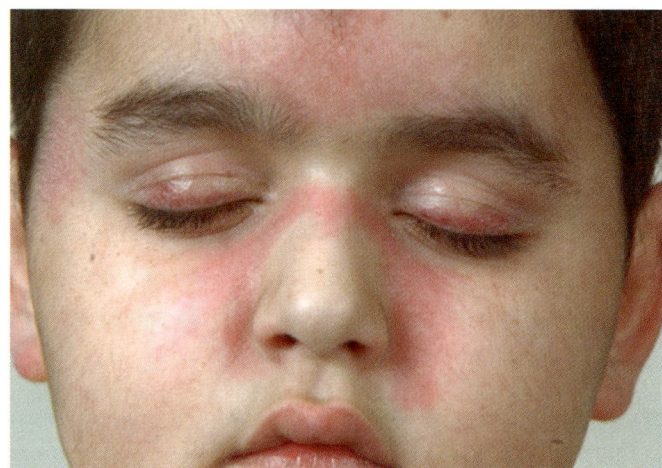

Fig. 17.8 Heliotrope rash in a child with juvenile dermatomyositis

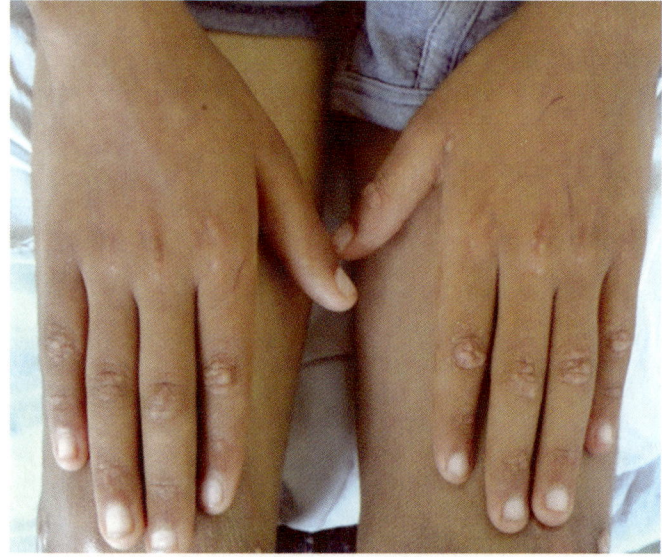

Fig. 17.9 Gottron papules in a child with juvenile dermatomyositis

involved. Gower sign may be positive. Anterior neck flexors are involved in severe cases. Palatal and pharyngeal muscle involvement can cause difficulty in deglutition, nasal regurgitation and nasal twang of speech. With typical skin and muscle features, diagnosis is not difficult.

Calcifications

At least 40% of children develop calcinosis at some point during the disease. It varies from discrete calcific nodules around the joints on the extensor surfaces to generalized calcinosis. Many patients have more difficulty with the calcium deposits than with the initial muscular inflammation.

Systemic Involvement

Less frequent findings include arthritis, and gastrointestinal complaints (gastrointestinal bleed, perforation). Dysphagia or regurgitation may result from palatal, pharyngeal, or esophageal muscular involvement.

Investigations

Certain investigations can help to confirm the muscle involvement and also help in monitoring of disease.

1. Muscle Enzymes

Creatine kinase (CK), aspartate transaminase, lactate dehydrogenase (LDH) and aldolase are usually raised in acute stage and start falling on treatment. Rise in enzymes on treatment can help predict a disease relapse before clinical features set in.

2. Imaging Studies

Magnetic resonance imaging (MRI) of proximal muscles especially thighs is frequently used to document objective evidence of muscle edema and inflammatory changes. Plain radiograph may reveal calcinosis in long bones/spine.

3. Autoantibodies

Since JDM is an autoimmune disease, various autoantibodies have been found in patients with JDM. However, these are not routinely used in clinical diagnosis or management of these patients. Anti-nuclear antibodies (ANA) are present in half of the cases. Rheumatoid factor is negative.

4. Inflammatory Parameters

Markers of acute inflammation like C-reactive protein and ESR are elevated.

5. Electromyography and Muscle Biopsy

These are invasive procedures and hence are not commonly used in children with typical skin and *muscle features of the disease.*

Diagnosis

Diagnosis is traditionally based on Bohan and Peter criteria (**Table 17.9**). However, since the advent of MRI, invasive tests like electromyography and muscle biopsy are not frequently used.

Table 17.9 Bohan and Peter Criteria for Diagnosis of Juvenile Dermatomyositis

1. Characteristic rashes of dermatomyositis
2. Symmetrical weakness, usually progressive, of the limb-girdle muscles
3. Elevation of serum levels of muscle-associated enzymes (creatine kinase, aldolase, lactate dehydrogenase, transaminases)
4. Electromyographic evidence of myopathy
5. Muscle biopsy evidence of myositis

Definite dermatomyositis: Rash plus three other criteria
Probable dermatomyositis: Rash plus two other criteria
Possible dermatomyositis: Rash plus one other criterion

Adapted from Bohan A, Peter JB. Polymyositis and dermatomyositis (parts 1 and 2). New Engl J Med 1975;292:344–7,403–7

Complications

Complications are seen in JDM in acute phase as well as in long-term.

Acute Complications

- Swallowing dysfunction
- Aspiration pneumonia
- Respiratory compromise due to respiratory muscle involvement and may be complicated further by aspiration pneumonia due to swallowing dysfunction
- Gastrointestinal hemorrhage due to vasculopathy

Long-term Complications

- *Calcinosis* (Fig. 17.10) It is seen as dystrophic calcification over the elbows, knee, digits and buttocks. There can be serious morbidity due to ulceration of the deposit, contractures and pain due to nerve entrapment.
- *Lipodystrophy* This is a late complication of JDM associated with progressive generalized loss of subcutaneous and

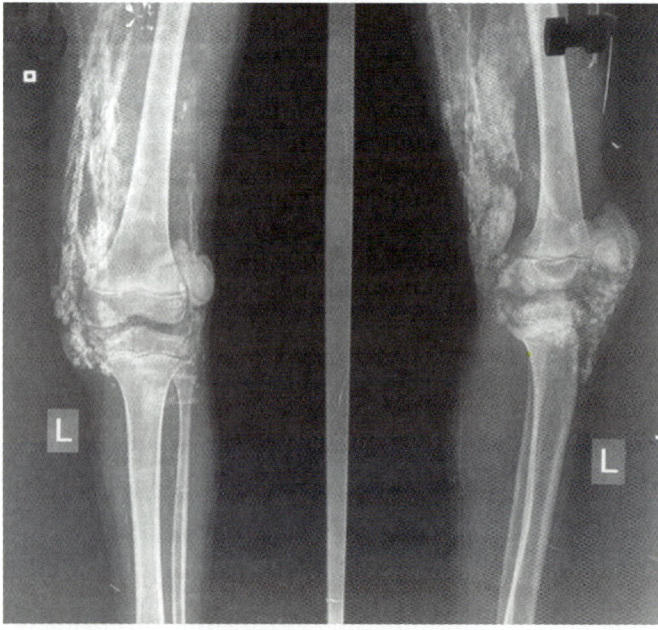

Fig. 17.10 Calcinosis cutis

visceral fat. It is usually associated with metabolic complications like hyperglycemia and derangement in serum lipids.

Differential Diagnosis

The differential diagnoses include muscular dystrophy, which can be differentiated on the basis of a selective muscular involvement, progression, and positive family history. Other differentials include congenital myopathies, and myasthenia gravis. Myositis can occur with viral infections, especially influenza B, Coxsackie B, and ECHO viruses and it is self-limiting condition.

Treatment	Juvenile Dermatomyositis

Corticosteroids are used to halt the inflammatory process. Use of steroids has reduced mortality of JDM from 33–40% to 2%. Steroids are started at high doses (methylprednisolone 30 mg/kg/d × 3 days) and then tapered gradually over several weeks with prednisolone (1 mg/kg/day) depending on response. Steroid sparing immunosuppressants are started upfront so that steroids can be tapered off quickly. Usual choice would be methotrexate which is given weekly at a dose of 15–20 mg/m^2. In more severe cases, one can use pulse cyclophosphamide.

Intravenous immunoglobulin (2 g/kg/month) has been used in treatment of refractory disease/rapidly progressive disease. Early aggressive therapy with steroids and steroid sparing agents helps in reducing risk of chronic complications like calcinosis.

Supportive Therapy

Besides immunosuppression, supportive care is very important. Children, who have poor gag reflex suggesting weakness of pharyngeal musculature, should be given nasogastric feeding with frequent oral suctions to prevent aspiration. Physiotherapy aims to prevent development of contractures and improve functional ability. Skin care is achieved by use of emollients, and sun protecting agents for photosensitive rash.

Revision Point

Juvenile Dermatomyositis

1. Juvenile dermatomyositis is the commonest idiopathic inflammatory myopathy of childhood.
2. Typical manifestations are related to skin and muscles. Heliotrope rash and Gottron papules are typical skin manifestations whereas proximal muscle involvement is the typical muscle disease.
3. Diagnosis is supported by markedly elevated muscle enzymes and suggestive MRI of involved muscles.
4. Early aggressive therapy with steroids and steroid sparing agents (usually methotrexate) is the mainstay of therapy.
5. Supportive therapy is vital for a good outcome.
6. Calcinosis and lipodystrophy are common complications of JDM.

Feldman BM, *et al*. Juvenile dermatomyositis and other idiopathic inflammatory myopathies of childhood. Lancet. 2008;371:2201–12.
Milone M. Diagnosis and management of immune-mediated myopathies. *Mayo Clin Proc.* 2017;92:826–37.

Case Study	Juvenile Dermatomyositis

A 10-year-old girl presented with difficulty in climbing stairs and getting up from sitting posture for last 2 months. This difficulty was insidiously progressive. She also had low grade fever. Examination findings were characteristic with heliotrope rash and Gottron papules. Weakness of trunk and proximal limbs was present with significant tenderness on palpation.

How sure are you about the diagnosis of JDM?

With typical skin features (Heliotrope rash and Gottron papules) and proximal muscle weakness, diagnosis of JDM does not seem to be in doubt. Muscle enzymes and MRI of thigh muscles will help in confirming the diagnosis. In presence of typical skin manifestations, electromyography and muscle biopsy are usually not needed. If skin features are absent, one needs to think of other causes of proximal muscle weakness like myopathy, muscle dystrophy, etc.

What acute emergencies can be seen in these children?

Respiratory compromise can occur in acute stage due to respiratory muscle involvement and aspiration pneumonia due to swallowing dysfunction. One must look for features such as neck flexor weakness, poor gag, and respiratory compromise at presentation. Poor gag warrants stoppage of oral feeding, starting nasogastric feeds, and frequent oral suctioning to prevent aspiration. Gastrointestinal hemorrhage due to vasculopathy is an uncommon emergency associated with significant mortality.

Papadopoulou C, Wedderburn LR. Treatment of Juvenile dermatomyositis: An update. *Paediatr Drugs*. 2017 May 26 [Epub ahead of print].
Thompson C, Piguet V, Choy E. The pathogenesis of dermatomyositis. *Br J Dermatol*. 2017 May 24. [Epub ahead of print].

17.8 VASCULITIS SYNDROMES

Vasculitis is defined as inflammation of vessel wall. For the sake of ease, we have classified vasculitis in three types:

- *Large vessels* Vessels like aorta and major branches arising from aorta; prototype condition being *Takayasu arteritis* (aortoarteritis)
- *Medium vessels* All vessels other than large and small vessels; prototype conditions being *Kawasaki disease, polyarteritis nodosa*
- *Small vessels* Small arteries in tissues, arterioles, capillaries and venules; prototype condition being *Henoch-Schonlein purpura* (HSP).

Clinical Presentation

Vessel involvement can be *localized* involving a few organs like skin, kidney, etc. or can be *systemic* involving many organs. Also, vasculitis can occur secondary to systemic conditions such as infections, malignancies, and rheumatological conditions like systemic lupus erythematosus.

Vasculitis can also be *acute* or *chronic*. The consequences of vasculitis depend on the type of vessel involved, area where vessels are involved, and severity of inflammation. Significant inflammation can cause ischemia of the tissue.

Vasculitis can cause nonspecific inflammatory symptoms like fever, anorexia and weight loss. Depending on type of vessel involved, clinical features can be as follows:

Box 17.2 Organ Specific Clinical Features of Vasculitis

- *Skin*: Palpable purpura, livedo reticularis
- *Musculoskeletal*: Myalgia/myositis, arthralgia/arthritis
- *Nervous system*: Mononeuritis multiplex, headache, stroke, tinnitus, reduced visual acuity, acute visual loss
- *Heart and arteries*: Myocardial infarction, hypertension, absent pulses, gangrene
- *Respiratory tract*: Nose bleeds, hemoptysis, lung infiltrates
- *Gastrointestinal tract*: Abdominal pain, bloody stool, perforation
- *Kidneys*: Glomerulonephritis, renal infarcts

1. *Large vessel vasculitis* Absent pulses, claudication, bruits, hypertension
2. *Medium vessel vasculitis* Skin rash, tender nodules, hypertension, abdominal angina, orchitis, gangrene, mononeuritis multiplex
3. *Small vessel vasculitis* Purpura, glomerulonephritis, mucosal ulcers, asthma, symptoms related to ear, nose, throat.

Organ specific symptoms and signs depend upon the organ involved **(Box 17.2)**.

Investigations

Investigations in a child with vasculitis depend on the type of vessel involved and area in which vessels are involved. Neutrophilic leukocytosis, thrombocytosis, raised erythrocyte sedimentation rate (ESR) and raised C-reactive protein are usual. However, they do not point to any specific vasculitis. Indirect clues can be seen on routine investigations like hematuria, proteinuria, deranged renal functions, and abnormal chest radiographs, in children with renal and pulmonary involvement, respectively.

Diagnosis

Diagnosis of vasculitis depends on demonstration of inflammation in vessel wall and hence is expected to be histopathological. Various tissue biopsies, depending on the organs involved, can be done to demonstrate vessel wall inflammation; however, this is not possible for large arteries because of the risks involved. *Histopathological diagnosis is required for small vessel and medium vessel vasculitis*. For large vessel vasculitis and some medium vessel vasculitis, diagnosis rests on vascular imaging, which can include angiography, ultrasound Doppler, and echocardiography.

Treatment

Management of vasculitis depends on type of vasculitis and will be discussed further with discussion of specific vasculitides.

17.9 KAWASAKI DISEASE

Kawasaki disease (KD) is an acute systemic medium vessel vasculitis of childhood with a tendency to cause coronary artery abnormalities. It was first reported from Japan in early 1960s by Dr Tomisaku Kawasaki as mucocutaneous lymph node syndrome. It has now been described worldwide and is now the leading cause of acquired heart disease in children.

Epidemiology

Japan has a maximum incidence of KD with rates of 240/1,00,000 children less than 5 years. Korea and Taiwan have reported the next high incidences. Whereas the incidence in USA (20 per 1,00,000 children less than 5 years) is static over years, Japan has been reporting increasing incidence rates over years. Incidence is not well known in Indian population.

Etiology

The exact etiology is unknown. Kawasaki disease appears to be a stereotyped pathological immune response to one or a variety of environmental or infectious triggers, to which certain individuals are predisposed by virtue of their genetic constitution. Eighty percent of affected cases are younger than the age of 5 years, with an average age of approximately 2 years and there is slight male preponderance. Reports from India have shown that 40% of affected children are above the age of 5 years.

Pathogenesis

Kawasaki disease is characterized by intensive T cell stimulation with activation of inflammatory cytokines and leukocyte recruitment. This leads to upregulation of proteolytic activity causing elastin degradation and vessel wall damage, which is responsible for characteristic coronary lesions seen in this disease.

Clinical Features

The diagnosis is entirely clinical. Characteristic features include fever, polymorphous exanthema, bilateral conjunctival congestion, changes in extremities, changes in lips and oral cavity, and cervical adenopathy.

- *Fever* is typically high grade (>39°C) with an abrupt onset and responds transiently to antipyretics. Usually fever persists for more than 5 days and can persist for more than 3 weeks, if not treated.
- *Rash* is usually a diffuse erythematous maculopapular rash which appears within first five days of illness.
- *Conjunctivitis* is typically bilateral, non-exudative (no discharge) and spares limbus (Fig. 17.11).
- *Changes in extremities* include diffuse non-pitting edema on the dorsum of hands and feet and characteristic periungual desquamation (Fig. 17.12) starting in late

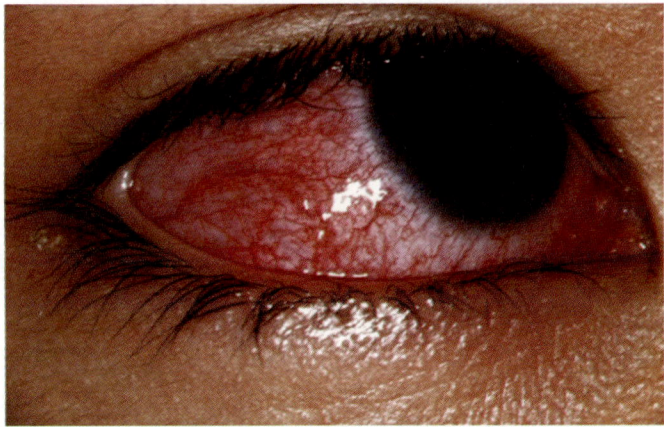

Fig. 17.11 Nonexudative conjunctivitis sparing limbus in a child with Kawasaki disease (KD)

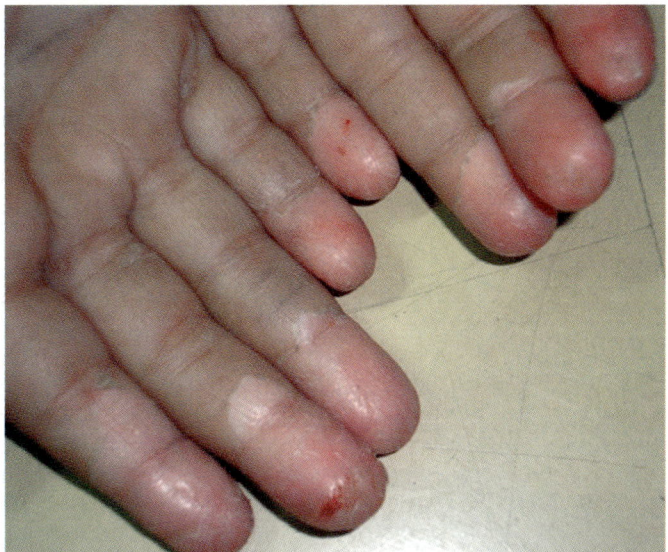

Fig. 17.12 Periungual desquamation in a child with Kawasaki disease

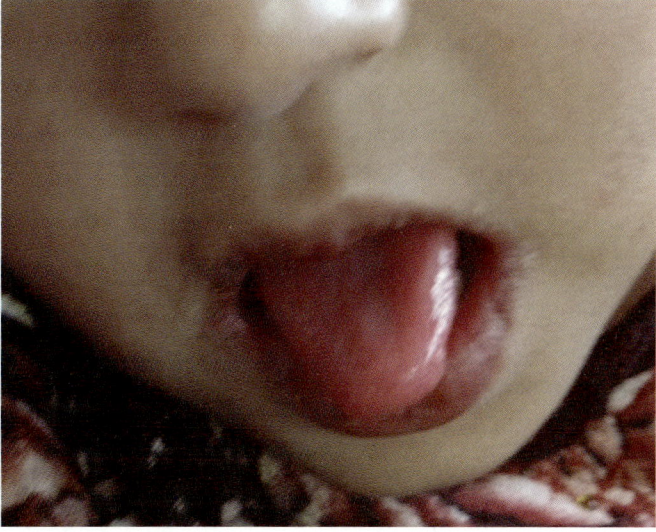

Fig. 17.14 Strawberry tongue and cracked lips in a child with Kawasaki disease

second or third week of illness. Perianal desquamation (Fig. 17.13) is also characteristic and usually precedes periungual desquamation.

- *Changes in lips and oral cavity* include strawberry tongue (Fig. 17.14) and cracking of lips.
- *Cervical adenopathy* is usually single, unilateral and non-tender and involves anterior cervical chain.

Table 17.10 describes the American Heart Association Diagnostic Criteria for KD. Besides these, other clinical features may be present and may help or confuse treating physician further. Irritability is usually extreme in infants to the extent that clinician may think of pyogenic meningitis. Aseptic meningitis is common in KD and responds briskly

Table 17.10 American Heart Association Diagnostic Criteria for Kawasaki Disease
Classic KD is diagnosed in the presence of fever for at least 5 days together with at least 4 of the 5 following principal clinical features:
1. Erythema and cracking of lips, strawberry tongue, and/or erythema of oral and pharyngeal mucosa
2. Bilateral bulbar conjunctival injection without exudate
3. Rash: Maculopapular, diffuse erythroderma, or erythema multiforme-like
4. Erythema and edema of the hands and feet in acute phase and/or periungual desquamation in subacute phase
5. Cervical lymphadenopathy (≥1.5 cm diameter), usually unilateral

Adapted from McCrindle BW, Rowley AH, Newburger JW, Burns JC, Bolger AF, Gewitz M; American Heart Association Rheumatic Fever, Endocarditis, and Kawasaki Disease Committee of the Council on Cardiovascular Disease in the Young; Council on Cardiovascular and Stroke Nursing; Council on Cardiovascular Surgery and Anesthesia; and Council on Epidemiology and Prevention. Diagnosis, treatment, and long-term management of Kawasaki Disease: A scientific statement for health professionals from the American Heart Association. Circulation. 2017;135:e927–e999.

to intravenous immunoglobulins (IVIg). Joint manifestations may include arthralgia and arthritis. Significant right hypochondriac pain can occur due to hydrops of gall bladder. Beau lines are frequently seen in convalescent phase (Fig. 17.15).

Incomplete Kawasaki Disease

Children with coronary artery involvement on 2D echo can be diagnosed as Kawasaki disease, even if less than 4 principal features are present. Experts now agree that *incomplete* cases do occur, usually in children less than 6 months. For diagnosis, fever plus 3 features are enough to establish the diagnosis. The rationale is that treatment is safe and effective; and failure to diagnose Kawasaki disease may have a significant negative impact on outcome.

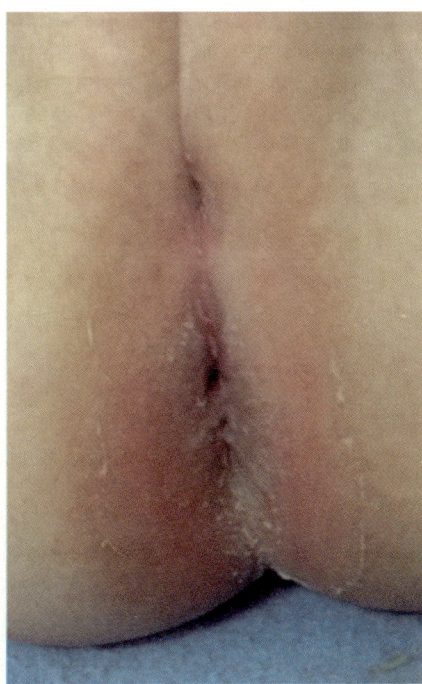

Fig. 17.13 Perianal desquamation in a child with Kawasaki disease

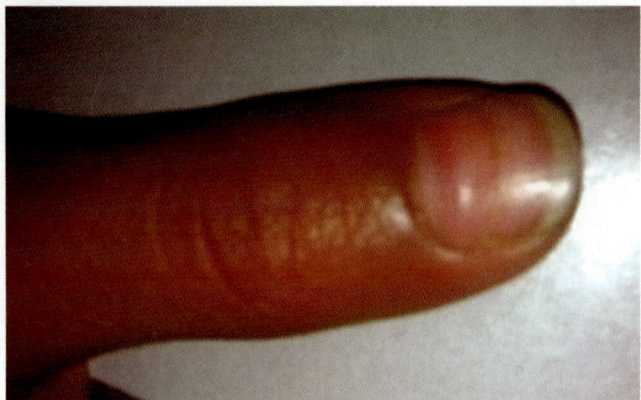

Fig. 17.15 Beau lines

Investigations

Acute phase is associated with various markers of inflammation which include neutrophilia, high ESR, high CRP, anemia, hypoalbuminemia, sterile pyuria (due to urethritis), and transaminitis. Cerebrospinal fluid analysis may reveal pleocytosis. None of these features are specific for KD. Thrombocytosis, which is described as a typical feature, is not seen before the end of second week of illness.

Echocardiography

Echocardiography is an important tool and is usually done at baseline and then after 6–8 weeks of illness. Another ECHO may be needed in second week of illness in children who do not show response to IVIg or have early coronary involvement. Coronary dilatation is described as Z-scores of ≥ 2.5 for internal diameters for both left anterior descending and right coronary arteries. However, coronary dilatation is usually not seen in first week of illness. There could be other suggestive findings in echocardiography like perivascular brightness, lack of tapering of vessels, low ejection fraction, mitral regurgitation and pericardial effusion. These findings may be useful in diagnosis especially in those infants where all the clinical features are not present (incomplete KD). A repeat echocardiography at 6–8 weeks of illness is useful in picking up residual coronary abnormalities and guiding further treatment.

Differential Diagnosis

Since the clinical features are relatively nonspecific, there are many differential diagnosis of KD. These include viral infections, Stevens-Johnson syndrome, toxin mediated syndromes, scarlet fever, leptospirosis, and hypersensitivity reactions to drugs. Exudative pharyngitis, exudative conjunctivitis, discrete intraoral lesions, bullous or vesicular rash, and diffuse lymphadenopathy should suggest an alternate diagnosis. Scarlet fever usually is not associated with conjunctivitis and shows a brisk response to antibiotics. Visceral involvement and hypotension is frequent in toxin mediated syndromes.

Treatment	Kawasaki Disease

Standard treatment of KD involves administration of intravenous immunoglobulins (IVIg) and aspirin. IVIg is given at a dose of 2 g/kg as a single dose infusion over 6–8 hours. Most patients show a brisk response to IVIg with defervescence and general well-being. Inflammatory parameters also show gradual improvement. IVIg has been shown to reduce the risk of coronary abnormalities from 25% to 3–5%, if given within first ten days of illness.

Aspirin is also given at a dose of 40–100 mg/kg/day till subsidence of inflammation. Once the child is afebrile and inflammatory parameters (CRP) show declining trend, dose of aspirin is reduced to antiplatelet doses (3–5 mg/kg/day). Aspirin is discontinued if the follow-up ECHO at 6–8 weeks is normal.

Prognosis

In the pre-IVIg era, about 25% children would go on to develop coronary abnormalities. Use of IVIg has reduced this risk to 3–5%. Coronary abnormalities can persist as ectasia or aneurysms. These aneurysms carry a significant risk of rupture, thrombosis, and stenosis and predispose the individual to ischemic events. Hence all patients who develop coronary abnormalities should be on life-long follow-up.

Case Study	Kawasaki Disease

A 1-year-old boy was brought to you with history of fever for 1 week. On examination, he has diffused maculopapular rash and red eyes without any discharge. Lips are red and cracked. Oral cavity also shows diffuse erythema. With a possibility of KD, he was investigated and found to have raised ESR, raised CRP, and neutrophilic leukocytosis. Ultrasound abdomen to look for gall bladder hydrops was normal. Urine microscopy was not contributory. Echocardiography did not reveal any coronary dilatation.

Does normal ECHO rule out possibility of KD?

No, coronary dilatation does not occur in all patients. Moreover, it is unusual to see coronary dilatation in first week of illness except in very sick patients. Normal ECHO does not rule out KD.

What will be the first line treatment for this child?

This child would need IVIg at a dose of 2 g/kg as single infusion. IVIg is known to reduce the risk of coronary complications. Aspirin is usually added in anti-inflammatory doses till subsidence of inflammation and then is reduced to antiplatelet doses.

Kawasaki Disease

1. Kawasaki disease is an acute systemic vasculitis which should be suspected in a child with unexpected fever for >5 days plus at least 4 of the following: unilateral cervical lymphadenopathy, nonvascular rash, edema/erythema of hands/feet, non-supportive conjunctivitis, and lesions of the oropharynx with strawberry tongue.
2. Timely recognition and management are important to reduce the risk of coronary complications.
3. No single diagnostic test is useful in the acute phase.
4. Intravenous immunoglobulin along with aspirin is the standard of care and most patients respond briskly to this treatment.
5. **Think of another diagnosis in presence of** exudative pharyngitis, exudative conjunctivitis, discrete intraoral lesions, bullous or vesicular rash, and diffuse lymphadenopathy.

Newburger JW. Kawasaki disease: State of the art. *Congenit Heart Dis*. 2017 Jun5. [Epub ahead of print].

Newburger JW. Kawasaki disease: Medical therapies. *Congenit Heart Dis*. 2017 Jun 5. [Epub ahead of print].

Son MBF, Newburger JW. Kawasaki disease. *Pediatr Rev*. 2013;34;151–162.

Yim D, Curtis N, Cheung M, Burgner D. An update on Kawasaki disease II: Clinical features, diagnosis, treatment and outcomes. *J Paediatr Child Health*. 2013;49:614–623.

17.10 HENOCH-SCHÖNLEIN PURPURA

Henoch-Schönlein purpura (HSP), also known as anaphylactoid purpura, is a multisystemic, IgA mediated, small vessel leukocytoclastic vasculitis. It is usually seen between the ages of 3 and 15 years and has a male preponderance. There is a seasonal trend in the occurrence with a noticeable peak observed in the months of October and November.

Etiology

Etiology of HSP is unknown however various triggers like infections, medications and vaccination have been implicated.

Pathogenesis

It is an immunoglobulin A (IgA) mediated disease as suggested by the deposition of IgA in various tissues. This may also explain the predilection of skin lesions in the lower extremities and buttocks in ambulatory children and sacrum along with buttocks and ears in infants as immune complexes tend to deposit and incite inflammation in dependent areas due to gravity. Vasculitis leads to extravasation of blood into the interstitial space resulting in edema and palpable purpura.

Pathology

The pathognomonic lesion is leukocytoclastic vasculitis and is seen in the dermal capillaries and postcapillary venules. Leukocytoclasis means breakdown of white blood cells in lesional tissue. Deposition of IgA is characteristic.

Clinical Features

HSP is a clinical diagnosis. It is diagnosed by a classic tetrad of (*i*) nonthrombocytopenic palpable purpura, (*ii*) arthritis/arthralgia, (*iii*) gastrointestinal, and (*iv*) renal involvement.

- *Skin involvement* is the most common presentation and occurs in the form of purpura, which are palpable (Fig. 17.7) and occur in crops. Purpuric lesions have a predilection for lower limbs and are not related to thrombocytopenia. The onset is acute but symptoms may appear sequentially resulting in delay in diagnosis. Involvement of the external genitalia is more common in boys and includes painless scrotal edema, purpura and acute onset edema of the glans penis or prepuce and acute testicular pain mimicking torsion.
- *Gastrointestinal involvement* can present as diffuse, acute, colicky abdominal pain. There may also be intussusception and gastrointestinal bleeding, which are most common emergencies in acute phase of disease.
- *Joints* may also be involved in the form of arthritis (joint swelling or pain with limitation on motion) or arthralgia (joint pain without joint swelling or limitation on motion). Joints are involved in 60–80% cases. Ankles and knees are most commonly affected. Arthritis occurs in 20–25% cases.
- *Renal involvement* can occur in 25–50% cases in the form of hematuria, proteinuria, deranged renal functions and hypertension. This is the most worrying chronic complication associated with HSP.

Diagnosis

Diagnosis of HSP is largely clinical **(Table 17.11)** and in case of typical skin lesions, one may not require skin biopsy. Skin biopsy shows leukocytoclastic vasculitis with predominant IgA deposits. In case of renal involvement, renal biopsy may show proliferative glomerulonephritis with IgA deposits.

Differential Diagnosis

Skin lesions are usually the first manifestation of HSP. Hence common differential diagnosis for purpuric lesions would include thrombocytopenia, where one has nonpalpable purpura.

If gastrointestinal manifestations are the first presentation, one needs to think of common causes of an acute surgical abdomen. One also should make an effort to undress the child and look for typical skin lesions of HSP in gluteal region and lower limbs.

Complications

- *Gastrointestinal complications* are common during acute stage of disease. Plain radiographs may show dilated bowel loops in children with abdominal symptoms. Ultrasound of the abdomen can demonstrate intussusception.
- *Acute testicular torsion* is another important complication during acute stage. Ultrasound may help confirm the diagnosis in a child with red tender scrotum.
- *Renal involvement* is usually seen within first six months of disease. This may be seen when all other manifestations of disease may have subsided which usually takes about 4–6 weeks. This is the most important long-term complication of HSP. Urine microscopy may show hematuria and proteinuria. Renal function test may also show raised blood urea and creatinine. Renal biopsy may be required in severe cases.

Table 17.11 Henoch-Schönlein Purpura EULAR/PRINTO/PRES Ankara 2008 Classification Definition

Purpura or petechiae with lower limb predominance and *at least one of the four following criteria*:
• Abdominal pain
• Histopathology: Typically leukocytoclastic vasculitis with predominant IgA deposit or proliferative glomerulonephritis with predominant IgA deposit
• Arthritis or arthralgia
• Renal involvement

Adapted from Ozen S, Pistorio A, Iusan SM, Bakkaloglu A, Herlin T, Brik R, and Paediatric Rheumatology International Trials Organisation (PRINTO). EULAR/PRINTO/PRES criteria for Henoch-Schönlein purpura, childhood polyarteritis nodosa, childhood Wegener granulomatosis and childhood Takayasu arteritis: Ankara2008. Part II: Final classification criteria. Ann Rheum Dis. 2010;69:798–806.

Investigations

Hemogram reveals normocytic normochromic anemia along with leukocytosis. Platelet count and ESR are mildly elevated. In patients with acute renal failure, urea and creatinine may be mildly elevated.

Urinalysis may show variable proteinuria and microscopic to gross hematuria. Serum IgA is elevated in 50–70% cases. Biopsy of skin lesions reveals acute leukocytoclastic vasculitis of involved capillaries and venules in the mid and upper dermis. Immunofluorescence microscopy shows perivascular IgA with occasional C3 and fibrinogen deposit. Patients of HSP do not require renal biopsy routinely unless complicated by nephrotic syndrome, acute nephritis with impaired renal function, or rapidly progressive renal failure.

Management

Most children require only supportive treatment as majority enter spontaneous remission. Analgesics (paracetamol or NSAIDs) are prescribed for pain and swelling associated with joint involvement. Steroids are indicated for severe gastrointestinal manifestations, ie, severe colic, gastro-intestinal bleed or acute abdomen. Oral predinosolone is given at the dose of 1–2 mg/kg per day for one week followed by tapering over the 2–3 weeks. Orchitis may also benefit from 2–3 weeks therapy of corticosteroids.

Severe renal manifestations including nephrotic syndrome, nephritic syndrome, or rapidly progressive glomerulonephritis may require long-term steroids or immunosuppressive (cyclophospamide/azathioprine) therapy. There is no evidence to suggest the role of steroids for preventing nephritic syndrome but children with minor urinary abnormalities (microscopic hematuria or non-nephrotic range proteinuria) should be followed up for 1 year to detect any progression.

Course and Prognosis

HSP is generally a benign disease with excellent prognosis. The average duration of disease is 4 weeks. Approximately 10–20%patients have recurrences which may recur within

Henoch-Schönlein Purpura

1. HSP is an acute small vessel vasculitis predominantly seen in childhood.
2. Diagnosis is clinical based on presence of typical palpable purpura in lower limbs. Other features like arthralgia/arthritis, gastrointestinal features and genitourinary features may be present.
3. Histopathology suggestive of leukocytoclastic vasculitis with IgA deposition on immunofluorescence is supportive.
4. Most children have self-limiting illness and need only supportive therapy.
5. Children with significant gastrointestinal involvement or genitourinary involvement respond briskly to steroids.
6. Steroids in acute phase do not reduce the risk of renal complications.
7. HSP nephritis is the most dreaded chronic complication of otherwise innocuous disease.

Case Study | **Henoch-Schönlein Purpura**

A 5-year-old boy presented with skin rash for 3 days. There was no history of fever. Examination revealed palpable purpura predominantly in lower limbs and arthritis of left ankle. Rest of the systemic examination was normal.

What investigations will you order in this child?

Hemogram is important as it will usually show normal or mild elevation in platelet count in HSP and will help rule out thrombocytopenic purpura. Baseline urine microscopic examination is helpful.

Would this child need a skin biopsy to confirm the diagnosis?

Skin biopsy will help confirm the diagnosis by showing leukocytoclastic vasculitis with predominant IgA deposition on immunofluorescence. However, it is not always required as HSP is usually a self-limiting disease and histopathology and immunofluorescence microscopy may not be easily available in all health care settings.

How will you counsel the parents and follow up this child?

Parents are usually worried because of the skin rash. One must counsel the parents regarding self-limiting nature of this disease. Also, it should be told that this rash can keep on appearing in crops for 4–6 weeks. Parents should be advised to seek urgent medical help in case of abdominal pain, blood in stools or abdominal distension. Periodic urine examination is required in all patients for at least six months to pick up renal involvement.

weeks and rarely up to 3–7 years. The long-term morbidity of HSP is predominantly associated with renal involvement. Around 5% of patients develop chronic nephritis and 5% of these may progress to end stage renal disease (ESRD) over 10–25 years period.

It is advisable to follow up the patients with HSP even with normal urinary findings for up to 6 months to detect any nephritis and those presenting with nephritis or nephrotic syndrome for 5 years.

Davin JC, Coppo R. Henoch-Schönlein purpura nephritis in children. *Nat Rev Nephrol.* 2014;10:563–73.

Trnka P. Henoch-Schönlein purpura in children. *J Paediatr Child Health.* 2013;49:995–1003.

Yang YH, Yu HH, Chiang BL. The diagnosis and classification of Henoch-Schönlein purpura: an updated review. *Autoimmun Rev.* 2014;13:355–8.

17.11 TAKAYASU ARTERITIS

Takayasu arteritis is prototype large vessel vasculitis seen in children. It was first described from Japan where it was described as "pulseless disease" (inability to palpate upper limb vessels) because of involvement of origins of vessels arising from arch of aorta. Pediatric disease accounts for 10–15% of all Takayasu arteritis patients. Overall, it is far less common than Kawasaki disease and HSP. Usual age at diagnosis is after the first decade and it is more common in girls. This is a chronic vasculitis leading to progressive stenosis of vessel lumen.

Clinical Features

Clinical manifestations depend on the site of vascular involvement and severity of stenosis. Stenosis of branches of arch of aorta leads to features of cerebral and retinal ischemia along with pulselessness of upper limbs. Organ-specific ischemic features may be seen like stroke, seizures and visual disturbances. This variant is more common in Japan. Stenosis of thoracoabdominal aorta and its branches like renal artery can manifest as severe hypertension (renal ischemia due to stenosis of renal artery or suprarenal aorta), reduced pulses in lower limbs and congestive heart failure. This variety is more common in Indian children. Typical pulseless disease is upper limbs is not seen unless branches of aortic arch are also involved. Hypertension is usually severe and may or may not be associated with differential pulses depending on the site involved. Cardiac dysfunction can occur due to severe hypertension and cardiomyopathy.

Symptoms of this disease can be subtle or sometimes alarming like accelerated hypertension and cerebral ischemia. Nonspecific features like fever, anorexia and weight loss are common. Claudication is not a common symptom, probably because of inability to express this symptom in childhood. Bruits can be heard because of irregular flow. Proximal pulses like brachial, carotid and femoral arteries should be looked for and reduced or absent pulses are important signs of proximal stenosis.

When to Suspect

In all children with hypertension, congestive heart failure, visual complaints and stroke/seizures/syncope, one must examine pulses in all four limbs as well as carotids. Blood pressure in all four limbs should be taken in case of hypertension. This basic examination is enough to make one think of this disease.

Diagnosis

Diagnosis of Takayasu arteritis is based on the criteria given by EULAR/PRINTO/PRES (**Table 17.12**). The gold standard for demonstrating typical arterial abnormalities is angiography. Angiography shows occlusion, stenosis (which is usually proximal and ostial), dilatation and occasionally aneurysms. Some other investigations like ultrasound to look for kidney size, Doppler to look for stenosis in carotids, abdominal aorta or renal arteries and echocardiography to look for cardiac dysfunction are useful.

Table 17.12 EULAR/PRINTO/PRES Ankara 2008 Classification Definition of Takayasu Arteritis
Angiographic abnormalities of the aorta or its main branches and pulmonary arteries showing aneurysm/dilatation (mandatory criterion) *Plus one of the five following criteria*:
1. Decreased peripheral artery pulse(s) or claudication of extremities
2. Four limb BP discrepancy
3. Bruits over the aorta or its major branches
4. Hypertension (related to childhood normative data)
5. Acute phase reactant

Adapted from Ozen S, Pistorio A, Iusan SM, Bakkaloglu A, Herlin T, Brik R, and Paediatric Rheumatology International Trials Organisation (PRINTO). EULAR/PRINTO/PRES criteria for Henoch-Schönlein purpura, childhood polyarteritis nodosa, childhood Wegener granulomatosis and childhood Takayasu arteritis: Ankara 2008. Part II: Final classification criteria. Ann Rheum Dis. 2010;69:798–806.

Differential Diagnosis

Coarctation of aorta is a common differential diagnosis and presents usually with hypertension in upper limbs, decreased pulses in lower limbs and radiofemoral delay. Collaterals are more common because of long duration of illness. Echocardiography and Doppler help in diagnosis. Angiography would show a discrete lesion in aorta in juxtaductal region and poststenotic dilatation.

Treatment	**Takayasu Arteritis**

Management aims at suppressing vessel wall inflammation and relieving distal ischemia. Steroids along with immuno-suppression are the mainstay to suppress inflammation. Relief of obstruction of vessel lumen in required in cases with significant distal ischemia and can be achieved by percutaneous or surgical revascularization procedures in a clear majority of children with carotid, thoracic/abdominal aorta or renal artery involvement.

Most patients also need supportive therapy for control of hypertension. Renovascular hypertension is usually severe and needs multiple antihypertensive agents. One must remember not to give angiotensin converting enzyme inhibitors to control hypertension if the patients have bilateral renal artery stenosis or critical suprarenal aortic stenosis, as this may precipitate renal failure.

Prognosis

It is a chronic disease with relapses and remissions. A monophasic course is seen in about 20% patients. Most patients would keep on having relapses. Adult survival rates

Case Study	**Takayasu Arteritis**

A 12-year-old girl was brought to emergency services with complaints of headache for last 1 week and one episode of seizure 12 hours back followed by unconsciousness. Examination revealed hypertension (BP 180/120 mmHg in right upper limb), no meningeal signs and no focal neurological signs. Rest of systemic examination was normal. Headache, seizure and altered sensorium were attributed to severe hypertension and aggressive antihypertensive therapy was started as per protocol. Meanwhile certain investigations were ordered to determine the cause of hypertension. Renal function tests were normal and urine dipstick showed 2+ proteinuria. Ultrasound of kidneys was ordered because of proteinuria and showed small left kidney with near absent blood flow in left renal artery on Doppler. Ultrasound Doppler also picked up additional blood flow abnormality in suprarenal aorta. Stenosis of suprarenal aorta and left renal artery were further confirmed by angiography; thus confirming a diagnosis of Takayasu arteritis.

What additional examination should have been done in this child?

Examination for proximal pulses especially carotids, brachials, and femorals could have given a clue in this child. In case of suprarenal aorta involvement, one may get reduced lower limb pulses. Blood pressure should have been taken in all four limbs. More than 10 mmHg difference in BP between limbs is an important clue to diagnosis. One should also look for bruits over major arteries and may find them over abdominal aorta and renal artery in such a case.

17

Takayasu Arteritis

1. Takayasu arteritis is a granulomatous large vessel arteritis of unknown etiology with resultant stenosis or occlusion of aorta and/or its major branches.
2. Clinical features are related to distal ischemia and effects thereof (renovascular hypertension, cardiac decompensation, seizures, syncope, stroke, visual manifestations). Claudication is not a common complaint in children.
3. Diagnosis is not difficult if suspected.
4. Conventional angiography is the gold standard for diagnosis.
5. Management is aimed at suppressing vessel wall inflammation and relieving distal ischemia. Inflammation is controlled by steroids and other steroid-sparing immunosuppressants. Relief of distal ischemia may need percutaneous or surgical revascularization procedures.

of 94–97% at 10–15 years have been achieved with immunosuppression and revascularization procedures. Higher mortality is seen however in children because of higher rate of congestive heart failure due both to hypertension and myocardial inflammation.

Johnston SL, Lock RJ, Gompels MM. Takayasu arteritis: A review. *J Clin Pathol*.2002;55:481–6.

Keser G, Direskeneli H, Aksu K. Management of Takayasu arteritis: A systematic review. *Rheumatology* (Oxford).2014;53:793–801

Numano F. The story of Takayasu arteritis.*Rheumatology* (Oxford). 2002;41:103–6.

Anju Gupta

Skin Disorders

Skin is a mirror of the human body where internal diseases may be reflected on the skin surface. Nearly one-third of the pediatric outpatient visits involve a dermatology complaint. In addition to the wide variety of primary skin disorders seen during childhood, the skin is often a marker of underlying systemic diseases and many hereditary syndromes. Besides identifying the primary and secondary skin lesions and studying their characteristics, it is vital to examine the hair, nails and mucosal surfaces.

18.1 SKIN LESIONS

Primary Lesions

- *Macules* are flat, circumscribed, non-palpable lesions that differ from the surrounding skin in terms of color. It can be of any shape or color (Fig. 18.1a). In some regions, macules larger than 1 cm are described as *patches*.
- *Papules* are palpable, elevated, circumscribed solid lesions less than 0.5–1 cm size (Fig. 18.1b); larger lesions are described as *nodules* (Fig. 18.1c).
- *Plaques* are elevated (Fig. 18.1d), circumscribed, flat-topped lesions; larger than 1 cm (Fig. 18.1e).
- *Vesicles* are elevated fluid filled lesions, *bullae* being larger than 1 cm.
- *Pustules* are well-circumscribed lesions containing purulent material.

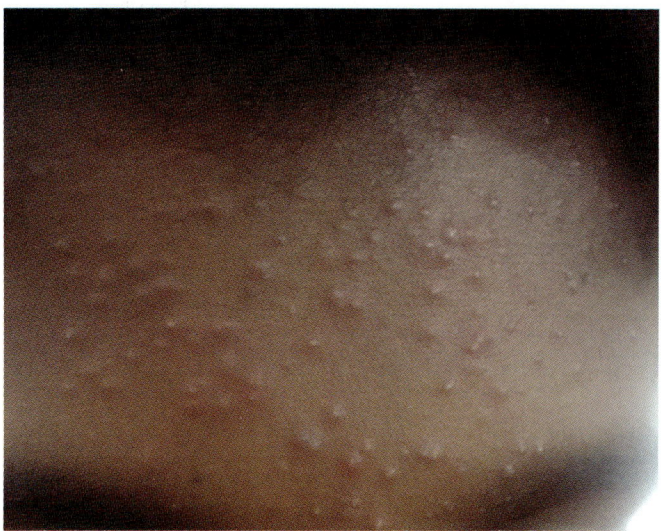

Fig. 18.1b Papules—palpable, elevated, circumscribed solid lesions less than 0.5–1 cm size. Some pustules (with yellow top) are also seen

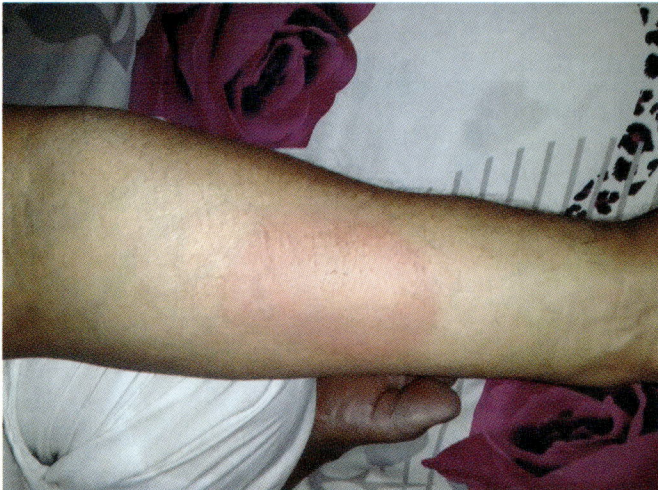

Fig. 18.1a Macule—circumscribed non-palpable lesion, appearing as red in the picture

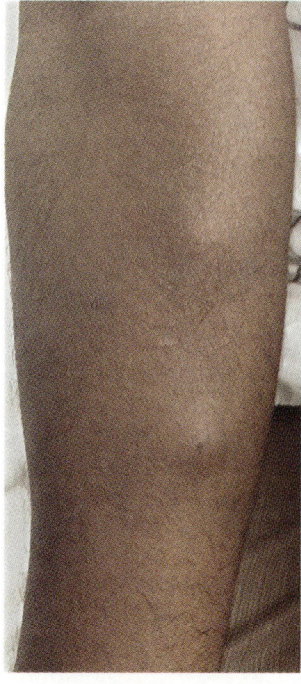

Fig.18.1c Nodule—elevated lesions larger than papules

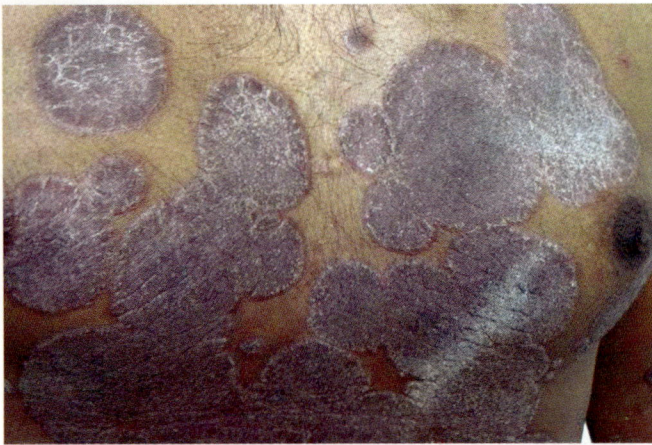

Fig. 18.1d Plaques—elevated, circumscribed, flat-topped lesions; larger than 1 cm

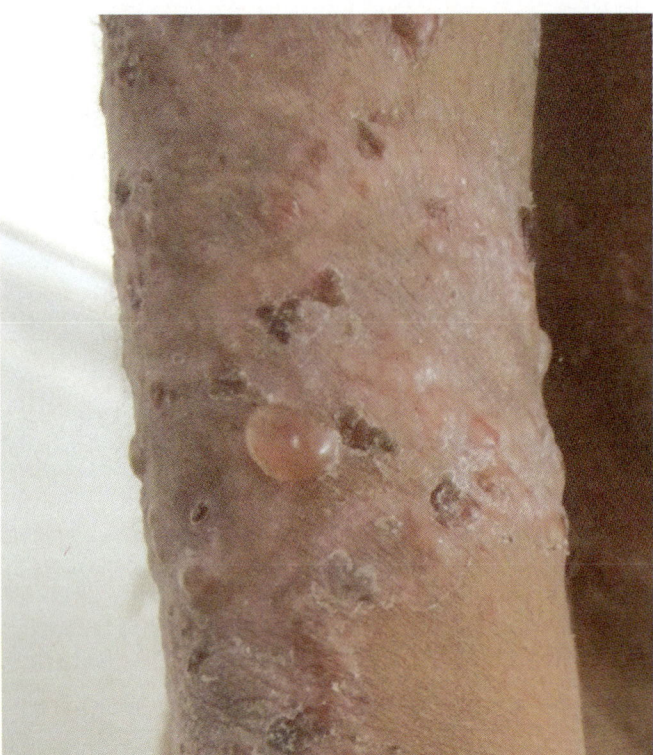

Fig.18.1e Bullae—elevated fluid filled lesions more than 1 cm in diameter

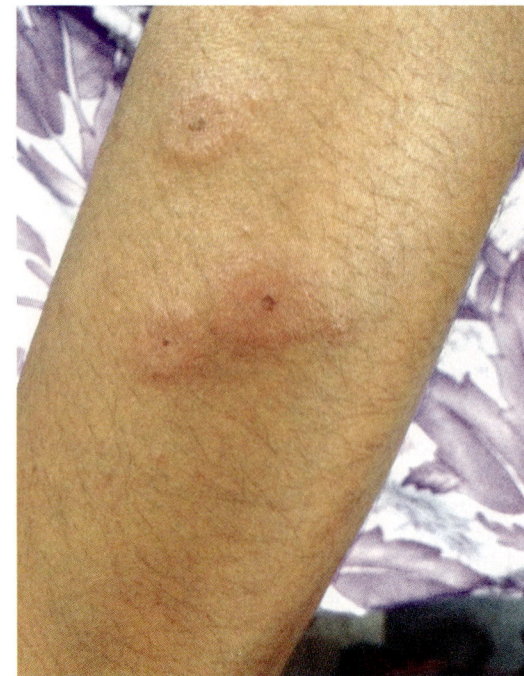

Fig.18.1f Target lesions—a central erythematous papule, macule, or vesicle; a surrounding area of pale edema; and a peripheral area of erythema

Secondary Lesions

These can evolve from primary lesions.

- *Scales* are flat plates or flakes of stratum corneum.
- *Erosion* is a break in the continuity of the epidermis.
- *Ulcers* signify a deeper involvement and extend into the dermis and tend to heal with scarring.
- *Fissures* are cracks in the skin (Fig. 18.1g).
- *Crusts* are dried up serum, exudates, blood or pus and epithelial debris on skin surface (Fig. 18.1h).
- *Lichenification* is thickening and hyperpigmentation of the skin with accentuation of skin markings caused by chronic scratching or inflammation (Fig. 18.1i).

- *Wheals* are transient, edematous and elevated flat topped lesions of various sizes, duration and configuration that represent dermal collection of edema fluid.
- *Cysts* are circumscribed, thick-walled lesions present deep in the skin which are covered by a normal skin and contain either fluid or semisolid material.
- *Petechiae* are punctate hemorrhagic spots approximately 1–2 mm in diameter; a macular area of hemorrhage more than 2 *mm diameter is called ecchymosis.*
- *Target lesions* These refer to a central erythematous papule, macule, or vesicle, a surrounding area of pale edema, and a peripheral area of erythema; commonly seen in erythema multiforme (Fig. 18.1f).

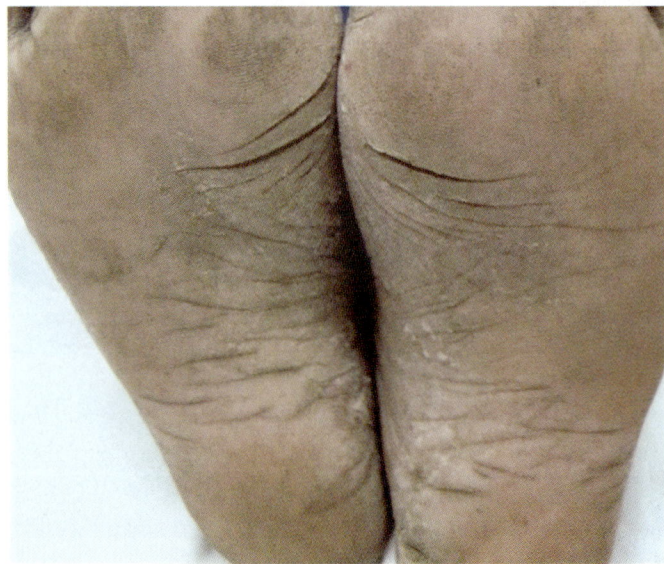

Fig. 18.1g Fissures—cracks in the skin

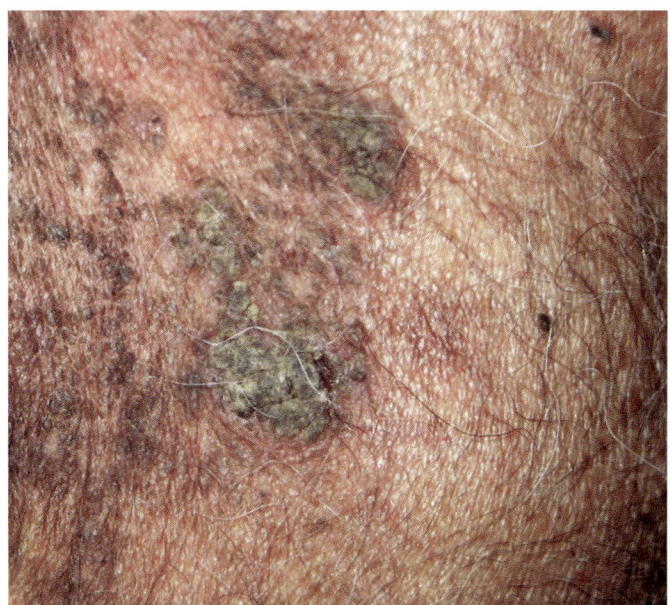

Fig. 18.1h Crust—dried up serum, exudates, blood or pus, and epithelial debris on skin surface

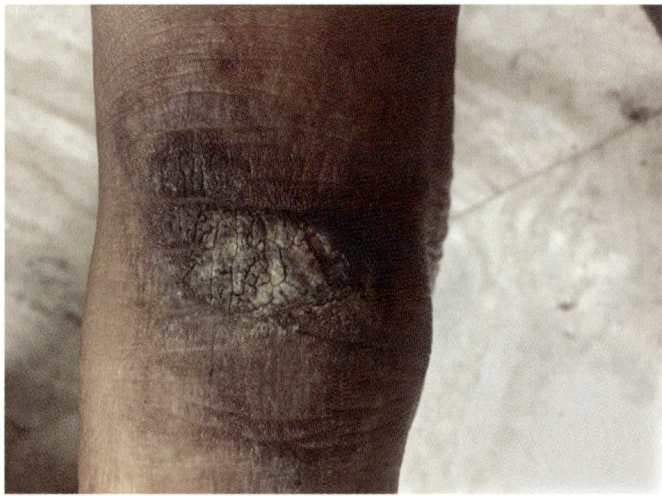

Fig.18.1i Lichenification—thickening and hyperpigmentation of the skin with accentuation of skin markings, caused by chronic scratching or inflammation

- *Scars* are end-stage lesions of inflammation which are formed by fibrous tissue and may be flat, depressed, or raised.
- *Comedone* is a plug of keratin or sebum in a dilated pilosebaceous opening. Commonly seen in acne vulgaris.

18.2 URTICARIA

Urticaria refers to an eruptive papular disorder of the skin characterized by transient, erythematous, edematous, pruritic swelling of the dermis, due to reversible exudation of plasma into the skin. The manifestations can last from a few minutes to 24 hours, before it resolves, leaving behind clinically normal skin. Urticaria is classified as *chronic* when it persists beyond 6 weeks duration.

Angioedema is a life-threatening manifestation of urticaria characterized by swelling of the subcutaneous or submucosal tissues; death can occur due to laryngeal disruption.

Anaphylaxis is a sudden, severe, life-threatening, systemic reaction often involving the skin due to mast cell mediator release.

Pathogenesis

Urticaria is due to a local increase of permeability of capillaries and small venules. It is due to the interplay of various mediators such as histamine, prostaglandins, leucotrienes, eosinophil, neutrophil chemotactic factors, etc. which in turn are stimulated to be released due to immunological or non-immunological stimuli.

The main causes of childhood urticaria are: Infections, (viral, streptococci group A or B infection, *Toxocara canis* infestation), drugs (penicillins, cephalosporins, NSAIDs, histamine liberating drugs such as codeine and radiocontrast products), food (eggs, cow's milk, nuts and peanuts, fish and seafood, food additives, fruits), insect bites (*hymenopteras*), physical stimuli (cold urticaria, solar urticaria, cholinergic urticaria and dermatographism), and idiopathic. Urticaria may also be associated with systemic diseases like systemic lupus erythematosus, juvenile arthritis, Kawasaki disease, lymphomas, leukemias or genetic disorders such as hereditary angioedema (types I and II), genetic hypo-complimentemia, and certain metabolic disorders.

Clinical Features

Wheals of variable size and shape develop on the skin, disappearing to leave behind a normal skin or a purpuric stain. The lesions have a white palpable center of edema with a variable halo of erythema. The size of the papules may be pin-point to large which may develop a polycyclic margin and spread at a rate of 1 cm or more per hour.

Angioedema may involve the mouth, lips, pharynx, and tongue; laryngeal obstruction can be an emergency. Anaphylaxis can occur and reach its peak after 5–30 minutes. Angioedema, hypotension, bronchospasm, and cardiac arrhythmias may be present in various combinations.

Differential Diagnosis

The main differential diagnosis is urticarial vasculitis—a type of small vessel leukocytoclastic vasculitis which may be associated with hypocomplementemia and other systemic manifestations, and where the wheals may last longer than 24 hours and may leave behind pigmentary changes unlike in urticaria. Hereditary angioedema and autoinflammatory syndromes presenting with urticarial rashes are other important differential diagnoses.

Treatment	Urticaria

It is important to remove the causative agent (if identified by careful history) or treat the systemic disease. H1 class antihistamines are the treatment of choice for urticaria. Non-sedating antihistamines can be given in children above 2 years of age. The use of classical antihistamines in older children is limited by their side-effects including sedation, anti-cholinergic properties, and paradoxical excitation. Treatment may have to be given from a few days to few months. In patients with angioedema or anaphylactic shock, subcutaneous adrenaline (0.01 mg/kg) is given. Corticosteroids are only given in severe cases. Hereditary angioedema is treated with purified C-1 inhibitor concentrate.

18.3 NAPKIN DERMATITIS

Napkin dermatitis is a contact dermatitis exclusively localized in the region covered by diapers in infants (Fig. 18.2). It is more common in artificially fed infants and those with poor perineal hygiene.

Pathogenesis

Multiple causative factors interplay with each other such as feces, urine, friction, moisture, temperature, chemical irritation, and diaper material. Fecal enzymes such as proteases and lipases act as irritants in an atmosphere of increased moisture and may possibly play an important role in the causation of napkin dermatitis. Prolonged contact with urine also induces an irritant erythema, which may break down to form erosions if untreated. *Candida albicans* infection may also play a role.

Clinical Features

The disorder involves convex surfaces such as buttocks, scrotal sac, mons pubis, or inner side of thigh. Alternatively, only flexures may be affected. There is presence of erythematous, glazed, well demarcated lesions on the diaper area.

Convex surfaces. The skin appears red, parchment like and scalded, which soon becomes infected giving rise to pustular erosions. Most often these lesions are due to contact dermatitis secondary to detergents used for cleaning the diaper.

Involvement of folds of skin. Retention of sweat makes the area moist and macerated. Constant rubbing of skin causes erosion and denudation of the skin. Bacteria grow easily in this environment and cause secondary infection. The lesions are generally sharply demarcated.

Differential Diagnosis

Diaper rash needs to be differentiated from candidiasis, acrodermatitis enteropathica, and other causes of contact dermatitis. Band-like erythematous lesions are attributed to contact dermatitis with elastic band at the diaper edges. Prickly heat or miliaria may also appear similar to diaper rash.

Treatment	Napkin Dermatitis

The aim is to keep the skin dry, along with use of barrier creams or emollients to restore normal epidermis. Parents have to be advised to frequently change the diaper as it becomes wet; and to expose the skin to air. Use of impervious or plastic underwear should be avoided. Lubricants such as petrolatum or barrier creams containing zinc oxide can be applied. A mild topical corticosteroid cream combined with an antibacterial or antifungal agent can be used for a short term, to treat the contact or irritant dermatitis.

Acute rash can be managed with cool wet compresses (using 1 teaspoonful of salt in a pint of water) intermittently for two or three days. When *Candida* infection is suspected, nystatin dusting powder or clotrimazole may be applied, locally.

18.4 TOXIC ERYTHEMA OF THE NEWBORN

Erythema toxicum neonatorum (ETN) or *toxic erythema of the newborn* is a benign, self-limited, asymptomatic skin condition. Usually appears in the first few days of life and is seen in about 50% of the neonates in all races.

The eruption is characterized by small, erythematous papules, vesicles, and occasionally, pustules. The lesions are usually surrounded by a distinctive diffuse, blotchy, erythematous halo (Fig. 18.3). They are most profuse on the trunk, particularly the anterior trunk, but also commonly appear on the face and proximal parts of the limbs, especially the thighs. Individual lesions are transitory, often disappearing within a day. The infant appears well, and unperturbed by the eruption.

No investigations or treatment is generally needed; if in doubt, cultures and smears from the pustules can be sent, to differentiate from bacterial pyoderma.

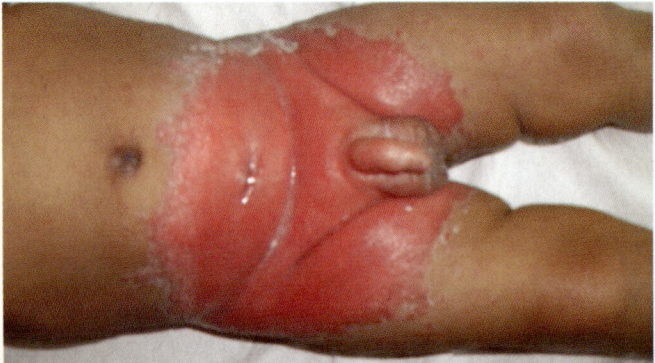

Fig. 18.2 Diaper dermatitis—presence of erythematous, glazed, well demarcated lesions on the diaper area

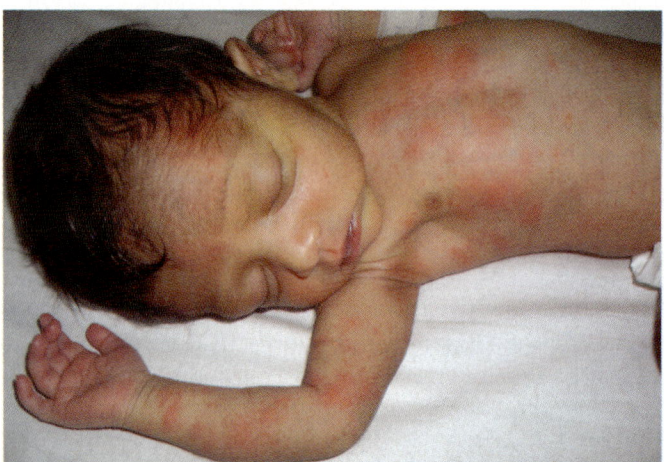

Fig. 18.3 Toxic erythema of the newborn (*Courtesy:* Prof. Ruchi Rai, Noida, UP)

18.5 SUBCUTANEOUS FAT NECROSIS OF THE NEWBORN

Subcutaneous fat necrosis of the newborn is an uncommon disorder characterized by firm, mobile, erythematous nodules and plaques over the trunk, arms, buttocks, thighs, and cheeks of full-term newborns. The precise cause is not known, but a variety of insults appear to have a role. These include birth asphyxia, maternal pre-eclampsia, maternal diabetes, obstetric trauma, hypothermia, and hypothermic cardiac surgery. Infants with subcutaneous fat necrosis usually appear well, which can be used to differentiate this condition from sclerema neonatorum—a kind of neonatal panniculitis that occurs in premature and small infants who are gravely ill and can result in death.

Clinical Features

Subcutaneous fat necrosis begins as an area of edema, usually between the second and third week of life and progresses to variably circumscribed nodules and plaques that have a deep, indurated feel, implying a panniculitis. The overlying skin may be flesh-colored, red, or purple and may look taut and shiny (Fig. 18.4). The lesions are not warm and are commonly seen on the trunk, arms, buttocks, thighs, or cheeks. As the lesions progress, they may become fluctuant and spontaneously drain necrotic fat.

Treatment	Subcutaneous Fat Necrosis

Treatment is generally not required, other than analgesia in some cases. Hypercalcemia tends to occur in around a quarter of all cases; it appears more frequently in infants with extensive disease, and almost exclusively when the trunk is affected.

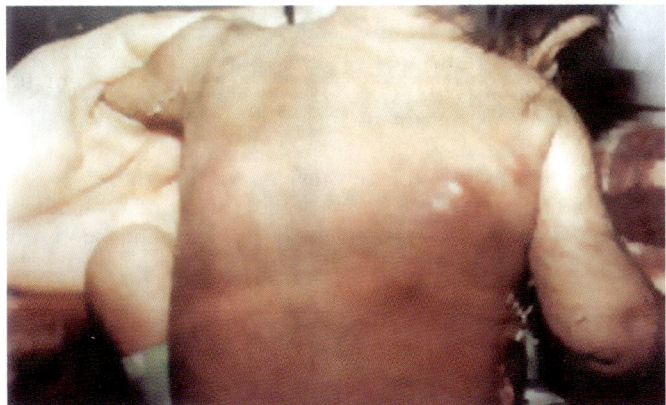

Fig. 18.4 Subcutaneous fat necrosis. Photograph showing multiple, reddish, nodular, swellings over the back in the right infrascapular area. Reproduced with permission: From Editor-in-Chief, Indian Pediatrics. Source: Lochan KK, Parmar GS. Subcutaneous fat necrosis of the newborn. Indian Pediatr. 2000;37:102. © Indian Pediatrics

18.6 BACTERIAL INFECTIONS—PYODERMA

A pyoderma is a superficial purulent infection of the skin (Fig. 18.5).
- *Primary pyoderma* occurs on normal skin, has a characteristic morphology and is initiated by a single organism.

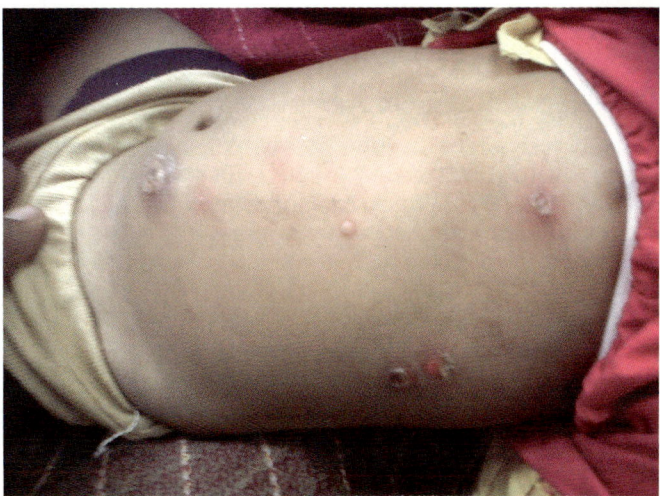

Fig. 18.5 Pyoderma: Most common non-bullous impetigo

These include impetigo, ecthyma, folliculitis, furuncle, carbuncle, erysipelas, cellulitis, and paronychia.
- *Secondary pyoderma* occurs on pre-existing skin lesions like cuts, eczema. They have a variable morphology and are caused by a variety of different organisms.

Staphylococcus aureus or group A streptococci (*Streptococcus pyogenes*) are responsible for most of the primary or secondary pyoderma. Staphylococci produce deeper lesions, which are more likely to be bullous. Streptococci produce thicker yellowish brown crusts. *Proteus, Klebsiella, Pseudomonas aeruginosa* and other organisms may also colonize the affected skin and cause nosocomial infections.

Impetigo

Impetigo is the most frequently diagnosed superficial bacterial skin infection involving the upper epidermis.
- *Non-bullous impetigo* occurs mainly on face and limbs. It begins as a reddish macule, turns into a transient flaccid vesicle, which ruptures, and the oozing fluid dries to form a honey-colored crust. Healing occurs without scar formation.
- *Bullous impetigo* appears as large fluid filled blisters, which rupture to form superficial erosions (Fig. 18.6). Face, palms, soles, and mucosa are involved.

Potential complications of impetigo include cellulitis, osteomyelitis, septic arthritis, pneumonia, and septicemia. Streptococcal infections can result in scarlet fever,

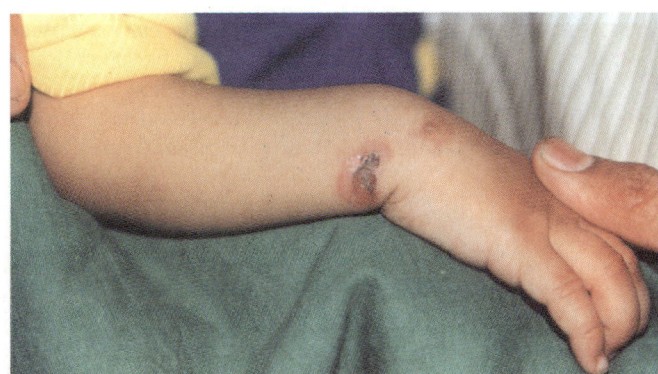

Fig. 18.6 Bullous impetigo. Erosions after rupture of bullae leaving a reddish raw base. Brown crusts are formed

18

lymphangitis, and lymphadenitis. Nephritogenic strains can result in post-streptococcal glomerulonephritis.

Infections of Hair and Dermis

- *Ecthyma* involves the lower epidermis and upper dermis and occurs on trauma prone sites. The lesions are characterized by a thick, brown, adherent crust.
- *Cellulitis* implies infection of the dermis and subcutaneous tissues. The affected area becomes red, edematous, and warm.
- *Folliculitis* is a superficial infection confined to the hair follicle and perifollicular structures.
- *Furuncle* (Fig. 18.7) refers to a deep infection manifesting as boils and abscesses around the hair follicles caused by virulent strains of staphylococci. There is severe perifollicular inflammation. The lesion is most commonly seen on buttocks, neck, face, and axillae.

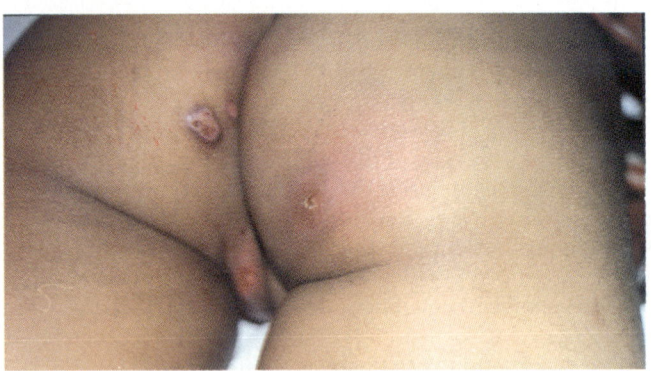

Fig. 18.7 Furuncle. A tender nodule with pus pointing on the surface

Treatment	Pyoderma

For self-limited pyodermas, simple measures such as removal of crusts with Condy's compresses or tepid water and careful washing with antibacterial soaps may be useful. Systemic oral antibiotics (erythromycin, cloxacillin, or cephalexin) limit the spread of infection and prevent complications. Topical application of 2% mupirocin ointment is comparable in efficacy to oral erythromycin and may be used for limited infections.

18.7 PARASITIC INFESTATIONS

Scabies

Scabies manifests as intensely pruritic skin lesions caused by the mite *Sarcoptes scabiei*. Incidence is higher in children younger than 2 years of age, but is fairly common in older children and young adults. It is transmitted by direct human contact and it is usual for other family members to be affected simultaneously.

Clinical Features

The cardinal symptom is pruritus, particularly severe at night time. Skin lesions are in the form of *burrows* (grayish thread-like tortuous lines due to burrowing of the itch mite into the epidermis), itchy papules, excoriations, nodules, vesiculo-pustules, eczematization, and secondary bacterial infection (Fig. 18.8). Burrows are found on the hands, particularly the finger webs and wrists. Other lesions are

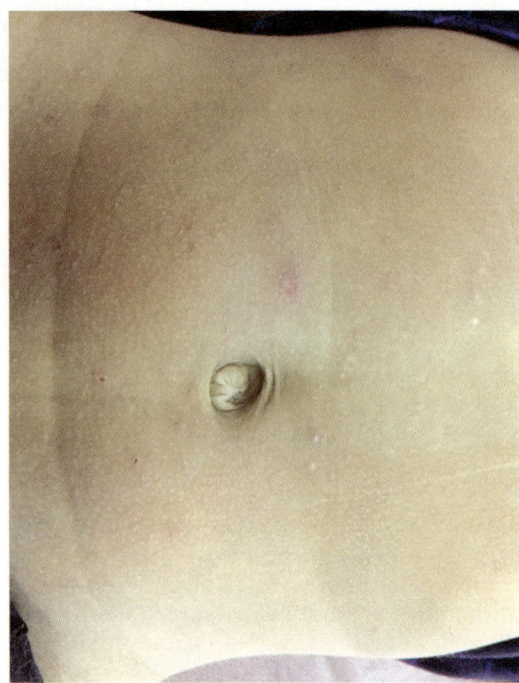

Fig. 18.8 Scabies—tiny excoriated papules on the abdomen

located in intertriginous areas, feet, axillary region, umbilicus, male genitalia, breast areolae in females, cubital, and popliteal regions. The head and neck can also be involved in infants.

Treatment	Scabies

Treatment of scabies includes elimination of mites, treatment of symptoms, and treatment of secondary infection. The most efficacious treatment for scabies is 5% permethrin topical cream in children beyond 2 months of age. A single application cures more than 90% children. There is no systemic toxicity. Permethrin is applied on the cool dry skin for a period of 8–12 hours (or 4 hours in infants) below the neck and followed by a bath after the period of application. 1% lindane and 5–10% crotamiton cream are other less efficacious therapies.

In children below 2 months of age, sulfur and crotamiton cream are safer yet less effective choices. The application can be repeated after one week in all cases.

Oral ivermectin (200 µg/kg body weight) given as a single dose or with a repeat dose after one week, can be given to children above 5 years of age. Topical ivermectin (0.5%) can also be used as a single application.

All members of the family should be treated concurrently even when there are no apparent skin lesions of scabies. After the treatment is completed, all clothes and bed linen should be boiled, put out in the sun and subjected to hot ironing.

Persistent itching can be treated with oral antihistamines. Secondary infections would require treatment with antistaphylococcal antibiotics.

Lice Infestation (Pediculosis)

Pediculosis or lice infestation in humans is caused by three species or subspecies of lice. *Pediculus humanus capitis*, the head louse; *Pediculus humanus corporis*, the body louse; and *Pthirus pubis*, the pubic or crab louse. Man is the only reservoir for the human louse.

Pediculosis capitis Itching over the scalp is the most common symptom. Scratching causes erosion of the scalp, redness, scaling, crusting, secondary infection and posterior cervical lymphadenopathy. Larval capsules which are cemented to the hair are called 'nits'. Infestation of eyelashes may cause redness, scaling and crusting.

Treatment	**Lice Infestation**

Permethrin is the most effective agent. Lindane shampoo is also useful. More than one application may be necessary for eliminating nits. Single application of ivermectin shampoo (0.5%) can also cure pediculosis. It is extremely important to wash and dry all clothing and bed linen; and clean combs and brushes with a pediculocide. Oral ivermectin is also being used in older children in recalcitrant cases.

18.8 VIRAL INFECTIONS

Non-genital Warts

Warts are benign proliferation of the epithelium of the skin and mucous membranes caused by human papillomavirus (HPV). Virus may spread by direct or indirect contact. Incubation period may vary from 3 months to several years.

Cutaneous non-genital warts include common skin warts, plantar warts, flat warts, and thread-like filiform warts over the neck and face (Fig. 18.9). Common warts are dome-shaped with conical projections and a rough surface. They are multiple, occurring on hands and under the nails. Black dots on warts may be due to small dermal vessel thrombosis. Plantar warts on the foot (Fig. 18.10) may be very painful. Flat warts found on face and extremities are small, flat topped, and multiple.

Treatment	**Non-genital Warts**

Treatment is designed to be cytodestructive. Topical daily application of keratolytic preparations (salicylic acid) or caustics (trichloroacetic acid) cures 80% of the warts within two months. More than 50% warts would disappear spontaneously without treatment in 2 years. Cryotherapy of warts with liquid nitrogen may be useful as a simple office procedure. Recalcitrant warts are treated with lasers or Interferon alpha injections.

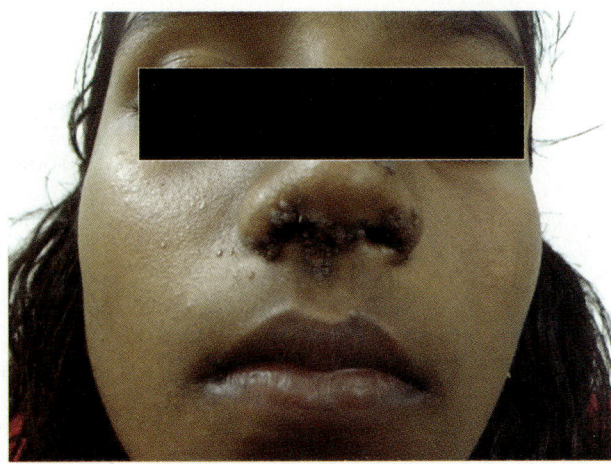

Fig. 18.9 Nasal warts in a girl

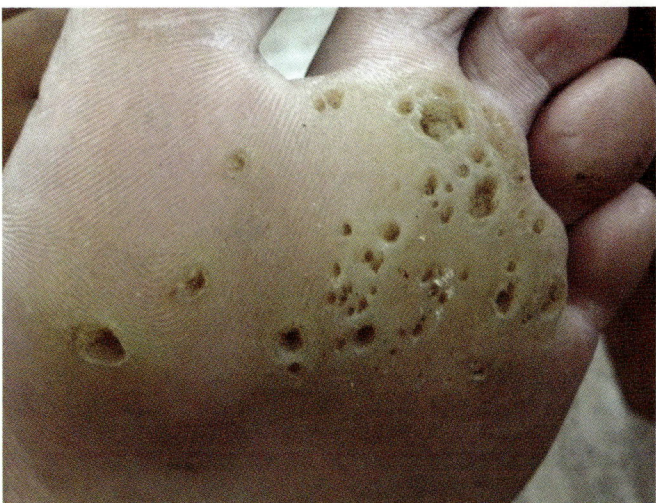

Fig. 18.10 Plantar warts

Molluscum Contagiosum

Molluscum contagiosum is caused by a type of poxvirus and characterized by well-circumscribed dome-shaped tiny pearly papules or nodules up to 1 cm in size, especially in intertriginous areas (Fig. 18.11). Most lesions are asymptomatic except those in perineum. Some lesions may disappear spontaneously but may persist elsewhere.

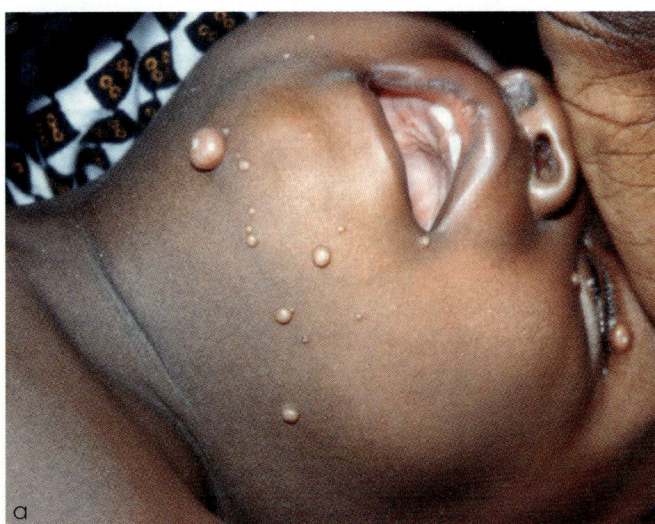

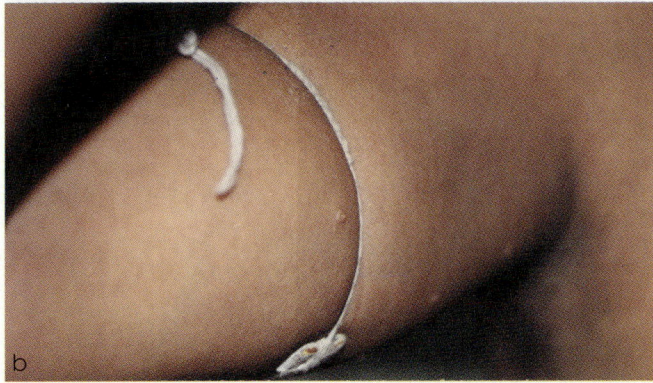

Fig. 18.11 Molluscum contagiosum. Pearly white umbilicated dome-shaped papules

18

Molluscum contagiosum is both contagious and autoinoculable.

| Treatment | Molluscum Contagiosum |

It is not always necessary to treat the lesions, as spontaneous resolution can occur; however the decision to treat has to be arrived after weighing each clinical situation. Individual lesions may be treated with curettage or application of trichloroacetic acid, phenol, potassium hydroxide, or cantharidin. Treatment is repeated each week until the lesions disappear. If the lesions do not improve within 4 weeks, it is not desirable to continue the treatment. Cryotherapy, electrocautery, or radiofrequency cautery, imiquimod or tretinoin cream, and laser therapy are the other therapeutic alternatives.

18.9 FUNGAL INFECTIONS

Superficial mycoses of the skin include candidiasis, tinea versicolor, and dermatophyte infections. A rapid diagnosis of fungal infection is possible with potassium hydroxide preparation or Wright's stain touch smear preparation of skin.

Candidiasis

Superficial infections with *Candida* species may present as oral thrush, diaper rash, vulvovaginitis, or paronychia (infection of nailbed). These infections may become severe with widespread systemic involvement in children on immunosuppressive drugs, after prolonged antibiotic therapy, or in acquired immunodeficiency syndrome.

Oral thrush Superficial infection of the oral mucosa with *Candida albicans* presents with curdy white plaques on the buccal mucosa and lateral borders of the tongue. These may gradually become confluent. There may be a white diamond-shaped area on dorsum of tongue with loss of papillae. Lesions may spread to the throat leading to serious dysphagia. Oral thrush is common in infancy and immuno-compromised patients.

Oral candidiasis can also present with denuded atrophic tongue, chronic atrophic inflamed mucous membranes, or persistent firm irregular white plaques on the cheek or tongue (Fig. 18.12).

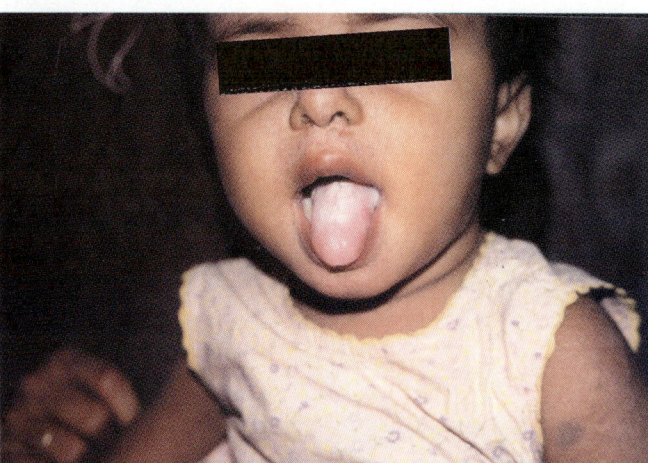

Fig. 18.12 Oral candidiasis

| Treatment | Oral Thrush |

Oral thrush responds quickly to topical treatment in infants. Nystatin oral suspension (100,000 IU/mL) or 1% clotrimazole mouth paint should be applied at 4–6 hours intervals for 5–7 days. Systemic therapy may have to be given in immuno-compromised patients with oral fluconazole or ketoconazole.

Candidal intertrigo It classically occurs in skin folds of obese children. It consists of extremely itchy, erythematous, scaly, flat-topped papules, which develop into a fringed irregular edge with pustules, which erode subsequently. Satellite lesions are also seen. Napkin candidiasis occurs in the moist skin of the buttocks and perianal area in infants.

Candidal paronychia There is swelling and redness of nailfold, followed by its detachment, loss of cuticle, or dystrophy.

Tinea Versicolor

Pityriasis versicolor is a mild, chronic superficial fungal infection of the skin caused by *Malassezia furfur* or *Pityrosporum ovale*. A hot humid climate, hyperhidrosis, and greasy skin favors the condition. The condition is characterized by multiple scaly, oval, macular, and patchy lesions of different sizes present over the upper trunk, proximal areas of the arms, neck, and lower abdomen (Fig. 18.13). The lesions may be hypopigmented or hyperpigmented. During summer, they fail to tan and in winters, they may appear to be relatively darker hence the word 'versicolor' is used.

| Treatment | Tinea Versicolor |

Treatment for this chronic condition includes application of 2.5% selenium sulfide shampoo over affected skin 15–20 minutes daily for 2–4 weeks or topical antifungals such as the imidazoles twice a day for 2–4 weeks. Recurrence is treated with oral fluconazole.

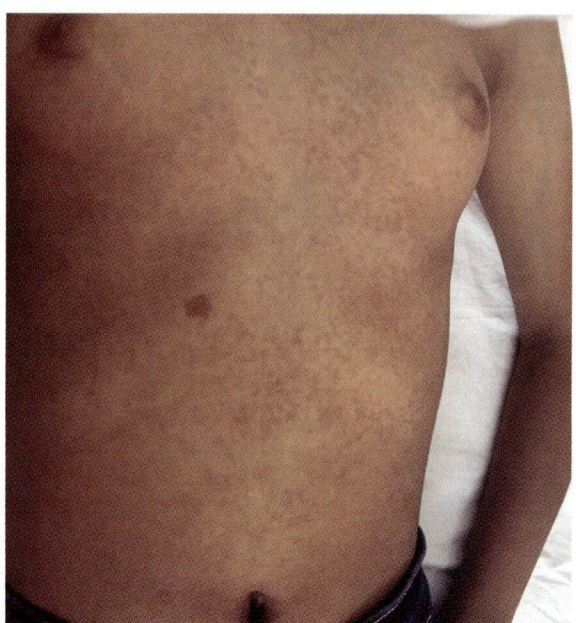

Fig. 18.13 Pityriasis versicolor—ill-defined hypo- and hyper-pigmented macules coalescing together

Dermatophytoses

Dermatophytes are aerobic fungi present in soil. These may be transmitted from animals or humans. Skin and hair infections are caused by *Microsporum, Trichophyton* and *Epidermophyton* species. Nail infection is caused by *Trichophyton* and *Epidermophyton* species.

Tinea Capitis

Tinea capitis presents as partial or complete areas of hair loss with minimal inflammatory features or discrete areas of alopecia studded with black dots (broken off hairs) or patchy or diffuse seborrheic dermatosis like scaling (Fig. 18.14). Some children may develop the inflammatory type of tinea capitis consisting of a boggy, inflammatory swelling, studded with follicular pustules (*kerion*), or yellow cup shaped crusts formed around hair (*favus*).

Treatment is with systemic griseofulvin for 6–8 weeks or oral terbinafine for 4 weeks.

Tinea Pedis

Tinea pedis may lead to a moccasin type of involvement of feet or may involve interdigital clefts of toes resulting in maceration, secondary infection, marked itching, and bad odor.

This is treated by agents that dry the web space. Aluminum chloride and gentian violet are used in addition to topical antifungal agent such as an azole preparation. Systemic antifungals are administered in extensive disease.

Tinea Unguium

There is infection of the distal and lateral nail plate with discoloration, thickening, and crumbling of nails (Fig. 18.15). Infection of nails is very resistant to treatment. Newly available topical preparations such as ciclopirox and natifine penetrate better in the nails.

Widespread eruptions or treatment failures of dermatophytoses may require systemic antifungal therapy with

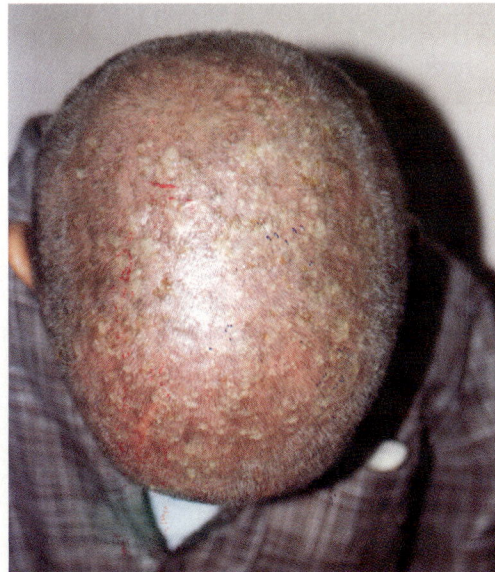

Fig. 18.14 Tinea capitis inflammatory type. Multiple patches of alopecia with follicular pustules and scaling

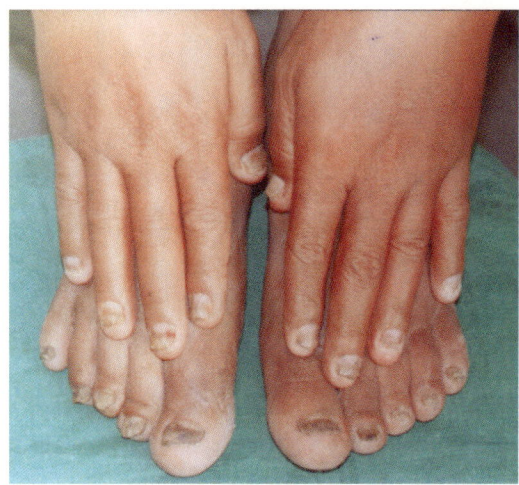

Fig. 18.15 Tinea unguium. Discoloration, thickening and crumbling of nails

terbinafine, griseofulvin, ketoconazole, fluconazole, or itraconazole for a longer duration.

18.10 BULLOUS DISORDERS

Children blister more often than adults because the thorny layer of their epidermis is relatively thinner and the connective tissue contains more soluble collagen and water.

Epidermolysis Bullosa

This is a group of inherited disorders characterized by spontaneous and post-traumatic bulla formation. Epidermolysis bullosa is inherited as autosomal recessive or autosomal dominant.

- *Autosomal dominant* presents with widespread blistering on hands, feet, elbows, and knees. Nails are dystrophic. Skin may show hyperkeratosis. Healing lesions leave behind scars.
- *Autosomal recessive* variety presents at birth. There is mild oral involvement. Nails become dystrophic. Severity ranges from mild disease restricted to extremities to extensive widespread involvement of the skin, mucosa, conjunctiva, cornea, and teeth. Patients with severe form succumb in 2–3 decades because of associated infection.

Therapy is largely supportive such as avoidance of trauma, use of soft and well-ventilated shoes, local care, cold compresses, topical antibiotics, systemic antibiotics and judicious use of hydrocortisone cream or a short course of steroids for severe blistering episodes.

Staphylococcal Scalded Skin Syndrome

Staphylococcal scalded skin syndrome (SSSS) is a potentially life-threatening yet treatable, toxin-mediated manifestation of localized infection with certain strains of staphylococci. It occurs mainly in infancy and early childhood up to the age of 5 years. The disease results from the effect of one of the two epidermolytic toxins, ET-A and ET-B.

Clinical Features

Localized infections leading to SSSS typically originate in the nasopharynx, umbilicus, urinary tract, conjunctivae and

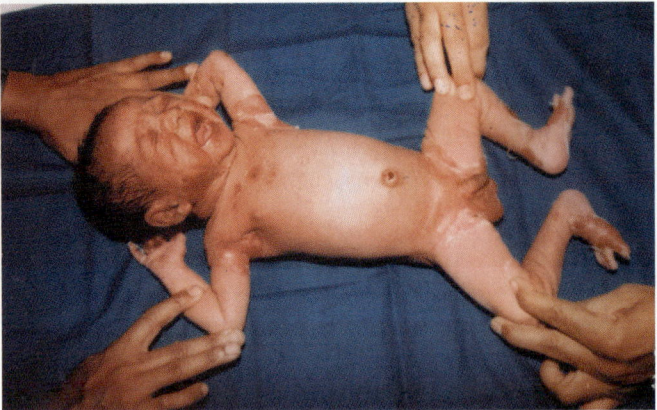

Fig. 18.16 Staphylococcal scalded skin syndrome. (*Courtesy:* Drs. VR Potdar and NV Potdar, Satara)

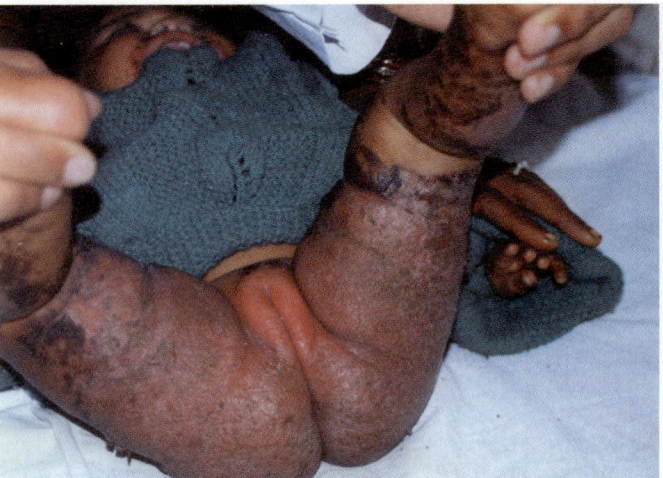

Fig. 18.17 Acrodermatitis enteropathica. Perineal and perianal symmetrical eczematous lesions

blood. The syndrome is ushered in by fever, irritability, generalized skin tenderness, and erythema. The redness is more marked in flexural and periorificial areas. Epidermis is cleavaged through the granular layer causing formation of flaccid bullae and erosions. This results in superficial denudation of the skin, easy disruption of skin with finger rubbing (*Nikolsky sign*), and skin tenderness. Disorder is more marked in flexures (Fig. 18.16). The denuded skin dries forming large flakes in one or two days. Healing is completed in 10–14 days. This may be confused with toxic epidermal necrolysis (*Lyell syndrome*).

Treatment **Staphylococcal Scalded Skin Syndrome**

Systemic penicillinase resistant antibiotics (cloxacillin, vancomycin) are the mainstay of therapy. Supportive skin care, good nutritional intake, saline compresses, and emollient application help in a quick recovery.

Erythema Multiforme

The most important characteristic is an acute target lesion, which may appear erythematous, macular, urticarial, papular, vesicular, or bullous. The lesions may either be localized to distal extremities or be generalized involving oral and genital mucosae and conjunctiva (*Stevens-Johnson syndrome*). Fever, chills and malaise with upper respiratory tract infection are usually associated.

Erythema multiforme is believed to be an immune complex disease in response to infections with a variety of agents, such as herpes simplex, coxsackievirus, echovirus, adenovirus, and mycoplasma. It can also occur secondary to several drugs. Spontaneous resolution might occur in 10–20 days.

Treatment   **Erythema Multiforme**

Antihistaminic drugs are prescribed to relieve itching. Topical compresses and soothing baths are given. Antibiotics are used if there is evidence of infection. Systemic steroids are likely to help in fulminant lesions. Care of conjunctiva and cornea is necessary to avoid residual scarring.

Acrodermatitis Enteropathica

This autosomal recessive disorder usually manifests in the first year of life. Deficiency in amount or function of a zinc binding ligandin is thought to be the causative mechanism.

Clinical manifestations include peripheral, acral, perioral, and perineal vesicular or eczematous skin lesions (Fig. 18.17) with loss or depigmentation of hair and chronic diarrhea. Ocular manifestations such as infection of lids and conjunctivae as well as corneal damage may be associated.

Treatment is aimed towards improving nutrition. Administration of zinc sulfate 50–100 mg per day orally brings about quick relief.

18.11 SEBORRHEIC DERMATITIS

Seborrheic dermatitis is a common inflammatory and scaly skin disease associated with the commensal lipophilic yeast *Pityrosporum ovale*. This is characterized by erythematous, scaly, symmetric eruption that is seen in hair-bearing and intertriginous regions. It is most common during the neonatal and adolescent periods.

Clinical Features

It is characterized by well defined papules and plaques of erythema covered with greasy scaling in regions of skin richly supplied with sebaceous glands—the face, scalp and upper trunk.

- Cradle cap or infantile seborrheic dermatitis in the neonate presents as a dirty, greasy plaque lesion over the scalp vertex (Fig. 18.18).
- Greasy scaling of the scalp or dandruff is a manifestation of seborrheic dermatitis which may be mild and can also occur alone.
- The skin eruption typically involves the nasolabial creases, cheeks, glabella, eyebrows, scalp, periauricular skin, central chest and upper back.
- Itching is not a prominent symptom except in patients with AIDS.

Treatment   **Seborrheic Dermatitis**

Topical therapy with antifungals including ketoconazole, miconazole, or clotrimazole is the mainstay of treatment. Selenium sulphide, tar, and salicyclic acid in shampoo forms have been used for dandruff. Mild topical corticosteroids such

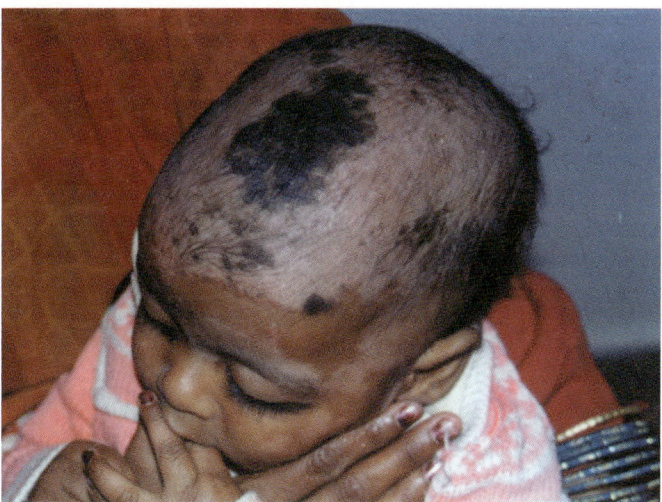

Fig. 18.18 Infantile seborrheic dermatitis

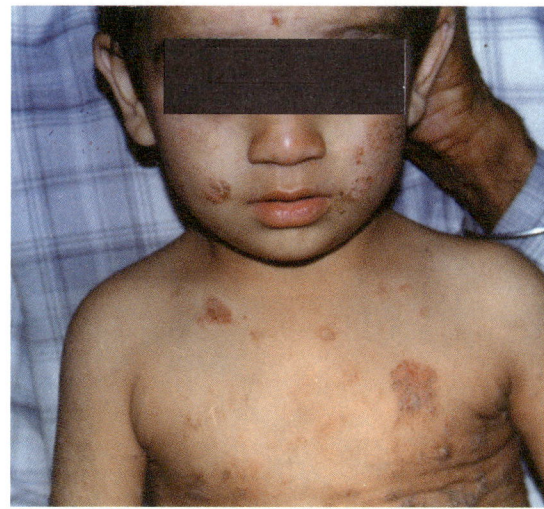

Fig. 18.19 Atopic dermatitis. Erythema, desquamation, papule formation and crusting

as hydrocortisone 1% cream or ointment can be used for face and flexures and high potency steroids could be used in an alcoholic solution for treatment of seborrheic dermatitis of the scalp.

18.12 ATOPIC DERMATITIS

Atopic dermatitis is a chronic relapsing dermatitis characterized by pruritus that may start by the age of 3 months. The onset may be delayed in some cases. The classical features are erythema, exudation, lichenification, and intense itching.

Pathogenesis

There is strong epidemiological association between atopic dermatitis, allergic rhinitis, asthma, and immune deficiency disorders such as Wiskott-Aldrich syndrome. It is now widely believed to be a late phase IgE-mediated reaction due to a constitutional anomaly in the immune system. The disorder may be triggered by an extrinsic allergen. Scratching of skin to relieve itching encourages entry of potential allergens such as resident flora of the skin, *viz.* staphylococci and even pneumococci. Factors released from inflamed skin perpetuate further changes in the dermal and circulating immune competent cells and set up a second vicious cycle.

Clinical Features

The earliest presentation before the age of 3 months may be like that of seborrheic dermatitis. Erythematous squamous lesions first appear on the scalp, behind the ears around the nose, buttock or genital region (Fig. 18.19). Itching may not be as pronounced. Most cases resolve in 4–6 weeks without leaving any residual sequel, but some patients go on to full-fledged infantile eczema by the age of 3–4 months.

Infantile eczema manifests as rosy erythema over the cheeks. There is brawny desquamation, small papule formation and some crusting. The skin folds behind the ear become fissured and neck creases appear sodden. These may be secondarily infected with *Candida*. Extensor surfaces of arms, legs and wrist may show dryness and scaling. Generally perioral, periorbital, and nasal regions are spared. Itching is marked. Buttocks generally escape because of

protective clothing. Most children show a resolution by the age of one or two years; but the illness may continue with remissions and exacerbations in few cases.

Flexural eczema As the age of the child advances, the lesions become more pronounced over the flexures of the elbows, knees, neck, and front of ankle. There is redness, scaling and lichenification.

Others Atopic dermatitis may also present with disseminated lesions as scattered round patches of scaling, lichenification and mild itching or as nummular eczema, with coin-shaped vesicular lesions with intense itching. Lesions may have a perifollicular distribution or skin may have a dry lusterless appearance.

Diagnostic Criteria

Hanifin and Rajka defined major and minor criteria for diagnostic accuracy of atopic dermatitis. Three major and three minor criteria should be present:

Major criteria
1. Pruritus
2. Distribution on the face and convexities in infants under the age of 2 years and over flexures in older children

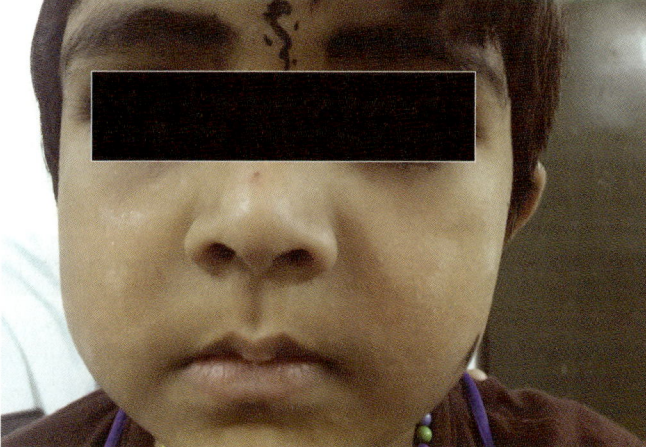

Fig. 18.20 Pityriasis alba on the cheeks—ill-defined hypo-pigmented macules

3. Tendency to chronicity
4. Personal or family history of atopy such as asthma, allergic rhinitis or atopic dermatitis.

Minor criteria Pityriasis alba (Fig. 18.20), delayed blanching to cholinergics, anterior subcapsular cataract, xerosis, ichthyosis vulgaris with accentuation over palmar creases, facial pallor/suborbital shadowing, infraorbital folds, keratoconus, recurrent skin infections, tendency to non-specific dermatosis of hand, and raised serum total IgE.

Consequently, Williams, et al. coordinated a UK attempt to refine the criteria of Hanifin and Rajka into a repeatable and validated set of diagnostic criteria. As per the UK diagnostic criteria, to qualify as a case of atopic dermatitis (eczema), the child must have the following.

An itchy skin condition plus three or more of the following:
1. Onset below age of 2 years
2. History of skin crease involvement
3. History of a generally dry skin
4. Personal history of other atopic disease
5. Visible flexural dermatitis

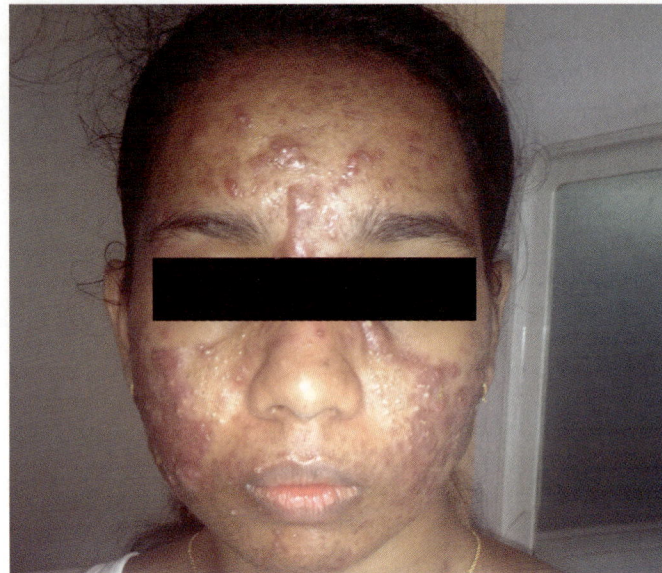

Fig. 18.21 Nodulocystic and keloidal acne

Treatment	Atopic Dermatitis

- General education and counseling regarding the condition is of paramount importance, atopic eczema being a chronic disease.
- Avoidance of the trigger factors, if clearly identified, is also as important as pharmacological treatment in some cases.
- The child should be gently bathed once or twice in a day using very small quantity of mild soap or non-soap cleanser in bath water. This is done to prevent drying of epidermis. After the bath, he or she should be patted dry with towel and emollients and topical medication should be applied on the still wet skin. The regular use of emollients softens the skin and reduces itch.

Drug Therapy

Systemic antibiotics such as cloxacillin or erythromycin may be given for 7–10 days if definite signs of secondary bacterial infection are present. A mild to moderately potent corticosteroid cream can be applied to relieve inflammation. Topical calcineurin inhibitors such as tacrolimus and pimecrolimus are used as second line therapy. Prophylactic treatment of staphylococcal carrier sites (nose, axillae and perineum) with topical antibiotics such as mupirocin ointment may be appropriate in patients with recurrent infected eczema. Antihistaminics relieve itching and also help in relieving the inflammation. Systemic steroid therapy is generally advisable only to control the severe flares, in the short term. Other immunomodulators like cyclosporine are being successfully used for a longer duration in very severe cases.

18.13 ACNE

Acne is a pleomorphic eruption usually seen on the face and trunk and rarely on arms, legs and buttocks. It is observed most commonly during adolescence but a rare variety may present during early infancy and persist for 1–5 years.

Early lesions are whiteheads or blackheads (*comedones*), which are seen 2 or 3 years before the development of classical signs of acne. The comedones may be infected with *Staphylococcus epidermidis* or *Propionibacterium acnes* resulting in formation of papules and pustules. Deeper lesions may lead to formation of nodular cysts and result in scarring (Fig. 18.21).

Pathogenesis

Acne results from the interplay of multiple factors acting at the level of the pilosebaceous unit which result in obstruction of the duct and subsequent inflammation. These factors include defects in keratinization resulting in plugging of the hair follicle, excess sebum production, the presence and activity of the commensal bacteria like *Propionibacterium acnes* and other factors resulting in inflammation. The increased production of sebum may be as a result of end organ hypersensitivity to androgens, which may be of gonadal or adrenal origin. Some lipids present in the sebum cause irritant dermatitis. Formation of comedones is also attributed to the lack of linoleic acid in the skin surface lipids. Colonization with *S. epidermidis* and *P. acnes* may set up inflammation in comedones.

Treatment	Acne

The child and adolescent should be psychologically prepared. Use of commercially advertised medicines should be discouraged. Comedonal or papular acne can be managed with topical application of clindamycin, erythromycin, or clarithromycin creams. Count of *P. acnes* and number of visible comedones can be reduced by the use of benzyl peroxide gel or cream (2.5%, 5% or 10%). Azaleic acid, a dicarboxylic acid derived from *P. ovale* is reported to be useful. Local application of retinoic acid reduces the number of non-inflamed lesions and ductal *P. acnes* count. It also helps to normalize the defect of keratinization.

Isoretinoin (13-*cis*-retinoic acid), 0.5 to 1.0 mg/kg per day, administered orally for 4 months improves acne in 85–90% adolescents. This should be used with caution in young married females for fear of possible teratogenicity.

18.14 VASCULAR LESIONS

Hemangioma

Hemangiomas are the most common benign tumors occurring in children. About 10% of infants at 1 year of age have hemangiomas. Hemangiomas are primarily composed of capillaries and are characterized by endothelial cell proliferation. These may either be superficial (*strawberry*) (Fig. 18.22) or deep (*cavernous*) (Fig. 18.23). Nearly two-thirds of hemangiomas are situated on the head and neck; 25% involve trunk and the rest are found on extremities. Lumbosacral hemangiomas may be associated with tethering of the spinal cord.

The natural course of the hemangiomas includes proliferative and involutional phases. The lesions proliferate rapidly during the first 6 months of life and then slowly during the second half of the first year. Thereafter, involution starts so that 50% of lesions resolve by 5 years, 70% by 7 years, and 90% by 9 years. Once resolved, residual changes such as hypopigmentation, atrophy, or scarring may occur. Bleeding, ulceration, and infection may occur, more often in the first six months of life.

Treatment	Hemangioma

Beta-blockers, most specifically propranolol, have been shown to induce involution of infantile hemangiomas and are now considered first-line treatment for problematic infantile hemangiomas. They are preferred over systemic steroids in the

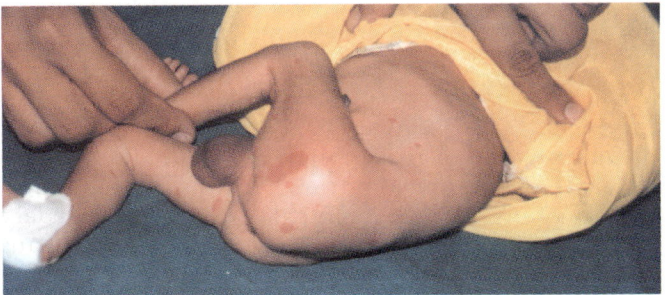

Fig. 18.22 Strawberry hemangioma in an infant

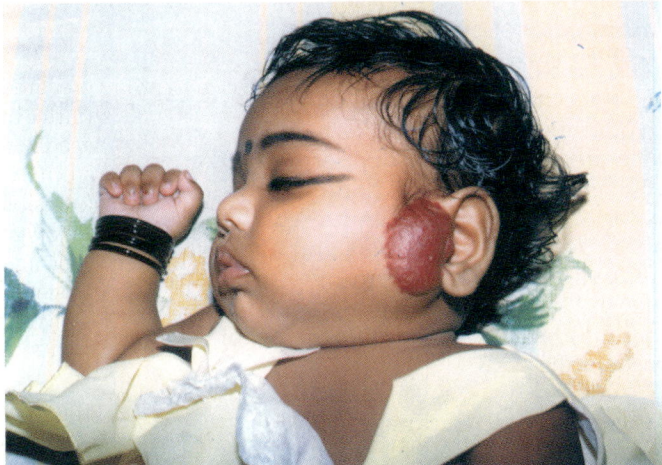

Fig. 18.23 Cavernous hemangioma (*Courtesy:* Dr. Newton Luiz, Kottayam)

treatment of complicated hemangiomas. Topical beta-blockers like timolol have been reported to be useful in the treatment of smaller, uncomplicated hemangiomas.

The 585 nm pulsed dye laser can be effective for treating superficial hemangiomas, particularly when they are treated early. Interferon 2-alpha is effective in blocking endothelial cell motility and proliferation *in vitro* and inhibiting the process of angiogenesis.

Salmon Patches

These are the commonest vascular lesions in infancy, also known as stork bites, angel's kisses or nevus flammeus neonatorum. These pale, pink to red macules are seen over the glabella, upper eyelids or neck in about 40% of all newborns. Most lesions fade by 1 to 2 years of age. Persistent lesions can be treated successfully with pulsed dye laser.

Port-wine Stains

These occur in 0.3% of all newborns and represent progressive ectasia of the superficial vascular plexus. These do not resolve spontaneously. These stains are typically pink in infancy, but may darken and develop vascular nodularity. Face is commonly involved, but these may occur anywhere on the body. Treatment is best achieved by 585 nm pulsed dye laser which destroys the blood vessels without damaging the surrounding tissues.

Sturge-Weber Syndrome

This is a vascular anomaly of the skin, choroid of the eye, and ipsilateral leptomeninges. The facial port-wine stain is distributed in the region of the trigeminal nerve. These patients may develop glaucoma and seizures. *Railroad* calcification in the occipital and temporal regions is characteristic in skull radiographs. MRI is the most sensitive technique for demonstrating cerebral lesions.

18.15 DISORDERS OF KERATINIZATION OR ICHTHYOSES

Ichthyoses are disorders of cornification in which abnormal differentiation and desquamation of the epidermis result in a defective epidermal barrier. Ichthyoses represent a large clinically and etiologically heterogeneous group of conditions that feature generalized scaling of the skin.

Clinical features, pattern of inheritance and structural, biochemical, and molecular abnormalities help to differentiate these disorders. Therapy is symptomatic and primarily aimed at reducing hyperkeratosis. Topical management consists of emollients, keratolytics, and retinoids. The most important types of this group of disorders are detailed below.

Ichthyosis Vulgaris

One of the commonest and mildest forms of ichthyosis, it is inherited in an autosomal dominant fashion. It occurs due to loss of function mutations in *filaggrin* gene. The disease is usually not evident at birth, and manifests during infancy or early childhood. Fine, white, flaky scales develop on the extremities, especially the extensor surfaces. The groin and flexural areas are usually spared. On the lower legs, the scales

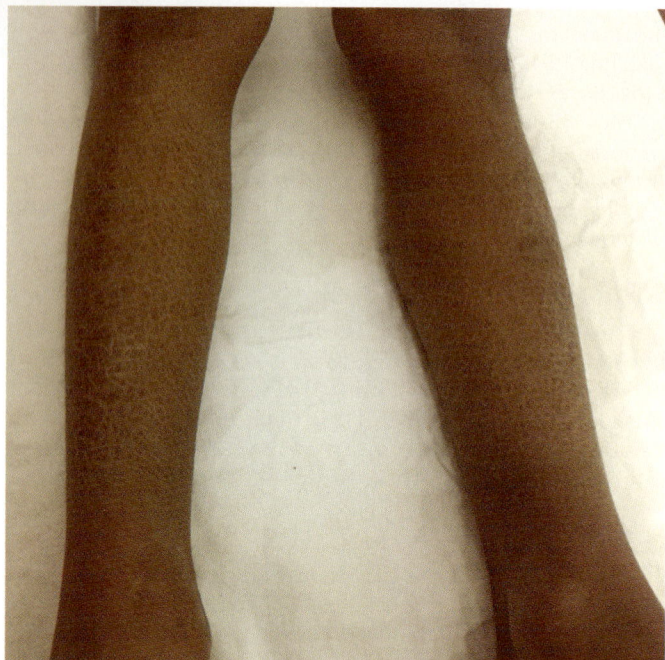

Fig. 18.24 *Ichthyosis vulgaris in a child*

are usually larger with an adherent center and detached, outward-turning edges (Fig. 18.24). Histopathology often reveals orthokeratotic hyperkeratosis with a reduced or absent granular layer.

X-linked Recessive Ichthyosis

This X-linked recessive disorder is transmitted by asymptomatic female carriers and almost exclusively affects boys and men. It is attributed to the deficiency of *steroid sulfatase* enzyme. The changes are usually evident from birth or the neonatal period itself. Large, dark polygonal scales are prominently seen on the trunk and extremities. The palms and soles are nearly always spared. Neck is usually involved, giving rise to the 'dirty neck appearance'; other flexures may or may not be involved. Histopathology often reveals a compact hyperkeratosis with a normal or increased granular layer.

Cryptorchidism and corneal opacities are the other features associated with this disorder.

Lamellar Ichthyosis

Lamellar ichthyosis is a genetically heterogenous ichthyotic disorder, inherited as an autosomal recessive trait, due to the deficiency of the enzyme *transglutaminase 1*. **Classic lamellar ichthyosis** is a severe disorder that is apparent at birth and persists throughout life, although milder variants also occur. Most affected neonates are encased in a collodion membrane (**collodion baby**). Over the first weeks of life, the collodion membrane is gradually replaced by generalized scaling, the scales are large, brown and plate-like that form a mosaic or bark-like pattern with minimal to no associated erythroderma. The scales are centrally attached and have raised borders, often leading to superficial fissures. Ectropion, eclabium may be associated. In a collodion baby, the membrane peels in 2–4 weeks and reveals the underlying condition.

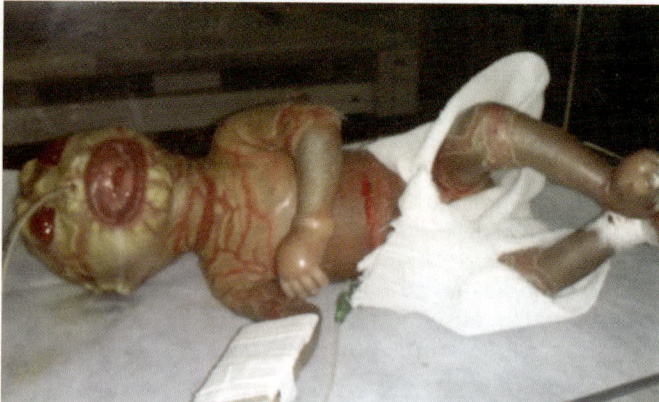

Fig. 18.25 Harlequin ichthyosis

Congenital ichthyosiform erythroderma or non-bullous ichthyosiform erythroderma is thought to be a milder variant of lamellar ichthyosis by many authors.

Harlequin Ichthyosis

Harlequin ichthyosis (HI) is the most severe type of congenital ichthyosis, caused by mutations in *ABCA12* gene. Neonates are born with armor-like skin (Fig. 18.25) which can considerably impair movement and the ability to drink and breath. Bilateral ectropion and clabium are present. A major problem in early infancy is susceptibility to infections, fluid and electrolyte imbalance. Respiratory problems are the major cause of death in neonates. The early initiation of systemic retinoids and improved supportive care have reduced the mortality in this disorder.

Syndromic Ichthyoses

This includes a very heterogenous group of conditions including Sjögren-Larsson syndrome, multiple sulfatase deficiency, Refsum syndrome, Conradi syndrome, Chanarin–Dorfman syndrome, KID syndrome, etc.

18.16 CUTANEOUS MANIFESTATIONS OF SYSTEMIC DISEASES

Gastrointestinal Diseases

Inflammatory Bowel Disease

Ulcerative colitis can have mucocutaneous manifestations in 30% patients. Aphthous ulcers, erythema nodosum, pyoderma gangrenosum (which is a non-infective focal ulcerative process with undermined borders and a floor covered by purulent discharge), and thrombophlebitis can occur. Crohn's disease can present with perianal fissures, abscesses, sinuses, fistulas and also aphthae, erythema nodosum, and pyoderma gangrenosum. Metastatic noncaseating granulomatous lesions may present as solitary or multiple plaques or nodules on perioral, perianal or other areas of the skin.

Malabsorption Syndrome

Skin manifestations due to malabsorption of the essential fatty acids include dryness, cracking and fissuring of the skin, psoriasiform rash, skin blistering, and pigmentation of the mucous membranes of the buccal cavity. Hair and nail loss are other features.

Chronic Liver Disease

Skin manifestations of chronic liver disease include jaundice, clubbing, diffuse hyperpigmentation, spider naevi, telangiectasia, palmar erythema, livedo reticularis and vasculitis. Purpuric rashes may occur due to vitamin K deficiency. Seborrhea and acneifom eruptions may occur on the upper extremities and Bier's spots can occur on lower extremities. The nail changes are absent.

Renal Diseases

In renal disease, the common manifestations are pruritus, dryness, fine scalp hair, and falling of axillary and pubic hair after puberty. In renal failure, pallor may occur due to anemia and hyperpigmentation may be due to increased melanocyte activity.

Thyroid Disease

Congenital Hypothyroidism

Cutaneous findings in congenital hypothyroidism are cool and dry skin, pronounced cutis marmorata, and a translucent pallor in the infant. The pallor is due to combined effects of anemia, poor peripheral perfusion, prolonged neonatal jaundice, and carotenemia. Due to deposition of glyco-saminoglycan in the skin and tongue, there is macroglossia and skin thickening. There is a characteristic facies consisting of thickened facial skin, protruding tongue, depressed nasal bridge and mild hypertelorism. Lusterless, slow-growing hair and nails, and delayed eruption of deciduous teeth are other findings.

Acquired Hypothyroidism

Long-standing acquired hypothyroidism will have cool dry skin with yellowish pallor, macroglossia, and skin thickening of face, over supraclavicular fossae, and around hands and feet. There is loss of lateral third of eyebrows and scalp and body hair are sparse, brittle and lusterless. Slow nail growth, along with brittleness and ridging are other findings.

Hyperthyroidism

Skin changes include a flushed appearance of the skin and a warm, clammy feel on palpation. Other uncommon findings are thinning of scalp hair, vitiligo, onycholysis, and hyperpigmentation. Pretibial myxedema occurs in less than 2% of children with Graves' disease. There is mucinous infiltration of the pretibial skin and also other sites such as posterior calves, thighs, arms, trunk, and dorsum of feet. The infiltration is in the form of yellow colored skin, red or brown non-pitting nodules, or plaques with dilated follicular orifices giving a *peau d' orange* appearance.

Cushing Disease

The skin findings are a plethoric face, purple striae, hyperpigmentation, hypertrichosis on the cheeks and forehead, skin fragility with poor wound healing, and purpura. Acneiform eruptions can also occur on face and upper trunk.

Addison Disease

Hyperpigmentation of the skin and mucosal surfaces occurs in patients with gradual onset of the diseases. The pigmentation is diffuse with accentuation on exposed areas, around new scars and over areas of friction or pressure. There is also darkening of existing melanocytic naevi and appearance of longitudinal pigmented bands in the nail plate. Postpubertal girls may have loss of pubic and axillary hair.

Diabetes Mellitus

Skin changes due to microangiopathy and neuropathy are never seen in prepubertal children. *Candida albicans* infection is common and can present as vulvovaginitis, balanitis, angular cheilitis, intraoral candidiasis, intertrigo and paronychia. Deep fungal infections, such as mucormycosis can rarely occur in poorly controlled diabetic children. Eruptive xanthomas due to hypertriglyceridemia can occur in children with poorly controlled type I diabetes mellitus. These are firm yellowish papules which may coalesce to form large plaques on buttocks, lumbosacral region, and extensor aspect of the limbs.

The typical skin findings which are characteristic of diabetes mellitus are limited joint mobility with waxy skin thickening which results in flexion contractions of proximal interphalangeal joints of the fourth and fifth finger. Necrobiosis lipoidica diabeticorum is located over the pretibial areas and is characterized as a well-defined, asymptomatic, erythematous papule or nodule which enlarges to produce a plaque with a raised rim and slightly depressed center. The center of the plaque may undergo atrophy and ulceration. Diabetic dermopathy is uncommon in children, but can present as reddish brown papules measuring less than 1–2 cm in diameter, which regress to produce depressed and slightly atrophic reddish brown macules which are found over pretibial area, arms, thighs and trunk.

The local side-effects of insulin therapy can be allergic reactions, development of soft tissue hypertrophy and the development of lipoatrophy or infections at injection sites.

Hypersensitivity Reactions to Drugs

Most drug-induced eruptions are in the form of mild morbilliform or exanthematous or urticarial eruptions and may resolve without complications on withdrawing the suspected agent. The diagnostic features of drug reactions on the skin include onset of the rash within 7–10 days after drug exposure, pruritus, peripheral spread and sometimes fever, arthralgia and lymphadenopathy. Eosinophilia is commonly seen. Common drugs causing various skin reactions are penicillins, sulfa drugs, cephalosporins, anticonvulsant, and aminoglycosides.

Drug Hypersensitivity Syndrome

This is a rare and serious syndrome and also known as DRESS (drug rash, eosinophilia, and systemic symptoms) syndrome. It is characterized by initial onset of fever, skin rash and possible involvement of internal organs (hepatitis). Hypersensitivity syndrome reaction (HSR) occurs mostly on first exposure to the drug after a period of 7–28 days. The offending drug is mostly an aromatic anticonvulsant (carbamazepine, phenobarbital, and phenytoin). The syndrome starts with fever, malaise followed by edema and swelling of the face. Pharyngitis and cervical lymphadenopathy are early features. The skin rash is diffuse, itchy, erythematous to urticarial eruption of coalescing plaques.

Laboratory investigations reveal eosinophilia, atypical lymphocytosis, hepatitis ranging from mild elevation of liver enzymes to frank hepatic failure. Systemic complications such as pneumonitis, interstitial nephritis and encephalitis can also occur.

The mechanism of development of this reaction involves a heritable defect in the epoxide hydrolase pathway of the anticonvulsants, which can lead to accumulation of toxic metabolites which react with lymphocytes.

Stevens-Johnson Syndrome and Toxic Epidermal Necrolysis

Stevens-Johnson syndrome (SJS) and toxic epidermal necrolysis (TEN) are the most severe forms of hypersensitivity reactions affecting the skin. Though rarer than in adults, these conditions can occur in children and can cause diagnostic dilemmas especially with viral illnesses like varicella and other drug reactions. Current terminology is based on maximal extent of epidermal detachment.

SJS indicates cases with epidermal necrolysis that involves less than 10% of the body surface area (Fig. 18.26), TEN with more than 30% (Fig. 18.27a and b), and overlap of SJS/TEN in between.

More than 100 drugs have been associated with these conditions, but only a small number are responsible for the majority of cases, especially in children. Common triggers include anticonvulsants, sulfonamides, and nonsteroidal anti-inflammatory drugs. Other reported triggers of SJS include chemicals, immunizations, *M. pneumoniae*, and viral infections.

Clinically, SJS and TEN are characterized by polymorphic lesions like erythematous macules, papules, plaque, vesicles, and bullae with positive Nikolsky sign. Oral, genital, and conjunctival mucosae are often involved in the form of erosion or ulceration. In children, the mortality rate is reported to be lower than in adults, but the incidence of long-term complications like scarring, ocular complications, etc. is more.

Serum Sickness Like Reactions

This is characterized by fever, rash, arthralgia, lymphadenopathy, 1–3 weeks after drug intake. The skin rash is urticarial to purpuric, well-defined coalescing plaques. Acral erythema and edema are other features. In contrast to true serum sickness; immune complexes, hypocomplementenemia, vasculitis, and renal lesions are absent. In children, the risk of serum sickness like reactions are more with cefaclor than with other antibiotics. Although the cause is not known, a toxic metabolite is suspected. These reactions typically occur after repeated drug exposures. Kawasaki disease, connective tissue diseases, and hypersensitivity syndrome should be considered in the differential diagnosis. Withdrawal of the offending drug and symptomatic treatment is required.

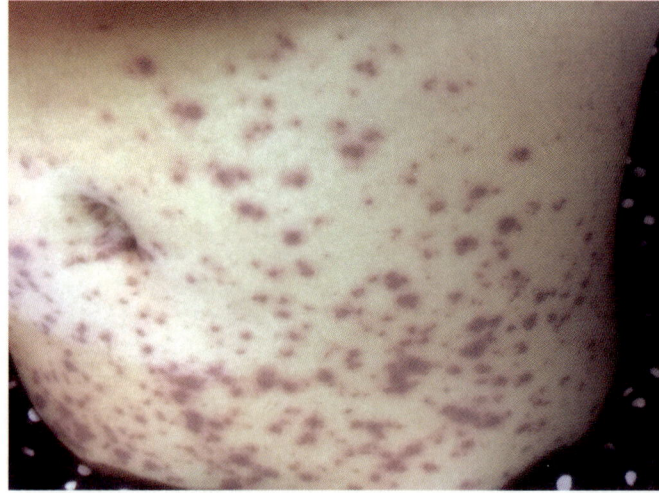

Fig. 18.26 Stevens-Johnson syndrome—charred lesions seen on the trunk of a young girl

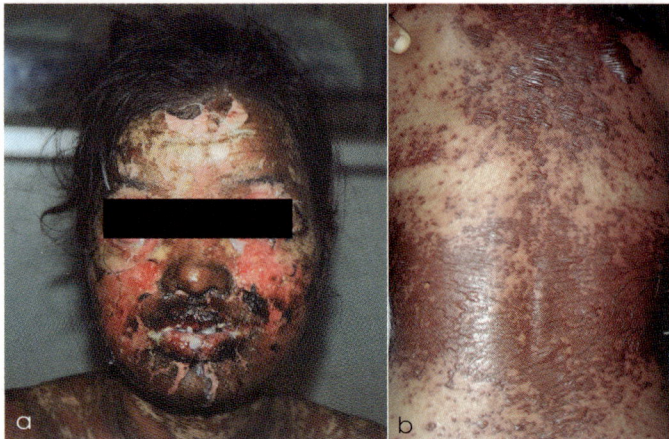

Fig. 18.27 Severe toxic epidermal necrolysis in a 16-year-old girl showing epidermal detachment, eye involvement, and hemorrhagic crusting of the lips

Akdis CA, Akdis M, Bieber T, *et al.* Diagnosis and treatment of atopic dermatitis in children and adults. European Academy of Allergology and Clinical Immunology/American Academy of Allergy, Asthma and Immunology/PRACTALL Consensus Report. *Allergy.* 2006:61:969–87.

Boul C, Groth D. Update: Treatment of viral warts in children. *Pediatr Dermatol.* 2011;28:217–29.

Kim RH, Armstrong AW. Current state of acne treatment: Highlighting lasers, photodynamic therapy and chemical peels. *Dermatology Online Journal.* 2011;17:2.

Lofgren S, Krol A. New therapies in pediatric dermatology. *Curr Opinion Pediatr.* 2011;23:399–402.

Menezes MD, McCarter R, Greene EA, Baumann NM. Status of propranolol for treatment of infantile haemangioma and description of a randomized clinical trial. *Ann Otol Rhinol Laryngol.* 2011;120:686–95.

Nutanson I, Steen CJ, Schwartz RA, Janigker CK. Pediculus humanus capitis: an update. *Acta Dermatovenereol Alp Paronica Adriat.* 2008;17:147–54.

Segal AR, Doherrty KM, Leggott J, Zlotoff B. Cutaneous reactions to drugs in children. *Pediatrics.* 2007;12: e1082–e1096.

Steinbach WJ. Antifungal agents in children. *Pediatr Clin North Am.* 2005;52:895–915.

Templer SJ, Brito MO. Bacterial skin and soft tissue infections. *Hospital Physician.* 2009;26:9–16.

Rashmi Sarkar, Soumya Jagadeesan, and Piyush Gupta

Ophthalmic Disorders

Eyes are the mirror to the whole body. Ocular symptoms in children can often be a reflection of various systemic disorders and may provide the first clue to the diagnosis. It is important for a pediatrician to be able to diagnose common ophthalmic diseases and decide when to refer to an ophthalmologist.

19.1 APPROACH TO COMMON SYMPTOMS

1. Red Eye

Common causes of a red eye include conjunctivitis, keratitis, keratoconjunctivitis, glaucoma, and uveitis. These diseases can occur in isolation or secondary to a systemic illness. Diagnostic approach to a child with red eye is shown in Fig. 19.1.

2. Discharge from the Eye

A causal relationship can be established based on the nature of discharge from the eye. Causes of and approach to a child with discharge from the eye is depicted in Fig. 19.2.

3. Itching/Eye Rubbing

Allergic conjunctivitis and seborrheic blepharitis are the most common causes of frequent rubbing or itching in the eyes. Other causes in younger children include foreign body (due to irritation), or an uncorrected refractive error (due to hazy view). A detailed examination is essential to rule out uncorrected refractive errors in all children with frequent rubbing of eyes. An approach to the diagnosis of frequent eye rubbing is illustrated in Fig. 19.3.

4. Decreased Vision

A child with decreased vision may never complain of it because that is the only vision he/she knows of. Additional symptoms to indicate decreased vision include frequent eye rubbing or infections, viewing through squeezed eyes to apply a pinhole effect, or a complaint from school teacher. Unilateral visual loss in a child is suspected, if the child's behavior changes on covering the normal eye. Blindness is difficult to establish clinically in a child under 3 months of age and sophisticated tests (visual evoked potentials, optokinetic nystagmus, and force choice preferential looking test) have to be conducted to determine the visual acuity. Visual acuity in an infant can be grossly ascertained by observing him/her reaching for objects and observing his interaction with parents. Between the ages of 1 and 3 years, a child is able to identify small objects of measured size. Beyond the age of 3 years, Snellen chart can be used for testing visual activity. Nystagmus in the first year of life also implies loss of visual acuity unless proven otherwise.

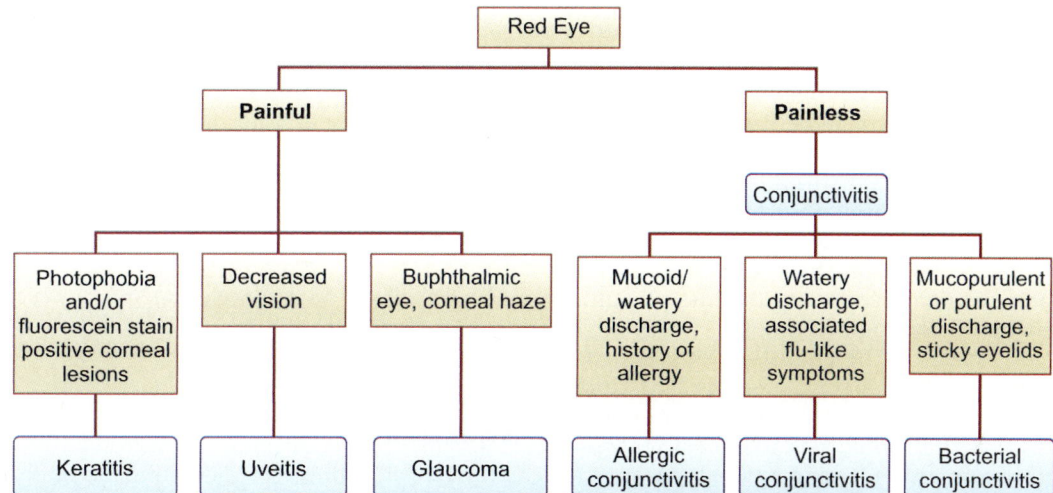

Fig. 19.1 Diagnostic approach to a child with red eye

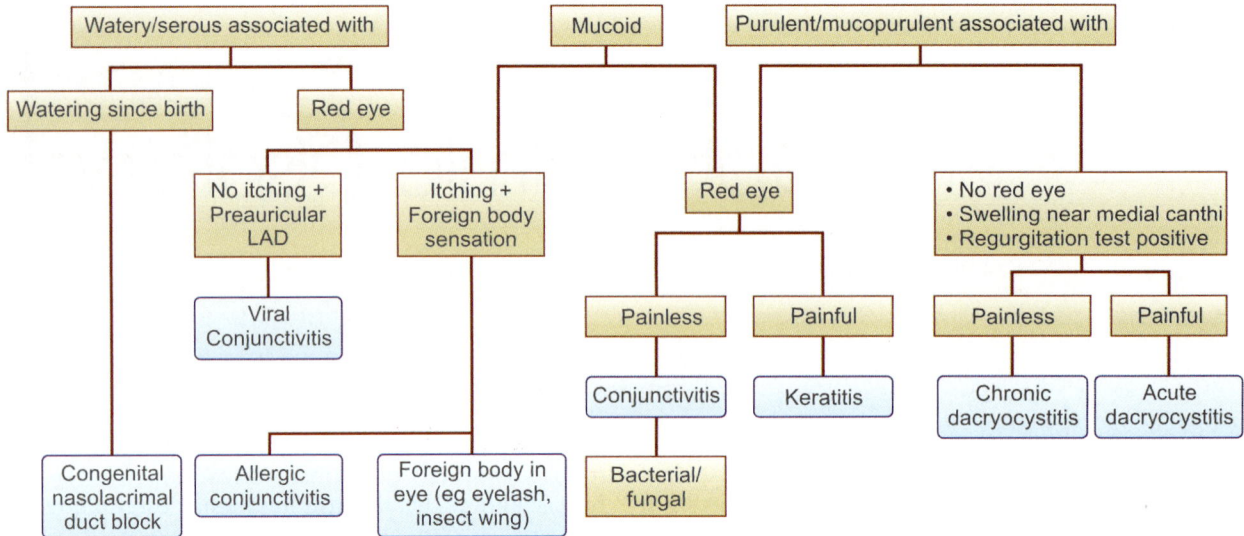

Fig. 19.2 Approach to a child with discharge from the eye

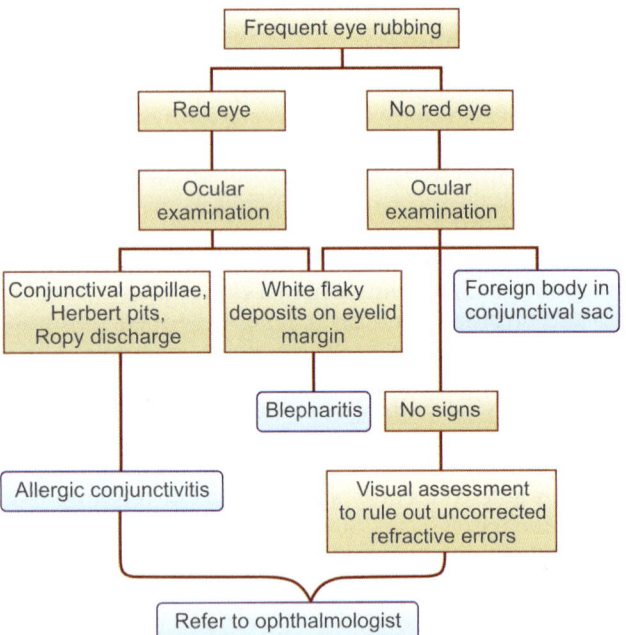

Fig. 19.3 Approach to the complaint of frequent eye rubbing

Approach to a child with low vision shown in Fig. 19.4. Common causes are discussed below.

• *Refractive errors* Normal eye is hypermetropic at birth by an average of 3 diopters. Refractive errors (myopia, hypermetropia, and astigmatism) thereafter should be recognized early and proper therapy be instituted. Uncorrected refractive errors in children cause sensory deprivation, which if prolonged, may result in strabismus (discussed later) and amblyopia (partial loss of sight in absence of any ophthalmologic findings).

• *Media opacities* These can be classified as (*a*) corneal opacities (due to keratomalacia, post-keratitis, post-traumatic, corneal dystrophies), (*b*) lenticular opacities presenting as a white reflex or leukocoria (cataract, retrolental fibroplasia), (*c*) hypopyon (pus in anterior chamber), (*d*) hyphema (blood in anterior chamber), and (*e*) other caused by uveitis, and vitreous hemorrhage.

• *Retinal diseases* Retinal detachment, retinitis pigmentosa, optic neuritis, papilledema, and retinal vascular occlusions all may lead to low vision.

19.2 COMMON ABNORMALITIES IN THE EYE

1. ORBIT

Look for abnormal protrusion of the eyeball (*proptosis*), retraction of the eye back into its orbit (*enophthalmos*), wide separation of the eyes (*hypertelorism*), and small palpebral fissures (*microphthalmos*). Palpate for any bony defects or swellings.

Proptosis

Proptosis can be objectively measured with Hertel's exophthalmometer. A simple way of clinically detecting proptosis is to stand behind a sitting child and ask him to tilt head upwards. In a normal eye, tips of cornea of both eyes should be visible to the examiner at the same time when viewed from above. Proptosis is said to be present in an eye *when the cornea in one eye is visible before that of the other eye.*

Proptosis may occur due to (*i*) diminished orbital volume as in craniosynostosis; or (*ii*) increase in the orbital tissue mass such as with malignant deposits, cavernous sinus thrombosis, orbital hemorrhage, and orbital cellulitis. Proptosis caused by thyrotoxicosis is multifactorial and is also known as *exophthalmos.*

Enophthalmos

It is caused by lesion of lower cervical and upper thoracic sympathetic nerve fibers, which supply the eyes. It usually occurs as a part feature of Horner syndrome; other manifestations being ptosis, absent ciliospinal reflex, anhidrosis, and miosis.

Hypertelorism

It can be determined by calculating the canthal index which is normally 38 in males and 38.5 in females (SD ±2.4). This index is increased in hypertelorism.

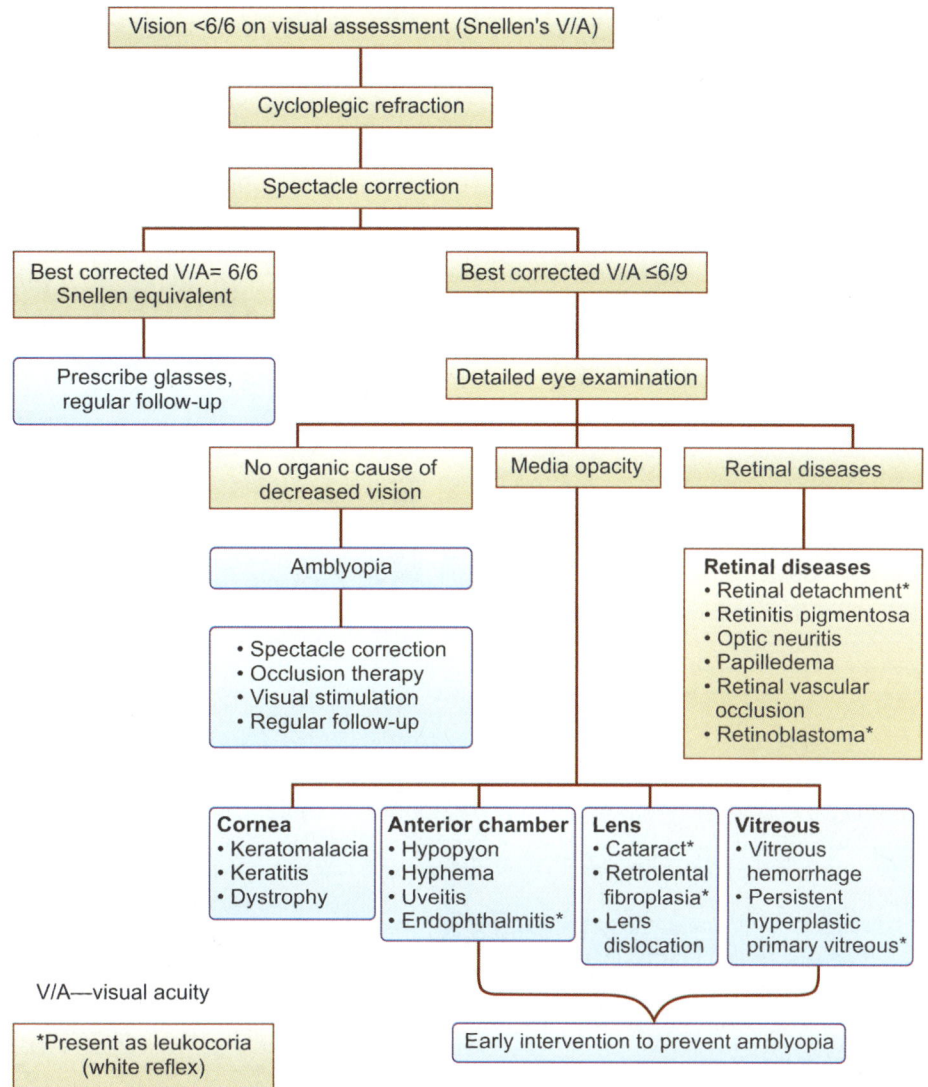

Fig. 19.4 Approach to decreased vision

Canthal index = [Inner canthal distance/Outer canthal distance] × 100

Microphthalmos and hypertelorism are frequently encountered in Down syndrome and intrauterine infections due to cytomegalovirus, rubella, or toxoplasma.

Telecanthus is said to be present when there is increased distance between the inner canthi only.

2. EYELIDS

Ptosis

Keep one hand firmly on the forehead to prevent action of the frontalis muscle and ask the child to lift the upper eyelid. Normally, the upper eyelid should cover about 2 mm of cornea below the upper limbus in primary gaze. Drooping of upper eyelid below this level is known as *ptosis*.

Ptosis may be *congenital* or *acquired* due to hemangioma (Sturge-Weber syndrome), plexiform neuroma (neurofibromatosis), myasthenia gravis (Fig. 19.5), Horner syndrome, lesions affecting the third nerve, lid tumors, and following drugs such as vincristine.

Other Lid Abnormalities

An upper lid that rests above the upper limbus is referred to as *lid retraction*. Inspect for inability to completely close the palpebral fissure (*lagophthalmos*). Lagophthalmos and lid retraction may occur as part of thyrotoxicosis. Also, look for lid inflammation (*blepharitis*), vascular anomalies (*nevus* or *telangiectasia*), and swelling of lid.

Notice the placement of the palpebral fissure. It is oblique, short and wide with the highest point at the center of the lid in Down syndrome (*mongoloid slant*). Another important lid anomaly in Down syndrome consists of skinfolds above the inner canthus (*epicanthic folds*).

Blepharophimosis syndrome (Fig. 19.6) is a congenital condition characterized by ptosis, blepharophimosis, telecanthus, and epicanthus inversus. It is mostly inherited as an autosomal dominant trait and may be associated with premature ovarian failure in type 1 cases.

3. LACRIMAL SYSTEM

Conjunctival irritation or unilateral watering of eye should indicate lacrimal involvement. Acute and bilateral

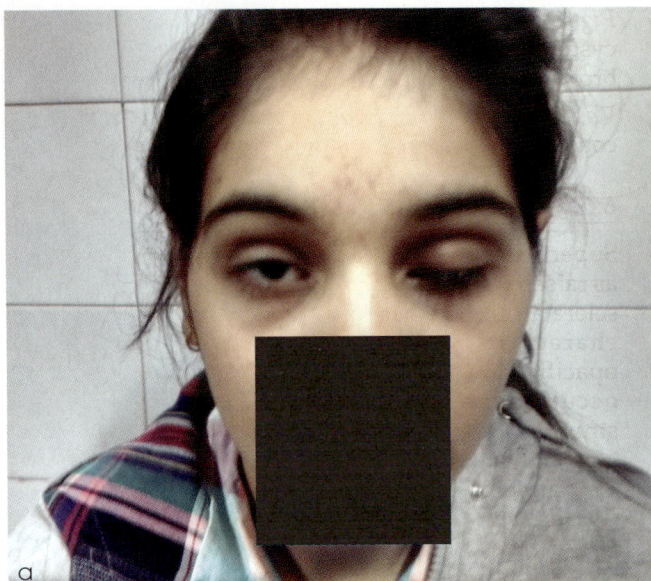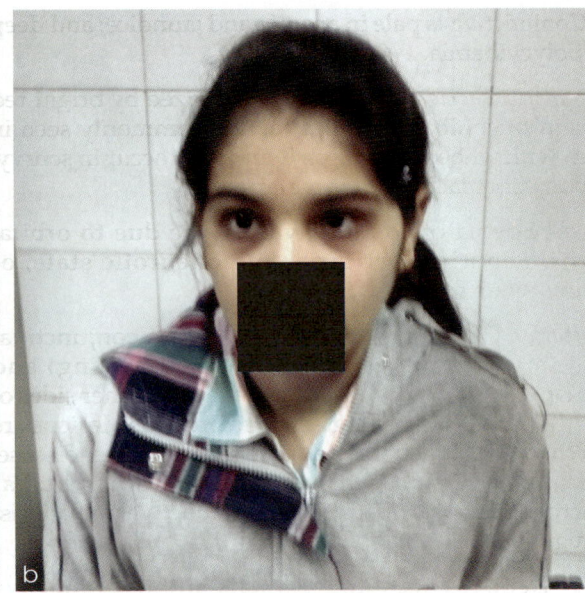

Fig. 19.5 Ocular myasthenia gravis: (a) Unilateral ptosis; (b) Ptosis corrected after applying ice for 2 minutes (*positive ice test*)

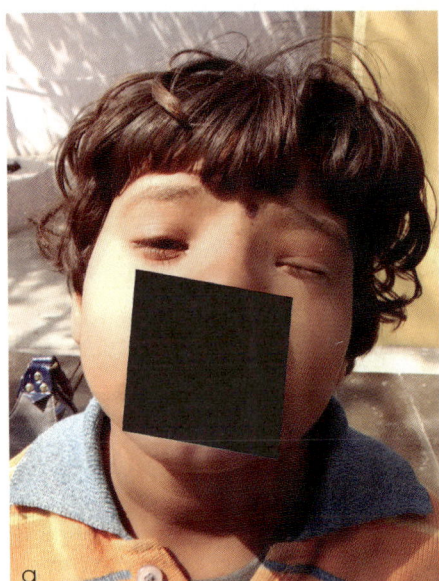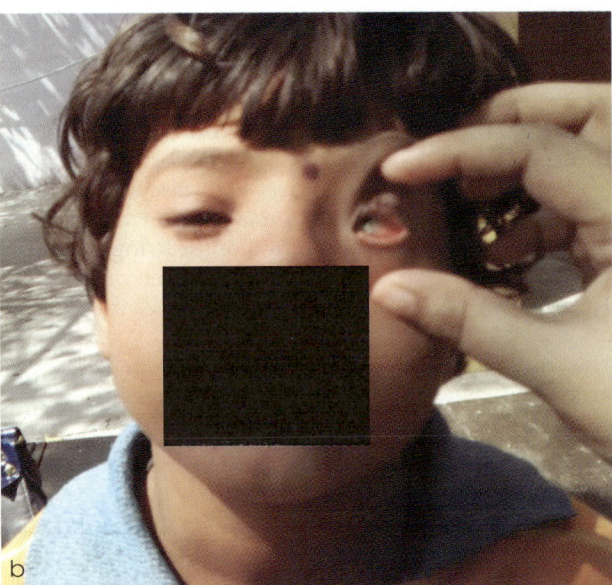

Fig. 19.6 (a) Blepharophimosis syndrome; (b) Nanophthalmic left eye. Also note raised eyebrows, chin lift, moderate ptosis right eye, complete ptosis left eye, and telecanthus

inflammation of lacrimal gland (*acute dacryoadenitis*) occurs in influenza, mumps, and infectious mononucleosis. *Chronic dacryoadenitis* is associated with syphilis, tuberculosis, and sarcoidosis.

Alacrima (dry eye) occurs in Riley-Day syndrome and ectodermal dysplasia. Deficiency of conjunctival mucus following Stevens-Johnson syndrome is another cause of alacrima. Tears are also reduced in dehydration. These conditions need immediate ophthalmic attention to prevent symblepharon/ankyloblepharon and visual loss due to corneal scarring.

Non-canalization of lacrimal passages lead to apparent increase in tears (*epiphora*) as in congenital block of nasolacrimal duct. Adequate sac massage (Criggler's hydrostatic sac massage) may result in re-canalization and alleviate need of surgery in more than 90% of cases.

4. CONJUNCTIVA

Conjunctivitis It may be observed as a part of generalized viral (measles, adenovirus) or bacterial (membranous conjunctivitis of Diphtheria) infections. It may at times be an allergic manifestation such as (*i*) endogenous, ie, phlyctenular conjunctivitis of tuberculosis and streptococcal infection; or (ii) exogenous, ie, vernal (allergic) conjunctivitis associated with eosinophilia. Conjunctivitis may be a component of Reiter disease (arthritis, urethritis, conjunctivitis). Pseudomembranous conjunctivitis occurs characteristically in Stevens-Johnson syndrome.

Color Conjunctiva is pale in anemia and jaundice; and deep red in polycythemia.

Subconjunctival hemorrhage It is characterized by bright red patches in the bulbar conjunctiva; it is commonly seen in children with whooping cough. It may also occur in scurvy, thrombocytopenia, injury, or malaria.

Chemosis Edema of conjunctiva may be due to orbital cellulitis, nephritis, urticaria, angioneurotic state, or cavernous sinus thrombosis.

Pigmentation Vitamin A deficiency causes conjunctival xerosis (manifesting as dryness and wrinkling) and triangular white dry patches on the outer and inner sides of the cornea (*Bitot spots*). Wedge-shaped brownish lesions are seen in chronic non-neuronopathic form of Gaucher disease. *Pingueculae* (whitish yellow elevated lesion on bulbar conjunctiva) and small black spots (conjunctival melanosis) are benign lesions.

Deposits Deposits of cystine crystals in the conjunctiva indicate the infantile variety of cystinosis. Surface nodules over conjunctiva may be seen in tuberculosis, leprosy, and syphilis. Conjunctival neurofibromas are found in neurofibromatosis.

5. CORNEA

Cornea has a diameter of 10 mm at birth that achieves the adult size of 12 mm by the end of second year of life. Corneal diameter of more than 13 mm is known as *megalocornea*. It is observed in Marfan syndrome and osteogenesis imperfecta.

Look for any corneal haze, opacity, pigmentation, scarring, or ulceration. *Kayser-Fleischer rings* (colored gray, green or golden brown) are located round the periphery of cornea in Wilson disease.

Conical cornea (*keratoconus*) is a feature of Down syndrome, Marfan syndrome, and osteogenesis imperfecta. The cornea is thin near the center and progressively bulges forwards.

Keratitis (Inflammation of Cornea)

Superficial keratitis Dendritic ulcers (branched ulcers with crenated edges) are seen in herpes simplex infection. This type of keratitis may also develop in Riley-Day syndrome.

Phlyctenular keratitis Corneal phlycten may be a manifestation of an allergic reaction to tubercular protein. A phlycten is a leash of capillaries leading from the scleral conjunctiva towards the limbus or over the cornea.

Interstitial keratitis Corneal opacities develop and generally remain as permanent stigmata of the congenital syphilis. Interstitial keratitis may also follow lesions due to tuberculosis or leprosy.

Opacities and Pigmentation

Haze Corneal haze at birth or during early infancy may be due to congenital anomaly, birth injury, or metabolic disorder including mucopolysaccharidosis, glycogen storage disease, and lipidosis. Full-fledged opacities are observed in mucopolysaccharidosis and glycogen storage disease.

Pigmentation Cystine deposits in the cornea are due to cystinosis, renal dwarfism, or Fanconi syndrome. Golden brown deposits near the limbus indicate alkaptonuria.

Vascularization Circumcorneal vascularization with conjunctivitis is a feature of advanced ariboflavinosis.

6. SCLERA

Superficial inflammation of the sclera (*episcleritis*) presents as raised congested nodules or a diffuse congestion at the sclera around the cornea. Deep inflammation (*scleritis*) is characterized by dusky ciliary congestion and opacification of cornea at the periphery. Episcleritis may occur as an allergic reaction to tuberculosis or streptococcal infection. Scleritis may be associated with connective tissue disorders such as polyarteritis nodosa, SLE, and rheumatoid arthritis.

Sclera becomes yellow in jaundice. *Blue sclera* (Fig. 19.7) is a feature of Marfan syndrome, osteogenesis imperfecta, and cutis hyperelastica. Blackish discoloration of sclera is due to accumulation of homogentisic acid in alkaptonuria (*ochronosis*).

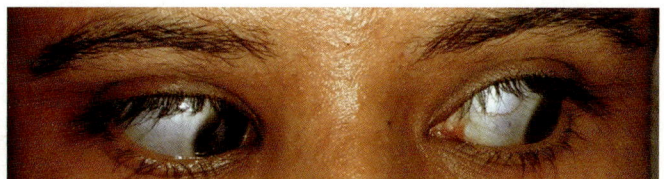

Fig . 19.7 Blue sclera (associated with hearing loss in this case)

7. UVEAL TRACT (IRIS, CILIARY BODY, CHOROID)

Compare irides for color difference (*heterochromia*). It may be congenital or acquired (*Horner syndrome*). Pink iris is a feature of complete albinism and blue characteristic of partial albinism.

Nodules over iris may be seen in neurofibromatosis. In Down syndrome, irides are speckled with whitish inclusions (*Brushfield spots*). Iris can also be involved in leukemic infiltration.

Examine for congenital absence of iris (*aniridia*). It may be associated with Wilms tumor.

Uveitis

Inflammation of anterior uveal tract (*iridocyclitis*) is intensly painful and characterized by a red eye, muddy iris, small irregular pupil with sluggish reaction to light. This condition can be observed in connective tissue disorders, juvenile rheumatoid arthritis, ankylosing spondylitis, tuberculosis, or may occur as a part of viral infections such as mumps, measles, and influenza. Granulomatous uveitis is seen in sarcoidosis and brucellosis.

Posterior uveal tract infection (*chorioretinitis*) is painless and recognized only on ophthalmoscopic examination as atrophic areas on the retina. It may be diffuse with sparing of macula in congenital cytomegaloviral infection while macula is particularly involved in chorioretinitis of congenital toxoplasmosis. Tuberculosis, syphilis, and rubella present with diffuse choroiditis.

19

8. PUPIL

- *Large pupils not reacting to light* are seen in atropine poisoning, after mydriatic drops, transtentorial herniation due to subdural hematoma, and raised intracranial tension.
- *Unilateral large pupil with poor reaction to light* (tonic pupil) is usually associated with familial dysautonomia (Riley-Day syndrome).
- *Small pupils* are characteristic of pontine hemorrhage, opium poisoning, barbiturate poisoning, Horner syndrome, and after instillation of pilocarpine drops.
- *Rhythmic dilatation and constriction of the pupil* is known as hippus; this may occur normally or in retrobulbar neuritis.

9. LENS

Common abnormalities in the lens include an opacity (*cataract*) or dislocation (*ectopia lentis*). Ectopia lentis is a feature of Marfan syndrome or homocystinuria. It can be diagnosed by tremulousness of the iris (*iridodonesis*) following an eye movement.

Causes of Cataract

- *Embryopathic* Congenital syphilis, congenital toxoplasmosis, congenital cytomegalovirus and congenital varicella infection. In congenital rubella, development of lens is inhibited at an early stage (lens is immune to rubella virus after 6 weeks of gestational age) so cataract at birth in such babies implies acquisition of maternal infection early in pregnancy.
- *Metabolic* Galactosemia (central oil droplet cataract), diabetes mellitus (snow flake opacities in posterior subcapsular region), Wilson disease (sunflower cataract), hypocalcemic tetany (lamellar cataract), cretinism (punctate subcapsular cataract), Lowe syndrome (cataract is universal), Fabry disease (sutural cataract), Mannosidosis (spoke like pattern) phenylketonuria, and homocystinuria.
- *Chromosomal disorders* Trisomy 21, trisomy 18, Cri-du-chat syndrome and Turner syndrome.
- *Physical agents* Trauma and radiation.
- *Malnutrition* Maternal or early infancy
- *Cataract of prematurity* Opacities occur in Y-distribution (10–2 o'clock position) of lens and disappear spontaneously.
- *Drugs* Corticosteroid, chlorpromazine, hypo- and hypervitaminosis D, tetracycline.
- *Others* Skeletal disorders like Hallerman-Streiff-Francois syndrome (membranous cataract) and Nance-Horan Syndrome, Marfan and Alport syndromes, myotonic dystrophy, Kartagener syndrome (dextrocardia, situs inversus, immobile cilia, bronchiectasis, sinusitis).
- *Causes within the eye* Retrolental fibroplasia, retinitis pigmentosa, retinal detachment, and uveitis.

10. OCULAR MOTILITY

Strabismus (squint)

Squint is defined as abnormality of ocular movements. The eyes deviate and the visual axis of the squinting eye is not directed at the object observed by the other eye. Transient strabismus is normal in the first four to six months of life and is attributed to physiologic hypermetropia. The strabismus is of two types:

Paralytic Type (non-concomitant)

This is due to weakness or paralysis of one or more of the extraocular muscles. There is limitation of movement, false orientation of the field of vision, dizziness and diplopia. Congenital paralytic strabismus is due to neuromuscular anomalies or birth trauma. Acquired lesions may be due to intracranial tumors, myasthenia gravis, central nervous system infections, polio encephalitis, neuronopathic Gaucher disease, diphtheria toxins, lead toxicity, botulism, thiamine deficiency, and fracture of the base of the skull.

Non-paralytic Type (concomitant)

This is the commoner variety. Diplopia never occurs. The movements of the individual ocular muscles are preserved. *It is due to the visual or ocular defect of the deviating eye.* The squint may be convergent or divergent.

Methods of Testing for Squint

- *Corneal light reflex test* (Hirschberg's reflex) is performed by shining a small light on the child's face and observing the reflection. In a normal eye, reflections are symmetric and well centered while in a squinting eye, the reflex is not well centered and the eye appears deviated. The degree of deviation can be measured by the amount of the prism needed to re-center the light reflex (prism bar reflex test).
- *Cover test* Patient is asked to look at a distant object. Alternatively, each eye is occluded by turn. If there is no movement of either eye, alignment is normal. When the fixating eye is occluded, the deviating eye will move inward in divergent squint and outward in convergent squint. In latent squint (heterophoria), occluded eye tends to deviate. Test should be performed both for distant and near vision and with glasses as well if the child is using them.

Treatment	Strabismus

Earliest possible diagnosis and treatment of a child with a squint is desirable as failure to do so may result in permanent amblyopia.

1. *To develop best possible and equal or near equal vision in both eyes*, it is essential that all refractory errors be corrected after accurate assessment of visual acuity and other associated conditions, such as cataract, be treated.
2. *Occlusion therapy* is recommended if the squinting eye is amblyopic so that the vision improves in the squinting eye by continuous exercise. For this purpose, normal eye has to be absolutely occluded for a duration depending on child's age and degree of amblyopia. However, if there is little improvement, it may be discontinued.
3. *Orthoptic training.* Specially designed visual exercises are advised to encourage the production of simultaneous and binocular vision, elimination of false projection and production of stereoscopic vision.
4. *Surgery* involves shortening, lengthening or repositioning of extraocular muscles and should be undertaken at earliest if other modalities fail.

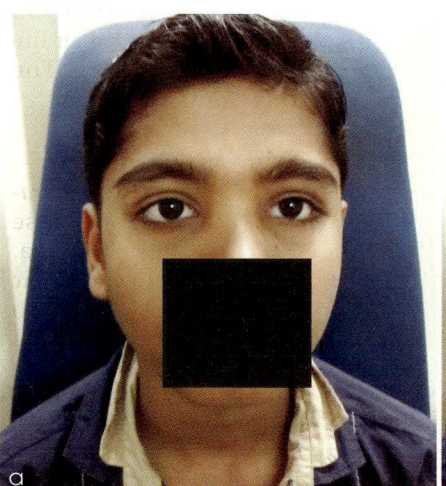 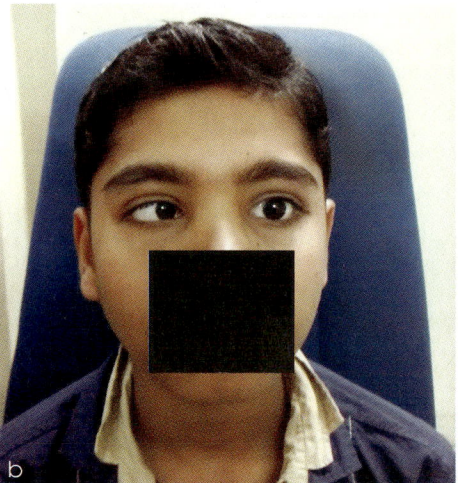 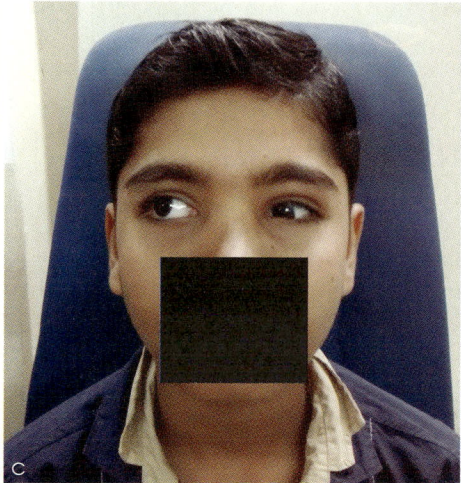

Fig. 19.8 Duannes retraction syndrome: (a) Slight face turn to left, no squint in primary gaze; (b) Limited abduction of left eye on left lateral gaze; and (c) Retraction of left globe on adduction of left eye

Nystagmus

It refers to involuntary, conjugate, and rhythmic oscillation of the eyeball. It may occur with lesions of internal ear, tumors of posterior fossa, and lesions affecting vestibular connections of brainstem and pons.

Opsoclonus

Sustained, irregular, multidirectional, and conjugate movement of the eyes is called *opsoclonus* and may be the first sign of an occult neuroblastoma or cerebellar infections.

Duanne Retraction Syndrome

It is an inherited disorder of ocular motility due to anomalous innervation of lateral rectus with 3rd cranial nerve resulting in limitation of abduction (type 1, Fig. 19.8), adduction (type 2), or both (type 3) along with globe retraction and narrowing of the palpebral fissure on adduction. Common symptom in such cases is diplopia but some children may be able to maintain a binocular single vision by assuming abnormal head posture.

11. BUPHTHALMOS

Congenital rise of intraocular pressure (IOP) prior to 3 years of age, resulting in a large eye due to stretching is known as buphthalmos (Fig. 19.9). It should be suspected whenever the anterioposterior diameter and the corneal diameter (>11 mm in less than 1 year age and >13 mm at any age) are increased in size along with the following coexisting features: (*i*) Corneal haze secondary to corneal edema, (*ii*) lacrimation, (*iii*) photophobia and blepharospasm, and (*iv*) blue sclera due to enhanced visualization of underlying uvea (secondary to scleral thinning).

Buphthalmos, when noticed by parents is usually a late sign of congenital glaucoma. Early in the course of disease, the parents may typically complain that the child prefers to keep head buried in pillows or on mothers shoulder (photophobia).

All children under 3 years of age suspected to be having raised IOP should undergo examination under general anesthesia for measurement of corneal diameter, IOP

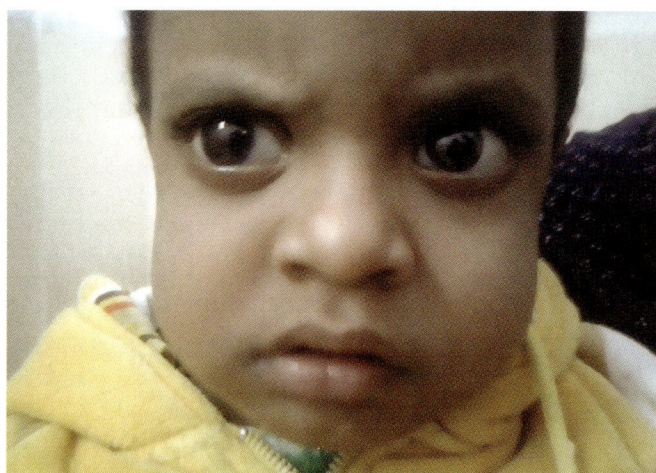

Fig. 19.9 Buphthalmos with a corneal diameter of 13.5 mm

measurement, gonioscopy (for visualization of angle of anterior chamber), and fundus evaluation to assess neuronal damage to retinal nerve fibers. In a co-operative child it can be done without general anesthesia.

Buphthalmos may be associated with (*i*) congenital rubella, (*ii*) trisomy 18,21, (*iii*) Marfan syndrome, (*iv*) homocystinuria, (*v*) mucopolysaccharidosis (Hurler), (*vi*) neurocutaneous syndromes, and (*vii*) prolonged steroid therapy.

12. VISUAL FIELD DEFECTS

Central field of vision is lost (*central scotoma*) in retrobulbar neuritis due to multiple sclerosis and vitamin B_{12} deficiency. *Bitemporal hemianopia* is usually due to a tumor of the pituitary gland or sella turcica. Concentric constriction of visual fields occurs in chronic papilledema, retinitis pigmentosa, and hysteria. Lead toxicity causes reduction in the peripheral vision. Visual field defects are to be checked by perimetry.

13. COLOR BLINDNESS

Congenital color blindness may be total or partial and is transmitted as an X-linked recessive trait. Acquired color vision defects can be caused by toxicity of drugs like ethambutol, barbiturates, streptomycin, and nalidixic acid or optic nerve diseases. Color vision is assessed by Ishihara charts.

14. NIGHT BLINDNESS

Night blindness is a feature of vitamin A and B₂ deficiency, quinine toxicity, Scheie syndrome, albinism, retinitis pigmentosa, and other pigmentary retinal dystrophies.

19.3 OCULAR MANIFESTATIONS OF VITAMIN DEFICIENCIES

- *Vitamin A deficiency* results in a syndrome of xerophthalmia that manifests as night blindness, conjunctival xerosis, bitot spots (Fig. 19.10), corneal xerosis, and corneal ulceration (keratomalacia). Keratomalacia is usually irreversible and results in corneal scarring or phthisis bulbi. Timely intervention and prompt therapy is the key to final outcome. Serum levels of retinol are below 12 mg/dL (*also* see *Chapter* 3).
- *Riboflavin deficiency* produces conjunctivitis and corneal vascularization.
- *Thiamine deficiency* results in ptosis, nystagmus, or extra-ocular muscular paralysis.
- *Vitamin C deficiency* Orbital or conjunctival hemorrhages are observed in scurvy.
- *Deficiency of vitamin D* in early infancy results in bilateral lamellar cataracts. They may even be seen in the neonatal period.

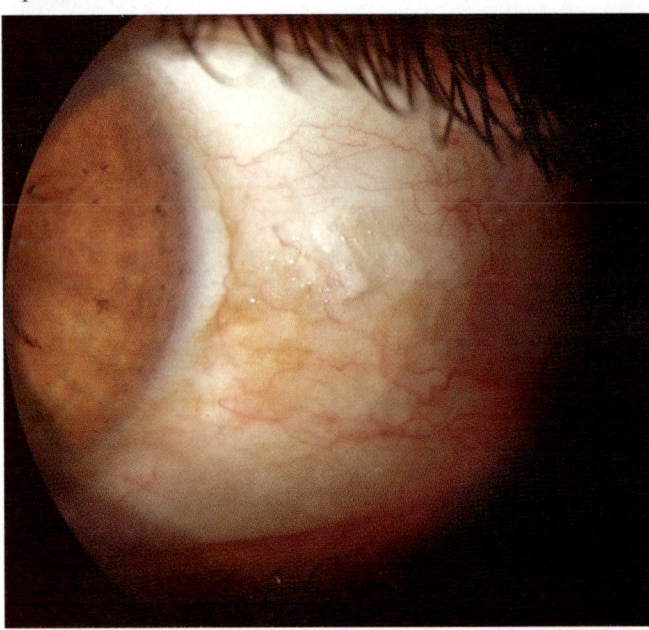

Fig. 19.10 Bitot spots seen as chalky-white lesion

19.4 FUNDUS EXAMINATION

Ophthalmoscopic examination of the fundus gives useful information on the state of optic disc, retina, and macula. Fundus changes are reflective of, and form an important association with severity and grade of many systemic diseases.

METHOD OF EXAMINATION

It is important to know how to do a fundus examination using a direct ophthalmoscope. It is helpful if the pupil is fully dilated with a mydriatic agent, but in a cooperative child, visualization of posterior pole is possible in undilated state. First find out the optic disc by tracing branched retinal vessels back to their origin. Normal optic disc is orange-yellow with well-defined margins. The vessels appear to emerge from the center of the disc forming a shallow depression called cup. The cup to disc ratio should be noted. In a normal eye it is 0.3:1. The vessel caliber, lumen, and arteriovenous crossings should be noted next. Then retina should be examined quadrant by quadrant. The last part to be examined is macula. The macula lies two disc diameters to the temporal side of the disc. Fovea appears as a bright reflex in the center of the macula and is studied by decreasing the intensity of light in the ophthalmoscope. Figure 19.11 depicts a normal fundus.

Following are a few indications of a fundus examination:
- Hypertension
- Diabetes mellitus
- Retinopathy of prematurity
- Night blindness (suspected retinitis pigmentosa)
- Raised intracranial tension (papilledema)
- Sudden severe visual loss (optic nerve disease, retinal detachment, retinal vascular occlusion)

HYPERTENSIVE RETINOPATHY

Generalized constriction and irregular narrowing of the arterioles are the first signs in the fundus. Hypertensive fundus is characteristic of long standing renal disease, coarctation of aorta, collagen diseases, and pheochromo-cytoma. Severity is traditionally classified in four grades:
- *Grade I* There is mild narrowing, sclerosis and tortuosity of retinal arteries.
- *Grade II* There is generalized irregular narrowing of the arteries along with sclerosis. Due to sclerosis, arteries become hard and press against the veins (*nipping* or *AV crossing phenomenon*).

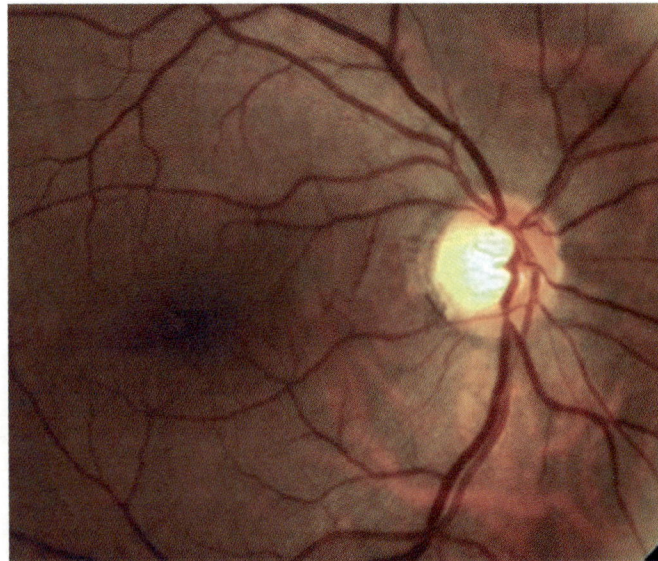

Fig. 19.11 Normal fundus

- *Grade III* Flame shaped hemorrhages, cotton wool spots and hard exudates are present in addition to grade II changes. Narrowed arteries become thick so as to reflect all the light and appear as white silvery lines (*Silver-wire appearance*).
- *Grade IV* Above changes are associated with papilledema.

DIABETIC RETINOPATHY

Retinopathy is present in 20% of juvenile diabetes mellitus after 10 years of known disease and in 45–60% after 20 years of known disease. Degree of control of diabetes is a more important factor than duration of diabetes for developing retinopathy.

Early changes (non-proliferative diabetic retinopathy) consist of (*i*) microaneurysm due to degeneration of the vessel walls, (*ii*) posterior polar hard exudates, (*iii*) punctate or round deep hemorrhages (dot and blot hemorrhages), and (*iv*) venous dilatation or beading.

Late variety is proliferative in nature and consists of (*i*) proliferation of connective tissue on retina and new vessel formation; and (*ii*) preretinal or vitreous hemorrhage. Retinal detachment and secondary glaucoma may follow.

At any stage macular edema may develop, characterized by thickening at macula, loss of foveolar reflex and hard exudates at or around macula.

PDR and clinically significant macular edema are indications for immediate ophthalmological intervention.

RETINOPATHY OF PREMATURITY (ROP)

This is a bilateral disease of at-risk premature infants with abnormal vascularization of retina after birth leading to fragile and leaky vessels, scarring, and finally detachment of retina.

Risk Factors

Predisposing factors include low birth weight, oxygen supplementation, sepsis, anemia, blood transfusions, respiratory distress, etc. In a premature newborn, retina is immature with poor vascularization and myelination. High oxygen concentration (hyperoxia) causes vasoconstriction and downregulation of vascular endothelial growth factor (VEGF) resulting in obliteration of vessels, halting of vessel migration, and capillary regression causing retinal ischemia. With growing eye and increased metabolic demands there is eventually an excessive VEGF production inciting neovascularization. New vessels are abnormal blood vessels which are fragile and can leak, scarring the retina and pulling it out of position. This may cause a retinal detachment. Retinal detachment is the main cause of visual impairment and blindness in ROP.

Grading of Severity

The severity of ROP, ranges from mild (stage I) to severe (stage V) and in location, from Zone I to Zone III (Fig. 19.12, **Box 19.1**). Blindness due to ROP is a preventable. All premature babies with risk factors should be screened for ROP by a specialist and should be referred for early intervention wherever required.

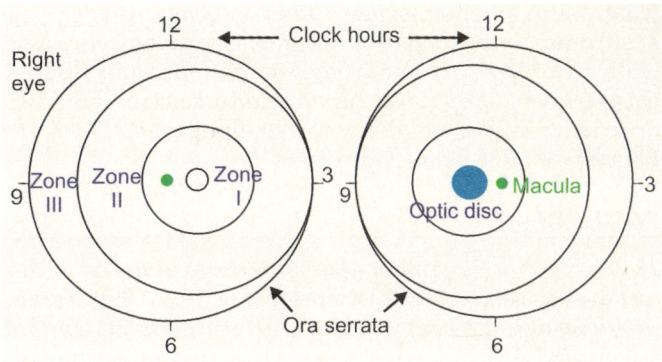

Fig. 19.12 Zones of ROP: *Zone I*: Contains optic disc and macula disc as centre, radius twice the distance between disc and macula (2 × 3 mm); *Zone II*: Outside zone I, with disc as centre circle with radius touching nasal ora serrata (anterior limit of retina); *Zone III*: Remaining temporal crescent of retina up to temporal ora serrata

Box 19.1 Grades of Retinopathy of Prematurity (ROP)
Stage I: Presence of a demarcation line between vascular and avascular regions of retina
Stage II: Ridge formed due to raise in demarcation line
Stage III: Extraretinal fibrovascular proliferation
Stage IV: Partial retinal detachment
Stage V: Total retinal detachment

Treatment   **Retinopathy of Prematurity**

The most effective proven treatments for ROP are laser therapy or cryotherapy. Laser therapy burns away the periphery of the retina, which has no normal blood vessels. In cryotherapy, freezing temperatures are applied to briefly touch spots on the surface of the eye that overlie the periphery of the retina. Both the treatment modalities destroy the peripheral areas of the retina, slowing or reversing the abnormal growth of blood vessels. Unfortunately, the treatments may also destroy some side vision. Both laser treatments and cryotherapy are indicated in Stage III with "plus disease." Other treatment options in later stages of the disease include scleral buckling (stages IV or V) and pars plana vitrectomy (stage V).

Recent studies have shown intravitreal anti-VEGF injections to be effective in reducing neovascularization in ROP eyes compared to laser therapy in terms of recurrence rates. The safety profile and exact dosing are still under investigation but the efficacy and less invasive nature of this intervention makes it a possible treatment of choice in near future.

RETINITIS PIGMENTOSA

It is a bilateral disease resulting in blindness by middle age. Rods are predominantly involved therefore the presenting complaint is night blindness. Field of vision is concentrically narrowed resulting in tube vision. Triad of arteriolar attenuation, bone spicule pigmentation (accumulation of dark brown or jet black spots assuming a bone corpuscle configuration), and waxy disc pallor on fundus examination is typical.

The disease may be *primary* or *secondary* to intrauterine infections (toxoplasmosis, rubella, CMV, syphilis) or drugs (chloroquin, phenothiazine). Other associations are Usher syndrome, Kearns-Sayre syndrome, Cockayne syndrome, Hallervorden-Spatz syndrome, neuronal ceroid lipofuschinoses, hereditary ataxia, Alport syndrome, cerebromacular degeneration, Refsum disease, abeta-lipoproteinemia, and Laurence-Moon-Biedl syndrome.

PAPILLEDEMA

This is a non-inflammatory passive edema at the optic disc due to increased intracranial tension (Fig. 19.13). Intracranial pressure could be raised due to (*i*) intracranial tumors, (*ii*) brain abscess, (*iii*) meningitis and encephalitis, (*iv*) intracranial hemorrhage, (*v*) hydrocephalus, (*vi*) pseudotumor cerebri, (*vii*) craniostenosis, (*viii*) cavernous sinus thrombosis, (*ix*) hypertension, and (*x*) hematological disorders including anemia, polycythemia, and leukemia. Increased intracranial pressure is transmitted to optic nerve via subarachnoid spaces leading to swelling of nerve fibers and secondary vascular changes.

Symptoms are generally absent initially with little visual disturbances. Episodes of transient obscuration of vision may be present. Long standing papilledema may result in a relative central scotoma and loss of peripheral field of vision.

The earliest features of papilledema include redness and blurring of margins of upper nasal quadrant of the disc. Later, blurring progresses to involve whole of the disc and progressive edema causes reduction in the size and ultimate obliteration of the physiological cup. Veins become congested and are engorged with the loss of pulsations. Finally there is elevation of disc above the retinal surface, so that a sharp bend in the retinal vessels can be observed as they dip down from swollen disc to the retina. In still late stages, edema extends to the macula producing a star or fan shaped figure. Peripapillary exudates and flame-shaped hemorrhages may also occur.

It is possible to measure the degree of edema by starting with a high plus lens and reducing the power of lens till

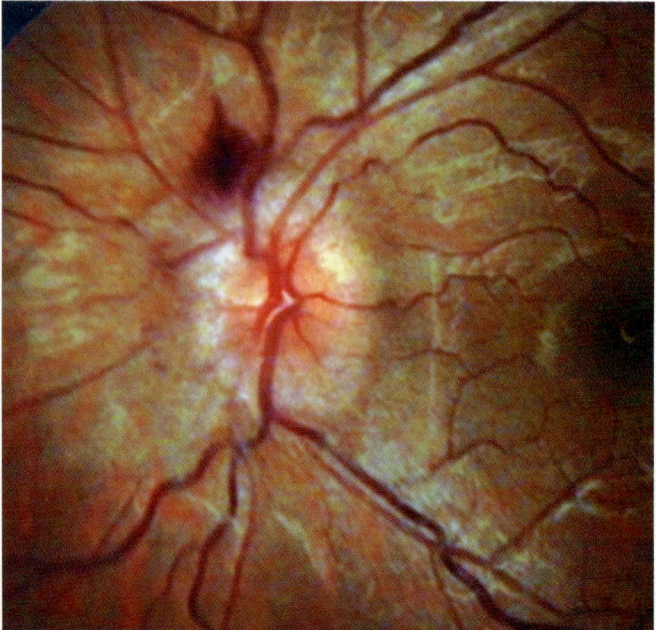

Fig. 19.13 Papilledema with superficial hemorrhages

center of the disc is in focus. The retina is then brought into focus by further reduction of the power of the lens. The difference indicates the degree of swelling of disc (1 mm swelling = 3 diopters).

OPTIC NEURITIS

Inflammation of optic nerve may be visible at the disc (*papillitis*, most common type of optic neuritis in children), may be associated with inflammation of retinal nerve fiber layer with macular star (*neuroretinitis*), or may not show any fundus changes at all (*retrobulbar neuritis*).

In *papillitis*, changes are more or less same as those in papilledema. Differentiating points being (i) decreased central vision, (ii) less swelling of the disc, (iii) less distension of retinal veins, (iv) hazy vitreous, retinal exudates, and (v) absence of other signs of raised intracranial pressure.

In *retrobulbar neuritis*, part of the optic nerve behind the eye is inflamed, therefore no fundus changes are seen and diagnosis is merely based on symptoms alone such as local pain, loss of vision and central scotoma. Lack of sustained constriction of the pupil to light is of greatest diagnostic significance.

Causes are (*a*) infective (acute meningitis, encephalitis, syphilis, typhoid, malaria, measles, and mumps); (*b*) demyelinating (multiple sclerosis, neuromyelitis optica, Schilder disease); (*c*) vitamin deficiency; and (*d*) drugs and chemicals (chlorpromazine, quinidine, ethambutol, phenothiazine, and lead).

OPTIC ATROPHY

This is a irreversible degeneration of optic disc in which disc becomes pale or white with reduction in the number of capillaries on the disc (less than seven, normal ≥10). It is of two types.

Primary Optic Atrophy

Atrophy occurs without any ophthalmoscopic evidence of previous local inflammation, papillitis, or papilledema; and is due to the disease of neurons proximal to optic disc. Clinically the disc is flat and white, sometimes with a blue or green tint and margins of the disc are well defined. Causes are optic neuritis, hereditary optic neuropathies, primary central nervous system disorders (microcephaly, hydrocephalus), craniosynostosis, pituitary tumors, homocystinuria, osteopetrosis, drugs and chemicals, (chloramphenicol, quinidine, chloroquine, lead), and following trauma.

Secondary Optic Atrophy

Disc is gray white in color and its edges are indistinct. It usually follows papillitis or papilledema and anterior ischemic optic neuropathy. In late stages, ophthalmological features of primary and secondary atrophy become indistinguishable.

VASCULAR OCCLUSION

Occlusion may either occur in *central retinal artery (CRAO)* or its *branch* (BRAO), or *central retinal vein* (CRVO) or its *branch* (BRVO). Vascular occlusions occur in of polycythemia, sickle cell disease (due to obstruction of capillaries by the sickled cells), and SC hemoglobinopathies.

Retinal Arterial Occlusion

Common causes of arterial occlusion are atherosclerosis related thrombi, carotid emboli, periarteritis, thrombophilic disorders, and sickling hemoglobinopathies. Clinical presentation ranges from being asymptomatic in BRAO to profound painless visual loss in CRAO. A pale optic disc and retina, marked constriction of retinal arteries with cattle trucking, and cherry red spot at macula are observed on fundus examination.

Retinal Venous Occlusion

Venous occlusions are *per se* uncommon under age of 50 years, hence presence of CRVO/BRVO should be investigated and treated aggressively. The causes include myeloproliferative disorders (polycythemia, myeloma), acquired hypercoagulable states (hyperhomocysteinemia), inherited hypercoagulable states (protein C and S deficiency, antithrombin deficiency, factor V leiden mutation, prothrombin gene mutation), periphlebitis (Behçet syndrome, sarcoidosis, Wegner granulomatosis, Goodpasture syndrome) or miscellaneous (chronic renal failure, Cushing syndrome, and dehydration. Presentation is variable ranging from asymptomatic (peripheral occlusion) to visual loss, field defects, and metamorphopsia. On retinal examination, engorged and tortuous retinal veins, edema of optic disc with flame shaped and dot blot hemorrhages are characteristic of CRVO (*tomato splashed appearance*).

RETINAL DETACHMENT

Separation of the retinal pigment epithelium layer (RPE), from the rest of the neurosensory retina is called retinal detachment. It may be *rhegmatogenous* (secondary to a full thickness break or tear in the sensory layer), *tractional* (secondary to a pull on the neurosensory retina by vitreoretinal adhesion bands as a result of trauma or proliferative diabetic retinopathy), *exudative* (secondary to intraocular tumors and inflammatory or vascular diseases of the retina), or *combined* mechanism.

The child may present with sudden painless decreased vision, floaters, or flashes of light. A typical history of curtain falling over the visual field may be elicited in older children. On examination a dirty white reflex on distant direct ophthalmoscopy is suggestive of RD, and indicates a dilated fundus examination, with an indirect ophthalmoscope.

RETINAL FEATURES IN PHAKOMATOSES

Nodular lesions, about the size of the disc, yellowish in color and refractile in nature are observed in tuberous sclerosis. Choroidal hemangiomas are described in Sturge-Weber syndrome. Multiple white small plaques occur in neurofibromatosis. Cystic angiomatous formations with large feeding vessels leading to massive exudates, hemorrhages, and retinal detachment, is seen in von Hippel-Lindau disease.

OTHER FINDINGS IN RETINA

Choroid tubercles Pale round choroid tubercles are seen near the disc in miliary tuberculosis.

Pepper and salt appearance Minute chorioretinal scars with pinpoint pigmentation is characteristic of congenital rubella infection.

Pigmentary degeneration of the macula This is observed in cerebromacular degeneration, Refsum disease, and due to drugs (chloroquine, phenothiazine, and lead toxicity).

Cherry red spot This is a round bright white area at the macula whose center is occupied by a cherry red circular spot. It is always bilateral and observed in case of Tay-Sachs disease (90% cases), Sandhoff variant (GM2 *type 2*) GM1 gangliosidoses, metachromatic leukodystrophy (sulfated lipidoses), Niemann-Pick disease, mucolipidosis (Farber disease), late infantile cerebromacular degeneration, and occlusion of central artery of retina.

Roth spots In about 40% of children with subacute bacterial endocarditis, round or oval hemorrhages with white center (*Roth spots*) are seen. Papilledema may be an associated feature.

Cyanosis of retina Dilated, dark, and tortuous veins along with scattered hemorrhages may be observed in congenital cyanotic heart disease and chronic pulmonary insufficiency.

Retinopathies of Hematopoietic System

- *Anemia* Fundus is pale; flame shaped hemorrhages may be present. Exudates, if present are wooly and small.
- *Polycythemia* Retinal veins are dilated and tortuous. Hemorrhages, edema, and papilledema are observed with increasing severity,
- *Leukemia* Retinal hemorrhages are characteristic. These are round with pale center. Venous dilatation may also be seen.

19.5 OCULAR MANIFESTATIONS OF SYSTEMIC DISODERS

These are summarized in **Table 19.1**.

Table 19.1 Eye Signs of Systemic Disease in Children		
Disorder	*Eye findings*	*Associated signs and symptoms*
Alkaptonuria	Blackish pigmentation of sclera at the limbus	Arthritis, dark black urine in presence of alkali
Ataxia telangiectasia	Partial ophthalmoplegia, nystagmus, tortuous bulbar conjunctival vessels	Recurrent pulmonary and sinus infections, ataxia, and telangiectasia of gastrointestinal tract
Cerebellar tumors	Diplopia, nystagmus, blindness, papilledema	Vomiting, ataxia, hypotonia, increasing head circumference

Contd...

Table 19.1 Eye Signs of Systemic Disease in Children (Contd.)

Disorder	Eye findings	Associated signs and symptoms
Cerebral palsy	Strabismus, amblyopia	Spasticity, dysphonia, and occasionally mental retardation
Corticosteroid toxicity	Glaucoma, cataract, possibly worsened herpetic corneal lesions, pseudotumor, papilledema	Growth retardation, increased susceptibility to various infections, osteoporosis, myopathy, moon face, central obesity, acne, fluid and electrolyte disturbances, edema, hyperglycemia
Craniopharyngioma	Field defects, diminished vision, optic atrophy	Suprasellar calcifications, diabetes insipidus
Cytomegalovirus infections	Diffuse peripheral chorioretinitis, optic atrophy	Microcephaly, periventricular calcifications, low birth weight, jaundice
Dermatomyositis	Exophthalmos, iritis, fluffy white retinal lesions, extraocular muscle palsy	Muscle weakness, pain, rash, dysphagia, angitis of muscle, skin and fat; elevated muscle enzymes
Diabetes mellitus	Diabetes can lead to retinopathy. Micro-aneurysms, hemorrhages, vasoproliferation, cataract	Insulin-dependent diabetes: Polyuria, polydipsia, ketoacidosis
Diphtheria	Paralysis of accommodation, occasionally ptosis and fourth or sixth nerve palsy, membraneous conjunctivitis	Gray membranous pharyngitis with paresis and cardiac toxicity
Duchenne muscular dystrophy	Occasional extraocular muscle palsy, rarely ophthalmoplegia	Profound muscle weakness, progressive wasting of muscle groups, pseudohypertrophy of gastrocnemii
Ehlers-Danlos syndrome	Blue sclera, epicanthal folds, keratoconus, ectopia lentis	Autosomal dominant inheritance, loose skin, kyphoscoliosis, decreased muscle tone, occasional spontaneous rupture of vessels
Encephalitis	Photophobia, occasionally extraocular muscle palsy, papillary abnormalities, ptosis	CNS signs of obtundation, coma, posturing, focal or generalized seizures, elevated CSF protein, CSF pleocytosis
Endocarditis, subacute bacterial	Retinal hemorrhages; Roth spots, bulbar and palpebral subconjunctival hemorrhages	Spiking fevers, new murmurs, occasionally congestive heart failure, embolic phenomena, sub-splinter hemorrhage
Frontal lobe tumors	Papilledema, rarely the Foster Kennedy syndrome (anosmia, optic atrophy with central scotoma and contralateral papilledema)	Central facial palsy, ataxia
Galactosemia	Cataract ("oil droplet" centrally located)	Hepatosplenomegaly, jaundice, vomiting, diarrhea, mental retardation; galactosuria (positive reducing substance in the urine)
Gaucher disease	Paralytic strabismus, pingueculae in chronic nonneuronopathic form	Splenomegaly, anemia, thrombocytopenia, leukopenia, growth failure. In the cerebral form, onset in infancy with cranial nerve palsy, spasticity
Glucose 6-phosphate dehydrogenase deficiency	Retinal and vitreous hemorrhages following acute hemolytic anemia, cataract	Acute hemolytic anemia following sulfonamide, antimalarial therapy, or fava bean ingestion
Herpes simplex infection	Keratoconjunctivitis; superficial punctate keratitis, dendritic ulcer; later scar formation, rarely hypopyon	Acute herpetic gingivostomatitis, eczema herpeticum, herpetic encephalitis
Homocystinuria	Dislocated lens; usually an inferior dislocation, myopia, cataract, retinal detachment	Mental retardation; occasionally presenting with hemiplegia, kyphoscoliosis, pectus excavatum, thromboembolic phenomena
Hurler disease	Glaucoma, cloudy cornea, retinal degeneration	Englarged skull anteroposterior diameter, short and broad mandible, mental retardation, hepatosplenomegaly, cardiac lesions

Contd...

Table 19.1 Eye Signs of Systemic Disease in Children (Contd.)

Disorder	Eye findings	Associated signs and symptoms
Hypertension	Retinopathy; arteriolar sclerosis. In children, only finding is focal arteriolar constriction, best seen in the nasal quadrants	Usually in children there is associated underlying pathology. Renal disease, Cushing syndrome, adrenogenital syndrome
Leukemia	Leukemic infiltrates: Sclera, conjunctivae, retina (usually with monocytic leukemia); fundoscopic signs of engorged veins and hemorrhages	Pallor, purpura, bleeding, leukoerythroblastic smear, leukemic infiltrates, adenopathy, splenomegaly (protean manifestations)
Lowe syndrome	Cataract, occasionally glaucoma	Aminoaciduria, glycosuria, albuminuria, vitamin-D resistant rickets, renal failure
Lupus erythematosus	Acute retinopathy; hyaline deposits, hemorrhages, macular edema	Butterfly malar rash, fever, splenomegaly, arthralgia, anemia and leukopenia, and hypertension
Marfan syndrome	Subluxated lenses: Occasionally sudden acute glaucoma	Long digits, long extremities, hyperextensibility, aortic aneurysms, kyphoscoliosis
Neurofibromatosis	Eyelid neuromas producing ptosis, exophthalmos secondary to orbital neurofibromas, occasional optic gliomas and meningiomas, glaucoma	More than 6 café au lait spots, skeletal abnormalities; cranial nerve and spinal nerve neurofibromas
Niemann-Pick disease	Macular red spots, occasionally vertical gaze palsies	Acute and chronic forms, hepatosplenomegaly; failure to thrive, hypotonia, and mental retardation; progressive
Reiter syndrome	Conjunctivitis and iritis, keratitis, and occasionally corneal scarring	Triad of conjunctivitis, urethritis, and arthritis in young men; rare in children
Rheumatic fever	Iritis, papillitis	Cardiac and joint signs, erythema marginatum, chorea
Rheumatoid arthritis	Anterior uveitis in 15 to 20% of juvenile rheumatoid arthritis patients	Spiking fevers, fleeting rash, symptoms in one or more joints; usually onset before age 10
Steven-Johnson syndrome	Acute, sometimes purulent conjunctivitis, often with pseudomembranes	Bullous erythematous lesions, often target like with mucosal involvement
Tay-Sachs disease	Cherry red macular spot, nystagmus (4 to 6 months), poor vision, optic atrophy	Apathy and abnormal startle response at 2 months, mental deterioration, seizures
Toxoplasmosis	Chorioretinitis; scarlike retinal lesions with distinct borders, often in macular area	Small for gestational age, microcephaly, diffuse intracranial calcifications, variable severity
Trisomy 21	Epicanthus, Mongolian slant occasionally; brushfield spots, cataract	Mongoloid facies, macroglossia, mental retardation
Vitamin B deficiency	Ptosis, ocular muscle palsy, nystagmus and glaucoma	Beriberi, peripheral polyneuropathy
Wilson disease	Kayser-Fleischer ring: A blue to greenish-brown ring in the periphery of the cornea	Autosomal recessive inheritance, tremor, tic like movements, progressive mental and behavioral changes

Eye Diseases in Children

1. Conjunctivitis, acute anterior uveitis, and acute congestive glaucoma are the most common causes of red eye.
2. It is important to rule out uncorrected refractive errors even with non-visual complaints like frequent rubbing of the eyes, repeated eye infections, or squint.
3. Media opacities and uncorrected refractive errors need to be addressed as soon as possible to prevent amblyopia.
4. Refer to an ophthalmologist if a neonate has large hazy cornea (buphthalmos), white reflex (cataract), mucopurulent discharge (ophthalmia neonatorum), or watering (congenital nasolacrimal duct block).
5. All hypertensive and diabetic children must undergo at least yearly fundus examination.
6. All preterm babies born ≥28 weeks of gestational age with any associated risk factor should be referred for ROP Screening within first 4 weeks of age. Smaller babies born <28 weeks gestation age or <1200 grams birth weight should be screened earlier, by 2–3 weeks of age.
7. Disc edema due to raised ICT is called papilledema. Earliest feature of papilledema on fundus examination is seen as blurring of disc margins.

BenEzra D, Cohen E, Maftzir G. Uveitis in children and adolescents.*Br J Ophthalmol*. 2005;89:444–8.

Committee on Practice and Ambulatory Medicine, Section on Ophthalmology.American Association of Certified Orthoptists; American Association for Pediatric Ophthalmology and Strabismus; American Academy of Ophthalmology.Eye examination in infants, children, and young adults by pediatricians.*Pediatrics*. 2003;111:902–7.

Creavin AL, Brown RD. Ophthalmic abnormalities in children with Down syndrome. *J PediatrOphthalmol Strabismus*. 2009;46:76–82.

Elder J. Pediatric Ophthalmology and Strabismus.*J Paediatr Child Health*. 2003;39:724.

Ellis FD. Selected pigmented fundus lesions of children. *J AAPOS*. 2005;9:306–14.

Friedman LS, Kaufman LM.Guidelines for pediatrician referrals to the ophthalmologist.*PediatrClin North Am*. 2003;50:41–53.

Gupta VP, Dhaliwal U, Sharma R, Gupta P, Rohatgi J. Retinopathy of prematurity—risk factors. *Indian J Pediatr*. 2004;71:887–92.

Kadayifcilar S, Eldem B, Tumer B. Uveitis in childhood.*J PediatrOphthalmol Strabismus*. 2003;40:335–40.

Kushner BJ. Pediatric ophthalmology in the new millennium.*Arch Ophthalmol*. 2000;118:1277–80.

Mac Cord Medina F, Silvestre de Castro R, *et al*. Management of dry eye related to systemic diseases in childhood and long term follow-up. *ActaOphthalmol Scand*. 2007 Jun 8; [Epub ahead of print].

Maida JM, Mathers K, Alley CL. Pediatric ophthalmology in the developing world.*CurrOpinOphthalmol*. 2008;19:403–8.

Mueller JB, McStay CM. Ocular infection and inflammation. *Emerg Med Clin North Am*. 2008;26:57–72.

Nielsen LS, Skov L, Jensen H.Visual dysfunctions and ocular disorders in children with developmental delay.I. prevalence, diagnoses and aetiology of visual impairment.*ActaOphthalmol Scand*. 2007;85:149–56.

O'Brien TP, JengBH, McDonald M, Raizman MB. Acute conjunctivitis: truth and misconceptions. *Curr Med Res Opin*. 2009;25:1953–61.

Prentiss KA, Dorfman DH. Pediatric ophthalmology in the emergency department.*Emerg Med Clin North Am*. 2008;26:181–98.

Reiff A. Ocular complications of childhood rheumatic diseases: uveitis. *CurrRheumatol Rep*. 2006;8:459–68.

Robbins SL, Christian WK, HertleRW, Granet DB.Vision testing in thepediatric population.*OphthalmolClin North Am*. 2003;16:253–67.

Seth D, Khan FI. Causes and management of red eye in pediatric ophthalmology.*Curr Allergy Asthma Rep*. 2011;11:212–9.

Sharma R, Gupta VP, Dhaliwal U, Gupta P. Screening for retinopathy of prematurity in developing countries. *J Trop Pediatr*. 2007;53:52–4.

Tingley DH. Vision screening essentials: screening today for eye disorders in the pediatric child. *Pediatr Rev*. 2007;28:54–61.

Payal Gupta, Srikanta Basu, and Piyush Gupta

Critical Care and Poisonings

20.1 SERIOUSLY ILL CHILD

The priority of triage should be to quickly identify the infants and children who may have impending respiratory, circulatory, or neurologic compromise; and prioritize manpower and resources so that these children receive appropriate and timely intervention in the emergency room. In the emergency room setting, it is important to recognize early changes in vital signs with frequent monitoring, keeping in mind the normal range (**Table 20.1**)

Table 20.1 Normal Range for Heart Rate, Respiratory Rate and Blood Pressure in Children

Ages	Heart rate (beats/minute)	Respiratory rate (breaths/minute)	Blood pressure (mm Hg) systolic/diastolic
Premature infants	120–170	40–70	55–75/35–45
0–3 months	100–150	35–55	65–85/45–55
3–6 months	90–120	30–45	70–90/50–65
6–12 months	80–120	25–40	80–100/55–65
1–3 years	70–110	20–30	90–105/55–70
3–6 years	65–110	20–25	95–110/60–75
6–12 years	60–95	14–22	100–120/60–75
>12 years	55–85	12–18	110–135/65–85

20.2 EMERGENCY TRIAGE ASSESSMENT AND TREATMENT

The World Health Organization (WHO) has developed guidelines for Emergency Triage Assessment and Treatment (ETAT). These guidelines outline the steps for immediate assessment of children with potentially life-threatening conditions that are generally encountered in a developing country setting.

Triage involves the immediate sorting of patients into *Emergency*, *Priority*, or *Non-Urgent* (Queue) categories based on their presenting signs and symptoms and availability of resources. The initial assessment includes a quick evaluation of patency of **A**irway, work of **B**reathing, adequacy of **C**irculation, presence of **C**oma, presence of **C**onvulsions, and assessment of **D**ehydration (ABCD).

ABCD ASSESSMENT

1. Airway and Breathing

Assessment for airway and breathing problems (Fig. 20.1) can be done by immediate inspection by looking, listening and feeling for air movement:
a. Is the child breathing?
b. Is the airway obstructed?
c. Is the child blue (or showing central cyanosis)?

Foreign body airway obstruction is an airway emergency that can be rapidly fatal, if not corrected immediately. For severe airway obstruction (ie, the child is unable to make a sound), perform sub-diaphragmatic abdominal thrusts (*Heimlich maneuver*) for a child until the object is expelled or the child becomes unresponsive. *For an infant*, deliver 5 back blows (slaps) followed by 5 chest thrusts repeatedly until the object is expelled or the victim becomes unresponsive. Abdominal thrusts are not recommended for infants because they may damage the relatively large and unprotected liver.

For the unresponsive child with a foreign body, look into the mouth before giving breaths and only if a foreign body is seen, then it should be removed. Blind finger sweeps should not be done as they may push the foreign body deeper.

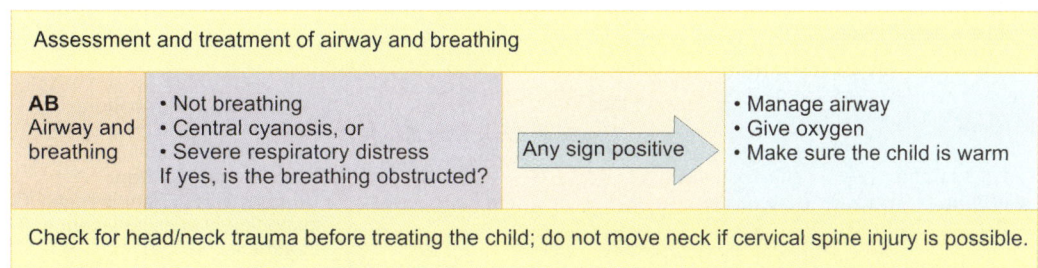

Fig. 20.1 Rapid assessment of airway and breathing

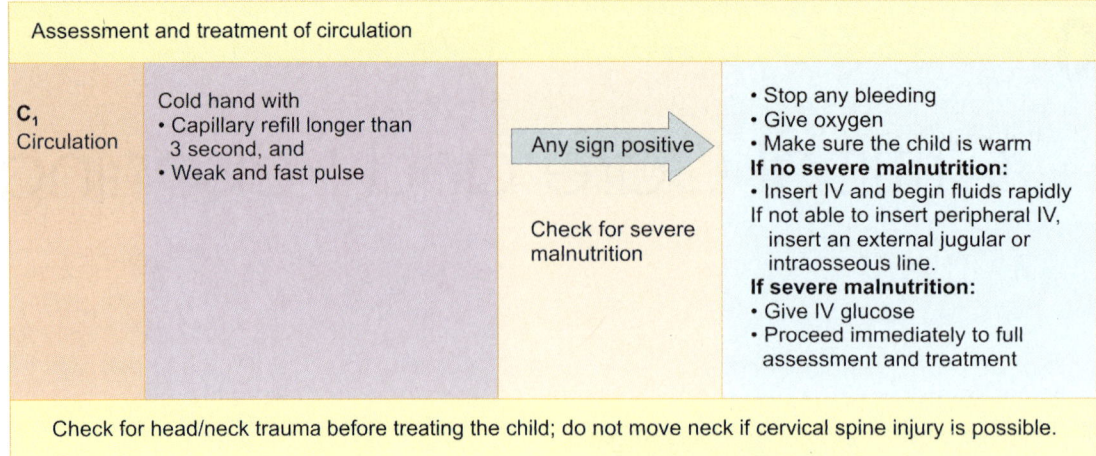

Fig. 20.2 Assessment of circulation and management of shock

2. Circulation

Adequacy of circulation (Fig. 20.2) can be assessed by touching the child:

a. Does the child have warm hands?

b. If hands are not warm, is the capillary refill time longer than 3 seconds?

c. Is the pulse fast and weak?

Measurement of blood pressure can also help in detection of early stages of shock. Hypotension is defined as systolic blood pressure less than the 5th percentile of normal for age, as per the cut-offs shown in **Table 20.2**.

Table 20.2 Cut-offs for Defining Hypotension in Different Age Groups	
Age	*Systolic blood pressure*
Term neonates (0–28 d)	<60 mm Hg
Infants (1–12 mo)	<70 mm Hg
Children (1–10 years)	<70 mm Hg + (2 × age in year)
Children (≥10 years)	<90 mm Hg

3. Consciousness

Assessment of consciousness can be done using the AVPU scale (**Box 20.1**), where the child can be assigned to one of the following categories: **A**lert, Responsive to **V**oice, Responsive to **P**ain, or **U**nresponsive

Table 20.3 Management of Coma and Convulsions	
Coma	*Convulsion*
If the child is unconscious you should • Manage the airway • Position the child (if there is a history of trauma, stabilize neck first) • Check the blood sugar • Give IV glucose	If the child is convulsing now you must • Manage the airway • Position the child • Check blood sugar • Give IV glucose • Give anticonvulsant

Box 20.1 AVPU Scale
1. **A**lert 2. Responsive to **V**oice 3. Responsive to **P**ain 4. **U**nresponsive

For patients with either coma or convulsions, immediate management **(Table 20.3)** includes proper positioning to manage the airway, and providing intravenous glucose, followed by treatment with anticonvulsant medication in case of active seizures.

4. Dehydration

Dehydration can be assessed (Fig. 20.3) by looking for the following:

a. Is the child unconscious or lethargic?

b. Does the child have sunken eyes?

c. Does a skin pinch go back very slowly?

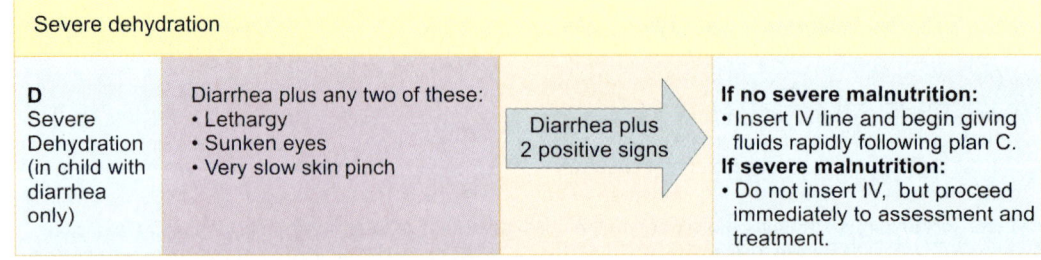

Fig. 20.3 Assessment and management of severe dehydration

TRIAGE

Triage in E (Emergency) Category

If the child has any one of the signs of ABCD assessment, then the child should be triaged to the Emergency (E) category and treatment should be started immediately. Since more than one intervention may have to be performed at the same time, it is recommended to involve several members of the team. A senior health care provider should be notified, and blood should be drawn for laboratory investigations (blood glucose, electrolytes, hemoglobin, and peripheral smear for malaria). If the child has had head or neck trauma, then immobilization of head and neck region should be initiated, while continuing to assess vital signs and provide ongoing treatment.

Triage in P (Priority) or Q (Queue) Category

For children without E signs, the health care provider should continue for assessment of Priority signs, which can be summarized by the mnemonic 3TPR-MOB (**Box 20.2**).

After completing the examination for priority signs, the child is assigned to Priority (P) or Queue (Non-Priority) category. Recognizing that many deaths in the hospital occur within 24 hours of admission, it is important to provide ongoing monitoring and support to the sickest children. Intravenous access should be obtained immediately; preferably with large bore intravenous cannula to provide fluid resuscitation, blood products, and medications. Obtain intraosseous access if IV access is not obtainable in a child less than 8 years of age.

Box 20.2 Assessment of Priority Signs

- **T**iny infant (less than 2 months of age)
- **T**emperature (fever)
- **T**rauma (or other surgical condition)
- Severe **P**allor
- **P**oisoning
- Severe **P**ain
- **R**estless, lethargy or irritability
- **R**espiratory distress
- Urgent **R**eferral (patient sent from another clinic/facility for treatment)
- Severe **M**alnutrition
- **O**edema of both feet
- Major **B**urns

Guideline: Updates on Paediatric Emergency Triage, Assessment and Treatment: Care of Critically-Ill Children. Geneva: World Health Organization; 2016.

20.3 PEDIATRIC BASIC LIFE SUPPORT (BLS)

Pediatric BLS comprises knowledge and skills that are necessary for providing life-sustaining support to an unresponsive child or infant in emergent situations, either outside or within the hospital setting. BLS can be performed even by a layman outside hospital setting; survival rates vary from 6% for children with cardiac arrest to 70% in those with respiratory arrest. Survival rates are better in hospital.

The International Liaison Committee on Resuscitation (ILCOR) revised and updated the recommendations for both pediatric basic and advanced life support in 2015. There are now separate algorithms for one-person (Fig. 20.4) and two-person (Fig. 20.5) CPR (cardiopulmonary resuscitation), and the rate of chest compression is now same for both children and adults (100–120 compressions per minute).

The emphasis of resuscitation is now aimed at early restoration of circulation and performing high quality chest compressions that provides blood flow to vital organs and helps to achieve return of spontaneous circulation. CAB (circulation-airway-breathing) approach is preferred over the traditional ABC approach. The sequence has been modified for witnessed sudden collapse where a cardiac etiology is the likely cause. In this situation, the one-rescuer algorithm emphasizes the early use of an Automated External Defibrillator (AED) to revert any shockable rhythms.

Sequence of BLS

The evaluation of any child who is found to be unresponsive should proceed in a sequential manner, as described in the BLS algorithm (Figs 20.4 and 20.5).

1. Verify Scene Safety

For rescuers performing CPR in an out-of-hospital setting, it is important to ensure the safety of the rescuer and the victim before proceeding (eg, motor vehicle accident victim lying in the middle of the road with oncoming traffic) and the victim should first be moved to a safe area.

2. Proper Positioning

Proper positioning of the child is of utmost importance. The child should be in a supine (face up) position on a flat, hard surface, such as a sturdy table, the floor, or the ground. If you must turn the victim, minimize turning or twisting of the head and neck to avoid causing damage to the spinal cord in case there is a cervical spine injury.

All pediatric trauma victims should have their necks immobilized before transport, by using a cervical collar (or any other modification such as keeping towels on both sides). The collar should be kept in place until cervical spine injury is definitively ruled out by radiologic imaging.

3. Call for Help/Activate Emergency Response

For single rescuer, it is important to call for help/activate the emergency response system. The 2015 guidelines emphasize the use of mobile phone technology in doing this while proceeding with evaluation of the patient. For two or more rescuers or in a healthcare setting, one person stays with the patient, while the second person calls for help/activates the emergency response system.

4. Check for Response

Check the responsiveness by gently tapping the victim and asking loudly, "Are you okay?" and then look for any movement. *If the child is responsive*, then check to see if the child has any injuries or needs medical assistance immediately. Also assess whether the child is breathing. If breathing is normal, cardiopulmonary resuscitation is not needed. *If the child is unresponsive*, feel for a pulse.

BLS healthcare provider
Pediatric cardiac arrest algorithm for single rescuer—2015 update

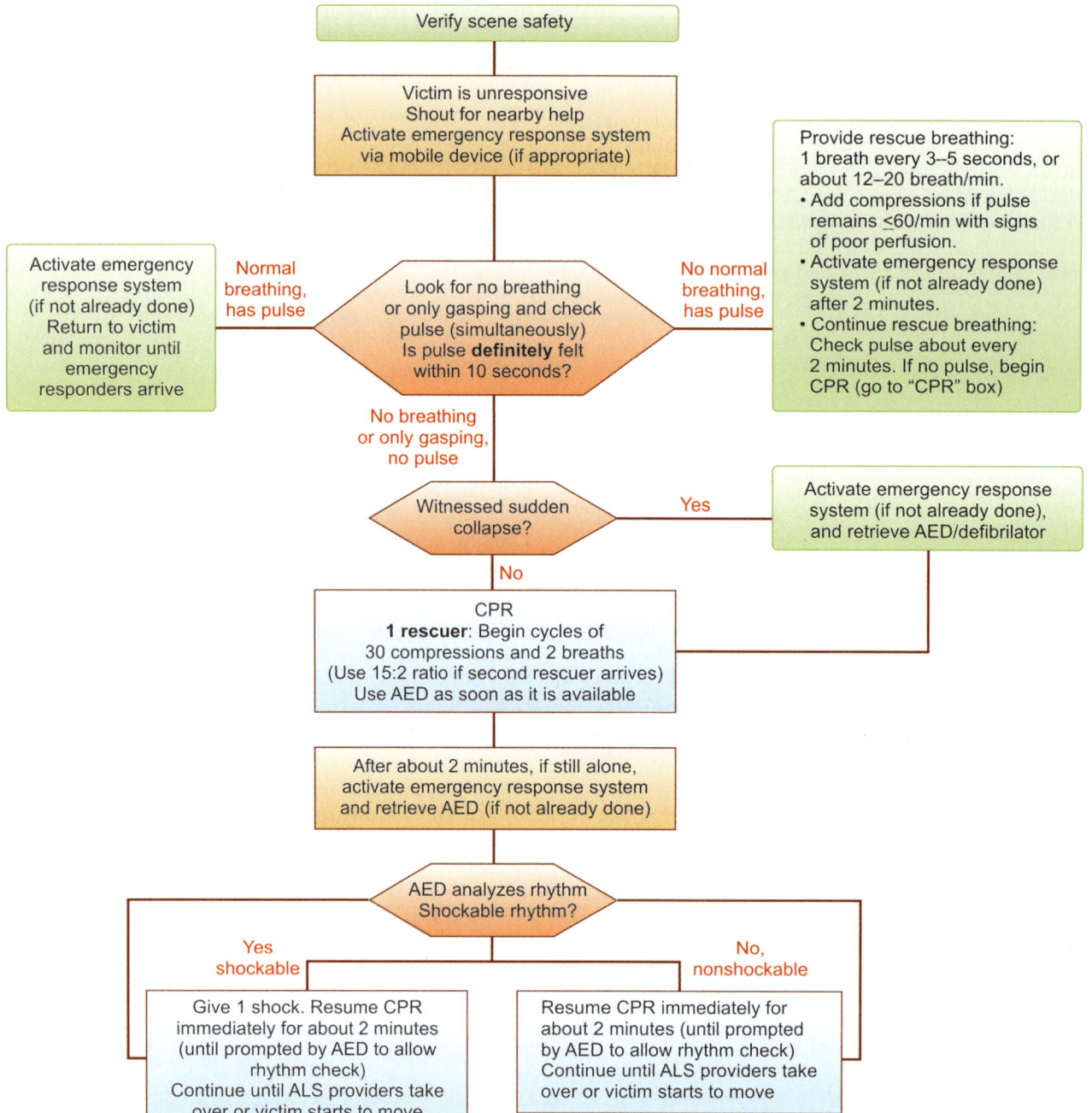

Fig. 20.4 Basic life support (BLS) healthcare provider pediatric cardiac arrest algorithm for single rescuer—2015 Update

5. Check for Breathing and Pulse

The 2015 guidelines emphasize the quick assessment of breathing and pulse of an unresponsive child within 10 seconds. If there is no breathing but pulse is present (brachial for an infant, carotid or femoral in a child), provide rescue breathing (1 breath every 3–5 seconds or 12–20 breaths/min) while continuing to assess the pulse every 2 minutes. However, if there is no breathing and no pulse is present, then immediately begin chest compressions.

- *No pulse* Start chest compressions
- *Pulse <60 per minute* Start chest compressions

- *Pulse ≥60 per min, inadequate breathing* Start rescue breathing 12–20 per minute until spontaneous breathing is present. Reassess pulse every 2 min, but take only 10 seconds to do so.

If pulse rate becomes <60/min despite adequate chest rise with rescue breaths, then chest compressions should also be initiated.

6. Chest Compressions

Chest compressions are initiated at a rate of 100 compressions per minute. First give 30 compressions, pushing hard enough

BLS healthcare provider
Pediatric cardiac arrest algorithm for 2 or more rescuers–2015 update

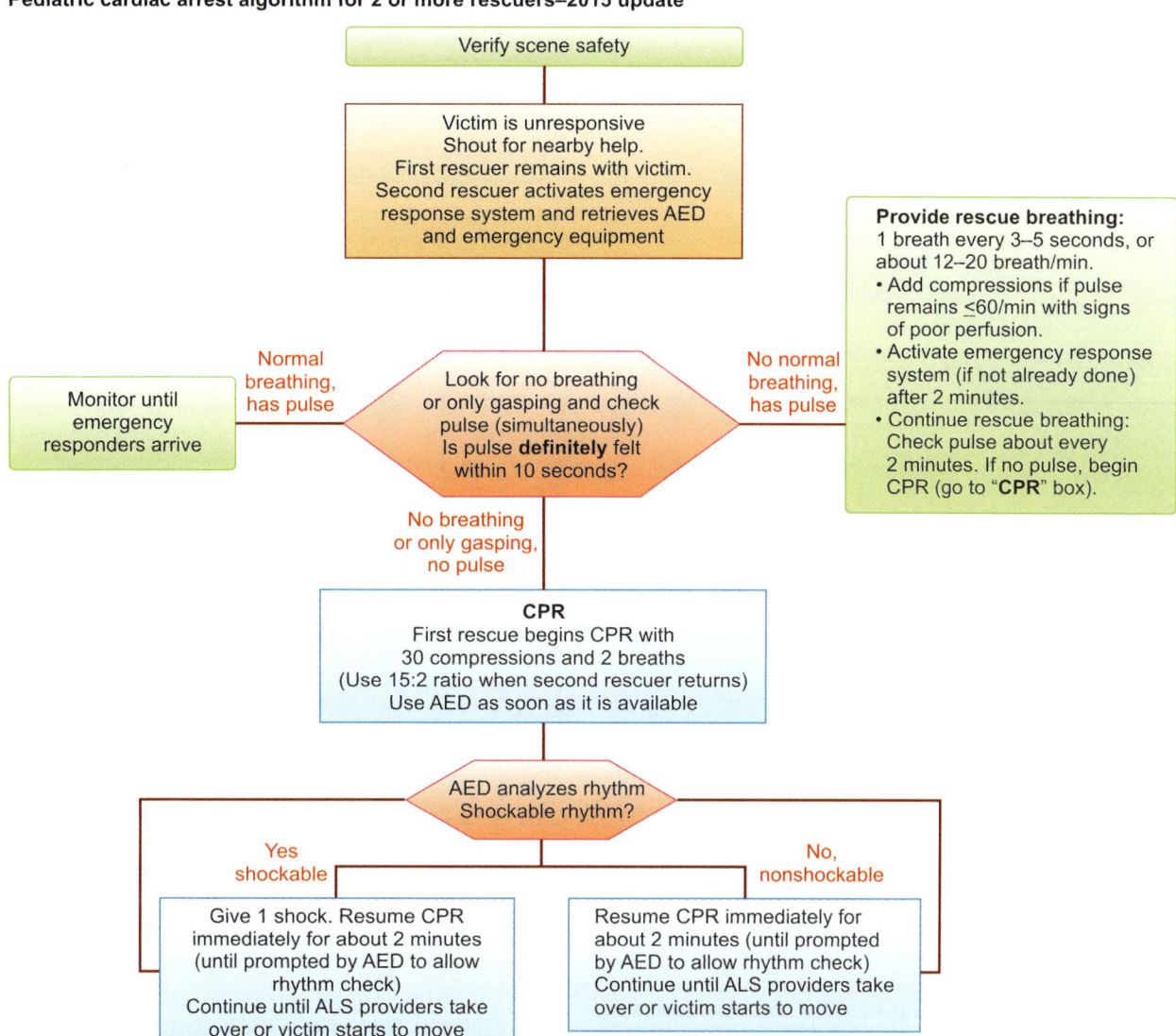

Fig. 20.5 Basic life support (BLS) healthcare provider pediatric cardiac arrest algorithm for two or more rescuers—2015 update

to depress the chest by one third of the anteroposterior diameter of the chest [1.5 inches (4 cm) in infants or 2 inches (5 cm) in children].

- *For infants* The 2-finger technique (compressing the sternum with 2 fingers just below the inter-nipple line in the midline) is preferred, if there is only 1 healthcare provider. The 2 *thumb-encircling hand technique* is used when there are 2 rescuers for the CPR. The 2-thumb technique produces higher coronary artery perfusion pressure and may generate higher systolic and diastolic pressures as compared to 2-finger technique.
- *Older children* Chest compression in older children is done with heel of one or both hands, as for adults.

Ensuring adequate chest recoil after chest compression will allow the heart to fill up with blood, which can then be pumped out to systemic circulation when the heart is squeezed during the subsequent compression. Better chest recoil is associated with a better prognosis because of increased coronary and cerebral perfusion. Techniques to lift

the heel of the hand following compression may improve chest recoil.

Any interruptions in chest compression should be avoided. If there is more than one rescuer, then chest compressions should be switched between both rescuers every 2 minutes to avoid fatigue, as it can impact the effectiveness of the compressions by reducing the coronary perfusion pressure.

Following the first 30 compressions, open the airway and give 2 rescue breaths, as detailed below.

7. Open the Airway and Ventilate

The next step (after 30 compressions) would be to open the airway using a *head tilt–chin lift maneuver* (Fig. 20.6) for both injured and non-injured victims. While maintaining an open airway, take no more than 10 seconds to check whether the victim is breathing: *Look* for rhythmic chest and abdominal movement, *listen* for exhaled breath sounds at the nose and mouth, and *feel* for exhaled air on your cheek. Periodic

20

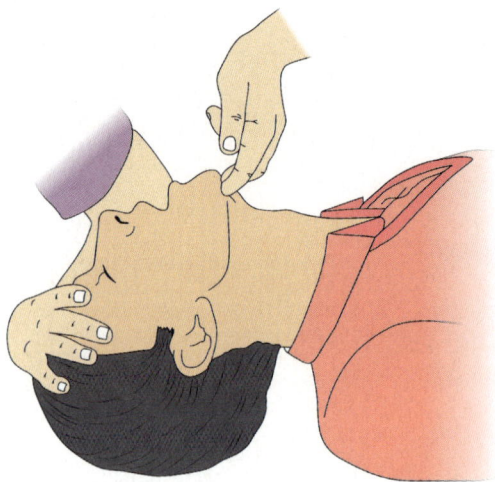

Fig. 20.6 Head tilt–chin lift maneuver

gasping, also called *agonal gasps,* is not synonymous with breathing.

If the child is *not breathing or has only occasional gasps,* maintain an open airway and give 2 breaths with bag and mask. Give mouth-to-mouth ventilation if bag and mask are not available. For providing rescue breaths in infants, it is recommended to use mouth-to-mouth-and-nose technique when bag and mask are not available. Make sure that the breaths are effective (ie, the chest rises). If the chest does not rise; reposition the head, make a better seal, and try again.

8. Co-ordinate Chest Compressions and Ventilation

One cycle of CPR for the single rescuer is 30 compressions and 2 breaths; and it is 15 compressions followed by 2 breaths for two rescuers. If the child has been intubated, there is no need for pausing. The person doing compression should continue at the rate of 100 per minute while the other rescuer can deliver 8–10 breaths per minute. Continue CPR for 5 cycles (about 2 minutes).

9. Defibrillation

An automated external defibrillator (AED) should be attached after 2 min of CPR to assess for the presence of any shockable rhythms. Once the AED is connected, it will display one ECG lead during resuscitation. Flat line on ECG suggests asystole, while Pulseless Electrical Activity (PEA) is defined as a rhythmic display of electrical activity other than ventricular fibrillation (VF) or ventricular tachycardia (VT) that does not produce a palpable arterial pulse. VF and pulseless VT are known as shockable rhythms because they would respond positively to defibrillation.

If no shockable rhythm is identified then CPR should continue for another 2 minutes, followed by another rhythm check. If shockable rhythm is identified, then CPR should resume after the shock has been delivered automatically by the AED. If a manual defibrillator is being used (preferred for infants), the first shock dose should be 2 joules/kg. This can be doubled (4 J/kg) if second dose is required. Resume CPR immediately after delivering the shock.

Atkins DL, Berger S, Duff JP, Gonzales JC, Hunt EA, Joyner BL, Meaney PA, Niles DE, Samson RA, Schexnayder SM. Part 11: Pediatric Basic Life Support and Cardiopulmonary Resuscitation Quality: 2015 American Heart Association Guidelines Update for Cardiopulmonary Resuscitation and Emergency Cardiovascular Care. *Circulation.* 2015; 132(18 Suppl 2): S519–25.

20.4 PEDIATRIC ADVANCED LIFE SUPPORT (PALS)

Most children become critically ill due to progressive respiratory failure or shock. Sudden cardiac arrest due to a primary cardiac cause is uncommon. Pediatric advanced life support (PALS) provides guidelines for advanced airway management and resuscitation in the hospital setting and delineates the approach for specific situations like bradycardia, tachyarrhythmias, and pulseless arrest. It also covers special resuscitation situations and post-resuscitation care. *While BLS is presented as a series of sequential events, ALS activities are performed simultaneously and in parallel.*

Rescuers in the team should be sufficiently trained to diagnose and manage respiratory failure and shock; perform rapid sequence intubation and ventilation; administer fluids, and drugs; and operate a defibrillator. The 2015 update for PALS provides additional recommendations for pre-arrest, intra-arrest, and post-arrest care. Pre-arrest care updates include establishment of medical emergency teams or rapid response teams in hospitals to improve outcomes, using Pediatric Early Warning Score (PEWS) to recognize and intervene for patients with higher likelihood of decline of their cardiorespiratory status.

Fluids and Drugs

- Evidence for limited resource settings suggest that the volume of isotonic crystalloid administered for resuscitation from septic shock should be limited (especially in settings where inotropic support and mechanical ventilation are not available).
- Use of atropine as a premedication in infants and children requiring emergency endotracheal intubation may be considered in specific situations where there is a higher risk of bradycardia.
- Treatment with extracorporeal membrane oxygenation (ECMO) may be considered for infants and children with myocarditis or dilated cardiomyopathy at risk for an impending cardiac arrest.
- The energy dose for defibrillation at 2 J/kg is safe and can be increased to 4 J/kg. Higher doses may be considered for refractory VF, but should not exceed 10 J/kg or the maximum adult dose. For management of out of hospital cardiac arrest patients, initial 2 days of hypothermia (32 to 34 deg C) may be considered and fever should be treated aggressively.
- For shock-refractory VF or pVT, lidocaine use may be considered.
- In post-arrest phase, use of parenteral fluids and inotropes and/or vasopressors should help maintain targeted measures of perfusion (such as blood pressure greater than 5th percentile for age).

Monitoring

- Use of a targeted PaO_2 strategy to maintain saturations between 94 and 100%, and limiting severe hypercapnia

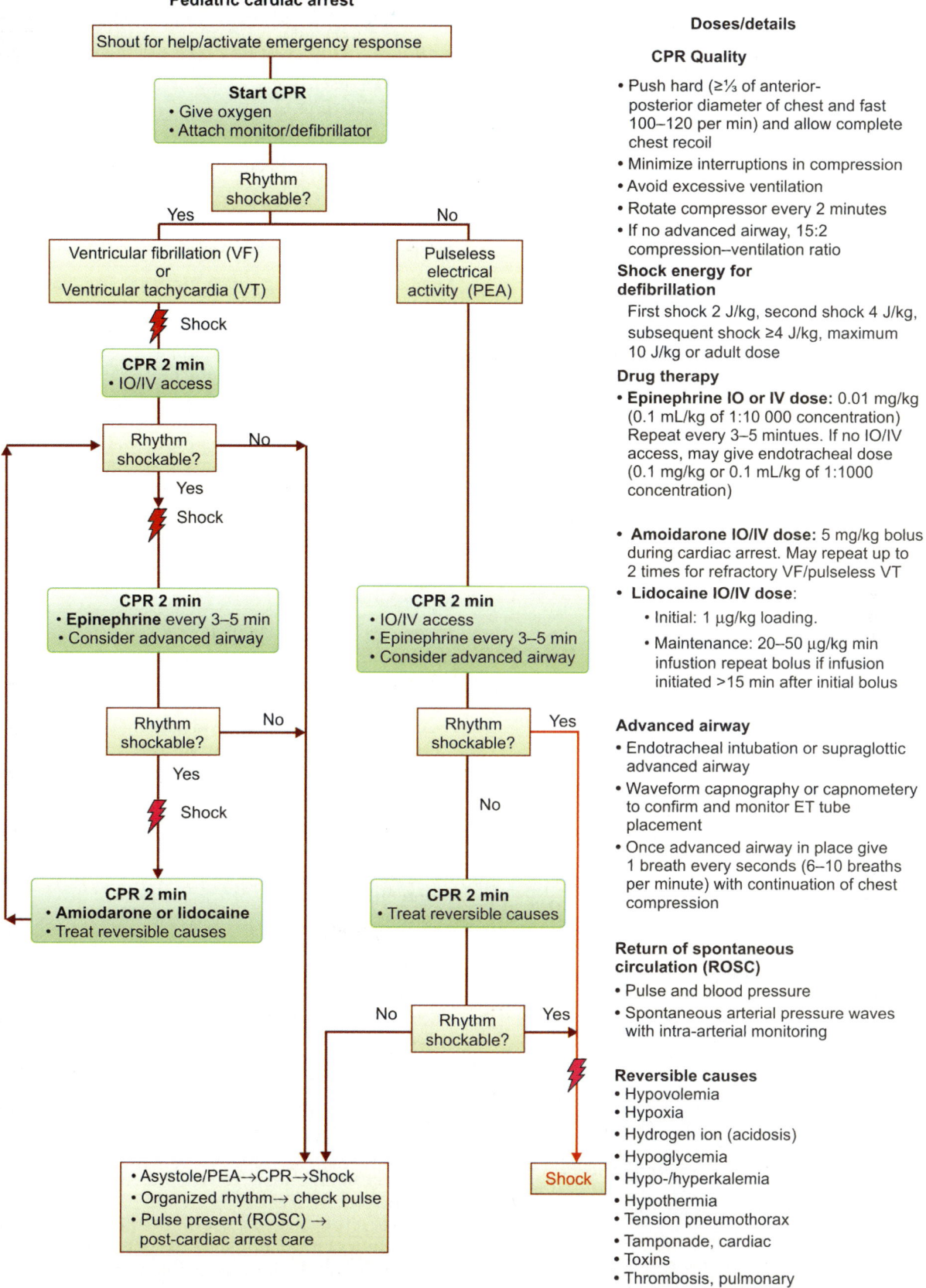

Pediatric cardiac arrest

Shout for help/activate emergency response

Start CPR
• Give oxygen
• Attach monitor/defibrillator

Rhythm shockable?

Yes — Ventricular fibrillation (VF) or Ventricular tachycardia (VT)

No — Pulseless electrical activity (PEA)

Shock

CPR 2 min
• IO/IV access

Rhythm shockable? — No

Yes

Shock

CPR 2 min
• **Epinephrine** every 3–5 min
• Consider advanced airway

CPR 2 min
• IO/IV access
• Epinephrine every 3–5 min
• Consider advanced airway

Rhythm shockable? — No

Yes

Shock

Rhythm shockable? — Yes

No

CPR 2 min
• **Amiodarone or lidocaine**
• Treat reversible causes

CPR 2 min
• Treat reversible causes

Rhythm shockable? — Yes

No

Shock

• Asystole/PEA→CPR→Shock
• Organized rhythm→ check pulse
• Pulse present (ROSC) → post-cardiac arrest care

Doses/details

CPR Quality
• Push hard (≥⅓ of anterior-posterior diameter of chest and fast 100–120 per min) and allow complete chest recoil
• Minimize interruptions in compression
• Avoid excessive ventilation
• Rotate compressor every 2 minutes
• If no advanced airway, 15:2 compression–ventilation ratio

Shock energy for defibrillation
First shock 2 J/kg, second shock 4 J/kg, subsequent shock ≥4 J/kg, maximum 10 J/kg or adult dose

Drug therapy
• **Epinephrine IO or IV dose:** 0.01 mg/kg (0.1 mL/kg of 1:10 000 concentration) Repeat every 3–5 mintues. If no IO/IV access, may give endotracheal dose (0.1 mg/kg or 0.1 mL/kg of 1:1000 concentration)

• **Amoidarone IO/IV dose:** 5 mg/kg bolus during cardiac arrest. May repeat up to 2 times for refractory VF/pulseless VT
• **Lidocaine IO/IV dose:**
  • Initial: 1 µg/kg loading.
  • Maintenance: 20–50 µg/kg min infustion repeat bolus if infusion initiated >15 min after initial bolus

Advanced airway
• Endotracheal intubation or supraglottic advanced airway
• Waveform capnography or capnometery to confirm and monitor ET tube placement
• Once advanced airway in place give 1 breath every seconds (6–10 breaths per minute) with continuation of chest compression

Return of spontaneous circulation (ROSC)
• Pulse and blood pressure
• Spontaneous arterial pressure waves with intra-arterial monitoring

Reversible causes
• Hypovolemia
• Hypoxia
• Hydrogen ion (acidosis)
• Hypoglycemia
• Hypo-/hyperkalemia
• Hypothermia
• Tension pneumothorax
• Tamponade, cardiac
• Toxins
• Thrombosis, pulmonary
• Thrombosis, coronary

Fig. 20.7 Pediatric cardiac arrest algorithm—2015 update. *Adapted from:* Circulation: 2010; 122:S876–S908.

(>50mm Hg) or hypocapnia (<30 mm Hg) can help to improve outcomes.

- During chest compressions, monitoring of end-tidal CO_2 ($ETCO_2$) can help to improve the quality of the CPR.
- While there are no known prognostic factors that help predict outcome, using blood pressure cut-offs in the presence of invasive hemodynamic monitoring during CPR can be considered.
- Neurologic outcomes can be predicted with use of electroencephalograms (EEGs) in the first 7 days, but there are no additional biomarkers to accurately predict outcomes.

Pulseless Arrest1

Figure 20.7 depicts an algorithm for the management of pulseless arrest in children. It is also important to recognize reversible causes of pulseless arrest such as tension pneumothorax, cardiac tamponade, severe hypovolemia, and other possible contributing factors, which can best be remembered as the **4H**—**h**ypoxia, **h**ypovolemia, **h**ypothermia, and **h**yper-/hypokalemia and metabolic disorders; and **4T**—**t**amponade, **t**ension pneumothorax, **t**oxins, **t**hromboembolism. Post-arrest care involves stabilization and transport of the patient to a tertiary care centre (if needed), with the goals of preservation of brain function, prevention of secondary organ injury, and assessment and treatment of the cause of illness.

For asystole and pulseless electrical activity, CPR should be continued with minimal interruption in the chest compressions. Once an endotracheal tube (or other advanced airway) has been placed, chest compressions should be continued at a rate of 100/min without stopping for ventilations. The second rescuer should provide one breath every 6 to 8 seconds (8 to 10 breaths per minute). Epinephrine may be given every 3 to 5 minutes and rhythm should be reassessed after every 2 minutes of CPR. Occasionally a shockable rhythm may be obtained for which defibrillation is attempted, followed by epinephrine (IV/IO or through tracheal tube), and then defibrillation again with higher energy (4J/kg each). Refractory cases may require anti-arrhythmic medications such as amiodarone, lidocaine, or magnesium, followed by repeat defibrillation. If rhythm is non-shockable, then CPR cycles with epinephrine should continue until return of spontaneous circulation (ROSC) or until it is decided to terminate efforts based on clinical situation.

Similarly, for ventricular fibrillation (VF) or pulseless ventricular tachycardia it is important to use an AED early in the course of resuscitation and then continue CPR for 2 minutes, followed by reassessment of rhythm and provision of shock as needed. The 2015 guidelines also emphasize the use of lidocaine or amiodarone in refractory patients.

de Caen AR, Berg MD, Chameides L, Gooden CK, Hickey RW, Scott HF, Sutton RM, Tijssen JA, Topjian A, van der Jagt ÉW, Schexnayder SM, Samson RA. Part 12: Pediatric Advanced Life Support: 2015 American Heart Association Guidelines Update for Cardiopulmonary Resuscitation and Emergency Cardiovascular Care. *Circulation*. 2015; 132(18 Suppl 2): S526–42.

Definition

Poisoning refers to all unintentional poisoning related deaths and non-fatal outcomes caused by exposure to noxious substances. Those which are intentional or for which the intent is undetermined as well as those resulting from reactions to drugs, are excluded as per ICD 10 criteria.

Etiology

Most of the poisonings in children are accidental in nature. The most common agents responsible for poisoning in South-East Asia are pesticides, kerosene, prescription drugs, and household chemicals. Chemical products, most often swallowed by children include household cleaners (bleach, detergents), fuel (kerosene, paraffin), cosmetics, medicines, paints and products for household repairs, and household pesticides. Bites and stings of animals and insects, and ingestion of poisonous plants and seeds also account for outdoor poisoning in children. Carbon monoxide poisoning can happen when fires, stoves, heaters or ovens are used in rooms and huts that do not have proper ventilation to let the gases out.

Exposure to Poison

Acute exposure is a single contact that lasts for seconds, minutes or hours, or several exposures over about a day or less. *Chronic exposure* is contact that lasts for many days, months or years.

A poison may get into the body through ingestion, inhalation (gas, vapors, dust, fumes, smoke, spray), skin contact (pesticides), or injection (bites and stings, drug injection).

Predisposing Factors

The peak age for childhood poisoning is between 1 and 3 years. As children become more mobile and curious, they come into contact with a variety of toxins in their environment. Hand-to-mouth activity and development of the pincer grasp in infants puts them at risk of ingesting potentially toxic substances.

- For children younger than 6 months, poisoning is unusual but may result from the inadvertent administration of an incorrect drug or drug dose by a parent, intentional administration of a drug by a parent or sibling, or passive exposure.
- Any poisoning in a child younger than 1 year of age should be carefully evaluated for possible child abuse or neglect.
- Unintentional ingestion is unusual after age 5 years, although it can result from mistaken consumption of any toxin from a mislabeled container.
- Between the ages of 5 and 9 years, poisoning may be a reflection of intrafamilial stress or suicidal intent.
- Beyond 9 years of age, overdose or poisoning frequently results either from a suicidal gesture or attempt, or from an adverse effect of drug abuse.
- Adolescents who enter the workplace may encounter hazardous chemicals, but may not have access to protective equipment or safety education.

Majority of the exposures occur at home. Preventive measures in the home environment can go a long way in reducing the overall morbidity of poisonings in children.

First Aid for Poisoning

A fast response is associated with better outcome of the affected person. There are some important initial steps to be followed without panicking and distressing the poisoned child **(Box 20.3)**. In minor poisoning, symptomatic and supportive treatment is generally not required, whereas for moderate or severe poisoning, advanced symptomatic and supportive treatment is always necessary.

Box 20.3 Poisoning First Aid: Do nots for Lay Persons

- DO NOT give an unconscious victim anything by mouth.
- DO NOT induce vomiting unless you are told to do so by the Poison Control Center or a doctor.
- DO NOT try to neutralize the poison with lemon juice or vinegar, or any other substance, unless you are told to do so by the Poison Control Center or a doctor. Do not apply any kind of potentially harmful herbal and folk remedies
- DO NOT use any "cure-all" type antidote.
- DO NOT wait for symptoms to develop if you suspect that someone has been poisoned.

For Ingested Poisons

- Remove the poison from the entry point. Wipe the affected area gently. Rinse with fresh water. Remove the clothes of the victim. Wash the eyes of the victim with fresh water and dry gently.
- Provoke vomiting only if the victim is conscious.
- If the victim vomits, protect the airway. Save the vomitus to allow identification of the poison.
- If the victim starts having convulsions, protect him/her from injury and give convulsion first aid.
- Reassure the victim and keep him/her comfortable. Position the victims on their left side while getting or awaiting medical help.

For Inhaled Poisons

- Open windows and doors to remove the fumes.
- Hold a wet cloth over your nose and mouth. Take several deep breaths of fresh air, then hold your breath as you go in.
- Take out the affected person from the toxic area to fresh air. Call for emergency help. Never attempt to rescue a victim without notifying others first.
- Avoid lighting a match stick as some gases may ignite.
- As necessary, perform first aid for skin burns, eye injuries (eye emergencies), or convulsions.
- If the victim vomits, protect the airway.

Treatment **Poisoning: General Principles**

Initial assessment of a patient with suspected but unknown toxic exposure should be aimed at treating the patient rather than treating the poison. The first priority is to assess airway and breathing, checking oxygen saturation by pulse oximetry and obtaining vital signs (pulse, respiratory rate, BP), and looking for any potential life threatening abnormality. Blood should be withdrawn for ABG, glucose, electrolytes, and also saved for

other studies. Urinary tract catheterization also needs to be done for urinary output monitoring and other studies.

Antidotes are available for very few commonly encountered poisons, and treatment is usually non-specific and symptomatic. In such cases, management consists of emergency first aid and stabilization measures, appropriate treatment to reduce absorption, measures to enhance life support, and followed by psychiatric counseling.

Figure 20.8 depicts a general approach to a child with poisoning.

1. Emergency Stabilization Measures

The unconscious patient should be transported in the head-down semi-prone position to minimize the risk of aspiration of gastric contents. A clear airway is established and ventilation is maintained. Potentially serious abnormalities such as metabolic acidosis, hyperkalemia, and hypoglycemia may require correction as a matter of urgency. Neurological assessment is done by calculating the Glasgow Coma Score (GCS). Monitor the vital signs every 5–15 minutes.

Contrary to popular belief, many poisons and drugs taken in overdose do not cause rapid loss of consciousness. Some of the presentations commonly seen with different intoxication are listed in **Table 20.4**.

Many drugs and poisons can cause convulsions, which, if recurrent, should be controlled with intravenous diazepam. Hypotension with peripheral circulatory failure is treated by correction of volume deficit, hypoxia, and acidosis. If adequate perfusion is not restored by these measures, the circulating volume should be increased by administration of a plasma expander intravenously. Cardiac arrhythmias are often improved or abolished by correction of hypoxia, acidosis, and electrolyte imbalance.

The next step should be to take a detailed history and perform physical examination. Aim is to try to identify the poison, or the toxidrome. Key to diagnosis of the toxidrome is provided in the next section.

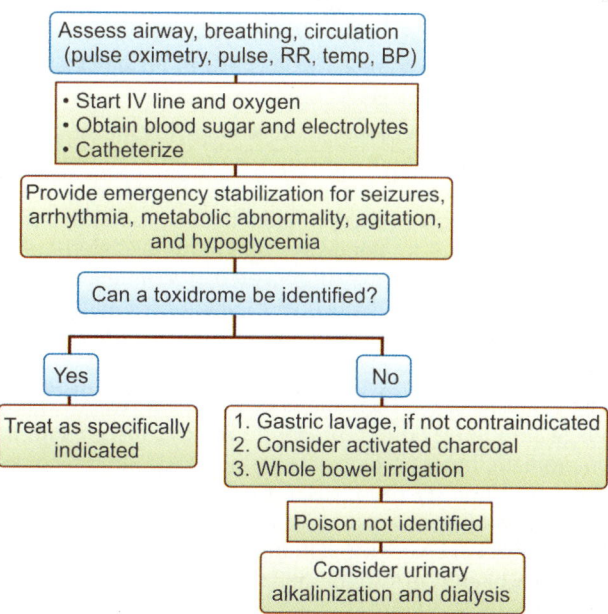

Fig. 20.8 A general approach to a child with poisoning

Table 20.4 Presenting Features of Common Poisonings
1. *Seizures* Organochlorines, chlorinated hydrocarbons, cocaine, isoniazid, phenothiazine, carbon monoxide, theophylline
2. *Respiratory compromise* Narcotics, organophosphates, barbiturate, benzodiazepines
3. *Cardiac arrythmias* Tricyclic antidepressants, amphetamine, aluminium phosphide, digitalis, theophylline, arsenic, cyanide, chloroquin
4. *Metabolic acidosis* Isoniazid, methanol, salicylates, phenformin, iron, cyanide
5. *GIT disturbances* Organophosphorus, arsenic, iron, lithium, mercury
6. *Cyanosis* Nitrobenzene compounds, aniline dyes, and dapsone

2. Removal of Toxin

The aim of decontamination procedures is to reduce the absorption of poison. It can be achieved by following measures.

Eye decontamination Ocular exposure to solvents, eg, hydrocarbons, detergents, alcohol, or corrosive agents require immediate local decontamination. This is achieved by copious irrigation with neutralizing solution (normal saline or water) for at least 30 minutes. Do not use acid or alkaline irrigating solution.

Dermal decontamination Absorption of organophosphorus and related compounds through cutaneous route can also be fatal. Remove all contaminated clothes and irrigate the whole body including nail, groin, skin-folds with water or saline as soon as possible after exposure and continue irrigating for at least 15 minutes. *Water should not be used to decontaminate skin in exposures to sodium and phosphorus.* In certain cases, specific agents may be indicated for skin decontamination (eg, mineral oil for elemental sodium, neosporin for super glue, and calcium gluconate for hydroflouric acid).

Gut Decontamination

This includes (*i*) gastric emptying; (*ii*) adsorbent administration; and (*iii*) catharsis. Gastric emptying is most effective within 1 hr of poisoning; it has some effect within 1–4 hr; it is ineffective when used at a late stage.

Emesis It is the preferred method of emptying the stomach in conscious children. Vomiting can be induced by administration of copious draughts of warm water. Syrup of ipecac may be used for inducing emesis in children older than 6 months in a single dose of 10 mL for 6–12 months age, and 15 mL for children above 1 year of age. The dose may be repeated in 20 minutes for those more than 1 year of age. Induction of vomiting is contraindicated in corrosive or kerosene poisoning and in comatose patients or those with absent gag reflex.

Gastric lavage If the vomiting does not occur quickly, gastric lavage should be done promptly to remove the poison. In a symptomatic but alert patient with minor ingestion, activated charcoal alone by mouth is sufficient for gastrointestinal decontamination.

The child is kept in the left lateral position with the head hanging over edge of the table and the face down. A large single lumen tube with multiple distal ports is necessary. A restraint is required for most children and mouth gag is placed in the mouth before the procedure. The catheter is passed gently and free end is dipped under water to make sure that the catheter is not in the airway. Generally tap water is used for lavage and four or five washes are done. The volume of each aliquot should be at least 10–15 mL/kg until clear. After the fluid has been instilled, it should be removed by gravity drainage or tube suction. Catheter is pinched before it is finally withdrawn or suction is maintained during withdrawal to prevent aspiration.

Gastric lavage should not be performed in children with poor gag reflex or corrosive ingestion. In kerosene poisoning, lavage may be done very cautiously if the child has consumed a large gulp of kerosene and is brought quickly to the hospital, otherwise it is better to avoid stomach wash.

Adsorbents An agent capable of binding to a toxic agent in the gut is known as adsorbent. Activated charcoal is the most widely used adsorbent. It is created by subjecting carbonaceous material eg, wood, coal, etc. to steam at 600–900°C and acid. For the comatose patient (Grades 3 or 4) with potentially serious overdose, gastric lavage is followed by administration of single dose of activated charcoal *via* an orogastric or nasogastric tube within 1–2 hours of ingestion.

Dose of activated charcoal administered should be at least 10 times the dose of ingested toxic material. The usual single dose is 1–2 g/kg for children and adults. Multiple dosing (1 g/kg every 2–6 h) is effective for poisoning with phenobarbitone, phenytoin, digitalis, and theophylline. In asymptomatic patient presenting early or without reliable history, 15–30 grams of activated charcoal may be used.

Catharsis Laxatives and purgatives may be given for poisoning with substances which do not cause corrosive action on gastrointestinal mucosa. Increased motility of the gut may reduce absorption. Commonly used cathartics include sorbitol and mannitol (1–2 g/kg), and magnesium or sodium sulfate (200–300 mg/kg). Do not give magnesium salt cathartics to children with renal failure.

Whole bowel irrigation (WBI) with polyethylene glycol electrolyte solution @ 0.5 L/hour for 4–6 hours should be considered for patients presenting after 2 h of enteric coated or sustained release drug ingestion including severe iron poisoning. Concurrent administration of activated charcoal and WBI may decrease the effectiveness of charcoal.

Use of gastric decontamination is highly individualized. It is not universal. American Academy of Clinical Toxicologists does not endorse the routine use of any form of gastric decontamination (ie, gastric lavage, ipecac administration, cathartics, whole bowel irrigation, single dose activated charcoal, etc.) for ingested poisons.

3. Specific Antidote Therapy

The antidotes may be physiological, chemical or physical. *Chemical antidotes* combine with the poison and render it innocuous. *Physiological antidotes* counteract the effects of the poison on the metabolism and physiological functions of the body and thus prevent its harmful effects. *Physical antidotes* prevent the contact of the poisonous substance with the target organ or adsorb the toxic components, thus preventing their toxicity.

Specific antidotes may be lifesaving but unfortunately they are not often available and are effective for less than 5% of poisoning

Table 20.5 Few Specific Antidotes	
Antidote/drug	*Indication*
Atropine (injection)	Organophosphates, carbamates (A1)
Amyl nitrite (inhalation)	Cyanides (A2)
Antidigoxin Fab (antibody fragments)	Digoxin (A1)
Acetylcysteine	Paracetamol (B1)
Beta-blockers	Sympathomimetics (A1), theophylline (B1)
Budesonide (inhalation)	Irritant gases
Calcium sodium edetate	Lead (C2)
Dicobalt edetate	Cyanides (A1)
Calcium gluconate	Hydrofluoric acid (A1)
Copper solution	Phosphorus white (yellow)
Diazepam	Chloroquin, organophosphates (A2)
Dimercaprol	Arsenic (B3), Mercury, heavy metals (C3)
Desferrioxamine	Iron (B1), aluminium (C2)
Flumazenil	Benzodiazepines (B1)
Ethanol	Methanol (A1)
Glucagon	Beta blockers (A1)
Glucose	Insulin (A1)
Methionine	Paracetamol (B1)
Methylene blue	Nitrites, nitrobenzene (A1)
Naloxone	Opioid analgesics (A1)
Neostigmine	Anticholinergic poisoning (B2)
Oxygen	Carbon monoxide (A1)
Penicillamine	Copper (C1)
Pralidoxime (injection)	Organophosphates (A1)
Polyethylene glycol 400 (topical)	Phenol
Physostigmine	Anticholinergics, tricyclic anti-depressants (A1)
Pyridoxine	Isoniazid (A2)
Sodium nitrite	Cyanide (A1)
Sodium nitroprusside	Ergotism (A1)
Sodium thiosulphate	Cyanide (A1)
Clotting factors	Warfarin (A1)

The classification in terms of urgency of availability (A, B, C) or proven effectiveness (1, 2, 3) is given next to the main indication.
A Required to be immediately available within 30 minutes.
B Required to be available within 2 hours.
C Required to be available within 6 hours.
1 Effectiveness well documented.
2 Widely used, not universally accepted as effective.
3 Questionable usefulness.

cases. When obtainable, they must be given without delay for maximum protective action. Some examples of antidotes and other drugs that may be needed are listed in **Table 20.5**.

Antidotes now considered obsolete include universal antidote for ingested poisons, acetazolamide for modification of urinary pH, ascorbic acid for methemoglobinemia, castor oil as cathartic, nalorphine for opiates, sodium chloride for emesis, and tannins for alkaloids.

4. Promotion of Excretion of Toxin
The efficiency of regimens for enhancement of drug elimination from the body can be predicted to a large extent if the physio-chemical properties, disposition, and pharmacokinetics of the substance are known. The fluid intake is increased to promote glomerular filtration and excretion of poison through the urine.

Forced diuresis Diuresis alone has relatively little effect on drug elimination because the renal clearance is proportional to the urine flow rate. In the case of drugs which are weak organic acids and bases, a much greater effect on clearance can be obtained by manipulation of the urine pH. The lipid solubility and hence tubular reabsorption of such acidic and basic drugs is decreased in alkaline and acidic urine, respectively; and their renal clearance is increased correspondingly. Theoretically for each change of one unit in urine pH, the renal clearance could change by a factor of 10. Urine pH is therefore much more important than urine flow rate.

20

- *Forced alkaline diuresis* is restricted largely to poisoning with phenobarbitone and salicylate, although much of the effect in lowering plasma salicylate concentrations result from hemodilution rather than increased urinary excretion. Raise the urinary pH to 7.5 for weak acids (eg, barbiturates, salicylates) with sodium bicarbonate.
- *Forced acidic diuresis* Maintain urinary pH to 5.5–6.5 in poisoning with weak bases, eg, tricyclic antidepressant and phenytoin, with ammonium chloride 4 g administered every two hourly through Ryle's tube.

Any form of forced diuresis is potentially dangerous. Forced diuresis is contraindicated in patients with cardiac and renal impairment; complications include water intoxication, disturbances of acid–base and electrolyte balance, left ventricular failure with pulmonary edema, and cerebral edema.

Hemodialysis, hemoperfusion, and peritoneal dialysis Drugs which can be removed reasonably effectively by hemoperfusion and hemodialysis include barbiturates, carbamazepine, salicylates, theophylline, dapsone, most antibiotics, lithium, chloral hydrate, methanol, and ethylene glycol. In general, hemoperfusion with coated charcoal or exchange resins is more effective than hemodialysis, although the latter may be preferred for simultaneous correction of acid–base and electrolyte balance (eg, in salicylate poisoning). Hemodialysis is also the method of choice for removal of methanol, ethylene glycol and lithium.

Peritoneal dialysis is much less effective and it is used rarely. It has the advantage that it does not require special facilities but may be complicated by fluid and electrolyte abnormalities, perforation, peritonitis, and adhesions.

Dialysis is not useful in poisoning with digitalis, antihistamines, belladonna alkaloids, opiates, etc.

Barry JD. Diagnosis and management of the poisoned child. *Pediatr Ann.* 2005;34:937–46.

Bond GR. The role of activated charcoal and gastric emptying in gastrointestinal decontamination: a state-of-the-art review. *Ann Emerg Med.* 2002;39:273–86.

Chyka PA, Seger D, Krenzelok EP, Vale JA; American Academy of Clinical Toxicology; European Association of Poisons Centres and Clinical Toxicologists. Position paper: Single-dose activated charcoal. *Clin Toxicol* (Phila). 2005;43:61–87.

Collee GG, Hanson GC. The management of acute poisoning. *Br J Anaesth.* 1993;70: 562–73.

Flomenbaum NE, Goldfrank LR. Principles of managing the poisoned or overdosed patient. *In*: Flomenbaum NE, Goldfrank LR, Hoffman RS, *et al* (Eds). Goldfrank's Toxicologic Emergencies. 8th Edition. New York: McGraw-Hill Professional;2006. p.42–50.

Gupta S, Taneja V. Poisoned child: emergency room management. *Indian J Pediatr.* 2003;70:S2–8.

Heard K. Gastrointestinal decontamination. *Med Clin North Am.* 2005;89:1067–78.

Manoguerra AS, Cobaugh DJ; Guidelines for the Management of Poisoning Consensus Panel. Guideline on the use of ipecac syrup in the out-of-hospital management of ingested poisons. *Clin Toxicol.* 2005;43:1–10.

Mofenson HC, Caraccio TR. Toxidromes. Compr Ther 1985;11:46–52.

Poisoning First Aid. MedlinePlus Medical Encyclopedia. Available from: http://www.nlm.nih.gov/medlineplus/ency/article/007579.htm. Accessed 7 July, 2012.

Poisonings: Overview. National Center for Injury Prevention and Control. Available from: http://www.cdc.gov/ncipc/factsheets/poisoning-overview.htm. Accessed 7 July, 2012.

Position paper: Cathartics. *J Toxicol Clin Toxicol.* 2004;42:243–53.

Position paper: Ipecac syrup. *J Toxicol Clin Toxicol.* 2004;42:133–43.

Position paper: Whole bowel irrigation. *J Toxicol Clin Toxicol.* 2004;42:843–54.

Ressel GW, AAP. AAP releases policy statement on poison treatment in the home. *Am Fam Physician.* 2004;69:741–2.

Vale JA, Kulig K; American Academy of Clinical Toxicology; European Association of Poisons Centres and Clinical Toxicologists. Position paper: gastric lavage. *J Toxicol Clin Toxicol.* 2004;42:933–43.

20.6 TOXIDROMES

Toxidrome refers to the group of signs and symptoms that consistently result from particular toxins. **Table 20.6** provides examples of some common toxidromes.

1. Sympathomimetic Syndrome

Etiology Prescription medications for asthma (albuterol, terbutaline, theophylline), decongestants (pseudoephedrine), ADHD medications (dextroamphetamine, methylpheni-

Table 20.6 Examples of Symptom Complexes/Toxidromes

Pupils	Respiration	Consciousness	Possible agent	Other associations
Pinpoint	↑↓	Coma	Organophosphorus insecticides, carbamates	Cholinergic: Bradycardia, wheeze, salivation
	↓	Coma	Opioids	Hypotension, hypothermia
	↓	Coma	Phenothiazines	Cardiac arrhythmia
Dilated	↑	Agitation, hallucination	Atropine	Anticholinergic: Fever, dry mucous membranes, flushing, urinary retention
	↓	Coma	Tricyclic antidepressants	Cardiac arrhythmia, seizures, hypotension
	↓	Coma	Sedatives, barbiturates	Hypotension, hypothermia, hyporeflexia
	↑	Agitation, hallucination	Theophylline, amphetamines	Seizures, tachycardia, hypertension, acidosis
Normal	↑	Coma	Uremia	Acidosis, hyperkalemia
	↑	Semi coma	Salicylates	Tinnitus, agitation, diaphoresis, alkalosis followed by acidosis

date), illicit drugs (amphetamines, cocaine, ecstasy), thyroid hormones, and monoamino-oxidase (MAO) inhibitors.

Clinical features Sympathomimetic toxic syndrome results from the activation of the sympathetic system, manifesting as tachycardia, hyperthermia, hypertension, mydriasis, agitation, and diaphoresis. End-organ effects include stroke, rhabdomyolysis, DIC, and psychosis which may progress to seizures and coma.

Treatment	Sympathomimetic Toxidrome

Management includes supportive measures in the form of hydration and active cooling for hyperthermia. Agitation, tachycardia and hypertension respond to benzodiazepine administration. For MDMA/ecstasy use by adolescents (used in rave parties), it is important to monitor serum sodium, as it can cause inappropriate ADH (antidiuretic hormone) secretion, leading to hyponatremia and presenting clinically as altered mental status and seizures.

2. Anticholinergic Toxic Syndrome

Etiology The most common cause is poisoning by *Datura stramonium* (jimson weed). Antihistaminics, and tricyclic antidepressants are the other incriminating agents. It blocks the action of acetylcholine at the muscarinic receptor sites.

Clinical manifestations include flushing, dry mucous membranes, mydriasis, delirium, and hyperthermia. The mnemonic for remembering these manifestations is *"Red as a beet, Dry as a bone, Blind as a bat, Mad as hatter, and Hot as hare."*

Treatment	Anticholinergic Toxidrome

Physostigmine (0.02 mg/kg, max 0.5 mg) is the antidote for anticholinergic toxicity, and it reversibly inhibits cholinesterases in both central and peripheral nervous system, allowing acetylcholine to accumulate and overcome the antimuscarinic effects. It should be used only if the following pre-conditions are satisfied: (*i*) Evidence of severe CNS and peripheral anticholinergic effects; (*ii*) normal QRS interval (<0.08 sec); (*iii*) no history of seizures; (*iv*) severe agitation, coma or cardiovascular instability unresponsive to other treatments, such as benzodiazepines; and (*v*) No history of ingestion of tricyclic antidepressants.

Physostigmine is infused slowly over 5 minutes. Additional doses may be necessary if symptoms reoccur, as its duration of action is 60 to 70 minutes.

3. Cholinergic Toxic Syndrome

Etiology The most common source of cholinergic exposure is ingestion or dermal exposure to pesticides; ie, organophosphates and carbamates. Other sources include muscarine-containing mushrooms, methacholine, carbachol, bethanechol, and nicotine alkaloids.

Clinical features These compounds render the enzyme acetylcholinesterase non-functional, by binding with it. As a result, acetylcholine can no longer be metabolized and accumulates leading to excessive stimulation of central and peripheral acetylcholine receptors, leading to altered mental status, diffuse muscle weakness, and excessive secretory activity. The mnemonic to remember its manifestations is: **DUMBELS** (for muscarinic effects)—**D**iarrhea, **U**rination, **M**iosis, **B**ronchorrhea, bronchospasm, **E**mesis, **L**acrimation, **S**ecretions; **CCC** (for central nicotinic effects)—Confusion, Coma, Convulsions.

- The route of exposure affects the temporal onset of symptoms, with respiratory route producing a rapid onset of systemic symptoms than dermal exposure.
- The initial presentation with dermal route may be muscle fasciculation and sweating whereas inhalational route may produce central effects, miosis, rapid onset of bronchospasm, bronchorrhea.
- Ingestion may produce nausea, vomiting and diarrhea prior to other features. Organophosphate induced delayed neuropathy can occur 2 to 3 weeks postexposure, presenting as profound weakness of the lower extremities. Another delayed manifestation that has been reported in children recovering from the cholinergic phase is bilateral vocal cord palsy after 1 to 4 days of exposure, requiring prolonged respiratory support.

Treatment	Cholinergic Toxidrome

Initial management consists of decontamination of skin, eyes, and gastrointestinal tract. Basic life support with support of the airway is initiated. Therapy is initiated with atropine (0.02 mg/kg IV every 5 to 10 minutes) for the reduction of secretions and bronchospasm.

Pralidoxime the specific antidote, is started (25–30 mg/kg infused over 30 minutes) and repeated in 4 to 6 hours, if there are persistent nicotinic symptoms.

4. Opioid Toxic Syndrome

Opioids are commonly used analgesics and drugs of abuse. Opioid toxidrome usually presents secondary to substance abuse (heroin). It is characterized by a clinical triad of respiratory depression, depressed mental status, and miosis.

Treatment	Opioid Toxidrome

Toxicologic screens remain positive 48 to 72 hours after ingestion. Naloxone is a competitive opioid antagonist that acts on mu, kappa, and delta receptors and can be used to rapidly reverse respiratory depression related to opiod toxicity.

5. Sedative-Hypnotic Toxic Syndrome

Sedative hypnotics (barbiturates, benzodiazepines, chloral hydrate), and alcohol may produce obtundation and coma, with normal vital signs at presentation with acute intoxication.

Setting There are three possible scenarios of exposure to these agents for the pediatric age groups: Firstly a young child with unintentional exposure, second group is that of children undergoing diagnostic or therapeutic procedures in the hospital setting, and thirdly adolescents may consume these drugs intentionally for suicidal intent or as drug abuse.

Clinical features Most patients present with altered mental status and relatively normal vital signs. As symptoms progress, bradycardia, hypotension, and hypothermia can occur due to CNS depression. Chloral hydrate may cause

20

Case Study | Unresponsive Child

A 2-year-old previously healthy male child is brought to the Emergency Room in an unresponsive state. The child had been playing unattended in his grandparents' room and was later found lying on the floor by his mother. Child is unresponsive, and Glasgow Coma Scale Score is 12.

What will you do now?

Assess Circulation, Airway, and Breathing (CAB). Assessment of vital signs along with immediate evaluation of circulatory state (peripheral pulses–presence and volume; skin perfusion by capillary refill time), patency of airway, and the rate and depth of breathing should be performed rapidly.

This child had HR of 100/min, adequate perfusion, no audible stridor, respiratory rate was 12/minute, and had good air entry on auscultation with no abnormal breath sounds. Blood pressure was 100/72 mm Hg, and pulse oximetry showed oxyhemoglobin saturation of 97%.

Do you need to perform any urgent laboratory tests?

Obtain blood sample for blood glucose and electrolytes.

His blood glucose value is 98 mg/dL, and his electrolytes are normal. Parents revealed that his grandmother's medication box was found open by his side and there were several pills on the floor. The child's grandmother has type 2 diabetes, hypertension and also takes sleeping pills at night. Grandmother's medication list includes—oral hypoglycemic agents, antihypertensive medications (beta-blocker and ACE inhibitor) and benzodiazepine.

Outline your further evaluation in view of this history?

Based on this information, we should consider accidental ingestion as the likely cause of the child's symptoms. Additional evaluations may include neurologic evaluation (assessment of pupils, muscle tone and tendon reflexes), heart rhythm evaluation and monitoring of body temperature and secretions.

This child had mildly dilated pupils that were reactive to light, normal heart rhythm, no increase in upper airway secretions, and body temperature was 36.8°C.

Can a toxidrome be identified?

Based on the history of sudden unresponsiveness accompanied by dilated reactive pupils, normal heart rate and rhythm, reduced respiratory rate and reduced body temperature, it is likely that the child has ingested a benzodiazepine.

nausea, vomiting, abdominal pain, and cardiac dysrhythmias. Some of these agents can produce fatal respiratory depression.

Treatment | Sedative-Hypnotic Toxidrome

- Activated charcoal use can reduce the serum half-lives of barbiturates such as phenobarbital and prevents absorption by adsorbing drug in the intestine.
- Multidose charcoal may interrupt enterohepatic recirculation and enhance elimination by enterocapillary exsorption. Theoretically, by constantly bathing the GI tract with charcoal, the intestinal lumen serves as a dialysis membrane for reverse absorption of drug from intestinal villous capillary blood into intestinal lumen, from where it can get adsorbed on to the

activated charcoal. An initial dose of 1 g/kg is recommended followed by 0.25 g/kg every 4 to 6 hours.

- Charcoal aqueous solutions are premixed with a cathartic (usually sorbitol 70%), so these patients should not be given additional doses of cathartic to prevent dehydration and electrolyte imbalances. There is anecdotal evidence for use of physostigmine for gamma hexabenzene toxicity but there is no proven antidote for it.
- Urinary alkalinization with sodium bicarbonate to a pH of 7.5 to 8.0 can hasten the renal excretion of phenobarbital, which is a weak acid and is excreted primarily from the kidneys. This can be done with an initial dose of 1 mEq/kg of sodium bicarbonate, followed by a continuous infusion. This usually requires close monitoring of urine pH and blood pH, trying to keep the former more than 7.5 and the latter less than 7.5 to prevent over-alkalinization. Alkalinization does not increase excretion of shorter acting agents as they are mostly metabolized by the liver.

Tarabar AF, Hoffman RS. Pediatric toxic syndromes (toxidromes). *In*: Erickson TB, Ahrens WR, Aks SE, *et al* (Eds). Pediatric Toxicology–Diagnosis and Management of the Poisoned Child, 1st Edition. New York: McGraw-Hill;2005. p.75–83.

20.7 SPECIFIC POISONS

1. Corrosive Poisoning

Corrosive poisonings in children have now surpassed kerosene oil poisoning as the most common cause of household accidental poisonings. This is due to common availability of toilet cleaner fluids in households. Pediatric acid and caustic ingestions often involve toddlers who find these solutions stored inappropriately in unsafe easy-to-open containers, and ingest small volumes in the course of their exploratory behaviors.

Epidemiology The most common acid containing agents that are accidentally ingested include toilet bowl cleaners (contain sulfuric or hydrochloric acid), anti-rust solutions (hydrofluoric, oxalic, and hydrochloric acids), swimming pool cleaners (hydrofluoric acid), and vinegar (acetic acid). Due to their unpleasant taste and odor, they get swallowed rapidly in smaller amounts and cause more gastric injury than esophageal injury.

Alkaline agents such as household cleaners (containing sodium hydroxide), drain openers, bleaches, toilet bowl cleaners and dishwashing detergents are generally swallowed in larger amounts, and cause more transmural injuries due to liquefactive necrosis. The epidemiology of corrosive injuries varies by country and the most prevalent household chemical agents that children have access to. *Data from limited case series published from various sites in India indicate that toilet bowl cleaner (acid) ingestion is one of the most common corrosive ingestion in the country.*

Pathogenesis In the first 3 to 4 days, the epithelium develops erythema, edema, ulceration, and necrosis; with associated bacterial invasion and tissue sloughing. After 4 days, neovascularization and fibroblast proliferation facilitate granulation and collagen cross linking. The tensile strength is lowest at this time and the risk of perforation is the highest. The healing process continues for 3 to 6 weeks after injury and causes fibrosis, contractures and cicatrisation, leading to strictures.

Ocular or dermal exposure may cause burns and scarring of varying severity. Inhalation injury can cause upper airway involvement with severe epiglottic and laryngeal edema and ulceration, or lower airway involvement with pneumonitis and impaired gas exchange. Children presenting with stridor have laryngeal involvement which can very quickly progress to life-threatening airway obstruction.

Clinical features The clinical progression of esophageal injury takes place in 3 stages, which correspond with the histopathologic changes. Children experience severe pain on contact with the solution, and they present with swelling of the lips, mouth and oropharynx, with drooling and refusal to drink. Retrosternal chest pain, hematemesis, or abdominal pain signifies esophageal or gastric injury. Fever, dyspnea, chest pain and subcutaneous emphysema herald the onset of mediastinitis. Other complications include peritonitis due to perforation of viscera, hemorrhage secondary to vessel erosion, aortoesophageal or tracheoesophageal fistulae, and pulmonary thrombosis.

Evaluation Chest X-ray should be done to rule out mediastinitis or esophageal perforation, and lateral view of neck to demonstrate laryngeal edema. Flexible endoscopic visualization of the upper GI tract in the first 48 hours is the cornerstone of management and is definitely indicated for any large volume ingestion, patient with severe respiratory distress, stridor, or hematemesis. In addition, presence of any two of the following symptoms—vomiting, prolonged drooling, abdominal pain, dysphagia and refusal to drink, are further indications for endoscopic evaluation.

Treatment	Corrosive Poisoning

A. Supportive Therapy
Any residual corrosive solution should immediately be removed from the patient's clothing, skin, and eyes by lavage with copious amounts of sterile saline. Emesis is contraindicated and charcoal use is ineffective, and it can induce emesis and obscure endoscopic visualization.

- *Neutralization* The process utilizes a weakly basic solution for acid ingestion, and *vice versa* for alkali ingestion, in an attempt to neutralize pH and minimize tissue damage. However, being an exothermic reaction, neutralization can exacerbate tissue injury, and its utility is limited as most damage occurs almost instantaneously after ingestion.
- *Dilution*, by administering a neutral solution such as water or milk, can minimize tissue contact and decrease transit time, without any thermal tissue damage. But clinical utility is limited to immediate use at home right after ingestion of small amounts in cooperative children only. There is a potential risk of perforation due to introduction of fluids into already injured esophageal tissue.
- *Steroids* Another controversial modality is the routine use of steroids, with the premise of reducing pathologic collagen cross-linking, shortening and cicatrization. Although children with first-degree injuries do not develop strictures, and those with third degree injury almost always progress to strictures, it is the children with second-degree injuries who have a variable outcome and have the greatest potential of benefit

from administration of methylprednisolone (2 mg/kg/day), or dexamethasone (1mg/kg/day), preferably within 24 hours of injury. Concomitant use of antibiotics is also recommended.

B. Specific Therapy
Specific therapy is recommended for hydrofluoric acid exposure, which is commonly found in cleaning, etching and rust removing products. After copious irrigation, topical application of calcium gluconate gel should be initiated, with minor burns requiring intradermal injection of 5% calcium gluconate, administered 0.5 cm to 1 cm away from the site of the burn. For severe burns, intra-arterial injection of calcium gluconate is recommended, and for oral ingestion, IV calcium and magnesium supplementation is given.

Prognosis

Esophageal stricture is the most common long-term adverse outcome. Gastric outlet obstruction and dysmotility may occur, in addition to scarring of other systems like the upper respiratory tract, face, or eyes. Longitudinal studies have shown 1000-fold increased risk of gastric and esophageal malignancies, occurring at an average of 40 years after the exposure. Children in whom endoscopy reveals significant lesions therefore need life-long surveillance.

2. Kerosene Oil Poisoning

Epidemiology The incidence of kerosene oil poisoning has declined recently, since it is not freely available now. Even then, kerosene oil is still used as fuel for cooking and lighting purposes due to shortage of cooking gas and electricity; moreover, kerosene oil is stored in soft drink and beer bottles which remain within easy reach of curious and prancing children.

Clinical features Most of the cases occur between 1 and 3 years of age. More than 70% children develop symptoms following ingestion of kerosene, with onset soon after to within 10 hours of ingestion. Respiratory symptoms occur as a result of chemical pneumonitis. Breathlessness, fever, cough, restlessness and abdominal distension are the common symptoms. Convulsions, coma, and cyanosis may occur infrequently.

Radiological changes may appear within an hour of ingestion and commonly consist of right basal infiltrates. Emphysema, pleural effusion and pneumatoceles have also been observed.

Prognosis Ingestion of more than 1 ounce of kerosene oil adversely affects the clinical and radiological profile. Severely malnourished children have extensive radiological changes and poor clinical outcome. Mortality ranges from 2–10%.

Treatment	Kerosene Oil Poisoning

The management is largely supportive and symptomatic. Gastric lavage is indicated only if the amount ingested is massive and the child is brought within 30 minutes of ingestion. Oxygen is administered for respiratory involvement. Antibiotics are given for secondary infection. Steroids have no role. Observation for at least 24 hours is essential even in an asymptomatic child.

3. Hydrocarbon Poisoning

Accidental ingestion of hydrocarbons is seen in young children, although they may be ingested by adolescents for suicidal attempts or inhaled for abuse. Viscosity, volatility and surface tension affect the type and extent of toxicity, but the main concern for these compounds is their pulmonary toxicity. Compounds with low viscosity and low surface tension (eg, mineral spirit, furniture polish, kerosene oil) have the greatest potential for causing aspiration.

There are three major classes of hydrocarbons:
- *Aliphatic* (straight chain compounds)—kerosene, gasoline, solvents, paint thinners.
- *Halogenated hydrocarbons*—carbon tetrachloride, trichloro-ethane.
- *Cyclic/aromatic compounds*—industrial solvents such as benzene, toluene, xylene.

Clinical Features

- *Lipoid pneumonia* is typically seen after high-viscosity hydrocarbon (mineral oil, liquid paraffin) ingestions, which produces more localized lung involvement with less inflammation, in contrast to low-viscosity compounds like kerosene. It can take several weeks to resolve and even after resolution of the acute insult, pulmonary dysfunction can persist for years. Systemic toxicity is not seen for volumes less than 1 to 2 mL/kg. Pulmonary edema and bacterial superinfection may occur later in the course.
- *Neurologic compromise* is frequent with aromatic hydrocarbons. Turpentine oil causes CNS depression, while halogenated and volatile hydrocarbons produce a euphoric state similar to alcohol intoxication.
- *Gastrointestinal symptoms* include nausea, vomiting, abdominal pain, and diarrhea, while chronic inhalation abuse can cause hematemesis.
- *Others* Fever is seen at presentation in 30% cases but does not initially correlate with infection and is probably of central origin. Most (75%) patients defervesce within 24 hours, but if it persists beyond 48 to 72 hours, bacterial superinfection should be considered.

Treatment	Hydrocarbon Poisoning

Asymptomatic children should be observed for 6 hours, before discharge. Symptomatic children should be admitted to the ICU and managed with supportive care, humidified oxygen, and nebulized β-agonists (for those with bronchospasm). Gastric lavage is not recommended, except for massive ingestions (exceeding 5 mL/kg) or when ingested solution contains dangerous additives such as benzene, toluene, heavy metals, camphor, pesticides, aniline or toxic compounds.

4. Household Poisoning

The household poisoning could either be a non-toxic ingestion or a toxic ingestion.
- *Non-toxic ingestion* is defined as that occurring after an individual consumes a non-edible product that usually does not produces symptoms, such as abrasives, adhesives, air fresheners, aluminium foils, antacids, baby products, cosmetics, candles, chalk, erasers, ball-point pen-ink, lipstick, and lubricants, etc.
- *Toxic ingestion* consists of consumption of either of the following: Soaps and detergents, shampoos, bleaches, disinfectants and deodorizers, acids and alkalis, boron compounds, cosmetics, nail polish remover (gamma butyrolactone), disk batteries, naphthalene moth balls, tobacco products, insecticides, pharmaceuticals, and paints.

Nearly 75% of poisoning episodes are due to ingestion of non-toxic substances which require reassurance to the children and their parents. Management of symptomatic toxic cases mostly involves supportive care and correct product identification. Once the product is identified, specific management relates to the nature of the principal chemical constituent.

5. Isoniazid (INH) Intoxication

Toxic effects of INH may be (i) directly due to the drug, ie, jaundice, SLE, arthralgia, altered sensorium, hemolysis, and hypersensitivity reactions; or (ii) due to pyridoxine depletion, manifesting as convulsions, peripheral neuropathy, demyelination, and inhibition of phenytoin metabolism. Lethal dose is >50 mg/kg. Gastric lavage is indicated. Patients are given 1 g of pyridoxine (vitamin B_6) for each gram of INH ingested. If amount of ingested INH is not known, administer 70 mg/kg of pyridoxine intravenously. The dose may be repeated if seizures recur. Use diazepam or phenobarbitone to control seizures. In severe cases with seizures not responding to treatment, hemodialysis may be necessary to save life.

6. Iron Intoxication

Ingestion of a number of tablets of ferrous sulphate may cause acute poisoning. Lethal dose is 300 mg/kg of iron. Severe vomiting and diarrhea occur. These may contain blood due to extensive gastrointestinal bleeding. The child may go into severe shock, hepatic and renal failure within a few hours or after a latent period of 1 to 2 days. Shock, coagulopathy (prothrombin index <50%), severe acidosis and acute liver failure are poor prognostic indicators.

Treatment	Iron Intoxication

Mainstay of management includes early decontamination of gut (gastric lavage/whole gut irrigation), desferrioxamine infusion, aggressive management of shock, and organ failure preferably in a PICU.

Stomach should be washed with sodium bicarbonate solution. An estimated ingestion of >60 mg/kg elemental iron, onset of symptoms, blood sugar >150 mg/dL, total leukocyte count >15,000 cu mm and serum iron concentration >500 μg/dL indicate severe toxicity and need chelation therapy with desferrioxamine IV at 15 mg/kg/hour until the serum iron is <300 μg/dL or till 24 hours after the child has stopped passing the characteristic 'vin rose' colored urine. Shock is corrected by infusion of fluids parenterally.

Appearance of "vin-rose" color urine following a dose of desferrioxamine may be helpful, but is not seen consistently after chelation therapy.

7. Lead Poisoning

Exposure to lead occurs from old lead based deteriorated house paint (in old houses) and dust and soil contaminated with lead such as from leaded gasoline, lead electrode plates from old automobile batteries, adulterated food, folk remedies, broken lead typesets scattered around old printing establishments. Food may be adulterated with colored metallic salts or the black collyrium used as *surma* may contain a proportion of black oxide of lead. Chronic lead intoxication occurs usually in children who eat non-edible substances (pica) and manifests as pain in abdomen and resistant anemia. Lead is deposited in the bones. Acute infections may mobilize lead from storage areas in bones and cause acute lead poisoning leading to acute lead encephalopathy. In these cases the child may be left with neurological sequelae.

Lead inhibits sulfhydryl enzymes and formation of heme. Heme precursors such as porphyrins accumulate in the blood and are excreted in the urine. Screening for lead intoxication is done by measuring zinc protoporphyrin or blood lead levels.

Treatment	Lead Poisoning

In symptomatic children, therapy is usually started with dimercaprol also called British anti-Lewisite (BAL) (75 mg/m^2 every 4 hourly IM). BAL may be stopped after 48 hours, while calcium disodium edetate is used for another 3 days but at a lower dosage of 50 mg/kg or 1000 mg/m^2 per 24 hours by continuous IV infusion. Maximum daily dose should not exceed 500 mg/kg. Stop BAL when blood lead level falls below 60 mg/dL. Give a second course of edetate alone if blood lead rebounds to 45–69 µg/dL. A second course of edetate in combination with BAL is recommended for rebound lead level of > 70 µg/dL. Wait for 5–7 days in between the two courses.

Aldridge MD. Acute iron poisoning: what every pediatric intensive care unit nurse should know. *Dimens Crit Care Nurs.* 2007;26:43–8.

American Academy of Pediatrics Committee on Injury, Violence, and Poison Prevention. Poison treatment in the home. American Academy of Pediatrics Committee on Injury, Violence, and Poison Prevention. *Pediatrics.* 2003;112:1182–5.

American Academy of Pediatrics. Committee on drugs. Treatment guidelines for lead exposure in children. *Pediatrics.* 1995; 96:155–60.

Baranwal AK, Singhi SC. Acute iron poisoning: management guidelines. *Indian Pediatr.* 2003;40:534–40.

Craft AW, Lawson GR, Williams H, et al. Accidental childhood poisoning with household products. *BMJ.* 1984;25:288–682.

Freudenthal W, Ralston M. Toxicity. Organophosphates. *EMedicine Journal* 2001;2:7.

Gupta P, Singh RP, Murali MV, *et al.* Kerosene oil poisoning-A childhood menace. *Indian Pediatr.* 1992;29:979–84.

Jayashree M, Singhi S, Gupta A. Predictors of outcome in children with hydrocarbon poisoning receiving intensive care. *Indian Pediatr.* 2006;43:715–9.

Lakshmi CP, Vijayahari R, Kate V, et al. A hospital based epidemiological study of corrosive alimentary injuries with particular reference to the Indian experience. *Nat Med J India.* 2013;26(1)31–6.

Lifsitz M, Shabak E, Sofer S. Carbamate and organophosphate poisoning in young children. *Pediatr Emerg Care.* 1999;15:1022–30.

Manoguerra AS, Erdman AR, Booze LL, *et al.* Iron ingestion: an evidence-based consensus guideline for out-of-hospital management. *Clin Toxicol.* 2005;43:553–70.

20.8 SNAKEBITE

Snakebite is a preventable public health hazard in tropical and subtropical countries, as snakes abound within dense vegetation and vast tracts of agricultural land. India has always been known as a land of exotic snakes. However, of the 2500–3000 species of snakes, only 500 belong to the 4 families of venomous snakes, of which only 200 species have caused death or permanent disability by biting humans.

Snakes generally do not bite unless provoked or cornered; usually as a mean of self-defense. Occasionally the bite may occur when the snake is inadvertently touched or trodden upon at night or in undergrowth. However, Asiatic kraits (*Bungarus* sp.) enter dwellings at night and bite people who are asleep. Common venomous snake species seen in India are: Cobra, Krait, Russell viper, and Saw scaled viper.

Clinical Features

Differentiating signs and symptoms due to envenoming from those due to fear and anxiety is an essential step in the management of snakebite. Since most of the suspected bites are due to non-venomous snakes, injudicious use of anti-snake venom can be avoided by proper clinical evaluation of the patients.

Cobra and Krait Bite

Neuroparalytic symptoms are characteristic of cobra and krait bites.

- Early *pre-paralytic symptoms* include repeated vomiting, contraction of the frontalis (before there is demonstrable ptosis), blurred vision, paraesthesiae especially around the mouth, hyperacusis, headache, dizziness, vertigo; and signs of autonomic nervous stimulation such as hypersalivation, congested conjunctivae and "goose-flesh."
- The earliest *paralytic symptoms* are in form of ptosis and external ophthalmoplegia, as ocular muscles are most sensitive to neuromuscular blockade. Later, the facial muscles, palate, jaws, tongue, vocal cords, neck muscles and muscles of deglutition, may become paralyzed. Intercostal muscles are affected before the limbs, diaphragm, and superficial muscles are paralyzed. Loss of consciousness and generalized convulsions may follow respiratory paralysis.

Death is usually due to respiratory paralysis, or due to upper airway obstruction caused by bulbar palsy, falling of paralyzed tongue or aspiration of vomitus.

Local symptoms are usually not prominent. Mild symptoms can be in form of local pain, burning sensation, local swelling and regional tender lymphadenopathy.

Viper Bites

Local signs and symptoms are more prominent, and consist of persistent bleeding from local site, hemorrhagic bleb/blister, ecchymotic edema, local tissue necrosis, and blood stained discharge from the wound. Local swelling may appear within 15 minutes and it spreads rapidly, sometimes involving the whole limb and adjacent trunk. There is associated pain, tenderness, and enlargement of regional lymph nodes.

Hemostatic abnormalities are characteristic. Persistent bleeding from the fang puncture wounds and from new injuries such as venepuncture sites and from old partially healed wounds may be the first clinical evidence of a bleeding diathesis. Spontaneous systemic hemorrhage is most often detected in the gingival sulci. Bleeding subsequently can occur from any site. Intracranial bleeding holds a grave prognosis.

Treatment	Snakebite

Snakebite is a medical emergency and the survival of the patient depends much on the appropriate first aid measures and immediate transportation to the nearest health facility. The first aid should be aimed at retarding systemic absorption of venom, preserve life, and prevent complications before the patient can receive medical care.

First Aid

1. *Reassurance* of the victim is essential, as most of them would certainly be terrified. It may also prevent neurogenic shock in an occasional patient due to extreme fear.
2. *Immobilization* of the bitten limb is the most important and effective first aid measure, which should be carried out in all cases of snakebite. It can be achieved using a splint or sling. If available, firm binding of the splint with a crepe bandage can be very effective. Keep the bitten limb below the victims' heart level so as to minimize blood returning to the heart and other organs of the body. Muscular contraction in the bitten limb will promote venous return and spread of venom, which should be avoided as far as possible.
3. Consider *pressure-immobilization* for bites by neurotoxic elapid snakes, including king cobra, kraits or sea snakes, to prevent life threatening respiratory paralysis. The aim is to contain the lymphatic spread of the venom. This is done by bandaging that begins 2 to 4 inches above the bite, winding around in overlapping turns and moving up towards the heart, then back down over the bite and past it towards hand or foot. The bandage is bound as tightly as for a sprained ankle, but not so tightly that the peripheral pulse (radial, posterior tibial, dorsalis pedis) is occluded or so loose that a finger cannot easily be slipped between its layers.
4. Immediate *transportation* of the patient to the nearest health clinic, dispensary or hospital where anti-snake venom is available and medical treatment can be given.
5. Since species diagnosis is critically important in the appropriate management of the patient, the snake should be taken along to hospital if it has already been killed. Snakes that appear to be dead should not be touched with the bare hands but carried in a bag or dangling across a stick. Some species (eg, *Hemachatus haemachatus*) sham death and even a severed head can inject venom by reflex action up to 1 hour.

Rejected or controversial first aid methods

Procedures that inflict further trauma or offer interference to the bite site are potentially harmful and should not be used. None of the following methods aimed at removing venom from the site of bite has received consistent support from the results of animal experiments.

1. Incision, excision, cauterization, amputation of the bitten digit as these can cause increased bleeding, secondary infection, injury to blood vessels, nerve and tendon and delayed wound healing. Moreover, all these procedures have not been proven to show benefit.
2. Suction by mouth, vacuum, or venom-ex apparatus, cooling with ice (cryotherapy) and electric shock, as it can cause tissue necrosis.
3. Instillation of chemical compounds, eg, potassium permanganate, which can potentiate local tissue necrosis.
4. The role of tourniquet, compression pads and bandages, in preventing systemic envenoming, remains controversial except for neurotoxic elapid bites. Tourniquets and other occlusive methods cause ischemia and gangrene (if applied for more than about 2 hours), damage to peripheral nerves (especially the lateral popliteal nerve), increased fibrinolytic activity, congestion, swelling, increased bleeding, increased local effects of venom and shock. It is also thought that the release of a tourniquet can lead to rapid development of life-threatening systemic envenoming.
5. Do not interfere with the bite wound as this may introduce infection, increase absorption of the venom and increase local bleeding.

Hospital Management

All patients with suspected snakebite, who are brought to the emergency, should be admitted. Rapid clinical assessment and immediate institution of appropriate treatment is the key to survival. If the snake can be diagnosed confidently as non-venomous, the patient can be discharged immediately after receiving a booster dose of tetanus toxoid. In case of suspected venomous snakebite, an IV line should be immediately secured and at least 10 vials of anti-snake venom should be procured and kept ready at hand.

After assessing the vitals of the patient, an evaluation for local or systemic signs and symptoms of envenoming should be carried out. If there are no features of envenoming, then the patient should be observed for a minimum of 24 hours before discharge. During the period of observation, the patient should be monitored hourly for ptosis, gingival bleed, local swelling, pulse rate and rhythm, respiratory rate, blood pressure, level of consciousness, and any other signs of envenoming.

Antisnake venom

The definitive therapy of snakebite is administration of anti-snake venom (ASV). In the management of snakebite, the most important clinical decision is whether or not to give anti-snake venom, for only a minority of snake-bitten patients need it, it may produce severe reactions, it is expensive and often in short supply. The ASV available in India, is a polyvalent preparation effective against the 4 common species found in India.

ASV administration criteria

ASV should not be used without evidence of systemic envenomation or severe local swelling. Signs of systemic envenomation include signs of spontaneous bleeding, ptosis, or a positive 20 minute whole blood clotting test (20 WBCT). Indications for antivenom therapy are listed in **Table 20.7**. Severe local symptoms are defined as swelling rapidly crossing a joint or involving half the bitten limb, in the absence of a tourniquet. For doing the 20 WBCT, take 2–3 mL of fresh venous blood of the victim in a clean, new and dry test tube. Leave it undisturbed for 20 minutes, and then gently tilt it. If the blood is still liquid this is evidence of coagulopathy (hypofibrinogenemia) and confirms that the biting species is Viperine. Cobras or Kraits do not cause anti-hemostatic symptoms.

The freeze dried powder is reconstituted with 10 mL saline. Antivenom infusion is administered IV at 20 mL/kg/h initially and slowed later. It can be given as:

- *Intravenous "push"* Reconstituted freeze-dried antivenom or undiluted liquid antivenom is given by slow intravenous injection (not more than 2 mL/minute).
- *Intravenous infusion* Reconstituted freeze-dried or undiluted liquid antivenom is diluted in approximately 5–10 mL of

Table 20.7 Indications for Antivenom Therapy

I. Systemic envenoming

- *Hemostatic abnormalities* Spontaneous systemic bleeding, coagulopathy or thrombocytopenia ($<100 \times 10^9$/liter)
- *Neurotoxic signs* Ptosis, external ophthalmoplegia, paralysis
- *Cardiovascular abnormalities* Hypotension, shock, cardiac arrhythmia, abnormal ECG
- *Acute renal failure* Oliguria/anuria, rising blood creatinine/urea
- *Hemoglobinuria/myoglobinuria* Dark brown urine, positive urine dipsticks, other evidence of intravascular hemolysis or generalized rhabdomyolysis (muscle aches and pains, hyperkalemia)
- Supporting laboratory evidence of systemic envenoming

II. Local envenoming

- Local swelling involving more than half of the bitten limb (in the absence of a tourniquet). Swelling after bites on the digits (toes and especially fingers)
- Rapid extension of swelling (beyond the wrist/ankle within few hours of bites on the hands/feet)
- Development of an enlarged tender lymph node draining the bitten limb

isotonic fluid per kg body weight (ie, 250–500 mL of saline or 5% dextrose) and is infused at a constant rate over a period of about 1 hour.

- Local administration of antivenom at the site of the bite is not recommended.

A starting dose of 50 mL (5 vials) of ASV is used for mild manifestations. Moderate and severe envenomation require 10 and 15 vials respectively in the initial phase.

In the past, hypersensitivity testing by intradermal or subcutaneous injections or intraconjunctival instillation of diluted anti-snake venom had been widely practiced. However, these tests delay the start of anti-snake venom treatment, are not without risk and have recently proved to have no predictive value for early (anaphylactic) or late (serum sickness type) anti-snake venom reactions. Keep adrenaline ready, lest anaphylaxis occurs.

Supportive measures in the form of neostigmine and mechanical ventilation in cobra bite and fresh frozen plasma or fresh blood transfusions in viper bite are other recommended adjunct therapy in the management of snakebite.

Adhisivam B, Mahadevan S. Snakebite envenomation in India: a rural medical emergency. *Indian Pediatr.* 2006;43:553–4.

Simpson ID. The pediatric management of snakebite the national protocol. *Indian Pediatr.* 2007;44:173–6.

Warrell DA. WHO/SEARO Guidelines for the clinical management of snake bite in the South East Asian Region. *Southeast Asian J Trop Med Public Health.* 1999;30:S 1,2.

20.9 SCORPION STING

Scorpion sting is an acute life-threatening emergency that usually occurs in the rural setting, and is known to have a mortality rate from 3–22%. Among the 86 species of scorpions in India, *Mesobuthus tamulus* and *Palamneus swammer-dami* are of medical importance and the former causes significant cardiovascular morbidity. Scorpions live in warm dry regions throughout India, especially areas with red soil and they live in crevices within dwellings, underground burrows, under logs or debris, paddy husk, sugarcane fields, coconut and banana plantations. They emerge mostly at night and most bites are in summer months, due to accidental contact.

Pathogenesis

Scorpion venoms are species-specific complex mixtures of short neurotoxic proteins (31–64 amino acid sequences), with important effects on voltage sensitive ion channels, which results in opening of sodium channel at presynaptic nerve terminals and inhibition of calcium dependant potassium channels. Stimulation of alpha receptors leads to hypertension, tachycardia, myocardial dysfunction, pulmonary edema and cold extremities. This autonomic storm is associated with other important metabolic changes such as suppression of insulin secretion, hyperglycemia, hyperkalemia, and accumulation of free fatty acids and free radicals; which is injurious to the myocardium.

Clinical Features

Systemic inflammatory response like syndrome is triggered following envenomation caused by scorpion species *Tityus serrulatus*, with increased levels of interleukin-6, IL-1α and IFN-γ in all patients. Direct neuronal toxicity leading to seizures, and DIC and microthrombi are also known to occur. Symptoms after scorpion sting progress to a maximal severity in about 5 hours and subside within a day or two.

- Features of cholinergic stimulation merge imperceptibly into those of adrenergic stimulation, with vomiting, salivation, sweating, priapism and bradycardia being the early diagnostic signs.
- Sweating and salivation persist for 6–13 hours, and increased oral secretions and bronchorrhea in the early cholinergic phase can worsen respiratory compromise.
- Pulmonary edema may develop within 30 minutes to three hours after a sting due to myocardial dysfunction.
- Central nervous system manifestations including encephalopathy, convulsions (within 1–2 hours of sting), hypertensive cerebral hemorrhage, stroke and central respiratory failure have been reported.

Treatment **Scorpion Sting**

Initial management is based on the severity of symptoms and vital signs at presentation. Pain management and adequate fluid therapy are essential supportive measures. Prazosin—a competitive postsynaptic alpha1, adrenoreceptor antagonist is the first line of management (dose 30 microgram/kg/dose), as it suppresses sympathetic outflow and activates venom-inhibited potassium channels. It decreases the preload, afterload, and blood pressure without increasing the heart rate, and counters vasoconstriction induced by endothelins through accumulation of cyclic GMP (cGMP). Prazosin should be repeated in the same dose at the end of 3 hours according to clinical response and then every 6 hours till extremities are warm, and dry and the peripheral veins are visible easily. The time lapse between the sting and administration of prazosin for symptoms of autonomic storm determines the outcome. There is no antivenom available for clinical use against the toxins of Indian scorpions.

Mahadevan S. Scorpion Sting. *Indian Pediatr*. 2000;37: 504–514.
World Health Organization. Guidelines for the Clinical management of snake bites in the South-East Asia Region. New Delhi: 2005.

20.10 DROWNING

Definition

Drowning is the process of experiencing respiratory impairment from submersion or immersion in liquid. Drowning outcomes are classified as (*i*) death, (*ii*) morbidity and (*iii*) no morbidity (2002 World Congress on Drowning).

Risk Factors

Children less than 5 years of age have the highest drowning mortality rates worldwide. Small children can drown in as little as one inch of water and are therefore at risk of drowning in wading pools, bathtubs, buckets, toilets, spas, and hot tubs. Approximately 10% of childhood drowning takes place in bathtubs, in the absence of adult supervision. Older children have drowning in swimming pools, lake or river. Infants drown when left unattended. Adolescent drowning frequently occurs in natural bodies of water and is associated with risk-taking behavior and intoxication.

Pathophysiology

Drowning typically begins with a period of panic, loss of the normal breathing pattern, breath holding, air hunger, and a struggle by the victim to stay above the water. Reflex inspiratory efforts eventually occur, leading to hypoxemia by either aspiration or reflex laryngospasm that occurs when water contacts the lower respiratory tract. Aspiration of more than 11 mL/kg of body weight must occur before blood volume changes occur, and more than 22 mL/kg before electrolyte changes take place. Since drowning victims aspirate no more than 3 to 4 mL/kg, the distinction between salt water and fresh water drowning is no longer considered important.

The major pathophysiologic changes are related to hypoxic-ischemic and reperfusion injuries. In general, there is decreased lung compliance, ventilation-perfusion mismatching and intrapulmonary shunting, leading to hypoxemia that causes diffuse organ dysfunction. Intrapulmonary shunting occurs due to a number of factors– bronchospasm, atelectasis, presence of aspirated water within alveolar space, infectious or chemical pneumonitis, and/or acute respiratory distress syndrome (ARDS). The resultant hypoxia, hypercarbia, and acidosis can decrease myocardial contractility, elevate pulmonary artery and systemic vascular resistance, and produce cardiac arrhythmias. The temperature of the water and the presence of contaminants also affect the outcome. Both salt water and fresh water wash out surfactant, and there is increased capillary endothelial permeability, which produces noncardiogenic pulmonary edema and ARDS.

Clinical Features

Survivors with drowning can be grouped into three categories depending on their severity of illness. *Category A* patients are awake and conscious. *Category B* victims are drowsy, have respiratory distress, cyanosis, and hypothermia. *Category C* patients are comatose, have central respiration and may be in decorticate, decerebrate, or flaccid state. Ultimately they have respiratory failure and apnea.

Treatment	Drowning

The net result of drowning is hypoxia, aspiration, and hypothermia. Initial resuscitation should be started immediately as described for basic life support protocol. Categories A and B patients require supportive care. Category C victims require advanced life support care. Also look for any injuries of spine or neck.

Diuretics are administered for pulmonary edema. Sodium bicarbonate may be given for metabolic acidosis. Steroids are not indicated. Convulsions are treated with diazepam and phenobarbital or phenytoin. Morphine is used for sedation in Category C patients. Supportive therapy for fluid electrolytes and control of infection is offered.

Hypothermia is managed by adequate warming. There is still controversy over what temperature range should be maintained in patients recovering from drowning. Hypothermia can reduce cerebral metabolism and therefore can possibly provide some neuroprotection from hypoxic injury, but at the same time no clear improvement in outcome has been demonstrated, and the treatment has been associated with an increased incidence of sepsis, probably secondary to cold-induced immuno-suppression. Euthermia is therefore desirable, as hyperthermia increases cerebral metabolic demands and lowers seizure threshold.

Antibiotics should be used only in cases of clinical pulmonary infection or if the victim was submerged in grossly contaminated water.

Mechanical ventilation may be needed for respiratory compromise and should be directed towards providing normocarbia and adequate oxygenation.

Prevention

Victims of drowning have a very slim chance of survival after immersion. The victim loses consciousness after approximately 2 minutes of immersion and irreversible brain damage can take place after 4–6 minutes. Therefore, prevention strategies are more important.

Prevention can be aimed at removing the hazard; drain unnecessary accumulations of water (pools, ponds, buckets). Fencing or barriers should be provided near water bodies. Children should be offered opportunity and encouraged to learn swimming. Parental education is a must to increase awareness of the need to supervise children, in proximity to water, both in and outside the home. Train the general community in resuscitation of drowning victims.

AAP Children's Health Topics: Water Safety. American Academy of Pediatrics. Available from: http://www.healthychildren.org/English/safety-prevention/at-play/Pages/Water-Safety-And-Young-Children.aspx. Accessed 1 July, 2012.

Burford AE, Ryan LM, Stone BJ, *et al*. Drowning and near-drowning in children and adolescents. *Pediatr Emerg Care*. 2005;21:612–6.

Drowning. Facts about injuries. Department of Injuries and Violence Prevention. Geneva: World Health Organization. Available from: *www.who.int/violence_injury_prevention/other-injury/drowning/en/*. Accessed 1 July, 2012.

Meyer RJ, Theodorou AA, Berg RA. Childhood drowning. *Pediatr Rev*. 2006;27:163–9.

Orlowski JP, Szpilman D. Drowning. Rescue, resuscitation, and reanimation. *Pediatr Clin North Am*. 2001;48:627–46.

van Beeck EF, Branche CM, Szpilman D, *et al*. A new definition of drowning: towards documentation and prevention of a global public health problem. *Bull WHO*; 2005;83:801–80.

20.11 BURNS

Definition

A burn occurs when some or all of the different layers of cells in the skin are destroyed by a hot liquid (scald), a hot solid (contact burns) or a flame (flame burns). Skin injuries due to ultraviolet radiation, radioactivity, electricity or chemicals, as well as respiratory damage resulting from smoke inhalation, are also considered to be burns (International Society for burn injuries).

Etiology

Fire related burns occur mainly either in the *home* or in the *workplace*. Kitchen is the most common place where children and women sustain burns. The risk factors associated with burns include cooking on open fires, explosion of pressure stoves, instability of small stoves, use of open fires to keep warm during winters and use of inflammable materials in housings and furnishings. Housing and clothing fires are the most severe events but not as frequent as scalds. Children are at risk from burns and fireworks-related injuries during festivals and celebrations.

First Aid in Burns

Application of cold water is the best first aid for burns. Stop the burning process by removing clothing. Apply cold water or allow the burned area to remain in contact with cold water for some time. In flame injuries, extinguish the flames by allowing the patient to roll on the ground or by applying a blanket, or using water or other fire extinguishing liquids. In chemical burns; remove or dilute the chemical agent by profusely irrigating with water.

Do not commence first aid before ensuring your own safety. Do not apply paste, oil, turmeric, raw cotton to the burnt area. Do not open the blisters. Do not apply any material directly to the wound as this increases the risk of infection. Avoid immediate application of topical medication.

Treatment	Burns

Estimate the burn size. The rule of nines does not apply to children less than 10 years. First degree burns are painful and erythematous without blistering. Second degree burns are characterized by blistering or a wet exudative wound. Deep second degree burns may be white and painless. Full thickness or third degree burns appear blanched and depressed and are painless.

- *Administer fluids* Establish IV line if more than 10% of skin is burnt. The total fluid need is estimated as follows: first 24 hours: $2 \, L/m^2$ of body surface area $+ 5 \, L/m^2$ of the estimated burnt surface area of the body; next 24 hours: $1.5 \, L/m^2$ of the total body surface area plus $3.5 \, L/m^2$ of the burnt surface. Alternatively, $10 \, L/m^2$ of the burnt surface may be given in first 48 hours (1/3 in 6 hours, 1/3 in 12 hours and 1/3 in 30 hours).

- *Type of fluids* To start, administer Ringer's lactate. Various types of other solutions are also recommended, eg, protein free electrolyte solutions of Ringer's lactate in 5% glucose solution $+ 12.5 \, g$ of albumin per liter of solution; OR a mixture of equal parts of Ringer's lactate solution and plasma.

- *Local care* Apply silver sulfadiazine ointment in thin layer over burns. Initial debridement should be limited to removing the loose hanging skin. Blisters are debrided only if they rupture spontaneously or become infected. Application of silver sulfadiazine should be stopped when epithelialization starts.

- *Supportive* Analgesics may be given to relieve pain. Tetanus immunoprophylaxis is given depending on the immune status of the child.

Prevention

Complications of burns include infection, airway obstruction, pneumonitis, ARDS, stress ulcers, skin contractures, heterotopic bone formation, and scarring. Primary prevention remains the best way of coping with the problem. Efforts should be directed at (*a*) improving environmental safety; and (*b*) changing the risk behavior.

Burns. Facts about injuries. Department of Injuries and Violence Prevention. Geneva: World Health Organization. Available from *www.who.int/violence_injury_prevention/other-injury/burns/en/*. Accessed 10 July 2014.

Finkelstein J. Pediatric burns. An overview. *Pediatr Clin North Am*.1992;39:1145.

Holland AJ. Pediatric burns: the forgotten trauma of childhood. *Can J Surg*. 2006;49:272–7.

Palmieri TL, Greenhalgh DG. Topical treatment of pediatric patients with burns: a practical guide. *Am J Clin Dermatol*. 2002;38:529–34.

Reed JL, Pomerantz WJ. Emergency management of pediatric burns. *Pediatr Emerg Care*. 2005;21:118–29.

20.12 SHOCK

Shock is defined as a state of circulatory dysfunction leading to inadequate cellular perfusion and tissue hypoxia. It results from inadequate blood flow and oxygen delivery to meet the metabolic demands of body tissues. Shock progresses over a continuum of severity, from a compensated to a decompen-sated state. In compensated shock, blood pressure remains normal; it is low in decompensated shock.

The effects of inadequate perfusion are reversible initially. However, prolonged oxygen deprivation leads to generalized cellular hypoxia and the disruption of critical biochemical processes, eventually resulting in cell membrane ion pump dysfunction, intracellular edema, inadequate regulation of intracellular pH, and cell death. These abnormalities are clinically manifested as end-organ damage, multi-system organ failure, and eventually death.

Pathophysiology

Shock is a progressive disorder. It usually evolutes through three stages *viz*. (*i*) compensated stage, (*ii*) uncompensated stage, and (*iii*) irreversible state **(Table 20.8)**.

Clinical parameter	Compensated	Uncompensated	Irreversible
Mental status	Agitation/confusion	Drowsiness	Unresponsive
Heart rate	Tachycardia	Marked tachycardia	Bradycardia
Respiration	Normal/mild tachypnea	Tachypnea/acidotic	Acidotic/apnea
Skin and capillary refill time	Increased with cold peripheral skin and decreased capillary return	Very slow capillary return and mottling	Cold and cyanotic
Urinary output	Adequate	Oliguria/anuria	Anuria
Blood pressure	Normal	Hypotension	Unrecordable

Table 20.8 Stages of Shock

Compensated Shock

Vital organ function (brain and heart) remain intact through sympathetic reflexes that increase systemic arterial resistance diverting blood away from non-essential tissues, constrict venous reservoir, increase systemic vascular resistance, and increase heart rate to maintain cardiac output. Primarily increasing the heart rate rather than stroke volume enhances the cardiac output in neonates and young children. In older children, it is the increased stroke volume that also augments cardiac output.

Signs of compensated shock are: Tachycardia, cool extremities, prolonged capillary refill (despite warm ambient temperature), weak peripheral pulses compared with central pulses; and normal blood pressure.

Uncompensated Shock

Compensatory mechanisms start failing. Due to tissue hypoperfusion, anaerobic metabolism sets in leading to lactic acidosis. Acidosis further depresses myocardium. There is failure of energy dependent Na^+–K^+ pump leading to hemostatic derangement and deterioration of lysosomal, mitochondrial and membrane functions. This ultimately results in abnormal capillary permeability, pooling of blood, and interstitial fluid loss. Following stasis, damaging chain reactions may be initiated in the kinin and coagulation pathways leading to bleeding tendencies. Chemical mediators that may play a role include histamine, serotonin, cytokines (tumor necrosis factor, interleukins), xanthine oxidase that generates oxygen derived free radicals, platelet activating factor (PAF), and bacterial toxins.

As compensatory mechanisms fail, signs of inadequate end-organ perfusion develop. These signs include: Hypotension; depressed mental status; decreased urine output; metabolic acidosis; tachypnea; and weak central pulses.

Irreversible shock It is characterized by severe damage to key organs like heart and brain; death occurs despite restoration of circulation. Pathophysiologically, the high-energy phosphate reserves are totally exhausted and body is said to have run out of energy.

Classification of Shock

Hypovolemic Shock

Acute hypovolemia is the most common cause of shock in pediatric practice. Diminished circulating blood volume results in decreased preload and hence decreases stroke volume and cardiac output. Intense vasoconstriction occurs as a compensatory mechanism. This coupled with hypo-

volemia, produces tissue ischemia, which impairs cellular metabolism and releases potent vasoactive mediators from injured cells *viz.* arachidonic acid metabolites, cytokines, and other vasoactive peptides. These alter myocardial contractility, vascular tone and membrane permeability.

Recovery depends on degree and rapidity with which hypovolemia develops and the patient's pre-existing status. Mortality is less than 10%, if diagnosed and treated at an early stage.

Cardiogenic Shock

Intravascular volume is normal or increased; cardiac dysfunction limits the cardiac output. As compensatory mechanisms are slowly overcome, the failing left ventricle leads to the cascade of raised left atrial pressure, increased pulmonary artery pressure, pulmonary edema, right ventricular overload, and cardiac failure.

Prognosis is generally poor in cardiogenic shock that is primarily cardiac in origin, eg, due to congenital heart disease, as compared to that occurring secondary to hypoxic ischemic injury.

Obstructive Shock

It results from inability to produce adequate cardiac output in the face of normal intravascular volume and myocardial contractility and usually indicates mechanical left ventricular outflow obstruction.

Distributive Shock

The cardiac output is characteristically high. However, the cardiac output is unevenly distributed leading to inadequate tissue perfusion in certain vascular beds. Low systemic vascular resistance results in enhanced skin blood flow and bounding peripheral pulses. Mismatch between tissue blood flow and requirement leads to relative ischemia and acidosis.

Septic shock It is a prototype of distributive shock and is usually caused by overwhelming gram negative bacteremia. It is said to be present when a patient with severe sepsis develops hypotension despite fluid administration; normotension can only be maintained with vasopressor agent support.

Dissociative Shock

It results from impaired oxygen utilization by cells despite normal perfusion. It is due to abnormal affinity of hemoglobin for oxygen preventing its release to tissues.

Various forms of pediatric shock and their etiology, and characteristics are summarized in **Table 20.9.**

Table 20.9 Classification and Description of Different Types of Shock

Type of shock	Common causes	Basic derangement	Distinctive features
1. Hypovolemic	• Diarrhea, vomiting • Hemorrhage • Renal losses • Capillary leak syndrome, ie, burns	Decreased circulating blood volume resulting in low cardiac output	Tachycardia and hypotension without signs of congestive heart failure or sepsis
2. Distributive	• Sepsis • Anaphylaxis • CNS/spinal injury • Drug intoxication	Maldistribution of regional blood flow, vasodilation, venous pooling and decreased preload. Cardiac output is high. Intravascular volume and myocardial contractility are normal	None, can present as any other form
3. Cardiogenic	• Severe congenital heart failure due to congenital or acquired heart disease • Myocarditis, cardiomyo-pathy, dysrhythmia • Following cardiac surgery • Anoxic and ischemic injuries • Metabolic derangement, ie, acidosis, hypoglycemia • Drug intoxication	Decreased myocardial contractility leading to low cardiac output. Intravascular volume is normal or increased	Gallop rhythm, raised jugular venous pressure, hepatomegaly, pulmonary edema
4. Obstructive	• Cardiac tamponade • Massive pulmonary embolus • Tension pneumothorax	Mechanical obstruction to ventricular flow leading to low cardiac output. Intravascular volume and myocardial contractility stay normal	Narrow pulse pressure, profound hypoxemia, low voltage ECG
5. Dissociative	• Methemoglobinemia • Carbon monoxide poisoning	Inappropriate release of oxygen from hemoglobin leading to poor perfusion. Cardiac output, intravascular volume and myocardial functions are intact	Signs of myocardial ischemia, chocolate colored blood, normal paO_2 but decreased saturation, elevated methemoglobin or carboxyhemoglobin

Diagnosis

Diagnosis is facilitated by a well taken history suggestive of infection, fluid loss, hemorrhage, heart disease, allergies, drug intake, trauma, previous illnesses, immune deficiency or congenital anomalies. Rapid circulatory assessment consists of evaluation of heart rate, pulse volume, capillary refill time, blood pressure, respiratory rate, skin appearance and temperature, mental status, and urinary output.

- *Cardiovascular status* Tachycardia is a compensatory mechanism. *Bradycardia* is a preterminal sign caused by hypoxia and acidosis. Low volume or *thready pulses* are an indicator of imminent decompensation. *Bounding pulses* may be observed in early septic shock.

- *Hypotension* is a late and often sudden sign of decompensated shock; if not reversed early, may lead to death. The lower limit of normal systolic pressure in children aged more than one year can be approximated by the following formula: 70 + (2 × age in years).

- *Skin changes* Mottling, pallor, cyanosis indicate poor perfusion. A core and toe temperature difference of more than 2°C is a sign of poor skin perfusion. *Slow capillary refill*

(> 3 seconds) after blanching pressure on palms/soles is an early sign of shock.

- *Mental status* Agitation and confusion alternating with *drowsiness* are the early features of ischemic brain injury. Infants may present with weak cry, hypotonia, irritability and inability to focus on parent's face.

- *Renal status* Urine output is an important parameter to monitor the progress of shock. Urine flow rate of less than 1 mL/kg/hr in children and 2 mL/kg/hr in infants suggest inadequate renal perfusion indicating prerenal failure, acute tubular necrosis or cortical necrosis.

- *Respiratory status* Acidosis due to poor tissue perfusion may lead to *deep rapid breathing*. Respiratory failure and *adult respiratory distress syndrome* (ARDS) are late manifestations of shock.

- *Hematological system* Bleeding may occur from various sites including both superficial (cutaneous) and deep (internal) hemorrhage. This suggests presence of coagulation abnormality such as *disseminated intravascular coagulation* associated with raised PT, PTTK, and thrombocytopenia.

20

• *GIT* Erosive gastritis, ischemic pancreatitis, and ischemic hepatitis indicate gastrointestinal involvement.

Laboratory Investigations

These are needed for two reasons: To ascertain the cause of shock; and to appraise the performance of different organ systems. Baseline investigations should include a complete blood count, platelet count, blood glucose, serum electrolytes, renal function tests, clotting screen, arterial blood gases and blood culture. Blood grouping should be obtained in case transfusion is needed. Estimation of blood lactate is a useful marker for assessing tissue perfusion. Examination of urine for specific gravity, albumin, sugar and cells is a must. Chest skiagram and EKG should also be obtained.

Treatment	Shock

Principles

1. Early recognition of shock state and prompt initiation of resuscitation.
2. Look for treatable cause such as cardiac tamponade, tension pneumothorax, etc.
3. Protect and support organ functions and complications.
4. Correction of any aggravating factors or deficiencies.
5. Continuous monitoring.

The management of shock in children is depicted in an algorithmic manner in Fig. 20.9. Initial management begins with assessment of the airway, breathing and circulatory status. It is important to secure the airway and ensure adequate breathing as all other interventions will fail, if adequate gas exchange and oxygen delivery cannot take place. The initial hour in the management of shock is the most crucial in determining the outcome and has therefore been called the 'Golden Hour.' Appropriate management with fluid boluses and ongoing assessment during this crucial period is of utmost importance.

A. Fluid Therapy

Administration of fluids for effective restoration of circulating volume is the key step in management of shock. The choice of fluids include crystalloids (normal saline, ringers lactate), and colloids (albumin, dextran, and blood products).

Crystalloids versus Colloids

Crystalloid solutions remain the initial fluid of choice for shock of undetermined etiology. The advantages of crystalloid include availability, low cost, and lack of exposure to blood products. These solutions contain large molecules that are relatively impermeable to the capillary membrane. This property leads to decreased extravasation and an increased percentage of the infused volume remaining intravascular. There is limited data on the superiority of colloids over crystalloids and there is not enough data for safety of colloid use in children. Therefore, use of crystalloids is recommended as the initial approach, and they should be combined with colloids in case of refractory hypovolemic shock.

Colloids are preferred in hypovolemic patients with renal, cardiac, and respiratory failure. Colloids are contraindicated in burns and severe capillary leaks. Large volumes of colloids can contribute to interstitial and pulmonary edema. Blood products are the preferred fluids in cases of trauma and hemorrhage.

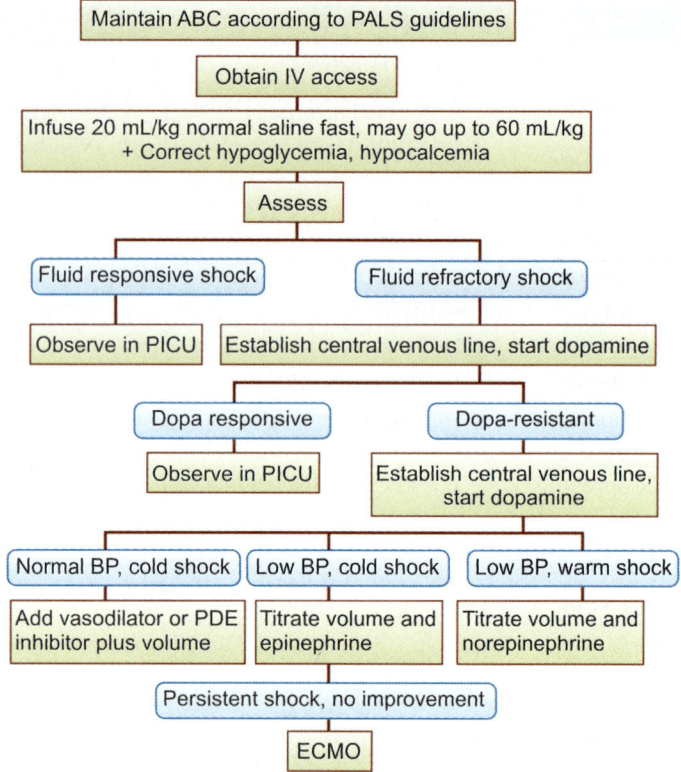

Fig. 20.9 Stepwise management of shock

Initial therapy

Initially, Ringer lactate solution or normal saline is given in a bolus of 20 mL/kg in less than 20 minutes and repeated according to response. Blood replacement therapy should begin immediately following hemorrhagic shock. A child with hypovolemic shock often requires 40–60 mL/kg during the first hour of therapy followed by reassessment of interstitial volume status and consideration of colloid for additional fluid replacement, as much as 200 mL/kg in the first few hours. Almost all patients with hypovolemic shock and one fourth of those with septic shock will respond to this management alone.

If the patient is still in shock at the end of the first hour of management, the diagnosis of fluid refractory shock is established and the patient should be started on inotropic support. The commonly used vasoactive medications and their doses are listed in **Table 20.10**.

CVP monitoring

Measurement of central venous pressure (CVP) should be carried out to decide the need for additional care. The normal CVP is to be maintained between 12 and 18 cm of water. If the CVP remains <10 cm of water, another fluid bolus of 10–20 mL/kg is administered. Dopamine infusion is started, if CVP is more than 15 cm of water. CVP between 10 and 15 cm is an indication for starting dopamine and considering dobutamine infusion. Persistent hypotension even after above measures necessitates continuous adrenaline infusion (0.1 to 2 μg/kg/min).

B. Vasopressor Therapy

Dopamine given in low dosages (1–5 μg/kg/min) acts as vasodilator to cerebral and renal beds; it is inotropic at 5–10 μg/kg/min and causes direct stimulation of β_1 receptors, thereby increasing cardiac contractility. Doses in excess of

Table 20.10 Vasoactive Medications

Agent (range)	Dose (range)	Site of action	Clinical effect
Dopamine	3–20 µg/kg/min	β, increasing α with increasing dose	Inotrope, vasoconstriction, chronotrope, increases peripheral vascular resistance (PVR)
Dobutamine	1–20 µg/kg/min	$\beta_2 > \beta_1$	Inotrope, vasodilation (beta2), decreases PVR
Epinephrine	0.01–1.0 µg/kg/min	β > α	Inotrope, chronotrope, vasoconstriction
Norepinephrine	0.01–1.0 µg/kg/min	α > β	Vasoconstriction, increases SVR, inotrope, chronotrope
Phenylephrine	0.1–0.5 µg/kg/min	α	Vasoconstriction, increases SVR
Amrinone	1–20 µg/kg/min	Type III phospho-diesterase inhibitor	Inotrope, chronotrope, vasodilator
Milrinone	0.25–1.0 µg/kg/min		
Nitroprusside	0.5–10 µg/kg/min	Vasodilator, arterial>venous	Decreases afterload
Vasopressin	0.0003–0.008 U/kg/min	V1 vascular receptor	Vasoconstriction, vasodilation of circle of Willis, stimulation of cortisol secretion

PVR—pulmonary vascular resistance, SVR—systemic vascular resistance

Case Study | Shock

A 5-year old child presented to the emergency room with history of fever, vomiting and diarrhea of two days' duration. His mother reported that he has had 15 watery stools (mixed with blood) and ongoing emesis and over the last 2 hours has become drowsier. Despite being fed oral rehydration solution by his mother with a spoon, he has not had any urine output for the past 4 hours and his extremities are pale and cool to touch. His vital signs are: Heart Rate: 160/min, Respiratory Rate: 18/min, Blood pressure: 88/54 mm Hg, oxyhemoglobin saturation: 91%. Capillary refill is >3 seconds and he is not responding to calling out his name.

Is this patient in compensated, uncompensated, or irreversible shock?
Based on his presentation with clear signs of reduced perfusion and oxygen delivery, this patient is clearly in an uncompensated stage of shock. Because of the rapid progression from compensated to uncompensated state due to his ongoing fluid losses, it is very important to start treatment promptly.

Based on the underlying etiology, what is the likely mechanism of shock?
This patient probably has a combination of septic (due to Gram-negative pathogens) and hypovolemic shock, which can be explained by the initial fever, bloody diarrhea and translocation of Gram-negative pathogens into the bloodstream, which was further complicated by the ongoing fluid losses from vomiting and diarrhea. Pediatric patients may lose a significant amount of fluids over a shorter span of time and become hypovolemic. Underlying medical conditions and concomitant sepsis can sometimes complicate the picture and require additional specific treatments. We could be dealing with *Shigella*, *Salmonella*, or *E.coli*.

Outline the initial management of this child
Initial management should be focused on rapid replacement of fluid volume by obtaining intravenous access. To improve oxygenation, additional supplemental oxygen should be initiated. Work up for sepsis and initiation of IV antibiotics should also be done as part of initial management. Close monitoring of mental status and urine output is necessary. Laboratory studies should include assessment of blood glucose and electrolytes and stool studies. If there are any concerns for this patient's inability to maintain adequate ventilation, then endotracheal intubation and mechanical ventilator support may be necessary until fluid replacement is completed.

10 µg/kg/min result in vasoconstriction due to α1 stimulation. Dobutamine is primarily an inotrope and vasodilator. Other vasoactive drugs that have been used in shock states include amrinone (inotrope), nitroprusside (vasodilator), and isoproterenol (inotrope and vasodilator).

Dopamine (10 µg/kg/min) is the preferred initial drug of choice. The infusion rate can be subsequently increased to 20 mg/kg/min. Dobutamine may be the ideal choice in patients with low output states such as congestive heart failure and cardiogenic shock. Combination of high dose dobutamine (5–20 µg/kg/min) with low dose dopamine (1–5 µg/kg/min) is also highly effective. Vasoactive drugs are tapered over 24 hours following stabilization of blood pressure and central venous pressure.

For patients in 'Warm Shock' norepinephrine may be the inotrope of choice. Vasopressin infusion is occasionally used for norepinephrine refractory patients with warm shock, as it does not use the alpha receptor and its efficacy is therefore not affected by ongoing alpha receptor down-regulation.

For patients who remain in a normotensive low cardiac output and high vascular resistance state despite epinephrine and nitrosovasodilator therapy, the use of milrinone (*if liver dysfunction is present*) or amrinone (*if renal dysfunction is present*) should be strongly considered.

C. Supportive Therapy
This includes general measures as well as specific care directed against multiple organ dysfunctions. Since oxygen delivery depends on the hemoglobin concentration, it should be

optimized and blood transfusion may be necessary. Infusion of packed red cells, fresh frozen plasma or platelets is mandatory, wherever indicated. H$_2$ antagonists are used for erosive gastritis, especially in the setting of hypovolemic shock. Mechanical ventilation is indicated for respiratory failure and ARDS. Renal complications are managed with appropriate fluids, diuretics, or dialysis. Role of steroids is not well established except in acute adrenal crisis with cardiovascular collapse.

Antibiotics should be started as soon as possible in suspected septic shock. Initial combination of a third generation cephalosporin such as ceftriaxone, and vancomycin provides a broad coverage against most Gram-positive and Gram-negative organisms.

Metabolic corrections Acidosis, hypoxia, hypoglycemia, hypocalcemia, hypokalemia, hyperkalemia, hyponatremia, etc. should be diagnosed and managed as per specific guidelines.
Newer therapies Agents directed towards blocking release/ counteracting the actions of endotoxins and cytokines have been tried. These include antitumor necrosis factor, anti-interleukin, and antiplatelet activating factors. Nitric oxide is an endogenous vasodilator that is believed to be responsible for hypotension in septic shock and causes some degree of myocardial depression. Trials are in progress using inhibitors of nitric oxide synthetase for treatment of shock. Shock refractory to all these measures may rarely require ECMO support until the underlying disease process can be controlled.

Carcillo JA, Fields AI, Task Force Committee Members. Clinical practice parameters for hemodynamic support of pediatric and neonatal patients in septic shock. *Crit Care Med*. 2002;30:1365–1378.

Cobb JP, Danner RL. Nitric oxide and septic shock. *JAMA*. 1996;275:1192–96.

McKiernan CA, Lieberman SA. Circulatory shock in children: An overview. Pedi*atr Rev*. 2005;26;451–460.

Singhi S. Management of shock. *Indian Pediatr*. 1999;36:265–88.

Tobias JD. Shock in children: the first 60 minutes. *Pediatr Ann*. 1996;25:330–8.

Social Pediatrics

21.1 INTRODUCTION TO CHILD HEALTH PROBLEMS

Child health and welfare forms the basis of development of any nation. Each year, approximately 27 million children are born in India, amounting to 20% of the total live births in the world. This makes India home to largest child population, significantly outnumbering China.

Children are now being recognized as individuals with independent rights and special needs. The overall health of children is affected by maternal health, socio-economic status, surrounding environment, and availability of health care facilities. The concept of child health care has shifted from treatment to prevention with holistic approach to take care of physical, physiological, intellectual, psychological, and social aspects to function properly for their age and sex. The emphasis is on care of 'whole child'.

A. STATUS OF CHILD SURVIVAL

Worldwide, around 6 million children are dying every year before reaching their fifth birthday (Unicef 2015); almost all (99%) of these deaths occur in low- and middle-income countries. About 27.4% of them have occurred in South-East Asia. Figure 21.1 highlights the major causes of under-5 mortality in the world. While prematurity, infection, and asphyxia together contribute to almost 85% of neonatal deaths; the major killers of children aged less than 5 years in the postneonatal age group include pneumonia, diarrhea, malaria, and measles.

About 35% of deaths in children have one or more of the three underlying risk factors: Underweight, micronutrient deficiency, and suboptimal breastfeeding. Undernutrition is the leading risk factor, causing 21% of deaths.

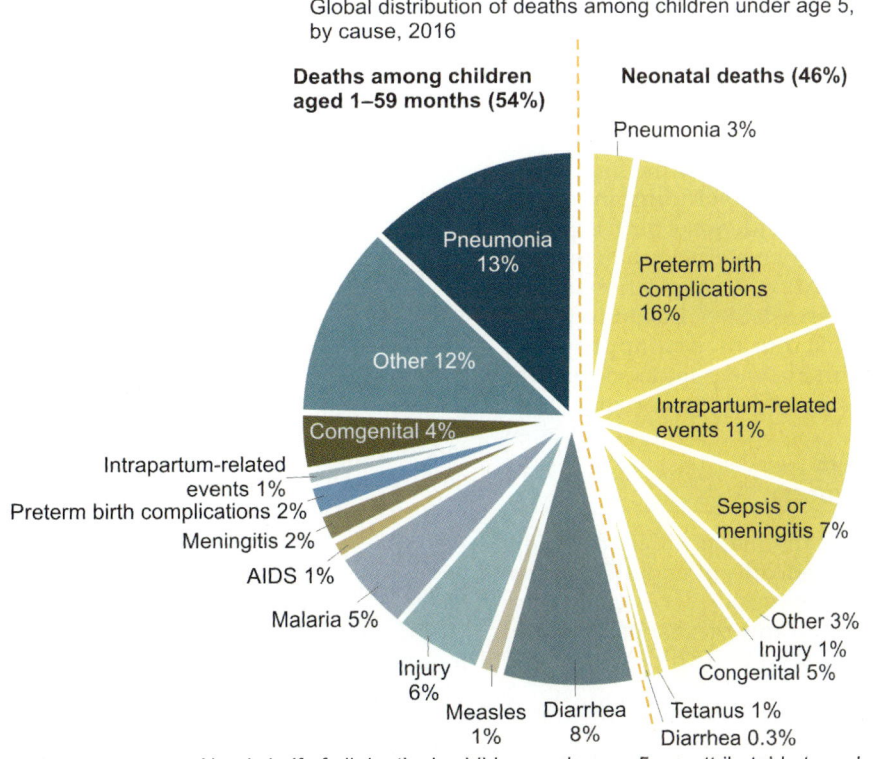

Global distribution of deaths among children under age 5, by cause, 2016

Deaths among children aged 1–59 months (54%)

Neonatal deaths (46%)

- Pneumonia 3%
- Preterm birth complications 16%
- Intrapartum-related events 11%
- Sepsis or meningitis 7%
- Other 3%
- Injury 1%
- Congenital 5%
- Tetanus 1%
- Diarrhea 0.3%

- Pneumonia 13%
- Other 12%
- Congenital 4%
- Intrapartum-related events 1%
- Preterm birth complications 2%
- Meningitis 2%
- AIDS 1%
- Malaria 5%
- Injury 6%
- Measles 1%
- Diarrhea 8%

Nearly half of all deaths in children under age 5 are attributable to undernutrition

Fig. 21.1 Causes of deaths children under-5 years. *Source:* UNICEF Report 2017. Levels and Trends in Child Mortality

B. CHILD HEALTH PROBLEMS IN THE NEONATAL PERIOD (FIRST 28 DAYS)

Around 2.6 million newborns die every year across the globe (2015 estimates), of which 0.76 are born in India. About 44% of deaths in children younger than 5 years occur within 28 days of birth—the neonatal period. Low birth weight—responsible for 35% of all newborn deaths—is the most important cause of death during first month after birth. Other important causes of neonatal mortality include birth asphyxia, sepsis, congenital anomalies, and neonatal tetanus.

1. Low Birth Weight

A newborn who weighs less than 2500 grams at birth is called a low birth weight (LBW). It is a key risk factor of adverse outcomes throughout life. As per WHO estimates, around 17 % of all newborns are LBW across the globe. In India, this figure increases to 30–35% out of which more than half are born at term. Approximately 75% of neonatal deaths and 50% of infant deaths occur in LBW newborns. LBW infants are prone to malnutrition, recurrent infections, and neurodevelopmental handicaps. They are also more likely to develop heart disease, diabetes mellitus, and stroke in later years of life.

2. Sepsis

Neonatal sepsis is the second most important cause of mortality in neonates accounting for around 27% of neonatal deaths. Neonatal infections and its associated manifestations may result in lifelong morbidities and neurodevelopmental delay, especially in preterms. It also contributes to increasing the burden of health services especially in a resource-poor setting like India.

3. Birth Asphyxia

Birth asphyxia is another important cause of neonatal deaths directly responsible for 23% of newborn deaths worldwide. Of these, 99% deaths occur in developing countries. The survivors may develop cerebral palsy with lifelong disabilities and may become a burden for the family and society. Etiology is multifactorial including maternal, uteroplacental, and fetal causes. Incidence of birth asphyxia can be lowered by improvement of maternal health in terms of managing anemia, malnutrition, and infections. Early identification and referral of high risk cases, training of health personnel in neonatal resuscitation, and appropriate transport of sick neonates can also help in decreasing the incidence of birth asphyxia and associated mortality.

C. PROBLEMS IN UNDER-FIVE CHILDREN (1 month–5 years)

Pneumonia and diarrhea are the major killers of young children contributing to 29% of deaths in under-5 children resulting in death of 2 million young lives each year. Malnutrition is the most important predisposing factor responsible for more than 50% of co-morbidities in under-5 children.

1. Pneumonia

Pneumonia is the most important cause of under-5 mortality, responsible for nearly 400,000 deaths in India, annually. Most important risk factors for pneumonia include low birth weight, malnutrition, inadequate breastfeeding, and overcrowding. Lack of appropriate treatment and timely care adds on to the disease related morbidity and mortality. Preventive measures like vaccination against diphtheria, *Streptococcus pneumoniae, H. influenzae*, pertussis and measles; exclusive breastfeeding; reduction of household air pollution, and control over overcrowding may help control the overall incidence of pneumonia in under-5 children.

2. Diarrhea

Diarrheal diseases are the second leading cause of under-5 mortality worldwide causing 11% of all childhood deaths. Most of these deaths occur in children of rural background in developing countries especially in Africa and South-Asia due to limited access to safe drinking water, sewage disposal, and unhygienic living conditions. Accessibility to safe water and food, proper sanitation and excreta disposal, hand washing, and exclusive breastfeeding can prevent most episodes of diarrhea.

3. Other Infections and Infestations

Other than pneumonia and diarrhea, the leading childhood infections include malaria, measles, diphtheria, pertussis, tuberculosis, typhoid, and dengue. HIV is emerging as another threat. Parasitic infestations including roundworm, hookworm, and giardiasis also add on to the morbidity of children. Malaria is still a main killer of under-five children, especially in Africa.

4. Malnutrition

Undernutrition is one of the most important causes of under-five mortality worldwide especially in developing countries where more than 50 million children under the age of five years are malnourished. Deficiency of macronutrients leads to protein-energy malnutrition (PEM) and severe acute malnutrition (SAM); while iron, iodine, and vitamin A are the major micronutrient deficiencies adding to the burden of undernutrition.

More than one-fourth of under-five children worldwide are underweight; and almost two-thirds of them live in Asia. Factors attributing to malnutrition include poverty, low birth weight, poor nutritional status of adolescent females and pregnant women, traditional beliefs and social taboos, and insufficient balanced diet. Undernutrition makes child more prone to infections and slows down recovery from acute illness. Mortality of severe acute malnutrition (SAM) may range from 30 to 50%. The overall prevalence of malnutrition in India was 36% in NFHS-4 (2015-2016) survey (under-five children with weight-for-age 2 Z score). There is an urgent need for stringent management strategies to decrease the related disease burden.

5. Accidental Injuries

Unintentional injuries are another important cause of morbidity and mortality among children all over the world. These include road-traffic accidents, poisonings, burns, drowning, suffocation, and falls. Most common accidental injuries in children less than 5 years include drowning and accidental poisonings. Road traffic accidents mostly affect children older than 5 years.

- Drowning is the third leading cause of unintentional death in children and youth worldwide.
- At least 5% of child drowning survivors have serious neurological damage.
- Poisoning is mostly accidental in children under 5 years of age. The common causes of poisoning in developing countries include corrosives (acids, alkalies), kerosene oil, household chemicals like insecticides, phenol, alkalis, naphthalene, and plant and plant products. In developed nations, principal causes of childhood poisoning involve pharmaceutical products and chemicals.

6. Disabilities and Handicaps

A handicapped child is the one who is not able to carry out his normal activities due to either physical, psychological, or social factors which may be the result of an impairment or disability that occurred during initial 5 years of life. Physical handicaps result from congenital defects, or acquired factors like disease or accidents and may result in blindness, paralysis, deaf mutism etc. Mental/psychological handicaps include global developmental delay and intellectual disability which may occur due to genetic causes like Down syndrome, hypothyroidism, congenital infections, and nutritional deficiencies during infancy. As per estimates, about 3% Indian children are handicapped.

Preventive measures include adequate nutrition, health education, and genetic counseling. Specific protective measures like vitamin A supplementation, immunization, and rubella vaccination can decrease the burden of handicapped children and improve the overall health infrastructure of country.

7. Child Abuse and Neglect

Child abuse is one of the major problems affecting children today. It includes not only physical but sexual, emotional abuse as well as social neglect. On an average, about 5–15 per 1000 children are abused by their family and employers. Physical and emotional abuse is more common amongst males while girls suffer from sexual abuse.

Overall preventive measures for health promotion in this transitional age group should include strengthening of primary health care infrastructure, consolidation and maintenance of immunization coverage, ensuring essential drug supply, early preschool education, and primary education facilities in underprivileged areas.

D. ADOLESCENT HEALTH

About 85% of the adolescent population resides in developing countries of South-East Asia and sub-Saharan region. Of late, many adolescent health issues have become the focus of health care providers. **Box 21.1** highlights various adolescent health problems.

To ensure holistic development of adolescent population, the Ministry of Health and Family Welfare launched *Rashtriya Kishor Swasthya Karyakram* (RKSK) on 7th January 2014 to reach out to 253 million adolescents—male and female, rural and urban, married and unmarried, in and out-of-school adolescents with special focus on marginalized and underserved groups. The objectives of RKSK are given in Fig. 21.2.

Box 21.1 Adolescent Health Issues

1. Nutritional disorders
   - Undernutrition
   - Anemia
   - Overweight and obesity
2. Infections
   - HIV/AIDS
   - STIs/STDs
3. Mental and psychiatric disorders
   - Substance abuse
   - Juvenile delinquency
   - Violence
   - Depression
   - Suicidal tendencies
4. Early marriages
5. Teenage/Unwanted pregnancies
6. Accidents/injuries

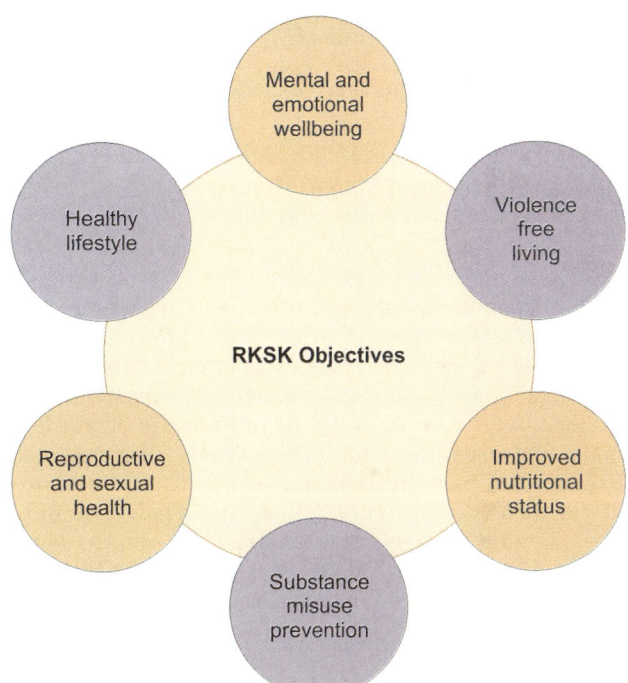

Fig. 21.2 Objectives of the Rashtriya Kishore Swasthya Karyakram. *Source:* Operational Framework: Translating strategies into programs, Rashtriya Kishore Swasthya Karyakram 2014, National Health Mission, Ministry of Health and Family Welfare, Government of India

21.2 INDICATORS OF CHILD HEALTH

Mortality indicators of child health recommended by WHO include perinatal mortality rate, neonatal mortality rate, infant mortality rate, postneonatal mortality rate, child mortality, and under-five mortality rate. Amongst these, perinatal mortality and neonatal mortality reflect the health of women and care during pregnancy and perinatal period, while infant mortality is one of the most sensitive indices of health and quality of living of a population.

21

A. UNDER-5 MORTALITY RATE

Under-5 mortality rate (U5MR) is defined as the probability of dying between birth and exactly five years of age expressed per thousand live births. This is an indicator of well-being of all children below the age of 5 years.

Over 5.9 million children under the age 5 years died in 2015, globally.

Current Status

India set a target of bringing down under five mortality to 42/1000 live birth by 2015. Under-5 mortality rate declined to 49/1000 live births in 2013 (SRS). However, NFHS-4 data (2015-2016) reported the under-5 mortality rate as 50 per 1000 live births. The trend of under-five mortality rate from 1990 to 2012 is shown in Fig. 21.3. The U5MR is higher in rural areas (56/1000) than urban areas (32/1000) at national level. Also, U5MR is higher in girls (53/1000) as compared to boys (47/1000).

Amongst the major states, the under five mortality rate was highest in Assam (73) and lowest in Kerala (12). States with under five mortality rate higher than the national level estimate in 2013 are Bihar (54), Chhattisgarh (53) and Rajasthan (57), Odisha (66), Uttar Pradesh (64), Madhya Pradesh (69) and Assam (73). Eleven states have achieved Millennium Development Goal-4 (<42 per 1000 live births) namely Andhra Pradesh, Delhi, Himachal Pradesh, Jammu & Kashmir, Karnataka, Kerala, Maharashtra, Punjab, Tamil Nadu, Telangana, and West Bengal.

Causes

Causes of deaths of under-5 children (2015) have been shown in Fig. 21.3. About 35% of deaths in children have one or more of the three underlying risk factors: Underweight, micronutrient deficiency, and inadequate breastfeeding.

Majority of the under-5 deaths in India are attributed to 4 major diseases: Respiratory infections, diarrhea, other infections and parasitic diseases, and malaria. Pneumonia and diarrhea account for 36% of all the deaths in children under-5 years of age. Most of these are deaths can be prevented by low cost preventive measures and treatment. Undernutrition is one of the major risk factors contributing to under-5 deaths.

In India, 54 million children under the age of 5 years are underweight, which constitutes to 37% of total underweight children in the world. Twenty five million under-5 children are wasted and 61 million are stunted in India which constitutes 31% and 28% of wasted and stunted in the world, respectively.

B. INFANT MORTALITY RATE (IMR)

It is the number of infant deaths in a year in relation to 1000 live births during the same period.

$$IMR = \frac{\text{Number of deaths in children less than 1 year of age in a year}}{\text{Total number of live births in a year}} \times 1000$$

The current IMR of India is 34 per thousand live births as per SRS 2017. Infant mortality is higher in girls as compared to boys. There is a wide variation in morbidity and mortality pattern of different regions in India. Madhya Pradesh and Assam have the highest infant mortality of 47 and 44, respectively. Goa has the lowest of 8 per 1,000 livebirths (SRS, 2016). Statewise IMR according to SRS, 2017 is depicted pictorially in Fig. 21.4.

Causes of Infant Deaths

Mortality is highest in the first few days of life. The causes of infant deaths in neonatal period (first 4 weeks of life) and postneonatal period (between 28 days and 365 days of life) differ significantly. In the neonatal period there are various endogenous factors attributing to high mortality. These include low birth weight, prematurity, congenital malformations, birth asphyxia, birth trauma and neonatal infections. The postneonatal mortality occurs due to exogenous factors like infections, eg, diarrhea, pneumonia, vaccine preventable diseases, faulty feeding practices, malnutrition and poor hygienic environment.

Low birth weight (birth weight <2.5 kg) is a major contributor to infant mortality. The factors causing low birth weight include maternal malnutrition, young maternal age (<18 years), high fertility rate, large family size and less spacing between pregnancies.

Prevention of Infant Deaths

Numerous strategies have been adopted by Government of India to reduce the infant and neonatal mortality in our country. Infant and child mortality rates reflect a country's quality of life and level of socio-economic development. Therefore, these can be used for monitoring and evaluating population, health programs and policies.

Preventive measures have to be aimed at improving the nutritional status of the mother, providing good and essential antenatal care, safe delivery, essential newborn care, promotion of breastfeeding, immunization, early detection of illness (achievable by growth monitoring) and their management, family planning, efficient services for reproductive and child health, provision of safe water, sanitation, improving the social and economic condition of the people and providing health education to the receptive audience.

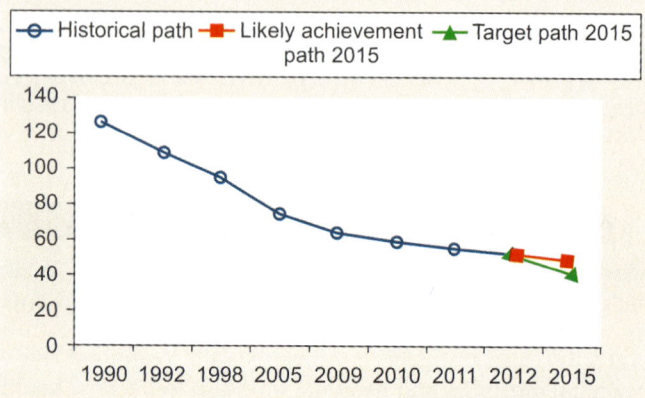

Fig. 21.3 Trend of under-five mortality rate in India. Source: SRS Report, September 2013, Registrar General of India

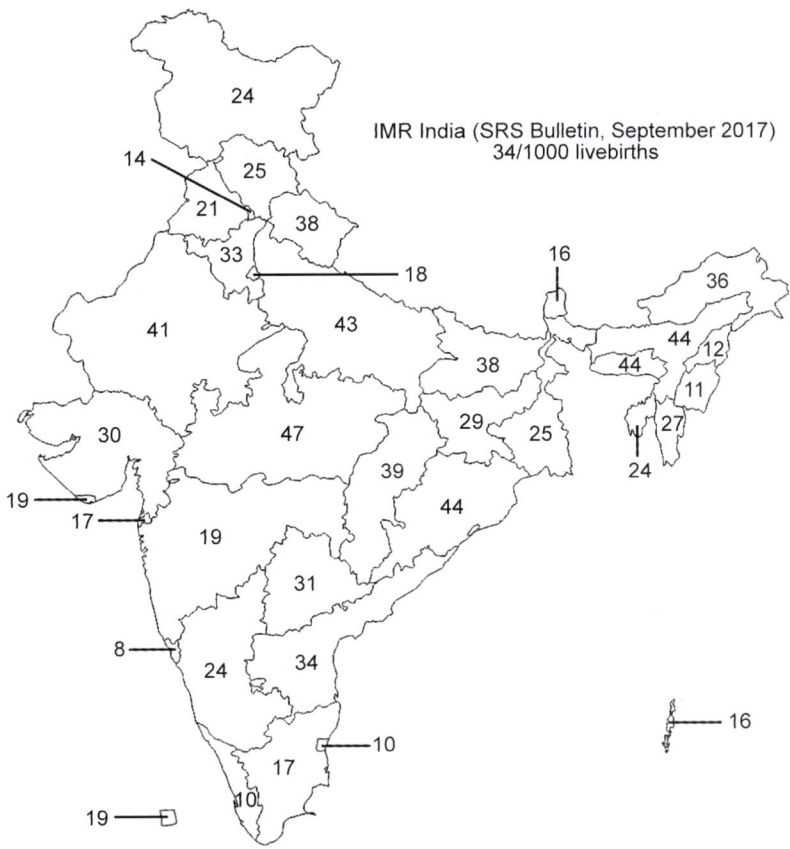

IMR India (SRS Bulletin, September 2017)
34/1000 livebirths

Fig. 21.4 Infant mortality rates in Indian States (SRS, 2017)

C. PERINATAL MORTALITY RATE (PMR)

Perinatal mortality rate refers to the number of deaths occurring in the perinatal period (includes stillbirths after 28 weeks of gestation plus the deaths occurring in the first seven days after birth) in a given year to the total number of births (live and still) in the same year. It is also expressed as rate per 1000 total births. For the purpose of inclusion in this rate, the stillbirth or live births should be either (i) >1000 g in weight, (ii) >28 weeks in gestation or if (i) and (ii) are not available, should measure 35 cm or more in length at birth.

$$PMR = \frac{\begin{array}{c}\text{Number of stillbirths + Deaths during}\\\text{the first week of life in a year}\end{array}}{\text{Total number of births in a year}} \times 1000$$

More than 5.5 million perinatal deaths occur each year worldwide; 3 million of these happen during late pregnancy and birth while 2.5 million newborn die in the first week. Africa has the highest PMR of 75 per 1000 total births. India has perinatal mortality rate of 24 per 1000 births (SRS, 2014). Perinatal mortality results from poor nutritional status of women, insufficient prevention of pregnancy related complications and few supervised deliveries. Some of these causes are rooted in the social, cultural and economic structure of the society.

D. NEONATAL MORTALITY RATE (NMR)

It is the number of neonatal deaths in relation to 1000 live births per year.

$$NMR = \frac{\begin{array}{c}\text{Number of deaths in neonates aged}\\\text{less than 28 days in a year}\end{array}}{\text{Total number of live births in a year}} \times 1000$$

Perinatal and neonatal mortality can be used as a measure of socio-economic development and for international comparisons. Of approximately 4.5 million infant deaths occurring annually, 2.6 million occur in the neonatal period; 98% of them in developing countries. Almost 65% of estimated 2.6 million neonatal deaths occur in the early neonatal period, ie, during first 7 days following birth. Thus, priority should be given to perinatal and neonatal problem in order to decrease infant mortality.

The current (2017) NMR of India is 25.6 per 1000 live births, much higher than the global average of 19 per 1000 live births. Given the current infant mortality and under-five mortality rates of 34 and 45 per 1000 live births respectively, about two-thirds of infant deaths and more than half of under-five child deaths in the country occur during the neonatal period. The NMR varies from 6 per 1000 livebirths in Kerala to 36 per 1000 livebirths in Odisha. The early neonatal mortality rate (ENMR)—deaths in the first week of life—is 20 per 1000 live births, while late NMR is 6 per 1000 livebirths. The first week of life alone accounts for 44% of total under-five child deaths. Causes of deaths in newborn have been discussed earlier in this Section.

E. STILLBIRTH RATE

It is the number of stillborn infants (after 28 weeks of gestation) related to the total number of births (live and still)

Table 21.1 Fertility, Mortality, and Other Health Indicators in India

Fertility indicators	
Crude birth rate	20.4 (SRS Statistical Report 2017)
General fertility rate	77.6 (SRS Statistical Report 2014)
Total fertility rate	2.3 (SRS Statistical Report2014)
Gross reproduction rate	1.1 (SRS Statistical Report 2014)
Natural growth rate	14.0 (SRS Bulletin2017)
Mortality indicators	
Crude death rate	6.4 (SRS 2017)
Infant mortality rate	34 (SRS 2017)
Neonatal mortality rate	26 (SRS Statistical Report 2014
Early neonatal mortality rate	20 (SRS Statistical Report 2014)
Late neonatal mortality rate	6 (SRS Statistical Report 2013)
Postneonatal mortality rate	12 (SRS Statistical Report 2013)
Perinatal mortality rate	24 (SRS Statistical Report 2014)
Stillbirth rate	4 (SRS Statistical Report 2014
Under-5 mortality rate	45 (SRS Statistical Report 2014)
Death rate for 5–15 years	0.7 (SRS Statistical Report 2014)
Maternal mortality ratio	167 (Maternal Mortality Ratio Bulletin 2013)
Life expectancy at birth	Males 67 year (2015)
	Females 70 year (2015
Immunization coverage	
BCG	91% (SOWC, UNICEF, 2016
DPT 3 doses	83% (SOWC, UNICEF, 2016)
OPV 3 doses	82% (SOWC, UNICEF, 2016)
Measles	83% (SOWC, UNICEF, 2016)
Vitamin A supplementation, full coverage (%)	61% (SOWC, UNICEF, 2016)
Nutrition indicators	
Under-5 suffering from	
Underweight (weight for age <–2 Z-score)	29% (SOWC, UNICEF, 2016
Wasting (weight for height <–2 Z-score)	15% (SOWC, UNICEF, 2016)
Stunting (height for age <–2 Z-score)	39% (SOWC, UNICEF, 2015)

Abbreviations: SRS, Sample Registration Survey; SOWC, State of the World Children Report.

Sources:

1. Maternal Mortality Ratio Bulletin 2011–13. Available at http://www.censusindia.gov.in/vital_statistics/mmr_bulletin_2011-13.pdf. Accessed on 5 August, 2017
2. Life expectancy at birth. Available at: http://www.who.int/countries/ind/en/. Accessed on 5 August, 2017
3. Govt. of India. SRS Bulletin, July 2016. Available at: http://www.censusindia.gov.in/vital_statistics/SRS_Bulletin_2014.pdf. Accessed on 5 August, 2017.
4. Govt. of India. SRS Statistical Report 2014. Available at: http://www.censusindia.gov.in/vital_statistics/SRS_Reports_2014.html. Accessed 5 August, 2017.
5. UNICEF. State of the World's Children Report 2016. Available from: https://www.unicef.org/sowc2016/. Accessed on 5 August, 2017
6. SRS Bulletin, September 2017.

during the same period. It is expressed in relation to 1000 total births.

$$= \frac{\text{Number of stillborn infants (in a year)}}{\text{Total number of births in the same year}} \times 1000$$

F. VITAL STATISTICS OF INDIA

Vital statistics are referred to a systemically collected and compiled data relating to vital events of life including birth, death, fertility, etc. These reflect the health profile of the community and form a basic tool for evaluating the adequacy of the health care delivery system.

In India, the main sources of vital statistics include the Census, registration records of vital events such as birth and deaths and Sample Registration System (SRS). Current status of various indicators related to mortality, fertility, life expectancy, family welfare program, literacy status, immunization coverage and nutrition status are summarized in **Table 21.1**.

21.3 CHILD HEALTH PROGRAMS

A. NATIONAL IMMUNIZATION PROGRAMS (EPI AND UIP)

Delivering effective and safe vaccines through an efficient delivery system is one of the most cost effective public health interventions. Immunization programs aim to reduce mortality and morbidity due to vaccine preventable diseases (VPDs).

Following the successful global eradication of smallpox in 1975 through effective vaccination programs and strengthened surveillance, the Expanded Program on Immunization (EPI) was launched in India in 1978 to control other VPDs. Initially, six diseases were selected: diphtheria, pertussis, tetanus, poliomyelitis, typhoid, and childhood tuberculosis. The aim was to cover 80% of all infants. Subsequently, the program was universalized and renamed as Universal Immunization Program (UIP) in 1985. Measles vaccine was included in the program and typhoid vaccine was discontinued.

The UIP envisaged achieving and sustaining universal immunization coverage in infants with three doses of DPT and OPV and one dose each of measles vaccine and BCG, and, in pregnant women, with two primary doses or one booster dose of TT. The UIP also required a reliable cold chain system for storing and transporting vaccines, and attaining self-sufficiency in the production of all required vaccines.

In 1992, the UIP became a part of the Child Survival and Safe Motherhood Program (CSSM), and in 1997, it became an important component of the Reproductive and Child Health Program (RCH). It continues to be an integral component of RMNCH+A strategy (launched 2013). The cold-chain system has been strengthened and training programs conducted extensively throughout the country. Intensified polio eradication activities were started in 1995-96 under the Polio Eradication Program, beginning with National Immunization Days (NIDs) and active surveillance for acute flaccid paralysis (AFP). The Polio Eradication Program was set up with the assistance of the National Polio Surveillance Project of WHO.

B. PROMOTION OF ORAL REHYDRATION THERAPY (ORT)

Diarrhea and the resultant dehydration still remain one of the leading causes of death among under-five children in India. Correct and timely use of oral rehydration therapy (ORT) can prevent a very large proportion of deaths due to diarrhea. Low-osmolarity ORS packets are available at all the public health facilities including PHCs and subcenters. ORS packets are being supplied as part of subcenter kits. Additionally, zinc supplementation is recommended to all children with acute diarrhea (to be given for 14 days).

C. IRON PROPHYLAXIS

Iron deficiency anemia is widely prevalent among young children. The National Family Health Survey-3 (NFHS-3, 2004-05) showed that nearly 3/4th children under the age of three years were anemic. Under the national program, Iron Folic Acid (IFA) tablets containing 20 mg of elemental iron and 0.1mg of folic acid are provided at the subcenter level. Current guidelines instruct the health worker to provide 100 tablets to clinically anemic children. Details of iron supplementation program are provided in the chapter on Nutrition.

D. VITAMIN A PROPHYLAXIS

Vitamin A deficiency, widely prevalent in preschool children, can lead to (nutritional) blindness. The national program seeks to administer five doses of vitamin A to all children under 3 years of age. The first dose (1 lakh units) is given at 9 months of age with measles vaccine. The second dose (2 lakh units) is given along with DPT/OPV booster. Subsequently, three doses are given (2 lakh units each) at six monthly intervals.

E. ARI CONTROL PROGRAM

Pneumonia is a leading cause of death of infants and young children in India accounting for about 20% of all under-five deaths. The ARI control strategy was developed in 1989. The health workers are being imparted training in practical skills in ARI management. Communication messages, a focus on recognition of symptoms and referral, are channeled through 'mother' meetings, interpersonal communication of female health workers and other units such as ICDS.

F. JANANI SHISHU SURAKSHA KARYAKRAM (JSSK)

This program was launched by Government of India in June 2011 to address the high neonatal mortality. The initiative entitles free delivery services including cesarean section to all pregnant women in public health institutions. All the expenses related to delivery in a public institution are borne by the government. A pregnant woman is entitled to free transportation from home to the government hospital. The woman is entitled to free medications, diagnostics, consumables, and free diet during her hospital stay, expected to be 3 days in case of normal delivery and 7 days in case of cesarean section. This program also entitles sick newborns accessing government hospitals for health care for 30 days after birth. There are also entitled to free treatment and free transportation in case if referrals. The entitlements given to pregnant woman and sick newborn are illustrated in **Box 21.2**.

Box 21.2 Entitlements given to Pregnant Women and Sick Newborn under *Janani Shishu Suraksha Karyakram* (JSSK)

A. *Entitlements given to pregnant women*
- Free and zero expense delivery and cesarean section
- Free drugs and consumables
- Free essential diagnostics (blood tests, urine tests, ultrasonography, etc.)
- Free diet during stay during health institutions (up to 3 days in case of normal delivery and 7 days in cesarean section)
- Free transport from home to health institution
- Free provision of blood
- Free transport between facilities in case of referrals
- Drop back from institution to home after 48 hours if stay
- Exemption from all kinds of user charges

B. *Entitlements to sick newborns*
- Free and expense free treatment
- Free drugs and consumables
- Free diagnostics
- Free provision of blood
- Free transport from home to health institution
- Free transport between facilities in referrals
- Drop back from institutions to home
- Exemption from all kinds of user charges

21

21.4 REPRODUCTIVE, MATERNAL, NEWBORN, CHILD, AND ADOLESCENT HEALTH (RMNCH+A) PROGRAM

Reproductive, maternal, and child health cannot be addressed in isolation as these are closely linked to the health status of the population. The health of an adolescent girl impacts pregnancy while the health of a pregnant woman impacts the health of the newborn and the child. Therefore,

Box 21.3 Priority Interventions Directed Toward Newborn and Child Care under RMNCH+A Program

1. Home-based newborn care and prompt referral
2. Facility-based care of sick newborns
3. Integrated management of common childhood illnesses (diarrhea, pneumonia, malaria)
4. Child nutrition and essential micronutrients supplementation
5. Immunization
6. Early identification and management of defects at birth, disease, deficiency and disability in children (1–18 years)

interventions are directed at various stages of life cycle, which should be mutually linked.

RMNCH+A strategy was launched for providing a comprehensive approach to improve child survival and safe motherhood, by targeting all the stakeholders in an integrated manner, under National Health Mission (Fig. 21.5). The priority interventions directed towards newborn and child care are depicted in **Box 21.3**.

A. HOME-BASED NEWBORN CARE AND PROMPT REFERRAL

At the national level, neonatal mortality accounts for almost 60% of the under-five mortality, most of which occurs in the first week of life. There is evidence that by providing home visits of community health workers in limited facility based areas to provide neonatal care, significantly reduces the neonatal mortality.

The home-based newborn care scheme, launched in 2011, provides for immediate postnatal care (especially in the cases of home delivery) and essential newborn care to all newborns up to the age of 42 days. Accredited social health activists

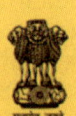
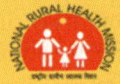

5 X 5 Matrix for High Impact RMNCH+A Interventions
To be Implemented with High Coverage and High Quality

Reproductive Health	**M**aternal Health	**N**ewborn Health	**C**hild Health	**A**dolescent Health
• Focus on spacing methods, particularly PPIUCD at high case load facilities • Focus on interval IUCD at all facilities including subcentres on fixed days • Home delivery of Contraceptives (HDC) and Ensuring Spacing at Birth (ESB) through ASHAs • Ensuring access to Pregnancy Testing Kits (PTK-"Nischay Kits") and strengthening comprehensive abortion care services • Maintaining quality sterilization services	• Use MCTS to ensure early registration of pregnancy and full ANC • Detect high risk pregnancies and line list including severely anemic mothers and ensure appropriate management • Equip Delivery points with highly trained HR and ensure equitable access to EmOC services through FRUs; Add MCH wings as per need • Review maternal, infant and child deaths for corrective actions • Identify villages with low institutional delivery and distribute Misoprostol to select women during pregnancy; incentivize ANMs for domiciliary deliveries	• Early initiation and exclusive breastfeeding • Home based newborn care through ASHA • Essential Newborn Care and resuscitation services at all delivery points • Special Newborn Care Units with highly trained human resource and other infrastructure • Community level use of Gentamicin by ANM	• Complementary feeding, IFA supplementation and focus on nutrition • Diarrhoea management at community level using ORS and Zinc • Management of pneumonia • Full immunization coverage • Rashtriya Bal Swasthya Karyakram (RBSK): screening of children for 4Ds (birth defects, development delays, deficiencies and disease) and its management	• Address teenage pregnancy and increase contraceptive prevalence in adolescents • Introduce community-based services through peer educators • Strengthen ARSH clinics • Roll out National Iron Plus Initiative including weekly IFA supplementation • Promote Menstrual Hygiene

Health Systems Strengthening
- Case load based deployment of HR at all levels
- Ambulances, drugs, diagnostics, reproductive health commodities
- Health Education, Demand Promotion & Behavior Change Communication
- Supportive supervision and use of data for monitoring and review, including scorecards based on HMIS
- Public grievances redressal mechanism; client satisfaction and patient safety through all round quality assurance

Cross-cutting Interventions
- Bring down out of pocket expenses by ensuring JSSK, RBSK and other free entitlements
- ANMs & Nurses to provide specialized and quality care to pregnant women and children
- Address social determinants of health through convergence
- Focus on un-served and underserved villages, urban slums and blocks
- Introduce difficult area and performance based incentives

Fig. 21.5 RMNCH+A 5 × 5 Matrix. *Source:* A strategic approach to reproductive, maternal, newborn, child and adolescent health in India. Ministry of Health and Family Welfare, Government of India, January 2013.

(ASHA) are trained and given incentive to provide special care to preterm and newborns; they are also trained in identification of illnesses, appropriate care, and referral through home visits.

B. FACILITY-BASED CARE OF SICK NEWBORNS

Special newborn care units (SNCU) have been established at district hospitals and tertiary care hospitals in order to strengthen care of low birth weight babies and sick newborns. Another smaller unit known as the Newborn Stabilization Unit (NBSU), which is a four-bedded unit providing basic level of sick newborn care, is being established at community health centers/first referral units. Provision of newborn care at these units increases the chances of survival for babies with health conditions requiring observation and stabilization. As part of the Janani Shishu Suraksha Karyakram, all newborns requiring facility-based newborn care up to 30 days receive diagnostics, drugs, and referral transport free of charge at these newborn care facilities.

Sick newborns discharged from health facilities should be followed up for developmental screening and early intervention. During these follow ups, counseling on exclusive breastfeeding, complementary feeding, monitoring of survival, growth monitoring, and screening for neurodevelopmental disorders (such as visual, hearing) must be included.

C. INTEGRATED MANAGEMENT OF COMMON CHILDHOOD ILLNESSES (DIARRHEA, PNEUMONIA, MALARIA)

Integrated Management of Childhood and Neonatal Illness (IMNCI) is an integrated strategy for both preventive and curative interventions adopted to address the most common causes of neonatal and child deaths in India. This is provided at all levels of care: At community (ASHA package), first level care (IMNCI) and referral level care (F-IMNCI). The strategy encompasses a range of interventions to prevent and manage the commonest major childhood illnesses which cause death. Details are provided in the next section.

D. CHILD NUTRITION AND ESSENTIAL MICRONUTRIENTS SUPPLEMENTATION

To reduce the prevalence of anemia among children, all children between the ages of 6 months to 5 years must receive iron and folic acid tablets or syrup (IFA) (as appropriate) for 100 days in a year as prevention. It is recommended to provide bi-weekly iron and folic acid supplementation for preschool children of 6 months to 5 years as part of the National Iron + initiative. ASHAs are given incentives to make home visits and to provide at least one dose per week under direct observation and educate the mothers about benefits of iron supplements and also how to administer it.

There is a provision for (*a*) weekly supplementation of iron and folic acid for children from 1st to 5th grades in government and government-aided schools; and (*b*) weekly supplementation for 'out of school' children (6–10 years) at anganwadi centers. Deworming (using albendazole syrup or tablet in single dose) is carried out every 6 months to reduce the intestinal parasite load.

Children between nine months to five years are also given six monthly doses of vitamin A. A child must receive nine doses of vitamin A by the 5th birthday.

The program also provides care to children with severe acute malnutrition (SAM) and this is mainly through facility-based care. Nutritional rehabilitation centers (NRCs) have been established for providing medical and nutritional care for children with SAM. The NRCs should be linked to community-based programs and to the Integrated Child Development Scheme (ICDS) for identification and referral of severely undernourished children.

E. IMMUNIZATION

Universal Immunization Program includes vaccines to prevent seven vaccine preventable diseases (tuberculosis, polio, diphtheria, pertussis, tetanus, measles, hepatitis B). Japanese encephalitis vaccine (JE vaccine) has been introduced in endemic districts in a campaign mode and also incorporated into the routine immunization program. The second dose of measles has been introduced and hepatitis B vaccine is now available in the entire country. Pentavalent vaccine, a combination vaccine (DPT + Hep-B + Hib) first introduced in two states (Kerala and Tamil Nadu), is now being expanded to cover the entire country. To strengthen routine immunization, newer initiatives include provision for autodisable (AD) syringes to ensure injection safety, support for alternate vaccine delivery from PHC to sub-centers as well as outreach sessions and mobilization of children to immunization session sites by ASHA.

F. CHILD HEALTH SCREENING AND EARLY INTERVENTION SERVICES

Rashtriya Bal Swasthya Karyakram (RBSK) is a new initiative aiming at early identification and early intervention to detect **4Ds** in children from birth to 18 years of age. These include **D**efects at birth, **D**eficiencies, **D**iseases, and **D**evelopmental delays including disabilities. Children 0–6 years age group will be specifically managed at District Early Intervention Center (DEIC) level while for 6–18 years age group, management of conditions will be done through existing public health facilities. DEIC will act as referral linkages for both the age groups.

Mechanisms for Screening at Community and Facility Level

Screening of children in RBSK is at two levels, community level and facility level. While facility-based newborn screening at PHC/CHC/DH, will be by the existing health manpower like Medical Officers, Staff Nurses and ANMs, the community level screening will be conducted by the mobile health teams at Anganwadi Centers and Government and Government aided Schools.

21.5 INTEGRATED MANAGEMENT OF CHILDHOOD AND NEONATAL ILLNESS (IMNCI)

Infant and childhood mortality are sensitive indicators of inequity and poverty. Surveys reveal that many sick children are not properly assessed and treated by these health providers, and that their parents are poorly advised. At first-level health facilities in low-income countries, diagnostic supports such as radiology and laboratory services are minimal or non-existent, and drugs and equipment are often scarce. Limited supplies and equipment, combined with an irregular flow of patients, leave doctors at this level with few opportunities to practise complicated clinical procedures. Instead, they often rely on history and signs and symptoms to determine a course of management that makes the best use of available resources.

Providing quality care to sick children in these conditions is a serious challenge. Yet how can this situation be reversed? Experience and scientific evidence show that improvements in child health are not necessarily dependent on the use of sophisticated and expensive technologies, but rather on effective strategies that are based on a holistic approach, are available to the majority of those in need, and which take into account the capacity and structure of health systems, as well as traditions and beliefs in the community.

Need for Integrated Approach

Many well-known prevention and treatment strategies have already proven effective for saving young lives. Childhood vaccinations have successfully reduced deaths due to measles. Oral rehydration therapy has contributed to a major reduction in diarrhea deaths. Effective antibiotics have saved millions of children with pneumonia. Prompt treatment of malaria has allowed more children to recover and lead healthy lives. Even modest improvements in breastfeeding practices have reduced childhood deaths.

While each of these interventions has shown great success, accumulating evidence suggests that a more integrated approach to managing sick children is needed to achieve better outcomes. Child health programs need to move beyond single diseases to addressing the overall health and well-being of the child. Because many children present with overlapping signs and symptoms of diseases, a single diagnosis can be difficult, and may not be feasible or appropriate. This is especially true for first-level health facilities where examinations involve few instruments, little or no laboratory tests, and no X-ray.

Integrated Management of Childhood Illness (IMCI) strategy, developed by World Health Organization in collaboration with UNICEF and many other agencies in mid-1990s, is a curative, preventive, and promotive strategy aimed at (i) reducing the death and frequency and severity of illness and disability, and (ii) contributing to improved growth and nutrition of under-five children. This strategy has been expanded in India to include neonatal care at home as well as in the health facilities and renamed as 'Integrated Management of Neonatal and Childhood Illness (IMNCI).'

IMNCI: Evidence-based Syndromic Approach

The IMNCI clinical guidelines target children less than 5 years old, the age group that bears the highest burden of deaths. The guidelines represent an evidence-based, syndromic approach to case management that supports the rational, effective and affordable use of drugs and diagnostic tools. In situations where laboratory support and clinical resources are limited, the syndromic approach is a more realistic and cost-effective way to manage patients. Careful

and systematic assessment of common symptoms, using well-selected reliable clinical signs, helps to guide rational and effective actions. An evidence-based syndromic approach can be used to determine: (a) Health problems the child may have; (b) severity of the child's illness; and (c) actions that can be taken to care for the child (eg, refer the child immediately, manage with available resources, or manage at home).

Principles of Integrated Care

Depending on a child's age, various clinical signs and symptoms differ in their degree of reliability and diagnostic value and importance. IMNCI clinical guidelines focus on neonates, infants as well as children up to 5 years of age. However, in view of similarities in the spectrum of illnesses, clinical signs and management protocols, the treatment guidelines have been broadly described under two age categories, ie, (i) young infants age up to 2 months, and (ii) children age 2 months up to 5 years.

The IMNCI guidelines are based on the following principles:
- All sick children under 5 years of age must be examined for conditions which indicate immediate referral or hospitalization.
- Children must be routinely assessed for major symptoms, nutritional and immunization status, feeding problems and other potential problems.
- Only a limited number of carefully selected clinical signs are used based on evidence of their sensitivity and specificity to detect disease.
- Based on the presence of selected clinical signs, the child is placed in a 'Classification'. Making a precise diagnosis is unnecessary.
- Classifications are color coded and suggest referral (pink), treatment in health facility (yellow), or management at home (green).
- IMNCI guidelines address most common, but not all pediatric problems.
- A limited number of essential drugs are used.
- Caretakers are actively involved in the treatment of children.
- Counseling of caretakers about home care including feeding, fluids and when to return to health facility, is an essential component of IMNCI strategy.

IMNCI Case Management Process

Depending on a child's age, various clinical signs and symptoms have different degrees of reliability and diagnostic value and importance. Therefore, the IMCI guidelines recommend case management procedures based on two age categories:
- Children age 2 months up to 5 years
- Young infants age 1 week up to 2 months

The case management of a sick child brought to a first-level health facility includes 4 important elements, listed below:
1. Assess the young infant/ child
2. Classify the illness, and Identify treatment
3. Referral, treatment or counseling of the child's caretaker (depending on the classification(s) identified);
4. Follow-up care.

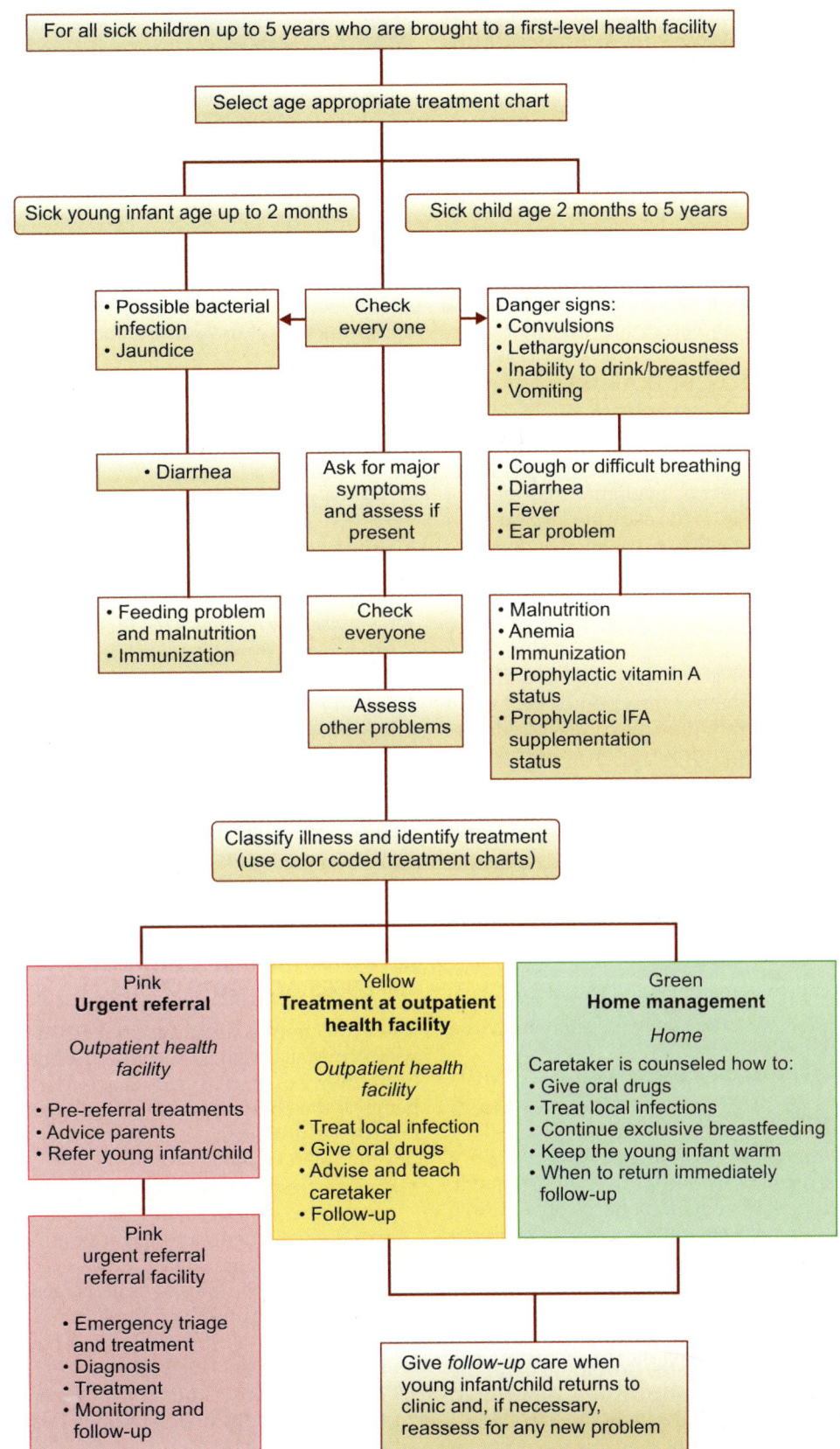

Fig. 21.6 IMNCI case management process

A summary of this case management process is pictorially depicted in Fig. 21.6.

Detailed descriptions are available in the IMNCI Chart booklet table (*see* Annexures).

21

21.6 CHILD ABUSE AND NEGLECT (CAN)

Child abuse is a state of physical, emotional and sexual ill treatment, neglect or negligent behavior that a child below the age of 18 years is subjected to in the society causing harm to the survival, health and development of the child.

According to World Health Organization, child abuse is most prevalent in children aged 0-4 years. An estimated 40 million children suffering from child neglect and abuse require social and health care. In 2005 National Crime Report Bureau, India reported 14,975 crime cases against children. These included child marriage and, genital mutilation in the name of traditional practices and economic exploitation.

A. DEFINITIONS RELATED TO CHILD ABUSE

1. Child Abuse or Maltreatment

It constitutes all forms of physical and/or emotional ill-treatment, sexual abuse, neglect or negligent treatment or commercial or other exploitation, resulting in actual or potential harm to the child's health, survival, development or dignity in the context of a relationship of responsibility, trust or power.

2. Physical Abuse

Physical abuse of a child is that which results in actual or potential physical harm from an interaction or lack of an interaction, which is reasonably within the control of a parent or person in a position of responsibility, power or trust.

3. Sexual Abuse

Child sexual abuse is the involvement of a child in sexual activity that he or she does not fully comprehend, is unable to give informed consent to, or for which the child is not developmentally prepared and cannot give consent, or that violate the laws or social taboos of society. This may include but is not limited to:

- Engagement of a child to engage in any unlawful sexual activity;
- Use of child in prostitution; and
- Use of children in pornographic materials.

4. Emotional Abuse

Emotional abuse includes the failure to provide a developmentally appropriate and supportive environment. Acts include restriction of movement, patterns of belittling, denigrating, scapegoating, threatening, scaring, discriminating, ridiculing, or other non-physical forms of hostile or rejecting treatment.

5. Neglect and Negligent Treatment

Neglect is the failure to provide for the development of the child in all spheres: Health, education, emotional development, nutrition, shelter and safe living conditions, in the context of resources reasonably available to the family or caretakers. It carries a high probability of causing harm to the child's physical, mental, spiritual, moral, or social development.

Child abuse can cause physical, emotional, and behavioral manifestations secondary to the abuse. This significantly

---

> **Box 21.4** Health Consequences of Child Abuse
>
> 1. *Physical consequences* Bruises/welts, fractures, scalds/burns, laceration, ocular injuries, poisoning, asphyxia
> 2. *Sexual consequences* STD, HIV/AIDS, unwanted pregnancy
> 3. *Emotional/Behavioral consequences* Hyperactivity, depression, poor school performance, somatic disorders, poor self esteem, eating disorders, drug/alcohol abuse
> 4. *Long term consequences* Depression, eating disorders, sleep disorders, developmental effects, risk taking behavior, self-destructive behavior, violent behavior, disability, infertility
> 5. *Fatal consequences* HIV/AIDS, infanticide, homicide, suicide

Source: Report of the Consultation on Child Abuse Prevention, WHO

increases the suffering and decreases the quality of life not only of the child but also their families. The health consequences of child abuse are listed in **Box 21.4**.

B. PREVENTION OF CHILD ABUSE

- *Primary prevention* It attempts to stop occurrence of abuse at the community level by educating the population about good parenting.
- *Secondary prevention* This includes targeting of high risk groups, eg, providing good parenting education to young parents who were abused in their childhood.
- *Tertiary prevention* This consists of providing protection to children who have undergone abuse and therapeutic care to parents who abuse their children.

It is seen that the benefits are more significantly apparent with success of primary and secondary prevention as the children are protected from being harmed in the first place. Preventive programs based on primary, secondary and tertiary preventive services have to be adapted at the community level to ensure full continuum of services.

C. PROTECTION OF CHILDREN FROM SEXUAL OFFENSES ACT, 2012 (POCSO)

The Protection of Children from Sexual Offenses Act, 2012 was formulated against sexual abuse and sexual exploitation of children less than 18 years of age. The Act regards the well-being of the child of paramount importance and ensures a healthy emotional, physical, social, and intellectual development of a child.

- It classifies sexual abuse into different categories as penetrative sexual assault, non-penetrative sexual assault, sexual harassment, and pornography. It deems a sexual assault to be "aggravated" under certain circumstances, such as when the abused child is mentally ill or when the abuse is committed by a person in a position of trust or authority *vis-à-vis* the child, like a family member, police officer, teacher, or doctor.
- People who traffic children for sexual purposes are also punishable under the provisions relating to abetment in the Act.
- The Act prescribes stringent punishment graded as per the gravity of the offence, with a maximum term of rigorous imprisonment for life, and fine.
- Under the Act, it is mandatory to report any sexual offense against children.

21.7 CHILD LABOR

Child labor is defined as work for which the child is too young, ie, work done below the required minimum age.

Data from UNICEF, World Bank and International Labor Organization (ILO) indicate that 168 million children between the age group of 5 and 18 years are subjected to child labor. Around 120 million of those are under the age of 14 years and around 30 million children in this age group specially girls, are forced to do unpaid household work in their own families.

Children under the age of 14 years are often forced to work for more than 18 hours. They are subjected to malnutrition, impaired vision, sitting for long hours in overcrowded places predisposing them to respiratory illnesses, tuberculosis and malignancies. Other extreme forms of prevalent child labor include forced and bonded labor, child soldiering, sexual exploitation and drug trafficking.

A. CHILD LABOR IN INDIA

According to NFHS-3 (2005-2006), nearly 12% children in the age group of 5–14 years work either for their own household or somebody else. Girls are more likely than boys to be doing chores and boys are more likely than girls to be working for someone other than family. Rural children are more likely to be engaged in household work as compared to urban children.

The major hazardous occupations engaging children in child labor are pan, bidi and cigarettes (21%), construction (17%), domestic workers (15%), and spinning and weaving (11%). The occupation wise distribution of children as per Census 2001 is given in Fig. 21.7.

B. NATIONAL POLICY ON CHILD LABOR

The Child Labor (Prohibition and Regulation) Act, 1986 prohibits employment of children below the age of 14 years. The State Government has the powers for enforcement of the provisions of the Act. The Union of India monitors the enforcement from time-to-time. Special drives on enforcement and awareness generation are also launched from time-to-time. During inspections and raids conducted under CLPRA, child labor are identified, rescued and rehabilitative measures are set forth in providing bridge education apart from vocational training with ultimate objective of mainstreaming them into the formal system of education.

21.8 STREET CHILDREN

Street children are commonly seen in all major urban cities of our country. Presence of children on streets reflects the lack of rehabilitation efforts as compared to the increasing magnitude of street population. It also indicates the magnitude of denial of basic rights of children.

A. CHILDREN *ON* AND *OF* STREET

According to UNICEF, street children are of several types:
  i. *Children on street* These children keep ties with their families, they return home at night and some of them attend school as well; a small number of them have actually left home and largely work on the streets. These live at home on urban areas or in the suburbs and contribute to the household economy through their engagement on the roadside activities such as eateries, workshops, and vending.
 ii. *Children of street* These children do not have functional family ties. These children are largely refugees, runaways, and displaced children and belong to the abandoned or neglected category.

B. MAGNITUDE OF THE PROBLEM

According to UNICEF and World Health Organization, the estimated number of street children is about 100 to 150 million in the world. UNICEF estimated that there are about 44 million working children in India, out of which 11 million are street children. Majority of children are in the age group between 11 and 15 years but a large percentage also belong to 6–10 years of age. Boys are more common than girls.

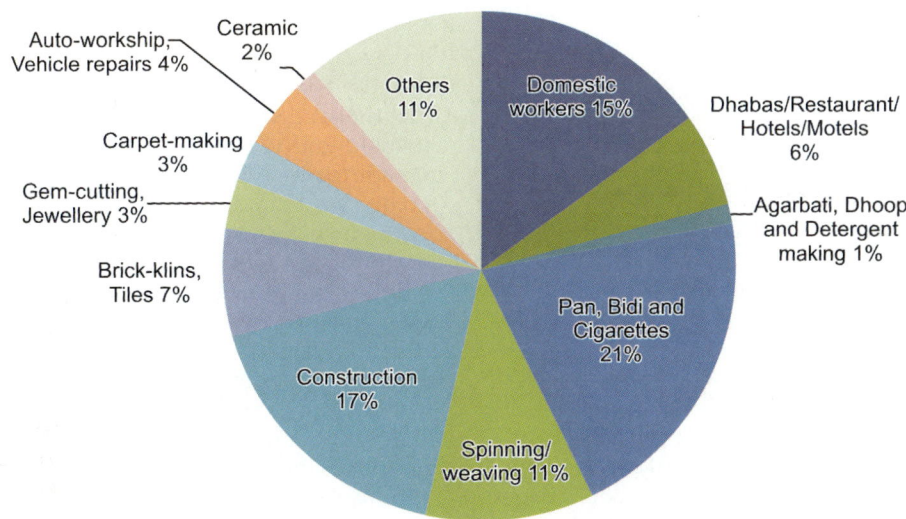

Fig. 21.7 Occupation wise distribution of child labor in India. *Source:* Census 2001

The most common causes attributing to it are poverty, rapid economic growth, urbanization, domestic violence, and breakdown of families.

C. IMPLICATIONS OF LIVING ON THE STREETS

- Street children are always exposed to violence, and live in difficulty health conditions, living and working conditions and have poor safety and security issues; therefore they are labeled as the "high risk" category.
- Street children are devoid of any emotional support, personal care and family support.
- They are exposed to substance abuse and sexual exploitation.
- These children are exposed to torture by their employers, police and society and may end up becoming criminals.

D. THE INTEGRATED CHILD PROTECTION SCHEME (ICPS)

The Integrated Child Protection Scheme is expected to create a system that will efficiently and effectively protect these children. The ICPS also provides preventive, statutory care and rehabilitation services to any vulnerable child. These include children of migrant families, families living in extreme poverty, lower castes, minorities, children with HIV, orphans, drug abusers, children of substance abusers, child beggars, trafficked or sexually exploited children, children of prisoners, and street and working children.

In order to reach out to all children, in particular to those in difficult circumstances, the Ministry of Women and Child Development proposes to combine its existing child protection schemes under one centrally sponsored scheme titled "Integrated Child Protection Scheme (ICPS)" for protecting children and preventing harm.

E. INTEGRATED PROGRAM FOR STREET CHILDREN

The purpose of this program is to provide support and develop awareness amongst the Government, NGO and community regarding the rights of the child. The objective is to facilitate withdrawal of street children and prevent their destitution. It provides nutrition, education, shelter, recreation facilities for street children and also seeks their protection against exploitation and abuse. This program mainly targets street children, children vulnerable to substance abuse and sexual exploitation like sex workers and pavement dwellers.

21.9 JUVENILE JUSTICE (CARE AND PROTECTION OF CHILDREN) ACT, 2015

Juvenile Justice (Care and Protection of Children) Act 2015 aims to replace the existing Act of 2000, so that juveniles in conflict with law in the age group 16–18 year involved in heinous crimes or offences, can be tried as adults. The new bill also introduces foster care in India.

In the Juvenile Justice Act (Care and Protection of Children) Act 2015 (JJB), a juvenile or child is defined as someone who has not completed 18 years of age. This not only protects the rights of children, but a person's rights when he/she was a child. For carrying out this act the state should create child protection units, whose officers ensure proper implementation of the Act.

This Act also emphasizes on the rehabilitation and social integration of children. It discusses certain non-institutional methods like adoption, foster care and sponsorship. The Act also allows children with special needs (mental or physical disease) to be given the necessary attention at an approved and appropriate institution.

The Integrated Child Protection Scheme (ICPS) and the Juvenile Justice Act, 2015 define vulnerability in two categories: (a) Children in need of care and protection; and (b) Children in conflict with law. A third category defined by ICPS is: Child in contact with law. These children are victims of crime or witnesses to crimes.

A. CHILDREN IN NEED OF CARE

Children in need of care and protection refer to children who:
- Do not have a home or shelter and have no means to obtain such an abode
- Reside with a person(s) who has threatened to harm them and is likely to carry out that threat, harmed other children and hence is likely to kill, abuse or neglect the child.
- Are mentally or physically handicapped, or have an illness, terminal or incurable disease and have no one to provide and care for them.
- Have a parent or guardian deemed unfit or unable to take care of the child.
- Are orphans, have no family to take care of them, or are runaway or missing whose parents cannot be located after a reasonable search period.
- Are being or are likely to be sexual, mentally, emotionally or physically abused, tortured or exploited.
- Are being trafficked or abusing drug substances.
- Are being abused for unthinkable gains or illegal activities.
- Are victims of arm conflict, civil unrest or a natural disaster.

The main aim is to bring the child back to his family or family environment after determining the safety of the environment.

B. CHILDREN IN CONFLICT WITH LAW

Children in conflict with law are juveniles who have allegedly committed a crime under the Indian Penal Code. After the necessary enquiry if the Juvenile Justice Board finds the child guilty, he is released after counseling and advice or made to pay a fine. There is no life imprisonment or death penalty for a child even if he is found guilty. If a juvenile runs away from an observation home he can be brought back without a warrant and without punishment. Cruelty against juveniles is a punishable offence. The Juvenile Justice Act also penalizes people who exploit children for different crimes. A person who employs children in hazardous industries, begging, or provides a child with drugs and alcohol is subjected to severe imprisonment and fine.

ICPS outlines that vulnerable children groups also include but are not limited to the following: Children of potentially vulnerable families, street and working children, child beggars, trafficked children, sexually assaulted children, children of socially excluded groups like extremely poor families, migrant families, minorities, scheduled castes, scheduled tribes and other backward classes, families subjected to or affected by discrimination, orphans, children infected and/or affected by HIV/AIDS, children of substance abusers, child drug abusers and children of prisoners.

A Strategic Approach to Reproductive, Maternal, Newborn, Child and Adolescent Health in India. New Delhi: Ministry of Health and Family Welfare, Government of India; 2013.

Belli PC, Bustreo F, Preker A. Investing in children's health: what are the economic benefits? Bull World Health Organ. 2005;83:777–84.

Integrated Child Development Services (ICDS) scheme. Ministry of Women and Child Development, Government of India. From: http://wcd.nic.in/icds.htm. Accessed on March 25, 2017.

MCEE-WHO Methods And Data Sources For Child Causes Of Death 2000–2015. http://www.who.int/healthinfo/global_burden_disease/ChildCOD_method_2000_2015.pdf. Accessed March 25, 2017.

Ministry of Health and Family Welfare. Integrated Management of Neonatal and Childhood Illness. Training Modules for Physicians. Chartbooklet. New Delhi: Ministry of Health and Family Welfare. Govt. of India; 2009.

Mission Indradhanush. Ministry of Health and Family Welfare, Government of India. Available from: http://www.missionindradhanush.in/. Accessed March 25, 2017.

National Plan of Action for Children 2016. Ministry of Women and Child Development, Government of India. Available from: http://wcd.nic.in/acts/national-plan-action-children-2016. Accessed March 25, 2017.

Operational Framework: Translating strategies into programs, Rashtriya Kishor Swasthya Karyakram 2014, National Health Mission, Ministry of Health and Family Welfare, Government of India. Available from: http://nrhm.gov.in/rashtriya-kishor-swasthya-karyakram.html. Accessed November 27 2016.

UNICEF. State of the World's Children Report 2016. Available from: https://www.unicef.org/sowc2016/. Accessed on November 24, 2016.

World Health Statistics 2015. Indicator compendium. http://www.who.int/gho/publications/world_health_statistics/2015/en/. Accessed March 25, 2017.

Piyush Gupta

Drug Therapy

22.1 ANTI-ARRHYTHMIC DRUGS

1. Adenosine

Intravenous; ampoule (3 mg/mL)

Indications: Supraventricular tachycardia: Children: 0.1–0.2 mg/kg rapid intravenous push over 1–2 seconds, may increase bolus dose by 0.05 mg/kg every 2 min till clinical response or maximum of 12 mg (0.25 mg/kg). Follow each dose with a normal saline flush.

Contraindications: 2nd and 3rd degree heart block or sick sinus syndrome.

Adverse effects: Bronchoconstriction, facial flushing, headache, chest pain, dyspnea, chest pain.

2. Atropine Sulfate *(Anticholinergic)*

Oral, intravenous, tablets (0.4 mg, 0.6 mg), ampoule (0.05, 0.1, 0.3, 0.4, 0.5, 0.8, 1 mg/mL)

Indications: Cardiac resuscitation: 0.02 mg/kg/dose IV every 5 min, maximum dose in children: 1 mg, in adolescents: 2 mg; *Pre-anesthesia dose:* Child: 0.01 mg/kg/dose SC/IV/IM, maximum dose 0.4 mg/dose; minimum dose: 0.1 mg/dose, may repeat q 4–6 h.

Contraindications: Glaucoma, tachyarrhythmias, thyrotoxicosis.

Adverse effects: Blurred vision, dry mouth, tachycardia, constipation, urinary retention.

3. Lignocaine Hydrochloride

Intravenous; 2% solution (20 mg/mL)

Indications: Tachyarrhythmia: Administer 1 mg/kg/dose IV slowly (can repeat in 5–10 minutes twice; maximum 3 mg/kg) loading followed by 20–50 µg/kg/min as maintenance.

Contraindications: Stokes-Adams attacks, SA, AV, or intraventricular heart block. Avoid lignocaine with epinephrine preparations

Adverse effects: Hypotension, asystole, seizures and respiratory arrest.

4. Phenytoin Sodium *(Sodium channel blocker; also an anticonvulsant)*

Intravenous, Oral; ampoule (50 mg/mL), syrup (125 mg/5 mL, 30 mg/5 mL), tablet (100 mg)

Indications: Anti-arrhythmic (secondary to digitalis intoxication): Loading dose 1.25mg/kg IV q 5 minutes (maximum 15 mg/kg); Maintenance dose in children 5–10 mg/kg/day q 12 h IV/PO.

Contraindications: Heart block or sinus bradycardia.

Adverse effects: Nystagmus, hypotension, Stevens-Johnson syndrome, rash, hepatitis, gingival hyperplasia, blood dyscrasia.

5. Propranolol *(Beta blocker)*

Oral, intravenous; tablet (10 mg), ampoule (1 mg/mL)

Indications: Supraventricular tachycardia: Oral: 0.25 mg/kg/dose q 6–8 h; Intravenous: 0.01–0.1 mg/kg/dose over 10–15 minutes, repeat q 6–8 h. *Thyrotoxicosis:* Neonates: 0.5 mg/kg/dose orally q 6 h; children: 0.5–1 mg/kg/dose orally q 6 h. *Migraine prophylaxis:* 0.5–2 mg/kg/day orally q 6–8 h.

Contraindications: Heart block, heart failure, and Raynaud syndrome.

6. Verapamil *(Calcium channel blocker)*

Oral, Intravenous; Tablet (40, 80 mg), ampoule (2.5 mg/mL) IV

Indications: Arrhythmia: Infants: 0.1–0.2 mg/kg IV over 2–3 minutes using continuous ECG monitoring. May repeat after 30 minutes; Children: IV 0.1–0.3 mg/kg, maximum dose: 5 mg. PO: 1–2 mg/kg/dose q 6–8 h.

Contraindications: Hypersensitivity, cardiogenic shock, severe CHF, sick-sinus syndrome or AV block. Avoid IV use in neonates and young infants due to apnea, bradycardia, and hypotension.

Adverse effects: Bradycardia, AV block, heart failure, hypotension, constipation, flushing, nausea.

Antidote: Calcium gluconate

22.2 ANTI-ASTHMATICS AND BRONCHODILATORS

1. Adrenaline *(Adrenergic agonist)*

Intravenous, subcutaneous, intramuscular, intratracheal; ampoule (1:1000 solution, 1 mL = 1 mg)

Indications: Cardiac arrest: 0.1 mL/kg of 1:10,000 diluted intravenous or intratracheal q 3–5 min. *Resuscitation in neonates:* 1:10,000 dilution 0.1–0.3 mL/kg IV q 3–5 min or 0.3–0.5 mL/kg ET. CPR in older children: 0.1 mg/kg IV/ET of

1:1000 dilution q 3–5 min. *Shock:* 0.05–0.5 µg/kg/min IV infusion. *Bronchodilation:* 1:1000 dilution, 0.01 mg/kg/dose SC, q 15 min × 3–4 doses. Nebulization: 0.5 mL/kg of 1:1000 solution diluted in 3 mL normal saline (Max dose in ≤4 years: 2.5 mL/dose and in older children: 5 mL/dose). *Anaphylaxis:* 0.01 mL/kg 1:1000 solution SC or IM, max 0.5 mL per dose.

Adverse effects: Tachycardia, restlessness, hypertension, tremors.

Remarks: Dilute in normal saline.

2. Aminophylline *(Methyl Xanthine)*

Oral, intravenous; syrup (20 mg/5 mL), ampoule (250 mg/10 mL)

Indications: Bronchospasm: 5 mg/kg IV loading over 30 min followed by 0.5 mg/kg/h: 6 wk–6 mo, 0.7 mg/kg/h: 6 mo–1 yr, 1 mg/kg/h: 1–9 yr, 0.9 mg/kg/h: 9–12 yr. *Apnea of prematurity:* 6 mg/kg IV/PO loading followed by 2.5 mg/kg/dose q 8–12 h.

Adverse effects: Arrhythmia, seizure, GERD.

Remarks: Narrow therapeutic range: 5–15 µg/mL.

3. Beclomethasone Dipropionate *(Inhaled Corticosteroid)*

Inhalational; MDI (50, 100, 200 µg/puff), rotacaps (100, 2000, 400 µg)

Indications: Bronchial asthma: 200–1000 µg/day in 2–4 divided doses.

Adverse effects: Hoarseness, oral candidiasis.

Contraindications: Not recommended in children <6 y.

Remarks: Rinse mouth after each use of MDI. Avoid using in doses exceeding the recommended doses.

4. Budesonide *(Inhaled corticosteroid)*

Inhalational; MDI (100, 200 µg/puff), rotacaps (100, 2000, 400 µg), nebulizing solution (250 µg/mL)

Indications: Bronchopulmonary dysplasia: 400 µg/kg inhaled twice daily. *Asthma:* Aerosol 1–12 yr: 50–400 µg; 12–18 yr: 200–400 µg, Nebulization: 3 mo–12 yr: 250–500 µg twice daily; 12–18 yr: 500 µg–1000 µg twice daily.

Adverse effects: Hoarseness, oral candidiasis.

Remarks: Rinse mouth after each use of MDI.

5. Formoterol Fumarate *(corticosteroid)*

Inhalational; MDI (25, 50, 125 µg/puff)

Indications: Asthma: MDI 50–500 µg/day in two divided doses.

Adverse effects: Oral thrush, dysphonia, dermatitis.

Remarks: Rinse mouth every time after use, cautious use in liver disease

6. Fluticasone Propionate *(Long Acting Beta Agonist: LABA)*

Inhalational: MDI (12 µg/puff); rotacaps (6 µg)

Indications: Asthma: MDI 50–500 µg/day in two divided doses.

Adverse effects: Tachycardia, headache, tremors, anxiety.

Remarks: Not to be used as monotherapy.

Contraindications: Avoid in patients with hyperthyroidism, diabetes, seizures, pheochromocytoma.

7. Ipratropium Bromide *(Anticholinergic)*

Inhalational; Nebulizing solution (250 µg/mL), MDI (20 µg/puff), <1 yr: 125 µg/dose, >1 yr: 250 µg/dose

Indications: Bronchospasm: Nebulized after dilution in 2–4 mL of saline and given over 10 minutes every 20 minutes for 3 doses followed by nebulization every 2–4 hours.

Contraindications: Glaucoma, intestinal obstruction, and achalasia.

8. Levosalbutamol *(Short Acting Beta Agonist: SABA)*

Oral, inhalational; syrup (1 mg/5 mL), nebulizing respules (0.31, 0.63, 1.2 mg/2.5 mL)

Indications: Bronchospasm: Oral: 0.05–0.1 mg/kg/dose 2–3 times/day, Nebulization: 0.075 mg/kg/dose.

Adverse effects: Tachycardia, tremors, hypokalemia but less severe than salbutamol.

9. Magnesium Sulfate

Intravenous; ampoule (50% sol; 1 mL=500 mg)

Indications: Asthma: 25–50 mg/kg/dose IV infusion.

Adverse effects: Respiratory depression if given in overdose.

Antidote: Calcium gluconate.

10. Montelukast Sodium *(Leukotriene Receptor Antagonist: LTRA)*

Oral; tablet (4 mg, 5 mg, 10 mg)

Indications: Bronchial asthma: 2–5 y: 4 mg once in the evening, 6–14 y: 5 mg once in the evening, >15 y: 10 mg once in the evening.

Adverse effects: Headache, dizziness, fatigue, elevated liver enzymes.

Contraindications: Chewable form not to be given in phenylketonuria.

11. Salbutamol *(SABA)*

Oral, inhalational; syrup (2 mg/5 mL), nebulizing solution (5 mg/mL), MDI (100 µg/puff)

Indications: Bronchospasm: Oral: 0.1–0.2 mg/kg/dose 2–3 times/day; Nebulization: 0.15 mg/kg/dose; minimum–1.25 mg; maximum–3 mg. *Acute exacerbation of asthma:* 2–4 puffs by MDI every 20 minutes followed by 2 puffs every 4–6 hrs.

Adverse effects: Tachycardia, tremors, hypokalemia.

12. Salmeterol *(LABA)*

Inhalational; MDI (25 µg/dose)

Indications: Asthma: 50–100 µg/day.

Contraindications: Not to be used as monotherapy. Not to be used in children < 4 yrs.

13. Terbutaline *(Beta-2 receptor agonist)*

Oral, Intravenous, Subcutaneous, Inhalational; Syrup (1.5 mg/mL), tablets (2.5, 5 mg), ampoule (0.5 mg/mL), MDI (250 µg/puff), nebulizing solution (10 mg/mL)

Indications: Bronchospasm: Oral: 0.05 mg/kg/dose (max 5 mg) 3 times/day, SC: 0.005–0.01 mg/kg/dose up to 4 times/day, Inhalational: 1–2 puffs of 250 µg q 6–8 h, Nebulization: 2.5 mg in children below 20 kg and 5 mg in children >20 kg.

Adverse effects: Tachycardia, arrhythmias, flushing, headache, tremors, hypokalemia.

Contraindications: Use cautiously in renal failure.

14. Theophylline *(Methylxanthine)*

Oral; tablets (100, 150, 200, 250, 400, 600 mg), syrup (80 mg/15 mL, 50 mg/5 mL)

Indications: Bronchospasm: 15–25 mg/kg/day q 8 h PO.

Adverse effects: Nausea, vomiting, abdominal pain, GERD, nervousness, arrhythmia, seizure, anorexia.

22.3 ANTIFUNGALS

1. Amphotericin B

Oral, intravenous; suspension (100 mg/mL), tablet (100 mg), Vial (50 mg/vial, liposomal: 10, 25, 50 mg)

Indications: Antifungal/anti-leishmanial: Start at 0.25 mg/kg and increase till 1 mg/kg/day OD as infusion in 5% dextrose, Liposomal 3–5 mg/kg/day OD.

Adverse effects: Nephrotoxic, IV administration may cause chills, fever, vomiting and headache, may premedicate with pethidine.

Remarks: Protect from light. Monitor serum potassium levels.

2. Clotrimazole

Topical application; Lotion, gel, mouth paint, powder, vaginal pessaries

Indications: Antifungal: Apply locally 3–4 times per day.

3. Fluconazole

Intravenous, oral; injection (200 mg/100 mL), tablet (50, 150 mg)

Indications: Antifungal: 3–6 mg/kg/day OD; in neonates, loading dose 12 mg/kg followed by 3–5 mg/kg/day OD.

Adverse effects: Nausea, vomiting, pain abdomen, itching, headache, dizziness.

Contraindications: Avoid in patients prone to arrhythmias or on cisapride and in hepatic/renal disease.

4. Griseofulvin

Oral; tablet (125, 250, 500 mg)

Indications: Antifungal: 10 mg/kg/day q 6–12 hours PO.

Adverse effects: Nausea, vomiting, diarrhea, headache, rash, dizziness, numbness, tingling.

Contraindications: Porphyria and hepatic disease.

5. Itraconazole

Oral, injection; capsule (100 mg), oral solution (10 mg/mL), Injection (10 mg/mL)

Indications: Antifungal: 200–400 mg/day q 12–24 h. Oral solution is used for treating oral candidiasis.

Adverse effects: Elevated liver enzymes, nausea, vomiting, convulsions, dry mouth, loss of appetite, mood disturbances, running nose, dizziness.

6. Ketoconazole

Topical, oral; cream, shampoo, tablet (200 mg), syrup (100 mg/5 mL)

Indications: Antifungal: 3.5–6.5 mg/kg/day OD.

Adverse effects: Nausea, vomiting, pruritis, raised liver enzymes, headache, fever.

Contraindications: Concomitant cisapride, terfenadine or astemizole.

7. Voriconazole

Intravenous, Oral; Vial (200 mg/vial), tablet (50, 200 mg)

Indications: Antifungal: Load 6 mg/kg IV q 12 h on day 1 followed by 4 mg/kg/day q 12 h. Consume 1 h before or 2 h after meals. *Aspergillosis, invasive candidemia:* 2–11 y: 9 mg/kg IV/PO every 12 h, >12 y: 6 mg/kg every 12 h IV/PO for 2 doses, followed by 4 mg/kg IV/PO every 12 h.

Adverse effects: Transient visual disturbances, hepatotoxicity, fever, rash, nausea, vomiting, abdominal pain, diarrhea, headache, peripheral edema and rarely cardiac arrhythmias.

22.4 ANTI-INFLAMMATORY, ANTIPYRETICS, AND ANALGESICS

1. Acetaminophen *(Paracetamol)*

Oral, intravenous; drops (150 mg/mL), syrup (125 mg/5 mL, 250 mg/5 mL), tablet (500 mg, 650 mg), ampoule (150 mg/mL)

Indications: Antipyretic: Oral: 10–15 mg/kg/dose q 4–6 h PO, Injection: 5 mg/kg IM single dose.

Remark: Excessive intake causes hepatic necrosis.

Antidote: In acute overdose N-acetylcysteine is the antidote.

2. Acetyl Salicylic Acid *(Aspirin: NSAID)*

Oral; Tablet (75 mg, 100 mg, 325 mg, 650 mg)

Indications: Fever: 10–15 mg/kg/dose 4–6 times/day. Anti-inflammatory dose: 80–100 mg/kg/day in 3–4 divided doses. Kawasaki: 25 mg/kg/dose QID. Antiplatelet dose: 3–5 mg/kg/day OD. Rheumatic fever: 100 mg/kg/day for 2–3 weeks followed by 60 mg/kg/day for the next 9–12 weeks.

Adverse effects: GI disturbance, headache, dizziness.

Contraindications: Do not use for treatment of varicella or flu like symptoms as it may cause Reye syndrome.

3. Codeine Phosphate *(Opioid analgesic)*

Oral; tablet (15 mg, 30 mg, 60 mg), syrup

Indications: Pain: 0.5–1 mg/kg/dose q 4–6 h, maximum 60 mg/dose. Cough: 1–1.5 mg/kg/24 h q 4–6 h.

Adverse effects: Constipation, drowsiness.

Contraindications: Postoperative pain after tonsillectomy/adenoidectomy.

4. Diclofenac Sodium *(NSAID)*

Oral, intramuscular; tablet (50 mg, 75 mg, 100 mg), injection (75 mg per 3 mL ampoule)

Indications: Anti-inflammatory: 1–3 mg/kg/day in 2–4 divided doses.

Adverse effects: Dizziness, headache, fluid retention, gastric bleeding or ulcer.

5. Fentanyl *(Opioid analgesic and sedative)*

Intravenous, oral; ampoule (50 µg/mL), oral lozenges (200, 300, 400 µg)

Indications: Narcotic: Infants 1–4 µg/kg/dose q 1–4 h IV; Continuous infusion 0.5–5 µg/kg/h, children 1–3 µg/kg/dose q 1–4 h IV; continuous infusion 1–5 µg/kg/h; PO 10–15 µg/kg/dose, max 400 µg/dose.

Adverse effects: Hypotension, bradycardia, GI upset, respiratory depression, biliary tract spasm.

Contraindications: Respiratory depression.

6. Ibuprofen *(NSAID)*

Oral, intravenous; syrup (100 mg/5 mL), tablet (200 mg), injection (10 mg/mL in 2 mL vials)

Indications: Fever/analgesia: 10–15 mg/kg/dose q 4–6 h, maximum 60 mg/kg/day. *Juvenile rheumatoid arthritis:* 30–70 mg/kg/d q 4–6 h, oral. *Ductus closure:* 10 mg/kg IV followed by 5 mg/kg IV every 24 h for 2 doses.

Adverse effects: Abdominal cramps, nausea, heartburn, fluid retention.

Contraindications: Active GI bleeding and ulceration.

7. Indomethacin *(NSAID)*

Oral, intravenous; capsule (25 mg, 50 mg), injection (1 mg vial)

Indications: Analgesia: 3 mg/kg/d q 8 h, oral. *Ductus closure in preterm neonate:* 0.2 mg/kg/dose IV 8 h for 3 doses.

Adverse effects: Abdominal cramps, nausea, heartburn.

Contraindications: Avoid in neonates with NEC, poor renal function, or active bleeding.

8. Mefenamic Acid *(NSAID)*

Oral; tablet (100 mg), capsule (250 mg, 500 mg), suspension (100 mg/5 mL, 50 mg/5 mL)

Indications: Arthritis: 25 mg/kg/d q 6 h. *Fever:* 3 mg/kg/dose.

Adverse effects: Diarrhea, skin rash and gastritis.

Remarks: Administer with food. Avoid in patients having seizures.

9. Morphine Sulfate *(Opioid Analgesic)*

Subcutaneous injection, occasionally intravenously; ampoule (10 mg, 15 mg, 25 mg per mL)

Indications: Analgesia: 0.1–0.2 mg/kg/dose SC, maximum 15 mg. Occasionally used for preoperative medication, postoperative pain, restlessness, pulmonary edema: IV 2–5 mg/dose, continuous infusion in neonates 0.01–0.02 mg/kg/h, infants and children 0.025–0.2 mg/kg/h.

Adverse effects: Constipation, blurred vision, headache, pain abdomen, confusion.

Antidote: Naloxone.

10. Naproxen *(NSAID)*

Oral; tablet (250 mg)

Indications: Analgesia: 5–7 mg/kg/dose q 8–12 h. JRA: 10–20 mg/kg/d q 12 h.

Adverse effects: Dizziness, rash, gastric irritation.

Contraindications: Peptic ulcer disease.

11. Pentazocine Hydrochloride *(Opioid analgesic)*

Oral, intravenous, intramuscular; tablet (25 mg; 15 mg pentazocin with 500 mg paracetamol), ampoule (30 mg/mL)

Indications: Analgesia: 0.5–1.0 mg/kg/d q 4 h oral, IM or IV (maximum dose 30 mg IV).

Contraindications: Raised intracranial tension, head injury.

Adverse effects: Blurred vision, constipation, confusion, nausea, vomiting.

12. Prednisolone *(Corticosteroid)*

Oral; tablets (5 mg, 10 mg, 20 mg), syrup (5 mg/5 mL)

Indications: Immunosuppression: 1–2 mg/kg/day q 6–12 h.

Adverse effects: Edema, hypertension, Cushing syndrome, peptic ulcer, hypothalamic pituitary-adrenal axis suppression.

22.5 ANTIBIOTICS

AMINOGLYCOSIDES

1. Amikacin Sulfate

Intravenous, intramuscular; vial (100, 250, 500 mg)

Indications: Antibiotic: 15–20 mg/kg/day q 8–12 h.

Contraindications: Dose adjustment in renal failure.

2. Gentamicin Sulfate

Intravenous, intramuscular; ampoule (10, 40 mg/mL)

Indications: Antibiotic: 5.0–7.5 mg/kg/day q 8–12 h.

Contraindications: Cautious use in patients receiving loop diuretics. Adjust dose in renal failure.

3. Kanamycin Sulfate

Intravenous, intramuscular; vial (500 mg, 1 g)

Indications: Antibiotic: 15 mg/kg/day q 8–12 h IM, IV given over 30–60 min; Used for MDR TB.

Remarks: Poor oral absorption. Given orally to treat bacterial overgrowth. Cautious use in renal derangement.

22

4. Streptomycin Sulfate

Intravenous, intramuscular; vial (750 mg, 1 g)

Indications: Antibiotic: 20–40 mg/kg/day q 12 h IV or single dose IM.

Contraindications: Aminoglycoside and sulfite hypersensitivity. Cautious use in with neuromuscular blocking agents, patients with vertigo, tinnitus, and neuromuscular disorders.

5. Tobramycin

Intravenous, intramuscular; vials (20 mg, 40 mg, 80 mg in 2 mL vial)

Indications: Antibiotic: 6–7.5 mg/kg/day q 8–12 h IV/ IM.

Contraindications: Avoid in myasthenia gravis or Parkinson's disease.

Adverse effects of aminoglycosides: Nephrotoxicity, hearing loss, vestibular toxicity

CEPHALOSPORINS

1. Cefazolin Sodium *(First Generation)*

Intravenous, intramuscular; Vial (250, 500 mg, 1g)

Indications: Antibiotic: 50–100 mg/kg/day q 6 h IV/IM

2. Cefepime *(Fourth Generation)*

Intravenous; vial (250, 500 mg, 1g)

Indications: Antibiotic: 100 mg/kg/day q 8–12 h IV/IM. Meningitis/serious infections: 150 mg/kg/d q 8 h.

3. Cefixime *(Third Generation)*

Oral; syrup (50 mg/5 mL), tablet (100, 200, 400 mg)

Indications: Antibiotic: 8–10 mg/kg/day q 12 h. Enteric fever: 15–20 mg/kg/day q 12 h.

4. Cefoperazone Sulbactam *(Third Generation)*

Intravenous; vial (1:1; 2:1, 500 mg, 1 g, 2 g)

Indications: Antibiotic: 80 mg/kg/day (1:1) q 6–12h. Serious infection: 160 mg/kg/day (2:1) divided 6–12 h.

Remarks: NOT recommended in meningitis

5. Cefotaxime Sodium *(Third Generation)*

Intravenous, intramuscular; Vial (250, 500 mg, 1 g)

Indications: Antibiotic: 100–150 mg/kg/day q 6–8 h. Meningitis: 200 mg/kg/day q 6 h IV, Neonate <7 days: 100 mg/kg/day q 12 h, > 7 days: 150 mg/kg/day q 8 h.

6. Cefpodoxime Proxetil *(Third Generation)*

Oral; syrup (50, 100 mg), tablet (100, 200 mg)

Indications: Antibiotic: 10 mg/kg/day q12 h.

7. Ceftazidime *(Third Generation)*

Intravenous, intramuscular; vial (250, 500 mg, 1 g)

Indications: Antibiotic: 100–150 mg/kg/day q 8 h, neonate < 7 days: 100 mg/kg/day q 12 h, > 7 days: 150 mg/kg/day q 8 h.

8. Ceftriaxone Sodium *(Third Generation)*

Intravenous, intramuscular; Vial (250, 500 mg, 1 g)

Indications: Antibiotic: 50–75 mg/kg/day q 12 h for AOM. Meningitis: 100 mg/kg/day q 12 h.

Remarks: Besides other side effects, also causes cholelithiasis (reversible), gall bladder sludging.

9. Cefuroxime Axetil *(Second Generation)*

Intravenous, oral; vial (250, 750 mg, 1.5 g), syrup (125 mg/5 mL), tablet (125, 250, 500 mg)

Indications: Antibiotic: Intravenous 75–150 mg/kg/day q 6–8 h, Oral 20–30 mg/kg/day q 12 h.

10. Cephalexin *(First Generation)*

Oral; syrup (125 mg/5 mL), tablet (125, 250 mg DT), capsule (250, 500 mg)

Indications: Antibiotic: 25–100 mg/kg/day q 6–8 h.

Adverse effects for cephalosporins: Nausea, vomiting, pain abdomen, deranged liver enzymes, false positive coombs test

Contraindications for cephalosporins: To use cautiously in renal disease/patients allergic to penicillin.

FLUOROQUINOLONES

1. Ciprofloxacin

Oral, intravenous; syrup (125 mg/5 mL), tablet (250, 500 mg), injection (200 mg/100 mL, 100 mg/50 mL)

Indications: Antibiotic: Intravenous 10–20 mg/kg/day q 8–12 h, Oral 20–30 mg/kg/day q 8–12 h.

Adverse effects: Rash, deranged liver enzymes, neutropenia, gynecomastia, diarrhea.

2. Gatifloxacin

Oral; Tablet (200, 400 mg)

Indications: Antibiotic: 10 mg/kg/dose OD oral.

Adverse effects: Dysglycemia

3. Levofloxacin

Intravenous, oral; tablet (250, 500 mg), injection (5 mg/mL)

Indications: Antibiotic: 10 mg/kg/dose OD oral or intravenous.

4. Nalidixic Acid

Oral; tablet (125, 500 mg), suspension (300 mg/5 mL)

Indications: Antibiotic: 50–55 mg/kg/day q 6–8 h.

Contraindications: Avoid in infants <3 months. Avoid in children with history of seizures, G-6-PD deficiency.

Adverse effects: Pseudotumor cerebri

5. Norfloxacin

Oral; tablet (100, 200, 400 mg), suspension (100 mg/5 mL)

Indications: Antibiotic: 10–15 mg/kg/day q 12 h.

Adverse effects: Arthropathy

6. Ofloxacin

Oral, intravenous; tablet (200, 400 mg), suspension (100 mg/ 5 mL), injection (200, 400 mg/100 mL)

Indications: Antibiotic: Oral 15 mg/kg/day q 12 h, Intravenous: 5–10 mg/kg/day q 12 h.

Adverse effects of fluoroquinolones: Nausea, vomiting, diarrhea, headache, insomnia, tendonitis.

Contraindications of fluoroquinolones: Avoid in hypersensitivity. To use cautiously in renal disease/liver disease.

MACROLIDES

1. Azithromycin

Oral, intravenous; tablets (250, 500 mg), suspension (100, 20 mg/5 mL), injection (500 mg)

Indications: Otitis media, community acquired pneumonia, tonsillitis: 10 mg/kg PO on day 1 followed by 5 mg/kg/day OD on days 2–5; alternately, give 30 mg/kg single dose PO. *Uncomplicated typhoid fever:* 20 mg/kg PO OD × 7 days. *M. avium complex prophylaxis:* 20 mg/kg/dose PO once a week.

Contraindications: Avoid use in infants <6 months of age.

2. Clarithromycin

Oral; tablets (250, 500 mg), syrup (125 mg/5 mL)

Indications: Antibiotic: 15 mg/kg/day q 12 h, PO. *M. avium* complex prophylaxis: 15 mg/kg/dose PO once a week.

Contraindications: Avoid use in infants < 6 months age. Not to be given in patients allergic to erythromycin and liver dysfunction.

Remarks: Adjust dose in renal failure. If creatinine clearance is < 50 mL/min, decrease dose by 50% and administer drug 12–24 h.

3. Erythromycin

Oral, intravenous; tablets (250, 500 mg), syrup (125 mg/5 mL), injection (1 g/vial)

Indications: Antibiotic: Intravenous 5 mg/kg/dose IV infusion over 8 h with normal saline or Ringer's lactate or intermittent bolus over 20–60 min every 6–8 h, oral 30–50 mg/kg/day q 6 h.

Contraindications: Avoid in patients on class 3/1a antiarrhythmics, those with QT prolongation, those susceptible to arrhythmias.

Adverse effects of macrolides: Nausea, vomiting, cholestasis, QT prolongation (specially with clarithromycin and erythromycin).

PENICILLINS

1. Amoxicillin

Oral; capsule (250, 500 mg), suspension (125 mg/5 mL), drops (50 mg/mL)

Indications: Antibiotic: 25–50 mg/kg/day q 8 h. Recurrent otitis media: 20 mg/kg/dose HS PO.

Contraindications: Dose adjustment in renal failure

2. Amoxicillin–Clavulanic Acid

Intravenous, oral; injection [150 mg (125 mg amox), 300 mg (250 mg amox), 600 mg (500 mg amox), 1200 mg (1000 mg amox)], tablet (250 mg amoxicillin with 125 mg clavulanate, 500 mg amoxicillin with 125 mg clavulanate), syrup (200 amox with 28.5 mg clavulanate/5 mL, 125 mg amox with 31.5 mg clavulanate)

Indications: Antibiotic: Oral 20–40 mg (amox base)/kg/day q 8–12 h, intravenous 50–100 mg (amox base)/kg/day q 6–8 h.

Contraindications: Dose adjustment in renal failure.

3. Ampicillin with Sulbactam

Intravenous, oral; vial (1 g ampicillin with 0.5 g sulbactam), tablet (375 mg containing 250 mg ampicillin)

Indications: Antibiotic: 100–200 mg/kg/day of ampicillin q 6 h IV.

Contraindications: Dose adjustment in renal failure.

4. Ampicillin Sodium Trihydrate

Oral, intravenous; capsule (250, 500 mg), syrup (125 mg/5 mL), injection (250, 500 mg)

Indications: Antibiotic: 100–200 mg/kg/day q 6 h IV or oral. *Meningitis:* 200–400 mg/kg/day q 4 h IV. *Enteric fever:* 200 mg/kg/day q 6 h oral.

Adverse effects: Interstitial nephritis, pseudomembranous enterocolitis.

Contraindications: Dose adjustment in renal failure

5. Cloxacillin

Oral, intravenous; capsule (250, 500 mg), syrup (125 mg/5 mL), vial (500 mg)

Indications: Antibiotic: 50–100 mg/kg/day q 6 h IV or PO (1 h before or 2 h after meals). *Meningitis:* 200 mg/kg/day q 4 h (maximum dose 4 g/day).

6. Penicillin G Aqueous

Oral, intravenous; tablet (2 lakh, 4 lakh, 8 lakh units), vial (5 lakh, 10 lakh units)

Indications: Antibiotic: 1–2 lakh units/kg/day IV infusion q 4–6 h. *Meningitis and endocarditis:* 2–3 lakh units/kg/day IM q 4 h (maximum dose 24 million U/day). *Rheumatic fever prophylaxis:* 2 lakh units (125 mg) BD.

Remarks: Administer 30 min before or 2 h after meals.

Adverse effects: Urticaria, hemolytic anemia, interstitial nephritis, Jarisch-Herxheimer reaction.

7. Penicillin G Benzathine

Intramuscular; vial (1.2, 2.4 million units)

Indications: Secondary prophylaxis of rheumatic fever: <6 years 0.6 MU IM every 21 days. > 6 years1.2 MU IM every 21 days.

Remarks: To be given only after test dose; can cause severe anaphylaxis. Never give IV as it may result in cardiac arrest and death.

Adverse effects: Urticaria, hemolytic anemia, interstitial nephritis, Jarisch-Herxheimer reaction.

22

8. Penicillin V *(Phenoxymethyl Penicillin)*

Oral; tablet (125, 250 mg)

Indications: Antibiotic: Infants 62.5–125 mg/dose q 6 h, < 5 years 125 mg/dose q 6 h, >5 years 250 mg/dose q 6 h. *Rheumatic fever prophylaxis:* 250 mg BD, < 5 years 125 mg BD, > 5 years 250 mg BD. (250 mg is equivalent to 4 lakh units).

Adverse effects: Urticaria, hemolytic anemia, interstitial nephritis, Jarisch-Herxheimer reaction.

9. Piperacillin

Intravenous, intramuscular; vial (1 g, 2 g, 4 g)

Indications: Antibiotic: 100–300 mg/kg/day q 4–6 h.

Adverse effects: Headache, bleeding, SJS.

Contraindications: Dose adjustment in renal failure.

10. Piperacillin–Tazobactam

Intravenous; vial (4 g of piperacillin with 500 mg of tazobactam)

Indications: Antibiotic: 300–400 mg/kg/day q 6–8 h. Dose based on piperacillin.

Adverse effects: Headache, bleeding, Stevens-Johnson syndrome.

Contraindications: Dose adjustment in renal failure.

11. Procaine Penicillin

Intramuscular; vial (4 lakh units/ vial)

Indications: Antibiotic: 25,000–50,000 units/kg/day single dose IM, neonates 50,000 units/kg/day IM.

Adverse effects: Urticaria, hemolytic anemia, interstitial nephritis, Jarisch-Herxheimer reaction. May cause seizures.

Remarks: To be given only after test dose; give as intramuscular only.

Adverse effects for penicillin group of drugs: Nausea, vomiting, diarrhea, stomach ache, rash, itching.

Contraindications for penicillin group of drugs: Contraindicated in hypersensitivity to penicillin.

MISCELLANEOUS ANTIBIOTICS

1. Chloramphenicol *(Chloromycetin)*

Oral, intravenous; capsule (250 mg, 500 mg), suspension (125 mg/5 mL), injection (1 g, 2 g vials)

Indications: Antibiotic: Oral 50–75 mg/kg/day q 8 h, intravenous 100 mg/kg/day q 6 h.

Adverse effects: Bone marrow suppression, grey baby syndrome at serum levels >50 mg/L.

2. Clindamycin Hydrochloride *(Lincosamide)*

Oral, intravenous; capsule (150,300 mg), injection (150 mg/mL)

Indications: Antibiotic: Oral 20–30 mg/kg/d div 6–8 h, Intravenous 20–40 mg/kg/d q 6–8 h.

3. Colistin Sulfate *(Polymyxin)*

Oral; suspension (25 mg/5 mL)

Indications: Antibiotic: 5–15 mg/kg/day q 6–8 h.

Adverse effects: Nephrotoxic, neurotoxic.

4. Colistimethate Sodium *(Colistin: Polymyxin E)*

Intravenous, intramuscular

Indications: Antibiotic: 2.5–5 mg/kg/day q 6–12 h IV of colistin base (1 mg of colistin base = 2.67 colistemethate sodium = 33,333 IU of colistemethate sodium). *Ventriculitis in neonates* may additionally be given intrathecally or intraventricularly as 2000 IU/kg/day.

Adverse effects: Nephrotoxic, neurotoxic.

5. Doxycycline *(Tetracycline)*

Oral; tablet (100 mg, 200 mg), syrup (25 mg, 50 mg/5 mL)

Indications: Antibiotic: 5 mg/kg/day q 12 h.

Adverse effects: GI symptoms, photosensitivity, hemolytic anemia, rash, skin manifestation, increased ICT.

Contraindications: Not recommended for children less than 8 years due to risk of tooth enamel hypoplasia.

6. Imipenem–Cilastatin *(Carbapenem)*

Intravenous, intramuscular; vials (250 mg, 500 mg)

Indications: Antibiotic: 60–100 mg/kg/day q 6 h.

Adverse effects: Pruritis, urticaria, GI symptoms, seizures, dizziness, hypotension, elevated LFTs, blood dyscrasias.

Remarks: It is the drug of choice for extended spectrum beta-lactamase producing microorganisms (ESBL).

7. Linezolid *(Oxazolidinone)*

Oral, intravenous; tablet (300 mg, 600 mg), injection (600 mg/300 mL)

Indications: Antibiotic: 10 mg/kg/dose q 12 h PO.

Adverse effects: Thrombocytopenia, diarrhea, nausea, vomiting, taste disturbances, oral thrush.

8. Meropenem *(Carbapenem)*

Intravenous; vials (500 mg, 1000 mg)

Indications: Sepsis: 60 mg/kg/day q 8 h. *Meningitis:* 120 mg/kg/day q 8 h. *Neonatal sepsis:* 20 mg/kg/dose q 12 h.

Adverse effects: Nausea, vomiting, rash, deranged liver enzymes.

9. Nitrofurantoin *(Nitrofuran)*

Oral; tablet (50 mg, 100 mg), syrup (25 mg/5 mL)

Indications: Antibiotic: 5–7 mg/kg/day q 6–8 h with meals, PO. Prophylaxis for UTI: 1–2 mg/kg/day HS.

Adverse effects: Nausea, hypersensitivity, vomiting, cholestatic jaundice, polyneuropathy and hemolytic anemia.

Contraindications: Avoid in G-6-PD deficiency.

10. Polymyxin

Oral, intravenous; injection (500,000 IU per vial, 1 mg = 10,000 IU)

Indications: Antibiotic for enteric infections: 5–15 mg/kg/day q 8 h PO. Systemic infections: 1.5–2.5 mg/kg/day q 12 h IV.

Meningitis/ventriculitis: 4 mg/kg/day q 8 h IV. Ventriculitis in neonates: May be additionally administered intrathecally or intraventricularly in a dose of 40,000 IU on alternate days for 7 days OR 20,000 IU once daily for 3 days followed by 25,000 IU on alternate days.

Adverse effects: Nephrotoxicity, drowsiness, dizziness, hypersensitivity, pain at injection site, neurotoxicity.

Contraindications: Avoid use with other neuromuscular relaxants or blockers.

11. Teicoplanin

Intravenous; vial (200 mg, 400 mg)

Indications: Antibiotic: 10 mg/kg/dose q 12 h for 3 doses followed by 10 mg/kg/dose 24 h.

Adverse effects: Fever, chills, allergic reactions, GI disturbances, headache, dizziness, "red-man" syndrome, disturbances in liver enzymes, renal impairment, ototoxicity, blood dyscrasias.

12. Trimethoprim–Sulfamethoxazole

Oral, Intravenous; Syrup (trimethoprim 40 mg, sulfamethoxazole 200 mg/5 mL), tablet (trimethoprim 20 mg/80 mg sulfamethoxazole 100 mg/400 mg)

Indications: Antibiotic: 5–8 mg/kg/day of trimethoprim q 12 h, 20–50 mg/kg/d of sulfamethoxazole q 12 h. Typhoid fever: 10 mg/kg/d q 12 h of trimethoprim. *Pneumocystis carinii* pneumonia: 20 mg/kg/d q 6–8 h of trimethoprim.

Adverse effects: Bleeding, rash, abdominal pain, fever, sore throat, cough, diarrhea.

Contraindications: Contraindicated if allergic to any ingredient in sulfamethoxazole/trimethoprim or to any other sulfonamide. Avoid in G-6-PD deficiency.

13. Vancomycin Hydrochloride

Intravenous, oral; vials (500 mg, 1 g), capsule (125 mg)

Indications: Sepsis: 10 mg/kg/dose q 6 h IV infusion. Meningitis: 15 mg/kg/dose q 6 h IV infusion. Pseudo-membranous enterocolitis: 40–50 mg/kg/day q 6–8 h PO.

Adverse effects: Nephrotoxicity, ototoxicity, red-man syndrome (flushing, hypotension, erythema), urticaria, thrombophlebitis, blood dyscrasia (neutropenia and thrombocytopenia), eosinophilia.

Remarks: Monitor renal functions, blood counts and auditory functions. Special precautions while giving with other nephrotoxic drugs like loop diuretics, aminoglycosides, amphotericin B, colistin and polymyxin B.

22.6 ANTICONVULSANTS

1. ACTH

Intramuscular, subcutaneous; vial (25, 40 units/mL), gel (40, 80 U/mL)

Indications: Infantile spasm and west syndrome: 20–40 units SC/IM daily for 4 weeks tapered over next 2 weeks.

Adverse effects: Hypersensitivity, side effects similar to steroids.

Contraindications: Similar to steroids.

2. Carbamazepine *(Dibenzazepine)*

Oral; tablet (200, 400 mg), syrup (100 mg/5 mL)

Indications: Partial, tonic-clonic, atonic, akinetic epilepsy, mesial temporal lobe epilepsy syndrome, trigeminal neuralgia, postherpetic neuralgia: 10–30 mg/kg/day q 8 h, PO. Initiate therapy at 30–50% of initial dose and increase over 5–7 days.

Adverse effects: Sedation, diplopia, Stevens-Johnson syndrome, urinary retention, aplastic anemia, liver dysfunction.

Remarks: Adjust dose in renal impairment. It may decrease activity of phenytoin, benzodiazepines, valproate and ethosuximide.

3. Clobazam *(Benzodiazepine)*

Oral; tablet (5, 10, 20 mg)

Indications: As an add on drug in complex partial, generalized tonic-clonic, generalized tonic, absence, myoclonic, atonic and Lennox-Gastaut syndrome: 0.3–1 mg/kg/day HS or divided in two doses. Febrile seizure prophylaxis: 0.5 mg/kg/dose 12 h for 48 h.

Adverse effects: Drowsiness, ataxia, constipation, insomnia, aggressive behavior.

Contraindications: Avoid in children below 3 years.

4. Clonazepam *(Benzodiazepine)*

Oral; tablet (0.25, 0.5, 1, 2 mg)

Indications: Atonic, akinetic epilepsy, resistant absence attacks, myoclonic seizures, infantile spasms and Lennox-Gastaut syndrome: Initially 0.01–0.03 mg/kg/24 h q 8–12 h, increase by 0.25–0.5 mg/24 h every 3–5 days to a maximum of 0.2 mg/kg/day.

Remarks: Therapeutic levels 20–80 ng/mL. Caution: Tachyphylaxis.

Contraindications: Contraindicated in severe liver disease and angle closure glaucoma.

Adverse effects: Drowsiness, thrombocytopenia, leucopenia, increased bronchial secretions.

5. Diazepam *(Benzodiazepine)*

Oral, intravenous, rectal; tablet (2.5, 5 mg), syrup (2 mg/5 mL), ampoule (5 mg/mL)

Indications: Status epilepticus: Intravenous: 0.2–0.5 mg/kg/dose, repeat at 3–5 min if needed (for 2–3 doses); maximum total dose < 5 years: 5 mg, > 5 years: 10 mg; per-rectal: 0.3–0.5 mg/kg/dose. Antianxiety, sedation, and muscle relaxation: Oral 0.1–0.3 mg/kg/day q 4–8 h adjusted according to clinical response. Neonatal tetanus: 0.5–5 mg/kg/dose IV q 2–4 h.

Adverse effects: Hypotension, respiratory depression.

Antidote: Flumazenil can revert sedation but not respiratory depression. 0.01 mg/kg IV (maximum 0.2 mg), then 0.005–0.01 mg/kg/min; maximum cumulative dose: 1 mg; may repeat after 20 min; maximum 3 mg/h.

6. Fosphenytoin *(Hydantoin)*

Intravenous; vial (50 mgPE/mL)

Indications: As substitute for oral phenytoin where intravenous phenytoin is not available/possible. Used in seizures occurring during neurosurgery, status epilepticus: Loading 15–20 mg/kg PE (not to exceed 3 mg PE/kg/min), maintenance dose 4–6 mg PE/kg/d IV/IM.

Adverse effects: Ataxia, rash, nystagmus, slurring of speech, tinnitus.

Remarks: 1.5 mg fosphenytoin = 1 mg phenytoin = 1 mg phenytoin equivalent (PE).

7. Gabapentin

Oral; capsules (300, 400 mg)

Indications: Add on therapy for partial seizures: 15–35 mg/kg/day q 8 h. Can increase over several days to 50 mg/kg/day.

Adverse effects: Somnolence, dizziness, ataxia, fatigue, nystagmus.

Contraindications: Adjust dose in renal impairment.

8. Lamotrigine

Oral; Tablet (5, 25, 50, 100 mg)

Indications: Partial seizures, generalized seizures, atypical absence, atonic generalized, tonic-clonic seizures: Started in low dose to lessen incidence of rash. Start at 0.6 mg/kg/day q 12–24 h for initial 2 weeks, followed by 1.2 mg/kg/day the next for 2 weeks followed by 5–15 mg/kg/day q 12 h. Maximum dose: 15 mg/kg/day or 400 mg/day.

Adverse effects: Ataxia, blurred vision, diplopia, dizziness, headache, rhinitis, rash, fever. *Contraindications:* Dose should be 1/4th in patients taking valproate.

9. Lorazepam *(Benzodiazepine)*

Oral, intravenous, intramuscular, per rectal; Tablet (1 mg, 2 mg), ampoule (2 mg/mL, 10 mg/mL).

Indications: Uncontrolled status epilepticus, anxiety and insomnia. Status epilepticus: 0.05–0.2 mg/kg/dose (maximum 4 mg) over 2–5 min IV or per rectal, may repeat after 10–15 min.

Adverse effects: Drowsiness, dizziness, blurred vision, muscle weakness, nausea, rash.

Remarks: Duration of action is longer than diazepam.

10. Midazolam *(Benzodiazepine)*

Intravenous, intramuscular, buccal; Vial (1 mg/mL in 5 mL and 10 mL vials, 5 mg/mL in 1 mL ampoule)

Indications: For status epilepticus, sedation during mechanical ventilation.

Status epilepticus: 0.2 mg/kg IV or IM bolus followed by 0.1–0.2 mg/kg/h. Sedation: Newborn-0.05–0.15 mg/kg q 1–2 h or 0.15–0.5 µg/kg/min as continuous infusion, children-0.05–0.2 mg/kg/dose q 1–2 h or 1–2 µg/kg/min as continuous infusion.

Adverse effects: Respiratory depression, hypotension, drowsiness.

11. Phenobarbitone Sodium

Intravenous, oral; Syrup (20 mg/5 mL), tablets (30, 60 mg), ampoule (200 mg/mL)

Indications: Neonatal seizures, tonic-clonic, akinetic, and partial seizures, may be used in febrile seizures: Loading dose 15–20 mg/kg IV over 15–20 min @ 1 mg/kg/min as slow IV bolus, may administer additional bolus 5 mg/kg/dose every 15–30 min up to a maximum of 30 mg/kg. Maintenance dose PO, IV in neonates: 3–5 mg/kg/day q 12 h, infants: 5–6 mg/kg/day q 12–24 h, Children (1–5 years) 6–8 mg/kg/day q 12–24 h, children (5–12 years) 4–6 mg/kg/day q 12–24 h, children (>12 years) 1–3 mg/kg/day q 12–24 h.

Adverse effects: Drowsiness, hypotension, respiratory depression, megaloblastic anemia, apnea, hepatitis.

Contraindications: Porphyria, severe respiratory disease with dyspnea or obstruction. Use with caution in hepatic or renal disease.

Remarks: Therapeutic levels: 15–40 µg/mL. Half-life varies with age: Neonates 45–100 h, infants 20–133 h, children 37–73 h.

12. Phenytoin Sodium

Intravenous, oral; tablet (50 mg, 100 mg), syrup (30 mg/5 mL), suspension (125 mg/5 mL), injection (25 mg/mL, 2 mL)

Indications: Tonic-clonic, atonic, akinetic, partial epilepsy: Loading dose: 15–20 mg/kg slow IV @ 1 mg/kg/min (IV dose should be diluted in normal saline and not dextrose, given slowly under cardiac monitoring). Maintenance dose-neonates: 5 mg/kg/24 h q 8–12 h, children: 5–8 mg/kg/24 h divided 12–24 h.

Adverse effects: Nystagmus, hypotension, Stevens-Johnson syndrome, rash, hepatitis, gingival hyperplasia, blood dyscrasia.

Contraindications: Porphyria and heart block.

13. Prednisolone

Oral; tablets (5 mg, 10 mg, 20 mg), syrup (5 mg/5 mL)

Indications: Infantile spasms: 2 mg/kg/day q 12 h × 2–6 weeks, taper over the next 4–12 weeks.

Adverse effects: Edema, hypertension, Cushing syndrome, peptic ulcer, hypothalamic pituitary-adrenal axis suppression.

Contraindications: Immunodeficiency, acute severe infection.

14. Pyridoxine

Intravenous, intramuscular, oral; tablet (25, 50, 100 mg), injection (100 mg/mL)

Indications: Pyridoxine dependent seizures: Loading 50–100 mg PO/IV followed by 50–100 mg/24 h PO. Drug induced neuritis: 1 mg/kg/24 h daily. Dietary deficiency: 5–15 mg/24 h for 3–4 weeks then half dose daily.

Adverse effects: Increased liver enzymes, decreased serum folic acid levels. Large intravenous doses can cause seizure.

15. Topiramate

Oral; tablet (25, 50, 100 mg)

Indications: As add on therapy for refractory partial seizures, primary generalized tonic clonic, absence seizures, Lennox-Gastaut syndrome: 1–3 mg/kg/24 h oral HS, increase by 1–3 mg/kg/day q 12 h in next 1–2 weeks till 5–10 mg/kg/day.

Adverse effects: Ocular side effects, oligohidrosis, hyperthermia, metabolic acidosis, suicidal tendency, neuropsychiatric disturbances.

Contraindications: Glaucoma.

16. Valproate Sodium

Oral, intravenous; tablet (200, 500 mg), syrup (200 mg/5 mL), injection (100 mg/mL)

Indications: Broad-spectrum anticonvulsant: Initial dose 10–15 mg/kg/day q 8–12 h, increase by 5–10 mg/kg every week up to maximum 60 mg/kg/day.

Adverse effects: Heptotoxicity, abdominal pain, alopecia, nausea, Reye's like syndrome, thrombocytopenia, tremor, vomiting, diarrhea, teratogen.

Contraindications: Avoid in children less than 2 years due to risk of hepatic failure.

Remarks: Therapeutic levels 50–100 µg/Ml.

17. Vigabatrin

Oral; tablet (500 mg)

Indications: Resistant partial seizures, infantile spasms due to tuberous sclerosis and Lennox-Gastaut syndrome: 20–40 mg/kg/day, maintenance 80–100 mg/kg/day q 8–12 h.

Adverse effects: Visual disturbances, arthralgia, confusion, depression, weight gain, cough, increase in seizures.

Contraindications: Children less than 3 months.

22.7 ANTIEMETICS

1. Chlorpromazine *(Phenothiazine)*

Oral, injection; Tablet (10, 25, 50, 100 mg), extended-release capsules (30, 75, 150, 200, 300 mg), syrup (10 mg/5 mL), suppository (25, 100 mg), injection (25 mg/mL)

Indications: Antiemetic: IM or IV 2.5–4 mg/kg/day q 6–8 h (Maximum dose: < 5 years: 40 mg/24 h, 5–12 years: 75 mg/24 h), PO 2.5–6 mg/kg/day q 4–6 h, PR 1 mg/kg/dose q 6–8 h.

Adverse effects: Drowsiness, jaundice, lowered seizure threshold, extrapyramidal/anticholinergic symptoms, hypotension, arrhythmias, neuroleptic malignant syndrome, bone marrow suppression.

Contraindications: Do not use simultaneously with carbamazepine.

2. Dimenhydrinate *(Antihistaminic)*

Oral, injection (intravenous, intramuscular); Tablet (50 mg), injection (50 mg/mL)

Indications: Antiemetic: 5 mg/kg/day q 6–8 h PO/IV/IM (maximum dose for children 2–6 years: 75 mg/day, 6–12 years: 150 mg/day).

Adverse effects: Drowsiness and anticholinergic side effects.

Contraindications: Not recommended in children < 2 years.

Remarks: Use recommended in management of prolonged vomiting of known etiology.

3. Domperidone *(Dopamine antagonist)*

Oral; Tablet (10 mg), syrup (5 mg/5 mL)

Indications: Antiemetic: 0.2–0.4 mg/kg/dose 6–8 hourly.

Adverse effects: Can cause gynecomastia in males and galactorrhea in females.

Contraindications: Prolactinoma, intestinal obstruction, prolonged QT interval.

4. Granisetron *(5-HT₃ Receptor antagonist)*

Intravenous, oral; Tablets (1 mg), injection (1 mg/mL)

Indications: Chemotherapy induced nausea and vomiting (CINV): Children 2 years and adults 10–20 mcg/kg/dose IV over 15–60 min before chemotherapy; may repeat 2–3 times after chemotherapy. Alternately, single dose of 40 mcg/kg/dose 15–60 min before starting chemotherapy. PO in adults 1 mg BD or 2 mg OD, started 1 h prior to chemotherapy.

Adverse effects: Hypertension, hypotension, arrhythmia, agitation, insomnia.

Contraindications: Use with caution in liver disease.

5. Metoclopramide Hydrochloride *(Prokinetic agent)*

Oral, intravenous; Tablet (10 mg), syrup (5 mg/5 mL), ampoule (5 mg/mL)

Indications: GER or GI dysmotility: Neonate- 0.03–0.1 mg/kg/dose 8 hourly, Children- 0.1–0.2 mg/kg/dose 8 hourly. Antiemetic effect: 1–2 mg/kg/dose q 2–6 h IV/IM/PO. CINV: 2–3 mg/kg/dose before and after chemotherapy.

Adverse effects: Headache, anxiety, depression, extra-pyramidal symptoms.

Remarks: Premedicate with diphenhydramine to reduce extrapyramidal side effects.

6. Ondansetron Hydrochloride *(5-HT₃ Receptor antagonist)*

Oral, intravenous, intramuscular; Tablet (4, 8 mg), syrup (4 mg/5 mL), ampoule (2 mg/mL)

Indications: Antiemetic: 0.15 mg/kg/dose q 6–8 h IV, 0.1–0.2 mg/kg/dose q 6–8 h PO. CINV: 0.15–0.45 mg/kg/dose at 30 min before and 4 and 8 h after emetogenic drugs.

Adverse effects: Side effects include bronchospasm, tachycardia, hypokalemia, seizures, constipation or diarrhea, transient increase in liver enzymes.

Contraindications: Avoid in QT syndrome.

7. Prochlorperazine *(Phenothiazine)*

Oral, intramuscular; tablets (5, 25 mg), injection (12.5 mg/mL)

Indications: Antiemetic: For >2 years old or body weight >10 kg, 0.4 mg/kg/day q 6–8 h oral. IM dose is half.

Adverse effects: Extrapyramidal symptoms or orthostatic hypotension can occur.

Contraindications: Avoid in children; do not use intravenously.

8. Promethazine Hydrochloride *(Antihistaminic: phenothiazine)*

Oral, intravenous, intramuscular, per-rectal; Tablet (10, 25 mg), elixir (5 mg/5 mL), ampoule (2 mL, 50 mg)

Indications: Motion sickness: 0.5 mg/kg/dose q 12 h PO; First dose 30 min before starting. Sedation/antiemetic: 0.25–1 mg/kg/dose q 4–6 h, PO, IM, IV or PR.

Adverse effects: Sedation, respiratory depression, blurred vision.

Contraindications: Avoid intravenous use, give slowly if required.

22.8 ANTIHELMINTHICS

1. Albendazole

Oral; syrup (200 mg/5 mL), tablet (200 mg, 400 mg).

Indications: For pinworms, roundworms, or hookworms: single oral dose of 200 mg in children aged 1–2 years and single oral dose of 400 mg in children > 2 years, to be repeated after 2 weeks for roundworms. Strongyloidosis, *H. nana* infection and taeniasis: 400 mg OD for 3 days. Giardiasis: 400 mg OD for 5 days. Trichinosis: 400 mg OD for 5 days. Neurocysticercosis: 15 mg/kg/d for 2–4 weeks with corticosteroids for 5 days to reduce edema. Albendazole is started on day 3 of steroids. Hydatid cyst: 400 mg BD for 4 weeks, to be taken with fatty meals, a total of 3 cycles repeated every 14 days for eradication of hydatid cysts.

Adverse effects: Nausea, vomiting, headache.

Contraindications: Albendazole is contraindicated in ocular and intraventricular cysticercosis.

2. Diethylcarbamazine

Oral; tablet (50 mg, 100 mg), syrup (120 mg/5 mL)

Indications: Filariasis: 6 mg/kg/day q 8h, oral, for 3–4 weeks; repeat course after 6 months. Tropical pulmonary eosinophilia and visceral larva migrans: 10 mg/kg/day, 8 h, oral for 4 weeks. Loeffler's pneumonia: 15 mg/kg/day, single daily dose, for 4 days.

Adverse effects: Fever, chills, nausea, joint pain, muscle ache, visual disturbances, itching, facial swelling, headaches.

Contraindications: Previous history of heart problems, gastrointestinal problems, and allergy.

3. Ivermectin

Oral; Tablet (6 mg)

Indications: Cutaneous larva migrans, scabies: 0.2 mg/kg, single oral dose. Strongyloidiasis: 0.2 mg/kg PO for 2 days. Onchocerciasis: 0.15 mg/kg oral single dose.

Adverse effects like diarrhea, nausea, vomiting, pruritis, dizziness, drowsiness.

Contraindications: Contraindicated in children <5 years age or weighing <15 kg.

4. Levamisole

Oral; Tablet (50 mg, 150 mg), syrup (50 mg/5 mL)

Indications: Ascariasis: 2 mg/kg/day PO single dose. Hookworm infestation: 50 mg q 6 h (4 doses); repeat course after 7 days.

Adverse effects: Leukopenia, agranulocytosis, thrombocytopenia, abdominal pain, nausea, headache, convulsions.

Contraindications: Pre-existing blood disorders, pregnancy and lactation and severe renal impairment.

5. Mebendazole

Oral; tablet (100 mg); suspension (100 mg/5 mL)

Indications: Ascariasis: 100 mg twice a day × 3 days. Enterobius infection: 100 mg single dose, repeat after 2 weeks. Tapeworms and mixed infections: 200 mg BD × 3 days; repeat course after 2–4 weeks. Hydatid cyst: 30 mg/kg/day q 8 h, oral, for 4 weeks.

Adverse effects: Diarrhea, abdominal cramp, rash, deranged liver enzymes.

Contraindications: Not recommended in children below 2 years. Should be taken with food.

6. Niclosamide

Oral; tablet (500 mg).

Indications: Taenia saginata, Taenia solium, Diphyllobothrium latum and *H. nana*: 1 g empty stomach followed by another dose after 1 hour, a brisk purgative is given after 2 hours of last dose. Dwarf tapeworm: Single dose as above followed by half dose for the next 6 days, use half of this dose in children <6 years.

Adverse effects: Nausea, vomiting, abdominal pain, constipation, itching, dizziness, skin rash, drowsiness, perianal itching, or an unpleasant taste.

7. Nitazoxanide

Oral; Tablet (100 mg, 500 mg); syrup 100 mg/5 mL

Indications: For ascariasis, Dwarf tapeworm: 100 mg BD × 3 d (2 to 3 years), 200 mg BD × 3 days (4 to 11 years), 500 mg BD × 3 d (>12 years).

Adverse effects: Abdominal pain, diarrhea, nausea, anorexia, flatulence, fever, pruritis.

8. Piperazine

Oral; tablet (500 mg), elixir (750 mg/5 mL)

Indications: Ascariasis: 75 mg/kg/day PO single dose on two consecutive nights (maximum dose 3.5 g/d). Enterobius: 65 mg/kg/day PO single dose × 7 days (maximum dose 2.5 g/d).

Adverse effects: Colicky pain, urticaria, bronchospasm.

Contraindications: Children with epilepsy due to risk of precipitating seizures.

9. Praziquantel

Oral; tablet (500 mg, 600 mg)

Indications: Neurocysticercosis: 50 mg/kg/day q 8 h, oral × 15 day with steroids to counter the raised intracranial tension. Tapeworm: 5–10 mg/kg, single dose. Schistosomiasis: 20 mg/kg/dose PO 8–12 hourly × 1 day.

Liverfluke: 25 mg/kg/dose q 8 h × 2 days. *H. nana*: 25 mg/kg PO single dose.

Adverse effects: Rash, headache, drowsiness, hyperglycemia.

Contraindications: Ocular and intraventricular cysticercosis.

10. Pyrantel Pamoate

Oral; tablet (250 mg), suspension (250 mg/5 mL)

Indications: Antihelminthic: 11 mg/kg single dose (maximum 1 g), repeat after 2 weeks. Hookworm: 11 mg/kg/dose, once daily × 3 days.

Adverse effects: Increased liver enzymes, abdominal cramps, rash.

Contraindications: Avoid in liver disease.

22.9 ANTIHISTAMINICS

1. Astemizole

Oral; tablet (10 mg), syrup (5 mg/5 mL)

Indications: Antihistaminic: 0.2 mg/kg OD (< 6 years), 5 mg OD (6–12 years), 10 mg OD (> 12 years).

Adverse effects: Can cause QT prolongation and life-threatening arrhythmias if given with drugs like erythromycin, itraconazole, ketoconazole, cimetidine, ciprofloxacin.

Contraindications: Avoid in liver disease.

Remarks: Avoid abrupt discontinuation. It has a long elimination half-life and is less sedating.

2. Cetirizine Dihydrochloride *(H1 antagonist)*

Oral; tablet (5 mg, 10 mg), syrup (5 mg/5 mL)

Indications: Antihistaminic: 2.5 mg BD or 5 mg OD (2–6 years), 5 to 10 mg OD (>6 years).

Adverse effects: Sedation, dryness of mouth, GI upset, headache.

Contraindications: Avoid in children < 2 years.

3. Chlorpheniramine Maleate *(H1 antagonist)*

Oral, parenteral (IV/IM/SC); Tablet (2, 4 mg), syrup (2 mg/5 mL), injection (10 mg/mL)

Indications: Antihistaminic: 0.35 mg/kg/day PO q 4–6 h or dose based on age bands as 1 mg/dose PO q 4–6 h, max 6 mg/24 h (2–6 years), 2 mg/dose PO q 4–6 h, max 12 mg/24 h (6–12 years), 4 mg/dose q PO 4–6 h, max 24 mg/24 h (>12 years). IV/IM/SC 5–20 mg once, max 40 mg/24 h.

Adverse effects: Sedation, dryness of mouth, blurred vision, urinary retention.

Contraindications: To be used with caution in children with asthma.

4. Cyproheptadine Hydrochloride *(H1 antagonist)*

Oral; tablet (2 mg, 4 mg), syrup (2 mg/5 mL)

Indications: Antihistaminic: 0.25–0.5 mg/kg/day q 8–12 h.

Adverse effects: Sedation, dryness of mouth, blurred vision, urinary retention.

Contraindications: Neonates and children suffering from asthma, glaucoma, or GI/GU obstruction, and therapy with MAO inhibitors.

5. Desloratadine *(H1 inverse antagonist)*

Oral; tablet (5 mg)

Indications: Antihistaminic: 1 mg OD (2–5 years), 2.5 mg OD (6–12 years).

Adverse effects: Dryness of mouth, tiredness, headache, tachycardia, sore throat.

6. Diphenhydramine Hydrochloride *(H1 antagonist)*

Oral, intravenous; Tablet (25 mg, 50 mg), syrup (12.5 mg/5 mL), injection (50 mg/mL, 10 mg/mL)

Indications: 1 mg/kg/dose PO q 6 h, max 300 mg/day.

Adverse effects: Nausea, vomiting, drowsiness, blurred vision.

Contraindications: Contraindicated in neonates, avoid in young children.

Remarks: Phenothiazine toxicity: 1 mg/kg intravenous.

7. Fexofenadine Hydrochloride *(H1 antagonist)*

Oral; tablet (30 mg, 120 mg, 180 mg), syrup (30 mg/5 mL)

Indications: Antihistaminic: 15 mg BD (6 months–2 years), 30 mg BD (2–12 years), 60 mg BD or 120 mg OD (>12 years).

Adverse effects: GI disturbances, drowsiness, fatigue.

Contraindications: Renal impairment.

8. Hydroxyzine Hydrochloride *(H1 antagonist)*

Oral, intramuscular; tablet (10 mg, 25 mg), syrup (10 mg/5 mL), injection (25 mg/mL)

Indications: Antihistaminic: 0.6 mg/kg/dose q 6 h PO, 0.5–1 mg/kg/dose q 6 h intramuscular.

Adverse effects: Dry mouth, drowsiness, tremor, convulsions, blurred vision, hypotension.

Contraindications: Do not use intravenously.

9. Loratadine *(H1 antagonist)*

Oral; tablet (5 mg, 10 mg), syrup (5 mg/5 mL)

Indications: Antihistaminic: 5 mg/24 h (< 30 kg), 10 mg/24 h (> 30 kg).

Adverse effects: Diarrhea, nervousness, fatigue, stomatits, rash, ear ache, viral infection, flu-like symptoms, dry mouth, headache, insomnia, somnolence.

Contraindications: Avoid in children with phenylketonuria

10. Pheniramine Maleate *(H1 antagonist)*

Oral, intramuscular, intravenous; tablet (25 mg, 50 mg), syrup (15 mg/mL), injection (22.75 mg/mL)

Indications: Antihistaminic: 0.5 mg/kg/day q 8 h PO, IM or IV.

Adverse effects: Dry mouth, constipation, CNS depression, bradycardia.

11. Promethazine Hydrochloride *(H1 antagonist)*

Oral, intramuscular, intravenous; tablet (10 mg, 25 mg), syrup (5 mg/mL), injection (25 mg/mL)

Indications: Allergy: 0.1 mg/kg/dose q 6–8 h PO/IM. Sedation/antiemetic: 1–2 mg/kg/single dose PO/IM.

Adverse effects: Sedation, respiratory depression, blurred vision.

Contraindications: Avoid intravenous use, give slowly if required.

22.10 ANTIHYPERTENSIVES

1. Amiloride *(Potassium sparing diuretic)*

Oral; tablet (2.5, 5 mg)

Indications: Hypertension: 0.4–0.625 mg/kg/day q 12–24 h.

Adverse effect: Hyperkalemia; rarely used alone because of risk of hyperkalemia. It has mild antihypertensive activity, used concomitantly with a thiazide diuretic.

Contraindication: Do not use in renal failure.

2. Amlodipine *(Calcium channel blocker)*

Oral, tablet (5 mg)

Indications: Antihypertensive: Starting dose 0.05 to 0.1 mg/kg/day, may increase to 0.3 to 0.4 mg/kg/day.

Adverse effects: Palpitations, dizziness, flushing, edema, dizziness.

Remarks: Titration should be done slowly, at 1 to 2 weeks intervals given once daily.

3. Atenolol *(Cardioselective beta-blocker)*

Oral; tablet (50, 100 mg)

Indications: Antihypertensive: 0.8–1.5 mg/kg/day (maximum 2 mg/kg/day).

Adverse effects: Hypotension, second or third degree block, lethargy, dizziness.

Contraindications: Pulmonary edema, cardiogenic shock.

Remarks: Should not be stopped suddenly, taper over 2 weeks.

4. Captopril *(Angiotensin converting enzyme inhibitor)*

Oral; tablet (12.5, 25, 50 mg)

Indications: Hypertension: Neonates-0.1–0.4 mg/kg/day PO q 6–24 h, children-initial dose: 0.3–0.5 mg/kg/dose q 8 h; titrate upward if needed, maximum 6 mg/kg/day q 8–12 h.

Contraindications: Use with caution in collagen vascular disease. Adjust dose in renal failure.

Adverse effect: May cause rash, proteinuria, neutropenia, angioedema, dysgeusia, hypotension and hyperkalemia.

5. Carvedilol *(Nonselective beta-blocker with alpha-blocking action)*

Oral; tablet (3.125, 6.25, 12.5, 25 mg)

Indications: Antihypertensive: 0.05 mg/kg/dose BD, increase every 2 weeks by 0.05 mg/kg/dose for the first increment and then 0.1 mg/kg/dose over 3 months till max 0.35 mg/kg/dose BD (Maximum: 25 mg BD).

Adverse effects: Hypotension, dizziness, AV block, arrhythmia.

Contraindications: To be used with caution in hepatic/renal disease, hyperthyroidism, diabetes, heart disease.

6. Clonidine Hydrochloride *(Central alpha-adrenergic agonist)*

Oral, injection, transdermal; tablet (100, 200, 300 μg), injection (100 μg/mL), transdermal patch (0.1, 0.2, 0.3 mg/24 h × 7 days)

Indications: Hypertension: 1–2 μg/kg/dose q 6 h; maximum 25 μg/kg/day.

Adverse effects: Dry mouth, dizziness, drowsiness, constipation, fatigue.

Remarks: Do not discontinue abruptly, taper gradually over 1 week.

7. Diazoxide *(Potassium channel activator)*

Injection, oral; ampoule (15 mg/mL), syrup (50 mg/mL), capsule (50 mg).

Indications: Hypertensive crisis: 1–3 mg/kg/dose IV up to maximum of 150 mg/dose, repeat q 5–15 min, then q 4–24 h. Hyperinsulinemic hypoglycemia: 8–15 mg/kg/24 h q 8–12 h (< 1 year), 3–8 mg/kg/day q 8–12 h (> 1 year).

Adverse effects: Hyponatremia, salt and water retention, GI disturbances, rash, ketoacidosis, hypertrichosis, arrhythmias.

8. Enalapril Maleate *(Angiotensin converting enzyme inhibitor)*

Oral; tablet (2.5, 5 mg)

Indications: Antihypertensive: Oral-0.1–0.5 mg/kg/day q 12–24 h, intravenous: 0.005–0.01 mg/kg/dose q 8–24 h.

Adverse effects: Nausea, diarrhea, headache, dizziness, hyperkalemia, hypoglycemia, hypersensitivity, cough and hypotension.

Contraindications: Bilateral renal artery stenosis.

9. Esmolol Hydrochloride *(Beta-1 selective adrenergic blocker)*

Intravenous; injection (10, 250 mg/mL)

Indications: Hypertension: 100–500 μg/kg IV over 1 min loading dose followed by maintenance dose 25–100 μg/kg/min infusion, may increase rate every 10 mins by 25–50 μg/kg/min up to 500 μg/kg/min.

Adverse effects: Congestive heart failure, hypotension, nausea, vomiting, bronchospasm.

Contraindications: Avoid in heart block first degree, heart failure, cardiogenic shock, sinus bradycardia.

10. Hydralazine Hydrochloride *(Arterial vasodilator)*

Oral, injection; tablet (10, 25, 50, 100 mg), oral liquid (1.25, 2, 4 mg/mL), ampoule (20 mg/mL)

Indications: Hypertensive crisis: 0.1–0.2 mg/kg/dose IM or IV q 4–6 h, maximum 20 mg/dose. *Chronic hypertension:* Start at 0.75–1 mg/kg/day PO q 6–12 h (maximum 25 mg/dose), can increase if needed to 5 mg/kg/day for infants and 7.5 mg/kg/day for older children.

Adverse effects: May cause reflex tachycardia, headache, hypotension, nausea, diarrhea, peripheral neuropathy.

Contraindications: Use with caution in severe renal and cardiac disease. Lupus like syndrome may be seen in patients with renal impairment.

11. Labetalol *(Adrenergic agonist (alpha and beta))*

Oral, intravenous; tablet (50, 100 mg), ampoule (5 mg/mL), suspension (10 mg/mL)

Indications: Hypertension: Oral 2 mg/kg/dose 12 h, maximum dose 40 mg/kg/d. *Hypertensive emergency:* IV 0.2–1 mg/kg/dose q 10 min, infusion 0.4–1 mg/kg/h to maximum of 3 mg/kg/h, can initiate with 0.2–1 mg/kg bolus, maximum 20 mg bolus.

Adverse effects: Blurred vision, dizziness, shortness of breath, tightness of chest.

Contraindications: Asthma, heart block, cardiogenic shock, pulmonary edema.

12. Methyldopa *(Alpha-2 receptor agonist)*

Oral, intravenous; tablet (250 mg), injection (50 mg/mL)

Indications: Hypertension: 5–40 mg/kg/day PO q 6–8 h. *Hypertensive crisis:* 2–4 mg/kg/dose IV to maximum of 5–10 mg/kg/dose IV 6–8 h.

Adverse effects: Positive Coombs test, GI disturbance, memory impairment, hepatitis, black tongue, orthostatic hypotension, fever, leukopenia and sedation.

Contraindications: Liver disease, pheochromocytoma, and depression.

13. Metoprolol *(Beta-1 receptor blocker)*

Oral; tablet (50,100 mg), injection (1 mg/mL)

Indications: Hypertension: Oral 1–5 mg/kg/day q 12 h, intravenous 0.1 mg/kg/dose

Adverse effects: Heart block, heart failure, bradyarrhythmias, dizziness, depression.

Contraindications: Congestive heart failure.

14. Minoxidil *(Direct vasodilator)*

Oral; tablet (2.5, 5, 10 mg)

Indications: Antihypertensive: Starting dose 0.2 mg/kg/day PO as single dose, increase by 0.1–0.2 mg/kg/day at 3-day intervals, can be increased till 5 mg/day.

Adverse effects: Can cause dizziness, CHF, pulmonary edema, pericardial effusion, Stevens-Johnson syndrome, leukopenia, and hypertrichosis (reversible).

Remarks: Usual effective dose: 0.25–1 mg/kg/day PO q 12–24 h. Maximum tolerated dose: 5 mg/kg/day or 50 mg/day.

15. Nifedipine *(Calcium channel blocker)*

Oral; Capsule (5, 10, 20 mg), tablet retard (20 mg), tablet (10 mg)

Indications: Hypertensive emergency/hypertension: 0.25–0.5 mg/kg/dose q 4–6 h (maximum 10 mg/dose). 300–500 µg/kg/dose sublingual for severe hypertension. *Hypertrophic cardiomyopathy:* 0.5–0.9 mg/kg/d q 6–8 h PO/SL.

Adverse effects: May cause hypotension, flushing, tachycardia, headache, dizziness and nausea.

Contraindications: Avoid concurrent beta blockers.

Remarks: For sublingual administration, capsule to be punctured and liquid expressed in mouth. Do not chew/crush sustained release tablets.

16. Propranolol *(Adrenergic blocking agent (beta blocker))*

Tablet (10, 40, 80 mg)

Indications: Hypertension: 0.5–1 mg/kg/day q 6–12 h, increase gradually if needed to a maximum 8 mg/kg/day.

Adverse effects: Hypoglycemia, hypotension, nausea, vomiting, depression, weakness, bronchospasm and heart block.

Contraindications: Avoid in bronchial asthma, heart block, congestive heart failure.

17. Sodium Nitroprusside *(Vasodilator)*

Intravenous; ampoule (50 mg/ampule)

Indications: Hypertensive crisis: 0.5–3 µg/kg/min as intravenous infusion, 50 mg dissolved in 1 liter of 5% dextrose to provide a concentration of 50 µg/mL.

Contraindications: Do not use in coarctation of aorta, arteriovenous shunts, raised intracranial tension, liver failure, congestive heart failure.

Adverse effects: Should not be used beyond 72 h as it gets converted to cyanide non-enzymatic mechanically and further to thiocyanate. Cyanide may result in methemoglobinemia and metabolic acidosis. Thiocyanate can cause seizures and psychosis.

18. Verapamil *(Calcium channel blocker)*

Oral, intravenous; tablet (40, 80, 120 mg), ampoule (2.5 mg/mL)

Indications: Hypertension: Oral 1–2 mg/kg/dose q 6–8 h, intravenous: 0.1–0.2 mg/kg/dose, give over 2–3 min under ECG monitoring.

Adverse effects: Bradycardia, AV block, heart failure, hypotension, constipation, flushing, nausea.

Contraindications: Hypersensitivity, cardiogenic shock, severe CHF, sick-sinus syndrome or AV block. Avoid in neonates due to a high-risk of heart block, apnea, bradycardia and hypotension. Do not use to treat SVT in infants.

Remarks: Antidote: calcium gluconate.

22.11 ANTIMALARIALS

1. Amodiaquine

Oral; tablet (200 mg base), suspension (150 mg base/5 mL)

Indications: Antimalarial: 10 mg/kg of base stat PO and then 5 mg/kg at 6 h, 24 h, 48 h, used in combination with artesunate.

Adverse effects: Hepatitis, agranulocytosis, peripheral neuropathy, corneal deposits.

2. Artemether *(Artemisin derivative)*

Oral, intramuscular; tablet (20 mg, 40 mg, 80 mg; in combination with lumefantrine), injection (80 mg/mL)

Indications: Severe and complicated malaria: 3.2 mg/kg IM on day 1 followed by 1.6 mg/kg daily for the next 6 days. *Uncomplicated P. falciparum malaria:* oral dose for fixed dose combination therapy (artemether 20 mg + lumefantrine 120 mg) is as 1 tablet BD for 3 days (5–14 kg), 2 tablet BD for 3 days (15–24 kg), 3 tablet BD for 3 days (25–34 kg), 4 tablet BD for 3 days (>34 kg).

Adverse effects: GI disturbances, agranulocytosis, bradycardia, first degree heart block.

Contraindications: Avoid use with other drugs known to prolong QT interval.

3. Artesunate *(Artemisin derivative)*

Intravenous, intramuscular, oral; vial (50 mg), tablet (50 mg, 100 mg, 200 mg) as part of artesunate combination therapy.

Indications: Oral 4 mg/kg/day OD for 3 days as part of artesunate combination therapy. *Severe and complicated malaria:* 2.4 mg/kg IV bolus or IM (loading dose) followed by 2.4 mg/kg IV or IM at 12 h and then OD for 6 days. *Chloroquine resistant malaria:* Artesunate 4 mg/kg OD × 3 days + sulfadoxine-pyrimethamine (25/1.25 mg/kg) on day 1, Artesunate 4 mg/kg OD × 3 days + mefloquine 25 mg/kg in two (15 +10) divided doses on day 2 and day 3 followed by single dose primaquine 0.75 mg/kg.

Adverse effects: Rash, agranulocytosis, first degree heart block, neurotoxicity, fever.

Remarks: The powder for injection should be reconstituted with 5% sodium bicarbonate and diluted in an equal volume of physiological saline or 5% (w/v) glucose. It should always be used immediately following reconstitution. If the solution is cloudy or a precipitate is present, the parenteral preparation should be discarded.

4. Chloroquine Phosphate

Oral; tablet 250(150 mg base), syrup (50 mg/5 mL)

Indications: Uncomplicated malaria: 10 mg/kg (base) followed by 5 mg/kg (base) after 6 h, 24 h and 48 h from first dose OR 10 mg/kg (base) followed by 10 mg/kg (base) after 24 h followed by 5 mg/kg (base) after 48 h from first dose.

Adverse effects: Nausea, vomiting, prolonged QT interval, blurred vision, increased liver enzymes, headache, vision abnormalities.

Remarks: To repeat dose if vomiting within 30 min of intake.

5. Lumefantrine

Oral; fixed dose combination with artemether (artemether 20 mg + lumefantrine 120 mg, artemether 40 mg + lumefantrine 240 mg).

Indications: Dose as mentioned under artemether.

6. Mefloquine Hydrochloride

Oral; tablet (250 mg)

Indications: Used as combination therapy with artesunate as 25 mg/kg divided as 15 mg/kg on day 1 and 10 mg/kg on day 2 OD. Used as single drug for prophylaxis as 3.5 mg/kg of base weekly.

Adverse effects: Co-administration of chloroquine with mefloquine increases the risk of seizures

Contraindications: Active depression, psychiatric disease, seizures.

7. Primaquine

Oral; tablet (2.5 mg, 7.5 mg, 15 mg)

Indications: Radical cure in P. vivax: 0.25 mg/kg OD for 14 days. *Gametocidal effect in P. falciparum:* 0.75 mg/kg single dose.

Adverse effects: Nausea, vomiting, pain abdomen, visual disturbances, headache.

Contraindications: Avoid in G6PD deficiency.

8. Pyrimethamine-sulfadoxine

Oral; tablet (25 mg pyrimethamine + 500 mg sulfadoxine), syrup (12.5 mg pyrimethamine+ 250 mg sulfadoxine/5 mL)

Indications: Chloroquine resistant uncomplicated P. falciparum malaria: 1.25 mg/kg pyrimethamine/25 mg/kg sulfadoxine as single dose with artesunate.

Adverse effects: Bone marrow suppression, glossitis, seizures, rash, photosensitivity.

Contraindications: Megaloblastic anemia.

9. Quinine Dihydrochloride

Intravenous; ampoule (300 mg/mL)

Indications: Severe malaria: Intravenous 20 mg/kg salt diluted in normal saline or 5% dextrose in a concentration of 1 mg/mL given as a loading dose over 4 h followed by 10 mg/kg/dose as in fusion over 4 h every 8 h for 7–10 days. Shift to oral therapy as soon as possible.

Adverse effects: Hypoglycemia, hypotension, cinchonism.

Remarks: Do not give rapidly or as bolus.

10. Quinine Sulfate

Oral; tablet (150, 300 mg salt)

Indications: Uncomplicated chloroquine resistant P. falciparum infections: Oral 10 mg/kg/dose of salt every 8 h. Used in combination with tetracycline (40 mg/kg/day q 6 h × 10 days), or clindamycin (20–40 mg/kg/day q 8 h × 3 days) or pyrimethamine (0.75 mg/kg/day q 12 h × 3 days), or sulfadiazine (150 mg/kg/day q 8 h × 6 days) to prevent drug resistance.

Adverse effects: Tinnitus, cinchonism, blurred vision, GI discomfort, nausea, vomiting.

Remarks: Do not crush the tablet. Do not eat empty stomach.

22.12 ANTIRETROVIRAL DRUGS

NUCLEOSIDE REVERSE TRANSCRIPTASE INHIBITORS (NRTIs)

1. Zidovudine (AZT/ZDV)

Oral, intravenous; capsules (100 mg), liquid (50 mg/5 mL), injection (10 mg/mL). Available also in combination with Lamivudine as combivir (tablets: 300 mg AZT + 150 mg 3TC). Daily dose 360 mg/m^2 to maximum 600 mg.

Indications: Antiretroviral: 12 mg/kg BD (4–9 kg), 9 mg/kg BD (<30 kg), 300 mg BD (>30 kg). Neonate 2 mg/kg/dose

QID PO or 1.5 mg/kg/dose QID IV over 60 min. Begin within 12 hours of birth and continue until 6 weeks of age.

Adverse effects: Side effects include anemia, neutropenia, headache, vomiting, neuropathy, anorexia, vomiting, hepatitis, lactic acidosis, myopathy.

2. Lamivudine (3TC)

Oral; tablets (150 mg, 300 mg), solution (5 mg/mL, 10 mg/mL).

Indications: Antiretroviral: 4 mg/kg/dose BID. Maximum 150 mg/dose. Available in fixed dose combination with lamivudine as combivir (300 mg AZT + 150 mg 3TC), or with abacavir (300 mg 3TC + 600 mg ABC), or both (150 mg 3TC + 300 mg AZT + 300 mg ABC).

Adverse effects: Common side effects are headache, fatigue, nausea, diarrhea, skin rash, pancreatitis, abdominal pain, peripheral neuropathy, decreased neutrophil count, and increased liver enzymes.

3. Stavudine (d4T)

Oral; capsules (15 mg, 20 mg, 30 mg, 40 mg), solution (1 mg/mL).

Indications: Antiretroviral: 1 mg/kg/dose BID. Maximum daily dose of 80 mg.

Adverse effects: Common side effects are headache, gastrointestinal discomfort, and rash. Peripheral neuropathy, pancreatitis, lactic acidosis, and raised liver enzymes may occur.

4. Didanosine (ddI)

Oral.

Indications: Antiretroviral: 180 mg/m^2/day divided into two doses. Maximum daily dose 400 mg.

Adverse effects: Side effects include headache, diarrhea, abdominal pain, pancreatitis, nausea, vomiting, peripheral neuropathy, dyselectrolytemias, hyperuricemia, increased liver enzymes, lactic acidosis, retinal pigmentation, CNS depression, rash/pruritus, myalgia, pancreatitis.

Remarks: Administer empty stomach.

5. Abacavir (ABC)

Oral; tablets (300 mg). Oral solution (20 mg/mL)

Indications: Antiretroviral: 8 mg/kg/dose BID.

Adverse effects: Life-threatening hypersensitivity reactions have been reported presenting as fever, skin rash, fatigue and gastrointestinal symptoms (nausea, vomiting, diarrhea or abdominal pain).

6. Zalcitabine (ddC)

Oral.

Indications: Antiretroviral: 0.01 mg/kg/dose TID.

Adverse effects: Common side effects are peripheral neuropathy, headache, malaise, gastrointestinal disturbances.

Contraindications: Use cautiously in patients with liver disease, pancreatitis, or severe myelosuppression. Adjust dose in renal disease.

7. Emtricitabine (FTC)

Oral; solution (10 mg/mL), capsule (200 mg).

Indications: Antiretroviral: 3 mg/kg OD (0–3 months), 6 mg/kg OD (3 months–17 years), (maximum dose 240 mg).

Adverse effects: Minimal toxicity. Severe hepatitis in children with hepatitis B co-infected persons.

NUCLEOTIDE REVERSE TRANSCRIPTASE INHIBITORS

Tenofovir (TDF)

Oral; tablet (150 mg, 200 mg, 250 mg, 300 mg).

Indications: Antiretroviral: Pediatric dose 8 mg/kg once daily.

Adverse effects: Asthenia, headache, diarrhea, nausea, vomiting, flatulence, renal insufficiency, decreased bone mineral density.

Contraindications: Not recommended in children aged <2 years.

NON-NUCLEOSIDE REVERSE TRANSCRIPTASE INHIBITORS

1. Efavirenz (EFV)

Oral; capsules (50 mg, 100 mg, 200 mg).

Indications: Antiretroviral: 15 mg/kg once a day. Maximum of 600 mg.

Adverse effects: Side effects include rash, granulocytopenias, hepatotoxicity and psychosis.

Contraindications: Usually not recommended in children < 3 years age/weight <10 kg.

2. Nevirapine (NVP)

Oral; tablets, syrup (10 mg/5 mL).

Indications: Antiretroviral: Start with 120 mg/m^2 once a day for initial 14 days followed by 120 mg/m^2/dose BID if no rash or other side effects. Maximum tolerated dose 400 mg/day.

For PMTCT: Birth weight < 2 kg 2 mg/kg PO started within 24 hours of birth and given for 6 weeks of life, birth weight 2–2.5 kg 10 mg, PO OD, birth weight > 2.5 kg 15 mg, PO OD.

Adverse effects: Side effects include nausea, pain abdomen, skin rash (can be life-threatening Stevens-Johnson type), granulocytopenia and hepatotoxicity. Discontinue if severe rash with fever, blistering, myalgias or mucositis occur.

Remarks: Nevirapine induces the metabolism of CYP4503AA to cause its own metabolism within 2–4 weeks of starting treatment. NVP decreases levels of indinavir, ritonavir, and saquinavir. Rifampicin and rifabutin decrease serum levels of NVP. NVP should be taken with food to decrease gastrointestinal irritation.

PROTEASE INHIBITORS

1. Nelfinavir (NFV)

Indications: Antiretroviral: Neonates 40 mg/kg/dose PO BID; children (>3 months) 25–30 mg/kg/dose PO TID, maximum 750 mg/dose.

2. Ritonavir (RTV)

Oral; solution (80 mg/mL), tablets (100 mg) available alone or in combination with other PIs.

Indications: The recommended dose of ritonavir varies and is specific to the drug combination selected. The major use of ritonavir is as an enhancer of other protease inhibitors (PIs) used in pediatric patients and in adolescents and adults.

Adverse effects: Gastrointestinal (GI) intolerance, nausea, vomiting, diarrhea, paresthesia (circumoral and extremities), hyperlipidemia, especially hypertriglyceridemia, hepatitis, asthenia, taste perversion, hyperglycemia, fat maldistribution, and rash.

3. Lopinavir/Ritonavir (LPVr)

Oral; solution (80 mg/20 mg LPV/r per mL; contains 42.4% alcohol by volume and 15.3% propylene glycol by weight/volume), tablets (100 mg/25 mg LPV/r, 200 mg/50 mg LPV/r).

Indications: Antiretroviral: Daily dose 460/115 mg/m^2 divided in 2 doses (maximum 800/200 mg per day) in ARV-naïve patients. 300 mg/75 mg per m^2 of BSA per dose twice daily (maximum dose 400 mg/100 mg twice daily). Preferred dose for treatment-experienced patients with possible decreased lopinavir susceptibility.

Adverse effects include diarrhea, headache, asthenia, nausea and vomiting, rash, and hyperlipidemia, especially hypertriglyceridemia, fat maldistribution.

Remarks: Can be administered without regard to food; administration with or after meals may enhance GI tolerability. Once-daily dosing is not recommended because of considerable variability in plasma concentrations in children aged <18 years and higher incidence of diarrhea.

4. Indinavir

Indications: Antiretroviral: If used, doses of 234–500 mg/m^2 BSA boosted with ritonavir have been tried.

Adverse effects include nausea, abdominal pain, headache, metallic taste, dizziness, asymptomatic hyperbilirubinemia, lipid abnormalities, pruritus, and rash, nephrolithiasis/urolithiasis with indinavir crystal deposits.

Contraindications: Not approved for use in infants. Generally avoided in children.

Remarks: Fasting increases absorption.

5. Saquinavir (SQV)

Indications: Antiretroviral: In children >2 years, dosing based on body weight and in combination with ritonavir as SQV 50 mg/kg + RTV 3 mg/kg BD (5–15 kg), SQV 50 mg/kg + RTV 2.5 mg/kg BD (15–40 kg), SQV 50 mg/kg + RTV 100 mg BD (>40 kg).

Contraindications: Not approved for use in infants. Generally avoided in children.

Remarks: Fatty meals increase absorption.

6. Atazanavir (ATV)

Oral.

Indications: Antiretroviral: Recommended in children >6 years. Dosing in combination with ritonavir and according to weight bands as ATV 150 mg + RTV 100 mg OD with food (15–20 kg), ATV 200 mg + RTV 100 mg OD with food (20–40 kg), ATV 300 mg + RTV 100 mg OD with food (>40 kg).

Adverse effects: Jaundice, prolonged PR interval, first-degree symptomatic atrioventricular (AV) block, nephrolithiasis, hyperglycemia, fat maldistribution, rash, raised liver enzymes.

7. Darunavir (DRV)

Oral; Tablets (75 mg, 150 mg, 400 mg, 600 mg, 800 mg), oral suspension (100 mg/mL).

Indications: Antiretroviral: Dosing according to weight band as DRV 200 mg + RTV 32 mg (10–11 kg), DRV 220 mg + RTV 32 mg (11–12 kg), DRV 240 mg + RTV 40 mg (12–13 kg), DRV 260 mg + RTV 40 mg (13–14 kg), DRV 280 mg + RTV 48 mg (14–15 kg), DRV 375 mg + RTV 48 mg (15–30 kg), DRV 450 mg + RTV 100 mg (30–40 kg), DRV 600 mg + RTV 100 mg (>40 kg).

Adverse effects: Skin rash, hepatitis, fat maldistribution, diarrhea, nausea, headache, and hyperlipidemia.

Contraindications: Not recommended in children <3 years or weight <10 kg because of risk of seizures.

Remarks: DRV should be administered with food.

8. Tipranavir

Oral; solution (100 mg/mL, with 116 International units (IU) vitamin E/mL), capsule (250 mg).

Indications: Antiretroviral: 375 mg/m^2 plus RTV 150 mg/m^2, both twice daily.

Adverse effects: Intracranial hemorrhage, skin rash, hepatitis, hyperglycemia, hyperlipidemia, fat maldistribution, nausea, vomiting and diarrhea.

Contraindications: Not approved for use in children aged <2 years.

Remarks: To be administered with food.

22.13 ANTITOXINS AND IMMUNOGLOBULINS

1. Anti-RhD Immunoglobulin

Intramuscular; vial (100, 250, 300, 350 μg).

Indications: Antenatal prophylaxis: 300 μg single dose IM at 28 weeks and 34 weeks of gestation or within 72 hours of delivery. *Abortion, amniocentesis, version:* 250 μg IM. *Immune thrombocytopenic purpura* 50–75 μg/kg IV single dose.

Adverse effects: Anaphylaxis rarely, fever, RBC breakdown (anemia), pain at injection site, headache.

Contraindications: Patients sensitive to other human immune globulin products may be sensitive to Anti-RhD immunoglobulin.

2. Anti-snake Venom (ASV)

Intravenous; vial (10 mL).

Indications: Mild envenomation: 5 vials, *moderate envenomation:* 5–15 vials, *severe envenomation:* 15–20 vials. Small children may require 1.5 times of this dose. Dilute the ASV in 250 mL of N/5 saline and given IV @ 20 mL/kg/hours. Sensitivity test (intradermal 0.02 mL of 1:10 diluted ASV) is necessary.

Adverse effects: Dyspnea, hypotension, urticaria, hypersensitivity.

3. Diphtheria Antitoxin (Equine)

Indications: For Schick test positive contacts: One dose of diphtheria toxoid should be given in one arm and 500–2000 U(IM) of diphtheria antitoxin in the other arm. Six weeks later, 3 doses of toxoid may be given monthly. *Therapeutic:* Intravenous ampoule (10,000; 20,000 U), pharyngeal/laryngeal 20,000–40,000 U IV, nasopharyngeal 40,000–60,000 U IV, extensive 80,000–1,20,000 U IV.
Remarks: Dilute the antitoxin in 1:20 isotonic sodium chloride solution and give at rate of 1mL/min.

4. Human High Dose Immunoglobulin

Intravenous, vial (0.5, 1, 2, 5 g).

Indications: Prophylaxis and treatment of life-threatening Gram-negative infections, immunodeficiency states, chronic ITP, Guillain-Barré syndrome, and Kawasaki disease: 400 mg/kg/day IV infusion over 6 hours × 5 days, or 1 g/kg/day IV infusion over 2 hours × 2 days, or 2 g/kg IV infusion over 10–12 hours as single dose.

Adverse effects: Headache, flushing, chills, myalgia, wheezing, tachycardia, lower back pain, nausea, and hypotension.

5. Human Normal Immunoglobulin

Intravenous, intramuscular; vial (10%, 16.5% in 1mL vial).

Indications: Primary immunodeficiency: 300–400 mg/kg intravenous once every 4 weeks. Attenuation of disease among close contacts: 0.3 mL/kg of 10% solution IM within 6 days of exposure to measles. Following exposure to hepatitis A 0.02–0.04 mL/kg of 10% solution IM.

Adverse effects: Headache, flushing, chills, myalgia, wheezing, tachycardia, lower back pain, nausea, and hypotension.

Remarks: No live vaccines to be given in next 6 weeks.

6. Human Hepatitis B Immunoglobulin (HBIG)

Intramuscular, intravenous; vial (160 mg/mL; 200 IU/mL).

Indications: Active immunization should be initiated simultaneously. The vaccine and HBIG should be administered in separate thighs. Newborn 0.5 mL intramuscular up to 72 hours of birth, preferably within 12 hours of birth. Children 0.06 mL/kg or 40 IU/kg, single dose intramuscular.

Adverse effects: Flu like symptoms, cold, nausea, vomiting, diarrhea, tremors, sore throat, rash.

7. Human Rabies Immunoglobulin

Intramuscular; vial (150 U/mL)

Indications: 20 U/kg, infiltrate in local site as much as possible, rest to be given intramuscular in gluteal region. If patient presents between 1 and 7 days, give the entire dose IM. Administer rabies vaccine simultaneously.

Adverse effects: Headache, fever, chills, nausea, vomiting, itching, rash, allergic reaction, or injection site reactions.

Remarks: To be given within 24 hours of bite. Perform prior intradermal testing for hypersensitivity.

8. Human Tetanus Immunoglobulin

Intramuscular; vial (250, 500 IU).

Indications: Tetanus prophylaxis: 250 IU IM, or 500 U if there is heavy contamination or > 24 hours have elapsed.
Treatment: 30–300 IU/kg IM, intrathecal 250–500 IU single dose.

Adverse effects: Local site reactions (pain, redness), flu like symptoms, hypersensitivity.

9. Respiratory Syncytial Virus (RSV) IG

Intravenous; vial (50 mg/mL).

Indications: For infants and children <2 years with bronchopulmonary dysplasia (BPD) who require oxygen, initiate RSV IG within 6 months before RSV season. May administer prophylactically in preterm infants (< 32 weeks) who do not have BPD. For those >28 weeks, consider till 12 months of age and for those with gestational age 29–32 weeks, may give RSV IG until 6 months of age. Dose is 750 mg/kg IV every 30 days.

Contraindications: Cyanotic congenital heart disease.

10. Varicella Zoster Immunoglobulin (VZIG)

Intramuscular; vial (125 U per vial).
Indications: Neonates of mother developing varicella 5 days before to 2 days after pregnancy, postnatally exposed preterm infants (>28 weeks) of susceptible mothers, hospitalized preterm infant born at < 28 weeks' gestation or birth weight <1 kg, immunocompromised children, susceptible pregnant women: 125 U for each 10 kg body weight IM, max 625 U, min 125 U. Give IM within 48 hours or at least 96 hours of exposure.

22.14 ANTIVIRAL DRUGS

1. Acyclovir

Oral, intravenous; tablet (200, 400, 800 mg), suspension (400 mg/5 mL), injection (250 mg).

Indications: Antiviral: Intravenous 10 mg/kg/dose q 8 h (to give for 14 days for HSV encephalitis),
Oral 20 mg/kg/dose q 6 h (to give for 5 days for varicella).
Adverse effects: Headache, insomnia, encephalopathy, increased liver enzymes, urticaria, arthralgia, rash.
Contraindications: Cautious use in renal impairment.

2. Amantadine Hydrochloride

Oral; capsule (100 mg), syrup (50 mg/5 mL).

Indications: Antiviral: 2–4 mg/kg/dose q 12 h. Maximum dose < 10 years: 150 mg/d, > 10 years: 200 mg/day.
Adverse effects: Dizziness, rash, mental instability, nausea, CHF, edema.

3. Foscarnet

Intravenous; injection (500 mg, 1 g).
Indications: CMV retinitis in AIDS: 60 mg/kg/dose q 8 h as slow IV infusion during induction phase followed by 90 mg/kg/dose OD IV infusion during maintenance phase.

22

Adverse effects: Seizures, hallucinations, peripheral neuropathy, renal failure, dyspnea, chest pain, fever, nausea, diarrhea.

Contraindications: Avoid in patients with renal diseases.

4. Ganciclovir

Oral, intravenous; capsule (250 mg), injection (500 mg).

Indications: CMV retinitis: 5 mg/kg/dose 12 hourly during induction phase followed by 5 mg/kg/dose OD during maintenance phase in immunocompromised host. For severe infections: 10 mg/kg/dose q 8 h IV for 14 days.

Adverse effects: Nephrotoxicity, neutropenia, thrombocytopenia, retinal detachment, confusion.

Remarks: Do not use subcutaneous or intramuscular route.

5. Isoprinosine *(Inosine pranobex)*

Oral; intramuscular; tablet (500 mg)

Indications: SSPE: 50–100 mg/kg/d q 12 h PO/IM.

Adverse effects: Transient elevation of uric acid levels in serum and urine, skin rash, GI disturbances, fatigue, nausea, arthralgia.

Oseltamivir *(Neuraminidase inhibitor)*

Oral; Capsule (30 mg, 45 mg, 75 mg), syrup (12 mg/mL).

Indications: Antiflu: <3 months: 12 mg BD; <15 kg: 30 mg BD; 15–23 kg: 45 mg BD; 23–40 kg: 60 mg BD; > 40 kg: 75 mg BD. For 5 days duration.

Adverse effects: Vomiting, diarrhea, headache, insomnia, seizures, neuropsychiatric disturbances.

Ribavirin

Oral; capsule (100 mg, 200 mg), syrup (50 mg/5 mL).

Indications: Antiviral: 10 mg/kg/day PO q 6–8 h.

Adverse effects: Anemia, psychiatric disturbances.

Contraindications: Pregnancy, hepatitis, heart disease, severe renal disease.

▌ 22.15 CARDIOTONICS

1. Adrenaline *(Epinephrine hydrochloride)*

Intravenous, subcutaneous, endotracheal; ampoule (1:1000; 1 mg/mL), dilute in normal saline.

Indications: Cardiac arrest: 0.1 mL/kg of 1:10,000 diluted intravenous or intratracheal q 3–5 min.

Resuscitation in neonates: Use 1:10,000 dilution 0.1–0.3 mL/kg IV q 3–5 min or 0.3–0.5 mL/kg ET. CPR in older children: use 1:1000 dilution 0.1 mg/kg IV/ET q 3–5 min. Shock: 0.05–0.5 μg/kg/min IV infusion. Bronchodilation: 1:1000 dilution, 0.01 mg/kg/dose SC, q 15 min × 3–4 doses. Nebulization: 0.5 mL/kg of 1:1000 solution diluted in 3 mL normal saline (Max dose in >4 years: 2.5 mL/dose and in older children: 5 mL/dose).

Adverse effects: Tachycardia, hypertension, arrhythmias, headache, nervousness, nausea, vomiting.

2. Amrinone *(Phosphodiesterase-3 Inhibitor)*

Intravenous; Injection (100 mg/20 mL).

Indications: Cardiovascular bipyridine, inotrope, vasodilator: 0.75 mg/kg IV bolus over 2–3 min followed by 3–5 μg/kg/min in newborns and 5–10 μg/kg/min in children as continuous infusion.

Adverse effect: Thrombocytopenia.

Contraindications: Amrinone is contraindicated in patients with hypertrophic cardiomyopathy. Avoid in patients with platelet counts below 50,000/mL.

Remarks: Amrinone should not be infused in dextrose-containing fluids, and the infusion solution should be protected from light. Furosemide should not be injected into intravenous lines carrying amrinone infusions because the drug forms a precipitate when added to amrinone solutions.

3. Digoxin *(Cardiac glycoside)*

Intravenous, oral; injection (0.5 mg/2 mL), tablet (0.25 mg), elixir (0.5 mg/mL).

Indications: Oral digitalizing dose preterm neonates: 0.04 mg/kg/day, term neonates: 0.06 mg/kg/day, <2 years: 0.04–0.05 mg/kg/day, > 2 years: 0.04 mg/kg/day; Parenteral dose: 2/3rds of oral dose—½ of digitalizing dose given stat, ¼th after 8 hours and ¼th after 16 hours. Daily maintenance dose ¼th of digitalizing dose.

Adverse effects: AV block, cardiac dysrhythmias.

Contraindications: Contraindicated in ventricular dysrhythmia; doses to be adjusted in renal failure.

Remarks: Calcium infusion in patients on digoxin can precipitate ventricular fibrillation.

4. Dobutamine *(Beta1 receptor agonist)*

Intravenous; vial (1 mL = 50 mg, 5 mL).

Indications: Inotrope: 5–20 μg/kg/min IV infusion.

Adverse effects: Arrhythmias, hypertension, tachycardia

Contraindications: IHSS .

Remarks: Do not mix with sodium bicarbonate.

5. Dopamine *(Vasopressor)*

Intravenous; ampoule (1 mL=40 mg, 5 mL).

Indications: Inotrope: 5–20 μg/kg/min.

Adverse effects: Arrhythmias, hypertension, vasoconstriction.

Remarks: Do not mix with sodium bicarbonate.

6. Milrinone *(Phosphodiesterase-3 inhibitor)*

Intravenous; injection (1 mg/mL).

Indications: Inotrope: Loading dose 50 μg/kg, continuous infusion 0.25–1 μg/kg/min.

Adverse effects: Dysarrhythmia, hypotension, hypokalemia, hepatitis.

Contraindications: Severe aortic stenosis, severe pulmonic stenosis, acute MI.

7. Norepinephrine *(Adrenaline: Sympathomimetic)*

Intravenous; ampoule (1 mg/mL).

Indications: Inotrope: 0.05–0.1 μg/kg/min. Maximum dose 2 mg/kg/min. To be given by central line only.

Adverse effects: Cardiac arrhythmia, headache.

Remarks: Extravasation causes severe tissue necrosis.

8. Vasopressin *(Antidiuretic hormone: Vasopressor)*

Intravenous, subcutaneous; Ampoule (20 U/mL)

Indications: Diabetes insipidus: 2.5–10 U/dose q 6–12 h subcutaneous. *Bleeding esophageal varices:* 0.002–0.01 U/kg/min continuous infusion. *Catecholamine refractory shock:* 0.3–2 U/kg/min.

Adverse effects: Water intoxication and hyponatremia, abdominal cramps, feeling of constant movement of self or surroundings, pale skin, throbbing headache, dizziness, sweating, trembling or shaking of the hands or feet, bronchospasm.

Contraindications: Contraindicated in heart failure, asthma, epilepsy.

22.16 DIURETICS

1. Acetazolamide *(Carbonic anhydrase inhibitor)*

Oral; tablet (250 mg).

Indications: Raised intracranial pressure: 50–70 mg/kg/day q 8 h. *Diuretic:* 5 mg/kg/dose q 8 h.

Adverse effects: Sedation, hypokalemia, acidosis, polyuria, decreased urate secretion.

Contraindications: Contraindicated in hepatic failure, renal failure.

2. Furosemide *(Loop diuretic)*

Oral, intravenous; tablet (40 mg), injection (20 mg/2 mL).

Indications: Diuretic: Neonates 0.5–1 mg/kg/dose q 8–24 h, maximum PO dose in newborn: 6 mg/kg/dose, maximum IV dose in newborn: 2 mg/kg/dose; children 0.5–2 mg/kg/dose q 6–12 h, max dose 6 mg/kg/dose, Continuous IV infusion 0.05–1 mg/kg/h.

Adverse effects: May cause hypokalemia, alkalosis, dehydration, hyperuricemia and increased calcium excretion. Prolonged use in preterm neonates can cause nephrocalcinosis. In the presence of renal disease, it can cause ototoxicity when used with aminoglycosides.

3. Hydrochlorthiazide *(Thiazide diuretic)*

Oral; tablet (25, 50 mg).

Indications: Diuretic: 2–4 mg/kg/day q 12 h, PO.

Adverse effects: Hyperuricemia, fluid and electrolyte disturbances.

4. Spironolactone *(Potassium sparing diuretic)*

Oral, tablets (25, 100 mg).

Indications: Diuretic: 2–3 mg/kg/day q 8–24 h, PO.

Adverse effects: Hyperkalemia, GI disturbance, rash, lethargy, dizziness, gynecomastia.

Contraindications: Contraindicated in renal failure, hyperkalemia.

Remarks: It is co-administered with thiazides.

5. Triamterene *(Potassium sparing diuretic)*

Oral; tablet (50 mg triamterene + 25 mg benzthiazide).

Indications: Diuretic: 2–4 mg/kg/day q 12 h, PO.

Adverse effects: Depletion of sodium, folic acid and calcium, nausea, vomiting, diarrhea, headache, dizziness, fatigue, dry mouth, palpitations.

Contraindications: It is contraindicated in renal failure, hyperkalemia.

22.17 MISCELLANEOUS DRUGS

1. Albumin

Intravenous; Human albumin 5% (250 mL), 20% (50 mL, 100 mL).

Indications: For *hypoproteinemia* and *acute hypovolemic shock:* 0.5–1 g/kg/dose IV over 2–4 h.

Adverse effects: Fluid overload, hypernatremia, hypersensitivity.

Contraindications: CHF, anemia.

2. Allopurinol *(Xanthine oxidase Inhibitor)*

Oral; Tablet (100 mg).

Indications: Hyperuricemia: 10 mg/kg/day q 8 h PO.

Adverse effects: Rash, neuritis, hepatotoxic, GI disturbances, bone marrow suppression.

Contraindications: Use cautiously in renal insufficiency.

3. Baclofen *(Muscle relaxant)*

Oral, intrathecal injection; tablet (10 mg, 25 mg), injection (0.5, 2 mg/mL).

Indications: Central muscle relaxant in severe chronic spasticity: 0.75–2 mg/kg/day oral q 8 h; dosage is increased over 3 days to get the desired effect or till maximum dose achieved if needed.

Max dose < 8 years: 40 mg/day; > 8 years: 60 mg/day.

Adverse effects: Drowsiness, fatigue, nausea, vertigo, psychiatric disturbances, urinary frequency, hypotonia, rash.

Contraindications: Use cautiously in children with seizure disorder, impaired renal function.

4. Caffeine Citrate *(Methylxanthine)*

Oral, intravenous; injection (20 mg/mL), oral solution (20 mg/mL)

Indications: Respiratory stimulant: 20 mg/kg intravenous infusion as loading followed by 10 mg/kg/day oral/intravenous maintenance after 24 hours.

Adverse effects: Tachycardia, neurologic and GI side effects.

Contraindications: Do not use in cardiac arrhythmias, do not use caffeine benzoate as it increases the risk of kernicterus.

5. Calcium Gluconate

Intravenous; injection (10% containing 100 mg/mL of calcium gluconate equivalent to elemental calcium of 8.9 mg/mL or 0.45 mEq/mL of Ca^{++}).

Indications: Hypocalcemia: 1–2 mL/kg/dose q 6 h, slow intravenous under cardiac monitoring, maintenance 2–4 mL/kg/day q 6 h. *Hyperkalemia:* 0.5 mL/kg over 5–10 min.

Adverse effects: Extravasation can cause tissue necrosis. Other side effects include hypotension, bradycardia.

Contraindications: Digitalized children.

6. Carnitine

Oral; tablet (330, 500 mg), syrup (50 mg/5 mL), injection (500 mg/2.5 L).

Indications: 50–100 mg/kg/day oral/intravenous q 8–12 h.

Adverse effects: Nausea, vomiting, diarrhea, pain abdomen, increased risk of seizures.

Contraindications: Caution in severe renal disease.

7. Deferasirox *(Iron chelating agent)*

Oral; tablet (125, 250, 500 mg).

Indications: Chelating agent: 20 mg/kg PO per day, dose may be titrated by increasing by 5–10 mg based on serum ferritin; if serum ferritin persistently > 2500 mcg/L, may increase up to maximum of 40 mg/kg per day.

Adverse effects: Increased risk of bleeding, kidney disease, GI upset.

Remarks: Tablet should not be chewed or swallowed whole but dispersed in apple or orange juice or in water before consumption. Preferably be taken empty stomach or 30 min prior to food.

8. Deferiprone *(Iron chelating agent)*

Oral, capsule (250 mg, 500 mg).

Indications: Chelating agent: 50–100 mg/kg/day q 6–12 h PO.

Adverse effects: Joint pain, agranulocytosis, zinc deficiency.

Contraindications: Do not use in pregnancy, breastfeeding, in patients having low TLC.

9. Desferrioxamine *(Iron chelating agent)*

Intravenous, subcutaneous; injection (500 mg).

Indications: Chelating agent for chronic iron overload: 20–40 mg/kg/day SC over 8–12 h using battery operated pump. *Acute iron poisoning:* IV 15 mg/kg/h OR 50 mg/kg/dose q 6 h.

Adverse effects: May cause flushing, erythema, hypotension, tachycardia, leg cramps, fever, hearing loss and cataracts.

Contraindications: Anuria, primary hemachromatosis.

10. Dextromethorphan

Oral; syrup (30 mg/5 mL).

Indications: Antitussive: 1–2 mg/kg/day q 8 h.

Adverse effects: Nausea, vomiting, dizziness.

Contraindications: Avoid in children less than 4 years.

11. Dicyclomine Hydrochloride *(Antispasmodic: Anticholinergic)*

Oral; Tablet (10, 20 mg), drops (10 mg/mL), syrup (10 mg/5 mL).

Indications: Infantile colic < 6 months: 5–10 drops 15 min before feeds, 6 months–2 years: 10–20 drops 15 min before feeds, >2 years: 1 mL every 6 hours.

Adverse effects: Tachycardia, dryness of mouth, GI disturbances.

Contraindications: Bowel obstruction.

12. Drotaverine Hydrochloride *(Phosphodiesterase-4 inhibitor)*

Oral; tablet (40 mg), syrup (20 mg/5 mL).

Indications: Antispasmodic: 1–6 years 20 mg TDS, > 6 years 40 mg TDS.

13. Erythropoietin

Intravenous, subcutaneous; injection (2000 IU, 4000 IU)

Indications: Chronic renal failure: 50–100 IU/kg SC 2–3 times/week. *Anemia of prematurity:* 25–100 IU/kg/dose SC 3 times per week for 8–12 weeks.

Adverse effects: Increased risk of thrombosis/stroke/cardiovascular event/death in those with Hb >11/CKD.

Remarks: Provide oral iron supplementation 2–3 mg/kg/d. Monitor for hypertension, blood urea, serum creatinine, hematocrit and clotting time. Peak effect in 2–3 weeks. Reduce dose when target attained or when hematocrit increases > 4 points in any 2 weeks period. SC route preferred to IV route.

14. Glucagon

Intramuscular, subcutaneous, intravenous; injection (1 mg).

Indications: Hypoglycemia: 0.5 mg (< 25 kg), 1 mg (> 25 kg).

Adverse effects: Nausea, vomiting, urticaria, respiratory distress.

15. Granulocyte Colony-stimulating Factor

Intravenous, subcutaneous; vial (300 µg).

Indications: To mobilize peripheral blood progenitor cells for hematopoietic stem cell transplantation and granulocytes for apheresis collection, and to decrease the duration of neutropenia after chemotherapy and to offset the neutropenia due to myelodysplasia, acquired immunodeficiency syndrome, and genetic disorders of granulocyte production: 5–10 µg/kg/day subcutaneous.

Adverse effects: Usually no adverse effects. Bone pain, local tenderness, nausea are the minor side effects.

16. Hyoscine Butylbromide *(Antispasmodic: Anticholinergic)*

Oral, intravenous, intramuscular; tablet (10 mg), injection (20 mg/mL)

Indications: 10 mg/dose q 8 h PO or 10–20 mg IV/IM bolus (6–12 years).

Adverse effects: Glaucoma, dry mouth, dry skin, blurred vision, diarrhea, palpitations, flushing, difficulty in urinating.

Contraindications: Glaucoma.

17. Lactulose

Oral; syrup (10 g/15 mL).

Indications: Constipation: 1–2 mL/kg/day q 6–8 h.

Adverse effects: Flatulence, belching, abdominal discomfort, cramps, nausea, vomiting, diarrhea

18. Lansoprazole *(Proton pump inhibitor)*

Oral; tablet (15, 30 mg)

Indications: Gastritis: 1 mg/kg/day.

Adverse effects: Headache, diarrhea, constipation, abdominal pain, nausea, drowsiness.

Contraindications: Contraindicated in patients with known severe hypersensitivity to any component of lansoprazole.

19. Magnesium Sulfate

Intravenous; ampoule (50%, 4 mEq/mL of elemental magnesium).

Indications: PEM: 2–3 mEq/kg/day. Bronchodilation: 25–50 mg/kg/dose as IV infusion.

Adverse effects and *Contraindications:* As mentioned previously.

20. Mannitol

Intravenous; 20% bottles (100 mL).

Indications: Raised intracranial tension: 5 mL/kg IV over 30 min (loading dose) followed by 2 mL/kg/dose q 6 h IV for 2 days.

Adverse effects: Electrolyte imbalance, circulatory overload.

Contraindications: Intracranial bleed, dehydration, pulmonary edema, severe renal disease.

21. Metronidazole

Oral, intravenous; syrup (200 mg/5 mL), tablet (200, 400 mg), vial (5 mg/mL).

Indications: Amebiasis: 30–50 mg/kg/day q 8 h for 10 days.

Trichomoniasis: 15 mg/kg/day q 8 h for 5 days. *Anaerobic infections:* 20 mg/kg/day q 8 hourly for 7–10 days.

Adverse effects: Nausea, vomiting, metallic taste, diarrhea, dry mouth.

Contraindications: Avoid in severe renal/hepatic disease.

22. Potassium Chloride

Oral, intravenous; injection (1 mL = 2 mEq), syrup (20 mEq/15 mL)

Indications: Hypokalemia: 1–2 mEq/kg/day q 8 h PO.

Adverse effects: Oral: GI upset, ulceration; intravenous: irritation, phlebitis, pain.

Remarks: Do not administer intravenous without dilution or rapidly as it may cause arrhythmias.

23. Ranitidine *(H1 receptor antagonist)*

Intravenous, oral; Injection (50 mg/2 mL), tablet (150 mg, 300 mg).

Indications: Gastritis: Intravenous 1–2 mg/kg/day q 12 h, oral 2–4 mg/kg/day q 12 h.

Adverse effects: Headache, drowsiness, arthralgia, fatigue.

Contraindications: Dose adjustment in severe renal disease.

24. Sodium Bicarbonate

Intravenous; Ampoule (7.5%, 10 mL; Contains 0.9 mEq/mL).

Indications: Metabolic acidosis: 1–2 mEq/kg/dose IV or calculate as [Base deficit × Weight × 0.6 = mEq or mL of 7.5% solution of sodium bicarbonate (total correction)].

Adverse effects: May cause hypernatremia, hypokalemia, hypomagnesemia, hypocalcemia, hyperreflexia, edema, and tissue necrosis (extravasation).

Contraindications: Do not mix with calcium, dobutamine or norepinephrine.

Remarks: To be diluted in distilled water or 5% dextrose in a dilution of 1:6 (1 part sodium bicarbonate and 6 parts of distilled water) and given as IV infusion; half the correction is given stat followed by the remaining in divided doses over the next 12–24 hours. Repeat blood gas as necessary. In neonates, it may be given as 1:3 dilution.

25. Ursodeoxycholic Acid

Oral; tablet (150 mg, 300 mg)

Indications: Cholelitholytic: 10–15 mg/kg/day q 8 h.

Adverse effects: Deranged liver enzymes, arthralgias, GI upset.

Contraindications: Contraindicated in bile stones, calcified cholesterol stones.

26. Zinc

Oral; syrup (10 mg/5 mL), capsules.

Indications: Diarrhea: 10 mg PO × 14 days (2–6 months), 20 mg PO for 14 days (6 months–5 years).

Adverse effects: Nausea, vomiting, leukopenia.

Remarks: Excessive zinc intake may cause copper deficiency.

Nidhi Bedi, and Pooja Dewan

1 Growth Tables (Birth to 18 Years)

Chart 1 Weight (kg) by Age of Boys, Percentile and Z scores, 0–5 years (WHO Standards)

Age		Percentiles							Z (SD) score					
Year	Month	3rd	15th	25th	50th	75th	85th	97th	−3Z	−2Z	−1Z	+1Z	+2Z	+3Z
	0	2.5	2.9	3.0	3.3	3.7	3.9	4.3	2.1	2.5	2.9	3.9	4.4	5.0
	0	2.5	2.9	3.0	3.3	3.7	3.9	4.3	2.1	2.5	2.9	3.9	4.4	5.0
	1	3.4	3.9	4.1	4.5	4.9	5.1	5.7	2.9	3.4	3.9	5.1	5.8	6.6
	2	4.4	4.9	5.1	5.6	6.0	6.3	7.0	3.8	4.3	4.9	6.3	7.1	8.0
	3	5.1	5.6	5.9	6.4	6.9	7.2	7.9	4.4	5.0	5.7	7.2	8.0	9.0
	4	5.6	6.2	6.5	7.0	7.6	7.9	8.6	4.9	5.6	6.2	7.8	8.7	9.7
	5	6.1	6.7	7.0	7.5	8.1	8.4	9.2	5.3	6.0	6.7	8.4	9.3	10.4
	6	6.4	7.1	7.4	7.9	8.5	8.9	9.7	5.7	6.4	7.1	8.8	9.8	10.9
	7	6.7	7.4	7.7	8.3	8.9	9.3	10.2	5.9	6.7	7.4	9.2	10.3	11.4
	8	7.0	7.7	8.0	8.6	9.3	9.6	10.5	6.2	6.9	7.7	9.6	10.7	11.9
	9	7.2	7.9	8.3	8.9	9.6	10.0	10.9	6.4	7.1	8.0	9.9	11.0	12.3
	10	7.5	8.2	8.5	9.2	9.9	10.3	11.2	6.6	7.4	8.2	10.2	11.4	12.7
	11	7.7	8.4	8.7	9.4	10.1	10.5	11.5	6.8	7.6	8.4	10.5	11.7	13.0
1	0	7.8	8.6	9.0	9.6	10.4	10.8	11.8	6.9	7.7	8.6	10.8	12.0	13.3
1	1	8.0	8.8	9.2	9.9	10.6	11.1	12.1	7.1	7.9	8.8	11.0	12.3	13.7
1	2	8.2	9.0	9.4	10.1	10.9	11.3	12.4	7.2	8.1	9.0	11.3	12.6	14.0
1	3	8.4	9.2	9.6	10.3	11.1	11.6	12.7	7.4	8.3	9.2	11.5	12.8	14.3
1	4	8.5	9.4	9.8	10.5	11.3	11.8	12.9	7.5	8.4	9.4	11.7	13.1	14.6
1	5	8.7	9.6	10.0	10.7	11.6	12.0	13.2	7.7	8.6	9.6	12.0	13.4	14.9
1	6	8.9	9.7	10.1	10.9	11.8	12.3	13.5	7.8	8.8	9.8	12.2	13.7	15.3
1	7	9.0	9.9	10.3	11.1	12.0	12.5	13.7	8.0	8.9	10.0	12.5	13.9	15.6
1	8	9.2	10.1	10.5	11.3	12.2	12.7	14.0	8.1	9.1	10.1	12.7	14.2	15.9
1	9	9.3	10.3	10.7	11.5	12.5	13.0	14.3	8.2	9.2	10.3	12.9	14.5	16.2
1	10	9.5	10.5	10.9	11.8	12.7	13.2	14.5	8.4	9.4	10.5	13.2	14.7	16.5
1	11	9.7	10.6	11.1	12.0	12.9	13.4	14.8	8.5	9.5	10.7	13.4	15.0	16.8
2	0	9.8	10.8	11.3	12.2	13.1	13.7	15.1	8.6	9.7	10.8	13.6	15.3	17.1
2	1	10.0	11.0	11.4	12.4	13.3	13.9	15.3	8.8	9.8	11.0	13.9	15.5	17.5
2	2	10.1	11.1	11.6	12.5	13.6	14.1	15.6	8.9	10.0	11.2	14.1	15.8	17.8
2	3	10.2	11.3	11.8	12.7	13.8	14.4	15.9	9.0	10.1	11.3	14.3	16.1	18.1
2	4	10.4	11.5	12.0	12.9	14.0	14.6	16.1	9.1	10.2	11.5	14.5	16.3	18.4
2	5	10.5	11.6	12.1	13.1	14.2	14.8	16.4	9.2	10.4	11.7	14.8	16.6	18.7
2	6	10.7	11.8	12.3	13.3	14.4	15.0	16.6	9.4	10.5	11.8	15.0	16.9	19.0
2	7	10.8	11.9	12.4	13.5	14.6	15.2	16.9	9.5	10.7	12.0	15.2	17.1	19.3
2	8	10.9	12.1	12.6	13.7	14.8	15.5	17.1	9.6	10.8	12.1	15.4	17.4	19.6
2	9	11.1	12.2	12.8	13.8	15.0	15.7	17.3	9.7	10.9	12.3	15.6	17.6	19.9
2	10	11.2	12.4	12.9	14.0	15.2	15.9	17.6	9.8	11.0	12.4	15.8	17.8	20.2
2	11	11.3	12.5	13.1	14.2	15.4	16.1	17.8	9.9	11.2	12.6	16.0	18.1	20.4
3	0	11.4	12.7	13.2	14.3	15.6	16.3	18.0	10.0	11.3	12.7	16.2	18.3	20.7
3	1	11.6	12.8	13.4	14.5	15.8	16.5	18.3	10.1	11.4	12.9	16.4	18.6	21.0
3	2	11.7	12.9	13.5	14.7	15.9	16.7	18.5	10.2	11.5	13.0	16.6	18.8	21.3
3	3	11.8	13.1	13.7	14.8	16.1	16.9	18.7	10.3	11.6	13.1	16.8	19.0	21.6
3	4	11.9	13.2	13.8	15.0	16.3	17.1	19.0	10.4	11.8	13.3	17.0	19.3	21.9
3	5	12.1	13.4	14.0	15.2	16.5	17.3	19.2	10.5	11.9	13.4	17.2	19.5	22.1
3	6	12.2	13.5	14.1	15.3	16.7	17.5	19.4	10.6	12.0	13.6	17.4	19.7	22.4
3	7	12.3	13.6	14.3	15.5	16.9	17.7	19.7	10.7	12.1	13.7	17.6	20.0	22.7
3	8	12.4	13.8	14.4	15.7	17.1	17.9	19.9	10.8	12.2	13.8	17.8	20.2	23.0
3	9	12.5	13.9	14.6	15.8	17.3	18.1	20.1	10.9	12.4	14.0	18.0	20.5	23.3
3	10	12.7	14.1	14.7	16.0	17.4	18.3	20.4	11.0	12.5	14.1	18.2	20.7	23.6
3	11	12.8	14.2	14.9	16.2	17.6	18.5	20.6	11.1	12.6	14.3	18.4	20.9	23.9
4	0	12.9	14.3	15.0	16.3	17.8	18.7	20.9	11.2	12.7	14.4	18.6	21.2	24.2
4	1	13.0	14.5	15.2	16.5	18.0	18.9	21.1	11.3	12.8	14.5	18.8	21.4	24.5
4	2	13.1	14.6	15.3	16.7	18.2	19.1	21.3	11.4	12.9	14.7	19.0	21.7	24.8
4	3	13.3	14.7	15.4	16.8	18.4	19.3	21.6	11.5	13.1	14.8	19.2	21.9	25.1
4	4	13.4	14.9	15.6	17.0	18.6	19.5	21.8	11.6	13.2	15.0	19.4	22.2	25.4
4	5	13.5	15.0	15.7	17.2	18.8	19.7	22.1	11.7	13.3	15.1	19.6	22.4	25.7
4	6	13.6	15.2	15.9	17.3	19.0	19.9	22.3	11.8	13.4	15.2	19.8	22.7	26.0
4	7	13.7	15.3	16.0	17.5	19.2	20.1	22.5	11.9	13.5	15.4	20.0	22.9	26.3
4	8	13.8	15.4	16.2	17.7	19.3	20.3	22.8	12.0	13.6	15.5	20.2	23.2	26.6
4	9	13.9	15.6	16.3	17.8	19.5	20.5	23.0	12.1	13.7	15.6	20.4	23.4	26.9
4	10	14.1	15.7	16.5	18.0	19.7	20.7	23.3	12.2	13.8	15.8	20.6	23.7	27.2
4	11	14.2	15.8	16.6	18.2	19.9	20.9	23.5	12.3	14.0	15.9	20.8	23.9	27.6
5	0	14.3	16.0	16.7	18.3	20.1	21.1	23.8	12.4	14.1	16.0	21.0	24.2	27.9

Chart 2 Weight (kg) by Age of Girls, Percentiles and Z (SD) Score for 0–5 years (WHO Standards)

| Age | | Percentiles | | | | | | | Z (SD) score | | | | | |
Year	Month	3rd	15th	25th	50th	75th	85th	97th	−3Z	−2Z	−1Z	+1Z	+2Z	+3Z
	0	2.4	2.8	2.9	3.2	3.6	3.7	4.2	2.0	2.4	2.8	3.7	4.2	4.8
	1	3.2	3.6	3.8	4.2	4.6	4.8	5.4	2.7	3.2	3.6	4.8	5.5	6.2
	2	4.0	4.5	4.7	5.1	5.6	5.9	6.5	3.4	3.9	4.5	5.8	6.6	7.5
	3	4.6	5.1	5.4	5.8	6.4	6.7	7.4	4.0	4.5	5.2	6.6	7.5	8.5
	4	5.1	5.6	5.9	6.4	7.0	7.3	8.1	4.4	5.0	5.7	7.3	8.2	9.3
	5	5.5	6.1	6.4	6.9	7.5	7.8	8.7	4.8	5.4	6.1	7.8	8.8	10.0
	6	5.8	6.4	6.7	7.3	7.9	8.3	9.2	5.1	5.7	6.5	8.2	9.3	10.6
	7	6.1	6.7	7.0	7.6	8.3	8.7	9.6	5.3	6.0	6.8	8.6	9.8	11.1
	8	6.3	7.0	7.3	7.9	8.6	9.0	10.0	5.6	6.3	7.0	9.0	10.2	11.6
	9	6.6	7.3	7.6	8.2	8.9	9.3	10.4	5.8	6.5	7.3	9.3	10.5	12.0
	10	6.8	7.5	7.8	8.5	9.2	9.6	10.7	5.9	6.7	7.5	9.6	10.9	12.4
	11	7.0	7.7	8.0	8.7	9.5	9.9	11.0	6.1	6.9	7.7	9.9	11.2	12.8
1	0	7.1	7.9	8.2	8.9	9.7	10.2	11.3	6.3	7.0	7.9	10.1	11.5	13.1
1	1	7.3	8.1	8.4	9.2	10.0	10.4	11.6	6.4	7.2	8.1	10.4	11.8	13.5
1	2	7.5	8.3	8.6	9.4	10.2	10.7	11.9	6.6	7.4	8.3	10.6	12.1	13.8
1	3	7.7	8.5	8.8	9.6	10.4	10.9	12.2	6.7	7.6	8.5	10.9	12.4	14.1
1	4	7.8	8.7	9.0	9.8	10.7	11.2	12.5	6.9	7.7	8.7	11.1	12.6	14.5
1	5	8.0	8.8	9.2	10.0	10.9	11.4	12.7	7.0	7.9	8.9	11.4	12.9	14.8
1	6	8.2	9.0	9.4	10.2	11.1	11.6	13.0	7.2	8.1	9.1	11.6	13.2	15.1
1	7	8.3	9.2	9.6	10.4	11.4	11.9	13.3	7.3	8.2	9.2	11.8	13.5	15.4
1	8	8.5	9.4	9.8	10.6	11.6	12.1	13.5	7.5	8.4	9.4	12.1	13.7	15.7
1	9	8.7	9.6	10.0	10.9	11.8	12.4	13.8	7.6	8.6	9.6	12.3	14.0	16.0
1	10	8.8	9.8	10.2	11.1	12.0	12.6	14.1	7.8	8.7	9.8	12.5	14.3	16.4
1	11	9.0	9.9	10.4	11.3	12.3	12.8	14.3	7.9	8.9	10.0	12.8	14.6	16.7
2	0	9.2	10.1	10.6	11.5	12.5	13.1	14.6	8.1	9.0	10.2	13.0	14.8	17.0
2	1	9.3	10.3	10.8	11.7	12.7	13.3	14.9	8.2	9.2	10.3	13.3	15.1	17.3
2	2	9.5	10.5	10.9	11.9	12.9	13.6	15.2	8.4	9.4	10.5	13.5	15.4	17.7
2	3	9.6	10.7	11.1	12.1	13.2	13.8	15.4	8.5	9.5	10.7	13.7	15.7	18.0
2	4	9.8	10.8	11.3	12.3	13.4	14.0	15.7	8.6	9.7	10.9	14.0	16.0	18.3
2	5	10.0	11.0	11.5	12.5	13.6	14.3	16.0	8.8	9.8	11.1	14.2	16.2	18.7
2	6	10.1	11.2	11.7	12.7	13.8	14.5	16.2	8.9	10.0	11.2	14.4	16.5	19.0
2	7	10.3	11.3	11.9	12.9	14.1	14.7	16.5	9.0	10.1	11.4	14.7	16.8	19.3
2	8	10.4	11.5	12.0	13.1	14.3	15.0	16.8	9.1	10.3	11.6	14.9	17.1	19.6
2	9	10.5	11.7	12.2	13.3	14.5	15.2	17.0	9.3	10.4	11.7	15.1	17.3	20.0
2	10	10.7	11.8	12.4	13.5	14.7	15.4	17.3	9.4	10.5	11.9	15.4	17.6	20.3
2	11	10.8	12.0	12.5	13.7	14.9	15.7	17.6	9.5	10.7	12.0	15.6	17.9	20.6
3	0	11.0	12.1	12.7	13.9	15.1	15.9	17.8	9.6	10.8	12.2	15.8	18.1	20.9
3	1	11.1	12.3	12.9	14.0	15.3	16.1	18.1	9.7	10.9	12.4	16.0	18.4	21.3
3	2	11.2	12.5	13.0	14.2	15.6	16.3	18.4	9.8	11.1	12.5	16.3	18.7	21.6
3	3	11.4	12.6	13.2	14.4	15.8	16.6	18.6	9.9	11.2	12.7	16.5	19.0	22.0
3	4	11.5	12.8	13.4	14.6	16.0	16.8	18.9	10.1	11.3	12.8	16.7	19.2	22.3
3	5	11.6	12.9	13.5	14.8	16.2	17.0	19.2	10.2	11.5	13.0	16.9	19.5	22.7
3	6	11.8	13.1	13.7	15.0	16.4	17.3	19.5	10.3	11.6	13.1	17.2	19.8	23.0
3	7	11.9	13.2	13.9	15.2	16.6	17.5	19.7	10.4	11.7	13.3	17.4	20.1	23.4
3	8	12.0	13.4	14.0	15.3	16.8	17.7	20.0	10.5	11.8	13.4	17.6	20.4	23.7
3	9	12.1	13.5	14.2	15.5	17.0	17.9	20.3	10.6	12.0	13.6	17.8	20.7	24.1
3	10	12.3	13.7	14.3	15.7	17.3	18.2	20.6	10.7	12.1	13.7	18.1	20.9	24.5
3	11	12.4	13.8	14.5	15.9	17.5	18.4	20.8	10.8	12.2	13.9	18.3	21.2	24.8
4	0	12.5	14.0	14.7	16.1	17.7	18.6	21.1	10.9	12.3	14.0	18.5	21.5	25.2
4	1	12.6	14.1	14.8	16.3	17.9	18.9	21.4	11.0	12.4	14.2	18.8	21.8	25.5
4	2	12.8	14.3	15.0	16.4	18.1	19.1	21.7	11.1	12.6	14.3	19.0	22.1	25.9
4	3	12.9	14.4	15.1	16.6	18.3	19.3	22.0	11.2	12.7	14.5	19.2	22.4	26.3
4	4	13.0	14.5	15.3	16.8	18.5	19.5	22.2	11.3	12.8	14.6	19.4	22.6	26.6
4	5	13.1	14.7	15.4	17.0	18.7	19.8	22.5	11.4	12.9	14.8	19.7	22.9	27.0
4	6	13.2	14.8	15.6	17.2	18.9	20.0	22.8	11.5	13.0	14.9	19.9	23.2	27.4
4	7	13.4	15.0	15.8	17.3	19.1	20.2	23.1	11.6	13.2	15.1	20.1	23.5	27.7
4	8	13.5	15.1	15.9	17.5	19.3	20.4	23.3	11.7	13.3	15.2	20.3	23.8	28.1
4	9	13.6	15.3	16.1	17.7	19.6	20.7	23.6	11.8	13.4	15.3	20.6	24.1	28.5
4	10	13.7	15.4	16.2	17.9	19.8	20.9	23.9	11.9	13.5	15.5	20.8	24.4	28.8
4	11	13.8	15.5	16.4	18.0	20.0	21.1	24.2	12.0	13.6	15.6	21.0	24.6	29.2
5	0	14.0	15.7	16.5	18.2	20.2	21.3	24.4	12.1	13.7	15.8	21.2	24.9	29.5

A

Chart 3 Length (cm) by Age of Boys and Girls Aged 0–2 Years (WHO Standards)

BOYS					Percentiles						Z (SD) score			
Age	(mo)	3rd	15th	25th	50th	75th	85th	97th	−3Z	−2Z	−1Z	+1Z	+2Z	+3Z
	0	46.3	47.9	48.6	49.9	51.2	51.8	53.4	44.2	46.1	48.0	51.8	53.7	55.6
	1	51.1	52.7	53.4	54.7	56.0	56.7	58.4	48.9	50.8	52.8	56.7	58.6	60.6
	2	54.7	56.4	57.1	58.4	59.8	60.5	62.2	52.4	54.4	56.4	60.4	62.4	64.4
	3	57.6	59.3	60.1	61.4	62.8	63.5	65.3	55.3	57.3	59.4	63.5	65.5	67.6
	4	60.0	61.7	62.5	63.9	65.3	66.0	67.8	57.6	59.7	61.8	66.0	68.0	70.1
	5	61.9	63.7	64.5	65.9	67.3	68.1	69.9	59.6	61.7	63.8	68.0	70.1	72.2
	6	63.6	65.4	66.2	67.6	69.1	69.8	71.6	61.2	63.3	65.5	69.8	71.9	74.0
	7	65.1	66.9	67.7	69.2	70.6	71.4	73.2	62.7	64.8	67.0	71.3	73.5	75.7
	8	66.5	68.3	69.1	70.6	72.1	72.9	74.7	64.0	66.2	68.4	72.8	75.0	77.2
	9	67.7	69.6	70.5	72.0	73.5	74.3	76.2	65.2	67.5	69.7	74.2	76.5	78.7
	10	69.0	70.9	71.7	73.3	74.8	75.6	77.6	66.4	68.7	71.0	75.6	77.9	80.1
	11	70.2	72.1	73.0	74.5	76.1	77.0	78.9	67.6	69.9	72.2	76.9	79.2	81.5
	12	71.3	73.3	74.1	75.7	77.4	78.2	80.2	68.6	71.0	73.4	78.1	80.5	82.9
	13	72.4	74.4	75.3	76.9	78.6	79.4	81.5	69.6	72.1	74.5	79.3	81.8	84.2
	14	73.4	75.5	76.4	78.0	79.7	80.6	82.7	70.6	73.1	75.6	80.5	83.0	85.5
	15	74.4	76.5	77.4	79.1	80.9	81.8	83.9	71.6	74.1	76.6	81.7	84.2	86.7
	16	75.4	77.5	78.5	80.2	82.0	82.9	85.1	72.5	75.0	77.6	82.8	85.4	88.0
	17	76.3	78.5	79.5	81.2	83.0	84.0	86.2	73.3	76.0	78.6	83.9	86.5	89.2
	18	77.2	79.5	80.4	82.3	84.1	85.1	87.3	74.2	76.9	79.6	85.0	87.7	90.4
	19	78.1	80.4	81.4	83.2	85.1	86.1	88.4	75.0	77.7	80.5	86.0	88.8	91.5
	20	78.9	81.3	82.3	84.2	86.1	87.1	89.5	75.8	78.6	81.4	87.0	89.8	92.6
	21	79.7	82.2	83.2	85.1	87.1	88.1	90.5	76.5	79.4	82.3	88.0	90.9	93.8
	22	80.5	83.0	84.1	86.0	88.0	89.1	91.6	77.2	80.2	83.1	89.0	91.9	94.9
	23	81.3	83.8	84.9	86.9	89.0	90.0	92.6	78.0	81.0	83.9	89.9	92.9	95.9
	24	82.1	84.6	85.8	87.8	89.9	91.0	93.6	78.7	81.7	84.8	90.9	93.9	97.0

GIRLS					Percentiles						Z (SD) score			
Age	(mo)	3rd	15th	25th	50th	75th	85th	97th	−3Z	−2Z	−1Z	+1Z	+2Z	+3Z
	0	45.6	47.2	47.9	49.1	50.4	51.1	52.7	43.6	45.4	47.3	51.0	52.9	54.7
	1	50.0	51.7	52.4	53.7	55.0	55.7	57.4	47.8	49.8	51.7	55.6	57.6	59.5
	2	53.2	55.0	55.7	57.1	58.4	59.2	60.9	51.0	53.0	55.0	59.1	61.1	63.2
	3	55.8	57.6	58.4	59.8	61.2	62.0	63.8	53.5	55.6	57.7	61.9	64.0	66.1
	4	58.0	59.8	60.6	62.1	63.5	64.3	66.2	55.6	57.8	59.9	64.3	66.4	68.6
	5	59.9	61.7	62.5	64.0	65.5	66.3	68.2	57.4	59.6	61.8	66.2	68.5	70.7
	6	61.5	63.4	64.2	65.7	67.3	68.1	70.0	58.9	61.2	63.5	68.0	70.3	72.5
	7	62.9	64.9	65.7	67.3	68.8	69.7	71.6	60.3	62.7	65.0	69.6	71.9	74.2
	8	64.3	66.3	67.2	68.7	70.3	71.2	73.2	61.7	64.0	66.4	71.1	73.5	75.8
	9	65.6	67.6	68.5	70.1	71.8	72.6	74.7	62.9	65.3	67.7	72.6	75.0	77.4
	10	66.8	68.9	69.8	71.5	73.1	74.0	76.1	64.1	66.5	69.0	73.9	76.4	78.9
	11	68.0	70.2	71.1	72.8	74.5	75.4	77.5	65.2	67.7	70.3	75.3	77.8	80.3
	12	69.2	71.3	72.3	74.0	75.8	76.7	78.9	66.3	68.9	71.4	76.6	79.2	81.7
	13	70.3	72.5	73.4	75.2	77.0	77.9	80.2	67.3	70.0	72.6	77.8	80.5	83.1
	14	71.3	73.6	74.6	76.4	78.2	79.2	81.4	68.3	71.0	73.7	79.1	81.7	84.4
	15	72.4	74.7	75.7	77.5	79.4	80.3	82.7	69.3	72.0	74.8	80.2	83.0	85.7
	16	73.3	75.7	76.7	78.6	80.5	81.5	83.9	70.2	73.0	75.8	81.4	84.2	87.0
	17	74.3	76.7	77.7	79.7	81.6	82.6	85.0	71.1	74.0	76.8	82.5	85.4	88.2
	18	75.2	77.7	78.7	80.7	82.7	83.7	86.2	72.0	74.9	77.8	83.6	86.5	89.4
	19	76.2	78.7	79.7	81.7	83.7	84.8	87.3	72.8	75.8	78.8	84.7	87.6	90.6
	20	77.0	79.6	80.7	82.7	84.7	85.8	88.4	73.7	76.7	79.7	85.7	88.7	91.7
	21	77.9	80.5	81.6	83.7	85.7	86.8	89.4	74.5	77.5	80.6	86.7	89.8	92.9
	22	78.7	81.4	82.5	84.6	86.7	87.8	90.5	75.2	78.4	81.5	87.7	90.8	94.0
	23	79.6	82.2	83.4	85.5	87.7	88.8	91.5	76.0	79.2	82.3	88.7	91.9	95.0
	24	80.3	83.1	84.2	86.4	88.6	89.8	92.5	76.7	80.0	83.2	89.6	92.9	96.1

A

Chart 4 Height by Age (cm) of Boys and Girls Aged 2–5 Years (WHO Standards)

BOYS		Percentiles							Z (SD) score					
Year	month	3rd	15th	25th	50th	75th	85th	97th	−3Z	−2Z	−1Z	+1Z	+2Z	+3Z
2	0	81.4	83.9	85.1	87.1	89.2	90.3	92.9	78.0	81.0	84.1	90.2	93.2	96.3
2	1	82.1	84.7	85.9	88.0	90.1	91.2	93.8	78.6	81.7	84.9	91.1	94.2	97.3
2	2	82.8	85.5	86.7	88.8	90.9	92.1	94.8	79.3	82.5	85.6	92.0	95.2	98.3
2	3	83.5	86.3	87.4	89.6	91.8	93.0	95.7	79.9	83.1	86.4	92.9	96.1	99.3
2	4	84.2	87.0	88.2	90.4	92.6	93.8	96.6	80.5	83.8	87.1	93.7	97.0	100.3
2	5	84.9	87.7	88.9	91.2	93.4	94.7	97.5	81.1	84.5	87.8	94.5	97.9	101.2
2	6	85.5	88.4	89.6	91.9	94.2	95.5	98.3	81.7	85.1	88.5	95.3	98.7	102.1
2	7	86.2	89.1	90.3	92.7	95.0	96.2	99.2	82.3	85.7	89.2	96.1	99.6	103.0
2	8	86.8	89.7	91.0	93.4	95.7	97.0	100.0	82.8	86.4	89.9	96.9	100.4	103.9
2	9	87.4	90.4	91.7	94.1	96.5	97.8	100.8	83.4	86.9	90.5	97.6	101.2	104.8
2	10	88.0	91.0	92.3	94.8	97.2	98.5	101.5	83.9	87.5	91.1	98.4	102.0	105.6
2	11	88.5	91.6	93.0	95.4	97.9	99.2	102.3	84.4	88.1	91.8	99.1	102.7	106.4
3	0	89.1	92.2	93.6	96.1	98.6	99.9	103.1	85.0	88.7	92.4	99.8	103.5	107.2
3	1	89.7	92.8	94.2	96.7	99.3	100.6	103.8	85.5	89.2	93.0	100.5	104.2	108.0
3	2	90.2	93.4	94.8	97.4	99.9	101.3	104.5	86.0	89.8	93.6	101.2	105.0	108.8
3	3	90.8	94.0	95.4	98.0	100.6	102.0	105.2	86.5	90.3	94.2	101.8	105.7	109.5
3	4	91.3	94.6	96.0	98.6	101.3	102.7	105.9	87.0	90.9	94.7	102.5	106.4	110.3
3	5	91.9	95.2	96.6	99.2	101.9	103.3	106.6	87.5	91.4	95.3	103.2	107.1	111.0
3	6	92.4	95.7	97.2	99.9	102.5	104.0	107.3	88.0	91.9	95.9	103.8	107.8	111.7
3	7	92.9	96.3	97.7	100.4	103.1	104.6	108.0	88.4	92.4	96.4	104.5	108.5	112.5
3	8	93.4	96.8	98.3	101.0	103.8	105.2	108.6	88.9	93.0	97.0	105.1	109.1	113.2
3	9	93.9	97.4	98.9	101.6	104.4	105.8	109.3	89.4	93.5	97.5	105.7	109.8	113.9
3	10	94.4	97.9	99.4	102.2	105.0	106.5	109.9	89.8	94.0	98.1	106.3	110.4	114.6
3	11	94.9	98.5	100.0	102.8	105.6	107.1	110.6	90.3	94.4	98.6	106.9	111.1	115.2
4	0	95.4	99.0	100.5	103.3	106.2	107.7	111.2	90.7	94.9	99.1	107.5	111.7	115.9
4	3	96.9	100.5	102.1	105.0	107.9	109.5	113.1	92.1	96.4	100.7	109.3	113.6	117.9
4	6	98.4	102.1	103.7	106.7	109.6	111.2	115.0	93.4	97.8	102.3	111.1	115.5	119.9
4	9	99.8	103.6	105.3	108.3	111.4	113.0	116.8	94.7	99.3	103.8	112.8	117.4	121.9
5	0	101.2	105.2	106.8	110.0	113.1	114.8	118.7	96.1	100.7	105.3	114.6	119.2	123.9

GIRLS		Percentiles							Z (SD) score					
Year	month	3rd	15th	25th	50th	75th	85th	97th	−3Z	−2Z	−1Z	+1Z	+2Z	+3Z
2	0	79.6	82.4	83.5	85.7	87.9	89.1	91.8	76.0	79.3	82.5	88.9	92.2	95.4
2	1	80.4	83.2	84.4	86.6	88.8	90.0	92.8	76.8	80.0	83.3	89.9	93.1	96.4
2	3	81.9	84.8	86.0	88.3	90.6	91.8	94.6	78.1	81.5	84.9	91.7	95.0	98.4
2	4	82.6	85.5	86.8	89.1	91.4	92.7	95.6	78.8	82.2	85.7	92.5	96.0	99.4
2	5	83.4	86.3	87.6	89.9	92.2	93.5	96.4	79.5	82.9	86.4	93.4	96.9	100.3
2	6	84.0	87.0	88.3	90.7	93.1	94.3	97.3	80.1	83.6	87.1	94.2	97.7	101.3
2	7	84.7	87.7	89.0	91.4	93.9	95.2	98.2	80.7	84.3	87.9	95.0	98.6	102.2
2	8	85.4	88.4	89.7	92.2	94.6	95.9	99.0	81.3	84.9	88.6	95.8	99.4	103.1
2	9	86.0	89.1	90.4	92.9	95.4	96.7	99.8	81.9	85.6	89.3	96.6	100.3	103.9
2	10	86.7	89.8	91.1	93.6	96.2	97.5	100.6	82.5	86.2	89.9	97.4	101.1	104.8
2	11	87.3	90.5	91.8	94.4	96.9	98.3	101.4	83.1	86.8	90.6	98.1	101.9	105.6
3	0	87.9	91.1	92.5	95.1	97.6	99.0	102.2	83.6	87.4	91.2	98.9	102.7	106.5
3	1	88.5	91.7	93.1	95.7	98.3	99.7	103.0	84.2	88.0	91.9	99.6	103.4	107.3
3	2	89.1	92.4	93.8	96.4	99.0	100.5	103.7	84.7	88.6	92.5	100.3	104.2	108.1
3	3	89.7	93.0	94.4	97.1	99.7	101.2	104.5	85.3	89.2	93.1	101.0	105.0	108.9
3	4	90.3	93.6	95.1	97.7	100.4	101.9	105.2	85.8	89.8	93.8	101.7	105.7	109.7
3	5	90.8	94.2	95.7	98.4	101.1	102.6	106.0	86.3	90.4	94.4	102.4	106.4	110.5
3	6	91.4	94.8	96.3	99.0	101.8	103.3	106.7	86.8	90.9	95.0	103.1	107.2	111.2
3	7	92.0	95.4	96.9	99.7	102.4	103.9	107.4	87.4	91.5	95.6	103.8	107.9	112.0
3	8	92.5	96.0	97.5	100.3	103.1	104.6	108.1	87.9	92.0	96.2	104.5	108.6	112.7
3	9	93.0	96.6	98.1	100.9	103.7	105.3	108.8	88.4	92.5	96.7	105.1	109.3	113.5
3	10	93.6	97.2	98.7	101.5	104.4	105.9	109.5	88.9	93.1	97.3	105.8	110.0	114.2
3	11	94.1	97.7	99.3	102.1	105.0	106.6	110.2	89.3	93.6	97.9	106.4	110.7	114.9
4	0	94.6	98.3	99.8	102.7	105.6	107.2	110.8	89.8	94.1	98.4	107.0	111.3	115.7
4	3	96.2	99.9	101.5	104.5	107.5	109.1	112.8	91.2	95.6	100.1	108.9	113.3	117.7
4	6	97.6	101.5	103.1	106.2	109.2	110.9	114.7	92.6	97.1	101.6	110.7	115.2	119.8
4	9	99.1	103.0	104.7	107.8	111.0	112.6	116.6	93.9	98.5	103.2	112.5	117.1	121.8
5	0	100.5	104.5	106.2	109.4	112.6	114.4	118.4	95.2	99.9	104.7	114.2	118.9	123.7

A

Chart 5 Weight (kg) for Length (cm) for Boys between 0 and 2 Years (WHO Reference Data) Percentiles and Z (SD) Scores

Length (cm)	Percentiles											Z (SD) score					
	1st	3rd	5th	15th	25th	50th	75th	85th	95th	97th	99th	−3Z	−2Z	−1Z	+1Z	+2Z	+3Z
45.0	2.0	2.1	2.1	2.2	2.3	2.4	2.6	2.7	2.9	2.9	3.0	1.9	2.0	2.2	2.7	3.0	3.3
45.5	2.1	2.1	2.2	2.3	2.4	2.5	2.7	2.8	2.9	3.0	3.1	1.9	2.1	2.3	2.8	3.1	3.4
46.0	2.1	2.2	2.3	2.4	2.5	2.6	2.8	2.9	3.0	3.1	3.3	2.0	2.2	2.4	2.9	3.1	3.5
46.5	2.2	2.3	2.3	2.5	2.5	2.7	2.9	3.0	3.1	3.2	3.4	2.1	2.3	2.5	3.0	3.2	3.6
47.0	2.3	2.4	2.4	2.5	2.6	2.8	3.0	3.1	3.2	3.3	3.5	2.1	2.3	2.5	3.0	3.3	3.7
47.5	2.3	2.4	2.5	2.6	2.7	2.9	3.0	3.1	3.3	3.4	3.6	2.2	2.4	2.6	3.1	3.4	3.8
48.0	2.4	2.5	2.6	2.7	2.8	2.9	3.1	3.2	3.4	3.5	3.7	2.3	2.5	2.7	3.2	3.6	3.9
48.5	2.5	2.6	2.6	2.8	2.9	3.0	3.2	3.3	3.5	3.6	3.8	2.3	2.6	2.8	3.3	3.7	4.0
49.0	2.6	2.7	2.7	2.9	2.9	3.1	3.3	3.4	3.6	3.7	3.9	2.4	2.6	2.9	3.4	3.8	4.2
49.5	2.6	2.7	2.8	2.9	3.0	3.2	3.4	3.5	3.8	3.8	4.0	2.5	2.7	3.0	3.5	3.9	4.3
50.0	2.7	2.8	2.9	3.0	3.1	3.3	3.5	3.7	3.9	4.0	4.1	2.6	2.8	3.0	3.6	4.0	4.4
50.5	2.8	2.9	3.0	3.1	3.2	3.4	3.6	3.8	4.0	4.1	4.2	2.7	2.9	3.1	3.8	4.1	4.5
51.0	2.9	3.0	3.1	3.2	3.3	3.5	3.8	3.9	4.1	4.2	4.4	2.7	3.0	3.2	3.9	4.2	4.7
51.5	3.0	3.1	3.2	3.3	3.4	3.6	3.9	4.0	4.2	4.3	4.5	2.8	3.1	3.3	4.0	4.4	4.8
52.0	3.1	3.2	3.3	3.4	3.5	3.8	4.0	4.1	4.4	4.5	4.6	2.9	3.2	3.5	4.1	4.5	5.0
52.5	3.2	3.3	3.4	3.6	3.7	3.9	4.1	4.3	4.5	4.6	4.8	3.0	3.3	3.6	4.2	4.6	5.1
53.0	3.3	3.4	3.5	3.7	3.8	4.0	4.3	4.4	4.6	4.7	4.9	3.1	3.4	3.7	4.4	4.8	5.3
53.5	3.4	3.5	3.6	3.8	3.9	4.1	4.4	4.5	4.8	4.9	5.1	3.2	3.5	3.8	4.5	4.9	5.4
54.0	3.5	3.6	3.7	3.9	4.0	4.3	4.5	4.7	4.9	5.0	5.3	3.3	3.6	3.9	4.7	5.1	5.6
54.5	3.6	3.8	3.8	4.0	4.2	4.4	4.7	4.8	5.1	5.2	5.4	3.4	3.7	4.0	4.8	5.3	5.8
55.0	3.7	3.9	4.0	4.2	4.3	4.5	4.8	5.0	5.3	5.4	5.6	3.6	3.8	4.2	5.0	5.4	6.0
55.5	3.9	4.0	4.1	4.3	4.4	4.7	5.0	5.1	5.4	5.5	5.8	3.7	4.0	4.3	5.1	5.6	6.1
56.0	4.0	4.1	4.2	4.4	4.6	4.8	5.1	5.3	5.6	5.7	5.9	3.8	4.1	4.4	5.3	5.8	6.3
56.5	4.1	4.3	4.3	4.6	4.7	5.0	5.3	5.4	5.7	5.9	6.1	3.9	4.2	4.6	5.4	5.9	6.5
57.0	4.2	4.4	4.5	4.7	4.8	5.1	5.4	5.6	5.9	6.0	6.3	4.0	4.3	4.7	5.6	6.1	6.7
57.5	4.4	4.5	4.6	4.8	5.0	5.3	5.6	5.8	6.1	6.2	6.5	4.1	4.5	4.9	5.7	6.3	6.9
58.0	4.5	4.6	4.7	5.0	5.1	5.4	5.7	5.9	6.2	6.4	6.6	4.3	4.6	5.0	5.9	6.4	7.1
58.5	4.6	4.8	4.9	5.1	5.3	5.6	5.9	6.1	6.4	6.5	6.8	4.4	4.7	5.1	6.1	6.6	7.2
59.0	4.7	4.9	5.0	5.2	5.4	5.7	6.0	6.2	6.6	6.7	7.0	4.5	4.8	5.3	6.2	6.8	7.4
59.5	4.8	5.0	5.1	5.4	5.5	5.9	6.2	6.4	6.7	6.9	7.2	4.6	5.0	5.4	6.4	7.0	7.6
60.0	5.0	5.1	5.2	5.5	5.7	6.0	6.3	6.5	6.9	7.0	7.3	4.7	5.1	5.5	6.5	7.1	7.8
60.5	5.1	5.3	5.4	5.6	5.8	6.1	6.5	6.7	7.1	7.2	7.5	4.8	5.2	5.6	6.7	7.3	8.0
61.0	5.2	5.4	5.5	5.8	5.9	6.3	6.6	6.8	7.2	7.4	7.7	4.9	5.3	5.8	6.8	7.4	8.1
61.5	5.3	5.5	5.6	5.9	6.1	6.4	6.8	7.0	7.4	7.5	7.8	5.0	5.4	5.9	7.0	7.6	8.3
62.0	5.4	5.6	5.7	6.0	6.2	6.5	6.9	7.1	7.5	7.7	8.0	5.1	5.6	6.0	7.1	7.7	8.5
62.5	5.5	5.7	5.8	6.1	6.3	6.7	7.0	7.3	7.6	7.8	8.1	5.2	5.7	6.1	7.2	7.9	8.6
63.0	5.6	5.8	5.9	6.2	6.4	6.8	7.2	7.4	7.8	8.0	8.3	5.3	5.8	6.2	7.4	8.0	8.8
63.5	5.7	5.9	6.0	6.3	6.5	6.9	7.3	7.5	7.9	8.1	8.4	5.4	5.9	6.4	7.5	8.2	8.9
64.0	5.8	6.0	6.2	6.5	6.6	7.0	7.4	7.7	8.1	8.2	8.6	5.5	6.0	6.5	7.6	8.3	9.1
64.5	5.9	6.1	6.3	6.6	6.8	7.1	7.6	7.8	8.2	8.4	8.7	5.6	6.1	6.6	7.8	8.5	9.3
65.0	6.0	6.3	6.4	6.7	6.9	7.3	7.7	7.9	8.3	8.5	8.9	5.7	6.2	6.7	7.9	8.6	9.4
65.5	6.1	6.4	6.5	6.8	7.0	7.4	7.8	8.1	8.5	8.7	9.0	5.8	6.3	6.8	8.0	8.7	9.6
66.0	6.2	6.5	6.6	6.9	7.1	7.5	7.9	8.2	8.6	8.8	9.1	5.9	6.4	6.9	8.2	8.9	9.7
66.5	6.3	6.6	6.7	7.0	7.2	7.6	8.1	8.3	8.8	8.9	9.3	6.0	6.5	7.0	8.3	9.0	9.9
67.0	6.4	6.7	6.8	7.1	7.3	7.7	8.2	8.4	8.9	9.1	9.4	6.1	6.6	7.1	8.4	9.2	10.0
67.5	6.5	6.8	6.9	7.2	7.4	7.9	8.3	8.6	9.0	9.2	9.6	6.2	6.7	7.2	8.5	9.3	10.2
68.0	6.6	6.9	7.0	7.3	7.5	8.0	8.4	8.7	9.2	9.3	9.7	6.3	6.8	7.3	8.7	9.4	10.3
68.5	6.7	7.0	7.1	7.4	7.7	8.1	8.5	8.8	9.3	9.5	9.8	6.4	6.9	7.5	8.8	9.6	10.5
69.0	6.8	7.1	7.2	7.5	7.8	8.2	8.7	8.9	9.4	9.6	10.0	6.5	7.0	7.6	8.9	9.7	10.6
69.5	6.9	7.1	7.3	7.6	7.9	8.3	8.8	9.1	9.5	9.7	10.1	6.6	7.1	7.7	9.0	9.8	10.8
70.0	7.0	7.2	7.4	7.7	8.0	8.4	8.9	9.2	9.7	9.9	10.3	6.6	7.2	7.8	9.2	10.0	10.9
70.5	7.1	7.3	7.5	7.8	8.1	8.5	9.0	9.3	9.8	10.0	10.4	6.7	7.3	7.9	9.3	10.1	11.1
71.0	7.2	7.4	7.6	8.0	8.2	8.6	9.1	9.4	9.9	10.1	10.5	6.8	7.4	8.0	9.4	10.2	11.2
71.5	7.3	7.5	7.7	8.1	8.3	8.8	9.3	9.6	10.1	10.3	10.7	6.9	7.5	8.1	9.5	10.4	11.3
72.0	7.4	7.6	7.8	8.2	8.4	8.9	9.4	9.7	10.2	10.4	10.8	7.0	7.6	8.2	9.6	10.5	11.5
72.5	7.5	7.7	7.9	8.3	8.5	9.0	9.5	9.8	10.3	10.5	11.0	7.1	7.6	8.3	9.8	10.6	11.6
73.0	7.5	7.8	8.0	8.4	8.6	9.1	9.6	9.9	10.4	10.7	11.1	7.2	7.7	8.4	9.9	10.8	11.8
73.5	7.6	7.9	8.0	8.4	8.7	9.2	9.7	10.0	10.6	10.8	11.2	7.2	7.8	8.5	10.0	10.9	11.9
74.0	7.7	8.0	8.1	8.5	8.8	9.3	9.8	10.1	10.7	10.9	11.4	7.3	7.9	8.6	10.1	11.0	12.1
74.5	7.8	8.1	8.2	8.6	8.9	9.4	9.9	10.3	10.8	11.0	11.5	7.4	8.0	8.7	10.2	11.2	12.2
75.0	7.9	8.2	8.3	8.7	9.0	9.5	10.1	10.4	10.9	11.2	11.6	7.5	8.1	8.8	10.3	11.3	12.3
75.5	8.0	8.2	8.4	8.8	9.1	9.6	10.2	10.5	11.0	11.3	11.7	7.6	8.2	8.8	10.4	11.4	12.5
76.0	8.0	8.3	8.5	8.9	9.2	9.7	10.3	10.6	11.2	11.4	11.9	7.6	8.3	8.9	10.6	11.5	12.6
76.5	8.1	8.4	8.6	9.0	9.3	9.8	10.4	10.7	11.3	11.5	12.0	7.7	8.3	9.0	10.7	11.6	12.7
77.0	8.2	8.5	8.7	9.1	9.4	9.9	10.5	10.8	11.4	11.6	12.1	7.8	8.4	9.1	10.8	11.7	12.8
77.5	8.3	8.6	8.7	9.2	9.5	10.0	10.6	10.9	11.5	11.7	12.2	7.9	8.5	9.2	10.9	11.9	13.0

A

Contd.

Chart 5 Weight (kg) for Length (cm) for Boys between 0 and 2 years (WHO Reference Data) Percentiles and Z (SD) Scores (Contd..)

Length					Percentiles								Z (SD) score				
(cm)	1st	3rd	5th	15th	25th	50th	75th	85th	95th	97th	99th	−3Z	−2Z	−1Z	+1Z	+2Z	+3Z
78.0	8.4	8.7	8.8	9.3	9.5	10.1	10.7	11.0	11.6	11.8	12.3	7.9	8.6	9.3	11.0	12.0	13.1
78.5	8.4	8.7	8.9	9.3	9.6	10.2	10.8	11.1	11.7	12.0	12.4	8.0	8.7	9.4	11.1	12.1	13.2
79.0	8.5	8.8	9.0	9.4	9.7	10.3	10.9	11.2	11.8	12.1	12.5	8.1	8.7	9.5	11.2	12.2	13.3
79.5	8.6	8.9	9.1	9.5	9.8	10.4	11.0	11.3	11.9	12.2	12.7	8.2	8.8	9.5	11.3	12.3	13.4
80.0	8.7	9.0	9.1	9.6	9.9	10.4	11.1	11.4	12.0	12.3	12.8	8.2	8.9	9.6	11.4	12.4	13.6
80.5	8.7	9.1	9.2	9.7	10.0	10.5	11.2	11.5	12.1	12.4	12.9	8.3	9.0	9.7	11.5	12.5	13.7
81.0	8.8	9.1	9.3	9.8	10.1	10.6	11.3	11.6	12.2	12.5	13.0	8.4	9.1	9.8	11.6	12.6	13.8
81.5	8.9	9.2	9.4	9.9	10.2	10.7	11.4	11.7	12.3	12.6	13.1	8.5	9.1	9.9	11.7	12.7	13.9
82.0	9.0	9.3	9.5	10.0	10.2	10.8	11.5	11.8	12.5	12.7	13.2	8.5	9.2	10.0	11.8	12.8	14.0
82.5	9.1	9.4	9.6	10.1	10.3	10.9	11.6	11.9	12.6	12.8	13.3	8.6	9.3	10.1	11.9	13.0	14.2
83.0	9.2	9.5	9.7	10.1	10.4	11.0	11.7	12.0	12.7	13.0	13.5	8.7	9.4	10.2	12.0	13.1	14.3
83.5	9.3	9.6	9.8	10.3	10.6	11.2	11.8	12.2	12.8	13.1	13.6	8.8	9.5	10.3	12.1	13.2	14.4
84.0	9.4	9.7	9.9	10.4	10.7	11.3	11.9	12.3	12.9	13.2	13.7	8.9	9.6	10.4	12.2	13.3	14.6
84.5	9.5	9.8	10.0	10.5	10.8	11.4	12.0	12.4	13.1	13.3	13.9	9.0	9.7	10.5	12.4	13.5	14.7
85.0	9.6	9.9	10.1	10.6	10.9	11.5	12.2	12.5	13.2	13.5	14.0	9.1	9.8	10.6	12.5	13.6	14.9
85.5	9.7	10.0	10.2	10.7	11.0	11.6	12.3	12.7	13.3	13.6	14.1	9.2	9.9	10.7	12.6	13.7	15.0
86.0	9.8	10.1	10.3	10.8	11.1	11.7	12.4	12.8	13.5	13.7	14.3	9.3	10.0	10.8	12.8	13.9	15.2
86.5	9.9	10.2	10.4	10.9	11.2	11.9	12.5	12.9	13.6	13.9	14.4	9.4	10.1	11.0	12.9	14.0	15.3
87.0	10.0	10.3	10.5	11.0	11.4	12.0	12.7	13.1	13.7	14.0	14.6	9.5	10.2	11.1	13.0	14.2	15.5
87.5	10.1	10.4	10.6	11.2	11.5	12.1	12.8	13.2	13.9	14.2	14.7	9.6	10.4	11.2	13.2	14.3	15.6
88.0	10.2	10.6	10.7	11.3	11.6	12.2	12.9	13.3	14.0	14.3	14.9	9.7	10.5	11.3	13.3	14.5	15.8
88.5	10.3	10.7	10.9	11.4	11.7	12.4	13.1	13.5	14.2	14.4	15.0	9.8	10.6	11.4	13.4	14.6	15.9
89.0	10.4	10.8	11.0	11.5	11.8	12.5	13.2	13.6	14.3	14.6	15.2	9.9	10.7	11.5	13.5	14.7	16.1
89.5	10.5	10.9	11.1	11.6	11.9	12.6	13.3	13.7	14.4	14.7	15.3	10.0	10.8	11.6	13.7	14.9	16.2
90.0	10.6	11.0	11.2	11.7	12.1	12.7	13.4	13.8	14.6	14.9	15.4	10.1	10.9	11.8	13.8	15.0	16.4
90.5	10.7	11.1	11.3	11.8	12.2	12.8	13.6	14.0	14.7	15.0	15.6	10.2	11.0	11.9	13.9	15.1	16.5
91.0	10.8	11.2	11.4	11.9	12.3	13.0	13.7	14.1	14.8	15.1	15.7	10.3	11.1	12.0	14.1	15.3	16.7
91.5	10.9	11.3	11.5	12.0	12.4	13.1	13.8	14.2	15.0	15.3	15.9	10.4	11.2	12.1	14.2	15.4	16.8
92.0	11.0	11.4	11.6	12.2	12.5	13.2	13.9	14.4	15.1	15.4	16.0	10.5	11.3	12.2	14.3	15.6	17.0
92.5	11.1	11.5	11.7	12.3	12.6	13.3	14.1	14.5	15.2	15.5	16.1	10.6	11.4	12.3	14.4	15.7	17.1
93.0	11.2	11.6	11.8	12.4	12.7	13.4	14.2	14.6	15.4	15.7	16.3	10.7	11.5	12.4	14.6	15.8	17.3
93.5	11.3	11.7	11.9	12.5	12.8	13.5	14.3	14.7	15.5	15.8	16.4	10.7	11.6	12.5	14.7	16.0	17.4
94.0	11.4	11.8	12.0	12.6	12.9	13.7	14.4	14.9	15.6	16.0	16.6	10.8	11.7	12.6	14.8	16.1	17.6
94.5	11.5	11.9	12.1	12.7	13.1	13.8	14.5	15.0	15.8	16.1	16.7	10.9	11.8	12.7	14.9	16.3	17.7
95.0	11.6	12.0	12.2	12.8	13.2	13.9	14.7	15.1	15.9	16.2	16.9	11.0	11.9	12.8	15.1	16.4	17.9
95.5	11.7	12.1	12.3	12.9	13.3	14.0	14.8	15.3	16.0	16.4	17.0	11.1	12.0	12.9	15.2	16.5	18.0
96.0	11.8	12.2	12.4	13.0	13.4	14.1	14.9	15.4	16.2	16.5	17.2	11.2	12.1	13.1	15.3	16.7	18.2
96.5	11.9	12.3	12.5	13.1	13.5	14.3	15.1	15.5	16.3	16.7	17.3	11.3	12.2	13.2	15.5	16.8	18.4
97.0	12.0	12.4	12.6	13.2	13.6	14.4	15.2	15.7	16.5	16.8	17.5	11.4	12.3	13.3	15.6	17.0	18.5
97.5	12.1	12.5	12.7	13.4	13.7	14.5	15.3	15.8	16.6	17.0	17.6	11.5	12.4	13.4	15.7	17.1	18.7
98.0	12.2	12.6	12.8	13.5	13.9	14.6	15.5	15.9	16.8	17.1	17.8	11.6	12.5	13.5	15.9	17.3	18.9
98.5	12.3	12.7	13.0	13.6	14.0	14.8	15.6	16.1	16.9	17.3	18.0	11.7	12.6	13.6	16.0	17.5	19.1
99.0	12.4	12.8	13.1	13.7	14.1	14.9	15.7	16.2	17.1	17.4	18.1	11.8	12.7	13.7	16.2	17.6	19.2
99.5	12.5	12.9	13.2	13.8	14.2	15.0	15.9	16.4	17.2	17.6	18.3	11.9	12.8	13.9	16.3	17.8	19.4
100.0	12.6	13.0	13.3	13.9	14.4	15.2	16.0	16.5	17.4	17.8	18.5	12.0	12.9	14.0	16.5	18.0	19.6
100.5	12.7	13.2	13.4	14.1	14.5	15.3	16.2	16.7	17.6	17.9	18.7	12.1	13.0	14.1	16.6	18.1	19.8
101.0	12.8	13.3	13.5	14.2	14.6	15.4	16.3	16.8	17.7	18.1	18.8	12.2	13.2	14.2	16.8	18.3	20.0
101.5	12.9	13.4	13.6	14.3	14.7	15.6	16.5	17.0	17.9	18.3	19.0	12.3	13.3	14.4	16.9	18.5	20.2
102.0	13.0	13.5	13.8	14.5	14.9	15.7	16.6	17.2	18.1	18.5	19.2	12.4	13.4	14.5	17.1	18.7	20.4
102.5	13.2	13.6	13.9	14.6	15.0	15.9	16.8	17.3	18.3	18.6	19.4	12.5	13.5	14.6	17.3	18.8	20.6
103.0	13.3	13.8	14.0	14.7	15.2	16.0	17.0	17.5	18.4	18.8	19.6	12.6	13.6	14.8	17.4	19.0	20.8
103.5	13.4	13.9	14.1	14.8	15.3	16.2	17.1	17.7	18.6	19.0	19.8	12.7	13.7	14.9	17.6	19.2	21.0
104.0	13.5	14.0	14.3	15.0	15.4	16.3	17.3	17.8	18.8	19.2	20.0	12.8	13.9	15.0	17.8	19.4	21.2
104.5	13.6	14.1	14.4	15.1	15.6	16.5	17.4	18.0	19.0	19.4	20.2	12.9	14.0	15.2	17.9	19.6	21.5
105.0	13.7	14.2	14.5	15.3	15.7	16.6	17.6	18.2	19.2	19.6	20.4	13.0	14.1	15.3	18.1	19.8	21.7
105.5	13.9	14.4	14.6	15.4	15.9	16.8	17.8	18.4	19.4	19.8	20.6	13.2	14.2	15.4	18.3	20.0	21.9
106.0	14.0	14.5	14.8	15.5	16.0	16.9	18.0	18.5	19.6	20.0	20.8	13.3	14.4	15.6	18.5	20.2	22.1
106.5	14.1	14.6	14.9	15.7	16.2	17.1	18.1	18.7	19.7	20.2	21.0	13.4	14.5	15.7	18.6	20.4	22.4
107.0	14.2	14.8	15.0	15.8	16.3	17.3	18.3	18.9	19.9	20.4	21.2	13.5	14.6	15.9	18.8	20.6	22.6
107.5	14.4	14.9	15.2	16.0	16.5	17.4	18.5	19.1	20.1	20.6	21.4	13.6	14.7	16.0	19.0	20.8	22.8
108.0	14.5	15.0	15.3	16.1	16.6	17.6	18.7	19.3	20.3	20.8	21.7	13.7	14.9	16.2	19.2	21.0	23.1
108.5	14.6	15.2	15.5	16.3	16.8	17.8	18.8	19.5	20.5	21.0	21.9	13.8	15.0	16.3	19.4	21.2	23.3
109.0	14.7	15.3	15.6	16.4	16.9	17.9	19.0	19.6	20.8	21.2	22.1	14.0	15.1	16.5	19.6	21.4	23.6
109.5	14.9	15.4	15.7	16.6	17.1	18.1	19.2	19.8	21.0	21.4	22.3	14.1	15.3	16.6	19.8	21.7	23.8
110.0	15.0	15.6	15.9	16.7	17.2	18.3	19.4	20.0	21.2	21.6	22.6	14.2	15.4	16.8	20.0	21.9	24.1

A

Chart 6 Weight (kg) for Length (cm) for Girls between 0 and 2 Years (WHO Reference Data) Percentiles and Z (SD) Scores

Length (cm)	Percentiles											Z score (SD)					
	1st	3rd	5th	15th	25th	50th	75th	85th	95th	97th	99th	−3Z	−2Z	−1Z	+1Z	+2Z	+3Z
45.0	2.0	2.1	2.1	2.2	2.3	2.5	2.6	2.7	2.9	2.9	3.1	1.9	2.1	2.3	2.7	3.0	3.3
45.5	2.1	2.2	2.2	2.3	2.4	2.5	2.7	2.8	3.0	3.0	3.2	2.0	2.1	2.3	2.8	3.1	3.4
46.0	2.1	2.2	2.3	2.4	2.5	2.6	2.8	2.9	3.1	3.1	3.3	2.0	2.2	2.4	2.9	3.2	3.5
46.5	2.2	2.3	2.3	2.5	2.6	2.7	2.9	3.0	3.2	3.2	3.4	2.1	2.3	2.5	3.0	3.3	3.6
47.0	2.3	2.4	2.4	2.6	2.6	2.8	3.0	3.1	3.3	3.3	3.5	2.2	2.4	2.6	3.1	3.4	3.7
47.5	2.4	2.4	2.5	2.6	2.7	2.9	3.1	3.2	3.4	3.4	3.6	2.2	2.4	2.6	3.2	3.5	3.8
48.0	2.4	2.5	2.6	2.7	2.8	3.0	3.2	3.3	3.5	3.5	3.7	2.3	2.5	2.7	3.3	3.6	4.0
48.5	2.5	2.6	2.7	2.8	2.9	3.1	3.3	3.4	3.6	3.7	3.8	2.4	2.6	2.8	3.4	3.7	4.1
49.0	2.6	2.7	2.7	2.9	3.0	3.2	3.4	3.5	3.7	3.8	3.9	2.4	2.6	2.9	3.5	3.8	4.2
49.5	2.7	2.8	2.8	3.0	3.1	3.3	3.5	3.6	3.8	3.9	4.1	2.5	2.7	3.0	3.6	3.9	4.3
50.0	2.7	2.8	2.9	3.1	3.2	3.4	3.6	3.7	3.9	4.0	4.2	2.6	2.8	3.1	3.7	4.0	4.5
50.5	2.8	2.9	3.0	3.2	3.3	3.5	3.7	3.8	4.0	4.1	4.3	2.7	2.9	3.2	3.8	4.2	4.6
51.0	2.9	3.0	3.1	3.2	3.4	3.6	3.8	3.9	4.2	4.3	4.4	2.8	3.0	3.3	3.9	4.3	4.8
51.5	3.0	3.1	3.2	3.4	3.5	3.7	3.9	4.0	4.3	4.4	4.6	2.8	3.1	3.4	4.0	4.4	4.9
52.0	3.1	3.2	3.3	3.5	3.6	3.8	4.0	4.2	4.4	4.5	4.7	2.9	3.2	3.5	4.2	4.6	5.1
52.5	3.2	3.3	3.4	3.6	3.7	3.9	4.2	4.3	4.6	4.7	4.9	3.0	3.3	3.6	4.3	4.7	5.2
53.0	3.3	3.4	3.5	3.7	3.8	4.0	4.3	4.4	4.7	4.8	5.0	3.1	3.4	3.7	4.4	4.9	5.4
53.5	3.4	3.5	3.6	3.8	3.9	4.2	4.4	4.6	4.9	5.0	5.2	3.2	3.5	3.8	4.6	5.0	5.5
54.0	3.5	3.6	3.7	3.9	4.0	4.3	4.6	4.7	5.0	5.1	5.3	3.3	3.6	3.9	4.7	5.2	5.7
54.5	3.6	3.7	3.8	4.0	4.2	4.4	4.7	4.9	5.2	5.3	5.5	3.4	3.7	4.0	4.8	5.3	5.9
55.0	3.7	3.9	3.9	4.1	4.3	4.5	4.8	5.0	5.3	5.4	5.7	3.5	3.8	4.2	5.0	5.5	6.1
55.5	3.8	4.0	4.0	4.3	4.4	4.7	5.0	5.2	5.5	5.6	5.8	3.6	3.9	4.3	5.1	5.7	6.3
56.0	3.9	4.1	4.2	4.4	4.5	4.8	5.1	5.3	5.6	5.8	6.0	3.7	4.0	4.4	5.3	5.8	6.4
56.5	4.0	4.2	4.3	4.5	4.7	5.0	5.3	5.5	5.8	5.9	6.2	3.8	4.1	4.5	5.4	6.0	6.6
57.0	4.1	4.3	4.4	4.6	4.8	5.1	5.4	5.6	5.9	6.1	6.3	3.9	4.3	4.6	5.6	6.1	6.8
57.5	4.3	4.4	4.5	4.8	4.9	5.2	5.6	5.7	6.1	6.2	6.5	4.0	4.4	4.8	5.7	6.3	7.0
58.0	4.4	4.5	4.6	4.9	5.0	5.4	5.7	5.9	6.2	6.4	6.7	4.1	4.5	4.9	5.9	6.5	7.1
58.5	4.5	4.6	4.7	5.0	5.2	5.5	5.8	6.0	6.4	6.5	6.8	4.2	4.6	5.0	6.0	6.6	7.3
59.0	4.6	4.8	4.9	5.1	5.3	5.6	6.0	6.2	6.6	6.7	7.0	4.3	4.7	5.1	6.2	6.8	7.5
59.5	4.7	4.9	5.0	5.2	5.4	5.7	6.1	6.3	6.7	6.9	7.2	4.4	4.8	5.3	6.3	6.9	7.7
60.0	4.8	5.0	5.1	5.4	5.5	5.9	6.3	6.5	6.9	7.0	7.3	4.5	4.9	5.4	6.4	7.1	7.8
60.5	4.9	5.1	5.2	5.5	5.6	6.0	6.4	6.6	7.0	7.2	7.5	4.6	5.0	5.5	6.6	7.3	8.0
61.0	5.0	5.2	5.3	5.6	5.8	6.1	6.5	6.7	7.2	7.3	7.6	4.7	5.1	5.6	6.7	7.4	8.2
61.5	5.1	5.3	5.4	5.7	5.9	6.3	6.7	6.9	7.3	7.5	7.8	4.8	5.2	5.7	6.9	7.6	8.4
62.0	5.2	5.4	5.5	5.8	6.0	6.4	6.8	7.0	7.4	7.6	8.0	4.9	5.3	5.8	7.0	7.7	8.5
62.5	5.3	5.5	5.6	5.9	6.1	6.5	6.9	7.2	7.6	7.8	8.1	5.0	5.4	5.9	7.1	7.8	8.7
63.0	5.4	5.6	5.7	6.0	6.2	6.6	7.0	7.3	7.7	7.9	8.3	5.1	5.5	6.0	7.3	8.0	8.8
63.5	5.5	5.7	5.8	6.1	6.3	6.7	7.2	7.4	7.9	8.0	8.4	5.2	5.6	6.2	7.4	8.1	9.0
64.0	5.6	5.8	5.9	6.2	6.4	6.9	7.3	7.5	8.0	8.2	8.5	5.3	5.7	6.3	7.5	8.3	9.1
64.5	5.7	5.9	6.0	6.3	6.6	7.0	7.4	7.7	8.1	8.3	8.7	5.4	5.8	6.4	7.6	8.4	9.3
65.0	5.8	6.0	6.1	6.5	6.7	7.1	7.5	7.8	8.3	8.5	8.8	5.5	5.9	6.5	7.8	8.6	9.5
65.5	5.9	6.1	6.2	6.6	6.8	7.2	7.7	7.9	8.4	8.6	9.0	5.5	6.0	6.6	7.9	8.7	9.6
66.0	6.0	6.2	6.3	6.7	6.9	7.3	7.8	8.0	8.5	8.7	9.1	5.6	6.1	6.7	8.0	8.8	9.8
66.5	6.1	6.3	6.4	6.8	7.0	7.4	7.9	8.2	8.7	8.9	9.3	5.7	6.2	6.8	8.1	9.0	9.9
67.0	6.1	6.4	6.5	6.9	7.1	7.5	8.0	8.3	8.8	9.0	9.4	5.8	6.3	6.9	8.3	9.1	10.0
67.5	6.2	6.5	6.6	7.0	7.2	7.6	8.1	8.4	8.9	9.1	9.5	5.9	6.4	7.0	8.4	9.2	10.2
68.0	6.3	6.6	6.7	7.1	7.3	7.7	8.2	8.5	9.0	9.2	9.7	6.0	6.5	7.1	8.5	9.4	10.3
68.5	6.4	6.7	6.8	7.2	7.4	7.9	8.4	8.6	9.2	9.4	9.8	6.1	6.6	7.2	8.6	9.5	10.5
69.0	6.5	6.7	6.9	7.3	7.5	8.0	8.5	8.8	9.3	9.5	9.9	6.1	6.7	7.3	8.7	9.6	10.6
69.5	6.6	6.8	7.0	7.3	7.6	8.1	8.6	8.9	9.4	9.6	10.0	6.2	6.8	7.4	8.8	9.7	10.7
70.0	6.7	6.9	7.1	7.4	7.7	8.2	8.7	9.0	9.5	9.7	10.2	6.3	6.9	7.5	9.0	9.9	10.9
70.5	6.7	7.0	7.1	7.5	7.8	8.3	8.8	9.1	9.6	9.9	10.3	6.4	6.9	7.6	9.1	10.0	11.0
71.0	6.8	7.1	7.2	7.6	7.9	8.4	8.9	9.2	9.8	10.0	10.4	6.5	7.0	7.7	9.2	10.1	11.1
71.5	6.9	7.2	7.3	7.7	8.0	8.5	9.0	9.3	9.9	10.1	10.5	6.5	7.1	7.7	9.3	10.2	11.3
72.0	7.0	7.3	7.4	7.8	8.1	8.6	9.1	9.4	10.0	10.2	10.7	6.6	7.2	7.8	9.4	10.3	11.4
72.5	7.1	7.4	7.5	7.9	8.2	8.7	9.2	9.5	10.1	10.3	10.8	6.7	7.3	7.9	9.5	10.5	11.5
73.0	7.2	7.4	7.6	8.0	8.3	8.8	9.3	9.6	10.2	10.4	10.9	6.8	7.4	8.0	9.6	10.6	11.7
73.5	7.2	7.5	7.7	8.1	8.3	8.9	9.4	9.7	10.3	10.6	11.0	6.9	7.4	8.1	9.7	10.7	11.8
74.0	7.3	7.6	7.8	8.2	8.4	9.0	9.5	9.9	10.4	10.7	11.2	6.9	7.5	8.2	9.8	10.8	11.9
74.5	7.4	7.7	7.8	8.3	8.5	9.1	9.6	10.0	10.5	10.8	11.3	7.0	7.6	8.3	9.9	10.9	12.0
75.0	7.5	7.8	7.9	8.3	8.6	9.1	9.7	10.1	10.7	10.9	11.4	7.1	7.7	8.4	10.0	11.0	12.2
75.5	7.6	7.8	8.0	8.4	8.7	9.2	9.8	10.2	10.8	11.0	11.5	7.1	7.8	8.5	10.1	11.1	12.3
76.0	7.6	7.9	8.1	8.5	8.8	9.3	9.9	10.3	10.9	11.1	11.6	7.2	7.8	8.5	10.2	11.2	12.4
76.5	7.7	8.0	8.2	8.6	8.9	9.4	10.0	10.4	11.0	11.2	11.7	7.3	7.9	8.6	10.3	11.4	12.5
77.0	7.8	8.1	8.2	8.7	9.0	9.5	10.1	10.5	11.1	11.3	11.8	7.4	8.0	8.7	10.4	11.5	12.6
77.5	7.9	8.2	8.3	8.8	9.1	9.6	10.2	10.6	11.2	11.4	11.9	7.4	8.1	8.8	10.5	11.6	12.8

A

Contd.

Chart 6 Weight (kg) for Length (cm) for Girls between 0 and 2 years (WHO Reference Data) Percentiles and Z (SD) Scores (Contd..)

Length (cm)	Percentiles											Standard deviation (SD) Z score					
	1st	3rd	5th	15th	25th	50th	75th	85th	95th	97th	99th	−3Z	−2Z	−1Z	+1Z	+2Z	+3Z
78.0	7.9	8.2	8.4	8.9	9.1	9.7	10.3	10.7	11.3	11.5	12.1	7.5	8.2	8.9	10.6	11.7	12.9
78.5	8.0	8.3	8.5	8.9	9.2	9.8	10.4	10.8	11.4	11.7	12.2	7.6	8.2	9.0	10.7	11.8	13.0
79.0	8.1	8.4	8.6	9.0	9.3	9.9	10.5	10.9	11.5	11.8	12.3	7.7	8.3	9.1	10.8	11.9	13.1
79.5	8.2	8.5	8.7	9.1	9.4	10.0	10.6	11.0	11.6	11.9	12.4	7.7	8.4	9.1	10.9	12.0	13.3
80.0	8.3	8.6	8.7	9.2	9.5	10.1	10.7	11.1	11.7	12.0	12.5	7.8	8.5	9.2	11.0	12.1	13.4
80.5	8.3	8.7	8.8	9.3	9.6	10.2	10.8	11.2	11.9	12.1	12.7	7.9	8.6	9.3	11.2	12.3	13.5
81.0	8.4	8.8	8.9	9.4	9.7	10.3	10.9	11.3	12.0	12.2	12.8	8.0	8.7	9.4	11.3	12.4	13.7
81.5	8.5	8.8	9.0	9.5	9.8	10.4	11.1	11.4	12.1	12.4	12.9	8.1	8.8	9.5	11.4	12.5	13.8
82.0	8.6	8.9	9.1	9.6	9.9	10.5	11.2	11.6	12.2	12.5	13.1	8.1	8.8	9.6	11.5	12.6	13.9
82.5	8.7	9.0	9.2	9.7	10.0	10.6	11.3	11.7	12.4	12.6	13.2	8.2	8.9	9.7	11.6	12.8	14.1
83.0	8.8	9.1	9.3	9.8	10.1	10.7	11.4	11.8	12.5	12.8	13.3	8.3	9.0	9.8	11.8	12.9	14.2
83.5	8.9	9.2	9.4	9.9	10.2	10.9	11.5	11.9	12.6	12.9	13.5	8.4	9.1	9.9	11.9	13.1	14.4
84.0	9.0	9.3	9.5	10.0	10.3	11.0	11.7	12.1	12.8	13.1	13.6	8.5	9.2	10.1	12.0	13.2	14.5
84.5	9.1	9.4	9.6	10.1	10.5	11.1	11.8	12.2	12.9	13.2	13.8	8.6	9.3	10.2	12.1	13.3	14.7
85.0	9.2	9.5	9.7	10.2	10.6	11.2	11.9	12.3	13.0	13.3	13.9	8.7	9.4	10.3	12.3	13.5	14.9
85.5	9.3	9.6	9.8	10.4	10.7	11.3	12.1	12.5	13.2	13.5	14.1	8.8	9.5	10.4	12.4	13.6	15.0
86.0	9.4	9.8	9.9	10.5	10.8	11.5	12.2	12.6	13.3	13.6	14.2	8.9	9.7	10.5	12.6	13.8	15.2
86.5	9.5	9.9	10.1	10.6	10.9	11.6	12.3	12.7	13.5	13.8	14.4	9.0	9.8	10.6	12.7	13.9	15.4
87.0	9.6	10.0	10.2	10.7	11.0	11.7	12.5	12.9	13.6	13.9	14.5	9.1	9.9	10.7	12.8	14.1	15.5
87.5	9.7	10.1	10.3	10.8	11.2	11.8	12.6	13.0	13.8	14.1	14.7	9.2	10.0	10.9	13.0	14.2	15.7
88.0	9.8	10.2	10.4	10.9	11.3	12.0	12.7	13.2	13.9	14.2	14.9	9.3	10.1	11.0	13.1	14.4	15.9
88.5	9.9	10.3	10.5	11.0	11.4	12.1	12.9	13.3	14.1	14.4	15.0	9.4	10.2	11.1	13.2	14.5	16.0
89.0	10.0	10.4	10.6	11.2	11.5	12.2	13.0	13.4	14.2	14.5	15.2	9.5	10.3	11.2	13.4	14.7	16.2
89.5	10.1	10.5	10.7	11.3	11.6	12.3	13.1	13.6	14.4	14.7	15.3	9.6	10.4	11.3	13.5	14.8	16.4
90.0	10.2	10.6	10.8	11.4	11.8	12.5	13.3	13.7	14.5	14.8	15.5	9.7	10.5	11.5	13.7	15.0	16.5
90.5	10.3	10.7	10.9	11.5	11.9	12.6	13.4	13.8	14.6	15.0	15.6	9.8	10.6	11.5	13.8	15.1	16.7
91.0	10.4	10.8	11.0	11.6	12.0	12.7	13.5	14.0	14.8	15.1	15.8	9.9	10.7	11.7	13.9	15.3	16.9
91.5	10.5	10.9	11.1	11.7	12.1	12.8	13.7	14.1	14.9	15.3	15.9	10.0	10.8	11.8	14.1	15.5	17.0
92.0	10.6	11.0	11.2	11.8	12.2	13.0	13.8	14.2	15.1	15.4	16.1	10.1	10.9	11.9	14.2	15.6	17.2
92.5	10.7	11.1	11.3	12.0	12.3	13.1	13.9	14.4	15.2	15.6	16.3	10.1	11.0	12.0	14.3	15.8	17.4
93.0	10.8	11.2	11.5	12.1	12.5	13.2	14.0	14.5	15.4	15.7	16.4	10.2	11.1	12.1	14.5	15.9	17.5
93.5	10.9	11.3	11.6	12.2	12.6	13.3	14.2	14.7	15.5	15.9	16.6	10.3	11.2	12.2	14.6	16.1	17.7
94.0	11.0	11.4	11.7	12.3	12.7	13.5	14.3	14.8	15.7	16.0	16.7	10.4	11.3	12.3	14.7	16.2	17.9
94.5	11.1	11.5	11.8	12.4	12.8	13.6	14.4	14.9	15.8	16.2	16.9	10.5	11.4	12.4	14.9	16.4	18.0
95.0	11.2	11.6	11.9	12.5	12.9	13.7	14.6	15.1	16.0	16.3	17.0	10.6	11.5	12.6	15.0	16.5	18.2
95.5	11.3	11.8	12.0	12.6	13.0	13.8	14.7	15.2	16.1	16.5	17.2	10.7	11.6	12.7	15.2	16.7	18.4
96.0	11.4	11.9	12.1	12.7	13.2	14.0	14.9	15.4	16.3	16.6	17.4	10.8	11.7	12.8	15.3	16.8	18.6
96.5	11.5	12.0	12.2	12.9	13.3	14.1	15.0	15.5	16.4	16.8	17.5	10.9	11.8	12.9	15.4	17.0	18.7
97.0	11.6	12.1	12.3	13.0	13.4	14.2	15.1	15.6	16.6	16.9	17.7	11.0	12.0	13.0	15.6	17.1	18.9
97.5	11.7	12.2	12.4	13.1	13.5	14.4	15.3	15.8	16.7	17.1	17.9	11.1	12.1	13.1	15.7	17.3	19.1
98.0	11.8	12.3	12.5	13.2	13.6	14.5	15.4	15.9	16.9	17.3	18.0	11.2	12.2	13.3	15.9	17.5	19.3
98.5	11.9	12.4	12.7	13.3	13.8	14.6	15.5	16.1	17.0	17.4	18.2	11.3	12.3	13.4	16.0	17.6	19.5
99.0	12.0	12.5	12.8	13.5	13.9	14.8	15.7	16.2	17.2	17.6	18.4	11.4	12.4	13.5	16.2	17.8	19.6
99.5	12.2	12.6	12.9	13.6	14.0	14.9	15.8	16.4	17.4	17.8	18.5	11.5	12.5	13.6	16.3	18.0	19.8
100.0	12.3	12.7	13.0	13.7	14.1	15.0	16.0	16.5	17.5	17.9	18.7	11.6	12.6	13.7	16.5	18.1	20.0
100.5	12.4	12.9	13.1	13.8	14.3	15.2	16.1	16.7	17.7	18.1	18.9	11.7	12.7	13.9	16.6	18.3	20.2
101.0	12.5	13.0	13.2	14.0	14.4	15.3	16.3	16.9	17.9	18.3	19.1	11.8	12.8	14.0	16.8	18.5	20.4
101.5	12.6	13.1	13.4	14.1	14.5	15.5	16.4	17.0	18.0	18.5	19.3	11.9	13.0	14.1	17.0	18.7	20.6
102.0	12.7	13.2	13.5	14.2	14.7	15.6	16.6	17.2	18.2	18.6	19.5	12.0	13.1	14.3	17.1	18.9	20.8
102.5	12.8	13.3	13.6	14.4	14.8	15.8	16.8	17.4	18.4	18.8	19.7	12.1	13.2	14.4	17.3	19.0	21.0
103.0	13.0	13.5	13.7	14.5	15.0	15.9	16.9	17.5	18.6	19.0	19.9	12.3	13.3	14.5	17.5	19.2	21.3
103.5	13.1	13.6	13.9	14.6	15.1	16.1	17.1	17.7	18.8	19.2	20.1	12.4	13.5	14.7	17.6	19.4	21.5
104.0	13.2	13.7	14.0	14.8	15.3	16.2	17.3	17.9	19.0	19.4	20.3	12.5	13.6	14.8	17.8	19.6	21.7
104.5	13.3	13.9	14.1	14.9	15.4	16.4	17.4	18.1	19.1	19.6	20.5	12.6	13.7	15.0	18.0	19.8	21.9
105.0	13.5	14.0	14.3	15.1	15.6	16.5	17.6	18.2	19.3	19.8	20.7	12.7	13.8	15.1	18.2	20.0	22.2
105.5	13.6	14.1	14.4	15.2	15.7	16.7	17.8	18.4	19.5	20.0	20.9	12.8	14.0	15.3	18.4	20.2	22.4
106.0	13.7	14.3	14.6	15.4	15.9	16.9	18.0	18.6	19.7	20.2	21.1	13.0	14.1	15.4	18.5	20.5	22.6
106.5	13.9	14.4	14.7	15.5	16.0	17.1	18.2	18.8	20.0	20.4	21.4	13.1	14.3	15.6	18.7	20.7	22.9
107.0	14.0	14.5	14.8	15.7	16.2	17.2	18.4	19.0	20.2	20.6	21.6	13.2	14.4	15.7	18.9	20.9	23.1
107.5	14.1	14.7	15.0	15.8	16.4	17.4	18.5	19.2	20.4	20.9	21.8	13.3	14.5	15.9	19.1	21.1	23.4
108.0	14.3	14.8	15.1	16.0	16.5	17.6	18.7	19.4	20.6	21.1	22.1	13.5	14.7	16.0	19.3	21.3	23.6
108.5	14.4	15.0	15.3	16.2	16.7	17.8	18.9	19.6	20.8	21.3	22.3	13.6	14.8	16.2	19.5	21.6	23.9
109.0	14.6	15.1	15.5	16.3	16.9	18.0	19.1	19.8	21.0	21.5	22.5	13.7	15.0	16.4	19.7	21.8	24.2
109.5	14.7	15.3	15.6	16.5	17.0	18.1	19.3	20.0	21.3	21.8	22.8	13.9	15.1	16.5	20.0	22.0	24.4
110.0	14.9	15.4	15.8	16.7	17.2	18.3	19.5	20.2	21.5	22.0	23.0	14.0	15.3	16.7	20.2	22.3	24.7

A

Chart 7 Weight (kg) for Height (cm) for Boys between 2 and 5 Years (WHO Reference Data) Percentiles and Z (SD) Scores

Height (cm)	Percentiles											Z (SD) score					
	1st	3rd	5th	15th	25th	50th	75th	85th	95th	97th	99th	−3Z	−2Z	−1Z	+1Z	+2Z	+3Z
65.0	6.2	6.4	6.5	6.8	7.0	7.4	7.9	8.1	8.5	8.7	9.1	5.9	6.3	6.9	8.1	8.8	9.6
65.5	6.3	6.5	6.6	6.9	7.1	7.6	8.0	8.2	8.7	8.9	9.2	6.0	6.4	7.0	8.2	8.9	9.8
66.0	6.4	6.6	6.7	7.1	7.3	7.7	8.1	8.4	8.8	9.0	9.3	6.1	6.5	7.1	8.3	9.1	9.9
66.5	6.5	6.7	6.8	7.2	7.4	7.8	8.2	8.5	8.9	9.1	9.5	6.1	6.6	7.2	8.5	9.2	10.1
67.0	6.6	6.8	6.9	7.3	7.5	7.9	8.4	8.6	9.1	9.3	9.6	6.2	6.7	7.3	8.6	9.4	10.2
67.5	6.7	6.9	7.0	7.4	7.6	8.0	8.5	8.7	9.2	9.4	9.8	6.3	6.8	7.4	8.7	9.5	10.4
68.0	6.8	7.0	7.1	7.5	7.7	8.1	8.6	8.9	9.3	9.5	9.9	6.4	6.9	7.5	8.8	9.6	10.5
68.5	6.8	7.1	7.2	7.6	7.8	8.2	8.7	9.0	9.5	9.7	10.0	6.5	7.0	7.6	9.0	9.8	10.7
69.0	6.9	7.2	7.3	7.7	7.9	8.4	8.8	9.1	9.6	9.8	10.2	6.6	7.1	7.7	9.1	9.9	10.8
69.5	7.0	7.3	7.4	7.8	8.0	8.5	9.0	9.2	9.7	9.9	10.3	6.7	7.2	7.8	9.2	10.0	11.0
70.0	7.1	7.4	7.5	7.9	8.1	8.6	9.1	9.4	9.9	10.1	10.5	6.8	7.3	7.9	9.3	10.2	11.1
70.5	7.2	7.5	7.6	8.0	8.2	8.7	9.2	9.5	10.0	10.2	10.6	6.9	7.4	8.0	9.5	10.3	11.3
71.0	7.3	7.6	7.7	8.1	8.3	8.8	9.3	9.6	10.1	10.3	10.7	6.9	7.5	8.1	9.6	10.4	11.4
71.5	7.4	7.7	7.8	8.2	8.4	8.9	9.4	9.7	10.2	10.5	10.9	7.0	7.6	8.2	9.7	10.6	11.6
72.0	7.5	7.8	7.9	8.3	8.5	9.0	9.5	9.8	10.4	10.6	11.0	7.1	7.7	8.3	9.8	10.7	11.7
72.5	7.6	7.8	8.0	8.4	8.6	9.1	9.7	10.0	10.5	10.7	11.1	7.2	7.8	8.4	9.9	10.8	11.8
73.0	7.7	7.9	8.1	8.5	8.7	9.2	9.8	10.1	10.6	10.8	11.3	7.3	7.9	8.5	10.0	11.0	12.0
73.5	7.8	8.0	8.2	8.6	8.8	9.3	9.9	10.2	10.7	11.0	11.4	7.4	7.9	8.6	10.2	11.1	12.1
74.0	7.8	8.1	8.3	8.7	8.9	9.4	10.0	10.3	10.9	11.1	11.5	7.4	8.0	8.7	10.3	11.2	12.2
74.5	7.9	8.2	8.4	8.8	9.0	9.5	10.1	10.4	11.0	11.2	11.7	7.5	8.1	8.8	10.4	11.3	12.4
75.0	8.0	8.3	8.4	8.9	9.1	9.6	10.2	10.5	11.1	11.3	11.8	7.6	8.2	8.9	10.5	11.4	12.5
75.5	8.1	8.4	8.5	9.0	9.2	9.7	10.3	10.6	11.2	11.4	11.9	7.7	8.3	9.0	10.6	11.6	12.6
76.0	8.2	8.5	8.6	9.0	9.3	9.8	10.4	10.7	11.3	11.6	12.0	7.7	8.4	9.1	10.7	11.7	12.8
76.5	8.2	8.5	8.7	9.1	9.4	9.9	10.5	10.8	11.4	11.7	12.1	7.8	8.5	9.2	10.8	11.8	12.9
77.0	8.3	8.6	8.8	9.2	9.5	10.0	10.6	10.9	11.5	11.8	12.3	7.9	8.5	9.2	10.9	11.9	13.0
77.5	8.4	8.7	8.9	9.3	9.6	10.1	10.7	11.0	11.6	11.9	12.4	8.0	8.6	9.3	11.0	12.0	13.1
78.0	8.5	8.8	8.9	9.4	9.7	10.2	10.8	11.1	11.7	12.0	12.5	8.0	8.7	9.4	11.1	12.1	13.3
78.5	8.5	8.8	9.0	9.5	9.7	10.3	10.9	11.2	11.9	12.1	12.6	8.1	8.8	9.5	11.2	12.2	13.4
79.0	8.6	8.9	9.1	9.5	9.8	10.4	11.0	11.3	12.0	12.2	12.7	8.2	8.8	9.6	11.3	12.3	13.5
79.5	8.7	9.0	9.2	9.6	9.9	10.5	11.1	11.4	12.1	12.3	12.8	8.3	8.9	9.7	11.4	12.4	13.6
80.0	8.8	9.1	9.3	9.7	10.0	10.6	11.2	11.5	12.2	12.4	12.9	8.3	9.0	9.7	11.5	12.6	13.7
80.5	8.9	9.2	9.3	9.8	10.1	10.7	11.3	11.6	12.3	12.5	13.0	8.4	9.1	9.8	11.6	12.7	13.8
81.0	8.9	9.3	9.4	9.9	10.2	10.8	11.4	11.8	12.4	12.6	13.1	8.5	9.2	9.9	11.7	12.8	14.0
81.5	9.0	9.3	9.5	10.0	10.3	10.9	11.5	11.9	12.5	12.8	13.3	8.6	9.3	10.0	11.8	12.9	14.1
82.0	9.1	9.4	9.6	10.1	10.4	11.0	11.6	12.0	12.6	12.9	13.4	8.7	9.3	10.1	11.9	13.0	14.2
82.5	9.2	9.5	9.7	10.2	10.5	11.1	11.7	12.1	12.7	13.0	13.5	8.7	9.4	10.2	12.1	13.1	14.4
83.0	9.3	9.6	9.8	10.3	10.6	11.2	11.8	12.2	12.9	13.1	13.6	8.8	9.5	10.3	12.2	13.3	14.5
83.5	9.4	9.7	9.9	10.4	10.7	11.3	12.0	12.3	13.0	13.3	13.8	8.9	9.6	10.4	12.3	13.4	14.6
84.0	9.5	9.8	10.0	10.5	10.8	11.4	12.1	12.5	13.1	13.4	13.9	9.0	9.7	10.5	12.4	13.5	14.8
84.5	9.6	9.9	10.1	10.6	10.9	11.5	12.2	12.6	13.3	13.5	14.1	9.1	9.9	10.7	12.5	13.7	14.9
85.0	9.7	10.1	10.2	10.7	11.1	11.7	12.3	12.7	13.4	13.7	14.2	9.2	10.0	10.8	12.7	13.8	15.1
85.5	9.8	10.2	10.3	10.9	11.2	11.8	12.5	12.8	13.5	13.8	14.3	9.3	10.1	10.9	12.8	13.9	15.2
86.0	9.9	10.3	10.5	11.0	11.3	11.9	12.6	13.0	13.7	13.9	14.5	9.4	10.2	11.0	12.9	14.1	15.4
86.5	10.0	10.4	10.6	11.1	11.4	12.0	12.7	13.1	13.8	14.1	14.6	9.5	10.3	11.1	13.1	14.2	15.5
87.0	10.1	10.5	10.7	11.2	11.5	12.2	12.9	13.2	13.9	14.2	14.8	9.6	10.4	11.2	13.2	14.4	15.7
87.5	10.2	10.6	10.8	11.3	11.6	12.3	13.0	13.4	14.1	14.4	14.9	9.7	10.5	11.3	13.3	14.5	15.8
88.0	10.3	10.7	10.9	11.4	11.8	12.4	13.1	13.5	14.2	14.5	15.1	9.8	10.6	11.5	13.5	14.7	16.0
88.5	10.5	10.8	11.0	11.5	11.9	12.5	13.2	13.6	14.4	14.6	15.2	9.9	10.7	11.6	13.6	14.8	16.1
89.0	10.6	10.9	11.1	11.7	12.0	12.6	13.4	13.8	14.5	14.8	15.4	10.0	10.8	11.7	13.7	14.9	16.3
89.5	10.7	11.0	11.2	11.8	12.1	12.8	13.5	13.9	14.6	14.9	15.5	10.1	10.9	11.8	13.9	15.1	16.4
90.0	10.8	11.1	11.3	11.9	12.2	12.9	13.6	14.0	14.8	15.1	15.6	10.2	11.0	11.9	14.0	15.2	16.6
90.5	10.9	11.2	11.4	12.0	12.3	13.0	13.7	14.1	14.9	15.2	15.8	10.3	11.1	12.0	14.1	15.3	16.7
91.0	11.0	11.3	11.5	12.1	12.4	13.1	13.9	14.3	15.0	15.3	15.9	10.4	11.2	12.1	14.2	15.5	16.9
91.5	11.0	11.4	11.6	12.2	12.5	13.2	14.0	14.4	15.2	15.5	16.1	10.5	11.3	12.2	14.4	15.6	17.0
92.0	11.1	11.5	11.7	12.3	12.7	13.4	14.1	14.5	15.3	15.6	16.2	10.6	11.4	12.3	14.5	15.8	17.2
92.5	11.2	11.6	11.8	12.4	12.8	13.5	14.2	14.7	15.4	15.7	16.3	10.7	11.5	12.4	14.6	15.9	17.3
93.0	11.3	11.7	11.9	12.5	12.9	13.6	14.4	14.8	15.6	15.9	16.5	10.8	11.6	12.6	14.7	16.0	17.5
93.5	11.4	11.8	12.0	12.6	13.0	13.7	14.5	14.9	15.7	16.0	16.6	10.9	11.7	12.7	14.9	16.2	17.6
94.0	11.5	11.9	12.1	12.7	13.1	13.8	14.6	15.0	15.8	16.1	16.8	11.0	11.8	12.8	15.0	16.3	17.8
94.5	11.6	12.0	12.2	12.8	13.2	13.9	14.7	15.2	16.0	16.3	16.9	11.1	11.9	12.9	15.1	16.5	17.9
95.0	11.7	12.1	12.4	12.9	13.3	14.1	14.9	15.3	16.1	16.4	17.1	11.1	12.0	13.0	15.3	16.6	18.1
95.5	11.8	12.2	12.5	13.1	13.4	14.2	15.0	15.4	16.2	16.6	17.2	11.2	12.1	13.1	15.4	16.7	18.3
96.0	11.9	12.3	12.6	13.2	13.6	14.3	15.1	15.6	16.4	16.7	17.4	11.3	12.2	13.2	15.5	16.9	18.4
96.5	12.0	12.4	12.7	13.3	13.7	14.4	15.2	15.7	16.5	16.9	17.5	11.4	12.3	13.3	15.7	17.0	18.6
97.0	12.1	12.5	12.8	13.4	13.8	14.6	15.4	15.9	16.7	17.0	17.7	11.5	12.4	13.4	15.8	17.2	18.8
97.5	12.2	12.7	12.9	13.5	13.9	14.7	15.5	16.0	16.8	17.2	17.9	11.6	12.5	13.6	15.9	17.4	18.9

Contd.

A

Chart 7 Weight (kg) for Height (cm) for Boys between 2 and 5 Years (WHO Reference Data) Percentiles and Z (SD) Scores (Contd..)

Height	Percentiles											Z (SD) score					
(cm)	1st	3rd	5th	15th	25th	50th	75th	85th	95th	97th	99th	−3Z	−2Z	−1Z	+1Z	+2Z	+3Z
98.0	12.3	12.8	13.0	13.6	14.0	14.8	15.7	16.1	17.0	17.3	18.0	11.7	12.6	13.7	16.1	17.5	19.1
98.5	12.4	12.9	13.1	13.8	14.2	14.9	15.8	16.3	17.2	17.5	18.2	11.8	12.8	13.8	16.2	17.7	19.3
99.0	12.5	13.0	13.2	13.9	14.3	15.1	15.9	16.4	17.3	17.7	18.4	11.9	12.9	13.9	16.4	17.9	19.5
99.5	12.7	13.1	13.3	14.0	14.4	15.2	16.1	16.6	17.5	17.8	18.5	12.0	13.0	14.0	16.5	18.0	19.7
100.0	12.8	13.2	13.5	14.1	14.5	15.4	16.2	16.7	17.6	18.0	18.7	12.1	13.1	14.2	16.7	18.2	19.9
100.5	12.9	13.3	13.6	14.2	14.7	15.5	16.4	16.9	17.8	18.2	18.9	12.2	13.2	14.3	16.9	18.4	20.1
101.0	13.0	13.4	13.7	14.4	14.8	15.6	16.5	17.1	18.0	18.4	19.1	12.3	13.3	14.4	17.0	18.5	20.3
101.5	13.1	13.6	13.8	14.5	14.9	15.8	16.7	17.2	18.2	18.5	19.3	12.4	13.4	14.5	17.2	18.7	20.5
102.0	13.2	13.7	13.9	14.6	15.1	15.9	16.9	17.4	18.3	18.7	19.5	12.5	13.6	14.7	17.3	18.9	20.7
102.5	13.3	13.8	14.1	14.8	15.2	16.1	17.0	17.6	18.5	18.9	19.7	12.6	13.7	14.8	17.5	19.1	20.9
103.0	13.4	13.9	14.2	14.9	15.3	16.2	17.2	17.7	18.7	19.1	19.9	12.8	13.8	14.9	17.7	19.3	21.1
103.5	13.6	14.0	14.3	15.0	15.5	16.4	17.3	17.9	18.9	19.3	20.1	12.9	13.9	15.1	17.8	19.5	21.3
104.0	13.7	14.2	14.4	15.2	15.6	16.5	17.5	18.1	19.1	19.5	20.3	13.0	14.0	15.2	18.0	19.7	21.6
104.5	13.8	14.3	14.6	15.3	15.8	16.7	17.7	18.2	19.2	19.7	20.5	13.1	14.2	15.4	18.2	19.9	21.8
105.0	13.9	14.4	14.7	15.4	15.9	16.8	17.8	18.4	19.4	19.9	20.7	13.2	14.3	15.5	18.4	20.1	22.0
105.5	14.0	14.5	14.8	15.6	16.1	17.0	18.0	18.6	19.6	20.1	20.9	13.3	14.4	15.6	18.5	20.3	22.2
106.0	14.2	14.7	15.0	15.7	16.2	17.2	18.2	18.8	19.8	20.3	21.1	13.4	14.5	15.8	18.7	20.5	22.5
106.5	14.3	14.8	15.1	15.9	16.4	17.3	18.4	19.0	20.0	20.5	21.3	13.5	14.7	15.9	18.9	20.7	22.7
107.0	14.4	14.9	15.2	16.0	16.5	17.5	18.5	19.1	20.2	20.7	21.5	13.7	14.8	16.1	19.1	20.9	22.9
107.5	14.5	15.1	15.4	16.2	16.7	17.7	18.7	19.3	20.4	20.9	21.7	13.8	14.9	16.2	19.3	21.1	23.2
108.0	14.7	15.2	15.5	16.3	16.8	17.8	18.9	19.5	20.6	21.1	22.0	13.9	15.1	16.4	19.5	21.3	23.4
108.5	14.8	15.3	15.6	16.5	17.0	18.0	19.1	19.7	20.8	21.3	22.2	14.0	15.2	16.5	19.7	21.5	23.7
109.0	14.9	15.5	15.8	16.6	17.1	18.2	19.3	19.9	21.1	21.5	22.4	14.1	15.3	16.7	19.8	21.8	23.9
109.5	15.1	15.6	15.9	16.8	17.3	18.3	19.5	20.1	21.3	21.7	22.7	14.3	15.5	16.8	20.0	22.0	24.2
110.0	15.2	15.8	16.1	16.9	17.5	18.5	19.7	20.3	21.5	22.0	22.9	14.4	15.6	17.0	20.2	22.2	24.4
110.5	15.3	15.9	16.2	17.1	17.6	18.7	19.9	20.5	21.7	22.2	23.1	14.5	15.8	17.1	20.4	22.4	24.7
111.0	15.5	16.1	16.4	17.2	17.8	18.9	20.1	20.7	21.9	22.4	23.4	14.6	15.9	17.3	20.7	22.7	25.0
111.5	15.6	16.2	16.5	17.4	18.0	19.1	20.3	20.9	22.1	22.6	23.6	14.8	16.0	17.5	20.9	22.9	25.2
112.0	15.7	16.3	16.7	17.6	18.1	19.2	20.5	21.1	22.4	22.9	23.9	14.9	16.2	17.6	21.1	23.1	25.5
112.5	15.9	16.5	16.8	17.7	18.3	19.4	20.7	21.4	22.6	23.1	24.1	15.0	16.3	17.8	21.3	23.4	25.8
113.0	16.0	16.6	17.0	17.9	18.5	19.6	20.9	21.6	22.8	23.4	24.4	15.2	16.5	18.0	21.5	23.6	26.0
113.5	16.2	16.8	17.1	18.1	18.7	19.8	21.1	21.8	23.1	23.6	24.6	15.3	16.6	18.1	21.7	23.9	26.3
114.0	16.3	17.0	17.3	18.2	18.8	20.0	21.3	22.0	23.3	23.8	24.9	15.4	16.8	18.3	21.9	24.1	26.6
114.5	16.5	17.1	17.5	18.4	19.0	20.2	21.5	22.2	23.5	24.1	25.2	15.6	16.9	18.5	22.1	24.4	26.9
115.0	16.6	17.3	17.6	18.6	19.2	20.4	21.7	22.4	23.8	24.3	25.4	15.7	17.1	18.6	22.4	24.6	27.2
115.5	16.8	17.4	17.8	18.7	19.4	20.6	21.9	22.7	24.0	24.6	25.7	15.8	17.2	18.8	22.6	24.9	27.5
116.0	16.9	17.6	17.9	18.9	19.5	20.8	22.1	22.9	24.3	24.8	25.9	16.0	17.4	19.0	22.8	25.1	27.8
116.5	17.1	17.7	18.1	19.1	19.7	21.0	22.3	23.1	24.5	25.1	26.2	16.1	17.5	19.2	23.0	25.4	28.0
117.0	17.2	17.9	18.3	19.3	19.9	21.2	22.5	23.3	24.7	25.3	26.5	16.2	17.7	19.3	23.3	25.6	28.3
117.5	17.4	18.0	18.4	19.4	20.1	21.4	22.8	23.6	25.0	25.6	26.7	16.4	17.9	19.5	23.5	25.9	28.6
118.0	17.5	18.2	18.6	19.6	20.3	21.6	23.0	23.8	25.2	25.8	27.0	16.5	18.0	19.7	23.7	26.1	28.9
118.5	17.7	18.4	18.7	19.8	20.4	21.8	23.2	24.0	25.5	26.1	27.3	16.7	18.2	19.9	23.9	26.4	29.2
119.0	17.8	18.5	18.9	20.0	20.6	22.0	23.4	24.2	25.7	26.3	27.5	16.8	18.3	20.0	24.1	26.6	29.5
119.5	17.9	18.7	19.1	20.1	20.8	22.2	23.6	24.5	26.0	26.6	27.8	16.9	18.5	20.2	24.4	26.9	29.8
120.0	18.1	18.8	19.2	20.3	21.0	22.4	23.8	24.7	26.2	26.8	28.1	17.1	18.6	20.4	24.6	27.2	30.1

A

Chart 8 Weight (kg) for Height (cm) for Girls between 2 and 5 Years (WHO Reference Data) Percentiles and Z (SD) Scores

Height	Percentiles											Standard deviation (SD) Z score					
(cm)	1st	3rd	5th	15th	25th	50th	75th	85th	95th	97th	99th	−3Z	−2Z	−1Z	+1Z	+2Z	+3Z
65.0	5.9	6.1	6.3	6.6	6.8	7.2	7.7	8.0	8.4	8.6	9.0	5.6	6.1	6.6	7.9	8.7	9.7
65.5	6.0	6.2	6.4	6.7	6.9	7.4	7.8	8.1	8.6	8.8	9.2	5.7	6.2	6.7	8.1	8.9	9.8
66.0	6.1	6.3	6.5	6.8	7.0	7.5	7.9	8.2	8.7	8.9	9.3	5.8	6.3	6.8	8.2	9.0	10.0
66.5	6.2	6.4	6.5	6.9	7.1	7.6	8.1	8.3	8.8	9.0	9.4	5.8	6.4	6.9	8.3	9.1	10.1
67.0	6.3	6.5	6.6	7.0	7.2	7.7	8.2	8.5	9.0	9.2	9.6	5.9	6.4	7.0	8.4	9.3	10.2
67.5	6.4	6.6	6.7	7.1	7.3	7.8	8.3	8.6	9.1	9.3	9.7	6.0	6.5	7.1	8.5	9.4	10.4
68.0	6.4	6.7	6.8	7.2	7.4	7.9	8.4	8.7	9.2	9.4	9.8	6.1	6.6	7.2	8.7	9.5	10.5
68.5	6.5	6.8	6.9	7.3	7.5	8.0	8.5	8.8	9.3	9.5	10.0	6.2	6.7	7.3	8.8	9.7	10.7
69.0	6.6	6.9	7.0	7.4	7.6	8.1	8.6	8.9	9.4	9.7	10.1	6.3	6.8	7.4	8.9	9.8	10.8
69.5	6.7	7.0	7.1	7.5	7.7	8.2	8.7	9.0	9.6	9.8	10.2	6.3	6.9	7.5	9.0	9.9	10.9
70.0	6.8	7.0	7.2	7.6	7.8	8.3	8.8	9.1	9.7	9.9	10.3	6.4	7.0	7.6	9.1	10.0	11.1
70.5	6.9	7.1	7.3	7.7	7.9	8.4	8.9	9.3	9.8	10.0	10.5	6.5	7.1	7.7	9.2	10.1	11.2
71.0	6.9	7.2	7.4	7.8	8.0	8.5	9.0	9.4	9.9	10.1	10.6	6.6	7.1	7.8	9.3	10.3	11.3
71.5	7.0	7.3	7.4	7.9	8.1	8.6	9.2	9.5	10.0	10.3	10.7	6.7	7.2	7.9	9.4	10.4	11.5
72.0	7.1	7.4	7.5	7.9	8.2	8.7	9.3	9.6	10.1	10.4	10.8	6.7	7.3	8.0	9.5	10.5	11.6
72.5	7.2	7.5	7.6	8.0	8.3	8.8	9.4	9.7	10.3	10.5	11.0	6.8	7.4	8.1	9.7	10.6	11.7
73.0	7.3	7.6	7.7	8.1	8.4	8.9	9.5	9.8	10.4	10.6	11.1	6.9	7.5	8.1	9.8	10.7	11.8
73.5	7.4	7.6	7.8	8.2	8.5	9.0	9.6	9.9	10.5	10.7	11.2	7.0	7.6	8.2	9.9	10.8	12.0
74.0	7.4	7.7	7.9	8.3	8.6	9.1	9.7	10.0	10.6	10.8	11.3	7.0	7.6	8.3	10.0	11.0	12.1
74.5	7.5	7.8	8.0	8.4	8.7	9.2	9.8	10.1	10.7	10.9	11.4	7.1	7.7	8.4	10.1	11.1	12.2
75.0	7.6	7.9	8.0	8.5	8.7	9.3	9.9	10.2	10.8	11.1	11.5	7.2	7.8	8.5	10.2	11.2	12.3
75.5	7.7	8.0	8.1	8.6	8.8	9.4	10.0	10.3	10.9	11.2	11.7	7.2	7.9	8.6	10.3	11.3	12.5
76.0	7.7	8.0	8.2	8.6	8.9	9.5	10.1	10.4	11.0	11.3	11.8	7.3	8.0	8.7	10.4	11.4	12.6
76.5	7.8	8.1	8.3	8.7	9.0	9.6	10.2	10.5	11.1	11.4	11.9	7.4	8.0	8.7	10.5	11.5	12.7
77.0	7.9	8.2	8.4	8.8	9.1	9.6	10.3	10.6	11.2	11.5	12.0	7.5	8.1	8.8	10.6	11.6	12.8
77.5	8.0	8.3	8.4	8.9	9.2	9.7	10.4	10.7	11.3	11.6	12.1	7.5	8.2	8.9	10.7	11.7	12.9
78.0	8.0	8.4	8.5	9.0	9.3	9.8	10.5	10.8	11.4	11.7	12.2	7.6	8.3	9.0	10.8	11.8	13.1
78.5	8.1	8.4	8.6	9.1	9.4	9.9	10.6	10.9	11.6	11.8	12.3	7.7	8.4	9.1	10.9	12.0	13.2
79.0	8.2	8.5	8.7	9.2	9.4	10.0	10.7	11.0	11.7	11.9	12.5	7.8	8.4	9.2	11.0	12.1	13.3
79.5	8.3	8.6	8.8	9.2	9.5	10.1	10.8	11.1	11.8	12.1	12.6	7.8	8.5	9.3	11.1	12.2	13.4
80.0	8.4	8.7	8.9	9.3	9.6	10.2	10.9	11.2	11.9	12.2	12.7	7.9	8.6	9.4	11.2	12.3	13.6
80.5	8.5	8.8	9.0	9.4	9.7	10.3	11.0	11.4	12.0	12.3	12.8	8.0	8.7	9.5	11.3	12.4	13.7
81.0	8.6	8.9	9.1	9.5	9.8	10.4	11.1	11.5	12.2	12.4	13.0	8.1	8.8	9.6	11.4	12.6	13.9
81.5	8.6	9.0	9.2	9.6	9.9	10.6	11.2	11.6	12.3	12.6	13.1	8.2	8.9	9.7	11.6	12.7	14.0
82.0	8.7	9.1	9.3	9.7	10.1	10.7	11.3	11.7	12.4	12.7	13.2	8.3	9.0	9.8	11.7	12.8	14.1
82.5	8.8	9.2	9.4	9.9	10.2	10.8	11.5	11.9	12.5	12.8	13.4	8.4	9.1	9.9	11.8	13.0	14.3
83.0	8.9	9.3	9.5	10.0	10.3	10.9	11.6	12.0	12.7	13.0	13.5	8.5	9.2	10.0	11.9	13.1	14.5
83.5	9.0	9.4	9.6	10.1	10.4	11.0	11.7	12.1	12.8	13.1	13.7	8.5	9.3	10.1	12.1	13.3	14.6
84.0	9.1	9.5	9.7	10.2	10.5	11.1	11.8	12.2	13.0	13.3	13.8	8.6	9.4	10.2	12.2	13.4	14.8
84.5	9.2	9.6	9.8	10.3	10.6	11.3	12.0	12.4	13.1	13.4	14.0	8.7	9.5	10.3	12.3	13.5	14.9
85.0	9.3	9.7	9.9	10.4	10.7	11.4	12.1	12.5	13.2	13.5	14.1	8.8	9.6	10.4	12.5	13.7	15.1
85.5	9.4	9.8	10.0	10.5	10.9	11.5	12.2	12.7	13.4	13.7	14.3	8.9	9.7	10.6	12.6	13.8	15.3
86.0	9.5	9.9	10.1	10.6	11.0	11.6	12.4	12.8	13.5	13.8	14.4	9.0	9.8	10.7	12.7	14.0	15.4
86.5	9.6	10.0	10.2	10.8	11.1	11.8	12.5	12.9	13.7	14.0	14.6	9.1	9.9	10.8	12.9	14.2	15.6
87.0	9.7	10.1	10.3	10.9	11.2	11.9	12.6	13.1	13.8	14.1	14.8	9.2	10.0	10.9	13.0	14.3	15.8
87.5	9.9	10.2	10.4	11.0	11.3	12.0	12.8	13.2	14.0	14.3	14.9	9.3	10.1	11.0	13.2	14.5	15.9
88.0	10.0	10.3	10.5	11.1	11.4	12.1	12.9	13.3	14.1	14.4	15.1	9.4	10.2	11.1	13.3	14.6	16.1
88.5	10.1	10.4	10.6	11.2	11.6	12.3	13.0	13.5	14.3	14.6	15.2	9.5	10.3	11.2	13.4	14.8	16.3
89.0	10.2	10.5	10.8	11.3	11.7	12.4	13.2	13.6	14.4	14.7	15.4	9.6	10.4	11.4	13.6	14.9	16.4
89.5	10.3	10.6	10.9	11.4	11.8	12.5	13.3	13.8	14.6	14.9	15.5	9.7	10.5	11.5	13.7	15.1	16.6
90.0	10.4	10.8	11.0	11.5	11.9	12.6	13.4	13.9	14.7	15.0	15.7	9.8	10.6	11.6	13.8	15.2	16.8
90.5	10.5	10.9	11.1	11.7	12.0	12.8	13.6	14.0	14.9	15.2	15.9	9.9	10.7	11.7	14.0	15.4	16.9
91.0	10.6	11.0	11.2	11.8	12.1	12.9	13.7	14.2	15.0	15.3	16.0	10.0	10.9	11.8	14.1	15.5	17.1
91.5	10.7	11.1	11.3	11.9	12.3	13.0	13.8	14.3	15.1	15.5	16.2	10.1	11.0	11.9	14.3	15.7	17.3
92.0	10.8	11.2	11.4	12.0	12.4	13.1	14.0	14.4	15.3	15.6	16.3	10.2	11.1	12.0	14.4	15.8	17.4
92.5	10.9	11.3	11.5	12.1	12.5	13.3	14.1	14.6	15.4	15.8	16.5	10.3	11.2	12.1	14.5	16.0	17.6
93.0	11.0	11.4	11.6	12.2	12.6	13.4	14.2	14.7	15.6	15.9	16.6	10.4	11.3	12.3	14.7	16.1	17.8
93.5	11.1	11.5	11.7	12.3	12.7	13.5	14.4	14.9	15.7	16.1	16.8	10.5	11.4	12.4	14.8	16.3	17.9
94.0	11.2	11.6	11.8	12.4	12.8	13.6	14.5	15.0	15.9	16.2	16.9	10.6	11.5	12.5	14.9	16.4	18.1
94.5	11.3	11.7	11.9	12.6	13.0	13.8	14.6	15.1	16.0	16.4	17.1	10.7	11.6	12.6	15.1	16.6	18.3
95.0	11.4	11.8	12.0	12.7	13.1	13.9	14.8	15.3	16.2	16.5	17.3	10.8	11.7	12.7	15.2	16.7	18.5
95.5	11.5	11.9	12.1	12.8	13.2	14.0	14.9	15.4	16.3	16.7	17.4	10.8	11.8	12.8	15.4	16.9	18.6
96.0	11.6	12.0	12.3	12.9	13.3	14.1	15.0	15.6	16.5	16.9	17.6	10.9	11.9	12.9	15.5	17.0	18.8
96.5	11.7	12.1	12.4	13.0	13.4	14.3	15.2	15.7	16.6	17.0	17.8	11.0	12.0	13.1	15.6	17.2	19.0
97.0	11.8	12.2	12.5	13.1	13.6	14.4	15.3	15.8	16.8	17.2	17.9	11.1	12.1	13.2	15.8	17.4	19.2
97.5	11.9	12.3	12.6	13.3	13.7	14.5	15.5	16.0	16.9	17.3	18.1	11.2	12.2	13.3	15.9	17.5	19.3

Contd.

A

Chart 8 Weight (kg) for Height (cm) for Girls between 2 and 5 Years (WHO Reference Data) Percentiles and Z (SD) Scores (Contd..)

Height (cm)	Percentiles											Z (SD) score					
	1st	3rd	5th	15th	25th	50th	75th	85th	95th	97th	99th	−3Z	−2Z	−1Z	+1Z	+2Z	+3Z
98.0	12.0	12.4	12.7	13.4	13.8	14.7	15.6	16.1	17.1	17.5	18.3	11.3	12.3	13.4	16.1	17.7	19.5
98.5	12.1	12.6	12.8	13.5	13.9	14.8	15.7	16.3	17.3	17.7	18.4	11.4	12.4	13.5	16.2	17.9	19.7
99.0	12.2	12.7	12.9	13.6	14.1	14.9	15.9	16.4	17.4	17.8	18.6	11.5	12.5	13.7	16.4	18.0	19.9
99.5	12.3	12.8	13.0	13.8	14.2	15.1	16.0	16.6	17.6	18.0	18.8	11.6	12.7	13.8	16.5	18.2	20.1
100.0	12.4	12.9	13.2	13.9	14.3	15.2	16.2	16.8	17.8	18.2	19.0	11.7	12.8	13.9	16.7	18.4	20.3
100.5	12.5	13.0	13.3	14.0	14.5	15.4	16.4	16.9	17.9	18.3	19.2	11.9	12.9	14.1	16.9	18.6	20.5
101.0	12.7	13.1	13.4	14.1	14.6	15.5	16.5	17.1	18.1	18.5	19.4	12.0	13.0	14.2	17.0	18.7	20.7
101.5	12.8	13.3	13.5	14.3	14.7	15.7	16.7	17.2	18.3	18.7	19.5	12.1	13.1	14.3	17.2	18.9	20.9
102.0	12.9	13.4	13.7	14.4	14.9	15.8	16.8	17.4	18.5	18.9	19.7	12.2	13.3	14.5	17.4	19.1	21.1
102.5	13.0	13.5	13.8	14.5	15.0	16.0	17.0	17.6	18.7	19.1	19.9	12.3	13.4	14.6	17.5	19.3	21.4
103.0	13.1	13.6	13.9	14.7	15.2	16.1	17.2	17.8	18.8	19.3	20.2	12.4	13.5	14.7	17.7	19.5	21.6
103.5	13.3	13.8	14.1	14.8	15.3	16.3	17.3	17.9	19.0	19.5	20.4	12.5	13.6	14.9	17.9	19.7	21.8
104.0	13.4	13.9	14.2	15.0	15.5	16.4	17.5	18.1	19.2	19.7	20.6	12.6	13.8	15.0	18.1	19.9	22.0
104.5	13.5	14.0	14.3	15.1	15.6	16.6	17.7	18.3	19.4	19.9	20.8	12.8	13.9	15.2	18.2	20.1	22.3
105.0	13.6	14.2	14.5	15.3	15.8	16.8	17.9	18.5	19.6	20.1	21.0	12.9	14.0	15.3	18.4	20.3	22.5
105.5	13.8	14.3	14.6	15.4	15.9	16.9	18.1	18.7	19.8	20.3	21.2	13.0	14.2	15.5	18.6	20.5	22.7
106.0	13.9	14.5	14.8	15.6	16.1	17.1	18.2	18.9	20.0	20.5	21.4	13.1	14.3	15.6	18.8	20.8	23.0
106.5	14.1	14.6	14.9	15.7	16.3	17.3	18.4	19.1	20.2	20.7	21.7	13.3	14.5	15.8	19.0	21.0	23.2
107.0	14.2	14.7	15.1	15.9	16.4	17.5	18.6	19.3	20.5	21.0	21.9	13.4	14.6	15.9	19.2	21.2	23.5
107.5	14.3	14.9	15.2	16.1	16.6	17.7	18.8	19.5	20.7	21.2	22.1	13.5	14.7	16.1	19.4	21.4	23.7
108.0	14.5	15.0	15.4	16.2	16.8	17.8	19.0	19.7	20.9	21.4	22.4	13.7	14.9	16.3	19.6	21.7	24.0
108.5	14.6	15.2	15.5	16.4	16.9	18.0	19.2	19.9	21.1	21.6	22.6	13.8	15.0	16.4	19.8	21.9	24.3
109.0	14.8	15.4	15.7	16.6	17.1	18.2	19.4	20.1	21.4	21.9	22.9	13.9	15.2	16.6	20.0	22.1	24.5
109.5	14.9	15.5	15.8	16.7	17.3	18.4	19.6	20.3	21.6	22.1	23.1	14.1	15.4	16.8	20.3	22.4	24.8
110.0	15.1	15.7	16.0	16.9	17.5	18.6	19.8	20.6	21.8	22.4	23.4	14.2	15.5	17.0	20.5	22.6	25.1
110.5	15.2	15.8	16.2	17.1	17.7	18.8	20.1	20.8	22.1	22.6	23.7	14.4	15.7	17.1	20.7	22.9	25.4
111.0	15.4	16.0	16.3	17.3	17.8	19.0	20.3	21.0	22.3	22.8	23.9	14.5	15.8	17.3	20.9	23.1	25.7
111.5	15.5	16.2	16.5	17.4	18.0	19.2	20.5	21.2	22.6	23.1	24.2	14.7	16.0	17.5	21.2	23.4	26.0
112.0	15.7	16.3	16.7	17.6	18.2	19.4	20.7	21.5	22.8	23.4	24.5	14.8	16.2	17.7	21.4	23.6	26.2
112.5	15.9	16.5	16.8	17.8	18.4	19.6	20.9	21.7	23.1	23.6	24.7	15.0	16.3	17.9	21.6	23.9	26.5
113.0	16.0	16.7	17.0	18.0	18.6	19.8	21.2	21.9	23.3	23.9	25.0	15.1	16.5	18.0	21.8	24.2	26.8
113.5	16.2	16.8	17.2	18.2	18.8	20.0	21.4	22.2	23.6	24.1	25.3	15.3	16.7	18.2	22.1	24.4	27.1
114.0	16.3	17.0	17.4	18.4	19.0	20.2	21.6	22.4	23.8	24.4	25.6	15.4	16.8	18.4	22.3	24.7	27.4
114.5	16.5	17.2	17.5	18.5	19.2	20.5	21.8	22.6	24.1	24.7	25.8	15.6	17.0	18.6	22.6	25.0	27.8
115.0	16.7	17.3	17.7	18.7	19.4	20.7	22.1	22.9	24.3	24.9	26.1	15.7	17.2	18.8	22.8	25.2	28.1
115.5	16.8	17.5	17.9	18.9	19.6	20.9	22.3	23.1	24.6	25.2	26.4	15.9	17.3	19.0	23.0	25.5	28.4
116.0	17.0	17.7	18.1	19.1	19.8	21.1	22.5	23.4	24.9	25.5	26.7	16.0	17.5	19.2	23.3	25.8	28.7
116.5	17.2	17.9	18.3	19.3	20.0	21.3	22.8	23.6	25.1	25.7	27.0	16.2	17.7	19.4	23.5	26.1	29.0
117.0	17.3	18.0	18.4	19.5	20.2	21.5	23.0	23.8	25.4	26.0	27.3	16.3	17.8	19.6	23.8	26.3	29.3
117.5	17.5	18.2	18.6	19.7	20.4	21.7	23.2	24.1	25.6	26.3	27.5	16.5	18.0	19.8	24.0	26.6	29.6
118.0	17.7	18.4	18.8	19.9	20.6	22.0	23.5	24.3	25.9	26.5	27.8	16.6	18.2	19.9	24.2	26.9	29.9
118.5	17.8	18.6	19.0	20.1	20.8	22.2	23.7	24.6	26.2	26.8	28.1	16.8	18.4	20.1	24.5	27.2	30.3
119.0	18.0	18.7	19.1	20.3	21.0	22.4	23.9	24.8	26.4	27.1	28.4	16.9	18.5	20.3	24.7	27.4	30.6
119.5	18.2	18.9	19.3	20.5	21.2	22.6	24.2	25.1	26.7	27.4	28.7	17.1	18.7	20.5	25.0	27.7	30.9
120.0	18.3	19.1	19.5	20.6	21.4	22.8	24.4	25.3	27.0	27.6	29.0	17.3	18.9	20.7	25.2	28.0	31.2

Chart 9 Head Circumference (cm) by Age Z (SD) Scores in Boys and Girls Aged 0–5 Years

Age					Boys							Girls			
Year	mo	−3SD	−2SD	−1SD	Median	+1SD	+2SD	+3SD	−3SD	−2SD	−1SD	Median	+1SD	+2SD	+3SD
0	0	30.7	31.9	33.2	34.5	35.7	37.0	38.3	30.3	31.5	32.7	33.9	35.1	36.2	37.4
	1	33.8	34.9	36.1	37.3	38.4	39.6	40.8	33.0	34.2	35.4	36.5	37.7	38.9	40.1
	2	35.6	36.8	38.0	39.1	40.3	41.5	42.6	34.6	35.8	37.0	38.3	39.5	40.7	41.9
	3	37.0	38.1	39.3	40.5	41.7	42.9	44.1	35.8	37.1	38.3	39.5	40.8	42.0	43.3
	4	38.0	39.2	40.4	41.6	42.8	44.0	45.2	36.8	38.1	39.3	40.6	41.8	43.1	44.4
	5	38.9	40.1	41.4	42.6	43.8	45.0	46.2	37.6	38.9	40.2	41.5	42.7	44.0	45.3
	6	39.7	40.9	42.1	43.3	44.6	45.8	47.0	38.3	39.6	40.9	42.2	43.5	44.8	46.1
	7	40.3	41.5	42.7	44.0	45.2	46.4	47.7	38.9	40.2	41.5	42.8	44.1	45.5	46.8
	8	40.8	42.0	43.3	44.5	45.8	47.0	48.3	39.4	40.7	42.0	43.4	44.7	46.0	47.4
	9	41.2	42.5	43.7	45.0	46.3	47.5	48.8	39.8	41.2	42.5	43.8	45.2	46.5	47.8
	10	41.6	42.9	44.1	45.4	46.7	47.9	49.2	40.2	41.5	42.9	44.2	45.6	46.9	48.3
	11	41.9	43.2	44.5	45.8	47.0	48.3	49.6	40.5	41.9	43.2	44.6	45.9	47.3	48.6
1	0	42.2	43.5	44.8	46.1	47.4	48.6	49.9	40.8	42.2	43.5	44.9	46.3	47.6	49.0
	1	42.5	43.8	45.0	46.3	47.6	48.9	50.2	41.1	42.4	43.8	45.2	46.5	47.9	49.3
	2	42.7	44.0	45.3	46.6	47.9	49.2	50.5	41.3	42.7	44.1	45.4	46.8	48.2	49.5
	3	42.9	44.2	45.5	46.8	48.1	49.4	50.7	41.5	42.9	44.3	45.7	47.0	48.4	49.8
	4	43.1	44.4	45.7	47.0	48.3	49.6	51.0	41.7	43.1	44.5	45.9	47.2	48.6	50.0
	5	43.2	44.6	45.9	47.2	48.5	49.8	51.2	41.9	43.3	44.7	46.1	47.4	48.8	50.2
	6	43.4	44.7	46.0	47.4	48.7	50.0	51.4	42.1	43.5	44.9	46.2	47.6	49.0	50.4
	7	43.5	44.9	46.2	47.5	48.9	50.2	51.5	42.3	43.6	45.0	46.4	47.8	49.2	50.6
	8	43.7	45.0	46.4	47.7	49.0	50.4	51.7	42.4	43.8	45.2	46.6	48.0	49.4	50.7
	9	43.8	45.2	46.5	47.8	49.2	50.5	51.9	42.6	44.0	45.3	46.7	48.1	49.5	50.9
	10	43.9	45.3	46.6	48.0	49.3	50.7	52.0	42.7	44.1	45.5	46.9	48.3	49.7	51.1
	11	44.1	45.4	46.8	48.1	49.5	50.8	52.2	42.9	44.3	45.6	47.0	48.4	49.8	51.2
2	0	44.2	45.5	46.9	48.3	49.6	51.0	52.3	43.0	44.4	45.8	47.2	48.6	50.0	51.4
	1	44.3	45.6	47.0	48.4	49.7	51.1	52.5	43.1	44.5	45.9	47.3	48.7	50.1	51.5
	2	44.4	45.8	47.1	48.5	49.9	51.2	52.6	43.3	44.7	46.1	47.5	48.9	50.3	51.7
	3	44.5	45.9	47.2	48.6	50.0	51.4	52.7	43.4	44.8	46.2	47.6	49.0	50.4	51.8
	4	44.6	46.0	47.3	48.7	50.1	51.5	52.9	43.5	44.9	46.3	47.7	49.1	50.5	51.9
	5	44.7	46.1	47.4	48.8	50.2	51.6	53.0	43.6	45.0	46.4	47.8	49.2	50.6	52.0
	6	44.8	46.1	47.5	48.9	50.3	51.7	53.1	43.7	45.1	46.5	47.9	49.3	50.7	52.2
	7	44.8	46.2	47.6	49.0	50.4	51.8	53.2	43.8	45.2	46.6	48.0	49.4	50.9	52.3
	8	44.9	46.3	47.7	49.1	50.5	51.9	53.3	43.9	45.3	46.7	48.1	49.6	51.0	52.4
	9	45.0	46.4	47.8	49.2	50.6	52.0	53.4	44.0	45.4	46.8	48.2	49.7	51.1	52.5
	10	45.1	46.5	47.9	49.3	50.7	52.1	53.5	44.1	45.5	46.9	48.3	49.7	51.2	52.6
	11	45.1	46.6	48.0	49.4	50.8	52.2	53.6	44.2	45.6	47.0	48.4	49.8	51.2	52.7
3	0	45.2	46.6	48.0	49.5	50.9	52.3	53.7	44.3	45.7	47.1	48.5	49.9	51.3	52.7
	1	45.3	46.7	48.1	49.5	51.0	52.4	53.8	44.4	45.8	47.2	48.6	50.0	51.4	52.8
	2	45.3	46.8	48.2	49.6	51.0	52.5	53.9	44.4	45.8	47.3	48.7	50.1	51.5	52.9
	3	45.4	46.8	48.2	49.7	51.1	52.5	54.0	44.5	45.9	47.3	48.7	50.2	51.6	53.0
	4	45.4	46.9	48.3	49.7	51.2	52.6	54.1	44.6	46.0	47.4	48.8	50.2	51.7	53.1
	5	45.5	46.9	48.4	49.8	51.3	52.7	54.1	44.6	46.1	47.5	48.9	50.3	51.7	53.1
	6	45.5	47.0	48.4	49.9	51.3	52.8	54.2	44.7	46.1	47.5	49.0	50.4	51.8	53.2
	7	45.6	47.0	48.5	49.9	51.4	52.8	54.3	44.8	46.2	47.6	49.0	50.4	51.9	53.3
	8	45.6	47.1	48.5	50.0	51.4	52.9	54.3	44.8	46.3	47.7	49.1	50.5	51.9	53.3
	9	45.7	47.1	48.6	50.1	51.5	53.0	54.4	44.9	46.3	47.7	49.2	50.6	52.0	53.4
	10	45.7	47.2	48.7	50.1	51.6	53.0	54.5	45.0	46.4	47.8	49.2	50.6	52.1	53.5
	11	45.8	47.2	48.7	50.2	51.6	53.1	54.5	45.0	46.4	47.9	49.3	50.7	52.1	53.5
4	0	45.8	47.3	48.7	50.2	51.7	53.1	54.6	45.1	46.5	47.9	49.3	50.8	52.2	53.6
	1	45.9	47.3	48.8	50.3	51.7	53.2	54.7	45.1	46.5	48.0	49.4	50.8	52.2	53.6
	2	45.9	47.4	48.8	50.3	51.8	53.2	54.7	45.2	46.6	48.0	49.4	50.9	52.3	53.7
	3	45.9	47.4	48.9	50.4	51.8	53.3	54.8	45.2	46.7	48.1	49.5	50.9	52.3	53.8
	4	46.0	47.5	48.9	50.4	51.9	53.4	54.8	45.3	46.7	48.1	49.5	51.0	52.4	53.8
	5	46.0	47.5	49.0	50.4	51.9	53.4	54.9	45.3	46.8	48.2	49.6	51.0	52.4	53.9
	6	46.1	47.5	49.0	50.5	52.0	53.5	54.9	45.4	46.8	48.2	49.6	51.1	52.5	53.9
	7	46.1	47.6	49.1	50.5	52.0	53.5	55.0	45.4	46.9	48.3	49.7	51.1	52.5	54.0
	8	46.1	47.6	49.1	50.6	52.1	53.5	55.0	45.5	46.9	48.3	49.7	51.2	52.6	54.0
	9	46.2	47.6	49.1	50.6	52.1	53.6	55.1	45.5	46.9	48.4	49.8	51.2	52.6	54.1
	10	46.2	47.7	49.2	50.7	52.1	53.6	55.1	45.6	47.0	48.4	49.8	51.3	52.7	54.1
	11	46.2	47.7	49.2	50.7	52.2	53.7	55.2	45.6	47.0	48.5	49.9	51.3	52.7	54.1
5	0	46.3	47.7	49.2	50.7	52.2	53.7	55.2	45.7	47.1	48.5	49.9	51.3	52.8	54.2

A

Table 10 Body Mass Index (BMI) by Age for Boys Aged 2–5 Years (WHO Standards)

BOYS	Percentiles									Z (SD) score					
Months	3rd	5th	15th	25th	50th	75th	85th	95th	97th	−3Z	−2Z	−1Z	+1Z	+2Z	+3Z
0.0	11.3	11.5	12.2	12.6	13.4	14.3	14.8	15.8	16.1	10.2	11.1	12.2	14.8	16.3	18.1
1.0	12.6	12.8	13.6	14.1	14.9	15.9	16.4	17.3	17.6	11.3	12.4	13.6	16.3	17.8	19.4
2.0	13.8	14.1	14.9	15.4	16.3	17.3	17.8	18.8	19.2	12.5	13.7	15.0	17.8	19.4	21.1
3.0	14.4	14.7	15.5	16.0	16.9	17.9	18.5	19.4	19.8	13.1	14.3	15.5	18.4	20.0	21.8
4.0	14.7	15.0	15.7	16.2	17.2	18.2	18.7	19.7	20.1	13.4	14.5	15.8	18.7	20.3	22.1
5.0	14.8	15.1	15.9	16.4	17.3	18.3	18.9	19.8	20.2	13.5	14.7	15.9	18.8	20.5	22.3
6.0	14.9	15.2	15.9	16.4	17.3	18.3	18.9	19.9	20.3	13.6	14.7	16.0	18.8	20.5	22.3
7.0	14.9	15.2	15.9	16.4	17.3	18.3	18.9	19.9	20.3	13.7	14.8	16.0	18.8	20.5	22.3
8.0	14.9	15.1	15.9	16.3	17.3	18.2	18.8	19.8	20.2	13.6	14.7	15.9	18.7	20.4	22.2
9.0	14.8	15.1	15.8	16.3	17.2	18.1	18.7	19.7	20.1	13.6	14.7	15.8	18.6	20.3	22.1
10.0	14.7	15.0	15.7	16.2	17.0	18.0	18.6	19.5	19.9	13.5	14.6	15.7	18.5	20.1	22.0
11.0	14.6	14.9	15.6	16.0	16.9	17.9	18.4	19.4	19.8	13.4	14.5	15.6	18.4	20.0	21.8
12.0	14.5	14.8	15.5	15.9	16.8	17.7	18.3	19.2	19.6	13.4	14.4	15.5	18.2	19.8	21.6
13.0	14.4	14.7	15.4	15.8	16.7	17.6	18.1	19.1	19.5	13.3	14.3	15.4	18.1	19.7	21.5
14.0	14.3	14.6	15.3	15.7	16.6	17.5	18.0	18.9	19.3	13.2	14.2	15.3	18.0	19.5	21.3
15.0	14.2	14.5	15.2	15.6	16.4	17.4	17.9	18.8	19.2	13.1	14.1	15.2	17.8	19.4	21.2
16.0	14.2	14.4	15.1	15.5	16.3	17.2	17.8	18.7	19.1	13.1	14.0	15.1	17.7	19.3	21.0
17.0	14.1	14.3	15.0	15.4	16.2	17.1	17.6	18.6	18.9	13.0	13.9	15.0	17.6	19.1	20.9
18.0	14.0	14.2	14.9	15.3	16.1	17.0	17.5	18.5	18.8	12.9	13.9	14.9	17.5	19.0	20.8
19.0	13.9	14.2	14.8	15.2	16.1	16.9	17.4	18.4	18.7	12.9	13.8	14.9	17.4	18.9	20.7
20.0	13.9	14.1	14.8	15.2	16.0	16.9	17.4	18.3	18.6	12.8	13.7	14.8	17.3	18.8	20.6
21.0	13.8	14.1	14.7	15.1	15.9	16.8	17.3	18.2	18.6	12.8	13.7	14.7	17.2	18.7	20.5
22.0	13.8	14.0	14.6	15.0	15.8	16.7	17.2	18.1	18.5	12.7	13.6	14.7	17.2	18.7	20.4
23.0	13.7	14.0	14.6	15.0	15.8	16.7	17.1	18.0	18.4	12.7	13.6	14.6	17.1	18.6	20.3
24.0	13.7	13.9	14.5	14.9	15.7	16.6	17.1	18.0	18.3	12.7	13.6	14.6	17.0	18.5	20.3

Years Months						BMI by Height									
2 0	13.9	14.2	14.8	15.2	16.0	16.9	17.4	18.3	18.7	12.9	13.8	14.8	17.3	18.9	20.6
2 1	13.9	14.1	14.8	15.2	16.0	16.9	17.4	18.3	18.6	12.8	13.8	14.8	17.3	18.8	20.5
2 2	13.8	14.1	14.7	15.1	15.9	16.8	17.3	18.2	18.6	12.8	13.7	14.8	17.3	18.8	20.5
2 3	13.8	14.0	14.7	15.1	15.9	16.8	17.3	18.2	18.5	12.7	13.7	14.7	17.2	18.7	20.4
2 4	13.8	14.0	14.7	15.1	15.9	16.7	17.2	18.1	18.5	12.7	13.6	14.7	17.2	18.7	20.4
2 5	13.7	14.0	14.6	15.0	15.8	16.7	17.2	18.1	18.4	12.7	13.6	14.7	17.1	18.6	20.3
2 6	13.7	13.9	14.6	15.0	15.8	16.7	17.2	18.0	18.4	12.6	13.6	14.6	17.1	18.6	20.2
2 7	13.7	13.9	14.5	15.0	15.8	16.6	17.1	18.0	18.4	12.6	13.5	14.6	17.1	18.5	20.2
2 8	13.6	13.9	14.5	14.9	15.7	16.6	17.1	18.0	18.3	12.5	13.5	14.6	17.0	18.5	20.1
2 9	13.6	13.8	14.5	14.9	15.7	16.6	17.0	17.9	18.3	12.5	13.5	14.5	17.0	18.5	20.1
2 10	13.5	13.8	14.4	14.9	15.7	16.5	17.0	17.9	18.2	12.5	13.4	14.5	17.0	18.4	20.0
2 11	13.5	13.8	14.4	14.8	15.6	16.5	17.0	17.9	18.2	12.4	13.4	14.5	16.9	18.4	20.0
3 0	13.5	13.7	14.4	14.8	15.6	16.5	17.0	17.8	18.2	12.4	13.4	14.4	16.9	18.4	20.0
3 1	13.5	13.7	14.4	14.8	15.6	16.4	16.9	17.8	18.1	12.4	13.3	14.4	16.9	18.3	19.9
3 2	13.4	13.7	14.3	14.7	15.5	16.4	16.9	17.8	18.1	12.3	13.3	14.4	16.8	18.3	19.9
3 3	13.4	13.6	14.3	14.7	15.5	16.4	16.9	17.7	18.1	12.3	13.3	14.3	16.8	18.3	19.9
3 4	13.4	13.6	14.3	14.7	15.5	16.4	16.8	17.7	18.1	12.3	13.2	14.3	16.8	18.2	19.9
3 5	13.3	13.6	14.2	14.7	15.5	16.3	16.8	17.7	18.0	12.2	13.2	14.3	16.8	18.2	19.9
3 6	13.3	13.6	14.2	14.6	15.4	16.3	16.8	17.7	18.0	12.2	13.2	14.3	16.8	18.2	19.8
3 7	13.3	13.5	14.2	14.6	15.4	16.3	16.8	17.7	18.0	12.2	13.2	14.2	16.7	18.2	19.8
3 8	13.3	13.5	14.2	14.6	15.4	16.3	16.8	17.7	18.0	12.2	13.1	14.2	16.7	18.2	19.8
3 9	13.2	13.5	14.2	14.6	15.4	16.3	16.8	17.6	18.0	12.2	13.1	14.2	16.7	18.2	19.8
3 10	13.2	13.5	14.1	14.5	15.4	16.2	16.7	17.6	18.0	12.1	13.1	14.2	16.7	18.2	19.8
3 11	13.2	13.5	14.1	14.5	15.3	16.2	16.7	17.6	18.0	12.1	13.1	14.2	16.7	18.2	19.9
4 0	13.2	13.4	14.1	14.5	15.3	16.2	16.7	17.6	18.0	12.1	13.1	14.1	16.7	18.2	19.9
4 1	13.2	13.4	14.1	14.5	15.3	16.2	16.7	17.6	18.0	12.1	13.0	14.1	16.7	18.2	19.9
4 2	13.2	13.4	14.1	14.5	15.3	16.2	16.7	17.6	18.0	12.1	13.0	14.1	16.7	18.2	19.9
4 3	13.1	13.4	14.0	14.5	15.3	16.2	16.7	17.6	18.0	12.1	13.0	14.1	16.6	18.2	19.9
4 4	13.1	13.4	14.0	14.4	15.3	16.2	16.7	17.6	18.0	12.0	13.0	14.1	16.6	18.2	19.9
4 5	13.1	13.3	14.0	14.4	15.3	16.2	16.7	17.6	18.0	12.0	13.0	14.1	16.6	18.2	20.0
4 6	13.1	13.3	14.0	14.4	15.3	16.2	16.7	17.6	18.0	12.0	13.0	14.0	16.6	18.2	20.0
4 7	13.1	13.3	14.0	14.4	15.2	16.2	16.7	17.6	18.0	12.0	13.0	14.0	16.6	18.2	20.0
4 8	13.1	13.3	14.0	14.4	15.2	16.1	16.7	17.6	18.0	12.0	12.9	14.0	16.6	18.2	20.1
4 9	13.0	13.3	14.0	14.4	15.2	16.1	16.7	17.6	18.0	12.0	12.9	14.0	16.6	18.2	20.1
4 10	13.0	13.3	13.9	14.4	15.2	16.1	16.7	17.6	18.0	12.0	12.9	14.0	16.6	18.3	20.2
4 11	13.0	13.3	13.9	14.4	15.2	16.1	16.7	17.7	18.1	12.0	12.9	14.0	16.6	18.3	20.2
5 0	13.0	13.3	13.9	14.3	15.2	16.1	16.7	17.7	18.1	12.0	12.9	14.0	16.6	18.3	20.3

A

Table 11 Body Mass Index (BMI) by Age for Girls Aged 2–5 Years (WHO Standards)

GIRLS	Percentiles									Z (SD) score					
Months	3rd	5th	15th	25th	50th	75th	85th	95th	97th	−3Z	−2Z	−1Z	+1Z	+2Z	+3Z
0	11.2	11.5	12.1	12.5	13.3	14.2	14.7	15.5	15.9	10.1	11.1	12.2	14.6	16.1	17.7
1	12.1	12.4	13.2	13.6	14.6	15.5	16.1	17.0	17.3	10.8	12.0	13.2	16.0	17.5	19.1
2	13.2	13.5	14.3	14.8	15.8	16.8	17.4	18.4	18.8	11.8	13.0	14.3	17.3	19.0	20.7
3	13.7	14.0	14.9	15.4	16.4	17.4	18.0	19.0	19.4	12.4	13.6	14.9	17.9	19.7	21.5
4	14.0	14.3	15.2	15.7	16.7	17.7	18.3	19.4	19.8	12.7	13.9	15.2	18.3	20.0	22.0
5	14.2	14.5	15.3	15.8	16.8	17.9	18.5	19.6	20.0	12.9	14.1	15.4	18.4	20.2	22.2
6	14.3	14.6	15.4	15.9	16.9	18.0	18.6	19.6	20.1	13.0	14.1	15.5	18.5	20.3	22.3
7	14.3	14.6	15.4	15.9	16.9	18.0	18.6	19.6	20.1	13.0	14.2	15.5	18.5	20.3	22.3
8	14.3	14.6	15.4	15.9	16.8	17.9	18.5	19.6	20.0	13.0	14.1	15.4	18.4	20.2	22.2
9	14.2	14.5	15.3	15.8	16.7	17.8	18.4	19.4	19.9	12.9	14.1	15.3	18.3	20.1	22.1
10	14.1	14.4	15.2	15.7	16.6	17.7	18.2	19.3	19.7	12.9	14.0	15.2	18.2	19.9	21.9
11	14.0	14.3	15.1	15.5	16.5	17.5	18.1	19.1	19.6	12.8	13.9	15.1	18.0	19.8	21.8
12	13.9	14.2	15.0	15.4	16.4	17.4	17.9	19.0	19.4	12.7	13.8	15.0	17.9	19.6	21.6
13	13.8	14.1	14.8	15.3	16.2	17.2	17.8	18.8	19.2	12.6	13.7	14.9	17.7	19.5	21.4
14	13.7	14.0	14.7	15.2	16.1	17.1	17.7	18.7	19.1	12.6	13.6	14.8	17.6	19.3	21.3
15	13.7	13.9	14.6	15.1	16.0	17.0	17.5	18.6	19.0	12.5	13.5	14.7	17.5	19.2	21.1
16	13.6	13.8	14.6	15.0	15.9	16.9	17.4	18.4	18.8	12.4	13.5	14.6	17.4	19.1	21.0
17	13.5	13.8	14.5	14.9	15.8	16.8	17.3	18.3	18.7	12.4	13.4	14.5	17.3	18.9	20.9
18	13.4	13.7	14.4	14.8	15.7	16.7	17.2	18.2	18.6	12.3	13.3	14.4	17.2	18.8	20.8
19	13.4	13.6	14.3	14.8	15.7	16.6	17.2	18.1	18.5	12.3	13.3	14.4	17.1	18.8	20.7
20	13.3	13.6	14.3	14.7	15.6	16.5	17.1	18.1	18.5	12.2	13.2	14.3	17.0	18.7	20.6
21	13.3	13.6	14.2	14.7	15.5	16.5	17.0	18.0	18.4	12.2	13.2	14.3	17.0	18.6	20.5
22	13.3	13.5	14.2	14.6	15.5	16.4	17.0	17.9	18.3	12.2	13.1	14.2	16.9	18.5	20.4
23	13.2	13.5	14.2	14.6	15.4	16.4	16.9	17.9	18.3	12.2	13.1	14.2	16.9	18.5	20.4
24	13.2	13.5	14.1	14.6	15.4	16.3	16.9	17.8	18.2	12.1	13.1	14.2	16.8	18.4	20.3

Years	Months	3rd	5th	15th	25th	50th	75th	85th	95th	97th	BMI by Height					
2	0	13.5	13.7	14.4	14.8	15.7	16.6	17.2	18.1	18.5	12.4	13.3	14.4	17.1	18.7	20.6
2	1	13.4	13.7	14.4	14.8	15.7	16.6	17.1	18.1	18.5	12.4	13.3	14.4	17.1	18.7	20.6
2	2	13.4	13.7	14.4	14.8	15.6	16.6	17.1	18.1	18.5	12.3	13.3	14.4	17.0	18.7	20.6
2	3	13.4	13.7	14.3	14.8	15.6	16.5	17.1	18.0	18.4	12.3	13.3	14.4	17.0	18.6	20.5
2	4	13.4	13.6	14.3	14.7	15.6	16.5	17.0	18.0	18.4	12.3	13.3	14.3	17.0	18.6	20.5
2	5	13.4	13.6	14.3	14.7	15.6	16.5	17.0	18.0	18.4	12.3	13.2	14.3	17.0	18.6	20.4
2	6	13.3	13.6	14.3	14.7	15.5	16.5	17.0	17.9	18.3	12.3	13.2	14.3	16.9	18.5	20.4
2	7	13.3	13.6	14.2	14.7	15.5	16.4	17.0	17.9	18.3	12.2	13.2	14.3	16.9	18.5	20.4
2	8	13.3	13.5	14.2	14.6	15.5	16.4	16.9	17.9	18.3	12.2	13.2	14.3	16.9	18.5	20.4
2	9	13.3	13.5	14.2	14.6	15.5	16.4	16.9	17.9	18.3	12.2	13.1	14.2	16.9	18.5	20.3
2	10	13.2	13.5	14.2	14.6	15.4	16.4	16.9	17.9	18.2	12.2	13.1	14.2	16.8	18.5	20.3
2	11	13.2	13.5	14.1	14.6	15.4	16.3	16.9	17.8	18.2	12.1	13.1	14.2	16.8	18.4	20.3
3	0	13.2	13.5	14.1	14.5	15.4	16.3	16.9	17.8	18.2	12.1	13.1	14.2	16.8	18.4	20.3
3	1	13.2	13.4	14.1	14.5	15.4	16.3	16.8	17.8	18.2	12.1	13.1	14.1	16.8	18.4	20.3
3	2	13.2	13.4	14.1	14.5	15.4	16.3	16.8	17.8	18.2	12.1	13.0	14.1	16.8	18.4	20.3
3	3	13.1	13.4	14.1	14.5	15.3	16.3	16.8	17.8	18.2	12.0	13.0	14.1	16.8	18.4	20.3
3	4	13.1	13.4	14.0	14.5	15.3	16.3	16.8	17.8	18.2	12.0	13.0	14.1	16.8	18.4	20.3
3	5	13.1	13.3	14.0	14.5	15.3	16.3	16.8	17.8	18.2	12.0	13.0	14.1	16.8	18.4	20.4
3	6	13.1	13.3	14.0	14.4	15.3	16.3	16.8	17.8	18.2	12.0	12.9	14.0	16.8	18.4	20.4
3	7	13.0	13.3	14.0	14.4	15.3	16.3	16.8	17.8	18.2	11.9	12.9	14.0	16.8	18.4	20.4
3	8	13.0	13.3	14.0	14.4	15.3	16.3	16.8	17.8	18.2	11.9	12.9	14.0	16.8	18.5	20.4
3	9	13.0	13.3	14.0	14.4	15.3	16.3	16.8	17.8	18.3	11.9	12.9	14.0	16.8	18.5	20.5
3	10	13.0	13.2	13.9	14.4	15.3	16.3	16.8	17.8	18.3	11.9	12.9	14.0	16.8	18.5	20.5
3	11	13.0	13.2	13.9	14.4	15.3	16.3	16.8	17.9	18.3	11.8	12.8	14.0	16.8	18.5	20.5
4	0	12.9	13.2	13.9	14.4	15.3	16.3	16.8	17.9	18.3	11.8	12.8	14.0	16.8	18.5	20.6
4	1	12.9	13.2	13.9	14.4	15.3	16.3	16.8	17.9	18.3	11.8	12.8	13.9	16.8	18.5	20.6
4	2	12.9	13.2	13.9	14.3	15.3	16.3	16.8	17.9	18.3	11.8	12.8	13.9	16.8	18.6	20.7
4	3	12.9	13.2	13.9	14.3	15.3	16.3	16.8	17.9	18.4	11.8	12.8	13.9	16.8	18.6	20.7
4	4	12.9	13.1	13.9	14.3	15.2	16.3	16.9	17.9	18.4	11.7	12.8	13.9	16.8	18.6	20.7
4	5	12.9	13.1	13.9	14.3	15.3	16.3	16.9	17.9	18.4	11.7	12.7	13.9	16.8	18.6	20.8
4	6	12.9	13.1	13.9	14.3	15.3	16.3	16.9	18.0	18.4	11.7	12.7	13.9	16.8	18.7	20.8
4	7	12.9	13.1	13.9	14.3	15.3	16.3	16.9	18.0	18.4	11.7	12.7	13.9	16.8	18.7	20.9
4	8	12.8	13.1	13.8	14.3	15.3	16.3	16.9	18.0	18.5	11.7	12.7	13.9	16.8	18.7	20.9
4	9	12.8	13.1	13.8	14.3	15.3	16.3	16.9	18.0	18.5	11.7	12.7	13.9	16.9	18.7	21.0
4	10	12.8	13.1	13.8	14.3	15.3	16.3	16.9	18.0	18.5	11.7	12.7	13.9	16.9	18.8	21.0
4	11	12.8	13.1	13.8	14.3	15.3	16.3	16.9	18.1	18.5	11.6	12.7	13.9	16.9	18.8	21.0
5	0	12.8	13.1	13.8	14.3	15.3	16.3	17.0	18.1	18.6	11.6	12.7	13.9	16.9	18.8	21.1

A

Table 12 Weight (kg) Centiles and Standard Deviation for Boys (5–18 Years): IAP Growth Charts 2015

Age (y)	3rd	10th	25th	50th	75th	90th	97th	SD
5.0	13.2	14.3	15.6	17.1	19.0	21.3	24.2	3.2
5.5	13.8	15.0	16.5	18.2	20.3	22.9	26.1	2.9
6.0	14.5	15.8	17.4	19.3	21.7	24.6	28.3	3.6
6.5	15.3	16.8	18.6	20.7	23.3	26.6	30.8	3.8
7.0	16.0	17.6	19.6	21.9	24.9	28.6	33.4	4.2
7.5	16.7	18.5	20.7	23.3	26.6	30.8	36.2	4.9
8.0	17.5	19.5	21.9	24.8	28.5	33.2	39.4	5.7
8.5	18.3	20.5	23.2	26.4	30.5	35.7	42.6	6.5
9.0	19.1	21.5	24.3	27.9	32.3	38.0	45.5	6.3
9.5	19.9	22.4	25.6	29.4	34.3	40.5	48.6	7.0
10.0	20.7	23.5	26.9	31.1	36.3	43.0	51.8	7.9
10.5	21.6	24.6	28.3	32.8	38.5	45.8	55.2	8.3
11.0	22.6	25.9	29.8	34.7	40.9	48.7	58.7	8.9
11.5	23.8	27.3	31.6	36.9	43.5	51.8	62.5	9.3
12.0	24.9	28.7	33.3	39.0	46.0	54.8	66.1	10.0
12.5	26.1	30.2	35.1	41.2	48.6	57.8	69.5	10.6
13.0	27.5	31.8	37.0	43.3	51.1	60.7	72.6	11.3
13.5	29.0	33.6	39.1	45.7	53.8	63.6	75.6	11.4
14.0	30.7	35.5	41.3	48.2	56.4	66.3	78.3	12.1
14.5	32.6	37.7	43.7	50.8	59.1	69.1	80.9	11.6
15.0	34.5	39.8	45.9	53.1	61.6	71.5	83.1	12.1
15.5	36.1	41.6	47.9	55.2	63.6	73.4	84.7	11.2
16.0	37.5	43.1	49.5	56.8	65.2	74.8	85.8	12.2
16.5	38.7	44.4	50.9	58.2	66.6	76.1	86.8	12.6
17.0	39.8	45.6	52.1	59.5	67.8	77.1	87.5	12.3
17.5	40.8	46.7	53.2	60.6	68.7	77.8	88.0	12.3
18.0	41.8	47.7	54.3	61.6	69.7	78.6	88.4	11.3

Table 13 *Weight (kg) Centiles and Standard Deviations for Girls (5–18 Years): IAP Growth Charts 2015*

Age (y)	3rd	10th	25th	50th	75th	90th	97th	SD
5.0	12.3	13.4	14.8	16.4	18.5	21.3	25.0	2.5
5.5	13.0	14.3	15.7	17.6	19.9	22.9	27.0	3.5
6.0	13.7	15.1	16.7	18.7	21.3	24.6	29.1	3.4
6.5	14.4	15.9	17.7	19.9	22.7	26.3	31.2	4.1
7.0	15.1	16.8	18.7	21.2	24.2	28.2	33.4	4.4
7.5	15.9	17.7	19.9	22.5	25.9	30.1	35.7	4.8
8.0	16.7	18.7	21.1	24.0	27.6	32.2	38.1	5.2
8.5	17.5	19.7	22.3	25.5	29.5	34.4	40.7	6.4
9.0	18.5	20.9	23.7	27.2	31.5	36.7	43.4	6.4
9.5	19.5	22.1	25.3	29.0	33.6	39.3	46.3	6.9
10.0	20.7	23.5	26.9	31.0	36.0	42.0	49.4	7.7
10.5	22.0	25.1	28.8	33.2	38.4	44.8	52.6	8.3
11.0	23.3	26.7	30.7	35.4	41.0	47.7	55.9	8.5
11.5	24.8	28.4	32.6	37.6	43.6	50.6	59.1	9.1
12.0	26.2	30.0	34.5	39.8	46.0	53.4	62.1	9.0
12.5	27.6	31.6	36.3	41.8	48.2	55.8	64.8	9.7
13.0	28.9	33.1	37.9	43.6	50.2	57.9	67.1	9.4
13.5	30.2	34.4	39.4	45.1	51.8	59.7	69.0	9.8
14.0	31.3	35.6	40.6	46.4	53.2	61.1	70.4	9.6
14.5	32.3	36.6	41.7	47.5	54.3	62.2	71.4	9.4
15.0	33.1	37.5	42.5	48.4	55.1	62.9	72.1	9.6
15.5	34.0	38.3	43.3	49.1	55.8	63.5	72.5	8.7
16.0	34.7	39.1	44.0	49.7	56.3	64.0	72.8	8.7
16.5	35.5	39.8	44.7	50.3	56.9	64.4	73.1	9.2
17.0	36.2	40.5	45.3	50.9	57.3	64.7	73.3	8.8
17.5	36.9	41.1	46.0	51.5	57.8	65.0	73.4	9.5
18.0	37.6	41.8	46.6	52.0	58.2	65.3	73.5	10.2

A

Table 14 *Height (cm) Centiles and Standard Deviation for Boys (5–18 Years): IAP Growth Charts 2015*

Age (y)	3rd	10th	25th	50th	75th	90th	97th	SD
5.0	99.0	102.3	105.6	108.9	112.4	115.9	119.4	5.7
5.5	101.6	105.0	108.4	111.9	115.4	119.0	122.7	5.3
6.0	104.2	107.7	111.2	114.8	118.5	122.2	126.0	5.6
6.5	106.8	110.4	114.0	117.8	121.6	125.4	129.3	5.5
7.0	109.3	113.0	116.8	120.7	124.6	128.6	132.6	5.9
7.5	111.8	115.7	119.6	123.5	127.6	131.7	135.9	5.7
8.0	114.3	118.2	122.3	126.4	130.5	134.8	139.1	6.3
8.5	116.7	120.8	124.9	129.1	133.4	137.8	142.2	6.1
9.0	119.0	123.2	127.5	131.8	136.3	140.7	145.3	6.4
9.5	121.3	125.6	130.0	134.5	139.1	143.7	148.3	6.4
10.0	123.6	128.1	132.6	137.2	141.9	146.6	151.4	6.8
10.5	125.9	130.5	135.2	139.9	144.7	149.5	154.4	6.5
11.0	128.2	133.0	137.8	142.7	147.6	152.5	157.5	7.6
11.5	130.7	135.6	140.6	145.5	150.5	155.6	160.6	7.3
12.0	133.2	138.3	143.3	148.4	153.5	158.6	163.7	8.1
12.5	135.7	141.0	146.2	151.4	156.5	161.7	166.8	7.9
13.0	138.3	143.7	149.0	154.3	159.5	164.7	169.9	9.0
13.5	140.9	146.4	151.8	157.2	162.4	167.6	172.7	8.4
14.0	143.4	149.0	154.5	159.9	165.1	170.3	175.4	9.0
14.5	145.8	151.5	157.0	162.3	167.6	172.7	177.7	7.8
15.0	148.0	153.7	159.2	164.5	169.7	174.8	179.7	7.9
15.5	150.0	155.7	161.2	166.5	171.6	176.5	181.4	6.6
16.0	151.8	157.4	162.9	168.1	173.1	178.0	182.7	7.2
16.5	153.4	159.1	164.5	169.6	174.5	179.3	183.8	6.7
17.0	155.0	160.6	165.9	171.0	175.8	180.4	184.8	6.9
17.5	156.6	162.1	167.3	172.3	177.0	181.5	185.8	6.1
18.0	158.1	163.6	168.7	173.6	178.2	182.5	186.7	6.9

Table 15 Height (cm) Centiles and Standard Deviations for Girls (5–18 Years): IAP Growth Charts 2015

Age (y)	3rd	10th	25th	50th	75th	90th	97th	SD
5.0	97.2	100.5	103.9	107.5	111.3	115.2	119.3	5.4
5.5	99.8	103.2	106.8	110.5	114.4	118.3	122.5	5.7
6.0	102.3	106.0	109.7	113.5	117.4	121.5	125.6	5.8
6.5	104.9	108.7	112.5	116.5	120.5	124.6	128.7	5.5
7.0	107.4	111.4	115.4	119.4	123.5	127.7	131.9	6.1
7.5	110.0	114.1	118.2	122.4	126.6	130.8	135.0	6.0
8.0	112.6	116.8	121.1	125.4	129.6	133.9	138.1	6.2
8.5	115.2	119.6	124.0	128.4	132.7	137.0	141.3	6.8
9.0	117.8	122.4	126.9	131.4	135.8	140.2	144.5	6.9
9.5	120.5	125.2	129.9	134.4	138.9	143.3	147.6	6.6
10.0	123.3	128.1	132.8	137.4	142.0	146.4	150.8	7.8
10.5	126.1	130.9	135.7	140.4	145.0	149.5	153.9	7.3
11.0	128.8	133.7	138.6	143.3	147.9	152.4	156.8	7.9
11.5	131.5	136.4	141.2	145.9	150.6	155.1	159.6	7.1
12.0	134.0	138.9	143.7	148.4	153.0	157.5	162.0	7.0
12.5	136.3	141.1	145.8	150.5	155.1	159.6	164.1	6.7
13.0	138.2	142.9	147.6	152.2	156.8	161.3	165.9	6.9
13.5	139.9	144.5	149.1	153.6	158.2	162.7	167.2	6.0
14.0	141.3	145.8	150.2	154.7	159.2	163.7	168.2	6.6
14.5	142.4	146.8	151.1	155.5	160.0	164.5	169.0	5.9
15.0	143.3	147.5	151.8	156.1	160.5	165.0	169.5	6.6
15.5	144.1	148.1	152.3	156.6	160.9	165.3	169.8	5.9
16.0	144.7	148.6	152.7	156.9	161.2	165.6	170.1	6.1
16.5	145.2	149.1	153.1	157.2	161.4	165.7	170.2	6.4
17.0	145.7	149.5	153.4	157.4	161.6	165.9	170.4	6.5
17.5	146.2	149.8	153.6	157.6	161.7	166.0	170.5	6.7
18.0	146.6	150.2	153.9	157.8	161.9	166.1	170.6	6.6

A

Table 16 *Body Mass Index Percentiles and Standard Deviations for Boys (5--18 Years): IAP Growth Charts 2015*

Age (y)	3rd	5th	10th	25th	50th	23rd (Eq 75)	27th (Eq 95)	SD
5.0	12.1	12.4	12.8	13.6	14.7	15.7	17.5	1.6
5.5	12.2	12.4	12.9	13.7	14.8	15.8	17.6	1.5
6.0	12.2	12.5	12.9	13.7	14.9	16.0	17.8	1.8
6.5	12.3	12.5	13.0	13.8	15.0	16.1	18.0	1.8
7.0	12.3	12.6	13.1	13.9	15.1	16.3	18.2	1.9
7.5	12.4	12.7	13.2	14.1	15.3	16.5	18.5	2.2
8.0	12.5	12.8	13.3	14.2	15.5	16.7	18.8	2.5
8.5	12.6	12.9	13.4	14.4	15.7	17.0	19.2	2.8
9.0	12.7	13.0	13.5	14.5	15.9	17.3	19.6	2.6
9.5	12.8	13.1	13.7	14.7	16.2	17.6	20.1	2.8
10.0	12.9	13.2	13.8	14.9	16.4	18.0	20.5	3.1
10.5	13.0	13.3	14.0	15.1	16.7	18.3	21.0	3.2
11.0	13.1	13.5	14.1	15.4	17.0	18.7	21.5	3.2
11.5	13.2	13.6	14.3	15.6	17.3	19.1	22.1	3.3
12.0	13.3	13.8	14.5	15.8	17.7	19.5	22.6	3.4
12.5	13.5	13.9	14.6	16.0	17.9	19.8	23.0	3.6
13.0	13.6	14.0	14.8	16.3	18.2	20.2	23.4	3.5
13.5	13.7	14.2	14.9	16.5	18.5	20.5	23.8	3.7
14.0	13.8	14.3	15.1	16.7	18.7	20.8	24.2	3.7
14.5	14.0	14.5	15.3	16.9	19.0	21.1	24.5	3.5
15.0	14.2	14.7	15.5	17.2	19.3	21.4	24.9	3.7
15.5	14.4	14.9	15.8	17.4	19.6	21.7	25.2	3.4
16.0	14.6	15.1	16.0	17.7	19.9	22.0	25.5	3.7
16.5	14.9	15.4	16.3	18.0	20.2	22.4	25.8	3.8
17.0	15.1	15.6	16.6	18.3	20.5	22.6	26.0	3.8
17.5	15.4	15.9	16.8	18.6	20.8	22.9	26.3	3.6
18.0	15.6	16.2	17.1	18.9	21.1	23.2	26.6	3.2

Table 17 *Body Mass Index Percentiles and Standard Deviations for Girls (5–18 Years): IAP Growth Charts 2015*

Age (y)	3rd	5th	10th	25th	50th	23rd (Eq 75)	27th (Eq 95)	SD
5.0	11.9	12.1	12.5	13.3	14.3	15.5	18.0	1.4
5.5	11.9	12.2	12.6	13.4	14.4	15.7	18.3	1.7
6.0	12.0	12.2	12.7	13.5	14.5	15.9	18.6	1.7
6.5	12.1	12.3	12.8	13.6	14.7	16.1	18.9	2.0
7.0	12.1	12.4	12.8	13.7	14.9	16.4	19.3	2.1
7.5	12.2	12.5	12.9	13.9	15.1	16.6	19.7	2.2
8.0	12.3	12.6	13.1	14.0	15.3	16.9	20.1	2.3
8.5	12.3	12.7	13.2	14.2	15.6	17.2	20.5	2.7
9.0	12.4	12.8	13.3	14.4	15.8	17.6	21.0	2.7
9.5	12.5	12.9	13.5	14.6	16.1	18.0	21.4	2.8
10.0	12.7	13.1	13.7	14.9	16.5	18.4	21.9	2.9
10.5	12.8	13.2	13.9	15.2	16.8	18.8	22.5	3.1
11.0	13.0	13.4	14.1	15.5	17.2	19.3	23.0	3.1
11.5	13.2	13.7	14.4	15.8	17.6	19.8	23.6	3.3
12.0	13.4	13.9	14.7	16.1	18.0	20.2	24.1	3.2
12.5	13.7	14.2	15.0	16.5	18.4	20.7	24.7	3.3
13.0	13.9	14.4	15.2	16.8	18.8	21.1	25.2	3.2
13.5	14.1	14.6	15.5	17.1	19.1	21.5	25.6	3.5
14.0	14.3	14.9	15.7	17.3	19.4	21.8	25.9	3.4
14.5	14.5	15.1	16.0	17.6	19.7	22.0	26.2	3.3
15.0	14.7	15.2	16.1	17.8	19.9	22.3	26.3	3.4
15.5	14.9	15.4	16.3	18.0	20.1	22.4	26.4	3.1
16.0	15.0	15.6	16.5	18.2	20.3	22.6	26.5	3.1
16.5	15.2	15.8	16.7	18.4	20.4	22.8	26.6	3.2
17.0	15.4	16.0	16.9	18.6	20.6	22.9	26.7	3.0
17.5	15.5	16.1	17.1	18.7	20.8	23.1	26.7	3.1
18.0	15.7	16.3	17.3	18.9	21.0	23.2	26.8	3.6

Source: IAP Growth Charts Committee. Indian Pediatrics 2015;52:47–55

A

2 Growth Standards for Newborns

International Standards for Size at Birth (Boys)

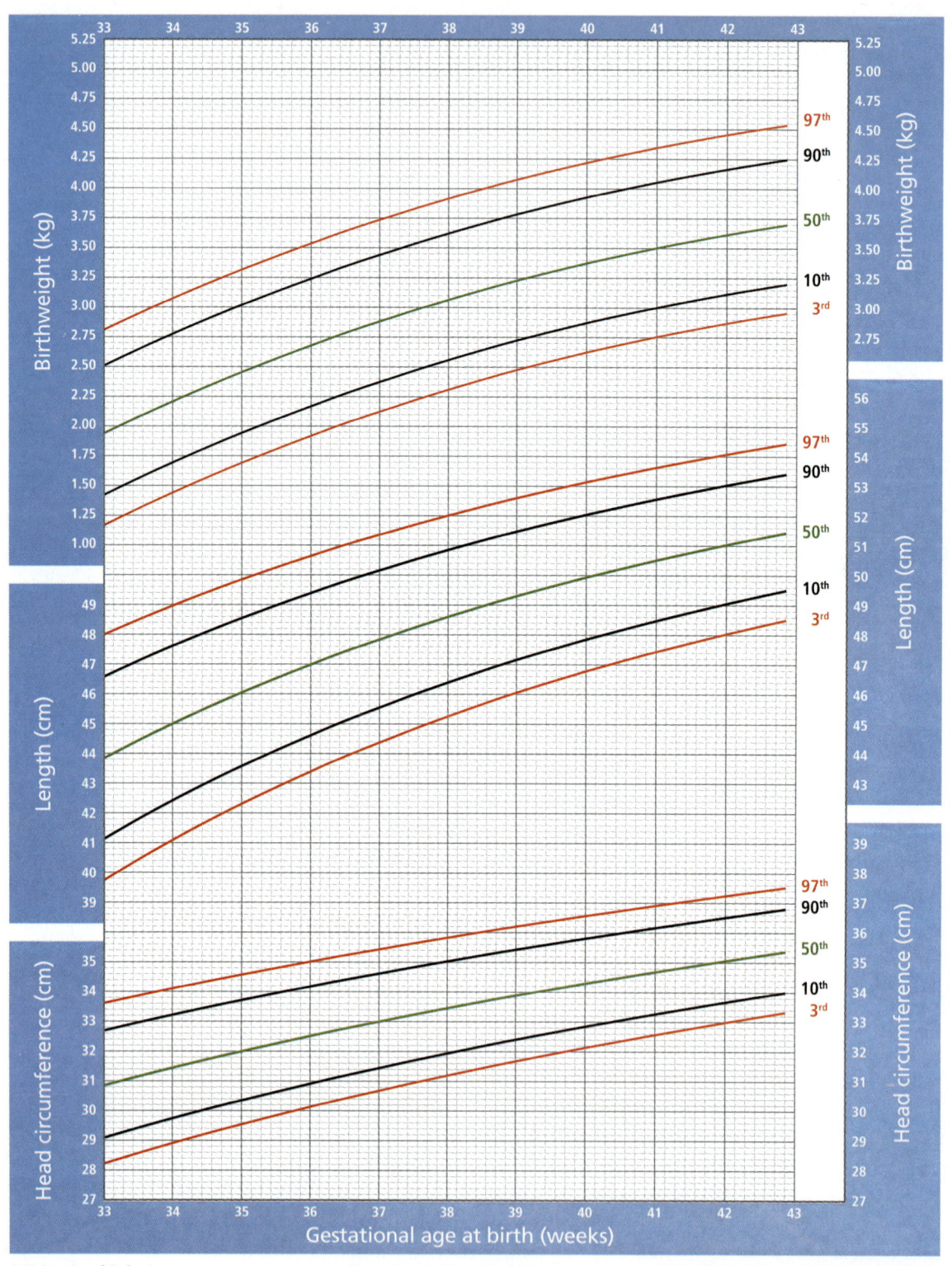

Gestational age at birth (weeks)

© University of Oxford   (Reproduced with permission)   Ref: Villar J et al. Lancet 2014; 384: 857-868

International Standards for Size at Birth (Girls)

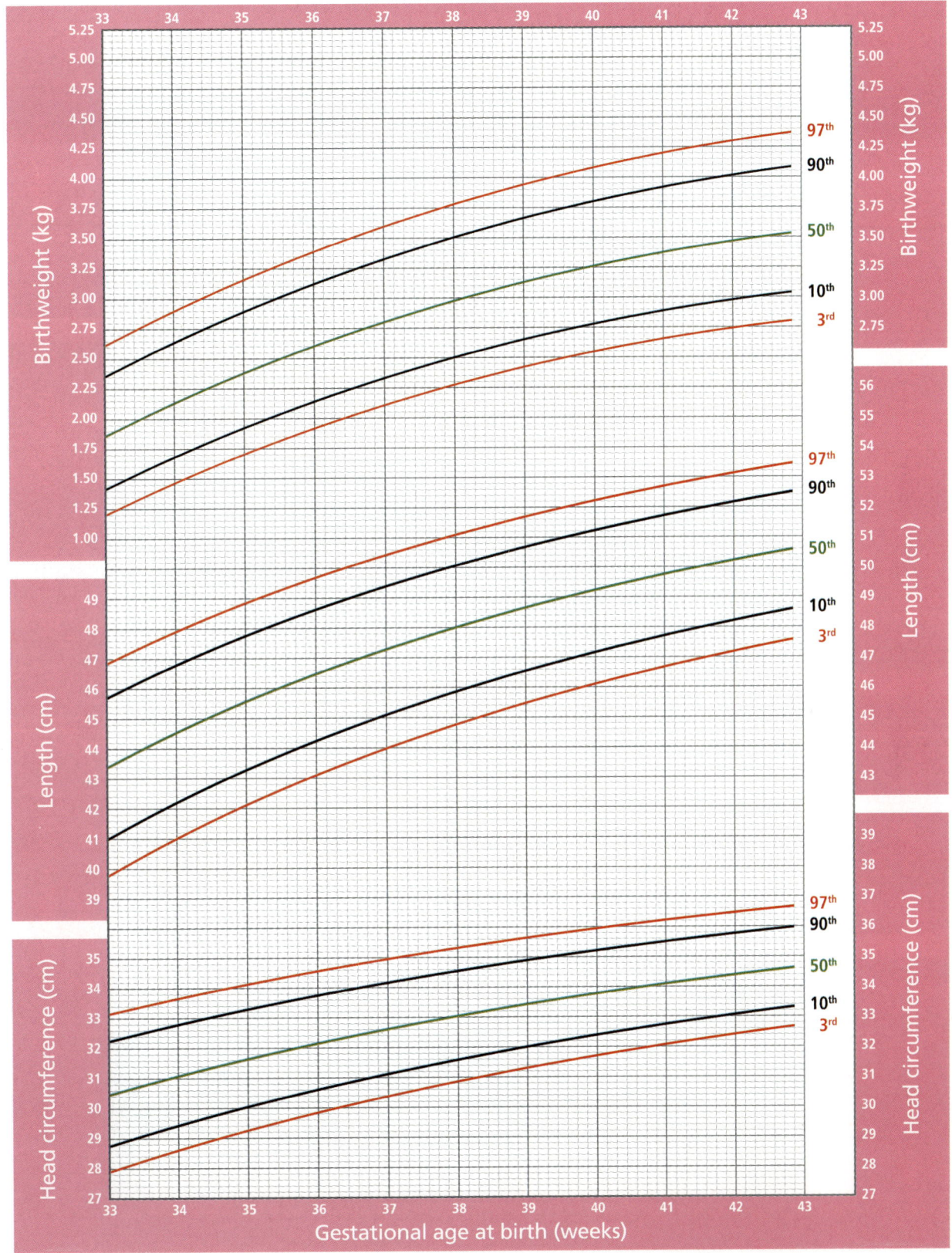

Gestational age at birth (weeks)

(Reproduced with permission)

Ref: Villar J et al. Lancet 2014; 384: 857-868

A

International Postnatal Growth Standards
for Preterm Infants (Boys)

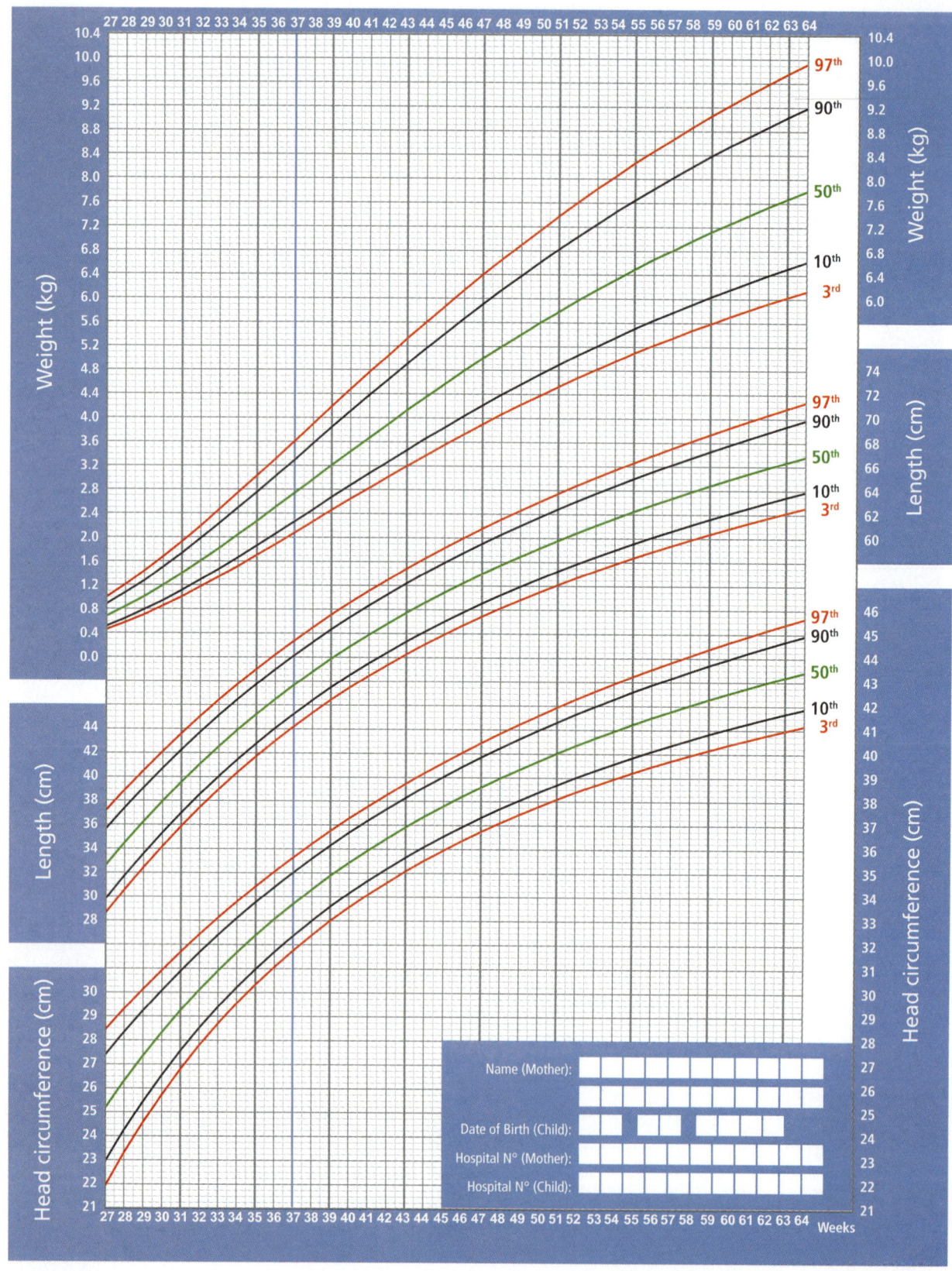

A

International Postnatal Growth Standards for Preterm Infants (Girls)

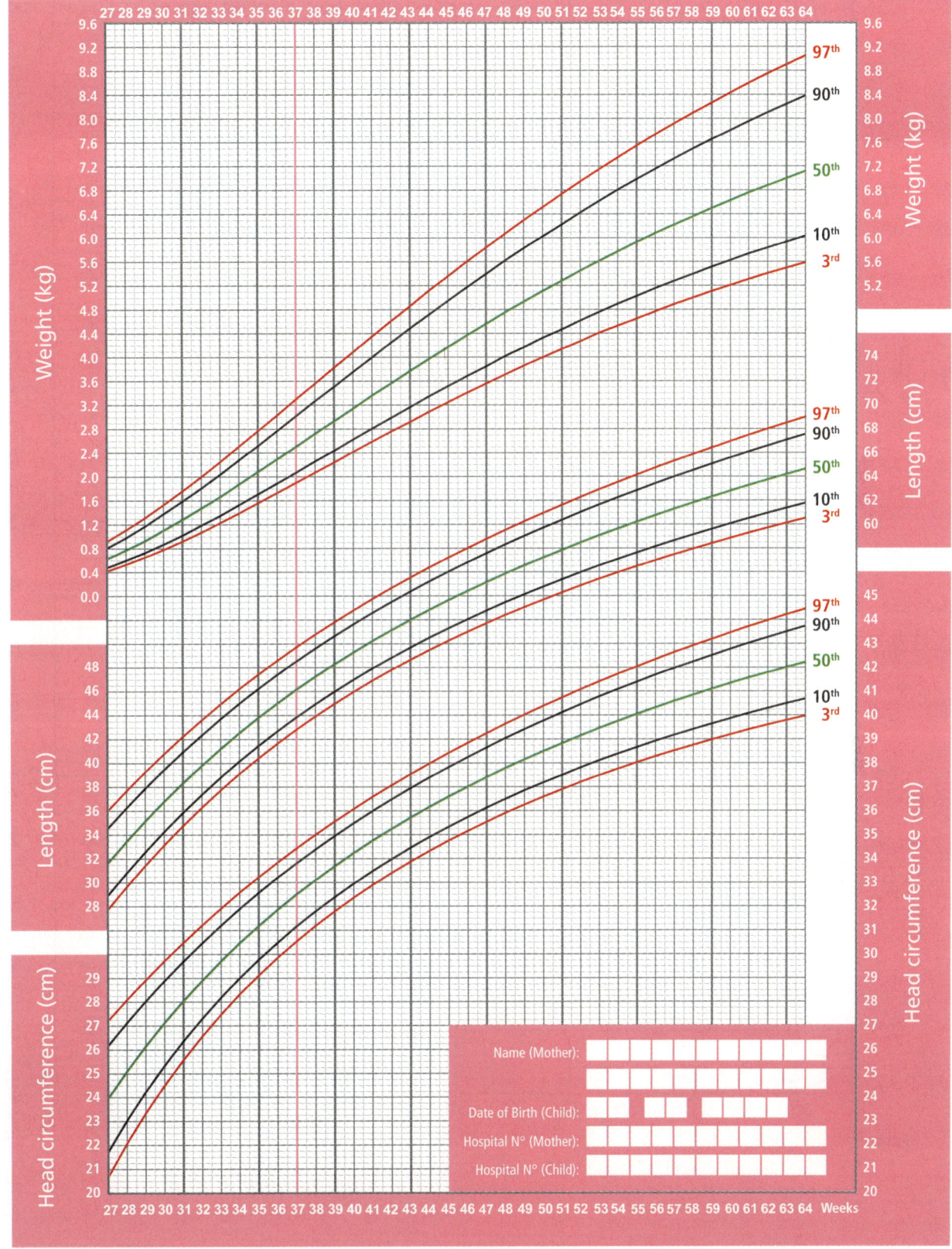

© University of Oxford   (Reproduced with permission)   Ref: Villar et al *Lancet Glob Heath* 2015;3:e681-91.

A

Fenton Growth Charts for Preterm Girls

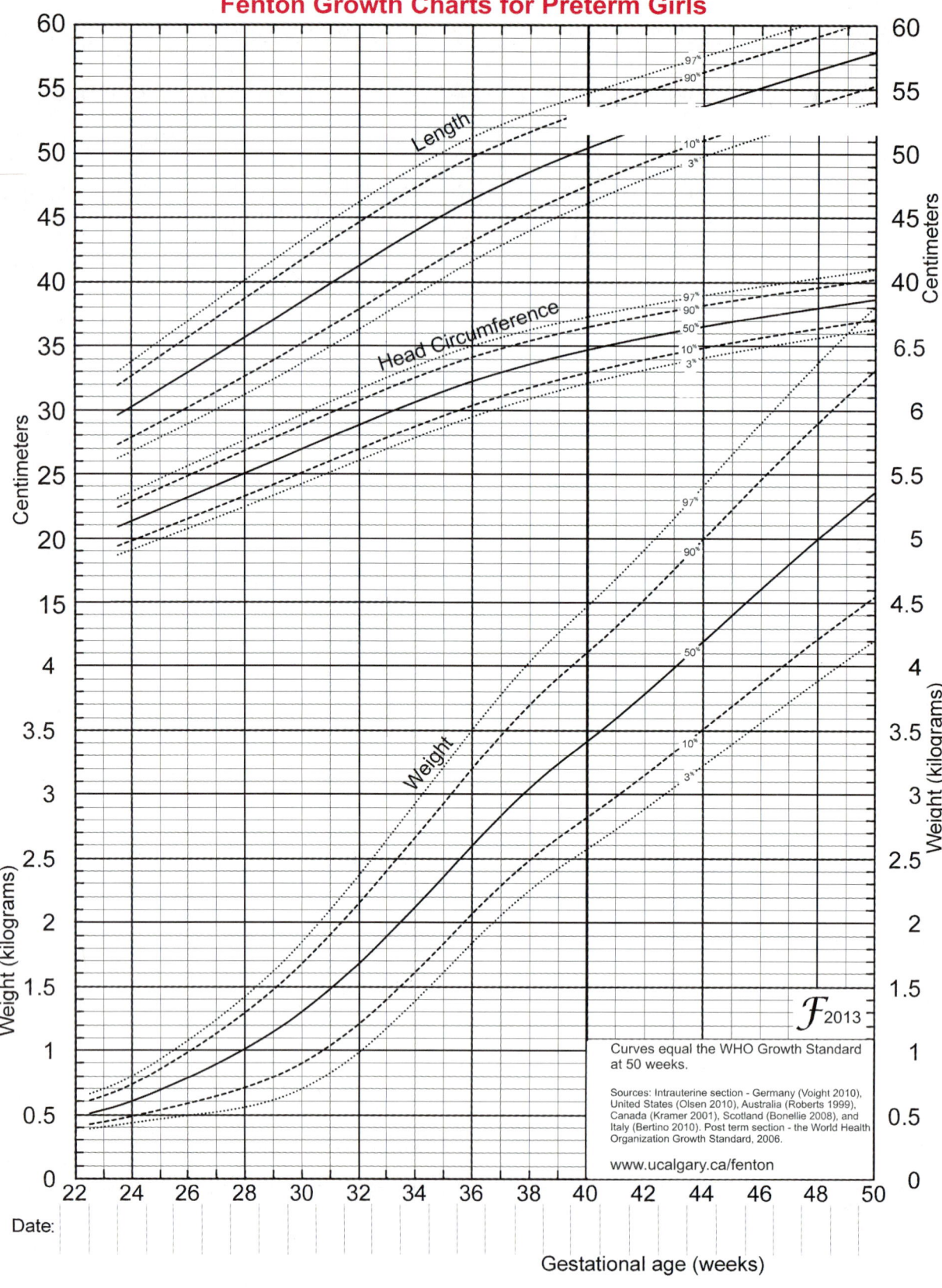

Fenton Growth Charts for Preterm Boys

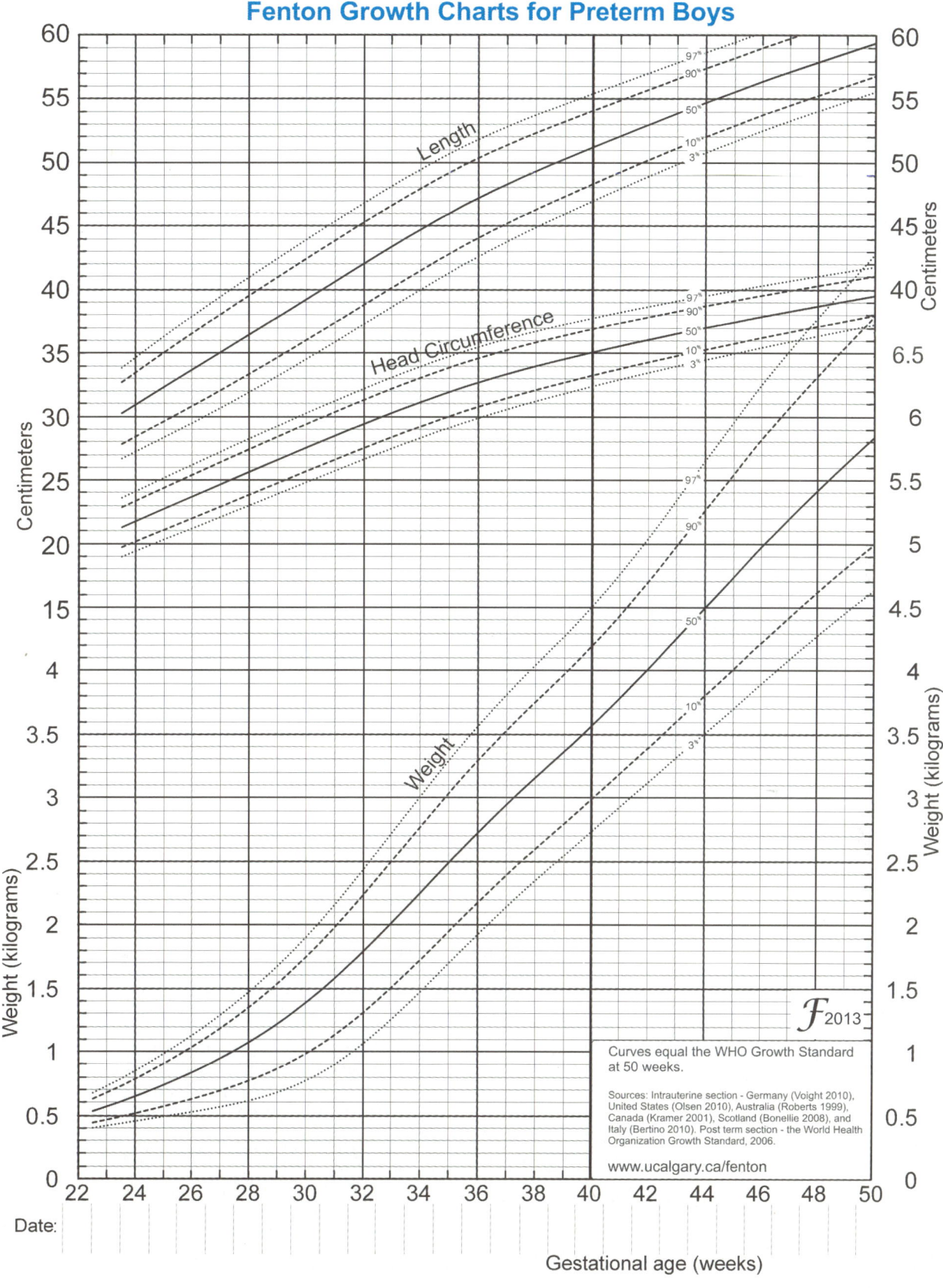

Date:

Gestational age (weeks)

$\mathcal{F}$2013

Curves equal the WHO Growth Standard at 50 weeks.

Sources: Intrauterine section - Germany (Voight 2010), United States (Olsen 2010), Australia (Roberts 1999), Canada (Kramer 2001), Scotland (Bonellie 2008), and Italy (Bertino 2010). Post term section - the World Health Organization Growth Standard, 2006.

www.ucalgary.ca/fenton

A

IMNCI Chart Booklet

Chart 1 ASSESS AND CLASSIFY THE SICK YOUNG INFANT AGE UP TO 2 MONTHS

ASSESS: Ask the mother what young infant's problems are? Use all boxes that match infant's symptoms

CLASSIFY: A child with a **Pink** classification needs **URGENT** attention, complete the assessment and pre-referral treatment immediately so that referral is not delayed. Check for possible bacterial infection/jaundice

ASK: • Has the infant had convulsions?

LOOK, LISTEN, FEEL:

- Count the breaths in one minute.
- Repeat the count if elevated.
- Look for severe chest indrawing.
- Look for nasal flaring.
- Look and listen for grunting.
- Look and feel for bulging fontanelle.

} Young infant must be calm

- Look for pus draining from the ear. • Look at the umbilicus. Is it red or draining pus?
- Look for skin pustules. Are there 10 or more skin pustules or a big boil?
- Measure axillary temperature (if not possible, feel for fever or low body temperature).
- See if the young infant is lethargic or unconscious.
- Look at the young infant's movements. Are they less than normal? • Look for jaundice? Are the palms and soles yellow?

Classify All Young Infants

SIGNS	CLASSIFY AS	IDENTIFY TREATMENT
• Convulsions or • Fast breathing (60 breaths per minute or more) or • Severe chest indrawing or • Nasal flaring or • Grunting or • Bugling fontanelle or • 10 or more skin pustules or a big boil or • If axillary temperature 37.5°C or above (or feels hot to touch) or temperature less than 35.5°C (or feels cold to touch) or • Lethargic or unconscious or • Less than normal movements.	**POSSIBLE SERIOUS BACTERIAL INFECTION**	• **Give first dose of intramuscular ampicillin and gentamicin.** • **Treat to prevent low blood sugar.** • **Warm the young infant by skin to skin contact if temperature less than 36.5°C (or feels cold to touch) while arranging referral.** • **Advise mother how to keep the young infant warm on the way to the hospital.** • **Refer URGENTLY to hospital*.**
• Umbilicus red or draining pus or • Pus discharge from ear or • <10 skin pustules.	**LOCAL BACTERIAL INFECTION**	• **Give oral cotrimoxazole or amoxicillin for 5 days.** • Teach mother to treat local infections at home. • Follow up in 2 days.

And if the infant has jaundice

• Palms and soles yellow or • Age <24 hours or • Age 14 days or more	**SEVERE JAUNDICE**	• **Treat to prevent low blood sugar.** • **Warm the young infant by skin to skin contact if temperature less than 36.5°C (or feels cold to touch) while arranging referral.** • **Advise mother how to keep the young infant warm on the way to the hospital.** • **Refer URGENTLY to hospital*.**
• Palms and soles not yellow	**JAUNDICE**	• Advise mother to give home care for the young infant. • Advise mother when to return immediately. • Follow up in 2 days.

And if the temperature is between 35.5°C and 36.4°C

• Temperature between 35.5°C–36.4°C	**LOW BODY TEMPERATURE**	• Warm the young infant using skin to skin contact for one hour and REASSESS. If no improvement, refer • Treat to prevent low blood sugar.

* If referral is not possible, treat the young infant and counsel the parents

Chart 2 YOUNG INFANT AGE UP TO 2 MONTHS

THEN ASK: Does the young infant has diarrhea?

1. **IF YES, ASK**
    * For how long? Is there blood in stool?
    LOOK AND FEEL
    * Look at the young infant's general condition. Is the infant lethargic or unconscious? Restless or irritable.
    * Look for sunken eyes.   • Pinch the skin of abdomen. Does it go back: Very slowly (longer than 2 seconds)? Slowly?
    What is diarrhea in a young infant?
    if the stools have changed from usual pattern and are many and watery (more water than fecal matter). The normal frequent or loose stools of a breastfed baby are not diarrhea.

Classify Diarrhea for Dehydration

SIGNS	CLASSIFY AS	IDENTIFY TREATMENT

Two of the following signs:
• Lethargic or unconscious.
• Sunken eyes.
• Skin pinch goes back very slowly.
	SEVERE DEHYDRATION	• **Give first dose of intramuscular ampicillin and gentamicin.**
		  –If infant also has low weight or another severe classification:
		    • **Refer URGENTLY to hospital with mother giving frequent sips of ORS on the way*.**
		    • **Advise mother to continue breastfeeding.**
		    • **Advise mother how to keep the young infant warm on the way to the hospital.**
		            OR
		• If infant does not have low weight or any other severe classification:
		  – Give fluid for severe dehydration (Plan C) and then refer to hospital after rehydration.

Two of the following signs:
• Restless, irritable
• Sunken eyes.
• Skin pinch goes back slowly.
	SOME DEHYDRATION	• **If infant also has low weight or another severe classification:**
		  – **Give first dose of intramuscular ampicillin and gentamicin.**
		  – **Refer URGENTLY to hospital with mother giving frequent sips of ORS on the way*.**
		  – **Advise mother to continue breastfeeding.**
		  – **Advise mother how to keep the young infant warm on the way to the hospital.**
		• If infant does not have low weight or another severe classification:
		  – Give fluids for some dehydration (Plan B)
		  – Advise mother when to return immediately.
		  – Follow up in 2 days.

• Not enough signs to classify as some or severe dehydration.	**NO DEHYDRATION**	• Give fluids to treat diarrhoea at home (Plan A) • Advise mother when to return immediately. • Follow up in 5 days if not improving.

And if Diarrhea is of 14 days or more

• Diarrhea lasting 14 days or more.	**SEVERE PERSISTENT DIARRHEA**	• Give first dose of intramuscular ampicillin and gentamicin if the young infant has low weight, dehydration or another severe classification. • Treat to prevent low blood sugar. • Advise how to keep infant warm on the way to the hospital. • Refer to hospital.*

And if there is blood in stool

• Blood in stool	**SEVERE DYSENTERY**	• Give first dose of intramuscular ampicillin and gentamicin if the young infant has low weight, dehydration or another severe classification. • Treat to prevent low blood sugar. • Advise how to keep infant warm on the way to hospital. • Refer to hospital.*

* *If referral is not possible, treat the young infant and counsel the mother.*

A

Chart 3 CHECK FOR FEEDING PROBLEM AND MALNUTRITION (Age up to 2 months)

ASK, LOOK, AND FEEL

- Is there any difficulty in feeding? Is the infant breastfed? Yes, how many times in 24 hours?
- Does the infant usually receive any other food or drink? If yes, how often?
- What do you use to feed the infant?
- **If AN INFANT:** Has any difficulty in feeding or is breastfeeding less than 8 times in 24 hours or is taking any other foods or drinks, or is low weight for age and has no indication to refer urgently to hospital.

LOOK, FEEL: Determine weight for age

ASSESS BREASTFEEDING: • Has the infant breastfed in the previous hour?

If the infant has not fed in the previous hour, ask the mother to put her infant to breast. Observe the breastfeed for 4 minutes. (If the infant was fed during the last hour, ask the mother if she can wait and tell you when the infant is willing to feed again).

Is the infant able to attach?   –   No attachment at all.   –   Not well attached. –   Good attachment.

TO CHECK THE ATTACHMENT, LOOK FOR: • Chin touching breast.   • Mouth wide open.   • Lower lip turned outward.
   • More areola visible above than below the mouth.
   (All of these signs should be present if the attachment is good).

- Is the infant suckling effectively (that is, slow deep sucks, sometimes pausing)?: not suckling at all,   Not suckling effectively, Suckling effectively.
   Clear a blocked nose if it interferes with breastfeeding.   • Look for ulcers or white patches in the mouth (Thrush).
- Does the mother have pain while breastfeeding? If yes look and feel for: Flat or inverted nipples, or sore nipples, engorged breasts or breast abscess.

Classify Feeding

SIGNS	CLASSIFY AS	IDENTIFY TREATMENT
• Not able to feed or • No attachment at all or • Not suckling at all or • Very low weight for age.	**NOT ABLE TO FEED POSSIBLE SERIOUS BACTERIAL INFECTION OR SEVERE MALNUTRITION**	• Give first dose of intramuscular ampicillin and gentamicin. • Treat to prevent low blood sugar. • Warm the young infant by skin to skin contact if temperature less than 36.5°C (or feels cold to touch) while arranging referral. • Advise mother how to keep the young infant warm on the way to the hospital. • Refer URGENTLY to hospital*.

• Not well attached to breast or
• Not suckling effectively or
• Less than 8 breastfeeds in 24 hours or
• Receives other foods or drinks or
• Thrush (ulcers or white patches in mouth) or
• Low weight for age
    OR
• Breasts or nipple problems
	FEEDING PROBLEM OR LOW WEIGHT FOR AGE	• If not well attached or not suckling effectively, teach correct positioning and attachment.
		• If breastfeeding less than 8 times in 24 hours, advise to increase frequency of feeding.
		• If receiving other foods or drinks, counsel mother about breastfeeding more, reducing other foods or drinks, and using a cup and spoon.
		  – If not breast feeding at all advise mother about giving locally appropriate animal milk and teach the mother to feed with a cup and spoon.
		• If thrush, teach the mother to treat thrush at home.
		• If low weight for age, teach the mother how to keep the young infant with low weight warm at home.
		• If breast or nipple problem, teach the mother to treat breast or nipple problems.
		• Advise mother to give home care for the young infant.
		• Advise mother when to return immediately.
		• Follow-up any feeding problem or thrush in 2 days.
		• Follow-up low weight for age in 14 days.

• Not low weight for age and no other signs of inadequate feeding.	**NO FEEDING PROBLEM**	• Advise mother to give home care for the young infant. • Advise mother when to return immediately. • Praise mother for feeding the infant well.

*   *If referral is not possible, treat the young infant and counsel the parents.*

A

Chart 4 ASSESS AND CLASSIFY THE SICK CHILD AGE 2 MONTHS UP TO 5 YEARS

ASK THE MOTHER WHAT THE CHILD'S PROBLEMS ARE?

- Determine if this is an initial or follow-up visit for this problem.
  - If follow-up visit, use the follow-up instructions on treat the child chart.
  - If initial visit, assess the child as follows:

CHECK FOR GENERAL DANGER SIGNS

ASK:

- Is the child able to drink or breastfeed?
- Does the child vomit everything?
- Has the child has convulsions?

LOOK:

- See if the child is lethargic or unconscious.

A child with any general danger sign needs urgent attention; complete the assessment and any pre-referral treatment immediately so that referral is not delayed.

THEN ASK ABOUT MAIN SYMPTOMS: Does the child have cough or difficult breathing?

IF YES, ASK: • For how long?

LOOK, LISTEN:

- Count the breaths in one minute.
- Look for chest indrawing.
- Look and listen for stridor.

(Child must be calm)

What is Fast breathing?

2–12 mo ≥50 breaths per min

1–5 yr ≥40 breaths per min

Classify Cough or Difficult Breathing

SIGNS	CLASSIFY AS	IDENTIFY TREATMENT (Urgent pre-referral-treatments are in bold print.)
• Any general danger sign or • Chest indrawing or • Stridor in calm child.	SEVERE PNEUMONIA OR VERY SEVERE DISEASE	• **Give first dose of injectable chloramphenicol (If not possible give oral amoxicillin).** • **Refer URGENTLY to hospital.***
• Fast breathing.	PNEUMONIA	• Give cotrimoxazole for 5 days. • Soothe the throat and relieve the cough with a safe remedy if child is 6 months or older. • Advise mother when to return immediately. • Follow-up in 2 days.
No signs of pneumonia or very severe disease.	NO PNEUMONIA COUGH OR COLD	• If coughing more than 30 days, refer for assessment. • Soothe the throat and relieve the cough with a safe home remedy if child is 6 months or older. • Advise mother when to return immediately. • Follow-up in 5 days if not improving.

* If referral is not possible, treat the child and counsel the mother/parents.

A

Chart 5 SICK CHILD AGE 2 MONTHS UP TO 5 YEARS

DOES THE CHILD HAVE DIARRHEA?

IF YES, ASK:

• For how long?

• Is there blood in the stool?

LOOK AND FEEL:

• Look at the child's general condition. Is the child lethargic or unconscious? Restless and irritable?

• Look for sunken eyes.

• Offer the child fluid. Is the child:

  – Not able to drink or drinking poorly?

  – Drinking eagerly, thirsty?

• Pinch the skin of the abdomen. Does it go back:

  – Very slowly (longer than 2 seconds)?

  – Slowly?

Classify Diarrhea for— Dehydration— Persistent Diarrhea and Dysentery

SIGNS	CLASSIFY AS	IDENTIFY TREATMENT

Two of the following signs:
• Lethargic or unconscious.
• Sunken eyes.
• Not able to drink or drinking poorly.
• Skin pinch goes back very slowly.
	SEVERE DEHYDRATION	• If child has no other severe classification.
		  – Give fluid for severe dehydration (Plan C).
		• **If child also has another severe classification:
		  Refer URGENTLY to hospital with mother giving frequent sips of ORS on the way*.
		  Advise the mother to continue breastfeeding.**
		• **If child is 2 years or older and there is cholera in your area, give doxycycline for cholera.**

Two of the following signs: • Restless, irritable • Sunken eyes • Drinks eagerly, thirsty • Skin pinch goes back slowly.	**SOME DEHYDRATION**	• Give fluid and food for some dehydration (Plan B). • **If child also has a severe classification: Refer URGENTLY to hospital with mother giving frequent sips of ORS on the way. Advise the mother to continue breastfeeding*.** • Advise mother when to return immediately. • Follow-up in 5 days if not improving.
Not enough signs to classify as some or severe dehydration.	**NO DEHYDRATION**	• Give fluid and food to treat diarrhoea at home (Plan A). • Advise mother when to return immediately. • Follow-up in 5 days if not improving.

And if Diarrhea 14 days or more

• Dehydration present.	**SEVERE PERSISTENT DIARRHEA**	• **Treat dehydration before referral unless the child has another severe classification.** • **Refer to hospital*.**
• No dehydration.	**PERSISTENT DIARRHEA**	• Advise the mother on feeding a child who has PERSISTENT DIARRHEA. • Give single dose of vitamin A. • Give zinc sulphate 20 mg daily for 14 days. • Follow-up in 5 days.

And if blood in stool

• Blood in the stool.	**DYSENTERY**	• **Treat for 5 days with cotrimoxazole.** • Follow-up in 2 days.

A

* If referral is not possible, treat the child and counsel the mother/parents.

Chart 6 SICK CHILD AGE 2 MONTHS UP TO 5 YEARS

DOES THE CHILD HAVE FEVER? (by history or feels hot or temperature 37.5°C or above)

IF YES: Decide Malaria Risk: High/Low

THEN ASK: • Fever for how long? • If more than 7 days, has fever been present everyday? • Has the child had measles within the last 3 months?

LOOK AND FEEL: • Look or feel for stiff neck. • Look and feel for bulging fontanelle. • Look for runny nose.

Look for signs of MEASLES: • Generalized rash and • One of these: cough, runny nose, or red eyes.

If the child has measles now or within the last 3 months: Look for mouth ulcers. Are they deep and extensive? Look for pus draining from the eye. Look for clouding of the cornea.

Classify Fever—High Malaria Risk Area

SIGNS	CLASSIFY AS	IDENTIFY TREATMENT
• Any general danger sign or • Stiff neck or • Bulging fontanelle.	**VERY SEVERE FEBRILE DISEASE**	• **Give first dose of IM quinine after making a blood smear.** • **Give first dose of IV or IM chloramphenicol (if not possible, give oral amoxicillin).** • **Treat the child to prevent low blood sugar.** • **Give one dose of Paracetamol in clinic for high fever (temp. 38.5°C or above)** • **Refer URGENTLY to hospital*.**
• Fever (by history or feels hot or temperature 37.5°C or above).	**MALARIA**	• **Give oral antimalarials for HIGH malaria risk area after making a blood smear.** • **Give one dose of paracetamol in clinic for high fever (temp. 38.5°C or above)** • Advise mother when to return immediately. • Follow-up in 2 days if fever persists. • If fever is present every day for more than 7 days, refer for assessment.

Low Malaria Risk Area

• Any general danger sign or • Stiff neck or • Bulging fontanelle.	**VERY SEVERE FEBRILE DISEASE**	• **Give first dose of IM quinine after making a blood smear.** • **Give first dose of IV or IM chloramphenicol (if not possible, give oral amoxicillin).** • **Treat the child to prevent low blood sugar.** • **Give one dose of paracetamol in clinic for high fever (temp. 38.5°C or above)** • **Refer URGENTLY to hospital*.**
• NO running nose and NO measles and NO other cause of fever.	**MALARIA**	• **Give oral antimalarials for LOW malaria risk area after making a blood smear.** • **Give one dose of paracetamol in clinic for high fever (temp. 38.5°C or above)** • Advise mother when to return immediately. • Follow-up in 2 days if fever persists. • If fever is present every day for more than 7 days, refer for assessment.
• Running nose PRESENT or • Measles PRESENT or • Other cause of fever PRESENT	**FEVER MALARIA UNLIKELY**	• **Give one dose of paracetamol in clinic for high fever (temp. 38.5°C or above).** • Advise mother when to return immediately. • Follow-up in 2 days if fever persists. • If fever is present every day for more than 7 days, refer for assessment.

If Measles Now Within Last 3 Months, Classify

• Any general danger sign or • Clouding of cornea or • Deep or extensive mouth ulcers.	**SEVERE COMPLICATED MEASLES**	• **Give first dose of vitamin A.** • **Give first dose of injectable chloramphenicol (if not possible, give oral amoxiycillin).** • **If clouding of the cornea or pus draining from the eye, apply tetracycline eye ointment.** • **Refer URGENTLY to hospital*.**
• Pus draining from the eye or • Mouth ulcers.	**MEASLES WITH EYE OR MOUTH COMPLICATIONS**	• Give first dose of vitamin A. • If pus draining from the eye, treat eye infection with tetracycline eye ointment. • If mouth ulcers, treat with gentian violet. • Follow-up in 2 days.
• Measles now or within the last 3 months.	**MEASLES**	• Give first dose of vitamin A.

* *If referral is not possible, treat the child and counsel the parents.*

A

THEN CHECK FOR ANEMIA

LOOK:
- Look for palmar pallor. Is it:
  - Severe palmar pallor?
  - Some palmar pallor?

Classify ANAEMIA

• Severe palmar pallor	**SEVERE ANEMIA**	• *Refer URGENTLY to hospital#.*
• Some palmar pallor	**ANEMIA**	• *Give iron folic acid therapy for 14 days.* • Assess the child's feeding and counsel the mother on feeding according to the FOOD box on the *COUNSEL THE MOTHER* chart. – If feeding problem, follow-up in 5 days. • Advise mother when to return immediately. • Follow-up in 14 days
• No palmar pallor	**NO ANEMIA**	• *Give prophylactic iron folic acid if child 6 months or older.*

THEN CHECK THE CHILD'S IMMUNIZATION *, PROPHYLACTIC VITAMIN A & IRON-FOLIC ACID SUPPLEMENTATION STATUS

IMMUNIZATION SCHEDULE:

AGE	VACCINE
Birth	BCG + OPV-0
6 weeks	DPT-1 + OPV-1 (+ HepB-1**)
10 weeks	DPT-2 + OPV-2 (+ HepB-2**)
14 weeks	DPT-3 + OPV-3 (+ HepB-3**)
9 months	Measles + Vitamin A
16–18 months	DPT Booster + OPV + Vitamin A
60 months	DT

PROPHYLACTIC VITAMIN A
Give a single dose of vitamin A:
100,000 IU at 9 months with measles immunization
200,000 IU at 16–18 months with DPT Booster
200,000 IU at 24 months
200,000 IU at 30 months
200,000 IU at 36 months

PROPHYLACTIC IFA

Give 20 mg elemental iron +100 mcg folic acid (one tablet of Pediatric IFA or 5 ml of IFA syrup or 1 ml of IFA drops) for a total of 100 days in a year after the child has recovered from acute illness if:

- The child 6 months of age or older, and
- Has not received Pediatric IFA tablet/syrup/drops for 100 days in last one year.

* A child who needs to be immunized should be advised to go for immunization the day vaccines are available at AW/SC/PHC
** Hepatitis B to be given wherever included in the immunization schedule

ASSESS OTHER PROBLEMS

MAKE SURE CHILD WITH ANY GENERAL DANGER SIGN IS REFERRED after first dose of an appropriate antibiotic and other urgent treatments.

Exception: Rehydration of the child according to Plan C may resolve danger signs so that referral is no longer needed.

\# *If referral is not possible, see the section **Where Referral Is Not Possible** in the module **Treat the Child**.*

A

Does the child have an ear problem?

IF YES, ASK:

- Is there ear pain?
- Is there ear discharge? If yes, for how long?

LOOK AND FEEL:

- Look for pus draining from the ear.
- Feel for tender swelling behind the ear.

Classify
EAR PROBLEM

• Tender swelling behind the ear.	**MASTOIDITIS**	➤ *Give first dose of injectable chloramphenicol (If not possible give oral amoxicillin).* ➤ *Give first dose of paracetamol for pain.* ➤ *Refer URGENTLY to hospital#.*
• Pus is seen draining from the ear and discharge is reported for less than 14 days, or • Ear pain.	**ACUTE EAR INFECTION**	➤ *Give cotrimoxazole for 5 days.* ➤ Give paracetamol for pain. ➤ Dry the ear by wicking. ➤ Follow-up in 5 days.
• Pus is seen draining from the ear and discharge is reported for 14 days or more.	**CHRONIC EAR INFECTION**	➤ Dry the ear by wicking. ➤ Follow-up in 5 days.
• No ear pain, and • No pus seen draining from the ear.	**NO EAR INFECTION**	No additional treatment.

If referral is not possible, see the section **Where Referral Is Not Possible** in the module **Treat the Child.**

THEN CHECK FOR MALNUTRITION

LOOK AND FEEL:

- Look for visible severe wasting.
- Look for edema of both feet.
- Determine weight for age.

Classify
NUTRITIONAL STATUS

• Visible severe wasting or • Edema of both feet.	**SEVERE MALNUTRITION**	• *Give single dose of Vitamin A.* • *Prevent low blood sugar.* • *Refer URGENTLY to hospital#.* • *While referral is being organized, warm the child.* • *Keep the child warm on the way to hospital.*
• Very low weight for age.	**VERY LOW WEIGHT**	• Assess and counsel for feeding. • Advise mother when to return immediately. • Follow-up in 30 days.
• Not very low weight for age and no other signs of malnutrition.	**NOT VERY LOW WEIGHT**	• If child is less than 2 years old, assess the child's feeding and counsel the mother on feeding according to the FOOD box on the *COUNSEL THE MOTHER* chart. - If feeding problem, follow-up in 5 days. • Advise mother when to return immediately.

A

Laboratory Values

THE NORMAL RANGE

Results of a laboratory test can be interpreted in terms of being normal or abnormal, and negative or positive only on the basis of already known *normal or reference values*. Normal values refer to those measurements which are usually central and around which most of the values lie in healthy individuals.

Almost all normal laboratory values are represented and expressed in a *reference range* and rarely in terms of a single measurement. For example, a large group of healthy children in the age group of 6–12 years may have an average hemoglobin level of 14 g/dL with the individual values ranging from 11.5 g/dL to 15.5 g/dL. In this case, the normal hemoglobin values in 6–12 years old are said to range between 11.5 g/dL and 15.5 g/dL, and not simply 14 g/dL. The normal or reference range is an integral part of all laboratory values because of considerable magnitude of inter-individual variability in the normal population. Variations in normal subjects occur due to a host of reasons, other than age and sex, which may include biological, genetic, environmental and chance factors apart from the interobserver and laboratory variability. In addition, the analytic method used in the laboratory is a major factor affecting the value obtained. All these sources are instrumental in creating a rather wide range of values that may be referred to for classifying an individual as having a normal or abnormal laboratory test.

The central values are measured in terms of mean, median and mode. Fortunately, these three measures generally coincide in most of the laboratory measurements in healthy individuals. The normal deviation around the mean is termed as standard deviation. In a typical Gaussian (bell shaped) distribution curve, 95% of the normal values lie between ±2 SD around the mean. However, certain laboratory values in normal individuals do not follow the Gaussian curve, making it difficult to assume all values within mean 2 SD as being normal. In such situation, the normal values are expressed in terms of a range covering 95% of values from a set of values found in a healthy population, excluding 2.5% each of the lowermost and uppermost values.

Most of the laboratory tests do not have any absolute or magic cut-off point for labeling their results as being normal and abnormal. For example, if normal range of values of serum urea nitrogen is 5–18 mg/dL in children, then 17 mg/dL carries an importance equivalent to a value of 19 mg/dL. Both these values are then termed *borderline*. Such borderline values can be present in healthy as well as sick subjects and should be interpreted cautiously.

UNITS OF MEASUREMENT

Laboratory estimates are usually expressed as conventional or traditional units. However, it may be appropriate to know the standard units referred to as the SI units. The International System of Units (abbreviated SI from French: *Le Système international d'unités*) is well accepted worldwide as a standard and modern form of metric measurement. For most parameters, the SI units are moles per liter, wherein mass is measured in moles and volume as liters.

Concentration in moles is the ratio of the weight in grams and the molecular weight.

To convert a value expressed in conventional units to a SI unit, we need to multiply by the conversion factor. For example, albumin 3 g/dL × 10 = 30 g/L. To convert from SI units to conventional units, we will need to divide the value by a conversion factor. For example, albumin 30 g/L = 30 ÷ 10 g/dL = 3 g/dL.

COMMON ABBREVIATIONS

Most of the commonly used units are written in an abbreviated from. A list of such units is given below in **Table A1**. Prefixes are used along with the units of length, capacity and mass **(Table A2)**.

Table A1 Abbreviations for Common Units		
Measure	*Unit name*	*Abbreviation*
Weight	gram	g
Length	meter	m
Capacity	liter	L
Pressure	millimeter of mercury	mm Hg
Enzyme activity	International unit	U
Volume	cubic millimeter	mm^3
Osmolality	mole	mol
Equivalent weight	milliequivalent	mEq

Table A2 Prefixes Used for Decimal Factors		
Prefix	*Symbol*	*Factor*
Mega	M	10^6
kilo	k	10^3
deci	d	10^{-1}
centi	c	10^{-2}
milli	m	10^{-3}
micro	u	10^{-6}
nano	n	10^{-9}
pico	p	10^{-12}
femto	f	10^{-15}

HEMATOLOGICAL VALUES

Parameter	Traditional or conventional units	Standard units (multiplication factor)
Blood volume	mL/kg	mL/kg (1.0)
At birth	61–100	61–100
Infants	73–78	73–78
1–3 years	74–82	74–82
4–6 years	80–86	80–86
7–18 years	83–90	83–90
Adults	68–88	68–88

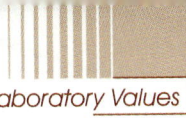

Erythrocyte sedimentation rate (ESR): Westergren method	mm/h	mm/h (1.0)
Neonate	0–4	0–4
Child	4–20	4–20
Adult males	0–10	0–10
Adult females	0–20	0–20

Hematocrit	%	% (1.0)
Birth	55 (45–65)	55 (45–65)
1 week	54 (43–66)	54 (43–66)
1–2 weeks	50 (42–66)	50 (42–66)
6 months–6 years	38 (33–42)	38 (33–42)
> 6-year males	46 (42–52)	46 (42–52)
> 6-year females	42 (37–47)	42 (37–47)

Hemoglobin (total) (Hgb)	g/dL	mmol/L (0.6206)
Birth	17 (14–20)	11.25 (8.68–12.41)
1 week	17 (13–21)	11.25 (8.06–13.06)
1–2 weeks	16.5 (13–20)	10.24 (8.06–12.41)
6 months–6 years	12 (10.5–14)	7.45 (6.15–8.68)
6–12 years	14 (11.5–15.5)	8.68 (7.14–9.62)
Adolescent males	16 (14–18)	9.93 (8.68–11.17)
Adolescent females	14 (12–16)	8.68 (7.45–9.93)
Hemoglobin A	≥95% of total Hgb	≥95% of total Hgb
Hemoglobin A_2	1.5–3.5% of total Hgb	1.5–3.5% of total Hgb
Hemoglobin A_{1c} (Glycated Hgb)	4.5–6.1% of total Hgb	4.5–6.1% of total Hgb

Hemoglobin fetal (Hgb F)	% of total Hgb	% of total Hgb
Neonate	60–90	60–90
Infant	2–59	2–59
Child	<2	<2
Adolescent	<2	<2
Adult	<2	<2
Methemoglobin	0–1.3% of total Hgb	0–1.3% of total Hgb

Mean corpuscular hemoglobin (MCH)	pg	pg
Birth	32–40	32–40
1 week	32–40	32–40
1–2 weeks	32–40	32–40
6 months–6 years	24–30	24–30
>6-year males	27–32	27–32
>6-year females	27–32	27–32

Mean corpuscular hemoglobin concentration (MCHC)	g/dL	g/L (10)
Birth	34–36	340–360
1 week	34–36	340–360
1–2 weeks	34–36	340–360
6 months–6 years	30–36	300–360
>6 year males	30–35	300–350
> 6 year females	30–35	300–350

Mean corpuscular volume (MCV)	fL	fL
Birth	94–118	94–118
1 week	88–104	88–104
1–2 weeks	86–106	86–106
6 months–6 years	76–88	76–88
>6-year males	76–98	76–98
>6-year females	76–96	76–96

Plasma volume	mL/kg	mL/kg (1.0)
At birth	33.5–49.5	33.5–49.5
Males	25–43	25–43
Females	28–45	28–45

Platelet count	$\times 10^3/mm^3$	$\times 10^9/L$
Birth	100–300	100–300
1 week–adults	150–450	150–450

Red blood cell count	$\times 10^6$ cells/mm^3	$\times 10^{12}$ cells/L(1.0)
Birth	3.7–6.5	3.7–6.5
2 weeks	3.9–5.9	3.9–5.9
2 months	3.1–4.3	3.1–4.3
6 months	3.8–4.9	3.8–4.9
1 year	3.9–5.1	3.9–5.1
2–6 years	3.9–5.0	3.9–5.0
6–12 years	3.9–5.2	3.9–5.2

Reticulocyte count	%	% (1.0)
Birth	5 (3–7)	5 (3–7)
2 weeks	2 (0–4)	2 (0–4)
months–6 years	1 (0–2)	1 (0–2)
6–12 years	0–2	0–2

White blood cell count	cells/mm^3	$\times 10^9$ cells/L (10^6)
Birth	18000 (9000–30000)	18 (9–30)
1 week	12000 (6000–22000)	12 (6–22)
2 weeks	12000 (5000–21000)	12 (5–21)
6 months–6 years	10000 (6000–15000)	10 (6–15)
>6 years	75000 (5000–10000)	7.5 (5–10)

Differential leukocyte count	Percentage of total WBC count	Percentage of total WBC count
Cord blood	N61 L31 E2 M6	N61 L31 E2 M6
0–12 weeks	N40 L48 E3 M9	N40 L48 E3 M9
3 months	N30 L63 E2 M5	N30 L63 E2 M5
6 months–6 years	N45 L48 E2 M5	N45 L48 E2 M5
7–12 years	N55 L38 E2 M7	N55 L38 E2 M7
Total neutrophil count	Cells/mm^3	$\times 10^6$ cells/L
Band cells	150–400	150–400
Segmented	3000–5800	3000–5800
Total lymphocyte count	cells/mm^3 1500–3000	$\times 10^6$ cells/L 1500–3000
Total monocyte count	cells/mm^3 285–500	$\times 10^6$ cells/L 285–500
Total eosinophil count	cells/mm^3 50–250	$\times 10^6$ cells/L 50–250
Total basophil count	cells/mm^3 15–50	$\times 10^6$ cells/L 15–50

A

MEASURES OF COAGULATION

Coagulation test	Value
Activated partial thromboplastin time (aPTT)	
Preterm neonate	35–100 s
Term neonate	35–70 s
1–5 years	24–36 s
6–10 years	26–36 s
11–16 years	26–37 s
Adult	27–40 s
Bleeding time (BT)	2–7 minutes
Clotting time (CT)	5–8 minutes
D-dimer	Positive titer = 1:8
Factor I/Fibrinogen	
Preterm neonate	1.2–3.8 g/L
Term neonate	1.5–3.5 g/L
Child	2.0–4.0 g/L
Adult	1.5–3.5 g/L
Fibrin degradation products (FDP)	207 (68–494) ng/L
Protein C (U/mL)	
Preterm neonate	0.28 (0.12–0.44)
Term neonate	0.35 (0.17–0.53)
1–5 years	0.66 (0.40–0.92)
6–10 years	0.69 (0.45–0.93)
11–16 years	0.83 (0.55–1.11)
Adult	0.96 (0.64–1.28)
Protein S Total (U/mL)	
Preterm neonate	0.26 (0.14–0.38)
Term neonate	0.36 (0.12–0.60)
1–5 years	0.86 (0.54–1.18)
6–10 years	0.78 (0.41–1.14)
11–16 years	0.72 (0.52–0.92)
Adult	0.81 (0.60–1.13)
Prothrombin time (PT)	
Preterm neonate	13–23 s
Term neonate	13–17 s
1–5 years	10.6–11.4 s
6–10 years	10.1–12.1 s
11–16 years	10.2–12.0 s
Adult	11.0–14.0 s
Reptilase time	
Preterm neonate	18–30 s
Term neonate	18–24 s
Adult	18–22 s
Thrombin time	
Preterm neonate	12–24 s
Term neonate	12–18 s
Adult	10–14 s

COAGULATION FACTORS (% OF NORMAL OR ADULT VALUE)

Coagulation factor	Preterm neonate	Term neonate	Children
Factor II	30–65	40–65	60–150
Factor V	50–100	50–100	60–150
Factor VII	20–150	40–70	60–150
Factor VIII	60–120	70–150	60–145
Factor IX	10–30	15–55	60–140
Factor X	10–45	20–55	60–130
Factor XI	10–50	15–70	65–135
Factor XII	20–50	25–70	65–150

SERUM BIOCHEMISTRY

Serum Proteins (g/dL)*

	Total proteins	Albumin	Globulins			
			α1	α2	β	γ
Preterm-neonate	4.3–7.6	3.0–4.2	0.1–0.5	0.3–0.7	0.3–1.2	0.3–1.4
Term neonate	4.6–7.7	2.5–5.0	0.1–0.3	0.3–0.5	0.2–0.6	0.8–1.2
1–7 years	6.1–7.9	4.0–5.0	0.2–0.4	0.5–0.8	0.5–0.8	0.3–1.2
> 7 years	6.4–8.2	3.4–5.0	0.2–0.3	0.4–1.0	0.5–1.1	0.5–1.8

*SI units: g/L, multiplication factor 10.

	Conventional units	SI units, multiplication factor
Ammonia (Heparinized venous sample on ice analyzed within 30 min)	µg/dL	µmol/L, 0.7
Neonate	90–150	64–107
0–2 months	79–129	56–92
>1 month	29–70	21–50
Adult	15–45	11–32

Bilirubin (serum), total		mg/dL	µmol/L, 17.1
Cord blood	Term	<2	<34
	Preterm	<2	<34
0–1 day	Term	<8	<137
	Preterm	<6	<103
1–2 days	Term	<12	<205
	Preterm	<8	<137
3–5 days	Term	<16	<274
	Preterm	<12	<205
Thereafter	Term	<2	<34
	Preterm	<1	<17
Adult		0.1–1.2	1.7–20.5
Bilirubin (serum), conjugated		0–0.4	0–8

Chloride (serum, heparinized plasma)	mEq/L	mmol/L, 1
Newborn	97–110	97–110
Thereafter	98–106	98–106

Creatinine (serum)	mg/dL	µmol/L, 90
Neonate	0.3–1.0	27–88
Infant	0.2–0.4	18–35
Child	0.3–0.7	27–62
Adolescent	0.5–1.0	44–88

C-reactive protein	mg/dL	mg/dL, 1
0–90 days	0.08–1.58	0.08–1.58
90 days–3 years		
Male	0.08–1.12	0.08–1.12
Female	0.05–0.79	0.05–0.79
4–10 years		
Male	0.06–0.79	0.06–0.79
Female	0.5–1.0	0.5–1.0
11–14 years		
Male	0.08–0.76	0.08–0.76
Female	0.06–0.71	0.06–0.71

Glucose (serum)	mg/dL	mmol/L, 0.0555
Preterm neonate	20–60	1.1–3.3
Term neonate	30–60	1.7–3.3

A

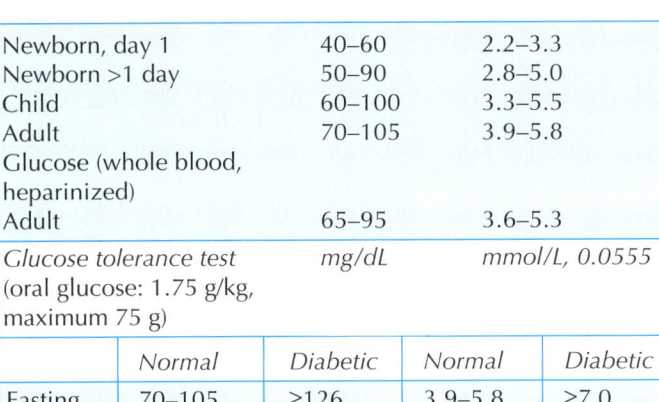

Newborn, day 1	40–60	2.2–3.3
Newborn >1 day	50–90	2.8–5.0
Child	60–100	3.3–5.5
Adult	70–105	3.9–5.8
Glucose (whole blood, heparinized)		
Adult	65–95	3.6–5.3

Glucose tolerance test (oral glucose: 1.75 g/kg, maximum 75 g)	mg/dL	mmol/L, 0.0555

	Normal	Diabetic	Normal	Diabetic
Fasting	70–105	≥126	3.9–5.8	≥7.0
60 min	120–170	≥200	6.7–9.4	≥11
90 min	100–140	≥200	5.6–7.8	≥11
120 min	70–120	≥200	3.9–6.7	≥11

Lactate	mmol/L	mmol/L, 1
Whole blood lactate		
1–12 months	1.1–2.3	1.1–2.3
1 year	0.8–1.5	0.8–1.5
7–15 years	0.6–0.9	0.6–0.9
Plasma lactate		
6 months–3 years	0.0–0.3	0.0–0.3

Serum lipids		
Cholesterol	mg/dL	mmol/L 0.0259
Cord blood	23–135	0.6–3.5
1–6 weeks	93–217	2.4–5.6
≥1 year	119–263	3.1–6.8

Phospholipids	mg/dL	g/L, 0.01
Cord blood	75–150	0.75–1.5
Neonate	170–250	1.7–2.5
>1 month	150–300	1.5–3.0

Total lipids	mg/dL	g/L, 0.01
Newborn	150–400	1.5–4.0
>1 month	400–1000	4.0–10.0

Free fatty acids	µEq/L	µmol/L
Newborn	250–1000	250–1000
>1 month	300–1450	300–1450

Pyruvate (whole blood)	mmol/L	mmol/L, 1
7–17 years	0.076 (±0.026)	0.076 (±0.026)

Urea (serum/plasma)	mg/dL	mmol/L, 0.357
Preterm neonate	3–25	1.1–9.0
Term neonate	3–12	1.1–4.3
Infant/child	5–18	1.8–6.4
Thereafter	7–18	2.5–6.4

Uric acid (serum)	mg/dL	mmol/L, 0.0595
	2–7	0.12–0.42

METALS AND BINDING PROTEINS

	Conventional units	SI units, multiplication factor
Serum ceruloplasmin	mg/dL	mg/L, 10
	21–53	210–530

Serum copper	µg/dL	µmoldd/L, 0.157
0–5 days	9–46	1.4–7.2
1–9 years	80–150	12.6–23.6
10–14 years	80–121	12.6–19
15–19 years	64–160	11.3–25.2
Serum folate	ng/mL	nmol/L, 2.265
	2.5–20	5.7–45.3

RBC folate	ng/mL RBCs	nmol/L cells
	150–450	340–1020

Serum iron	µg/dL	µmol/L, 0.179
Term neonate	100–250	18–45
Infant	40–100	7–18
Child	50–120	9–22
Adult, male	65–175	12–30
Adult, female	50–170	9–30

Total iron binding capacity (TIBC)	µg/dL	µmol/L, 0.179
Term neonate	150–200	26.8–35.8
Infant	200–400	35.8–71.6
Child	250–500	44.8–89.5
Adolescent	300–600	53.7–107.4
Adult	250–425	44.8–76.1

Serum transferrin	mg/dL	g/L, 0.01
Term neonate	130–275	1.3–2.75
Infant	200–360	2.0–3.6
Child	200–360	2.0–3.6
Adolescent	220–400	2.2–4.0
Adult	220–400	2.2–4.0

Serum ferritin	ng/mL	µg/L, 1
Term neonate	25–200	25–200
Infant	50–600	50–600
Child	7–140	7–140
Adolescent	7–140	7–140
Adult, male	20–250	20–250
Adult, female	10–120	10–120

Serum magnesium	mg/dL	mmol/L, 0.411
0–6 days	1.2–2.6	0.48–1.05
7 days–2 years	1.6–2.6	0.65–1.05
2–14 years	1.5–2.3	0.60–0.95

Blood lead	µg/dL	µmol/L, 4.8
Children	<10	<48
Adults	<40	<192
Toxic	≥70	≥336

Serum zinc	µg/dL	µmol/L, 0.153
	70–150	10.7–22.9

SERUM ENZYMES

Enzyme	Reference value
Amylase 1–19 years	U/L 30–100
Aldolase	U/L
10 months– 2 years	3.4–11.8
2–16 years	1.2–8.8

A

Alkaline phosphatase	U/L
Preterm neonate	Up to 1500
Term neonate	Up to 700
Infants	250–1000
2–5 years	250–850
6–7 years	250–1000
8–9 years	250–750
10–11 years, male	250–730
10–11 years, female	250–950
12–13 years, male	275–875
12–13 years, female	200–730
Acid phosphatase	0–0.8 U/L

Alanine aminotransferase (ALT,SGPT)	U/L
0–7 days	25–100
8–30 days	22–71
1–3 years	20–60
3–9 years	15–50
10–15 years	10–40

Aspartate aminotransferase (AST,SGOT)	U/L
0–7 days	25–100
8–30 days	22–71
1–3 years	20–60
3–9 years	15–50
10–15 years	10–40

Antistreptolysin O (ASO) titers*	Todd units
2–5 years	120–160
6–9 years	240
10–12 years	320
α1-Antitrypsin	0.93–2.24 g/L

Creatine kinase	U/L
Newborn	10–200
Adult	20–200

Creatine kinase isoenzymes	CKMB	CKBB
Cord blood	0.3–3.1%	0.3–10.5%
0–24 hours	1.7–7.9%	3.6–13.4%
72–100 hours	1.4–5.9%	5.1–13.3%
Older	0–2%	0
Gastrin	< 100 ng/L	
Glucose 6 phosphate dehydrogenase (G6PD)Adult**	3.4–8.0 U/g hemoglobin or 1.16–2.72 U/mL RBC	

γ-glutamyl transferase (GGT)	U/L
<3 weeks	0–130
3 weeks–3 months	4–120
>3 months, boy	5–65
>3 months, girl	5–35
1–15 years	0–23
Adult, male	11–50
Adult, female	7–32

Lactate dehydrogenase (LDH)	U/L
< 1 years	170–580
1–9 years	150–500
10–19 years	120–330

Lactate Dehydrogenase, Isoenzymes (% total)	
LD1 heart	24–34%
LD2 heart, RBCs	35–45%
LD3 muscle	15–25%

LD4 liver, trace muscle	4–10%
LD5 liver, muscle	1–9%
Lipase	U/L
1–18 years	145–216

*4× rise in paired serial specimens is significant.
**Values are 50% higher in newborns.

NORMAL ACID–BASE STATUS AND ELECTROLYTES

	Conventional units	SI units, multiplication factor
Anion gap	mEq/L	mmol/L, 1
[Sodium-(Chloride+Bicarbonate)]	7–16	7–16
Base excess	mmol/L	mmol/L
Newborn	–10 to –2	–10 to –2
Infant	–7 to –1	–7 to –1
Child	–4 to +2	–4 to +2
Older	–3 to +3	–3 to +3
Bicarbonate, serum	mEq/L	mmol/L, 1
Arterial	21–28	21–28
Venous	22–29	22–29
Calcium, total, serum	mg/dL	mmol/L, 0.25
< 24 hours	9.0–10.6	2.3–2.65
24–48 hours	7.0–12.0	1.75–3.0
4–7 days	9.0–10.9	2.25–2.73
Child	8.8–10.8	2.2–2.7
Calcium, ionized, serum	mg/dL	mmol/L, 0.25
< 24 hours	4.3–5.1	1.07–1.2
24–48 hours	4.0–4.7	71.0–1.17
Child	4.8–4.92	1.12–1.23
Carbon dioxide, total (tCO₂)	mmol/L	mmol/L, 1
Cord	14–22	14–22
Newborn	13–22	13–22
Infant	20–28	20–28
Child	20–28	20–28
Carbon dioxide partial pressure, arterial (PaCO₂)	mm Hg	kPa, 0.1333
Newborn	27–40	3.6–5.3
Infant	27–41	3.6–5.5
Thereafter, males	35–48	4.7–6.4
Thereafter, females	32–45	4.3–6.0
Chloride, serum	mEq/L	mmol/L
	95–106	95–106
Osmolarity, serum	mosm/L	mosm/L
	275–290	275–290
Oxygen partial pressure (PaO₂), arterial	mm Hg	kPa, 0.1333
Birth	8–24	1.1–3.2
5–10 min	33–75	4.4–10
30 min	31–85	4.1–11.3
>1 hour	55–80	7.3–10.6
1 day	54–95	7.2–12.6
Thereafter	83–108	11–14.4

A

Oxygen saturation (SaO$_2$), arterial	%	Fraction saturation, 0.01
Newborn	85–90	0.85–0.90
Thereafter	95–99	0.95–0.99
pH, arterial		
Birth	7.11–7.36	7.11–7.36
24 hours	7.3–7.45	7.3–7.45
Older	7.35–7.45	7.35–7.45
Potassium, serum	*mEq/L*	*mmol/L, 1*
<2 months	3–7	3–7
2–12 months	3.5–6	3.5–6
>12 months	3.5–5	3.5–5
Sodium, serum	*mEq/L*	*mmol/L*
Newborn	134–146	134–146
<1 year	139–144	139–144
Child	138–145	138–145

HORMONES IN SERUM AND URINE

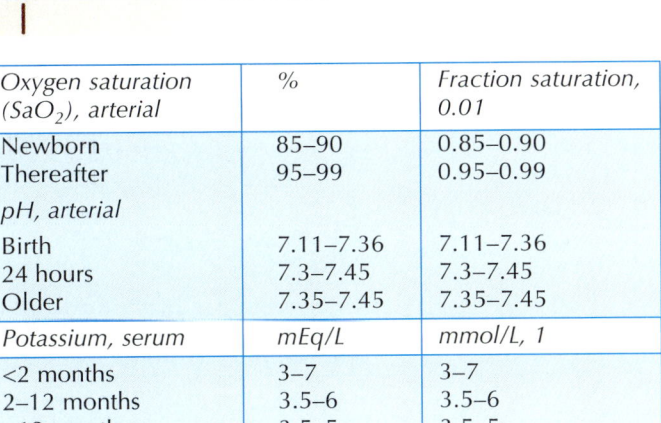

	Conventional units	SI units, multiplication factor
Adrenocorticotrophic hormone (ACTH), plasma	pg/mL	ng/L, 1
Cord blood	130–160	130–160
1–7 days postnatal	100–140	100–140
Adult		
Morning	25–100	25–100
Evening	< 50	< 50
Aldosterone, plasma/serum	*ng/dL*	*nmol/L, 1*
1–12 months	5–90	1.4–2.5
1–2 years	7–54	0.19–1.5
2–10 years	3–35	0.1–0.97
10–15 years	2–22	0.1–0.6
Aldosterone, urine	*µg/24 hours*	*nmol/24 hours, 2.78*
Newborn	0.5–5	1.39–13.9
4–10 years	1–8	2.78–22.2
Older	3–19	8.3–52.8
Antidiuretic hormone (ADH), plasma varies with plasma osmolarity (mosm/kg)	pg/mL	pg/mL, 1
270–280	<1.5	<1.5
280–285	<2.5	<2.5
285–290	1–5	1–5
290–295	2–7	2–7
295–300	4–12	4–12
Calcitonin, plasma	*pg/mL*	*pmol/L, 0.28*
Newborn	70–348	19.6–97.4
Males	3–26	0.8–7.2
Females	2–17	0.6–4.7
Catecholamines, serum	*µg/24 hours*	*µg/24 hours, 1*
Dopamine	100–440	100–440
Epinephrine	<15	<15
Norepinephrine	15–86	15–86
Metanephrines	<0.4	<0.4
Normetanephrines	<0.9	<0.9
Homovanillic acid (HVA)	0–10	0–10
Vanillyl mandelic acid (VMA)	2–10	2–10

Cortisol, plasma	µg/dL	nmol/L, 27.59
Newborn	1–24	28–662
Adults		
Morning 8 am	5–23	138–635
Evening 4 pm	3–15	82–413
Night 8 pm	Less than 50% of morning level	Less than 50% of morning level
Cortisol, free, urine	*µg/24 hours*	*nmol/24 hours, 2.75*
Child	2–27	5.5–74.2
Adolescent	5–55	13.7–151.25
Dehydroepiandrosterone (DHEA) sulfate, serum	*µg/dL*	*nmol/L, 2.714*
Newborn	1.7–3.6	4.6–9.7
Prepubertal	0.1–0.6	0.27–1.6
Men	1.4–7.9	3.7–21.4
Women	0.7–4.5	1.9–12.2
Dihydrotestosterone (DHT), serum	*ng/dL*	–
Prepubertal, males	<3–13	
Prepubertal, females	<3–10	
Tanner 2, males	5–17	
Tanner 2, females	4–12	
Tanner 3, males	7–35	
Tanner 3, females	9–21	
Tanner 4, males	12–52	
Tanner 4, females	9–23	
Tanner 5, males	13–17	
Tanner 5, females	<3–36	
Adults, males	30–100	
Adults, females	6–33	
Estradiol, serum	*pg/mL*	*pmol/L, 3.571*
Prepubertal	<25	< 89.2
Men	6–44	21.4–157.1
Women	15–260 (luteal)	53.6–928.5
	10–200 (follicular)	35.7–714.2
	120–375 (midcycle)	428.5–1339.1
Gonadotropins, serum	*mIU/mL*	–
FSH		
Prepubertal	0–2.8	
Men	1.4–14.4	
Women, follicular	3.7–12.9	
LH		
Prepubertal	0–1.6	
Men	1–10.2	
Women, follicular	0.9–14	
Growth hormone, plasma	*ng/mL*	*µg/L, 1*
1 day	5–53	5–53
1 week	5–27	5–27
1–12 months	2–10	2–10
Child	0.7–6	0.7–6
Adult	0.7–6	0.7–6

5-Hydroxy indoleacetic acid (HIAA), urine	mg/24 hours	–
17-Hydroxy-corticosteroid, urine	2–8 mg/24 hours	
Infant	0–1.0	
Child	1.0–5.6	
Adult, male	3–10	
Adult, female	2–8	
17-Hydroxy-progesterone, serum	ng/L	ng/L, 1
Prepubertal		
Males	0–81	0–81
Females	0–92	0–92
Adult		
Males	36–154	36–154
Females	15–102 (follicular) 150–386 (luteal)	15–102 (follicular) 150–386 (luteal)
17-Ketosteroids, urine	mg/24 hours	–
<1 month	<2.0	
1 month–5 years	<0.5	
6–8 years	1.0–2.0	
Men	9–22	
Women	5–15	
Insulin, plasma (12 hours fasting)	μU/mL	pmol/L, 7.14
Newborn	3–20	21–143
Thereafter	7–24	50–171
Prolactin, serum	μg/L	pmol/L, 42.5
Male	<15	<652
Female	<20	<850
Parathormone, serum	pg/mL	pg/mL, 1
Intact	<10–65	<10–65
C-terminal	50–340	50–340
N-terminal	4–19	4–19
Renin activity, plasma	nmol/L/hour	nmol/L/hour, 1
0–6 days	2.8–79	2.8–79
6 days–1 years	6.4–27.2	
2–4 years	1.5–22.6	
5–9 years	1.8–7.2	
10–15 years	0.7–7.8	6.4–27.21.5–
22.61.8–7.20.7–7.8		
Testosterone, total, serum	ng/dL	nmol/L, 0.0347
Prepubertal	10–20	0.3–0.6
Men	275–875	9.5–30.4
Women	23–75	7.9–2.6
Pregnant females	35–195	1.2–6.7
Thyroxine (T_4), serum	ng/dL	pmol/L, 13
Free T_4		
1–10 days	0.6–2.0	7.8–26
> 10 days	0.7–1.7	9.1–22.1

Total T_4, by RIA	μg/dL	pmol/L, 13
Cord	6.6–17.5	85.8–227.5
1–3 days	11.0–21.5	143–279.5
1–4 weeks	8.2–16.6	106.6–215.8
1–12 months	7.2–15.6	93.6–202.8
1–5 years	7.3–15.0	94.9–195
6–10 years	6.4–13.3	83.2–172.9
11–15 years	5.6–11.7	72.8–152.1
16–20 years	4.2–11.8	54.6–153.4
21–50 years	4.3–12.5	56–162.5
Triiodothyronine (T_3), serum, by RIA	ng/dL	nmol/L, 0.015
Cord	14–86	0.2–1.3
1–3 days	100–38	1.5–5.7
1–4 week	099–310	1.5–4.6
1–12 months	102–264	1.5–3.9
1–5 years	105–269	1.6–4.1
6–10 years	94–241	1.4–3.6
11–15 years	83–213	1.2–3.2
16–20 years	80–210	1.2–3.1
21–50 years	70–204	1.0–3.1
Thyroid stimulating hormone (TSH), serum	μIU/mL	–
Cord	<2.5–17.4	
1–3 days	<2.5–13.3	
1–4 weeks	0.6–10.0	
1–15 years	0.6–6.3	
16–50 years	0.2–7.6	
Thyoxine-binding globulin (TBG), serum	mg/dL	mg/L, 10
Cord	0.7–4.7	7–47
1–3 days	–	–
1–4 weeks	0.5–4.5	5–45
1–12 months	1.6–3.6	16–36
1–15 years	1.3–2.8	13–28
16–20 years	1.4–2.6	14–26
21–50 years	1.2–2.4	12–24
T3, reverse, serum	ng/dL	–
Newborn	90–250	
Children	10–50	
Adult	10–50	

NORMAL URINARY VALUES

Volume	mL
Neonate	50–300
Infant	350–550
Child	500–1000
Adolescent	700–1400
Specific gravity	
24 hours	1.015–1.025
After fluid restriction for 12 hours	> 1.025
Osmolality	mosm/kg
24 hours	50–1400
After fluid restriction for 12 horus	>850

A

pH	
Neonate	5–7
Child	4.5–8
Cell count	Cells/hpf
Red blood cells	0–2
White blood cells	0–5
Epithelial cells	A few
Bacteria	0–20 in centrifuged specimen
Casts	Per hpf
Hyaline casts	0–1
RBC, WBC, epithelial casts	Absent
Ammonia	$mEq/min/m^2$
2–12 months	4–20
1–16 years	6–16
Creatinine	mg/kg/24 hours
Newborns	7–10
Children	20–30
Adult males	21–26
Adult females	16–22
Glomerular filtration rate	$mL/min/1.73\ m^2$
Neonate <34 weeks' gestation	11 (11–15)
2–8 days	20 (15–28)
4–28 days	50 (40–65)
30–90 days	
Neonate >34 weeks' gestation	39 (17–60)
2–8 days	47 (26–68)
4–28 days	58 (30–86)
30–90 days	7 (39–114)
1–6 months	103 (49–157)
6–12 months	127 (62–1910)
12–19 months	127 (89–165)
2 years–adult	
Growth hormone	
2.2–13.3 years (Tanner 1)	0.4–6.3 ng/24 hours (0.9–12.3 ng/g creatinine)
10.3–14.6 years (Tanner 2)	0.8–12.0 ng/24 hours (1.0–14.1 ng/g creatinine)
11.5–15.3 years (Tanner 3)	1.7–20.4 ng/24 hours (1.9–17.0 ng/g creatinine)
12.7–17.1 years (Tanner 4)	1.5–18.2 ng/24 hours (1.3–14.4 ng/g creatinine)
13.5–19.9 years (Tanner 5)	1.2–14.5 ng/24 hours (0.8–11.0 ng/g creatinine)
Porphyrins	
α-Aminolevulinic acid	0–7 mg/24 hours (0–53.4 mol/24 hours)
Porphobilinogen	0–2 mg/24 hours (0–8.8 mol/24 hours)
Coproporphyrin	0–160 mg/24 hours (0–244 mol/24 hours)
Uroporphyrin	0–26 mg/24 hours (0–31 mol/24 hours)
Sodium	
24 hours sample	41—115 mmol/24 hours
Spot sample	>20 mmol/L

Potassium	mmol/L
24 hours sample	10–60
Chloride	mmol/24 hours
Infant	2–10
Child	15–40
Calcium	
24 hours sample	100–250 mg (2.5–6.2 mmol)
Calcium: creatinine	(mg/mg ratio)
<7 months	0.86
7–18 months	0.6
19 months–6 years	0.42
Adults	0.22
Protein	mg/24 hours
Total (24 hours)	
At rest	50–80
Following exercise	Up to 250
Glucose	
Qualitative estimation	Nil
Quantitative estimation	0.5 g/24 hours
Galactose	mg/dL
Neonate	<60
Child	14
Copper	mg/mol creatinine
	0.36–7.56
Coproporphyrin	µg/24 hours
	34–234
Total free catecholamines	µg/24 hours
0–1 year	10–15
1–5 years	15–40
6–15 years	20–80
Homovanillic acid (HVA)	mg/g creatinine
0–1 year	<32.2
2–4 years	<22
5–19 years	<14
Vanillyl mandelic acid (VMA)	mg/g creatinine
0–1 year	<18.8
2–4 years	<11.0
5–19 years	<8.0
Mucopolysaccharides	µg/g creatinine
0–2 years	<50
2–4 years	<25
4–15 years	<20

Hemoglobin, bilirubin, ketones, myoglobin, porphobilinogen and glucose are undetectable in normal urine by qualitative tests.

CEREBROSPINAL FLUID

Opening pressure	mm Hg
Newborn	80–110
Infant/child	<200
Respiratory variation	5–10
WBC count	Cells/mm³
Preterm mean (range)	9 (0–25), 57% polymorphs

A

Term mean (range) Child	8 (0–22), 61% polymorphs 0–7, 0% polymorphs
Glucose*	mg/dL
Preterm mean (range) Term mean (range) Child	50 (24–63) 52 (34–119) 40–80
Protein	mg/dL
Preterm mean (range) Term mean (range) Child	115 (65–150) 90 (20–170) 5–40
Lactic acid dehydrogenase	U/L
	20 (5–30), or about 10% of serum value
Myelin basic protein	ng/mL< 4
Chloride	mmol/L
	118–132
Lactate	mmol/L
	0.8–2.4

*CSF glucose is at least 50–70% of corresponding blood sugar.

STOOL SPECIMEN

pH	7.0–7.5
Fecal fats (Measured over 72 hours)	g/24 hours
Breastfed infant 0–6 years	<1 <2
Fecal bile acids	mg/24 hours
	120–225
Fecal α1 antitrypsin	mg/g of stool
Breastfed infant Top fed infant 6 months–4 years Occult blood	<4.4 <2.9 < 1.7 Negative (< 2 mL/24 hours in 100–200 g of stool)
Ova and cysts	Nil

AMNIOTIC FLUID

α Fetoprotein	µg/mL
15 weeks gestation	13.5 ± 3.42
16 weeks gestation	11.7 ± 3.38
17 weeks gestation	10.3 ± 3.03
18 weeks gestation	9.5 ± 3.22
19 weeks gestation	7.1 ± 2.85
20 weeks gestation	5.0 ± 2.45
Creatinine	mg/dL
	>2 (after term gestation)
Lecithin	mg/dL
Lecithin/sphingomyelin (LS ratio)	>0.1 indicates fetal lung maturity >2:1 indicates fetal lung maturity
Total bilirubin	mg/dL
28 weeks' gestation 40 weeks' gestation	<0.075 <0.025

SWEAT

Sweat Chloride Test	
Value	Interpretation
<40 mmol/L 40–60 mmol/L ≥60 mmol/L	Normal Borderline Cystic fibrosis

SERUM VITAMIN LEVELS

Vitamin	Conventional units	SI units
Vitamin A/Retinol	µg/dL	µmol/L
Newborn	35–75	1.22–2.62
Child	30–80	1.05–2.79
Adult	30–65	1.05–2.27
Vitamin B_1/Thiamine	µg/dL	µmol/L
	5.3–7.9	0.16–0.23
Vitamin B_2/Riboflavin	µg/dL	µmol/L
	3.7–13.7	98–363
Vitamin B_6/Pyridoxine	ng/mL	nmol/L
	5–24	30–144
Vitamin B_{12}/Cobalamin	pg/mL	pmol/L
	130–785	96–579
Vitamin C/Ascorbic acid	mg/dL	µmol/L
	0.2–2	11.4–113.6
Vitamin D_2	pg/mL	pmol/L
	24–65	58–156
Vitamin D_3/Calcitriol	pg/mL	pmol/L
	25–45	60–108
Vitamin E	mg/dL	µmol/L
	5–20	10.7–22.9
Folate, serum	ng/mL	nmol/L
	>1.9	>4.3

SERUM IMMUNOGLOBULIN LEVELS

Age	IgG (mg/dL)	IgM (mg/dL)	IgA (mg/dL)	IgE (IU/mL)
Cord blood (term)	1121 (636–1606)	1.3 (6.3–25)	2.3 (1.4–3.6)	-
1 month	503 (251–906)	45 (20–87)	13 (1.3–53)	-
6 month	407 (215–704)	62 (35–102)	25 (8.1–68)	2.68 (0.44–16.3)
1 year	679 (345–1213)	93 (43–173)	44 (14–123)	3.49 (0.80–15.2)
2 years	685 (424–1051)	95 (48–168)	47 (14–123)	3.03 (0.31–29.5)
3 years	728 (441–1135)	104 (47–200)	66 (22–159)	1.80 (0.19–16.9)
4–5 years	780 (463–1236)	99 (43–196)	68 (25–154)	8.58 (1.07–68.9)
6–8 years	915 (633–1280)	107 (48–207)	90 (33–202)	12.89 (1.03–161.3)
9–10 years	1007 (608–1572)	121 (52–242)	113 (45–236)	23.66 (0.98–570.6)
Adult	994 (639–1349)	156 (56–352)	171 (70–312)	13.2 (1.53–114.0)

Values expressed in mean (95% CI). *Immunoglobulin D:* Newborn: 0 mg/dL; Thereafter: 0-8 mg/dL.

A

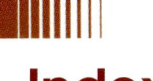

Index